MISCH'S

CONTEMPORARY IMPLANT DENTISTRY

FOURTH EDITION

MISCH'S

CONTEMPORARY IMPLANT DENTISTRY

Randolph R. Resnik, DMD, MDS

Clinical Professor
Department of Graduate Periodontology and Oral Implantology
Kornberg School of Dentistry-Temple University
Philadelphia, Pennsylvania

Adjunct Professor
University of Pittsburgh School of Dental Medicine
Graduate Prosthodontics
Pittsburgh, Pennsylvania

Clinical Professor
Department of Oral & Maxillofacial Surgery
Allegheny General Hospital
Pittsburgh, Pennsylvania

Surgical Director/Chief of Staff
Misch International Implant Institute
Beverly Hills, Michigan

ELSEVIER

Previous editions copyrighted 2008, 1999, and 1993.

Library of Congress Control Number: 2020930388

Executive Content Strategist: Alexandra Mortimer
Content Development Manager: Rebecca Gruliow
Content Development Specialist: Anne Snyder
Publishing Services Manager: Julie Eddy
Senior Project Manager: Abigail Bradberry
Design Direction: Maggie Reid

Printed in Canada

Last digit is the print number: 9   8   7   6   5   4   3   2   1

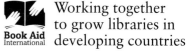

Contributors

Martha Warren Bidez, PhD*
Professor
Department of Biomedical Engineering
University of Alabama at Birmingham
Birmingham, Alabama
   Chapter 6 Clinical Biomechanics in Implant Dentistry

Diana Bronstein, DDS, MS
Associate Director of Predoctoral Periodontology
Nova Southeastern University
Ft. Lauderdale, Florida
   Chapter 42 Implant Maintenance: Long-term Implant Success

Grant Bullis, MBA
Vice President and General Manager, Implants
Prismatik Dentalcraft
Glidewell Laboratories
Newport Beach, California
   Chapter 3 Functional Basis for Dental Implant Design

C. Stephen Caldwell, DDS
Private Practice
El Paso, Texas
Misch International Implant Institute
Surgical Faculty Member
Detroit, Michigan
   Chapter 36 Particulate Membrane Grafting/Guided Bone Regeneration
   Chapter 38 Intraoral Autogenous Bone Grafting

Joseph E. Cillo, Jr., DMD, MPH, PhD, FACS
Associate Professor of Surgery
Residency Program Director
Director of Research
Division of Oral & Maxillofacial Surgery
Allegheny General Hospital
Pittsburgh, Pennsylvania
   Chapter 13 Dental Implant Infections

John M. Conness, DDS, FAGD, DICOI
Ottawa, Illinois

David J. Dattilo, DDS
Director
Oral and Maxillofacial Surgery
Allegheny General Hospital
Pittsburgh, Pennsylvania
   Chapter 39 Extraoral Bone Grafting for Implant Reconstruction

Kevan S. Green, DMD
Clinical Professor
Department of Periodontology and Oral Implantology
Kornberg School of Dentistry-Temple University
Philadelphia, Pennsylvania
Periodontist, Private Practice
Philadelphia, PA

Mayuri Kerr, BDS, MS
Clinical Affairs Manager
Glidewell Dental
Irvine, California
   Chapter 2 Terminology in Implant dentistry
   Chapter 9 Dental Implant Surfaces

Jack E. Lemons, PhD*
Professor
Department of Prosthodontics, Surgery, and Biomedical Engineering
University of Alabama at Birmingham
Birmingham, Alabama
   Chapter 5 Biomaterials for Dental Implants

Carl E. Misch, DDS, MDS, PhD (HC)*
Clinical Professor and Past Director
Oral Implant Dentistry
Temple University
Kornberg School of Dentistry
Department of Periodontics and Implant Dentistry
Philadelphia, Pennsylvania
Adjunct Professor
University of Alabama at Birmingham
School of Engineering
Birmingham, Alabama
Founder
Misch International Implant Institute
Beverly Hills, Michigan
   Chapter 1 Rationale for Dental Implants
   Chapter 6 Clinical Biomechanics in Implant Dentistry
   Chapter 7 Stress Treatment Theorem for Implant Dentistry
   Chapter 8 Treatment Planning: Force Factors Related to Patient Conditions
   Chapter 16 Available Bone and Dental Implant Treatment Plans
   Chapter 17 Prosthetic Options in Implant Dentistry
   Chapter 18 Bone Density: A Key Determinant for Treatment Planning
   Chapter 19 Treatment Plans Related to Key Implant Positions and Implant Number
   Chapter 20 Treatment Plans for Partially and Completely Edentulous Arches in Implant Dentistry

* deceased

Chapter 21 Preimplant Prosthodontic Factors Related to Surgical Treatment Planning
Chapter 23 Treatment Planning for the Edentulous Posterior Maxilla
Chapter 24 The Edentulous Mandible: Fixed Versus Removable Prosthesis Treatment Planning
Chapter 25 The Edentulous Maxilla: Fixed versus Removable Treatment Planning
Chapter 28 Ideal Implant Positioning
Chapter 29 Maxillary Anterior Implant Placement
Chapter 33 Immediate Load/Restoration in Implant Dentistry
Chapter 37 Maxillary Sinus Anatomy, Pathology, and Graft Surgery
Chapter 38 Intraoral Autogenous Bone Grafting

Francine Misch-Dietsh, DMD, MDS
Clinical Adjunct Professor
Department of Periodontology and Oral Implantology
Kornberg School of Dentistry-Temple University
Philadelphia, Pennsylvania
Chapter 5 Biomaterials for Dental Implants
Chapter 21 Preimplant Prosthodontic Factors Related to Surgical Treatment Planning

Neil I. Park, DMD
Vice President of Clinical Affairs
Glidewell Dental
Newport Beach, California
Chapter 2 Terminology in Implant Dentistry
Chapter 9 Dental Implant Surfaces
Chapter 22 Single and Multiple Tooth Replacement: Treatment Options

Ralph Powers, DDS
Adjunct Clinical Professor
Medical Diagnostics and Translational Science
Old Dominion University
Norfolk, Virginia, Consultant
Dental Education
Ralph Powers LLC
Chesapeake, Virginia
Chapter 35 Bone Substitutes and Membranes

Christopher R. Resnik, DMD, MDS
Prosthodontist
University of Pittsburgh
Pittsburgh, Pennsylvania
Chapter 26 Basic Surgical Techniques and Armamentarium

Randolph R. Resnik, DMD, MDS
Clinical Professor
Department of Periodontology and Oral Implantology
Kornberg School of Dentistry-Temple University
Philadelphia, Pennsylvania
Adjunct Professor
Department of Graduate Prosthodontics
University of Pittsburgh School of Dental Medicine
    Pittsburgh, Pennsylvania
Clinical Professor
Department of Oral & Maxillofacial Surgery
Allegheny General Hospital

Pittsburgh, Pennsylvania
Surgical Director/Chief of Staff
Misch International Implant Institute
Beverly Hills, Michigan
Chapter 1 Rationale for Dental Implants
Chapter 5 Biomaterials for Dental Implants
Chapter 7 Stress Treatment Theorem for Implant Dentistry
Chapter 8 Treatment Planning: Force Factors Related to Patient Conditions
Chapter 10 Medical Evaluation of the Dental Implant Patient
Chapter 11 Radiographic Evaluation in Oral Implantology
Chapter 14 Pharmacology in Implant Dentistry
Chapter 15 Interactive Computed Tomography and Dental Implant Treatment Planning
Chapter 16 Available Bone and Dental Implant Treatment Plans
Chapter 17 Prosthetic Options in Implant Dentistry
Chapter 18 Bone Density: A Key Determinant for Treatment Planning
Chapter 19 Treatment Plans Related to Key Implant Positions and Implant Number
Chapter 20 Treatment Plans for Partially and Completely Edentulous Arches in Implant Dentistry
Chapter 21 Preimplant Prosthodontic Factors Related to Surgical Treatment Planning
Chapter 22 Single and Multiple Tooth Replacement: Treatment Options
Chapter 23 Treatment Planning for the Edentulous Posterior Maxilla
Chapter 24 The Edentulous Mandible: Fixed Versus Removable Prosthesis Treatment Planning
Chapter 25 The Edentulous Maxilla: Fixed versus Removable Treatment Planning
Chapter 26 Basic Surgical Techniques and Armamentarium
Chapter 27 Implant Placement Surgical Protocol
Chapter 28 Ideal Implant Positioning
Chapter 29 Maxillary Anterior Implant Placement
Chapter 30 Mandibular Anatomic Implications for Dental Implant Surgery
Chapter 31 Dental Implant Complications
Chapter 32 Immediate Implant Placement Surgical Protocol
Chapter 33 Immediate Load/Restoration in Implant Dentistry
Chapter 34 Atraumatic Tooth Extraction and Socket Grafting
Chapter 37 Maxillary Sinus Anatomy, Pathology, and Graft Surgery
Chapter 40 The Use of Botox and Dermal Fillers in Oral Implantology

Robert J. Resnik, MD, MBA
Internal Medicine
Cary Adult Medicine
Cary, North Carolina
Chapter 10 Medical Evaluation of the Dental Implant Patient

W. Eugene Roberts, DDS, PhD, DHC (Med)
Professor Emeritus of Orthodontics
Indiana University School of Dentistry
Indianapolis, Indiana
Chapter 4 Bone Physiology, Metabolism, and Biomechanics

Mohamed Sharawy, BDS, PhD
Professor
Department of Oral Biology and Diagnostic Sciences
Dental College of Georgia at Augusta University
Augusta Georgia
Chapter 12 Applied Anatomy for Dental Implants

Amanda M. Sheehan, DDS, DICOI, FAGD
Waterford, Michigan
Chapter 40 The Use of Botox and Dermal Fillers in Oral Implantology

Jon B. Suzuki, DDS, PhD, MBA
Professor Emeritus of Microbiology and Immunology (School of Medicine)
Professor Emeritus of Periodontology and Oral Implantology (School of Dentistry)
Temple University School of Medicine
Philadelphia, Pennsylvania
Clinical Professor, Department of Periodontics, University of Maryland
Clinical Professor, Department of Periodontics, Nova Southeastern University
Clinical Professor, Department of Graduate Prosthodontics, University of Washington
Chapter 34 Atraumatic Tooth Extraction and Socket Grafting
Chapter 41 Peri-Mucositis and Peri-Implantitis Diagnosis, Classification, Etiologies, and Therapies
Chapter 42 Implant Maintenance: Long-term Implant Success

Kevin R. Suzuki, DMD, MS
Associate Professor
Graduate Periodontics
Temple University School of Dentistry
Philadelphia, Pennsylvania
Affiliate Professor
Predoctoral Periodontics
University of Washington School of Dentistry
Seattle, Washington
Chapter 41 Peri-Mucositis and Peri-Implantitis Diagnosis, Classification, Etiologies, and Therapies

Foreword

After 50 years of involvement in dental implant evaluation and research and 47 years of clinical implant practice, I feel greatly honored as well as having a substantial professional responsibility to provide the Foreword to *Misch's Contemporary Implant Dentistry* authored by Dr. Randolph R. Resnik. Why? This book should, simply put, have an incalculable influence on dentistry for years to come.

Since 1972 I have also served continuously on the Executive Committee of the International Congress of Oral Implantologists (ICOI). Today, the ICOI is one of the largest implant societies in the world. For many years, Dr. Carl E. Misch and I were Co-Chairman of the ICOI. Since his death, I have acted as CEO. ICOI's mission has always been to promote worldwide dental implant education, research and international fraternity.

Having known Dr. Randy Resnik for many years, I can assure you that he is a shining example of a multi-talented individual who has pursued these goals and has dedicated his life to oral implantology/implant dentistry and expanding the impact of the Contemporary Implant Dentistry texts.

Because of his extensive teaching and mentoring background, he appreciates like few others the "gestalt" of oral implantology/implant dentistry. With the exponential growth of this field, fueled by exceptional professional acceptance and growing consumer awareness, Dr. Resnik has been able to thoughtfully identify the numerous sources of complications that can occur and propose many solutions. Further, he makes a strong case that dental implants are for the many, not just the privileged few. In this view several clinicians around the world are attempting to influence manufacturers to lower the price of implants or the required number of implants used in specific cases to increase their availability to patients and yet obtain satisfactory results.

Having spent many hours discussing the question with Dr. Resnik, I can assure you that he feels, as I do, that implants are the purview of generalists as well as specialists worldwide. What determines the elements of treatment that individual practitioners do should be determined by how well they train, by how much they are committed to lifelong education, and by how well they are influenced by mentors who are open, honest and caring, such as Dr. Resnik.

Several aspects of *Misch's Contemporary Implant Dentistry* have to be emphasized so that casual reading is not encouraged. There are eight sections with 42 chapters, all of which have been updated. Further, approximately 20 chapters are brand new and present in-depth multiple new topics. Dr. Resnik is very aware of how much and how fast the field of oral implantology/implant dentistry is changing. To this end, Dr. Resnik has asked multiple colleagues, researchers and specialists to contribute their knowledge.

Misch's Contemporary Implant Dentistry, authored by Dr. Randolph R. Resnik, is a classic guide for the student and the young practitioner and a valuable reference for well-experienced clinicians.

With great personal and professional respect,
Kenneth W. M. Judy, DDS, FAGD, FACD, MICD
CEO & Co-Chairman, ICOI
Clinical Professor, *New York University College of Dentistry*, New York, New York
Clinical Professor Department of Oral Implantology, Dental Medicine Section of Oral, Diagnostic and Rehabilitation Sciences, Division of Prosthodontics, *Columbia University College of Dental Medicine*, New York, New York

To my wife Diane, and children Christopher and Allison, for their patience and understanding along with enriching my life.

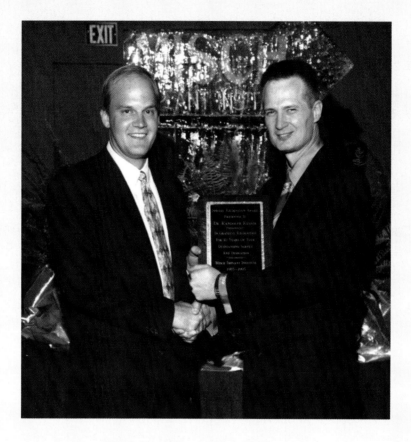

Carl E. Misch Dedication

The sign of a true genius is someone who has the innate ability to foresee what the future beholds. This is reflective of Dr. Carl E. Misch's life. Over 30 years ago, he was responsible for pioneering the foundation and protocols that are universally utilized today in the mainstream field of dental implantology. He had the unbelievable foresight to develop these concepts, usually against much resistance, to unprecedented perfection. When Carl, like other gifted geniuses, leave this life, the accomplishments they achieved reveal the true impact they have made on our daily lives.

Carl will always be known as one of the true "fathers" in implant dentistry, as most techniques and procedures today are based on his original principles and classifications. He had more to do with the inception, evolution and current theories of today's implant dentistry than any other practitioner in the field. He dedicated his life's work to the field of implant dentistry and worked painlessly every day to achieve these accomplishments.

Carl had a singular focus toward the understanding that if properly utilized, dental implants would have significant positive impacts on the health of the population at large. His passion was centered on perfecting the clinical outcomes of implant patients and his vision allowed implant dentistry to become a reality. He

was a true innovator that has led to dental implants becoming the standard of care in dentistry even though he went against the odds and encountered much resistance.

Carl will be remembered as the consummate clinician, researcher, educator and father. He lived and taught what he believed, teaching right up to the end of his life. He was relentless and determined to further implant dentistry in the medical community. Not only did he continue teaching every one of us about dental implantology, he was also imparting further wisdom with his love for life. Carl was able to stimulate a renaissance in oral implantology that will continue to impact the field forever.

That is the beauty of life. Certain geniuses come along with great gifts. The best of these decide to dedicate their lives to sharing those gifts with others. That is a great description of Dr. Carl E. Misch, and I, as well as the rest of our profession, will never forget him. His legacy will live on in the clinicians he has educated, the teachers he has influenced, and the patients who will benefit from his tireless and profound work.

Carl, thank you for allowing me to continue your legacy. You are truly missed and you are in our thoughts every day. Rest in peace, my friend!

Preface

The use of dental implants in the field of dentistry has become a widely acceptable treatment modality to rehabilitate patients with edentulous sites. Dental implant clinicians and researchers continue to dedicate a significant amount of time and resources to the future development of the field. The global dental implant market continues to grow at an unprecedented rate, expected to exceed 7.0 billion by 2024. With an ever-increasing public awareness of the benefits of dental implantology, the popularity of dental implant rehabilitation will continue to increase for the future. A growing number of the population experience partial or complete edentulism, and the dental implant is now the preferred method of choice to replace a single, multiple, or completely edentulous sites. Therefore, it is imperative the dental implant clinician have a strong foundation of the accepted principles for treatment planning, radiographic evaluation, surgical procedures, prosthetic rehabilitation and postoperative care.

In the fourth edition of Contemporary Implant Dentistry, the underlying theme of past editions is clearly maintained with respect to the science-based concept of implant dentistry. This new edition is a comprehensive overview of all surgical aspects of implant dentistry, which include eight sections and 42 chapters. Each chapter in this book is specifically written to be related to all other chapters in the text with the concept of consistent and predictable care as the priority. The fourth edition has nearly tripled in size from the first edition written in the early 1990s. New chapters on treatment planning, implant surgery, pharmacology, medical evaluation, immediate placement and immediate loading, bone grafting techniques, Botox and dermal fillers, and the treatment of peri-implant disease have been added to this fourth edition.

The first part of the fourth edition Contemporary Implant Dentistry is related to the scientific basis for dental implants. It presents the rationale for the use of dental implants as inert replacements for missing teeth and why biomechanics play such a significant role in the treatment planning process. A comprehensive outline of the terminology is explained with clear and concise examples. Science based research is used as the basis for discussing implant design and biomaterials, along with the physiologic bone response to these materials.

The second part of this book discusses the biomechanical properties which relate to the dental implant process. The pioneering stress theorem concepts postulated by Dr. Carl Misch are the basis for these chapters as the various force factors which dental implants are exposed to are presented. The effects of these forces along with how different implant surfaces relate to the stresses are discussed in detail.

The third part of Contemporary Implant Dentistry provides information concerning the related basic sciences of oral implantology. The medical evaluation chapter details medical conditions and medications which have direct and indirect effects on the short and long-term success of dental implants. The radiographic evaluation chapter allows the reader to have a comprehensive understanding of normal anatomy as well as anatomic and pathologic variants related to dental implantology. An updated pharmacology chapter encompasses all prophylactic and therapeutic medications related to pre- and postoperative care of dental implants. And lastly, applied anatomy of the head and neck is discussed with an overview on possible infectious episodes that may result from dental implant treatment.

The fourth part of Contemporary Implant Dentistry is based upon all aspects of the treatment planning process. The pioneering classifications from Dr. Carl Misch including available bone, prosthetic options, key implant positions and bone density are updated. A new chapter added to this section details the use of interactive cone beam computerized tomography (CBCT) in the treatment planning process. Valuable treatment planning concepts are discussed with a generic protocol for the use of CBCT.

The fifth part of Contemporary Implant Dentistry discusses generalized treatment planning concepts related to anatomical regions within the oral cavity. Single , multiple, and fully edentulous treatment planning principles are presented according to anatomic areas in the anterior and posterior maxilla and mandible. The edentulous treatment planning process for fixed versus removable prostheses are compared with respect to anatomic areas in the maxilla and mandible.

The sixth part of Contemporary Implant Dentistry is dedicated to the implant surgery process. A new chapter related to surgical techniques entails basic surgical principles and protocols, as well as the armamentarium required in the field of oral implantology. Various surgical protocols are discussed related to the specific anatomy in the maxilla and mandible. In addition, a full array of possible complications of implant surgery with respect to etiology, management, and prevention is presented. And lastly, new classifications and protocols related to immediate implant placement surgery along with immediate loading techniques are explained in science- and research-based techniques.

The seventh part of Contemporary Implant Dentistry discusses all aspects of soft and hard tissue rehabilitation. A detailed chapter explains guidelines and techniques for atraumatic extraction and socket grafting. A new chapter specifically discussing the available bone substitutes and membranes, with advantages and disadvantages based on science and the latest research is presented. In addition, updated and comprehensive bone grafting chapters on guided tissue regeneration, maxillary sinus augmentation, intraoral bone grafts, and extraoral techniques are included in this part. And lastly, a new chapter related to the use of Botox and dermal fillers is added to this section which includes the use for esthetic and functional aspects of oral implantology.

The last section of Contemporary Implant Dentistry is related to the postoperative care, specifically the treatment of peri-implant disease with an emphasis on treatment protocols. The last chapter includes a detailed protocol and treatment techniques on the maintenance of dental implants.

In summary, Contemporary Implant Dentistry has been used over the years as a textbook for dental schools, dental residents, postgraduate programs, lab technicians, general dentists, and dental specialists. The translations into many languages has shown the popularity and acceptance of this textbook in the field of oral implantology worldwide. The fourth edition of this textbook comprehensively updates the reader on all aspects of dental implantology with the goal of elevating the educational standards through a science-based approach.

Randolph R. Resnik, DMD, MDS

Acknowledgments

I would like to express my sincere gratitude for the many individuals who helped shape my career and provided the foundation for the writing of this book. First and foremost, I would never have had the ambition, aspiration, and discipline to write this book if not for the two mentors in my life, my late father, Dr. Rudolph Resnik, and the true pioneer in oral implantology, Dr. Carl E. Misch. My father was the perfect role model, educator, clinician, and a true pioneer in the field of fixed prosthetics. He was my hero and best friend, and the number one reason I am where I am today. His endless support and encouragement motivated me to give 100% to every endeavor that I ever pursued.

Secondly, Dr. Carl Misch was not only my mentor, but also a very close friend. His endless energy and ability to foresee the future of oral implantology and its impact on dentistry allowed me to be at the forefront of this challenging profession. His dedication and contributions to the field of oral implantology are unprecedented and will never be forgotten. The scientific basis for his classifications and principles will be an integral component in the field forever.

I would also like to acknowledge the thousands of doctors, whom over the past 30 years, have attended my various lectures, symposiums and especially the past graduates of the Misch International Implant Institute. It is through their inquisitiveness and ambition to learn that has empowered me to write the Fourth Edition of Contemporary Implant Dentistry. They have given me the determination and desire to raise the standard of care in our profession and elevate implant dentistry to the next level.

I am sincerely thankful to all the additional chapter authors for sharing their expertise with the writing of this book. Their dedication to implant dentistry, and especially their friendship and personal support to me, is greatly appreciated: Dean Jon Suzuki, Steven Caldwell, Robert Resnik, Christopher Resnik, David Datillo, Joseph Cillo, Neil Park, Grant Bullis, Mauri Kerr, Amanda Sheehan, Kevin Suzuki, Diana Bronstein, Ralph Powers, Francine Misch- Dietsh, and Mohamed Sharowry.

A special note of thanks to the staff at Elsevier Publishing for their, encouragement, enthusiasm and guidance with the content of this book. In particular, Content Strategist, Alexandra Mortimer and Senior Content Development Specialist, Anne E. Snyder, for their dedication and endless hours of work in the development and creativity of this book. Without their help, this book would never have come to fruition.

At last but not least, I would like to thank my family, for their support and encouragement they gave me during this project, despite the sacrifice and burden it often imposed on them. My wife, Diane, who's unwavering support always gives me the strength to succeed. So proud of both of my children, Christopher, currently in a residency program at the University of Pittsburgh and soon to be third generation Prosthodontist and my beautiful daughter, Allison, who is currently in medical school at Georgetown University.

Contents

PART I

Scientific Basis

1

Rationale for Dental Implants

RANDOLPH R. RESNIK AND
CARL E. MISCH

The goal of modern dentistry is to restore the patient to normal contour, function, comfort, esthetics, speech, and health by removing a disease process from a tooth or replacing teeth with a prosthesis. What makes implant dentistry unique is the ability to achieve this goal, regardless of the atrophy, disease, or injury of the stomatognathic system.[1] However, the more teeth a patient is missing, the more challenging this task becomes. As a result of continued research, diagnostic tools, treatment planning, implant designs, advanced materials, and techniques, predictable success is now a reality for the rehabilitation of many challenging clinical situations.

The impact of dental implants has surely affected the field of dentistry in the United States. The number of dental implants placed in the United States has increased more than 10-fold from 1983 to 2002, and another fivefold from 2000 to 2005. More than 1 million dental implants are inserted each year and the industry is expected to be a $10 billion industry in 2020.[2,3] More than 90% of interfacing surgical specialty dentists currently provide dental implant treatment on a routine basis in their practices, 90% of prosthodontists restore implants routinely, and more than 80% of general dentists have used implants to support fixed and removable prostheses, compared with only 65% 15 years ago.[4-7]

Despite these figures demonstrating implants are incorporated into dentistry more than ever before, there is still a great deal of room for continued growth. Utilization of dental implants varies widely in different countries. For example, it is estimated that the number placed each year per 10,000 people is 230 for Israel (the greatest number); 180 for South Korea and Italy; 140 for Spain and Switzerland; 100 for Germany; 60 each for Brazil, the Netherlands, and the United States; 50 for Japan and France; 40 for Canada and Australia; and Taiwan and the United Kingdom, at 20 per year, use implants less often. The six countries with the greatest use of implants (five in Europe and South Korea) accounted for more than half the total market growth from 2002 to 2007. A long-term growth of 12% to 15% is expected in the future in most countries using implants at this time (Fig. 1.1).

The percentage of teeth replaced with an implant, rather than traditional fixed or removable prostheses, also dramatically varies by country. In countries such as Israel, Italy, and South Korea, 30% to 40% of teeth replaced incorporate a dental implant. In Spain, Switzerland, Germany, and Sweden, 20% to 26% of restorations to replace teeth are supported by an implant, whereas in Brazil and Belgium approximately 13% to 16% of restorations use an implant. Surprisingly, the United States, Japan, France, and Canada use implants in 10% or fewer of the teeth replaced, however this number is increasing (Fig. 1.2).[8]

Increasing Demand for Dental Implants

The increased need and use of implant-related treatments result from the combined effect of several factors, including (1) patients living longer, (2) age-related tooth loss, (3) patients are more socially active and esthetic conscious, (4) a higher incidence of partial and complete edentulism, (5) conventional prosthesis complications, and (6) the inherent advantages of implant-supported restorations.

Patients Living Longer

According to the literature, age is directly related to every indicator of tooth loss[9,10]; therefore the aging population is an important factor to consider in implant dentistry. When Alexander the Great conquered the ancient world, he was only 17 years old. However, life expectancy at that time was only 22 years of age. From 1000 BCE to CE 1800, life span remained less than 30 years (Fig. 1.3). The latest statistics from the National Center for Health Statistics show that the average American life expectancy is approximately 78.6 years, with women (81.1 years) living approximately 5 years longer than men (76.1 years). The group older than age 65 is projected to increase from 12% in 2000 to more than 20% of the population before 2025 (Fig. 1.4).[11]

In addition, not only is the percentage of the population over 65 years increasing, but the overall population as a whole is increasing. The population in 2000 was 282 million and is projected to increase 49% to 420 million by 2050. Considering the effect of both a population increase and a greater percentage of that population being older than age 65, a dramatic overall increase in patient numbers can be expected. In 2003, 35 million people were older than age 65. This number is expected to increase 87% by 2025, resulting in almost 70 million people being older than age 65[9] (Fig. 1.5). Because older people are more likely to be missing teeth, the need for implant dentistry will dramatically increase over the next several decades.

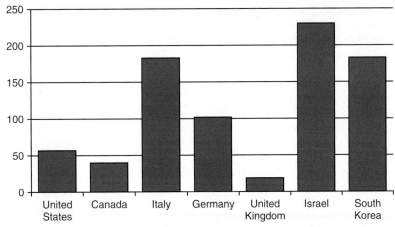

• **Fig. 1.1** Implant used to replace teeth varies by country. Estimated implant use per 10,000 people per year is greatest in Israel, South Korea, and Italy. (From Misch CE. Rationale for dental implants. In: Misch CE, ed. *Dental Implant Prosthetics*. 2nd ed. St Louis: Mosby; 2015.)

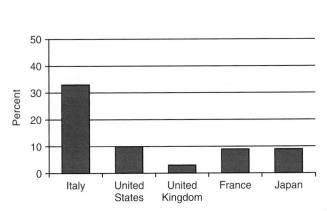

• **Fig. 1.2** Implant versus nonimplant tooth replacement (percentage) varies greatly by country. In the United States only 1 of every 10 teeth replaced incorporates an implant. (From Misch CE. Rationale for dental implants. In: Misch CE, ed. *Dental Implant Prosthetics*. 2nd ed. St Louis: Mosby; 2015.)

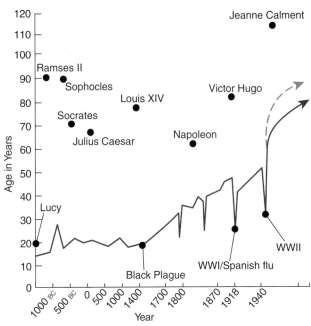

• **Fig. 1.3** Average life expectancy remained approximately 20 to 30 years for several hundred years of human civilization. Since the late 18th century, there has been a gradual increase in life span. (Redrawn from *Le Figaro Magazine*, Paris, 2004.)

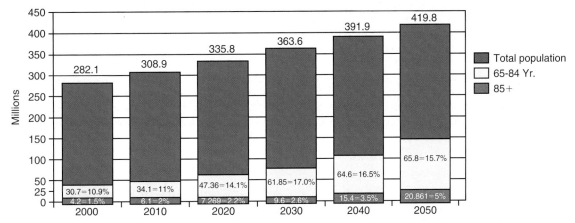

• **Fig. 1.4** By 2050, 20.7% of the population will be older than age 65. In addition to the increasing percentage of 65 year olds, the population is also increasing. As a result, 34.9 million people were older than 65 in 2000, and 86.6 million people will reach this milestone by 2050.

Life expectancy has increased significantly past the age of retirement. A 65 year old person can now expect to live more than 20 additional years, and an 80-year-old person can expect to live 9.5 more years[10] (Fig. 1.6). Women represent two-thirds of the population older than age 65. It is not unusual for a 70-year-old patient to ask, "Is it worth it for me to spend a lot of money to repair my mouth at my age?" The response should be very positive because the patient's life expectancy will extend for two more decades on average, and his or her current oral situation will normally become worse if not corrected.

Over 69% of Americans between 35 and 44 years have at least one missing tooth. According to the National Center for Health Statistics, 91% of the people in the United States aged 20 to 64 had dental caries in their permanent teeth. The National Health and Nutrition Examination survey estimated that approximately 42% of the children aged 2 to 11 years have tooth caries, and over 23% are left untreated. The National Institute of Dental and Craniofacial Research has determined that tooth loss in American adults begins between the ages of 35 and 45, and more than 24% of adults older than 74 years are completely edentulous.[12]

Age-Related Tooth Loss

The aging process directly affects the oral cavity with negative consequences. As the tooth enamel wears away, teeth become more vulnerable to disease processes and eventual tooth loss. Many medications directly affect the teeth, especially causing xerostomia. Xerostomia not only weakens the teeth, but also results in hard and soft tissue loss. Therefore, a direct correlation between the aging process and tooth loss exists.

The posterior regions of the oral cavity are the most common areas for single-tooth loss[13] (Fig. 1.7). The first molars are the first permanent teeth to erupt in the mouth and, unfortunately, are often the first teeth lost as a result of decay, failed endodontic therapy, or fracture (usually after endodontics).

The molar teeth are vitally important for maintenance of the arch form and proper occlusal schemes. In addition, the adult patient often has one or more crowns as a consequence of previous larger restorations required to repair the integrity of the tooth. Longevity reports of crowns have yielded very disparate results. The mean life span at failure has been reported as approximately 10.3 years. Other reports range from a 3% failure rate at 23 years to a 20% failure rate at 3 years. The primary cause of failure of the crown is caries followed by periodontal disease and endodontic therapy.[14] The tooth is at risk for extraction as a result of these complications, which are the leading causes of single posterior tooth loss in the adult (Fig. 1.8, Fig. 1.9).[15]

Researchers have found a direct correlation of tooth loss in the elderly population exhibiting physical and mental decline. The data showed that subjects who had lost all their natural teeth performed approximately 10% worse in both memory and mobility (walking) than counterparts with natural teeth. Usually, tooth loss is less with patients of higher socioeconomic status. However, in this study, the link between total tooth loss and mobility (slower walking speed) remained significant when all variables were taken into consideration.

Patients More Socially Active and Esthetic Conscious

With patients living longer, their social pleasures, including dining and dating, are continuing into their elderly years. In the past, treatment of elderly patients emphasized nonsurgical approaches and palliative treatment. Today, the full scope of dental services for elderly patients is increasing in importance to both the public and the profession because of the increasing age of our society. Studies have shown that

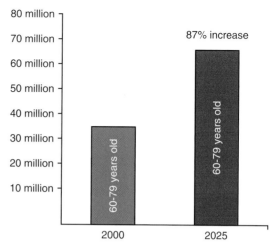

• **Fig. 1.5** Adult population older than the age of 60 years will increase by 87% from the year 2000 to the year 2025. (From Misch CE. Rationale for dental implants. In: Misch CE, ed. *Dental Implant Prosthetics*. 2nd ed. St Louis: Mosby; 2015.)

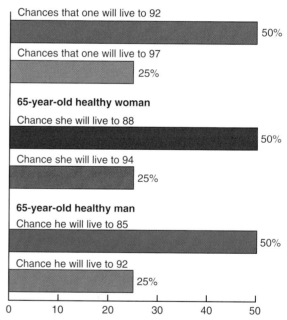

• **Fig. 1.6** When a person reaches age 65 years, he or she may often feels an investment in health is less appropriate. A 65-year-old healthy woman will live 23 more years 50% of the time and 29 more years 25% of the time. Her present oral condition will become worse during this extended time frame if treatment is not rendered.

elderly patients that are more socially active will have a slower progression of health declines than elderly people who become less socially active. Engaging older people have been shown to be more motivated to maintain their health than their less-engaged peers. Therefore with patients living longer, patient education is vitally important as the demand for more comprehensive dental implant treatment will be most definitely increasing in the future to maintain social activity.

Higher Prevalence of Partial and Complete Edentulism

Partial Edentulism

Currently, the prevalence of partial edentulism in the general population has resulted in an increased need for dental implants.

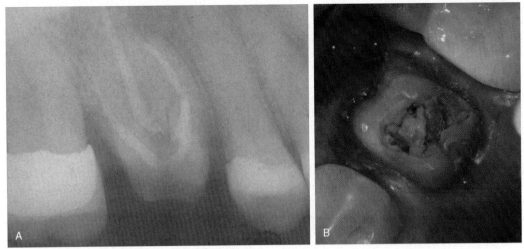

• **Fig. 1.7** (A and B) The most common tooth to be lost is the first molar. Approximately 80% of the time, the adjacent teeth are unrestored or have minimal restorations.

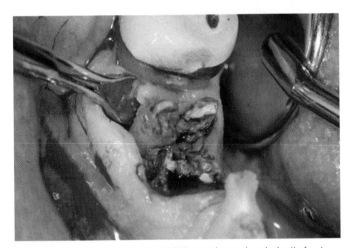

• **Fig. 1.8** Posterior molar tooth exhibiting caries and endodontic fracture, which are two of the most common complications leading to an unrestorable tooth.

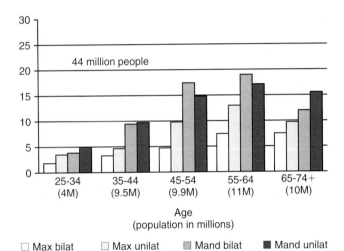

• **Fig. 1.10** There are more than 44 million people in the United States missing at least one quadrant of posterior teeth (most often in the mandible). (From Misch CE. Rationale for dental implants. In: Misch CE, ed. *Dental Implant Prosthetics*. 2nd ed. St Louis: Mosby; 2015.)

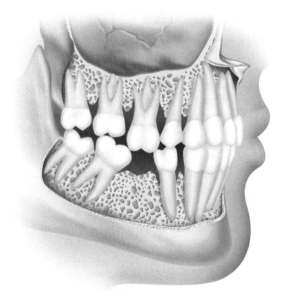

• **Fig. 1.9** Posterior missing tooth is a frequent occurrence in a general practice. The most common single tooth missing is the first molar. which results in many dental arch complications. (From Misch CE. Rationale for dental implants. In: Misch CE, ed. *Dental Implant Prosthetics*. 2nd ed. St Louis: Mosby; 2015.)

Various studies have shown this pattern to be as high as 48% of the population. Many variables which have been associated this increase include gender, ethnicity, and chronic disease. In addition, adults exhibiting partial edentulism were 22.6% more likely to be from rural areas and 31.5% from depressed locations.[16]

As stated previously, the most common missing teeth are have been shown to be molars.[17] Partial free-end edentulism is of particular concern because in these patients, teeth are often replaced with removable partial prostheses. Implant placement in the posterior regions is often challenging because of the location of the maxillary sinus and the mandibular canal. Mandibular free-end edentulism frequency is greater than its maxillary counterpart in all age groups. Unilateral free-end edentulism is more common than bilateral edentulism in both maxillary and mandibular arches in the younger age groups (ages 25–44). About 13.5 million persons in these younger age groups have free-end edentulism in either arch (Fig. 1.10).

In 45- to 54-year-old patients, 31.3% have mandibular free-end edentulism, and 13.6% have free-end edentulism in the maxillary arch. Approximately 9.9 million persons in the 45- to 54-year-old group have at least one free-end edentulous quadrant, and almost half of these have bilateral partial edentulism. The pattern of posterior edentulism evolves in the 55- to 64-year-old group, in which 35% of mandibular arches show free-end edentulism compared with 18% of maxillary arches. As a result, approximately 11 million individuals in this age group are potential candidates for implants. An additional 10 million show partial free-end edentulism at age 65 or older. Additional US survey studies have documented approximately 44 million people to have at least one quadrant of posterior missing teeth. For example, if each of these arches requires three implants to support a fixed prosthesis, 132 million implants, added to the 192 million for edentulous patients, would be required.[18-20]

Total Edentulism

Although the percentage of patients with total edentulism is decreasing because of the baby-boomer population, the total number of patients exhibiting edentulism that will require treatment will increase in the future. In the past, full arch extractions were mainly indicated because of the combined pathologic processes of dental caries, periodontal disease, or as a method to reduce the costs associated with dental treatment. However, because of the high success rate of dental implants today, it is not uncommon for full-mouth extractions to be completed when teeth are questionable, especially in anticipation of future implant placement. Similar to other pathologic outcomes of disease, the occurrence of total loss of teeth is directly related to the age of the patient. The rate of edentulism increases approximately 4% per 10 years in early adult years and increases to more than 10% per decade after age 70.[21]

The average total edentulous rate worldwide is approximately 20% at age 60, although there is wide disparity between the countries with the highest and lowest rates. For example, in the 65- to 74-year age group, the total edentulous rate in Kenya and Nigeria was 0%, whereas the Netherlands and Iceland have a 65.4% and 71.5% rate, respectively. The edentulous Canadian rate was 47% at ages 65 to 69 and 58% from ages 70 to 98 (with Quebec at 67% for those older than age 65 compared with Ontario with a 41% rate).[22]

In the United States the comparison of edentulism from 1957 to 2012 decreased from 19% to 5%. Income is often related to education and may also play a role in the rate of edentulism in the United States from 1988 to 1994, studies reported an edentulous rate of 22% for those with less than 8 years of education, 12% for those with 9 to 11 years of school, 8% for those with 12 years of school, and 5% for individuals with more than 12 years of education.

Studies show that edentulism in the United States is rarely seen in high-income individuals. The level of education is inversely proportional to edentulism. Geographically, edentulism was found to be highest in states that are bordered by the Appalachian Mountains and the Mississippi Delta. The lowest prevalence was found in California, Connecticut, Hawaii, and Minnesota. The prevalence in southern states is nearly twice that in western states (Fig. 1.11).[23]

In the National Institute of Dental Research national surveys, the occurrence of total edentulism (absence of teeth) of a single arch (35 times more frequent in the maxilla) was slight in the 30- to 34-year-old age group, but it increased at around age 45 to 11% and then remained constant after 55 years at approximately 15% of the adult population. A total of approximately 12 million individuals in the United States have edentulism in one arch, representing 7% of the adult population overall. With the passing of generations born in the mid-20th century, the rate of decline in edentulism is projected to slow, reaching approximately 2.6% by the year 2050. This continuing decline, however will be offset by population aging. The projected number of edentulous people in

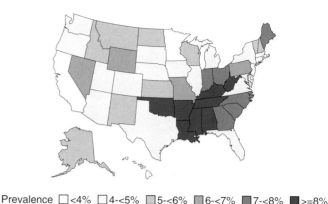

Prevalence ☐<4% ☐4-<5% ☐5-<6% ☐6-<7% ■7-<8% ■>=8%

Fig. 1.11 Age-standardized edentulism prevalence among adults aged ≥25 years in the United States in 2010. (From Slade GD, Akinkugbe AA, Sanders, AE. Projections of U.S. edentulism prevalence following 5 decades of decline. *J Dent Res.* 2014;93(10):959–965.)

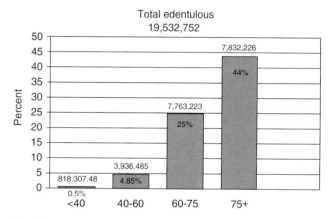

Total edentulous
19,532,752

Population 163,607,356   81,165,640   31,052,895   17,800,513
Total population = 298 million

Fig. 1.12 The US population completely edentulous rate ranges from 5% for 40 year olds to 44% for those older than age 75. As a result, 20 million people (10.5% of the population) in the United States have no teeth. An additional 12 million people (7% of the adult population) have no maxillary teeth opposing at least some mandibular teeth.

2050 will be approximately 8.6 million. This will be 30% lower than the 12.2 million edentulous people in 2010.[23]

The present younger population is benefiting from today's advanced knowledge and restorative techniques. Edentulism has been noted in 5% of employed adults aged 40 to 44, gradually increasing to 26% at age 65, and almost 44% in seniors older than age 75 (Fig. 1.12).[24] As expected, older persons are more likely to be missing all their teeth. Gender was not found to be associated with tooth retention or tooth loss once adjustments were made for age. The percentages of one- or two-arch edentulism translate into more than 30 million people, or about 17% of the entire US adult population. To put these numbers in perspective, 30 million people represent approximately the entire US African American population, or the entire population of Canada. Although the edentulism rate is decreasing every decade, the elderly population is rising so rapidly that the adult population in need of one or two complete dentures will actually increase from 33.6 million adults in 1991 to 37.9 million adults in 2020. The total number of edentulous arches is estimated at 56.5 million in 2000, 59.3 million in 2010, and 61 million in 2020. Complete edentulism, therefore, remains a significant concern, and affected patients often

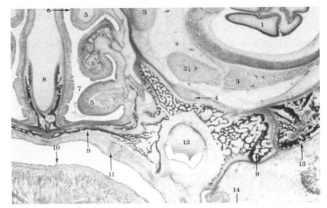

• **Fig. 1.13** The alveolar bone forms as a result of the tooth root formation. When no tooth root is present, the alveolar process does not form (i.e., ectodermal dysplasia when partial or complete anodontia of both primary and secondary teeth occurs).

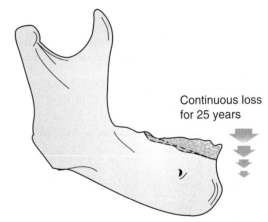

Continuous loss for 25 years

• **Fig. 1.14** After the initial extraction of teeth, studies have shown the average first-year bone loss is more than 4 mm in height and 30% in crestal bone width. Although the rate of bone loss is slower after the first year, the bone loss is continuous throughout life.

require dental implant treatment to solve several related problems. For example, to show the need for implant treatment with the edentulous group, if four implants were used to help support each complete edentulous arch in 2000, a total of 226 million implants would have been required. However, only approximately 1 million implants were inserted for all patient treatment (partially or completely edentulous) that year. Almost 70% of dentists spend less than 1% to 5% of their treatment time on edentulous patients, leaving a great unfulfilled need for implant dentistry.[25]

When the partially edentulous figures are added to the complete edentulous percentages, almost 30% of the adult US population are candidates for a complete or partial removable prosthesis. The need for additional retention, support and stability, and the desire to eliminate a removable prosthesis are common indications for dental implants. As a result, 74 million adults (90 million arches) are potential candidates for dental implants. Because a minimum of five appointments is required to implant and restore a patient, every US dentist would need approximately 20 appointments every month for 20 years to treat the present posterior partial and complete edentulous population with implant-supported prostheses. The population's evolution to an increased average age, combined with the existing population of partially and completely edentulous patients, guarantees implant dentistry's future for several generations of dentists.

In the elderly population, tooth loss is more common. The baby-boomer population in the United States is the major purchaser of elective plastic surgery and antiaging procedures and medications. This generation is destined to be the most affluent older generation ever in the United States, and they will inherit the largest inflation-adjusted transfer of wealth in history at approximately $10 trillion.[26] This propensity for discretionary spending has fueled unprecedented growth in implant dentistry during the last decade, and it is expected to continue. The 65-year-plus population in the United States is expected to increase at annual rates of 1.5% to 3% from 2010 through 2035. The population of 65+ age group will increase from 12.4% of the population in 2000 to 20.6% in 2050.[27,28]

Anatomic Consequences Of Edentulism

Hard Tissue Loss. Basal bone forms the dental skeletal structure, contains most of the muscle attachments, and begins to form in the fetus before teeth develop (Box 1.1). Alveolar bone first appears when the Hertwig root sheath of the tooth bud evolves (Fig. 1.13). The alveolar bone does not form in the absence of primary or secondary tooth development. The close relationship between the tooth and the alveolar process continues throughout life. Wolff's law (1892) stated that bone remodels in relationship to the forces applied. Every time the function of bone is modified, a definite change occurs in the internal architecture and external configuration.[29,30] In dentistry, the consequences of complete edentulous and remaining bone volume was noted by Misch in 1922, in which he described the skeletal structure of a 90-year-old woman without teeth for several decades.[31]

Bone requires stimulation to maintain its form and density. Roberts and colleagues[32] reported that a 4% strain to the skeletal system maintains bone and helps balance the resorption and formation phenomena. Teeth transmit compressive and tensile forces to the surrounding bone. These forces have been measured as a piezoelectric effect in the imperfect crystals of durapatite that compose the inorganic portion of bone. When a tooth is lost, the lack of stimulation to the residual bone causes a decrease in trabeculae and bone density in the area, with loss in external width, then height, of the bone volume.[32] There is a 25% decrease in the width of bone during the first year after tooth loss and an overall 4-mm decrease in height during the first year after extractions for an immediate denture. In a pioneering longitudinal 25-year study, demonstrated continued bone loss during this time span; in comparing the bone loss of the maxilla to the mandible, a fourfold greater loss was observed in the mandible (Fig. 1.14).[33] Although, initially the mandibular bone height is twice that of the maxilla, maxillary bone loss is very significant in the long-term edentulous patient. In fact, maxillary implant placement and bone graft procedures may be more challenging in comparison to the mandible.

Prostheses also contribute to bone loss. In general, a tooth is necessary for the development of alveolar bone, and stimulation of this bone is required to maintain its density and volume. A removable denture (complete or partial) does not stimulate and maintain bone; rather, it accelerates bone loss. The load from mastication is transferred to the bone surface only and not the entire bone. As a result, blood supply is reduced and total bone volume loss occurs. This issue, which is of utmost importance, has been observed but not addressed until recently in traditional dentistry. Most often dentists overlook the insidious bone loss that will occur after tooth extraction. Therefore, it is imperative patients be educated about the anatomic changes and the potential consequences of continued bone loss. The bone loss accelerates when the patient wears a poorly fitting soft tissue–borne prosthesis. Patients do not understand that bone is being lost over time and at a greater rate beneath poorly fitting dentures (Fig. 1.15). Patients infrequently return for follow-up visits for evaluation of their edentulous condition; instead, they will return for a repair of the prosthesis. Hence the traditional method of tooth replacement (e.g. removable prosthesis) often affects bone loss in a manner not sufficiently considered by the doctor and the patient. Bone loss has been shown to increase with the use of a poorly fitting soft tissue–borne prosthesis. Patients should be informed of periodic evaluations to reline or fabricate a new prosthesis (Fig. 1.16).

Preventive dentistry has traditionally emphasized methods to decrease tooth loss. No predictable therapy had been accepted by the profession to avoid the bone changes resulting from tooth loss. Today, the profession must consider the loss of both teeth and bone. The loss of teeth causes remodeling and resorption of the surrounding alveolar bone and eventually leads to atrophic edentulous ridges. The rate and amount of bone loss may be influenced by such things as gender, hormones, metabolism, parafunction, and ill-fitting dentures (Box 1.2). Yet almost 40% of denture wearers have been wearing an ill-fitting prosthesis for more than 10 years. Patients wearing dentures day and night place greater forces on the hard and soft tissues, which accelerates bone loss. Nonetheless, studies have shown that approximately 80% of dentures are worn both day and night.[34] Atrophic edentulous ridges are associated with anatomic problems that often impair the predictable results of traditional dental therapy (Fig. 1.17; Box 1.3).

Loss of bone in the maxilla or mandible is not limited to alveolar bone; portions of the basal bone also may be resorbed, especially in the posterior aspect of the mandible in which severe resorption may result in catastrophic bone loss.[35] The contents of the mandibular canal or mental foramen eventually become dehiscent and serve as part of the support area of the prosthesis. As a result, acute pain and transient to permanent nerve impairment of the areas supplied by the mandibular nerve are possible. The body of the mandible is also at increased risk of pathologic fracture, even under very low impact forces. The mandibular fracture causes the jaw to shift to one side and makes stabilization and an esthetic result most difficult to obtain during treatment of the fracture.

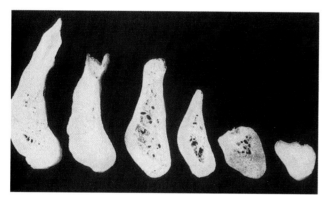

• **Fig. 1.15** Atwood described six different stages of resorption in the anterior mandible. Stage 1 represents the tooth and surrounding alveolar process and basal bone. Stages II and III illustrate the initial residual ridge after tooth loss. Stages IV to VI primarily describe a continuous loss in length of anterior residual bone.

• **BOX 1.2** **Factors Effecting Rate and Amount of Bone Loss**

- Gender
- Medications
- Hormones
- Age
- Metabolism
- Bone Quality
- Parafunction (Increased Biting Force)
- Ill-fitting prosthesis
- Facial type (brachiocephalic versus dolichocephalic)
- Time period dentures are worn
- Past History of Dental Disease

Modified from Misch CE. Rationale for dental implants. In: Misch CE, ed. Dental Implant Prosthetics. 2nd ed. St Louis: Mosby; 2015.

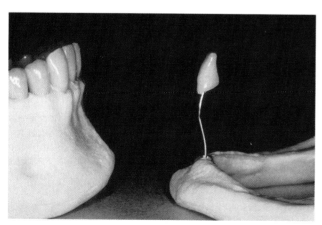

• **Fig. 1.16** Loss of bone height in the mandible may be significant resulting in loss of function. This vertical bone loss has a large impact on restoring the patient back to dental health. The patient should understand that to restore the hard and soft tissue loss, more extensive treatment is usually indicated.

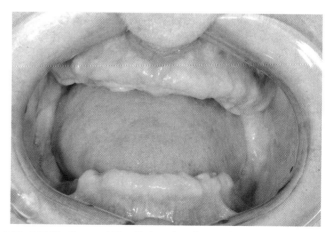

• **Fig. 1.17** Maxillary and Mandibular edentulous arches depicting irregular bone resorption with varying degrees of quality soft tissue (i.e. attached tissue).

In the maxilla, extensive bone loss can also be problematic. In some cases, the complete anterior ridge and even the anterior nasal spine may be resorbed in the maxilla, causing pain and an increase in maxillary denture movement during function. Masticatory forces generated by short facial types (brachiocephalics) can be three to four times that of long facial types (dolichocephalics). Short facial–type patients are at increased risk for developing severe atrophy.

Many of these similar conditions exist in the partially edentulous patient wearing a removable soft tissue–borne prosthesis (e.g. removable partial denture) (Fig. 1.18). In addition, the natural abutment teeth, on which direct and indirect retainers are designed, experience significant lateral forces. Because these teeth are often compromised by deficient periodontal support or large restorations, the resultant forces may be damaging. These forces may result in an increase in mobility of the removable prosthesis and greater soft tissue support. These conditions often will lead to accelerated the bone loss in the edentulous regions (see Box 1.3).

Soft Tissue Consequences. As bone loses width, then height, then width and height again, the attached gingiva gradually decreases. A very thin attached tissue usually lies over the advanced atrophic mandible or maxilla. The increased zones of nonkeratinized gingiva are prone to abrasions caused by the overlaying prosthesis. In addition, unfavorable high muscle attachments and hypermobile tissue often complicate the situation (Fig. 1.19).

As the bone resorbs from Division A to Division B, the resultant narrow residual ridge will often cause discomfort when pressure (from a prosthesis) is applied to the ridge. This often occurs in the posterior mandible, as atrophy may cause a prominent mylohyoid and internal oblique ridges covered by thin, movable, unattached mucosa. In severe atrophy cases the anterior residual alveolar process will continue to resorb, and the superior genial tubercles (which are approximately 20 mm below the crest of bone when teeth are present) eventually become the most superior aspect of the anterior mandibular ridge. This results in excessive movement of the prosthesis during function or speech. This condition is further compromised by the vertical movement of the distal aspect of the prosthesis during contraction of the mylohyoid and buccinator muscles and the anterior incline of the atrophic mandible compared with that of the maxilla.[36]

The thickness of the mucosa on the atrophic ridge is also related to the presence of systemic disease and the physiologic changes that accompany aging. Conditions such as hypertension, diabetes, anemia, and nutritional disorders have a deleterious effect on the vascular supply and soft tissue quality under removable prostheses. These disorders result in a decreased oxygen tension to the basal cells of the epithelium. Surface cell loss occurs at the same rate, but the cell formation at the basal layer is slowed. As a result, the

---

• BOX 1.3   Edentulous Patient Complications

- Continued loss of supporting bone width
- Prominent mylohyoid and internal oblique ridges with increased sore spots
- Progressive decrease in keratinized mucosa surface
- Prominent superior genial tubercles with sore spots and increased denture movement
- Muscle attachment near crest of ridge
- Elevation of prosthesis with contraction of mylohyoid and buccinator muscles serving as posterior support
- Forward movement of prosthesis from anatomic inclination (angulation of mandible with moderate to advanced bone loss)
- Thinning of mucosa, with sensitivity to abrasion
- Loss of basal bone
- Possible Nerve Impairment from dehiscent mandibular neurovascular canal
- More active role of tongue in mastication
- Effect of bone loss on esthetic appearance of lower third of face
- Increased risk of mandibular body fracture from advanced bone loss
- Loss of anterior ridge and nasal spine, causing increased denture movement and sore spots during function

---

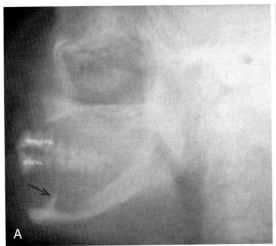
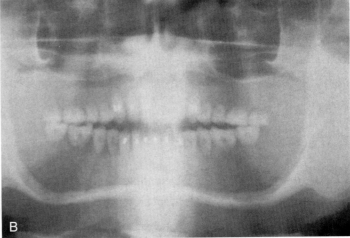

• **Fig. 1.18** (A) Lateral cephalogram of a patient demonstrates the restored vertical dimension of occlusion with a denture. However, because of the advanced basal bone loss in the mandible, the superior genial tubercles (red arrow) are positioned above the residual anterior ridge. The body of the mandible is only a few millimeters thick, and the mandibular canal is completely dehiscent. In the maxillary anterior ridge, only the nasal spine remains (not the original alveolar ridge), and the posterior maxillary bone is very thin because of basal bone loss at the crest and the pneumatization of the maxillary sinus. (B) A denture may restore the vertical dimension of the face, but the bone loss of the jaws can continue until the basal bone becoems pathologically thin.

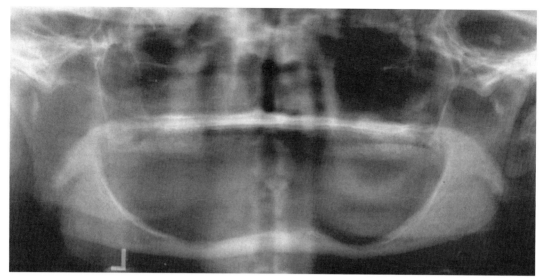

● **Fig. 1.19** Resorption of an edentulous mandible may result in dehiscence of the mandibular canal and associated nerve impairment. In addition, a conventional removable prosthesis is often difficult to wear because of the associated discomfort from the exposed nerve. The soft tissue is often thin and is usually hypersensitive, especially if the patient is wearing a conventional removable prosthesis

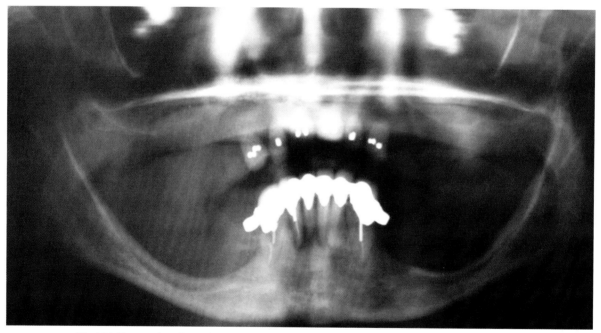

● **Fig. 1.20** Panoramic radiograph exhibiting extensive mandibular posterior atrophy. Note that the anterior teeth have maintained the bone in the anterior mandible and has resulted in the degradation of the pre-maxilla (Combination Syndrome). Wearing of a mandibular class I removable partial denture has escalated the posterior bone loss.

thickness of the surface tissues gradually decreases. Therefore, soft tissue irritation usually results.

The tongue of the patient with edentulous ridges often enlarges to accommodate the increase in space formerly occupied by teeth. At the same time, the tongue is used to limit the movements of the removable prostheses and takes a more active role in the mastication process. As a result, the removable prosthesis decreases in stability. The decrease in neuromuscular control, often associated with aging, further compounds the problems of traditional removable prosthodontics. The ability to wear a denture successfully may be largely a learned, skilled task. The aged patient who recently became edentulous may lack the motor skills needed to adjust to the new conditions (Fig. 1.20; Box 1.4).

• BOX 1.4   Soft Tissue Consequences of Edentulism

- Attached, keratinized gingiva is lost as bone is lost
- Unattached mucosa for denture support causes increased soft spots
- Thickness of tissue decreases with age, and systemic disease causes more sore spots for dentures
- Tongue increases in size, which decreases denture stability
- Tongue has more active role in mastication, which decreases denture stability
- Decreased neuromuscular control of jaw in the elderly

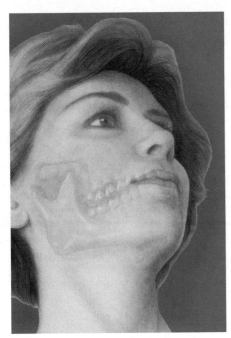

● **Fig. 1.21** Esthetics of the inferior third of the face are related to the position of the teeth and include the muscles that attach to the bone.

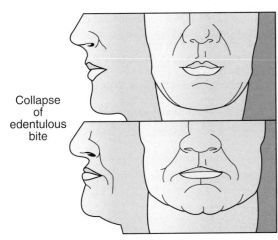

Collapse
of
edentulous
bite

● **Fig. 1.22** Long term denture use leads to many soft tissue changes. The loss of vertical dimension results in many changes, including a closed bite, a mandible that rotates forward, a receding maxilla, reverse smile line, increased number and depth of lines in the face, more acute angle between the nose and the face, loss of vermilion border in the lips, jowls, and witch's chin from loss of muscle attachment.

Esthetic Consequences. The facial changes that naturally occur in relation to the aging process can be accelerated and potentiated by the loss of teeth. Several esthetic consequences result from the loss of alveolar bone (Figs. 1.21 and 1.22). A decrease in facial height from a collapsed vertical dimension results in several facial changes. The loss of the labiomental angle and deepening of vertical lines in the area create a harsh appearance. As the vertical dimension progressively decreases, the occlusion evolves toward a pseudo class III malocclusion. As a result, the chin rotates forward and creates a prognathic facial appearance (Fig. 1.23). These conditions result in a decrease in the horizontal labial angle at the corner of the lips, and the patient appears unhappy when the mouth is at rest. Short facial types suffer higher bite forces, greater bone loss, and more dramatic facial changes with edentulism compared with others.

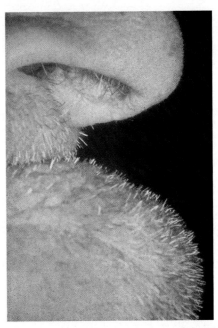

● **Fig. 1.23** Loss of bone height can lead to a closed bite with rotation of the chin anterior to the tip of the nose.

A thinning of the vermilion border of the lips results from the poor lip support provided by the prosthesis and the loss of muscle tone; its retruded position is related to the loss of premaxilla ridge and the loss of tonicity of the muscles involved in facial expression. Sutton et. al. evaluated 179 white patients at different stages of jaw atrophy, the collapse of the lips and circumoral musculature.[37] The contraction of the orbicularis oris and buccinator muscles in the patient with moderate to advanced bone atrophy displaces the modiolus and muscles of facial expression medially and posteriorly. As a result, a narrowing of the commissure, inversion of the lips, and hollowing of the cheeks are very characteristic findings (Fig. 1.24).[37] Women often use one of two techniques to hide this cosmetically undesirable appearance: either no lipstick and minimal makeup, so that little attention is brought to this area of the face, or lipstick drawn on the skin over the vermilion border to give the appearance of fuller lips. A deepening of the nasolabial groove and an increase in the depth of other vertical lines in the upper lip are related to normal aging but are accelerated with bone loss. This usually is accompanied by an increase in the columella-philtrum angle and can make the nose appear larger than if the lip had more support (Fig. 1.25). The maxillary lip naturally becomes longer with age as a result of gravity and loss of muscle tone, resulting in less of the anterior teeth shown when the lip is at rest. This has a tendency to "age" the smile, because the younger the patient, the more the teeth show in relation to the upper lip at rest or when smiling. Loss of muscle tone is accelerated in the edentulous patient, and the lengthening of the lip occurs at a younger age.

The attachments of the mentalis and buccinator muscles to the body and symphysis of the mandible also are affected by bone atrophy. The tissue sags, producing "jowls" or a "witch's chin." This effect is cumulative because of the loss in muscle tone with the loss of teeth, the associated decrease in bite force, and the loss of bone in the regions in which the muscles used to attach.

Patients usually are unaware the hard and soft tissue changes are from the loss of teeth. Studies have shown that 39% of denture patients have have been wearing the same prosthesis for more than 10 years.[35] Therefore the consequences of tooth loss is a slow process and must be explained to the partially or completely edentulous patient during the early phases of treatment (Box 1.5).

Conventional Prosthesis Complications

Fixed Partial Denture Morbidity

In the past, the most common treatment option to replace a posterior single tooth was a three-unit fixed partial denture (FPD). This type of restoration can be fabricated within a very short period of time and usually satisfies the criteria of normal contour, comfort, function, esthetics, speech, and health. Because of these benefits, a FPD has been the treatment of choice for the last 6 decades. This is a widely accepted procedure within the profession. Hard and soft tissue considerations in the missing site are minimal. Every dentist is familiar with the procedure, and it is widely accepted by the profession, patients, and dental insurance companies. In the United States, approximately 70% of the population is missing at least one tooth. Almost 30% of those aged 50 to 59 examined in a US National Survey exhibited either single or multiple edentulous

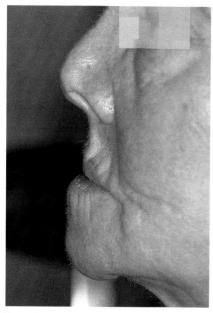

• **Fig. 1.24** This patient has severe bone loss in the maxilla and mandible. Although she is wearing her 15-year-old dentures, the facial changes are significant. The loss of muscle attachments lead to ptosis of the chin (witch's chin), loss of vermilion border (lipstick is applied to the skin), reverse lip line (decrease in horizontal angles), increased vertical lines in the face and lips, increased lip angle under the nose, and a lack of body in the masseter and buccinator muscles.

• **BOX 1.5** **Esthetic Consequences of Bone Loss**

- Decreased facial height
- Loss of labiomental angle
- Deepening of vertical lines in lip and face
- Chin rotates forward giving a prognathic appearance
- Decreased horizontal labial angle of lip, which makes the patient look unhappy
- Loss of tone in muscles of facial expression
- Thinning of vermilion border of the lips from loss of muscle tone
- Deepening of nasolabial groove
- Increase in columella-philtrum angle
- Increased length of maxillary lip, so less teeth show at rest and smiling, which ages the smile
- Ptosis of buccinator muscle attachment, which leads to jowls at side of face
- Ptosis of mentalis muscle attachment, which leads to "witch's chin"

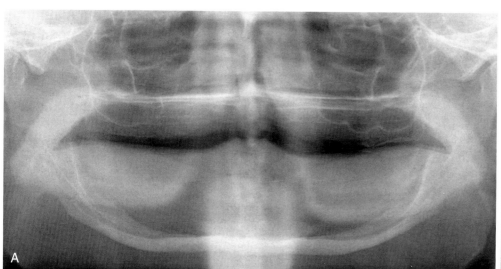
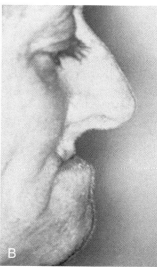

• **Fig. 1.25** (A) Panoramic radiograph of a 68-year-old female. The maxillary arch has severe atrophy and almost complete basal bone loss, including most of the nasal spine. The maxillary sinuses are completely pneumatized. The mandible exhibits severe atrophy with associated nerve dehiscence (B) Profile view. Note the maxillary bone loss effect: the lack of vermilion border of the lip, deep labial folds, and the columella-philtrum angle. The lower lip has a normal vermilion border and the muscles to the lower jaw are still attached, providing a normal contour.

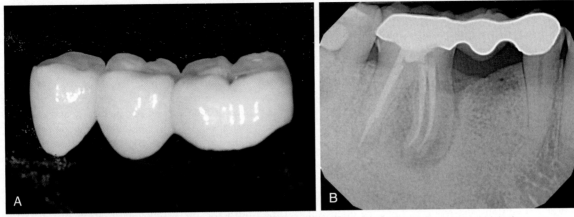

● **Fig. 1.26** (A) Three-unit fixed partial denture is the most common method to replace missing teeth in the posterior regions of the jaws. (B) Three-unit fixed partial dentures have an increased possibility of recurrent decay or fracture with a poorer long-term success rate than an implant supported prosthesis.

spaces bordered by natural teeth.[38] However, there exist many inherent complications with FPDs. A three-unit FPD also presents survival limitations to the restoration and, more importantly, to the abutment teeth.[39] In an evaluation of 42 reports since 1970, Creugers and colleagues[15] calculated a 74% survival rate for FPDs for 15 years. The mean life spans of 9.6 to 10.3 years have been reported by Walton and colleagues[40] and Schwartz colleagues,[41] respectively. However, reports are very inconsistent, with as little as 3% loss over 23 years to 20% loss over 3 years. Caries and endodontic failure of the abutment teeth are the most common causes of prostheses failure. Up to 15% of abutment teeth for an FPD require endodontic therapy compared with 3% of nonabutment teeth that have crown preparations. The long-term periodontal health of the abutment teeth, including bone loss, may also be at greater risk.[39] Unfavorable outcomes of FPD failure include both the need to replace the failed prosthesis and the loss of an abutment and the need for additional pontics and abutment teeth in the replacement bridge. The abutment teeth of an FPD may be lost at rates as high as 30% within 14 years. Approximately 8% to 12% of the abutment teeth holding an FPD are lost within 10 years. The most common reason for single-tooth loss is endodontic failure or fracture of a tooth (usually after endodontic therapy).[42] Because 15% of abutment teeth require endodontics, and root canal therapy may be 90% successful at the 8-year mark, abutment teeth are at increased risk of loss. In addition, abutment teeth are more prone to caries when splinted together with an intermediary pontic. Individual crowns have decay rates below 2%; however, the risk of caries in abutment teeth is approximately 20%, mainly because the pontic region acts as a plaque reservoir. The carious lesion at the crown margin may cause structural failure, even if endodontic treatment is possible (Fig. 1.26). Almost 80% of abutments prepared for a three-unit FPD have no existing or only minimal restorations.[33] Rather than removing sound tooth structure and crowning two or more teeth, increasing the risk of decay and endodontic therapy (and splinting teeth together with pontics, which have the potential to cause additional tooth loss), a dental implant may replace the single tooth with a very high success rate (Box 1.6).

Therefore even though an FPD is an accepted treatment in dentistry, many inherent complications may develop. When evaluating partially edentulous spaces, a treatment option for replacement with a dental implant should always be included in the possible options presented to the patient.

● **BOX 1.6** **Single-Tooth Replacement—Fixed Partial Denture**

- Estimated mean life span of FPD (50% survival) reported at 10 years
- Caries most common cause of FPD failure
- 15% of FPD abutments require endodontics
- Failure of abutment teeth of FPD 8% to 12% at 10 years and 30% at 15 years
- 80% of teeth adjacent to missing teeth have no or minimal restoration
- Possible esthetic issues

FPD, Fixed partial denture.

Removable Partial Denture Morbidity

Removable soft tissue–borne partial dentures (RPD's) have one of the lowest patient acceptance rates in dentistry. Half the patients with a removable partial denture chew better without the prosthesis. A 44-year Scandinavian study revealed that only 80% of patients were wearing such prostheses after 1 year. The number further decreased to only 60% of the free-end partial dentures worn by the patients after 4 years.[43,44]

Wetherall et. al. reported a 60% tolerance and success in a 5-year distal extension RPD study. After 10 years, this was reduced to 35%[45] Wilding et. al. showed that very few partial dentures survived more than 6 years.[46] Although one of five US adults has had a removable prosthesis of some type, 60% reported at least one problem with it.[47] Reports of removable partial dentures indicate that the health of the remaining dentition and surrounding oral tissues often deteriorates. In a study that evaluated the need for repair of an abutment tooth as the indicator of failure, the survival rate of conventional removable partial dentures was 40% at 5 years and 20% at 10 years.[43,45] Those patients wearing the partial dentures often exhibit greater mobility of the abutment teeth, greater plaque retention, increased bleeding on probing, higher incidence of caries, speech inhibition, taste inhibition, and noncompliance of use. A report by Shugars and colleagues found abutment tooth loss for a removable partial denture may be as high as 23% within 5 years and 38% within 8 years.[39] Aquilino and colleagues reported a 44% abutment tooth loss within 10 years for a removable partial denture.[48] In addition, it should be noted that those patients wearing an RPD will accelerate bone loss

- Low survival rate: 60% at 4 years
- Low survival rate: 35% at 10 years
- Morbidity of abutment teeth: 60% at 5 years and 80% at 10 years
- Increased mobility, plaque, bleeding on probing, and caries of abutment teeth
- 44% abutment tooth loss within 10 years
- Accelerated bone loss in edentulous region if wearing removable partial denture

in the soft tissue support regions. Therefore alternative therapies that improve oral conditions and maintain bone are often warranted (Box 1.7).

Complete Denture Morbidity

Masticatory function is an important factor when discussing complete denture function. The difference in maximum occlusal forces recorded in a person with natural teeth and one who is completely edentulous is dramatic. In the first molar region of a dentate person, the average force has been measured at 150 to 250 pounds per square inch (psi).[49] A patient who grinds or clenches the teeth may exert a force that approaches 1000 psi. The maximum occlusal force in the edentulous patient has been shown to be reduced to less than 50 psi. The longer patients are edentulous, the less force they are able to generate. Patients wearing complete dentures for more than 15 years may have a maximum occlusal force of 5.6 psi.[50]

As a result of decreased occlusal force and the instability of the denture, masticatory efficiency also decreases with tooth loss. Within the same 15-year time frame, 90% of the food chewed with natural teeth fits through a No. 12 sieve; this is reduced to 58% in the patient wearing complete dentures.[51] The 10-fold decrease in force and the 40% decrease in efficiency affects the patient's ability to chew. In persons with dentures, 29% are able to eat only soft or mashed foods,[52] 50% avoid many foods, and 17% claim they eat more efficiently without the prosthesis. A study of 367 denture wearers (158 men and 209 women) found that 47% exhibited a low masticatory performance.[53] Lower intakes of fruits, vegetables, and vitamin A by women were noted in this group. These patients took significantly more medications (37%) compared with those with superior masticatory ability (20%), and 28% were taking medications for gastrointestinal disorders. The reduced consumption of high-fiber foods could induce gastrointestinal problems in edentulous patients with deficient masticatory performance. In addition, the coarser bolus may impair proper digestive and nutrient extraction functions.[54] There are systemic consequences from patients wearing conventional dentures. The literature includes several reports suggesting that a compromised dental function causes poor swallowing and masticatory performance, which in turn may influence systemic changes favoring illness, debilitation, and shortened life expectancy.[55-59] In a study evaluating the ability to eat fruit, vegetables, and other dietary fiber in edentulous subjects, 10% claimed difficulty, and blood tests demonstrated reduced levels of plasma ascorbate and plasma retinol compared with dentate subjects. These two blood tests are correlated with an increased risk of dermatologic and visual problems in aging adults.[60] In a study, the masticatory performance and efficiency in denture wearers were compared with dentate individuals. This report noted that when appropriate connections were made for different performance norms and levels, the chewing efficiency of

a denture wearer was less than one-sixth of a person with teeth. Several reports in the literature correlate a patient's health and life span to dental health.[61] Poor chewing ability may be a cause of involuntary weight loss in old age, with an increase in mortality. In contrast, persons with a substantial number of missing teeth were more likely to be obese.[62] After conventional risk factors for strokes and heart attacks were accounted for, there was a significant relationship between dental disease and cardiovascular disease, with the latter still remaining as the major cause of death. It is logical to assume that restoring the stomatognathic system of these patients to a more normal function may indeed enhance the quality and length of their lives.[63-65]

When patients wear a removable prosthesis, there exists a significant psychological component to the associated drawbacks of the prosthesis. The psychological effects of total edentulism are complex and varied and range from very minimal to a state of neuroticism. Although complete dentures are able to satisfy the esthetic needs of many patients, there are those who feel their social life is significantly affected.[66] They are concerned with kissing and romantic situations, especially if a new partner in a relationship is unaware of their oral handicap. Fiske and colleagues,[66] in a study of interviews with edentulous subjects, found tooth loss was comparable to the death of a friend or loss of other important parts of a body in causing a reduction of self-confidence ending in a feeling of shame or bereavement.

One dental survey of edentulous patients found 66% were dissatisfied with their mandibular complete dentures. Primary reasons were discomfort and lack of retention causing pain and discomfort.[67] Past dental health surveys indicated that only 80% of the edentulous population are able to wear both removable prostheses all the time.[68] Some patients wear only one prosthesis, usually the maxillary, whereas others are able to wear their dentures for short periods only. In addition, approximately 7% of patients are not able to wear their dentures at all and become "oral invalids." They rarely leave their home environment and when they feel forced to venture out, the thought of meeting and talking to people when not wearing their teeth is unsettling.

A report of 104 completely edentulous patients seeking treatment was performed by Misch.[53] Of the patients studied, 88% claimed difficulty with speech, with one-fourth having great difficulty. As a consequence, it is easy to correlate the reported increase with concern relative to social activities. Awareness of movement of the mandibular denture was cited by 62.5% of these patients, although the maxillary prosthesis stayed in place most of the time at almost the same percentage. Mandibular discomfort was listed with equal frequency as movement (63.5%), and surprisingly, 16.5% of the patients stated they never wear the mandibular denture.

In comparison, the maxillary denture was uncomfortable half as often (32.6%), and only 0.9% were seldom able to wear the prosthesis. Function was the fourth most common problem reported by these 104 denture wearers. Half the patients avoided many foods, and 17% claimed they were able to masticate more effectively without the prostheses. The psychological effects of the inability to eat in public can be correlated with these findings. Other reports agree that the major motivating factors for patients to undergo treatment were related to the difficulties with eating, denture fit, and discomfort. The psychological need of the edentulous patient is expressed in many forms. For example, in 1970, Britons used approximately 88 tons of denture adhesive.[69] In 1982, more than 5 million Americans used denture adhesives (Ruskin Denture Research Associates: AIM study, unpublished

- Bite force is decreased from approximately 200 to 50 psi
- 15-year denture wearers have reduced bite force to 6 psi
- Masticatory efficiency is decreased
- Lack of proprioception
- Higher incidence of gastrointestinal disorders
- Patients life span may be decreased
- Food selection is limited
- Psychological factors

psi, *Pounds per square inch.*

• BOX 1.9 Advantages of Implant-Supported Prostheses

- Maintain bone
- Restore and maintain occlusal vertical dimension
- Maintain facial esthetics (muscle tone)
- Improve esthetics (teeth positioned for appearance versus decreasing denture movement)
- Improve phonetics
- Improve occlusion
- Improve/regain oral proprioception (occlusal awareness)
- Increase prosthesis success
- Improve masticatory performance/maintain muscles of mastication and facial expression
- Reduce size of prosthesis (eliminate palate, flanges)
- Provide fixed versus removable prostheses
- Improve stability and retention of removable prostheses
- Increase survival times of prostheses
- No need to alter adjacent teeth
- More permanent replacement
- Improve psychological health
- Overall health improved

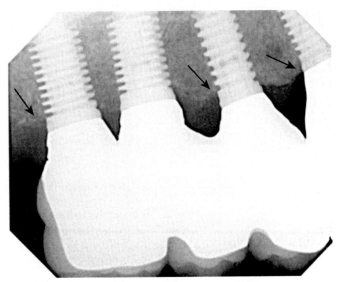

• **Fig. 1.27** Note the long term bone maintenance around the multiple splinted implants.

data, 1982), and a report shows that in the United States, more than $200 million is spent each year on denture adhesives, representing 55 million units sold.[70] The patient is often willing to accept the unpleasant taste, need for recurring application, inconsistent denture fit, embarrassing circumstances, and continued expense for the sole benefit of increased retention of the prosthesis. Clearly the lack of retention and psychological risk of embarrassment in the denture wearer with removable prostheses is a concern the dental profession must address (Box 1.8).

Advantages of Implant-Supported Prostheses

The use of dental implants to provide support for prostheses offers many advantages compared with the use of FPDs or removable soft tissue–borne restorations (Box 1.9).

Maintenance of Bone

A primary reason to consider dental implants to replace missing teeth is the maintenance of alveolar bone (Fig. 1.27). The dental implant placed into the bone serves both as an anchor for the prosthesis and as one of the effective maintenance procedures in dentistry. Stress and strain may be applied to the bone surrounding the implant. As a result, the decrease in trabeculation and loss of bone that occurs after tooth extraction is reversed. There is an

increase in bone trabeculae and density when the dental implant is inserted and functioning. The overall volume of bone is also maintained with a dental implant. Even grafts of iliac crest bone to the jaws, which usually resorb without dental implant insertion within 5 years, are instead stimulated and maintain overall bone volume and implant integration. An endosteal implant can maintain bone width and height as long as the implant remains healthy and stimulates the bone within physiologic limits.[71]

The benefit of bone maintenance is especially noteworthy in the maxillary edentulous arch. Rather than using implants only in the edentulous mandibular arch, because the main mechanical denture problems are in this arch, the maxillary arch should also be addressed. Once implant prostheses are placed to support and retain the mandibular restoration, the bone in the maxillary region continues to be lost and eventually the patient may complain of loss of retention and inability of the maxillary denture to function. The loss of facial esthetics is most often first noted in the maxillary arch, with the loss of vermilion border of the lip, increased length of the maxilla lip, and lack of facial bone support. Implants should be used to treat the continued bone loss and prevent the later complications found in the maxillary arch.

A mandibular denture often moves when the mylohyoid and buccinator muscles contract during speech or mastication. The teeth are often positioned for denture stability rather than where natural teeth usually reside. With implants, the teeth may be positioned to enhance esthetics and phonetics rather than in the neutral zones dictated by traditional denture techniques to improve the stability of a prosthesis. The features of the inferior third of the face are closely related to the supporting skeleton. When vertical bone is lost, the dentures only act as "oral wigs" to improve the contours of the face. The dentures become bulkier as the bone resorbs, making it more difficult to control function, stability, and retention. With implant-supported prostheses, the vertical dimension may be restored, similar to natural teeth. In addition, the implant-supported prosthesis allows a cantilever of anterior teeth for ideal soft tissue and lip contour and improved appearance in all facial planes. This occurs without the instability that usually occurs when an anterior cantilever is incorporated in a traditional denture. The facial profile may be enhanced for the long term with implants, rather than deteriorating over the years, which can occur with traditional dentures.

Occlusion Stability

Occlusion is difficult to establish and stabilize with a completely soft tissue–supported prosthesis. Because the mandibular prosthesis may move as much as 10 mm or more during function, proper occlusal contacts occur by chance, not by design,[72,73] but an implant-supported restoration is stable. The patient can more consistently return to centric-relation occlusion rather than adopt variable positions dictated by the prosthesis' instability. Proprioception is awareness of a structure in time and place. The receptors in the periodontal membrane of the natural tooth help determine its occlusal position. Although endosteal implants do not have a periodontal membrane, they provide greater occlusal awareness than complete dentures. Patients with natural teeth can perceive a difference of 20 μm between the teeth, whereas implant patients can determine a 50-μm difference with rigid implant bridges compared with 100 μm in those with complete dentures (either uni- or bilateral).[74]

Occlusal Awareness

As a result of improved occlusal awareness, the patient functions in a more consistent range of occlusion. With an implant-supported prosthesis, the direction of the occlusal loads is controlled by the restoring dentist. Horizontal forces on removable prostheses accelerate bone loss, decrease prosthesis stability, and increase soft tissue abrasions. Therefore the decrease in horizontal forces that are applied to implant restorations improves the local parameters and helps preserve the underlying soft and hard tissues.

Masticatory Efficiency

In a randomized clinical trial by Kapur and colleagues, the implant group of patients demonstrated a higher level of eating enjoyment and improvement of speech, chewing ability, comfort, denture security, and overall satisfaction.[75] The ability to eat several different foods among complete denture versus mandibular overdenture patients was evaluated by Awad and Feine.[76] The implant overdenture was superior for eating not only harder foods, such as carrots and apples, but also softer foods, such as bread and cheese.[76] Geertman and colleagues evaluated complete denture wearers with severely resorbed mandibles before and after mandibular implant overdentures. The ability to eat hard or tough foods significantly improved.[77,78]

General Health

Researchers at McGill University in Montreal evaluated blood levels of complete denture patients and mandibular implant prostheses 6 months after treatment. Within this rather short period, implant patients had higher B$_{12}$ hemoglobin (related to iron increase) and albumin levels (related to nutrition). These patients also had greater body fat in their shoulders and arms, with decreased body fat in their waists.[79]

Higher Success in Comparison To Other Treatments

The success rate of implant prostheses varies, depending on a host of factors that change for each patient. However, compared with traditional methods of tooth replacement, the implant prosthesis offers increased longevity, improved function, bone preservation, and better psychological results. According to 10-year survival surveys of fixed prostheses on natural teeth, decay is indicated as the most frequent reason for replacement; survival rates are approximately 75%.[42]

In the partially edentulous patient, independent tooth replacement with implants may preserve intact adjacent natural teeth as abutments, further limiting complications such as decay or endodontic therapy, which are the most common causes of fixed prosthesis failure. A major advantage of the implant-supported prosthesis is that the abutments cannot decay and never require endodontics. The implant and related prosthesis can attain a 10-year survival of more than 90%.

Increased Biting Force

The maximum occlusal force of a traditional denture wearer ranges from 5 to 50 psi. Patients with an implant-supported fixed prosthesis may increase their maximum bite force by 85% within 2 months after the completion of treatment. After 3 years, the mean force may reach more than 300%, compared with pretreatment values. As a result, an implant prosthesis wearer may demonstrate a force similar to that of a patient with a fixed restoration supported by natural teeth. Chewing efficiency with an implant prosthesis is greatly improved compared with that of a soft tissue–borne restoration. The masticatory performance of dentures, overdentures, and natural dentition was evaluated by Rissin and colleagues.[51] The traditional denture showed a 30% decrease in chewing efficiency; other reports indicated a denture wearer has less than 60% of the function of people with natural teeth. The supported overdenture loses only 10% of chewing efficiency compared with natural teeth. These findings are similar with implant-supported overdentures. In addition, rigid, implant-supported fixed bridges may function the same as natural teeth.

Nutrition

Beneficial effects such as a decrease in fat, cholesterol, and the carbohydrate food groups have been reported, as well as significant improvement in eating enjoyment and social life.[80,81] Stability and retention of an implant-supported prosthesis are great improvements over soft tissue–borne dentures. Mechanical means of implant retention are far superior to the soft tissue retention provided by dentures or adhesives and cause fewer associated problems. The implant support of the final prosthesis is variable, depending on the number and position of implants, yet all treatment options demonstrate significant improvement to the patients health.[82,83]

Phonetics

Phonetics may be impaired by the instability of a conventional denture. The buccinator and mylohyoid muscles may flex and propel the posterior portion of the denture upward, causing clicking, regardless of the vertical dimension.[73] As a result, a patient in whom the vertical dimension is collapsed may still produce clicking sounds during speech. Often the tongue of the denture wearer is flattened in the posterior areas to hold the denture in position. The anterior mandibular muscles of facial expression may be tightened to prevent the mandibular prosthesis from sliding forward. The implant prosthesis is stable and retentive and does not require these oral manipulations. The implant restoration allows reduced flanges or palates of the prostheses. This is of special benefit to the new denture wearer who often reports discomfort with the bulk of the restoration. The extended soft tissue coverage also affects the taste of food, and the soft tissue may be tender in the extended regions. The palate of a maxillary prosthesis may cause gagging in some patients, which can be eliminated in an implant-supported overdenture or fixed prosthesis.

Psychological Health

Patients treated with implant-supported prostheses judge their overall psychological health as improved by 80% compared with their previous state while wearing traditional, removable prosthodontic prostheses. This group perceived the implant-supported prosthesis as an integral part of their body.[84] For example, Raghoebar and colleagues evaluated 90 edentulous patients in a randomized multi-center study.[85] Five years after treatment, a validated questionnaire targeted patient esthetic satisfaction, retention, comfort, and the ability to speak and eat with either a complete mandibular denture, complete mandibular denture with vestibuloplasty, or mandibular two-implant overdenture. Implant overdentures had significantly higher ratings, whereas no significant difference was found between the two complete-denture groups.[85] Geertman et al. reported similar results comparing chewing ability of conventional complete dentures with mandibular implant overdentures (Box 1.10).[78,86]

The Future of Implant Dentistry

The future of oral implantology is very positive and is expected to continue as one of the fastest and largest growth areas in medicine. The compound annual growth rate (CAGR) for dental implants is expected to grow at an annual rate of 9.7% through 2020, which is supported by improvement in techniques, technology, and materials.[87]

Techniques

Advancements in surgical procedures have had a significant impact on the field of oral implantology. Understanding bone density and modifications in surgical techniques has allowed an increase in success rates in poorer bone qualities. Modification of the bone using new techniques similar to osseodensification now can improve the quality of bone. With more biomechanically advantageous implant designs and the use of resonance frequency analysis (RFA), immediate implant placement and loading protocols have become more predictable. The RFA technology allows for the clinician to measure the bone-to-implant contact (Implant Stability Quotation), which is more accurate and predictable than subjective techniques. The use of better bone substitutes has allowed for predictable bone regeneration procedures to restore the hard and soft tissue loss from extractions. The ability to use bone growth factors (e.g., bone morphogenic proteins [BMPs]) increases the predictability of these procedures.

Technology

Technological advances have had a significant effect on the field of implant dentistry. The use of computerized tomography, mainly cone beam computerized tomography (CBCT), has changed the way clinicians plan and design implant cases. Faster, more efficient, low-radiation scanning machines allow the clinician to virtually plan the implant case with remarkable accuracy. New computer-aided design/computer-aided manufacturing (CAD/CAM) technology associated with CBCT scans allow clinicians to plan, design, and mill the entire case from provisionalization to the final prosthesis in the office setting.

The advent and accuracy of intraoral scanning technologies has risen to a level that has made conventional impression techniques almost obsolete. From a simple digital scan of the area of interest, the image data may be exported to a laboratory for fabrication and design of custom abutments, provisional restorations, and final restorations. Final casts or models may be fabricated via CAD/CAM milling or three-dimensional (3D) printing techniques. In-office 3D printers have given the clinician the luxury of printing models and prostheses in their offices, which is fast and simple.

Materials

One of the major advances in implant dentistry that will have a lasting effect on implant dentistry is the use of zirconia. This material allows the clinician to have a more predictable prosthetic option, which results in fewer and less maintenance and complication issues. The use of CAD/CAM to fabricate zirconia prostheses provides superior marginal integrity, fracture resistance, and flexural strength never seen in dentistry before. Zirconia is used for implant prosthetics and as a dental implant material. Major implant manufacturers are now creating zirconia implant options, showing a significant trend and a real presence of increased use of zirconia in the implant world.

Summary

The goal of modern dentistry is to return patients to oral health in a predictable fashion. The partial and complete edentulous patient may be unable to recover normal function, esthetics, comfort, or speech with a traditional prosthesis. The patient's function when wearing a denture may be reduced to one-sixth of that level formerly experienced with natural dentition; however, an implant prosthesis may return the function to near-normal limits. The esthetics of the edentulous patient are affected as a result of muscle and bone atrophy. Continued bone resorption leads to irreversible facial changes. An implant prosthesis allows normal muscle function, and the implant stimulates the bone and maintains its dimension in a manner similar to healthy natural teeth. As a result, the facial features are not compromised by lack of support, as is often required for removable prostheses. In addition, implant-supported restorations are positioned in relation to esthetics, function, and speech, not in neutral zones of soft tissue support. The soft tissues of the edentulous patients are tender from the effects of thinning mucosa, decreased salivary flow, and unstable or unretentive prostheses. The implant-retained restoration does not require soft tissue support and improves oral comfort. Speech is often compromised with soft tissue–borne prostheses because the tongue and perioral musculature may be compromised to limit the movement of the mandibular prosthesis. The implant prosthesis is stable and retentive without the efforts of the musculature. An implant-supported prostheses offers a more predictable treatment course than traditional prosthetic restorations. The profession and the public are becoming increasingly aware of this dental discipline. Manufacturers' sales are increasing and expected to increase in the future at an alarming rate. Almost all professional dental journals now publish refereed reports on dental implants. All US dental schools now teach implant dentistry, and this discipline has become an integral part of most specialty programs. The future of implant dentistry is very exciting with unlimited expansion via technology and development. Implant dentistry has become the ideal and primary option for tooth replacement.

References

1. Tatum OH. *The Omni Implant System*. Birmingham, AL: Alabama Implant Congress; 1988.
2. National Institutes of Health consensus development conference statement on dental implants. *J Dent Educ*. 1988;52:686–691.
3. Millenium Research Group report. *US Markets for Dental Implants 2006*. USDI; 2006.
4. Stillman N, Douglass CW. Developing market for dental implants. *J Am Dent Assoc*. 1993;124:51–56.
5. Watson MT. Implant dentistry: a 10-year retrospective report. *Dental Products Report*. 1996;30:26–32.
6. Watson MT. Specialist's role in implant dentistry rooted in history: a survey of periodontists and maxillofacial surgeons. *Dental Products Report*. 1997;31:14–18.
7. Reis-Schmidt T. Surgically placing implants—a survey of oral maxillofacial surgeons and periodontists. *Dental Products Report*. 1998;32:26–30.
8. *Bernstein Research*. London: Sanford Bernstein and Col., LLC; 2011:104.
9. Census 2000 Data on Aging. http://www.aoa.gov/prof/statistics/census2000/census2000.asp. Accessed July 14, 2007.
10. Health, United States, 2004, Life expectancy at 65 and 75 years. http://www.cdc.gov/nchshus.htm. Accessed July 14, 2007.
11. Murdock SH, Hogue MN. Current patterns and future trends in the population of the United States: implications for dentists and the dental profession in the 21st century. *J Am Coll Dent*. 1998;65:29–38.
12. https://www.grandviewresearch.com/industry-analysis/dental-implants-market.
13. Palmqvist S, Swartz B. Artificial crowns and fixed partial dentures 18 to 23 years after placement. *Int J Prosthodont*. 1993;6:279–285.
14. Priest GF. Failure rates of restorations for single tooth replacements. *Int J Prosthodont*. 1996;9:38–45.
15. Paddock, Catharine. "Tooth loss in seniors linked to mental and physical decline." Medical News Today. *MediLexicon, Intl.*, 22 Dec. 2014. Web. 29 Apr. 2019.
16. Saman DM, Lemieux A, Arevalo O, et al. A population-based study of edentulism in the US: does depression and rural residency matter after controlling for potential confounders? *BMC Public Health*. 2014;14:65.
17. Hirschfeld L, Wasserman B. A long term survey of tooth loss in 600 treated periodontal patients. *J Periodontol*. 1978;49:225–237.
18. Weintraub JA, Bret BA. Oral health status in the United States: tooth loss and edentulism. *J Dent Ed*. 1988;49:368–378.
19. Meskin LH, Brown LJ, Brunelle JA. Patterns of tooth loss and accuracy of prosthodontic treatment potential in U.S. employed adults and seniors. *Gerodontics*. 1988;4:126–135.
20. Redford M, Drury TF, Kingman A, et al. Denture use and the technical quality of dental prostheses among persons 18-74 years of age: United States, 1988-1991. *J Dent Res*. 1996;75(Spec No):714–725.
21. Mojon P. The world without teeth: demographic trends. In: Feine JS, Carlsson GE, eds. *Implant Overdentures: the Standard of Care for Edentulous Patients*. Carol Stream, IL: Quintessence; 2003.
22. Health Promotion Survey Canada. Statistics Canada, 1990, record number 3828. http://www.statcan. Accessed July 14, 2007.
23. Slade GD, Akinkugbe AA, Sanders AE. Projections of U.S. edentulism prevalence following 5 decades of decline. *J Dent Res*. 2014;93:959–965.
24. Centers for Disease Control, and Prevention (US). *Surveillance for Dental Caries, Dental Sealants, Tooth Retention, Edentulism, and Enamel Fluorosis: United States, 1988-1994 and 1999-2002*. Vol. 54. Department of Health and Human Services, Centers for Disease Control and Prevention; 2005.
25. Doug CW, Shih A, Ostry L. Will there be a need for complete dentures in the United States in 2020? *J Prosthet Dent*. 2002;87:5–8.
26. Otwell T, Reported by China R. *Schoenberger for Forbes, November 19, 2002*. Rose, DDS, MD: Also Louis F; 2000. from multiple sources.
27. National Institute on Aging. US Population aging 65 years and older: 1990 to 2050. www.nia.nik.gov/Researchinformation/ConferencesAndMeeetings/WorkshopReport/Figure4.htm. Accessed September 3, 2009.
28. Babbush CA, Hahn JA, Krauser JT, et al. *Dental Implants: The Art and Science*. 2nd ed. St Louis: Elsevier; 2010.
29. Wolff J. *The Laws of Bone Remodeling*. Berlin: Springer; 1986 (Translated by Maquet P, Furlong R; originally published in 1892).
30. Murray PDF. *Bones: a Study of the Development and Structure of the Vertebrae Skeleton*. Cambridge: Cambridge University Press; 1936.
31. Misch J. *Lehrbuch Der Grenzgebiete Der Medizin und Zahnheilkunde*. Leipzig, Germany: FC Vogel; 1922.
32. Roberts WE, Turley PK, Brezniak N, et al. Implants: bone physiology and metabolism. *Cal Dent Assoc J*. 1987;15:54–61.
33. Tallgren A. The reduction in face height of edentulous and partially edentulous subjects during long-term denture wear: a longitudinal roentgenographic cephalometric study. *Acta Odontol Scand*. 1966;24:195–239.
34. Marcus P, Joshi A, Jones J, et al. Complete edentulism and denture use for elders in New England. *J Prosthet Dent*. 1996;76:260–265.
35. Gruber H, Solar P, Ulm C. *Maxillomandibular Anatomy and Patterns of Resorption During Atrophy. Endosseous Implants: Scientific and Clinical Aspects*. Berlin: Quintessence; 1996:29–63.
36. Hickey JC, Zarb GA, Bolender CL, eds. *Boucher's Prosthodontic Treatment for Edentulous Patients*. 10th ed. St Louis: Mosby; 1990:3–27.
37. Sutton DN, Lewis BR, Patel M, et al. Changes in facial form relative to progressive atrophy of the edentulous jaws. *Int J Oral Maxillofac Surg*. 2004;33(7):676–682.
38. Bloom B, Gaft HC, Jack SS. *National Center for Health Statistics. Dental Services and Oral Health. United States, 1989. Vital Health Stat. 10(183)*. DHHS Pat No (PAS) 93-1511. Washington, DC: U.S. Government Printing Office; 1992.
39. Shugars DA, Bader JD, White BA, et al. Survival rates of teeth adjacent to treated and untreated posterior bounded edentulous spaces. *J Am Dent Assoc*. 1998;129:1085–1095.
40. Walton JN, Gardner FM, Agar JR. A survey of crown and fixed partial denture failures, length of service and reasons for replacement. *J Prosthet Dent*. 1986;56:416–421.
41. Schwartz NL, Whitsett LD, Berry TG. Unserviceable crowns and fixed partial dentures: life-span and causes for loss of serviceability. *J Am Dent Assoc*. 1970;81:1395–1401.
42. Goodacre CJ, Bernal G, Rungcharassaeng K. Clinical complications in fixed prosthodontics. *J Prosthet Dent*. 2003;90:31–41.
43. Koivumaa KK, Hedegard B, Carlsson GE. Studies in partial denture prostheses: I. An investigation of dentogingivally-supported partial dentures. *Suom Hammaslaak Toim*. 1960;56:248–306.
44. Carlsson GE, Hedegard B, Koivumaa KK. Studies in partial denture prosthesis. IV. Final results of a 4-year longitudinal investigation of dentogingivally supported partial dentures. *Acta Odontol Scand*. 1965;23(5):443–472.
45. Wetherell J, Smales R. Partial dentures failure: a long-term clinical survey. *J Dent*. 1980;8:333–340.
46. Wilding R, Reddy J. Periodontal disease in partial denture wearers—a biologic index. *J Oral Rehab*. 1987;14:111–124.
47. Vermeulen A, Keltjens A, Vant'hof M, et al. Ten-year evaluation of removable partial dentures: survival rates based on retreatment, not wearing and replacement. *J Prosthet Dent*. 1996;76:267–272.
48. Aquilino SA, Shugars DA, Bader JD, et al. Ten-year survival rates of teeth adjacent to treated and untreated posterior bounded edentulous spaces. *J Prosthet Dent*. 2001;85:455–460.
49. Howell AW, Manley RS. An electronic strain gauge for measuring oral forces. *J Dent Res*. 1948;27:705.
50. Carr A, Laney WR. Maximum occlusal force levels in patients with osseointegrated oral implant prostheses and patients with complete dentures. *Int J Oral Maxillofac Implants*. 1987;2:101–110.

51. Rissin L, House JE, Manly RS, et al. Clinical comparison of masticatory performance and electromyographic activity of patients with complete dentures, overdentures and natural teeth. *J Prosthet Dent.* 1978;39:508–511.

52. Carlsson GE, Haraldson T. Functional response. In: Brånemark PI, Zarb GA, Albrektsson T, eds. *Tissue Integrated Prostheses: Osseointegration in Clinical Dentistry.* Chicago: Quintessence; 1985.

53. Misch LS, Misch CE. Denture satisfaction: a patient's perspective. *Int J Oral Implant.* 1991;7:43–48.

54. Feldman RS, Kapur KK, Alman JE, et al. Aging and mastication: changes in performance and in the swallowing threshold with natural dentition. *J Am Geriatr Soc.* 1980;28:97–103.

55. Chen MK, Lowenstein F. Masticatory handicap, socio-economic status and chronic conditions among adults. *J Am Dent Assoc.* 1984;109:916–918.

56. Hildebrandt GH, Dominguez BL, Schock MA, et al. Functional units, chewing, swallowing and food avoidance among the elderly. *Prosthet Dent.* 1997;77:588–595.

57. Joshipura KJ, Wilkett WC, Douglass CW. The impact of edentulousness on food and nutrient intake. *J Am Dent Assoc.* 1996;127:459–467.

58. Sheiham A, Steele JC, Marcenes W, et al. The impact of oral health on stated ability to eat certain food; findings from the National Diet and Nutrition Survey of Older People in Great Britain. *Gerontology.* 1999;16:11–20.

59. Sheiham A, Steele JG, Marcenes W, et al. The relationship among dental status, nutrient intake, and nutritional status in older people. *J Dent Res.* 2001;80:408–413.

60. Krall E, Hayes C, Garcia R. How dentition status and masticatory function affect nutrient intake. *J Am Dent Assoc.* 1998;129:20–23.

61. Kapur KK, Soman SD. Masticatory performance and efficiency in denture wearers. *J Prosthet Dent.* 1964;14:687–694.

62. Sheiham A, Steele JG, Marcenes W, et al. The relationship between oral health status and body mass index among older people: a national survey of older people in Great Britain. *Br Dent J.* 2002;192:703–706.

63. Loesche WJ. Periodontal disease as a risk factor for heart disease. *Compend Contin Educ Dent.* 1994;15:976–992.

64. Carlsson GE. Masticatory efficiency: the effect of age, the loss of teeth, and prosthetic rehabilitation. *Int Dent J.* 1984;34:93–97.

65. Gunne HS, Wall AK. The effect of new complete dentures on mastication and dietary intake. *Acta Odontol Scand.* 1985;43:257–268.

66. Fiske J, Davis DM, Frances C, et al. The emotional effects of tooth loss in edentulous people. *Br Dent J.* 1998;184:90–93.

67. Berg E. The influence of some anamnestic demographic and clinical variables on patient acceptance of new complete dentures. *Acta Odontol Scand.* 1984;42:119–127.

68. Bergman B, Carlsson GE. Clinical long-term study of complete denture wearers. *J Prosthet Dent.* 1985;53:56–61.

69. Stafford GD. Denture adhesives: a review of their use and composition. *Dent Pract.* 1970;21:17–19.

70. Pinto D, ed. *Chain Drug Review.* 1998;20:46.

71. Zarb G, Schmitt A. The edentulous predicament. I: a prospective study of the effectiveness of implant-supported fixed prostheses. *J Am Dent Assoc.* 1996;127:59–72.

72. Sheppard IM. Denture base dislodgement during mastication. *J Prosthet Dent.* 1963;13:462–468.

73. Smith D. The mobility of artificial dentures during comminution. *J Prosthet Dent.* 1963;13:834–856.

74. Lundqvist S, Haraldson T. Occlusal perception of thickness in patients with bridges on osteointegrated oral implants. *Scand J Dent Res.* 1984;92:88.

75. Kapur KK, Garrett NR, Hamada MO, et al. Randomized clinical trial comparing the efficacy of mandibular implant supported overdentures and conventional dentures in diabetic patients. Part III: comparisons of patient satisfaction. *J Prosthet Dent.* 1999;82:416–427.

76. Awad MA, Feine JJ. Measuring patient satisfaction with mandibular prostheses. *Community Dent Oral Epidemiol.* 1998;26:400–405.

77. Geertman ME, Boerrigter EM, van't Hof MA, et al. Two-center clinical trial of implant-retained mandibular overdentures versus complete dentures—chewing ability. *Community Dent Oral Epidemiol.* 1996;24:79–84.

78. Geertman ME, Van Waas MA, van't Hof MA, et al. Denture satisfaction in a comparative study of implant-retained mandibular overdenture: a randomized clinical trial. *Int J Oral Maxillofac Implants.* 1996;11:194–2000.

79. McGill University. *Health and Nutrition Letter.* 2003;(2)21.

80. Humphries GM, Healey T, Howell RA, et al. The psychological impact of implant-retained mandibular prostheses: a cross-sectional study. *Int J Oral Maxillofac Implants.* 1995;10:437–444.

81. Meijer HJ, Raghoebar GM, van't Hof MA, et al. Implant-retained mandibular overdentures compared with complete dentures; a 5 years' follow up study of clinical aspects and patient satisfaction. *Clin Oral Implants Res.* 1999;10:238–244.

82. Harle TH, Anderson JD. Patient satisfaction with implant supported prostheses. *Int J Prosthodont.* 1993;6:153–162.

83. Wismeijer D, van Waas MA, Vermeeren JI, et al. Patient satisfaction with implant-supported mandibular overdentures: a comparison of three treatment strategies with ITI-dental implants. *Int J Oral Maxillofac Surg.* 1997;26:263–267.

84. Grogono AL, Lancaster DM, Finger IM. Dental implants: a survey of patients' attitudes. *J Prosthet Dent.* 1989;62:573–576.

85. Raghoebar GM, Meijer HJ, Stegenga B, et al. Effectiveness of three treatment modalities for the edentulous mandible: a five-year randomized clinical trial. *Clin Oral Implants Res.* 2000;11:195–201.

86. Kapur KK. Veterans Administration cooperative dental implant study—comparisons between fixed partial dentures supported by blade-vent implants and removable partial dentures. Part III: comparisons of masticatory scores between two treatment modalities. *J Prosthet Dent.* 1991;65:272–283.

87. http://www.researchandmarkets.com/publication/mdjieps/global_market_study_on_dental_implants_asia.

2

Terminology in Implant Dentistry

NEIL I. PARK AND MAYURI KERR

The terminology used in implant dentistry is distinct, in many ways, from the terms and nomenclature used in other disciplines of clinical dentistry. Much of the instrumentation used in the placement and restoration of dental implants has been developed for those specific purposes and will be new to clinicians entering the field. There is also an extensive variation in types of implants and their designs, as well as surgical techniques used for site preparation, implant placement, and restoration. This chapter presents an overview to familiarize the reader with many of the terms used in implant dentistry.

Generic and Proprietary Terminology

As treatment with dental implants gained widespread acceptance in the 1980s and 1990s, several manufacturers developed instruments and components for commercial distribution. These companies also developed proprietary naming systems for their various components that were usually different, and sometimes conflicting, from one manufacturer to another. For example, Nobelpharma, the Swedish company formed to commercialize Professor Brånemark's treatment methods, discouraged the use of the term *implant*, preferring to call its anchoring devices *fixtures*, to differentiate them from the previous generation of dental implants.

Because these companies have been actively involved in sponsoring educational programs to bring new users to implant dentistry, these varying and conflicting terms have the potential to create confusion for clinicians and laboratory technicians attempting to treat patients with these products. Although it is appropriate for commercial manufacturers to develop proprietary names for product developments and refinements that are differentiated from the competition and protected by intellectual property laws, such situations of true product differentiation are increasingly rare. This chapter will present a generic nomenclature system for instruments and components that has developed over time and entered common usage in the literature. Every effort will be made to maintain consistency with published terms from sources such as the *Glossary of Implant Dentistry* from the International Congress of Oral Implantologists (ICOI) and the *Glossary of Prosthodontic Terms* from the American College of Prosthodontists (ACP). The ICOI document is a glossary developed specifically for terms used in implantology. ICOI released *Glossary III* to the public in 2017 as a digital document intended to allow changes and additions as clinicians and researchers provide suggestions in the years to come.[1] The *Glossary of Prosthodontic Terms,* now in its ninth edition, was first published by the Academy of Denture Prosthetics in 1956. The editors of the ninth edition sought to develop the glossary consistent with the spoken vernacular, and they have produced a highly useful document.[2]

Osseointegration

Although dental implants in varying forms have been used in the replacement of missing teeth for many years, current scientifically based concepts and treatment protocols owe their origins to the pioneering work of Per-Ingvar Brånemark, who was a Swedish physician and researcher (Fig. 2.1). Brånemark and colleagues first described *osseointegration* as direct contact between an implant and living bone at the light microscope level (Fig. 2.2).[3] He found this accidentally in 1952 while studying blood flow in the rabbit femur using titanium chambers inserted into the bony tissue; over time the chambers became firmly affixed to the bone and could not be removed. A bond was found between the bone and the titanium surface. In fact, when fractures occurred during the experiment, they were always found between bone and bone, never between the bone and the implant.[4] This definition of osseointegration was intended to distinguish the treatment method described by the Brånemark group from previously reported implant methods that frequently resulted in a soft tissue interface between the implant and supporting bone. The Swedish group presented clinical evidence resulting from a treatment protocol with specified instrumentation, drilling methods, cooling requirements, insertion techniques, and prosthetic loading protocols designed to minimize heating and denaturation of the bone. Together these protocols resulted in the regeneration of bone, rather than replacement with fibrous soft tissue, around the implant. The result was a treatment method that provided the patient with a bone-anchored prosthesis that restored function and could be maintained over a long period of time.

Other authors have proposed definitions of osseointegration that may be more useful in the clinical setting. The description of osseointegration as "a process whereby clinically asymptomatic rigid fixation of alloplastic materials is achieved, and maintained, in bone during functional loading"[5] provides specific parameters for the clinical assessment of implants in situ.

Osseointegration is also referred to as *secondary stability.* When implants are surgically placed, they rely on the *macrostructure,*

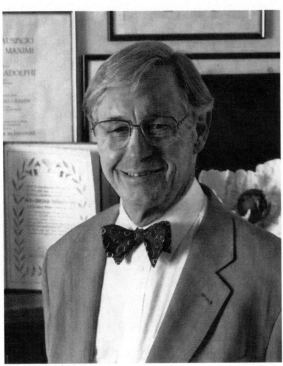

• **Fig. 2.1** Per-Ingvar Brånemark. (From Garg A. *Implant Dentistry: A Practical Approach*. 2nd ed. St Louis: Mosby; 2010.)

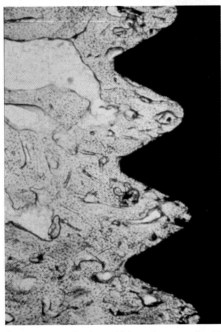

• **Fig. 2.2** Brånemark described osseointegration as a direct bone-implant interface viewed under the power of light microscopy. (From Misch CE. Generic root form component terminology. In: Misch CE, ed. *Dental implant prosthetics*. St Louis: Elsevier Mosby; 2015.)

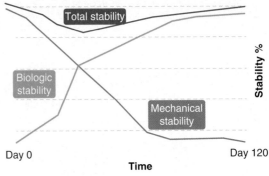

Stability of implant over time

Total stability

Biologic stability

Mechanical stability

Day 0

Day 120

Time

Stability %

• **Fig. 2.3** Implant stability graph.

(Fig. 2.3). The period between primary and secondary stability in which inadequate total stability exists is referred to as the ***stability dip.*** Implant manufacturers attempted to reduce the duration and magnitude of this stability dip by improving the mechanical and surface characteristics of the implant, and by altering the drilling protocol.[6]

The biomechanical concept of secondary stability, or osseointegration, of dental implants has been characterized as a structural and functional connection between newly formed bone and the implant surface.[7] Osseointegration is comprised of a cascade of complex physiologic mechanisms similar to direct fracture healing.[8] The secondary stability of a dental implant largely depends on the degree of new bone formation at the bone-to-implant interface. At the end of the remodeling phase, about 60% to 70% of the implant surface is in contact with bone.[9] This is termed ***bone-to-implant contact (BIC)*** and is widely used in research to measure the degree of osseointegration.[6,10]

In 1986, Albrektsson and colleagues proposed the following criteria for an implant to be regarded as clinically successful[11]:
1. The unattached implant exhibits no clinical mobility.
2. Radiography demonstrates no evidence of radiolucency between implant and bone.
3. Marginal bone loss is less than 0.2 mm annually after the first year of service.
4. Absence of persistent pain, discomfort, or infection.

Albrektsson and colleagues proposed that these criteria (with a success rate of 85% at the end of a 5-year observation period and 80% at the end of a 10-year period) should be the minimum acceptable levels for a treatment method to be considered successful.[11]

Determination of Stability

Primary stability is an important factor in implant survival. Without primary stability, the implant may experience micromotion during the healing process, which may compromise the osseointegration process. Two methods are commonly used to determine primary stability. ***Insertion torque*** is the rotational force recorded during the surgical insertion of a dental implant into the prepared site, and it is expressed in Newton centimeters.[1] Although helpful in forming a clinical impression of initial stability, this measurement can be influenced by implant macrostructure and the comparative relationship between that design and the shape of the surgical osteotomy.

In an effort to more accurately report the primary stability of an implant, a technique using ***resonance frequency analysis***

or overall shape of the implant, combined with the surgical protocol to provide ***primary stability,*** which is an initial level of mechanical or frictional stability in the bone. As the bone heals, the process of osseointegration produces secondary stability, which is responsible for the long-term success of the implant. During the bone remodeling process after implant placement, primary stability decreases while secondary stability increases from new bone formation

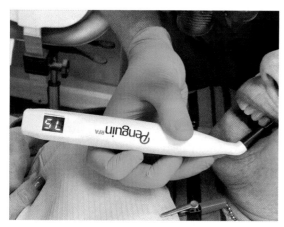

• **Fig. 2.4** Resonance frequency analysis using the Penguin RFA. (Integration Diagnostics Sweden AB, Göteborg, Sweden.)

(RFA) was introduced in the late 1990s.[12] RFA stability measurements essentially apply a bending load, which mimics the clinical load and direction and provides information about the stiffness of the implant–bone junction.[13] Implant Stability Quotient (ISQ) is a measurement (based on a scale from 1–100) of the lateral stability of the dental implant, which serves as a surrogate for the degree of stability achieved. Fig. 2.4 shows the Penguin RFA (Integration Diagnostics Sweden AB, Göteborg, Sweden) device and its use clinically.

Devices such as the Osstell (Osstell AB, Göteborg, Sweden) and the Penguin RFA that measure ISQ can be used in the clinical setting to assess the stability of an implant and, most significantly, to determine the changes in stability over time.

Other methods to determine implant stability have been proposed, such as **percussion testing** and **reverse torque testing.** The percussion test involves the tapping of a mirror handle or other instrument against the implant carrier and judging stability by the sound. **Reverse torque testing** is the application of a reverse or unscrewing torque to the implant at the time of abutment connection. The latter two methods have not been shown to produce reliable results and are no longer commonly recommended.[13]

Types of Dental Implants

Endosseous Implants

An **endosteal** or **endosseous** dental implant is designed for placement into the alveolar or basal bone of the mandible or maxilla while maintaining the body of the implant within the bone. There are two basic types of endosseous implants, **blade** and **root form** (Fig. 2.5).

In contrast to earlier designs, such as the **periosteal** or **transosteal** (which are discussed in later sections of this chapter), in which one implant is usually fabricated to treat the entire arch, endosseous implants are individual units. This design provides the opportunity for the clinician to vary the number and size of the implants placed in the patient to maximize use of the supporting anatomy and to properly support the prosthetic reconstruction. This allows significantly greater flexibility in treatment planning and in the design of the prosthesis and provides better options for long-term maintenance, as well as for dealing with any future complications. Endosseous implants are currently the most widely used implant types.

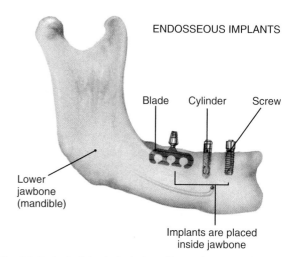

ENDOSSEOUS IMPLANTS

• **Fig. 2.5** Endosteal implant design. Shown here are three different endosseous implant designs. Notice that all of the designs are implanted directly within the bone. Although the blade design has fallen out of use, the cylinder and screw-shaped versions continue to be the most widely placed implant designs in use today. (From Sakaguchi RL, Powers JM, eds. *Craig's Restorative Dental Materials*. 14th ed. St Louis: Mosby; 2019.)

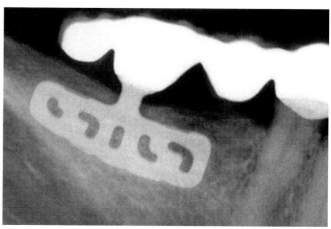

• **Fig. 2.6** Radiograph of a blade implant supporting the distal aspect of a mandibular fixed partial denture. (From White SN, Sabeti MA. History of Single Implants. In: Torabinejad M, Sabeti MA, Goodacre CJ, eds. *Principles and Practice of Single Implant and Restorations*. Philadelphia: Saunders; 2014.)

Modern endosseous implants are designed with a macrostructure that optimizes initial stability and a **microstructure,** or surface texture, which promotes osseointegration. Similarly, the recommended surgical and restorative protocols are designed to promote and maintain primary stability and osseointegration of the implant.

Blade Implants

Blade implants are endosseous implants with a flat shape and are available in one-piece and two-piece designs (Fig. 2.6). Popularized by Linkow, the original blade was constructed from a CrNiVa alloy, but titanium alloy, aluminum oxides, and vitreous carbon materials have also been used. Cranin, Rabkin, and Garfinkel reported the outcome of 952 blades placed in 458 patients. The 5-year success rate was 55%. Smithloff and Fritz reported the outcome of 33 Linkow blades inserted in 22 patients (5 maxillae and 28 mandibles), with a 5-year success rate estimated at 42% to

66%. Ten-year results did not exceed a 50% success rate. Armitage found a 49% 5-year survival in a clinical study of 77 blade-vent implants[11] (Fig. 2.7).

With the widespread utilization and high success rates of root-form implants, overall usage of blade implants has decreased,[14] but they remain available from several manufacturers and find usage in the narrow bony ridge as an option for horizontal bone grafting.

Cylinder Implants

A *cylinder or press-fit implant* is an endosseous design consisting of a straight cylinder that is pushed or tapped into the surgical osteotomy (Fig. 2.8). Cylinder implants gained widespread popularity in the late 1980s to early 1990s because of their simple surgical placement protocol. Primary stability of these designs relies on a highly roughened surface texture to increase frictional resistance to dislodgement from the bone. Surfaces used for these implants included hydroxyapatite (HA), titanium plasma spray (TPS), and small metal balls sintered to the surface of the implant. These implants are used infrequently today because the highly roughened surfaces are associated with increased risk of peri-implant complications and because of improvements in other implant designs and surgical protocols.

Screw-Shaped Implants

Screw-shaped implants, in which the implant body exhibits screw threads throughout most or all its length, have become the most commonly used implant design. Current designs feature improved primary stability and simplified surgical placement protocols that have enabled thousands of practitioners globally, after receiving the required training and experience, to successfully treat millions of patients worldwide.

The original Brånemark implant was a *parallel-walled* design, featuring an implant body that maintained the same diameter throughout its length. Current designs feature a *tapered screw* design, in which the diameter of the implant body decreases toward the apex (Fig. 2.9).

One-Piece versus Two-Piece

The *two-piece* implant design consists of an *implant body,* which provides anchorage within the bone, and a *platform,* which provides a connection. This connection is used to join the implant to various instruments and components and, finally, to an abutment or prosthesis. A one-piece implant, as seen in Fig. 2.10, has an abutment as part of the implant.

Small Diameter Implants

Small diameter implants (SDIs), often called *mini-implants* (Fig. 2.11), are screw-shaped implants with diameters from 1.8 to 2.9 mm and lengths ranging from 10 to 18 mm. The primary indication for SDIs is for treating patients with thin residual ridges that do not allow the placement of standard implants of 3.0 mm and greater and as a treatment alternative to lateral ridge augmentation.

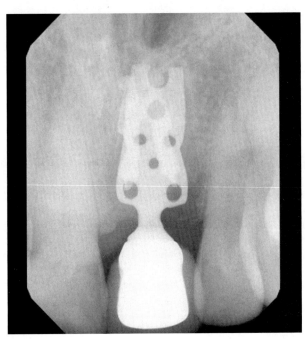

• **Fig. 2.7** Radiograph of blade implant with significant bone loss.[14]

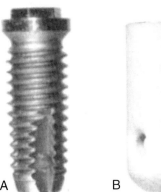 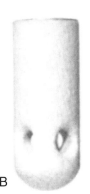 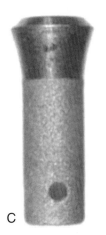 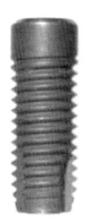

A   B   C   D

• **Fig. 2.8** Diagram showing a wide range of implant macro designs. (A) Brånemark solid screw implant. (B) straight flange intramobile cylinder press-fit implant. (C) flared flange in International Team of Implantology press-fit implant. (D) straight flange in a solid screw Astra implant. (From Huang YS, McGowan T, Lee R, Ivanovski S. Dental implants: biomaterial properties influencing osseointegration. *Comp Biomater.* 2017;7:[II]:444–466.)

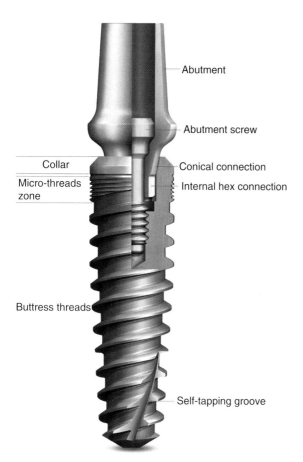

• **Fig. 2.9** Structure of an implant.

Abutment

Abutment screw

Collar

Conical connection

Micro-threads zone

Internal hex connection

Buttress threads

Self-tapping groove

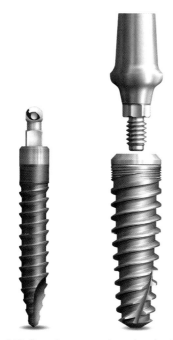

• **Fig. 2.10** One-piece versus two-piece implants.

SDIs are usually a one-piece design and, in addition to thin ridge cases, have been used for retention of provisional restorations during implant healing and as orthodontic anchorage devices.

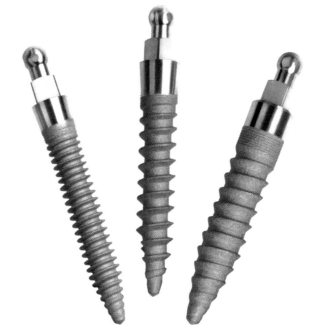

• **Fig. 2.11** One-piece mini-implants.

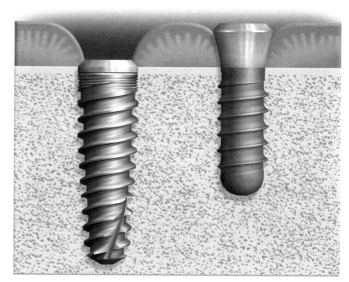

• **Fig. 2.12** Bone-level versus tissue-level implant.

Bone-Level versus Tissue-Level Implants

Most root-form implants can be described as ***bone-level implants,*** because they are designed to be placed with the collar at or near the bone crest. This design provides additional flexibility for creation of the soft tissue emergence profile of the implant restoration. Implants that are designed for placement with the collar at or near the soft tissue margin are referred to as ***tissue-level*** implants (Fig. 2.12).

In 1961, Gargiulo and colleagues theorized that the vertical dimension of the dentogingival junction, comprised of sulcus depth (SD), junctional epithelium (JE), and connective tissue attachment (CTA), is a physiologically formed and stable dimension, subsequently called ***biologic width,*** and that this unit forms at a level dependent on the location of the crest of the alveolar bone.[15] Tissue-level implants were developed to increase the distance of the implant–abutment interface from the bone surface to provide the required biologic width. Bone-level designs were later developed with conical connections and platform shifts, which serve similar goals.[16]

Implant Macrostructure

Implant macrostructure, or overall shape, is designed to optimize precise placement, initial stability within the bone, and distribution of forces within the bone. The predominating macrostructure for root-form endosseous implants is the screw shape, which includes the parallel-sided screw and the tapered screw (Fig. 2.13).

- The parallel-sided screw was documented extensively by Brånemark and colleagues and was considered to be the standard design

for many years. The surgical protocol for placing this implant shape included graduated drills of increasing diameter and usually ended with a tapping or thread-forming instrument that created threads that complemented the threads of the implant. Later, self-tapping implants were developed with a more aggressive apical shape that did not require this thread-forming step. For self-tapping designs, the surgical protocol normally dictated an osteotomy that conformed to the inner diameter of the screw, allowing the threads to cut their way in the bone during insertion.

- The tapered screw design was developed to provide two advantages over the parallel-sided implant: increased initial stability and anatomic conformity. A tapered screw implant design can provide improved primary stability because it condenses bone in areas of reduced bone quality.[17] Tapered screw implants also distribute occlusal forces to adjacent bone to a greater degree than parallel walled types.[18] Additionally, the anatomic shape of this design makes perforation of the buccal and lingual bony walls less likely to occur[19] and creates a more favorable opportunity to safely position the implant between adjacent tooth roots. Schiegnitz and colleagues found that the tapered design demonstrated greater primary implant stability than cylindrical implants.[20] In experimental groups, tapered implants were found to have better primary stability than parallel-sided implants.[21,22]

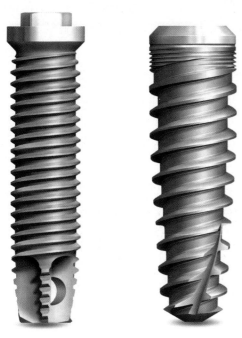

- **Fig. 2.13** Parallel-sided screw-shaped implant (left) and the tapered screw design (right). Comparison of the two designs illustrated design refinements made from approximately 1988 to 2015.

Implant Threads

Dental implants on the market today come in several different thread configurations; they can be understood using screw design terminology from engineering. The **crest** is the outer surface of the thread, and it joins the two sides of the thread. The diameter measured around the crest is the **outer diameter (OD)** of the implant. The **root** is the inner surface of the thread, and it joins the two sides of the thread. The diameter measured around the root is the **inner diameter (ID)** of the implant. The **helix angle** describes the angulation between the wall of the thread and the perpendicular axis. The **pitch** is the distance between two adjacent threads. Greater pitch is considered to be more aggressive in cutting through bone. The lead is the axial distance that the implant is inserted with one complete turn (Fig. 2.14).

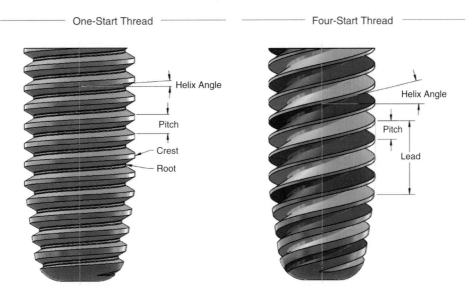

- **Fig. 2.14** Demonstrating the difference in lead depending on the threads. (From Bullis G, Abai S. Form and function of implant threads in cancellous bone. *Inclusive Mag.* 2013;4[1].)

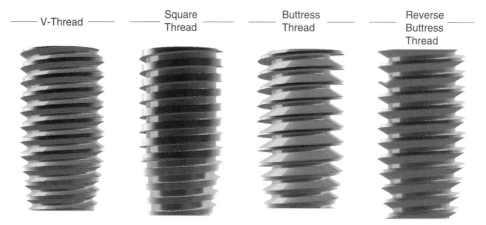

——— V-Thread ———   Square Thread   Buttress Thread   Reverse Buttress Thread

● **Fig. 2.15** Types of implant macrothreads. (From Bullis G, Abai S. Form and function of implant threads in cancellous bone. *Inclusive Mag.* 2013;4[1].)

The geometry of the threads themselves influences stress distribution around the implant. Deeper threads seem to improve primary stability, particularly in bone of poor quality.[23]

V-threads, square threads, and buttress threads are dental implant thread forms with a long history of successful use. These threads serve to dissipate occlusal loads into the bone surrounding the implant; however, they differ in form, inherent strength, and in how they transmit forces. V-threads are strong, but they transmit more shear forces to the surrounding bone. Square-thread forms transmit occlusal forces with less shear force than V-threads. Buttress threads minimize shear forces in a manner similar to square threads, and they combine excellent primary stability with the best features of both V- and square-thread forms (Fig. 2.15).[23]

The original Brånemark parallel-sided threaded implant was designed for placement into an osteotomy in which negative threads had been created during the surgical protocol using a ***screw tap instrument*** as a ***threadformer***. Later, ***self-tapping implants*** were introduced, primarily for use in bone of lower density to improve the primary stability of the implant. With a non–self-tapping implant, the osteotomy is prepared to a size approaching the OD of the implant, whereas with a self-tapping implant the osteotomy is prepared to the approximate size of the inner diameter of the implant.

Most implants in use today feature the tapered screw design that has a self-tapping feature, which eliminates the need for tapping in all but the most dense bone.

Microthreads

Microthreads are a series of threads of small pitch placed in the crestal or collar portion of the implant. Microthreads help spread forces from the collar of the implant and can assist with the maintenance of crestal bone height.[21,24]

Implant Surfaces

Implant microstructure refers to the surface structure, or degree of surface roughness, of the dental implant. The surface structure of dental implants is critical for adhesion and differentiation of cells during the bone remodeling process.[6]

After the machining of a titanium or titanium alloy implant, contact with air causes the immediate development of a titanium oxide surface on the implant. Until the late 1980s, further surface treatments were rarely performed. Since that time, several surface

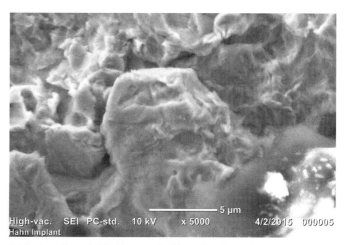

High-vac.   SEI PC-std.   10 kV   x 5000   4/2/2015   000005
Hahn Implant

● **Fig. 2.16** Resorbable blast media blasted surface of the Hahn tapered implant.

modifications have been developed in an effort to modify the surface roughness of the implant to promote the process of osseointegration, particularly with poor bone quality.[6]

These modifications can be divided into ***subtractive*** and ***additive*** processes, depending on whether material is removed or deposited on the implant surface in the development of the surface. Commonly used scientific parameters to describe the surface roughness are the two-dimensional (2D) ***Ra*** (profile roughness average) and the three-dimensional (3D) ***Sa*** (area roughness average).[25] Although the ideal surface roughness is undetermined, according to Albrektsson and Wennerberg,[26] *Ra* in the range of 1 to 2 μm seems to provide the optimal degree of roughness to promote osseointegration. Pits, grooves, and protrusions characterize the microtopography and set the stage for biologic responses at the bone-to-implant interface. The modifications of microtopography contribute to an increase in surface area. Studies have shown increased levels of BIC for microrough surfaces.[25,27]

Subtractive processes include the following:
1. Etching with acid
2. Blasting with an abrasive material, such as silicon or HA; blasting with HA, known as ***resorbable blast media (RBM)***, is particularly advantageous because, unlike with grit or sandblasting, any particles remaining on the surface are resorbable (Fig. 2.16)
3. Treatment with lasers

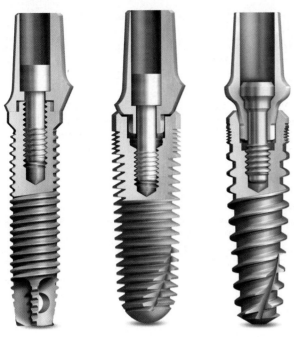

• **Fig. 2.17** External versus internal implant–abutment connections.

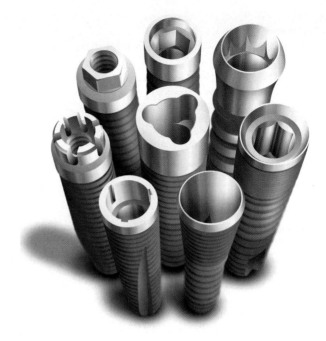

• **Fig. 2.18** Various connection types.

Additive processes share the same goal of modifying the implant surface to a moderately rough degree, and they include:
1. HA coating
2. TPS
3. Anodization to thicken the titanium oxide surface

Implant Platforms and Connections

Connection Type

Implant connections are defined by the geometry of the connecting elements. The Brånemark implant design features an *external hex* on the implant, which mates with an *internal hex* on the abutment. In contrast, *internal connection* implants feature a chamber within the implant body to which an external projection of the abutment can engage (Fig. 2.17). Commonly used internal connections include hexagon, octagon, and trichannel, and many of these include a conical interface as part of their internal geometry (Fig. 2.18).

External hex designs are less commonly used today because of the mechanical and restorative advantages of internal connections. Screw loosening is a risk for external hex connections because greater lateral forces are transferred to the connection screw and because preload of the screw is the only force that resists occlusal forces.[28-30]

The IMZ implant, which is no longer manufactured, was distinguished by an intramobile element (IME) that included a Delrin spacer designed for placement between the implant and abutment. The design was thought to reduce the mechanical stress on the implant, but clinical experience over time resulted in the discontinuation of the design.

Platform Switched versus Platform Matching

Traditional implant designs, such as the Brånemark external hex, maintained the same diameter from the implant collar to the portion of the abutment that connects to the implant in a design known as a *butt-joint* or *platform matched.* With the advent of the internal

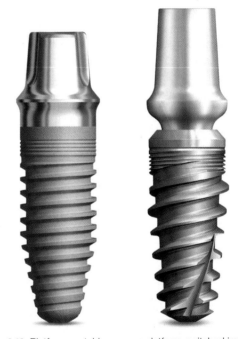

• **Fig. 2.19** Platform-matching versus platform-switched implants.

conical connection, it became possible to create a stable implant–abutment connection while reducing the diameter of the abutment. The situation in which the abutment is narrower than the implant at the connection is termed *platform switching* (Fig. 2.19). Platform switching has been shown to be beneficial in reducing bone loss around the implant, and it allows a greater volume of soft tissue at the implant–abutment interface to help achieve soft tissue esthetics.[31,32]

Surgical Protocols

Three different surgical protocols have been used for two-piece implant systems: *one stage, two stage,* and *immediate restoration.*

Using the standard, or two-stage protocol, the implant body, with a *cover screw,* is submerged below the soft tissue until the initial bone healing has occurred. During a *second-stage surgery,* the soft tissues are reflected to attach a component that passes from the implant connection, through the soft tissue, and enters the oral cavity. With the one-stage surgical approach, the surgeon places the implant body and a *temporary healing abutment,* which emerges through the soft tissue. During the restorative process, the healing abutment is replaced so that the prosthetic abutment or restoration can be connected, eliminating the need for a second surgery.

With the immediate restoration approach, the implant body and a prosthetic abutment are both placed at the initial surgery. A provisional restoration is then attached to the abutment.

Immediate Placement after Extraction versus Placement in Healed Sites

The standard protocol promulgated by Brånemark and colleagues dictated that after tooth extraction the site should be allowed to heal before implant placement. Pioneering work by Hahn and others showed high success rates for implants placed into the alveolus immediately after tooth extraction. A procedure known as the *emergency implant* was developed and popularized as a method used to provide an immediate implant replacement for a nonrestorable tooth.[33]

Bone Grafting

Insufficient bone volume may result from atrophy after tooth extraction, trauma, congenital deficiency, or surgical resection. Because an adequate volume of bone in the surgical site is an inviolable prerequisite for successful implant placement, *bone augmentation* techniques have been developed to facilitate implant treatment that would otherwise not be an option for some patients. *Site preparation* refers to bone grafting procedures performed before implant placement, whereas simultaneous grafting refers to procedures performed at the same time as implant placement. There are numerous alternative techniques and various agents and biomaterials currently used to augment bone for various indications.

Materials for Grafting

Materials used to augment bone volume include (Box 2.1):

Autogenous bone grafts are harvested from an adjacent or remote site in the same patient and used to build up the deficient area. Because of their osteogenic potential and low patient risk,

autogenous grafts are considered the ideal bone grafting material.

Allografts are bone grafts harvested from cadavers of the same species and processed to remove contamination and antigenic potential. The grafts are supplied by specially licensed tissue banks in particulate or block form.

Xenografts are bone grafts derived from nonhuman sources. Grafts from bovine, porcine, or equine sources are highly processed to completely remove the organic content.

Alloplastic graft material are synthetic bone substitutes, including calcium phosphates and bioactive glasses.

Table 2.1 lists considerations in selecting a bone grafting material.

Bone Augmentation Techniques

Guided bone regeneration (GBR) uses *barrier membranes* to protect bony defects from the rapid ingrowth of soft tissue cells so that bone progenitor cells may develop bone uninhibited. Ingrowth of soft tissue may disturb or totally prevent osteogenesis in a defect or wound. Examples of membranes used in this technique include *collagen* and *expanded polytetrafluoroethylene (PTFE).* Membranes are referred to as *resorbable* or *nonresorbable,* depending on whether they require a subsequent surgery for removal (Figs. 2.20 and 2.21).

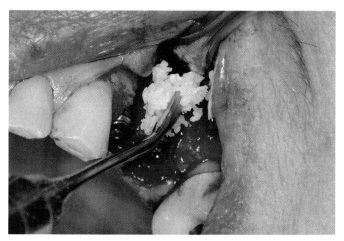

• **Fig. 2.20** Bone graft material placement.

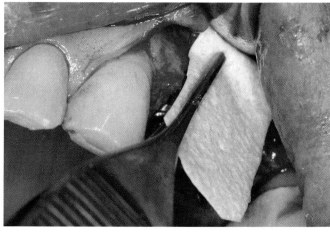

• **Fig. 2.21** Membrane placement for guided bone regeneration.

TABLE 2.1 Bone Graft Material Considerations

Graft type	Advantages	Disadvantages	Healing			Space Maintenance	Resorption Time	Indications
			Osteogenesis	Osteoinductive	Osteoconductive			
Autograft	• Gold standard • Nonimmunogenic • Predictable	• Requires second surgical site • Limited availability • Additional skill set required • Resorbs quickly	+	+	+	+	Medium to fast	All deficient areas
Demineralized allograft	• Osteoinductive qualities • No second surgical site • Readily available • Predictable	• Immunogenicity • Slight potential for disease transmission • Cultural concerns • Not for large graft sites	−	+	+	−	Fast	GBR, socket, sinus grafts
Mineralized allograft	• No second surgical site • Readily available • Predictable	• Potential immunogenicity • Slight potential for disease transmission • Cultural concerns • Not for large graft sites	−	−	+	+	Medium to slow	GBR, socket, sinus grafts
Xenograft	• No second surgical site • Readily available	• Increased inflammatory response • Slow resorption • Only osteoconductive • Immunogenicity • Potential for disease transmission • Cultural concerns • Not for large graft sites	−	−	+	+	Medium to slow	GBR, socket, sinus grafts
Alloplast	• No disease transmission • No immunogenicity • Greater acceptance • No second surgical site • Readily available	• Resorption • Unpredictability • Not for large graft sites	−	−	+	+	Fast to slow	Larger defects, sinus grafts

GBR, Guided bone regeneration.
From Resnik RR. Bone substitutes in oral implantology. *Chairside Mag.* 2017;12(3).

Some surgical techniques used to augment bone volume include only grafting, inlay grafting, ridge expansion, and socket-shield technique.

Onlay grafting describes a technique of applying the graft material over the defective area to increase width or height of the implant site.

With *inlay grafting,* a section of the jaw is surgically separated and graft material is sandwiched between two sections.

In *ridge expansion* techniques, the alveolar ridge is split longitudinally and parted to allow placement of an implant or graft material in the void.[35]

The *socket-shield* technique (Fig. 2.22) is designed to maintain the volume and contours of hard and soft tissue to optimize implant placement after tooth extraction. The technique involves preserving the buccal part of the root and placing an implant lingual to it. The gap between the implant and bone is filled with graft material and the area is allowed to heal[36] (Fig. 2.23).

Sinus Augmentation

The posterior maxilla is an area that frequently lacks adequate bone volume for implant placement. Several predictable techniques have been developed to graft bone to augment the sinus floor to accommodate dental implant insertion.

Maxillary sinus floor augmentation (MSFA), using the *lateral window technique,* was originally developed by Tatum in the mid-1970s and was later described by Boyne and James in 1980. This surgical intervention is still the most frequently used method to enhance the alveolar bone height of the posterior part of the maxilla before or in conjunction with implant placement.[37] The *crestal sinus lift* or *sinus bump* consists of raising the sinus floor and inserting graft material through the osteotomy.[38]

Bone Graft Properties

Bone grafts can be described as *osteogenic, osteoinductive,* and *osteoconductive* based on their contribution to bone healing. These properties of bone grafts directly affect the success or failure of graft incorporation, and the selection of the proper grafting protocol.[34]

Osteogenesis is the ability of the graft to produce new bone, and it is a property found only in fresh autogenous bone and in bone marrow cells.[39]

Osteoconduction is the property of the graft to serve as a scaffold for viable bone healing. Osteoconduction allows for the ingrowth of neovasculature and the infiltration of osteogenic precursor cells into the graft site. Osteoconductive properties are found in cancellous autografts and allografts, demineralized bone matrix, HA, collagen, and calcium phosphate.[39]

Osteoinduction is the ability of graft material to induce stem cells to differentiate into mature bone cells. This process is typically associated with the presence of bone growth factors within the graft material or as a supplement to the bone graft. Bone morphogenic proteins and demineralized bone matrix are the principal osteoinductive materials. Autograft and allograft bone also have some osteoinductive properties.[39]

The ideal bone-graft substitute is biocompatible, bioresorbable, osteoconductive, osteoinductive, structurally similar to bone, easy to use, and cost-effective.

Surgical Instrumentation

Dental implants are designed and sold as *implant systems* that include a *surgical instrumentation kit* with drills designed for the surgical protocol for that specific implant system. Depending on the

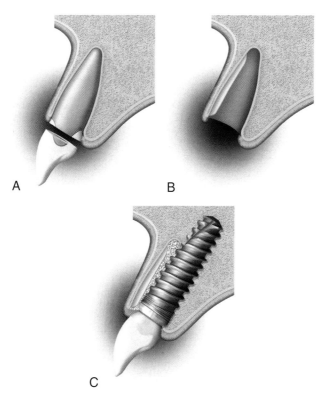

• **Fig. 2.22** Stages of the socket-shield technique. (A) Crown sectioned. (B) Removal of the root, keeping the buccal "shield" intact. (C) Socket is grafted and the implant is placed.

manufacturer, surgical instrumentation kits include an assortment of **drills, drivers, wrenches, screw taps,** and **implant mounts** (Fig. 2.24).

Implant Drills

Implant drills are rotary cutting instruments that are used to create an osteotomy in bone. They are made of various materials, including surgical stainless steel, titanium alloy, and ceramics. When used in the proper sequence with the recommended rotary speed, torque, and irrigation, the drills are designed to create the correct size and shape of the osteotomy, providing initial stability without causing mechanical or thermal damage to the bone.[40]

Drivers

Various drivers are included in the surgical kit, depending on the manufacturer. Screws used in the course of implant treatment are engaged with hexed, slotted, or unigrip drivers.

Implant Mounts

Some systems require an implant mount to be attached to the implant to enable placement with the correct instrumentation. An implant mount serves to facilitate the delivery of a dental implant to the surgical site, and it can be used to rotate the implant to the correct depth. The implant mount is then removed from the implant to obtain visual confirmation of the position.

Other implant systems incorporate a direct-drive feature, in which an instrument engages directly into the implant, allowing for a simpler procedure and better vision during implant placement (Fig. 2.25).

Wrenches

Surgical kits include a ratchet wrench or **torque wrench** to place the implant. A torque wrench or torque driver is a manual instrument used to apply a specific amount of torque when placing an implant or prosthetic screw. A **torque controller** refers to an electronic machine designed for the same purpose. A torque wrench is recommended to ensure the application of a force that conforms to the manufacturer's recommendation.

Implant Components

The **cover screw,** sometimes called a **healing screw,** is a component used to occlude the connection of the implant while submerged during a two-stage procedure (Fig. 2.26).

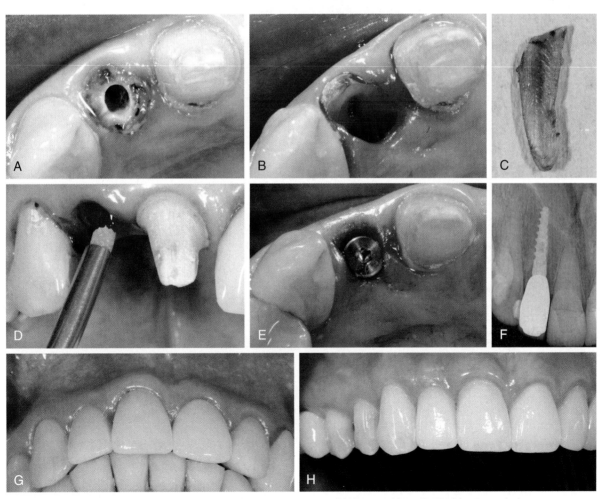

• **Fig. 2.23** Clinical case using the socket-shield technique. (A) Unrestorable tooth #7 with crown missing. (B) Removal of bulk of the root while retaining the buccal shield in the socket. (C) Extracted root. (D) Bone graft material placed in the socket. (E) Implant placed in grafted socket. (F) Radiograph of Hahn implant with definitive restoration. (G and H) Intraoral views of Hahn implant with BruxZir crown on #7. Note maintenance of ideal gingival margin.

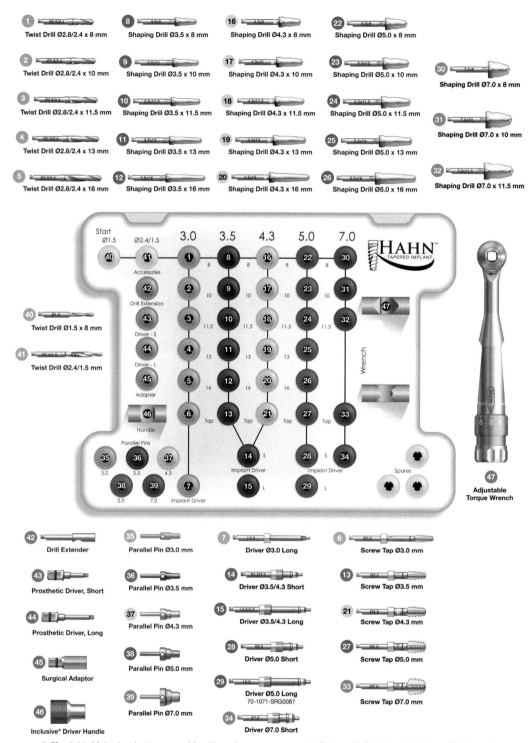

① Twist Drill Ø2.8/2.4 x 8 mm
② Twist Drill Ø2.8/2.4 x 10 mm
③ Twist Drill Ø2.8/2.4 x 11.5 mm
④ Twist Drill Ø2.8/2.4 x 13 mm
⑤ Twist Drill Ø2.8/2.4 x 16 mm

⑧ Shaping Drill Ø3.5 x 8 mm
⑨ Shaping Drill Ø3.5 x 10 mm
⑩ Shaping Drill Ø3.5 x 11.5 mm
⑪ Shaping Drill Ø3.5 x 13 mm
⑫ Shaping Drill Ø3.5 x 16 mm

⑯ Shaping Drill Ø4.3 x 8 mm
⑰ Shaping Drill Ø4.3 x 10 mm
⑱ Shaping Drill Ø4.3 x 11.5 mm
⑲ Shaping Drill Ø4.3 x 13 mm
⑳ Shaping Drill Ø4.3 x 16 mm

㉒ Shaping Drill Ø5.0 x 8 mm
㉓ Shaping Drill Ø5.0 x 10 mm
㉔ Shaping Drill Ø5.0 x 11.5 mm
㉕ Shaping Drill Ø5.0 x 13 mm
㉖ Shaping Drill Ø5.0 x 16 mm

㉚ Shaping Drill Ø7.0 x 8 mm
㉛ Shaping Drill Ø7.0 x 10 mm
㉜ Shaping Drill Ø7.0 x 11.5 mm

⑳ Twist Drill Ø1.5 x 8 mm
㊶ Twist Drill Ø2.4/1.5 mm

㊷ Drill Extender
㊸ Prosthetic Driver, Short
㊹ Prosthetic Driver, Long
㊺ Surgical Adaptor
㊻ Inclusive® Driver Handle

㉟ Parallel Pin Ø3.0 mm
㊱ Parallel Pin Ø3.5 mm
㊲ Parallel Pin Ø4.3 mm
㊳ Parallel Pin Ø5.0 mm
㊴ Parallel Pin Ø7.0 mm

⑦ Driver Ø3.0 Long
⑭ Driver Ø3.5/4.3 Short
⑮ Driver Ø3.5/4.3 Long
㉘ Driver Ø5.0 Short
㉙ Driver Ø5.0 Long 70-1071-SRG0087
㉞ Driver Ø7.0 Short

⑥ Screw Tap Ø3.0 mm
⑬ Screw Tap Ø3.5 mm
㉑ Screw Tap Ø4.3 mm
㉗ Screw Tap Ø5.0 mm
㉝ Screw Tap Ø7.0 mm

㊼ Adjustable Torque Wrench

• **Fig. 2.24** Hahn implant surgery kit with various components. (Prismatik Dentalcraft, Irvine, California.)

A ***healing abutment*** is a component that connects to the dental implant and protrudes through the soft tissue. It can be connected to the implant at the second-stage surgical procedure, or it can be inserted at the time of implant placement to eliminate the need for a second surgery. This component has also been referred to as a ***healing collar, permucosal extension, permucosal abutment,*** or ***healing cuff*** (Fig. 2.27). Healing abutments are typically provided as stock components with a cylindrical shape, but they also can be customized for the specific case (Fig. 2.28). Healing abutments are typically left in place temporarily until the soft tissue has healed sufficiently to allow restoration of the implant. At that time, the healing abutment is removed, providing access to the restorative platform of the implant (Fig. 2.29).

Guided Surgery

A *surgical guide,* or *surgical template* (Figs. 2.30–2.32), is a device created for a specific case to assist the surgeon in placing the implants in the intended location. Guided surgery involves the use of a guide that directs placement of the implant. Fig. 2.30 illustrates the components of the Hahn guided surgery kit. Before the availability of 3D imaging digital data, guides were created based on a diagnostic wax-up of the final restoration and an approximate transfer of data from radiographs and intraoral examination. Currently, surgical guides are most commonly created from cone beam computerized tomography (CBCT) data, using dedicated software to digitally plan the case and design the surgical guide (Fig. 2.33).

Implant Restorations

Loading Protocols

The restoration of dental implants consists of the procedures needed for the connection of a prosthesis to one or more implants.

Restoration is accomplished using one of these basic loading protocols:

1. *Conventional loading:* Restoration occurs after the initial bone and soft tissue healing process, usually in 3 to 6 months, depending on bone density.
2. *Immediate loading:* A prosthesis is connected at the time of implant placement. This is usually a provisional restoration that is replaced with a definitive restoration after implant and soft tissue healing.
3. *Early loading:* The prosthesis connection occurs from 2 to 3 weeks after implant placement. This is considered to be a less predictable loading protocol because the restoration is sometimes placed during the stability dip, which is the period of lowest implant stability.
4. *Delayed loading:* The prosthesis is connected 6 to 12 months after implant placement. This method is often chosen in poor-quality bone and in situations in which primary stability cannot be achieved during surgical placement.

A summary of loading protocols is provided in Table 2.2.[41]

Standardized and Custom Components

Implant restorative components are said to be *standardized* when they are stock parts produced by the implant manufacturer.

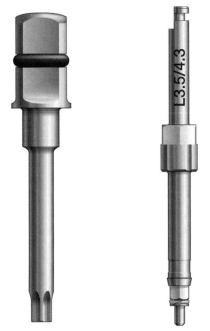

• **Fig. 2.25** Hand driver (left) and rotary driver (right).

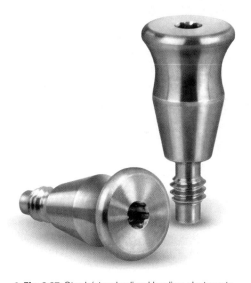

• **Fig. 2.27** Stock/standardized healing abutments.

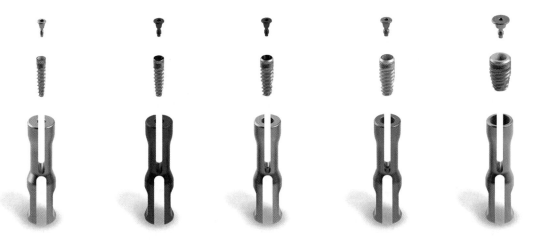

• **Fig. 2.26** Hahn implant with holder and cover screw.

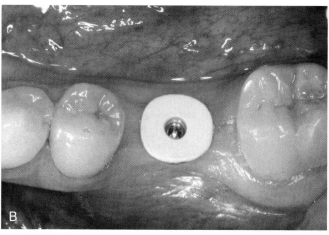

• **Fig. 2.28** (A) Custom healing abutment with ideal contours. (B) Healing abutment connected after implant placement.

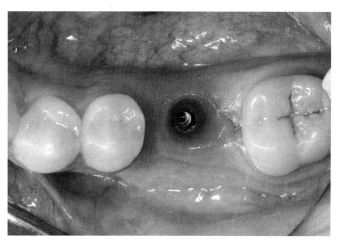

• **Fig. 2.29** Removing the custom healing abutment reveals an ideal soft tissue cuff around the implant.

Custom components are designed and fabricated for a specific site in the same way that restorations are customized for a specific patient.

Impression Procedures

Impressions for implant restorations can be accomplished at the implant level or at the abutment level. ***Implant-level impressions*** are made by attaching a standardized ***implant-level impression coping*** directly to the implant and capturing that position in an impression. Implant-level impression copings are specific to the implant brand, platform diameter, and connection design. A cast is produced by attaching an ***implant analog*** to the impression coping and pouring the impression with dental stone. The implant analog is a standardized component that reproduces the implant platform and connection. From this, a cast is produced on which the doctor or technician may (1) select the appropriate standardized abutment to attach to the implant analog; (2) design and fabricate a custom abutment using the cast; or (3) fabricate an ***implant-level prosthesis,*** which attaches directly to the implant.

Abutment-level impressions are made intraorally after a standardized or custom abutment has been attached directly to the implant. If a custom abutment is used, then the abutment-level impression is very similar to an impression made for a typical fixed prosthesis, capturing the shape, position, and marginal detail of the custom abutment. In the case of a standardized abutment, an ***abutment-level impression coping,*** which is also a standardized component, is sometimes used.

Implant components are said to be ***engaging or nonengaging*** depending on how they connect with the implant connection. Engaging components fit into the hex, octagon, or cams of the implant, preventing rotation after screw clamping. Nonengaging components bypass the antirotation feature of the implant to reduce the difficulty of engagement for multi-implant prostheses.

Impression Techniques

There are two major techniques used for making impressions using impression copings. Each method is facilitated by a specific coping design. In the ***transfer*** or ***closed-tray*** technique, the impression coping has a tapered shape and is attached to the implant or abutment, and it remains attached when the impression is removed from the mouth. The copings are then removed from the mouth and inserted into the impression. Analogs are attached to the impression copings before or after insertion, and the cast is poured[42] (Fig. 2.34).

With the ***pick-up*** or ***open-tray*** technique, the impression coping features squares or other retentive elements and is attached to the implant or abutment before the impression is made. The screws, which retain the impression copings, project through the impression tray and are loosened before impression removal. The impression copings are removed with the impression, analogs are connected, and the cast is poured[42] (Fig. 2.35).

Scanning abutments, or ***scan bodies,*** are used when making digital impressions of implants using an intraoral scanner (Fig. 2.36). The scanning abutment is attached to the implant before the digital scan, and it is recognized by the scanning or design software to indicate the correct implant position.

An ***implant verification jig (IVJ)*** is a device used to verify the accuracy of the master cast for an implant restoration. It consists of pick-up impression copings embedded in an acrylic framework and sectioned between the implants. The clinician then attaches each section to the implant, fuses the sections together intraorally, and provides the device to the laboratory for model verification (Fig. 2.37).

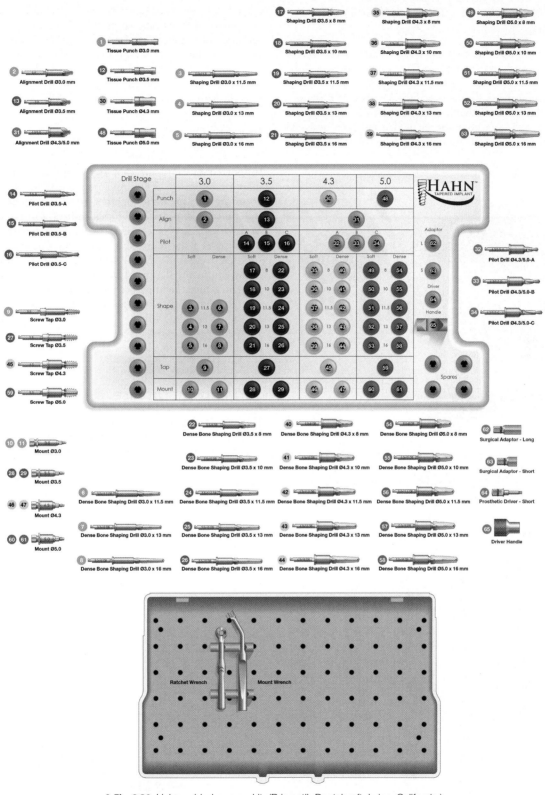

• **Fig. 2.30** Hahn guided surgery kit. (Prismatik Dentalcraft, Irvine, California.)

Screw-Retained versus Cement-Retained Restorations

Fixed implant restorations may be ***screw retained*** or ***cement retained.*** For a screw-retained restoration, the prosthesis can be attached to the implant directly, or indirectly, through the use of a standardized abutment. Cement-retained restorations may use a standardized abutment that has been modified for the specific case or, more commonly, a custom abutment that has been designed for the specific case. Custom abutments can be fabricated using a

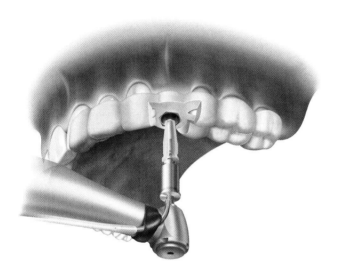

• **Fig. 2.31** Guide created for the Hahn guided surgery kit. Note the hex sleeve placed in a three-dimensional position to direct the surgical drills and implant and the windows to ensure a tooth-supported guide has seated completely.

castable abutment, or through a computer-aided design (CAD)/ computer-aided manufacturing (CAM) process, and can be produced from titanium, gold alloy, or milled zirconia with a titanium base (Figs. 2.38–2.43). Implant components are machined to close tolerances to ensure a precise fit, as seen in Fig. 2.44, which shows a computed tomographic (CT) scan of a Hahn implant with a stock abutment (Fig. 2.45).

Implant Overdenture

An ***implant overdenture*** is a full-arch prosthesis retained or supported by implants that is removable by the patient for daily maintenance. The implants may be unattached, or ***free-standing,*** or ***splinted*** together to increase the capacity for the prosthesis to resist biomechanical forces. ***Overdenture attachments*** are mechanical devices used to provide retention between the removable prosthesis and the implants. For splinted overdenture cases, the attachments are normally incorporated into the design of the splinting bar. For free-standing implants, the attachments are often in the form of an abutment that attaches directly to the implant, such as a ball or Locator attachment (Fig. 2.46).

Temporary abutments are standardized components embedded in the provisional prosthesis that are screw retained to the implant (Fig. 2.47).

Peri-implant Disease

Peri-implant disease refers to inflammatory reactions found in the soft and hard tissues surrounding an implant, and it is a well-reported complication of implant treatment. ***Peri-implant mucositis*** refers to the presence of inflammation in the soft tissue surrounding an implant with no signs of lost supporting bone. ***Peri-implantitis*** describes an inflammatory process

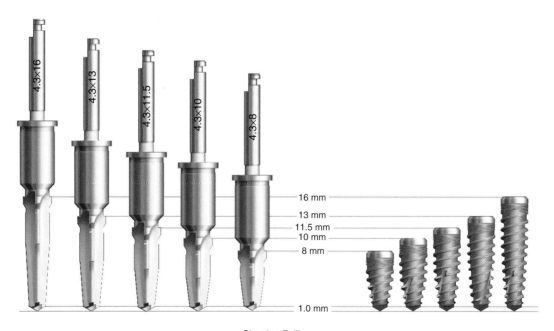

Shaping Drills

• **Fig. 2.32** Hahn guided surgery drills are designed with a cuff that fits precisely into the guide sleeve and eliminates the need for a spoon to hold the drill in place. Each drill is matched with the corresponding implant height.

around an implant, characterized by soft tissue inflammation and loss of supporting bone[43-45] (Fig. 2.48). Tissue loss from peri-implantitis can result in the failure of implants and the associated prosthesis.

Other Types of Implants

Based on the site of implantation, there are three main types of dental implants: eposteal, transosteal, and endosseous. A fourth

type of implant depends on extraoral anchorage, such as the zygomatic arch and the pterygoid process.

Eposteal Implants

Eposteal implants receive their primary support from contact against the remaining bone of the jaw.

The *subperiosteal implant* is the eposteal implant system that has received the greatest amount of usage and study in this

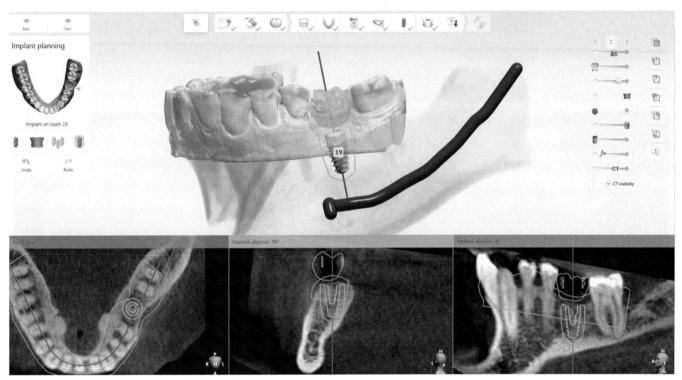

• **Fig. 2.33** Three-dimensional imaging data is used to plan the surgical guide.

TABLE 2.2 Loading Strategies for Dental Implants

Immediate loading	Enhanced primary stability	Loading is temporally irrelevant with respect to osseointegration	Implant placement with primary stability and prosthetic loading occurs at the same clinical visit
Early loading	Primary stability	Loading after onset of osteogenesis, before attaining osseointegration	Implant loading occurs 2–3 weeks[a] after implant placement
Conventional loading	Primary stability	Loading after osteogenesis and woven bone remodeling to load-bearing lamellar bone	Implants are loaded 3–6 months after healing in a submerged or nonsubmerged mucosal orientation
Delayed loading	Stability limited	Loading after protracted period and process of bone formation involving low-density or augmented bone	Loading 6–12 months after implants are placed without primary stability, when implants are placed into bone of low density, and when implants are placed into extraction sockets or concomitant with bone grafting without significant primary stability

[a]Rapid loading should not perturb initial healing (blood clot formation, cellular infiltration, and onset of epithelialization; approximately 2–3 weeks of healing). Provisionalization infers no occlusal contact for restoration of unsplinted implants.

From Cooper LF, De Kok IJ, Rojas-Vizcaya F, Pungapong P, Chang KH. The immediate loading of dental implants. *Inclusive Mag.* 2011;2(2).

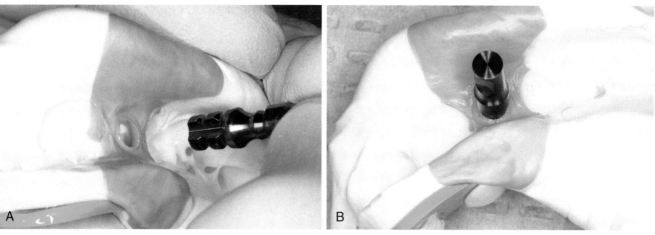

● **Fig. 2.34** (A) Implant analog aligned for seating in a closed-tray impression. (B) Impression with implant analog seated and ready for pouring of cast.

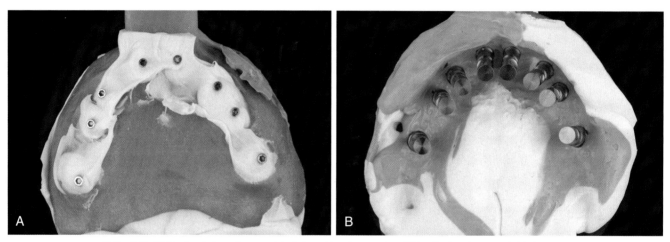

● **Fig. 2.35** (A) Occlusal view of a completed closed-tray impression. (B) Implant analogs seated in impression and ready for pouring of cast.

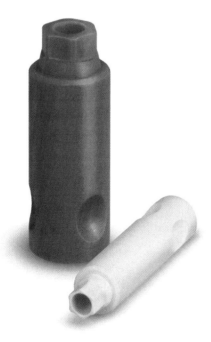

● **Fig. 2.36** Scanning abutments are attached to implants to make a digital impression using an intraoral scanner.

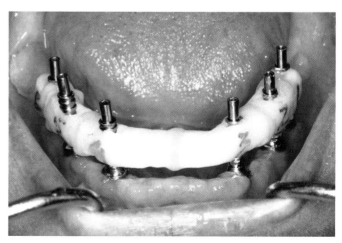

● **Fig. 2.37** Individual sections of the laboratory-provided implant verification jig are connected to the multiunit abutments and luted together, ensuring an accurate recording of the interimplant positions in the final impression.

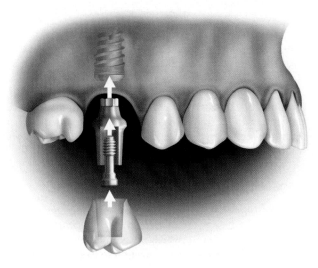

• **Fig. 2.38** Cement-retained crown.

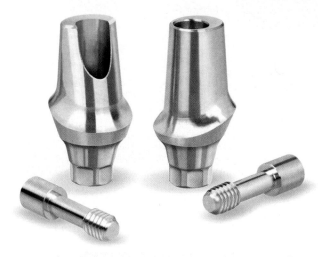

• **Fig. 2.41** Standardized abutments for cemented restorations. Provided by implant manufacturers, these abutments are modified by the clinician or laboratory for the specific case.

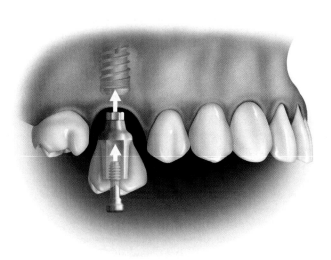

• **Fig. 2.39** Screw-retained crown.

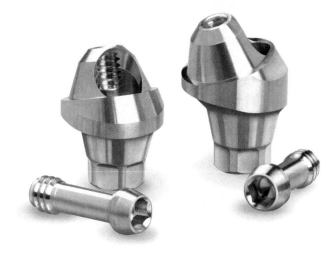

• **Fig. 2.42** Multiunit abutments with screws. These standardized abutments are used for screw-retained multiple unit restorations.

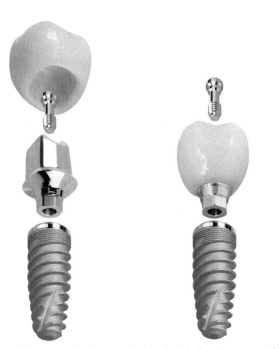

• **Fig. 2.40** Cement-retained crown with implant (left) and screw-retained crown (right).

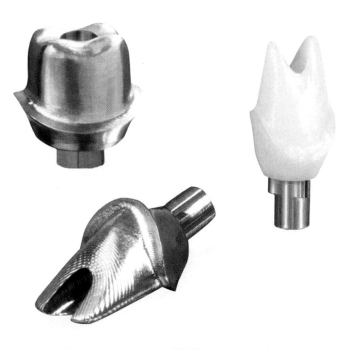

• **Fig. 2.43** Computer-aided design (CAD)/computer-aided manufacturing (CAM) custom abutments. Left to right, posterior milled titanium abutment, anterior milled titanium abutment, and hybrid milled zirconia bonded to titanium abutment base.

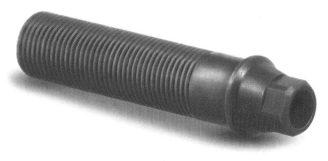

• **Fig. 2.44** Plastic burnout pattern for a castable abutment.

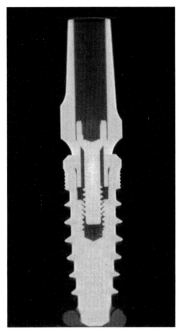

• **Fig. 2.45** Cross-sectional view from computer tomographic data of Hahn implant with stock abutment. Note the precise fit and machining.

category. Introduced by Dahl in 1943, with additional contributions from Goldberg and Gershkoff[46] and Linkow and Ghalili,[47] the subperiosteal implant is used principally for treatment of the edentulous mandible. The predominant treatment method involves two surgical interventions. During the first surgery, the operator reflects the oral mucosa and periosteum to uncover the bony edentulous alveolar process and the surrounding basal mandibular bone. While this tissue is reflected, an impression is made of the denture-bearing area. The surgical incision is then sutured, and a custom frame is fabricated, usually from a cobalt-chromium alloy. In a second surgical procedure, this frame is placed subperiosteally with several projections through the mucosa for attachment of the prosthesis. Fixed or removable prostheses can then be connected to these transmucosal posts.

Subperiosteal implants have been used for treatment of the edentulous mandible and maxilla. However, the best results have been reported for treatment of the edentulous mandible because of the greater bone density and resulting capacity to support the load of the prosthesis. Subperiosteally anchored implants are not considered to be osseointegrated implants, but they are intended to gain support by resting on the residual bony ridge (Fig. 2.49).

The *ramus frame,* another eposteal implant design, has also received significant clinical documentation. This is a one-piece implant, used in the mandible only, with right and left posterior extensions that are surgically placed into the corresponding right and left ascending rami, and an anterior foot, which is surgically placed in the bone of the symphysis (Fig. 2.50). Because long-term results for ramus frame and subperiosteal implants are less favorable than those from root-form implants, these designs are not currently considered as the first option for treatment of the edentulous arch.[4,11,37,47-49]

Transosteal Implants

Transosteal implants are a group of implant designs that pass completely through the bone. The *transmandibular implant (TMI)* refers to a design in which posts are inserted through the mandible in an inferior-superior direction to fixate a metal framework on which the prosthesis is attached. Implants included in this category include the *Smooth Staple* implant and the *Bosker.* These systems were developed specifically for the extremely atrophied mandible. In published studies, the majority of the patients treated had an anterior mandibular bone height of less than 12 mm.[50-53] The TMI is inserted through an extraoral approach, with the baseplate fixed to the inferior border of the mandible with the cortical screws. The transosseous posts, connected to the baseplate, perforate the mandible and the oral mucosa and are connected to each other with a bar equipped with two distal cantilevers. Three months after placement, an implant-supported overdenture is usually constructed. The completed prosthesis is retained by clips held in the mandibular denture. The clips engage bar segments, which are a part of the implant superstructure, and provide the necessary retention for the overdenture[54] (Fig. 2.51).

The TMI has been shown to be a successful clinical solution to prosthetic rehabilitation of patients with severe mandibular atrophy. In a study of 1356 patients over a period of 13 years, the implants show a consistent success rate of 96.8%.[50]

Studies comparing the TMI with endosseous implants[55,56] showed no significant differences between the two systems after 1 year,[55] but thereafter significantly more complications were reported with the TMI system. After 6 years, a survival rate of 97% was reported for the endosseous implants versus a survival rate of 72% for the TMI group.[57] In the highly resorbed mandible, short endosseous implants perform significantly better than the TMI.[56]

The staple bone implant system was developed as an alternative to subperiosteal frames because of the major complications that were encountered in the clinical application of subperiosteal frames.[58] The staple bone implant consists of a baseplate with two or four (parallel) transosseous pins and from two to five retentive pins (or screws) to stabilize the baseplate to the inferior border. The implant is made of a titanium alloy to allow for osseointegration. To prevent overloading of this implant system, a tissue-supported overdenture is fabricated with stress-breaking attachments to the implant. The mandibular staple bone implant has been evaluated in several retrospective studies that have reported survival rates of between 86% and 100%.[56,59-61]

Zygomatic and Pterygoid (Tubero-Pterygo-Maxillary) Implants

Although prosthetic treatment with osseointegrated implants is a predictably successful treatment method, in many cases severe maxillary atrophy remains a clinical challenge.[62] The success rate for root-form implants placed in the nongrafted severely resorbed

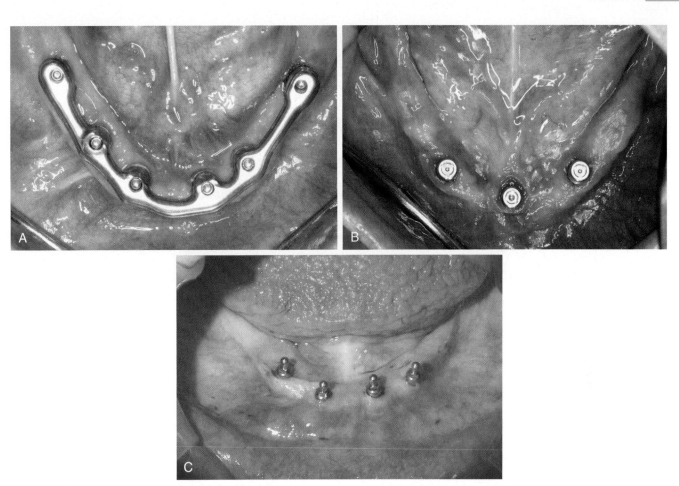

• **Fig. 2.46** Types of overdenture attachments. (A) Bar. (B) Locator. (C) Ball.

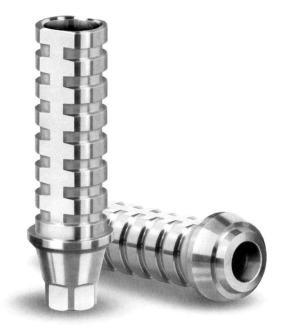

• **Fig. 2.47** Temporary abutments.

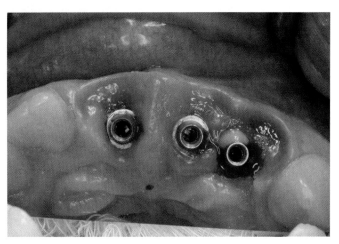

• **Fig. 2.48** Inflammation and purulent discharge around these maxillary implants are indicative of peri-implantitis. (From Wingrove SS, Horowitz RA. Peri-implant disease: prevention, diagnosis and nonsurgical treatment. *Inclusive Mag.* 2014;5[1].)

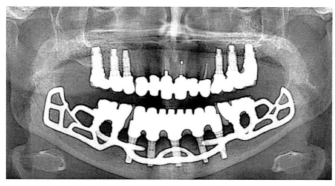

• **Fig. 2.49** Circumferential Subperiosteal Implant: Subperiosteal implant which is a custom implant which directly is supported by the mandibular cortical bone, supports bilateral edentulous spaces.

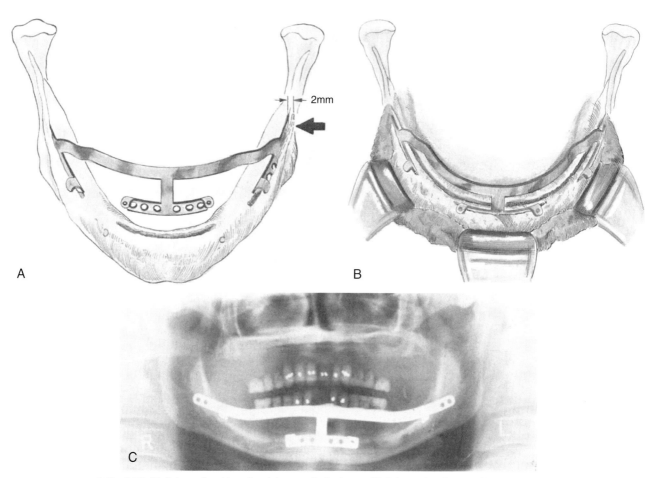

• **Fig. 2.50** (A) Schematic of insertion into mandibular bone. (B) Schematic of ramus frame seated into bone. (C) Radiograph of ramus frame mandibular implant. (From Lemons JE, Misch CE. Dental implantation. In: Ratner BD, Hoffman A, Schoen F, Lemons J, eds. *Biomaterials Science*. 3rd ed. Waltham, MA: Academic Press; 2013.)

posterior maxilla is approximately 85%.[62] In these cases, implants placed in the zygomatic and pterygoid processes may offer patients an opportunity to have full arch prostheses by finding anchorage outside the maxilla.

The ***zygomatic implant*** enables the clinician to provide support for a maxillary prosthesis by anchoring implants in facial bone of sufficient volume and density. The technique involves the placement of implants of 50 mm or longer, extending from the maxilla to the zygomatic process. Several techniques have been proposed, with some involving a transosseous drilling path, and others remaining lateral to the sinus. Because of the challenges of limited direct vision and risks of associated anatomic structures, specialized training and careful technique are required for placement of this implant design. Because of the greater length of these implants, a significant error can result from even a small deviation from the intended drilling path.[62] The zygomatic implant has been established as a valuable treatment option for the patient with a highly resorbed maxilla. Angled abutments, as well as angled implant collars and prosthetic connections, have been developed to facilitate the fabrication of screw-retained prostheses supported by this type of implant (Fig. 2.52).

Clinical studies of the zygomatic implant show high rates of clinical success. Chrcanovic and colleagues published a review of studies on zygomatic implants. The 68 studies described 4556 zygomatic implants in 2161 patients, with only 103 failures (12-year Cumulative Survival Rate CSR, 95.21%). The survival rates reported suggest that zygomatic implants can successfully support immediate loading when patient selection and loading protocols are carefully controlled. The protocol dictated the prosthetic connection of all maxillary implants with a rigid connector, which results in a favorable load distribution, particularly important for immediate or early loading.[63]

Pterygoid implants were introduced as another method of maximizing the usable bone for placement of implants in the posterior maxilla. First described by Tulasne in 1989, the pterygoid implant is intended to pass through the maxillary tuberosity and pyramidal process of palatine bone and then engage the pterygoid process of the sphenoid bone. Implants used in this technique usually range from 15 to 20 mm. The implant enters in the maxillary first or second molar region and follows an oblique mesiocranial direction proceeding posteriorly toward the pyramidal process. It subsequently proceeds upward between both wings of the pterygoid processes and finds anchorage in the pterygoid or scaphoid fossa of the sphenoid bone (Fig. 2.53).

The advantages of using pterygoid implants are the availability of dense cortical bone for engagement of the implant and the potential to avoid the need for augmentation of the maxillary sinus and other grafting procedures. This may shorten the treatment time and allow immediate loading of the pterygoid implant. Increasing implant anchorage in the posterior maxilla also allows for a prosthesis with greater posterior extensions, eliminating the need for distal cantilevers. The disadvantages of the pterygoid

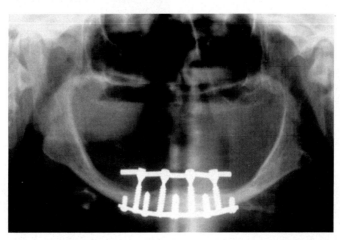

• **Fig. 2.51** Panoramic radiograph of a one-piece transosseous implant consisting of a metal plate located on the inferior border of the mandible, five posts that are placed into the mandible, and four posts that pass through the mandible. A bar has been attached to the four posts to provide retention and stability for a mandibular implant overdenture. (From White SN, Sabeti MA. History of single implants. In: Torabinejad M, Sabeti MA, Goodacre CJ, eds. *Principles and Practice of Single Implant and Restorations.* Philadelphia: Saunders; 2014.)

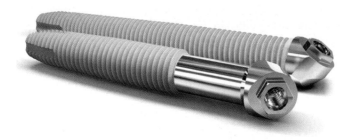

• **Fig. 2.52** Zygomatic implants (Southern Implants, Centurion, South Africa). Note the angled connection.

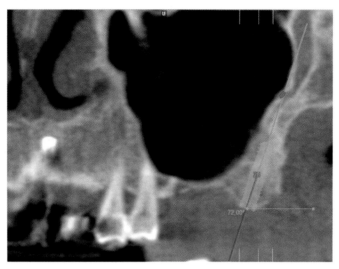

• **Fig. 2.53** Virtual implant placement following the pterygoid bone corridor. The mesiodistal inclination (panoramic view) is shown. (From Rodriguez X, Lucas-Taulé E, Elnayef B, et al. Anatomical and radiological approach to pterygoid implants: a cross-sectional study of 202 cone beam computed tomography examinations. *Int J Oral Maxillofac Surg.* 2016;45[5]:636–640.)

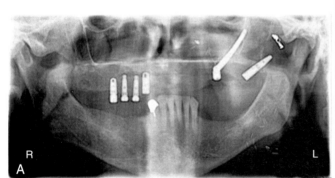
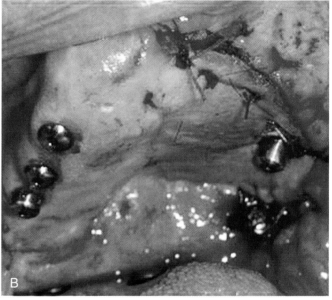

• **Fig. 2.54** (A) Zygoma implant plus pterygoid implant with contralateral conventional implants. (B) Zygoma implant and pterygoid implants penetrating the radial forearm flap for reconstruction after left maxillectomy. (From Dierks EJ, Higuchi KW. Zygoma implants in a compromised maxilla. In: Baheri SC, Bell RB, Ali H, eds. *Current Therapy in Oral Maxillofacial Surgery.* Amsterdam: Elsevier; 2012. Courtesy David Hirsch, New York.)

implant are technique sensitivity associated with the procedure, proximity to vital anatomic structures, and access difficulty for clinicians and patients.[64] The success rate for pterygoid implants has been reported from 71% to nearly 100%.[65] Fig. 2.54 shows conventional, pterygoid and zygomatic implants in the patient's upper jaw.

Tuberosity implants originate at the most distal aspect of the maxillary alveolar process and may engage the pyramidal process.[66] There is some lack of consistency in the literature regarding the terminology associated with implants placed in this region. The terms "pterygoid implants," "pterygomaxillary

implants," and "tuberosity implants" are sometimes used interchangeably. The pterygoid implant has been defined as "implant placement through the maxillary tuberosity and into the pterygoid plate," and authors using the term pterygomaxillary implant are likely referring to implants placed in this complex, which involves the maxillary tuberosity, pyramidal process of palatine bone, and pterygoid plates. In contrast, the maxillary tuberosity is defined as "the most distal aspect of the maxillary alveolar process," and significant differences exist between pterygoid and tuberosity implants (Fig. 2.55). Pterygoid implants originate at the tuberosity, and a major portion

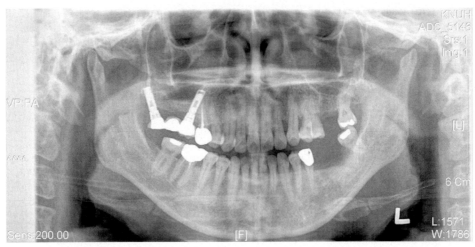

• **Fig. 2.55** Two implants were placed in the left maxilla, one in the tuberosity region and the other in the first molar region, and splinted with a ceramometal fixed bridge. (From Park YJ, Cho SA. Retrospective chart analysis on survival rate of fixtures installed at the tuberosity bone for cases with missing unilateral upper molars: a study of 7 cases. *J Oral Maxilllofac Surg.* 2010;68[6]:1338–1344.)

of the tuberosity body and apex is embedded in dense cortical bone of the pterygoid plates and pyramidal process of palatine bone, whereas tuberosity implants originate at the most distal aspect of the maxillary alveolar process and may engage the pyramidal process. Because the tuberosity region is predominantly composed of dense bone, the difference in bony support for a pterygoid implant and a tuberosity implant can be significant.[64]

Conclusion

A specific set of terms has been developed within the field of dental implantology to describe the instruments, components, and techniques used in clinical and laboratory practice. The basic terms have been described in this chapter, and, for further information, the reader is advised to consult the *Glossary of Implant Dentistry* (ICOI) and the *Glossary of Prosthodontic Terms* (ACP).

References

1. International Congress of Oral Implantologists. *Glossary of Implant Dentistry III*. Fairfield, NJ: ICOI; 2017:209.
2. Driscoll CF, Freilich MA, Guckes AD, et al. The glossary of prosthodontic terms: ninth edition. *J Prosthet Dent.* 2017;117(5S):e1–e105. https://doi.org/10.1016/j.prosdent.2016.12.001.
3. Tagliareni JM, Clarkson E. Basic concepts and techniques of dental implants. *Dent Clin North Am.* 2015;59(2):255–264. https://doi.org/10.1016/J.CDEN.2014.10.005.
4. Abraham CM. A brief historical perspective on dental implants, their surface coatings and treatments. *Open Dent J.* 2014;8:50–55.
5. Zarb G, Albrektsson T. Osseointegration: a requiem for the periodontal ligament. *Int J Periodontics Restor Dent.* 1991;11(2):1–88.
6. Smeets R, Stadlinger B, Schwarz F, et al. Impact of dental implant surface modifications on osseointegration. *Biomed Res Int.* 2016;2(1):1–15.
7. Albrektsson T, Jacobsson M. Bone-metal interface in osseointegration. *J Prosthet Dent.* 1987;57(5):597–607. https://doi.org/10.1016/0022-3913(87)90344-1.
8. von Wilmowsky C, Moest T, Nkenke E, et al. Implants in bone: part I. A current overview about tissue response, surface modifications and future perspectives. *Oral Maxillofac Surg.* 2014;18(3):243–257. https://doi.org/10.1007/s10006-013-0398-1.
9. Schwartz Z, Nasazky E, Boyan BD. Surface microtopography regulates osteointegration: the role of implant surface microtopography in osteointegration. *Alpha Omegan.* 2005;98(2):9–19.
10. von Wilmowsky C, Moest T, Nkenke E, et al. Implants in bone: part II. Research on implant osseointegration. *Oral Maxillofac Surg.* 2014;18(4):355–372. https://doi.org/10.1007/s10006-013-0397-2.
11. Albrektsson T, Zarb G, Worthington P, Eriksson AR. The long-term efficacy of currently used dental implants: a review and proposed criteria of success. *Int J Oral Maxillofac Implants.* 1986;1(1):11–25.
12. Meredith N, Alleyne D, Cawley P. Quantitative determination of the stability of the implant-tissue interface using resonance frequency analysis. *Clin Oral Implants Res.* 1996;7(3):261–267. https://doi.org/10.1034/j.1600-0501.1996.070308.x.
13. Sennerby L, Meredith N. Implant stability measurements using resonance frequency analysis: biological and biomechanical aspects and clinical implications. *Periodontol 2000.* 2008;47:51–66.
14. Kosinski T. Implant therapy: then and now. *Incl Mag.* 2014;5(1).
15. Gargiulo AW, Wentz FM, Orban B. Dimensions and relations of the dentogingival junction in humans. *J Periodontol.* 1961;32(3):261–267. https://doi.org/10.1902/jop.1961.32.3.261.
16. Esfahrood ZR, Kadkhodazadeh M, Gholamin P, et al. Biologic width around dental implants: an updated review. *Biol Width Around Dent Implant.* 2016;5(2).
17. Martinez H, Davarpanah M, Missika P, et al. Optimal implant stabilization in low density bone. *Clin Oral Implants Res.* 2001;12(5):423–432.
18. Glauser R, Sennerby L, Meredith N, et al. Resonance frequency analysis of implants subjected to immediate or early functional occlusal loading. Successful vs. failing implants. *Clin Oral Implants Res.* 2004;15(4):428–434. https://doi.org/10.1111/j.1600-0501.2004.01036.x.
19. Garber DA, Salama H, Salama MA. Two-stage versus one-stage—is there really a controversy? *J Periodontol.* 2001;72(3):417–421. https://doi.org/10.1902/jop.2001.72.3.417.
20. Schiegnitz E, Al-Nawas B, Tegner A, et al. Clinical and radiological long-term outcome of a tapered implant system with special emphasis on the influence of augmentation procedures. *Clin Implant Dent Relat Res.* 2016;18(4):810–820. https://doi.org/10.1111/cid.12338.

21. Wilson TG, Miller RJ, Trushkowsky R, Dard M. Tapered implants in dentistry. *Adv Dent Res*. 2016;28(1):4–9. https://doi.org/10.1177/0022034516628868.

22. Glauser R. Implants with an oxidized surface placed predominately in soft bone quality and subjected to immediate occlusal loading: results from an 11-year clinical follow-up. *Clin Implant Dent Relat Res*. 2016;18(3):429–438. https://doi.org/10.1111/cid.12327.

23. Bullis G, Abai S. Form and function of implant threads in cancellous bone. *Incl Mag*. 2013;4(1).

24. Al-Thobity AM, Kutkut A, Almas K. Microthreaded implants and crestal bone loss: a systematic review. *J Oral Implantol*. 2017;43(2):157–166. https://doi.org/10.1563/aaid-joi-D-16-00170.

25. Dohan Ehrenfest DM, Coelho PG, Kang BS, et al. Classification of osseointegrated implant surfaces: materials, chemistry and topography. *Trends Biotechnol*. 2010;28(4):198–206. https://doi.org/10.1016/j.tibtech.2009.12.003.

26. Albrektsson T, Wennerberg A. Oral implant surfaces: part 1—review focusing on topographic and chemical properties of different surfaces and in vivo responses to them. *Int J Prosthodont*. 2004;17(5):536–543.

27. Fischer K, Stenberg T. Prospective 10-year cohort study based on a Randomized Controlled Trial (RCT) on implant-supported full-arch maxillary prostheses. part 1: sandblasted and acid-etched implants and mucosal tissue. *Clin Implant Dent Relat Res*. 2012;14(6):808–815. https://doi.org/10.1111/j.1708-8208.2011.00389.x.

28. Burguete RL, Johns RB, King T, Patterson EA. Tightening characteristics for screwed joints in osseointegrated dental implants. *J Prosthet Dent*. 1994;71(6):592–599.

29. Haack JE, Sakaguchi RL, Sun T, Coffey JP. Elongation and preload stress in dental implant abutment screws. *Int J Oral Maxillofac Implants*. 1995;10(5):529–536.

30. Schwarz MS. Mechanical complications of dental implants. *Clin Oral Implants Res*. 2000;11(suppl 1):156–158.

31. Martini AP, Freitas AC, Rocha EP, et al. Straight and angulated abutments in platform switching. *J Craniofac Surg*. 2012;23(2):415–418. https://doi.org/10.1097/SCS.0b013e31824b9c17.

32. Rossi F, Zavanelli AC, Zavanelli RA. Photoelastic comparison of single tooth implant-abutment-bone of platform switching vs conventional implant designs. *J Contemp Dent Pr*. 2011;12(2):124–130. https://doi.org/10.5005/jp-journals-10024-1021.

33. Hahn J. Single-stage, immediate loading, and flapless surgery. *Clin J Oral Implantol*. 2000;193(3):193–198. https://doi.org/10.1563/1548-1336(2000)026<0193:SILAFS>2.3.CO;2.

34. Resnik RR. Bone substitutes in oral implantology. *Chairside Mag*. 2018;12(3).

35. Esposito M, Grusovin MG, Felice P, et al. The efficacy of horizontal and vertical bone augmentation procedures for dental implants: a cochrane systematic review. In Chiappelli F, (eds). *Evidence-Based Pract Towar Optim Clin Outcomes*. 2010:195–218. https://doi.org/10.1007/978-3-642-05025-1_13.

36. Al-dary HH. The socket shield technique a case report. *Smile Dent J*. 2013;8(1):32–36.

37. Starch-Jensen T, Aludden H, Hallman M, et al. A systematic review and meta-analysis of long-term studies (five or more years) assessing maxillary sinus floor augmentation. *Int J Oral Maxillofac Surg*. 2018;47(1):103–116. https://doi.org/10.1016/j.ijom.2017.05.001.

38. Danesh-Sani SA, Loomer PM, Wallace SS. A comprehensive clinical review of maxillary sinus floor elevation: anatomy, techniques, biomaterials and complications. *Br J Oral Maxillofac Surg*. 2016;54:724–730. https://doi.org/10.1016/j.bjoms.2016.05.008.

39. Kalfas IH. Principles of bone healing. *Neurosurg Focus*. 2001;10(4):1–4. https://doi.org/10.3171/foc.2001.10.4.2.

40. Brisman DL. The effect of speed, pressure, and time on bone temperature during the drilling of implant sites. *Int J Oral Maxillofac Implants*. 1997;11(1):35–37.

41. Cooper LF, et al. The immediate loading of dental implants. *Inclusive Mag*. 2011;2(2).

42. Lee H, So JS, Hochstedler JL, Ercoli C. The accuracy of implant impressions: a systematic review. *J Prosthet Dent*. 2008;100(4):285–291. https://doi.org/10.1016/S0022-3913(08)60208-5.

43. Lindhe J, Meyle J, Group D of European Workshop on Periodontology. Peri-implant diseases: Consensus Report of the Sixth European Workshop on Periodontology. *J Clin Periodontol*. 2008;35(suppl 8):282–285. https://doi.org/10.1111/j.1600-051X.2008.01283.x.

44. Zitzmann NU, Berglundh T. Definition and prevalence of peri-implant diseases. *J Clin Periodontol*. 2008;35(suppl 8):286–291. https://doi.org/10.1111/j.1600-051X.2008.01274.x.

45. Wingrove SS, Horowitz RA. Peri-Implant disease: prevention, diagnosis and nonsurgical treatment. *Incl Mag*. 2014;5(1).

46. Goldberg NI, Gershkoff A. The implant lower denture. *Dent Dig*. 1949;55(11):490–494.

47. Linkow LI, Ghalili R. Critical design errors in maxillary subperiosteal implants. *J Oral Implantol*. 1998;24(4):198–205. https://doi.org/10.1563/1548-1336(1998)024<0198:CDEIMS>2.3.CO;2.

48. Stellingsma C, Vissink A, Meijer H, Raghoebar G. Implantology and the severely resorbed edentulous mandible. *Crit Rev Oral Biol Med*. 2004;15(4):240–248.

49. Reddy Vootla N, Reddy KV. Osseointegration-key factors affecting its success-an overview. *IOSR J Dent Med Sci*. 2017;16(4):2279–2861. https://doi.org/10.9790/0853-1604056268.

50. Bosker H, Jordan RD, Sindet-Pedersen S, Koole R. The transmandibular implant: a 13-year survey of its use. *J Oral Maxillofac Surg*. 1991;49(5):482–492.https://doi.org/10.1016/0278-2391(91)90171-H.

51. Bosker H, van Dijk L. The transmandibular implant: a 12-year follow-up study. *J Oral Maxillofac Surg*. 1989;47(5):442–450. https://doi.org/10.1016/0278-2391(89)90275-9.

52. Bosker H. The transmandibular implant (TMI) for mandibular reconstruction. *J Oral Maxillofac Surg*. 1991;49(8):21. https://doi.org/10.1016/0278-2391(91)90501-C.

53. Maxson B, Sindet-Pedersen S, Tideman H, et al. Multicenter follow-up study of the transmandibular implant. *J Oral Maxillofac Surg*. 1989;47(8):785–789.

54. Unger JW, Crabtree DG. The transmandibular implant: prosthodontic treatment considerations. *J Prosthet Dent*. 1991;66(5):660–664. https://doi.org/10.1016/0022-3913(91)90449-7.

55. Geertman ME, Boerrigter EM, Van Waas MA, van Oort RP. Clinical aspects of a multicenter clinical trial of implant-retained mandibular overdentures in patients with severely resorbed mandibles. *J Prosthet Dent*. 1996;75(2):194–204.

56. Stellingsma C, Vissink A, Meijer HJA, et al. Implantology and the severely resorbed edentulous mandible. *Crit Rev Oral Biol Med*. 2004;15(4):240–248.

57. Meijer HJA, Geertman ME, Raghoebar GM, Kwakman JM. Implant-retained mandibular overdentures: 6-year results of a multicenter clinical trial on 3 different implant systems. *J Oral Maxillofac Surg*. 2001;59(11):1260–1268. https://doi.org/10.1053/JOMS.2001.27512.

58. Small IA. Chalmers J. Lyons memorial lecture: Metal implants and the mandibular staple bone plate. *J Oral Surg*. 1975;33(8):571–585.

59. Small IA, Misiek D. A sixteen-year evaluation of the mandibular staple bone plate. *J Oral Maxillofac Surg*. 1986;44(1):60–66.

60. Small IA. The fixed mandibular implant: a 6-year review. *J Oral Maxillofac Surg*. 1993;51(11):1206–1210.

61. Meijer HJ, Van Oort RP, Raghoebar GM, Schoen PJ. The mandibular staple bone plate: a long-term retrospective evaluation. *J Oral Maxillofac Surg*. 1998;56(2):141–145. discussion 145-6.

62. Vrielinck L, Politis C, Schepers S, et al. Image-based planning and clinical validation of zygoma and pterygoid implant placement in patients with severe bone atrophy using customized drill guides. Preliminary results from a prospective clinical follow-up study. *Int*

J Oral Maxillofac Surg. 2003;32(1):7–14. https://doi.org/10.1054/ijom.2002.0337.

63. Chrcanovic BR, Albrektsson T, Wennerberg A. Survival and complications of zygomatic implants: an updated systematic review. *J Oral Maxillofac Surg.* 2016;74(10):1949–1964. https://doi.org/10.1016/j.joms.2016.06.166.

64. Bidra AS, Huynh-Ba G. Implants in the pterygoid region: a systematic review of the literature. *Int J Oral Maxillofac Surg.* 2011;40(8):773–781. https://doi.org/10.1016/j.ijom.2011.04.007.

65. Candel E, Peñarrocha D, Peñarrocha M. Rehabilitation of the atrophic posterior maxilla with pterygoid implants: a review. *J Oral Implantol.* 2012;38(S1):461–466. https://doi.org/10.1563/AAID-JOI-D-10-00200.

66. Lopes LFdTP, da Silva VF, Santiago JF, et al. Placement of dental implants in the maxillary tuberosity: a systematic review. *Int J Oral Maxillofac Surg.* 2015;44(2):229–238. https://doi.org/10.1016/j.ijom.2014.08.005.

3

Functional Basis for Dental Implant Design

GRANT BULLIS

Dental implant therapy is a widely accepted treatment method for restoring chewing function in partially or fully edentulous patients. Treatment planning for dental implants requires consideration of the type of prosthesis, bone density, occlusion, function, bone volume, and any medically compromising factors.[1,2] Compromised bone density, large occlusal loads, and/or parafunction require greater implant support for the desired treatment outcome.[3-5] When compromising factors exist, the implant treatment plan must be adjusted to mitigate them to the maximum extent possible. Mitigation options include bone grafting,[6,7] lateral compression with osteotomes to improve bone density at the time of surgery,[8] implant site localization in conjunction with prosthesis design to minimize unfavorable occlusal loads,[9,10] and use of dental implants with attributes that address these compromising factors.[11]

Implant designs have progressed over time from the early press-fit blade designs, to press-fit cylinders, and finally to the straight and tapered threaded implants that comprise the majority of implant designs today. Press-fit cylinders are relatively easy to place because they do not have external threads that have to be advanced into the implant site. This ease of placement, however, comes with some compromise in primary stability and lower bone-implant contact relative to a threaded implant of comparable length and diameter. The surgical placement of press-fit blade implants in thin alveolar crests is also often easier than threaded implants because bone grafting can be avoided, and the surgical technique is relatively simple and can be performed with standard instruments.[12]

The aforementioned implant designs have high osseointegration success rates before loading; however, reported long-term success rates in function can be significantly lower (Table 3.1).[13-15] With this in mind, implant design should be predicated around addressing potential complications that may arise during function. Marginal bone loss after uncovering or loading of the implant is the most frequently reported complication in the dental literature. In a study conducted at the Brånemark Clinic in Gothenburg, Sweden, 28% of the 662 patients with implant-supported prostheses in function at least 5 years exhibited progressive bone loss to the level of three or more threads on at least one implant.[16] Bone quality, implant diameter, and implant length also contribute to implant failure rates after loading with softer bone, smaller diameter, and shorter implants exhibiting higher failure rates related to inadequate support relative to the load placed on these implants in function.[17,18] Because some percentage of restorative situations will present with soft bone and/or compromised bone volume, the design of the implant should compensate for these loading conditions.

Implant survival and marginal bone maintenance can vary greatly between implant designs. In a clinical report on the success of 43 consecutively placed Core-Vent Implants examined and followed from 3 months to 4 years, Malmqvist et al.[19] reported a success rate of 37.2%. A total of 11 implants were removed, 9 because of progressive vertical bone loss and 2 because of fractures. The vertical bone loss was calculated for the 32 remaining implants. Twenty-eight implants demonstrated a bone loss of more than 2 mm, and 16 showed a loss of more than one-third of the implant height.[19]

A study of 550 one-piece Nobel Direct implants by Albrektsson et al.[20] found a 10.7% average failure rate after 1 year from placement, with significant crestal bone loss on many of the remaining implants. Implant design contributed to the high failure rates of these implants relative to their peers (Table 3.2). Another study by Ormianer et al.[21] evaluated marginal bone loss using three dental implant thread designs with differences in thread pitch, lead, and helix angle. These implants had the same material and surfaces. The mean bone loss observed was between 1.90 and 2.02 mm for the single lead V-thread and double-lead progressive thread implants, respectively (Table 3.3). The overall implant survival rate was 96.3%. The remainder of this chapter applies biomechanical principles to dental implant design to improve short- and long-term outcomes and minimize complications. The function, form, and materials considered in the design of modern, threaded implants are examined in detail.

Function and Implant Design

Dental implants provide support for the prosthesis and transfer the occlusal forces to the supporting bone. The transfer of the forces to the supporting bone is determined by the resultant force transferred from the prosthesis to the implant and the amount of implant area available to transfer the force to the supporting bone. Implants have features designed to provide transfer occlusal forces to the bone and provide a secure, stable prosthetic connection (Fig. 3.1).

Besides the transfer of occlusal forces into the supporting bone, dental implants have features that facilitate the correct position of prefabricated and customized prosthetics, provide a mechanism

TABLE 3.1 Implant Long-Term Success Rates in Function

Study Author(s)	Implant Type	Time Period	Success Rate
Bodine and Yanase	Subperiosteal	15 years	54%
Cranin, Rabkin, Garfinkel	Blade	5 years	55%
Smithloff and Fritz	Blade	10 years	~50%
Armitage	Blade	5 years	50%
McCoy	Cylinder	5 years	31%

From Albrektsson T, Zarb G, Worthington P, Eriksson AR. The long-term efficacy of currently used dental implants: a review and proposed criteria of success. *Int J Oral Maxillofac Implants.* 1986;1:11-25.

TABLE 3.2 Reported Failure Rates of Nobel Direct One-Piece Implants

Implant Diameter	Number of Implants	Number Lost	Failure Rate
3 mm	55	11	20%
3.5 mm	68	8	12%
4.3 mm	287	8	3%
5.0 mm	60	8	13%
Not specified	80	24	30%
All diameters	550	59	11%

From Albrektsson T, Gottlow J, Meirelles L, Östman PO, Rocci A, Sennerby L. Survival of Nobel Direct implants: an analysis of 550 consecutively placed implants at 18 different clinical centers. *Clin Implant Dent Relat Res.* 2007;9:65-70.

for insertion into the implant site, contribute to the seal stability and strength of the prosthetic connection, and aid in the correct identification of restorative components for the specific prosthetic connection. Combining features that are robust for their intended use helps to minimize complications during the surgical placement of implants and long after they are in function.[22,23]

Occlusal Forces and Implant Design

Force Type

Bone response to occlusal forces varies with the magnitude and the direction of the forces applied. Occlusal forces along the axis of the implant result in primarily compressive loading of the supporting bone. Nonaxial occlusal forces that are transverse to the implant axis result in significant tensile and shear forces (Fig. 3.2). Prosthesis design plays an important role in the transmission of occlusal forces to the implant and then to the supporting bone. Prostheses with cantilevered designs will transmit more tensile forces to the bone adjacent to the implant.[24,25] Bone is best able to resist loads that place it in compression, less resistant to tensile forces, and significantly less resistant to shear forces.[26] Because bone is strongest when resisting compression forces, implant design should facilitate compressive transfer of occlusal forces to

bone.[27] Load transfer to the supporting bone is most efficiently accomplished by the implant surfaces perpendicular to the axis of the implant. These surfaces transfer compressive and tensile forces to the bone. Implant surfaces that are not perpendicular or parallel to the implant axis will transfer shear forces, along with compressive and tensile forces, to the supporting bone (Fig. 3.3).

Force Magnitude

Bite force varies with the region of the mouth, muscularity, and the type of dentition. Observed mean bite forces in the molar region where forces are highest approach 200 psi for men and 135 psi for women with significant variation.[28] For some individuals, average bite forces can approach 1000 psi in the posterior regions.[29] Using a larger number of implants also helps distribute the bite forces.[30] These large bite forces require implant designs and materials robust enough to withstand peak and sustained forces of these magnitudes. Currently, titanium and titanium alloys provide the best strength properties without unacceptable compromises in other areas, such as biocompatibility.

Force Direction

As forces that diverge from the axis of the implant, the load-bearing capabilities of the supporting bone are compromised. The greater the divergence of the direction of the load from the implant axis, the greater the stresses at the implant-bone interface. Vertical loading of angled implants significantly increases the compressive stress values in the cervical region of the angled implants relative to those in axially loaded vertical implants.[31] The nonisotropic behavior of bone under different loading conditions further exacerbates the adverse effect of angled loads of bone. The tensile, compressive, shear, and ultimate strength of bone vary with the direction of the occlusal load applied to the bone.[32] Ideally, the implant should be placed with the implant axis loaded as near to vertical as possible to minimize shear and tensile force transmission to the interface between the bone and the implant. Prosthesis design, such as the avoidance of excessive distal cantilevers, that minimizes nonaxial load transfer to the implant and supporting bone also helps to minimize the stress to the components in the restoration. This also decreases the risk for force-related complications.

Force Duration

The duration of bite forces is widely distributed. Under ideal conditions the teeth come together during swallowing and eating, but only briefly. A study by Sheppard et al.[33] indicated that there is no tooth contact during most of the time spent in mastication. Approximately 19.5% of the time required for mastication was involved in possible tooth contacts for three foods.[33] The total time varies with the amount of mastication; however, it is estimated to be less than 30 minutes per day.[34] Bruxism increases force duration and is considered to be a contributing factor of dental implant and prosthetic complications and dental implant failure.[35]

Implant Geometry

Implant Shape

As mentioned previously, forces applied to the implant can be evaluated in magnitude, duration, type, and direction. The area over which the forces are applied serves to transmit the forces to the supporting bone. The larger the implant surface available for force transmission, the lower the stress experienced by the implant system and vice versa.

TABLE 3.3 Mean Bone Loss and Survival Rate of V-Thread and Double-Lead Progressive Thread Implants

Implant	Thread Type	Thread Pitch	Thread Lead	Implant Qty	Implant Survival	Bone loss (mm)
SPI	Progressive	1.05 mm	2.1 mm	388	96.6%	2.02 (±1.70)
DFI	Progressive	0.6 mm	1.2 mm	911	95.9%	2.10 (±1.73)
Arrow	V-shape	Not stated	Not stated	62	100.0%	1.90 (±1.40)
All				1361	96.3%	

From Ormianer Z, Matalon S, Block J, Kohen J. Dental implant thread design and the consequences on long-term marginal bone loss. *Implant Dent.* 2016;25:471-477.

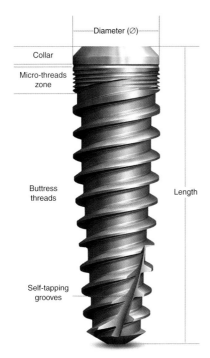

• **Fig. 3.1** Illustration of the macrofeatures of a contemporary dental implant. *(Image courtesy of Glidewell Dental, Newport Beach, California)*

The surface area of the implant that participates in the transmission of occlusal forces to the supporting bone can be characterized as the area beneath the alveolar crest. Of that surface area, the surface area that participates in compressive load dissipation is most beneficial. Compressive load dissipation best serves to dissipate occlusal forces because bone is best able to resist compressive loads.[26] The bone-implant contact area available for occlusal force distribution in compression is therefore the most effective area for force transfer to the supporting bone.

Force transfer is not uniform across crestal and trabecular bone. Crestal bone stresses are highest when crestal bone thickness is less than 2 mm.[36] This distribution of occlusal stresses to the cortical bone dictates that the implant design in the cortical bone region suitably distributes occlusal forces to the surrounding bone without detrimental overload.[37-42]

Below the cortical region of the dental implant, implant geometry has a direct effect on the implant surface area and occlusal load distribution. In this region, trabecular bone is responsible for dissipating the remaining occlusal forces. The implant shape in the trabecular region reflects the need to transmit occlusal forces to the supporting bone in compression to the greatest extent possible. The shape of the implant, along with the implant length and

diameter, all contribute to the area available to transmit forces in a compressive manner to bone in contact with the implant. This is particularly important with poor-quality bone because the area of the bone in direct contact with the implant is compromised by the lower bone density. As bone density decreases, more implant surface area is required to dissipate occlusal forces.[11]

Different implant survival rates and amounts of marginal bone loss may be directly related to different implant shapes. The shape of the implant relates to the surface area involved in the transfer of forces to the supporting bone. Any geometric features that extend outward from the axis of the implant may transfer stresses to the bone under load (Fig. 3.4).

Vandamme et al.[43] installed a repeated sampling bone chamber with a central implant in the tibia of 10 rabbits and performed highly controlled loading experiments with cylindrical and screw-shaped implants. They concluded that well-controlled immediate implant loading accelerates tissue mineralization at the bone-implant interface. Adequate bone stimulation via mechanical coupling may account for the larger bone response around the screw-type implant compared with the cylindrical implant. Implant shape was a contributing factor.

Ormianer and Palti[44] studied long-term performance of tapered screw implants placed in patients with a variety of potentially compromising clinical variables. They found that tapered implants maintained crestal bone levels even in clinically compromised conditions. Concerns that tapered implant designs may be more prone to crestal bone loss than cylinder designs were unsupported by the results of their study.[44]

Atieh et al.[45] reviewed the implant stability of tapered and parallel-walled dental implants. Their analysis showed greater implant stability at insertion and after 8 weeks, but the difference was not statistically significant. Failure rates were not significantly different between the two implant shapes. Marginal bone loss, however, was significantly less for the tapered implants compared with the parallel-walled implants.

Implant Diameter

For a given implant length, increasing the implant diameter will increase the implant surface area that is available for force transfer to the bone. Provided there is sufficient bone volume, a larger diameter implant is better able to resist occlusal forces, particularly in the molar region. Nevertheless, implant diameter alone is not a predictor of better clinical success in all situations. In a 5-year retrospective study of clinical results, Krennmair et al.[46] studied the survival and success rates of 541 CAMLOG tapered implants of 3.8, 4.3, and 5/6 mm placed and restored. The failure rates were 3.7%, 1.4%, and 1.0% for the respective implant diameters. There was no difference in the observed peri-implant marginal bone resorption among the implant diameters.[46]

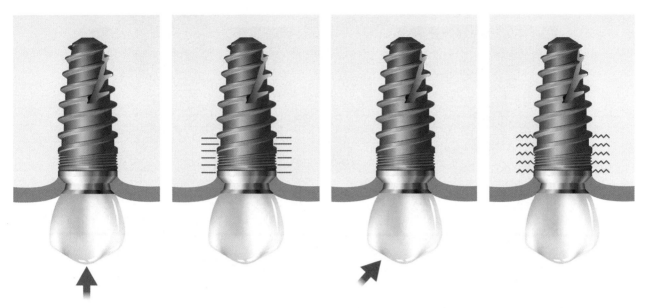

• **Fig. 3.2** Force transfer to supporting bone from axial and nonaxial forces. *(Image courtesy of Glidewell Dental, Newport Beach, California)*

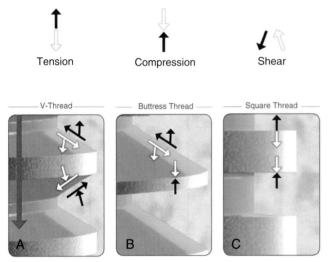

• **Fig. 3.3** Diagrams of Force Transmission by Different Implant Thread Types. (A) V-thread: the direction of forces applied by V-form screw threads. (B) Buttress thread: the direction of forces applied by buttress-form screw threads. (C) Square thread: the direction of forces applied by square-form threads. *(Image courtesy of Glidewell Dental, Newport Beach, California)*

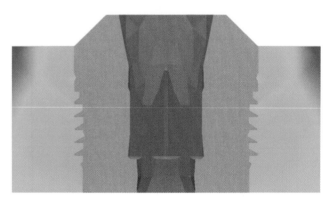

• **Fig. 3.4** Geometric features that extend outward from the axis of the implant transfer stresses to the surrounding bone. *(Image courtesy of Glidewell Dental, Newport Beach, California)*

Javed and Romanos[47] reviewed literature regarding the influence of implant diameter on long-term survival of dental implants placed in the posterior maxilla. Their study examined threaded, rough-surfaced dental implants with diameters ranging between 3.0 and 5.5 mm, and follow-up periods and cumulative survival rates ranging between 5 and 15 years and 80.5% and 100%, respectively. They concluded that "the role of implant diameter on long-term survival of dental implants placed in posterior maxilla is secondary. A well-designed surgical protocol, achievement of sufficient primary stability at the time of implant placement, and pre- and postsurgical oral hygiene maintenance visits are critical factors that influence the long-term survival of dental implants placed in posterior atrophic maxilla."

Olate et al.[48] studied the influence of implant diameter and length on early implant failure. They examined 1649 implants in 650 patients from three different manufacturers. All of the implants were of cylindrical shape and similar surface (acid-etched). The implants were placed in all regions of the mouth. The early survival rate was 96.2% for all implants, with wide implants (2.7%) experiencing lower losses than regular (3.8%) and narrow (5.5%) implants. Short implants (6–9 mm) related to the largest (9.9%) incidence rate of early implant loss.

Wider implants decrease stress at the bone-implant interface. Conversely, smaller-diameter implants show increased stress at this interface. Stress is force divided by the cross-sectional area the force is acting on. For implants of a given length and geometry, wider implants have more surface area to occlusal forces to act on and thus lower stress. This is most pronounced with implants smaller than 4 mm in diameter (Fig. 3.5). Smaller-diameter implants with shorter implants lengths have significantly less surface area to distribute forces to the supporting bone (Fig. 3.6). This unfavorable combination should be avoided to the extent possible, particularly in the posterior region, where bite forces are greater.

Besides decreased stress at the bone-implant interface, wider implants are generally more resistant to fracture from occlusal overload and fatigue conditions. Prosthetics are fastened to the implant by means of an abutment screw, which extends internally

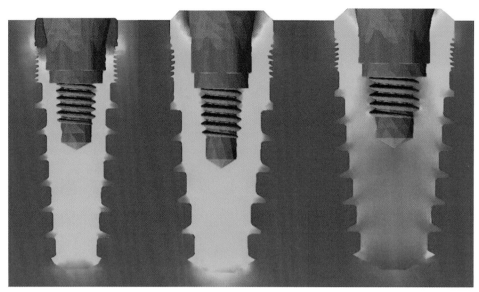

• **Fig. 3.5** Stresses around 10-mm length implants of 3.5-, 4.3-, and 5.0-mm diameters. Note the significant decline in stress as diameter increases to more than 3.5 mm. *(Image courtesy of Glidewell Dental, Newport Beach, California)*

	3.5 x 10 mm	3.5 x 16 mm	5.0 x 10 mm	5.0 x 16 mm
HAHN TAPERED IMPLANT	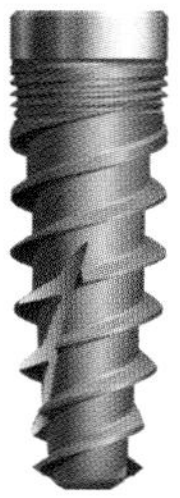	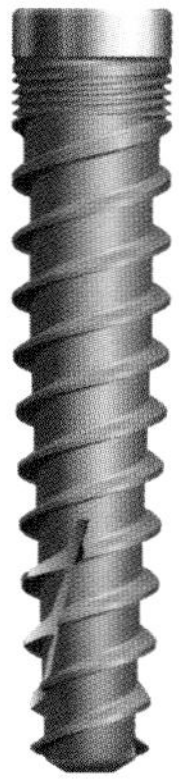	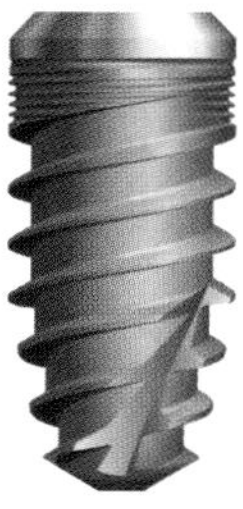	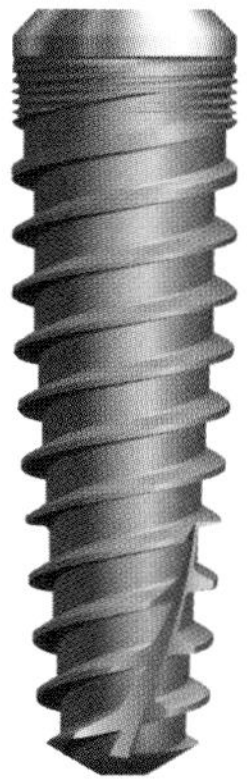
Surface Area	137.84 mm²	208.93 mm²	271.93 mm²	320.89 mm²

• **Fig. 3.6** There is a large variation in surface area among implant lengths and diameters. *(Image courtesy of Glidewell Dental, Newport Beach, California)*

into the implant and engages the internal threads of the implant. The screw receiving bore inside the implant removes material and increases stress on the implant because the cross-sectional area acted on by occlusal forces is reduced. After accounting for the loss of area for the abutment screw bore, wider implants will still have more cross-sectional area (wall thickness) than narrower implants, lower stress, and more fracture resistance (Fig. 3.7).

Most modern implant designs also use the prosthetic connection geometry to insert the implant into the implant site. The insertion tool or fixture transmits stress to the connection geometry, which can deform the connection or lead to fracture of the implant in the connection region (Fig. 3.8). Wider-diameter implants with greater wall thickness are most resistant to implant fractures of this nature.

In a retrospective study of 2670 patients consecutively treated with implant-supported prostheses, Chrcanovic et al.[49] analyzed anatomic, patient, and implant-related factors as explanatory variables to implant fracture. They analyzed 44 fractured implants from a total population of 10,099 and found implant diameter to be a strong explanatory variable related to the probability of implant fracture. For every 1-mm increase in implant diameter, there was a 96.9% decrease in the probability of implant fracture (Table 3.4). Other factors such as direct adjacency to cantilevers and bruxism increased the probability of implant fracture by 247.6% and 1819.5%, respectively. Wider implants offer increased resistance to the stresses encountered in these clinical situations when prosthesis design and parafunctional habits are not optimal.

Implant Length

Implant length is another parameter to consider in implant design. Along with implant diameter, implant length affects the

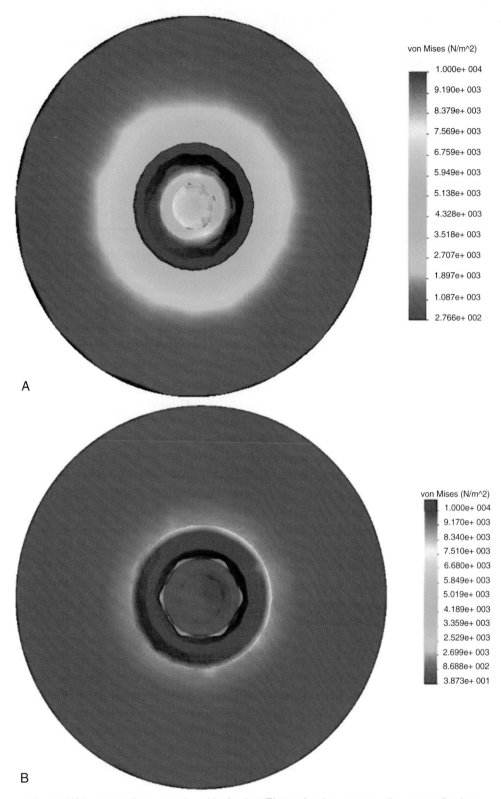

von Mises (N/m^2)

1.000e+ 004
9.190e+ 003
8.379e+ 003
7.569e+ 003
6.759e+ 003
5.949e+ 003
5.138e+ 003
4.328e+ 003
3.518e+ 003
2.707e+ 003
1.897e+ 003
1.087e+ 003
2.766e+ 002

A

von Mises (N/m^2)

1.000e+ 004
9.170e+ 003
8.340e+ 003
7.510e+ 003
6.680e+ 003
5.849e+ 003
5.019e+ 003
4.189e+ 003
3.359e+ 003
2.529e+ 003
2.699e+ 003
8.688e+ 002
3.873e+ 001

B

• **Fig. 3.7** With more surface area, the wider implant (B) transfers less stress to the surrounding bone (shown as blue circular perimeter) than the narrower implant (A). *(Image courtesy of Glidewell Dental, Newport Beach, California)*

stability and the transfer of forces to the surrounding bone. In a study of 2907 implants from placement to 36 months, Winkler et al.[50] studied the implant survival and stability for implants with lengths varying from 7 to 16 mm. Survival rates varied from 66.7% for 7-mm length implants to 96.4% for 16-mm length

implants. Shorter implants had statistically lower survival rates compared with longer implants.

Conversely, a prospective clinical study with 1 to 10 years of follow-up by Mangano et al.[51] of 215 locking taper implants (8 mm) supporting single-tooth crowns in the posterior region

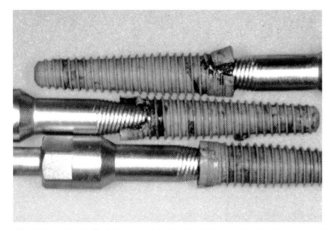

• **Fig. 3.8** Implants that fractured during insertion and had to be removed. *(Image courtesy of Glidewell Dental, Newport Beach, California)*

TABLE 3.4 **Factors Influencing Probability of Implant Fracture**

Factor	Change in Probability of Implant Fracture
Use of stronger grades of titanium	−72.9%
Bruxism	+1819.5%
Directly adjacent to cantilever	+247.6%
1 mm increase in implant length	+22.3%
1 mm increase in implant diameter	−96.9%

From Chrcanovic BR, Kisch J, Albrektsson T, Wennerberg A. Factors influencing the fracture of dental implants. *Clin Implant Dent Relat Res.* 2018;20:58-67. https://doi.org/10.1111/cid.12572

showed an implant survival rate greater than 98%. Marginal bone loss was 0.31 (±0.24), 0.43 (±0.29), and 0.62 (±0.31) mm at the 1-, 5-, and 10-year follow-up session.

Another study by Ding et al.[52] used a finite element mandibular model to evaluate the effects of diameter and length on stress distribution of the alveolar crest around immediate loading of Straumann implants with diameters ranging from 3.3 to 4.8 mm and length ranging from 6 to 14 mm. The implants were loaded vertically and obliquely, and the stresses and strains in the surrounding cortical bone were evaluated. Under both vertical and oblique loading conditions, maximal values were recorded in the 3.3 × 10 mm implant configuration, the second-highest values in the 4.1 × 6 mm implant configuration, and the lowest values in the 4.8 × 10 mm implant configuration. Increasing the diameter and length of the implant decreased the stress and strain on the alveolar crest; however, diameter had a more significant effect than length to relieve the crestal stress and strain concentration. The 10-mm length of the 3.3-mm implant was not sufficient to compensate for the larger diameter of the 4.1-mm implant despite the 4.1-mm implant having 4 mm less length.

Greater implant length is beneficial in decreasing stress and strain in the supporting bone; however, a larger implant diameter is more effective (Fig. 3.9). Implant length alone may be insufficient to compensate for diameter, particularly if bone quality is poor. For example, a 7.0 × 8.0 mm Hahn implant has approximately 20% more surface area than a 5.0 × 10.0 mm implant.

Implant Features

Implant Collar

The implant collar serves as the transition area between the prosthesis and the body of the implant. Its design dictates the placement of the prosthetic interface relative to the bone and gingival tissue surrounding the implant site, as well as stress distribution into the surrounding cortical bone. These characteristics make the implant collar a critical implant feature with important implications for the long-term success of the implant restoration.

Implant collars designed for a supragingival prosthetic connection are characterized by an extended region above the implant threads that protrudes above the gingival tissue (Fig. 3.10). The surface of the collar is typically smoother than the threaded region of the implant body, and the diameter of the collar region is larger than the body of the implant below it. Because the collar is designed to position the prosthetic platform above tissue height, there is little to no need for healing abutments and tissue-forming components.

Collars for bone-level implants have subgingival design considerations. Because of the curvature of the osseous crest, the crestal bone interface for bone level implants can vary at the time of placement (Fig. 3.11). Unless the implant placement is significantly subcrestal, some portion of the implant collar will be supracrestal and in contact with the gingival tissue immediately after surgical placement. In an animal study of tissue reactions to plaque formation after ligature removal of commercially available implants exposed to experimental peri-implantitis, Albouy et al.[54] found that spontaneous progression of experimentally induced peri-implantitis occurred at implants with different geometry and surface characteristics. The progression was most pronounced at implants with an anodized (TiUnite) surface. In another animal study of the progression of peri-implantitis around implants with different surface roughness, Berglund et al.[55] found that the progression of peri-implantitis, if left untreated, is more pronounced at implants with a moderately rough surface than at implants with a polished surface. The upper region of the implant collar may be transosteal after placement, and roughened surfaces in this region can leave the implant more vulnerable to the progression of peri-implantitis. A machined rather than roughened surface at the upper region of the implant collar is more beneficial during the epithelial wound-healing process[56] (Fig. 3.12).

Although animal studies have shown bone formation in the crestal region despite the presence of significant circumferential defects at the time of implantation,[57,58] at the crestal bone level, and below, the implant collar helps to seal the implant site against fibrous tissue encapsulation and bacterial contamination. Initial bone-implant contact is improved with an implant collar at least the same diameter or slightly larger than the body of the implant. Petrie and Williams[59] studied the influence of diameter, length, and taper on strains in the alveolar crest, and found a strong correlation between increased implant diameter leading to reduced stresses in the crestal region. Taper in the implant collar region was found to increase crestal bone stress because it reduced the diameter and surface area in contact with the cortical bone. The distribution of stress at the crestal area is dictated by the surface area of the implant collar (Fig. 3.13).

An implant with a slightly larger collar surface area reduces stress in the crestal region compared with the implant with the smaller collar.

Besides the diameter and surface texture of the implant collar, features in the collar region of the implant that have been

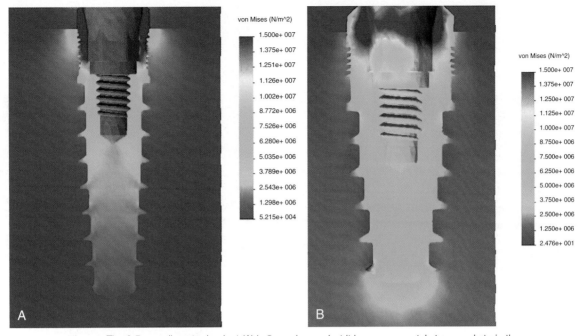

von Mises (N/m^2)

(A)
1.500e+ 007
1.375e+ 007
1.251e+ 007
1.126e+ 007
1.002e+ 007
8.772e+ 006
7.526e+ 006
6.280e+ 006
5.035e+ 006
3.789e+ 006
2.543e+ 006
1.298e+ 006
5.215e+ 004

(B)
1.500e+ 007
1.375e+ 007
1.250e+ 007
1.125e+ 007
1.000e+ 007
8.750e+ 006
7.500e+ 006
6.250e+ 006
5.000e+ 006
3.750e+ 006
2.500e+ 006
1.250e+ 006
2.476e+ 001

• **Fig. 3.9** The 3.5-mm diameter implant (A) is 3 mm longer, but it has more crestal stress and strain than the 4.3-mm implant (B). *(Images courtesy of Glidewell Dental, Newport Beach, California)*

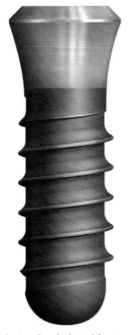

• **Fig. 3.10** Typical implant collar designed for supragingival (tissue level) implant. *(Image courtesy of Glidewell Dental, Newport Beach, California)*

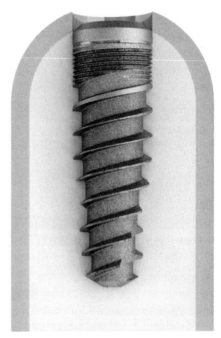

• **Fig. 3.11** Bone-level implant placement varies according to width and curvature of the crestal ridge. *(Image courtesy of Glidewell Dental, Newport Beach, California)*

attributed with preserving crestal bone levels include microthreads and platform switching. These features were created to improve the dissipation of occlusal loads in the crestal bone region and to mitigate complications related to biologic width development during and subsequent to the implant wound healing process.

Microthreads in the implant collar region have been shown to help maintain marginal bone levels.[60,61] In an animal study of implants with and without microthreads in the marginal region connected to fixed partial dentures in the mandibles of beagle dogs, Abrahamsson and Berglundh[62] observed that the degree of bone-implant contact within the marginal portion of the implants was significantly higher at the test (microthread) implants (81.8%) than at the control implants (72.8%). Using axisymmetric finite element analysis, Hansson and Werke[63] analyzed the effect of variations of the size and the profile of the thread of an axially loaded, screw-shaped bone implant on the magnitude of the stress peaks in cortical bone. They found that very small threads of a favorable profile can be quite effective at distributing stress in the cortical bone region and that the shape of the thread profile has a profound effect on the magnitude of the stresses in the bone. Hudieb et al.[64] conducted a finite element analysis of the magnitude and

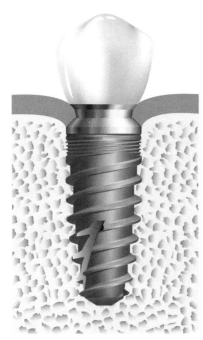

• **Fig. 3.12** Implant collar with machined upper region beneficial for epithelial wound healing. *(Image courtesy of Glidewell Dental, Newport Beach, California)*

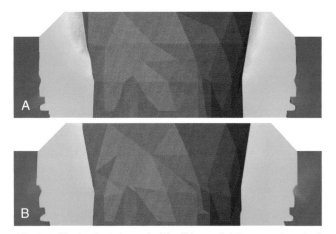

• **Fig. 3.13** The implant shown in (A) will have slightly more stress in the crestal region compared with the same implant with a slightly larger collar and more surface area to dissipate loads (B). *(Image courtesy of Glidewell Dental, Newport Beach, California)*

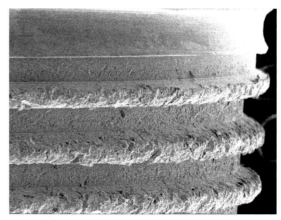

• **Fig. 3.14** Scanning electron microscopy image of microthreads in the implant collar region with a resorbable blast media surface. *(Image courtesy of Glidewell Dental, Newport Beach, California)*

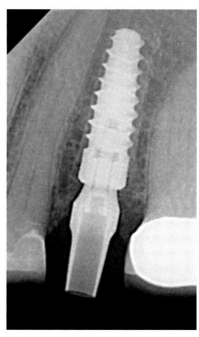

• **Fig. 3.15** Radiograph showing the platform shift between the implant collar outer diameter and the prosthetic connection. *(Image courtesy of Glidewell Dental, Newport Beach, California)*

direction of mechanical stress of a microthreaded implant relative to the same implant design without microthreads. The analysis showed that regardless of the loading angle, principal stresses at the bone-implant interface of the microthread model were always perpendicular to the lower flank of each microthread. Whereas in the implant without microthreads, stresses were affected by the loading angle and directed obliquely to the bone-implant interface, resulting in higher shear stress. The lower shear-stress component of the microthreaded implant in this simulation was an explanatory biomechanical variable for crestal bone preservation in implants with microthreads (Fig. 3.14).

Platform shifting, or the use of abutments with a diameter less than the implant collar, is thought to be beneficial to the preservation of marginal bone levels[65] and to provide a biomechanical advantage in osseointegrated implants by shifting the stress concentration area away from the cervical bone-implant interface with

an inverse relationship between the amount of implant-abutment diameter mismatch and cortical bone stress concentration.[66,67] There has not been a conclusive correlation between platform switching and implant placement relative to the crestal bone level. With delayed loading, differences in crestal and subcrestal placement of platform-switched implants have not been significant after up to 36 months of follow-up for soft tissue parameters and crestal bone levels[68] (Fig. 3.15).

Canullo et al.[69] evaluated the microbiota associated with implants restored with and without platform switching. They found no statistically significant differences between groups for any of the species of peri-implant microbiota. The results of their study suggest that the difference in preservation of marginal bone levels between implants restored with platform switching and traditionally restored implants is not associated with differences in the peri-implant microbiota. Rocha et al.[70] evaluated differences in the clinical performance and crestal bone levels between identical implants restored with single crowns with either platform-matched or platform-switched abutments after 3 years. This study found that platform-switching restorations showed a significant effect in the preservation of marginal bone levels compared with platform-matching restorations. Platform switching has a beneficial effect when it comes to the preservation of marginal bone levels; however, the biological and/or biomechanical processes underlying platform switching are not fully understood at this time.

Implant Prosthetic Connection

There are many different designs for implant-abutment prosthetic connections. They can be characterized as external and internal connection types by the position of the connection geometry relative to the body of the implant. External prosthetic connections, mostly hexagonal, place the connection external to the implant body. Internal implant connections have the connection geometry inside the implant body. Both types of connections have a history of safe and effective use, and are well documented in the clinical literature.[71,72]

The prosthetic connection has multiple functions. It serves as the junction between the implant and the prosthesis, as the feature used to transmit the insertion forces required to place the implant into the osteotomy, and to orient the corresponding mating feature geometry of prosthetic components. In most contemporary implant designs, the prosthesis is fastened to the implant by an abutment screw. Because loads pass from the prosthesis to the implant at the prosthetic connection, the connection design must be strong enough to withstand any clinically relevant forces.[73] Implant diameter and cross section and the abutment screw also have a significant effect on the overall strength of the prosthetic connection[74,75] (Fig. 3.16).

External prosthetic connections were the first prosthetic connections in wide use on screw-type implants. The Brånemark external hex implant, with its 0.7-mm-tall external hex, was designed

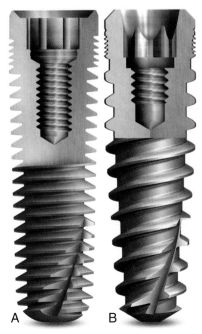

• **Fig. 3.16** (A and B) Implant connections. (*Images courtesy of Glidewell Dental, Newport Beach, California*)

to connect to a fixture mount for placement of the implant and then connect to a transmucosal element of a restoration for an edentulous arch. The external hex connection worked well for this treatment modality; however, it was not ideal when used for single-crown and partially edentulous restorations because the abutment screw was subjected to more lateral loading than in splinted restorations, and increasing the height of the external hex to provide more resistance to lateral loads interfered with angled abutments.[76-78]

Internal prosthetic connection implants were developed to overcome some of the complications arising from the use of external hex implants in partially edentulous cases. The desire for a stronger, more stable implant connection led to the development of the internal connection implants in wide use today. One of the first internal connection designs to be widely adopted was an internal hex connection below a 45-degree lead-in bevel. The internal hex design is still in wide use more than 30 years after it was first developed.[79] The design of the internal hex connection mitigated some of the inherent challenges of the external hex connection, such as angled abutments, and the lead-in bevel stabilized the connection better against tipping forces, reducing the incidence of screw loosening.[80]

Another internal prosthetic connection that is widely used is the conical implant connection. The conical connection is deeper within the implant body, and the angle of the abutment interface is smaller. The conical connection interface area improves abutment stability, fit, and seal performance.[81] Caricasulo et al.[82] reviewed the influence of implant-abutment connection to peri-implant bone loss and found that conical connections exhibited lower peri-implant bone loss in the short to medium term compared with external connections. Quaresma et al.[83] conducted a finite element analysis of an internal hexed connection implant and a conical connection implant. They found that the conical connection implant connected to a solid, internal, conical abutment put lower stresses on the alveolar bone and prosthesis, and greater stresses on the abutment relative to the internal hexed connection implant. Hansson[84] used finite element analysis to study the distribution of stresses in supporting bone for conical connection implants placed at the level of the marginal bone. He found that the peak bone stresses resulting from an axial load arose farther down in the bone, with the conical implant-abutment interface at the level of the marginal bone. Conical prosthetic connections provide a stable abutment connection, lower peak bone stresses when placed at the level of the marginal bone, and a high resistance to axial loads.[85]

Implant Threads

Most dental implants are of the threaded cylinder and tapered threaded cylinder types. Study of threaded implant bodies retrieved from patients shows a greater bone-implant contact from the coronal region of the implant to the first bone-implant contact and a greater percentage of bone-implant contact compared with non-threaded cylinder implants.[86] The threads of the implant increase the surface area available to distribute occlusal forces into the supporting bone, and they transmit more of the forces in compression and less in shear than nonthreaded cylindrical implants. Because the bone is strongest in compression, this lessens the potential for occlusal overload at the bone-implant interface, potentially leading to microfractures and subsequent osteoclastogenesis.[63] The threads of the implant are important for achieving primary stability, particularly in sites with poor bone density, as well as dissipating forces during the healing period and throughout the life of the restoration. The geometric characteristics of the thread influence how stresses are transferred from the implant to the bone. Sufficient initial contact with surrounding bone is important to facilitate primary stability of the implant. Macroenhancements to the surface area of the implant from the thread geometry itself increase potential bone apposition and both the primary and secondary stability of the implant. Implant threads can be described by their thread shape, thread pitch, and thread depth. These thread parameters vary significantly between implants, and there are many possible combinations of these parameters (Fig. 3.17).

Thread Pitch

Thread pitch can be defined as the distance from a point on one thread to a corresponding point on the adjacent thread, measured parallel to the axis. Thread lead is the axial distance that the implant advances in one complete turn. For a single-start thread, thread pitch and thread lead are the same. For multiple-start threads the lead is a multiple of the pitch. For a two-start thread the lead is twice the pitch. A three-start thread has a lead that is three times the pitch (Fig. 3.18). Although the implant advances farther into the bone axially for each revolution on implants with multiple start threads, the surface area is not increased because the pitch remains the same.

Smaller thread pitch increases surface area and is thought to improve stress distribution in the surrounding bone. Orsini et al.[87] tested implants with a 0.5-mm pitch and 1.7-mm pitch for osseointegration after 0 days and 4 and 8 weeks in a sheep iliac crest model. Their findings showed that initial mechanical anchorage and subsequent early endosseous integration in low-density bone could be improved by a reduction of thread pitch. The smaller thread pitch increased bone-implant contact and primary stability from the time of implant placement, and exhibited a higher quantity of newly deposited bone and a more regular and mature geometric distribution of bone tissue at the interface. Their research suggests that, all other factors being equal, a thread pitch less than 1.7 mm is more optimal for primary stability and osseointegration.

However, because of the interaction between thread pitch, thread form, and thread depth, the optimum thread pitch for stress distribution in cortical and cancellous bone may vary. Hassan et al.[88] used three-dimensional (3D) finite element analysis to investigate the influence of the number of threads in the neck of the implant on implant-cortical bone interface stresses. Overall, their analysis showed that stress was highest in the cortical bone at the neck of implant and lowest in the cancellous bone regardless of the number of threads in contact with cortical bone. On the other hand, reducing the number of threads in the neck resulted in a decrease in the developed stresses in both types of bones. The developed stresses around the bone decreased gradually in cortical bones and dramatically in cancellous bones when the number of threads decreased in the neck of the implant.[88]

Kong et al.[89] evaluated the effects of the implant thread pitch on the maximum von Mises stresses in jaw bones and the implant-abutment complex using a finite element method. The thread pitches used in the analysis ranged from 0.5 to 1.6 mm. Their results suggested that under axial load, the maximum equivalent stresses in cortical bone, cancellous bone, and implant-abutment complex decreased by 6.7%, 55.2%, and 22.3%, respectively, with the variation of thread pitch, and 2.7%, 22.4%, and 13.0%, respectively, under buccolingual load. When thread pitch

One-Start Thread

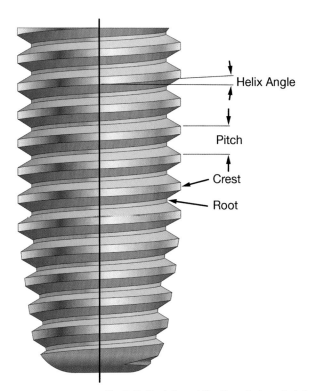

Four-Start Thread

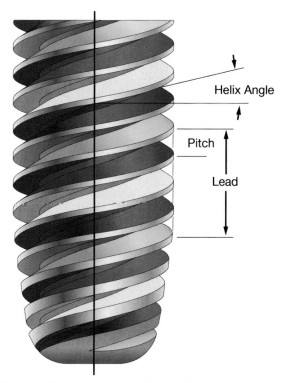

• **Fig. 3.17** Depiction of the thread characteristics of screw-type dental implants, including helix angle, pitch, lead, crest, and root. (*Image courtesy of Glidewell Dental, Newport Beach, California*)

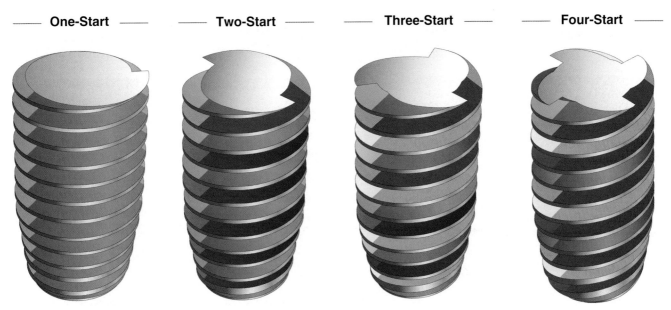

One-Start — **Two-Start** — **Three-Start** — **Four-Start**

• **Fig. 3.18** Depiction of the difference between single-thread and multiple-thread dental implants. (*Image courtesy of Glidewell Dental, Newport Beach, California*)

exceeded 0.8 mm, minimum stresses were obtained. Their data indicated that cancellous bone was more sensitive to thread pitch than cortical bone, thread pitch played a greater role in protecting dental implant under axial load than under buccolingual load, and thread pitch exceeding 0.8 mm was the optimal selection for a threaded implant by biomechanical consideration.[89]

In another finite element analysis conducted for 3D optimization and sensitivity analysis of dental implant thread parameters, Geramizadeh et al.[90] found that a thread pitch of 0.808 mm in the implant body area was optimal for stress distribution. This thread pitch parameter was for a V-shaped thread and agrees closely with the analysis by Kong et al.[89] Optimal thread pitch parameters may vary according to the thread shape. Lan et al.[91] conducted an analysis of alveolar bone stress around implants with different thread designs and pitches in the mandibular molar area. Their analysis showed that an optimal thread pitch was 1.2 mm for a triangular-thread implant, and a trapezoidal-threaded implant with thread pitch of 1.6 mm had the lowest stress value among trapezoidal-threaded implants. Each thread shape had a unique optimal thread pitch concerning lower concentration of bone stress.[91]

Thread pitch also relates to the placement torque and time required to place the implant. Implants with more threads also require more revolutions to place the implant. It will therefore take more time to insert implants with more threads, and placement will require more force in dense bone. Thread pitch is a factor that affects both primary stability and initial healing of the implant site. It is part of the overall implant thread parameters in combination with thread shape and thread depth. Varying the thread pitch affects stress distribution, primary stability, and the quantity and quality of osseointegration.

Thread Shape

Thread shape is another geometric characteristic that has bearing on the distribution of forces into the supporting bone. Thread forms in dental implant designs include square, V-form, buttress, and reverse buttress (Fig. 3.19). These thread shapes are not exclusive to dental implants. They were adapted from existing thread shapes developed for other purposes. V-form threads were developed for general-purpose fastener applications. Square and buttress threads were developed to repeatedly move machine parts against heavy loads.[92] Square and buttress threads have the flank of the thread, which transfers force to the bone, nearly perpendicular to the thread axis, whereas reverse-buttress threads have the nearly perpendicular flank oriented in reverse relative to square and buttress threads. Dental implant applications dictate the need for a thread form optimized for long-term function (load transmission) under occlusal, intrusive (the opposite of pullout) load directions. The buttress or square thread provides an optimized surface area for intrusive, compressive load transmission. Many contemporary implant designs use a buttress thread for compressive load transmission (Hahn Tapered, Inclusive Tapered, Implant Direct), and a few implant designs have incorporated a square thread design (Ankylos, Biohorizons).

As with thread pitch, thread shape does not act in isolation at the bone-implant interface. Other factors such as the implant shape, thread pitch, thread depth, and load type also influence the stress transfer to the bone surrounding the implant.[91] Much of the published literature concerning the direct and indirect effects of thread shape on implant performance takes the form of literature searches and finite element analysis. Eraslan and İnan[93] conducted a 3D finite element analysis on the effect of thread design on stress distribution in a solid screw implant. They analyzed the maximum stress concentrations of V-thread, buttress, reverse buttress, and square thread designs in cortical and cancellous bone regions under a 100-N static load applied to the occlusal surface of the abutment. The results of their analysis showed that stress concentration at cortical bone (18.3 MPa) was higher than cancellous bone (13.3 MPa), and stress concentration at the first thread (18 MPa) was higher than other threads (13.3 MPa). The study showed that the use of different thread form designs did not affect the von Mises stress concentration at the supporting bone structure. However, thread shape did affect compressive stress.

Geng et al.[94] performed a finite element analysis of four thread-form configurations in a stepped screw implant. They analyzed V-thread, thin-thread, and two square-thread forms of different width under oblique loading. Their results indicated that a

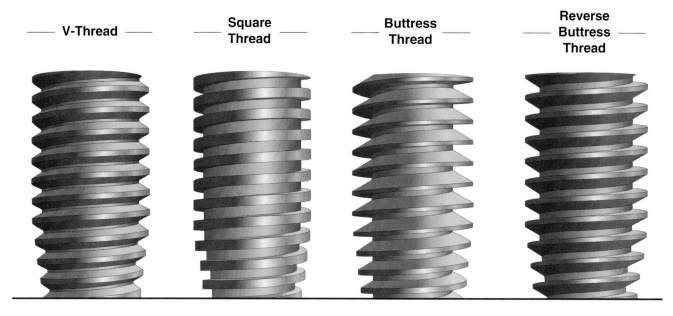

V-Thread	Square Thread	Buttress Thread	Reverse Buttress Thread

For example:
- Brånemark System® (Nobel Biocare)
- Screw-Vent® (Zimmer Dental)
- Certain® (Biomet 3i)

For example:
- External Implant System (BioHorizons)

For example:
- Inclusive® Tapered Implant (Glidewell Dental)
- Straumann® Standard (Straumann USA, LLC)

For example:
- NobelReplace® (Nobel Biocare)

• **Fig. 3.19** Thread shapes of dental implants (V-thread, square, buttress, and reverse buttress). (*Image courtesy of Glidewell Dental, Newport Beach, California*)

V-thread and large square thread were the optimal thread shapes for their experimental stepped screw implant.[94] Force direction affected the stress distribution of the thread shapes evaluated in this study. McAllister et al.[95] conducted a multicenter clinical trial for a 2-year evaluation of a variable-thread tapered implant in extraction sites with immediate temporization. Their results indicated that variable-thread shape tapered implants are a safe and effective immediate postextraction tooth replacement treatment option under immediate load conditions.[95] Arnhart et al.[96] conducted a randomized, controlled, multicenter trial aimed at comparing two versions of a variable-thread dental implant design with a standard tapered dental implant design in cases of immediate functional loading for 36 months after loading. Their results showed stable or improving bone levels for all treatment groups after the initial bone remodeling seen during the first 3 months after placement. The variable-thread implants showed results comparable with those of standard tapered implants with reverse buttress threads in cases of immediate function.[96] Finite element analysis simulations have shown similar stress concentrations in the supporting bone among different thread shapes under occlusal loading and favorable stress distribution for V-shape and square threads under oblique loads. Actual human clinical trials of immediately loaded implants showed very good performance of variable and reverse buttress thread shapes after 3 years in function. Because of their thread flanks transfer forces to the bone nearly perpendicular to the implant axis, buttress and square thread shapes have an optimal implant thread shape under axial load conditions.

Thread Depth

The thread depth is measured as the distance between the root and the crest of the thread. Thread depth directly affects the compressive load-bearing surface of the inferior flank of the implant thread. The deeper the thread, the larger the surface area available

for compressive force transfer to the supporting bone (Fig. 3.20). Implant wall thickness relative to thread depth is a consideration, particularly for smaller-diameter implants, because increasing the distance between the root and crest of the thread comes at the expense of cross-sectional thickness and will affect the strength of the implant body. Increasing thread depth also increases the insertion torque and primary stability in low-density bone because it increases initial bone-implant contact. In denser bone the increased insertion torque of implants with greater thread depth may require the use of a bone tap to fully seat the implant.

In a study of the effect of thread depth on the mechanical properties of dental implants, Lee et al.[97] tested implants with four different thread depths and found that implants with deeper thread depth had higher mean insertion torque values but not lower compressive strength. The thread depth in the implants of this study was increased by increasing the major diameter of the implant body and not by reducing the minor diameter at the root of the threads. This maintained a similar cross section and resultant compressive strength between implants. For the implant with the deepest thread depth (1.1 mm), doubling the density of the bone also nearly doubled the required insertion torque.

In a finite element analysis study of the effects of thread depth and width on an immediately loaded cylinder implant, Ao et al.[98] found that thread depths greater than 0.44 mm and widths between 0.19 and 0.23 mm caused the lowest stresses in moderately dense bone. Thread depth had a greater effect than thread width on bone stress and implant primary stability than thread width. Insertion force was not a component of this study. Table 3.5 shows the relative gain in surface area attributable to increasing the implant major diameter rather than decreasing the thread minor diameter to increase the depth of thread. Either method will increase the thread depth; however, increasing the major diameter of the implant creates more surface area in contact with bone and available to dissipate forces. Decreasing the minor diameter of the

Standard
Hahn™ Tapered Implant
3.5x10 mm

1.2X
Hahn™ Tapered Implant
3.5x10 mm

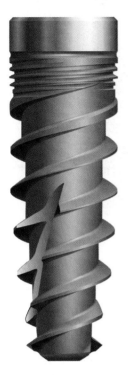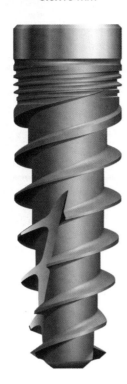

Increased implant thread depth by
1.2X increases functional surface
area from 137.84 mm² to 187.44 mm².

• **Fig. 3.20** Increasing the implant thread depth also increases the functional surface area. The implant on the right has an implant thread depth that increases the functional surface area by a multiple of 1.2 (137.84–182.32 mm²). (*Image courtesy of Glidewell Dental, Newport Beach, California*)

TABLE 3.5	Relative Gain in Implant Surface Area Attributable to Increasing the Implant Major Diameter for Implants of the Same Length		
Implant Diameter	Implant Length	Surface Area	% Increase
3.5 mm	10 mm	137.84 mm²	-
5.0 mm	10 mm	271.93 mm²	97%

implant thread also reduces the wall thickness and strength of the implant, and should be avoided.

Implant Apical Region

The apical region of the implant has features to facilitate insertion into the osteotomy and initiate engagement of the implant threads with the surrounding bone. The tip of the implant is tapered to allow some of the axial length of the implant to enter the implant site before the threads come into contact with the walls of the osteotomy (Fig. 3.21). This makes it easier to keep the implant axis aligned with the axis of the osteotomy and is more comfortable for the patient because it does not require the patient to open his or

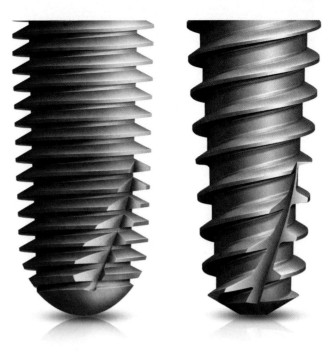

• **Fig. 3.21** Tapered apical ends of implants. (*Image courtesy of Glidewell Dental, Newport Beach, California*)

her mouth as much. The implant taper typically matches the apical portion of the implant drill used to prepare the hole, with the exception of some small-diameter implants that are designed to be placed deeper than the implant site is drilled to improve primary stability. The apical end of conventional implants should be flat to rounded in shape to minimize the probability of perforating sinus membranes during placement. The apical end on small-diameter implants typically tapers to a sharp point to advance into the bone below the implant hole without further site preparation (Fig. 3.22).

The apical region may include a hole or slot feature through the implant body for bone to grow into and increase anchorage against torsional forces, such as healing abutment and healing screw removal and tightening of screws used to fasten the prosthesis to the implant. These features are still found on some implant designs in use today, such as the Zimmer Screw-Vent implant; however, their use has declined in favor of other features that serve the same purpose. More often the apical region of the implant incorporates flat regions or grooves circumferentially arranged on the implant body and originating in the apical region to stabilize the implant against rotation and aid in insertion. During the healing phase, bone will grow against these regions, forming an interlocking matrix that resists rotation. These features also help with the tapping of the implant threads into the wall of the osteotomy. As the threads advance, they create small bone chips that accumulate in these features instead of building up on the bottom of the implant site or being forced into the wall of the osteotomy, resulting in difficulty in seating the implant to depth or increased insertion forces. Incorporating an angled or helical tapping feature in the apical region of the implant further improves the tapping performance because the cutting forces are distributed over a larger region (Figs. 3.23 and 3.24).

Implant Materials

Materials suitable for dental implants and their prosthetic components must meet several specific criteria. The material must be

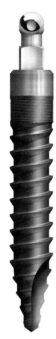

• **Fig. 3.22** Implant apical regions on small-diameter implants. (*Image courtesy of Glidewell Dental, Newport Beach, California*)

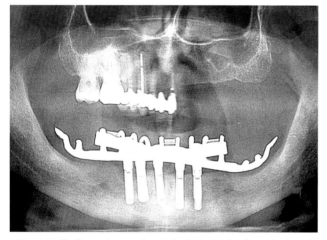

• **Fig. 3.23** Radiograph showing hole features in the apical end of Steri-Oss implants. (*Image courtesy of Glidewell Dental, Newport Beach, California*)

biocompatible and capable of functioning indefinitely without causing damage or degradation of the surrounding bone and tissues. It must also have sufficient tensile and compressive strength to resist forces encountered during function and parafunction over long periods. Further, implant materials require excellent fracture toughness and fatigue resistance to cyclic loading. Finally, materials used in dental implants must have adequate resistance to corrosion and wear, and should have a modulus of elasticity as close as practical to that of the surrounding bone (Fig. 3.25).

Biocompatibility

A number of materials are suitable for dental implants from a biocompatibility standpoint. Currently, commercially pure titanium, titanium alloys, and zirconia (zirconium dioxide, ZrO_2) ceramic implants are the representative biomaterials in wide use for dental

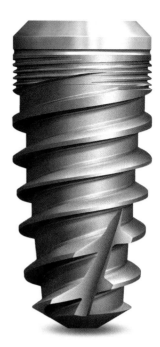

• **Fig. 3.24** Implant with helical self-tapping feature designed to reduce tapping force and collect bone chips. (*Image courtesy of Glidewell Dental, Newport Beach, California*)

implant applications. Commercially pure titanium has the longest history of use for dental implant applications, and its biocompatibility with bone and soft tissues is well established.[100] Titanium alloys, mostly titanium alloyed with varying amounts of aluminum, vanadium, niobium, and zirconium, also exhibit excellent biocompatibility for dental implant applications.[101,102] The most often used titanium alloy is grade 5 titanium, which contains 6% aluminum and 4% vanadium as alloying elements.[103] Although it is not used as frequently as titanium and titanium alloys, zirconia has been proven to be biocompatible in vitro and in vivo; it has interesting microstructural properties; and it is osseoconductive.[104]

Strength

Tensile, compressive, and fatigue strength properties vary between commercially pure titanium, titanium alloy, and zirconia ceramic materials. Titanium and titanium alloy specifications are defined in ASTM International specification B348.[103] The specifications for commercially pure titanium are described by grades 1 through 4, and alloy titanium specifications are described by grades 5 and above. Grade 4 titanium is more than twice as strong as grade 1 titanium, and grade 5 titanium is more than 60% stronger than grade 4 titanium. Grade 23 is a higher-purity form of grade 5 titanium with better fatigue properties. The mechanical properties of titanium grades 1, 4, 5, and 23 are summarized in Table 3.6. Zirconia has much larger compressive strength than titanium; however, it has relatively poor tensile strength, and it is vulnerable to bending loads.[104,105] The ultimate strength of a material determines the amount of load it can withstand before yielding or breaking. Titanium and zirconia implant materials have sufficient ultimate strength to resist clinically relevant loads provided the implant cross section is sufficient. However, more implants fail because of fatigue fractures than from loads that exceed the ultimate strength of the material. Fatigue strength, the maximum cyclical load that the implant and restoration can withstand

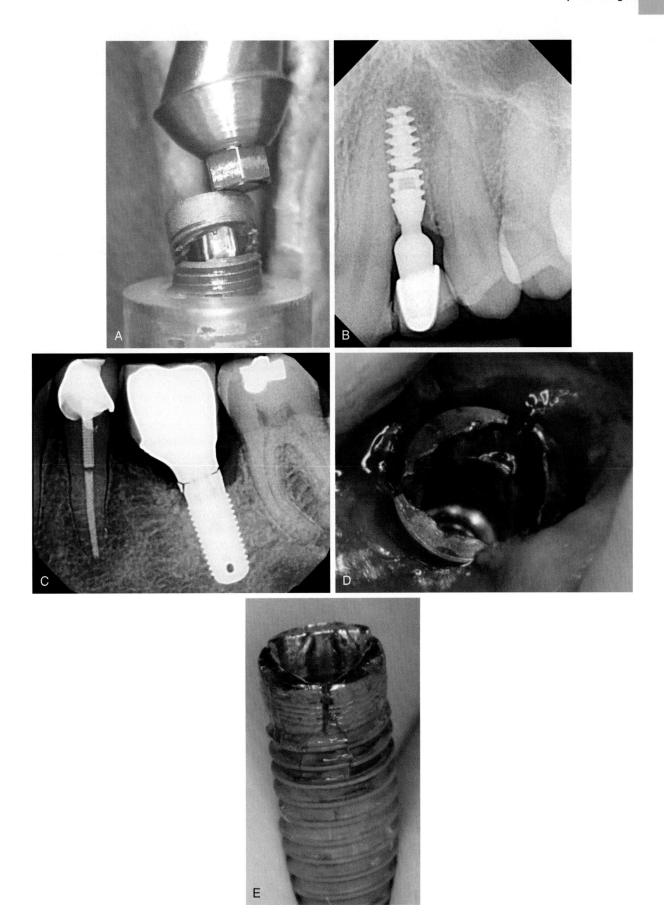

• **Fig. 3.25** (A) Implant fracture caused by fatigue (sustained loading). (B and C) Implant neck fracture. (D and E) Tri-lobe design implant fracture. (*A: Image courtesy of Glidewell Dental, Newport Beach, California*)

TABLE 3.6	The Mechanical Properties of Titanium Grades 1, 4, 5, and 23	
Titanium Grade	Modulus of Elasticity	Tensile Strength, min
Grade 1	100 GPa	240 MPa
Grade 4	105 GPa	550 MPa
Grade 5	109 GPa	895 MPa
Grade 23	114 GPa	828 MPa

Min, minimum. From ASTM International. *ASTM B348-13, Standard Specification for Titanium and Titanium Alloy Bars and Billets.* West Conshohocken, PA: ASTM International; 2013; www.astm.org.

repeatedly without failure or loss of function, is the more relevant property. Fatigue strength relates to material strength; however, it is affected to a large degree by loading conditions such as cantilever length, force direction, among others. It is important to determine the fatigue limit of the implant in combination with its premanufactured prosthetic components to ensure that it will have sufficient strength to function reliably for the patient. Fatigue limits are established by in vitro dynamic testing usually in accordance with the ISO 14801 standard for dynamic loading test for endosseous dental implants.[106]

Corrosion Resistance

Titanium and its alloys have outstanding corrosion resistance under physiologic environmental conditions. They spontaneously form a passive titanium oxide passive film at the surface that resists corrosion very well in the oral environment and immediately reforms if it is damaged or removed by mechanical means.[107] Zirconia ceramic is essentially inert in the oral environment and not susceptible to metallic corrosion. However, zirconia is susceptible to low-temperature degradation. Zirconium dioxide has three crystalline states: monoclinic at room temperature, tetragonal above 1170°C, and cubic above 2100°C.[108] Dental zirconia is stabilized in the tetragonal state by addition of yttrium oxide. The tetragonal crystalline state is responsible for the high strength and fracture toughness of Y-TZP (yttrium oxide stabilized tetragonal zirconium dioxide polycrystals) materials. Contact with water can transform zirconia from the stronger tetragonal phase to the weaker monoclinic phase, resulting in a reduction in strength of the affected area. The degradation-related failure of the Prozyrs femoral heads in 2001 to 2002 is one well-known example.[109] Careful attention to technique is suggested when handling and adjusting zirconia implants and prosthetics.[110]

Modulus of Elasticity

When the modulus of elasticity of the implant and the surrounding bone are not matched, the stress transfer between the implant and the bone is compromised. The mean modulus of elasticity (a measure of stiffness) of dense cortical bone is approximately 16 GPa,[111] compared with the mean modulus of grade 4 commercially pure titanium (105 GPa), grade 5 (Ti-6Al-4V) (109 GPa), and grade 23 (Ti-6Al-4V ELI) (114 GPa). In comparison, zirconia ceramic is very stiff (200 GPa) and may have a higher potential for relative motion or disuse atrophy related to stress shielding at the bone-implant interface. Loading zirconia implants after

osseointegration is complete[112] has been suggested as a mitigating measure to reduce the possibility of crestal bone loss.

At this time, titanium alloys remain the best biomaterial for dental implants. They possess the best combination of biocompatibility, strength, corrosion resistance, and fatigue performance under repetitive loading. They have a long history of safe and effective use that is well documented in the dental literature, and they are suitable for use in all regions of the mouth and all treatment modalities.

Functional Basis for Dental Implant Design

Dental implants transfer forces from the prosthesis to the supporting bone, and the form of dental implants follows this basic function. Dental implant designs have progressed from early subperiosteal, blade type, and press-fit cylinder implants to the straight and tapered threaded implants of today. Their design remains an area of intense activity even now, decades after success rates in the upper 90th percentile are considered the norm. The form and design features of these implants relate to the knowledge base of what was known and believed to be effective and clinically sound at the time. Because force transfer is central to the function of dental implants, their form has evolved to make this ever more efficient and predictable. A functional basis for dental implant design blends current advances in dental technology with proven principles. The form of an implant designed on this basis has features that are briefly described in this section.

For the implant shape a tapered implant body is more advantageous because it is beneficial for implant stability at the time of insertion (primary stability) and marginal bone-level maintenance. As for implant diameter, wider is better, provided the bone volume exists. All other factors (such as length) being equal, wider implants have more surface area to dissipate stress at the bone-implant interface, and they are more resistant to fracture than narrower implants with the same connection geometry due to their increased cross section. Implant length is another parameter where more is generally better when it comes to stress distribution into the supporting bone. However, increasing implant diameter is more effective at decreasing stress and strain in the supporting bone.

The implant collar is important because it dictates the placement of the prosthetic interface relative to the bone and the gingival tissue surrounding the implant, as well as stress distribution into the cortical bone. Because the upper region of the implant collar may be transosteal after placement, and rougher surfaces in this region can leave the implant more vulnerable to peri-implantitis, a machined rather than roughened surface at the upper region of the implant collar is more beneficial during the epithelial wound-healing process. The implant collar should be at least the same diameter or slightly larger than the implant to improve initial bone-implant contact and to help seal the implant site against fibrous tissue encapsulation and bacterial contamination. The collar region should also have microthreads to help distribute stress in the cortical bone region and maintain marginal bone levels. When the cross section of the implant permits, platform shifting should be used in order to shift the stress area away from the bone-implant interface. Current knowledge of prosthetic connections suggests that an internal prosthetic connection provides the best functionality. Of the internal prosthetic connection types in use today, the conical prosthetic connection possesses the best feature set. Conical prosthetic connections provide a stable abutment connection, lower peak bone stresses when placed at the level of the marginal bone, and a high resistance to axial loads.

Implant threads are important for achieving primary stability, particularly in sites with poor bone quality and for dissipating stresses at the bone-implant interface during the healing period and throughout the life of the restoration. Study of the effect of thread pitch on the primary stability, osseointegration, and stress distribution into the surrounding bone suggests that a thread pitch between 0.8 and 1.6 mm is optimal, depending on the thread shape and depth. Buttress and square thread shapes transfer forces to the bone nearly perpendicular to the implant axis and are the optimal thread shapes under axial load conditions. Increasing thread depth also increases the functional surface area available for compressive force transfer into the supporting bone and improves primary stability at the expense of some increase in insertion force. Thread depths greater than 0.4 mm appear to be the most beneficial for reducing stress in moderately dense bone.

The implant apical region should be tapered to facilitate insertion into the osteotomy and initial engagement of the implant threads. The apical end should be rounded or flat to minimize the probability of perforating membranes during placement. It will have flat regions or grooves circumferentially arranged on the implant body to stabilize the implant against rotation after healing and to aid in insertion. Titanium alloys still have the best mechanical and biocompatibility properties for dental implants, and their use is recommended.

Summary

Dental implants provide support for the prosthesis and transfer the occlusal forces to the supporting bone. The design of the dental implant has to take into account primary stability, insertion forces, stress transfer to the surrounding bone, strength, fatigue resistance, and biocompatibility. The dental implants of today address all of these factors in some capacity, and advances in dental technology suggest there are more improvements yet to come.

References

1. Scully C, Hobkirk J, D Dios P. Dental endosseous implants in the medically compromised patient. *J Oral Rehabil.* 2007;34:590–599. https://doi.org/10.1111/j.1365-2842.2007.01755.x.
2. Gaviria L, Salcido JP, Guda T, Ong JL. Current trends in dental implants. *J Korean Assoc Oral Maxillofac Surg.* 2014;40(2):50–60. https://doi.org/10.5125/jkaoms.2014.40.2.50.
3. Chrcanovic BR, Albrektsson T, Wennerberg A. Reasons for failures of oral implants. *J Oral Rehabil.* 2014;41:443–476. https://doi.org/10.1111/joor.12157.
4. Lobbezoo F, Brouwers JE, Cune M, Naeije M. Dental implants in patients with bruxing habits. *J Oral Rehabil.* 2006;33:152–159. https://doi.org/10.1111/j.1365-2842.2006.01542.x.
5. Raghoebar GM, Meijer HJ, Slot W, Slater JJ, Vissink A. A systematic review of implant-supported overdentures in the edentulous maxilla, compared to the mandible: how many implants? *Eur J Oral Implantol.* 2014;7(suppl 2):S191–S201. Review.
6. Bazrafshan N, Darby I. Retrospective success and survival rates of dental implants placed with simultaneous bone augmentation in partially edentulous patients. *Clin Oral Impl Res.* 2014;25:768–773. https://doi.org/10.1111/clr.12185.
7. Rammelsberg P, Schmitter M, Gabbert O, Bermejo JL, Eiffler C, Schwarz S. Influence of bone augmentation procedures on the short–term prognosis of simultaneously placed implants. *Clin Oral Impl Res.* 2011;23(10):1232-1237. https://doi.org/10.1111/j.1600-0501.2011.02295.x
8. Shayesteh YS, Khojasteh A, Siadat H, et al. A Comparative study of crestal bone loss and implant stability between osteotome and conventional implant insertion techniques: a randomized controlled clinical trial study. *Clin Implant Dent Relat Res.* 2013;15:350–357. https://doi.org/10.1111/j.1708-8208.2011.00376.x.
9. Cooper LF. Prosthodontic complications related to non-optimal dental implant placement. In: *Dental Implant Complications.* S. J. Froum; 2015. https://doi.org/10.1002/9781119140474.ch24.
10. Duyck J, Oosterwyck H, Sloten J, Cooman M, Puers R, Naert I. Magnitude and distribution of occlusal forces on oral implants supporting fixed prostheses: an *in vivo* study. *Clin Oral Impl Res.* 2000;11:465–475. https://doi.org/10.1034/j.1600-0501.2000.011005465.x.
11. Tada S, Stegaroiu R, Kitamura E, Miyakawa O, Kusakari H. Influence of implant design and bone quality on stress/strain distribution in bone around implants: a 3-dimensional finite element analysis. *Int J Oral Maxillofac Implants.* 2003;18:357–368.
12. Dal Carlo L, Pasqualini ME, Carinci F, et al. A brief history and guidelines of blade implant technique: a retrospective study on 522 implants. *Annals Oral Maxillofacial Surg.* 2013;1(1):3.
13. Albrektsson T, Zarb G, Worthington P, Eriksson AR. The long-term efficacy of currently used dental implants: a review and proposed criteria of success. *Inter J Oral Maxillofacial Implants.* 1986;1:11–25.
14. Golec TS, Krauser JT. Long-term retrospective studies on hydroxyapatite coated endosteal and subperiosteal implants. *Dent Clin North Am.* 1992;36:39–65.
15. McGlumphy EA, Peterson LJ, Larsen PE, et al. Prospective study of 429 hydroxyapatite-coated cylindric omniloc implants placed in 121 patients. *Int J Oral Maxillofac Implants.* 2003;18:82–92.
16. Fransson C, Lekholm U, Jemt T, Berglundh T. Prevalence of subjects with progressive bone loss at implants. *Clin Oral Impl Res.* 2005;16:440–446. https://doi.org/10.1111/j.1600-0501.2005.01137.x.
17. Turkyilmaz I, McGlumphy EA. Influence of bone density on implant stability parameters and implant success: a retrospective clinical study. *BMC Oral Health.* 2008;8:32. https://doi.org/10.1186/1472-6831-8-32.
18. Winkler S, Morris HF, Ochi S. Implant survival to 36 months as related to length and diameter. *Annals Periodontol.* 2000;5:22–31. https://doi.org/10.1902/annals.2000.5.1.22.
19. Malmqvist JP, Sennerby L. Clinical report on the success of 47 consecutively placed Core-Vent implants followed from 3 months to 4 years. *Int J Oral Maxillofac Implants.* 1990;5:53.
20. Albrektsson T, Gottlow J, Meirelles L, Östman P, Rocci A, Sennerby L. Survival of nobeldirect implants: an analysis of 550 consecutively placed implants at 18 different clinical centers. *Clin Implant Dent Relat Res.* 2007;9:65–70. https://doi.org/10.1111/j.1708-8208.2007.00054.x.
21. Ormianer Z, Matalon S, Block J, Kohen J. Dental implant thread design and the consequences on long-term marginal bone loss. *Implant Dent.* 2016;25:471–477.
22. Almeida EO, Freitas AC, Bonfante EA, Marotta L, Silva NR, Coelho PG. Mechanical testing of implant-supported anterior crowns with different implant/abutment connections. *Inter J Oral Maxillofacial Impl.* 2013;28(1):103–108.
23. Mangano C, Iaculli F, Piattelli A, Mangano F. Fixed restorations supported by Morse-taper connection implants: a retrospective clinical study with 10–20 years of follow-up. *Clin Oral Impl Res.* 2015;26:1229–1236. https://doi.org/10.1111/clr.12439.
24. Kim Y, Oh TJ, Misch CE, Wang HL. Occlusal considerations in implant therapy: clinical guidelines with biomechanical rationale. *Clin Oral Implants Res.* 2005;16(1):26–35.
25. Lindquist LW, Rockler B, Carlsson GE. Bone resorption around fixtures in edentulous patients treated with mandibular fixed tissue-integrated prostheses. *J Prosthet Dent.* 1988;59(1):59–63.
26. Misch CE, Qu Z, Bidez MW. Mechanical properties of trabecular bone in the human mandible: implications for dental implant treatment planning and surgical placement. *J Oral Maxillofac Surg.* 1999;57:700–706.
27. Lemons J. Biomaterials in implant dentistry. In: Misch CE, ed. *Contemporary Implant Dentistry.* St Louis: Mosby; 1993.

28. Waltimo A, Könönen M. A novel bite force recorder and maximal isometric bite force values for healthy young adults. *European J Oral Sci*. 1993;101:171–175. https://doi.org/10.1111/j.1600-0722.1993.tb01658.x.

29. Gibbs CH, Mahan PE, Mauderli A, Lundeen HC, Walsh EK. Limits of human bite strength. *J Prosthetic Dent*. 1986;56(2):226–229.

30. Duyck J, Oosterwyck H, Sloten J, Cooman M, Puers R, Naert I. Magnitude and distribution of occlusal forces on oral implants supporting fixed prostheses: an in vivo study. *Clin Oral Implant Res*. 2000;11:465–475. https://doi.org/10.1034/j.1600-0501.2000.011005465.x.

31. Canay S, Hersek N, Akpinar I, Aşik Z. Comparison of stress distribution around vertical and angled implants with finite-element analysis. *Quintessence Int*. 1996;27(9):591–598.

32. O'Mahony AM, Williams JL, Spencer P. Anisotropic elasticity of cortical and cancellous bone in the posterior mandible increases peri-implant stress and strain under oblique loading. *Clin Oral Implants Res*. 2001;12:648–657. https://doi.org/10.1034/j.1600-0501.2001.120614.x.

33. Sheppard IM, Markus N. Total time of tooth contacts during mastication. *J Prosthetic Dent*. 12(3):460–463.

34. Graf H. Bruxism. *Dent Clin North Am*. 1969;13:659–665.

35. Zhou Y, Gao J, Luo L, Wang Y. Does bruxism contribute to dental implant failure? *Clin Impl Dent Related Res*. 2016;18:410–420. https://doi.org/10.1111/cid.12300.

36. Chen Q, Chen X, Shan Y, Ding X, Huiming W. Influence of thickness of cancellous bone and cortical bone in stress distribution in vicinity of an implant. *J Jilin University (Medicine ed)*. 2016;42(2):204–209.

37. Negri B, Calvo Guirado JL, Maté Sánchez de Val JE, et al. Peri-implant tissue reactions to immediate nonocclusal loaded implants with different collar design: an experimental study in dogs. *Clin. Oral Impl. Res*. 2014;25:e54–e63.

38. Abrahamsson I, Berglundh T. Tissue characteristics at microthreaded implants: an experimental study in dogs. *Clin Impl Dent Relat Res*. 2006;8:107–113.

39. Ormianer Z, Palti A. Retrospective clinical evaluation of tapered screw-vent implants: results after up to eight years of clinical function. *J Oral Implantol*. 2008; (3):150–160. https://doi.org/10.1563/1548-1336(2008)34[150:RCEOTS]2.0.CO;2.

40. Talwar BS. A Focus on soft tissue in dental implantology. *J Indian Prosthodont Soc*. 2012;12(3):137–142. https://doi.org/10.1007/s13191-012-0133-x.

41. Goswami M. Comparison of crestal bone loss among two implant crest module designs. *Med J Armed Forces India*. 2009;65:319–322.

42. Hansson S, Werke M. The implant thread as a retention element in cortical bone: the effect of thread size and thread profile: a finite element study. *J Biomechanics*. 36(9):1247–1258.

43. Vandamme K, Naert I, Geris L, Sloten JV, Puers R, Duyck J. Influence of controlled immediate loading and implant design on peri-implant bone formation. *J Clin Periodontol*. 2007;34:172–181. https://doi.org/10.1111/j.1600-051X.2006.01014.x.

44. Ormianer Z Palti A. Long-term clinical evaluation of tapered multi-threaded implants: results and influences of potential risk factors. *J Oral Implantol*. 2006;32(6):300–307.

45. Atieh MA, Alsabeeha N, Duncan WJ. Stability of tapered and parallel-walled dental implants: a systematic review and meta-analysis. *Clin Implant Dent Relat Res*. 2018;20:634–645. https://doi.org/10.1111/cid.12623.

46. Krennmair G, Seemann R, Schmidinger S, Ewers R, Piehslinger E. Clinical outcome of root-shaped dental implants of various diameters: 5-year results. *Int J Oral Maxillofac Implants*. 2010;25(2):357–366. 20369096.

47. Javed F, Romanos GE. Role of implant diameter on long-term survival of dental implants placed in posterior maxilla: a systematic review. *Clin Oral Invest*. 2015;19(1):1–10. https://doi.org/10.1007/s00784-014-1333-z.

48. Olate S, Lyrio MC, de Moraes M, Mazzonetto R. Moreira RW. Influence of diameter and length of implant on early dental implant failure. *J Oral Maxillofacial Surg*. 2010;68(2):414–419. https://doi.org/10.1016/j.joms.2009.10.002.

49. Chrcanovic BR, Kisch J, Albrektsson T, Wennerberg A. Factors influencing the fracture of dental implants. *Clin Implant Dent Relat Res*. 2018;20:58–67. https://doi.org/10.1111/cid.12572.

50. Winkler S, Morris HF, Ochi S. Implant survival to 36 months as related to length and diameter. *Annals Periodontol*. 2000;5:22–31. https://doi.org/10.1902/annals.2000.5.1.22.

51. Mangano FG, Shibli JA, Sammons RL, Iaculli F, Piattelli A, Mangano C. Short (8-mm) locking-taper implants supporting single crowns in posterior region: a prospective clinical study with 1-to 10-years of follow-up. *Clin Oral Impl Res*. 2014;25:933–940. https://doi.org/10.1111/clr.12181.

52. Ding X, Liao S, Zhu X, Zhang X, Zhang L. Effect of diameter and length on stress distribution of the alveolar crest around immediate loading implants. *Clin Implant Dent Relat Res*. 2009;11:279–287. https://doi.org/10.1111/j.1708-8208.2008.00124.x.

53. Deleted in review.

54. Albouy J, Abrahamsson I, Persson LG, Berglundh T. Spontaneous progression of peri-implantitis at different types of implants. An experimental study in dogs. I: clinical and radiographic observations. *Clin Oral Impl Res*. 2008;19:997–1002. https://doi.org/10.1111/j.1600-0501.2008.01589.x.

55. Berglundh T, Gotfredsen K, Zitzmann NU, Lang NP, Lindhe J. Spontaneous progression of ligature induced peri-implantitis at implants with different surface roughness: an experimental study in dogs. *Clin Oral Impl Res*. 2007;18:655–661. https://doi.org/10.1111/j.1600-0501.2007.01397.x.

56. Atsuta I, Ayukawa Y, Furuhashi A, et al. Epithelial sealing around rough surface implants. *Clin Implant Dent Relat Res*. 2014;16:772–781. https://doi.org/10.1111/cid.12043.

57. Yoon H, Choi J, Jung U, et al. Effects of different depths of gap on healing of surgically created coronal defects around implants in dogs: a pilot study. *Journal of Periodontol*. 2008;79:355–361. https://doi.org/10.1902/jop.2008.070306.

58. Jung U, Kim C, Choi S, Cho K, Inoue T, Kim C. Healing of surgically created circumferential gap around non-submerged-type implants in dogs: a histomorphometric study. *Clin Oral Impl Res*. 2007;18:171–178. https://doi.org/10.1111/j.1600-0501.2006.01310.x.

59. Petrie CS, Williams JL. Comparative evaluation of implant designs: influence of diameter, length, and taper on strains in the alveolar crest. *Clin Oral Impl Res*. 2005;16:486–494. https://doi.org/10.1111/j.1600-0501.2005.01132.x.

60. Lee D, Choi Y, Park K, Kim C, Moon I. Effect of microthread on the maintenance of marginal bone level: a 3-year prospective study. *Clin Oral Impl Res*. 2007;18:465–470. https://doi.org/10.1111/j.1600-0501.2007.01302.x.

61. Calvo–Guirado JL, Gómez–Moreno G, Aguilar–Salvatierra A, Guardia J, Delgado–Ruiz RA, Romanos GE. Marginal bone loss evaluation around immediate non–occlusal microthreaded implants placed in fresh extraction sockets in the maxilla: a 3–year study. *Clin Oral Impl Res*. 2015;26:761–767. https://doi.org/10.1111/clr.12336.

62. Abrahamsson I, Berglundh T. Tissue characteristics at microthreaded implants: an experimental study in dogs. *Clin Implant Dent Relat Res*. 2006;8:107–113. https://doi.org/10.1111/j.1708-8208.2006.00016.x.

63. Hansson S, Werke M. The implant thread as a retention element in cortical bone: the effect of thread size and thread profile: a finite element study. *J Biomech*. 2003;36(9):1247–1258. https://doi.org/10.1016/s0021-9290(03)00164-7.

64. Hudieb MI, Wakabayashi N, Kasugai S. Magnitude and direction of mechanical stress at the osseointegrated interface of the microthread implant. *J Periodontol*. 2011;82(7):1061–1070. https://doi.org/10.1902/jop.2010.100237.

65. Atieh MA, Ibrahim HM, Atieh AH. Platform switching for marginal bone preservation around dental implants: a systematic review

and meta-analysis. *J Periodontol.* 2010;81:1350–1366. https://doi .org/10.1902/jop.2010.100232.

66. Maeda Y, Miura J, Taki I, Sogo M. Biomechanical analysis on platform switching: is there any biomechanical rationale? *Clin Oral Implant Res.* 2007;18:581–584. https://doi.org/10.1111/ j.1600-0501.2007.01398.x.

67. Pessoa RS, Bezerra FJ, Sousa RM, Vander Sloten J, Casati MZ, Jaecques SV. Biomechanical evaluation of platform switching: different mismatch sizes, connection types, and implant protocols. *J Periodontol.* 2014;85:1161–1171. https://doi.org/10.1902/ jop.2014.130633.

68. Al Amri MD, Al-Johany SS, Al Baker AM, Al Rifaiy MQ, Abduljabbar TS, Al-Kheraif AA. Soft tissue changes and crestal bone loss around platform-switched implants placed at crestal and subcrestal levels: 36-month results from a prospective split-mouth clinical trial. *Clin Oral Impl Res.* 2017;28:1342–1347.

69. Canullo L, Quaranta A, Teles RP. The microbiota associated with implants restored with platform switching: a preliminary report. *J Periodontol.* 2010;81:403–411. https://doi.org/10.1902/ jop.2009.090498.

70. Rocha S, Wagner W, Wiltfang J, et al. Effect of platform switching on crestal bone levels around implants in the posterior mandible: 3 years results from a multicentre randomized clinical trial. *J Clin Periodontol.* 2016;43:374–382. https://doi.org/10.1111/ jcpe.12522.

71. Buser D, Mericske-stern R, Pierre Bernard JP, et al. Long-term evaluation of non-submerged ITI implants. Part 1: 8–year life table analysis of a prospective multi-center study with 2359 implants. *Clin Oral Implants Res.* 1997;8:161–172. https://doi .org/10.1034/j.1600-0501.1997.080302.x.

72. Dierens M, Vandeweghe S, Kisch J, Nilner K, De Bruyn H. Long-term follow-up of turned single implants placed in periodontally healthy patients after 16–22 years: radiographic and peri-implant outcome. *Clin Oral Implants Res.* 2012;23:197–204. https://doi .org/10.1111/j.1600-0501.2011.02212.x.

73. Dittmer S, Dittmer MP, Kohorst P, Jendras M, Borchers L, Stiesch M. Effect of implant-abutment connection design on load bearing capacity and failure mode of implants. *J Prosthodontics.* 2011;20:510–516. https://doi.org/10.1111/j.1532-849X.2011. 00758.x.

74. Hansson S. Implant-abutment interface: biomechanical study of flat top versus conical. *Clin Implant Dent Relat Res.* 2000;2:33–41. https://doi.org/10.1111/j.1708-8208.2000.tb00104.x.

75. Bordin D, Witek L, Fardin VP, Bonfante EA, Coelho PG. Fatigue failure of narrow implants with different implant-abutment connection designs. *J Prosthodontics.* 2018;27:659–664. https://doi .org/10.1111/jopr.12540.

76. Binon P. The effect of implant/abutment hexagonal misfit on screw joint stability. *Int J Prosthodontics.* 1996;9:149–160.

77. Binon P, Sutter F, Beaty K, Brunski J, Gulbransen H, Weiner R. The role of screws in implant systems. *Int J Oral Maxillofac Implants.* 1994;9:48–63.

78. Jorneus L, Jemt T, Carlsson L. Loads and designs of screw joints for single crowns supported by osseointegrated implants. *Int J Oral Maxillofac Implants.* 1992;7:353–359.

79. Niznick G. The implant abutment connection: the key to prosthetic success. *Compendium.* 1991;12(12):932–938.

80. Khraisat A, Abu-Hammad O, Dar-Odeh N, Al-Kayed AM. Abutment screw loosening and bending resistance of external hexagon implant system after lateral cyclic loading. *Clin Implant Dent Relat Res.* 2004;6:157–164. https://doi.org/10.1111/j.1708-8208.2004 .tb00216.x.

81. Schmitt CM, Nogueira-Filho G, Tenenbaum HC, et al. Performance of conical abutment (Morse Taper) connection implants: a systematic review. *J Biomed Mater Res Part A.* 2014;102A:552–574.

82. Caricasulo R, Malchiodi L, Ghensi P, Fantozzi G, Cucchi A. The influence of implant–abutment connection to peri-implant bone loss: a systematic review and meta-analysis. *Clin Implant Dent Relat Res.* 2018;20:653–664. https://doi.org/10.1111/cid.12620.

83. Quaresma SE, Cury PR, Sendyk WR, Sendyk C. A finite element analysis of two different dental implants: stress distribution in the prosthesis, abutment, implant, and supporting bone. *J Oral Implant.* 2008;34:1–6.

84. Hansson S. A conical implant-abutment interface at the level of the marginal bone improves the distribution of stresses in the supporting bone. An axisym-metric finite element analysis. *Clin Oral Implants Res.* 2003;14(3):286–293.

85. Hansson S. Implant–abutment interface: biomechanical study of flat top versus conical. *Clin Implant Dent Relat Res.* 2000;2:33–41. https://doi.org/10.1111/j.1708-8208.2000.tb00104.x.

86. Bolind PK, Johansson CB, Becker W, Langer L, Sevetz EB, Albrektsson TO. A descriptive study on retrieved non-threaded and threaded implant designs. *Clin Oral Implants Res.* 2005;16:447–455. https://doi.org/10.1111/j.1600-0501.2005.01129.x.

87. Orsini E, Giavaresi G, Trirè A, Ottani V, Salgarello S. Dental implant thread pitch and its influence on the osseointegration process: an in vivo comparison study. *Int J Oral Maxillofacial Implants.* 2012;27(2):383–392.

88. Hassan M, El-Wakad M, Bakr EM. Effect of the number of dental implant neck threads in contact with the cortical bone on interface stresses using finite element method. *Proceedings of the ASME 2013 International Mechanical Engineering Congress and Exposition. Volume 3A: Biomedical and Biotechnology Engineering.* San Diego, California. 2013. V03AT03A061. https://doi.org/10.1115/IMECE2013-63822.

89. Kong L, Zhao Y, Hu K, et al. Selection of the implant thread pitch for optimal biomechanical properties: a three-dimensional finite element analysis. *Adv Eng Software.* 2009;40:474–478. https://doi .org/10.1016/j.advengsoft.2008.08.003.

90. Geramizadeh M, Katoozian H, Amid R, Kadkhodazadeh M. Three-dimensional optimization and sensitivity analysis of dental implant thread parameters using finite element analysis. *J Korean Assoc Oral Maxillofac Surg.* 2018;44(2):59–65. https://doi.org/10.5125/jka-oms.2018.44.2.59.

91. Lan TH, Du JK, Pan CY, et al. Biomechanical analysis of alveolar bone stress around implants with different thread designs and pitches in the mandibular molar area. *Clin Oral Invest.* 2012;16:363. https://doi.org/10.1007/s00784-011-0517-z.

92. Oberg E, Jones F, Horton H, Ryffel H, Green R, McCauley C. *Machinery's Handbook.* 25th ed. New York: Industrial Press, Inc; 1996.

93. Eraslan O, İnan Ö. The effect of thread design on stress distribution in a solid screw implant: a 3D finite element analysis. *Clin Oral Investig.* 2009;14:411–416.

94. Geng JP, Ma QS, Xu W, Tan KB, Liu GR. Finite element analysis of four thread-form configurations in a stepped screw implant. *J Oral Rehabil.* 2004;31:233–239.

95. McAllister BS, Cherry JE, Kolinski ML, Parrish KD, Pumphrey DW, Schroering RL. Two-year evaluation of a variable-thread tapered implant in extraction sites with immediate temporization: a multicenter clinical trial. *Int J Oral Maxillofac Implants.* 2012;27:611–618.

96. Arnhart C, Kielbassa AM, Martinez-de Fuentes R, et al. Comparison of variable-thread tapered implant designs to a standard tapered implant design after immediate loading. A 3-year multicentre randomised controlled trial. *Eur J Oral Implantol.* 2012;5:123–136.

97. Lee SY, Kim SJ, An HW, et al. The effect of the thread depth on the mechanical properties of the dental implant. *J Advanced Prosthodontics.* 2015;7(2):115–121. http://doi.org/10.4047/jap.2015.7.2.115.

98. Ao J, Li T, Liu Y, et al. Optimal design of thread height and width on an immediately loaded cylinder implant: a finite element analysis. *Comput Biol Med.* 2010;40:681–686.

99. Deleted in review.

100. Albrektsson T, Brånemark PI, Hansson HA. J. Lindström. Osseointegrated titanium implants:requirements for ensuring a long-lasting, direct bone-to-implant anchorage in man. *Acta Orthop Scand.* 1981;52(2):155–170. https://doi.org/10.3109/17453678108991776.

101. Williams DF. *Biocompatibility of Clinical Implant Materials.* Vol. 1. Boca Raton, FL: CRC Press; 1981.

102. Luckey HA, Kubli Jr F. *Titanium Alloys in Surgical Implants*. Philadelphia: ASTM STP 796; 1983.

103. *ASTM B348-13, Standard Specification for Titanium and Titanium Alloy Bars and Billets*. West Conshohocken, PA: ASTM International; 2013. www.astm.org.

104. Hisbergues M, Vendeville S, Vendeville P. Zirconia: established facts and perspectives for a biomaterial in dental implantology. *J Biomed Mater Res*. 2009;88B:519–529. https://doi.org/10.1002/jbm.b.31147.

105. Osman RB, Swain MV. A critical review of dental implant materials with an emphasis on titanium *versus* zirconia. *Materials*. 2015;8(3):932–958. http://doi.org/10.3390/ma8030932.

106. ISO 14801. *Fatigue Test for Endosseous Dental Implants*; 2003.

107. Brunette DM, Tengvall P, Textor M, Thomsen P, eds. *Titanium in Medicine: Material Science, Surface Science, Engineering, Biological Responses and Medical Applications*. Springer Science & Business Media; 2012.

108. Lughi V, Sergo V. Low temperature degradation -aging- of zirconia: a critical review of the relevant aspects in dentistry. *Dent Mater*. 2010;26:807–820.

109. Chevalier J. What future for zirconia as a biomaterial? *Biomaterials*. 2006;27:535–543.

110. Manicone PF, Iommetti PR, Raffaelli L. An overview of zirconia ceramics: basic properties and clinical applications. *J Dent*. 2007;35(11):819–826.

111. Choi K, Kuhn JL, Ciarelli MJ, Goldstein SA. The elastic moduli of human subchondral, trabecular, and cortical bone tissue and the size-dependency of cortical bone modulus. *J Biomechanics*. 1990;23(11):1103–1113.

112. Akagawa Y, Ichikawa Y, Nikai H, Tsuru H. Interface histology of unloaded and early loaded partially stabilized zirconia endosseous implant in initial bone healing. *J Prosthetic Dent*. 1993;69(6):599–604.

4

Bone Physiology, Metabolism, and Biomechanics

W. EUGENE ROBERTS

Consistent success with implant-supported prostheses requires a thorough knowledge of the physiology, metabolism, and biomechanics of bone as a tissue, and bones as musculoskeletal organs. Bone is a vital mineralized tissue, and bones are unique morphologic organs composed of calcified and soft tissues that provide structural and metabolic support for a wide variety of interactive functions (Fig. 4.1).

Understanding the clinical manipulation of bone begins with an appreciation of the fundamental genetic and environmental mechanisms of osseous development and adaptation. The genome codes for growth factors, ischemic agents, vascular induction/invasion mechanisms, and mechanically induced inflammation. These biological mechanisms interact with the physical factors of diffusion limitation and mechanical loading to produce bone morphology (Fig. 4.2). Fundamental principles control the quality and quantity of bone that directly and indirectly supports stomatognathic function. A firm grasp of the modern concepts of bone physiology, metabolism, and biomechanics is an essential prerequisite for innovative clinical practice. These principles are an objective basis for designing a realistic treatment plan that has a high probability of meeting the esthetic and functional expectations of the patient.

Bone is a dynamic structure that is adapting constantly to its environment. Because the skeleton is the principal reservoir of calcium, bone remodeling (physiologic turnover) performs a critical life support role in mineral metabolism (Fig. 4.3). Collectively, bones are essential elements for locomotion, antigravity support, and life-sustaining functions such as mastication. Mechanical adaptation of bone is the physiologic basis of stomatognathic reconstruction with implant-supported prostheses. A detailed knowledge of the dynamic nature of bone physiology and biomechanics is essential to enlightened clinical practice.

Osteology

In defining the physiologic basis of orthodontics, the initial consideration is bone morphology (osteology) of the craniofacial complex. Via the systematic study of a personal collection of more than 1000 human skulls, Spencer Atkinson[1] provided the modern basis of craniofacial osseous morphology as it relates to the biomechanics of stomatognathic function. A frontal section of an adult skull shows the bilateral symmetry of bone morphology and functional loading (Figs. 4.4 and 4.5). Because the human genome contains genes to pattern the structure of only half of the body, the contralateral side is a mirror image. Consequently, normal development of the head is symmetric. Thus unilateral structures are on the midline, and bilateral structures are equidistant from it. As shown in Fig. 4.5, the vertical components of the cranium tend to be loaded in compression (negative stress), and the horizontal components are loaded in tension (positive stress). From an engineering perspective, the internal skeletal structure of the midface is similar to that of a ladder: vertical rails loaded in compression connected by rungs loaded in tension. This is one of the most efficient structures for achieving maximal compressive strength with minimal mass in a composite material.

Differential Osteology of the Maxilla and Mandible

Although equal and opposite functional loads are delivered to the maxilla and mandible, the maxilla transfers stress to the entire cranium, whereas the mandible must absorb the entire load. Consequently, the mandible is much stronger and stiffer than the maxilla. A midsagittal section through the incisors (Fig. 4.6) and a frontal section through the molar region (Fig. 4.7) show the distinct differences in the osseous morphology of the maxilla and mandible. The maxilla has relatively thin cortices that are interconnected by a network of trabeculae (see Figs. 4.4, 4.6, and 4.7). Because it is loaded primarily in compression, the maxilla is structurally similar to the body of a vertebra.

The mandible, however, has thick cortices and more radially oriented trabeculae (see Figs. 4.6 and 4.7). The structural array is similar to the shaft of a long bone and indicates that the mandible is loaded predominantly in bending and torsion. This biomechanical impression based on osteology is confirmed by in vivo strain gauge studies in monkeys. Hylander[2,3] demonstrated substantial bending and torsion in the body of the mandible associated with normal masticatory function (Fig. 4.8). A clinical correlation consistent with this pattern of surface strain is the tendency of some humans to form tori in the areas of maximal bending and torsion (Fig. 4.9). The largest tori are on the side on which the individual habitually chews (preferential working side).

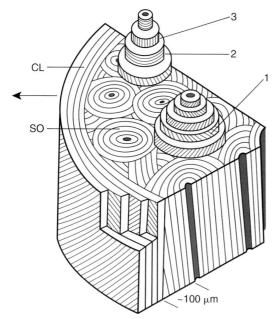

• **Fig. 4.1** Schematic drawing of a wedge of a cortical bone that is growing to the left demonstrates the morphology of circumferential lamellae *(CL)* and secondary osteons *(SO)*. Depending on the mechanical loading at the time the matrix is formed, bone lamellae may have a collagen orientation that is an alternating bias *(1)* or alternating horizontal *(2)* and vertical *(3)* orientations. (From Roberts WE, Hartsfield Jr JK. Bone development and function: genetic and environmental mechanisms. *Semin Orthod.* 2004;10:100–122.)

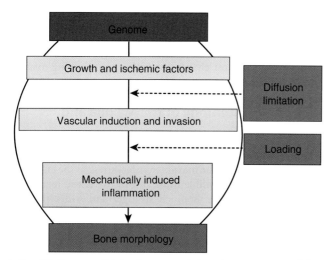

• **Fig. 4.2** Genome dictates bone morphology by a sequence of three genetic mechanisms: (1) growth and ischemic factors, (2) vascular induction and invasion, and (3) mechanically induced inflammation. The latter two are influenced by two major physical influences: (1) diffusion limitation for maintaining viable osteocytes and (2) mechanical loading history. (From Roberts WE, Hartsfield Jr JK. Bone development and function: genetic and environmental mechanisms. *Semin Orthod.* 2004;10:100–122.)

Temporomandibular Articulation

The temporomandibular joint (TMJ) is the principal adaptive center for determining the intermaxillary relationship in all three planes of space. Fig. 4.10 shows optimal skeletal development consistent with normal morphology of the TMJ. Fig. 4.11 shows aberrant skeletal and dental relationships consistent with degeneration of the fossa and mandibular condyle (i.e., the enlarged

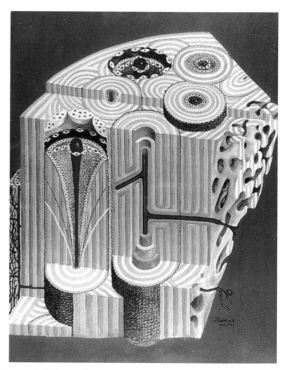

• **Fig. 4.3** Artist's rendition of the dynamic principles of cortical bone remodeling produced by the renowned dental illustrator Rolando De Castro. Remodeling is a vascularly mediated process of bone turnover that maintains the integrity of structural support and is a source of metabolic calcium. Osteoblasts are derived from preosteoblasts circulating in the blood, and perivascular mesenchymal cells give rise to osteoblasts. Note the three colored chevrons (yellow, green, and orange) progressively marking the mineralization front of the evolving second osteon that is moving superiorly on the left. (From Roberts WE, Arbuckle GR, Simmons KE. What are the risk factors of osteoporosis? Assessing bone health. *J Am Dent Assoc.* 1991;122:59–61.)

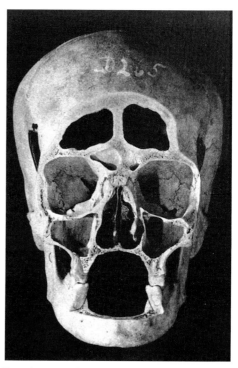

• **Fig. 4.4** Frontal section of a human skull in the plane of the first molars. (From Atkinson SR. Balance: the magic word. *Am J Orthod.* 1964;50:189.)

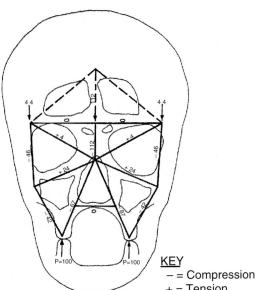

KEY
− = Compression
+ = Tension
P = Assumed load
applied to upper
jaw, bilaterally

Approximate stress
Diagram of skull section D265

• **Fig. 4.5** Two-dimensional vector analysis of stress in the frontal section of the human skull depicted in Fig. 4.4. Relative to a bilateral biting force of 100 arbitrary units, the load is distributed to the vertical components of the midface as compressive (negative) stress. The horizontal structural components are loaded in tension. In a nongrowing individual the stress across the midpalatal suture is 0. When masticating, loads increase and the midpalatal suture is subjected to a tensile load, resulting in an increase in maxillary width. (From Atkinson SR. Balance: the magic word. *Am J Orthod.* 1964;50:189.)

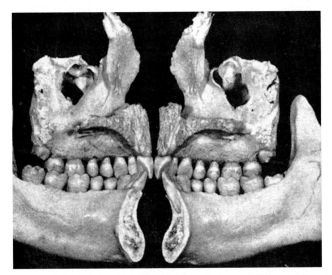

• **Fig. 4.6** Midsagittal section of a human skull shows that the maxilla primarily is composed of trabecular (spongy) bone. The opposing mandible has thick cortices connected by relatively coarse trabeculae. (From Atkinson SR. Balance: the magic word. *Am J Orthod.* 1964;50:189.)

mushroom shape of the condylar process, the roughened topography of the articulating surfaces, the loss of articular cartilage and subchondral plate). Progressive degeneration or hyperplasia of one or both mandibular condyles may result in substantial

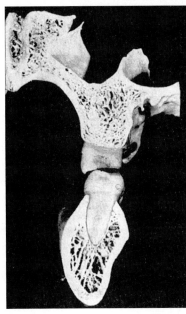

• **Fig. 4.7** Frontal section of the maxilla and mandible in the plane of the first molars. Because it transmits masticatory loads to the entire cranium, the maxilla has thin cortices connected by relatively fine trabeculae. The mandible, however, is loaded in bending and torsion; therefore it is composed of thick cortical bone connected by coarse, oriented trabeculae. (From Atkinson SR. Balance: the magic word. *Am J Orthod.* 1964;50:189.)

intermaxillary discrepancies in the sagittal, vertical, and frontal dimensions. Adaptation of the TMJ allows for substantial growth change to occur without disturbing the intermaxillary relationship of the dentition (e.g., class I occlusion remains class I). In the adult years the intermaxillary relationship continues to change but at a slower rate. The face lengthens and may rotate anteriorly as much as 10 mm over the adult lifetime.[4] The mandible adapts to this change by lengthening and maintaining the intermaxillary dental relationship (Fig. 4.12). However, if the TMJs of an adult undergo bilateral degenerative change, whether symptomatic or not, the mandible can decrease in length, resulting in a shorter, more convex face (Fig. 4.13).

Within physiologic limits, the TMJ has remarkable regenerative and adaptive capabilities, allowing for spontaneous recovery from degenerative episodes (Fig. 4.14). Unlike other joints in the body, the TMJ has the ability to adapt to altered jaw structure and function. After a subcondylar fracture, the condylar head is pulled medially by the superior pterygoid muscle and resorbs. If the interocclusal relationship is maintained, a new condyle forms from the medial aspect of the ramus and assumes normal function. Unilateral subcondylar fractures usually result in regeneration of a new functional condyle with no significant deviation of the mandible.[5] However, about one-fourth of subcondylar fractures result in a mandibular deviation toward the injured side, resulting in an asymmetric class II malocclusion with a midline deviation. Another sequela of mandibular trauma is internal derangement such as a unilateral closed lock (a condyle distally displaced relative to the disk). If the range of motion is reduced in a growing patient, the compromised function may inhibit mandibular growth, resulting in a cant of the occlusal plane. Progressive dysfunction and pain may ensue, particularly when associated with occlusal trauma. Reestablishing normal bilateral function allows the compromised condyle or condyles to adapt favorably.

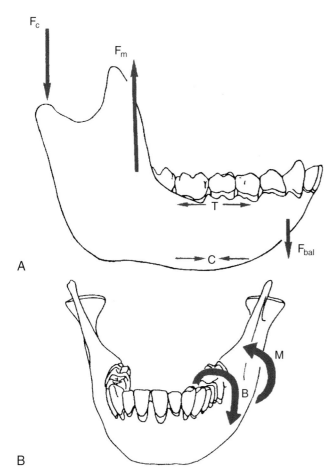

A

B

● **Fig. 4.8** Stress patterns in the primate mandible during unilateral mastication. F_c and F_m are the condylar reaction and the resultant muscle forces on the balancing side, respectively. F_{bal} is the force transmitted through the symphysis from the balancing to the working side. T and C indicate the location of tensile stress and compressive stress, respectively. (A) During the power stroke, the mandibular corpus on the balancing side is bent primarily in the sagittal plane, resulting in tensile stress along the alveolar process and compressive stress along the lower border of the mandible. (B) On the working side, the corpus is twisted primarily about its long axis (it also experiences direct shear and is slightly bent). The muscle force on this side tends to evert the lower border of the mandible and invert the alveolar process *(curved arrow M)*. The twisting movement associated with the bite force has the opposite effect *(curved arrow B)*. The portion of the corpus between these two twisting movements experiences maximal twisting stress. (From Hylander WL. Patterns of stress and strain in the macaque mandible. In: Carlson DS, ed. *Craniofacial Biology.* Ann Arbor, MI: Center for Human Growth and Development;1981.)

Bone Physiology

The morphology of bone has been well described, but its physiology is elusive because of the technical limitations inherent in the study of mineralized tissues. Accurate assessment of the orthodontic or orthopedic response to applied loads requires time markers (bone labels) and physiologic indexes (DNA labels, histochemistry, and in situ hybridization) of bone cell function. Systematic investigation with these advanced methods has defined new concepts of clinically relevant bone physiology.

Specific Assessment Methodology

Physiologic interpretation of the response to applied loads requires the use of specially adapted methods, as follows:

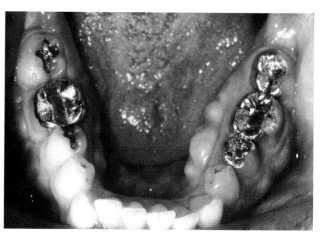

● **Fig. 4.9** Occlusal view of the mandibular dentition of a male patient with extensive buccal and lingual tori. Note that the exostoses are most extensive in the area of the second premolar and first molar, which is the area of maximal torsion in the posterior segment of the mandible.

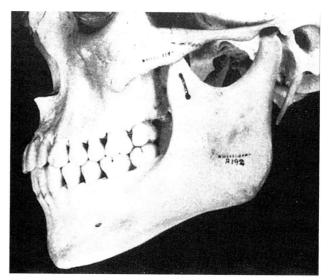

● **Fig. 4.10** Adult human skull with ideal occlusion and osseous form of the maxilla and mandible. Note the ideal anatomic form of the condyle and articular fossa of the temporomandibular joint. (From Atkinson SR. Balance: the magic word. *Am J Orthod.* 1964;50:189.)

- Mineralized sections are an effective means of accurately preserving structure and function relationships.[6]
- Polarized light birefringence detects the preferential orientation of collagen fibers in the bone matrix.[7]
- Fluorescent labels (e.g., tetracycline) permanently mark all sites of bone mineralization at a specific point in time (anabolic markers).[7]
- Microradiography assesses mineral density patterns in the same sections.[8]
- Autoradiography detects radioactively tagged precursors (e.g., nucleotides, amino acids) used to mark physiologic activity.[9-11]
- Nuclear volume morphometry differentially assesses osteoblast precursors in a variety of osteogenic tissues.[12]
- Cell kinetics is a quantitative analysis of cell physiology based on morphologically distinguishable events in the cell cycle (i.e., DNA synthesis [S] phase, mitosis, and differentiation-specific change in nuclear volume).[12,13]
- Finite-element modeling is an engineering method of calculating stresses and strains in all materials, including living tissue.[14-17]

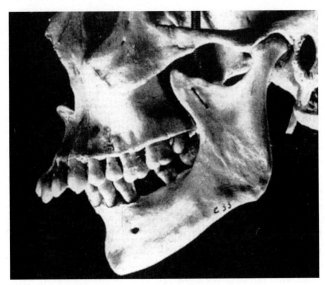

• **Fig. 4.11** Adult human skull with a severe class II malocclusion. Note the degeneration of the temporomandibular joint (i.e., the large, mushroom-shaped condyle and the enlarged, roughened articular fossa). (From Atkinson SR. Balance: the magic word. *Am J Orthod.* 1964;50:189.)

- Microelectrodes inserted in living tissue such as the periodontal ligament (PDL) can detect electrical potential changes associated with mechanical loading.[13,18]
- Backscatter emission is a variation of electron microscopy that assesses relative mineral density at the microscopic level in a block specimen.[19]
- Microcomputed tomography is an in vitro imaging method for determining the relative mineral density of osseous tissue down to a resolution of approximately 5 μm (about the size of an osteoblast nucleus).[20]
- Microindentation testing is a method for determining the mechanical properties of bone at the microscopic level.[21]

Mineralized Sections

Fully mineralized specimens are superior to routine demineralized histologic sections for most critical analyses of teeth, periodontium, and supporting bone because fully mineralized specimens experience less processing distortion. Furthermore, the inorganic mineral and organic matrix can be studied simultaneously.[6-8,22] For tissue-level studies, Sections 100 mm thick are appropriate because they can be studied by means of several analytic methods. Even without bone labels, microradiographic images of polished mineralized sections provide substantial information about the strength, maturation, and turnover rate of cortical bone (Fig. 4.15A). Reducing the thickness of the section to less than 25 mm considerably enhances cellular detail and resolution of bone labels. Specific stains are useful for enhancing the contrast of cellular and extracellular structures. The disadvantages of thin mineralized sections are (1) bone labels quench more rapidly, and (2) tissue density is inadequate for microradiographic analysis.

Polarized Light

Birefringence of polarized light (see Fig. 4.15B) has particular biomechanical significance. The lamellar fringe patterns revealed with polarized light indicate the preferential collagen orientation within the matrix.[23] Most lamellar bone has alternating layers of collagen fibers at right angles. However, two specialized collagen configurations can be seen in the same or adjacent osteons: (1)

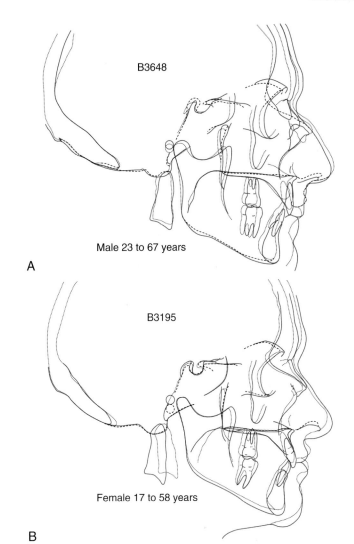

• **Fig. 4.12** (A) Superimposed cephalometric tracings of a male patient at ages 23 and 67 years (black and red tracings, respectively). Note the downward and forward growth of the mandible and the substantial increase in the length of the face. The nasal form was altered by a rhinoplasty in the intervening years. (B) Superimposed cephalometric tracings of an adult female at ages 17 and 58 years (black and red tracings, respectively). Note the downward growth of the mandible and the substantial increase in length of the face. (From Behrents RG. Adult facial growth. In: Enlow DH, ed. *Facial growth.* 3rd ed. Philadelphia: WB Saunders; 1990.)

longitudinally aligned collagen fibers efficiently resist tension, and (2) transverse or circumferential collagen fibers are preferential supports for compression.[24] Loading conditions at the time of bone formation appear to dictate the orientation of the collagen fibers to best resist the loads to which the bone is exposed. The important point is that bone formation can adapt to different loading conditions by changing the internal lamellar organization of mineralized tissue.

Fluorescent Labels

Administered in vivo, calcium-binding labels are anabolic time markers of bone formation. Histomorphometric analysis of label incidence and interlabel distance is an effective method of determining the mechanisms of bone growth and functional adaptation (see Fig. 4.15C). Because they fluoresce at different wavelengths (colors), six bone labels can be used: (1) tetracycline (10 mg/kg,

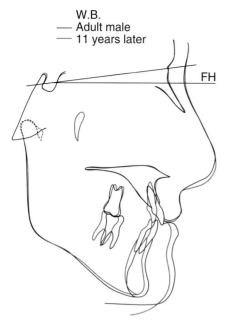

• **Fig. 4.13** Superimposed cephalometric tracings of a middle-aged man over an 11-year period. Although the soft tissue changes are similar to those seen in other adult males (see Fig. 4.12A), the less prominent mandible and more convex skeletal profile are consistent with a shortened mandible. This man had a history of bilateral temporomandibular internal derangement that progressed to crepitus. However, despite the substantial change in facial form and occlusal compensation, no appreciable pain was reported.

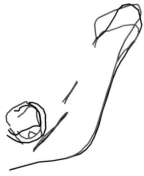

• **Fig. 4.14** Superimposed tracings of a series of panoramic radiographs documenting the degeneration of a mandibular condyle between 13.5 and 18 years of age. Between the ages of 18 and 25.5 years, the degenerative condyle "grew," restoring the original length of the mandible. (From Peltola JS, Kononen M, Nystrom M. A follow-up study of radiographic findings in the mandibular condyles of orthodontically treated patients and associations with TMD. *J Dent Res.* 1995;74:1571.)

bright yellow), (2) calcein green (5 mg/kg, bright green), (3) xylenol orange (60 mg/kg, orange), (4) alizarin complexone (20 mg/kg, red), (5) demeclocycline (10 mg/kg, gold), and (6) oxytetracycline (10 mg/kg, dull or greenish yellow). The multiple-fluorochrome method (sequential use of a variety of different colored labels) is a powerful method of assessing bone growth, healing, functional adaptation, and response to applied loads.[7,25]

Microradiography

High-resolution images require polished sections approximately 100 mm thick. Differential radiographic attenuation shows that new bone is less mineralized than mature bone. Newly formed bone matrix is osteoid and requires about 1 week of maturation to become mineralized bone matrix. Depending on the collagen configuration of the bone matrix, osteoblasts deposit 70% to 85% of the eventual mineral complement by a process called *primary mineralization*.[7,24] Secondary mineralization (mineral maturation) completes the maturation process in about 8 months by a crystal growth process (see Fig. 4.15D). Because the strength of bone tissue is related directly to mineral content, the stiffness and strength of an entire bone depends on the distribution and relative degree of mineralization of its osseous tissue.[26] The initial strength of new bone is the result of the cell-mediated process of primary mineralization, but its ultimate strength is dictated by secondary mineralization, which is the physiochemical process of crystal growth. This concept has important clinical value in orthodontics. Fully mineralized lamellar bone (i.e., bone in steady state with respect to modeling and remodeling) is expected to be less susceptible to relapse tendencies than its woven and composite bone predecessors.[6,27] After active orthodontic therapy, retaining dental corrections for at least 6 to 8 months is important to allow for mineral maturation of the newly formed bone (Fig. 4.16).

Endosseous implants can be placed in the nasal bones of rabbits to serve as anchorage units to load the nasal suture. Slow sutural expansion (Fig. 4.17) produces high-quality lamellar bone along the osseous margins of the suture and the periosteal (superior) surface of the nasal bones (Fig. 4.18). Compression of the nasal bones (see Fig. 4.17A) is manifested by resorption along the margins of the suture (Fig. 4.19). Compressive and tensile loading of the suture are associated with extensive bone modeling and remodeling of the adjacent bones. Sutural adaptation to physiologic and therapeutic loads is associated with a regional acceleration of modeling and remodeling in the adjacent bones.

The PDL is the adaptive connective tissue interface between a tooth and its supporting bone. The overall quality and relative maturation of alveolar bone supporting a rat maxillary molar is shown by a microradiographic image of a histologic section (Fig. 4.20A). If the same section is viewed with fluorescent light, the pattern of osteogenic activity in the bone directly supporting the PDL is visible. Sharp labels mark lamellar bone, and diffuse labels indicate woven bone. Extensive turnover (remodeling) of the alveolar process is shown by uptake of internal labels (Fig. 4.20B). These data reveal that the entire alveolar process responds to tooth movement. Uncoupled anabolic and catabolic modeling occurs along bone surfaces that border the periosteum and PDL. Remodeling (coupled foci of bone resorption and formation) is the process of internal turnover and adaptation.

To a limited extent the temporal fossa can adapt to growth and functional loading, primarily in an anteroposterior direction, but the principal site of skeletal growth and adaptation is the mandibular condyle. In one study, multifluorochrome labeling and microradiography were used to compare bone in growing adolescent rabbits (Fig. 4.21) with that in adult female rabbits who had completed growth (Fig. 4.22). The adolescent primary spongiosa, the layer of endochondral bone immediately beneath the articular cartilage, is predominantly woven bone (marked by the diffuse labels in Fig. 4.22). More inferiorly, the primary spongiosa is remodeled to secondary spongiosa (broad, distinct labels). Progressing deeper into the secondary spongiosa (trabecular bone),

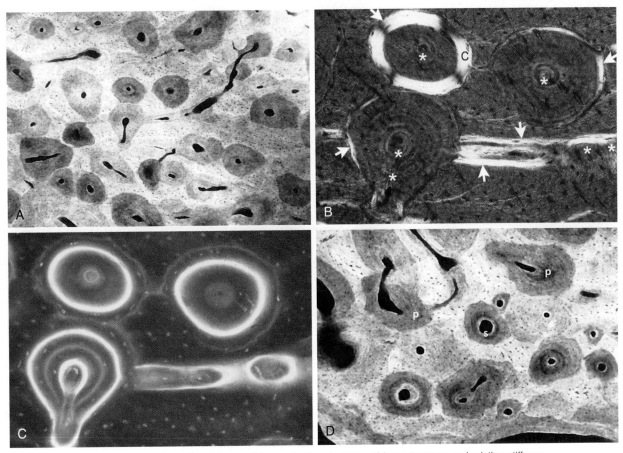

• **Fig. 4.15** (A) Microradiography provides a physiologic index of bone turnover and relative stiffness. The more radiolucent (dark) osteons are the youngest, the least mineralized, and the most compliant. Radiodense (white) areas are the oldest, most mineralized, and rigid portions of the bone. (B) Polarized light microscopy shows the collagen fiber orientation in bone matrix. Lamellae with a longitudinally oriented matrix *(C)* are particularly strong in tension, whereas a horizontally oriented matrix (dark) has preferential strength in compression *(arrows,* resorption arrest lines; *asterisks,* vascular channels). (C) Multiple fluorochrome labels administered at 2-week intervals demonstrate the incidence and rates of bone formation. (D) This microradiograph shows an array of concentric secondary osteons (haversian systems) characteristic of rapidly remodeling cortical bone. Primary *(p)* and beginning secondary *(s)* mineralization are more radiolucent and radiodense, respectively. (From Roberts WE, Garetto LP, Katona TR. Principles of orthodontic biomechanics; metabolic and mechanical control mechanisms. In: Carlson DS, Goldstein S, eds. *Bone Biodynamics in Orthodontic and Orthopedic Treatment.* Ann Arbor, MI: Center for Human Growth and Development; 1992. Craniofacial Growth Series; vol. 27.)

continuing remodeling of lamellar bone is shown by the sharp labels (see Fig. 4.21). This progressive pattern of bone modeling and remodeling is characteristic of the skeletal mechanism of long bone growth.

In contrast, the nongrowing condyles of adult animals have a much thinner subchondral plate composed primarily of woven bone (see Fig. 4.22). The supporting metaphysis is composed entirely of secondary spongiosa. Bone-label uptake documents a high rate of remodeling of lamellar bone.

These data suggest that the mandibular condyle has a high rate of remodeling consistent with heavy functional loading. All things considered, the substantial histologic variance of functioning condyles in adolescent and adult animals indicates that the TMJ is highly adaptable. However, the presence of woven bone and diffuse labels in the thin subchondral plate of adults suggests that the mandibular condyle may be fragile and susceptible to degenerative changes if overloaded. Nevertheless the high rate of physiologic activity in the mandibular condyle of young and old animals may

explain the remarkable ability of this joint to heal and even regenerate after injury (see Fig. 4.14).

Microindentation, Backscatter Imaging, and Microcomputed Tomography

Huja and colleagues[21] developed a microindentation method for determining the material properties of bone in a block specimen and demonstrated that the lamellar bone within 1 mm of the surface of an implant is more compliant than the supporting bone of the jaw. Polarized microscopy demonstrates the more irregular collagen pattern of the compliant lamellar bone near the interface (Fig. 4.23). Backscatter emission imaging[19] recently has been refined as a high-resolution method for assessing the bone mineral density and surface topography patterns of the osseous interface of dental implants (Fig. 4.24). In another important technologic advancement, Yip and colleagues[20] developed a special tuning sequence for the microcomputed tomography that allows three-dimensional detection of bone mineral density patterns to a

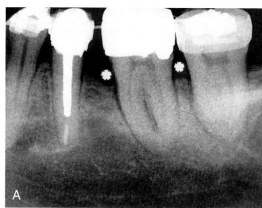
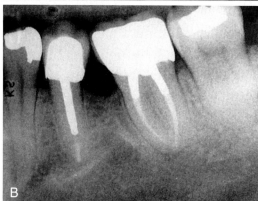

• **Fig. 4.16** Periapical radiographs comparing bone maturation at the end of active orthodontic treatment and 2 years later. (A) At the end of treatment, large amorphous areas of relatively immature bone can be seen. (B) After retention and restorative treatment, including endodontics, distinct definition of cortices and trabeculae is evident. (From Roberts WE, Garetto LP, Katona TR. Principles of orthodontic biomechanics; metabolic and mechanical control mechanisms. In: Carlson DS, Goldstein S, eds. *Bone Biodynamics in Orthodontic and Orthopedic Treatment*. Ann Arbor, MI: Center for Human Growth and Development; 1992. Craniofacial Growth Series; vol. 27.)

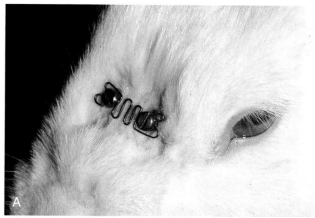
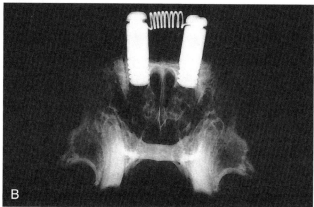

• **Fig. 4.17** (A) Endosseous implants in rabbit nasal bones are loaded in tension to expand the suture between the nasal bones. (B) Radiograph of a postmortem specimen of rabbit maxilla and nasal bones shows two bilateral endosseous implants used as abutments for a coil spring that delivers a compressive load across the internasal suture. (From Don MT. *Orthopedic Anchorage with Endosseous Implants in Rabbit Nasal Bones.* [master's thesis]. San Francisco: University of the Pacific; 1988.)

resolution of 5 mm (Fig. 4.25). Furthermore, this exciting new method can detect bone-remodeling foci within intact specimens (Fig. 4.26) and can differentiate between primary and secondary lamellar bone along the metallic surfaces of endosseous implants. Collectively, these new methods have been valuable for assessing the material properties and mineral density of bone integrating endosseous implants that are used for orthodontic and dentofacial orthopedic anchorage. However, these advanced technologies offer the promise of considerably exceeding the capability of previous histologic methods for defining the adaptive response of the oral and craniofacial structures to therapeutic loads.

Autoradiography

Radioactive precursors for structural and metabolic materials can be detected in tissue by coating histologic sections with a nuclear track emulsion. By localizing radioactive disintegrations, one can determine the location of the radioactive precursors (Fig. 4.27). Specific radioactive labels for proteins, carbohydrates, and nucleic acids are injected at a known interval before tissue sampling is done. Qualitative and quantitative assessment of label uptake is a physiologic index of cell activity. The autoradiographic labeling procedures most often used in bone research are ^{3}H-thymidine labeling of cells synthesizing DNA (S-phase cells) and ^{3}H-proline

labeling of newly formed bone matrix. Bromodeoxyuridine immunocytochemistry, a nonradioactive method of labeling S-phase cells in vivo (Fig. 4.28), shows promise of becoming an important bone cell kinetic method of the future.[14]

Nuclear Volume Morphometry

Measuring the size of the nucleus is a cytomorphometric procedure for assessing the stage of differentiation of osteoblast precursor cells. This method has been particularly useful for assessing the mechanism of osteogenesis in orthodontically activated PDLs (Fig. 4.29). Preosteoblasts (C and D cells) have significantly larger nuclei than committed osteoprogenitor (A') cells or their less differentiated precursors (A cells). The B-cell compartment is a group of fibroblast-like cells that appear to have little or no osteogenic potential.[28] Careful cytomorphometric assessment of the size of the nucleus (Fig. 4.30) has proved to be an effective means of determining the relative differentiation of PDL and other bone-lining cells.

Classification of Bone Tissue

Orthodontic tooth movement involves a cytokine-mediated bone adaptation response similar to wound healing; therefore tooth movement is a good experimental model for understanding the types of bone formed during the postoperative bone

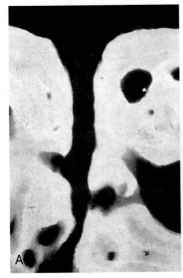
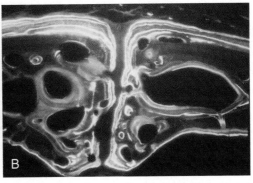

• **Fig. 4.18** (A) Microradiograph of the superficial portion of an internasal suture loaded in tension shows smooth bone surfaces consistent with bone apposition. (B) Fluorescent light photomicrograph of rabbit nasal bones loaded in tension shows bone-modeling and remodeling patterns associated with mechanical expansion of the suture. Bone-forming surfaces were labeled with fluorescent dyes at weekly intervals. The superior portion of the labeled suture corresponds to the microradiograph in (A). (From Don MT. *Orthopedic Anchorage with Endosseous Implants in Rabbit Nasal Bones.* [master's thesis]. San Francisco: University of the Pacific; 1988.)

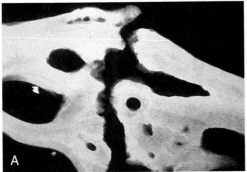
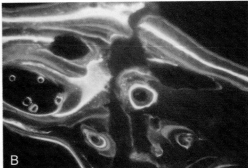

• **Fig. 4.19** (A) Microradiograph of an internasal suture loaded in compression shows scalloped bone surfaces consistent with bone resorption. (B) Fluorescent light photomicrograph of rabbit nasal bones loaded in compression shows bone modeling and remodeling patterns associated with mechanical contraction of the suture. Bone-forming surfaces were labeled with fluorescent dyes at weekly intervals. (From Don MT. *Orthopedic Anchorage with Endosseous Implants in Rabbit Nasal Bones.* [master's thesis]. San Francisco: University of the Pacific; 1988.)

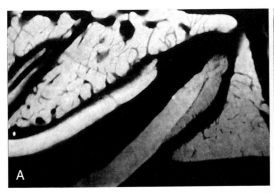
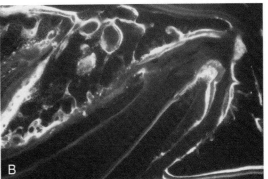

• **Fig. 4.20** (A) Microradiograph of a midsagittal section through the mesial root of a rat maxillary first molar shows the varying degrees of mineralization of the alveolar bone and the tooth root. (B) Fluorescent light photomicrograph of the corresponding section shows the bone modeling and remodeling patterns associated with extrusion and distal (left) tipping of the root. (From Shimizu KA. The *Effects of Hypofunction and Hyperfunction on the Supporting Structures of Rat Molar Teeth*. [master's thesis]. San Francisco: University of the Pacific; 1987.)

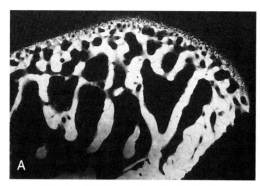
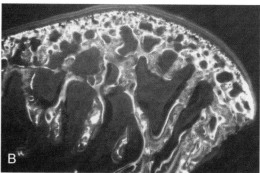

● **Fig. 4.21** (A) Microradiograph of a frontal section through the mandibular condyle of a young, growing rabbit reveals that the superior cortical plate (primary spongiosa) is composed of relatively porous, primary cortical bone that is supported by a secondary spongiosa of lamellar trabeculae. (B) Fluorescent light photomicrograph of the corresponding section shows that the superior cortical plate is composed primarily of woven bone (indistinct labels). The supporting trabeculae are composed of remodeling trabecular bone (sharp labels). (From Larsen SJ. *The Influence of Age on Bone Modeling and Remodeling.* [master's thesis]. San Francisco: University of the Pacific; 1986.)

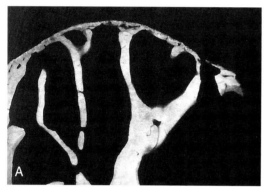
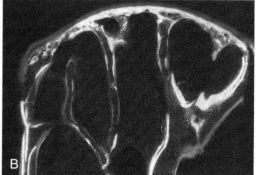

● **Fig. 4.22** (A) Microradiograph of a frontal section through the mandibular condyle of a mature adult rabbit shows that the superior cortical plate (primary spongiosa) is composed of a thin layer of porous primary bone supported by a secondary spongiosa of lamellar trabeculae. (B) Fluorescent light photomicrograph of the corresponding section shows that the superior cortical plate is composed primarily of woven bone (indistinct labels). The supporting trabeculae are composed of remodeling trabecular bone (sharp labels). (From Larsen SJ. *The Influence of Age on Bone Modeling and Remodeling.* [master's thesis]. San Francisco: University of the Pacific; 1986.)

modeling and long-term remodeling response to bone manipulative therapy. The first bone formed is relatively immature woven bone (Fig. 4.31). Woven bone is compacted to form composite bone (primary osteons) and subsequently is remodeled to lamellar bone. To appreciate the biologic mechanism of bone healing and adaptation, the practitioner must have knowledge of bone types.

Woven Bone

Woven bone varies considerably in structure; it is relatively weak, disorganized, and poorly mineralized. However, it serves a crucial role in wound healing by (1) rapidly filling osseous defects; (2) providing initial continuity for fractures, osteotomy segments, and endosseous implants; and (3) strengthening a bone weakened by surgery or trauma. The first bone formed in response to wound healing is the woven type. Woven bone is not found in the adult skeleton under normal, steady-state conditions; rather, it is compacted to form composite bone, remodeled to lamellar bone, or rapidly resorbed if prematurely loaded.[8,29] The functional limitations of woven bone are an important aspect of orthodontic retention (see Fig. 4.16), as well as postoperative healing of implants and orthognathic surgery segments.[30]

Lamellar Bone

Lamellar bone, a strong, highly organized, well-mineralized tissue, makes up more than 99% of the adult human skeleton. When new lamellar bone is formed, a portion of the mineral component (hydroxyapatite) is deposited by osteoblasts during primary mineralization (see Fig. 4.15D). Secondary mineralization, which completes the mineral component, is a physical process (crystal growth) that requires many months. Within physiologic limits, the strength of bone is related directly to its mineral content.[24,26] The relative strengths of different histologic types of osseous tissue are such that woven bone is weaker than new lamellar bone, which is weaker than mature lamellar bone.[30] Adult human bone is almost entirely comprised of the remodeled variety: secondary osteons and spongiosa.[7,8,24] The full strength of lamellar bone that supports an endosseous implant is not achieved until about 1 year postoperatively. This is an important consideration in planning the functional loading of an implant-supported prosthesis.

Composite Bone

Composite bone is an osseous tissue formed by the deposition of lamellar bone within a woven bone lattice, which is a process called *cancellous compaction.*[6,31] This process is a rapid means of

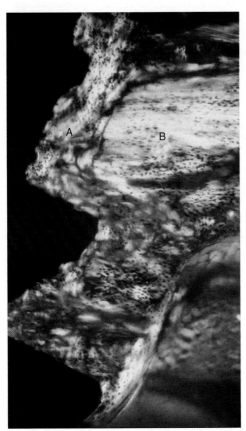

• **Fig. 4.23** Polarized illumination photomicrograph shows the healed interface of a titanium implant in rabbit cortical bone. Note the layer of newly formed lamellar bone *(A)* formed by multidirectional remodeling within about 1 mm of the implant surface. Compare the more compliant layer of primarily mineralized lamellar bone *(A)* with the fully mineralized lamellar bone *(B)* supporting the interfacial layer.

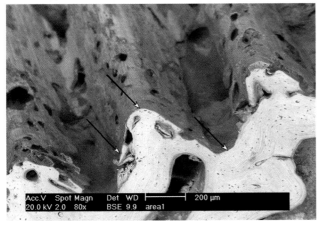

• **Fig. 4.24** Backscatter emission imaging of the bone surface immediately adjacent to an implant (removed) reveals the mineral density of surface topography of the rapidly remodeling interfacial layer. (From Huja SS, Roberts WE. Mechanism of osseointegration: characterization of supporting bone with indentation testing and backscattered imaging. *Semin Orthod.* 2004;10:162–173.)

producing relatively strong bone in a short period.[26] Composite bone is an important intermediary type of bone in the physiologic response to functional loading (see Fig. 4.31), and it usually is

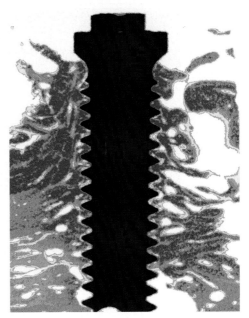

• **Fig. 4.25** Microcomputed tomography of a section through an implant placed in canine cortical bone reveals a broad array of mineralized tissues. The original gray-level distribution has been color coded gold, blue, red, and yellow to demonstrate decreasing levels of mineral density. The method can resolve structures as small as an osteoblast. (From Yip G, Schneider P, Roberts WE. Micro-computed tomography: high resolution imaging of bone and implants in three dimensions. *Semin Orthod.* 2004;10:174–187.)

the predominant osseous tissue for stabilization during the early process of postoperative healing. When the bone is formed in the fine compaction configuration, the resulting composite of woven and lamellar bone forms structures known as *primary osteons.* Although composite bone may be high-quality, load-bearing osseous tissue, it is eventually remodeled into secondary osteons.[7,30]

Bundle Bone

Bundle bone is a functional adaptation of lamellar structure to allow attachment of tendons and ligaments. Perpendicular striations, called *Sharpey's fibers,* are the major distinguishing characteristics of bundle bone. Distinct layers of bundle bone usually are seen adjacent to the PDL (see Fig. 4.31) along physiologic bone-forming surfaces.[32] Bundle bone is the mechanism of ligament and tendon attachment throughout the body. First-generation blade implants were thought to form a ligamentous attachment to bone, which was deemed a *pseudoperiodontium.* However, histologic studies could not demonstrate any bundle bone attaching fibrous connective tissue to bone at the interface. Because the fibrous tissue encapsulation had no physiologic role, it was actually scar tissue, which was equivalent to a nonunion in a failed facture repair.

Skeletal Adaptation: Modeling and Remodeling

Skeletal adaptation to the mechanical environment is achieved through changes in (1) bone mass, (2) geometric distribution, (3) matrix organization, and (4) collagen orientation of the lamellae. In addition to these adaptive mechanisms that influence bone formation, the mechanical properties of osseous structures change as a result of maturation, function, aging, and pathologic processes.

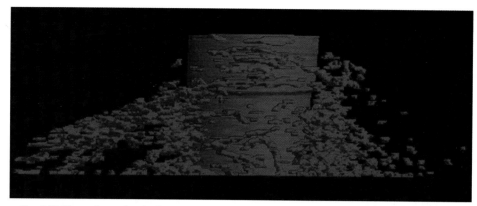

• **Fig. 4.26** Three-dimensional microcomputed tomography view of the peri-implant radiolucent areas reveals an uneven distribution of vascular areas and remodeling foci. This image of the cervical half of a cylindric implant is consistent with the intense bone-remodeling pattern focused within the center of the endosseous portion. This image was tuned to demonstrate less-mineralized structures: internal vascularity including remodeling foci (cutting/filling cones). (From Yip G, Schneider P, Roberts WE. Microcomputed tomography: high resolution imaging of bone and implants in three dimensions. *Semin Orthod.* 2004;10:174–187.)

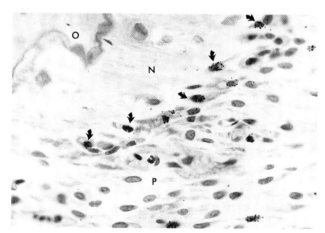

• **Fig. 4.27** At 56 hours after initiation of orthodontic force, new bone *(N)* is forming on the original *(O)* alveolar bone surface. The ³H-thymidine–labeled osteoblasts *(arrows)* are derived from preosteoblasts in the periodontal ligament *(P)* (×450).

A few physiologic and pathologic examples are (1) secondary mineralization, (2) mean bone age, (3) fatigue damage, and (4) loss of vitality (pathologic hypermineralization).[33]

Trabecular and cortical bone grow, adapt, and turn over by means of two fundamentally distinct mechanisms: modeling and remodeling. In bone modeling, independent sites of resorption and formation change the form (shape, size, or both) of a bone. In bone remodeling, a specific, coupled sequence of resorption and formation occurs to replace previously existing bone (Fig. 4.32). The mechanism for internal remodeling (turnover) of dense compact bone involves axially oriented cutting and filling cones (Fig. 4.33).[6] From an orthodontic perspective the biomechanical response to tooth movement involves an integrated array of bone-modeling and remodeling events (Fig. 4.34A). Bone modeling is the dominant process of facial growth and adaptation to applied loads such as headgear, rapid palatal expansion, and functional appliances. Modeling changes can be seen on cephalometric tracings (see Fig. 4.34B), but remodeling events, which usually occur at the same time, are apparent only at the microscopic level.

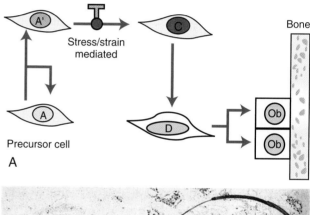

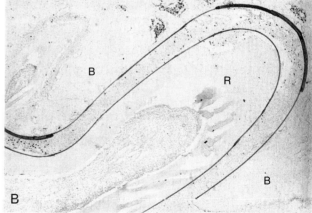

• **Fig. 4.28** (A) Histogenesis sequence of osteoblasts *(Ob)*. Precursor cells, located around blood vessels in the periodontal ligament (PDL), migrate toward bone as they differentiate through several stages (A→A′→C→D→Ob) to become alveolar bone-forming cells (Ob). The A′→C step is believed to be mediated by stress and strain. (B) The area between the lines is the PDL; *R,* root, *B,* bone. The 5-bromo-2′-deoxyuridine (BDU) is a thymidine analog taken up by cells in the PDL (dark dots) in which the nuclei are synthesizing DNA. BDU-labeled regions in the PDL are adjacent to areas of eventual bone formation (thick line segments). The BDU immunohistochemically labeled pattern of cells in the PDL of a young control rat is consistent with proliferation supporting tooth eruption. (Adapted from Katona TR, Paydar NH, Akay HU, Roberts WE. Stress analysis of bone modeling response to rat molar orthodontics. *J Biomech.* 1995;28:27–38.)

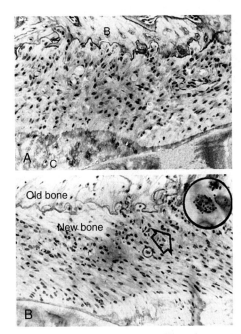

• **Fig. 4.29** (A) Bone *(B)*, periodontal ligament *(P)*, and cementum *(C)* in the control periodontium of a young adult rat (6–8 weeks of age) (×100). (B) At 56 hours after application of force, new bone is noted; a ³H-thymidine–labeled preosteoblast is selected from the periodontal ligament *(circle)* and magnified to 1000 times in the upper right corner (×100) *(large arrow* indicates the zoom in magnification to show cellular detail).

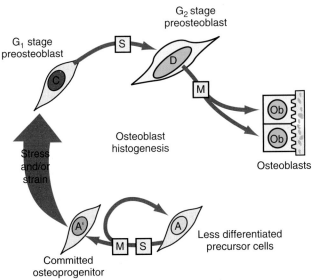

• **Fig. 4.30** Frequency distribution of nuclear volume for fibroblast-like cells in unstimulated rat periodontal ligament. A, A′, C, and D cells are a morphologic classification based on peaks in the distribution curve. The osteoblast histogenesis sequence is a progression of five morphologically and kinetically distinguishable cells. The process involves two DNA S phases *(S)* and two mitotic *(M)* events. (Redrawn from Roberts WE, Morey ER. Proliferation and differentiation sequence of osteoblast histogenesis under physiologic conditions in rat periodontal ligament. *Am J Anat.* 1985;174:105.)

True remodeling usually is not imaged on clinical radiographs,[34] but it can be detected with clinical scintillation scans. Constant remodeling (internal turnover) mobilizes and redeposits calcium by means of coupled resorption and formation: bone is resorbed and redeposited at the same site. Osteoblasts, osteoclasts, and possibly their precursors are thought to communicate by chemical messages known as *coupling factors.* Transforming growth factor β is thought to be a coupling factor.[35]

Cortical Bone Growth and Maturation

Enlow[31] sectioned human skulls and histologically identified areas of surface apposition and resorption. The overall patterns of bone modeling ("external remodeling") helped define the mechanisms of facial growth. Although the method could not distinguish between active and inactive modeling sites, it was adequate for determining the overall direction of regional activity in the maxilla and mandible. This method of osseous topography was a considerable advance in the understanding of surface modeling of facial bones.

Melsen[36] used microradiographic images of mineralized sections to extend the capability of the osseous topography method. Patterns of primary and secondary mineralization (as described in Fig. 4.15) identified active appositional sites and provided a crude index of bone formation rates. Through the systematic study of autopsy specimens of 126 normal males and females from birth to 20 years of age, the most stable osseous structures in the anterior cranial base of growing children and adolescents were defined anatomically (Fig. 4.35A). This research established that the three most stable osseous landmarks for superimposition of cephalometric radiographs are (1) the anterior curvature of the sella turcica, (2) the cribriform plate, and (3) the internal curvature of the frontal bone (see Fig. 4.35B). In effect, this research established the gold standard for reliable superimposition on the anterior cranial base. This information is valuable for implantologists because a superimposed tracing of serial cephalometric radiographs is the most reliable means for determining when postadolescent growth is complete. The latter is essential for treatment planning implant placement during the late adolescent and early adult periods.

Roberts and colleagues[6,7,25] introduced simultaneous use of multiple fluorochrome labels and microradiography to assess modeling and remodeling patterns over extended periods of time. Noorda[37] applied these methods for a three-dimensional assessment of subcondylar growth of the mandible of adolescent rabbits. Twenty-week-old rabbits (early adolescents) were labeled every 2 weeks with a rotating series of six different multifluorochrome labels for 18 weeks. Cross sections of the subcondylar region (Fig. 4.36A) were superimposed on original, oldest-labeled, and newest-labeled bone according to fluorescent time markers (see Fig. 4.36B). Because all three sections were at the same relative level at a point in time, superimposition on original (unlabeled) bone and the oldest-labeled bone (see Fig. 4.36C) provided an index of the relative amounts of bone resorbed and formed as the mandible grew superiorly (see Fig. 4.36D). This method provides the most accurate assessment to date of cortical bone drift over time. The major mechanism of the increase in interramal width during adolescent growth in rabbits is lateral drift of the entire subchondral region.

The Noorda study also produced important quantitative data on the rates of surface modeling (apposition and resorption) of primary bone (Fig. 4.37). During the last 18 weeks of growth to adult stature, the surface apposition rate decreased from more than 25 μm/day to less than 5 μm/day (Fig. 4.38A). The secondary osteon census peaked at about 8 to 10 weeks (see Fig. 4.38B). Therefore under conditions of relatively rapid growth, primary cortical bone is remodeled to secondary osteons in about

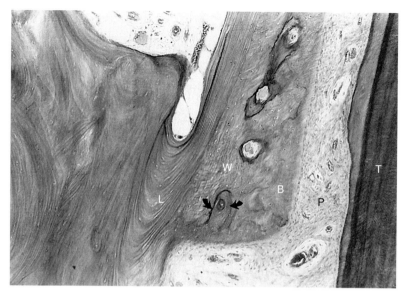

• **Fig. 4.31** Section of human periodontium from the lower first molar region shows a typical histologic response to orthodontic tooth movement. With respect to the mature lamellar bone *(L)* on the left, the tooth *(T)* is being moved to the right. The first bone formed adjacent to the periodontal ligament *(P)* is of the woven type *(W)*. Subsequent lamellar compaction forms primary osteons of composite bone *(arrows)*. Bundle bone *(B)* is formed where ligaments, such as the periodontal ligament, are attached. (From Roberts WE, Turkey PK, Breznia KN, Fielder PJ. Implants: bone physiology and metabolism. *CDA J.* 1987;15:54–61.)

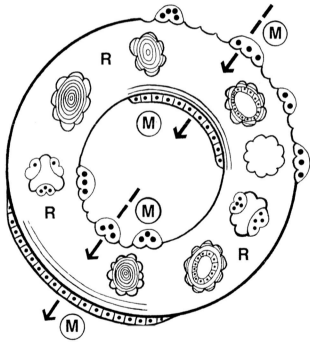

• **Fig. 4.32** Schematic cross section of cortical bone shows surface modeling *(M)*, which is the process of uncoupled resorption and formation. Remodeling *(R)* is the turnover of existing bone. (From Roberts WE, Garetto LP, DeCastro RA. Remodeling of devitalized bone threatens periosteal margin integrity of endosseous titanium implants. *J Indiana Dent Assoc.* 1989; 68:19–24.)

2 months. Remodeling therefore is a time-dependent maturation of primary cortical bone.[6,7]

There is little long-term documentation of the bone remodeling response to functional loading of implant-supported restorations. The same methods used for defining the growth and development of the rabbit mandible would provide valuable new information for the field of implantology.

Cutting and Filling Cones

The rate at which cutting and filling cones progress through compact bone is an important determinant of turnover. The progression is calculated by measuring the distance between initiation of labeled bone-formation sites along the resorption arrest line in longitudinal sections.[6] Using two fluorescent labels administered 2 weeks apart in adult dogs, the velocity was 27.7 ± 1.9 mm/day (mean ± SEM [standard error of the mean], *n* = 4 dogs, 10 cutting and filling cones sampled from each). At this speed, evolving secondary osteons travel about 1 mm in 36 days. Newly remodeled secondary osteons (formed within the experimental period of the dog study) contained an average of 4.5 labels (administered 2 weeks apart); the incidence of resorption cavities is about one-third the incidence of labeled osteons.[25] These data are consistent with a remodeling cycle of about 12 weeks in dogs,[25] compared with 6 weeks in rabbits[6] and 17 weeks in humans.[7,8] This relationship is useful for extrapolating animal data to human applications. More recent experimental studies have shown that new secondary osteons may continue to fix bone labels for up to 6 months, indicating that terminal filling of the lumen is slow.[38]

Traumatic or surgical wounding usually results in intense but localized modeling and remodeling responses. After an osteotomy or placement of an endosseous implant, callus formation and resorption of necrotic osseous margins are modeling processes; however, internal replacement of the devitalized cortical bone surrounding these sites is a remodeling activity. In addition, a gradient of localized remodeling disseminates through the bone adjacent to any invasive bone procedure. This process, called *regional acceleratory phenomenon,* is an important aspect of postoperative healing.[8,39]

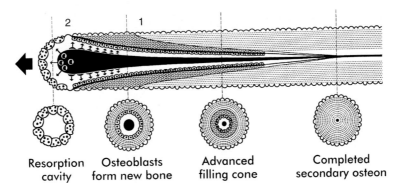

• **Fig. 4.33** The cutting/filling cone has a head of osteoclasts that cut through the bone and a tail of osteoblasts that form a new secondary osteon. The velocity through bone is determined by measuring between two tetracycline labels *(1 and 2)* administered 1 week apart. (Adapted from Roberts WE, Garetto LP, Arbuckle GR, Simmons KE, DeCastro, RA. What are the risk factors of osteoporosis? Assessing bone health. *J Am Dent Assoc.* 1991;122:59–61.)

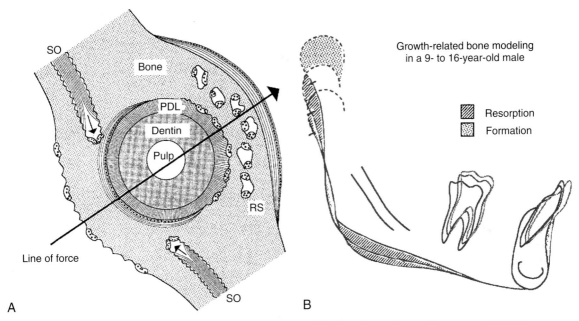

• **Fig. 4.34** (A) Orthodontic bone modeling, or site-specific formation and resorption, occurs along the periodontal ligament (PDL) and periosteal surfaces. Remodeling, or turnover, occurs within alveolar bone along the line of force on both sides of the tooth. (B) Orthopedic bone modeling related to growth in an adolescent male involves several site-specific areas of bone formation and resorption. Although extensive bone remodeling (i.e., internal turnover) also is underway, it is not evident in cephalometric radiographs superimposed on stable mandibular structures. (SO = Secondary Osteon, BM = Bone Remodeling)

Modeling and remodeling are controlled by an interaction of metabolic and mechanical signals. Bone modeling is largely under the integrated biomechanical control of functional applied loads (Table 4.1). However, hormones and other metabolic agents have a strong secondary influence, particularly during periods of growth and advanced aging. Paracrine and autocrine mechanisms, such as local growth factors and prostaglandins, can override the mechanical control mechanism temporarily during wound healing.[40] Remodeling responds to metabolic mediators such as parathyroid hormone (PTH) and estrogen, primarily varying the rate of bone turnover (Box 4.1). Bone scans with ^{99}Te-bisphosphate, a marker of bone activity, indicate that the alveolar processes, but not the basilar mandible, have a high remodeling rate.[41,42] Uptake of the marker in alveolar bone is similar to uptake in trabecular

bone of the vertebral column. The latter is known to remodel at a rate of about 20% to 30% per year compared with most cortical bone, which turns over at a rate of 2% to 10% per year.[43] Metabolic mediation of continual bone turnover provides a controllable flow of calcium to and from the skeleton.

Structural and Metabolic Fractions

The structural fraction of cortical bone is the relatively stable outer portion of the cortex; the metabolic fraction is the highly reactive inner aspect (Fig. 4.39A). The primary metabolic calcium reserves of the body are found in trabecular bone and the endosteal half of the cortices. Analogous to orthodontic wires, the stiffness and strength of a bone are related directly to its cross-sectional area. Diaphyseal rigidity quickly is enhanced by adding a

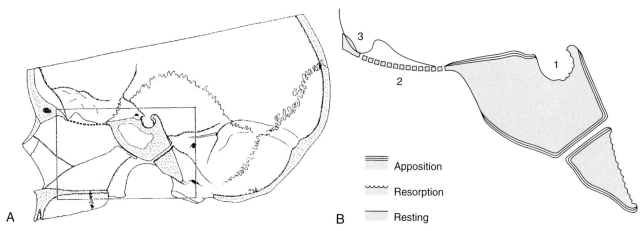

• **Fig. 4.35** (A) Schematic drawing of a skull showing the tissue block removed at autopsy from a series of growing children and adolescents from birth to 20 years of age. (B) Diagrammatic representation of the bone-modeling patterns of the cranial base in growing children. Histologic and microradiographic analysis established that the three most stable anatomic landmarks are *(1)* the anterior curvature of the sella turcica, *(2)* the cribriform plate, and *(3)* the internal curvature of the frontal bone. (From Melsen B. The cranial base. *Acta Odontol Scand.* 1974;32[suppl 62]:S103.)

circumferential lamella at the periosteal surface. Even a thin layer of new osseous tissue at the periosteal surface greatly enhances bone stiffness because it increases the diameter of the bone. In engineering terms, cross-sectional rigidity is related to the second moment of the area. The same general relationship of round wire diameter and stiffness (strength) is well known to orthodontists. The rigidity of a wire increases as the fourth power of diameter.[44] Therefore when a relatively rigid material (bone or wire) is doubled in diameter, the stiffness increases 16 times.

The addition of new osseous tissue at the endosteal (inner) surface has little effect on overall bone strength. Structurally, the long bones and mandible are modified tubes, which is an optimal design for achieving maximal strength with minimal mass.[26] Within limits, loss of bone at the endosteal surface or within the inner third of the compacta has little effect on bone rigidity. The inner cortex can be mobilized to meet metabolic needs without severely compromising bone strength (see Fig. 4.39B); this is the reason patients with osteoporosis have bones with a normal diameter but thin cortices. Even under severe metabolic stress, the body follows a cardinal principle of bone physiology: *maximal strength with minimal mass.*[45]

Bone Metabolism

Restoration of esthetics and function with implant-supported prostheses requires substantial bone manipulation. The biomechanical response to altered function and applied loads depends on the metabolic status of the patient. Bone metabolism is an important aspect of clinical medicine that is directly applicable to implant dentistry. This section discusses the fundamentals of bone metabolism with respect to clinical practice.

The skeletal system is composed of highly specialized mineralized tissues that have structural and metabolic functions. Structurally, lamellar, woven, composite, and bundle bone are unique types of osseous tissue adapted to specific functions. Bone modeling and remodeling are distinct physiologic responses to integrated mechanical and metabolic demands. Biomechanical manipulation of bone is the physiologic basis of stomatognathic reconstruction.

However, before addressing dentofacial considerations, the clinician must assess the patient's overall health status. Implantology is bone-manipulative therapy, and favorable calcium metabolism is an important consideration. Because of the interaction of structure and metabolism, a thorough understanding of osseous structure and function is fundamental to patient selection, risk assessment, treatment planning, and retention of desired dentofacial relationships.[45,46]

Bone is the primary calcium reservoir in the body (Fig. 4.40). Approximately 99% of the calcium in the body is stored in the skeleton. The continual flux of bone mineral responds to a complex interaction of endocrine, biomechanical, and cell-level control factors that maintain the serum calcium level at about 10 mg/dL (10 mg%).

Calcium homeostasis is the process by which mineral equilibrium is maintained. Maintenance of serum calcium levels at about 10 mg/dL is an essential life-support function. Life is thought to have evolved in the sea; calcium homeostasis is the mechanism of the body for maintaining the primordial mineral environment in which cellular processes evolved.[45]

Calcium metabolism is one of the fundamental physiologic processes of life support. When substantial calcium is needed to maintain the critical serum calcium level, bone structure is sacrificed (see Fig. 4.40). The alveolar processes and basilar bone of the jaws also are subject to metabolic bone loss.[47] Even in cases of severe skeletal atrophy, the outer cortex of the alveolar process and the lamina dura around the teeth are preserved. This preservation is analogous to the thin cortices characteristic of osteoporosis.

Calcium homeostasis is supported by three temporally related mechanisms: (1) rapid (instantaneous) flux of calcium from bone fluid (which occurs in seconds), (2) short-term response by osteoclasts and osteoblasts (which extends from minutes to days), and (3) long-term control of bone turnover (over weeks to months) (Fig. 4.41). Precise regulation of serum calcium levels at about 10 mg/dL is essential for nerve conductivity and muscle function. A low serum calcium level can result in tetany and death. A sustained high serum calcium level often is a manifestation of hyperthyroidism and some malignancies. Hypercalcemia may lead to kidney stones and dystrophic calcification of soft tissue.

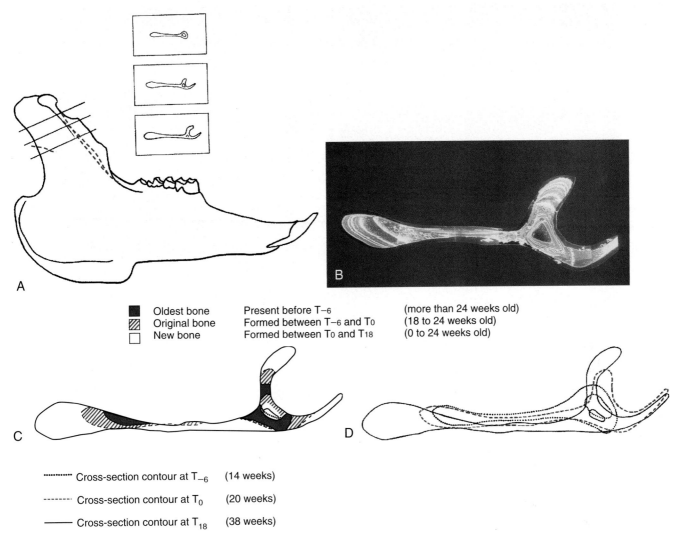

Oldest bone — Present before T−6 — (more than 24 weeks old)
Original bone — Formed between T−6 and T0 — (18 to 24 weeks old)
New bone — Formed between T0 and T18 — (0 to 24 weeks old)

⋯⋯⋯ Cross-section contour at T_{-6} (14 weeks)

------ Cross-section contour at T_0 (20 weeks)

—— Cross-section contour at T_{18} (38 weeks)

• **Fig. 4.36** (A) Schematic drawing of a rabbit mandible showing the plane of sectioning in the subcondylar region of the ramus. (B) Fluorescent light photomicrographs of the most inferior section are arranged in a composite. The weekly deposition of bone labels over 4 months shows the patterns of bone modeling and remodeling associated with the growth and development of the subcondylar region. (C) Based on the uptake of bone labels, the age of specific areas in a given cross section can be determined accurately. (D) Because the subcondylar region of the ramus is growing superiorly, superimposition of the three sections on the oldest bone gives an estimation of the patterns of bone resorption (catabolic modeling) associated with growth of the mandibular ramus. (From Noorda CB. *Modeling and Remodeling in the Cortical Bone of Both Growing and Mature Rabbits.* [master's thesis]. San Francisco: University of the Pacific; 1986.)

Normal physiology demands precise control of the serum calcium level.[45,46,48]

Instantaneous regulation of calcium homeostasis is accomplished in seconds by selective transfer of calcium ions into and out of bone fluid (see Fig. 4.41B). Bone fluid is separated from extracellular fluid by osteoblasts or relatively thin bone-lining cells (the latter are thought to be atrophied remnants of osteoblasts). A decrease in the serum calcium level stimulates secretion of PTH, which enhances transport of calcium ions from bone fluid into osteocytes and bone-lining cells. The active metabolite of vitamin D (1,25-dihydroxy-cholecalciferol [1,25-DHCC])

enhances pumping of calcium ions from bone-lining cells into the extracellular fluid. By means of this sequence of events, calcium is transported across the bone-lining cells, resulting in a net flux of calcium ions from bone fluid to extracellular fluid. Within physiologic limits, support of calcium homeostasis is possible without resorption of bone. Radioisotope studies have confirmed that bone contains a diffuse mineral component that can be mobilized or redeposited without osteoblastic and osteoclastic activity.[24] However, a sustained negative calcium balance can be compensated for only by removing calcium from bone surfaces.[45,46]

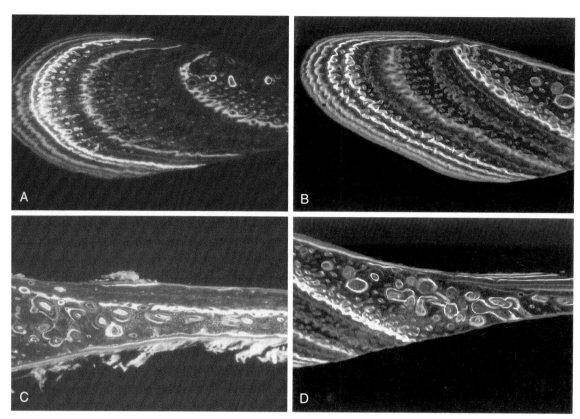

• **Fig. 4.37** (A) Fluorescent microscopy of weekly bone labels shows the patterns of anabolic modeling (bone apposition) in a rabbit. Note the diminishing space between the labels as growth slows and the animal achieves an adult skeletal form. (B) A similar section from another rabbit in the same study shows the consistency of the growth pattern. (C) In the first rabbit, the adjacent microscopic field shows several sites of bone remodeling in primary cortical bone formed about 6 to 12 weeks earlier. (D) In the second rabbit, the adjacent microscopic field shows a consistent pattern of remodeling of new cortical bone at about 6 to 12 weeks after formation. (From Noorda CB. *Modeling and Remodeling in the Cortical Bone of Both Growing and Mature Rabbits.* [master's thesis]. San Francisco: University of the Pacific; 1986.)

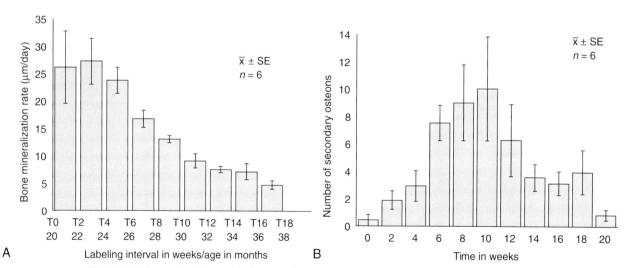

• **Fig. 4.38** (A) Age-related changes in the rate of periosteal apposition that occur in the posterior border of the mandibular ramus of the rabbit. Note the progressive decrease in the rate of periosteal bone apposition as the adolescent animals mature. (B) Remodeling of new cortical bone. The highest incidence of remodeling to secondary osteons occurs when new cortical bone is 6 to 12 weeks old. (From Noorda CB. *Modeling and Remodeling in the Cortical Bone of Both Growing and Mature Rabbits.* [master's thesis]. San Francisco: University of the Pacific; 1986.) (SE = Standard Error)

TABLE 4.1 Control Factors for Bone Modeling

Factor	Peak Load in Microstrain ($\mu\varepsilon$)[a]
Mechanical[b]	
Disuse atrophy	<200
Bone maintenance	200–2500
Physiologic hypertrophy	2500–4000
Pathologic overload	>4000
Endocrine	
Bone metabolic hormones: PTH, vitamin D, calcitonin	
Growth hormones: somatotropin, IGF-I, IGF-II	
Sex steroids: testosterone, estrogen	
Paracrine and autocrine	
Wide variety of local agents	

[a]$\mu\varepsilon$ = percent deformation × 10^{-4}.

[b]Frost's mechanostat theory.

IGF, Insulin-like growth factor; *PTH*, parathyroid hormone.

From Frost HM. Skeletal structural adaptations to mechanical usage [SATMU]. 2. Redefining Wolff's law: the remodeling problem. *Anat Rec.* 1990;226:414.

• BOX 4.1 Control Factors for Bone Remodeling

Metabolic
Parathyroid hormone: ↑ activation frequency
Estrogen: ↓ activation frequency

Mechanical
<1000 $\mu\varepsilon$: more remodeling
>2000 $\mu\varepsilon$: less remodeling

Short-term control of serum calcium levels affects rates of bone resorption and formation within minutes through the action of the three calcific hormones: PTH, 1,25-DHCC, and calcitonin. Calcitonin, a hormone produced by interstitial cells in the thyroid gland, is believed to help control hypercalcemia by transiently suppressing bone resorption. PTH, acting in concert with 1,25-DHCC, accomplishes three important tasks: (1) it enhances osteoclast recruitment from promonocyte precursors,[49] (2) it increases the resorption rate of existing osteoclasts, and (3) it may suppress the rate at which osteoblasts form bone.[45,46]

Long-term regulation of metabolism has profound effects on the skeleton. Biomechanical factors (e.g., normal function, exercise, posture, habits), noncalcific hormones (e.g., sex steroids, growth hormone), and the metabolic mechanisms previously discussed (see Figs. 4.40 and 4.41) dictate mass, geometric distribution, and the mean age of bone (Fig. 4.42). Mass and geometric distribution of bone are influenced strongly by load history (biomechanics) and sex hormone status. PTH is the primary regulator of the frequency of remodeling (Box 4.2). Because the adult skeleton is composed almost entirely of secondary (remodeled) bone, the PTH-mediated activation frequency determines mean bone age. Bone age is an important determinant of fragility because old bone presumably has been weakened by fatigue damage.[45,46]

Calcium Conservation

Calcium conservation is the aspect of bone metabolism that involves preservation of skeletal mass. A failure in calcium conservation because of one problem or a combination of metabolic and biomechanical problems may leave a patient with inadequate bone mass for reconstructive dentistry.

The kidney is the primary calcium conservation organ in the body. Through a complex series of excretion and endocrine functions, the kidney excretes excess phosphate while minimizing the loss of calcium (see Figs. 4.40 and 4.41A). A patient with impaired renal function often is a high risk for osseous manipulative procedures such as endosseous implants or orthognathic surgery. Because of its components of secondary hyperparathyroidism and impaired vitamin D metabolism, kidney disease may result in poor bone quality, which is a condition often referred to as *renal osteodystrophy*.[45,46,50]

Absorption from the small intestine is the primary source of exogenous calcium and phosphate. Phosphate is absorbed passively and rarely is deficient. Optimal calcium uptake, however, requires an active absorption mechanism. A unique factor involved in the gut absorption process is calcium-binding protein, which is formed in response to the active metabolite of vitamin D.[51] Common clinical profiles associated with poor calcium absorption include a diet deficient in dairy products, vitamin D deficiency, liver disease, and kidney problems.[16,45,46]

Under normal physiologic conditions, the body expends about 300 mg of calcium per day, primarily as a result of secretory processes in the intestines and kidneys. To maintain the serum calcium level, this 300-mg deficit must be recovered by absorption from the gut. However, absorption of calcium from the gut depends on vitamin D and is only about 30% efficient. If less than about 300 mg/day of calcium is absorbed from the intestine, the serum calcium level drops, PTH secretion ensues, and the necessary calcium is removed from the bones (see Fig. 4.40).

Positive calcium balance normally occurs during the growing period and for about 10 years thereafter. The skeletal mass of prepubertal children can be enhanced with regular calcium supplements.[52] Peak skeletal mass is attained between 25 and 30 years. After the early adult years, natural aging is associated with a slightly negative calcium balance that progressively erodes bone volume throughout life. Zero calcium balance (see Fig. 4.40) is the ideal metabolic state for maintaining skeletal mass. Preservation of bone requires a favorable diet, endocrine balance, and adequate exercise.[45,46]

Diet

Animal studies have documented endosteal bone loss of the alveolar processes of dogs maintained on a low-calcium diet.[47] These

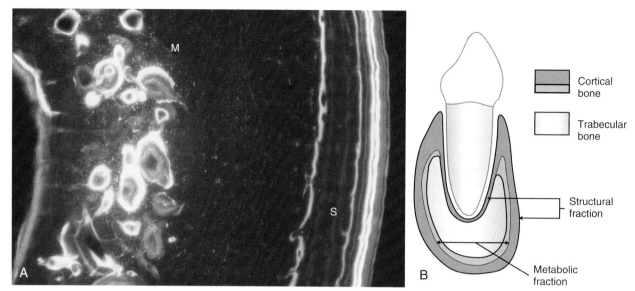

• **Fig. 4.39** (A) Structural *(S)* and metabolic *(M)* fractions of cortical bone are revealed by multiple fluoro-chrome labeling of a rabbit femur during the late growth and early adult periods. Continuing periosteal bone formation (right) contributes to structural strength, and high remodeling of the endosteal half of the compacta provides a continual supply of metabolic calcium. (B) Structural and metabolic fractions of bone in the mandible. (From Roberts WE, Garetto LP, Katona TR. Principles of orthodontic biomechanics; metabolic and mechanical control mechanisms. In: Carlson DS, Goldstein S, eds. *Bone Biodynamics in Orthodontic and Orthopedic Treatment.* Ann Arbor, MI: Center for Human Growth and Development; 1992. Craniofacial Growth Series; vol. 27.)

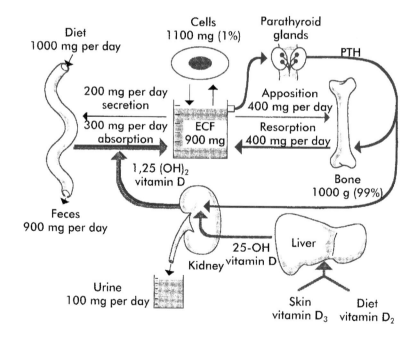

• **Fig. 4.40** Calcium metabolism is a complex physiologic process. Maintaining zero calcium balance requires optimal function of the gut, parathyroid glands, bone, liver, and kidneys. Parathyroid hormone (PTH) and the active metabolite of vitamin D, 1,25 dihydroxycholecalciferol, are the major hormones involved. (From Roberts WE, Garetto LP, Katona TR. Principles of orthodontic biomechanics; metabolic and mechanical control mechanisms. In: Carlson DS, Goldstein S, eds. *Bone Biodynamics in Orthodontic and Orthopedic Treatment.* Ann Arbor, MI: Center for Human Growth and Development; 1992. Craniofacial Growth Series; vol. 27.) (ECF = Extracellular Fluid)

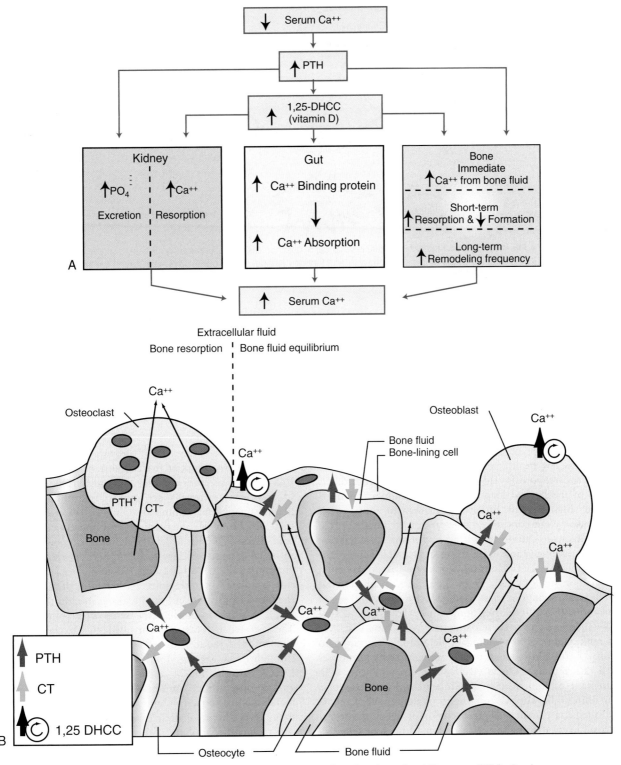

• **Fig. 4.41** (A) Flowchart of calcium homeostasis shows the roles of parathyroid hormone (PTH); vitamin D; and the kidneys, gut, and bone in maintaining serum calcium levels. Note that bone has immediate, short-term, and long-term responses. (B) PTH, the active metabolite of vitamin D (1,25 DHCC), and calcitonin (CT) play active roles in transporting ionic calcium (Ca^{++}) between the bone fluid and extracellular fluid compartments. This is the mechanism of immediate homeostatic control of the serum calcium level. (Redrawn from Roberts WE, Simmons KE, Garetto LP, DeCastro RA. Bone physiology and metabolism in dental implantology: risk factors for osteoporosis and other metabolic bone diseases. *Implant Dent.* 1992;1:11–21.)

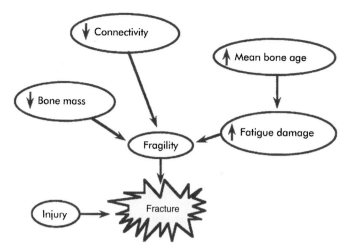

• **Fig. 4.42** Structural integrity (fracture resistance) of osseous tissue is affected by bone mass, connectivity (geometric distribution), mean bone age, and fatigue damage. Fragile bone may be fractured by normal functional loads or minor injuries.

data indicate that a low-calcium diet may have severe effects on the bones of the oral cavity. In adult humans the current recommended daily allowance of calcium is 1000 to 1500 mg/day (Table 4.2). Growing adolescents, pregnant or lactating women, and particularly pregnant teenagers, need as much as 1500 mg/day. Postmenopausal women who are not receiving estrogen replacement therapy should get 1500 mg of calcium per day. In the United States dairy products supply about 70% of dietary calcium. As previously mentioned, dietary phosphate deficiency is a rare problem.[16,27,45,46]

Obesity has few health benefits; however, it is a protective factor against osteoporosis. This most probably is a result of the high rates of mechanical loading needed to support an overweight body. Slight stature, however, is a risk factor for osteoporosis. Because weight control is a concern for the population at risk, the calcium-to-calorie ratio is an important consideration in dietary counseling (Table 4.3). The most favorable dairy products with respect to the calcium-to-calorie ratio are nonfat milk; part-skim mozzarella cheese; Swiss cheese; and plain, low-fat yogurt. Typical servings of these products have about 300 mg of calcium and 100 to 200 calories. Some adults avoid milk because of intolerance to lactose. These patients often assume that they have a milk allergy, which should be determined according to symptoms. Lactose intolerance usually is manifested by an upset stomach rather than a classic anaphylaxis. Even patients who are intolerant of milk usually can tolerate cultured products such as buttermilk, cheese, and yogurt. Calcium supplements are indicated if a patient is allergic to milk or fails to achieve a calcium-sufficient diet for any other reason. Other foods, particularly green, leafy vegetables (e.g., turnip greens, spinach), contain substantial amounts of calcium, but the calcium is tightly bound and little ionic calcium is absorbed. In effect, to consume adequate calcium in a diet that excludes dairy products is difficult.[45,46] Calcium supplements of many varieties are available in pharmacies and health food stores, and most supplements provide adequate calcium when used as directed. However, consumers should beware of toxic contaminants in some natural supplements, such as bone meal and dolomite, which may contain significant amounts of lead, arsenic, or other heavy metals.

Among the least expensive, readily tolerated supplements are calcium carbonate (e.g., Tums, calcium-rich Rolaids). To determine the amount of elemental calcium in a supplement, consumers must remember to use the molecular weight. For instance, calcium carbonate is only 40% calcium, which means that a 500-mg tablet provides only 200 mg of calcium.[45,46]

Endocrinology

Peptide hormones (e.g., PTH, growth hormone, insulin, calcitonin) bind receptors at the cell surface and may be internalized with the receptor complex. Steroid hormones (e.g., vitamin D, androgens, estrogens) are lipid soluble and pass through the plasma membrane to bind receptors in the nucleus.[45,46] PTH increases serum calcium by direct and indirect vitamin D–mediated effects. Vitamin D (cholecalciferol) originally was thought to be an essential dietary factor. However, vitamin D is not a vitamin at all; it is a hormone. Cholecalciferol is synthesized in skin irradiated by ultraviolet light, hydroxylated in the liver at the No. 25 position, and then hydroxylated in the kidney at the No. 1 position to produce the active metabolite 1,25-DHCC. The last step is feedback controlled; hydroxylation at the No. 1 position is induced by a low serum calcium level, probably through PTH (see Fig. 4.40). Clinically a major effect of 1,25-DHCC is induction of active absorption of calcium from the gut. Because of the complexity of vitamin D synthesis and the metabolic pathway, calcium absorption may be inhibited at many levels. Some of these inhibitors are (1) lack of skin exposure to adequate sunlight of the proper wavelength; (2) failure to consume vitamin D through the diet, thereby not compensating for the lack of vitamin D synthesis; (3) a genetic defect in the skin; (4) liver disease; and (5) kidney failure.[45,46]

Sex hormones have profound effects on bone. Androgens (testosterone and other anabolic steroids) build and maintain musculoskeletal mass. The primary hypertrophic effect of androgens is to increase muscle mass. The anabolic effect on bone is a secondary biomechanical response to increase loads generated by the enhanced muscle mass. Estrogen, however, has a direct effect on bone; it conserves skeletal calcium by suppressing

• BOX 4.2   Temporomandibular Discrepancies: A Case Study

A 52-year-old man sought treatment for a long history of facial pain, occlusal dysfunction, and an internal derangement of the right mandibular condyle (see figures). Intracapsular surgery was performed on the right temporomandibular joint (TMJ) accelerated, the pain increased, and a progressive anterior open bite malocclusion developed. Masticatory function deteriorated, and an internal derangement of the left TMJ was noted. Bilateral intracapsular surgery was performed to restore "normal jaw function." After the second surgical procedure, the patient suffered for 10 years with chronic pain and progressive bilateral degeneration of both TMJs. Orthodontic and orthotic (splint) therapy failed to relieve the pain and functional debilitation. The patient declined further treatment was managed with pain medication. From a physiologic perspective, intracapsular surgery usually is contraindicated because it inhibits the natural ability of the joint to adapt to changing biomechanical demands. The TMJ is a remarkably regenerative and adaptive joint if its physiologic limits are respected.

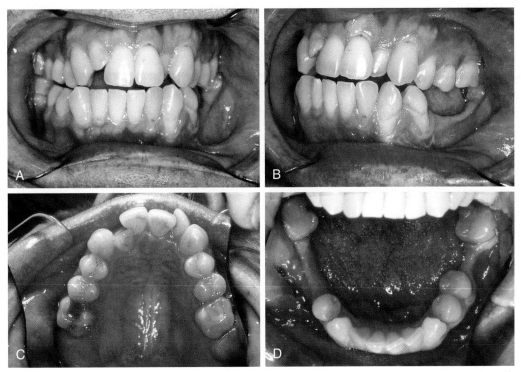

(A) Frontal view, (B) lateral view, (C) maxillary occlusal view, and (D) mandibular occlusal view of the dentition of a 52-year-old man with a partly edentulous open bite malocclusion. Note the atrophic extraction sites and gingival recession. (From Roberts WE. Adjunctive orthodontic therapy in adults over 50 years of age: clinical management of compensated, partially edentulous malocclusion. *J Indiana Dent Assoc.* 1997;76:33–41.)

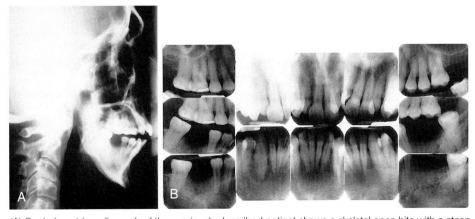

(A) Cephalometric radiograph of the previously described patient shows a skeletal open bite with a steep mandibular plane and a relatively short ramus. The thin symphyseal cortex is consistent with a systemic osteopenia. (B) A full-mouth radiographic survey shows a generalized lack of cortical bone at the alveolar crest and a pattern of indistinct lamina dura and trabeculae. This generalized ground-glass approach of the alveolar bone is consistent with high-turnover metabolic bone disease. (From Roberts WE. Adjunctive orthodontic therapy in adults over 50 years of age: clinical management of compensated, partially edentulous malocclusion. *J Indiana Dent Assoc.* 1997;76:33–41.)

TABLE 4.2 Dietary Calcium Recommendations

Group	Age	Dosage (mg/day)
Infants	Birth–6 months	400
	6–12 months	600
Children	1–5 years	800
	6–10 years	800–1200
Adolescents and young adults	11–24 years	1200–1500
Men	25–65 years	1000
Women	25–50 years	1000
Pregnant or lactating	—	1200–1500
Postmenopausal		
Receiving estrogen replacement therapy	—	1000
Not receiving estrogen replacement therapy	—	1500
Men and women	>65 years	1500

From National Institutes of Health. *Consensus statement: optimal calcium intake;* 1994.

TABLE 4.3 Calcium and Calorie Content of Common Dairy Products

Product	Calcium (mg)	Calories	Ratio (calcium:calories)
Milk			
Whole, 3.3% fat, 1 cup	291	150	1.9:1
Low-fat, 2% fat, 1 cup	297	120	2.5:1
Buttermilk, 1 cup	285	100	2.8:1
Skim milk, 0% fat, 1 cup[a]	302	85	3.6:1
Cheese			
American, pasteurized process, 1 ounce	174	104	1.7:1
Cheddar, 1 ounce	204	115	1.8:1
Cottage, creamed, 4% fat, 1 cup	135	235	0.6:1
Cottage, low-fat, 2%, 1 cup	155	205	0.8:1
Monterey Jack, 1 ounce	212	106	2.0:1
Mozzarella, part-skim, 1 ounce[a]	207	80	2.6:1
Swiss, 1 ounce[a]	272	105	2.6:1
Yogurt			
Plain, low-fat, 8 ounces	415	145	2.9:1
Plain, nonfat, 8 ounces[a]	452	125	3.6:1
Fruit, low-fat, 8 ounces	345	230	1.5:1

[a]Food or foods with most favorable calcium-to-calorie ratios in each category.

Data provided by the American Dairy Association.

the activation frequency of bone remodeling.[53] At menopause, enhanced remodeling activation increases turnover.[54] Because a slight negative calcium balance is associated with each remodeling event, a substantial increase in the turnover rate can result in rapid bone loss, leading to symptomatic osteoporosis. Even young women are susceptible to significant bone loss if the menstrual cycle (menses) stops.[55] Bone loss is a common problem in women who have low body fat and who exercise intensely (e.g., running, gymnastics) and in women who are anorexic.[56] Clearly, estrogen protects the female skeleton from bone loss during the childbearing years. Lack of menses in women of any age is a high-risk factor for the development of osteoporosis later in life.[45,46]

Estrogen replacement therapy is widely recommended for calcium conservation and the prevention of osteoporosis in postmenopausal women.[57,58] A major concern of many patients and of some physicians is the relationship of estrogen therapy to the incidence and progression of breast cancer.[59] It generally is accepted that estrogen replacement therapy increases the risk of breast cancer by about 2% but decreases the risk of osteoporosis, heart disease, colon cancer, and Alzheimer's disease by as much as 50%. For many women, estrogen replacement therapy remains a wise health measure.

The antiestrogen tamoxifen is used to treat some forms of breast cancer. Fortunately, in postmenopausal women, tamoxifen has a beneficial effect on bone similar to that of estrogen.[60] Recently raloxifene (Evista) has been shown to reduce the risk of osteoporosis and heart disease without increasing the risk of breast cancer. Some studies have even shown a substantial anticancer protective effect.[61]

Skeletal Compromise

Skeletal health is related to diet, exercise, lifestyle, and proper functioning of numerous organ systems. To provide optimal support over a broad spectrum of conditions, the skeletal system has evolved complex mechanical, endocrine, and cell-level regulatory mechanisms. A failure of one or more of these homeostatic mechanisms can result in metabolic bone disease. Low skeletal mass and/or poor osteogenic capability may make some patients poor candidates for orthodontic or orthognathic procedures. Skeletally compromised patients who seek unrelated dental treatment provide dentists with unique diagnostic opportunities. Timely medical referral of individuals with high-risk profiles can result in substantial health benefits. If osteopenia is confirmed, corrective medical therapy can be started before the onset of the debilitating symptoms associated with osteoporosis.[45,46]

The concept of structural and metabolic fractions (see Fig. 4.39) has considerable clinical significance. The dietary requirement for calcium increases during the growing years. A high dietary calcium intake (1200 mg/day) is essential during the adolescent period (see Table 4.2) to provide structural strength without compromising the metabolic reserve. Pregnancy and lactation before the age of 19 may be precipitating factors for osteopenia later in life. Multiple births during the teenage years are of particular concern. Under these circumstances, young women may fail to deposit sufficient skeletal reserves to withstand the sustained negative calcium balance that follows menopause.[45,46,61]

Although the metabolic fraction of cortical bone can make a substantial contribution, the major source of serum calcium under steady-state conditions is trabecular bone. The primary reason for this is the differential remodeling rates. Cortical bone turns over about 2% to 10% per year, whereas trabecular bone, which is much more active, remodels at 20% to 30% per year.[62] Because it is more labile, trabecular bone is more susceptible to loss under conditions of negative calcium balance. For this reason, patients with osteoporosis have a tendency to suffer structural failure at sites primarily dependent on trabecular bone: the spine (compression fracture), the wrist (Colles' fracture), and the hip (femoral neck fracture). Degenerative changes in the TMJ have not been related directly to skeletal atrophy. However, some relationship is likely because these problems tend to affect the same high-risk group (postmenopausal women).[45,46,63]

Women depend on estrogen to maintain skeletal mass. Lack of normal menses, even in young women, usually indicates an estrogen deficiency and probable negative calcium balance. Numerous national and international consensus conferences[64,57] have recommended that most postmenopausal white and Asian women should be treated with estrogen to prevent osteoporosis. Surveys indicate that some physicians fail to prescribe estrogen for their postmenopausal patients[65]; however, the most common problem is the failure of many women to comply despite the recommendations of their physicians. For this reason many women in Western society are estrogen deficient. About 20% will develop frank osteoporosis, and as many as 50% will have some signs or symptoms.[46] All health care providers should be concerned particularly about the skeletal status of postmenopausal white and Asian women. However, even low-risk groups, such as men and black women, have an incidence of osteoporosis that approaches 5%. Osteopenia and osteoporosis therefore are significant health risks for almost everyone. Bone metabolic evaluation is an important diagnostic concern for all patients being considered for dental implants or any other bone-manipulative therapy.[16,45,66]

Metabolic Bone Disease

Osteoporosis is a generic term for low bone mass (osteopenia). The most important risk factor for the development of osteoporosis is age: after the third decade, osteopenia is related directly to longevity. Other high-risk factors are (1) a history of long-term glucocorticoid treatment, (2) slight stature, (3) smoking, (4) menopause or dysmenorrhea, (5) lack of or little physical activity, (6) low-calcium diet, (7) excessive consumption of alcohol, (8) vitamin D deficiency, (9) kidney failure, (10) liver disease (cirrhosis), and (11) a history of fractures. These risk factors are effective in identifying 78% of those with the potential for osteopenia.[61,67] This is a particularly good screening method for skeletally asymptomatic dental patients. However, one must realize that more than 20% of individuals who eventually develop osteoporosis have a negative history for known risk factors. Any clinical signs or symptoms of low bone mass (e.g., low radiographic density of the jaws, thin cortices, excessive bone resorption) are grounds for referral. A thorough medical workup, including bone mineral density measurement, usually is necessary to establish the diagnosis of osteopenia. The term *osteoporosis* usually is reserved for patients with evidence of fracture or other osteoporotic symptoms. The treatment of metabolic bone diseases such as osteoporosis depends on the causative factors. Physicians specifically trained in bone metabolism best handle medical management of these often complex disorders.[45,46]

Because the loss of teeth is an important risk factor for osteoporosis, dental patients, especially adult women, are at high risk for developing osteoporosis. A sampling of all adult female dental patients at a midwestern dental school showed that about 65% were at high risk for developing osteoporosis (estrogen deficient or had at least two other risk factors).[68]

See Box 4.1 for a relevant case study.

Biomechanics

Gravitational loads have a substantial influence on normal skeletal physiology. Osteoblast differentiation that leads to new bone formation is stimulated by mechanical loading[12] but inhibited by weightlessness.[28,69] Space flight studies have established that gravity helps maintain skeletal mass.[70,71] A substantial part of the physiologic loading of the mandible is related to antigravity posturing. In erect posture, gravity tends to open the mouth; muscular force is used to hold the mouth closed. Apparently, growth of the rat mandibular condyle may be inhibited during space flight because of weightlessness and the decrease in functional loading.[72] Gravity may prove to be an important factor in the secondary growth mechanism of the mandible.

Mechanical loading is essential to skeletal health. Control of most bone modeling (see Table 4.1) and some remodeling processes are related to strain history, which usually is defined in microstrain ($\mu\varepsilon$).[73] Repetitive loading generates a specific response, which is determined by the peak strain.[74-78] In an attempt to simplify the often conflicting data, Frost[79] proposed the mechanostat theory. Reviewing the theoretical basis of this theory, Martin and Burr[24] proposed that (1) subthreshold loading of less than 200 $\mu\varepsilon$ results in disuse atrophy, manifested as a decrease in modeling and an increase in remodeling; (2) physiologic loading of about 200 to 2500 $\mu\varepsilon$ is associated with normal, steady-state activities; (3) loads exceeding the minimal effective strain (about 2500 $\mu\varepsilon$) result in a hypertrophic increase in modeling and a concomitant decrease in remodeling; and (4) after peak strains exceed about 4000 $\mu\varepsilon$, the structural integrity of bone is threatened, resulting in pathologic overload. Fig. 4.43 is a representation of the mechanostat. Many of the concepts and microstrain levels are based on experimental data.[24] The strain range for each given response probably varies between species and may be site specific in the same individual.[16,24,74,76,78] However, the mechanostat provides a useful clinical reference for the hierarchy of biomechanical responses to applied loads.

Normal function helps build and maintain bone mass. Suboptimally loaded bones atrophy as a result of increased remodeling frequency and inhibition of osteoblast formation.[80] Under these conditions, trabecular connections are lost and cortices are thinned from the endosteal surface. Eventually the skeleton is weakened until it cannot sustain normal function. Assuming that the negative calcium balance is corrected and adequate bone structure remains, patients with a history of osteoporosis or other metabolic bone disease are viable candidates for reconstructive dental procedures. The crucial factor is the residual bone mass in the area of interest after the disease process has been arrested (Fig. 4.44).

When flexure (strain) exceeds the normal physiologic range, bones compensate by adding new mineralized tissue at the periosteal surface. Adding bone is an essential compensating mechanism because of the inverse relationship between load (strain magnitude) and the fatigue resistance of bone.[81] When loads are less

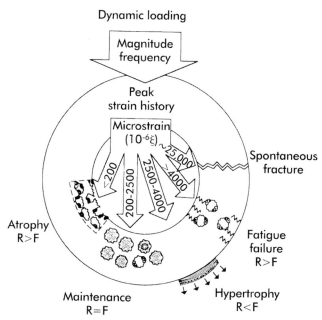

• **Fig. 4.43** Mechanostat concept of Frost as defined by Martin and Burr. Bone formation *(F)* and resorption *(R)* are the modeling phenomena that change the shape and/or form of a bone. The peak strain history determines whether atrophy, maintenance, hypertrophy, or fatigue failure occurs. Note that the normal physiologic range of loading (maintenance *R = F*) is only at less than 10% of maximal bone strength (spontaneous fracture). Fatigue damage can accumulate rapidly at greater than 4000 $\mu\varepsilon$.

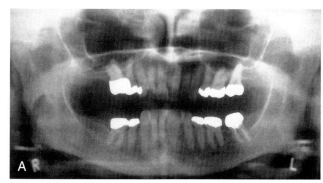

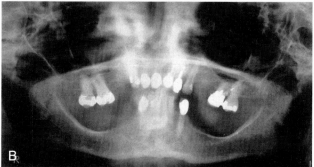

• **Fig. 4.44** Two postmenopausal females with systemic osteopenia present widely varying patterns of lower posterior bone loss. (A) Alveolar bone in the buccal segments is well preserved by functional loading of natural teeth. (B) Severe resorption of the alveolar process and basilar mandible has occurred in the absence of adequate functional loading. (From Roberts WE. Fundamental principles of bone physiology, metabolism and loading. In: Naert I, van Steenberghe D, Worthington P, eds. *Osseointegration in Oral Rehabilitation: an Introductory Textbook.* London: Quintessence; 1993.)

than 2000 με, lamellar bone can withstand millions of loading cycles, more than a lifetime of normal function. However, increasing the cyclic load to 5000 με (about 20% of the ultimate strength of cortical bone) can produce fatigue failure in 1000 cycles, which is achieved easily in only a few weeks of normal activity. Repetitive overload at less than one-fifth of the ultimate strength of lamellar bone (25,000 με, or 2.5% deformation) can lead to skeletal failure, stress fractures, and shin splints.

From a dental perspective, occlusal prematurities or parafunction may lead to compromise of periodontal bone support. Localized fatigue failure may be a factor in periodontal clefting, alveolar recession, tooth oblation (cervical ditching), or TMJ arthrosis. Guarding against occlusal prematurities and excessive tooth mobility, while achieving an optimal distribution of occlusal loads, are important objectives for orthodontic treatment. The human masticatory apparatus can achieve a biting strength of more than 2200 N, or more than 500 pounds of force.[82,83] Because of the high magnitude and frequency of oral loads, functional prematurities during reconstructive treatment could contribute to isolated incidences of alveolar clefting (Fig. 4.45A) and root resorption (see Fig. 4.45B). Excessive tooth mobility should be monitored carefully. Prevention of occlusal prematurities is a particular concern in treating periodontally compromised teeth.

Sutures

The facial sutures are important mediators of skeletal adaptation to craniofacial growth and biomechanical therapy. Expansion of the midpalatal suture often is a key objective in dentofacial orthopedic treatment. Although the potential for sutural expansion has been appreciated since the middle of the 19th century, Haas[84] introduced the modern clinical concepts of rapid palatal expansion in the last half of the 20th century. Despite the long history of this important clinical procedure, little was known of the cell kinetics of osteogenesis and the bone remodeling response associated with it. Sutures and the PDL were widely assumed to have similar mechanisms of osseous adaptation.

Chang and colleagues[85,86] compared the osteogenic reaction in the expanded midpalatal suture with orthodontically induced osteogenesis in the PDL of adjacent incisors (Figs. 4.46–4.49). The widened PDL resulted in direct osteogenic induction of new bone, whereas the adjacent expanded suture experienced hemorrhage, necrosis, and a wound-healing response. Vascular invasion of the blood clot in the expanded suture was a prerequisite for new bone formation. Chang and colleagues[85] also defined the angiogenic capillary budding process associated with the propagation of perivascular osteogenic cells (Fig. 4.50). After its vascularity had been reestablished, the expanded midpalatal suture and adjacent widened PDL produced new osteoblasts by the same mechanism. Pericytes, the osteogenic cells that are perivascular to the venules (Fig. 4.51), are the cells of origin for preosteoblasts.[85,86] The role of perivascular cells in the origin of PDL osteoblasts first was reported in 1987.[87] Over the last decade a number of investigators have reported the same mechanism for the production of osteoblasts throughout the body. Doherty and colleagues[88] recently reviewed the literature and provided evidence that vascular pericytes express osteogenic potential in vivo and in vitro. What is now clear is that perivascular osteogenesis is not a mechanism unique to the PDL and sutures; rather, it is the source of osteoblasts all over the body under a variety of osteogenic conditions. Parr and colleagues[89] used an innovative endosseous implant mechanism (see Fig. 4.17) to expand the nasal bones in young adult rabbits with forces from 1 to 3 N. Injection of multiple fluorochrome bone labels documented the bone-modeling and remodeling

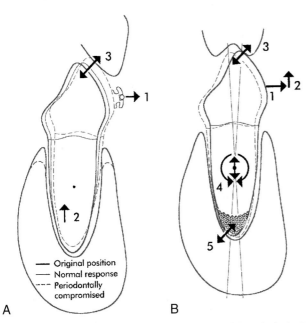

• **Fig. 4.45** (A) A moderate load in the buccal direction *(1)* results in tipping displacement of the crown. In the absence of vertical constraint, a normal healthy tooth would be expected to extrude slightly because of the inclined plane effect of the root engaging the tapered alveolus *(2)*. As a result of diminished bone support and destruction of restraining collagen fibers at the alveolar crest, a periodontally compromised tooth may tip and extrude considerably more. Depending on the occlusion, this displacement may cause an occlusal prematurity *(3)*. (B) Orthodontic tipping *(1)* with an extrusive component *(2)* may produce an occlusal prematurity *(3)* and mobility *(4)*. An individual tooth in chronic occlusal trauma is expected to fatigue the root apex continuously. This combination of physical failure in a catabolic environment may lead to progressive root resorption *(5)*.

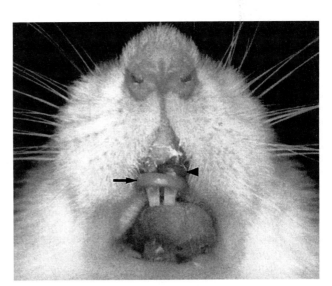

• **Fig. 4.46** Expansion appliance placed on the maxillary incisors of a rat. A 1-mm-diameter elastomeric ring *(arrowhead)* was fitted into the left incisor; a 2-mm-diameter elastomeric ring *(arrow)* encircled both incisors, 2 mm from cutting edges. The 2-mm ring constricts the incisors, whereas the interproximal elastic elicits a parallel separation of the interpremaxillary suture. (From Chang HN, Garetto LP, et al. Angiogenesis and osteogenesis in an orthopedically expanded suture. *Am J Orthod Dentofacial Orthop.* 1997;3:382–390.)

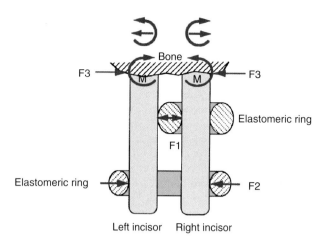

• **Fig. 4.47** Forces *(F)* and moments *(M)* on a tooth. F1 and F2 were produced by inner and outer elastomeric rings, respectively. This illustration of the device demonstrates the formation of a couple that resulted in parallel separation of the interpremaxillary suture. As measured in a pilot study using a Dontrix tension gauge, the outer elastomeric ring exerted about 200 g of initial separation force (F2), of which 90 g remained at the end of day 3. This force level (90 g) is suitable for premaxillary expansion in rats. (From Chang HN, Garetto LP, Potter RH, et al. Angiogenesis and osteogenesis in an orthopedically expanded suture. *Am J Orthod Dentofacial Orthop.* 1997;3:382–390.)

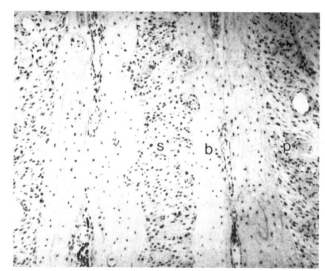

• **Fig. 4.49** Photomicrograph of a sagittal section of the interpremaxillary suture, showing the relationship of expanded suture *(s)*, alveolar bone *(b)*, and periodontal ligament *(p)*. (Stained with hematoxylin and eosin; original magnification ×40.) (From Chang HN, Garetto LP, Potter RH, et al. Angiogenesis and osteogenesis in an orthopedically expanded suture. *Am J Orthod Dentofacial Orthop.* 1997;3:382–390.)

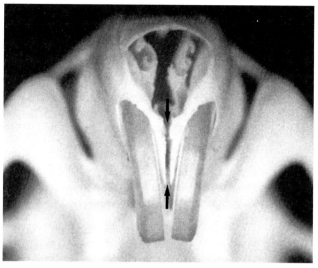

• **Fig. 4.48** Dry skull, expanded as illustrated in Fig. 4.55, shows parallel separation of the interpremaxillary suture *(arrow)*. (From Chang HN, Garetto LP, Potter RH, et al. Angiogenesis and osteogenesis in an orthopedically expanded suture. *Am J Orthod Dentofacial Orthop.* 1997;3:382–390.)

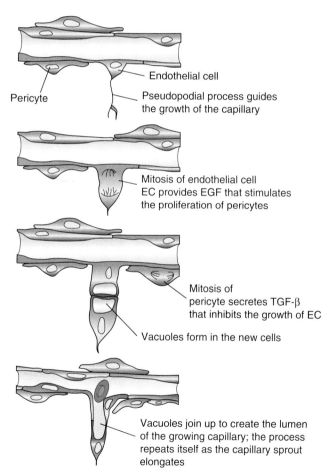

• **Fig. 4.50** Angiogenesis involves a well-defined sequence of capillary budding followed by an extension of the perivascular network of pericytes, which are the source of osteoprogenitor cells. *EC,* Endothelial cell; *EGF,* epidermal growth factor; *TGF-β,* transforming growth factor β. (Redrawn from Chang HN, Garetto LP, Katona TR, Potter RH, Roberts WE. Angiogenic induction and cell migration in an orthopedically expanded maxillary suture in the rat. *Arch Oral Biol.* 1996;41:985–994.)

reactions that occurred not only adjacent to the suture but also throughout the nasal bones. Expansion of a suture results in a regional adaptation of adjacent bones similar to the postoperative regional acceleratory phenomenon that is characteristic of bone wound healing.[24] Parr and colleagues[89] described the bone formation rate and mineral apposition rate for new bone formed in the suture (Figs. 4.52–4.54). Sutural expansion, relative to load decay, is shown for repeatedly reactivated 1- to 3-N loads (Fig. 4.55). Osseointegrated implants were excellent abutments for sutural expansion mediated by loads as large as 3 N.

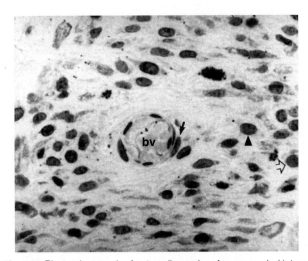

• **Fig. 4.51** Photomicrograph of autoradiography of an expanded interpremaxillary suture, showing blood vessel *(bv)* and paravascular cells. Note the relationship of pericyte *(solid arrow)*, fibroblast-like cells *(arrowhead)*, and mature osteoblast *(open arrow)* lining the suture-bone interface. (Stained with hematoxylin and eosin; original magnification ×400.) (From Chang HN, Garetto LP, Potter RH, et al. Angiogenesis and osteogenesis in an orthopedically expanded suture. *Am J Orthod Dentofacial Orthop.* 1997;3:382–390.)

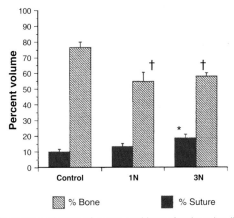

• **Fig. 4.53** Volume percent of suture and bone for three loading groups (mean ± SEM); an asterisk *(*)* indicates significant difference in the percentage of sutural expansion from the control at $p < 0.05$; a dagger *(†)* indicates significant difference in the percentage of bone from the control at $p < 0.05$. (From Parr JA, Garetto LP, Wohlford ME, Arbuckle GR, Roberts WE. Sutural expansion using rigidly integrated endosseous implants: an experimental study in rabbits. *Angle Orthod.* 1978;67:283–290.)

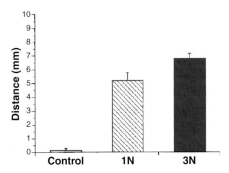

• **Fig. 4.52** Expansion of the suture between the nasal bones of a rabbit (see Fig. 4.17A) is expressed as the mean difference of initial and final measurements between implants for the three loading groups (mean ± SEM, all groups significant at $p < 0.05$). (From Parr JA, Garetto LP, Wohlford ME, Arbuckle GR, Roberts WE. Sutural expansion using rigidly integrated endosseous implants: an experimental study in rabbits. *Angle Orthod.* 1978;67:283–290.)

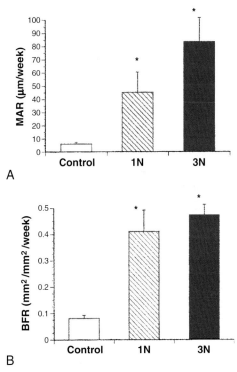

• **Fig. 4.54** (A) Mineral apposition rate (MAR). (B) Bone formation rate (BFR) was calculated at the suture during the final 6 weeks of loading for three loading groups (mean ± SEM; an asterisk *[*]* indicates significant difference from the control at $p < 0.05$). (From Parr JA, Garetto LP, Wohlford ME, Arbuckle GR, Roberts WE. Sutural expansion using rigidly integrated endosseous implants: an experimental study in rabbits. *Angle Orthod.* 1978;67:283–290.)

Overall, expanded sutures are less efficient at initiating osteogenesis because of postactivation necrosis. However, after a wound-healing response has occurred to reestablish sutural vitality, the vascularly mediated origin of osteoblasts is the same as for the PDL and other skeletal sites. Expansion of a suture results in a regional acceleration of bone adaptive activity, which allows for extensive adaptation of the affected bones to new biomechanical conditions. These results indicate that sutural expansion within physiologic limits is a clinically viable means of repositioning the bones of the craniofacial complex to improve esthetics and function. With respect to fundamental bone physiology, sutural expansion is similar to surgically mediated distraction osteogenesis.

Using sequential labels of ^{3}H-thymidine and bromodeoxyuridine in rabbits, Sim[90] demonstrated that the osteoblast histogenesis sequence for evolving secondary osteons was a perivascular process (Fig. 4.56) similar to that previously demonstrated for the PDL[91] and the intermaxillary suture.[85,86] The Sim data confirmed the hypothesis that the perivascular connective tissue cells proliferate and migrate along the surface of the invading capillaries or venules. Fig. 4.57 is a three-dimensional perspective of a remodeling foci (cutting/filling cone) in cortical bone, which

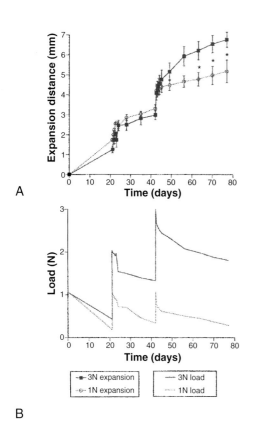

A

B

• **Fig. 4.55** (A) Sutural expansion measured as an increase in the distance between implants. The slope of this curve is the rate of sutural expansion; 3 N is significantly greater than 1 N at these time points $p < 0.05$. (B) Load on the suture as a function of time. Load was calculated using the formula $F = kx$, where k is the spring constant and x is the distance between implants. As sutural expansion occurs, force decays. Loads were placed at day 0 and adjusted at days 21 and 42. (From Parr JA, Garetto LP, Wohlford ME, Arbuckle GR, Roberts WE. Sutural expansion using rigidly integrated endosseous implants: an experimental study in rabbits. *Angle Orthod.* 1978;67:283–290.)

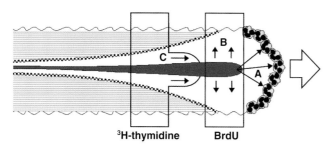

• **Fig. 4.56** Cutting/filling cone in rabbit cortical bone shows the intravascular origin of osteoclasts (A). The perivascular proliferation and migration away for the perivascular surface (B) is demonstrated by bromodeoxyuridine (BrdU) labeling and nuclear volume morphometry. A sequence of ^{3}H-thymidine labels from 2 to 72 hours before sacrifice and nuclear morphometric analysis revealed migration of proliferating perivascular cells in the direction of vascular invasion (C). These data demonstrate the perivascular origin of osteoblasts in evolving secondary osteons. (From Sim Y. *Cell Kinetics of Osteoblast Histogenesis in Evolving Rabbit Secondary Haversian Systems Using a Double Labeling Technique with ^{3}H-thymidine and Bromodeoxyuridine.* [doctoral thesis]. Indianapolis: Indiana University School of Dentistry; 1995.)

demonstrates that perivascular cells, near the head of the proliferating blood vessel, are the source of osteoblasts for the filling cone. Confirmation of a perivascular origin of osteoblasts in PDL,

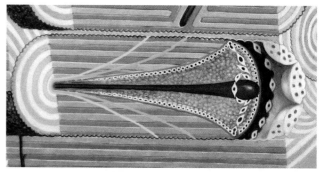

• **Fig. 4.57** Evolving secondary osteon, moving to the right, shows a head of multinucleated osteoclasts (right), followed by a layer of mononuclear cells secreting cement substance (blue) to cover the scalloped resorption arrest line. The perivascular osteogenic cells proliferate and differentiate to osteoblasts, which form the new secondary osteon. Three sequential colored bone labels (yellow, green, and orange) allow the calculation of the velocity of the cutting/filling cone through cortical bone.

sutures, and cortical bone remodeling foci strongly suggests that all osteoblasts, at least in the peripheral skeleton, are derived from perivascular precursors. These data suggest that less differentiated osteogenic cells grow along the surface of bone-related blood vessels (capillaries and venules) as they invade blood clots or other connective tissue spaces in preparation for osteogenesis. From a clinical perspective, the perivascular origin of osteoblasts confirms an important surgical principle: preservation of the blood supply is essential for optimal healing of bone.

Implant-Anchored Orthodontics

A major problem in orthodontics and facial orthopedics is anchorage control.[30] Undesirable movement of the anchorage units is a common problem that limits the therapeutic range of biomechanics.[92] An important application of the basic principles of bone physiology is the use of rigid endosseous implants for orthodontic and orthopedic anchorage. Animal studies[25] and clinical trials of custom orthodontic devices[34] have established that rigidly integrated implants do not move in response to conventional orthodontic and orthopedic forces. These devices are opening new horizons in the management of asymmetry, mutilated dentition, severe malocclusion, and craniofacial deformity.[93]

A preclinical study in dogs tested the anchorage potential of two prosthetic-type titanium implants: (1) a prototype of an endosseous device with a cervical post, asymmetric threads, and an acid-etched surface and (2) a commercially available implant with symmetric threads (Fig. 4.58). Based on label incidence (Fig. 4.59A) and the relative number of new osteons in microradiographs (see Fig. 4.59B), the rate of bone remodeling near the implant was higher compared with the basilar mandible only a few millimeters away.[94] Compared with titanium implants with a smooth surface, the degree of remodeling at the interface is greater for threaded implants placed in a tapped bone preparation.[30] This may be related to the increased resistance of threaded implants to torsional loads over time.[95]

Direct bone apposition at the endosseous interface results in rigid fixation (osseointegration).[96] From an anchorage perspective, a rigid endosseous implant is the functional equivalent of an ankylosed tooth. Complete bony encapsulation is not necessary for an implant to serve as a rigid anchorage unit. The crucial feature is indefinite maintenance of rigidity despite continuous orthodontic loads. Over time, orthodontically loaded implants achieve

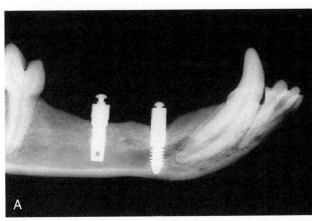
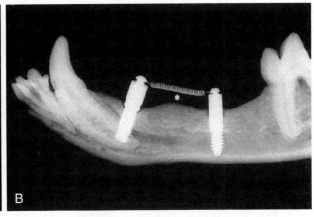

• **Fig. 4.58** (A) Two titanium implants of different design were placed in the partly edentulous mandible of young adult dogs. (B) After 2 months of unloaded healing, a 3-N compressive load was applied between the implants for 4 months. Increased periosteal apposition *(*)* was noted between the implants of some dogs. None of the rigidly integrated fixtures was loosened by the continuous load superimposed on function. (From Roberts WE, Helm FR, Marshall KJ, Gongloff RK. Rigid endosseous implants for orthodontic and orthopedic anchorage. *Angle Orthod.* 1989;59:247–256.)

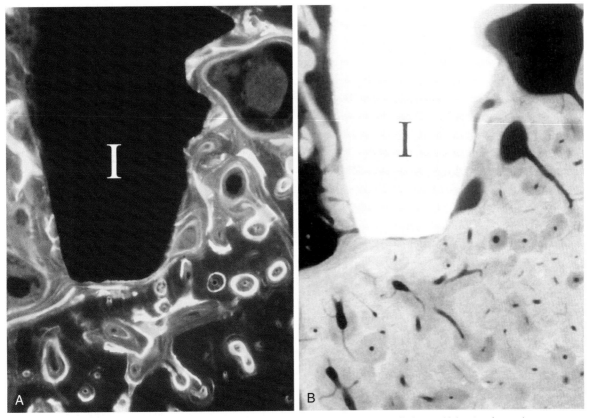

• **Fig. 4.59** (A) Multiple fluorochrome labels in bone adjacent to an implant *(I)* show a high rate of remodeling at the bone-implant surface. (B) Microradiographic image of the same section shows direct bone contact on the surface of the implant. (From Roberts WE, Garotto LP, Katona TR. Principle of orthodontic biomechanics: metabolic and mechanical control mechanisms. In: Carlson DS, Goldstein SA, eds. *Bone Biodynamics in Orthodontic and Orthopedic Treatment.* Ann Arbor, MI: University of Michigan Press; 1992.)

a greater fraction of direct osseous interface.[34,95] From an orthodontic and orthopedic perspective, titanium implants can resist substantial continuous loads (1–3 N superimposed on function) indefinitely. Histologic analysis with multiple fluorochrome labels and microradiography confirm that rigidly integrated implants do not move relative to adjacent bone (see Fig. 4.59).[25] By definition, maintaining a fixed relationship with supporting bone is true osseous anchorage. Endosseous (osseointegrated) implants are well suited to many demanding orthodontic applications.[30,34]

Routine use of rigid implants for prosthetic or orthodontic applications requires that fixtures are placed between or near the roots of teeth. Inadvertent impingement on the PDL and the root of an adjacent tooth still may provide an acceptable result (Fig. 4.60). Cementum repair occurs where the root is cut, the PDL

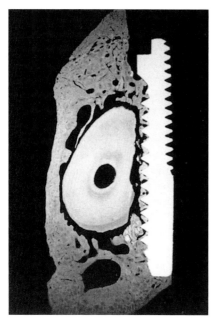

• **Fig. 4.60** Endosseous implant inadvertently impinged on the root of a canine. The implant successfully integrated with bone and served as a rigid anchor for orthopedic loading. (From Roberts WE, Helm FR, Marshall KJ, Gongloff RK. Rigid endosseous implants for orthodontic and orthopedic anchorage. *Angle Orthod.* 1989;59:247–256.)

reorganizes, and the implant surface is integrated rigidly with osseous tissue. No evidence exists of ankylosis of the tooth.[25]

Retromolar Implant Anchorage

The isolated loss of a lower first molar with a retained third molar is a common problem. Rather than extract the third molar and replace the first molar with a three-unit bridge, mesial translation of second and third molars to close the edentulous spaces often is preferable (Fig. 4.61). The first case with long-term follow-up has been published.[34] Because of the increasing incidence of progressive bone loss and fatigue fracture associated with single-tooth implants in lower first and second molar areas, the orthodontic option for mesially translating the molars to close the space is increasing in popularity.

External Abutment Mechanism

An anchorage wire that is secured to a retromolar implant can be used to intrude and protract mandibular second and third molars to close an atrophic first molar extraction site (see Fig. 4.61B).[16] The tipping and extrusion of residual lower molars limits potential orthodontic repositioning. Rigid retromolar implants offer a unique capability for intrusion and alignment. Fig. 4.62 demonstrates the mechanics for achieving three-dimensional control to intrude the third molar to the plane of occlusion and translate

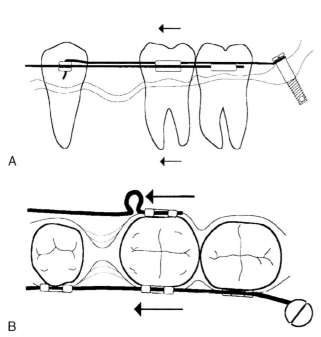

• **Fig. 4.61** (A) Mechanics of using a retromolar implant with an external abutment as anchorage to stabilize the premolar anterior to an extraction site. (B) Using buccal and lingual mechanics to balance the load and shield the periosteum in the extraction site, the atrophic extraction site is closed without periodontal compromise of any of the adjacent teeth. (From Roberts WE, Garotto LP, Katona TR. Principle of orthodontic biomechanics: metabolic and mechanical control mechanisms. In: Carlson DS, Goldstein SA, eds. *Bone Biodynamics in Orthodontic and Orthopedic Treatment.* Ann Arbor, MI: University of Michigan Press; 1992.)

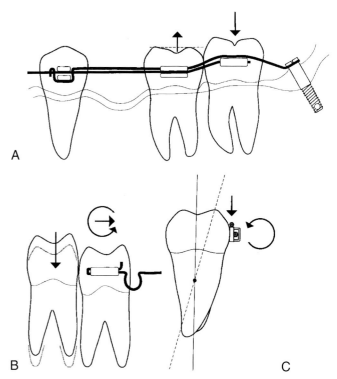

• **Fig. 4.62** (A) The mechanics of intruding a third molar with implant anchorage before space closure. (B) Removable lingual arch prevents extrusion of the second molar. (C) Because the intrusive force on the third molar is buccal to the center of resistance, the tooth tends to tip buccally. This problem is controlled by placing lingual crown torque in the rectangular wire inserted in the tube. (From Roberts WE, Garotto LP, Katona TR. Principle of orthodontic biomechanics: metabolic and mechanical control mechanisms. In: Carlson DS, Goldstein SA, eds. *Bone Biodynamics in Orthodontic and Orthopedic Treatment.* Ann Arbor, MI: University of Michigan Press; 1992.)

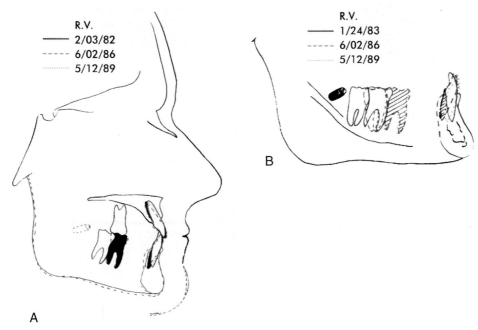

• **Fig. 4.63** (A) Pretreatment, finish, and 3-year postretention cephalometric tracings document 10 to 12 mm of molar translation to close an atrophic first molar extraction site. (B) Mandibular superimposition shows the mesial movement of the second and third molars, as well as lingual root torque of the lower incisors. (From Roberts WE, Marshall KJ, Mozsary PG. Rigid endosseous implant utilized as anchorage to protract molars and close an atrophic extraction site. *Angle Orthod.* 1990;60:135–152.)

both teeth mesially. Cephalometric tracings (Fig. 4.63) document the more than 10 mm of mesial translation and its stability. Panoramic radiographs show the initial alignment (Fig. 4.64A) and the final space closure (see Fig. 4.64B). Clinical details are published.[34]

Histologic analysis of implants recovered after completion of treatment has revealed important information about the continuous remodeling process that maintains the rigid integration and anchorage value of the endosseous device. Two intravital bone labels, administered within 2 weeks of implant recovery, have shown a continuing high rate of bone remodeling (more than 500% per year) within 1 mm of the implant surface (see Fig. 4.64C–D). This biological mechanism apparently is the means by which rigid osseous integration is maintained indefinitely.[8,34] If no fracture is present at the implant interface or in its supporting bone, rigid implants are not moved by orthodontic loads.[6,25,34] Well-integrated endosseous implants remain rigid despite continued remodeling of the bone supporting them because only a portion of the osseous resorbed interface is turned over at any given time.[34] Fig. 4.65 shows the mechanics for mesial translation of molars to close an edentulous space when a premolar is congenitally missing. Rigid endosseous implants show great promise for considerably extending the therapeutic possibilities of orthodontics and dentofacial orthopedics.

Internal Abutment Mechanism

The 0.019 × 0.025-inch titanium-molybdenum alloy anchorage wire (Ormco Corporation, Orange, California) is secured to the endosseous implant when the implant is placed (Fig. 4.66). A 7 to 10 × 3.75-mm Brånemark implant (Nobel Biocare, Gothenburg, Sweden) is placed in the retromolar area 3 to 5 mm buccal and distal to the terminal molar. The end of the anchorage wire is bent into a circle and firmly attached to the implant with a standard healing cap (Figs. 4.67 and 4.68). This "internal abutment" approach offers a number of advantages over the original external abutment method as follows:

- Minimal surgery: no postoperative uncovering is required.
- Less expense: only one surgical procedure is needed, and no transmucosal abutment is required.
- Better hygiene: wire exiting in the depth of the buccal fold requires little or no periodontal maintenance.
- Immediate loading: no healing period is necessary.
- More versatile intrusive force: control of the intrusive load on the mandibular molars is easier.

Nineteen years of experience with the internal abutment mechanism (Fig. 4.69) has established its utility as an implant anchorage mechanism for managing edentulous spaces in the mandibular buccal segments.[97-100]

Indirect anchorage with a retromolar implant is proving to be useful for closing missing second premolar spaces in growing children. However, an increased tendency for soft tissue irritation exists if the anchorage wire is positioned in the depth of the mucobuccal fold (Fig. 4.70A). When the wire is repositioned to just under the brackets of the molars (see Fig. 4.70B), soft tissue irritation ceased to be a problem and the second molar space was closed in about 10 months.

Mini-Implants for Orthodontic Anchorage

Kanomi[101] introduced a series of miniscrews as miniature implants for orthodontic anchorage. Although some of the

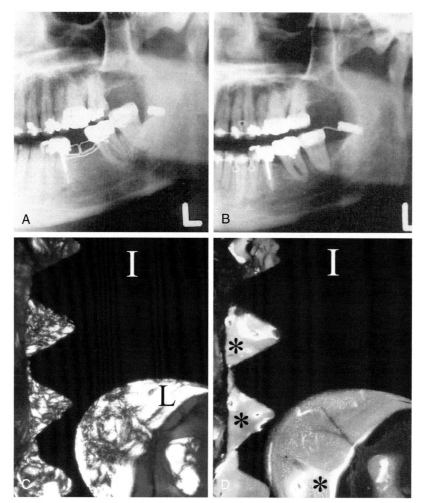

• **Fig. 4.64** (A) Panoramic radiograph of the initial buccal alignment before an implant is uncovered. (B) Panoramic radiograph of the closed extraction site. (C) Polarized light microscopy of lamellar bone *(L)* around the implant *(I)* recovered after completion of treatment. (D) Two demeclocycline labels *(*)* in bone adjacent to the implant *(I)* document the high rate of bone remodeling that apparently is the mechanism for long-term maintenance of rigid osseous fixation (osseointegration). (From Roberts WE, Marshall KJ, Mozsary PG. Rigid endosseous implant utilized as anchorage to protract molars and close an atrophic extraction site. *Angle Orthod.* 1990;60:135–152.)

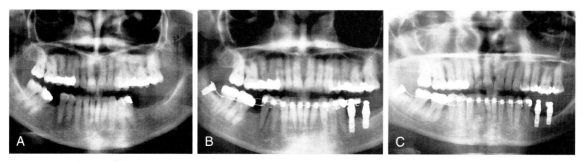

• **Fig. 4.65** This 44-year-old female has a partly edentulous mandibular arch and a long history of temporomandibular dysfunction and pain. (A) A progress radiograph shows restoration of occlusion in the left mandibular buccal segment with implants. (B) The molars on the right side are being intruded and rotated mesially with the retromolar implant anchorage mechanism. (C) By the end of active treatment, the mandibular curve of Spee has flattened and ideal alignment of the residual dentition has been achieved. (From Epker BN, Stella JP, Fish LC: *Dentofacial Deformities: Integrated Orthodontic and Surgical Correction.* Vol. 4. 2nd ed. St Louis: Mosby; 1999.)

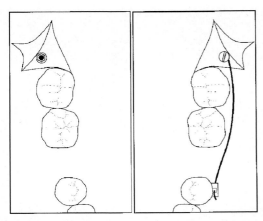

• **Fig. 4.66** Drawing on the left shows the soft tissue flap design for placing a retromolar anchorage implant distal to a mandibular right third molar. The drawing on the right illustrates the attachment of the 0.019 × 0.025-inch titanium-molybdenum alloy wire to the implant with a standard cover screw. Note that the free end of the passive anchorage wire is inserted into the vertical slot of a bracket bonded to the buccal surface of a mandibular left second premolar. (From Epker BN, Stella JP, Fish LC: *Dentofacial Deformities: Integrated Orthodontic and Surgical Correction.* Vol. 4. 2nd ed. St Louis: Mosby; 1999.)

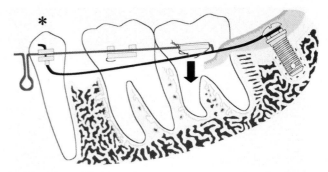

• **Fig. 4.68** Schematic drawing of the implant anchorage mechanism shows an internal abutment (i.e., the titanium-molybdenum alloy anchorage wire) attached to the endosseous base with the cover screw (healing cap). The anchorage wire passes through the mucosa in the depth of the buccal fold on the buccal aspect of the terminal molar. Extrusion of the molars during axial alignment and space closure is controlled by the intrusive force *(arrow)* generated by ligating the molar bracket to the anchorage wire with a steel ligature. Sagittal anchorage for mesial movement of the molars is achieved by inserting the passive anchorage wire into the vertical tube of a bracket anterior to the extraction site (*). To achieve unidirectional space closure, the "keyhole" vertical loop is activated by pulling the arch wire at the distal of the terminal molar and bending it down. (Redrawn from Epker BN, Stella JP, Fish LC: *Dentofacial Deformities: Integrated Orthodontic and Surgical Correction.* Vol. 4. 2nd ed. St Louis: Mosby; 1999.)

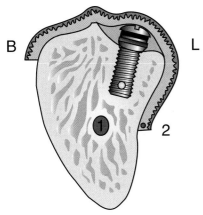

• **Fig. 4.67** (A) Cross section of the mandible distal to the third molar shows that the retromolar implant is inclined buccally *(B)*. Using the shelf of bone on the lingua *(L)*, the 7- to 10-mm implant is oriented toward the inferior alveolar nerve *(1)* and away from the lingual nerve *(2)*. (Redrawn from Epker BN, Stella JP, Fish LC: *Dentofacial Deformities: Integrated Orthodontic and Surgical Correction.* Vol. 4. 2nd ed. St Louis: Mosby; 1999.)

nonintegrated titanium screws served as adequate anchorage units, some loosened and failed during treatment. A new series of osseointegrated mini-implants was developed and tested in animals.[43] Deguchi and colleagues[102] found that 97% of 96 implants placed in eight dogs successfully integrated, and 100% of the implants that achieved osseointegration were successful as anchorage units. Clinical use of these simple devices has produced some impressive results. Fig. 4.71 documents the treatment of a 15-year-old girl with a gummy smile and bimaxillary protrusion. Four first premolars were extracted and the maxillary

anterior segment was intruded with mini-implant anchorage (see Fig. 4.71A–B). Comparison of frontal smile photographs pretreatment (see Fig. 4.71C) and posttreatment (see Fig. 4.71D) demonstrate the effective anchorage of the mini-implants. Fig. 4.71E is a cephalometric superimposition that demonstrates intrusion of the maxillary anterior segment and a horizontal vector of mandibular growth. Clearly, miniscrews are effective osseous anchorage for some types of malocclusion.

Summary

Bone physiologic, metabolic, and cell kinetic concepts have important clinical applications in all phases of stomatognathic reconstruction: implant surgery, orthodontics, prosthodontics, and long-term functional loading. The application of fundamental concepts is limited only by the knowledge and imagination of the clinician. Modern clinical practice is characterized by a continual evolution of methods based on fundamental and applied research.

Acknowledgments

This research was supported by the National Institute of Dental Research (part of the National Institutes of Health [NIH]) grants DE09237 and DE09822, NASA-Ames grants NCC 2-594 and NAG 2-756, and private donors through the Indiana University Foundation. The author gratefully acknowledges the assistance of faculty and staff members at the University of the Pacific School of Dentistry and Indiana University School of Dentistry. Ryuzo Kanomi provided the material on mini-implants for orthodontic anchorage.

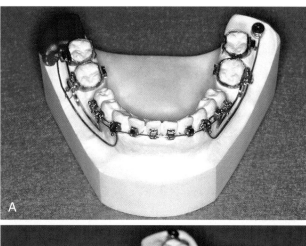
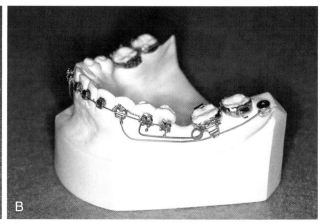
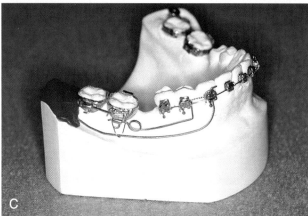

• **Fig. 4.69** (A) Mock-up demonstrates retromolar implant anchorage. Orthodontic mechanics are designed to align mandibular second and third molars and close the edentulous spaces by translating the molars mesially. The left retromolar implant shows the relationship of the fixture to supporting bone (surgical view). The right implant is covered with wax to simulate the closure of soft tissue over the implant with the titanium-molybdenum alloy anchorage wire attached. (B) Mechanics are shown for mesial root movement of the second molar into the first molar extraction site. Note that the mesial arm on the root spring is immediately adjacent to the first premolar bracket to prevent the second molar from moving distally as it is positioned upright. To prevent space from opening mesial to the first premolar, a steel ligature ("rope tie") connects the first premolar to the canine. A steel ligature connecting the bracket of the second molar to the titanium-molybdenum alloy anchorage wire controls molar extrusion. (C) Similar mechanics as shown in (B) are used for simultaneous alignment of both molars. A rectangular arch wire segment connects the two molars. Extrusion is controlled by tying the second molar to the anchorage wire with a steel ligature.

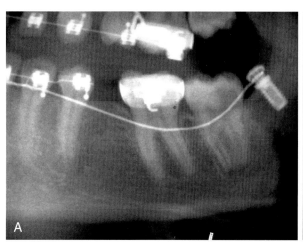
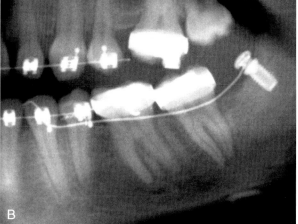

• **Fig. 4.70** (A) Postoperative panoramic radiograph reveals a retromolar implant to be used for indirect anchorage to close the space caused by a missing second premolar in an 11-year-old girl. Note that the anchorage wire is positioned too far apically. (B) A panoramic radiograph shows the rapid space closure associated with mesial movement of the molars. Note the anchorage wire has been repositioned just under the molar brackets to lessen soft tissue irritation.

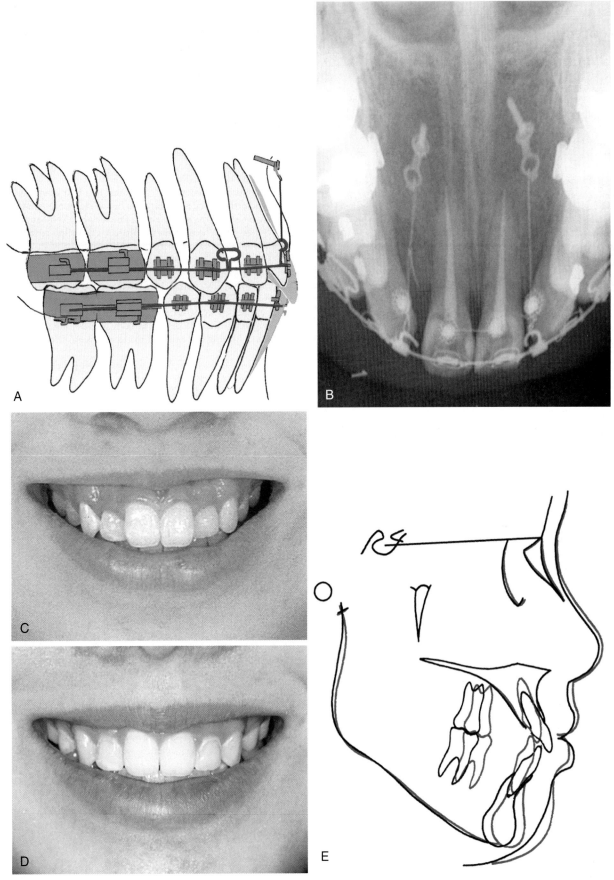

• **Fig. 4.71** (A) Drawing of space closure mechanics demonstrates the use of a mini-implant apical to the central incisors to intrude the maxillary anterior segment. (B) An occlusal radiograph shows the two miniscrews apical to the maxillary incisors. (C) Pretreatment photograph of a 15-year-old girl reveals a gummy smile. (D) Posttreatment photograph shows a pleasant smile line with ideal gingival exposure. (E) Pretreatment *(black)* and posttreatment *(red)* tracings of cephalometric radiographs are superimposed on the anterior cranial base. Note the intrusion of the maxillary anterior incisors and the horizontal component to mandibular growth. (Courtesy Ryuzo Kanomi.)

References

1. Atkinson SR. Balance: the magic word. *Am J Orthod*. 1964;50:189.
2. Hylander WL. Mandibular function in Galago crassicaudatus and Macaca fasicularis: an in vivo approach to stress analysis. *J Morphol*. 1979;159:253.
3. Hylander WL. Patterns of stress and strain in the macaque mandible. In: Carlson DS, ed. *Craniofacial Biology*. Ann Arbor, Mich: Center for Human Growth and Development; 1981.
4. Behrents RG. Adult facial growth. In: Enlow DH, ed. *Facial Growth*. 3rd ed. Philadelphia: WB Saunders; 1990.
5. Pead MJ, Lanyon LE. Indomethacin modulation of load-related stimulation of new bone formation in vivo. *Calcif Tissue Int*. 1989;45:34.
6. Roberts WE, Smith RK, Zilberman Y, et al. Osseous adaptation to continuous loading of rigid endosseous implants. *Am J Orthod*. 1984;86:95.
7. Roberts WE, Turley PK, Brezniak N, et al. Implants: bone physiology and metabolism. *CDA J*. 1987;15:54.
8. Roberts WE. Bone tissue interface. *J Dent Educ*. 1988;52:804.
9. Roberts WE. Advanced techniques for quantitative bone cell kinetics and cell population dynamics. In: Jaworski ZFG, ed. *Proceedings of the First Workshop on Bone Morphometry*. Ottawa: University of Ottawa Press; 1976.
10. Roberts WE, Chase DC, Jee WSS. Counts of labeled mitoses in orthodontically stimulated periodontal ligament in the rat. *Arch Oral Biol*. 1974;19:665.
11. Roberts WE, Jee WSS. Cell kinetics of orthodontically stimulated and nonstimulated periodontal ligament in the rat. *Arch Oral Biol*. 1974;19:17.
12. Roberts WE, Mozsary PG, Klingler E. Nuclear size as a cell kinetic marker for osteoblast differentiation. *Am J Anat*. 1982;165:373.
13. Roberts WE, Ferguson DJ. Cell kinetics of the periodontal aligament. In: Norton LA, Burstone CJ, eds. *The Biology of Tooth Movement*. Boca Raton, Fla: CRC Press; 1989.
14. Katona TR, et al. Stress analysis of bone modeling response to rat molar orthodontics. *J Biomech*. 1995;28:27.
15. Rapperport DJ, Carter DR, Schurman DJ. Contact finite element stress analysis of porous ingrowth acetabular cup implantation, ingrowth, and loosening. *J Orthop Res*. 1987;5:548.
16. Roberts WE, Garetto LP, Katona TR. Principles of orthodontic biomechanics: metabolic and mechanical control mechanisms. In: Carlson DS, Goldstein SA, eds. *Bone Biodynamics in Orthodontic and Orthopedic Treatment*. Ann Arbor, Mich: University of Michigan Press; 1992.
17. Siegele D, Dr-Ing US. Numerical investigations of the influence of implant shape on stress distribution in the jaw bone. *Int J Oral Maxillofac Implants*. 1989;4:333.
18. Roberts WE, Smith RK, Cohen JA. Change in electrical potential within periodontal ligament of a tooth subjected to osteogenic loading. In: Dixon A, Sarnat B, eds. *Factors and Mechanisms Influencing Bone Growth*. New York: Alan R Liss; 1982.
19. Huja SS, Roberts WE. Mechanism of osseointegration: characterization of supporting bone with indentation testing and backscattered imaging. *Semin Orthod*. 2004;10:162–173.
20. Yip G, Schneider P, Roberts WE. Micro-computed tomography: high resolution imaging of bone and implants in three dimensions. *Semin Orthod*. 2004;10:174–187.
21. Huja SS, Katona TR, Moore BK, et al. Microhardness and anisotropy of the vital osseous interface and endosseous implant supporting bone. *J Orthop Res*. 1998;16:54–60.
22. Roberts WE, Poon LC, Smith RK. Interface histology of rigid endosseous implants. *J Oral Implantol*. 1986;12:406.
23. Ascenzi A, Baschieri P, Benvenuti A. The bending properties of single osteons. *J Biomech*. 1990;8:763.
24. Martin RB, Burr DB. *Structure, Function, and Adaptation of Compact Bone*. New York: Raven Press; 1989.
25. Roberts WE, et al. Rigid endosseous implants for orthodontic and orthopedic anchorage. *Angle Orthod*. 1989;59:247.
26. Currey JD. *The Mechanical Adaptations of Bones*. Princeton, NJ: Princeton University Press; 1984.
27. Roberts WE. Rigid endosseous anchorage and tricalcium phosphate (TCP)-coated implants. *Calif Dent Assoc J*. 1984;12:158.
28. Roberts WE, Morey ER. Proliferation and differentiation sequence of osteoblast histogenesis under physiological conditions in rat periodontal ligament. *Am J Anat*. 1985;174:105.
29. Keeting PE, et al. Lack of a direct effect of estrogen on proliferation and differentiation of normal human osteoblast-like cells. *J Bone Miner Res*. 1992;7:S369.
30. Roberts WE, Garetto LP, Simmons KE. Endosseous implants for rigid orthodontic anchorage. In: Bell WH, ed. *Surgical Correction of Dentofacial Deformities*. Vol. 2. Philadelphia: WB Saunders; 1992.
31. Enlow DH. *Facial Growth*. 3rd ed. Philadelphia: WB Saunders; 1990.
32. Colditz GA, Stampfer MJ, Willett WC, et al. Prospective study of estrogen replacement therapy and risk of breast cancer in postmenopausal women. *J Am Dent Assoc*. 1990;264:2648.
33. Roberts WE, Garetto LP, DeCastro RA. Remodeling of devitalized bone threatens periosteal margin integrity of endosseous titanium implants with threaded or smooth surfaces: indications for provisional loading and axially directed occlusion. *J Indiana Dent Assoc*. 1989;68:19.
34. Roberts WE, Marshall KJ, Mozary PG. Rigid endosseous implant utilized as anchorage to protract molars and close an atrophic extraction site. *Angle Orthod*. 1990;60:135.
35. Mundy GR, Bonewald LF. Transforming growth factor beta. In: Gowen M, ed. *Cytokines and Bone Metabolism*. Boca Raton, Fla: CRC Press; 1992.
36. Melsen B. The cranial base. *Acta Odontol Scand*. 1974;32:1.
37. Noorda CB. *Modeling and Remodeling in the Cortical Bone of Both Growing and Adult Rabbits [Master's Thesis]*. San Francisco: University of the Pacific; 1986.
38. Brockstedt H, Bollerslev J, Melsen F, et al. Cortical bone remodeling in autosomal dominant osteopetrosis: a study of two different phenotypes. *Bone*. 1996;18:67.
39. Frost HM. The regional acceleratory phenomenon: a review. *Henry Ford Hosp Med J*. 1983;31:3.
40. Roberts WE, Garetto LP. Physiology of osseous and fibrous integration. *Alpha Omegan*. 1992;85:57.
41. Jeffcoat MK, Williams RC, Kaplan ML, et al. Nuclear medicine techniques for the detection of active alveolar bone loss. *Adv Dent Res*. 1987;1:80.
42. Reddy MS, English R, Jeffcoat MK, et al. Detection of periodontal disease activity with a scintillation camera. *J Dent Res*. 1991;70:50.
43. Ohmae M, Saito S, Morohashi T, et al. A clinical and histological evaluation of titanium mini-implants as anchors for orthodontic intrusion in the beagle dog. *Am J Orthod Dentofacial Orthop*. 2001;119:489–497.
44. Nikolai RJ. *Bioengineering Analysis of Orthodontic Mechanics*. Philadelphia: Lea & Febiger; 1985.
45. Roberts WE, Garetto LP, Arbuckle GR, et al. What are the risk factors of osteoporosis? Assessing bone health. *J Am Dent Assoc*. 1991;122:59–54.
46. Roberts WE, Simmons KE, Garetto LP, et al. Bone physiology and metabolism in dental implantology: risk factors for osteoporosis and other metabolic bone diseases. *Implant Dent*. 1992;1:11.
47. Midgett RJ, Shaye R, Fruge JF. The effect of altered bone metabolism on orthodontic tooth movement. *Am J Orthod*. 1981;80:256.
48. Rhodes R, Pflanzer R. *Human Physiology*. Philadelphia: WB Saunders; 1989.
49. Holtrop ME, Raisz LG, Simmons HA. The effects of parathyroid hormone, colchicine, and calcitonin on the ultrastructure and the activity of osteoclasts in organ culture. *J Cell Biol*. 1974;60:346.
50. Malluche HH, Faugere MC. Renal bone disease 1990: an unmet challenge for the nephrologist. *Kidney Int*. 1990;38:193.

51. Carter DR, Smith DJ, Spengler DM, et al. Measurement and analysis of in vivo bone strains on the canine radius and ulna. *J Biomech*. 1980;13:27.
52. Johnston CC, Miller JZ, Slemenda CW, et al. Calcium supplementation and increases in bone mineral density in children. *N Engl J Med*. 1992;327:82.
53. Frost HM. *Bone Remodeling and Its Relationship to Metabolic Bone Diseases*. Springfield, Ill: Charles C Thomas; 1973.
54. Heaney RP. Estrogen-calcium interactions in postmenopause: a quantitative description. *Bone Miner*. 1990;11:67.
55. Drinkwater BL, Nilson K, Chesnut CH, et al. Bone 3rd. mineral content of amenorrheic and eumenorrheic athletes. *N Engl J Med*. 1984;311:277.
56. Rigotti NA, Neer RM, Skates SJ, et al. The clinical course of osteoporosis in anorexia nervosa. *JAMA*. 1991;265:1133.
57. Consensus conference report on osteoporosis. *J Am Dent Assoc*. 1984;252:799.
58. Eriksen EF, Mosekilde L. Estrogens and bone. *J Bone Miner Res*. 1990;7:273.
59. Enrich JB. The postmenopausal estrogen/breast cancer controversy. *JAMA*. 1992;268:1900.
60. Love RR, Mazess RB, Barden HS, et al. Effects of tamoxifen on bone mineral density in postmenopausal women with breast cancer. *N Engl J Med*. 1992;326:852.
61. Slemenda CW, et al. Predicators of bone mass in premenopausal women. *Ann Intern Med*. 1990;112:96.
62. Parfitt AM. The physiological and clinical significance of bone histomorphometric data. In: Recker RR, ed. *Bone Histomorphometry: Techniques and Interpretation*. Boca Raton, Fla: CRC Press; 1983.
63. Heaney RP. Calcium, bone health in osteoporosis. In: Peck WA, ed. *Bone and Mineral Research*. Amsterdam: Elsevier Science; 1986.
64. Christiansen C. Consensus development conference: prophylaxis and treatment of osteoporosis. *Am J Med*. 1991;90:107.
65. Grisso JA, Baum CR, Turner BJ. What do physicians in practice do to prevent osteoporosis? *J Bone Miner Res*. 1990;5:213.
66. Roberts WE, Arbuckle GR, Katona TR. Bone physiology of orthodontics: metabolic and mechanical control mechanisms. In: Witt E, Tammoscheit U-G, eds. *Symposion der Deutschen Gesellschaft für Kieferorthopadie*. Munich: Urban & Vogel; 1992.
67. Johnston CC. Osteoporosis: extent and cause of the disease. *Proc Soc Exp Biol Med*. 1989;191:258.
68. Becker AR, Handick KE, Roberts WE, et al. Osteoporosis risk factors in female dental patients. *J Indiana Dent Assoc*. 1997;76:15.
69. Roberts WE, Mozsary PG, Morey ER. Suppression of osteoblast differentiation during weightlessness. *Physiologist*. 1981;24(suppl 6):S75.
70. Morey ER, Baylink DJ. Inhibition of bone formation during space flight. *Science*. 1978;201:1138.
71. Simmons DJ, Russell JE, Winter F, et al. Effect of space flight on the non-weight-bearing bones of rat skeleton. *Am J Physiol*. 1983;244:319.
72. Jackson CB, Roberts WE, Morey ER. Growth alterations of the mandibular condyle in Spacelab-3 rats (abstract). *ASGSB Bull*. 1988;1:33.
73. Cowin SC. *Bone Mechanics*. Boca Raton, Fla: CRC Press; 1989.
74. Lanyon LE. Control of bone architecture by functional load bearing. *J Bone Miner Res*. 1992;7:S369.
75. Riggs BL. Overview of osteoporosis. *West J Med*. 1991;154:63.
76. Rubin CT, Lanyon LE. Regulation of bone mass by mechanical strain magnitude. *Calcif Tissue Res*. 1985;37:411.
77. Rubin CT, Lanyon LE. Osteoregulatory nature of mechanical stimuli: function as a determinant for adaptive modeling in bone. *J Orthop Res*. 1987;5:300.
78. Rubin CT, McLeod KJ, Bain SD. Functional strains and cortical bone adaptation: epigenetic assurance of skeletal integrity. *J Biomech*. 1990;23:43.
79. Frost HM. Skeletal structural adaptations to mechanical usage (SATMU). 2. Redefining Wolff's law: the remodeling problem. *Anat Rec*. 1990;226:414.
80. Frost HM. *Intermediary organization of the skeleton*. Vol. 1. Boca Raton, Fla: CRC Press; 1986.
81. Carter DR. Mechanical loading history and skeletal biology. *J Biomech*. 1987;20:1095.
82. Brunski JB. Forces on dental implants and interfacial stressed transfer. In: Laney WR, Tolman DE, eds. *Tissue Integration in Oral, Orthopedic, and Maxillofacial Reconstruction*. Chicago: Quintessence; 1992.
83. Brunski JB, Shalak R. Biomechanical considerations. In: Worthington P, Brånemark PI, eds. *Advanced Osseointegration Surgery*. Chicago: Quintessence; 1992.
84. Haas AJ. The treatment of maxillary deficiency by opening the midpalatal suture. *Angle Orthod*. 1965;35:200–217.
85. Chang HN, Garetto LP, Katona TR, et al. Angiogenic induction and cell migration in an orthopaedically expanded maxillary suture in the rat. *Arch Oral Biol*. 1996;41:985–994.
86. Chang HN, Garetto LP, Potter RH, et al. Angiogenesis and osteogenesis in an orthopedically expanded suture. *Am J Orthod Dentofacial Orthop*. 1997;111:382–390.
87. Roberts WE, Wood HB, Chambers DW, et al. Vascularly oriented differentiation gradient of osteoblast precursor cells in rat periodontal ligament: implications for osteoblast histogenesis and periodontal bone loss. *J Periodontal Res*. 1987;22:461.
88. Doherty MJ, Ashton BA, Walsh S, et al. Vascular pericytes express osteogenic potential in vitro and in vivo. *J Bone Miner Res*. 1998;13:828.
89. Parr JA, Garetto LP, Wohlford ME, et al. Sutural expansion using rigidly integrated endosseous implants. *Angle Orthod*. 1997;67:283.
90. Sim Y. *Cell Kinetics of Osteoblast Histogenesis in Evolving Rabbit Secondary Haversian Systems Using a Double Labeling Technique with 3H-Thymidine and Bromodeoxyuridine [Doctoral Thesis]*. Indianapolis: Indiana University School of Dentistry; 1995.
91. Roberts WE, Wood HB, Chambers DW, et al. Vascularly oriented differentiation gradient of osteoblast precursor cells in rat periodontal ligament: implications for osteoblast histogenesis and periodontal bone loss. *J Periodontal Res*. 1987;22:461–467.
92. Arbuckle GR, Nelson CL, Roberts WE. Osseointegrated implants and orthodontics. *Oral Maxillofac Surg Clin North Am*. 1991;3:903.
93. Goodacre CJ, Brown DT, Roberts WE, et al. Prosthodontic considerations when using implants for orthodontic anchorage. *J Prosthet Dent*. 1997;77:162.
94. Helm FR, et al. Bone remodeling response to loading of rigid endosseous implants [abstract]. *J Dent Res*. 1987;66:186.
95. Albrektsson T, Jacobsson M. Bone-metal interface in osseointegration. *J Prosthet Dent*. 1987;60:75.
96. Brånemark P-I. Osseointegration and its experimental background. *J Prosthet Dent*. 1983;50:399.
97. Roberts WE. Dental implant anchorage for cost-effective management of dental and skeletal malocclusion. In: 2rd ed. Epker BN, Stella JP, Fish LC, eds. *Dentofacial Deformities*. Vol. 4. St Louis: Mosby; 1999.
98. Roberts WE, Arbuckle GR, Analoui M. Rate of mesial translation of mandibular molars utilizing implant-anchored mechanics. *Angle Orthod*. 1996;66:331.
99. Roberts WE, Hartsfield JK. Multidisciplinary management of congenital and acquired compensated malo-cclusions: diagnosis, etiology and treatment planning. *Indiana Dent Assoc J*. 1997;76:42.
100. Roberts WE, Nelson CL, Goodacre CJ. Rigid implant anchorage to close a mandibular first molar extraction site. *J Clin Orthod*. 1994;28:693.
101. Kanomi R. Mini-implant for orthodontic anchorage. *J Clin Orthod*. 1997;31:763–767.
102. Deguchi T, Takano-Yamamoto T, Kanomi R, et al. The use of small titanium screws for orthodontic anchorage. *J Dent Res*. 2003;82:377–381.

5

Biomaterials for Dental Implants

JACK E. LEMONS, FRANCINE MISCH-DIETSH, AND
RANDOLPH R. RESNIK

Compatibility of Surgical Biomaterials and the Role of Synthetic Materials

The biocompatibility profiles of synthetic substances (biomaterials) used for the replacement or augmentation of biological tissues have always been a critical concern within the health care disciplines. Special circumstances are associated with dental implant prosthetic reconstruction of the oral-maxillofacial areas because the devices extend from the mouth, across the protective epithelial zones, and onto or into the underlying bone. The functional aspects of use also include the transfer of force from the occlusal surfaces of the teeth through the crown and bridge and neck-connector region of the implant into the implant for interfacial transfer to the supporting soft and hard tissues. This situation represents a complex series of chemical and mechanical environmental conditions.

This most critical aspect of biocompatibility is, of course, dependent on the basic bulk and surface properties of the biomaterial. All aspects of basic manufacturing, finishing, packaging and delivering, sterilizing, and placing (including surgical placement) must be adequately controlled to ensure clean and nontraumatizing conditions. The importance of these considerations has been reemphasized through the concept and practice of osteointegration of endosteal root form implant systems.

The disciplines of biomaterials and biomechanics are complementary to the understanding of device-based function. The physical, mechanical, chemical, and electrical properties of the basic material components must always be fully evaluated for any biomaterial application, because these properties provide key inputs into the interrelated biomechanical and biological analyses of function. It is important to separate the roles of macroscopic implant shape from the microscopic transfer of stress and strain along biomaterial–tissue interfaces. The macroscopic distribution of mechanical stress and strain is predominantly controlled by the shape and form of the implant device. One important material property related to design (shape and form) optimization is the elastic strain (one component of the elastic modulus) of the material.

The localized microscopic strain distribution is controlled more by the basic properties of the biomaterial (e.g., surface chemistry, microtopography, modulus of elasticity) and by whether the biomaterial surface is attached to the adjacent tissues. Engineering

analyses of implant systems include optimization considerations related both to the design and to the biomaterial used for construction. Therefore the desire to positively influence tissue responses and to minimize biodegradation often places restrictions on which materials can be used safely within the oral and tissue environments. Designs are often evolved for specific biomaterials because of the imposed environmental or restorative conditions.

Bulk Properties

History of Materials and Designs

Over the past several decades, definitions of material biocompatibilities have evolved and reflect an ever-changing opinion related to philosophies of surgical implant treatment. In general the definition of biocompatibility has been given as an appropriate response to a material (biomaterial) within a device (design) for a specific clinical application.[1] Metallic and nonmetallic implantable materials have been studied in the field of orthopedics since the turn of the twentieth century.[2-7]

In the 1960s emphasis was placed on making the biomaterials more inert and chemically stable within biological environments. The high-purity ceramics of aluminum oxide (Al_2O_3), carbon, and carbon-silicon compounds and extra-low interstitial–grade alloys are classic examples of these trends. In the 1970s biocompatibility was defined in terms of minimal harm to the host or to the biomaterial. The importance of a stable interaction then moved into central focus for both the research and the clinical communities. In the 1980s the focus transferred to bioactive substrates intended to positively influence tissue responses, whereas most recently emphasis on chemically and mechanically anisotropic substrates combined with growth (mitogenic) and inductive (morphogenic) substances. Today many biomaterials are being constituted, fabricated, and surface modified to directly influence short- and long-term tissue responses. Bioactive coatings on most classes of biomaterials have continued to evolve from human clinical trials to acceptable modalities of surface preparation, and research focus has shifted to combinations of active synthetic and biological implants.

Of interest, dental implants have significantly influenced these trends. In the 1960s dental devices were recognized as being in a research and development phase, and critical longitudinal reviews of clinical applications were strongly recommended.[8] During this time, longevity studies of various devices demonstrated that the longest duration of clinical applications were for orthopedic prostheses. In the 1980s controlled clinical trials showed that dental implants provided functional longevities that exceeded most other types of functional tissue replacement modalities.[9,10] Clearly, these clinical studies have strongly influenced both the research and development and the clinical application processes. Presently the exponential growth of implant use and related scientific reports support the views expressed by early visionaries several decades ago.

The evolution of any implant modality is a multipart story in which significant roles have been played by biomaterials; biomechanical analyses of designs, tissues, and function; wound healing along interfaces; surgical methods to minimize mechanical, chemical, and thermal trauma; prosthodontic and periodontal restorative and maintenance treatment modalities; and protocols for controlled multidisciplinary clinical trials. The interdependence of all phases of basic and applied research should be recognized. All interrelate and must evolve to provide a level of better understanding of the basic physical and biological phenomena associated with the implant systems before the longer clinical outcomes will be fully described.

Evaluations of endosteal and subperiosteal dental implants raise interesting questions with respect to the interrelationships between material and design selection. Opportunities exist to select a material from a number of systems, such as metals, ceramics, carbons, polymers, or composites. In addition, only the available anatomic dimensions and the requirement to attach some form of intraoral restorative device limit implant shape and form (design). Because of the wide range of biomaterial properties demonstrated by the classes of materials available, it is not advisable to fabricate any new implant design without a thorough biomechanical analysis. Another approach now often used is to determine a specific design based on clinical considerations and then to select the biomaterial of choice from computer-based analyses. The safety of these combinations can then be demonstrated through laboratory and animal investigations. Controlled clinical trials following prospective protocols, of course, provide the final evaluation for both safety and effectiveness. Long-term success is thus determined clinically in investigator follow-up studies and is clearly an area that should be emphasized for many available dental implant systems.

Research and Development

Basic studies within the physical and biological sciences have been supportive of the development of surgical implant systems. One example is the continued progress from materials that have been available for industrial applications to the new classes of composites that have evolved for biomedical applications. This same situation exists within a broad area; for example, surface science and technology, mechanics and biomechanics of three-dimensional structures, pathways and processes of wound healing along biomaterial interfaces, and the description of the first biofilms that evolve on contact with blood or tissue fluids.[11-14] The progressive move from materials to quantitatively characterized biomaterials has been extremely important to the biomedical applications of surgical implants. Dental implant investigations now play a leadership role within selected areas of this overall process, and all phases of medicine and dentistry should benefit.

Physical, Mechanical, and Chemical Requirements for Implant Materials

Physical and Mechanical Properties

Forces exerted on the implant material consist of tensile, compressive, and shear components. As for most materials, compressive strengths of implant materials are usually greater than their shear and tensile counterparts. A hypothesis that dental implants are less affected by alternating stresses than implants of the cardiovascular and locomotor systems because of the significantly lower number of loading cycles must be qualified because of the special concern that dental implants are considerably smaller in physical dimension. All fatigue failures obey mechanical laws correlating the dimensions of the material to the mechanical properties of said material.[11,15] In addition, when present, parafunction (nocturnal and/or diurnal) can be greatly detrimental to longevity because of the mechanical properties, such as maximum yield strength, fatigue strength, creep deformability, ductility, and fracture. Limitations of the relevance of these properties are mainly caused by the variable shape and surface features of implant designs. A recurring problem exists between the mechanical strength and deformability of the material and the recipient bone. A different approach to match more closely the implanted material and hard tissue properties led to the experimentation of polymeric, carbonitic, and metallic materials of low modulus of elasticity.[16,17]

Because bone can modify its structure in response to forces exerted on it, implant materials and designs must be designed to account for the increased performance of the musculature and bone in jaws restored with implants. The upper stress limit decreases, with an increasing number of loading cycles sometimes reaching the fatigue limit after 10^6 to 10^7 loading cycles.[11,15,18] In other words, the higher the applied load, the higher the mechanical stress—and therefore the greater the possibility for exceeding the fatigue endurance limit of the material.

In general the fatigue limit of metallic implant materials reaches approximately 50% of their ultimate tensile strength.[11,18] However, this relationship is applicable only to metallic systems, and polymeric systems have no lower limit in terms of endurance fatigue strength. Ceramic materials are weak under shear forces because of the combination of fracture strength and no ductility, which can lead to brittle fracture. Metals can be heated for varying periods to influence properties, modified by the addition of alloying elements or altered by mechanical processing such as drawing, swagging, or forging, followed by age or dispersion hardening, until the strength and ductility of the processed material are optimized for the intended application.

The modifying elements in metallic systems may be metals or nonmetals. A general rule is that constitution or mechanical process hardening procedures result in an increased strength but also invariably correspond to a loss of ductility. This is especially relevant for dental implants. Consensus standards for metals (ASTM International [formerly American Society for Testing and Materials], International Standardization Organization [ISO], American Dental Association) require a minimum of 8% ductility to minimize brittle fractures. Mixed microstructural-phase hardening of austenitic materials with nitrogen (e.g., stainless steels) and the increasing purity of the alloys seem most indicated to achieve maximum strength and maintain this high level of possible plastic deformation.[1,15,19-23]

Corrosion and Biodegradation

Corrosion is a special concern for metallic materials in dental implantology, because implants protrude into the oral cavity, where electrolyte and oxygen compositions differ from that of tissue fluids. In addition, the pH can vary significantly in areas below plaque and within the oral cavity. This increases the range of pH that implants are exposed to in the oral cavity compared with specific sites in tissue.[24-29]

Plenk and Zitter[15] state that galvanic corrosion (GC) could be greater for dental implants than for orthopedic implants. Galvanic processes depend on the passivity of oxide layers, which are characterized by a minimal dissolution rate and high regenerative power for metals such as titanium. The passive layer is only a few nanometers thick and is usually composed of oxides or hydroxides of the metallic elements that have greatest affinity for oxygen. In reactive group metals such as titanium, niobium, zirconium, tantalum, and related alloys, the base materials determine the properties of the passive layer. The stability zones of the oxides of passivable elements cover the redox potentials and pH values typical of the oral environment. However, titanium, tantalum, and niobium oxides cover a markedly larger zone of environmental stability compared with chromium oxides.

The risk for mechanical degradation, such as scratching or fretting of implanted materials, combined with corrosion and release into bone and remote organs has been previously considered. For example, investigators such as Laing,[30] Willert et al.,[31] and Lemons[32,33] have studied extensively the corrosion of metallic implants. Steinemann[34] and Fontana and Greene[35] have presented many of the basic relationships specific to implant corrosion. Mears[26] addressed concerns about GC and studied the local tissue response to stainless steel and cobalt-chromium-molybdenum (Co-Cr-Mo), and showed the release of metal ions in the tissues. Williams[36] suggested that three types of corrosion were most relevant to dental implants: (1) stress corrosion cracking (SCC), (2) GC, and (3) fretting corrosion (FC).

Stress Corrosion Cracking

The combination of high magnitudes of applied mechanical stress plus simultaneous exposure to a corrosive environment can result in the failure of metallic materials by cracking, where neither condition alone would cause the failure. Williams[36] presented this phenomenon of SCC in multicomponent orthopedic implants. Others hypothesized that it may be responsible for some implant failures in view of high concentrations of forces in the area of the abutment–implant body interface.[37-39] Most traditional implant body designs under three-dimensional finite-element stress analysis show a concentration of stresses at the crest of the bone support and cervical third of the implant. This tends to support potential SCC at the implant interface area (i.e., a transition zone for altered chemical and mechanical environmental conditions). This has also been described in terms of corrosion fatigue (i.e., cyclical load cycle failures accelerated by locally aggressive medium). In addition, nonpassive prosthetic superstructures may incorporate permanent stress, which strongly influences this phenomenon under loaded prostheses (Fig. 5.1A and 5.1B).[37,40,41]

GC occurs when two dissimilar metallic materials are in contact and are within an electrolyte, resulting in current flowing between the two. The metallic materials with the dissimilar potentials can have their corrosion currents altered, thereby resulting in a greater corrosion rate (Fig. 5.1C). FC occurs when a micromotion and rubbing contact occur within a corrosive environment (e.g., the perforation of the passive layers and shear-directed loading along adjacent contacting surfaces). The loss of any protective film can result in the acceleration of metallic ion loss. FC has been shown to occur along implant body–abutment–superstructure interfaces.

Normally the passive oxide layers on metallic substrates dissolve at such slower rates that the resultant loss of mass is of no mechanical consequence to the implant. A more critical problem is the irreversible local perforation of the passive layer that chloride ions often cause, which may result in localized pitting corrosion. Such perforations can often be observed for iron-chromium-nickel-molybdenum (Fe-Cr-Ni-Mo) steels that contain an insufficient amount of the alloying elements stabilizing the passive layer (i.e., Cr and Mo) or local regions of implants that are subjected to abnormal environments. Even ceramic oxide materials are not fully degradation resistant. Corrosion-like behavior of ceramic materials can then be compared with the chemical dissolution of the oxides into ions or complex ions of respective metallic oxide substrates. An example of this is the solubility of Al_2O_3 as alumina or titanium oxide as titanium. This statement is generally valid; however, most metallic oxides and nonmetallic substrates have amorphous hydroxide-inclusive structures, whereas bulk ceramics are mostly crystalline. The corrosion resistance of synthetic polymers, in contrast, depends not only on their composition and structural form but also on the degree of polymerization. Unlike metallic and ceramic materials, synthetic polymers are not only dissolved but also penetrated by water and substances from biological environments. The resulting degree of alteration depends on the material property conditions for the manufactured component.

Toxicity and Consideration

Toxicity is related to primary biodegradation products (simple and complex cations and anions), particularly those of higher atomic weight metals. Factors to be considered include: (1) the amount dissolved by biodegradation per time unit, (2) the amount of material removed by metabolic activity in the same time unit, and (3) the quantities of solid particles and ions deposited in the tissue and any associated transfers to the systemic system. For example, the quantity of elements released from metals during corrosion time (e.g., grams per day) can be calculated by using the following formula[15]:

$$TE \left(\frac{g}{day}\right) = \frac{TEA\,(\%) \times CBR\,(g/cm^2 \times day) \times IS\,(cm^2)}{100}$$

where TE = toxic element; TEA = toxic elements in alloy; CBR = corrosion biodegradation; and IS = implant surface.

It is of little importance for the formula whether the metallic substrate is exposed because the passive layer is dissolved. The critical issue is that the surface represents the "finished" form of the implant. The formula is also valid for ceramic materials and for substances transferred from synthetic polymers. Therefore it appears that the toxicity is related to the content of the materials' toxic elements and that they may have a modifying effect on corrosion rate.[15]

The transformation of harmful primary products is dependent on their level of solubility and transfer. It is known that chromium and titanium ions react locally at low concentrations, whereas cobalt, molybdenum, or nickle can remain dissolved at higher relative concentrations, and thus may be transported

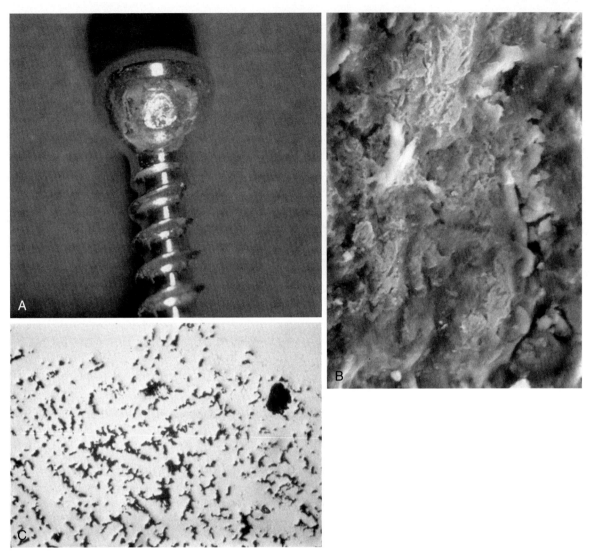

● **Fig. 5.1** (A) Stainless-steel (316L) fracture fixation screw showing crevice corrosion after 1 year in vivo (approximately ×5). (B) Microscopic characteristics of cobalt alloy root form surface showing environmental degradation (approximately ×100). (C) As-polished microstructure of cobalt alloy subperiosteal showing porosity associated with galvanically assisted corrosion (approximately ×100).

and circulated in body fluids. Several studies have documented the relative toxicity of titanium and its various alloys. Lemons[32] reported on the formation of electrochemical couples as a result of oral implant and restorative procedures, and stressed the importance of selecting compatible metals to be placed in direct contact with one another in the oral cavity to avoid the formation of adverse electrochemical couples. The electrochemical behavior of implanted materials has been instrumental in assessing their biocompatibility.[42] Zitter and Plenk[43] have shown that anodic oxidation and cathodic reduction take place in different spaces but must always balance each other through charge transfer. This has been shown to impair both cell growth and transmission of stimuli from one cell to another. Therefore an anodic corrosion site can be influenced by ion transfer but also by other possibly detrimental oxidation phenomena. Charge transfer appears to be a significant factor specific to the biocompatibility of metallic biomaterials. Passive layers along the surfaces of titanium, niobium, zirconium, and tantalum increase resistance to change-transfer processes by isolating the substrate from the electrolyte, in addition to providing a higher resistance to ion transfers. In contrast, metals based on iron, nickel, or cobalt are not as resistant to transfers through the oxide-like passive surface zones.

Metals and Alloys

To date, most of the dental implant systems available within the United States are constructed from metals or alloys. These materials are reviewed in this chapter by separating the metals and alloys according to their elemental compositions, because a growing proportion have modified surface characteristics.

Several organizations have provided guidelines for the standardization of implant materials.[44] ASTM Committee F4 (ASTM F4) and ISO (ISOTC 106, ISOTR 10541) have provided the basis for such standards.[19,20] To date a multinational survey by ISO indicated that titanium and its alloy are mainly used. The most widely used nonmetallic implants are oxidic, carbonitic, or graphitic oxide-like materials.[45] The major groups of implantable materials for dentistry are titanium and alloys, cobalt chromium alloys, austenitic Fe-Cr-Ni-Mo steels, tantalum, niobium and zirconium alloys, precious metals, ceramics, and polymeric materials.

TABLE 5.1 Engineering Properties of Metals and Alloys Used for Surgical Implants

Material	Nominal Analysis (w/o)	Modulus of Elasticity GN/m² (psi × 10⁶)	Ultimate Tensile Strength MN/m² (ksi)	Elongation to Fracture (%)	Surface
Titanium	99⁺Ti	97 (14)	240–550 (25–70)	>15	Ti oxide
Titanium-aluminum-vanadium	90Ti-6Al-4V	117 (17)	869–896 (125–130)	>12	Ti oxide
Cobalt-chromium-molybdenum (casting)	66Co-27Cr-7Mo	235 (34)	655 (95)	>8	Cr oxide
Stainless steel (316L)	70Fe-18Cr-12Ni	193 (28)	480–1000 (70–145)	>30	Cr oxide
Zirconium	99⁺Zr	97 (14)	552 (80)	20	Zr oxide
Tantalum	99⁺Ta	—	690 (100)	11	Ta oxide
Gold	99⁺Au	97 (14)	207–310 (30–45)	>30	Au
Platinum	99⁺Pt	166 (24)	131 (19)	40	Pt

Minimum values from the American Society for Testing and Materials Committee F4 documents are provided. Selected products provide a range of properties.

GN/m², Giganewton per meter squared; *ksi*, thousand pounds per inch squared; *MN/m²*, meganewton per meter squared; *w/o*, weight percent.

Titanium and Titanium-6 Aluminum-4 Vanadium

This reactive group of metals and alloys (with primary elements from reactive group metallic substances) form tenacious oxides in air or oxygenated solutions. Titanium oxidizes (passivates) on contact with room-temperature air and normal tissue fluids. This reactivity is favorable for dental implant devices. In the absence of interfacial motion or adverse environmental conditions, this passivated (oxidized) surface condition minimizes biocorrosion phenomena. In situations in which the implant would be placed within a closely fitting receptor site in bone, areas scratched or abraded during placement would repassivate in vivo. This characteristic is one important property consideration related to the use of titanium for dental implants.[37,46-48] Some reports show that the oxide layer tends to increase in thickness under corrosion testing[48] and that breakdown of this layer is unlikely in aerated solutions.[49]

Bothe et al.[50] studied the reaction of rabbit bone to 54 different implanted metals and alloys, and showed that titanium allowed bone growth directly adjacent to the oxide surfaces. Leventhal[51] further studied the application of titanium for implantation. Beder and Eade,[52] Gross and Gold,[53] Clarke and Hickman,[54] and Brettle[55] were able to expand indications of these materials. In all cases, titanium was selected as the material of choice because of its inert and biocompatible nature paired with excellent resistance to corrosion.[1,56-60]

Specific studies in the literature have addressed the corrosion of titanium implants. Unfortunately most are for in vitro and unloaded conditions, and few identify precisely the type of titanium and titanium surface studied.

The general engineering properties of the metals and alloys used for dental implants are summarized in Table 5.1. Titanium shows a relatively low modulus of elasticity and tensile strength compared with most other alloys. The strength values for the wrought soft and ductile metallurgic condition (normal root forms and plate form implants) are approximately 1.5 times greater than the strength of compact bone. In most designs in which the bulk dimensions and shapes are simple, strength of this magnitude is adequate. Because fatigue strengths are normally 50% weaker or less than the corresponding tensile strengths, implant design criteria are decidedly important. The creation of sharp corners or thin sections must be avoided for regions loaded under tension or shear conditions. The modulus of elasticity of titanium is five times greater than that of compact bone, and this property places emphasis on the importance of design in the proper distribution of mechanical stress transfer. In this regard, surface areas that are loaded in compression have been maximized for some of the newer implant designs. Four grades of unalloyed titanium and titanium alloy are the most popular. Their ultimate strength and endurance limit vary as a function of their composition.

The alloy of titanium most often used is titanium-aluminum-vanadium. The wrought alloy condition is approximately six times stronger than compact bone and thereby affords more opportunities for designs with thinner sections (e.g., plateaus, thin interconnecting regions, implant-to-abutment connection screw housing, irregular scaffolds, porosities). The modulus of elasticity of the alloy is slightly greater than that of titanium, being about 5.6 times that of compact bone. The alloy and the primary element (i.e., titanium) both have titanium oxide (passivated) surfaces. Information has been developed on the oxide thickness, purity, and stability as related to implant biocompatibilities.[9,14,19] In general, titanium and alloys of titanium have demonstrated interfaces described as *osteointegrated* for implants in humans. In addition, surface conditions in which the oxide thickness has varied from hundreds of angstroms of amorphous oxide surface films to 100% titania (titanium dioxide [TiO$_2$] rutile form ceramic) have demonstrated osteointegration.

The possible influences of aluminum and vanadium biodegradation products on local and systemic tissue responses have been reviewed from the perspectives of basic science and clinical applications.[61] Extensive literature has been published on the corrosion rate of titanium within local tissue fluids[62-64] and the peri-implant accumulation of "black particles."[65] A few adverse effects have been reported.[66] Increased titanium concentrations were found in both peri-implant tissues and parenchymal organs,[67,68] mainly the lung, and much lesser concentrations in the liver, kidney, and spleen.[25,66-70] However, alloy compositions were not well defined or controlled. Corrosion and mechanical wear have been suggested as possible causes.[48,67,68] Authors who still caution about the applicability of these results to the presently available titanium alloys have developed other alloys using iron, molybdenum, and other elements as primary alloying agents.[17] More recently, several new titanium alloys of higher strength have been introduced.[33,71]

Although many basic science questions remain, clinical applications of these alloys in dental and orthopedic surgical systems have been very positive, especially in light of improved strength, and the titanium alloys have not demonstrated significant numbers of identifiable negative sequelae.[19] Electrochemical studies support the selection of conditions in which elemental concentrations would be relatively low in magnitude.[11] Electrochemically, titanium and titanium alloy are slightly different in regard to electromotive and galvanic potentials compared with other electrically conductive dental materials. Results of these electrochemical potentials and how they relate to in vivo responses have been published previously.[9,42,63] In general, titanium- and cobalt-based systems are electrochemically similar; however, comparative elements imitating the conditions in an aeration cell revealed that the current flow in titanium and titanium alloys is several orders of magnitude lower than that in Fe-Cr-Ni-Mo steels or Co-Cr alloys.[15] Gold-, platinum-, and palladium-based systems have been shown to be noble, and nickel-, iron-, copper-, and silver-based systems are significantly different (subject to galvanic coupling and preferential in vivo corrosion).

Mechanically, titanium is much more ductile (bendable) than titanium alloy. This feature has been a favorable aspect related to the use of titanium for endosteal plate form devices. The need for adjustment or bending to provide parallel abutments for prosthetic treatments has caused manufacturers to optimize microstructures and residual strain conditions. Coining, stamping, or forging followed by controlled annealing heat treatments are routinely used during metallurgic processing. However, if an implant abutment is bent at the time of implantation, then the metal is strained locally at the neck region (bent), and the local strain is both cumulative and dependent on the total amount of deformation introduced during the procedure. This is one reason, other than prior loading fatigue cycling, why reuse of implants is not recommended. In addition, mechanical processes can sometimes significantly alter or contaminate implant surfaces. Any residues of surface changes must be removed before implantation to ensure mechanically and chemically clean conditions.

The emerging techniques to cast titanium and titanium alloys remain limited for dental implant application because of high melting points of the elements and propensity for absorption of oxygen, nitrogen, and hydrogen, which may cause metallic embrittlement. A high vacuum or ultrapure protective gas atmosphere allows the production of castings in titanium and its alloys at different purity levels,[72,73] although microstructures and porosity are relatively unfavorable related to fatigue and fracture strengths.[9,32] Typical strengths of cast commercially pure titanium grade 2 and titanium-6 aluminum-4 vanadium (Ti-6Al-4V) after heat treatment and annealing can be in the range of those of wrought titanium alloys used for dental implants.[74]

Cobalt-Chromium-Molybdenum–Based Alloy

The cobalt-based alloys are most often used in an as-cast or cast-and-annealed metallurgic condition. This permits the fabrication of implants as custom designs such as subperiosteal frames. The elemental composition of this alloy includes cobalt, chromium, and molybdenum as the major elements. Cobalt provides the continuous phase for basic properties; secondary phases based on cobalt, chromium, molybdenum, nickel, and carbon provide strength (four times that of compact bone) and surface abrasion resistance (see Table 5.1); chromium provides corrosion resistance through the oxide surface; and molybdenum provides strength and bulk corrosion resistance. All of these elements are critical, as is their concentration, which emphasizes the importance of controlled casting and fabrication technologies. Also included in this alloy are minor concentrations of nickel, manganese, and carbon. Nickel has been identified in biocorrosion products, and carbon must be precisely controlled to maintain mechanical properties such as ductility. Surgical alloys of cobalt are not the same as those used for partial dentures, and substitutions should be avoided.

In general the as-cast cobalt alloys are the least ductile of the alloy systems used for dental surgical implants, and bending of finished implants should be avoided. Because many of these alloy devices have been fabricated by dental laboratories, all aspects of quality control and analysis for surgical implants must be followed during alloy selection, casting, and finishing. Critical considerations include the chemical analysis, mechanical properties, and surface finish as specified by the ASTM F4 on surgical implants and the American Dental Association.[19,21] When properly fabricated, implants from this alloy group have been shown to exhibit excellent biocompatibility profiles.

Iron-Chromium-Nickel–Based Alloys

The surgical stainless-steel alloys (e.g., 316 low carbon [316L]) have a long history of use for orthopedic and dental implant devices. This alloy, as with titanium systems, is used most often in a wrought and heat-treated metallurgic condition, which results in a high-strength and high-ductility alloy. The ramus blade, ramus frame, stabilizer pins (old), and some mucosal insert systems have been made from the iron-based alloy.

The ASTM F4 specification for surface passivation was first written and applied to the stainless-steel alloys.[19] In part, this was done to maximize corrosion-biocorrosion resistance. Of the implant alloys, this alloy is most subject to crevice and pitting biocorrosion, and care must be taken to use and retain the passivated (oxide) surface condition. Because this alloy contains nickel as a major element, use in patients allergic or hypersensitive to nickel should be avoided. In addition, if a stainless-steel implant is modified before surgery, then recommended procedures call for repassivation to obtain an oxidized (passivated) surface condition to minimize in vivo biodegradation.

The iron-based alloys have galvanic potentials and corrosion characteristics that could result in concerns about galvanic coupling and biocorrosion if interconnected with titanium, cobalt, zirconium, or carbon implant biomaterials.[75-77] In some clinical conditions, more than one alloy may be present within the same dental arch of a patient. For example, if a bridge of a noble or a base-metal alloy touches the abutment heads of a stainless-steel and titanium implant simultaneously, then an electrical circuit would be formed through the tissues. If used independently, where the alloys are not in contact or not electrically interconnected, then the galvanic couple would not exist, and each device could function independently. As with the other metal and alloy systems discussed, the iron-based alloys have a long history of clinical applications. Long-term device retrievals have demonstrated that, when used properly, the alloy can function without significant in vivo breakdown. Clearly, the mechanical properties and cost characteristics of this alloy offer advantages with respect to clinical applications.

Other Metals and Alloys

Many other metals and alloys have been used for dental implant device fabrication. Early spirals and cages included tantalum, platinum, iridium, gold, palladium, and alloys of these metals. More recently, devices made from zirconium, hafnium, and tungsten have been evaluated.[15,78,79] Some significant advantages of these reactive group metals and their alloys have been reported, although large numbers of such devices have not been fabricated in the United States.

Gold, platinum, and palladium are metals of relatively low strength, which places limits on implant design. In addition, cost-per-unit weight and weight-per-unit volume (density) of the device along the upper arch have been suggested as possible limitations for gold and platinum. These metals, especially gold because of nobility and availability, continue to be used as surgical implant materials. For example, the Bosker endosteal staple design represents use of this alloy system.[80]

Ceramics and Carbon

Ceramics are inorganic, nonmetallic, nonpolymeric materials manufactured by compacting and sintering at elevated temperatures. They can be divided into metallic oxides or other compounds. Oxide ceramics were introduced for surgical implant devices because of their inertness to biodegradation, high strength, physical characteristics such as color and minimal thermal and electrical conductivity, and a wide range of material-specific elastic properties.[81,82] In many cases, however, the low ductility or inherent brittleness has resulted in limitations. Ceramics have been used in bulk forms and more recently as coatings on metals and alloys.

Aluminum, Titanium, and Zirconium Oxides

High-strength ceramics from aluminum, titanium, and zirconium oxides have been used for the root form, endosteal plate form, and pin type of dental implants.[83] The overall characteristics of these ceramics are summarized in Table 5.2. The compressive, tensile, and bending strengths exceed the strength of compact bone by three to five times. These properties, combined with high moduli of elasticity, and especially with fatigue and fracture strengths, have resulted in specialized design requirements for these classes of biomaterials.[19,84] For example, the fabrication of a subperiosteal

device from a high ceramic should not be done because of the custom nature of these devices, the lower fracture resistance, and the relative cost for manufacturing. The aluminum, titanium, and zirconium oxide ceramics have a clear, white, cream, or light-gray color, which is beneficial for applications such as anterior root form devices. Minimal thermal and electrical conductivity, minimal biodegradation, and minimal reactions with bone, soft tissue, and the oral environment are also recognized as beneficial compared with other types of synthetic biomaterials. In early studies of dental and orthopedic devices in laboratory animals and humans, ceramics have exhibited direct interfaces with bone, similar to an osteointegrated condition with titanium. In addition, characterization of gingival attachment zones along sapphire root form devices in laboratory animal models has demonstrated regions of localized bonding.[9,85-89]

Although the ceramics are chemically inert, care must be taken in the handling and placement of these biomaterials. Exposure to steam sterilization results in a measurable decrease in strength for some ceramics; scratches or notches may introduce fracture initiation sites; chemical solutions may leave residues; and the hard and sometimes rough surfaces may readily abrade other materials, thereby leaving a residue on contact. Dry-heat sterilization within a clean and dry atmosphere is recommended for most ceramics.

One series of root form and plate form devices used during the 1970s resulted in intraoral fractures after several years of function.[90] The fractures were initiated by fatigue cycling, where biomechanical stresses were along regions of localized bending and tensile loading. Although initial testing showed adequate mechanical strengths for these polycrystalline alumina materials,[91] the long-term clinical results clearly demonstrated a functional design-related and material-related limitation. This illustrates the need for controlled clinical investigation to relate basic properties to in vivo performance. The established chemical biocompatibilities, improved strength and toughness capabilities of sapphire and zirconia, and the basic property characteristics of high ceramics continue to make them excellent candidates for dental implants.

Bioactive and Biodegradable Ceramics Based on Calcium Phosphates

Bone Augmentation and Replacement

The calcium phosphate ($CaPO_4$) materials (i.e., calcium phosphate ceramics [CPCs]) used in dental reconstructive surgery include a wide range of implant types and thereby a wide range of clinical applications. Early investigations emphasized solid and porous particulates with nominal compositions that were

TABLE 5.2 Engineering Properties of Some Inert Ceramics Used as Biomaterials

Material	Modulus of Elasticity GN/m² (psi × 10⁶)	Ultimate Bending Strength MPa (ksi)	Surface
Aluminum oxide polycrystalline	372 (54)	300–550 (43–80)	Al_2O_3
Single crystal (sapphire)	392 (56)	640 (93)	Al_2O_3
Zirconium oxide zirconia (PSZ)	195–210 (28–30)	500–650 (72–94)	ZrO_2
Titanium oxide (titania)	280 (41)	69–103 (10–15)	TiO_2

These high ceramics have 0% permanent elongation at fracture.

GN/m², Giganewton per meter squared; *ksi*, thousand pounds per inch squared; *MPa*, megapascal.

relatively similar to the mineral phase of bone ($Ca_5[PO_4]_3OH$). Microstructural and chemical properties of these particulates were controlled to provide forms that would remain intact for structural purposes after implantation. The laboratory and clinical results for these particulates were most promising and led to expansions for implant applications, including larger implant shapes (e.g., rods, cones, blocks, H-bars) for structural support under relatively high-magnitude loading conditions.[92,93] In addition, the particulate size range for bone replacements was expanded to both smaller and larger sizes for combined applications with organic compounds. Mixtures of particulates with collagen, and subsequently with drugs and active organic compounds such as bone morphogenetic protein, increased the range of possible applications. These types of products and their uses have continued to expand significantly.[93-96]

Endosteal and Subperiosteal Implants

The first series of structural forms for dental implants included rods and cones for filling tooth-root extraction sites (ridge retainers)[97] and, in some cases, load-bearing endosteal implants.[98] Limitations in mechanical property characteristics soon resulted in internal reinforcement of the CPC implants through mechanical (central metallic rods) or physicochemical (coating over another substrate) techniques.[99,100] The numbers of coatings of metallic surfaces using flame or plasma spraying (or other techniques) increased rapidly for the CPCs.[93] The coatings have been applied to a wide range of endosteal and subperiosteal dental implant designs, with an overall intent of improving implant surface biocompatibility profiles and implant longevities (they are addressed later in this chapter).[101-103]

Advantages and Disadvantages

Box 5.1 summarizes the advantages and disadvantages of CPCs. The recognized advantages associated with the CPC biomaterials are as follows[104]:

1. chemical compositions of high purity and of substances that are similar to constituents of normal biological tissue (calcium, phosphorus, oxygen, and hydrogen);
2. excellent biocompatibility profiles within a variety of tissues, when used as intended;

3. opportunities to provide attachments between selected CPC and hard and soft tissues;
4. minimal thermal and electrical conductivity plus capabilities to provide a physical and chemical barrier to ion transport (e.g., metallic ions);
5. moduli of elasticity more similar to bone than many other implant materials used for load-bearing implants;
6. color similar to bone, dentin, and enamel; and
7. an evolving and extensive base of information related to science, technology, and application

Some of the possible disadvantages associated with these types of biomaterials are as follows:

1. variations in chemical and structural characteristics for some currently available implant products;
2. relatively low mechanical tensile and shear strengths under condition of fatigue loading;
3. relatively low attachment strengths for some coating-to-substrate interfaces;
4. variable solubilities depending on the product and the clinical application (The structural and mechanical stabilities of coatings under in vivo load-bearing conditions—especially tension and shear—may be variable as a function of the quality of the coating.);
5. alterations of substrate chemical and structural properties related to some available coating technologies; and
6. expansion of applications that sometimes exceed the evolving scientific information on properties.

Critical to applications are the basic properties of these substances. Table 5.3 provides a summary of some properties of bioactive and biodegradable ceramics. In general these classes of bioceramics have lower strengths, hardness, and moduli of elasticity than the more chemically inert forms previously discussed. Fatigue strengths, especially for porous materials, have imposed limitations with regard to some dental implant designs. In certain instances, these characteristics have been used to provide improved implant conditions (e.g., biodegradation of particulates). Calcium aluminates, sodium-lithium invert glasses with $CaPO_4$ additions (Bioglass or Ceravital), and glass ceramics (AW glass ceramic) also provide a wide range of properties and have found extended applications.[96,100]

Bioactive Ceramic Properties

Physical properties are specific to the surface area or form of the product (block, particle), porosity (dense, macroporous, microporous), and crystallinity (crystalline or amorphous). Chemical properties are related to the calcium-phosphate ratio, composition, elemental impurities (e.g., carbonate), ionic substitution in atomic structure, and the pH of the surrounding region. These properties, plus the biomechanical environment, all play a role in the rate of resorption and the clinical application limits of the materials.

The atomic relationships of the basic elements, stoichiometric ratios, and the normal chemical names for several characterized CPCs are provided in Table 5.4. The general family of apatites has the following formula:

$$M_{10}^{2+}(XO_4^{3})_6 Z_2^{1}$$

Often apatite atomic ratios are nonstoichiometric; that is, 1 mol apatite may contain fewer than 10 mol metallic ions (M^{2+}) and fewer than 2 mol anions Z^{-1}.[105] The number of XO retains a number of 6. Multiple metals and anions can be substituted within

BOX 5.1	Advantages and Disadvantages of Calcium Phosphate Ceramics	
Advantages	**Disadvantages**	
• Chemistry mimics normal biological tissue (C, P, O, H)	• Variable chemical and structural characteristics (technology and chemistry related)	
• Excellent biocompatibility	• Low mechanical tensile and shear strengths under fatigue loading	
• Attachment between calcium phosphate ceramics and hard and soft tissues	• Low attachment between coating and substrate	
• Minimal thermal and electrical conductivity	• Variable solubility	
• Moduli of elasticity closer to bone than many other implantable materials	• Variable mechanical stability of coatings under load-bearing conditions	
• Color similar to hard tissues	• Overuse	
• Extensive research		

this formulation. Most important, the relative physical, mechanical, and chemical properties of each final $CaPO_4$ material, including each of the apatites, are different from one another.[89,95] In addition, the microstructure of any final product (solid structural form or coating) is equally important to the basic properties of the substance alone. The crystalline monolithic hydroxyapatite (HA) (fired ceramic $Ca_{10}[PO_4]_6[OH]_2$) of high density and purity (50 maximum ppm impurities) has provided one standard for comparison related to implant applications. The ratio of calcium to phosphorus of $Ca_{10}(PO_4)_6(OH)_2$ is 1.67, and the ceramic can be fully crystalline. Considerable differences exist between the synthetic HA ceramics that are produced by elevated temperature processing and biological apatites (HAs).[105] Biological apatites contain trace amounts of CO_3^2, sodium, magnesium, fluorine, and chlorine ions. These exist in varying ratios and distributions, and of course are only one phase of calcified tissues.

The crystalline tricalcium phosphate ($bCa_3[PO_4]_2$) (TCP) ceramic has also provided a high-purity (<50 ppm maximum impurities) biomaterial for comparison with other products. National standard specifications related to the basic properties and characteristics of both HA and TCP have been published.[19] These two compositions have been used most extensively as particulates for bone augmentation and replacement, carriers for organic products, and coatings for endosteal and subperiosteal implants.

One of the more important aspects of the CPCs relates to the possible reactions with water. For example, hydration can convert other compositions to HA; also, phase transitions among the various structural forms can exist with any exposure to water. This has caused some confusion in the literature, in that some CPCs have been steam autoclaved for sterilization purposes before surgical implantation. Steam or water autoclaving can significantly change the basic structure and properties of CPCs (or any bioactive surface), and thereby provide an unknown biomaterial condition at the time of implantation. This is to be avoided through the use of presterilized or clean, dry heat or gamma sterilized conditions.

Forms, Microstructures, and Mechanical Properties

Particulate HA, provided in a nonporous (<5% porosity) form as angular or spherically shaped particles, is an example of a crystalline, high-purity HA biomaterial[106] (Fig. 5.2A). These particles can have relatively high compressive strengths (up to 500 MPa), with tensile strengths in the range of 50 to 70 MPa. Usually, dense

---

TABLE 5.3 **Properties of Bioactive and Biodegradable Ceramics**

Material	Modulus of Elasticity GPa (psi × 10⁶)	Ultimate Bending Strength MPa (ksi)	Surface
Hydroxyapatite	40–120 (6–17)	40–300 (6–43)	$Ca_{10}(PO_4)_6(OH)_2$
Tricalcium phosphate	30–120 (4–17)	15–120 (2–17)	$Ca_3(PO_4)_2$
Bioglass or Ceravital	40–140 (6–20)	20–350 (3–51)	$CaPO_4$
AW ceramic	124 (18)	213 (31)	$CaPO_4 + F$
Carbon	25–40 (4–6)	150–250 (22–36)	C
Carbon-silicon (low-temperature isotropic)	25–40 (4–6)	200–700 (29–101)	CSi

These ceramics and carbons have 0% permanent elongation at fracture.

GPa, Gigapascal; *ksi*, thousand pounds per inch squared; *MPa*, megapascal.

TABLE 5.4 **Names, Formulae, and Atomic Ratios for Some Calcium Phosphate Materials**

Mineral or General Name	Formula	Ca:P Ratio	Applications
Monetite (DVP)	$CaHPO_4$	1	Nonceramic bone substitute particulate
Brushite (DCPD)	$CaHPO_4 2H_2O$	1	Phase of some $CaPO_4$ biomaterials
Octacalcium phosphate (OCP)	$Ca_8(HPO_4)_2(PO_4)\ 5H_2O$	1.33	Phase of some $CaPO_4$ biomaterials
Whitlockite (WH)	$Ca_{10}(HPO_4)(PO_4)_6$	1.43	Phase of some $CaPO_4$ biomaterials
Beta-tricalcium phosphate (b-TCP)	$Ca_3(PO_4)_2$	1.48	Biodegradable $CaPO_4$ ceramic for bone substitute and coatings; also a phase of some $CaPO_4$ biomaterials
Defective hydroxyapatite (DOHA) biomaterials	$Ca_9(HPO_4)(PO_4)_5(OH)$	1.5	Component of some $CaPO_4$ biomaterials
Hydroxyapatite (HA)	$Ca_{10}(PO_4)_6(OH)_2$	1.67	Major mineral phase of bone; when fired as a ceramic, named HA

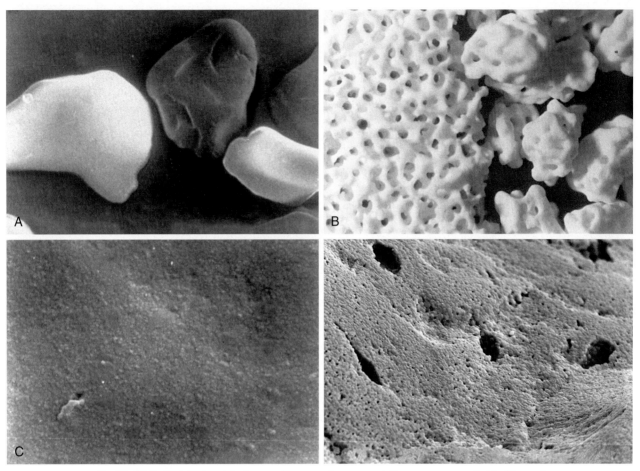

• **Fig. 5.2** (A) Particulate dense hydroxyapatite presents as a crystalline nonporous material with angular or spherical particles. (B and C) Macroporous (B) and microporous (C) particulate offer the advantage of increased surface area per unit volume, which facilitates solution and cell-mediated resorption. (*Courtesy Ceramed Corp, Denver, CO*)

polycrystalline ceramics consisting of small crystallites exhibit the highest mechanical strength, apart from monocrystalline ceramics free of defects (e.g., single-crystal sapphire implants). Ceramics are brittle materials and exhibit high compressive strengths compared with tensile strengths. However, less resistance to tensile and shear stresses limit their application as dental implants because of mechanical constraints of implant form and volume. Nonresorbable, "bioinert" ceramics exhibiting satisfactory load-bearing capability are limited to dense monocrystalline and polycrystalline aluminum, zirconium, and titanium oxide ceramics. These same mechanical characteristics exist for the solid portions of several porous HA particulates and blocks. The macroporous (>50 mm) or microporous (<50 mm) particulates have an increased surface area per unit volume. This provides more surface area for solution- and cell-mediated resorption under static conditions and a significant reduction in compressive and tensile strengths (Figs. 5.2B, 5.2C, and 5.3). The porous materials also provide additional regions for tissue ingrowth and integration (mechanical stabilization), and thereby a minimization of interfacial motion and dynamic (wear-associated) interfacial breakdown. The strength characteristics after tissue ingrowth would then become a combination of the ceramic and the investing tissues.[107]

A number of the CPCs are phase mixtures of HA and TCP, whereas some compounds are composites or mechanical mixtures with other materials[93] (see Table 5.4). These classes of bioactive ceramics, including glasses, glass ceramics, mixtures of ceramics,

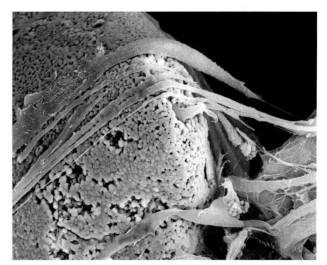

• **Fig. 5.3** Scanning electron microscopy of cells, which actively endocytosed fragments of granules (×1500). (*Courtesy Ceramed Corp, Denver, CO*)

combinations of metals and ceramics, or polymers and ceramics, exhibit a wide range of properties. In general, these biomaterials have shown acceptable biocompatibility profiles from laboratory and clinical investigations. Bulk-form implant designs made from CPCs, which were contraindicated for some implant designs because of poor mechanical performance, have found a wide range of indications as coatings of stronger implant materials.

The coatings of CPCs onto metallic (cobalt- and titanium-based) biomaterials have become a routine application for dental implants. For the most part these coatings are applied by plasma spraying, have average thickness between 50 and 70 mm, are mixtures of crystalline and amorphous phases, and have variable microstructures (phases and porosities) compared with the solid portions of the particulate forms of HA and TCP biomaterials.[93,108] At this time, coating characteristics are relatively consistent, and the quality-control and stricter quality-assurance programs from the manufacturers have greatly improved the consistency of coated implant systems. (A more detailed discussion of surface treatment options is presented in the next section.)

Concerns continue to exist about the fatigue strengths of the $CaPO_4$ coatings and coating–substrate interfaces under tensile and shear loading conditions. There have been some reports of coating loss as a result of mechanical fracture, although the numbers reported remain small.[89] This has caused some clinicians and manufacturers to introduce designs in which the coatings are applied to shapes (geometric designs) that minimize implant interface shear or tensile loading conditions (e.g., porosities, screws, spirals, plateaus, vents). From theoretic considerations, the coating of mechanically protected areas seems most desirable.

Density, Conductivity, and Solubility

Bioactive ceramics are especially interesting for implant dentistry because the inorganic portion of the recipient bone is more likely to grow next to a more chemically similar material. The bioactive (bioreactive) categorization includes $CaPO_4$ materials such as TCP, HA, calcium carbonate (corals), and calcium sulfate–type compounds and ceramics. A chemical-biochemical contact between the host bone and grafted material may be developed, as well as a possible stimulus of bone activity.[95] Their limitations have been associated with the material forms that have lower strengths (i.e., similar to or less than bone).[95]

The very technique-sensitive fabrication steps related to phase transition and thermal expansion during cooling might cause the final product of $CaPO_4$-type coatings to be more or less resorbable. In addition, the original categories of resorbable versus nonresorbable for these materials must be carefully weighed as a function of their particle size, porosity, chemical structure, and environmental exposure conditions.

Dissolution characteristics of bioactive ceramics have been determined for both particulates and coatings.[109,110] In general, solubility is greater for TCP than for HA. Each increase relative to increasing surface area per unit volume (porosity) and the CPC solubility profiles depend on the environment (e.g., pH, mechanical motion). If one considers a uniform material chemistry, then the larger the particle size is, the longer the material will remain at an augmentation site. Thus 75-mm particles will be resorbed more rapidly than 3000-mm particles.

In addition, the porosity of the product affects the resorption rate. Tofe et al.[111] reported on the porosity of dense, macroporous, and microporous $CaPO_4$. Some of the dense HA lacks any macroporosity or microporosity within the particles. The longest resorption rate occurred with the dense nonporous HA type because osteoclasts may attack only the surface and cannot penetrate the nonporous material. Macroporous $CaPO_4$ (e.g., corallin

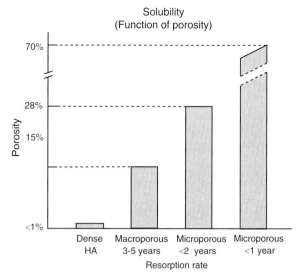

Fig. 5.4 Diagram of solubility of hydroxyapatite in function of percent porosity.

HA) demonstrated 100-mm or 500-mm pores, which comprised 15% or more of the total material volume. Minimal porosity was found in the HA bulk material that surrounded the large pores. Microporous apatites often have their origin in bovine or human bone. The porosity observed in these materials is approximately 5 mm or less and comprises less than 28% of the total volume. The pores or holes are regions where blood components and organic materials can reside when placed within bone, and they represent the regions where living material existed before the processing of the implant material. The greater the porosity is, the more rapid is the resorption of the graft material. For example, clinical observation shows dense crystalline forms of HA may last longer than 15 years in the bone, the macroporous 5 years, and the microporous HA as short as 6 months (Fig. 5.4).

The crystallinity of HA also affects the resorption rate of the material. The highly crystalline structure is more resistant to alteration and resorption. An amorphous product has a chemical structure that is less organized with regard to atomic structure. The hard or soft tissues of the body are more able to degrade the components and resorb the amorphous forms of grafting materials. Thus crystalline forms of HA are found to be very stable over the long term under normal conditions, whereas the amorphous structures are more likely to exhibit resorption and susceptibility to enzyme- or cell-mediated breakdown.[112] Therefore, in general, the less crystalline the material, the faster its resorption rate.[92,93,95,112,113]

The purity of the HA bone substitutes may also affect the resorption rate. The resorption of the bone substitute may be cell or solution mediated. Cell-mediated resorption requires processes associated with living cells to resorb the material, similar to the modeling and remodeling process of living bone, which demonstrates the coupled resorption and formation process. A solution-mediated resorption permits the dissolution of the material by a chemical process. Impurities or other compounds in bioactive ceramics, such as calcium carbonate, permit more rapid solution-medicated resorption, which then increases the porosity of the bone substitute. Although the coralline HA does not demonstrate micropores along the larger holes, the HA may have carbonates incorporated within the material, which hastens the resorption process.

The pH in the region in which the bone substitutes are placed also affects the rate of resorption. As the pH decreases (e.g., because of chronic inflammation or infection), the components of living bone, primarily $CaPO_4$, resorb by a solution-mediated process (i.e., they become unstable chemically).

The $CaPO_4$ coatings are nonconductors of heat and electricity. This can provide a relative benefit for coated dental implants, where mixtures of conductive materials may be included in the overall prosthetic reconstruction. In combination with color (off-white), these properties are considered to be advantageous.

In most applications within bone, solubilities are higher during the first few weeks, then decrease with continued in vivo exposure and the apposition of mineralized structures.[109,110] However, some investigators have shown situations in which osteoclastic resorption has removed localized zones of $CaPO_4$ coatings.[114] This raises interesting questions about long-term in vivo stabilities. At this time, clinical results have been favorable, and expanded applications have continued.

Current Status and Developing Trends

The CPCs have proved to be one of the more successful high technology–based biomaterials that have evolved most recently. Their advantageous properties strongly support the expanding clinical applications and the enhancement of the biocompatibility profiles for surgical implant uses. Within the overall theme for new-generation biomaterials to be chemically (bonding to tissue) and mechanically (nonuniform, multidirectional properties) anisotropic, the CPCs could be the biomaterial surfaces of choice for many device applications.[115,116]

Carbon and Carbon Silicon Compounds

Carbon compounds are often classified as *ceramics* because of their chemical inertness and absence of ductility; however, they are conductors of heat and electricity. Extensive applications for cardiovascular devices, excellent biocompatibility profiles, and moduli of elasticity close to that of bone have resulted in clinical trials of these compounds in dental and orthopedic prostheses. One two-stage root replacement system (Vitredent) was quite popular in the early 1970s.[10] However, a combination of design, material, and application limitations resulted in a significant number of clinical failures and the subsequent withdrawal of this device from clinical use.

Ceramic and carbonitic substances continue to be used as coatings on metallic and ceramic materials. Advantages of coatings as mentioned in an earlier section include tissue attachment; components that are normal to physiologic environments; regions that serve as barriers to elemental transfer, heat, or electrical current flow; control of color; and opportunities for the attachment of active biomolecules or synthetic compounds. Possible limitations relate to mechanical strength properties along the substrate–coating interface; biodegradation that could adversely influence tissue stabilities; time-dependent changes in physical characteristics; minimal resistance to scratching or scraping procedures associated with oral hygiene; and susceptibility to standard handling, sterilizing, or placing methodologies. Greater uses of surface-coated dental implants have been developed by the research and development communities.

Zirconia

The use of ceramic implants has been available in implant dentistry. since the 1970's. These types of implants never gained acceptance because they were at a biomechanical disadvantage and clinically had a poor success rate. However, today a new type of implant made out of zirconia has recently been introduced into dental implantology as an alternative to titanium implants.

Initially zirconia was used in medicine with orthopedic procedures for total hip replacements, artificial hips, and finger and acoustic implants. In the 1990s, zirconia was introduced to dentistry for fabrication of endodontic posts, crown and bridge prostheses, esthetic orthodontic brackets, and custom implant abutments.[117] Zirconia possesses many advantages over titanium in its biologic, esthetic, mechanical, and optical properties, as well as its inherent biocompatibility and low plaque affinity. This zirconia-based material has been shown to have improved flexural strength and fracture resistance over early versions of ceramic implants.[118] Even though zirconia implants are becoming more popular, they have become extremely controversial. Zirconia implants have been plagued by high fracture rates. Since receiving U.S. Food and Drug Administration approval in 2011, zirconia dental implants have been touted as the next generation of dental implants. Zirconia implants initially were used in cases of metal-free dentistry, mainly for patients with known metal allergies or hypersensitivities. The prevalence rate of titanium allergy has been estimated to be approximately 0.6%.[119] Originally, zirconia implants were available only as a one-piece implant, but the introduction of two-piece zirconia implants now allows for abutments to be fully customized, creating the best outcomes.

Zirconia Chemical Composition

Zirconia implants are fabricated from a shiny, gray-white metal named zirconium, which has an atomic number of 40 and is symbolized in the periodic table as Zr. Zirconia is the oxide form of zirconium, which was first isolated in an impure form by Jöns Jacob Berzelius in 1824. The pure form of zirconia occurs in two basic forms: (1) crystalline zirconia, which is soft, white, and ductile; and the (2) amorphous form, which is bluish-black and powdery in nature. The powder form of zirconia is refined and treated at high temperatures to produce an optically translucent form of crystalline zirconia. There exist three crystalline phases with zirconia implants: monoclinic (m), tetragonal (t), and cubic (c). The monoclinic phase of zirconia exists at room temperature and is stable for up to approximately 1170°C. At greater than 1170°C, the monoclinic phase changes to tetragonal phase with approximately 5% decrease in volume. At 2370°C, the cubic phase starts to appear. Upon cooling, a tetragonal-to-monoclinic transformation with a 3% to 4% increase in volume takes place for about 100°C until 1070°C. Unfortunately, the increase in volume and resultant expansion without a mass transfer on cooling generates stress and causes it to become unstable at room temperature[120] (Fig. 5.5).

Therefore to minimize this phenomenon and to generate a partially stabilized zirconia (PSZ) with stable tetragonal and/or cubic phases, various stabilizing oxides [16 mol% magnesia (MgO), 16 mol% of limestone (CaO), or 8 mol% yttria (Y_2O_3)] are added in the fabrication of zirconia implants.[121] This martensitic-like phase transformation significantly increases the crack and fracture toughness, and the longevity of zirconia endosseous implants.[122] Today the most common type of ceramic implants is produced from yttria-stabilized tetragonal zirconia polycrystal.

In addition, other variants of zirconia implants being studied include 12Ce-TZP (ceria-stabilized zirconia) and alumina-toughened zirconia. Alumina has also been added to yttria-stabilized tetragonal zirconia polycrystal in small quantities (0.25 wt%) that results in a tetragonal zirconia polycrystal with alumina. This new zirconia form significantly improves the durability and stability of zirconia crystals along with minimizing degradation of

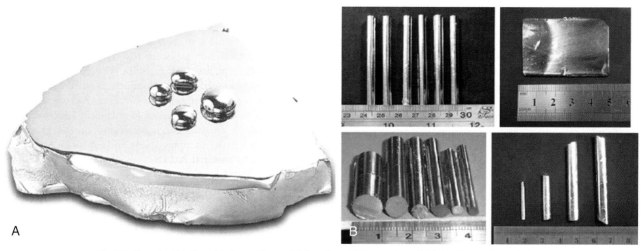

• **Fig. 5.5** Zirconia: (a) is the oxide form of the metal zirconium, (b) Zirconia is available in different size and shapes for use in implant dentistry. (*From Telford M. The case for bulk metallic glass. Materials Today. 2004;7:36–43.*)

the zirconia.[123,124] Most significantly, research has shown that implants without alumina, when exposed to the oral cavity, have a survival rate of 50%, whereas implants with alumina have a much greater survival rate of approximately 87% to 100%.[125]

Physical Properties. The physical properties of zirconia implants are dependent on many factors, including the composition, crystalline structure, polymorphic structure, percentage of stabilizing metal oxide, aging process, and the macrodesign and microdesign of the implant.[126,127] An ideal grain size (0.2–0.6 µm) should be used to retain the tetragonal phase of the material, to minimize the degradation or aging of zirconia. Watanabe et al.[128] reported that too small of a grain size results in a less stable material. However, a larger grain size (e.g., >1 µm) exhibits a decrease in strength with an increased amount of tetragonal-monoclinic transformation.[128]

Surface Roughness. Many studies have shown that zirconia with a moderately rough surface is advantageous in attracting osteoblasts and osseointegration.[129,130] By modifying the zirconia surface into a microrough surface, acceleration of the osseointegration process results. Currently, sandblasting followed by acid etching is the method of choice in adjusting the zirconia surface.[130] In addition, the zirconia surface may be chemically modified, which increases the hydrophilicity of the material.[131]

Types of Zirconia Implants

Zirconia implants are classified as either one piece or two piece. The one-piece implant consists of an implant and abutment as a single unit. The two-piece is similar to traditional implant, where the abutment may be screwed or cemented in place.[132] Currently, most available research has been completed for one-piece zirconia implants, which show superior mechanical properties relative to two-piece implants[133] (Fig. 5.6).

Fracture Resistance. In early studies, zirconia implants exhibited high rates of fractures in preclinical animal studies using canine mandibles. In two different studies, Thoma et al.[134,135] reported a higher incidence of zirconia implant fractures before and after loading in comparison with titanium implants. The fracture resistance of zirconia implants is dependent on many variables, but most importantly on the occlusal load and physical characteristics of the abutment. Numerous studies have shown the flexural strength (900–1200 MPa), fracture toughness (8–10 MPa-m$^{1/2}$), and static fracture strength (725–850 N).[136]

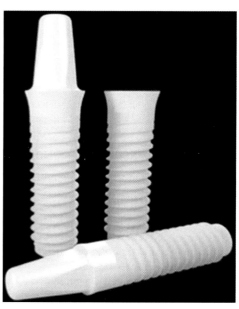

• **Fig. 5.6** Two different types of zirconia implants: one piece and two piece.

When comparing the fracture resistance, the type (i.e., one or two piece) of zirconia implant must be determined. Kohal et al.[137] compared the mechanical properties and effect of occlusal loading on one- and two-piece zirconia implants. They concluded that the fracture strength was less for two-piece zirconia, both under loaded and unloaded conditions. Therefore two-piece zirconia implants are becoming more popular; however, they have an increased morbidity.[137]

The type and extent of modification of the zirconia implant influences the fracture resistance. Kohal et al.[137] evaluated the effects of cyclic loading and finish line design on the fracture strength of one-piece zirconia implants. They concluded that a chamfer finish line along with cyclic loading decrease the fracture strength of zirconia implants.[137] When circumferential preparation was completed, a depth of 0.5 mm on the zirconia abutments was better than 0.6 and 0.7 mm. Each increase in preparation depth of 0.2 mm decreases the fracture load by 68 N, and aging and chewing simulations decrease the fracture load to 102 N.[138,139]

Spies et al.[140] reported on the fracture resistance of different types of two-piece zirconia implant systems (e.g., bonded and screwed) and single-piece zirconia implants after the process of thermomechanical cycling under an aqueous environment. The results showed that both screwed and bonded two-piece zirconia implants had a significant decreased fracture resistance and were weak and susceptible to fracture[140] (Fig. 5.7).

Osseointegration. Zirconia-based implants are advantageous because they exhibit excellent osseointegration qualities. Zirconia is chemically inert, with minimal local or systemic adverse reactions. They possess enhanced cell adhesion, favorable tissue responses, and excellent biocompatibility with the surrounding hard and soft tissues. There exists numerous animal and human studies that have verified that new mature bone forms around zirconia implants with minimal inflammation and abundance of active osteoblasts.[141-143] Several in vitro and in vivo studies have shown zirconia possesses osteoconductive features with no cytotoxic or mutagenic effects on the bone and fibroblasts after implantation.[144-146] When evaluating osseointegration differences of titanium and zirconia implants, most studies show little difference between the two implant materials. Scarano et al.[147] showed an excellent bone response to zirconia implants at 4 weeks with bone–implant contact of 68.4%. Dubruille et al.[148] compared the bone implant contact in titanium, alumina, and zirconia implants. They concluded no statistically significant difference between the three types of implants (i.e., 68% for alumina, 64.6% for zirconia, and 54% for titanium). Hoffman et al.[149] showed at 2 weeks postinsertion, zirconia implants had a higher degree of bone apposition (54%–55%) compared with titanium implants (42%–52%). However, at 4 weeks, titanium had a higher bone–implant contact (68%–91%) in comparison with zirconia (62%–80%).

Zirconia Implant Success Studies
Unfortunately few clinical studies exist on the long-term success of zirconia implants. Oliva et al.[150] reported on the first zirconia implant study involving 100 implants with different surface roughness. There overall success rate approached 98%. Osman et al.[151] evaluated the 1-year success of one-piece zirconia implants compared with titanium implants with conventional loading protocols. No difference in success rates in the mandible was seen; however, in the maxilla a significant difference was seen (i.e., titanium, 72%; zirconia, 55% success rate).

Devji et al.[152] conducted a metaanalysis of patients treated with only zirconia implants and found an average implant survival rate of 95.6% after 12 months, with an expected decrease of 0.05% per year for 5 years (0.25% after 5 years). After 1 year the marginal bone loss around zirconia implants was favorable at 0.79 mm.

Narrow-diameter zirconia implants have not proven to be predictable in clinical studies because success rates have been unfavorable. Various studies have shown up to a 30% incidence rate of fracture with zirconia implants.[153]

In summary, zirconia dental implants are a new and exciting development in implant dentistry. The limited preliminary studies are positive, showing less inflammation in the peri-implant tissues, less biofilm accumulation, and a favorable bone–implant contact. In addition, they exhibit excellent esthetics and are ideal for patients who exhibit metal sensitivities or who prefer a metal-free option. However, there is room for further technical progress of currently available zirconia implant systems. Two-piece zirconia implant systems are ideal; however, they are still technically challenging because of limitations in the material. Zirconia dental implants have the potential to become the future ideal alternative to titanium alloy dental implants (Boxes 5.2 and 5.3).

Polymers and Composites

The use of synthetic polymers and composites continues to expand for biomaterial applications. Fiber-reinforced polymers offer advantages in that they can be designed to match tissue properties, can be anisotropic with respect to mechanical characteristics, can be coated for attachment to tissues, and can be fabricated at relatively low cost. Expanded future applications for dental implant systems, beyond inserts for damping force transfers such as those

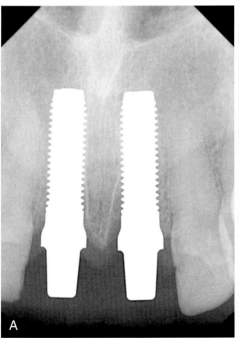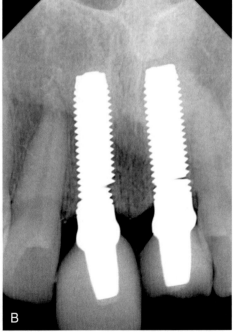

● **Fig. 5.7** Zirconia Implant Fracture. One of the most significant disadvantages of zirconia implants to date is the high fracture rate. (A) Immediate postinsertion radiograph depicting #8 and #9 zirconia implants. (B) Radiograph showing the fracture of both zirconia implants within 1 year of insertion.

used in the IMZ (Interpore, Inc.) and Flexiroot (Interdent Corp.) systems, are anticipated as interest continues in combination synthetic and biological composites.

Structural Biomedical Polymers

The more inert polymeric biomaterials include polytetrafluoroethylene (PTFE), polyethylene terephthalate, polymethylmethacrylate (PMMA), ultra-high-molecular-weight polyethylene, polypropylene, polysulfone, and polydimethylsiloxane (or silicone rubber). These are summarized in Table 5.5. In general the polymers have lower strengths and elastic moduli, and higher elongations to fracture compared with other classes of biomaterials. They are thermal and electrical insulators, and when constituted as a high-molecular-weight system without plasticizers, they are relatively resistant to biodegradation. Compared with bone, most polymers have lower elastic moduli with magnitudes closer to soft tissues.

Polymers have been fabricated in porous and solid forms for tissue attachment, replacement, and augmentation, and as coatings

> ### • BOX 5.2   Advantages of Zirconia Implants
>
> - More esthetically pleasing
> - Retains less plaque and calculus in comparison with titanium (less biofilm)
> - Excellent flexural strength and fracture toughness
> - Favorable and possibly better bone–implant contact in comparison with titanium
> - Does not undergo corrosion
> - No piezoelectric current with dissimilar metals
> - Thermally nonconductive

> ### • BOX 5.3   Disadvantages of Zirconia Implants
>
> - Clinical studies into long-term success are limited
> - One-piece implants require a load-free healing period
> - One-piece implants may require modification depending on positioning
> - Modification leads to reduction of physical properties of material
> - Lack of research on two-piece zirconia abutments
> - Slightly higher fracture rates than titanium

for force transfer to soft tissue and hard tissue regions. Cold-flow characteristics and creep and fatigue strengths are relatively low for some classes of polymers (e.g., silicone rubber and PMMA) and have resulted in some limitations. In contrast, some are extremely tough and fatigue-cycle resistant (e.g., polypropylene, ultra-high-molecular-weight polyethylene, PTFE) and afford opportunities for mechanical force transfer within selected implant designs. Most uses have been for internal force distribution connectors for osteointegrated implants, where the connector is intended to better simulate biomechanical conditions for normal tooth functions. The indications for PTFE have grown exponentially recently because of the development of membranes for guided tissue regeneration techniques. However, PTFE has a low resistance to contact abrasion and wear phenomena.

Composites

Combinations of polymers and other categories of synthetic biomaterials continue to be introduced. Several of the more inert polymers have been combined with particulate or fibers of carbon, Al_2O_3, HA, and glass ceramics. Some are porous, whereas others are constituted as solid-composite structural forms.[154,155]

In some cases, biodegradable polymers, such as poly vinyl alcohol, polylactides or glycolides, cyanoacrylates, or other hydratable forms have been combined with biodegradable $CaPO_4$ particulate or fibers.[156] These are intended as structural scaffolds, plates, screws, or other such applications. Biodegradation of the entire system, after tissues have adequately reformed and remodeled, has allowed the development of significantly advantageous procedures such as bone augmentation and peri-implant defect repairs.

In general, polymers and composites of polymers are especially sensitive to sterilization and handling techniques. If intended for implant use, then most cannot be sterilized by steam or ethylene oxide. Most polymeric biomaterials have electrostatic surface properties and tend to gather dust or other particulate if exposed to semiclean air environments. Because many can be shaped by cutting or autopolymerizing in vivo (PMMA), extreme care must be taken to maintain quality surface conditions of the implant. Porous polymers can be deformed by elastic deformation, which can close open regions intended for tissue ingrowth. In addition, cleaning of contaminated porous polymers is not possible without a laboratory environment. In this regard, talc or starch on surgical

TABLE 5.5   Engineering Properties of Polymers (Some Medical Grades)

Material	Modulus of Elasticity GPa (Psi × 10^5)	Ultimate Tensile Strength MPa (ksi)	Elongation to Fracture (%)
PTFE	0.5–3 (0.07–4.3)	17–28 (2.5–4)	200–600
PET	3 (4.3)	55 (8)	50–300
PMMA	3 (4.3)	69 (10)	2–15
PE	8 (1.2)	48 (7)	400–500
PP	9 (1.3)	35 (5)	500–700
PSF	3.5 (5)	69 (10)	20–100
SR	0.1 (0.014)	5 (1.1)	300–900
POM	3 (4.3)	70 (10.1)	10–75

Polymer properties exhibit a wide range depending on processing and structure. These values have been taken from general tables.

GPa, Gigapascal; *ksi*, thousand pounds per inch squared; *MPa*, megapascal; *PE*, polyethylene; *PET*, polyethylene terephthalate; *PMMA*, polymethylmethacrylate; *POM*, polyoxymethylene (IME insert); *PP*, polypropylene; *PSF*, polysulfone; *PTFE*, polytetrafluoroethylene; *SR*, silicone rubber.

gloves, contact with a towel or gauze pad, or the touching of any contaminated area must be prevented for all biomaterials.

Long-term experience, excellent biocompatibility profiles, ability to control properties through composite structures, and properties that can be altered to suit the clinical application make polymers and composites excellent candidates for biomaterial applications, as the constant expansion of the applications of this class of biomaterials can verify.

Inserts and Intramobile Elements

Relatively low moduli of elasticity (compared with metals and ceramics), high elongations to fracture, and inherent toughness have resulted in use of selected polymers for connectors or interpositional spacers for dental implants. One popular polymer insert system was included in Table 5.5 for general reference purposes. The most significant limitation has been the polymeric materials' resistance to cyclical-load creep and fatigue phenomena. Retrieved transfer systems, in some clinical retrievals, have shown significant plastic deformation and fracture.[157] Although the desire to achieve such a stress-damping effect seems well founded, the inadequate long-term performance of the materials and high time and cost associated with maintenance of these devices have limited their field of application, and they are used less today than during the previous decade.

Future Areas of Application

Synthetic substances for tissue replacement have evolved from selected industrial-grade materials such as metals, ceramics, polymers, and composites. This situation offers opportunities for improved control of basic properties. The simultaneous evolution of the biomechanical sciences also provides optimization of design and material concepts for surgical implants. Knowledge of tissue properties and computer-assisted modeling and analyses also supports the present developments. The introduction of anisotropy with respect to mechanical properties; chemical gradients from device surface to center, with bonding along the tissue interfaces; and control of all aspects of manufacturing, packaging, delivering, placing, and restoring enhance the opportunities for optimal application and, it is hoped, device treatment longevities. Health care delivery would benefit from better availability and decreased per-unit costs.

Combinations to provide compositions with bioactive surfaces, the addition of active biomolecules of tissue-inductive substances, and a stable transgingival attachment mechanism could improve device systems. An integrated chemical and physical barrier at the soft tissue transition region would, at least theoretically, enhance clinical longevities. Devices that function through bone or soft tissue interfaces along the force-transfer regions could be systems of choice, depending on the clinical situation.[9]

Unquestionably, the trend for conservative treatment of oral diseases will continue. Thus it can be anticipated that dental implants will frequently be a first-treatment option. Therefore increased use of root-form systems is to be expected. Clearly the true efficacy of the various systems will be determined by controlled clinical studies with 10- to 20-year follow-up periods, which include statistically significant quantitative analyses.

Surface Characteristics

Many aspects of biocompatibility profiles established for dental surgical implants have been shown to depend on interrelated biomaterial, tissue, and host factors. For discussion purposes, the biomaterial characteristics can be separated into categories associated with either: (1) surface or (2) bulk properties. In general, the biomaterial surface chemistry (purity and critical surface tension for wetting), topography (roughness), and type of tissue integration (osseous, fibrous, or mixed) can be correlated with shorter- and longer-term in vivo host responses. In addition, the host environment has been shown to directly influence the biomaterial-to-tissue interfacial zone specific to the local biochemical and biomechanical circumstances of healing and longer-term clinical aspects of load-bearing function. The interfacial interaction between recipient tissues and implanted material are limited to the surface layer of the implant and a few nanometers into the living tissues. The details of the integration (hard or soft tissue) and force transfer that results in static (stability) or dynamic (instability or motion) conditions have also been shown to significantly alter the clinical longevities of intraoral device constructs.

Many of the conference proceedings cited have focused on biomaterial-to-tissue interfacial interactions, which strongly supports the value of scrutinizing the surface characteristics of dental implants. This was one consistent recommendation from the 1978 and 1988 consensus conferences on the benefit and risk aspects of dental implant-based clinical treatments.[9,10,158]

The synthetic biomaterials used for the construction of dental implants and the associated abutments that contact subepithelial zones of oral tissues can be classified into *metallic, ceramic,* and *surface-modified* (coated, reacted, or ion-implanted) groups. It has long been recognized that synthetic biomaterials should be mechanically and chemically clean at the time of surgical placement. Surface properties are chemical in nature and have been described in terms of atomic structural characteristics with extensions to the subatomic scale. These characteristics are critical to the surface composition, corrosion resistance, cleanliness, surface energy, flexure, and tendency to interact, such as the ability to denature proteins. Surface characteristics are the theme of this section, with emphasis on metallic, ceramic, and surface-modified dental implant biomaterials.

Surface Characterization and Tissue Interaction

Metal and Alloy Surfaces

Standard grades of alpha (unalloyed) titanium and alpha-beta and beta-base alloys of titanium exist with an oxide surface at normal temperatures, with ambient air or normal physiologic environments that act as oxidizing media. A formation of a thin oxide exists via dissociation of and reactions with oxygen or other mechanisms such as oxygen or metal ion diffusion from and to the metallic surface, especially for titanium. Independent from the fabrication process, the oxide is primarily TiO_2, with small quantities of Ti_2O_3 and TiO, with some minor variable stoichiometry.[159-163] This thin layer of amorphous oxide will rapidly re-form if removed mechanically. Surface properties are the result of this oxide layer and differ fundamentally from the metallic substrate.[63,160] Therefore the oxidation parameters such as temperature, type and concentration of the oxidizing elements, and eventual contaminants all influence the physical and chemical properties of the final implant product. The type of oxide on surgical implants is primarily amorphous in atomic structure (brookite) if formed in normal-temperature air or tissue fluid environments, and is usually very adherent and thin in thickness dimensions (<20 nm). In contrast, if unalloyed titanium (alpha) substrates (titanium grades 1–4) are processed at elevated temperatures (above approximately 350° C [660° F]) or anodized in organic acids at higher voltages (above 200 mV), then the oxide forms a crystalline atomic structure (rutile or anatase) and can be 10 to 100 times thicker. The grain structure of the metal and the oxidation process also condition the microstructure and morphology of the surface oxides. Porosity, density, and general homogeneity of the substrate are all related to this process. Low-temperature thermal oxides are relatively homogeneous and dense[164]; with increasing temperatures they become more heterogeneous and more likely to exhibit porosity as scale formations, and some have glass-like surface oxide conditions (semicrystalline).[162,164]

Depending on the mechanical aspects of polishing and the chemical and electrochemical aspects of cleaning and passivating, these amorphous or crystalline oxides can exhibit microscopically smooth or rough topographies at the micrometer level. However, surface macroscopic roughness is normally introduced into the substrate beneath the oxide zone by mechanical (grinding), particulate blasting (resorbable blast media or other), or chemical (acid-etching) procedures. The surface topography and roughness obtained by such techniques is characteristic of each fabrication process.[11,165] The oxide dimension (thickness) along these rougher surfaces remains relatively constant and within nanometer dimensional thicknesses under normal temperature and environmental exposure conditions.

The titanium alloys used for dental implant components include microstructural phases of alpha and beta or room temperature–stabilized beta (only). The alpha-phase surface regions of the alloy are similar to unalloyed titanium in atomic arrangement (close-packed hexagonal), whereas the beta phases demonstrate a different atomic structure (body-centered cubic) and elemental chemistry. However, the beta-phase oxide formation kinetics, chemistry, dimensions, and environmental stabilities are relatively similar to the alpha-phase regions. Electrochemical investigations have shown that the alpha- and beta-phase oxides provide substrate coverage and a high degree of chemical and biochemical inertness (resistance to corrosion and ion transfer) for titanium and alloys of titanium. Both titanium and Ti-6Al-4V have been reported to contain small amounts of titanium nitride along their surface oxide.[161,166,167] Ions, carbon, and substances other than alloying elements may be picked up in the oxide through the preparation process, similar to that found at the surface of commercially pure titanium.[163,168-171] Nevertheless, in the cases of titanium and titanium alloy, the oxide layer grows homogeneously, and a well-controlled inert coating of very stable insoluble oxide normally contacts the living tissues.

Considerable research has been conducted on the roles of alloying elements in titanium alloys and how these elemental compositions may influence oxide properties and host tissue compatibility. This is dependent on the amount of the ions available to the tissues and relative rates of ion transfers, which could result in host tissue toxicity. In general, adequately processed and finished titanium alloys have shown integration with bone and soft tissue environments for a wide range of dental and medical implant devices. Surface analysis studies have shown that the titanium alloy exhibits a similar oxide layer and as such is able to interact with surrounding bone in ways that are similar to unalloyed titanium.[172] Predictable results can be achieved with titanium alloy implant with a similar degree of bone integration.[173] In addition, electrochemical measurements of corrosion and ion release rates strongly support the chemical-biochemical stability properties of titanium alloys.

Some reports have expressed concerns because titanium alloy surface oxides contain significant amounts of alloying elements and exhibit different morphology and crystallization.[166,174-177] Aluminum in particular has been reported in both the outermost and the innermost layers. At the innermost layer, it was found especially overmixed phases (alpha and beta) grains of the alloy.[166] The different surface oxides are then argued to be responsible for a "lesser" quality of osseointegration in particular because of the potential of corrosion products that contain aluminum and vanadium.[178-180] The orthopedic and dental literature specific to in vivo animal and human studies have also documented long-term success with titanium alloys that demonstrated close physical adaption of the bone to the surface of the alloy.[181-188]

Tissue Interactions

Oxide modification during in vivo exposure has been shown to result in increased titanium oxide layer thickness of up to 200 nm.[189-191] The highest oxide growth area corresponded to a bone marrow site, whereas the lowest growth was associated with titanium in contact with cortical regions of bone. Increased levels of calcium and phosphorus were found in the oxide surface layers and seemed to indicate an active exchange of ions at the interface. Hydrogen peroxide environmental conditions have been shown to interact with Ti and form a complex gel.[192-194] "Titanium gel conditions" are credited with attractive in vitro properties such as low apparent toxicity, inflammation, bone modeling, and bactericidal characteristics. The authors restricted their studies to commercially pure titanium exclusively and not titanium alloys.

Other elements interacting with the surface layer of several implanted materials are calcium and phosphorus,[195,196] exhibiting a $CaPO_4$ structure somewhat similar to apatite on the titanium surface. However, the low percentage of these elements along the material surface indicates this was the result of transfer and adsorption of these elements from tissue fluids, not an osteointegration process per se. The surface biointeraction processes may be slow or activated by local reactions, and may cause ion release and oxide alteration of the substrate. Local and systemic increases of the ion concentration have been reported.[197,198] In vitro studies showed that both titanium and titanium alloy were released in measurable quantities of the substrate elements at the surface.[23,199] Especially high rates of ion release were observed in ethylenediamine tetraacetic acid and sodium citrate solutions, and varied as a function of the corroding medium.[199] Ion release corresponds to an oxide layer thickness growth with inclusions of calcium, phosphorus, and sulfur in particular. This is especially a concern for larger orthopedic or porous implants, where such ion release may be a part of the origin of implant failure and allergic reactions, and has even proposed to be a local or systemic reason for the formation of tumors. In addition, free-titanium ions have been shown to inhibit the growth of HA crystals (i.e., the mineralization of calcified tissues at the interface).[200-202]

Integration With Titanium and Alloys

Although titanium is known to exhibit better corrosion resistance, independent of the surface preparation, in vivo and in vitro studies have shown that titanium may interact with the recipient living tissues over several years. This interaction results in the release of small quantities of corrosion products even though a thermodynamically stable oxide film exists.

Several studies have concentrated on the behavior of titanium and titanium alloys in simulated biological environments. Williams[36] cautioned that although titanium can demonstrate excellent properties of its tenacious oxide film, it is usually not sufficiently stable to prevent wear and galling in bearing systems under load. Some situations have resulted in metal-to-metal contact and local welding.

Solar et al.[203] stated that under static conditions, titanium and titanium alloy should withstand exposure to physiologic chlorine solutions at body temperature indefinitely but would be susceptible to oxide changes caused by mechanical micromotion.

Bundy et al.[204] exposed implant alloys simultaneously to tensile stress and corrosive environments (stress-applied conditions). In vivo, stainless-steel and titanium alloy demonstrated crack-like features when loaded to yield stress and then reimplanted under laboratory conditions for 8 weeks. Crack-like features also were seen in stainless-steel and titanium alloy loaded to or beyond the yield stress and subsequently electrochemically polarized for 38 weeks in the in vitro part of the study. None of the samples actually failed by completely cracking, but the authors presumed that it would have occurred with a longer exposure time, as previously suggested.[36,205]

Geis Gerstorfer and Weber[39] used linear polarization methods to show that titanium showed minimal breakdown in simulated tissue fluids, whereas Ni-Ti showed rapid breakdown of passivity with increased chlorine product–related concentrations in unbuffered solutions. Therefore body fluids could be responsible for the dissolution of some metallic passive oxide films.[206]

Lemons[75] studied single-stage solid implants modified by bending or cutting, and showed that damage could increase corrosion.

Rostoker and Pretzel[207] studied couple corrosion in vitro for alloys and found that dissimilar metals in a combined prosthesis did not create a regional breakdown of the titanium passive layer. A second in vivo study evaluated couple and crevice corrosion of prosthetic alloys in vertebral muscles of dogs for 30 weeks (non-load-bearing, nonosseointegrated).[208] It was concluded that metals of superior corrosion resistance, such as titanium alloy, and wrought cobalt alloys can be combined with titanium alloy in one prosthesis to provide superior mechanical performance without creating additional corrosion. However, repeated oxide breakdown such as sustained abrasion was likely to damage the corrosion resistance of an alloy for any type of coupling.

Results from Thompson et al.[209] did not predict accelerated corrosion for titanium alloy coupled to carbon for galvanic couples under static conditions.

Marshak and colleagues[210,211] studied the potential for existence of SCC, GC, and FC in an in vitro study of titanium alloy and gold alloy abutment implants and abutment complexes simultaneously submitted to a laterally oriented 10-kg loading and a simulated tissue fluid solution at 37°C. SCC was studied in the most likely area, that is, the screw-to-abutment connection, which was under constant and simultaneous tension and compression stresses. These studies showed possibilities for interactions at contact regions between the cast gold and titanium alloy and components under selected environmental conditions.

Cohen and Burdairon[212] showed that odontologic fluoride gels, which create an acidic environment, could lead to the degradation of the titanium oxide layer and possibly inhibit the osseointegration process. Deposits consistent with the presence of GC by-products were detected on various surfaces of the experimental metal.[213,214] Liles et al.[215] investigated the GC between titanium and seven crown and bridge alloys in 1% sodium chloride (NaCl) solution. The nonprecious Ni-Co complex was likely to trigger GC. Clinically this means that in the short term, the presence of the surface impurities such as iron found on some implant parts, as well as other contaminants related to the machining process, could result in loss of bone and integration in crestal areas exposed to corrosion products. The long-term presence of corrosion reaction products and ongoing corrosion could also lead to fracture of the affected alloy–abutment interface, the abutment, or possibly the implant body itself. This combination of stress and corrosion, possibly together with factors associated with bacteria, could be one of the reasons why implants fail at the local or individual levels rather than in a generalized fashion.[216] Protocols for manufacturing and cleaning prosthetic titanium parts (specifically abutments that contact the implant body) appear less stringent than those for implant bodies. This should not be the case, and the same standards should be applied to both implant body and prosthetic components. In addition, the short and longer clinical implications of the potential GC effect could be ideally nullified by the use of electrochemically compatible alloys for the superstructure.

Cobalt and Iron Alloys

The alloys of cobalt (Vitallium) and iron (surgical stainless steel—316L) exhibit oxides of chromium (primarily Cr_2O_3 with some suboxides) under normal implant surface–finishing conditions after acid or electrochemical passivation. These chromium oxides, as with titanium and alloys, result in a significant reduction in chemical activity and environmental ion transfers. Under normal conditions of acid passivation, these chromium oxides are relatively thin (nanometer dimensions) and have an amorphous atomic structure. The oxide atomic spatial arrangement can be converted to a crystalline order by elevated temperature or electrochemical exposures.

The chromium oxides on cobalt and iron alloys are microscopically smooth, and again, roughness is usually introduced by substrate processing (grinding, blasting, or etching). Because these oxides, similar to titanium oxides, are very thin (nanometer dimensions), the reflected light color of the alloys depends on the metallic substrate under the oxide.[33] However, as mentioned earlier, the titanium, cobalt, and iron metallic systems depend on the surface reaction zones with oxygen (oxides) for chemical and biochemical inertness.

The cobalt and iron alloy bulk microstructures are normally mixtures of the primary alloy phases with regions of metallic carbides distributed throughout the material.[33,56,76,77] Along the surfaces the chromium oxide covers the matrix phase (metallic regions), whereas the carbides stand as secondary components (usually as mounds above the surface) at the microscopic level. In contrast with homogenization-annealed alloys, the as-cast cobalt alloys exhibit multiphasic characteristics within their microstructure, with relatively extensive regions of the alloy surfaces occupied by complex metallic carbides. Thus tissue-to-oxide and tissue-to-metallic carbide zones could be used to describe tissue integration of cobalt alloy. This is uniquely different compared with titanium implant biomaterials, where tissue-to-oxide regions predominate at the interface.[76,77]

The iron-based alloy chromium oxide and substrate are more susceptible to environmental breakdown, in comparison with cobalt- and titanium-based biomaterials. This has been discussed in the literature related to crevice and pitting corrosion biodegradation phenomena for stainless-steel implant systems.[59,76,77] In general, if stainless steel implant surfaces are mechanically altered during implantation, or if the construct introduces an interface that is subjected to biomechanical fretting, then the iron alloy will biodegrade in vivo, and the fatigue strength of surgical stainless steel can be significantly decreased in a corrosive environment.[217] In some cases this has resulted in implant loss. However, in the absence of surface damage, the chromium oxides on stainless steel biomaterials have shown excellent resistance to breakdown, and multiple examples of tissue and host biocompatibility have been shown for implants removed after long-term (beyond 30 years in vivo) implantations.

Dental implants and implant abutments have also been fabricated from gold alloy, with many abutments fabricated from palladium or Co-Cr-Ni-Mo alloys.[37] The minimally alloyed gold and palladium systems are noble electrochemically and do not depend on surface oxides for chemical and biochemical inertness. This would be the case for the high noble alloys (major compositions of gold, platinum, palladium, iridium, and ruthenium). However, some palladium alloys and other lower noble element content alloys gain chemical and biochemical inertness from complex metallic surface oxides.[37] As mentioned earlier, the multicomponent (wrought) cobalt-based alloys, as with other base-metal systems, depend on chromium oxide surface conditions for inertness. In general the noble-metal alloys do not demonstrate the same characteristics of tissue interaction compared with the base-metal (Ti and Co alloy) systems. The ultrastructural aspects of tissue integration have not been extensively investigated for noble-alloy systems, although some have presented results describing osteointegration of gold alloys. The noble alloys, when used in a polished condition, are resistant to debris accumulation on a relative basis compared with other alloys. This has been listed as an advantage for their use in intraoral abutment systems. In addition, mechanical finishing of the more noble alloys can result in a high degree of polish and a minimal concern about damaging or removing surface oxides.

Ceramics

Al_2O_3 ceramics have been extensively investigated related to surface properties and how these properties relate to bone and soft tissue integration.[92,93,104-116,154] Al_2O_3 ceramics are fully oxide materials (bulk and surface), thereby affording advantages related to tissue interface–related investigation. In addition, studies have included the polycrystalline (alumina) and single-crystalline (sapphire) forms of the oxide structure. These forms have introduced very different surface roughness values for the same material substrate plus bulk properties where ion transfer and electrochemical phenomena are minimal influences. Bone and soft tissue integration have been demonstrated for this oxide material over the long term in humans and laboratory animals. Direct relationships have been established between the interfacial events of tissue integration for metallic surface oxides of titanium and chromium and the Al_2O_3 systems. As mentioned previously, surface quality can be directly correlated with tissue integration and clinical longevity. Because the Al_2O_3 ceramics are crystalline and extend throughout the surface and bulk zones, biomechanical instabilities do not alter the chemical aspects of biomaterial properties. (No electrochemical change is introduced if the surface is removed.) Ceramic coatings (e.g., Al_2O_3) have been shown to enhance the corrosion resistance and biocompatibility of metal implants, in particular surgical stainless steel and Ni-Cr, Co-Cr alloys.[218] However, the Ni-Cr and steel alloys can be subject to crevice corrosion. Studies in orthopedics caution that the Al_2O_3 coating may cause a demineralization phenomenon caused by a high local concentration of substrate ions in the presence of metabolic bone disease.[219] This remains to be established within the use of Al_2O_3 implants for clinical applications.

Hydroxyapatite

In addition to the bulk Al_2O_3 biomaterials, $CaPO_4$-based ceramic or ceramic-like coatings have been added to titanium and cobalt

alloy substrates to enhance tissue integration and biocompatibility. These coatings, for the most part, are applied by plasma spraying small-size particles of crystalline HA ceramic powders. The process of coating and the coating dimensions and property characteristics are addressed further in the next section.

The surface topography is characteristic of the preparation process. Variations in the roughness and porosity of the surface (<100 mm) can be categorized in function of the surfacing process. Machined implants exhibit an irregular surface with grooves, ridges, and pits, including a nanometer scale.[220,221] Proponents of such a surface argue that it is the most conducive to cell attachment[159-161] (Fig. 5.8).

Surface roughening by particulate blasting can be achieved by different media. Sandblasting provides irregular rough surfacing with <10-mm scales and a potential for impurity inclusions. Researchers used a titanium alloy Ti-6Al-4V to improve the mechanical properties and elected to electropolish the surface to reduce surface roughness to be only in the 0.1-mm scale by controlled removal of the surface layer by dissolution.[220,222,223] Titanium implants may be etched with a solution of nitric and hydrofluoric acids to chemically alter the surface and eliminate some types of contaminant products (Fig. 5.9). The acids rapidly attack metals other than titanium, and these processes are electrochemical in nature. Proponents of this technique argue that implants treated by sandblasting and acid etch provide superior radiographic bone densities along implant interfaces compared

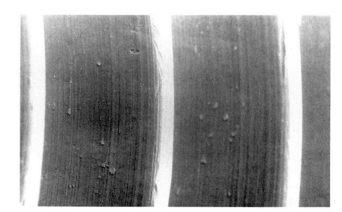

• **Fig. 5.8** Machined surfaces exhibit an irregular surface with grooves, ridges, and pits, including a nanometer scale. *(Brånemark fixture, Nobel Biocare)*

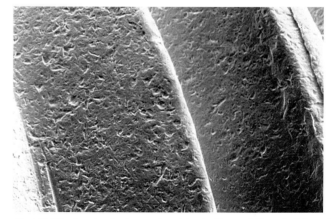

• **Fig. 5.9** Titanium implants may be etched with a solution of nitric and hydrofluoric acids. *(Screw-vent implant, Zimmer)*

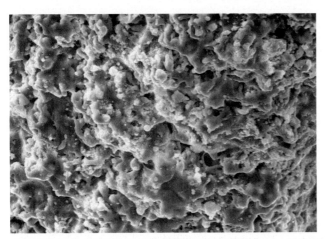

● **Fig. 5.10** Resorbable blast media provide a comparable roughness to alumina grit blast finish, which can be rougher than machined or etched surfaces. *(D2 Maestro implant, BioHorizons)*

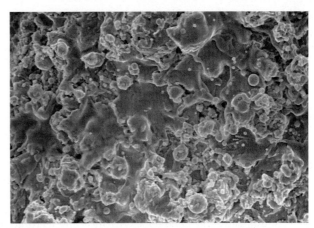

● **Fig. 5.11** Titanium plasma-sprayed surfaces result in increased total surface area, which may introduce a dual physical and chemical anchor system and increase load-bearing capability (scanning electron microscopy of BioHorizons D3 implant; ×500).

with titanium plasma-sprayed surfaces.[224] Recently, concerns have been expressed regarding embedded media from glass beading (satin finish) and grit blasting (alumina Al_2O_3), and a possible risk for associated osteolysis caused by foreign debris.[225,226] Ricci et al.[226] reported on failed retrieved implants that exhibited extensive surface inclusions consisting of silicon and/or Al_2O_3-related product, which were also present in the surrounding tissues. A relatively new process (resorbable blast media) has been said to provide a comparable roughness to an alumina grit blast finish, which can be a rougher surface than the machined, glass-beaded, or acid-etched surfaces (Fig. 5.10).[227]

Porous and Featured Coatings

The implant surface may also be covered with a porous coating. These may be obtained with titanium or HA particulate–related fabrication processes. Examples of coatings and processes for producing surface-modified implants are summarized in the following sections.

Titanium Plasma Sprayed

Porous or rough titanium surfaces have been fabricated by plasma spraying a powder form of molten droplets at high temperatures. At temperatures in the order of 15,000°C, an argon plasma is associated with a nozzle to provide very high-velocity (600 m/sec) partially molten particles of titanium powder (0.05- to 0.1-mm diameter) projected onto a metal or alloy substrate.[63,228] The plasma-sprayed layer after solidification (fusion) is often provided with a 0.04- to 0.05-mm thickness. When examined microscopically, the coatings show round or irregular pores that can be connected to each other (Fig. 5.11). Hahn and Palich[229] first developed these types of surfaces and reported bone ingrowth in titanium hybrid powder plasma spray–coated implants inserted in animals. Karagianes and Westerman[230] assessed the suitability of porous titanium and titanium alloy to achieve bone–implant bonding characteristics in miniature swine and likened it to a three-dimensional surface. Kirsch[157] conducted histologic studies for plasma flame-sprayed particulate titanium coating root form specimen (IMZ) implanted and integrated to the bone in dogs, with complete integration reported at 6 weeks. In animal experiments and histologic studies, Schroeder et al.[231] concluded that the rough and porous surfaces showed a three-dimensional, interconnected

configuration likely to achieve bone–implant attachment for stable anchorage. Other animal studies concluded that a porous titanium surface from various fabrication methods may increase the total surface area (up to several times), produce attachment by osteoformation, enhance attachment by increasing ionic interactions, introduce a dual physical and chemical anchor system, and increase the load-bearing capability 25% to 30%.[100,157,232-237] In vitro studies of fibroblast attachment conducted by Lowenberg et al.[238] showed superior attachment to surface-ground titanium alloy disks compared with porous titanium but with a better cell orientation on porous forms of titanium.

In 1981 Clemow et al.[239] showed that the rate and percentage of bone ingrowth into the surface was inversely proportional to the square root of the pore size for sizes greater than 100 mm and that the shear properties of the interface were proportional to the extent of bone ingrowth. The optimum pore size for bone ingrowth was determined in a study of cobalt-base alloy porous implants inserted in canine femurs. The optimum pore size was deduced from the maximum fixation strength measurements. These surface porosities ranged from 150 to 400 mm and coincidentally correspond to surface feature dimensions obtained by some plasma-spraying processes.[240-243] In addition, porous surfaces can result in an increase in tensile strength through ingrowth of bony tissues into three-dimensional features. High shear forces determined by the torque-testing methods and improved force transfer into the peri-implant area have also been reported.[244,245]

In 1985 at the Brussels Osseointegration Conference, the basic science committee did not present results that showed any major differences between smooth, rough, or porous surfaces regarding their ability to achieve osseointegration. However, proponents of porous surface preparations reported that there have been results showing faster initial healing compared with noncoated porous titanium implants and that porosity allows bone formation within the porosities even in the presence of some micromovement during the healing phase.[246,247] Such surfaces were also reported to allow the successful placement of shorter-length implants compared with noncoated implants. The basic theory was based on increased area for bone contact. Reports in the literature caution about cracking and scaling of coatings because of stresses produced by elevated temperature processing[248,249] and risk for accumulation of abraded material in the interfacial zone during implanting of titanium plasma-sprayed implants. It may be indicated to restrict the limit of coatings in lesser bone densities that cause less frictional torque transfer during the implant placement process. In addition, the present technology allows metallurgic bonding of coatings and a high resistance against mechanical separation of the coating, with many coating test values exceeding the published standard requirements.[250]

Hydroxyapatite Coating

HA coating by plasma spraying was brought to the dental profession by deGroot.[92] Kay et al.[251] used scanning electron microscopy and spectrographic analyses to show that the plasma-sprayed HA coating could be crystalline and could offer chemical and mechanical properties compatible with dental implant applications. Block et al.[252] and Thomas et al.[253] showed an accelerated bone formation and maturation around HA-coated implants in dogs compared with noncoated implants. HA coating can also reduce the corrosion rate of the same substrate alloys.[254] Researchers measured the HA coating thickness after retrieval from specimens inserted in animals for 32 weeks, and it showed a consistent thickness of 50 mm, which is in the range advocated for manufacturing.[19,89,255,256] The bone adjacent to the implant has been reported to be better organized than with other implant materials and with a higher degree of mineralization.[257] In addition, numerous histologic studies have documented the greater surface area of bone apposition to the implant in comparison with uncoated implants,[252,258,259] which may enhance the biomechanics and initial load-bearing capacity of the system. HA coating has been credited with enabling HA-coated titanium or titanium alloy implants to obtain improved bone–implant attachment compared with machined surfaces.

Studies also demonstrated that the HA–bone attachment is superior to the HA–implant interface.[253,255,256] However, proponents of such surfaces report excellent reliability of HA-coated implants.[260,261] The most significant result is the increase in bone penetrations, which enhances fixation in areas of limited initial bone contact.[37,40,41,262] However, controversies still exist, and some authors caution that HA coatings do not necessarily represent an advantage for the long-term prognosis of the system.

Implants of solid sintered HA have been shown to be susceptible to fatigue failure.[98,256,263] This situation can be altered by the use of a CPC coating along metallic substrates. Although several methods may be used to apply CPC coatings, the majority of commercially available implant systems are coated by a plasma spray technique. A powdered crystalline HA is introduced and melted by the hot, high-velocity region of a plasma gun and propelled onto the metal implant as a partially melted ceramic (Fig. 5.12).[108,228] One of the concerns regarding CPC coatings is the strength of the bond between the CPC and the metallic substrate. Investigative ion beam–sputtering coating techniques for CPC or CPC-like nonresorbable coatings to varied substrates appear to produce dense, more tenacious, and thinner coatings (a few micrometers), which would minimize the problem of poor shear strength and fatigue at the coating–substrate interface.[108] Recent reports have introduced a new type of treatment for coatings, which appear primarily amorphous in nature, and further in vivo studies are needed to determine tissue response.[264,265] Other investigations include developing new biocompatible coatings based on TCP or titanium nitride.[266]

It has been shown that the plasma-spraying technique can alter the nature of the crystalline ceramic powder and can result in the

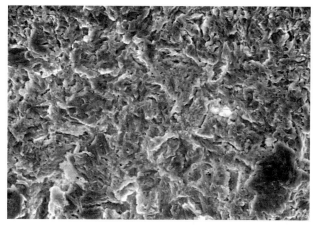

● **Fig. 5.12** Hydroxyapatite (HA) coatings on implant surface provide several clinical properties because of the osteoconductive properties of HA (scanning electron microscopy of BioHorizons D4 implant; ×500).

deposition of a variable percentage of a resorbable amorphous phase.[267] A dense coating with a high crystallinity has been listed as desirable to minimize in vivo resorption. In addition, the deposited CPC may be partially resorbed through remodeling of the osseous interface.[28,268,269] It is therefore wise to provide a biomechanically sound substructure design[267,268] that is able to function under load-bearing conditions to compensate for the potential loss of the CPC coating over years. In addition, the CPC coatings may resorb in infected or chronic inflammation areas. Animal studies also show reductions in coating thickness after in vivo function.[270] One advantage of CPC coatings is that they can act as a protective shield to reduce potential slow ion release from the Ti-6Al-4V substrate.[271] In addition, the interdiffusion between titanium and calcium (and phosphorus and other elements) may enhance the coating substrate bond by adding a chemical component to the mechanical bond.[269,272-275]

When these coatings were introduced in the 1990's., many researchers expressed concerns about the biomechanical and gingival sulcus area biochemical stabilities. It was recommended that national and international standards for these coatings be developed, in part to provide detailed description of coating properties using consistent and uniform (standardized) test methods. Initial national standards were developed for *Beta Tricalcium Phosphate for Surgical Implantation by the ASTM Committee F4* (ASTM F4-1088). A standard specification for *Composition of Ceramic Hydroxyapatite for Surgical Implants* (ASTM F4-1185) was developed, and additional standards have been more recently approved, including *Glass and Glass-Ceramic Biomaterials for Implantation* (ASTM F4-1538), *Standard Test Method for Tension Testing of Calcium Phosphate Coatings* (ASTM F4-1501 F1147-05), *Standard Test Method for Calcium Phosphate Coatings for Implantable Materials* (ASTM F4-1609), *Test Method for Bending and Shear Fatigue Testing of Calcium Phosphate Coatings on Solid Metallic Substrates* (ASTM F4-1659 1160), and a *Standard Test Method for Shear Testing of Calcium Phosphate Coatings* (ASTM F4-1658 1044).[19] Additional standards being developed at the task-group level with ASTM F4 include *Calcium Phosphate Coating Crystalline Characteristics, Mechanical Requirements for Calcium Phosphate Coatings,* and *Environmental Stability of Calcium Phosphate Coatings F1926.* An additional standard on anorganic bone (ASTM F4-1581) has also been established within the ceramics subcommittee of ASTM F4.[19] These national and related international standards

(ISO) should provide basic property information for $CaPO_4$ materials and coatings. This information should prove most useful as longer-term investigations on biocompatibility are conducted for dental implant systems.

In addition, national and international standards have been established for the surgical implant alloys, bulk ceramics, and surface finishing of metallic biomaterials. The concerns related to $CaPO_4$ coatings have focused on: (1) the biomechanical stability of the coatings and coating–substrate interface under in vivo conditions of cyclic loading, and (2) the biochemical stability of these coatings and interfaces within the gingival sulcus (especially in the presence of inflammation or infection) and during enzymatic processes associated with osteoclasis remodeling of the bone–coating interfacial zones. Some of these questions were addressed at an ASTM symposium on $CaPO_4$ coatings, and some researchers related that the longer-term clinical studies (less than 10 years' experience) do not support reasons for concern. It will be interesting to reevaluate these questions and answers after 20 years of clinical experience.

Other Surface Modifications

Surface modification methods include controlled chemical reactions with nitrogen or other elements or surface ion implantation procedures. The reaction of nitrogen with titanium alloys at elevated temperatures results in titanium nitride compounds being formed along the surface. These nitride surface compounds are biochemically inert (like oxides) and alter the surface mechanical properties to increase hardness and abrasion resistance. Most titanium nitride surfaces are gold in color, and this process has been used extensively for enhancing the surface properties of industrial and surgical instruments.[19] Increased hardness, abrasion, and wear resistance can also be provided by ion implantation of metallic substrates. The element most commonly used for surface ion implantation is nitrogen. Electrochemically the titanium nitrides are similar to the oxides (TiO_2), and no adverse electrochemical behavior has been noted if the nitride is lost regionally. The titanium substrate reoxidizes when the surface layer of nitride is removed. Nitrogen implantation and carbon-doped layer deposition have been recommended to improve the physical properties of stainless steel without affecting its biocompatibility.[276] Again, questions could be raised about coating loss and crevice corrosion.

Surface Cleanliness

A clean surface is an atomically clean surface with no other elements than the biomaterial constituents. Contaminants can be particulates, continuous films (e.g., oil, fingerprints), and atomic impurities or molecular layers (inevitable) caused by the thermodynamic instability of surfaces. Even after reacting with the environment, surfaces have a tendency to lower their energy by binding elements and molecules. The typical composition of a contaminated layer depends on atmospheres and properties of surface. For example, high-energy surfaces (metals, oxides, ceramics) usually tend to bind more to this type of monolayer than polymers and carbon (amorphous).

In the earlier times of dental implantology, no specific protocol for surface preparation, cleaning, sterilization, and handling of the implants was established.[277] Researchers have respectively demonstrated adverse host responses caused by faulty preparation and sterilization, omission to eliminate adsorbed gases, and organic and inorganic debris.[159,160,174,278] According to Albrektsson,[177] implants that seem functional may fail even after years of

function, and the cause may be attributed to improper ultrasonic cleaning, sterilization, or handling during the surgical placement.

A systematic study of contamination layers is not available. Lausmaa et al.[161] showed that titanium implants had large variations in carbon contamination loads (20%–60%) in the 0.3- to 1-nm thickness range, attributed to air exposure and residues from cleaning solvents and lubricants used during fabrication. Trace amounts of Ca, P, N, Si, S, Cl, and Na were noted from other studies.[169,170,278-280] Residues of fluorine could be attributed to passivation and etching treatments; Ca, Na, and Cl to autoclaving; and Si to sand and glass-beading processes.

Surface Energy

Measurements of surface property values of an implant's ability to integrate within bone include contact angle with fluids, local pH, and surface topography. These are often used for the determination of surface characteristics. Numerous studies were conducted to evaluate liquid, solid, and air contact angles, wetting properties, and surface tensions as criteria to assess surface cleanliness, because these parameters have been shown to have a direct consequence on osseointegration.[12,281,282] An intrinsically high surface energy is said to be most desirable. High surface energy implants showed a threefold increase in fibroblast adhesion, and higher-energy surfaces such as metals, alloys, and ceramics are best suited to achieve cell adhesion.[12] Surface tension values of 40 dyne/cm and higher are characteristic of very clean surfaces and excellent biological integration conditions.[281] A shift in contact angle (increase) is related to the contamination of the surface by hydrophobic contaminants and decreases the surface tension parameters. Because a spontaneously deposited, host-dependent conditioning film is a prerequisite to the adhesion of any biological element, it is suggested that the wetting of the surface by blood at the time of placement can be a good indication of the high surface energy of the implant.[281]

Passivation and Chemical Cleaning

ASTM International (ASTM B600, ASTM F-86) specifications for final surface treatment of surgical titanium implants require pickling and descaling with molten alkaline base salts. This is often followed by treatment with a solution of nitric or hydrofluoric acid to decrease and eliminate contaminants such as iron. Iron or other elements may contaminate the implant surface as a result of the machining process. This type of debris can have an effect of demineralizing the bone matrix.[283,284] However, these finishing requirements remain very general. Studies of fibroblast attachment on implant surfaces showed great variations, depending on the different processes of surface preparation. Inoue et al.[181] showed that fibroblasts developed a capsule or oriented fibrous attachment following the grooves in titanium disks. Contact angles are also greatly modified by acid treatment or water rinsing.[285] Machining operations, polishing, texturing process, residual chemical deposits, and alloy microstructure all inadvertently affect the surface composition. In addition, many ways exist to intentionally modify the surface of the implant. They include conventional mechanical treatment (sandblasting), wet or gas chemical reaction treatment, electroplating or vapor plating, and ion beam processing, which leaves bulk properties intact and has been newly adapted to dentistry from thin film technology. Preliminary studies by Schmidt[286] and Grabowski et al.[287] showed modified fibroblast adhesion on nitrogen and carbon-ion implanted titanium. A general rule has been that cleaner is better.

Sterilization

Manipulation with bare fingers or powdered gloves, tap water, and residual vapor-carried debris from autoclaving can all contaminate implant surfaces. Baumhammers,[277] in a scanning electron microscopy study of dental implants, showed contamination of the surface with acrylic materials, powder from latex gloves, and bacteria. Today, in most cases, the manufacturer guarantees precleaned and presterilized implants with high-technology procedures, with the implants ready to be inserted. If an implant needs to be resterilized, then conventional sterilization techniques are not normally satisfactory. It appears at the present time that no sterilization medium is totally satisfactory for all biomaterials and designs. Metal or alloy constituents, inorganic and organic particles, corrosion products, polymers, and precipitates can be absorbed at the surface throughout the manufacturing, polishing, cleaning, sterilization, packaging, and storage processes. Baier et al.[12] correlated the usual type of contaminant found in relation to the sterilization technique used. Baier and Meyer[281] showed that steam sterilization can cause deposits of organic substances resulting in poor tissue adhesion. Doundoulakis[169] submitted titanium samples to different sterilization techniques, concluded the adverse effect of steam sterilization and degradative effect of endodontic glass bead sterilizers, found that dry heat sterilization leaves organic deposits on the surface, and suggested that ultraviolet (UV) light sterilization may become a good alternative after further evaluation. In addition, accelerated oxide growth on titanium may occur with impurity contamination leading to surface discoloration.[32,159,288] In a study by Keller et al.,[289] corrosion products and films from autoclaving, chemicals, and cytotoxic residues from solutions were identified at the surface of implants submitted to sterilization. They suggested that alteration of the titanium surface by sterilization methods may in turn affect the host response and adhesive properties of the implant. In contrast, Schneider et al.[290] compared the surface of titanium plasma-sprayed and HA-coated titanium implants after steam or ethylene dioxide sterilization using energy-dispersive radiograph analysis and concluded that these techniques do not modify the elemental composition of the surface. Keller and colleagues[291] studied the growth of fibroblasts on disks of commercially pure titanium sterilized by autoclaving, ethylene oxide, ethyl alcohol, or solely passivated with 30% nitric acid, and concluded that sterilization seems to inhibit cell growth, whereas passivation does not.

Presently, proteinaceous deposits and their action as films can be best eliminated by the radiofrequency glow discharge technique (RFGDT), which seems to be a suitable final cleaning procedure. The implants are treated within a controlled noble-gas discharge at very low pressure. The gas ions bombard the surface and remove surface atoms and molecules, which are absorbed onto it or are constituents of it. However, the quality of the surface treated depends on the gas purity. Baier and Glantz[292] showed that RFGDT is good for cleaning and, at the same time, for granting a high-energy state to the implant, which is related to improved cell adhesion capabilities. Thinner, more stable oxide films and cleaner surfaces have been reported with RFGDT plus improved wettability and tissue adhesion.[292-294] The principal oxide at the surface is unchanged by the RFGDT process.[295] A decrease in bacteria contamination on HA-coated implant surfaces was reported after RFGDT,[296] and studies suggest that RFGDT may enhance calcium and/or phosphate affinity because of an increase in elemental zone at the surface resulting in the formation of amorphous $CaPO_4$ compounds.[294]

Recently a modified UV light sterilization protocol was shown to enhance bioreactivity, which was also effective for eliminating some biological contaminants. Singh and Schaaf[297] assessed the quality of UV light sterilization and its effects on irregularly shaped objects, and they established its effectiveness on spores and its ability to safely and rapidly clean the surface and to grant high surface energy. Hartman et al.[298] submitted implants to various pretreatment protocols (RFGDT, UV light, or steam sterilization) and inserted them in miniature swine. Although RFGDT- and UV-sterilized implants showed rapid bone ingrowth and maturation, steam-sterilized implants seemed to favor thick collagen fibers at the surface. In contrast, Carlsson et al.[299] inserted implants in rabbits and compared the performances of conventionally treated implants with implants treated with RFGDT, found similar healing responses, and further cautioned that the RFGDT process produces a much thinner oxide layer at the surface of the implant and may deposit silica oxide from the glass envelope.

Adequate sterilization of clean, prepackaged dental implants and related surgical components has resulted in an ever-expanding use of gamma radiation procedures. Because gamma radiation sterilization of surgical implants is a well-established methodology within the industry, facilities, procedures, and standards are well known. Most metallic systems are exposed to radiation doses exceeding 2.5 Mrad, where the packaging and all internal parts of the assembly are sterilized. This is an advantage in that components remain protected, clean, and sterile until the inner containers are opened within the sterile field of the surgical procedure. The healing screws, transfer elements, wrenches, and implants are all exposed to the gamma sterilization, which reduces opportunities for contamination.

Some ceramics can be discolored and some polymers degraded by gamma radiation exposures. The limits are known for classes of biomaterials, and all types of biomaterials can be adequately sterilized within the industry. Systems control, including prepackaging and sterilization, has been an important part of the success of dental implantology.

Summary

In the 1960s dental implantology as a clinical discipline was judged by some to be rather disorganized, and treatments provided were often said to be not as successful as hospital-based orthopedic and cardiovascular surgery procedures. One part of this opinion related to the use of standard intraoral dental materials for implants plus general dental operatories for surgical activities (e.g., no gloves, high-speed drills, tap water). The biomaterials discipline evolved rapidly in the 1970s. Successful uses of synthetic biomaterials have been based on experience within the field of dental implantology. The basis for many of the newer and more clinically successful surgical reconstructions evolved within dentistry, with some now recognized as the most successful types of musculoskeletal reconstructive surgery. The biomaterials discipline therefore has evolved significantly since the 1990's, and synthetic biomaterials are now constituted, fabricated, and provided to health care professionals as mechanically and chemically clean devices that have a high predictability of success when used appropriately within the surgical disciplines. This chapter on biomaterials has been separated into sections related to bulk and surface properties of biomaterials, and emphasis has been placed on the published literature on how these biomaterial properties relate to interactions at the tissue interface.

Surface characterization and working knowledge about how surface and bulk biomaterial properties interrelate to dental implant biocompatibility profiles represent an important area in implant-based reconstructive surgery. This chapter has provided summary information on surface and bulk properties for metallic, ceramic, and surface-modified biomaterials. The authors strongly recommend the reference material listed, in addition to a desire to have investigators always provide biomaterial surface and bulk property information as a component of any research studies on tissue response (biocompatibility) profiles.

Acknowledgments

In 1970 Jack E. Lemons was attending his first American and International Associations for Dental Research (AADR/IADR) meeting and was introduced to Ralph Phillips within a group discussion on dental materials. Phillips quickly determined that Lemons knew little about the "dental" and some about the "materials." Phillips included Lemons in the interactions with carefully placed and directed questions and comments so that he was not excluded. This happened repeatedly over the years, until Lemons had the opportunity to reverse the exchange after making a presentation on behalf of the AADR/IADR Dental Materials Group on basic biocompatibility testing, with Phillips as the overview discussant. This opportunity was to coordinate and help direct some of the emerging exchanges among those experienced in the material and biological sciences. Subsequently, ongoing interactions with Phillips fostered many wonderful times with colleagues, students, and friends throughout the world.

The contents of this chapter represent a later stage, in which Lemons provided written comments and opinions about implant biomaterials as one extension of dental biomaterials. This chapter is dedicated in part to Phillips's memory, and most especially to their long-term friendship. The dental implant field, in the authors' opinion, will benefit from a continuation of a multidisciplinary approach to the science, technology, and applications. We wish that Ralph could have continued, and we certainly will miss his counsel.

References

1. Williams DF, ed. *Biocompatibility of Clinical Implant Materials.* Vol. 1. Boca Raton, Fla: CRC Press; 1981.
2. Zierold AA. Reaction of bone to various metals. *Arch Surg.* 1924;9:365.
3. Menegaux GA. Action cytotoxique de quelques metaux sur le tissu osseux cultive en vie ralentie. *Presse Med.* 1935;42:1.
4. Venable CS, Stuck WG, Beach A. The effects on bone of the presence of metals based upon electrolysis, an experimental study. *Ann Surg.* 1939;105:917–938.
5. Ludwigson DC. Today's prosthetic metals. *J Metals.* 1964;16.
6. Williams DF, Roaf R. *Implants in Surgery.* London: WB Saunders; 1973.
7. Weissman SL. Models for systemic effects of implants. *Nat Spec Pub.* 1997;472:28.
8. Natiella J, Armitage JJ, Meenaghan M, et al. Current evaluation of dental implants. *J Am Dent Assoc.* 1972;84:1358.
9. Rizzo AA, ed. Proceedings of the 1988 consensus development conference on dental implants. *J Dent Educ.* 1988;52:678–827.
10. Dental implants: benefit and risk, PHS No 81-1531. In: Schnitman PA, Shulman LB, eds. *Proceedings of the Harvard-National Institute of Dental Research Conference.* Boston 1980.
11. Von Recuum A, ed. *Handbook of Biomaterials Evaluation.* New York: Macmillan; 1986.
12. Baier R, Meyer A, Natiella J, et al. Surface properties determine bioadhesive outcomes. *J Biomed Mater Res.* 1984;18:337–355.
13. Baier R, Shafrin E, Zisman WA. Adhesion: mechanisms that assist or impede it. *Science.* 1968;162:1360.
14. Davies JE, ed. *The Bone-Biomaterial Interface.* Toronto: University of Toronto Press; 1991.
15. Plenk H, Zitter H. Material considerations. In: Watzek G, ed. *Endosseous Implants: Scientific and Clinical Aspects.* Chicago: Quintessence; 1996.
16. Zitter H, Plenk H. The electrochemical behavior of metallic implant materials as an indicator of their biocompatibility. *J Biomed Mater Res.* 1987;21:881–896.
17. Zwicker U, Breme J, Etzold U. *Titanwerkstoffe mit niedrigem elastizitatsmodul aus gesinterten titanlegierungspulvern, Vortage der 7. Sitzung d. DVM-Arbeitskreises Implantate am 18.11 1986.* Bundesanstalt fur Material prufung. Berlin; 1986: 47–58.
18. Zitter H, Maurer KL, Gather T, et al. Implantatwerkstoffe. *Berg und Hüttenmänn Monatshefte.* 1990;135:171–181.
19. American Society for Testing and Materials. *Surgical and Medical Devices.* Vol. 14.01. Philadelphia: American Society for Testing and Materials; 1996.
20. *International Standards Organization, Standard References.* Philadelphia: ANSI-USA; 1996.
21. *American Dental Association.* Chicago: Standards; 1996.
22. Williams DF. *Biocompatibility of Orthopaedic Implants.* Vol. 1. Boca Raton, Fla: CRC Press; 1982.
23. Ducheyne P, Hastings GW, eds. *Functional Behavior of Orthopaedic Materials.* Vols. 2. Boca Raton, Fla: CRC Press; 1984.
24. Till T, Wagner G. Uber elektrochemische untersuchungen an verschiedenen metallischen Zahnreparaturmaterialien. *ZWR.* 1971;80:334–339.
25. Ferguson AB, Laing PG, Hodge ES. The ionization of metal implants in living tissues. *J Bone Joint Surg Am.* 1960;42A:77–90.
26. Mears DC. Electron probe microanalysis of tissues and cells from implant areas. *J Bone Joint Surg.* 1966;48B:567.
27. Geis-Gerstorfer J, Weber H, Sauer KH. In vitro substance loss due to galvanic corrosion in Ti implant/Ni-Cr super-construction systems. *Int J Oral Maxillofac Implants.* 1989;4:119–123.
28. Jarcho M. Retrospective analysis of hydroxyapatite development for oral implant applications. *Dent Clin North Am.* 1992;36:19–36.
29. Ogus WI. Research report on implantation of metals. *Dent Dig.* 1951;57:58.
30. Laing P. The significance of metallic transfer in the corrosion of orthopaedic screws. *J Bone Joint Surg Am.* 1958;40:853–869.
31. Willert H, Buchhorn G, Semlitsch M. Particle disease due to wear of metallic alloys. In: Morrey B, ed. *Biological, Material and Mechanical Considerations of Joint Replacement.* New York: Raven Press; 1993.
32. Lemons JE. Dental implant retrieval analyses. *J Dent Educ.* 1988;52:748–756.
33. Lemons JE, Morrey BF. Metals and alloys for devices in musculoskeletal surgery. In: *Joint Replacement Arthroplasty.* Edinburgh: Churchill Livingstone; 1991.
34. Steinemann S. Tissue compatibility of metals from physico-chemical principles. In: Kovaks P, Istephanous N, eds. *Compatibility of Biomechanical Implants, Electrochem Society.* Vol. 94-15. San Francisco: Conference Proceedings; 1994:1–14.
35. Fontana M, Greene N. *Corrosion Engineering.* New York: McGraw-Hill; 1967.
36. Williams DF. Titanium as a metal for implantation. *J Med Eng Technol.* 1977;1(195–202):266–270.
37. Lemons JE. Biomaterial considerations for dental implants. I. Metals and alloys, Alabama Academy of General Dentistry sponsored symposium on dental implants. *J Oral Implantol.* 1975;4:503–515.

38. Van Orden A, Fraker A, Ruff, et al. Surface preparation and corrosion of titanium alloys for surgical implants. In: Luckey H, Kublic F, eds. *ASTM STP 796*. Philadelphia: American Society for Testing and Materials; 1981.

39. Geis Gerstorfer J, Weber H. Corrosion resistance of the implant materials contimet 35, memory and Vitallium in artificial physiological fluids. *Int J Oral Maxillofac Implants*. 1988;3:135–139.

40. Skalak R. Biomechanical considerations in osseointegrated prostheses. *J Prosthet Dent*. 1983;49:843–848.

41. Spector M. Biocompatibility in orthopaedic implants. In: Williams DF, ed. *Biocompatibility of Materials*. Boca Raton, Fla: CRC Press; 1984.

42. Lemons JE, Lucas LC, Johansson B. Intraoral corrosion resulting from coupling dental implants and restorative metallic systems. *Implant Dent*. 1992;1:107–112.

43. Zitter H, Plenk Jr H. The electrochemical behavior of metallic implant materials as an indicator of their biocompatibility. *J Biomed Mater Res*. 1987;21:881–896.

44. Newesely H. Der stand der normung bei dentalimplan-taten, vortrage des arbeitskreises implantate, berichsband d. 5 sitzung d. dtsch verb f. materialforschung u prufung ev. 1984:53–55.

45. *International Standardization Organization Technical Report 10451: Dental Implants—State of the art—Survey of Materials* Geneva; 1991.

46. Lautenschlager EP, Sarker NK, Acharaya A, et al. Anodic polarization of porous metal fibers. *J Biomed Mater Res*. 1974;8:189–191.

47. Rae T. The biological response to titanium and titanium aluminum vanadium alloy particles. *Biomaterials*. 1986;7:3036.

48. Solar RJ, Pellack SR, Korostoff E. In vitro corrosion testing of titanium surgical implant alloys. *J Biomed Mater Res*. 1979;13:217–250.

49. Hoar TP, Mears DC. Corrosion-resistant alloys in chlorine solution: materials for surgical implants. *Proc R Soc Lond B Biol Sci*. 1966;A294:486.

50. Bothe RE, Beaton LE, Davenport HA. Reaction of bone to multiple metallic implants. *Surg Gynecol Obstet*. 1940;71:598–602.

51. Leventhal GS. Titanium, a metal for surgery. *J Bone Joint Surg*. 1951;33:473–474.

52. Beder OE, Eade G. An investigation on tissue tolerance to titanium metal implants in dogs. *Surgery*. 1956;39:470.

53. Gross PP, Gold L. The compatibility of Vitallium and austanium in completely buried implants in dogs. *Oral Surg*. 1957;10:769.

54. Clarke EG, Hickman J. An investigation into the correlation between the electrical potential of metals and their behavior in biological fluids. *J Bone Joint Surg*. 1963;35B:467.

55. Brettle JA. Survey of the literature on metallic surgical implants. *Injury*. 1976;2:26.

56. Lemons JE, Niemann KMW, Weiss AB. Biocompatibility studies on surgical grade Ti, Co and Fe base alloys. *J Biomed Mater Res*. 1976;10:549.

57. Lemons JE, ed. *Quantitative Characterization and Performance of Porous Implants for Hard Tissue Application, ASTM STP 953*. Philadelphia: American Society for Testing and Materials; 1987.

58. Lucas LC, Lemons JE, Lee J et al. *In Vitro Corrosion Characteristics of Co-Cr-Mo/Ti-6Al-4V/Ti Alloys*. Paper presented at the American Society for Testing Materials, Symposium on Quantitative Characteristics of Porous Materials for Host Tissues; 1978.

59. Lucas LC, Bearden LF, Lemons JE. Ultrastructural examinations of in vitro and in vivo cells exposed to solutions of 316L stainless steel. In: Fraker A, Griffin C, eds. *ASTM STP 859*. Philadelphia: American Society for Testing and Materials; 1985.

60. Van Orden AC. Corrosive response of the interface tissue to 316L stainless steel, titanium base alloys and cobalt base alloys. In: McKinney RV, Lemons JE, eds. *The Dental Implant*. San Diego: PSG Co; 1985.

61. Lang B, Mossie H, Razzoog M. *International Workshop: Biocompatibility, Toxicity and Hypersensitivity to Alloy Systems Used in Dentistry*. Ann Arbor, University of Michigan Press; 1985.

62. Steinemann S. Corrosion of surgical implants—in vivo and in vitro tests. In: Winter GD, Jeray JL, deGroot K, eds. *Evaluation of biomaterials*. Chichester, England: Wiley; 1980.

63. Steinemann SG, Perren SM, Muller ME. Titanium alloys as metallic biomaterials. In: Lutjering G, Zwicker U, Bunk W, eds. *Proceedings of the 5th International Conference on Titanium*. Dtsch Gesf Materialkunde eV. 1985;2:1327–1334.

64. Steinemann SG. Corrosion of titanium and titanium alloys for surgical implants. In: Lutering G, Zwicker U, Bunk W, eds. *Proceedings of the 5th International Conference on Titanium*. Dtsch Gesf Materialkunde eV. 1985;2:1373–1379.

65. Hillmann G, Donath K. Licht und elektronemikro-sko-pische untersuchung zur biostabilitat dentaler titanim-plantate. *Z Zahnarztl Implantol*. 1991;7:170–177.

66. Schliephake H, Neukam FW, Urban R. Titanbelastung parenchymatoser organe nach insertion von titanschrau-benimplantaten. *Z Zahnarztl Implantol*. 1989;5:180184.

67. Schliephake H, Reiss G, Urban R, et al. Freisetzung von titan aus schraubenimplantaten. *Z Zahnarztl Implantol*. 1991;6:6–10.

68. Woodman JL, Jacobs JJ, Galante JO, et al. Metal ion release from titanium-based prosthetic segmental replacement of long bones in baboons. A long-term study. *J Orthop Res*. 1984;1:421–430.

69. Ferguson AB, Akahoshi Y, Laing PG, et al. Characteristics of trace ion release from embedded metal implants in the rabbit. *J Bone Joint Surg*. 1962;44:317–336.

70. Osborn JF, Willich P, Meenen N. The release of titanium into human bone from a titanium implant coated with plasma-sprayed titanium. In: Heimke G, Solesz U, Lee AJC, eds. *Advances in Biomaterials*. Amsterdam: Elsevier; 1990.

71. Semlitsch M, Staub F, Weber H. Development for biocom-patible high strength titanium-aluminum-niobium alloy surgical implants. *Biomed Tech (Berl)*. 1985;30:334–339.

72. Newman JR, Eylon D, Thorne JK. Titanium and tita-nium alloys. In: Stefanescu D, Kurz W, eds. *Metals Handbook*. Vol. 15. 9th ed. Metals Park, Ohio: ASM International; 1988.

73. Ott D. Giessen von titan im dentallabor. *Metall*. 1990;44:366–369.

74. Soom U. Reines titan in der zahnmedizin und zahntechnik: anwendungsbereiche in der implantologie und der prothetik. *Swiss Dent*. 1987;8:27–32.

75. Lemons JE. Surface conditions for surgical implants and biocompatibility. *J Oral Implantol*. 1977;7:362–374.

76. Lucas LC, Buchanan RA, Lemons JE. Investigations on the galvanic corrosion of multialloy total hip prostheses. *J Biomed Mater Res*. 1981;15. 753–747.

77. Lucas LC, Buchanan RA, Lemons JE, et al. Susceptibility of surgical cobalt-base alloy to pitting corrosion. *J Biomed Mater Res*. 1982;16:799–810.

78. *Proceedings of the Third World Biomaterials Congress 11*. Kyoto, Japan: Society for Biomaterials; 1988.

79. Brown SA, Lemons JE, eds. *Medical Applications of Titanium and its Alloys: the Material and Biological Issues, STP 1272*. Ann Arbor, Mich: American Society for Testing and Materials; 1996.

80. Bosker H, Kijk L. Het transmandibulaire implantaat. *Ned Tijdschr Tandheelkd*. 1983;90:381–389.

81. Hench LL, Ethridge EC. *Biomaterials, an Interfacial Approach*. New York: Academic Press; 1982.

82. Vincenzini P, ed. *Ceramics in Surgery*. Amsterdam: Elsevier; 1983.

83. Sandhaus S. *Nouveaux Aspects de L'implantologie, L'Implant CBS Suisse*. Lausanne, Switzerland: Sandhaus; 1969.

84. Heimke G, Schulte W, d'Hoedt B, et al. The influence of fine surface structures on the osseo-integration of implants. *Int J Artif Organs*. 1982;5:207–212.

85. McKinney Jr RV, Lemons JE. *The Dental Implant*. Littleton, Mass: PSG Publishing; 1985.

86. Steflic D, Sisk A, Parr G, et al. HVEM and conventional electron microscopy of interface between bone and endosteal dental implants. *J Biomed Mater Res*. 1992;26. 529–245.

87. McKinney R, Steflic D, Koth D, et al. The scientific basis for dental implant therapy. *J Dent Educ.* 1988;52:696–705.
88. Koth DL, McKinney Jr RV. The single crystal sapphire endosteal dental implant. In: Hardin JF, ed. *Clark's Clinical Dentistry.* Philadelphia: JB Lippincott; 1981.
89. Horowitz F, Parr J, eds. *Characterization and Performance of Calcium Phosphate Coatings for Implants, ASTM STP 1196.* Philadelphia: American Society for Testing and Materials; 1994.
90. Brose M, et al. Six year evaluation of submerged alumina dental root implants in humans (IADR abstract 56). *J Dent Res.* 1987;66:113.
91. Driskell TS. Development and application of ceramics and ceramic composites for implant dentistry. In: Young FA, Hulbert DF, eds. *Materials for Implant Dentistry.* New York: Gordon & Breach; 1970.
92. deGroot K, ed. *Bioceramics of Calcium Phosphate.* Boca Raton, Fla: CRC Press; 1983.
93. Ducheyne P, Lemons JE, eds. *Bioceramics: Material Characteristics Versus in Vivo Behavior.* New York: New York Academy of Science; 1988.
94. Koeneman J. Workshop on characterization of calcium phosphate materials. *J Appl Biomater.* 1990;1:79.
95. LeGeros RZ. Calcium phosphate materials in restorative dentistry: a review. *J Dent Res.* 1988;68:164–180.
96. Yamamuro T, Hench L, Wilson J, eds. *Handbooks of Bioactive Ceramics.* Vols. 1 and 2. Boca Raton, Fla: CRC Press; 1990.
97. Kent J, et al. Augmentation of deficient edentulous alveolar ridges with dense polycrystalline hydroxylapatite (abstract 3.8.2). In: *Final Program and Book of Abstracts.* Vienna: First World Biomaterials Congress, Society for Biomaterials; 1980.
98. dePutter C, deGroot K, Sillevis-Smitt P. Transmucosal apatite implants in dogs. *Trans Soc Biomater.* 1981;9:115.
99. English C. Cylindrical implants. *J Calif Dent Assoc.* 1988;16:17–40.
100. Hench LL, Clark AE. Adhesion to bone. In: Williams DF, ed. *Biocompatibility of Orthopaedic Implants.* Vol. 2. Boca Raton, Fla: CRC Press; 1982.
101. Ducheyne P, Healy K, Black J et al. The effects of HA coatings on the metal ion release from porous titanium and Cr-Co alloys. Paper presented at the *Thirteenth Annual Meeting of the Society for Biomaterials.* San Francisco; 1987.
102. Ducheyne P, Martens M. Apatite materials. Clinical and morphological evaluation of custom made bioreactive glass coated canine hip prosthesis. *J Biomed Mater Res.* 1984;18:1017–1030.
103. Ducheyne P, Hench LL, Kagan A, et al. Effect of hydroxyapatite impregnation on skeletal bonding of porous coated implants. *J Biomed Mater Res.* 1987;14:225–237.
104. Lemons JE. Hydroxylapatite coatings. *Clin Orthop Relat Res.* 1988;235:220–223.
105. Driessens F. Formation and stability of calcium phosphates in relation to phase composition of the mineral in calcified tissues. In: deGroot K, ed. *Bioceramics of Calcium Phosphates.* Boca Raton, Fla: CRC Press; 1983.
106. Jarcho M. Calcium phosphate ceramics as hard tissue prostheses. *Clin Orthop Relat Res.* 1981;157:259–278.
107. Hjorting-Hansen E, Worsaae N, Lemons LE. Histological response after implantation of porous hydroxylapatite ceramics in humans. *Int J Oral Maxillofac Implants.* 1990;5:255.
108. Lacefield WC. The coating of hydroxylapatite onto metallic and ceramic implants. In: *Proceedings of the Twelfth Annual Meeting of the Society for Biomaterials.* St Paul, Minn; 1986.
109. Cook SD, et al. Variables affecting the interface strength and histology of hydroxylapatite coated implant surfaces. *Trans Soc Biomater.* 1986;9:14.
110. Lee DR, Lemons J, LeGeros RZ. Dissolution characterization of commercially available hydroxylapatite particulate. *Trans Soc Biomater.* 1989;12:161.
111. Tofe AJ, Watson BA, Bowerman MA. Solution and cell mediated resorption of grafting materials. *J Oral Implantol.* 1991;17:345 (abstract).
112. Jarcho M, Bolen CH, Thomas MB, et al. Hydroxyapatite synthesis and characterization in dense polycrystalline form. *J Mater Sci Mater Med.* 1976;11:2027–2035.
113. Wang S, Lacefield WR, Lemons JE. Interfacial shear strength and histology of plasma sprayed and sintered hydroxyapatite implants in vivo. *Biomaterials.* 1996;17:1965–1970.
114. Gross U, et al. Biomechanically optimized surface pro-files by coupled bone development and resorption at hydroxylapatite surfaces. *Trans Soc Biomater.* 1990;13:83.
115. Lemons JE. Ceramics: past, present and future. *Bone.* 1996;19(suppl):121S–128S.
116. Oonishi H, Aoki H, Sawai K. *Bioceramics.* St Louis: EuroAmerica; 1989.
117. Sivaraman K, Chopra A, Narayan AI, et al. Is zirconia a viable alternative to titanium for oral implant? A critical review. *J Prosthodont Res.* 2018;62(2):121–133.
118. Pieralli S, Kohal RJ, Lopez Hernandez E, et al. Osseointegration of zirconia dental implants in animal investigations: a systematic review and meta-analysis. *Dent Mater.* 2018;34(2):171–182.
119. Sicilia A, Cuesta S, Coma G, et al. Titanium allergy in dental implant patients: a clinical study on 1500 consecutive patients. *Clin Oral Impl Res.* 2008;19:823–835.
120. Christel P, Meunier A, Heller M, et al. Mechanical properties and short term in-vivo evaluation of yttrium-oxide-partially-stabilized zirconia. *J Biomed Mater Res.* 1989;23:45–61.
121. De Aza AH, Chevalier J, Fantozzi G, et al. Crack growth resistance of alumina, zirconia and zirconia toughened alumina ceramics for joint prostheses. *Biomaterial.* 2002;23:937–945.
122. Ardlin BI. Transformation-toughened zirconia for dental inlays, crowns and bridges: chemical stability and effect of low-temperature aging on flexural strength and surface structure. *Dent Mater.* 2002;18(8):590–595.
123. Ross IM, Rainforth WM, McComb DW, et al. The role of trace additions of alumina to yttria-tetragonal zirconia polycrystals (Y-TZP). *Scr Mater.* 2017;45:653–660.
124. Li LF, Watanabe R. Influence of a small amount of Al2O3 addition on the transformation of Y2O3-partially stabilized ZrO2 during annealing. *J Mater Sci.* 1997;32:1149–1153.
125. Andreiotelli M, Wenz HJ, Kohal RJ. Are ceramic implants a viable alternative to titanium implants? A systematic literature review. *Clin Oral Implants Res.* 2009;4:32–47.
126. Guazzato M, Albakry M, Quach L, Swain MV. Influence of grinding, sandblasting, polishing and heat treatment on the flexural strength of a glass-infiltrated alumina-reinforced dental ceramic. *Biomater.* 2004;25:2153–2160.
127. Piconi C, Maccauro G. Zirconia as a ceramic biomaterial. *Biomaterials.* 1999;20:1–25.
128. Watanabe M, Iio S, Fukuura I. *Ageing Behaviour of Y-TZP. Science and Technology of Zirconia II, Advances in Ceramics.* Columbus. OH: The American Ceramic Society, Inc.; 1984:391–398.
129. Sivaraman K, Chopra A, Narayan AI, Balakrishnan D. Is zirconia a viable alternative to titanium for oral implant? A critical review. *J Prosthodont Res.* 2017;62(2):121–133.
130. Hafezeqoran A, Koodaryan R. Effect of zirconia dental implant surfaces on bone integration: a systematic review and meta-analysis. *Biomed Res Int.* 2017;9246721.
131. Bacchelli B, Giavaresi G, Franchi M, et al. Influence of a zirconia sandblasting treated surface on peri-implant bone healing: an experimental study in sheep. *Acta Biomater.* 2009;5(6):2246–2257.
132. Kohal RJ, Finke HC, Klaus G. Stability of prototype two-piece zirconia and titanium implants after artificial aging: an in vitro pilot study. *Clin Implant Dent Relat Res.* 2009;11(4):323–329.
133. Kohal RJ, Wolkewitz M, Tsakona A. The effects of cyclic loading and preparation on the fracture strength of zirconium-dioxide implants: an in vitro investigation. *Clin Oral Implants Res.* 2011;22:808–814.
134. Thoma DS, Benic GI, Muñoz F, et al. Histological analysis of loaded zirconia and titanium dental implants: an experimental study in the dog mandible. *J Clin Periodontol.* 2015;42:967–975.

135. Thoma DS, Benic GI, Muñoz F, et al. Marginal bone-level alterations of loaded zirconia and titanium dental implants: an experimental study in the dog mandible. *Clin Oral Implants Res.* 2016;27:412–420.

136. Pabst W, Havrda J, Gregorová E, et al. Alumina toughened zirconia made by room temperature extrusion of ceramic pastes. *J Am Ceram Soc.* 2000;44:41–47.

137. Kohal RJ, Finke HC, Klaus G. Stability of prototype two piece zirconia and titanium implants after artificial aging: an in vitro pilot study. *Clin Implant Dent Relat Res.* 2009;11:323–329.

138. Joo HS, Yang HS, Park SW, et al. Influence of preparation depths on the fracture load of customized zirconia abutments with titanium insert. *J Adv Prosthodont.* 2015;3:183–190.

139. Silva N, Coelho PG, Fernandes C, et al. Reliability of one-piece ceramic implant. *J Biomed Mater Res B Appl Biomater.* 2009;88:419–426.

140. Spies BC, Nold J, Vach K, Kohal RJ. Two-piece zirconia oral implants withstand masticatory loads: an investigation in the artificial mouth. *J Mech Behav Biomed Mater.* 2016;53:1–10.

141. De Medeiros RA, Vechiato-Filho AJ, Pellizzer EP, et al. Analysis of the peri-implant soft tissues in contact with zirconia abutments: an evidence-based literature review. *J Contemp Dent Pract.* 2013;14(3):567–572.

142. Akagawa Y, Ichikawa Y, Nikai H, Tsuru H. Interface histology of unloaded and early loaded partially stabilized zirconia endosseous implant in initial bone healing. *J Prosthet Dent.* 1993;69:599–604.

143. Nevins M, Camelo M, Nevins ML, Schupbach P, Kim DM. Pilot clinical and histologic evaluations of a two-piece zirconia implant. *Int J Periodontics Restorative Dent.* 2011;31:157–163.

144. Stadlinger B, Hennig M, Eckelt U, Kuhlisch E, Mai R. Comparison of zirconia and titanium implants after a short healing period: a pilot study in minipigs. *Int J Oral Maxillofac Surg.* 2010;39:585–592.

145. Depprich R, Ommerborn M, Zipprich H, et al. Behavior of osteoblastic cells cultured on titanium and structured zirconia surfaces. *Head Face Med.* 2008;4:29.

146. Cranin AN, Schnitman PA, Rabkin SM, Onesto EJ. Alumina and zirconia coated vitallium oral endosteal implants in beagles. *J Biomed Mater Res.* 1975;9:257–262.

147. Scarano A, Di Carlo F, Quaranta M, Piattelli A. Bone response to zirconia ceramic implants: an experimental study in rabbits. *J Oral Implantol.* 2003;29:8–12.

148. Dubruille JH, Viguier E, Le Naour G, et al. Evaluation of combinations of titanium, zirconia, and alumina implants with 2 bone fillers in the dog. *Int J Oral Maxillofac Implants.* 1999;14:271–277.

149. Hoffmann O, Angelov N, Gallez F, et al. The zirconia implant bone interface: a preliminary histologic evaluation in rabbits. *Int J Oral Maxillofac Implants.* 2008;23:691–695.

150. Oliva J, Oliva X, Oliva JD. One-year follow-up of first consecutive 100 zirconia dental implants in humans: a comparison of 2 different rough surfaces. *Int J Oral Maxillofac Implants.* 2007;22:430–435.

151. Osman RB, Morgaine KC, Duncan W, Swain MV, Ma S. Patients' _perspectives on zirconia and titanium implants with a novel distribution supporting maxillary and mandibular overdentures: a qualitative study. *Clin Oral Implants Res.* 2016;25:587–597.

152. Devji T. Survival rates and marginal bone loss of zirconia implants are promising, but more evidence on long-term outcomes is needed. *J Am Dent Assoc.* 2017;148(9):e128.

153. Gupta S. Zirconia vs titanium implants–deciding factors. *J Dent Oral Disord Ther.* 2016;4(4):1–2.

154. Hollinger JO, Battistone GC. Biodegradable bone repair materials. *Clin Orthop Relat Res.* 1986;20:290–305.

155. Lemons JE. Phase boundary interactions for surgical implants. In: Rubin LE, ed. *Biomaterials in Reconstructive Surgery.* St Louis: Mosby; 1983.

156. Andrade JD. The interface between physics, materials, science and biology. *Trans Soc Biomater.* 1989;12:6.

157. Kirsch A. The two phase implantation method using IMZ intramobile cylinder implant. *J Oral Implantol.* 1983;11:197–210.

158. Albrektsson T, Isidor F. Consensus report of session V. In: Lang NP, Karring T, eds. *Proceedings of the 1st European Workshop on Periodontology.* London: Quintessence; 1993.

159. Kasemo B. Biocompatibility of titanium implants: surface science aspects. *J Prosthet Dent.* 1983;49:832–837.

160. Kasemo B, Lausmaa J. Metal selection and surface characteristics. In: Brånemark PI, ed. *Tissue Integrated Prostheses, Osseointegration in Clinical Dentistry.* Chicago: Quintessence; 1985.

161. Lausmaa J, Kasemo B, Mattson H. Surface spectroscopic characterization of titanium implant materials. *Appl Surf Sci.* 1990;44:133–146.

162. Samsonov GV. *The Oxide Handbook.* New York: IFI Plenum; 1973.

163. Ong JL, Lucas LC, Connatser RW, et al. Spectroscopic characterization of passivated titanium in a physiological solution. *J Mater Sci Mater Med.* 1995;6:113–119.

164. Radegran G, Lausmaa J, Rolander U, et al. Preparation of ultrathin oxide windows on titanium for TEM analysis. *J Electron Miscrosc Tech.* 1991;19:99–106.

165. Smith DC, Piliar RM, Chernecky R. Dental implant materials. I. Some effects of preparative procedures on surface topography. *J Biomed Mater Res.* 1991;25:1045–1068.

166. Ask M, Lausmaa J, Kasemo G. Preparation and surface spectroscopic characterization of oxide films Ti6A14V. *Appl Surf Sci.* 1988;35:283–301.

167. Ask M, Rolander U, Lausmaa J, et al. Microstructure and morphology of surface oxide films Ti6A14V. *J Mater Res.* 1990;5:1662–1667.

168. Mausli PA, Block PR, Geret V, et al. Surface characteristics of titanium and titanium alloys. In: Christel P, Meunier A, Lee AJC, eds. *Biological and Biochemical Performance of Biochemicals.* Amsterdam: Elsevier; 1986.

169. Doundoulakis JH. Surface analysis of titanium after sterilization: role in implant-tissue interface and bioadhesion. *J Prosthet Dent.* 1987;58:471–478.

170. Binon P, Weir D, Marshall S. Surface analysis of an original Brånemark implant and three related clones. *Int J Oral Maxillofac Implants.* 1992;7:168–175.

171. Kilpadi DV, Lemons JE. Surface energy characterization of unalloyed titanium implants. *J Biomed Mater Res.* 1995;29:1469.

172. Parr GR, Gardner LK, Toth RW. Titanium: the mystery metal of implant dentistry, dental material aspects. *J Prosthet Dent.* 1985;54:410–414.

173. Anderson G, Gaechter G, Rostoker W. Segmental replacement of long bones in baboons using a fiber implant. *J Bone Joint Surg.* 1978;60:31.

174. Kasemo B, Lausmaa J. Biomaterials and implant surface: on the role of cleanliness, contamination and preparation procedures. *J Biomed Mater Res B Appl Biomater.* 1988;22A2:145–158.

175. Mausli PA, Simpson JP, Burri G, et al. Constitution of oxides or titanium alloys for surgical implants. In: de Putter C, ed. *Implant Materials in Biofunction.* Amsterdam: Elsevier; 1988.

176. Smith DC, Pilliar KM, Mattson JB, et al. Dental implants materials. II. Preparative procedures and spectroscopic studies. *J Biomed Mater Res.* 1991;25:1069–1084.

177. Albrektsson T. Bone tissue response. In: Brånemark PI, Zarb GA, Albrektsson T, eds. *Tissue Integrated Prostheses—Osseointegration in Clinical Dentistry.* Chicago: Quintessence; 1985.

178. Johansson CB, Albrektsson T, Ericson LE, et al. A qualitative comparison of the cell response to commercially pure titanium and Ti6A14V implants in the abdominal wall of rats. *J Mater Sci Mater Med.* 1992;3:126–136.

179. Johansson C, Hansson HA, Albrektsson T. Qualitative interfacial study of bone and tantalum, niobium or commercially pure titanium. *Biomaterials.* 1990;11:277.

180. Johansson C, Lausmaa J, Ask M, et al. Ultrastructural differences of the interface zone between bone and Ti-6Al-4V or commercially pure titanium. *J Biomed Eng.* 1989;11:3.

181. Inoue T, Box JE, Pilliar RM, et al. The effect of the surface geometry of smooth and porous coated titanium alloy on the orientation of fibroblasts in vitro. *J Biomed Mater Res.* 1987;21:107–126.

182. Brunette DM. The effects of implant surface topography on the behavior of cells. *Int J Oral Maxillofac Implants.* 1988;3:231.

183. Lum L, Beirne O, Dillinges M, et al. Osseointegration of two types of implants in non human primates. *J Prosthet D1988ent.* 1988;60:700–705.

184. Small IA, Helfrick IF, Stines AV. The fixed mandibular implant. In: Fonseca RJ, Davis WH, eds. *Reconstructive Preposthetic Oral and Maxillofacial Surgery.* 2nd ed. Philadelphia: WB Saunders; 1995.

185. Smith DC, Piliar RM, McIntyre NS. Surface characteristics of dental implant materials. In: Kawahara H, ed. *Oral Implantology and Biomaterials.* Amsterdam: Elsevier; 1989.

186. Small IA, Misiek D. A sixteen year evaluation of the mandibular stable bone plate. *J Oral Maxillofac Surg.* 1986;44:60–66.

187. Walker C, Aufdemorte TB, McAnear JT, et al. The mandibular staple bone plate, a 5½ year follow-up. *J Am Dent Assoc.* 1987;114:189–192.

188. Morris HF, Manz MC, Tarolli JH. Success of multiple endosseous dental implant designs to second stage surgery across study sites. *J Oral Maxillofac Surg.* 1997;55:76–82.

189. McQueen D, Sundgren JE, Ivarson B, et al. Auger electron spectroscopy studies of titanium implants. In: Lee AJC, Albrektsson T, Brånemark PI, eds. *Clinical Applications of Biomaterials.* New York: John Wiley & Sons; 1982.

190. Sundgren JE, Bodo P, Lundstrom I, et al. Auger electron spectroscopic studies of stainless-steel implants. *J Biomed Mater Res.* 1985;19:663–671.

191. Sundgren JE, Bodo P, Lundstrom I. Auger electron spectroscopic studies of the interface between human tissue and implants of titanium and stainless steel. *J Colloid Interface Sci.* 1986;110:9–20.

192. Tengvall P, Elwing H, Sjoqvist L, et al. Interaction between hydrogen peroxide and titanium: a possible role in the biocompatibility of titanium. *Biomaterials.* 1989;10:118–120.

193. Tengvall P. *Titanium-Hydrogen Peroxide Interaction with Reference to Biomaterial Applications [Dissertation].* Linkoping, Sweden: University of Linkoping; 1990.

194. Tengvall P, Lindstrom I. Physicochemical considerations of titanium as biomaterial. *Clin Mater.* 1992;9:115–134.

195. Hanawa T. Titanium and its oxide film: a substratum for formation of apatite. In: Davies JE, ed. *The Bone-Biomaterial Interface.* Toronto: Toronto University Press; 1991.

196. Hanawa T, Ota M. Calcium phosphate naturally formed on titanium in electrolyte solution. *Biomaterials.* 1991;12:767–774.

197. Jacobs JJ, Skipor AK, Black J, et al. Release and excretion of metal in patients who have total hip-replacement component made of titanium-base alloy. *J Bone Joint Surg.* 1991;73A:1475–1486.

198. Lugowski SJ, Smith DC, McHugh AD, et al. Release of metal ions from dental implant materials in vivo: determinations of Al, Co, Cr, Mo, Ni, V, and Ti in organ tissue. *J Biomed Mater Res.* 1991;25:1443–1458.

199. Bruneel N, Helsen JA. In vitro stimulation of biocom-patibility of Ti-6A1-4V. *J Biomed Mater Res.* 1988;22:203–214.

200. Ducheyne P, Williams G, Martens M. In vivo metal-ion release from porous titanium fiber material. *J Biomed Mater Res.* 1984;18:293–308.

201. Healy KE, Ducheyne P. The mechanisms of passive dissolution of titanium in a model physiological environment. *J Biomed Mater Res.* 1992;26:319–338.

202. Blumenthal NC, Cosma V. Inhibition of apatite formation by titanium and vanadium ions. *J Biomed Mater Res.* 1989;23:13–22.

203. Solar RJ, Pollack SR, Korostoff E. In vitro corrosion testing of titanium surgical implant alloys, an approach to understanding titanium release from implants. *J Biomed Mater Res.* 1979;13:217.

204. Bundy KJ, Marck M, Hochman RF. In vivo and in vitro studies of stress-corrosion cracking behavior of surgical implant alloys. *J Biomed Mater Res.* 1993;17:467.

205. Jones RL, Wing SS, Syrett BC. Stress corrosion cracking and corrosion fatigue of some surgical implant materials in a physiological saline environment. *Corrosion.* 1978;36:226–236.

206. Meachim ZG, Williams DF. Changes in non osseous tissue adjacent to titanium implants. *J Biomed Mater Res.* 1973;7:555–572.

207. Rostoker W, Pretzel CW. Coupled corrosion among alloys for skeletal prostheses. *J Biomed Mater Res.* 1974;8:407–419.

208. Rostoker W, Galante JO, Lereim P. Evaluation of couple crevice corrosion by prosthetic alloys under in vivo conditions. *J Biomed Mater Res.* 1979;12:823.

209. Thompson NG, Buchanan RA, Lemons JE. In vitro corrosion of Ti-6A1-4V and 316 stainless steel when galvanically coupled with carbon. *J Biomed Mater Res.* 1979;13:35.

210. Marshak BL, Ismail Y, Blachere J, et al. Corrosion between titanium alloy implant components and substructure alloy. *J Dent Res.* 1992;71:723 (abstract).

211. Marshak BL. *An in Vitro Study of Corrosion at the Implant Abutment Interface* [master's thesis]. Pittsburgh: University of Pittsburgh; 1994.

212. Cohen F, Burdairon G. Corrosive properties of odon-tologic fluoride containing gels against titanium. *J Dent Res.* 1992;71:525 (abstract).

213. Wig P, Ellingsen JE, Videm K. Corrosion of titanium by fluoride. *J Dent Res.* 1993;72:195 (abstract).

214. Rozenbaijer N, Probster L. Titanium surface corrosion caused by topical fluorides. *J Dent Res.* 1993;72:227 (abstract).

215. Liles A, Salkend S, Sarkar N. Galvanic corrosion between titanium and selected crown and bridge alloys. *J Dent Res.* 1993;72:195 (abstract).

216. Luthy H, Strub JR, Scharer P. Analysis of plasma flame-sprayed coatings on endosseous oral titanium implants exfoliated in man: preliminary results. *Int J Oral Maxillofac Implants.* 1987;2:197–202.

217. Morita M, Hayashi H, Sasada T, et al. The corrosion fatigue properties of surgical implants in a living body. In: de Putter C, et al., ed. *Implant Materials in Biofunction.* Vol. 8. Amsterdam: Elsevier; 1988.

218. Sella C, Martin JC, Lecoeur J, et al. Biocompatibility and corrosion resistance in biological media of hard ceramic coatings sputter deposited on metal implants. *Mater Sci Eng A Struct Mater.* 1991;139:49–57.

219. Toni A, Lewis CG, Sudanese A, et al. Bone demineralization induced by cementless alumina coated femoral stems. *J Arthrop.* 1994;9:435–441.

220. Baro AM, Garcia N, Miranda A, et al. Characterization of surface roughness in titanium dental implants measured with scanning tunneling microscopy at atmospheric pressure. *Biomaterials.* 1986;17:463–467.

221. Olin H, Aronssoid BO, Kasemo B, et al. Scanning tunneling microscopy of oxidized titanium surfaces in air. *Ultramicroscopy.* 1992;42–44:567–571.

222. Niznick GA. The core-vent implant system. *J Oral Implantol.* 1982;10:379.

223. Niznick GA. Comparative surface analysis of Brånemark and core-vent implants. *J Oral Maxillofac Surg.* 1987;45.

224. Cochran DL, Nummikoski PV, Higginbottom FL, et al. Evaluation of an endosseous titanium implant with a sandblasted and acid etched surface in the canine mandible: radiographic results. *Clin Oral Implants Res.* 1996;7:240–252.

225. Clarke A. Particulate debris from medical implants. In: John KR St, ed. *ASTM STP 1144.* Philadelphia: American Society for Testing and Materials; 1992.

226. Ricci JL, Kummer FJ, Alexander H, et al. Embedded particulate contaminants in textured metal implant surfaces. *J Appl Biomater.* 1992;3:225–230.

227. Technical data on the RBM surface roughening treatment. *Southfield, Mich: Bio–Coat Inc.* 1996.

228. Hermann H. Plasma spray deposition processes. *MRS Bull.* 1988:60–67.

229. Hahn H, Palich W. Preliminary evaluation of porous metal surfaced titanium for orthopaedic implants. *J Biomed Mater Res.* 1970;4:571–577.

230. Karagianes MT, Westerman RE. Development and evaluation of porous ceramic and titanium alloy dental anchors implanted in miniature swine. *J Biomed Mater Res Symp.* 1974;8:391–399.

231. Schroeder A, Van der Zypen E, Stich H, et al. The reactions of bone, connective tissue and epithelium to endosteal implants with titanium sprayed surfaces. *J Maxillofac Surg.* 1981;9:15–25.

232. Young FA, Spector M, Kresch CH. Porous titanium endosseous dental implants in rhesus monkeys: micro-radiography and histological evaluation. *J Biomed Mater Res.* 1979;13:843–856.

233. Deporter DA, Watson PA, Pilliar RM, et al. A histological assessment of the initial healing response adjacent to porous surfaced titanium alloy dental implants in dogs. *J Dent Res.* 1986;5:1064–1070.

234. Deporter DA, Watson PA, Pilliar RM, et al. A histological evaluation of a functional endosseous, porous-surfaced, titanium alloy dental implant in the dog. *J Dent Res.* 1988;67:1990–1995.

235. Deporter DA, Watson PA, Pilliar RM, et al. A histological comparison in the dog of porous-coated versus threaded dental implant. *J Dent Res.* 1990;69:1138–1145.

236. Pilliar RM, Deporter DA, Watson PA, et al. Dental implant design effect on bone remodeling. *J Biomed Mater Res.* 1991;25:467–483.

237. Deporter DA, Watson PA, Pilliar RM, et al. A prospective clinical study in humans of an endosseous dental implant partially covered with a powder-sintered porous coating: 3 to 4 year results. *Int J Oral Maxillofac Implants.* 1996;11:87–95.

238. Lowenberg BF, Pilliar RM, Aubin JE, et al. Migration, attachment and orientation of human gingival fibroblasts to root slices, naked and porous surfaces titanium alloy discs and zircalloy discs in vitro. *J Dent Res.* 1987;66:1000–1005.

239. Clemow AJT, Weinstein AM, Klawitter JJ, et al. Interface mechanics of porous titanium implants. *J Biomed Mater Res.* 1981;1:73–82.

240. Hulbert SF, Morrison S, Klawitter JJ. Tissue reactions to three ceramics of porous and nonporous structures. *J Biomed Mater Res.* 1972;6:347–374.

241. Hulbert SF, Cooke FW, Klawitter JJ, et al. Attachment of prostheses to the musculoskeletal system by tissue ingrowth. *J Biomed Mater Res.* 1973;7:1–23.

242. Bobyn JD, Pilliar RM, Cameron HU, et al. The optimum pore size for the fixation of porous surfaced metal implants by the ingrowth of bone. *Clin Ortop Relat Res.* 1980;150:263–270.

243. Predecki P, Auslaender BA, Stephan JE, et al. Attachment of bone to threaded implants by ingrowth and mechanical interlocking. *J Biomed Mater Res.* 1972;6:401–412.

244. Claes L, Hutzschenreutet O, Pholer V, et al. Lose-momente von corticaliszugschrauben in abhangigkeit von implantationszeit und oberflachebeschaffenheit. *Arch Orthop Unfallchir.* 1976;85:155–159.

245. Proceedings of an International Congress, Brussels. Tissue integration. In: Van Steenberghe D, ed. *Oral and Maxillo-Facial Reconstruction.* Amsterdam: Excerpta Medica; 1985.

246. Maniatopoulos C, Pilliar RM, Smith DC. Threaded vs porous surface designs for implant stabilization in bone-endodontic implant model. *J Biomed Mater Res.* 1986;20:1309–1333.

247. Pilliar RM, Lee J, Maniatopoulos C. Observations on the effect of movement on bone in growth into porous surface implants. *Clin Orthop.* 1986;208:108–113.

248. Moser W, Nentwig GH. Zur problematik von titan-spritzbeschichtungen. *Z Zahnarztl Implantol.* 1987;3:282–285.

249. Watzek G, Danhel-Mayhauser M, Matejka M et al. *Experimental Comparison of Brånemark and Tps Dental Implants in a Sheep Model, Abstract 50.* Paper presented at the UCLA Symposium on Implants in the Partially Edentulous Patient. Palm Springs: Calif; 1990.

250. American Society for Testing and Materials. *Standard Specification for Titanium and Titanium 6Al4V alloy Powders for Coating of Surgical Implants. ASTM F 1580.* Philadelphia: American Society for Testing and Materials; 1995.

251. Kay JF, Jarcho M, Logan G, et al. The structure and properties of HA coatings on metal. In: *Proceedings of the Twelfth Annual Meeting of the Society for Biomaterials*; 1986.

252. Block MS, Kent JN, Kay JF. Evaluation of hydroxylapatite-coated titanium dental implants in dogs. *J Oral Maxillofac Surg.* 1987;45:601–607.

253. Thomas KA, Kay JF, Cook SD, et al. Effect of surface microtexture and hydroxylapatite coating on the mech-anical strengths and histologic profiles of titanium implant materials. *J Biomed Mater Res.* 1987;21:1395–1414.

254. Griffin CD, Kay JF, Smith CL. The effect of hydroxylapatite coatings on corrosion of Co-Cr alloy In: *Proceedings of the Thirteenth Annual Meeting of the Society for Biomaterials.* San Francisco; 1987.

255. Cook SD, Kay JF, Thomas KA, et al. Interface mechanics and histology of titanium and HA coated titanium for dental implant applications. *Int J Oral Maxillofac Implants.* 1987;2:15–22.

256. Geesink RGT, deGroot K, Klein CPAT. Bonding of bone to apatite coated implants. *J Bone Joint Surg.* 1988;70B:17–22.

257. Thomas KA, Jay JF, Cook SD, et al. The effect of surface macrotexture and hydroxylapatite coating on the mechanical strengths and histologic profiles of titanium implant materials. *J Biomed Mater Res.* 1987;21:1395–1414.

258. Meffert RM, Block MS, Kent JN. What is osseointegration? *Int J Periodontics Restorative Dent.* 1987;4:9–21.

259. Block MS, Finger IM, Fontenot MG, et al. Loaded hydroxylapatite coated and grit blasted titanium implants in dogs. *Int J Oral Maxillofac Implants.* 1989;4:219–224.

260. Kent JN, Block MS, Finger IM, et al. Biointegrated hydroxylapatite coated dental implants. 5 year observations. *J Am Dent.* 1990;121:138–144.

261. Jensen R, Jensen J, Krauser JT, et al. Hydroxylapatite coated dental implants. *New Dent.* 1989;68:14–25.

262. Kaufmann J, Ricci JL, Jaffe W, et al. Bone attachment to chemically textured titanium alloy with and without HA coating. In: *Proceedings of the Twenty-Third Annual Meeting of the Society for Biomaterials.* New Orleans, La; 1997.

263. deGroot K, Geesink R, Klien C, et al. Plasma sprayed coatings of hydroxyapatite. *J Biomed Mater Res.* 1987;21:1375–1381.

264. Wolke JGC, deGroot K, Jansen JA. Initial wound healing around subperiosteal RF magnetron sputtered Ca-P implants. In: *Proceedings of the Twenty-Third Annual Meeting of the Society for Biomaterials.* New Orleans, La; 1997.

265. Kim YK, Kim S, Lee JH. Interfacial shear strength of laser treated hydroxylapatite layer on titanium alloy In: *Proceedings of the Twenty-Third Annual Meeting of the Society for Biomaterials.* New Orleans, La; 1997.

266. Gerner BT, Barth E, Albrektsson T, et al. Comparison of bone reactions to coated tricalcium phosphate and pure titanium dental implants in the canine iliac crest. *Scand J Dent Res.* 1988;96:143–148.

267. Kay JF. Calcium phosphate coatings for dental implants current status and future potential. *Dent Clin North Am.* 1992;36:1–18.

268. Klien CPAT, deGroot K. Histology of hydroxylapatite coatings. *J Dent Res.* 1989;68:863.

269. Meffert RM. How to treat ailing and failing implants. *Implant Dent.* 1992;1:25–33.

270. Caulier H, Vercaigne S, Naert I, et al. The effect of Ca-P plasma sprayed coatings on the initial bone healing of oral implants and experimental study in the goat. *Biomed Mater Res.* 1997;34:121–128.

271. Ducheyne P, Healy KE. The effect of plasma sprayed calcium phosphate ceramic coatings on the metal ion release from porous titanium and cobalt chrome alloys. *J Biomed Mater Res.* 1988;22:1127–1163.

272. Filiggi MJ, Coombs NA, Pilliar RM. Characterization of the interface in the plasma sprayed HA coating/Ti6A14V implant system. *J Biomed Mater Res.* 1991;25:1211–1229.

273. Tufecki E, Brantley WA, Mitchell JC, et al. Microstructures of plasma sprayed HA coated Ti6A14V dental implants. *Int J Oral Maxillofac Implants.* 1997;12:25–31.

274. Lewandrowski JA, Johnson CM. Structural failure of osseointegrated implants at the time of restoration, a clinical report. *J Prosthet Dent.* 1989;62:127–129.

275. Krauser J, Berthold P, Tamary I, et al. A scanning electron microscopy study of failed endosseous root formed dental implants. *J Dent Res.* 1991;70:274 (abstract).

276. Bordji K, Jouzeau JY, Mainand D, et al. Evaluation of the effect of three surface treatments on the biocompatibility of 316 stainless steel using human differentiated cells. *Biomaterials.* 1996;17:491–500.

277. Baumhammers A. Scanning electron microscopy of conta-minated titanium implants following various cleaning techniques. *J Oral Implantol.* 1975;6:202–209.

278. Baier RE, Meyer AE, Akers CK, et al. Degradative effects of conventional steam sterilization on biomaterial surfaces. *Biomaterials.* 1982;3:241–244.

279. Grobe GL, Baier RE, Gardella J et al. *Relation of Metal Inter-Face Properties to Broad Adhesive Success.* Paper presented at The Third International Conference on Environment Degradation of Engineering Materials: Pennsylvania State University; 1987.

280. Smith DC. Surface characterization of implant materials. Biological implication. In: Davies JB, ed. *The Bone Bio-Material Interface.* Toronto: Toronto University Press; 1991.

281. Baier RE, Meyer AE. Implant surface preparation. *Int J Oral Maxillofac Implants.* 1988;3:3–19.

282. Baier RE, Meenaghan MA, Hartman LC, et al. Implant surface characteristics and tissue interaction. *J Oral Implantol.* 1988;13:594–605.

283. American Society for Testing and Materials. *B 600-74, Standard Recommended Practice for Descaling and Cleaning Titanium and Titanium Alloy Surfaces.* Philadelphia: American Society for Testing and Materials; 1985.

284. American Society for Testing and Materials. *F-86-84: Standard Practice for Surface Preparation and Marking of Metallic Surgical Implants.* Philadelphia: American Society for Testing and Materials; 1985.

285. Keller JC, Stanford CM, Wightman JP, et al. Characterization of commercially pure titanium surfaces. *J Biomed Mater Res.* 1994;28:939–946.

286. Schmidt FA. Surface modification by ion implantation. *Naval Res Lab Rev.* 1985:69–79.

287. Grabowski KS, Gossett CR, Young FA, et al. Cell adhesion to ion implanted surfaces. In: *Proceedings of the Materials Research Society Symposium;* 1987.

288. Lausmaa J, Kasemo B, Hannson S. Accelerated oxide growth on titanium implants during autoclaving caused by fluorine contamination. *Biomaterials.* 1985;6:23–27.

289. Keller JC, Draughn RA, Wightman JP, et al. Characterization of sterilized commercially pure titanium surfaces. *Int J Oral Maxillofac Implants.* 1990;5:360–366.

290. Schneider R, Olson RA, Krizan KB. Sterilization effects on the surface of coated implants [abstract]. *J Dent Res.* 1989;68.

291. Stanford CM, Keller JC, Solvrsh M. Bone cell expression on titanium surfaces is altered by sterilization treatments. *J Dent Res.* 1994;73:1061–1071.

292. Baier RE, Glantz PO. Characterization of oral in vivo films formed on different types of solid surfaces. *Acta Odontol Scand.* 1988;36:289–301.

293. Baier RE. *Improved Passivation of Implantable Biomaterials by Glow Discharge Process.* Paper presented at the Surfaces in Biomaterials Symposium: Minneapolis, Minn; 1991:9–11.

294. Walivaraza B, Aronsson BO, Rodahl M, et al. Titanium with different oxides in vitro studies of protein adsorption and contact activation. *Biomaterials.* 1994;15:827–834.

295. Kawahara D, Ong JL, Raikar GN, et al. Surface characterization of radio frequency glow discharged and auto-claved titanium surfaces. *Int J Oral Maxillofac Implants.* 1996;11:435–442.

296. Moreira M. *Radio Frequency Glow Discharge Treatment as an Alternative for Cleaning and Sterilizing Dental Implants [Master's Thesis].* Birmingham, Ala: University of Alabama; 1993.

297. Singh S, Schaaf NG. Dynamic sterilization of titanium implants with UV light. *Int J Oral Maxillofac Implants.* 1989;4:139–146.

298. Hartman LC, Meenaghan MA, Schaaf MG, et al. Effects of pretreatment sterilization and cleaning methods on materials properties and osseoinductivity of a threaded implant. *Int J Oral Maxillofac Implants.* 1989;4:11–18.

299. Carlsson LV, Albrektsson T, Berman C. Bone response to plasma cleaned titanium implants. *Int J Oral Maxillofac Implants.* 1989;4:199–204.

PART II

Biomechanical Properties of Dental Implants

6

Clinical Biomechanics in Implant Dentistry

MARTHA WARREN BIDEZ AND CARL E. MISCH[†]

The discipline of biomedical engineering, which applies engineering principles to living systems, has unfolded a new era in diagnosis, treatment planning, and rehabilitation in patient care. One aspect of this field, biomechanics, concerns the response of biological tissues to applied loads. Biomechanics uses the tools and methods of applied engineering mechanics to search for structure–function relationships in living materials.[1] Advancements in prosthetic, implant, and instrumentation design have been realized because of mechanical design optimization theory and practice.[2] This chapter provides fundamental concepts and principles of dental biomechanics as they relate to long-term success of dental implants and restorative procedures.

Loads Applied to Dental Implants[i]

Dental implants are subjected to occlusal loads when placed in function. Such loads may vary dramatically in magnitude, frequency, and duration depending on the patient's parafunctional habits. Passive mechanical loads also may be applied to dental implants during the healing stage because of mandibular flexure, contact with the first-stage cover screw, and second-stage permucosal extension.

Perioral forces of the tongue and circumoral musculature may generate low but frequent horizontal loads on implant abutments. These loads may be of greater magnitude with parafunctional oral habits or tongue thrust. Finally, application of nonpassive prostheses to implant bodies may result in mechanical loads applied to the abutment, even in the absence of occlusal loads. So many variables exist in implant treatment that it becomes almost impossible to compare one treatment philosophy with another. However, basic units of mechanics may be used to provide the tools for the consistent description and understanding of such physiologic (and nonphysiologic) loads. Two different approaches may render a similar short-term result; however, a biomechanical approach can still determine which treatment renders more risk over the long term.

Mass, Force, and Weight

Mass, a property of matter, is the degree of gravitational attraction the body of matter experiences. As an example, consider two cubes composed of hydroxyapatite (HA) and commercially pure

titanium, respectively. If the two cubes are restrained by identical springs, then each spring will deflect by a certain amount relative to the attraction of gravity for the two cubes. The two spring deflections in this example can be made equal by removing part of the material from the titanium cube. Even though the cubes are of completely different composition and size, they can be made equivalent with respect to their response to the pull of gravity. This innate property of each cube that is related to the amount of matter in physical objects is referred to as *mass*. The unit of mass in the metric (International System of Units) system is the kilogram (kg); in the English system, it is the pound mass (lbm).[3]

In 1687, Sir Isaac Newton described a force in what is now referred to as *Newton's laws of motion*.[3] In his second law, Newton stated that the acceleration of a body is inversely proportional to its mass and directly proportional to the force that caused the acceleration. The familiar relation expresses this law:

$$F = ma$$

where F is force (newtons [N]), m is mass (kg), and a is acceleration (meters per second squared [m/s^2]). In the dental implant literature, force commonly is expressed as kilograms of force. The gravitational constant ($a = 9.8$ m/s^2) is approximately the same at every location on Earth; therefore mass (kilograms) is the determining factor in establishing the magnitude of a static load.

Weight is simply a term for the gravitational force acting on an object at a specified location. Weight and force can be expressed by the same units, newtons or pound force (lbf). If a titanium cube is considered as though placed on the moon, then its weight (force caused by gravity) is different from its weight on the Earth. The mass in the cube has not changed, but the *acceleration caused by gravity* has changed. Recalling Sir Isaac Newton's work, an apple weighs approximately 1 N (0.225 lbf). The reader will find the conversion factors in Box 6.1 useful.[4]

Forces

Forces may be described by magnitude, duration, direction, type, and magnification factors. Forces acting on dental implants are referred to as *vector quantities;* that is, they possess magnitude and direction. Restated, to state simply that "a force of 75 lb exists on the distal abutment" is not sufficient. The more correct statement is "a force of 75 lb exists on the distal abutment directed axially along the long axis of the implant body." The dramatic influence of load direction on implant longevity and bone maintenance is discussed later in this chapter and in other chapters. Typical maximum bite force magnitudes exhibited by adults are affected by age, sex, degree of edentulism, bite location, and especially parafunction[5-9] (Table 6.1).

A force applied to a dental implant rarely is directed absolutely longitudinally along a single axis. In fact, three dominant clinical loading axes exist in implant dentistry: (1) mesiodistal, (2) faciolingual, and (3) occlusoapical (Fig. 6.1). A single occlusal contact most commonly results in a three-dimensional occlusal force. Importantly, this three-dimensional force may be described in terms of its component parts (fractions) of the total force that are directed along the other axes. For example, if an occlusal scheme on an implant restoration is used that results in a large magnitude of force component

directed along the faciolingual axis (lateral loading), then the implant is at extreme risk for fatigue failure (described later in this chapter). The process by which three-dimensional forces are broken down into their component parts is referred to as *vector resolution* and may be used routinely in clinical practice for enhanced implant longevity.

Components of Forces (Vector Resolution)

Occlusion serves as the primary determinant in establishing load direction. The position of occlusal contacts on the prosthesis directly influences the type of force components distributed throughout the implant system.

The dentist should visualize each occlusal contact on an implant restoration in its component parts. Consider the example of a restored dental implant subjected to a premature contact during occlusion. When the contact is broken down into its component parts directed along the three clinical loading axes, a large, potentially dangerous lateral component is observed. Occlusal adjustments consistent with implant protective occlusion to eliminate the premature contact minimize the development of such dangerous load components.

Angled abutments also result in development of dangerous transverse force components under occlusal loads in the direction of the angled abutment. Implants should be placed surgically to provide for mechanical loading down the long axis of the implant body to the maximum extent possible. Angled abutments are used to improve esthetics or the path of insertion of a restoration, not to determine the direction of load.

Three Types of Forces

Forces may be described as compressive, tensile, or shear. Compressive forces attempt to push masses toward each other. Tensile

---

> ● BOX **6.1** **Useful Conversion Factors**

Mass
  1 kg = 2.205 lbm
  1 lbm = 0.45 kg
Force
  1 N = 1 kg(m/s^2) = 0.225 lbf
  1 lbf = 4.448 N
Area
  1 m^2 = 10.764 sq ft
  1 sq ft = 0.093 m^2
  1 sq in = 6.452 × 10^{-4} m^2
Pressure[a]
  1 lbf/sq in (psi) = 144 lbf/sq ft = 6894.8 Pa = 6.89 kPa = 0.0069 MPa
  1 Pa = 1 N/m^2 = 1.450 × 10^{-4} psi = 0.021 lbf/sq ft

[a]Stress uses these same units of measurement.
lbf, Pounds force; lbm, pound mass; psi, pounds per square inch.

> TABLE 6.1 **Maximum Bite Force**

Reference	Age (year)	Number	Incisor	Canine	Premolar	Molar (N)	Comments
Braun et al.[a]	26–41	142	—	—	—	710	Between premolar and molar; male subjects 789 N; female subjects 596 N
van Eijden[b]	31.1 (±4.9)	7	—	323–485 N	424–583 N	475–749	Second premolar and second molar, left and right (male subjects only)
Dean et al.[c]	Adult	57	150 N	—	—	450	Converted from figures
Bakke et al.[d]	21–30	20	—	—	—	572	Measured in left and right first molar
	31–40	20	—	—	—	481	—
	41–50	20	—	—	—	564	—
	51–60	17	—	—	—	485	—
	61–70	8	—	—	—	374	—
Braun et al.[e]	18–20	–	—	—	—	176	First molar or first premolar

[a]Braun S, Bantleon H-P, Hnat WP, et al. A study of bite force. 1. Relationship to various physical characteristics. *Angle Orthod*. 1995;65:367–372.
[b]van Eijden TMGJ. Three-dimensional analyses of human bite-force magnitude and moment. *Arch Oral Biol*. 1991;36:535–539.
[c]Dean JS, Throckmorton GS, Ellis EE, at al. A preliminary study of maximum voluntary bite force and jaw muscle efficiency in preorthognathic surgery patients. *J Oral Maxillofac Surg*. 1992;50:1282–1288.
[d]Bakke M, Holm B, Jensen L, et al. Unilateral, isometric bite force in eight- to eighty-eight year old women and men related to occlusal factors. *Second J Dent Res*. 1990;98:149–158.
[e]Braun S, Hnat WP, Freudenthaler JW, et al. A study of maximum bite force during growth and development. *Angle Orthod*. 1996;66:261–264.

• **Fig. 6.1** Forces are three-dimensional, with components directed along one or more clinical coordinate axes: mesiodistal, faciolingual, and occlusoapical (vertical).

TABLE 6.2	Cortical Bone Strengths in Human Femur Specimens	
Type of Force Applied	**Strength (MPa)[a]**	**Load Direction/ Comments**
Compressive	193.0 (13.9)	Longitudinal
	173.0 (13.8)	30° off axis
	133.0 (15.0)	60° off axis
	133.0 (10.0)	Transverse
Tensile	133.0 (11.7)	Longitudinal
	100.0 (8.6)	30° off axis
	60.5 (4.8)	60° off axis
	51.0 (4.4)	Transverse
Shear	68.0 (3.7)	Torsion

[a]Standard deviations are listed in parentheses.

From Reilly DT, Burstein AH. The elastic and ultimate properties of compact bone tissue. *J Biomech.* 1975;8:393.

F = resultant force

F_N = normal component

F_S = shear or tangential component

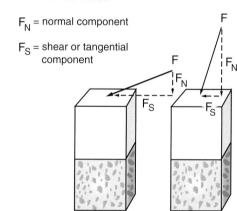

• **Fig. 6.2** Force can be resolved into a combination of normal and shear force components in a given plane. Depending on the direction of load application, the same magnitude of force has different effects.

forces pull objects apart. Shear forces on implants cause sliding. Compressive forces tend to maintain the integrity of a bone–implant interface, whereas tensile and shear forces tend to distract or disrupt such an interface. Shear forces are most destructive to implants and bone compared with other load modalities. In general, compressive forces are accommodated best by the complete implant-prosthesis system. Cortical bone is strongest in compression and weakest in shear (Table 6.2).[10] Additionally, cements and retention screws, implant components, and bone–implant interfaces all accommodate greater compressive forces than tensile or shear. For example, whereas the compressive strength of an average zinc-phosphate dental cement is 83 to 103 MPa (12,000–15,000 pounds per square inch [psi]), the resistance to tension and shear is significantly less (500 psi) (Fig. 6.2).

The implant body design transmits the occlusal load to the bone. Threaded or finned dental implants impart a combination of all three force types at the interface under the action of a single occlusal load. This "conversion" of a single force into three different types of forces is controlled completely by the implant geometry. The prevalence of potentially dangerous tensile and shear forces in threaded or finned implants may be controlled optimally through careful engineering design. Cylinder implants in particular are at highest risk for harmful shear loads at the implant–tissue interface under an occlusal load directed along the long axis of the implant body. As a consequence, cylinder implants require a coating to manage the shear stress at the interface through a more uniform bone attachment along the implant length. Bone loss adjacent to cylindrical implants and coating degradation result in a mechanically compromised implant.

Offset loading on single-tooth or multiple-abutment restorations results in moment (bending) loads (described later under the section "Force Delivery and Failure Mechanisms"). As a result, an increase in tensile and shear force components is often found. Compressive forces typically should be dominant in implant prosthetic occlusion.

Multiple abutment restorations, particularly with distal cantilevers, produce a remarkably complex load profile in the prosthesis and in the bone–implant interface. These clinical realities underscore the need for optimizing dental implant design to provide the maximum functional surface area to dissipate such forces.

Stress

The manner in which a force is distributed over a surface is referred to as *mechanical stress.* Thus the familiar relation defines stress:

$$\sigma = F/A$$

where σ is stress (pounds per square inch; pascals), F is force (newtons; pound force), and A is area (square inches; square meters). The internal stresses that develop in an implant system and surrounding biological tissues under an imposed load may have a significant influence on the long-term longevity of the implants in vivo. As a general rule, a goal of treatment planning should be to minimize and evenly distribute mechanical stress in the implant system and the contiguous bone.

The magnitude of stress depends on two variables: (1) force magnitude and (2) cross-sectional area over which the force is dissipated. It is rare that a dentist can control the force magnitude completely. The magnitude of the force may be decreased by reducing these significant magnifiers of force: cantilever length, offset loads, and crown height. Night guards to decrease nocturnal parafunction; occlusal materials that decrease impact force; and overdentures, rather than fixed prostheses, that can be removed at night are further examples of force reduction strategies. The functional surface area over which the force is distributed, however, is controlled completely through careful treatment planning.

A *functional cross-sectional* area is defined as that surface that participates significantly in load bearing and stress dissipation. This area may be optimized by (1) increasing the number of implants for a given edentulous site and (2) selecting an implant geometry that has been designed carefully to maximize functional cross-sectional area. An increase in functional surface area serves to decrease the magnitude of mechanical stress imposed on the prosthesis, implant, and biological tissues.

Stress components are described as normal (perpendicular to the surface and given the symbol σ) and shear (parallel to the surface and given the symbol τ). One normal stress and two shear stresses act on each plane (x, y, z); therefore $\tau_{xy} = \tau_{yx}$, $\tau_{yz} = \tau_{zy}$, and $\tau_{xz} = \tau_{zx}$. Thus any three-dimensional element may have its stress state completely described by three normal stress components and three shear components.

The question arises as to what are the peak stresses or maximum stresses that an implant and the surrounding interfacial tissues experience. Peak stresses occur when the stress element is positioned in a particular orientation (or geometric configuration) in which all shear-stress components are zero. When an element is in this configuration, the normal stresses are given a particular name, *principal stresses,* and are indicated as σ_1, σ_2, and σ_3. By convention, maximum principal (σ_1) stresses represent the most positive stresses (typically peak tensile stresses) in an implant or tissue region and minimum principal (σ_3) stresses, which are the most negative stresses (typically peak compressive stresses). Sigma 2 (σ_2) represents a value intermediate between σ_1 and σ_3. Determination of these peak normal stresses in a dental implant system

and tissues may give valuable insight regarding sites of potential implant fracture and bone atrophy.

Deformation and Strain

A load applied to a dental implant may induce deformation of the implant and surrounding tissues. Biological tissues may be able to interpret deformation or a manifestation thereof and respond with the initiation of remodeling activity.

The deformation and stiffness characteristics of the materials used in implant dentistry, particularly the implant materials, may influence interfacial tissues, ease of implant manufacture, and clinical longevities. Elongation (deformation) of biomaterials used for surgical dental implants ranges from 0 for aluminum oxide ceramics to up to 55 for annealed 316 L stainless steel[11] (Table 6.3). Related to deformation is the concept of strain, which is a parameter believed to be a key mediator of bone activity.

Under the action of a tensile force (F), the straight bar (of original gauge length, l_0) undergoes elongation to a final length ($l_0 + \Delta1$) (Fig. 6.3). Engineering strain, which is unitless, is defined as elongation per unit length and is described as:

$$\varepsilon = \frac{1 - l_0}{l_0} = \frac{\Delta 1}{l_0}$$

where Δl is elongation, l_0 is original gauge length, and l is final length after elongation, Δl. Shear strain, γ, describes the change in a right angle of a body or stress element under the action of a pure shearing load. All materials (biological and nonbiological) are characterized by a maximum elongation possible before permanent deformation or fracture results. Furthermore, biological materials exhibit strain-rate dependence in that their material properties (e.g., modulus of elasticity, ultimate tensile strength) are altered as a function of the rate of loading (and subsequent deformation rate).

Experimental observation also has demonstrated that lateral strain also accompanies axial strain under the action of an axial load. Within an elastic range (defined later in this section), these two strains are proportional to one another as described by Poisson's ratio, μ. For tensile loading:

$$\mu = \frac{\text{Lateral Strain}}{\text{Axial Strain}}$$

The material and mechanical properties described provide for the determination of implant-tissue stress-strain behavior according to established relationships in solid-mechanics theory.[12]

Stress-Strain Relationship

A relationship is needed between the applied force (and stress) that is imposed on the implant and surrounding tissues and the subsequent deformation (and strain) experienced throughout the system. If any elastic body is subjected experimentally to an applied load, then a load versus deformation curve can be generated (Fig. 6.4A). Dividing the load (force) values by the surface area over which they act and the change in the length by the original length produces a classic engineering stress-strain curve (see Fig. 6.4B). Such a curve provides for the prediction of how much strain will be experienced in a given material under the action of an applied load. The slope of the linear (elastic) portion of this curve is referred to as the *modulus of elasticity (E),* and its value indicates the stiffness of the material under study.

TABLE 6.3   Mechanical Properties of Selected Surgical Implant Biomaterials

| Property | Ti (Wrought) | Ti-Al-V (Wrought) | Co-Cr-Mo (Cast) | CO ALLOY (WROUGHT) | |
				Annealed	Cold Worked
Density (g/mL)	—	4.5	8.3	9.2	9.2
Hardness (Vickers)	R_b100	—	300	240	450
Yield strength	170–480	795–827	490	450	1050
MPa	(25–70)	(115–120)	71	(62)	(152)
Ultimate tensile strength	240–550	860–896	690	950	1540
MPa	(35–80)	(125–130)	(100)	(138)	(223)
Elastic modulus					
GPa	96	105–117	200	230	230
(psi × 10^3)	(14)	(15–17)	(29)	(34)	(34)
Endurance limit (fatigue)					
MPa	—	170–240	300	—	240–490
(psi × 10^3)	—	(24.6–35)	(43)	—	(35–71)
Elongation %	15–24	10–15	8	30–45	9

psi, Pounds per square inch.

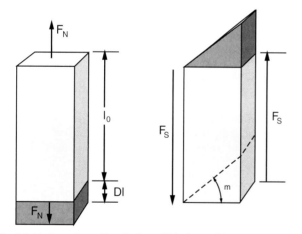

• **Fig. 6.3** Under action of tensile force (F_N), the straight bar originally l_0 is elongated by an amount Δl. Engineering strain ε is the deformation per unit length. Shear strain γ is the change in a right angle of a body or stress element under action of a pure shearing load (F_S).

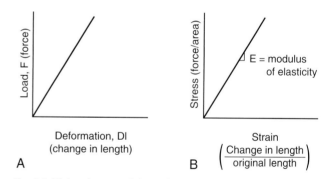

• **Fig. 6.4** (A) Load versus deformation curve may be generated for any elastic body experimentally subjected to a load. (B) Dividing load values by the surface area and the deformation of the original gauge length of the specimen produces a stress-strain curve.

The closer the modulus of elasticity of the implant resembles that of the contiguous biological tissues, the less the likelihood of relative motion at the tissue–implant interface. The cortical bone is at least five times more flexible than titanium. As the stress magnitude increases, the relative stiffness difference between bone and titanium increases. As the stress magnitude decreases, the stiffness difference becomes much less. Restated, the viscoelastic bone can stay in contact with more-rigid titanium more predictably when the stress is low. In terms of full-arch kinematics, the practitioner should consider that the mandible flexes toward the midline on opening. A prosthesis and implant support system that is splinted from molar to molar must provide similar movement if the interface is to remain intact.

Once a particular implant system (i.e., a specific biomaterial) is selected, the only way for an operator to control the strain experienced by the tissues is to control the applied stress or change the density of bone around the implant (Fig. 6.5). Such stress (force/area) may be influenced by the implant design, size, implant number, implant angulation, and restoration. The macrogeometry of the implant (i.e., the amount and orientation of functional surface area available to dissipate loads) has a strong influence on the nature of the force transfer at the tissue–implant interface. Surgical grafting procedures may increase the quantity and quality of bone and allow placement of a larger implant with more bone contiguous to the interface implant. The applied stress is also influenced by the restoration, including the size of

BIOMATERIAL							
Fe-Cr-Ni 316-L		C-Si	Al₂O₃		UHMW Polyethylene	PMMA	PTFE
Annealed	Cold Worked		Sapphire	Alumina			
7.9 170–200	7.9 300–350	1.5–2.0	3.99	3.9 HV23.000	0.94 D65	1.2 M60–M100	2.2 D50–D65
240–300 (35–44)	700–800 (102–116)	—	—	—	—	—	—
600–700 (87–102)	1000 (145)	350–517 (51–75)	480 (70)	400 (58)	21–44 (3.0–6.4)	55–85 (8.0–12.3)	14–34 (2–5)
200 (29)	200 (29)	28–34 (4.0–4.9)	414 (60)	380 (55.1)	1 (0.145)	2.4–33 (0.3480–479)	0.4 (0.058)
300 (43)	230–280 (33.3–40.6)	—	—	—	—	—	—
35–55	7–22	0	0	0	400	2–7	200–400

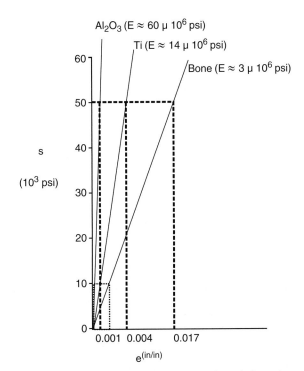

• **Fig. 6.5** Once a particular implant system is selected, the only way to control strain (ε) on tissues is to control applied stress (σ). The greater the magnitude of stress applied to the system, the greater the difference in strain between implant material and bone. *E,* Modulus of elasticity.

occlusal tables, stress breakers, use of overdenture versus fixed prosthesis, and occlusal contact design. Generally, the greater the magnitude of stress applied to a dental implant system, the greater the difference in strain between the implant material and bone. In such cases, the implant is less likely to stay attached to the bone, and the probability of fibrous tissue ingrowth into the interfacial region to accommodate the range of difference becomes greater. The density of bone is related not only to the

bone strength but also to the modulus of elasticity (stiffness). The stiffer the bone, the more rigid it is; the softer the bone, the more flexible the bone. Therefore the difference in stiffness is less for commercially pure titanium (or its alloy) and division 1 dense bone compared with titanium and division 4 soft bone. Decreasing stress in softer bone is more important for two primary reasons: (1) to reduce the resultant tissue strains resulting from the elasticity difference and (2) because softer bone exhibits a lower ultimate strength.

Hooke's law is the name given to the relationship between stress and stain; in its simplest form, the law is described mathematically as the following:

$$\sigma = E\varepsilon$$

where σ is normal stress (pascal or pounds per square inch), E is the modulus of elasticity (pascal or pounds per square inch), and ε is normal strain (unitless). A similar relationship exists for shear stress and shear strain, where the constant of proportionality is the modulus of rigidity *(G)* expressed by the following:

$$\tau = G\gamma$$

where τ is shear stress (pascal or pounds per square inch), G is the modulus of rigidity (pascal or pounds per square inch), and γ is shear strain (unitless).

Impact Loads

When two bodies collide in a small interval of time (fractions of a second), large reaction forces develop. Such a collision is described as *impact.* In dental implant systems subjected to occlusal implant loads, deformation may occur in the prosthodontic restoration, in the implant itself, and in the contiguous interfacial tissues. The nature of the relative stiffness of these components in the overall implant system largely controls the response of the system to impact load. The higher the impact load, the greater the risk of implant and bridge failure and bone fracture.

Rigidly fixed implants generate a higher interfacial impact force with occlusion compared with natural teeth, which possess a

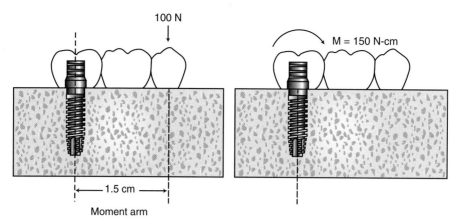

• **Fig. 6.6** Moment of a force is defined as a vector *(M)*, the magnitude of which equals the product of the force magnitude multiplied by the perpendicular distance (moment arm) from the point of interest to the line of action of the force.

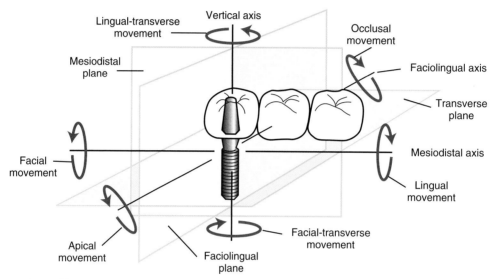

• **Fig. 6.7** Moment loads tend to induce rotations in three planes. Clockwise and counterclockwise rotations in these three planes result in six moments: lingual-transverse, facial-transverse, occlusal, apical, facial, and lingual.

periodontal ligament. Soft tissue–borne prostheses have the least impact force because the gingival tissues are resilient. Occlusal material fracture is a significant complication of fixed prostheses on natural teeth. The incidence of occlusal material fracture is greater on implants and may approach rates as high as 30%.

Various methods have been proposed to address the issue of reducing implant loads. Skalak[13] has suggested the need for using acrylic teeth along with osteointegrated fixtures partially to mitigate high-impact loads that might damage bony tissues adjacent to the implant. Weiss[14] has proposed that a fibrous tissue–implant interface provides for physiologic shock absorption in a fashion similar to that exhibited by a functioning periodontal ligament. At least one implant design has attempted to incorporate shock absorption capability in the design itself by the use of an "intramobile element" of lower stiffness compared with the rest of the implant.[15] Misch[16] has advocated an acrylic provisional restoration with a progressive occlusal loading to improve the bone–implant interface before the final restoration, occlusal design, and masticatory loads are distributed to the system. Only limited data exist concerning impact forces on natural dentition and tooth-supported bridgework.[17,18]

Force Delivery and Failure Mechanisms

The manner in which forces are applied to implant restorations within the oral environment dictates the likelihood of system failure. The duration of a force may affect the ultimate outcome of an implant system. Relatively low-magnitude forces, applied repetitively over a long time, may result in fatigue failure of an implant or prosthesis. Stress concentrations and, ultimately, failure, may develop if insufficient cross-sectional area is present to dissipate high-magnitude forces adequately. If a force is applied some distance away from a weak link in an implant or prosthesis, then bending or torsional failure may result from moment loads. An understanding of force delivery and failure mechanisms is critically important to the implant practitioner to avoid costly and painful complications.

Moment Loads

The moment of a force about a point tends to produce rotation or bending about that point. In Fig. 6.6, the moment is defined as a vector *(M)* (vectors are described in terms of magnitude and direction), the magnitude of which equals the product of the force magnitude multiplied by the perpendicular distance (also called the *moment arm*) from the point of interest to the line of action of the force. This imposed moment load is also referred to as a *torque* or *torsional load* and may be destructive to implant systems. Torques or bending moments imposed on implants because of, for example, excessively long cantilever bridge or bar sections may result in interface breakdown, bone resorption, prosthetic screw loosening, or bar or bridge fracture. The negative effect of cantilevers has been reported for more than 30 years.[19,20] Proper restorative design must include consideration of forces and the moment loads caused by those forces.

Clinical Moment Arms

A total of six moments (rotations) may develop about the three clinical coordinate axes previously described (occlusoapical, faciolingual, and mesiodistal) (Fig. 6.7). Such moment loads induce microrotations and stress concentrations at the crest of the alveolar ridge at the implant–tissue interface, which lead inevitably to crestal bone loss.

Three clinical moment arms exist in implant dentistry: (1) occlusal height, (2) cantilever length, and (3) occlusal width.

Minimization of each of these moment arms is necessary to prevent unretained restorations, fracture of components, crestal bone loss, or complete implant system failure.

Occlusal Height

Fig. 6.8 shows that the occlusal height serves as the moment arm for force components directed along the faciolingual axis such as working or balancing occlusal contacts, tongue thrusts, or in passive loading by cheek and oral musculature (see Fig. 6.8B), as well as force components directed along the mesiodistal axis (see Fig. 6.8C).

In division A bone, initial moment load at the crest is less than in division C or division D bone because the crown height is greater in division C and division D bone. Treatment planning must take into account this initially compromised biomechanical environment (Table 6.4). The moment contribution of a force component directed along the vertical axis is not affected by the occlusal height because no effective moment arm exists. Offset occlusal contacts or lateral loads, however, introduce significant moment arms (see Fig. 6.8E).

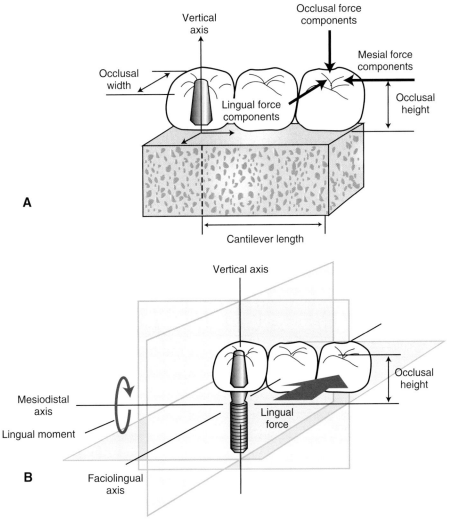

• **Fig. 6.8** (A) Three clinical moment arms contribute to torsional (moment) loads on dental implants: occlusal height, occlusal width, and cantilever length. (B) Occlusal height serves as moment arm for force components directed along faciolingual axis and

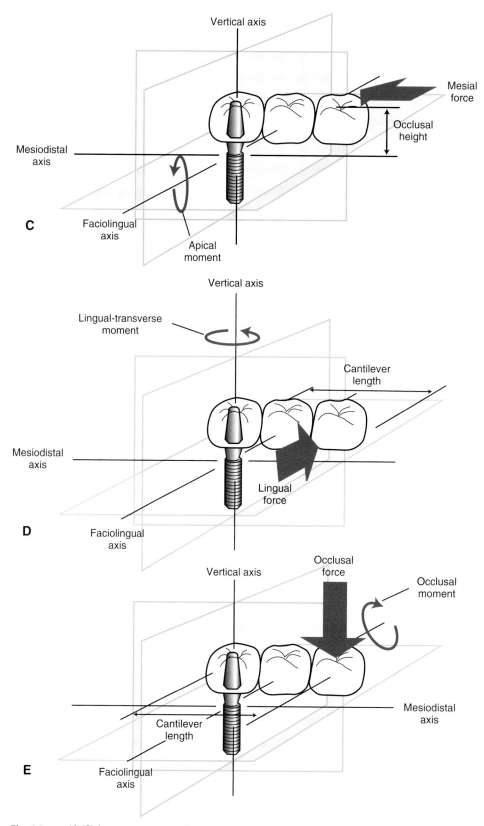

Fig. 6.8, cont'd (C) force components directed along mesiodistal axis. (D) Lingual force component also may induce twisting moment about the implant neck if applied through the cantilever length. (E) Moment of force along the vertical axis is not affected by occlusal height because its effective moment arm is zero if positioned centrically.

TABLE 6.4	Moment Load at Crest, Division A Bone When Subjected to Forces Shown in Fig. 6.3						
INFLUENCES ON MOMENT		**IMPOSED MOMENTS (N/MM) AT IMPLANT CROWN–CREST INTERFACE**					
Occlusal Height (mm)	Cantilever Length (mm)	Lingual	Facial	Apical	Occlusal	Facial-transverse	Lingual-transverse
10	10	100	0	50	200	0	100
10	20	100	0	50	400	0	200
10	30	100	0	50	600	0	300
20	10	200	0	100	200	0	100
20	20	200	0	100	400	0	200
20	30	200	0	100	600	0	300

Cantilever Length

Large moments may develop from vertical axis force components in prosthetic environments designed with cantilever extensions or offset loads from rigidly fixed implants. A lingual force component also may induce a twisting moment about the implant neck axis if applied through a cantilever length (see Fig. 6.8D).

An implant with a cantilevered mesobar extending 1 to 3 cm has significant ranges of moment loads. A 100-N force applied directly over the implant does not induce a moment load or torque because no rotational forces are applied through an offset distance. This same 100-N force applied 1 cm from the implant results in a 100 N-cm moment load. Similarly, if the load is applied 2 cm from the implant, then a 200 N-cm torque is applied to the implant-bone region, and at 3 cm a 300 N-cm moment load results. For comparison, recall that implant abutments typically are tightened with 30 N-cm of torque.

Cantilever prostheses attached to splinted implants result in a complex load reaction. In its simplest form, a class 1 lever action may be expressed. If two implants 10 mm apart are splinted together, and a 20-mm distal cantilever is designed with a 100-N load, then the following forces result. The 100-N load is resisted with a 200-N tensile force by the mesial implant, and the distal implant acts as a fulcrum with a 300-N compressive load (Fig. 6.9A). If the position and amount of distal load remain the same, but the distal implant is positioned 5 mm anterior, then the resultant loads on the implants change (see Fig. 6.9B). The anterior implant must resist a 500-N tensile force, and the distal, fulcrum implant receives a 600-N compressive force. Therefore the tensile force is increased 2.5 times on the anterior implant, whereas the compressive force is increased twofold. Because bone and screws are weaker under the action of tensile forces, both implants become more at risk for complications.

Similar principles regarding class 1 lever forces apply to cantilever loads with anterior splinted implants placed on a curve with distal extended prostheses. The Nobel Biocare (Zurich, Switzerland) prosthetic protocol uses four to six anterior implants placed in front of the mental foramen or maxillary sinuses and uses a full-arch fixed prosthesis with cantilevered segments.[21-23] Specific cantilever lengths are not stated, although two to three premolars are recommended. The cantilever length is suggested to be reduced when four rather than six implants are used to support the restoration[24] or when implants are in the softer bone of the maxilla.[25] A line is drawn from the distal of each posterior implant. The distance

to the center of the most anterior implant is called the *anteroposterior distance* (A-P spread).[26] The greater the A-P spread is between the center of the most anterior implant or implants and the most distal aspect of the posterior implants, the smaller the resultant loads on the implant system from cantilevered forces because of the stabilizing effect of the A-P distance. According to Misch,[25] the amount of stress applied to the system determines the length of this distal cantilever. Because stress equals force divided by area, both aspects must be considered. The magnitude and direction of force are determined by parafunction, crown height, masticatory dynamics, gender, age, and arch location. The functional surface area is determined by the number of implants, width, length, design, and bone density, which determines the area of contact and bone strength. Clinical experiences suggest that the distal cantilever should not extend 2.5 times the A-P spread under ideal conditions (e.g., parafunction absent or five division A implants). One of the greatest determinants for the length of the cantilever is the magnitude of the force. Patients with severe bruxism should not be restored with any cantilevers, regardless of other factors.

A square arch form involves smaller A-P spreads between splinted implants and should have shorter length cantilevers. A tapered arch form has the largest distance between anterior and posterior implants and may have the longest cantilever design. The maxilla has less dense bone than the mandible and more often has an anterior cantilever with the prosthesis. As a result, more distal implants may be required in the maxilla to increase the A-P spread for the anterior or posterior cantilever than in the mandible, and sinus augmentation may be required to permit posterior placement of the implant.

Occlusal Width

Wide occlusal tables increase the moment arm for any offset occlusal loads. Faciolingual tipping (rotation) can be reduced significantly by narrowing the occlusal tables or adjusting the occlusion to provide more centric contacts.

In summary, a vicious, destructive cycle can develop with moment loads and result in crestal bone loss. As crestal bone loss develops, occlusal height automatically increases. With an increased occlusal height moment arm, the faciolingual microrotation and rocking increases and causes even more crestal bone loss. Unless the bone increases in density and strength, the cycle continues to spiral toward implant failure if the biomechanical environment is not corrected.

Fatigue Failure

Fatigue failure is characterized by dynamic, cyclic loading conditions. Four fatigue factors significantly influence the likelihood of fatigue failure in implant dentistry: (1) biomaterial, (2) macrogeometry, (3) force magnitude, and (4) number of cycles.

Fatigue behavior of biomaterials is characterized graphically in what is referred to as an *S-N curve* (a plot of applied stress versus number of loading cycles) (Fig. 6.10A). If an implant is subjected to an extremely high stress, then only a few cycles of loading can be tolerated before fracture occurs. Alternatively, an infinite number of loading cycles can be maintained at low stress levels. The stress level below which an implant biomaterial can be loaded indefinitely is referred to as its *endurance limit.* Titanium alloy exhibits a higher endurance limit compared with commercially pure titanium (see Fig. 6.10B).

The geometry of an implant influences the degree to which it can resist bending and torsional loads and ultimately fatigue fracture. Implants rarely, if ever, display fatigue fracture under axial compressive loads. Morgan and colleagues[27] reported fatigue fractures of Brånemark dental implants (Nobel Biocare, Zurich, Switzerland) caused by cyclical buccolingual loads (lateral loading) in an area of weak bending strength within the fixture (i.e., reduced moment of inertia [defined later]). The fracture of the implant body occurred in three of the patients studied, and fracture of the abutment screws for the Brånemark implant occurred in less than three patients. Fifteen acrylic or composite tooth fractures occurred on 10 to 20 of the fixed prostheses supported by implants over a 1- to 5-year period.[28-31]

The geometry also includes the thickness of the metal or implant. The fatigue fracture is related to the fourth power of the thickness difference. A material two times thicker in wall thickness is approximately 16 times stronger. Even small changes in thickness can result in significant differences. Often the weak link in an implant body design is affected by the difference in the inner and outer diameter of the screw and the abutment screw space in the implant.[32]

To the extent that an applied load (stress) can be reduced, the likelihood of fatigue failure is reduced. As described previously, the magnitude of loads on dental implants can be reduced by careful consideration of arch position (i.e., higher loads in the posterior compared with anterior mandible and maxilla), elimination of moment loads, and increase in surface area available to resist an applied load (i.e., optimize geometry for functional area or increase the number of implants used).

Finally, fatigue failure is reduced to the extent that the number of loading cycles is reduced. Thus aggressive strategies to eliminate parafunctional habits and reduce occlusal contacts serve to protect against fatigue failure.

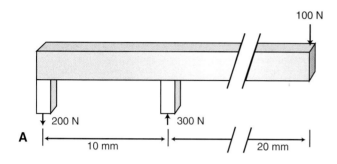

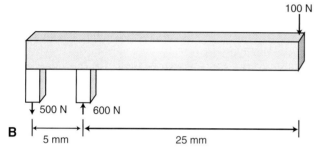

• **Fig. 6.9** (A) If two implants are designed 10 mm apart and splinted together with a 20-mm distal cantilever, then a 100-N load is resisted by a 200-N force by the mesial implant, and the distal implant acts as a fulcrum with a 300-N load. (B) If implants are 5 mm apart, then the anterior implant must resist a 500-N force and the distal fulcrum implant receives a 600-N force.

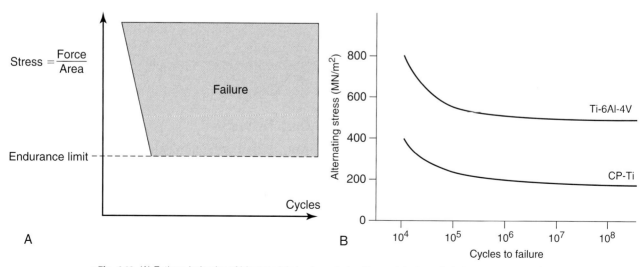

• **Fig. 6.10** (A) Fatigue behavior of biomaterials is characterized by a plot of applied stress versus number of loading cycles (an S-N curve). (B) Endurance limit defines the stress level below which an implant biomaterial may be loaded indefinitely without failure. Titanium alloy is two to four times stronger in fatigue conditions compared with commercially pure titanium.

Moment of Inertia

Moment of inertia is an important property of cylindrical implant design because of its importance in the analysis of bending and torsion. The bending stress in a cylinder is given by the following equation:

$$\sigma = \frac{My}{I}$$

where M is moment (newton-centimeters), y is the distance from the neutral axis of bending (centimeters), and I is the moment of inertia (centimeters to the fourth power).

Root-form implants have varying cross-sectional geometries. The root-form implant may be modeled as a hollow circle because a channel exists in the implant body to allow for abutment screw engagement. In the distal (apical) region of a root-form implant, the cross-sectional geometry may more closely represent a solid circle. In some designs, vents that penetrate transversely through the cross-sectional geometry may interrupt the apical geometry.

The bending stress (and likelihood of bending fracture) decreases with an increasing moment of inertia. Consider the mathematical formulations for the solid versus hollow cylindrical cross-sectional geometry:

Solid circle (cylinder in the middle region) : $4\,I = \pi R^4$

Hollow circle (cylinder in apical region) : $4\,I = \pi R^4 - R_i^4$

where R is the outer radius (centimeters), and R_i is the inner wall radius (centimeters).

Summary

The most common complications in implant-related reconstruction are related to biomechanical conditions. Implant healing failures may result from micromovement of the implant from too much stress. Early crestal bone loss may be related to occlusal overload conditions. Prostheses or abutment screws may become loose from bending or moment forces. Implant or component fracture may occur from fatigue conditions. Prosthesis failure may result from all of the foregoing or bending fracture resistance. In addition, the manifestation of biomechanical loads on dental implants (moments, stress, and strain) controls the long-term health of the bone–implant interface. Knowledge of basic biomechanical principles is thus required for the dentist.

References

1. Schmid-Schonbein GW, Woo SL-Y, Zweifack BW, et al. *Frontiers in Biomechanics*. New York: Springer-Verlag; 1986.
2. National institutes of health consensus development conference statement on dental implants. *J Dent Educ*. 1988;52(824–827):13–15.
3. Higdon A. Dynamics. *Engineering Mechanics*. Vol. 2. Englewood Cliffs, NJ: Prentice-Hall; 1976.
4. Baumeister T, Avallone EA, Baumeister T, et al. *Marks' Standard Handbook for Mechanical Engineers*. 8th ed. New York: McGraw-Hill; 1978.
5. Braun S, Bantleon H-P, Hnat WP, et al. A study of bite force. I. Relationship to various physical characteristics. *Angle Orthod*. 1995;65:367–372.
6. van Eijden TMGJ. Three-dimensional analyses of human bite-force magnitude and moment. *Arch Oral Biol*. 1991;36:535–539.
7. Dean JS, Throckmorton GS, Ellis EE, et al. A preliminary study of maximum voluntary bite force and jaw muscle efficiency in preorthognathic surgery patients. *J Oral Maxillofac Surg*. 1992;50:1284–1288.
8. Bakke M, Holm B, Jensen L, et al. Unilateral, isometric bite force in eight- to eighty-eight year old women and men related to occlusal factors. *Scand J Dent Res*. 1990;98:149–158.
9. Braun S, Hnat WP, Freudenthaler JW, et al. A study of maximum bite force during growth and development. *Angle Orthod*. 1996;66:261–264.
10. Reilly DT, Burstein AH. The elastic and ultimate properties of compact bone tissue. *J Biomech*. 1975;8:393.
11. Lemons JE, Bidez MW. Biomaterials and biomechanics in implant dentistry. In: McKinney RV, ed. *Endosteal Dental Implants*. St Louis: Mosby; 1991.
12. Timoshenko SP, Goodier JN. *Theory of Elasticity*. 3rd ed. New York: McGraw-Hill; 1970.
13. Skalak R. Biomedical considerations in osseointegrated prostheses. *J Prosthet Dent*. 1983;49:843–848.
14. Weiss CW. Fibro-osteal and osteal integration: a comparative analysis of blade and fixture type dental implants supported by clinical trials. *J Dent Educ*. 1988;52:706–711.
15. Kirsch A. The two-phase implantation method using IMZ intramobile cylinder implants. *J Oral Implantol*. 1983;11:197–210.
16. Misch CE. Progressive bone loading. *Pract Periodontics Esthetic Dent*. 1990;2:27–30.
17. Salis SG, Hood JA, Stokes AN, et al. Impact-fracture energy of human premolar teeth. *J Prosthet Dent*. 1987;58:43–48.
18. Saunders WP. The effects of fatigue impact forces upon the retention of various designs of resin-retained bridgework. *Dent Mater*. 1986;3:85–89.
19. Schweitzer JM, Schweitzer RD, Schweitzer J. Free end pontics used on fixed partial dentures. *J Prosthet Dent*. 1968;20:120–138.
20. Crabb HSM. A reappraisal of cantilever bridgework. *J Oral Rehabil*. 1974;1:3–17.
21. Brånemark PI, Zarb GA, Albrektsson T. *Tissue Integrated Prostheses*. Chicago: Quintessence; 1985.
22. Zarb GA, Schmitt A. The longitudenal clinical effectiveness of osseointegrated dental implants, the Toronto study. III. Problems and complications encountered. *J Prosthet Dent*. 1990;64:185–194.
23. Taylor R, Bergman G. *Laboratory Techniques for the Brånemark System*. Chicago: Quintessence; 1990.
24. Rangert B, Jemt T, Jorneus L. Forces and moments on Brånemark implants. *Int J Oral Maxillofac Implants*. 1989;4:241–247.
25. Misch CE. Cantilever length and its relationship to bio-mechanical stress. In: *Misch Implant Institute Manual*. Dearborn: Mich: Misch International Implant Institute; 1990.
26. English C. The critical A-P spread. *Implant Soc*. 1990;1:2–3.
27. Morgan MJ, James DF, Pilliar RM. Fractures of the fixture component of an osseointegrated implant. *Int J Oral Maxillofac Implants*. 1993;8:409–413.
28. Lekholm U, Adell R, Brånemark PI. Complications. In: Brånemark PI, Zarb GA, Albrektsson T, eds. *Tissue Integrated Prostheses*. Chicago: Quintessence; 1985.
29. Lekholm U, van Steenberghe D, Herman D. Osseointegrated implants in the treatment of partially edentulous jaws: a prospective 5-year multicenter study. *Int J Oral Maxillofac Implants*. 1994;9:627–635.
30. Quirynen M, Naert I, van Steenberghe D, et al. The cumulative failure rate of the Brånemark system in the overdenture, the fixed partial, and the fixed full prosthesis design: a prospective study in 1,273 fixtures. *J Head Neck Pathol*. 1991;10:43–53.
31. Naert I, Quirynen M, van Steenberghe D, et al. A six-year prosthodontic study of 509 consecutively inserted implants for the treatment of partial edentulism. *J Prosthet Dent*. 1992;67:236–245.
32. Boggan RS, Strong JT, Misch CE, et al. Influences of hex geometry and geometric table width on static and fatigue strength of dental implants. *J Prosthet Dent*. 1999;82:436–440.

7

Stress Treatment Theorem for Implant Dentistry

CARL E. MISCH AND RANDOLPH R. RESNIK

The field of dentistry is a unique aspect of medicine, blending science and art form. Some aspects of the dental field emphasize the art form, such as in dental esthetics, which deals with tooth color and shape to enhance a patient's smile and overall appearance. These may be separated into a biologic component and a biomechanic component. For general dentists, the biological aspects of oral health are well emphasized. Common complications related to the natural dentition are primarily of biological origins, with periodontal diseases, caries, and endodontic problems as examples.[1-4]

When evaluating failures of tooth-supported prostheses, a combination of biological and biomechanical factors exist. The four most common complications for a typical three-unit fixed prostheses are (1) caries, (2) endodontic involvement, (3) unretained prosthesis, and (4) material fracture.[5,6] The biological complications occur with greater frequency (11%–22%), compared with the biomechanical (7%–10%), but the clinician should have a strong foundation for both aspects. The field of implant dentistry most often involves the replacement of teeth. When implant complications are reported, the vast majority of problems are related to the implant sciences rather than esthetics.[7] But, unlike natural teeth, the biological aspects of implant dentistry have relatively few complications. For example, the development of a direct bone–implant interface is largely biological. Most recent reports indicated that the surgical phase of implants form a successful interface more than 95% of the time, regardless of the implant system used.[7] Hence the biological aspect of the field is very predictable. The most common implant-related complications are biomechanical in nature and occur after the implant is loaded. A literature review focusing on implant failure indicated these problems primarily occur within 18 months of initial implant loading. Most early implant loading failures occur in the softest bone types (16% failure). These failures are typically caused by biomechanical factors because poorer-quality bone is too weak for the occlusal forces applied to the implants (Fig. 7.1).[8-20]

The most common complications that do not lead to the failure of the implant are also biomechanical problems. Implant overdentures have been shown to have attachment fracture or complication (30%) and removable-prosthesis fracture (12%). With implant-supported fixed prostheses, abutment or prosthetic screw loosening has been shown to encompass 34% of prosthetic complications[21] and a complication rate of 40% after 5 years.[22] In addition, implant components (2%–4%) and even implant bodies may

fracture (1%–2%) (Box 7.1). In summary, mechanical complications far outnumber biological implant problems.[7,20] Any complex engineering structure will fail at its "weakest link," and dental implant structures are no exception. A general concept in engineering is to determine the causes of complications and develop a system to reduce the conditions that cause the problems. The most common etiologic factors for implant-related complications are centered around stress. Thus the overall treatment plan should (1) assess the greatest force factors in the system and (2) establish mechanisms to protect the overall implant-bone-prosthetic system.

Biomechanical Overload

Surgical Failure

There are many reasons for the failure of an implant to integrate initially with the bone. The primary causes of early failure relate to excessive heat during the preparation of the osteotomy or excessive pressure at the implant–bone interface at the time of implant insertion (Fig. 7.2).[23] The excessive pressure (i.e., pressure necrosis) at implant insertion is observed most often in more dense bone (e.g., D1 or D2) with a greater thickness of cortical bone. An additional cause of surgical failure is micromovement of the implant while the developing interface is established (Fig. 7.3). A fractured arm is immobilized to prevent movement at the fracture site to decrease the risk of a fibrous nonunion. Movement as little as 20 microns has been reported to cause a fibrous interface to form at the fracture site. Brunski observed a fibrous tissue interface development when a dental implant moved more than 100 microns during initial healing.[24] The original Brånemark protocol used a two-stage surgical approach for the most part to avoid any undue pressure.[25,26] One of the main reasons for this concept was to place the implant at or below the crestal bone region to decrease the risk of implant movement during initial bone healing. Schroeder also suggested an unloaded healing period on implants, although the implant was placed at or slightly above the gingival tissues.[27] Occlusal forces applied to an interim removable prosthesis over a healing implant may also cause incision line opening of the soft tissue and delay soft tissue healing.[28] These occlusal forces may also affect the marginal bone around the developing implant site. Transferring these forces to an overlying soft tissue–borne prosthesis may cause micromovement of the implant–bone interface, whether the implant is healing below or

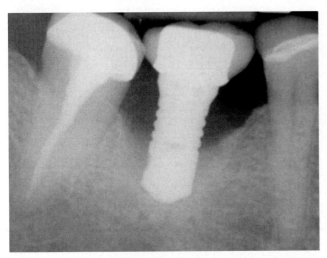

• **Fig. 7.1** Majority of early implant failures occur within 18 months after prosthetic loading and are related to poor-quality bone.

above the gingival tissues. Stresses applied to a healing implant increase the risk of complications. On the other hand, multicenter clinical reports indicate that an experienced surgeon may obtain rigid fixations after surgical placement 99% of the time.[29] The surgical component of implant failure is often the lowest risk associated with the overall implant treatment.

Early Loading Failure

On occasion, an implant may fail shortly after it has initially "integrated" to the bone. Before failure, the implant appears to have rigid fixation, and all clinical indicators are within normal limits. However, once the implant is loaded, the implant becomes mobile shortly thereafter. This has been termed *early loading failure* by Jividen and Misch.[9] The cause of early loading failure is usually excessive stress for the bone–implant interface, which has been

documented in many studies. Isidor and colleagues allowed eight implants to integrate in monkey jaws.[30] Crowns were attached to the healed implants with excessive premature occlusal contacts. Over a 20-month period, six of eight implants failed (Fig. 7.4). In these same animals, eight integrated implants with no occlusal loads had strings placed in the marginal gingiva to increase the amount of plaque retention. None of these implants failed over the next 20 months. The authors concluded that in this animal model, biomechanical occlusal stress was a greater risk factor for early implant failure than the biological component of bacterial plaque.[30,31]

The morbidity of early loading failure is worse for the implant clinician than when a surgical failure occurs because the patient may lose confidence in the restoring dentist. In addition, there exists a significant financial and time commitment. Early loading failure is directly related to the amount of force applied to the prosthesis[8,24,32-35] and the density of the bone around the implants,[7,10-14,36] and it may affect up to 15% of implant restorations.[6-11] Early implant failure from biomechanical overload, as high as 40%, has been reported in the softest bone types.[13] No reports in the literature correlate such high incidence extreme with early implant failure rates related to the biological width-related complications observed in the field.

Impact of Occlusal Overload on Mechanical Components

Screw Loosening

Abutment-screw loosening has been shown to be the most common dental implant prosthetic complication, accounting for up to 33% of all postimplant prosthodontic issues.[37] The incidence of screw loosening with single implant crowns has been reported as high as 59.6% within 15 years of placement.[38] Unfortunately, screw loosening may cause many complications that contribute to crestal bone loss, screw fracture, implant fracture, or implant failure. Although screw loosening may occur in any area of the oral cavity, studies have shown the overwhelming majority of loosened screws occur in the maxillary and mandibular molar areas (~63%) and with single implant-crown restorations (~75%).[39]

Biomechanical forces are a significant etiologic factor with respect to screw loosening. When a screw is tightened (torque), it will elongate, which produces tension or preload within the screw joint. The preload exerts a force that leaves the screw joint in compression and promotes a springlike effect. The preload applied also has an associated elastic recovery that is transferred to the abutment and implant, pulling them together and creating a clamping force (i.e., equal in magnitude to the elongation and elastic recovery).[40]

For a screw to remain tight, the clamping force must be greater than the separating forces. Most often, these separating forces are in the form of external forces that act on a screw joint. Although these forces are termed joint-separating forces, they are the same forces that place the implant at risk for implant failure, crestal bone loss, and component fracture. When the external joint-separating forces are greater than the force holding the screws together (the clamping force), the screw will become loose. These external forces may result from many factors, including parafunction, excessive crown height, masticatory dynamics, prosthesis position in the dental arch, and opposing dentition. In addition, conditions that magnify or increase external forces include cantilevers, angled loads, and poor occlusal designs (Fig. 7.5).

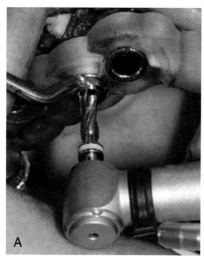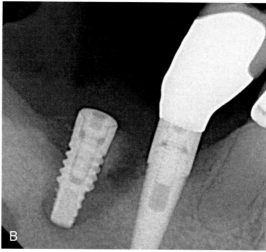

• **Fig. 7.2** Early surgical failures. (A) Excessive heat is a common etiologic factor in the early failure of implants. A common problem is related to guided surgery, which results in compromised irrigation to the surgical site. This is especially common in more dense bone (e.g., D1 or D2). (B) Radiograph of early implant failure resulting from overheating the bone. A radiolucent area (necrotic bone) is usually present around the implant interface.

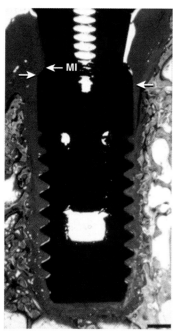

• **Fig. 7.3** Micromovement of a developing bone–implant interface may cause fibrous tissue to form around an implant rather than a bone–implant interface. Excessive stresses to an implant may cause overload and failure. This implant had occlusal overload, which resulted in fibrous tissue formation around the implant (From Isidor F. Loss of osseointegration caused by occlusal load of oral implants: a clinical and radiographic study in monkeys. *Clin Oral Implants Res.* 1996; 7:143–152.)

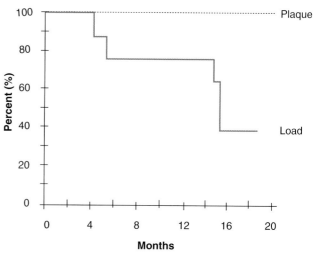

• **Fig. 7.4** Premature occlusal contacts caused six of eight integrated implants to fail within 18 months. Strings in the sulcus and excessive plaque accumulation caused no failure during this period. (From Isidor F. Loss of osseointegration caused by occlusal load of oral implants: a clinical and radiographic study in monkeys. *Clin Oral Implants Res.* 1996; 7:143–152.)

Implant Component Biomechanical Complications

Materials follow a fatigue curve, which is related to the number of cycles and the intensity of the force. There is a force so great that one cycle causes a fracture (e.g., karate blow to a piece of wood). However, if a lower force magnitude repeatedly hits an object, it will still fracture. The wire coat hanger that is bent does not break the first time, but repeated bends will fracture the material, not because the last bend was more forceful, but because of fatigue. Indeed, when the patient says he soaked his bread in coffee and then placed it in his mouth before the porcelain/abutment screw/cement seal/cantilevered prostheses fracture, it may have been "the straw that broke the camel's back."

Prosthesis screw fracture has been noted in both fixed-partial and complete-fixed prostheses, with a mean incidence of 4% and a range of 0% to 19%[7] (Fig. 7.6). Abutment screws are usually larger in diameter and therefore fracture less often, with a mean incidence of 2% and a range of 0.2% to 8% (Fig. 7.7). Metal framework fractures also have been reported in an average of 3% of fixed-complete and overdenture restorations, with a range of 0% to 27% (Fig. 7.8). Implant body fracture has the least incidence of this type of complication, with an occurrence of 1% (Fig. 7.9). This condition is reported with more frequency in long-term fixed prostheses and may even account for the majority of long-term failures. Prosthetic material complications for fixed prostheses have been shown to have a 33% rate at 5 years and 67% after 10 years.[41] Prostheses-related fractures far outnumber implant component fractures.

Uncemented restorations (or worse, partially uncemented prostheses) occur most often when chronic loads are applied to the cement interface or when shear forces are present (as found with cantilevers). Cement strengths are weakest in shear loads. For example, zinc phosphate cement may resist a compressive force of 12,000 pounds per square inch (psi) but can only resist a shear force of 500 psi. It is interesting to note that bone is also strongest to compression and 65% weaker to shear forces. A similar scenario relative to shear load is found with porcelain or other occlusal materials. As a consequence, the evaluation, diagnosis, and modification of treatment plans related to stress conditions are of considerable importance. Therefore once the implant dentist has identified the sources of additional force on the implant system, the treatment plan is altered in an attempt to minimize their negative effect on the longevity of the implant, bone, and final restoration.

Marginal Bone Loss

Crestal bone loss has been observed around the permucosal portion of dental implants for decades. It has been described in the crestal region of successfully osteointegrated implants regardless of surgical approaches. It can range from loss of marginal bone to complete failure of the implant[17,25,42,43] and dramatically decreases after the first year (Box 7.2). For the one-piece blade implants, this phenomenon was described as a "saucerization" and occurred after implant loading.[42]

Occlusal Trauma: Bone Loss

Adell and colleagues[25] were the first to quantify and report marginal bone loss. The study also indicated greater magnitude and occurrence of bone loss during the first year of prosthesis loading, averaging 1.2 mm during this time frame, with a range of 0 to 3 mm. This report measured bone loss from the first thread as the 0-mm baseline, not from the original level of crestal bone

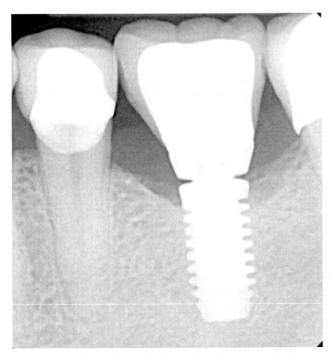

• **Fig. 7.5** Risk of screw loosening is greatest for single-implant crowns most commonly from biomechanical force. A loose screw may lead to prosthesis failure and peri-implant disease if not corrected.

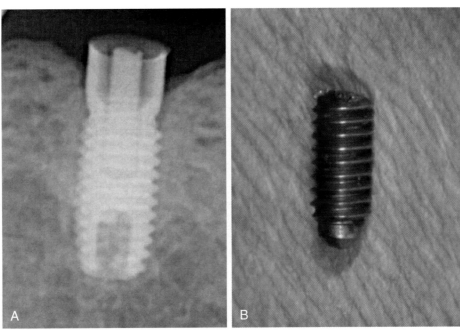

• **Fig. 7.6** Screw fracture. (A) prosthesis screw fractured, which leads to difficulty in removal. (B) Fractured retrieved screw.

at insertion, which was 1.8 mm above this baseline point. Thus the actual first-year crestal bone loss averaged 3.3 mm around the implants observed (Fig. 7.10). Years subsequent to the first showed an average of 0.05- to 0.13-mm bone loss per year. Other studies report an average first-year bone loss of 0.93 mm, with a range from 0.4 to 1.6 mm and a mean loss of 0.1 mm after the first year.[33,34] The early crestal bone loss has been observed so frequently that proposed criteria for successful implants often do not even include the first-year bone loss amount.[44]

The initial transosteal bone loss around an implant forms a V-shaped or a U-shaped pattern, which has been described as *ditching* or *saucerization* around the implant. The current hypotheses

for the cause of crestal bone loss have ranged from reflection of the periosteum during surgery, preparation of the implant osteotomy, the position of the "microgap" between the abutment and implant body, micromovement of the abutment components, bacterial invasion, the establishment of a biological width, and factors of stress.[17,25,43-48]

An understanding of the causes of marginal crestal bone loss around dental implants and early implant failure is critical in preventing such occurrences, fostering long-term peri-implant health, and improving long-term implant success rates and, foremost, implant prosthesis success. Marginal crestal bone loss may influence esthetics because the height of the soft tissue (e.g.,

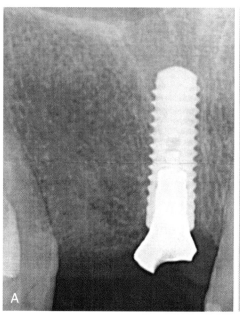
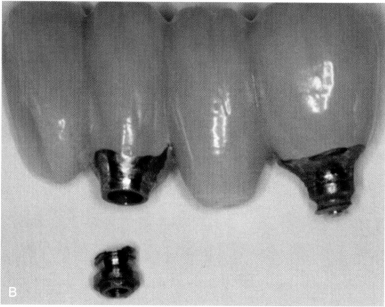

• **Fig. 7.7** Abutment fracture. (A) most commonly fractured from overpreparation of the abutment and biomechanical force. (B) abutment fracture on a splinted implant prosthesis.

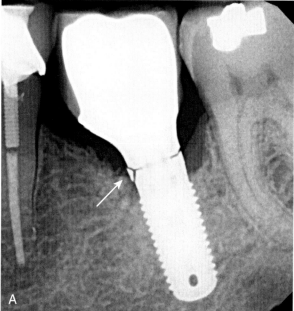
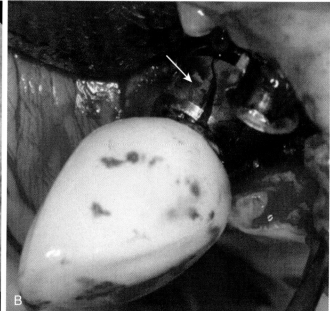

• **Fig. 7.8** Implant body fracture. (A and B) Implant neck fracture because of a concentration of force at the crestal area.

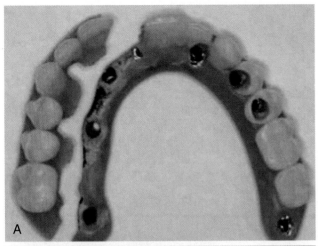

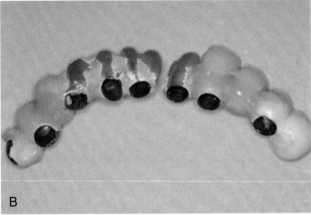

• **Fig. 7.9** Prosthesis fracture. (A) Hybrid fixed prosthesis fracture. (B) Full-arch fixed porcelain fused to metal framework fracture.

• BOX 7.2   Effects of Crestal Bone Loss

- Early implant failure (especially in soft bone or short implants)
- Crestal bone loss may have an occlusal stress component
- Prosthetic-screw loosening
- Abutment-screw loosening
- Restorative material fracture
- Unretained cemented restoration
- Prosthetic framework fracture
- Overdenture attachment adjustments
- Acrylic base fracture of overdentures
- Overdenture attachment fracture
- Abutment screw fracture
- Implant body fracture
- Esthetic complications
- Peri-implant disease

---

interdental papilla) is directly related to the marginal bone. If the tissue shrinks as a consequence of the bone loss, the emergence profile of the crown elongates and the papilla may disappear next to the adjacent tooth or implant. If the soft tissue does not shrink, then the increase in pocket depth may be related to the presence of anaerobic bacteria and peri-implantitis.

Over the years, the cause of marginal bone loss has kept the implant community busy with academic debates and clinical studies. However, clinical consequences are such that all phases of

implant dentistry, from diagnosis and treatment planning to the final stages of occlusion and prosthesis delivery, must focus on its reduction or elimination.

Periosteal Reflection Hypothesis

Periosteal reflection causes a transitional change in the blood supply to the crestal cortical bone. Ninety percent of the arterial blood supply and 100% of the venous return are associated with the periosteum in the long bones of the body.[49] When the periosteum is reflected off the crestal bone, the cortical bone blood supply is affected dramatically, causing osteoblast death on the surface from trauma and lack of nutrition. These events have fostered the periosteal reflection theory as a cause for early bone loss around an endosteal implant.

Although crestal bone cells may die of the initial trauma of periosteal reflection, the blood supply is reestablished once the periosteum regenerates. Cutting cones develop from monocytes in the blood and precede new blood vessels into the crestal regions of bone. Osteoblasts then are able to remodel the crestal bone anatomy.[50] Composite bone forms rapidly on periosteal surfaces to restore its original condition. In addition, the underlying trabecular bone is also a vascular source because its blood supply often is maintained in spite of crestal periosteal reflection. The greater the amount of trabecular bone under the crestal cortical bone, the less crestal bone loss is observed.[51] To place the implant in sufficient available bone, an implant ridge is usually 5 mm or wider at the crest. As a result, trabecular bone is readily available to assist in cortical blood supply and remodeling around the implants. The cortical bone is remodeled to its original contour, without significant loss of height.

The periosteal reflection theory would lead to a generalized horizontal bone loss of the entire residual ridge reflected and not the localized ditching pattern around the implant that typically is observed. In addition, generalized bone loss already would be directly noticeable at the second-stage uncovery of the implant body, 4 to 8 months after stage I implant placement surgery. Yet generalized bone loss rarely is observed at the second-stage uncovery surgery (Fig. 7.11). Therefore the periosteal reflection hypothesis does not appear as a primary causal agent of marginal crestal bone loss around an implant.

Implant Osteotomy Hypothesis

Preparation of the implant osteotomy has been reported as a causal agent of early implant bone loss. Bone is a labile organ and is sensitive to heat. The implant osteotomy causes trauma to the bone in immediate contact with the implant, and a devitalized bone zone of about 1 mm is created around the implant. A renewed blood supply and cutting cones are necessary to remodel the bone at the interface. The crestal region is more susceptible to bone loss during initial repair because of its limited blood supply and the greater heat generated in this denser bone, especially with the less efficient cutting of countersink drills used in this region.[51-53] This condition supports implant osteotomy preparation as a causal agent for marginal crestal bone loss around the implant.

However, if heat and trauma during implant osteotomy preparation were responsible for marginal crestal bone loss, the effect would be noticeable at the second-stage uncovery surgery 4 to 8 months later. The average bone loss of 1.5 mm from the first thread is not observed at stage II uncovery. In fact, bone often has grown over the first-stage cover screw, especially when level

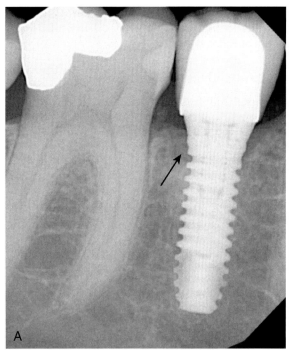
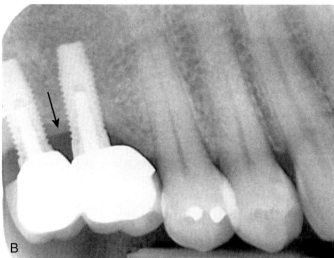

• **Fig. 7.10** Marginal bone loss. (A and B) Marginal bone loss around the crestal portion of an implant often occurs during the first year of occlusal loading.

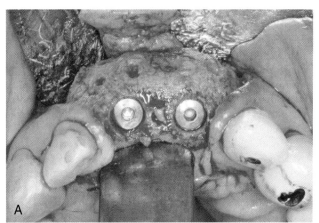
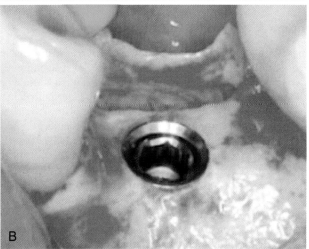

• **Fig. 7.11** Stage II uncovery. (A and B) Marginal bone level at stage II surgery is variable (i.e., minimal crestal bone loss, bone at the top of the implant, bone overgrowth of the cover screw). The bone loss has been attributed to the reflection of the periosteum or the osteotomy preparation.

or slightly countersunk below the bone. Reports in the literature indicated different surgical trauma causes and numbers for bone loss. For example, Manz[54] observed that bone loss at second-stage surgery ranged from 0.89 to 0.96 mm regardless of the bone density. Hoar and colleagues[55] reported only 0.2-mm bone loss at stage II uncovery. The surgical system or approach may influence these data, but usually this bone loss remains minimal. One should remember that these are averages of bone loss reported. Therefore if 2 mm of bone loss is found on one implant, and the next nine implants exhibit no bone loss, the average bone loss would be 0.2 mm. Most implants at stage II uncovery do not demonstrate any bone loss. Therefore the implant osteotomy hypothesis for marginal crestal bone loss cannot be primarily responsible for this routinely observed phenomenon.

Autoimmune Response of Host Hypothesis

The primary cause of bone loss around natural teeth is bacteria induced. Repeat studies demonstrated that bacteria are the causative element for vertical defects around teeth. Occlusal trauma may accelerate the process, but trauma alone is not deemed a determining factor.[56] The implant gingival sulcus in the partially edentulous implant patient exhibits a bacterial flora similar to that of natural teeth.[1] A logical assumption is that if implants are similar to teeth, then the marginal implant bone loss is caused primarily by bacteria, with occlusal factors playing a contributing or accelerating role.

In a prospective study of 125 implants, Adell and colleagues[43] reported 80% of implant sulcular regions were without inflammation. Lekholm and colleagues[57] found that deep gingival pockets around implants were not associated with crestal bone loss, yet the marginal crestal bone loss to the first thread of screw-type implants is a common radiologic finding. If bacteria were the causal agent for the initial bone loss, why does most bone loss occur the first year (1.5 mm) and less (0.1 mm) each successive year? The implant sulcus depth (SD) progressively increases from the early bone loss, impairing hygiene and making anaerobic bacteria more likely the cause of bacteria-related bone loss. If bacteria are responsible for 1.5-mm early crestal bone loss, what local environmental changes occur to reduce their effect by 15 times after the first year?[25] The bacteria autoimmune theory cannot explain the marginal bone loss condition when it follows the pattern most often reported.

Although the bacteria theory does not explain adequately the marginal crestal bone loss phenomenon, this does not mean that bacteria are not a major contributor to bone loss around an implant. Threads and porous implant surfaces exposed to bacteria are reported to cause a more rapid loss of bone around an implant.[57] Poor hygiene also is reported to accelerate the bone loss observed around endosteal implants[58,59] (Fig. 7.12). To state that bacteria are never involved in marginal bone loss around an implant would be incorrect. Bone loss often is associated with bacteria as a causal agent. However, when most bone loss occurs in the first year and less bone loss is observed afterward, the hypothesis of bacteria as the primary causal agent for the early crestal bone loss cannot be substantiated.

Biological Width Hypothesis

The sulcular regions around an implant and around a tooth are similar in many respects. The rete peg formation within the attached gingiva and the histologic lining of the gingiva within the sulcus are similar in implants and teeth. A free gingival margin forms around an implant with nonkeratinized sulcular epithelium, and the epithelial cells at its base are similar to the functional epithelial cells described with natural teeth.[60] However, a fundamental difference characterizes the base of the gingival sulcus.

For a natural tooth, an average biological width of 2.04 mm exists between the depth of the sulcus and the crest of the alveolar bone (Fig. 7.13). It should be noted the biological "width" is actually a height dimension with a greater range in the posterior region compared with the anterior region and may be greater than 4 mm in height. In teeth, it is composed of a connective tissue (CT) attachment (1.07-mm average) above the bone and a junctional epithelial attachment (0.97-mm average) at the sulcus base, and the most consistent value between individuals is the CT attachment.[61-63]

The biological width allows gingival fibers and hemidesmosomes to establish direct contact with the natural tooth and acts as a barrier to the bacteria in the sulcus to the underlining periodontal tissues. When a crown margin invades the biological width, the crestal bone recedes to reestablish a favorable environment for the gingival fibers.[64,65]

Many surgical protocols recommend the placement of endosteal implants at or below the crest of the ridge during the first-stage surgery. The abutment-to-implant body connection may be compared with a crown margin. Berglundh and colleagues[66] observed 0.5 mm of bone loss below the implant-abutment connection within 2 weeks after stage II uncovery and abutment connection in dogs (Fig. 7.14). Lindhe and colleagues[67] reported an inflammatory CT extending 0.5 mm above and below this implant-abutment connection. Wallace and Tarnow[68,69] stated that the biological width also occurs with implants and may contribute to some of the marginal bone loss observed. The biological width theory seems attractive to explain the lack of bone loss from the first stage of surgery and the early bone loss seen within the first year after the second-stage abutment placement. However, it should be noted that the biological width in implants, as reported,

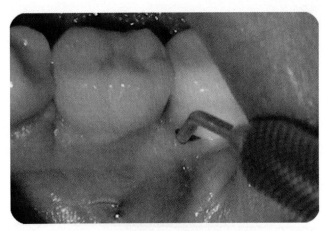

• **Fig. 7.12** Exudate around an implant is more likely to be present when the probing depth is greater than 5 mm because the biofilm is difficult to remove.

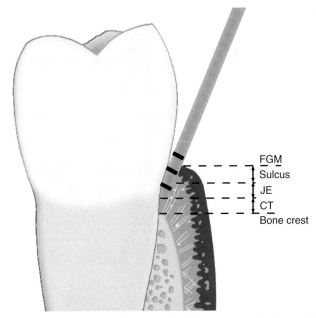

• **Fig. 7.13** Biological width of a natural tooth has a connective tissue (CT) zone that inserts into the cementum of the tooth. A periodontal probe will penetrate the sulcus and the junctional epithelial attachment. *FGM,* Free gingival margin; *JE,* junctional epithelium.

often includes the SD, whereas the natural tooth biological width does not include the SD.

Eleven different gingival fiber groups are observed around a natural tooth: dentogingival (coronal, horizontal, and apical), alveologingival, intercapillary, transgingival, circular, semicircular, dentoperiosteal, transseptal, periosteogingival, intercircular, and intergingival. At least six of these gingival fiber groups insert into the cementum of the natural tooth: the dentogingival (coronal, horizontal, and apical), dentoperiosteal, transseptal, circular, semicircular, and transgingival fibers. In addition, some crestal fibers from the periodontal fiber bundles also insert into the cementum above the alveolar bone.[63] However, in a typical implant gingival region, only two of these gingival fiber groups and no periodontal fibers are present (Fig. 7.15). These fibers do not insert into the implant body below the abutment margin as they do into the

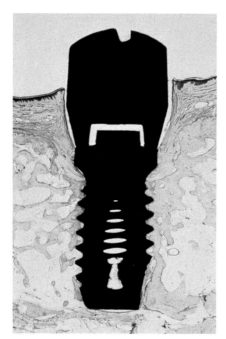

• **Fig. 7.14** Bone levels recede to at least 0.5 mm around an abutment to implant connection after the implant extends through the soft tissue, regardless of whether the implant is loaded. (Courtesy Steve Wallace.)

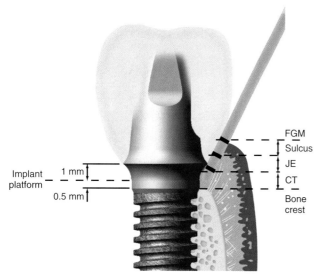

• **Fig. 7.15** There are primarily two soft tissue fiber groups around an implant: circular fibers and crestal bone fibers. Neither of these fiber types insert into the implant or the abutment. The peri-implant probe penetrates the sulcus, junctional epithelial attachment, and most of the connective tissue (CT) zone. *FGM,* Free gingival margin; *JE,* junctional epithelium.

cementum of natural teeth.[62,70] Instead, the collagen fibers in the CT attachment around an implant run parallel to the implant surface, not perpendicular, such as with natural teeth.[71,72] The gingival and periosteal fiber groups are responsible for the CT attachment component of the biological width around teeth, and these are not present around the transosteal region of an implant. Therefore the CT attachment around the abutment-implant connection cannot be compared with the CT attachment of a tooth.

James and Keller[70] were first to begin a systematic scientific study to investigate the biological seal phenomenon of the soft tissue around dental implants. Hemidesmosomes help form a basal lamina–like structure on the implant, which can act as a biological seal. However, collagenous components of the linear body cannot physiologically adhere to or become embedded into the implant body as they do in the cementum of the tooth.[73] The hemidesmosomal seal only has a circumferential band of gingival tissue to provide mechanical protection against tearing.[74] Therefore the biological seal around dental implants can prevent the migration of bacteria and endotoxins into the underlying bone. It is unable, however, to constitute a junctional epithelial attachment component of the biological width similar to the one found with natural teeth. The amount of early crestal bone loss therefore seems unlikely to be solely the result of the remodeling of the hard and soft tissues to establish a biological width below an abutment connection. No CT attachment zone or components of the linear body are embedded into an implant. The importance, amount, and mechanism for these anatomic structures require further investigation.

The crevice between the cover screw and the implant body during initial healing is similar to the crevice of the abutment-implant connection. Yet bone can grow over the cover screw, and therefore the crevice, in and of itself, may not be the cause of bone loss. The crevice between the implant and the abutment connection has been called a microgap. The actual dimension of this connection is usually 0 mm and has a direct metal-to-metal connection. However, when the crevice is exposed to the oral environment, bone loss is usually observed for at least 0.5 mm below the connection.[74-76]

The biological width hypothesis cannot fully explain the several millimeters of marginal crestal bone loss, which also has been observed readily with one-stage implants that extend through the tissue at the initial implant placement surgery and have no abutment-implant connections. For example, plate form (blade) implants, transosteal implants, pins, one-piece screw implants, and even subperiosteal implants, demonstrate the marginal crestal bone loss phenomenon. It is true that bone loss does occur around an exposed abutment-implant connection placed below the bone and is observed within 2 to 4 weeks once the connection is exposed to the oral environment. The bone loss often occurs before the implant is loaded with the prosthesis. It is logical to call this marginal bone loss the *biological width.*

The primary question remains, when the surgeon places the implant-abutment connection below the bone: How much bone loss is from the implant biological width, and therefore out of the influence of the dental practitioner? Several reports in the literature note implant macro- and microgeometry may affect the biological width dimensions or the amount of early crestal bone loss.[33,34,55,77-80]

The bone loss to the first thread observation implies that the amount of bone loss is similar for different implant designs. However, the first thread is a different distance from the abutment margin for several implant designs. A smooth, polished 4-mm collar below the bone has been associated with greater bone loss than a smooth 2-mm collar below the bone. The implant biological width concept does not explain completely the total amount of vertical bone loss observed. In addition, the amount of bone loss from the biological width occurs within 1 month, whether the implant is loaded or not, and is related to the crest module implant design and the position of the abutment-implant connection in relation to the bone but is unrelated to the density of the bone. The concept does not explain why greater crestal bone loss often is observed in soft bone compared with denser bone after loading, nor does it explain the higher implant failure rates in lesser-quality bone after loading.

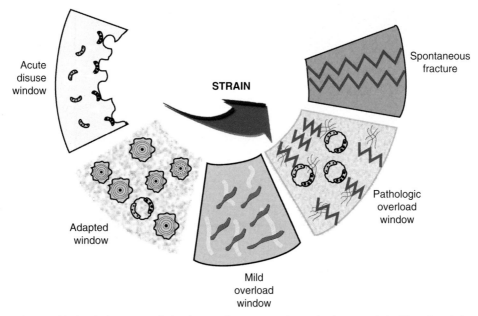

• **Fig. 7.16** Mechanical stress applied to bone cells causes a change in shape or strain. The microstrains may trigger the release of cytokines and bone resorption.

Occlusal Trauma

Marginal bone loss on an implant may be from occlusal trauma.[45] *Occlusal trauma* may be defined as an injury to the attachment apparatus as a result of excessive occlusal force.[1] There is controversy as to the role of occlusion in the bone loss observed after an implant prosthesis delivery.[8] Some articles stated that peri-implant bone loss without implant failure is primarily associated with biological formations or complications.[16-18] Other authors suggested a correlation of crestal bone loss to occlusal overload.[8,45,47,81,82] The determination of the etiology of bone loss around dental implants is needed to minimize its occurrence and foster long-term peri-implant health that may ultimately determine implant prosthesis survival.

The association of occlusal trauma and bone loss around natural teeth has been debated since Karolyi claimed a relationship in 1901.[82] A number of authors concluded trauma from occlusion is a related factor in bone loss, although bacteria is a necessary agent.[83-88] On the other hand, Waerhaug and many others stated there is no relationship between occlusal trauma and the degree of periodontal tissue breakdown.[89-91] According to Lindhe and colleagues, "trauma" from occlusion cannot induce periodontal tissue breakdown.[92] However, occlusal trauma may lead to tooth mobility that can be transient or permanent. By extrapolation of this rationale, several authors have also concluded that occlusal trauma is not related to marginal bone loss around a dental implant.[16-18] To establish a further correlation between marginal bone loss and occlusal overload, related articles from cellular biomechanics, engineering principles, mechanical properties of bone, physiology of bone, implant design biomechanics, animal studies, and clinical reports were procured.[45]

Cellular Biomechanics

Bone remodeling at the cellular level is controlled by the mechanical environment of strain.[93] *Strain* is defined as the change in length divided by the original length, and the units of strain are given in percentages. The amount of strain in a material is directly related to the amount of stress applied.[94] Occlusal stress applied through the implant prosthesis and components can transmit stress to the bone–implant interface.[93] The amount of bone strain at the bone–implant interface is directly related to the amount of stress applied through the implant prosthesis. Mechanosensors in bone respond to minimal amounts of strain, and microstrain levels 100 times less than the ultimate strength of bone may trigger bone remodeling[95] (Fig. 7.16).

One of the earliest remodeling theories for a direct relationship between stress and the magnitude of bone remodeling was proposed by Kummer in 1972.[96] More recently, Frost reported on the cellular reaction of bone to different microstrain levels.[97,98] He observed that bone fractures at 10,000 to 20,000 microstrain units (1%–2% deformation). However, at levels 20% to 40% of this value (4000 units), bone cells may trigger cytokines to begin a resorption response. In other words, excessive bone strain may result in physical fracture, and it may cause bone cellular resorption. Therefore the hypothesis that occlusal stresses beyond the physiologic limits of bone may result in strain in the bone significant enough to cause bone resorption is plausible from a cellular biomechanics standpoint. To date, bone-cellular studies have not replicated this bone condition next to a dental implant. However, cytokines in the bone–implant interface tissue obtained from failed hip replacement devices leading to bone loss have been reported in humans.[99]

Engineering Principles

The relationship between stress and strain determines the modulus of elasticity (stiffness) of a material.[94] The modulus conveys the amount of dimensional change in a material for a given stress level. The modulus of elasticity of a tooth is similar to cortical bone. Dental implants are typically fabricated from titanium or its alloy. The modulus of elasticity of titanium is 5 to 10 times greater than that of cortical bone (Fig. 7.17). An engineering principle called the *composite beam analysis* states that when two materials of different elastic moduli are placed together

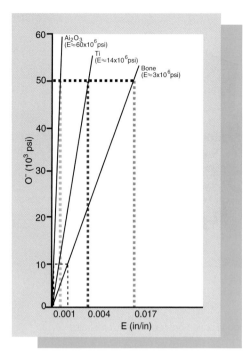

• **Fig. 7.17** Modulus of elasticity is greater for titanium (Ti) compared with bone. When stress is plotted on the Y-axis and strain on the X-axis, the modulus of elasticity can be obtained. Titanium is 5 to 10 times more rigid than cortical bone.

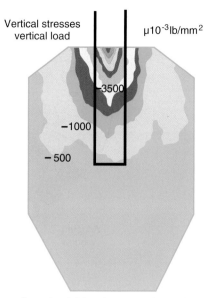

• **Fig. 7.18** Three-dimensional finite-element analysis of a titanium implant in a bone model after axial loading. The V-shape pattern of strain is greatest at the crestal region and decreases in intensity as the stress is dissipated throughout the implant length.

with no intervening material and one is loaded, a stress contour increase will be observed in which the two materials first come into contact.[100] In an implant–bone interface, these stress contours are of greater magnitude at the crestal bone region. This phenomenon was observed in both photoelastic and three-dimensional finite-element analysis studies when implants were loaded within a bone simulant.[101-104] These authors noted that the marginal bone loss observed clinically and radiographically around implants follows a pattern similar to the stress contours in these reports.

Bone Mechanical Properties

Bone density is directly related to the strength and elastic modulus of bone.[105] In denser bone, there is less strain under a given load compared with softer bone. As a result, there is less bone remodeling in denser bone compared with softer bone under similar load conditions.[97] A decrease in bone remodeling can result in a reduction of bone loss (Fig. 7.18). In a prospective human study, Manz observed that the amount of marginal bone loss next to an implant was related to the density of bone.[54] The initial peri-implant bone loss from implant insertion to uncovery was similar for all bone qualities. However, 6 months after prosthesis delivery, the additional radiographic-observed peri-implant bone loss ranged from 0.68 mm for quality 1 to 1.1 mm for quality 2-type bone, 1.24 mm for quality 3-type bone, and 1.44 mm for quality 4-type bone (Fig. 7.19). In other words, the more dense the bone, the less peri-implant bone loss was observed after prosthesis delivery. A clinical report by Appleton and colleagues[106,107] demonstrated that progressively loaded single-tooth implants in the first premolar region of human beings exhibited greater bone density increase in the crestal half of the implant interface and less marginal bone loss compared with nonprogressively loaded implants in the same jaw

region and even the same patient on the contralateral side without progressive loading. Because an increase in bone density is related to bone strength, elastic modulus, bone remodeling, and a decrease in marginal bone loss, these entities may be related to each other.

Animal Studies

Several animal studies in the literature demonstrated the ability of bone tissue to respond to a dental implant. For example, Hoshaw and colleagues inserted dental implants into a dog femur perpendicular to the axis of the long bone and perpendicular to the direction of the osteons.[108,109] After applying a tensile load to the implants for only 5 days, the bone cells reorganized to follow the implant-thread pattern and resist the load. This unique bone pattern was only observed for 3 to 4 mm around the implants. Crestal bone loss was also noted around these implants and explained as stress overload. To rearrange its osteal structure, bone must remodel.

Miyata placed crowns on integrated dental implants with no occlusal contacts (control group), and premature interceptive occlusal contacts of 100, 180, and 250 mm in a monkey animal model.[110-112] After 4 weeks of premature occlusal loads, the implants were removed in a block section and evaluated. The crestal bone levels for 100-mm and control implants with no loading were similar. However, statistically significant crestal bone loss was observed in the 180-mm group (Fig. 7.20). The 250-mm group experienced two to three times the bone loss of the crowns with moderate prematurities (Fig. 7.21).

Duyck used a dog model to evaluate the crestal bone loss around screw-type dental implants with no loads (controls), static loads, and dynamic loads.[113] The dynamic-loaded implants were the only group to demonstrate crestal bone loss. Because the only variable in these two studies was the intensity or type of occlusal load applied to the implants, these animal reports implied that dynamic occlusal loading may be a factor in crestal bone loss around rigid fixated dental implants.

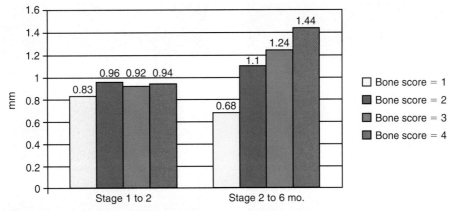

• **Fig. 7.19** Mean peri-implant vertical bone change for study intervals by bone quality score. Many observed that the amount of bone loss from stage I to stage II was similar, regardless of bone quality. However, after 6 months of loading, the amount of marginal bone loss was directly related to the quality of the bone, with type 4 bone (the softest bone) exhibiting the greatest bone loss. (From Manz MC. Radiographic assessment of peri-implant vertical bone loss: DICRG Interim Report No 9. *J Oral Maxillofac Surg.* 1997;55(12 Suppl):62–71.)

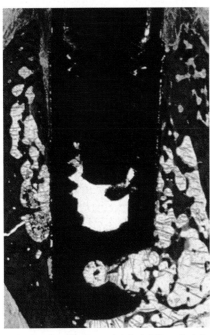

• **Fig. 7.20** Miyata and colleagues loaded integrated implants for 4 weeks with premature contacts on crowns of 100, 180, and 250 mm. The implants with 180-mm premature contacts demonstrate a V-shaped crestal bone loss. (From Miyata T, Kobayashi Y, Araki H, et al. The influence of controlled occlusal overload on peri-implant tissue. Part 3: a histologic study in monkeys. *Int J Oral Maxillofac Implants.* 2000;15:425–431.)

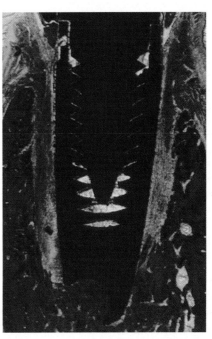

• **Fig. 7.21** Implants with 250-mm premature contacts demonstrated greater bone loss than the 180-mm group. The 250-mm premature contact for 4 weeks lost the most bone. The higher stresses resulted in more crestal bone loss. (From Miyata T, Kobayashi Y, Araki H, et al. The influence of controlled occlusal overload on peri-implant tissue. Part 3: a histologic study in monkeys. *Int J Oral Maxillofac Implants.* 2000;15:425–431.)

Clinical Reports

Clinical reports have shown an increase in marginal bone loss around implants closest to a cantilever used to restore the lost dentition[114-116] (Fig. 7.22). Cantilever length and an increase in occlusal stress to the nearest abutment are directly related[117] and point to the fact that the increase in marginal bone loss may be related to occlusal stress. Quirynen and colleagues evaluated 93 implant patients with various implant restorations and concluded that the amount of crestal bone loss was definitely associated with occlusal loading.[33] These authors also reported increased crestal bone loss

around implants in patients with no anterior occlusal contacts and parafunctional habits in full-arch fixed prostheses in both jaws.[33,34] These clinical reports did not provide statistical analyses to demonstrate a clear link between occlusal stress and bone loss. However, they indicated a consensus by some authors that occlusal overload may be related to the incidence of peri-implant bone loss around the cervical aspect of an implant. In fact, in a study of 589 consecutive implants, Naert and colleagues suggested that overload from parafunctional habits may be the most probable cause of implant loss and marginal bone loss after loading.[118]

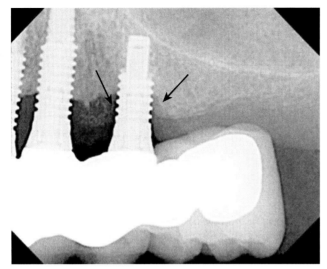

• **Fig. 7.22** Cantilevers on fixed partial dentures have been shown to increase the marginal bone loss on the implant next to the cantilever.

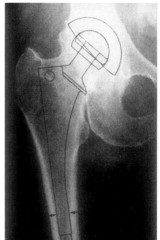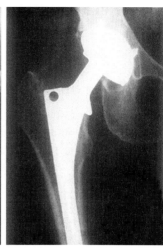

• **Fig. 7.23** Bone loss around orthopedic implants (osteolysis) is primarily caused by mechanical stress to the bone–implant interface.

Rangert and colleagues have noted that occlusal loads on an implant may act as a bending moment, which increases stress at the marginal bone level and can cause implant body fracture.[35] Before the fracture of the implant body, marginal bone loss was noted in this retrospective clinical evaluation. The same stress that caused implant fracture is the logical cause of the peri-implant bone loss before the event.

Rosenberg and colleagues found microbial differences in implant failures from both overload and biological complications.[81] Uribe and colleagues presented the case of a mandibular implant crown with a marginal peri-implantitis and osseous defect.[119] Histologic analysis revealed an infiltrate and a central zone of dense fibroconnective tissue with scanty inflammatory cells. According to the authors, this finding differed from chronic inflammatory tissue associated with infectious peri-implantitis and can be directly related to occlusal overload.

A clinical report by Leung and colleagues observed radiographic angular crestal bone loss to the seventh thread around one of two implants supporting a fixed prosthesis in hyperocclusion 2 weeks after prosthesis delivery.[120] The prosthesis was removed, and over the next few months radiographic observation showed that the crestal defect was repaired to almost the initial level, without any surgical or drug intervention. The prosthesis was then seated with proper occlusal adjustment. The bone levels stabilized at the second thread of the implant and remained stable over the next 36 months. This report indicated bone loss from occlusal overload is not only possible but may even be reversible when found early in the process. Therefore although no prospective clinical study to date has clearly demonstrated a direct relationship between stress and bone loss without implant failure, several practitioners agreed that a causal relationship may exist.

Discussion

Limited marginal bone loss during the first year of function after stage II surgery has been observed around the permucosal portion of dental implants for decades.[25,43] Hypotheses for the causes of crestal bone loss have included the reflection of the periosteum during surgery, preparation of the implant osteotomy, level of the microgap between the abutment and implant body, bacterial

invasion, the establishment of a biological width, the implant crest module design, and occlusal overload (Fig. 7.23).[8,45,47,121]

The fact that occlusal overload may be an etiology for crestal bone loss does not mean other factors are not present. For example, the microgap position of the implant platform and abutment and the biological width often affect the marginal bone during the first month after the implant becomes permucosal.[54] However, the clinician has certain variables under their control that may influence the amount of peri-implant bone loss. The position of the microgap in relation to the bony crest and the implant crest module design are primarily under the control of the implant surgeon. On the other hand, the autoimmune or bacterial response of the patient, the biological width, and the patient response to the surgical trauma of implant placement are variables often escaping the control of the dentist. Once the final prosthesis is delivered to the patient, many events responsible for marginal bone loss have already occurred, whereas others such as occlusal overload and its relationship to the quality of bone persist. Occlusal overload is one factor most in control of the restoring dentist. If a relationship between occlusal overload and crestal bone loss exists, approaches to decrease stress to an implant interface appear appropriate.

A puzzling element in the relationship between occlusal force and peri-implant bone loss is the lack of continued bone loss until the implant fails. Implant crown height may be measured from the occlusal plane to the crest of the bone. The crown height is a vertical cantilever, which may magnify the stresses applied to the prosthesis. As a result of the greater crown height from the vertical bone loss, occlusal overload will be increased after crestal bone loss occurs. Therefore if occlusal loading forces can cause crestal bone loss, the resulting increased moment forces should further promote the loss of bone until the implant fails, yet most clinical studies indicate the rate of bone loss decreases after the first year of loading and is minimal thereafter. There are two reasons the bone levels may become stable after initial marginal bone loss, even when the cause is from occlusal overload: bone physiology and implant design mechanics.

Bone Physiology

The bone is less dense and weaker at stage II implant surgery than it is 1 year later after prosthetic loading.[122] Bone is 60% mineralized at 4 months and takes 52 weeks to complete its mineralization.[123]

Partially mineralized bone is weaker than fully mineralized bone. In addition, the microscopic organization of bone progresses during the first year. Woven bone is unorganized and weaker than lamellar bone, which is organized and more mineralized. Lamellar bone develops several months after the woven bone repair has replaced the devitalized bone caused by the surgical insertion trauma around the implant.[122] The occlusal stress levels may be high enough to cause woven bone microfracture or overload during the first year, but the increase in bone strength achieved after complete mineralization and organization may be able to resist the same stress levels during the subsequent years.

Because functional forces are placed on an implant, the surrounding bone can adapt to the stresses and increase its density, especially in the crestal half of the implant body during the first 6 months to 1 year of loading.[123] In a histologic and histomorphometric study of bone, Piatelli and colleagues reported reactions to unloaded and loaded nonsubmerged implants in monkeys (Figs. 7.24 and 7.25). The bone changed from a fine trabecular pattern after initial healing to a more dense and coarse trabecular pattern after loading, especially in the crestal half of the implant interface.[124] Hoshaw loaded threaded implants in dogs with a tensile load and noted that the fine trabecular bone pattern became coarse trabecular bone around the implant.[108,109] In addition, the bone reorganized to a more favorable condition to assist the direction and type of occlusal load (Fig. 7.26).

Fine trabecular bone is less dense than coarse trabecular bone.[122] Because the density of bone is directly related to its strength and elastic modulus, the crestal bone strength and biomechanical mismatch between titanium and bone may diminish gradually during the functional loading phase. In other words, the stresses applied to the peri-implant bone may be great enough to cause bone resorption during the first year because bone strains are greatest at the crest. However, the stresses applied below the crest of bone are of less magnitude and may correspond to the physiologic strain that allows the bone to gain density and strength. As a result, the occlusal load that causes bone loss initially (overload) is not great enough to cause continued bone loss once the bone matures and becomes more dense.

A clinical report by Appleton and colleagues demonstrated that progressively loaded single-tooth implants in the first premolar region of humans exhibited less bone loss and greater bone density increase in the crestal half of the implant interface compared with nonprogressively loaded implants in the same jaw region, and even in the same patient on the contralateral side (Fig. 7.27).[106,107] Marginal bone loss is less in the mandible compared with the maxilla in several clinical reports. The bone is denser in the mandible than the maxilla. The reduced crestal bone loss that has been reported in the mandible, in greater bone densities, and in progressively loaded implants points to the fact that stress/strain is a primary etiology of crestal bone loss after the implant is loaded. Therefore the stresses at the crest of the ridge may cause microfracture or overload during the first year, and the change in bone strength after loading and mineralization is complete alters the stress/strain relationship and reduces the risk of microfracture during the following years.[125]

Implant Design Biomechanics

Implant design may affect the magnitude or type of forces applied to the bone–implant interface. A smooth collar at the crest module may transmit shear forces to the bone. Bone is strongest under compressive forces, 30% weaker under tensile loads, and 65%

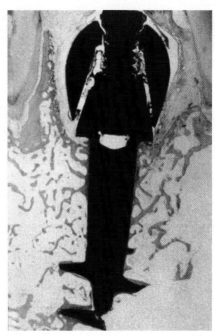

• **Fig. 7.24** In evaluating the bone around an implant after healing in a monkey model, a fine trabecular pattern is noted. (From Piatelli A, Ruggeri A, Franchi M, et al. An histologic and histomorphometric study of bone reactions to unloaded and loaded nonsubmerged single implants in monkeys: a pilot study. *J Oral Implantol.* 1993;19(4):314–320.)

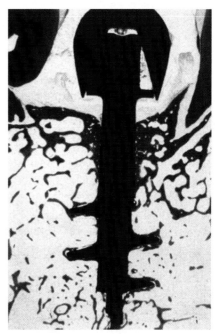

• **Fig. 7.25** Once the implant is loaded, the fine trabecular bone became coarse trabecular bone, especially at the crestal region. When the stresses are too great, bone loss occurs. When the stresses are within the physiologic range, the bone density increases. (From Piatelli A, Ruggeri A, Franchi M, et al. An histologic and histomorphometric study of bone reactions to unloaded and loaded nonsubmerged single implants in monkeys: a pilot study. *J Oral Implantol.* 1993;19(4):314–320.)

weaker to shear forces.[126] Bone may heal to the smooth metal collar of the implant crest module from the time of implant insertion to implant uncovery; but placed under loading conditions,

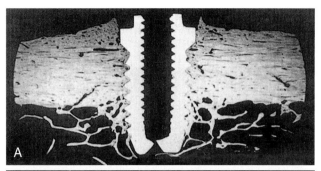

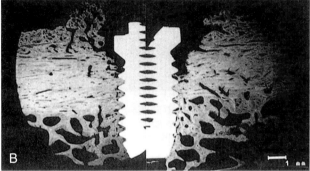

• **Fig. 7.26** Researchers loaded threaded implants in dog tibiae and noted that the (A) fine trabecular bone in the apical region became (B) coarse trabecular after loading. In addition, crestal bone loss was observed on the loaded implant. (From Hoshaw SJ, Brunski JB, Cochran GVB: Mechanical loading of Brånemark fixtures affects interfacial bone modeling and remodeling, *Int J Oral Maxillofac Implants* 9:345–360, 1994.)

the weaker shear interface is more likely to overload the bone. The first thread or a roughened surface condition of the implant is where the type of force changes from primarily shear to compressive or tensile loads. Therefore in many situations the 35% to 65% increase in bone strength, through changes from shear to compressive and/or tensile loads, is sufficient to halt the bone-loss process. This may be one of the reasons why implant designs with a 2-mm smooth collar above the first thread and a 4-mm smooth collar above the first thread lose bone to this "first thread" landmark.[127] (A previous review addressed the range of bone loss with different implant designs.[128-130]) Because implant crest module designs may affect the amount of bone loss, and the implant design contributes to the force transfer of the bone–implant interface, the stress-related theory for one of the etiologies of crestal bone loss is further enhanced.

Literature from cellular biomechanics, engineering principles, differences in bone loss related to bone density, animal studies, and clinical reports all substantiate that occlusal overload may be an etiology of peri-implant bone loss. Literature related to orthopedic joint replacement devices clearly indicate biomechanical stress and overload contribute to bone loss at the implant interface. The increase in bone mineralization and organization during the first year, the increase in bone density at the implant interface, and the type of force changes at the first thread of the implant body all are factors that may halt the bone loss phenomenon after the initial marginal loss. Although this occlusal overload concept does not negate other factors related to marginal bone loss, it is more clinician dependent than most other parameters. Treatment plans that emphasize occlusal stress reduction to the prosthesis are therefore mandated.

Biomechanical Stress Effects on Treatment Planning

Understanding the relationships of stress and related complications provides a basis for a consistent treatment system. The clinical success and longevity of endosteal dental implants as load-bearing abutments are controlled largely by the biomechanical milieu in which they function.[127,131] The stress treatment theorem, developed by the Dr. Carl E. Misch, states that most all treatment related to the science of implant dentistry should be centered around the biomechanical aspects of stress.[131]

Stress-related conditions that affect the treatment planning in implant dentistry include the bone volume lost after tooth loss, bone quality decrease after tooth loss, complications of surgery, implant positioning, initial implant interface healing, initial loading of an implant, implant design, occlusal concepts, prosthesis fixation, marginal bone loss, implant failure, component fracture, prosthesis fracture, and implant fracture. Biomechanical parameters are excellent predictors of increased risks because they are objective and can be measured. One can not only predict which condition presents greater stress, and therefore greater risk, but also how much the risk is increased. A risk factor is not an absolute contraindication, but it significantly increases the complication rate. With so many variables, success or failure in implant dentistry is often a complex subject and not necessarily an exact science, but this does not mean a method cannot be established to decrease the risk. Greater forces in one aspect of treatment do not always equal implant failure or complications, especially because so many factors are involved, including the density of bone around the implant. Yet the risks may be considerably reduced

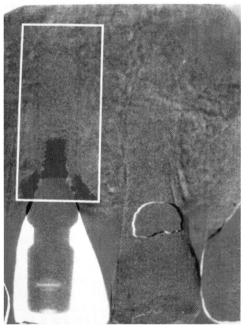

• **Fig. 7.27** Researchers observed in humans that less crestal bone loss and an increase in bone density were present around implants progressively loaded in the maxillary first premolar region. (From Appleton RS, Nummikoski PV, Pigno MA, et al. A radiographic assessment of progressive loading on bone around single osseointegrated implants in the posterior maxilla. *Clin Oral Implants Res.* 2005;16(2):161–167.)

by decreasing the overall stress to the overall system. To assess the increase in risk factors, each factor is considered separately. The goal is to decrease the overall risk. Understanding the relationships of stress and related complications provides a basis for a consistent treatment system. The stress-treatment theorem has evolved into a particular sequence of treatment planning (Box 7.3).

Prosthesis Design

When partially and completely edentulous patients seek implant treatment, their goal is to obtain teeth; therefore it is imperative the clinician visualize the prosthesis before the selecting the foundation (the implants). This is often termed "top-down" treatment planning. The design of the prosthesis is related to a number of factors with the number and position being of utmost importance. For example, if an inadequate number of implants are placed, then the final prosthesis is at risk from biomechanical stress. If the positions of the implants are not ideal, then the final prosthesis is compromised because of potential biomechanical stress issues.

Patient Force Factors

It is crucial the implant clinician take into consideration specific force factors related to the patient. There are numerous force factors to consider: (1) bruxism, (2) clenching, (3) tongue thrust, (4) crown height space, (5) masticatory dynamics, and (6) the opposing arch. The forces applied to the prosthesis also differ by their (1) magnitude, (2) duration, (3) type, and (4) predisposing factors (e.g., cantilevers).

Some patient force factors are more important than others. For example, severe bruxism is the most significant factor and, on a risk scale from 1 to 10, is a 10.[132] Forces from bruxism are often the most difficult forces to contend with on a long-term basis.[132,133] As a result of this condition, marginal implant bone loss, unretained abutments, and fatigue fractures of implants or prostheses are more likely. The increase in force magnitude and duration is a significant problem. A bruxing patient is at higher risk in two ways. The magnitude of the force increases because the muscles become stronger and the number of cycles on the prosthetic components is greater as a result of the parafunction. Eventually some component of the system will break if the occlusal disease cannot be reduced in intensity or duration.

The second-highest risk factor is severe clenching, which is a 9 on the risk scale. Cantilevers, including crown height, are next on the list, followed by masticatory muscle dynamics. The position of the implant in the arch is followed by the direction of load, with a risk of 5. These numbers are arbitrary because they are influenced by the other force factors. For example, angled forces greater than 30 degrees to the implant body are more damaging than a crown height of 20 mm with a long axis load.[134-136] The clinician should

---

> ### • BOX 7.3   Stress Treatment Theorem Sequence of Treatment Planning
>
> 1. Prosthesis design
> 2. Patient force factors
> 3. Bone density in implant sites
> 4. Key implant positions and number
> 5. Implant size
> 6. Available bone
> 7. Implant design

---

evaluate the number of force conditions and their influencing severity factors. As the overall number increases, the risks increase, and the overall treatment plan should be modified to decrease the increased force or by increasing the area of support.

Bone Density

The density of bone is directly related to the strength of the bone.[105,137] Misch and colleagues have reported on the biomechanical properties of four different densities of bone in the jaws.[105] Dense cortical bone is 10 times stronger than the soft, fine trabecular bone. D2 bone is approximately 50% stronger than D3 bone. In addition, the stiffness of the bone is affected by the bone density. Young's modulus for compact bone is 10 times larger than that for cancellous bone. The denser the bone, the stiffer the bone, and there is less biomechanical mismatch to titanium during loading.

Therefore in poorer bone qualities that are susceptible to biomechanical stress, the concept of progressive bone loading may be implemented. Progressive bone loading changes the amount and density of the implant–bone contact. The bone is given time to respond to a gradual increase in occlusal load. This increases the quantity of bone at the implant interface, improves the bone density, and improves the overall support system mechanism.

Key Implant Positions and Implant/Abutment Number

Key Implant Positions

In any prostheses, there are implant positions that are more important from a stress management perspective. In one- or two-unit prostheses, an implant should be placed in each prospective tooth position, without a cantilever crown contour in any direction (e.g., facial, lingual, mesial, distal). In a three- to four-unit restoration, the most important abutments are the terminal abutments. If a terminal abutment is not present, a cantilever is created, which magnifies the stress to the rest of the support system. Cantilevers are a force magnifier and represent a considerable risk factor in implant support, screw loosening, crestal bone loss, fracture, and any other item negatively affected by force.[134,136,138] Therefore the goal of implant position should be to eliminate cantilevers whenever possible, especially when other force factors are increased.

In a 5- to 14-unit prosthesis, intermediary abutments are also important to limit the edentulous spans to less than three pontics. A three-pontic prosthesis flexes 18 times more than a two-pontic prosthesis, whereas a two-pontic restoration flexes eight times more than a one-pontic prosthesis.

The canine is an important implant position whenever the canine and two adjacent teeth are missing. Therefore when the two premolars, a first premolar and lateral, or a lateral and a central, are missing next to a canine, a canine implant is warranted. In addition, the ideal occlusion for an implant prosthesis is implant-protected occlusion. This entails disoccluding off the canine; therefore an implant in this position has significant occlusion benefits.

For fixed full-arch prostheses, the arches may be divided into sections. An edentulous mandible may be divided into three sections from a biomechanical perspective: the anterior (canine to canine) and the bilateral posterior regions (premolar and molars). A key implant position is one implant in each region, or at least three key implants.

The edentulous maxilla is divided in five regions: the anterior (laterals and centrals), bilateral canines, and the bilateral posterior (premolar and molars). A key implant position is one implant in each region, or at least five key implants.

Treatment plans should incorporate methods to reduce stress and minimize its initial and long-term complications. The definition of *stress* is force divided by the functional area over which it is applied. One biomechanical approach to decrease stress is to increase the surface area of the implant support system.[134] The overall stress to the implant system may be reduced by increasing the area over which the force is applied. The most effective method to increase the surface area of implant support is by increasing the number of implants used to support a prosthesis (Fig. 7.28).

Splinting

The concept of splinting is controversial in implant dentistry. Studies by Bidez and Misch demonstrated that force distributed over three abutments results in less localized stress to crestal bone than two abutments.[139] This study applied only to implants that are splinted together. Therefore the number of pontics should be reduced and the number of implant abutments should be increased whenever forces are increased compared with a treatment plan for an ideal patient with minimal force factors.[136,138,140-142] The retention of the prosthesis is also improved with a greater number of splinted abutments. This approach also decreases the incidence of unretained restorations and restorative material fracture. The overall amount of stress to the system is reduced, and the marginal ridges on the implant crowns are supported by the connectors of the splinted crowns, with resulting compressive forces rather than shear loads on the restorative material.

Common clinical sense indicates that it is better to err with one extra implant than to err with too few. One implant too few, and the entire treatment, along with the prosthesis, may fail. One implant too many rarely will be problematic. Because of the associated morbidity of too few implants (i.e., loss of the prosthesis, financial costs, loss of patient confidence), top-down treatment planning should always be adhered to (Fig. 7.29).

Implant Size

An excessive implant length is not critical at the crestal bone interface but it is critical for initial stability and the overall amount of bone–implant interface. The increased length also provides resistance to torque or shear forces when abutments are screwed into place. However, the additional length does little to decrease the stress that occurs at the transosteal region around the implant at the crest of the ridge during occlusal loading.[143-145] Therefore excessive implant length is not as effective in decreasing stress from force factors.

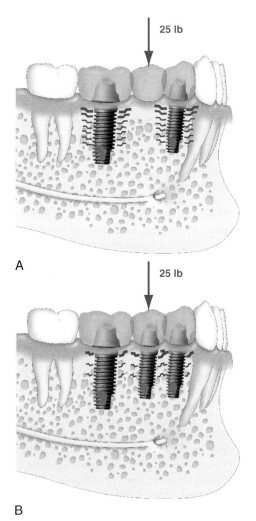

• **Fig. 7.28** Increasing the implant number is an effective method to decrease the stress to each component in the system. (A) Two implants supporting a three-unit prosthesis have more stress to the implant interface than (B) three implants supporting a similar restoration. The additional implant also decreases the pontic number and increases the retention of the prosthesis.

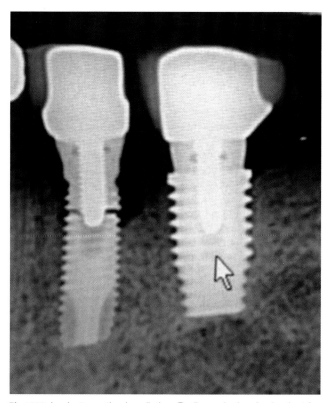

• **Fig. 7.29** Implant prosthesis splinting. Radiograph showing implant fracture in a patient with parafunction. Most likely if the implants were splinted, then the implant body fracture would not have occurred.

On the other hand, with improper biomechanical management, shorter implants may have higher failure rates after loading.[146,147] Therefore the initial treatment plan should use implants with lengths that are related to the amount of force expected, bone density, and patient-related force factors. Ideally, softer bone types require longer implants than denser bone. The surface area of each implant is directly related to the width of the implant. Wider root form implants have a greater area of bone contact than narrow implants (of similar design), which is a result of their increased circumferential bone contact areas. Each 0.25-mm increase in implant diameter may increase the overall surface area approximately 5% to 10% in a cylinder implant body. Bone augmentation in width may be indicated to increase implant diameter by 1 mm when force factors are greater than ideal. In addition, it has been suggested that an increase in implant diameter may be more effective than implant staggering to reduce stress.[148,149]

It is interesting to note that the natural teeth are narrower in the anterior regions of the mouth, in which the amount of force generated is less. The natural teeth increase in diameter in the premolar region and again in the molar region as the amount of force increases, with a total 300% surface area increase from the lower anterior teeth to the maxillary molars. The length of natural teeth roots does not increase from anterior to posterior regions of the arch, but their cross section does. The supplemental implant support gained from the greater diameter decreases stress and the likelihood of implant fracture and it reduces the force to the abutment screw, which results in less screw loosening.

Available Bone

Once the previous steps to the treatment plan sequence have been determined, the available bone in the potential implant sites is evaluated. If adequate bone is present to position the preselected implant number, size, and design, the treatment sequence proceeds to the next factor. If available bone is not present, then bone augmentation or modification is required. If these options are not possible, then the sequence of treatment is begun again, starting from the prosthesis design.

In the past, the available bone was the first condition evaluated and the treatment would proceed based on the number and position of implants, with little regard to size or design. This approach often led to the high complication rates related to increased stress conditions.

Implant Design

Implant macrodesign may affect surface area even more than an increase in width. A cylinder (bullet-shaped) implant provides 30% less surface area than a conventional threaded implant of the same size. Strong and colleagues have identified 11 different variables that affect the overall functional surface area of an implant.[150] A threaded implant with 10 threads for 10 mm has more surface area than one with five threads. A thread depth of 0.2 mm has less surface area than an implant with 0.4 mm. Therefore implant design be one of the easiest methods to increase surface area significantly and decrease overall risk to the implant interface.

In addition to the stress theorem and relative sequence of treatment plan, corollaries have been developed to facilitate the selection of the most appropriate therapy (Box 7.4).

• BOX 7.4 **Stress Treatment Theorem Corollaries**

A. Patients want teeth, not implants. The advantages and disadvantages of fixed versus removable should be discussed in detail with the patient.
B. If you had (1) ideal bone conditions, (2) optimal patient economic conditions, (3) optimal training, and (4) no time limitation, what would the treatment plan be?
C. Do not compromise a long-term prosthesis for a 3- to 6-month delay in treatment or the addition of an extra implant.
D. Understand the difference between *can* versus *should*.
E. When in doubt, overengineer the foundation (e.g., increase implant number increase surface area).
F. When two or more approaches may obtain a similar result, use the least invasive and least complicated to achieve a predictable result.
G. When two or more methods may obtain a similar result, use the least expensive yet predictable method when developing the treatment plan.
H. When two or more approaches may obtain a similar result, use the most predictable rather than the fastest method.
I. Time is a factor in treatment only when all other factors are equal.
J. The patient with economic limitations cannot afford complications.
K. Apply primarily compressive loads when possible at the following levels:
   1. Restorative material
   2. Cement
   3. Abutment
   4. Screw
   5. Implant body
   6. Implant–bone interface
L. If you do not understand biomechanical stress, it will lead to psychological stress.
M. It is often necessary to modify the mouth or modify the mind of the patient.
N. It is better to see the back of the patient's head once than it is to see their face over and over again

---

Summary

An understanding of the etiology of the most common implant complications has led to the development of a stress-based treatment plan theorem. Once the implant clinician has identified the sources of forces on the implant system, the treatment plan may be designed to minimize their potential effect on the implant, bone, and final prosthesis. Under these conditions, a consistent solution is an increase in implant–bone surface area. Additional implants are the solution of choice to decrease stress, along with an increase in implant width or height (i.e., poor bone density). In addition, the reduced pontic area helps to dissipate stresses more effectively to the bone structure, especially at the crest. The retention of the final prosthesis or superstructure is further improved with additional implant abutments. Therefore a number of variables and factors should be considered to reduce the morbidity of the implant process with respect to biomechanical stress.

References

1. Rams TE, Roberts TW, Tatum Jr H, et al. The subgingival microflora associated with human dental implants. *J Prosthet Dent.* 1984;5:529–539.
2. MacDonald JB. The etiology of periodontal disease. Bacteria as part of a complex etiology. *Dent Clin North Am.* 1960;11:699–703.
3. Waerhaug J. Subgingival plaque and loss of attachment in periodontosis as evaluated on extracted teeth. *J Periodontol.* 1977;48:125–130.

4. Priest GF. Failure rates of restorations for single tooth replacements. *Int J Prosthodont.* 1996;9:38–45.

5. Goodacre CJ, Bernal G, Rungcharassaeng K, et al. Clinical complications in fixed prosthodontics. *J Prosthet Dent.* 2003;90:31–41.

6. Creugers NH, Kayser HF, Van't Hof MA. A meta analysis of durability data on conventional fixed bridges. *Community Dent Oral Epidermiol.* 1994;22:448–452.

7. Goodacre CJ, Bernal G, Rungcharassaeng K. Clinical complications with implants and implant prostheses. *J Prosthet Dent.* 2003;90:121–132.

8. Oh T-J, Yoon J, Misch CE, et al. The cause of early implant bone loss: myth or science? *J Periodontol.* 2002;73:322–333.

9. Jividen G, Misch CE. Reverse torque testing and early loading failures—help or hindrance. *J Oral Implantology.* 2000;26:82–90.

10. Jemt T, Lekholm U, Adell R. Osseointegrated implants in the treatment of partially edentulous patients: a preliminary study on 876 consecutively placed fixtures. *Int J Oral Maxillofac Implants.* 1989;4:211–217.

11. Gunne J, Jemt T, Linden B. Implant treatment in partially edentulous patients: a report on prostheses after 3 years. *Int J Prosthodont.* 1994;7:143–148.

12. Lekholm U, Adell R, Lindhe J, et al. Marginal tissue reactions at osseointegrated titanium fixtures. II. A cross sectional retrospective study. *Int J Oral Maxillofac Surg.* 1986;15:53–61.

13. Jaffin R, Berman C. The excessive loss of Brånemark fixtures in type IV bone: a 5 year analysis. *J Periodontol.* 1991;62:2–4.

14. van Steenberghe D, Lekholm U, Bolender C. The applicability of osseointegrated oral implants in the rehabilitation of partial edentulism: a prospective multicenter study on 558 fixtures. *Int J Oral Maxillofac Implants.* 1990;5:272–281.

15. Esposito M, Hirsch J-M, Lekholm U, et al. Biological factors contributing to failures of osseointegrated oral implants. II. Etiopathogenesis. *Eur J Oral Sci.* 1998;106:721–764.

16. Lang NP, Wilson TG, Corbet EF. Biological complications with dental implants: their prevention, diagnosis and treatment. *Clin Oral Implants Res.* 2000;11(suppl):146–155.

17. Tonetti MS, Schmid J. Pathogenesis of implant failures. *Periodontology.* 1994;2000(4):127–138.

18. Heitz-Mayfield LJ, Schmid B, Weigel C, et al. Does excessive occlusal load affect osseointegration? An experimental study in the dog. *Clin Oral Impl Res.* 2004;15:259–268.

19. Johns RB, Jemt T, Heath MR, et al. A multicenter study of overdentures supported by Brånemark implants. *Int J Oral Maxillofac Implants.* 1992;4:187–194.

20. Bragger U, Aeschlimann S, Burgin W, et al. Biological and technical complications and failures with fixed partial dentures (FPD) on implants and teeth after four to five years of function. *Clin Oral Implants Res.* 2001;12:26–34.

21. Kourtis SG, Sotiriadou S, Voliotis S, et al. Private practice results of dental implants. Part I: survival and evaluation of risk factors—Part II: surgical and prosthetic complications. *Implant Dent.* 2004;13(4):373–385.

22. Kallus T, Bessing C. Loose gold screws frequently occur in full-arch fixed prostheses supported by osseointegrated implants after 5 years. *Int J Oral Maxillofac Implants.* 1994;9(2):169–178.

23. Eriksson RA, Albrektsson T. The effect of heat on bone regeneration: an experimental study in the rabbit using the bone growth chamber. *J Oral Maxillofac Surg.* 1984;42:705–711.

24. Brunski JB, Moccia Jr AF, Pollack SR, et al. The influence of functional use of endosseous implants on the tissue implant interface. II. Clinical aspects. *J Dent Res.* 1979;58:1970–1980.

25. Adell R, Lekholm U, Rockler B, et al. A 15 year study of osseointegrated implants in the treatment of the edentulous jaw. *Int J Oral Surg.* 1981;10:387–416.

26. Albrektsson T, Zarb GA, Worthington P, et al. The long-term efficacy of currently used dental implants: a review and proposed criteria of success. *Int J Oral Maxillofac Impl.* 1986;1:11–25.

27. Schroeder A, Mawglen G, Sutter F. Hohlzylinderimplantat: Typ-f zur prothesen-retention bei zahnlosen Kafer. *SSO Schweiz Monatsschr Zahnheilk.* 1983;93:720–733.

28. Smedberg JL, Lothigius E, Bodin I, et al. A clinical and radiological two-year follow-up study of maxillary overdentures on osseointegrated implants. *Clin Oral Implants Res.* 1993;4:39–46.

29. Kline R, Hoar J, Beck GH, et al. A prospective multicenter clinical investigation of a bone quality-based dental implant system. *Implant Dent.* 2002;11:1–8.

30. Isidor F. Loss of osseointegration caused by occlusal load of oral implants: a clinical and radiographic study in monkeys. *Clin Oral Implants Res.* 1996;7:143–152.

31. Isidor F. Histological evaluation of peri-implant bone at implant subjected to occlusal overload or plaque accumulation. *Clin Oral Implant Res.* 1997;8:1–9.

32. Bidez MW, Misch CE. Forces transfer in implant dentistry: basic concepts and principles. *J Oral Implantol.* 1992;18:264–274.

33. Quirynen M, Naert I, van Steenberghe D. Fixture design and overload influence on marginal bone loss and fixture success in the Brånemark implant system. *Clin Oral Implants Res.* 1992;3:104–111.

34. Van Steenberghe D, Tricio J, Van den Eynde, et al. Soft and hard tissue reactions towards implant design and surface characteristics and the influence of plaque and/or occlusal loads. In: Davidovitch Z, ed. *The Biological Mechanism of Tooth Eruption, Resorption and Replacement by Implants.* Boston: Harvard Society for the Advancement of Orthodontics; 1994.

35. Rangert B, Krogh PHJ, Langer B, et al. Bending overload and implant fracture: a retrospective clinical analysis. *Int J Oral Maxillofac Implants.* 1995;10:326–334.

36. Snauwaert K, Duyck J, van Steenberghe D, et al. Time dependent failure rate and marginal bone loss of implant supported prostheses: a 15-year follow up study. *Clin Oral Invest.* 2000;4:13–20.

37. Kourtis SG, Sotiriadou S, Voliotis S, et al. Private practice results of dental implants. Part I: survival and evaluation of risk factors—Part II: surgical and prosthetic complications. *Implant Dent.* 2004;13(4):373–385.

38. Jemt T. Single implants in the anterior maxilla after 15 years of follow-up: comparison with central implants in the edentulous maxilla. *Int J Prosthodont.* 2008;21(5):400–408.

39. Kirov D, Stoichkov B. Factors affecting the abutment screw loosening. In: *Journal of IMAB–Annual Proceeding (Scientific Papers).* 2017;23:1505–1509.

40. Mar 40inucci T. *Influence of Repeated Tightening and Loosening of the Prosthetic Screw in Micromovements Abutment/Implant [Master's Thesis].* Coimbra, Portugal: University of Coimbra; 2013.

41. Papaspyridakos P, Chen C-J, Chuang S-K, et al. A systematic review of biologic and technical complications with fixed implant rehabilitations for edentulous patients. *Int J Oral Maxillofac Implants.* 2012;27(1):102–110.

42. Linkow LI. Statistical analyses of 173 patients. *J Oral Implants.* 1974;4:540–562.

43. Adell R, Lekholm U, Rockler B, et al. Marginal tissue reactions at osseointegrated titanium fixtures (1). A 3-year longitudinal prospective study. *Int J Oral Maxillofac Surg.* 1986;15:39–52.

44. Albrektsson T, Zarb GA, Worthington P, et al. The long-term efficacy of currently used dental implants: a review and proposed criteria of success. *Int J Oral Maxillofac Implants.* 1986;1:11–25.

45. Misch CE, Suzuki JB, Misch-Dietsh FD, et al. A positive correlation between occlusal trauma and peri-implant bone loss: literature support. *Implant Dent.* 2005;14:108–114.

46. Glossary of prosthodontic terms. 7th ed. *J Prosthet Dent.* 1999;81:1–141.

47. Misch CE. Early crestal bone loss etiology and its effect on treatment planning for implants. 2. Dental Learning Systems Co, Inc. *Postgrad Dent;* 1995:3–17.

48. van Steenberghe D. A retrospective multicenter evaluation of the survival rate of osseointegrated fixtures supporting fixed partial prostheses in the treatment of partial edentulism. *J Prosthet Dent.* 1989;61:217–223.

49. Rhinelander FW. Circulation of bone. In: Bourne GH, ed. *The Biochemistry and Physiology of Bone.* New York: Academic Press; 1972.

50. Roberts WE, Smith RK, Zilberman Y, et al. Osseous adaptation to continuous loading of rigid endosseous implants. *Am J Orthodont.* 1984;86:95–111.

51. Wilderman MN, Pennel BM, King K, et al. Histogenesis of repair following osseous surgery. *J Periodontol.* 1970;41:551–565.

52. Haider R, Watzek G, Plenk H. Effects of drill cooling and bone structure on IMZ implant fixation. *Int J Oral Maxillofac Impl.* 1993;8:83–91.

53. Brisman EL. The affect of speed, pressure and time on bone temperature during the drilling of implant sites. *Int J Oral Maxillofac Impl.* 1996;11:35–37.

54. Manz MC. Radiographic assessment of peri-implant vertical bone loss: DIRG implant report No 9. *J Oral Maxillofac Surg.* 1997;55(suppl 5):62–71.

55. Hoar JE, Beck GH, Crawford EA, et al. Prospective evaluation of crestal bone remodeling of a bone density based dental system. *Comp Cont Educ Dent.* 1998;19:17–24.

56. Glickman I, Samelos JB. Effect of excessive forces upon the pathway of gingival inflammation in humans. *J Periodontol.* 1965;36:141–147.

57. Lekholm U Ericsson I, Adell R, et al. The condition of the soft tissues of tooth and fixture abutments supporting fixed bridges; a microbiological and histological study. *J Oral Clin Periodontol.* 1986;13:558–562.

58. Kent JN, Homsby CA. Pilot studies of a porous implant in dentistry and oral surgery. *J Oral Surg.* 1972;30:608.

59. Becker W, Becker BE, Newman MG, et al. Clinical and microbiologic findings that may contribute to dental implant failure. *Int J Oral Maxillofac Impl.* 1990;5:31–38.

60. Koutsonikos A. Implants: success and failure—a literature review. *Ann R Australas Coll Dent Surg.* 1998;14:75–80.

61. Gargiulo AW, Wentz FM, Orban B. Dimensions and relations of the dentogingival junction in humans. *J Periodontol.* 1961;32:261–267.

62. Vacek JS, Gher ME, Assad DA, et al. The dimensions of the human dentogingival junction. *Int J Perio Rest Dent.* 1994;14:155–165.

63. Rateitschak KJ, ed. *Color Atlas of Dental Medicine.* Stuttgart, Germany: Thieme; 1989.

64. Maynard JS, Wilson RD. Physiologic dimensions of the periodontium significant to the restorative dentist. *J Periodontol.* 1979;50:170–174.

65. Tarnow D, Stahl S, Maner A, et al. Human gingival attachment: responses to subgingival crown placement marginal remodeling. *J Clin Periodontol.* 1986;13:563–569.

66. Berglundh T, Lindhe J, Erricsson I, et al. The soft tissue barrier at implants and teeth. *Clin Oral Implants Res.* 1991;2:81–90.

67. Lindhe J, Berglundh T, Ericsson I, et al. Experimental breakdown of peri-implant and periodontal tissues. A study in the beagle dog. *Clin Oral Implants Res.* 1992;3:9–16.

68. Wallace S, Tarnow D. *The Biologic Width Around Implants.* Munich, Germany: International Congress Oral Implant Meeting; 1995.

69. Wallace SS. Significance of the biologic width with respect to root form implants. *Dent Impl Update.* 1994;5:25–29.

70. James RA, Keller EE. A histopathological report on the nature of the epithelium and underlying connective tissue which surrounds oral implant. *J Biomed Mat Res.* 1974;8:373–383.

71. Gould TRL, Westbury L, Brunette DM. Ultrastructural study of the attachment of human gingival to titanium in vivo. *J Prosthet Dent.* 1984;52:418–420.

72. Hansson HA, Albrektsson T, Brånemark PI. Structural aspects of the interface between tissue and titanium implants. *J Prosthet Dent.* 1983;50:108–113.

73. McKinney RV, Steflik DE, Koth DL. Evidence for a junctional epithelial attachment to ceramic dental implants: a transmission electronmicroscopic study. *J Periodontol.* 1985;56:579–591.

74. Barboza EP, Caúla AL, Carvalho WR. Crestal bone loss around submerged and exposed unloaded dental implants: a radiographic and microbiological descriptive study. *Implant Dent.* 2002;11:162–169.

75. Weber HP, Buser D, Donath K, Fiorellini JP, et al. Comparison of healed tissue adjacent to submerged and non-submerged unloaded titanium dental implants: a histometric study in beagle dogs. *Clin Oral Implants Res.* 1996;7:11–19.

76. Cochran DL, Hermann JS, Schenik RS, et al. Biologic width around titanium implants: a histometric analysis of the implanto-gingival junction around unloaded and loaded nonsubmerged implants in the canine mandible. *J Periodontol.* 1997;68:186–198.

77. Abrahamsson I, Berglundh T, Wennstrom J, et al. The peri-implant hard and soft tissue characteristics at different implant systems: a comparative study in dogs. *Clin Oral Implants Res.* 1996;7:212–219.

78. Hermann JS, Buser D, Schenk RK, et al. Crestal bone changes around titanium implants: a histometric evaluation of unloaded non-submerged and submerged implants in the canine mandible. *J Periodontol.* 2000;71:1412–1424.

79. Jung YC, Han CH, Lee KW. A 1-year radiographic evaluation of marginal bone around dental implants. *Int J Oral Maxillofac Implants.* 1996;11:811–818.

80. Wiskott HW, Belser UC. Lack of integration of smooth titanium surfaces: a working hypothesis based on strains generated in the surrounding bone. *Clin Oral Implants Res.* 1999;10:429–444.

81. Rosenberg ES, Torosian JP, Slots J. Microbial differences in 2 clinically distinct types of failures of osseointegrated implants. *Clin Oral Implants Res.* 1991;2:135–144.

82. Karolyi M. Beobachtungen über Pyorrhea alveolaris. *Osterenorichisch-Ungarische viertel jahresschrift fur Zahnheilkunde.* 1991;17:279.

83. Glickman I. Clinical significance of trauma from occlusion. *J Am Dent Assoc.* 1965;70:607–618.

84. Macapanpan LC, Weinmann JP. The influence of injury to the periodontal membrane on the spread of gingival inflammation. *J Dent Res.* 1954;33:263–272.

85. Posselt U, Emslie RD. Occlusal disharmonies and their effect on periodontal diseases. *Internat Dent J.* 1959;9:367–381.

86. Fleszar TJ, Knowles JW, Monson EC, et al. Tooth mobility and periodontal therapy. *J Clin Periodont.* 1980;7:495–505.

87. Bergett F, Ramfjord S, Nissle R, et al. A randomized trial of occlusal adjustment in the treatment of periodontitis patients. *J Clin Periodontol.* 1992;19:381–387.

88. Belting CM, Gripta OP. The influence of psychiatric disturbances on the severity of periodontal diseases. *J Periodont.* 1961;32:219–226.

89. Waerhaug J. The infrabony pocket and its relationship to trauma from occlusion and subgingival plaque. *J Periodontol.* 1979;50:355–365.

90. Lordahl A, Scher O, Waerhaug J, et al. Tooth mobility and alveolar bone resorption as a function of occlusal stress and oral hygiene. *Acta Odontol Scand.* 1959;17:61–77.

91. Baer P, Kakehashi S, Littleton NW, et al. Alveolar bone loss and occlusal wear. *J Am Soc Periodontics.* 1963:11–98.

92. Lindhe J, Nyman S, Ericsson I. Trauma from occlusion. In: Lindhe J, ed. *Clinical Periodontology and Implant Dentistry.* 4th ed. Oxford: Blackwell; 2003.

93. Cowin SC, Hegedus DA. Bone remodeling I: theory of adaptive elasticity. *J Elasticity.* 1976;6:313–326.

94. Bidez MW, Misch CE. Force transfer in implant dentistry: basic concepts and principles. *Oral Implantol.* 1992;18:264–274.

95. Cowin SC, Moss-Salentijn L, Moss ML. Candidates for the mechanosensory system in bone. *J Biomechan Engineer.* 1991;113:191–197.

96. Kummer BKF. Biomechanics of bone: Mechanical properties, functional structure, functional adaptation. In: Fung YC, Perrone H, Anliker M, eds. *Biomechanics: Foundations and Objectives.* Englewood Cliffs: Prentice-Hall; 1972.

97. Frost HM. Bone "mass" and the "mechanostat": a proposal. *Anat Rec.* 1987;219:1–9.

98. Frost HM. Bone's mechanostat: a 2003 update. *The Anatomical Record Part A.* 2003;275A:1081–1101.

99. Chiba J, Rubash JE, Kim KJ, et al. The characterization of cytokines in the interface tissue obtained from failed cementless total hip arthroplasty with and without femoral osteolysis. *Clin Orthop.* 1994;300:304–312.

100. Baumeister T, Avallone EA. *Marks' Standard Handbook of Mechanical Engineers.* 8th ed. New York: McGraw-Hill; 1978.

101. Bidez M, McLoughlin S, Lemons JE. FEA investigations in plate-form dental implant design. In: *Proceedings of the First World Congress of Biomechanics.* San Diego, Calif.; 1990.

102. Misch CE. A three dimensional finite element analysis of two blade implant neck designs [Master's Thesis]. Pittsburgh: University of Pittsburgh; 1989.

103. Bidez MW, Misch CE. Issues in bone mechanics related to oral implants. *Implant Dent.* 1992;1:289–294.

104. Kilamura E, Slegaroui R, Nomura S, et al. Biomechanical aspects of marginal bone resorption around osseointegrated implants: consideration based in a three dimensional finite element analysis. *Clin Oral Implant Res.* 2004;15:401–412.

105. Misch CE, Qu M, Bidez MW. Mechanical properties of trabecular bone in the human mandible: implications of dental implant treatment planning and surgical placement. *J Oral Maxillofac Surg.* 1999;57:700–706.

106. Appleton RS, Nummikoski PV, Pigmo MA, et al. Peri-implant bone changes in response to progressive osseous loading. *J Dent Res.* 1997;76:412. [special issue].

107. Appleton RS, Nummikoski PV, Pigno MA, et al. A radiographic assessment of progressive loading on bone around single osseointegrated implants in the posterior maxilla. *Clin Oral Implants Res.* 2005;16:161–167.

108. Hoshaw S. *Investigation of Bone Remodeling and Remodeling at a Loaded Bone-Implant Interface [Thesis].* Troy, NY: Rensselaer Polytechnic Institute; 1992.

109. Hoshaw SJ, Brunski JB, Cochran GVB. Mechanical loading of Brånemark fixtures affects interfacial bone modeling and remodeling. *Int J Oral Maxillofac Implants.* 1994;9:345–360.

110. Miyata T, Kobayashi Y, Araki H, et al. An experimental study of occlusal trauma to osseointegrated implants: part 2. *Jpn Soc Periodont.* 1997;39:234–241.

111. Miyata T, Kobayashi Y, Araki H, et al. The influence of controlled occlusal overload on peri-implant tissue: a histologic study in monkeys. *Int J Oral Maxillofac Implants.* 1998;13:677–683.

112. Miyata T, Kobayashi Y, Araki H, et al. The influence of controlled occlusal overload on peri-implant tissue. Part 3: a histologic study in monkeys. *Int J Oral Maxillofac Implants.* 2000;15:425–431.

113. Duyck J, Ronold HJ, Oosterwyck HV, et al. The influences of static and dynamic loading on marginal bone reactions around osseointegrated implants: an animal experimental study. *Clin Oral Implant Res.* 2001;12:207–218.

114. Lindquist JW, Rockler B, Carlsson GE. Bone resorption around fixtures in edentulous patients treated with mandibular fixed tissue integrated prostheses. *J Prosthet Dent.* 1988:59–63.

115. Shackleton JL, Carr L, Slabbert JC. Survival of fixed implant-supported prostheses related to cantilever lengths. *J Prosthet Dent.* 1994;71:23–26.

116. Wyatt CC, Zarb GA. Bone level changes proximal to oral implants supporting fixed partial prostheses. *Clin Oral Implants Res.* 2002;13:62–68.

117. Duyck J, Van Oosterwyck H, Van der Sloten J, et al. Magnitude and distribution of occlusal forces on oral implants supporting fixed prostheses: an in vivo study. *Clin Oral Implants Res.* 2000;11:465–475.

118. Naert I, Quirynen M, Van Steenberghe D, et al. A study of 589 consecutive implants supporting complete fixed prostheses. Part II: prosthetic aspects. *J Prosthet Dent.* 1992;68:949–956.

119. Uribe R, Penarrocha M, Sanches JM, et al. Marginal peri-implantitis due to occlusal overload: a case report. *Med Oral.* 2004;9:159–162.

120. Leung KC, Chew TW, Wat PY, et al. Peri-implant bone loss: management of a patient. *Int J Oral Maxillofac Implant.* 2001;16:273–277.

121. Misch CE, Bidez MW. Occlusion and crestal bone resorption etiology and treatment planning strategies for implants. In: Mc Neill C, ed. *Science and Practice of Occlusion.* 1st ed. Chicago: Quintessence; 1997.

122. Roberts WE, Turley DK, Brezniak N, et al. Bone physiology and metabolism. *J Calif Dent Assoc.* 1987;54:32–39.

123. Roberts WE, Garetto LP, De Castro RA. Remodeling of devitalized bone threatens periosteal margin integrity of endosseous titanium implants with threaded or smooth surfaces: indications for provisional loading and axially directed occlusion. *J Indiana Dent Assoc.* 1989;68:19–24.

124. Piatelli A, Ruggeri A, Franchi M, et al. An histologic and histomorphometric study of bone reactions to unloaded and loaded non-submerged single implants in monkeys: a pilot study. *J Oral Implant.* 1993;19:314–319.

125. Rotter BE, Blackwell R, Dalton G. Testing progressive loading of endosteal implants with the periotest—a pilot study. *Implant Dent.* 1996;5:28–32.

126. Reilly DT, Burstein AH. The elastic and ultimate properties of compact bone tissue. *J Biomech.* 1975;8:393–405.

127. Misch CE. Stress factors: influence on treatment planning. In: Misch CE, ed. *Dental Implant Prosthetics.* St Louis: Elsevier; 2005.

128. Zechner W, Trinki N, Watzek G, et al. Radiographic follow-up of peri-implant bone loss around machine-surfaced and rough-surfaced interforaminal implants in the mandible functionally loaded for 3 to 7 years. *Int J Oral Maxillofac Implants.* 2004;19:216–222.

129. Karousis IK, Brägger U, Salvi G, et al. Effect of implant design on survival and success rates of titanium oral implants: a 10 year prospective cohort study of the ITI dental implant system. *Clin Oral Implant Res.* 2004;15:8–17.

130. Taylor TD, Belser U, Mericke-Stern RI. Prosthodontics considerations. *Clin Oral Implants Res.* 2000;11:101–107.

131. Misch CE. Consideration of bio mechanical stress in treatment with dental implants. *Dent Today.* 2007;25:80–85.

132. Misch CE. The effect of bruxism on treatment planning for dental implants. *Dent Today.* 2002;9:76–81.

133. Misch CE. Clenching and its effect on implant treatment plans. *Oral Health.* 2002:11–21.

134. Misch CE, Bidez MW. Implant protected occlusion, a biomechanical rationale. *Compend Cont Educ Dent.* 1994;15:1330–1342.

135. Cehreli MC, Iplikcioglu H, Bilir OG. The influence of the location of load transfer on strains around implants supporting four unit cement-retained fixed prostheses: in vitro evaluation of axial versus off-set loading. *J Oral Rehabil.* 2002;29:394–400.

136. Duyck J, Naert I. Failure of oral implants—etiology, symptoms and influencing factors. *Clin Oral Investig.* 1998;2:102–114.

137. Thomsen JS, Ebbesen EN, Mosekilde L. Relationships between static histomorphometry and bone strength measurements in human iliac crest bone biopsies. *Bone.* 1998;22:153–163.

138. Sennerby L, Roos J. Surgical determinants of clinical success of osseointegrated oral implants: a review of the literature. *Int J Prosthodont.* 1998;11:408–420.

139. Bidez MW, Misch CE. The biomechanics of inter-implant spacing. In: *Proceedings of the 4th International Congress of Implants and Biomaterials in Stomatology.* Charleston, SC; 1990.

140. Bidez MW, Misch CE. Issues in bone mechanics related to oral implants. *Implant Dent.* 1992;1:289–294.

141. Borchers L, Reichart P. Three dimensional stress distribution around dental implants at different stages of interface development. *J Dent Res.* 1994;62:155–159.

142. Naert I, Koutsikakis G, Duyck J, et al. Biologic outcome of implant-supported restoration in the treatment of partial edentulism. Part 1: a longitudinal clinical evaluation. *Clin Oral Implants Res*. 2002;13:381–389.

143. Weinberg LA, Kruger B. An evaluation of torque on implant/prosthesis with staggered buccal and lingual offset. *Int J Oral Maxillofac Implants*. 1996;16:253.

144. Lum LB, Osier JF. Load transfer from endosteal implants to supporting bone: an analysis using statics. *J Oral Implant*. 1992;18:343–353.

145. Lum LB. A biomechanical rationale for the use of short implants. *J Oral Implant*. 1991;17:126–131.

146. Misch CE, Steigenga J, Barboza E, et al. Short dental implants in posterior partial edentulism: a multicenter retrospective 6-year case series study. *J Periodontol*. 2006;77:1340–1347.

147. Misch CE. Short dental implants: a literature review and rationale for use. *Dent Today*. 2005;26:64–68.

148. Sertgoz A, Guvener S. Finite element analysis of the effect of cantilever and implant length on stress distribution on implant supported prosthesis. *J Prosthet Dent*. 1996;75:165–169.

149. Sato Y, Shindoi N, Hosokawa R, et al. A biomechanical effect of wide implant placements and offset placements of three implants in the partially edentulous region. *J Oral Rehab*. 2000;27:15–21.

150. Strong JT, Misch CE, Bidez MW, et al. Functional surface area: threadform parameter optimization for implant body design. *Compend Cont Educ Deat*. 1998;19:19–25.

8

Treatment Planning: Force Factors Related to Patient Conditions

RANDOLPH R. RESNIK AND CARL E. MISCH†

Biomechanic stress is a significant risk factor in implant dentistry. Its magnitude is directly related to force. As a result an increase in any dental force factor magnifies the risk for stress-related complications. Various patient conditions place different amounts of force in magnitude, duration, type, and direction. In addition, several factors may multiply or increase the effect of these other conditions. Once the prosthesis option and key implant positions are determined, the potential force levels that will be exerted on the prosthesis should be evaluated and accounted for to modify the overall treatment plan. Several factors observed during the dental evaluation predict additional forces on future implant abutments. The initial implant survival, loading survival, marginal crestal bone loss, incidence of abutment or prosthetic screw loosening, unretained restorations, porcelain fracture, and component fracture are all influenced by the force factors.

Box 8.1 includes primary patient factors that affect the stress environment of the implant and prosthesis.

Bite Force

The greatest natural forces exerted against teeth, and thus against implants, occur during mastication.[1,2] These forces are primarily perpendicular to the occlusal plane in the posterior regions, are of short duration, occur only during brief periods of the day, and range from 5 to 44 pounds for natural teeth. The actual force on each tooth during function has been recorded on strain gauges in inlays.[3] A force of 28 psi was needed to chew a raw carrot, and 21 psi was needed to chew meat. The actual time during which chewing forces are applied on the teeth was about 9 minutes each day.[4] The perioral musculature and tongue exert a more constant, yet lighter horizontal force on the teeth or on implants. These forces reach 3 to 5 psi during swallowing.[5] A person swallows 25 times per hour while awake and 10 times per hour while sleeping, for a total of 480 times each day.[4] Therefore natural forces against teeth are primarily in their long axis, less than 30 psi, and for less than 30 minutes for all normal forces of deglutition and mastication (Box 8.2). Forces of mastication placed on implant-supported bridges have been measured in a similar range as natural teeth.

The maximum bite force differs from mastication force, varies widely among individuals, and depends on the state of the dentition and masticatory musculature. There have been many attempts to quantify the normal maximum bite force. In 1681 Borelli suspended weights on a thread over the molars while the mandible was open. The maximum load recorded for which the person was still able to close ranged from 132 to 440 lb. A force of 165 lb was recorded on a gnathodynamometer, the first instrument to record occlusal force; the gnathodynamometer was developed by Patrick and Dennis in 1892. Black[6] improved this early design and recorded average forces of approximately 170 lb. More recent studies indicate normal maximum vertical biting forces on teeth or implants can range from 45 to 550 psi.[7-22] The forces on the chewing side and the opposite side appear very similar in amplitude (Table 8.1).[8]

Awawdeh et al.[23] evaluated maximum bite force in endodontically treated teeth versus natural, vital teeth. They showed the maximum biting force was significantly higher in root-canaled teeth in comparison with vital natural teeth. The loss of the mechanoreceptor-mediated protective mechanism allows for the increased biting force. Therefore caution should be exercised when an implant prosthesis opposes an endodontically treated tooth because protective modifications need to be addressed in the occlusion and prosthesis design.[23]

In summary, maximum biting forces are not expressed quantitatively or qualitatively by patients. The implant clinician must take into consideration various factors that may dictate a higher biting force and therefore could increase risks for occlusal overload to the implant and implant prosthesis.

Parafunction

Parafunctional forces on teeth or implants are characterized by repeated or sustained occlusion and have long been recognized as harmful to the stomatognathic system.[24-26] These forces are also most damaging when applied to implant prostheses.[18] For example, the lack of rigid fixation during healing is often a result of parafunction from soft tissue–borne prostheses overlying the submerged implant. The most common cause of both early and late implant

---

†Deceased.

• BOX 8.1 | Patient Force Factors

• BOX 8.1   Patient Force Factors

- Parafunction
  - Bruxism
  - Clenching
  - Tongue thrust
- Crown height space
- Masticatory dynamics
- Opposing arch position
- Opposing arch composition

• BOX 8.2   Normal Forces Exerted on Teeth

Bite Forces
- Perpendicular to occlusal plane
- Short duration
- Brief total period (9 min/day)
- Force on each tooth: 20 to 30 psi
- Maximum bite force: 50 to 500 psi

Perioral Forces
- More constant
- Lighter
- Horizontal
- Maximum when swallowing (3–5 psi)
- Brief total swallow time (20 min/day)

failure after successful surgical fixation is the result of parafunction. Such complications occur with greater frequency in the maxilla because of a decrease in bone density and an increase in the resulting moment of force.[27] The presence of these conditions must be carefully noted during the early phases of treatment planning.

Nadler[25] has classified the causes of parafunction or nonfunctional tooth contact into the following six categories:

1. Local
2. Systemic
3. Psychological
4. Occupational
5. Involuntary
6. Voluntary

Local factors include tooth form or occlusion, as well as soft tissue changes such as ulcerations or pericoronitis. Systemic factors include cerebral palsy, epilepsy, and drug-related dyskinesia. Psychological causes occur with the greatest frequency and include the release of emotional tension or anxiety.[28] Occupational factors concern professionals such as dentists, athletes, and precision workers, as well as the seamstress or musician who develops altered oral habits. The fifth cause of parafunctional force is involuntary movement that provokes bracing of the jaws, such as during lifting of heavy objects or sudden stops while driving. Voluntary causes include chewing gum or pencils, bracing the telephone between the head and shoulder, and pipe smoking.

The parafunctional groups presented in this chapter are divided into bruxism, clenching, and tongue thrust or size. The dental literature usually does not identify bruxism and clenching as separate entities. Although several aspects of treatment are similar, their diagnosis and treatment are in some ways different. As such, they will be presented as different entities in this discussion. The magnitude of parafunction may be categorized as absent, mild, moderate, or severe. Bruxism and clenching are the most critical factors to evaluate in any implant reconstruction. No long-term success will be obtained with severe parafunction of bruxism or clenching. Therefore the clinician should always try to diagnose the presence of these conditions.

This does not mean that patients with moderate and severe parafunction cannot be treated with implants. For example, a physician treats a patient with uncontrolled diabetes. However, the patient may lose his or her vision or require an amputation treatment. Unsuccessful treatment of the patient with diabetes may not be the fault of the physician. Not recognizing diabetes in the presence of obvious signs and symptoms, of course, is another issue. Because the patient with moderate-to-severe parafunction represents so many additional risks in implant dentistry, one must be aware of these conditions and the methods to reduce their noxious effects on the entire implant-related system.

Bruxism

Bruxism primarily includes the horizontal, nonfunctional grinding of teeth. The forces involved are in significant excess of normal physiologic masticatory loads. Bruxism may affect the teeth, muscles, joints, bone, implants, and prostheses. These forces may occur while the patient is awake or asleep, and may generate increased force on the system several hours per day. Bruxism is the most common oral habit.[25] Sleep clinic studies have evaluated nocturnal bruxism and found approximately 10% of those observed had obvious movement of the mandible with occlusal contacts.[29,30] More than half of these patients had tooth wear affecting esthetics. Only 8% of these patients were aware of their nocturnal bruxism, and only one quarter of the patients' spouses were aware of the nocturnal habit. Muscle tenderness in the morning was observed less than 10% of the time.[31] A study on bruxing patients with implants showed 80% of sleep bruxism occurred during light sleep stages but did not cause arousal.[32] Therefore patients with bruxism may or may not have obvious tooth wear affecting esthetics; may brux nocturnally, but their bed partners do not know most of the time; rarely have muscle tenderness when they are awake; and are usually unaware of their oral habit. In other words, nocturnal bruxism is sometimes difficult to diagnose.[33] Multiple studies have also shown a direct correlation between stress and bruxism.[34,35]

The maximum biting force of bruxing patients is greater than average. Just as an experienced weight lifter can lift more weight, the patient constantly exercising the muscles of mastication develops a greater bite force. For example, a man who chews paraffin wax for an hour each day for a month can increase the bite force from 118 to 140 psi within 1 week. Chewing gum, bruxism, and clenching may accomplish the same feat. Eskimos, with a very tenacious diet and who chew their leather to soften it before fabrication of clothing, have maximum bite forces of more than 300 psi. A 37-year-old patient with a long history of bruxism recorded a maximum bite force of more than 990 psi (four to seven times normal).[36] Fortunately the bite force does not continue to increase in most bruxing patients. When muscles do not vary their exercise regimen, their size and function adjust to the dynamics of the situation. As a result the higher bite forces and muscle size usually do not continue in an unending spiral.

Diagnosis

Bruxism does not necessarily represent a contraindication for implants, but it does dramatically influence treatment planning. The first step is to recognize the condition before the treatment is rendered. The symptoms of this disorder, which may be ascertained by a dental history, may include repeated headaches, a history of fractured teeth or restorations, repeated uncemented restorations, and jaw discomfort upon awakening.[24,37] Therefore

TABLE 8.1	Mean Maximum Biting Force Recorded on Natural Teeth or Implants	
Authors	**Natural Teeth Dental Implants**	**Mean Maximum Masticatory Force**
Carr and Laney, 1987[a]	Conventional denture	59 N
	Implant-supported prostheses	112.9N
Morneburg and Proschel, 2002[b]	Implant-supported three-unit FPD	220 N
	Single implant: anterior	91 N
	Single implant: posterior	12 N
Fontijn-Tekamp et al., 1998[c]	Implant-supported prostheses	(unilateral)
	Molar region	50–400 N
	Incisal region	25–170 N
Mericske-Stern and Zarb 1996[d]	Complete denture/implant-supported prostheses	35–330 N
van Eijden, 1991[e]	Canine	469 ± 85 N
	Second premolar	583 ± 99 N
	Second molar	723 ± 138 N
Braun et al., 1995[f]	Natural teeth	738 ± 209 N (male > female)
Raadsheer et al., 1999[g]	Male teeth	545.7 N
	Female teeth	383.6 N

Comparison of available studies examining masticatory forces generated under varying loading condition. Study results are reported in Newtons (N) of force unless otherwise indicated. Differences between male and female force generation are noted in applicable studies.

FPD, Fixed partial dentures.

[a]Carr AB, Laney WR. Maximum occlusal forces in patients with osseointegrated oral implant prostheses and patients with complete dentures. *Int J Oral Maxillofac Impl.* 1987;2:101–108.

[b]Morneburg TR, Proschel PA. Measurement of masticatory forces and implant loads: a methodologic clinical study. *Int J Prosthodont.* 2002;15:20–27.

[c]Fontijn-Tekamp FA, Slageter AP, van't Hof MA, et al. Bite forces with mandibular implant-retained overdentures. *J Dent Res.* 1998;77:1832–1839.

[d]Mericske-Stern R, Assal P, Buergin W. Simultaneous force measurements in three dimensions on oral endosseous implants in vitro and vivo: a methodological study. *Clin Oral Implants Res.* 1996;7:378–386.

[e]van Eijden TM. Three dimensional analyses of human bite force magnitude and moment. *Arch Oral Biol.* 1991;36:535–539.

[f]Braun S, Bantleon HP, Hnat WP, et al. A study of bite force. Part I: relationship to various physical characteristics. *Angle Orthod.* 1995;65:367–372.

[g]Raadsheer MC, van Eijden TM, van Ginkel FC, et al. Contribution of jaw muscle size and craniofacial morphology to human bite force magnitude. *J Dent Res.* 1999;87:31–42.

when the patient is aware of muscle tenderness or the spouse is conscious of the nocturnal condition, the diagnosis is readily obtained. However, many patients do not attribute these problems to excessive forces on the teeth and report a negative history. A lack of these symptoms does not negate bruxism as a possibility.

Fortunately, many clinical signs warn of excessive grinding. The signs of bruxism include an increase in size of the temporal and masseter muscles (these muscles along with the external pterygoid may be tender), deviation of the lower jaw on opening, limited occlusal opening, increased mobility of teeth, cervical abfraction of teeth, fracture of teeth or restorations, and uncemented crowns or fixed prostheses. However, the most accurate and easiest way to diagnose bruxism is to evaluate the wearing of teeth. Not only is this the simplest method to determine bruxism in an individual patient, it also allows the disorder to be classified as absent, mild, moderate, or severe (Figs. 8.1 through 8.3). No anterior wear patterns in the teeth signify an absence of bruxism. Mild bruxism has slight wearing of anterior teeth but is not a cosmetic compromise. Moderate bruxism has obvious anterior incisal wear facets but no posterior occlusal wear pattern. Severe bruxism has minimal to absent incisal guidance from excessive wear, and posterior wearing of the teeth is obvious.

Nonfunctional wear facets on the incisal edges may occur on both natural or replacement teeth, especially in the mandible and

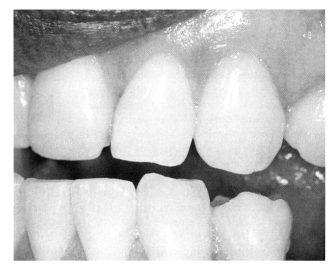

• **Fig. 8.1** A patient has mild bruxism exhibiting a wear facet (incisal edge) on the mandibular canine and the slight notch in the maxillary lateral incisor.

maxillary canines, and there may be notching of the cingulum in the maxillary anterior teeth. Isolated anterior wear is usually of little significance if all posterior teeth contacts can be eliminated in excursions.

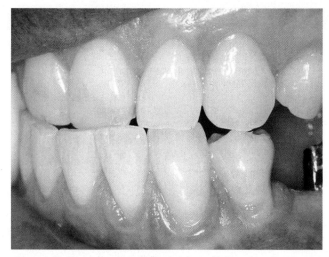

• **Fig. 8.2** Patients usually will grind their teeth in a specific, repeated movement of the mandible. When the opposing wear facets of the teeth are in contact, one should note the occlusal position of the teeth. The patient shown in Fig. 8.1 has a working contact on the mandibular premolar with the maxillary canine in this engram position (green arrow). The slight cervical abfraction of the mandibular first premolar is a consequence of the parafunction. The patient's posterior teeth should not occlude in this excursive position to decrease the amount of force on the anterior teeth.

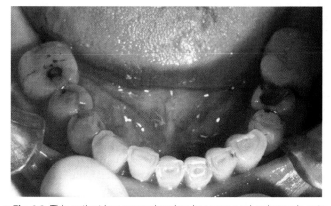

• **Fig. 8.3** This patient has severe bruxism because occlusal wear is anterior and posterior. Because of the excessive wear, the incisal guidance should be reestablished before a maxillary arch fixed reconstruction.

Tooth wear is most significant when found in the posterior regions, and it may changes the intensity of bruxism from the moderate to the severe category. Posterior wear patterns are more difficult to manage, because this usually is related to a loss of anterior guidance in excursions; once the posterior teeth contact in excursive jaw positions, greater forces are generated.[38] The masseter and temporalis muscles contract when posterior teeth contact. With incisal guidance and an absence of posterior contact, two-thirds of these muscles do not contract, and as a consequence the bite force is dramatically reduced. However, when the posterior teeth maintain contact, the bite forces are similar in excursions, as during posterior biting. Therefore in the patient with severe bruxism, the occlusal plane, the anterior incisal guidance, or both may need modification to eliminate all posterior contacts during mandibular excursions before the implant restoration.

Bruxing patients often repeat mandibular movements, which are different from border movements of the mandible and are in one particular direction. As a result the occlusal wear is very specific and primarily on one side of the arch, or even on only a few teeth

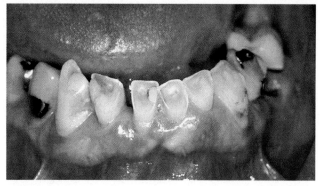

• **Fig. 8.4** This patient exhibits an engram pattern of bruxism primarily toward the left canine to central incisors. The right canine and lateral incisor have far fewer wear facets. This "pathway of destruction" is specific.

(Fig. 8.4). This engram pattern usually remains after treatment. If the restoring dentist reestablishes incisive guidance on teeth severely affected by an engram bruxing pattern, the incidence of complications on these teeth will be increased. The most common complications on teeth restored in this "pathway of destruction" are porcelain fracture, uncemented prostheses, and root fracture.[37] When implants support the crowns in the pathway of destruction, the implant may fail, fracture, or have crestal bone loss, abutment screw loosening, material fracture, or unretained restorations.[39-42] If the patient continues the severe bruxism pattern, the question is not whether but when and which complications will occur. The dentist should inform the patient that these habits will cause these problems. Treatment may be rendered to repair these problems, but there will be complications if the bruxism is not reduced.

Bruxism changes normal masticatory forces by the magnitude (higher bite forces), duration (hours rather than minutes), direction (lateral rather than vertical), type (shear rather than compression), and magnification (four to seven times normal).[36,43-45] The method to restore severe bruxism may be problematic, even when the desire is primarily cosmetic. As the anterior teeth wear, they often erupt, and the overall occlusal vertical dimension (OVD) remains unchanged. In addition, the alveolar process may follow the eruption of the tooth. As such, when the anterior teeth are restored for esthetics (or to obtain an incisal guidance), the reduced crown height cannot be increased merely by increasing the height of the crown to an average dimension. Instead, the following guidelines are suggested:

1. Determine the position of the maxillary incisor edge of the anterior teeth. They may be acceptable (if eruption occurred as they wore) or need greater coronal length to correct related incisal wear.
2. Determine the desired occlusal vertical dimension (OVD). This is not an exact dimension and may exist at several different positions without consequence. However, like most factors, there is a range that is patient specific and does follow guidelines. The most common methods to determine this dimension relate to facial measurements, closest speaking space, physiologic rest position, speech, and esthetics. This is one of the most important steps. If the vertical dimension is collapsed because of anterior and posterior occlusal wear, much more rehabilitation is required. This condition is observed more often when bruxism is severe, the anterior incisal guidance was lost, and as a consequence, the severe bruxism wear is increased due to an increase in force factors. The accelerated occlusal wear may cause a loss of OVD. The OVD is rarely decreased when incisal

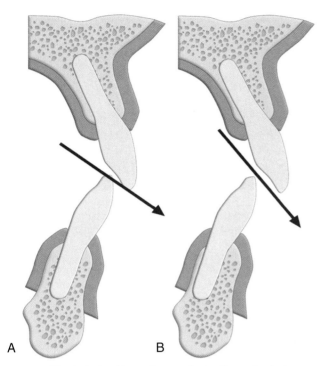

A   B

• **Fig. 8.5** The incisal guidance for a patient with moderate-to-severe bruxism should be shallow (A), not deep (B) to reduce the force on the anterior teeth during excursive movement of the mandible.

- Overeruption of teeth
- Gingiva and bone move with teeth
- Curved or concave gingival line in relation to horizon
- Can occur in any teeth in the mouth
- Etiology
  - Uncoupled anterior teeth (i.e., Class II malocclusion)
  - Supereruption secondary to incisal wear
  - Supereruption secondary to lack of opposing teeth
  - Developmental cant

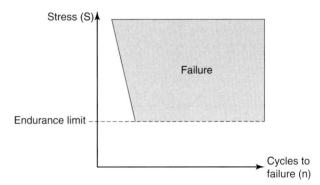

• **Fig. 8.6** On a fatigue curve for a material, stress corresponds to the vertical axis and cycles to failure to the horizontal axis. A point exists at which the stress is so great that the material breaks with only one cycle. When the stress is low enough, the material will not break, regardless of the number of cycles. The stress amount at the highest point of this safe zone is called the *endurance limit*. Patients with parafunction increase the amount of stress to the implant-prosthetic system and increase the number of the cycles for the higher levels. Fatigue failures are therefore common.

guidance is still present, because the posterior teeth maintain the dimension and the anterior teeth have sufficient time to erupt because the forces are less and the wear rate is slower.

3. Evaluate and restore the position of the lower anterior teeth where necessary. In the past, several authors have stated that a reconstruction begins with the lower anterior teeth. The mandibular arch cannot be restored until the maxillary anterior teeth and OVD are established. Many esthetic and speech guidelines are available to help the restoring dentist with the position of the maxillary anterior teeth. For example, when a dentist begins the restoration of a completely edentulous patient, the maxillary anterior wax rim position is often first determined for similar reasons.

The position of the lower anterior teeth should contact the lingual surfaces of the maxillary anterior teeth at the established OVD, and the amount of vertical overlap of the maxillary incisal edge and the angle of the incisal contacts in protrusive movements of the mandible determines the angle and height of the anterior guidance. This dimension must be greater than the condylar disc assembly (the angle of the eminentia) so the posterior teeth will separate during mandibular excursions.

In patients with moderate-to-severe bruxism, the height of the vertical overjet and the angle of incisal guidance should not be extreme, because the amount of the force on the anterior abutments, cement seals, and restortaive material is directly related to these conditions (Fig. 8.5). In other words, the greater the incisal overjet, the greater the distance between the posterior teeth in excursions, and the greater the force generated on the anterior teeth during this movement. In patients with severe bruxism the intensity of the force should be reduced because the duration of the force is increased.

When anterior tooth wear is accompanied by tooth eruption and maintenance of the OVD, and alveolar bone in the region has extruded toward the incisal plane (dentoalveolar extrusion), the incisal edges of the teeth should not be elevated. Instead, the

alveolar bone and cervical regions should be reduced, and crown lengthening should be performed on the teeth before their restoration. This is most often necessary in the mandibular anterior region but may be observed in any region of the mouth after long-term severe bruxism. Usually there exist anterior wear and extrusion with no posterior wear (i.e., posterior teeth maintain the vertical dimension). In addition, endodontic therapy may be required to allow proper anterior tooth preparation (Box 8.3). Crown lengthening and associated procedures are not necessary when the vertical dimension has been reduced in relation to the incisal wear. Instead, the teeth may be prepared in their present state. The restoration restores the OVD and reestablishes anterior incisal guidance.

4. The posterior plane of occlusion is then determined. This may be accomplished by using first the maxillary arch or the posterior mandibular arch. However, it is best if the same bilateral posterior quadrants are addressed at the same time, so that the posterior plane may be parallel to the horizontal plane. The maxillary posterior region is most often determined first in the completely edentulous patient.

Fatigue Fractures

The increase in duration of the force is a significant problem. Materials follow a fatigue curve, which is affected by the number of cycles and the intensity of the force (Fig. 8.6).[46-48] A force can be so great that one cycle causes a fracture (e.g., a karate blow to a piece of wood). However, if a lower force magnitude repeatedly hits an object, the object will still fracture. For example, the

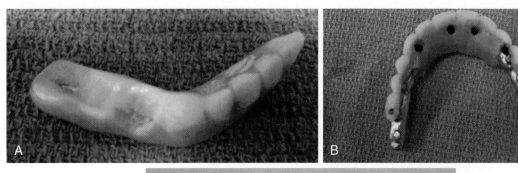

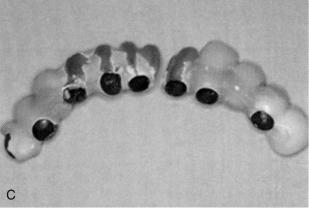

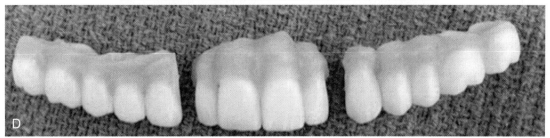

● **Fig. 8.7** (A and B) FP-3 hybrid (acrylic + metal) prostheses exhibiting significant wear from parafunctional habits. (C) Porcelain fused to metal FP-3 showing metal framework fracture and porcelain fracture. (D) Zirconia framework fracture resulting from parafunctional habits.

wire coat hanger that is bent does not break the first time, but repeated bends will fracture the material, not because the last bend was more forceful but because of fatigue. A bruxing patient is at greater risk for fatigue fractures for two reasons: The magnitude of the forces increases over time as the muscles become stronger, and the number of cycles increases on the prosthetic components. Eventually, one of the components (i.e., implant, screw, abutment, prosthesis) will break if the parafunction cannot be reduced in intensity or duration (Fig. 8.7). No long-term prosthetic result is expected in patients with severe bruxism. Therefore once the implant dentist has identified the sources of additional force on the implant system, the treatment plan is altered in an attempt to minimize the negative effect on the longevity of the implant, bone, and final restoration. All elements able to reduce stress should be considered.

Occlusal Guards to Determine Direction of Force

The cause of bruxism is multifactorial and may include occlusal disharmony.[49] When an implant reconstruction is considered in a bruxing patient, occlusal analysis is warranted. Premature and posterior contacts during mandibular excursions increase stress conditions. An elimination of eccentric contacts may allow recovery of periodontal ligament health and muscle activity within 1 to 4 weeks. Occlusal harmony does not necessarily eliminate

bruxism, but this is no reason not to perform an occlusal analysis and eliminate the premature contacts. No study demonstrates an increase in parafunction after occlusal adjustment. Therefore the ability to decrease the risk for occlusal overload on particular teeth and the added benefit of perhaps reducing parafunction is warranted in almost every patient diagnosed with a parafunctional habit of bruxism or clenching.

The term *night guard* is often used to describe this type of prosthesis. However, this prosthesis should be termed an *occlusal guard*, as a night guard may be misconstrued to be used only at night. The occlusal guard can be a useful diagnostic tool to evaluate the influence of occlusal disharmony on nocturnal bruxism. The Michigan occlusal guard exhibits even occlusal contacts around the arch in centric relation occlusion and provides posterior disocclusion with anterior guidance in all excursions of the mandible.[50] This device may be fabricated with 0.5 to 1 mm colored acrylic resin on the occlusal surface. After 4 weeks of nocturnal wear, if the patient wears this device for an additional month or more, the influence of occlusion on the bruxism may be directly observed. There are no premature contacts while the device is worn; however, if the colored acrylic is still intact, the nocturnal parafunction has been reduced or eliminated.[51] Therefore occlusal reconstruction or modification may proceed. If the colored acrylic on the occlusal guard is ground through, an occlusal adjustment will have little influence

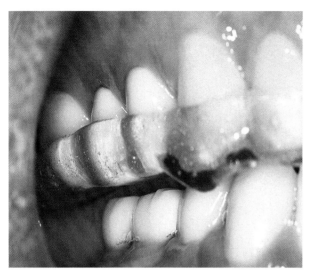

• **Fig. 8.8** A night guard for a partially edentulous patient restored with implants may be designed to transfer the force to the implant prosthesis. When the implant prosthesis is in the opposing arch to the guard, there are no occlusal contacts in centric or during excursion with the guard in place.

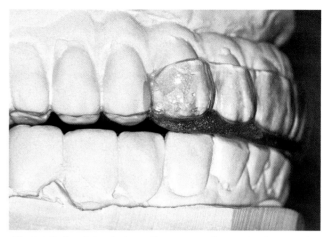

• **Fig. 8.9** Full-arch implant prostheses opposing each other may have only anterior occlusal contact in centric and during mandibular excursions with the guard in place.

on decreasing this parafunctional habit. The occlusal guard is still indicated to relieve stresses during nocturnal parafunction, but the treatment plan should account for the greater forces.

Forces from bruxism are the most difficult to address on a long-term basis. Education and informed consent of the patient are helpful to gain cooperation in eliminating or reducing the noxious effects. If the opposing arch is a soft tissue–supported removable prosthesis, the effects of the nocturnal habit may be minimized if the patient removes the prosthesis at night. The use of a occlusal guard is helpful for a patient with a fixed prosthesis, to transfer the weakest link of the system to the removable acrylic device.[52] Centric contacts in centric relation occlusion and anterior-guided disocclusion of the posterior teeth in excursions are strongly suggested on the occlusal guard, which may be designed to fit the maxilla or mandible.

Unlike teeth, implants do not extrude in the absence of occlusal contacts. As a result, in partially edentulous patients, the maxillary occlusal guard can be relieved around the implant crowns so the remaining natural teeth bear the entire load. For example, for a maxillary implant restoration, the night guard is hollow so no occlusal force is transmitted to the implant crown. When the restoration is in the mandible, the occluding surfaces of the maxillary occlusal guard are relieved over the implant crowns so no occlusal force is transmitted to the implants (Fig. 8.8).

A mandibular posterior cantilever on a full-arch implant prosthesis may also be taken out of occlusion with a maxillary night guard. When a posterior quadrant of implants supports a fixed prosthesis in the maxilla opposing mandibular teeth, a soft reline material is placed around the implant crowns to act as a stress relief element and decrease the impact force on the restoration (Fig. 8.9). When full-arch implant restorations are opposing each other, the night guard provides solely anterior contacts during centric occlusion and mandibular excursions. Thus the parafunctional force is reduced on the anterior teeth/implants and eliminated in the posterior regions.

Clenching

Clenching is a habit that generates a constant force exerted from one occlusal surface to the other without any lateral movement. The habitual clenching position does not necessarily correspond to centric occlusion. The jaw may be positioned in any direction before the static load; therefore a bruxing and clenching combination may exist. The clench position most often is in the same repeated position and rarely changes from one period to another. The direction of load may be vertical or horizontal. The forces involved are in significant excess of normal physiologic loads and are similar to bruxism in amount and duration; however, several clinical conditions differ in clenching.

Diagnosis

Many clinical symptoms and signs warn of excessive grinding. However, the signs for clenching are often less obvious. The forces generated during clenching are directed more vertically to the plane of occlusion, at least in the posterior regions of the mouth. Wearing of the teeth is usually not evident; therefore clenching often escapes notice during the intraoral examination. As a result the dentist must be more observant to the diagnosis of this disorder.[26,49,52]

Many of the clinical signs of clenching often resemble bruxism. When a patient has a dental history of muscle tenderness on awakening or tooth sensitivity to cold, parafunction is strongly suspected. In the absence of tooth wear, clenching is the prime suspect. Tooth mobility, muscle tenderness or hypertrophy, deviation during occlusal opening, limited opening, stress lines in enamel, cervical abfraction, and material fatigue (enamel, enamel pits, porcelain, and implant components) are all associated clinical signs of clenching. All of these conditions may also be found in the bruxing patient. However, enamel wear has such a strong correlation to bruxism that it is the primary and often the only factor needed to evaluate for bruxism. The clenching patient has the "sneaky disease of force." Therefore particular attention is paid to diagnose this disorder from less obvious clinical conditions.

A physical examination for the implant candidate should include palpation of the muscles of mastication. The masseter and temporalis muscles are easily examined at the initial appointment. Hyperactive muscles are not always tender, but tender muscles in the absence of trauma or disease is a sign of excess use or incoordination among muscle groups. The lateral pterygoid muscle is more often overused by the bruxing or clenching patient but is difficult to palpate. The ipsilateral medial pterygoid muscle provides more reliable information in this region. It acts as the antagonist to the lateral pterygoid in hyperfunction and, when tender, provides a good indicator of overuse of the lateral pterygoid.[49]

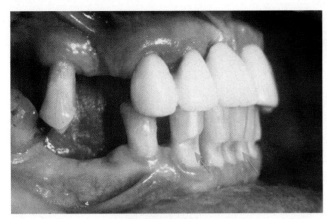

• **Fig. 8.10** Clenching habits are more difficult to diagnose because occlusal wear is often absent. This clenching patient has cervical abfraction of the mandibular anterior teeth. Cervical abfraction (green arrows) is often misdiagnosed as toothbrush abrasion.

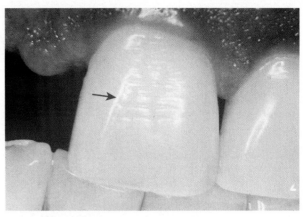

• **Fig. 8.11** This patient has horizontal abfraction lines (red arrow) in the enamel from clenching.

Muscle evaluation for clenching also includes deviation during opening the jaw, limited opening, and tenderness of the temporomandibular joint. Deviation to one side during opening indicates a muscle imbalance on the same side.[49] Limited opening is easily evaluated and may indicate muscular imbalance or degenerative joint disease. The normal opening should be at least 40 mm from the maxillary incisal edge to the mandibular incisal edge in an Angle's Class I patient, taking into consideration an overjet or overlap. If any horizontal overjet or overlap exists, its value in millimeters is subtracted from the 40-mm minimum opening measurement.[53] The range of opening without regard for overlap or overjet has been measured in the range of 38 to 65 mm for men and 36 to 60 mm for women, from incisal edge to edge.[54]

Increased mobility of teeth may be an indication of a force beyond physiologic limits, bone loss, or their combination. This requires further investigation in regard to parafunction and is important if an implant may be placed in the region of the mobile teeth. The rigid implant may receive more than its share of occlusal force when surrounded by mobile teeth. Fremitus, a vibration type of mobility of a tooth, is often present in the clenching patient. To evaluate this condition, the dentist's finger barely contacts the facial surface of one tooth at a time and feels for vibrations while the patient taps the teeth together. Fremitus is symptomatic of local excess occlusal loads.

Cervical erosion is primarily a sign of parafunctional clenching or bruxism (Fig. 8.10). In the past, Black analyzed the eight most popular theories for gingival ditching of the teeth, finding all inconclusive. This observation has frequently been called *toothbrush abrasion*. McCoy[55] has reported this condition on every other tooth, only one tooth, and even on the teeth of some animals. Parafunction was the common link among patients presenting with this condition.[55] The notched appearance of the cervical portion of the tooth directly correlates with the concentration of forces shown in three-dimensional finite analysis[56] and photoelasticity studies.[57] Abfraction of teeth was also observed in cats, rats, and marmosets and was described in the literature as early as 1930.[58] A study of a noninstitutionalized older human population revealed that cervical abrasion was present in 56% of the participants.[59]

Other signs of enamel or occlusal material fatigue encountered in bruxing or clenching patients include occlusal invaginations or pits, stress lines in enamel, stress lines in alloy restorations or acrylic (lines of Luder), and material fracture (Fig. 8.11). Fremitus can be noticed clinically on many cervically eroded, nonmobile teeth. Not all gingival erosions are caused by parafunction. However,

when present, the occlusion should be carefully evaluated along with other signs of excess force. If excessive forces appear to be the cause, the condition is referred to as cervical abfraction.[60]

Clenching patients may also suffer from masseter hypertrophy. This may be easily diagnosed via radiographic identification of an antegonial notch. Because of the excessive parafunctional habits, the angle of the mandible "notches" or resorbs because of excess force applied from the masseter muscle. The insertion of the masseter muscle is in the lateral aspect of the ramus (angle of the mandible) (Fig. 8.12).

A common clinical finding of clenching is a scalloped border of the tongue (Fig. 8.13). The tongue is often braced against the lingual surfaces of the maxillary teeth during clenching, exerting lateral pressures and resulting in the scalloped border. This braced tongue position may also be accompanied by an intraoral vacuum, which permits a clench to extend for a considerable time, often during sleep.

Fatigue Fractures

An increase in force magnitude and duration is a significant problem, whether by bruxism or clenching. The fatigue curve previously presented for bruxism also applies to clenching. In addition, the clenching patient may suffer from a phenomenon called *creep*, which also results in fracture of components. Creep occurs in a material when an increasing deformation is expressed as a function of time, when subjected to a constant load (Fig. 8.14). Although the cycles of load may not be present to affect the deformation of a material, the constant force is still able to cause fracture. In other words, something will break if the continued force is not abated or at least reduced in intensity or duration (Fig. 8.15). This condition may also occur in bone, which may result with implant mobility and failure. All elements to reduce the excessive force of clenching and its consequence should be considered.

Clenching affects the treatment plan in a fashion similar to bruxism. However, the vertical forces are less detrimental than horizontal forces, and alteration of the anterior occlusal scheme is not as critical as with the bruxing patient. Occlusal guards are also less effective. However, a hard acrylic shell and softer, resilient liner night guard, which is slightly relieved over the implants, is often beneficial to a clenching patient. Unlike teeth, implants do not extrude. As a result the occlusal guard can be relieved around an intermediate implant, and the teeth bear the entire load. In a full-arch or quadrant implant restoration, the night guard provides a biomechanical advantage to reduce the impact of the force during clenching (Fig. 8.16).[61]

A common cause of implant failure during healing is parafunction in a patient wearing a soft tissue–supported prosthesis over a

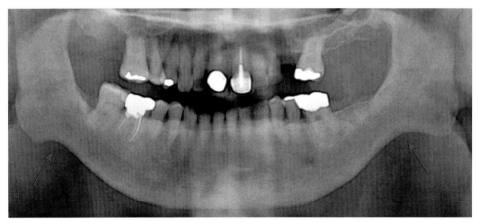

• **Fig. 8.12** Panoramic radiographic depicting extensive antegonial notching (red arrows) resulting from masseter hypertrophy from parafunctional habits.

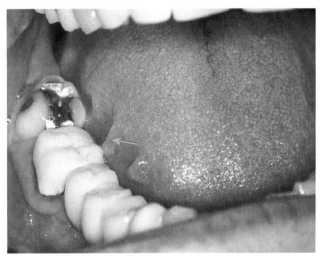

• **Fig. 8.13** A scalloped border of the tongue (green arrow) most often is found in a clenching patient. To maintain the force between the teeth, a vacuum is created in the mouth, and the impression of the lingual contours of the upper teeth is seen on the tongue.

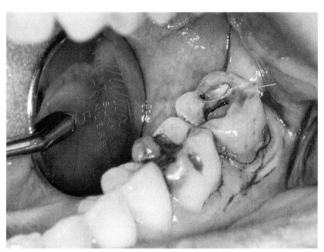

• **Fig. 8.15** The patient exhibits clenching, diagnosed from the enlarged size of the masseter and temporalis muscles. The mandibular second molar has fractured from mesial to distal. Note the slight abfraction on the distal buccal root of the first mandibular molar (green arrow).

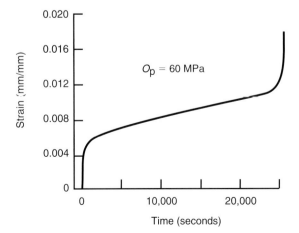

• **Fig. 8.14** A creep curve for materials is created, placing strain on the vertical axis and time on the horizontal axis when a constant load is applied. This is a creep curve for bone at a load of 60 MPa. The bone changes shape (i.e., strain) at the initial stress condition and then at an increasing amount over time until the material breaks.

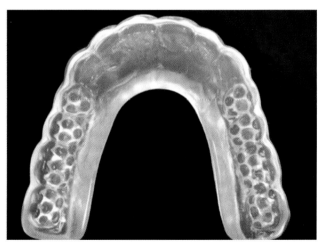

• **Fig. 8.16** A night guard with a rigid acrylic shell and a soft resilient liner can decrease stress during clenching episodes.

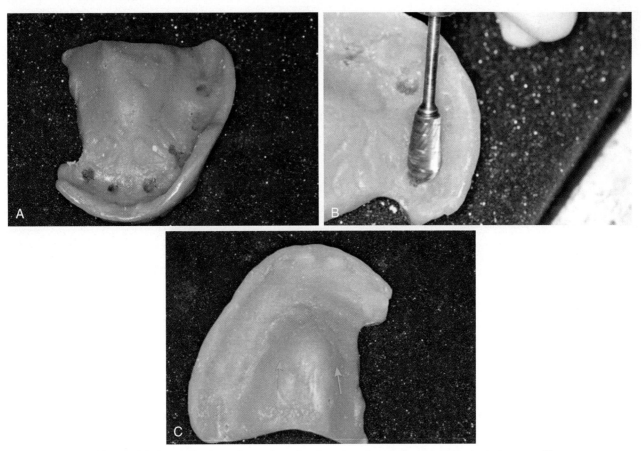

• **Fig. 8.17** Interim prosthesis requires surface alteration when placed immediately after implant surgery. (A) Existing prosthesis. (B) Area over implant sites modified with a barrel bur. (C) Final altered prosthesis; note the stress-bearing areas are not adjusted (green arrows).

submerged implant. The tissue overlying the implant is compressed during the parafunction. The premature loading may cause micromovement of the implant body in the bone and may compromise osteointegration. When an overlying soft tissue–borne restoration exerts pressure as a result of parafunction, pressure necrosis causes soft tissue dehiscence over the implant. This condition is not corrected by surgically covering the implant with soft tissue, but the soft tissue support region of the prosthesis over the implant should be generously relieved during the healing period whenever parafunction is noted. A removable partial denture over a healing implant is especially of concern. The acrylic between the soft tissue–borne region and metal substructure is usually less than 1 mm thick. Removing the thin acrylic region over the implant is often insufficient. Instead, a 6-mm-diameter hole through the metal substructure should be prepared. With a full complete interim prosthesis, the implants should be hollowed out followed by removing the flanges in the area. Any pressure on the implant or bone graft leads to an increased morbidity (Figs. 8.17 and 8.18).

Treatment Planning for Bruxism and Clenching (Table 8.2)

To combat the detrimental effects of bruxism or clenching, numerous modifications to the standard treatment protocols may be implemented.

Progressive Bone Loading

The time intervals between prosthodontic restoration appointments may be increased to provide additional time to produce

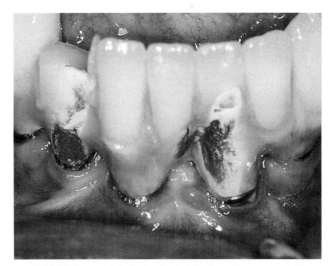

• **Fig. 8.18** This patient fractured the porcelain on her fixed mandibular implant–supported restoration. The cervical regions were the primary sites of fracture because the patient had a clenching habit.

load-bearing bone around the implants through progressive bone-loading techniques.[62] By using the progressive bone-loading technique, poorer bone density may be transformed into better quality bone, which is more ideal for adapting to excessive occlusal loads.

Greater Surface Area

Anterior implants that are subjected to parafunctional forces are problematic because they are usually are have nonaxial or shear forces

TABLE 8.2	Bruxism Versus Clenching	
	Bruxism	Clenching
Force direction	Horizontal, nonfunctional grinding	Mainly vertical
Type of force	Shear	Compression
Force magnification	4–7 times normal	———————
Tooth wear	Yes	Less common
Wear facets	Yes, on incisal edges	Less common
	Notching on the cingulum of maxillary anterior teeth	
Headaches	Common	Less common
Fractured teeth/restorations	Common	Less common
Uncemented restorations	Common	Less common
Abfraction of teeth	Less common	Common
Fremitus	Common	Common
Incisal guidance	Absent in severe cases	Present
Muscle weakness upon awakening	Yes	Yes
Muscle hypertrophy	Significant	Moderate
Masseter, temporalis tenderness	Yes	Sometimes
Scalloped tongue	Not common	Very common
Deviation upon opening	Yes	Yes

applied to them. The use of wider-diameter implants or an additional number of implants (i.e., greater surface area) should be treatment planned to counteract this excessive force.

Occlusion

With parafunctional habits, the occlusion must be strictly designed and monitored. Ideally the patient should be maintained in a canine-guided occlusion, as long as the canines are healthy. Mutually protected occlusion, with additional anterior implants or teeth-distributing forces, is developed if the implants are in the canine position or if this tooth is restored as a pontic. The elimination of posterior lateral occlusal contacts (i.e., nonaxial loading) during excursive movements is recommended when opposing natural teeth or an implant or tooth-supported fixed prosthesis. The anterior teeth may be modified to re-create the proper incisal guidance and avoid posterior interferences during excursions. This is beneficial in two aspects. First, lateral forces dramatically increase stress at the implant–bone interface, and the elimination of posterior contacts diminishes the negative effect of angled forces during bruxism. Second, with the presence of posterior contacts during excursions, almost all fibers of the masseter, temporalis, and the external pterygoid muscles contract and place higher forces on the anterior teeth/implants. Kinsel et al.[63] showed patients exhibiting bruxism and with no night guard had approximately seven times the rate of porcelain fracture. Alderman et al.[26] related that during occlusal excursions in the absence of posterior contacts, fewer fibers of the temporalis and masseter muscles are stimulated, and the forces applied on the anterior implant/teeth system are reduced by as much as two-thirds.

Prosthesis Design

The prosthesis may be designed to improve the distribution of stress throughout the implant system with centric vertical contacts aligned with the long axis of the implant whenever possible. Narrow posterior occlusal tables to prevent inadvertent lateral forces and to decrease the occlusal forces are beneficial.[64] Enameloplasty of the cusp tips of the opposing natural teeth is indicated to help improve the direction of vertical forces within the guidelines of the intended occlusion (i.e., improve plane of occlusion). Newer occlusal materials (e.g., zirconia), wider implant bodies, harder cement types (e.g., resin versus zinc oxide), titanium alloy implant bodies, and more implants splinted together are all beneficial.

Occlusal Guard

The most important treatment for a patient with parafunctional habits is the use of an occlusal guard. Ideally patients should wear a hard, processed acrylic occlusal guard during times of parafunctional activity. The guard will absorb the majority of the parafunctional forces, reducing the damaging forces to the implant system. Patients should also be instructed to wear the guard during any time they might exhibit parafunction, such as stressful time periods, driving, and working at a computer.

Tongue Thrust and Size

Parafunctional tongue thrust is the unnatural force of the tongue against the teeth during swallowing.[65] A force of approximately 41 to 709 g/cm^2 on the anterior and lateral areas of the palate has been recorded during swallowing.[66] In orthodontic movement, a few grams of constant force is sufficient to displace teeth. Six different types of tongue thrust have been identified: anterior, intermediate, posterior, and either unilateral or bilateral may be found, and in most any combination (Figs. 8.19 and 8.20). A common question is which came first, the aberrant tongue position or the misalignment

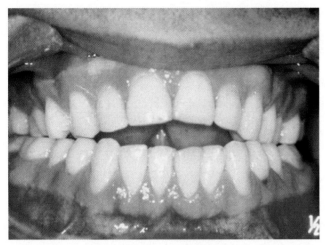

• **Fig. 8.19** Six different types of tongue-thrust habits have been classified. This patient has an anterior tongue thrust and as a result does not have anterior guidance.

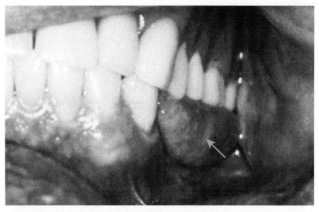

• **Fig. 8.21** This patient has a maxillary complete denture and no posterior mandibular teeth. The patient has developed a posterior tongue position to support the denture and prevent it from dropping posteriorly when the patient occludes (green arrow). This tongue will adapt easily to a mandibular posterior implant prosthesis.

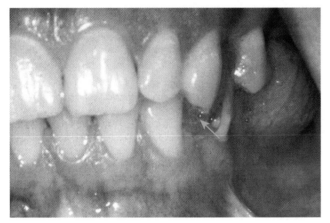

• **Fig. 8.20** This patient has a unilateral posterior tongue thrust. When the patient swallows, the tongue is forced between the maxillary canine and first premolar (green arrow), the mandibular lateral incisor and canine, and the posterior edentulous regions in both arches. Posterior one-stage implants would receive an immediate horizontal load. The patient will feel that the implant prosthesis is constricting the tongue.

of teeth? Regardless, this condition can contribute to implant healing and prosthetic complications. Although the force of tongue thrust is of lesser intensity than in other parafunctional forces, it is horizontal in nature and can increase stress at the permucosal site of the implant. This is most critical for one-stage surgical approaches in which the implants are in an elevated position at initial placement and the implant interface is in an early healing phase. The tongue thrust may also contribute to incision line opening, which may compromise both the hard and soft tissues.

A tongue thrust habit may lead to tooth movement or mobility, which is of consequence when implants are present in the same quadrant. If the natural teeth in the region of the tongue thrust were lost as a result of an aberrant tongue position or movement, the implants are at increased risk during initial healing and early prosthetic loading. If the remaining teeth exhibit increased mobility, the implant prosthesis may be subject to increased occlusal loads. To evaluate anterior tongue thrust, the doctor holds the lower lip down, irrigates water into the mouth with the water syringe, and asks the patient to swallow. A normal patient forms a vacuum in the mouth, positions

the tongue on the anterior aspect of the palate, and is able to swallow without difficulty. A patient with an anterior tongue thrust is not able to create the vacuum needed to swallow when the lower lip is retracted, because the seal and vacuum for the patient are achieved between the tongue and the lower lip. As a consequence the patient is unable to swallow while the lower lip is withdrawn.

A posterior tongue thrust is evaluated by retracting one cheek at a time away from the posterior teeth/edentulous region with a mirror, injecting water into the mouth with a water syringe, and asking the patient to swallow. Visual evidence of the tongue during deglutition may also be accompanied by pressure against the instrument and confirms a lateral force. The posterior tongue thrust may occur in patients wearing a maxillary denture opposing a Kennedy Class I mandibular arch, without a mandibular prosthesis replacing the posterior teeth. Under these conditions the maxillary denture often loses valve seal and drops posteriorly, as only anterior teeth contact. To limit this problem, the patient extends the lateral aspect of the tongue into the edentulous region to prevent the maxillary denture from dislodgement (Fig. 8.21).

A potential prosthetic complication for a patient with a lateral tongue thrust is the complaint of inadequate room for the tongue once the mandibular implants are restored. A prosthetic mistake is to reduce the width of the lingual contour of the mandibular teeth. The lingual cusp of the restored mandibular posterior teeth should follow the curve of Wilson and include proper horizontal overjet to protect the tongue during function. A reduction in the width of the posterior teeth often increases the occurrence of tongue biting and may not dissipate with time. Rather than being a short-term inconvenience, the prosthesis may need to be refabricated. The restoring dentist should identify the tongue position before treatment and inform the patient about the early learning curve for the tongue once the teeth are delivered on the implants.

Even in the absence of tongue thrust, the tongue often accommodates to the available space, and its size may increase with the loss of teeth. As a result, a patient not wearing a mandibular denture often has a larger-than-normal tongue. The placement of implants and prosthetic teeth in such a patient results in an increase in lateral force, which may be continuous. This patient complains of inadequate room for the tongue and may bite it during function.

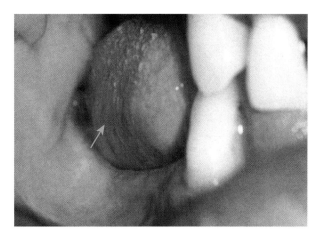

• **Fig. 8.22** When a patient has missing teeth and no prosthetic replacement, such as a complete or partial denture, the tongue often increases in size (green arrow). Although the tongue does not transfer an active lateral force during swallowing, prosthetic complications of tongue biting are at a greater risk.

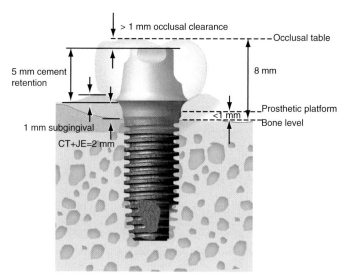

• **Fig. 8.23** The crown height space is measured from the occlusal plane to the crest of the bone.

However, this condition is usually short-lived, and the patient eventually adapts to the new intraoral condition (Fig. 8.22).

A common complication occurs when patients are missing teeth and no interim prosthesis is worn. This can be especially problematic on the mandibular arch because the tongue will gradually increase in size. After implant restoration, whether a removable or fixed prosthesis, the patient will often report a "crowded" tongue with insufficient space. This usually will take weeks to months for the patient to adapt. If the patient refuses to wear the interim prosthesis socially, he or she can be instructed to wear it during the day to allow for better adaptation.

Treatment Planning for Tongue Thrust and Size

Even in the absence of tongue thrust, the tongue often accommodates to the available space, and its size may increase with the loss of teeth. As a result a patient who is not wearing a mandibu-lar denture often has a larger-than-normal sized tongue. The placement of implants and prosthetic teeth in such a patient results in an increase in lateral force, which may be continuous. The patient then complains of inadequate room for the tongue and may bite it during function. However, this condition is usually short-lived, and the patient eventually adapts to the new intraoral condition.

However, it has been observed that a fixed restoration is more advantageous for this type of patient. If the patient has an RP-5 prosthesis, it should be turned into an RP-4. An RP-5 restoration is much less stable in patients with tongue thrust or size issues, and patient complaints are more common with removable restorations in general.

Crown Height Space

The interarch distance is defined as the vertical distance between the maxillary and mandibular dentate or dentate arches under specific conditions (e.g., the mandible is at rest or in occlusion).[67] A dimension of only one arch does not have a defined term in prosthetics; therefore Misch proposed the term *crown height space* (CHS).[68]

The CHS for implant dentistry is measured from the crest of the bone to the plane of occlusion in the posterior region and the incisal edge of the arch in question in the anterior region (Fig.

8.23; Box 8.4). In the anterior regions of the mouth the presence of a vertical overbite means the CHS is larger in the maxilla than the space from the crest of the ridge to the opposing teeth's incisal edge. In general, when the anterior teeth are in contact in centric occlusion, there is a vertical overbite. The anterior mandibular CHS is therefore usually measured from the crest of the ridge to the mandibular incisal edge. However, the anterior maxillary CHS is measured from the maxillary crestal bone to the maxillary incisal edge, not the occlusal contact position.

The ideal CHS needed for a fixed implant prosthesis should range between 8 and 12 mm. Monolithic zirconia has been shown to be successful with as little as 8-mm interocclusal space. For most other types of restorative materials, space greater than 10 mm is usually indicated. This measurement accounts for the biological width, abutment height for cement retention or prosthesis screw fixation, occlusal material strength, esthetics, and hygiene considerations around the abutment crowns. Removable prostheses often require a CHS greater than 12 mm for denture teeth and acrylic resin base strength, attachments, bars, and oral hygiene considerations.[69,70] For a bar overdenture, approximately 15 mm is usually necessary, especially if being restored with acrylic/denture teeth prosthesis.

Biomechanic Consequences of Excessive Crown Height Space

Mechanical complication rates for implant prostheses are often the highest of all complications reported in the literature.[42,71] Mechanical complications are often caused by excessive stress applied to the implant–prosthetic system. Implant failure may occur from overload and result in prosthesis failure and bone loss around the failed implants. Implant body fracture may result from fatigue loading of the implant at a higher force, but occurs at less incidence than most complications. The higher the force, the fewer the number of cycles before fracture, so the incidence increases. Crestal bone loss may also be related to excessive forces and often occurs before implant body fracture. Occlusal material fracture rates may increase as the force to the restoration is increased. The risk for fracture to the opposing prosthesis increases with an average of 12% in implant overdentures opposing a denture.[71] With resin veneer implant fixed partial dentures, 22% of the veneers fractured. Clips or attachment fractures in overdentures may average 17%. Fracture of the framework or substructure may also occur as a result of an increase in biomechanical forces.

Force magnifiers are situations or devices that increase the amount of force applied and include a screw, pulley, incline plane, and lever.[46] The biomechanics of CHS are related to lever mechanics. The properties of a lever have been appreciated since the time of Archimedes, 2000 years ago. The issues of cantilevers and implants were demonstrated in the edentulous mandible, where the length of the posterior cantilever directly related to complications or failure of the prosthesis.[42] Rather than a posterior cantilever, the CHS is a vertical cantilever when any lateral or cantilevered load is applied, and therefore is also a force magnifier.[47,48] As a result, because CHS excess increases the amount of force, any of the mechanical-related complications related to implant prostheses may also increase (Fig. 8.24).

When the direction of a force is in the long axis of the implant, the stresses to the bone are not magnified in relation to the CHS. However, when the forces to the implant are placed on a cantilever, or a lateral force is applied to the crown, the forces are magnified in direct relationship to the crown height. Bidez and Misch[47,48] evaluated the effect of a cantilever on an implant and its relation to crown height. When a cantilever is placed on an implant, there are six different potential rotation points (i.e., moments) on the implant body (Fig. 8.25 and Table 8.3). When the crown height is increased from 10 to 20 mm, two of these six moments are increased 200%. A cantilevered force may be in any direction: facial, lingual, mesial, or distal. Forces cantilevered to the facial and lingual direction are often called *offset loads*. The bone width

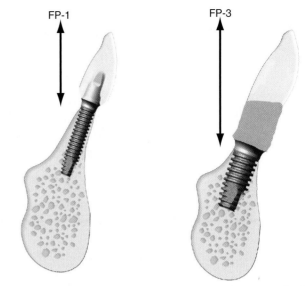

Fig. 8.24 The Crown Height Space Is a Vertical Cantilever. The FP-3 prosthesis on the right will deliver greater stresses to the implant compared with the implant on the left. Therefore a wider-diameter implant is of benefit to support the implant restoration on the right.

decrease is primarily from the facial aspect of the edentulous ridge. As a result, implants are often placed more lingual than the center of the natural tooth root. This condition often results in a restoration cantilevered to the facial. When the available bone height is also decreased, the CHS is increased. Therefore the potential length of the implant reduced in excessive CHS conditions, and the implant position results in offset loads.

An angled load to a crown will also magnify the force applied to the implant. A 12-degree force to the implant will be increased by 20%. This increase in force is further magnified by the crown height. For example, a 12-degree angle with a force of 100 N will result in a force of 315 N/mm on a crown height of 15 mm.[47] Maxillary anterior teeth are usually at an angle of 12 degrees or more to the occlusal planes. Even implants placed in an ideal position are usually loaded at an angle. Maxillary anterior crowns are often longer than any other teeth in the arch, so the effects of crown height cause greater risk.

The angled force to the implant also may occur during protrusive or lateral excursions, as the incisal guide angle may be 20 degrees or more. Anterior implant crowns will therefore be loaded at a considerable angle during excursions, compared with the long axis position of the implant. As a result, an increase in the force to maxillary anterior implants should be compensated for in the treatment plan.

Most forces applied to the osteointegrated implant body are concentrated in the crestal 7 to 9 mm of bone, regardless of implant design and bone density.[72] Therefore implant body height is not an effective method to counter the effects of compromised crown height. In other words, crown/root ratio is a prosthetic concept that may guide the restoring dentist when evaluating a natural tooth abutment. The longer the natural tooth root, the shorter the crown height, which acts as a lever to rotate the tooth around an axis located two-thirds down the root. However, the crown height/implant ratio is not a direct comparison. Crown height is a vertical cantilever that magnifies any lateral or cantilever force in either a tooth- or an implant-supported restoration. However, this condition is not improved by increasing implant length to dissipate stresses, unless in very poor bone quality. The implant

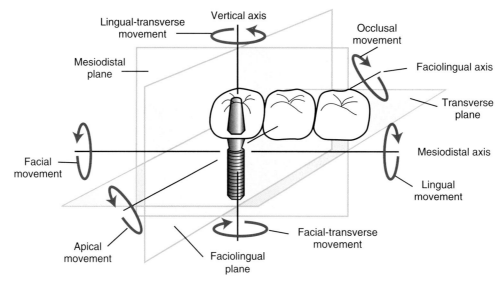

• **Fig. 8.25** Moment Loads Tend to Induce Rotations in Three Planes. Clockwise and counterclockwise rotations in these three planes result in six moments: lingual-transverse, facial-transverse, occlusal, apical, facial, and lingual.

TABLE 8.3   Moment Load at Crest, Division A Bone When Subjected to Forces Shown in Fig. 8.25

INFLUENCES ON MOMENT		IMPOSED MOMENTS (N/MM) AT IMPLANT CROWN–CREST INTERFACE					
Occlusal Height (mm)	Cantilever Length (mm)	Lingual	Facial	Apical	Occlusal	Facial Transverse	Lingual Transverse
10	10	100	0	0	200	0	100
10	20	100	0	0	400	0	200
10	30	100	0	0	600	0	300
20	10	200	0	100	200	0	100
20	20	200	0	100	400	0	200
20	30	200	0	100	600	0	300

does not rotate away from the force in relation to implant length. Instead, it captures the force at the crest of the ridge. The greater the CHS, the greater number of implants usually required for the prosthesis, especially in the presence of other force factors. This is a complete paradigm shift to the concepts advocated originally, with many implants in greater available bone and small crown heights and fewer implants with greater crown heights in atrophied bone (Figs. 8.26 and 8.27).

The CHS increases when crestal bone loss occurs around the implants. An increased CHS may increase the forces to the crestal bone around the implants and increase the risk for crestal bone loss. This in turn may further increase both the CHS and the moment forces to the entire support system, resulting in screw loosening, crestal bone loss, implant fracture, and implant failure.

The vertical distance from the occlusal plane to the opposing landmark for implant insertion is typically a constant in an individual. Therefore as the bone resorbs, the crown height becomes larger, but the available bone height decreases (Fig. 8.28). An indirect relationship is found between the crown and implant height. Moderate bone loss before implant placement may result in a crown height–bone height ratio greater than 1, with greater lateral forces applied to the crestal bone than in abundant bone (in which the crown height is less). A linear relationship exists between the applied load and internal stresses.[73,74] Therefore the greater the load applied, the greater the tensile and compressive stresses transmitted at the bone interface and to the prosthetic components. And yet many implant treatment plans are designed with more implants in abundant bone situations and fewer implants in atrophied bone volume. The opposite scenario should exist. The lesser the bone volume, the greater the crown height and the greater the number of implants indicated.

Excessive Crown Height Space

CHS greater than 15 mm is excessive; it is primarily the result of the vertical loss of alveolar bone from long-term edentulism. Other causes may include genetics, trauma, periodontal disease, and implant failure (Box 8.5). Treatment of excessive CHS before implant placement may include orthodontic and surgical methods. Orthodontics in partially edentulous patients is the method of choice, because other surgical or prosthetic methods are usually more costly and have greater risks for complications. Several

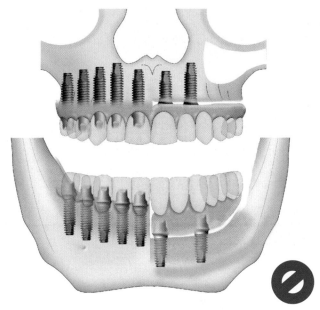

• **Fig. 8.26** In the past, treatment plans included more implants in abundant bone and fewer implants in less available bone. However, crown height increases as bone height decreases, and this approach creates unfavorable mechanics and is less ideal.

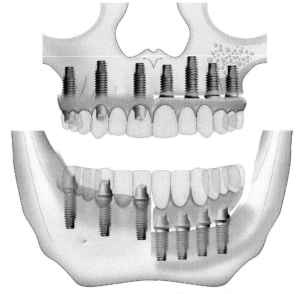

• **Fig. 8.27** Crown height is a force magnifier to any lateral load or horizontal cantilever. Therefore when available bone height decreases, more implants should be inserted and cantilever length reduced.

advanced surgical techniques may also be considered, including block onlay bone grafts, particulate bone grafts with titanium mesh or barrier membranes, interpositional bone grafts, and distraction osteo-genesis. A staged approach to reconstruction of the jaws is often preferred to simultaneous implant placement, especially when large-volume gains are required. Significant vertical bone augmentation may even require multiple surgical procedures.

In case of excessive CHS, bone augmentation may be preferred to prosthetic replacement. Surgical augmentation of the residual ridge height will reduce the CHS and improve implant biomechanics. Augmentation will often permit the placement of wider body implants with the associated benefit of increased surface area. Although prosthetics is the most commonly used option to

address excess CHS, it should be the last choice. Using gingival colored prosthetic materials (pink porcelain zirconia or acrylic resin) on fixed restorations or changing the prosthetic design to a removable restoration should often be considered when restoring excessive CHS (Fig. 8.29).

In the maxilla a vertical loss of bone results in a more palatal ridge position. As a consequence, implants are often inserted more palatal than the natural tooth position. Removable restorations have several advantages under these clinical circumstances. The removable prosthesis does not require embrasures for hygiene. The removable restoration may be removed during sleep to decrease the effects of an increase in CHS on nocturnal parafunction. The removable restoration may improve the lip and facial support, which is deficient because of the advanced bone loss. The overdenture may have sufficient bulk of acrylic resin to decrease the risk for prosthesis fracture. The increase in CHS permits denture tooth placement without infringement of the substructure.

Soft tissue support in addition to implant-supported removable implant restorations with an excessive CHS are recommended when it is not possible to overengineer the implant support system. A rigid overdenture has identical requirements to a fixed prosthesis because it is rigid during function. Misch[76] describes the "hidden cantilever" beyond the cantilevered bar with a rigid implant overdenture. When the overdenture has no movement during function, the cantilever does not stop at the end of the cantilevered substructure but ends at the last occlusal contact position on the prosthesis, often the distal of a second molar.

The position and type of overdenture attachments may render an overdenture rigid during function, even in the absence of distal cantilevers on the bar. For example, when three anterior implants are splinted together and a Hader clip is used to retain the prosthesis, if the Hader clips are placed at angles to the midline, the attachments have limited movement and result in a rigid overdenture during function. Misch[76] suggests the prosthesis movement, not the individual attachment movement, should be evaluated. Excessive CHS with overdentures are situations that benefit from a prosthesis designed to have more than one direction of movement.

The ideal CHS for a fixed prosthesis is between 8 and 12 mm, accounting for an ideal 3 mm of soft tissue, 2 mm of occlusal material thickness, and a 5 mm or greater abutment height. A CHS greater than 12 mm may be of concern in fixed restorations. The replacement teeth are elongated and often require the addition of gingival tone materials in esthetic regions (Fig. 8.30). The greater impact force on implants compared with teeth, combined with the increased crown height, creates increased moment forces on implants and risks for component and material fracture. These problems are especially noted when associated with less favorable biomechanics on cantilevered sections of fixed restorations.[42,71]

A CHS greater than 15 mm means a large amount of metal must be used in the substructure of a traditional fixed restoration to keep porcelain to its ideal 2-mm thickness (Fig. 8.31). Fine-tuning techniques for traditional fixed restorations allowed Dabrowsky[77] to manufacture and monitor multiple full-mouth, cement-retained prostheses with a large CHS, delivered in various centers across the United States. Controlling surface porosities of metal substructures after casting as their different parts cool at different rates becomes increasingly difficult. Furthermore, when the casting is reinserted into the oven to bake the porcelain, the heat is maintained within the casting at different rates, so the porcelain cools in different regions at different rates.[78] If not controlled properly, both these factors increase the risk for porcelain fracture after loading.[79] For excessive CHS, considerable weight of the

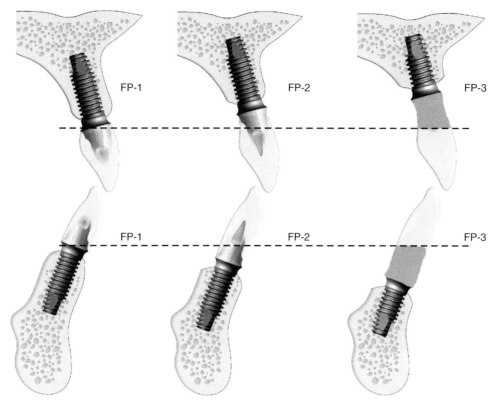

• **Fig. 8.28** As the crown height increases, the available bone height decreases. This is especially noteworthy in the maxillary arch, as the initial available bone height is less than in the mandible. As a consequence, shorter implants in the maxilla are a common occurrence.

• BOX 8.5 Excessive Crown Height Space

1. Excessive CHS increases mechanical complications in fixed prostheses.
2. The need for gingival replacement procedures should be evaluated before implant placement for fixed restorations.
3. Metal and porcelain shrinkage is a more significant problem in traditional fixed prosthetic cases.
4. Hybrid FP-3 fixed prostheses with denture teeth, metal substructure, and acrylic resin are indicated.
5. Overdentures are recommended in completely edentulous patients with RP-4 and RP-5.
6. The implant support for RP-4 should be as great as that for a fixed prosthesis.
7. When designing a RP-5, there should be adequate soft tissue support (i.e., maxilla: crest of ridge and horizontal palate; mandible: buccal shelf).
8. In overdentures, there may be two different components of the CHS: the distance from the crest of the bone to the height of the attachment and the distance from the attachment to the occlusal plane.

CHS, crown height space.

---

prosthesis (approaching 3 oz of alloy) may affect maxillary trial placement appointments, because the restoration does not remain in place without the use of adhesive. Noble metals must be used to control alloy's heat expansion or corrosion; therefore the costs of such implant restorations have dramatically increased. Proposed methods to produce hollow frames to alleviate these problems, including the use of special custom trays to achieve a passive fit, will double or triple the labor costs.[80]

An alternative method of fabricating fixed prostheses in situations of CHSs of 15 mm or greater is the fixed complete denture or hybrid prosthesis, with a smaller metal framework, denture teeth, and acrylic resin to join these elements together (Fig. 8.32). The reduced metal framework compared with a porcelain-to-metal fixed prosthesis exhibits fewer dimensional changes and may more accurately fit the abutments, which is important for a screw-retained restoration. It is less expensive to fabricate than a porcelain-to-metal fixed prosthesis, is highly esthetic (premade denture teeth), easily replaces teeth and soft tissue in appearance, and is easier to repair if fracture occurs. Because resin acts as an intermediary between the teeth and metal substructure, the impact force during dynamic occlusal loading may also be reduced. In addition, a hybrid prosthesis (acrylic/denture teeth) is far lighter than a metal-based prosthesis, which is advantageous in cases with excessive interocclusal space. Therefore this type of fixed prosthesis is often indicated for implant restorations with a large CHS. On occasion, undercontoured interproximal areas are designed by the laboratory in such restorations to assist oral hygiene and have been referred to as "high water" restorations. This is an excellent method in the mandible; however, it results in food entrapment, affects air flow patterns, and may contribute to speech problems in the anterior maxilla.

Because an increase in the biomechanical forces are in direct relationship to the increase in CHS, the treatment plan of the implant restoration should consider stress-reducing options whenever the CHS is increased. Methods to decrease stress include:[6,8,70]

1. Shorten cantilever length.
2. Minimize offset loads to the buccal or lingual.
3. Increase the number of implants.
4. Increase the diameters of implants.
5. Design implants to maximize the surface area of implants.
6. Fabricate removable restorations that are less retentive and incorporate soft tissue support.

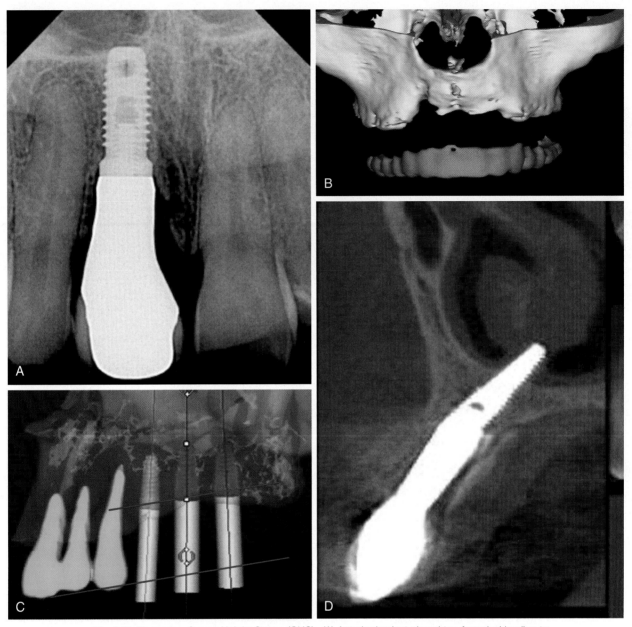

• **Fig. 8.29** Excessive Crown Height Space (CHS). (A) Anterior implant placed too far apical leading to FP-3 prosthesis along with compromising the adjacent bone levels. (B) Edentulous maxillary arch displaying excessive hard and soft tissue loss. (C) Maxillary posterior is a common area for excessive CHS because of the vertical bone loss that is associated with this area. (D) Maxillary cuspid implant placed with an excessive CHS that perforated the nasal cavity.

7. Remove the removable restoration during sleeping hours to reduce the noxious effects of nocturnal parafunction.
8. Splint implants together, whether they support a fixed or removable prosthesis.
9. Narrow occlusal table (buccal-lingually).
10. Minimal cusp height on prosthesis.
11. Mutually protected if opposing fixed teeth.
12. Occlusal contacts centered over implants and eliminatd over cantilevers.

Because CHS is a considerable force magnifier, the greater the crown height, the shorter the prosthetic cantilever that should extend from the implant support system. In CHS greater than 15 mm, no cantilever should be considered, unless all other force factors are minimal. The occlusal contact intensity should be reduced on any offset load from the implant support system. Occlusal contacts in centric relation occlusion may even be eliminated on the most posterior aspect of a cantilever. In this way a parafunction load may be reduced, because the most cantilevered portion of the prosthesis is loaded only during functional activity (such as chewing).

Masticatory Dynamics (Patient Size, Gender, Age, and Skeletal Position)

Masticatory muscle dynamics are responsible for the amount of force exerted on the implant system. Several criteria are included under this heading: patient size, gender, age, and skeletal position.[9,11,16,21,81-84]

The size of the patient can influence the amount of bite force. Large, athletic men can generate greater forces; patients of weak physical condition often develop less force than athletic patients (Fig. 8.33). In general the forces recorded in women are approximately 20 lb less than those in men. In a clinical report by van Steenberghe et al.,[85] partially edentulous men have a 13% implant failure rate compared with 77% for women. In a report by Wyatt and Zarb,[86] first-year radiograph bone loss was positively correlated with male sex, younger age, and implants supporting a distal extension prosthesis. Older patients record lower bite forces than young adults. In addition, the younger patient lives longer and requires the additional implant support for the prosthesis for a longer time. (An 80-year-old patient will need implant support for far fewer years than a 20-year-old, all other factors being equal.)

The skeletal arch position may influence the amount of maximum bite force. The brachiocephalic, with a stout head shape, may generate three times the bite force compared with a regular head shape. This is especially noteworthy when accompanied by moderate-to-severe bruxism or clenching. The maximum bite force decreases as muscle atrophy progresses throughout years of edentulism. A maximum occlusal force of 5 psi may be the result of 15 years without teeth.[82] This force may increase 300% in the 3 years after implant placement.[21,22,82-84] Therefore sex, muscle mass, exercise, diet, state of the dentition, physical status, and age all influence muscle strength, masticatory dynamics, and maximum bite force.

The skeletal Class III patient is primarily a vertical chewer and generates vertical forces with little excursive movement. However, some patients appear "pseudo–Class III" as a result of anterior bone resorption or loss of posterior support and collapse of the vertical dimension with an anterior rotation of the mandible. These patients do exhibit lateral excursive movements when the incisal edge position is restored to its initial position.

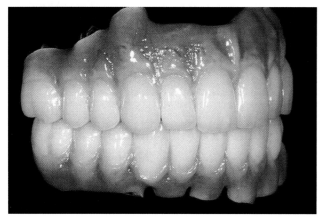

• **Fig. 8.30** When the crown height space is greater than 12 mm, pink (porcelain, acrylic, zirconia) is often used to replace the soft tissue drape in the prosthesis.

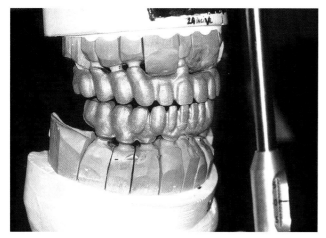

• **Fig. 8.31** Porcelain thickness for fixed prostheses should not be greater than 2 mm. When the crown height space is greater than 15 mm, the amount of metal in the substructure may be extensive.

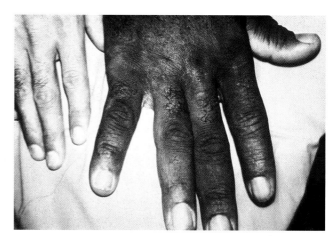

• **Fig. 8.33** Masticatory dynamics are affected by the size of the patient (larger persons generally have greater bite forces).

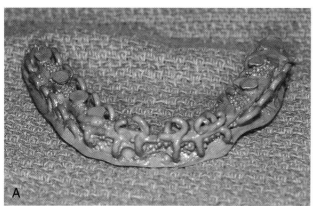
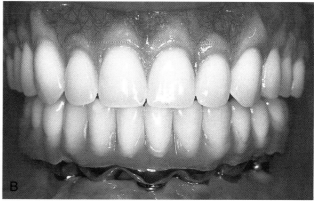

• **Fig. 8.32** (A) A metal framework for a hybrid prosthesis composed of metal, acrylic, and denture teeth presents several advantages for fixed prostheses with a crown height space greater than 15 mm. (B) Denture teeth are then added to the metal substructure.

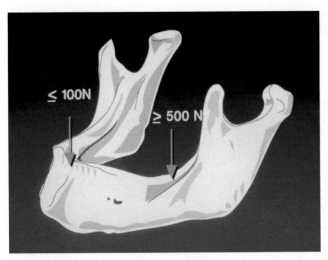

Fig. 8.34 The maximum bite forces are greater in the posterior regions of the jaws compared with the anterior regions (approximately 5:1).

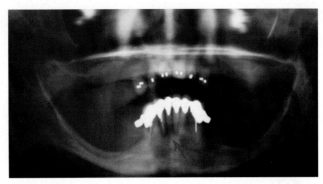

Fig. 8.35 Mandibular anterior passive eruption leading to extrusion of the anterior segment (red arrow) and destruction of the premaxilla and hypertrophy of the maxillary posterior area (combination syndrome). A common incorrect treatment includes attempting bone grafting in the posterior mandible, which often leads to a neurosensory impairment. Ideally implants may be inserted after extraction of the mandibular teeth and associated osteoplasty.

As a general rule the implant treatment plan should reduce other force magnifiers when masticatory musculature dynamics increase. For example, a cantilever length should be reduced in cases of elevated masticatory dynamics. A crown height may be reduced by bone augmentation. The prosthesis may be made removable so nocturnal bruxism is reduced (if they do not wear their prosthesis). The implant number, size, and design may also be increased to increase the surface area of load.

Arch Position

The maximum biting force is greater in the molar region and decreases as measurements progress anteriorly. Maximum bite forces in the anterior incisor region correspond to approximately 35 to 50 psi, and those in the canine region range from 47 to 100 psi, whereas those in the molar area vary from 127 to 250 psi (Fig. 8.34).[8] Mansour et al.[87] evaluated occlusal forces and moments mathematically using a Class III lever arm, the condyles being the fulcrum and the masseter and temporalis muscles supplying the force. Similar figures were obtained by mathematical calculation and by direct measurement. In addition, the forces at the second molar were 10% higher than at the first molar, indicative of a range from 140 to 275 psi.

In a study by Chung et al.[88] with 339 implants in 69 patients in function for an average of 8.1 years (range of 3–24 years) the posterior implants (even with keratinized mucosa) showed a 3.5-fold greater average bone loss per year than anterior implants.

The anterior biting force is decreased in the absence of posterior tooth contact and greater in the presence of posterior occlusion or eccentric contacts.[38,89] Besides the mechanical properties of a Class III lever function, there also is a biological component to increased bite force in the posterior regions. When the posterior teeth are in contact, the large masticatory muscles contract. When the posterior teeth are not in contact, two-thirds of the temporalis and masseter muscles do not contract their fibers. As a consequence the bite force is reduced.

In the anterior regions with less force the anterior natural tooth roots are smaller in diameter and root surface area compared with posterior teeth. Yet in implant dentistry, we often alter the implant length primarily and place longer implants in the anterior region and shorter implants in the posterior regions (or cantilever off the anterior implants, which results in posterior bite forces magnified by the cantilever length). This approach should be corrected to conform to biomechanics similar to that observed with natural teeth. In other words, implants in the posterior regions should often be of greater diameter, especially in the presence of additional force factors. The greater increase in natural tooth surface area occurs in the molar region, with a 200% increase compared with the premolars. Hence the larger implant diameter is especially considered in the molar region.

The edentulous bone density varies in function of arch position. The natural teeth are surrounded by a thin cortical plate of bone and periodontal complex, which is similar for all teeth and arch positions. However, after the teeth are lost, the bone density in the edentulous site is different for each region of the mouth. The posterior regions, in general, form less bone density after tooth loss than the anterior regions. The mandibular anterior implant sites benefit from denser bone than the maxillary anterior implant sites. The denser the bone, the greater its resistance to stress applied at the implant–bone interface. In other words, the edentulous bone density is inversely related to the amount of force generally applied in that arch position. As a result the posterior maxilla is the most at-risk arch position, followed by the posterior mandible, and then the anterior maxilla. The most ideal region is the mandibular anterior.

Opposing Arch

Natural teeth transmit greater impact forces through occlusal contacts than soft tissue–borne complete dentures. In addition, the maximum occlusal force of patients with complete dentures is limited and may range from 5 to 26 psi.[82] The force is usually greater in recent denture wearers and decreases with time. Muscle atrophy, thinning of the oral tissues with age or disease, and bone atrophy often occur in the edentulous patient as a function of time.[90] Some denture wearers may clench on their prosthesis constantly, which may maintain muscle mass. However, this condition usually accelerates bone loss. Implant overdentures improve the masticatory performance and permit a more consistent return to centric relation occlusion during function. The maximum force generated in an implant prosthesis is related to the amount of tooth or implant supporting the opposing arch (Figs. 8.35 and 8.36).[12,82,83]

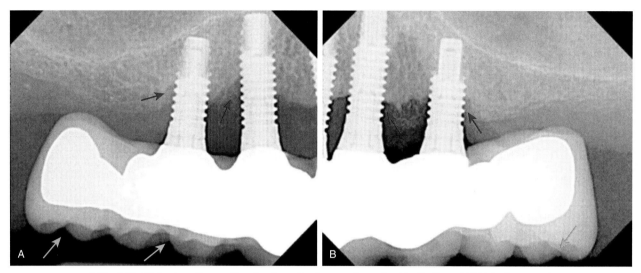

• **Fig. 8.36** Bilateral cantilever with a fixed prosthesis opposing natural teeth. (A and B) Note the associated bone loss (red arrows) because of the significant cantilever and large cusp heights (green arrows) leading to shear forces.

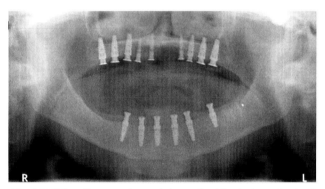

• **Fig. 8.37** When the opposing arch has a fixed implant prosthesis, the bite forces are greatest. The decrease in proprioception results in higher forces during function and parafunction. In this patient a posterior implant was placed on the mandible to counteract the excessive forces.

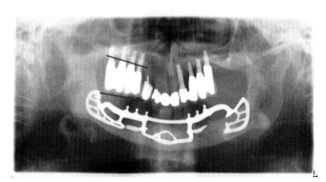

• **Fig. 8.38** Excessive maxillary crown height with mandibular subperiosteal implant leading to bone loss and failure of the subperiosteal implant.

A complete implant fixed prosthesis does not benefit from proprioception as do natural teeth, and patients bite with a force four times greater than with natural teeth. Thus the highest forces are created with implant prostheses (Fig. 8.37). In addition, premature contacts in occlusal patterns or during parafunction on the implant prostheses do not alter the pathway of closure, because occlusal awareness is decreased with implant prostheses compared with natural teeth.[17,18] Therefore continued stress increases can be expected to occur with the implant restoration.

Partial denture patients may record forces intermediate between that of natural teeth and complete dentures, depending on the location and condition of the remaining teeth, muscles, and joints. In the partially edentulous patient with implant-supported fixed prostheses, force ranges are more similar to those of natural dentition, but lack of proprioception may magnify the load amount during parafunctional activity.

As a consequence of the opposing arch affecting the intensity of forces applied to an implant prosthesis, the treatment plan may be modified to reduce the risk for overload. Rarely should the opposing arch be maintained in a traditional denture to decrease the stress to the implant arch. Instead, the implant arch should be designed to compensate for the higher stresses expected from an implant-supported opposing arch (Fig. 8.38).

Summary

Patient force factors are highly variable from one person to another. An implant foundation should be designed to support the load and resist the stresses of the prosthesis. An ideal treatment plan may be established relative to the number and position of missing teeth. The treatment plan is then modified dependent on the force factors of the individual patient.

It is far more advantageous to overengineer the amount of support necessary for a prosthesis. If just one too few or too small an implant is used, implant bone loss, fracture, and failure may occur. As a general rule, the best way to reduce the risk for biomechanical overload is to add additional implants.

The five most important force factors related to patient conditions were presented in this chapter. Of these, parafunction is the predominant element to account for in the treatment plan. On a scale of 1 to 10, severe bruxism is a 10; an excessive CHS can double a force, and therefore is a 7 on the importance scale. Severe masticatory dynamics can also double a force component and result in a 7 on this scale. Position of the abutment in the arch determines the magnitude of force and is a 1 or 2 when in the mandibular anterior region, a 3 or 4 in the maxillary anterior, a 5 in the posterior mandible, and a 6 or 7 in the posterior maxilla (because bone density is most ideal in the anterior mandible and least biomechanically favorable in the posterior maxilla). Direction of load under ideal implant placement conditions is a factor of 3 or 4 in the maxillary anterior regions. The other arch positions may have a more ideal direction of load, unless cantilever loads are positioned on the implant restoration. The opposing arch under typical treatment conditions is the least important force component modifier. A complete implant restoration may be a factor of 3, natural teeth a factor of 2, and an opposing soft tissue–supported denture a factor of 1.

References

1. Picton DC, Johns RB, Wills DJ, et al. The relationship between the mechanisms of tooth and implant support. *Oral Sci Rev*. 1971;5:3–22.
2. Picton DC. The effect of external forces on the peri-dontium. In: Melcher AH, Bowen WH, eds. *Biology of the Periodontium*. London: Academic Press; 1969.
3. Scott I, Ash MM. A six-channel intra-oral transmitter for measuring occlusal forces. *J Prosthet Dent*. 1966;16:56.
4. Graf H. Bruxism. *Dent Clin North Am*. 1969;13:659–665.
5. Proffit WR. The facial musculature in its relation to the dental occlusion. In: Carlson DS, McNamara JA, eds. Muscle adaptation in the craniofacial region. *Proceedings of Symposium, Craniofacial Growth Series, Monograph 8*. Ann Arbor, Mich: University of Michigan; 1978.
6. Black GV. An investigation of the physical characters of the human teeth in relation to their diseases, and to practical dental operations, together with the physical characters of filling materials. *Dent Cosmos*. 1895;37:469.
7. Craig RG. *Restorative Dental Materials*. 6th ed. St Louis: Mosby; 1980.
8. Carlsson GE. Bite force and masticatory efficiency. In: Kawamura Y, ed. *Physiology of Mastication*. Basel, Switzerland: Karger; 1974.
9. Ingervall B, Helkimo E. Masticatory muscle force and facial morphology in man. *Arch Oral Biol*. 1978;23:203–206.
10. Helkimo E, Carlsson GE, Helkimo M. Bite force and state of dentition. *Acta Odontol Scand*. 1977;35:297–303.
11. Lassila V, Holmlund J, Koivumaa KK. Bite forces and its correlations in different denture types. *Acta Odontol Scand*. 1985;43:127–132.
12. Haraldson T, Carlsson GE. Bite force and oral function in patients with osseointegrated implants. *Scand J Dent Res*. 1977;85:200–208.
13. van Eijden TM. Three dimensional analyses of human bite force magnitude and moment. *Arch Oral Biol*. 1991;36:535–539.
14. Lindquist LW, Carlsson GE. Long-term effects on chewing with mandibular fixed prostheses on osseointegrated implants. *Acta Odontol Scand*. 1985;43:39–45.
15. Lundgren D, Laurell L, Falk J, et al. Distribution of occlusal forces in a dentition unilaterally restored with a bridge construction supported on osseointegrated titanium implants. In: van Steenberghe D, ed. *Tissue Integration in Oral and Maxillo-Facial Reconstruction*. Brussels: Excerpta Medica; 1985.
16. Braun S, Bantleon HP, Hnat WP, et al. A study of bite force. Part I: relationship to various physical characteristics. *Angle Orthod*. 1995;65:367–372.
17. Haraldson T, Zarb GA. A 10-year follow-up study of the masticatory system after treatment with osseointegrated implant bridges. *Scand J Dent Res*. 1988;96:243–252.
18. Falk J, Laurell L, Lundgren D. Occlusal interferences and cantilever joint stress in implant supported prostheses occluding with complete dentures. *Int J Oral Maxillofac Impl*. 1990;5:70–77.
19. Richter EJ. In vivo vertical forces on implants. *Int J Oral Maxillofac Impl*. 1995;10:99–108.
20. Falk H. On occlusal forces in dentitions with implants supported fixed cantilever prostheses. *Swed Dent J*. 1990;69:1–40.
21. Raadsheer MC, van Eijden TM, van Ginkel FC, et al. Contribution of jaw muscle size and craniofacial morphology to human bite force magnitude. *J Dent Res*. 1999;87:31–42.
22. Morneburg TR, Proschel PA. Measurement of masticatory forces and implant loads: a methodologic clinical study. *Int J Prosthodont*. 2002;15:20–27.
23. Awawdeh L, Hemaidat K, Al-Omari W. Higher maximal occlusal bite force in endodontically treated teeth versus vital contralateral counterparts. *J Endod*. 2017;43(6):871–875.
24. Ramfjord SP, Ash MM. *Occlusion*. 4th ed. Philadelphia: WB Saunders; 1995.
25. Nadler SC. Bruxism, a clinical and electromyographic study. *J Am Dent Assoc*. 1961;62:21.
26. Alderman MM. Disorders of the temporomandibular joint and related structures. In: Burket LW, ed. *Oral Medicine*. 6th ed. Philadelphia: JB Lippincott; 1971.
27. Jaffin R, Berman C. The excessive loss of Brånemark fixtures in type IV bone: a 5-year analysis. *J Periodontol*. 1991;62:2–4.
28. Fischer WF, O'Toole ET. Personality characteristics of chronic bruxers. *Behav Med*. 1993;19:82–86.
29. Lavigne GJ, Montplaisir JY. Restless legs syndrome and sleep bruxism: prevalence and association among Canadians. *Sleep*. 1994;17:739–743.
30. Glass EG, McGlynn FD, Glaros AG, et al. Prevalence of TM disorder symptoms in a major metropolitan area. *Cranio*. 1993;11:217–220.
31. Ohayon MM, Li KK, Guilleminault C. Risk factors for sleep bruxism in the general population. *Chest*. 2002;119:453–461.
32. Tosun T, Krabuda C, Cuhadaroglu C, et al. Evaluation of sleep bruxism by polysomnographic analysis in patients with dental implants. *Int J Oral Maxillofac Imp*. 2003;18:286–292.
33. Thorpy MD, Broughton RJ, Cohn MA, et al., eds. *The International Classification of Sleep Disorders, Revised: Diagnostic and Coding Manual*. Westchester, Ill: American Academy of Sleep Medicine; 2001.
34. Ohayon MM, Li K, Guilleminault C. Risk factors for sleep bruxism in the general population. *Chest*. 2001;119(1):53–61.
35. Abekura H, Tsuboi M, Okura T, et al. Association between sleep bruxism and stress sensitivity in an experimental psychological stress task. *Biomed Res*. 2011;32(6):395–399.
36. Gibbs CH, Mahan PE, Mauderli A, et al. Limits of human bite force. *J Prosthet Dent*. 1986;56:226–229.
37. Glaros AG, Rao SM. Effects of bruxism: a review of the literature. *J Prosthet Dent*. 1977;38:149–157.
38. Williamson EH, Lundquist DO. Anterior guidance: its effect on electromyographic activity of temporal and masseter muscles. *J Prosthet Dent*. 1983;49:816–823.
39. Del Valle V, Faulkner G, Walfaardt J. Craniofacial osseointegrated implant-induced strain distribution: a numerical study. *Int J Oral Maxillofac Impl*. 1997;12:200–210.
40. Ishigaki S, Nakano T, Yamada S, et al. Biomechanical stress in bone surrounding an implant under simulated chewing. *Clin Oral Implant Res*. 2002;14:97–102.
41. Oh T, Yoon J, Misch CE, et al. The cause of early implant bone loss: myth or science? *J Periodontol*. 2002;73:322–333.
42. Bragger U, Aeschlimann S, Burgin W, et al. Biological and technical complications and failures with fixed partial dentures (FPD) on implants and teeth after four to five years of function. *Clin Oral Impl Res*. 2001;12:26–43.
43. Misch CE, Palattella A. Bruxism and its effect on treatment plans. *Int Mag Oral Implant*. 2002;2:6–18.
44. Mericske-Stern R, Assal P, Buergin W. Simultaneous force measurements in three dimensions on oral endosseous implants in vitro and vivo: a methodological study. *Clin Oral Implants Res*. 1996;7:378–386.
45. Choy E, Kydd WL. Bite force duration: a diagnostic procedure for mandibular dysfunction. *J Prosthet Dent*. 1988;60:365–368.
46. Bidez MW, Misch CE. Force transfer in implant dentistry: basic concepts and principles. *Oral Implantol*. 1992;18:264–274.
47. Bidez MW, Misch CE. Issues in bone mechanics related to oral implants. *Implant Dent*. 1992;1:289–294.

48. Misch CE, Bidez MW. Biomechanics in implant dentistry. In: Misch CE, ed. *Contemporary Implant Dentistry*. St Louis: Mosby; 1993.

49. Dawson PE. *Differential Diagnosis and Treatment of Occlusal Problems*. 2nd ed. St Louis: Mosby; 1989.

50. Rateitschak KJ, ed. *Color Atlas of Dental Medicine*. Stuttgart: Thieme; 1989.

51. Sheikholescham A, Riise C. Influence of experimental interfering occlusal contacts on the activity of the anterior temporal and masseter muscles during submaximal and maximal bite in the intercuspal position. *J Oral Rehabil*. 1983;10:207–214.

52. Misch CE. Clenching and its effects on implant treatment plans. *Oral Health*. 2002;92:11–24.

53. Tanaka TT. Recognition of the pain formula for head, neck, and TMJ disorders: the general physical examination. *Calif Dent Assoc J*. 1984;12:43–49.

54. Mezitis M, Rallis G, Zachariades N. The normal range of mouth opening. *J Oral Maxillofac Surg*. 1989;47:1028–1029.

55. McCoy G. The etiology of gingival erosion. *J Oral Implantol*. 1982;10:361–362.

56. Selna LG, Shillingburg HT, Kerr PA. Finite element analysis of dental structure asymmetric and plane stress idealizations. *J Biomed Mater Res*. 1975;9:235–237.

57. Hood JAA. Experimental studies on tooth deformation: stress distribution in Class V restorations. *N Z Dent J*. 1968;68:116–131.

58. DuPont GA, DeBowers LJ. Comparison of periodontics and root replacement in cat teeth with resorptive lesions. *J Vet Dent*. 19:71–75; erratum in *J Vet Dent*. 2002;19:230.

59. Hand ASJ, Hunt A, Reinhardt JW. The prevalence and treatment implications of cervical abrasion in the elderly. *Gerodontics*. 1986;2:167–170.

60. Grippo JO. Abfractions: a new classification of hard tissue lesions of teeth. *J Esthet Dent*. 1991;3:14–19.

61. Perel M. Parafunctional habits, nightguards, and root form implants. *Implant Dent*. 1994;3:261–263.

62. Misch CE. Progressive bone loading. *Dent Today*. 1995;14(1):80–83.

63. Kinsel RP, Lin D. Retrospective analysis of porcelain failures of metal ceramic crowns and fixed partial dentures supported by 729 implants in 152 patients: patient-specific and implant-specific predictors of ceramic failure. *J Prosthet Dentistry*. 2009;101(6):388–394.

64. Misch CE, Bidez MW. Implant protected occlusion, a biomechanical rationale. *Compend Cont Educ Dent*. 1994;15:1330–1342.

65. Kydd WL, Toda JM. Tongue pressures exerted on the hard palate during swallowing. *J Am Dent Assoc*. 1962;65:319.

66. Winders RV. Forces exerted on the dentition by the peri-oral and lingual musculature during swallowing. *Angle Orthod*. 1958;28:226.

67. The glossary of prosthodontic terms. *J Prosthet Dent*. 1999;81:39–110.

68. Misch CE, Misch-Dietsh F. Pre-implant prosthodontics. In: Misch CE, ed. *Dental Implant Prosthetics*. St Louis: Mosby; 2005.

69. Misch CE, Goodacre CJ, Finley JM, et al. Consensus conference panel report: crown-height space guidelines for implant dentistry—part 1. *Implant Dent*. 2005;14:312–318.

70. Misch CE, Goodacre CJ, Finley JM, et al. Consensus conference panel report: crown-height space guidelines for implant dentistry—part 2. *Implant Dent*. 2006;15:113–121.

71. Goodacre CJ, Bernal G, Rungcharassareng K, et al. Clinical complications with implants and implant prostheses. *Prosthet Dent*. 2003;90:121–132.

72. Misch CE, Bidez MW. Occlusion and crestal bone resorption: etiology and treatment planning strategies for implants. In: McNeill C, ed. *Science and Practice of Occlusion*. Chicago: Quintessence; 1997.

73. Kakudo Y, Amano N. Dynamic changes in jaw bones of rabbit and dogs during occlusion, mastication, and swallowing. *J Osaka Univ Dent Soc*. 1972;6:126–136.

74. Kakudo Y, Ishida A. Mechanism of dynamic responses of the canine and human skull due to occlusal, masticatory, and orthodontic forces. *J Osaka Univ Dent Soc*. 1972;6:137–144.

75. Jensen OT, Cockrell R, Kuhlke L, et al. Anterior maxillary alveolar distraction osteogenesis: a prospective 5-year clinical study. *Int J Oral Maxillofac Implants*. 2002;17:507–516.

76. Misch CE. Screw-retained versus cement-retained implant-supported prostheses. *Pract Perio Esthet*. 1995;7:15–18.

77. Dabrowsky T. *Personal Communication*; 2005.

78. Bidger DV, Nicholls JI. Distortion of ceramometal fixed partial dentures during the firing cycle. *J Prosthet Dent*. 1981;45:507–514.

79. Bertolotti RL, Moffa JP. Creep rate of porcelain-bonding alloys as a function of temperature. *J Dent Res*. 1980;59:2062–2065.

80. Bryant RA, Nicholls JI. Measurement of distortion in fixed partial dentures resulting from degassing. *J Prosthet Dent*. 1979;42:515–520.

81. Howell AH, Bruderold F. Vertical forces used during chewing of food. *J Dent Res*. 1950;29:133.

82. Carr AB, Laney WR. Maximum occlusal forces in patients with osseointegrated oral implant prostheses and patients with complete dentures. *Int J Oral Maxillofac Impl*. 1987;2:101–108.

83. Carlsson GE, Haraldson T. Functional response in tissue-integrated prostheses osseointegration. In: Brånemark PI, Zarb GA, Albrektsson T, eds. *Clinical Dentistry*. Chicago: Quintessence; 1985.

84. Fontijn-Tekamp FA, Slageter AP, van't Hof MA, et al. Bite forces with mandibular implant-retained overdentures. *J Dent Res*. 1998;77:1832–1839.

85. van Steenberghe D, Lekholm U, Bolender C, et al. Applicability of osseointegrated oral implants in the rehabilitation of partial edentulism: a prospective multicenter study on 558 fixtures. *Int J Oral Maxillofac Implants*. 1990;5:272–281.

86. Wyatt CC, Zarb Z. Bone level changes proximal to oral implants supporting fixed partial prostheses. *Clin Oral Impl Res*. 2002;13:162–168.

87. Mansour RM, Reynik RJ, Larson PC. In vivo occlusal forces and moments: forces measured in terminal hinge position and associated moments. *J Dent Res*. 1975;56:114–120.

88. Chung DM, Oh TJ, Shotwell B, et al. *Significance of Keratinized Mucosa in Maintenance of Dental Implants with Different Surface Conditions [Master's Thesis]*. Ann Arbor: Mich: University of Michigan; 2005.

89. Belser UC. The influence of altered working side occlusal guidance on masticatory muscles and related jaw movement. *J Prosthet Dent*. 1985;53:406–413.

90. Michael CG, Javid NS, Colaizzi FA, et al. Biting strength and chewing forces in complete denture wearers. *J Prosthet Dent*. 1990;3:549–553.

9

Dental Implant Surfaces

NEIL I. PARK AND MAYURI KERR

Introduction

Successful oral rehabilitation with dental implants is dependent on the interrelationship of the following key determinants of life-long osseointegration, presented by Albrektsson and colleagues:[1]

1. The status of the implant bed: The patient must exhibit a state of general health that will support the healing process. In addition, bone of sufficient quality and quantity is required.
2. The surgical technique: Successful treatment requires the use of proven surgical principles as well as the instruments, equipment, and techniques appropriate for the specific implant system.
3. Long-term loading: After successful implant placement, protocols for prosthesis design, selection of restorative materials, occlusal relationships, esthetics, and maintenance must be followed to support the long-term health of the implants.
4. Biocompatibility of the implant material: Dental implants must be constructed of materials that will be tolerated by the patient and not generate significant antigenic responses. Although commercially pure titanium (cpTi) and titanium alloys predominate, there are other materials, most notably zirconia, that are also used.
5. Implant macrostructure, or overall design of the implant: Although many different implant designs have been studied and used, the most widely used designs have converged to favor a tapered screw shape with an internal connection.
6. Implant microstructure, or surface: The surface of the implant and the response elicited from the patient's soft and hard tissues is the topic of this chapter. The surface structure of dental implants has proven to be critical for adhesion and differentiation of cells during the bone remodeling process essential to osseointegration.[2]

It is important to note that each of these factors is critical in treatment success; no single factor in isolation should be considered the keystone or most important determinant. In addition, it is notable that the last three determinants are controlled by the manufacturer of the implant, whereas the first three factors depend on patient characteristics and the skill of the treatment team. Although this chapter will deal with the macroscopic and microscopic nature of the implant surface and discuss its role in osseointegration and survival of dental implants, it is important to place this topic in the proper context of the overall treatment.

Surface Roughness

The process of osseointegration begins with the interaction of the cells in the immediate area with the implant surface. The surface roughness of dental implants has a significant effect on the process of osseointegration; it is crucial in the formation of bone because, although fibroblasts and epithelial cells adhere more strongly to smooth surfaces, rougher surfaces enhance the adhesion and differentiation of osteoblastic cells allowing for the deposition of bone.[3,4]

Osseointegration is a series of coordinated events, which include cell proliferation, transformation of osteoblasts, and bone formation. All of these are affected by different surface topographies.[5,6] Commonly used scientific parameters to describe the surface roughness are the two-dimensional Ra (profile roughness average) and the three-dimensional Sa (area roughness average).[7] Ra and Sa are considered to be valid and reliable parameters of surface roughness and are commonly used to describe the magnitude of the pits and fissures on implant surfaces. Ra is the arithmetic mean deviation of a linear profile, and Sa is the corresponding three-dimensional deviation. Surface roughness measurements are divided into the categories of smooth, minimally rough, moderately rough, and rough surfaces (Table 9.1).[8]

Smooth (Sa 0–0.4 μm) and minimally rough (Sa 0.5–1 μm) surfaces show weaker bone integration than rougher surfaces. Moderately rough (Sa 1–2 μm) surfaces showed stronger bone responses than rough (Sa > 2 μm) in some studies 43. Although the ideal surface roughness is undetermined, according to Albrektsson and Wennerberg,[9] moderately rough surfaces with Sa in the range of 1 to 2 μm seem to provide the optimal degree of roughness to promote osseointegration.

Structural features in the extracellular matrix are on the nanometer scale, and it is thought that biomaterials that mimic this environment might more effectively promote the processes of bone regeneration.[10] As nanotechnology advances, nanoscale surfaces have been introduced in dentistry as well. Nanotechnology involves materials with a surface roughness range between 1 and 100 nm, which are thought to influence the adsorption of proteins, adhesion of osteoblastic cells, and therefore the rate of osseointegration (Fig. 9.1).[11-14]

Review of Implant Surfaces

After the machining of a cpTi or titanium alloy implant, contact with air causes the immediate development of a titanium oxide surface on the implant. The first generation of osseointegrated dental implants, such as the Bränemark System (Nobel Biocare, Kloten, Switzerland), featured this surface. After being manufactured, these implants are subjected to cleaning, decontamination, and sterilization procedures. Scanning electron microscopy analysis showed that the surfaces of machined implants have grooves, ridges, and marks from the tools used for their manufacturing. These surface defects provide mechanical resistance through bone interlocking. Treatment performed with this type of surface requires a longer healing time between surgery and implant loading and should follow the original protocol suggested by Bränemark, with a 3- to 6-month healing time before loading.[15]

Until the late 1980s, further surface treatments were rarely performed. Since that time, several surface modifications have been developed in an effort to modify the surface roughness of the implant to promote the process of osseointegration, particularly in poor bone quality.[2]

Pits, grooves, and protrusions characterize the microtopography and contribute to an increase in surface area. Studies have shown increased levels of bone-to-implant contact (BIC) for microrough surfaces.[7,16] These modifications can be divided into subtractive and additive processes, depending on whether material is removed or deposited on the implant surface in the development of the surface.

Subtractive Processes

Etching with Acid

Acid treatment of a titanium implant removes the surface oxide and any contamination resulting in a clean and homogenous surface. The acids used include hydrochloric acid, sulfuric acid,

TABLE 9.1	Classification of Rough Surfaces	
Surface Roughness Category	**Sa Range**
Smooth	0–0.4 μm
Minimally rough	0.5–1 μm
Moderately rough	1–2 μm
Maximally rough	>2 μm

hydrofluoric acid, and nitric acid. Acid etching of titanium and titanium alloy implants results in uniform roughness with micro pits ranging in size from 0.5 to 2 μm, and an increase in surface area. Acid treatment of implant surfaces enhances osseointegration through improved migration and retention of osteogenic cells at the implant surface.[17]

Blasting with an Abrasive Material

Blasting the implant surface with hard ceramic particles projected through a nozzle at high velocity is another method of surface roughening. Different surface roughnesses can be achieved based on the size of the blasting media particles. Several materials have been used, including alumina, titanium oxide, and hydroxyapatite (HA). Wennerberg and colleagues compared blasted surfaces with different roughnesses and compared them with turned surfaces.[9,18-20] The blasted surfaces demonstrated a stronger bone response than the turned implants in rabbit bone.

Some blasting techniques involve the use of a resorbable blast media (RBM) that is biocompatible, such as HA, β-tricalcium phosphate ceramic particles, and biphasic calcium phosphates (CaPs). These biomaterials are resorbable, creating a textured surface. In the event that some of the blasting media remains on the implant surface, the media is resorbed during the healing process without affecting the biocompatibility.[8] Several studies have reported that the extent of the BIC in RBM implants is greater than that in machined implants.[21-23]

Implants with the RBM surface treatment, in which HA is used as the blast media, offer particular advantages because, unlike blasting with aluminum oxide, grit, or sand, any particles remaining on the surface are resorbable and do not affect healing in the immediate vicinity because of the presence of foreign particles. HA is also a component of bone; thus blasting with HA is not only biocompatible and resorbable but also osteoinductive. This produces a surface in the moderately rough category with an Sa of 1.49, which is in Wennerberg's recommended range of roughness. Blasting with alumina particles in the size range of 25 to 75 μm results in mean surface roughness in the range 0.5 to 1.5 μm,[18,24,25] whereas roughness in the range of 2 to 6 μm is

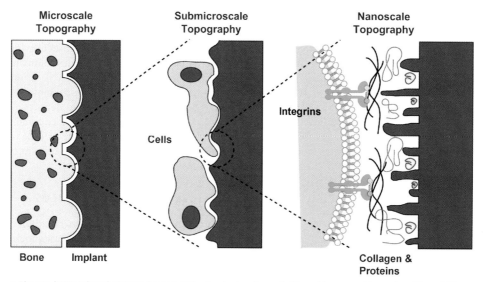

• **Fig. 9.1** Interactions between bone and the implant surface at different topographic scales. (From Gittens RO, McLachlan T, Olivares-Navarrette R, et al. The effects of combined micron-/submicron-scale surface roughness and nanoscale features on cell proliferation and differentiation. *Biomaterials.* 2011;32(13):3394–3403.)

reported for surfaces blasted with particles sized between 200 and 600 μm.[26,27] Use of fine particle size glass particles of 150 to 230 μm results in relatively smooth surface with an Ra value of 1.36 μm, whereas the use of coarse alumina particles of 200 to 500 μm provides a much rougher surface with an Ra value of 5.09 μm (Fig. 9.2).[28,29]

Treatment with Lasers

Lasers can also be used to modify implant surfaces by using an ablation technique. During laser ablation, the substrate material vaporizes and forms a crater. Depending on the material properties, a resolidified material forms a rim along the periphery of the crater. Laser ablation technology results in titanium surface microstructures with increased hardness, corrosion resistance, and purity with a standard roughness and thicker oxide layer.[30,31] Biological studies evaluating the role of titanium ablation topography and chemical properties showed the potential of the surface to orient osteoblast cell attachment and control the direction of ingrowth.[12,32]

Additive Processes

Additive processes share the same goal, which is to roughen the implant surface to accelerate osseointegration, particularly in lower bone densities:

Hydroxyapatite Coating and Titanium Plasma Spraying

Plasma spraying is an industrial technique in which the desired coating, in powder form, is injected through a plasma torch to melt the powder and shoot it onto the substrate surface, in which it is deposited and fuses with the surface. Plasma-sprayed coatings can be deposited with thicknesses ranging from a few micrometers to a few millimeters.

Plasma spraying has been used for applying titanium and HA coatings on the surfaces of titanium implants. This serves to roughen the surface of the implant, usually into the range of Ra 7 μm. This was considered to be an improvement over the machined surface because of the increased BIC. Additional studies[33] found that HA-coated implants stimulated bone growth during the healing phase (Table 9.2).

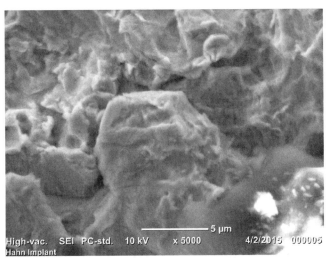

High-vac. SEI PC-std. 10 kV x 5000 4/2/2015 000005
Hahn Implant

• **Fig. 9.2** Resorbable blast media surface of the Hahn tapered implant. (From http://www.Hahnimplant.com.)

Despite the healing advantages found with HA-coated implants, in recent years they have fallen out of favor because of increased risk of complications. Implant failure can be caused by microbial infection and occlusal trauma.[35-37] It has been suggested that HA-coated implants are more susceptible to bacterial colonization than uncoated implants or natural teeth.[38] Enhanced growth of biofilm on HA-coated implant surfaces may result from the increased roughness, which then contributes to peri-implantitis.[39,40]

If marginal bone loss occurs, it will lead to the HA surface implant becoming exposed to the oral environment with resultant contamination. In this case it would also be more difficult for the patient to maintain the implant, resulting in increased risk of peri-implant disease.[41,42] Another concern associated with HA-coated implants is dissolution of the HA layer or fracture of the HA coating–titanium interface, which leads to loss of the coating with subsequent implant mobility and loss.[39,43-45]

Overall, there are major concerns with the use of plasma-sprayed coatings. In the case of both HA and titanium plasma spray (TPS)–coated implants, the surface roughness is at a higher level than the moderately rough that is currently considered optimal. Such rough surfaces are also thought to contribute to the spread of peri-implantitis when the surface is exposed to the oral cavity and facilitates the formation and retention of plaque. As with the HA coatings, delamination of the titanium particles in TPS implants has been observed leading to mobility and eventual loss of the implants.

Oxidation or Anodization

Although all cpTi and titanium alloy implants develop an oxide layer on exposure to air, oxidized implants have been subjected to additional treatment to significantly thicken this layer. In the process of anodic oxidation, the titanium surface to be treated serves as the anode in an electrolytic cell with acid solutions serving as the electrolyte. The thickness of the oxide layer is controlled by altering the voltage and the electrolyte solution.

After such treatment, the surface oxide increases from an approximately 5-nm thickness to 3 μm or more. A positive correlation was found between increasing height deviation of the treated surface and implant healing when oxidized implants prepared at different voltages were compared. This means that implants with a thicker oxidation layer had greater BIC compared with those with a thinner oxide layer. However, an oxide layer greater than 3 μm in thickness did not cause any further increase in bone implant contact (Table 9.3).[46]

Biological Responses and Interaction with the Implant Surface

Osseointegration of a dental implant after placement into a prepared osteotomy follows three stages of repair:[12] (1) initial formation of a blood clot, (2) cellular activation, and (3) cellular response.[47] After implant placement, blood components interact with dental implant surfaces, leading to the adsorption of plasma proteins such as fibrin on the implant surface. The migration of bone cells necessary for osseointegration then occurs through the fibrin clot. The ability of an implant surface design to retain fibrin during the wound contraction phase of healing is critical in determining whether the migrating cells will reach the implant. Bone cells reach the implant surface by migration through fibrin and other early structural matrix proteins and lay down bone on the implant surface itself. Moderately rough and rough surfaces

TABLE 9.2	Different Techniques to Deposit Hydroxyapatite Coating[34]			
Technique	**Thickness**	**Advantages**		**Disadvantages**
Plasma spraying	$<20\ \mu m$	Rapid deposition; sufficiently low cost; fast bone healing, less risk for coating degradation		Poor adhesion, alternation of HA structure caused by the coating process; nonuniformity in coating density; extreme high temperature up to 1200°C, phase transformation and grain grow of substance caused by high-temperature procedure; increase in residual stress; unable to produce complete crystalline HA coating
Thermal spraying	$30–200\ \mu m$	High deposition rates; low cost		Line-of-sight technique; high temperatures induce decomposition; rapid cooling produces amorphous coatings; lack of uniformity; crack appearance; low porosity; coating spalling and interface separation between the coating and the substrate
Sputter coating	$0.5–3\ \mu m$	Uniform coating thickness on flat substrates; dense coating; homogenous coating; high adhesion		Line-of-sight technique; expensive and time-consuming; produces amorphous coatings; low crystallite, which accelerates the dissolution of the film in the body
Pulsed laser deposition	$0.05–5\ mm$	Coating that is crystalline and amorphous; coating that is dense and porous; ability to produce wide range of multilayer coatings from different materials; ability to produce high crystalline HA coating; ability to restore complex stoichiometry; high degree of control on deposition parameters		Line-of-sight technique; expensive and time-consuming; produces amorphous coating; low crystalline, which accelerates the dissolution of the film in the body line-of-sight technique splashing or particle deposition; needs surface pretreatment; lack of uniformity
Dip coating	$<1\ \mu m$	Inexpensive; coatings applied quickly; can coat complex substrates; high surface uniformity; good speed of coating		Requires high sintering temperatures; thermal expansion mismatch; crack appearance
Sol-gel	$0.1–2.0\ \mu m$	Can coat complex shapes; low processing temperatures; relatively cheap because coatings are very thin; simple deposition method; high purity; high corrosion resistance; fairly good adhesion		Some processes require controlled atmosphere processing; expensive raw materials; not suitable for industrial scale; high permeability; low wear resistance; hard to control the porosity
Electrophoretic deposition	$0.1–2.0\ mm$	Uniform coating thickness; rapid deposition rates; can coat complex substrates; simple setup, low cost, high degree of control on coating morphology and thickness; good mechanical strength; high adhesion for n-HA		Difficult to produce crack-free coatings; requires high sintering temperatures; HA decomposition during sintering stage
Hot isostatic pressing	$0.2–2.0\ mm$	Produces dense coatings; produces net-shape ceramics; good temperature control; homogeneous structure; high uniformity; high precision; no dimensional or shape limitation		Cannot coat complex substrates; high temperature required; thermal expansion mismatch; elastic property differences; expensive; removal/interaction of encapsulation material
Ion beam–assisted deposition	$<0.03\ \mu m$	Low temperature process; high reproducibility and reliability; high adhesion; wide atomic intermix zones are coating-to-substrate interface		Crack appearance on the coated surface

HA, Hydroxyapatite.

From Mohseni E, Zalnezhad E, Bushroa AR. Comparative investigation on the adhesion of hydroxyapatite coating on Ti-6Al-4V implant: a review paper. *Int J Adhes*. 2014;40:230–257.

promote this activity by providing surface features with which fibrin can become entangled and by increasing the available surface area for fibrin attachment.[48] This leads to greater BIC and improved osseointegration. Implant surface properties also have the potential to alter ionic interactions, protein adsorption, and cellular activity at the implant surface (Fig. 9.3).[49]

Bone cell migration and bone formation observed on titanium implant surfaces are also thought to be related to the similarity between the microroughness of the surface and the pit irregularities found in natural bone surfaces resulting from osteoclast activity.[50,51]

After implant placement, remodeling of the surrounding bone occurs by osteoclastic activity, which removes some of the existing bone around the implant. The natural surface of the demineralized bone matrix created by osteoclast resorption processes is rough and pitted. This becomes the recipient surface for new bone formation. Submicron scale features $<1\ \mu m$ with undercuts allow the deposition of bone matrix, micron scale surface features $<10\ \mu m$ mimic a single osteoclast resorption pit, and macroscale cavities $>10\ \mu m$ are similar to resorption activity of one or more osteoclasts.[52-54] As with natural bone, osteoblasts find these surface irregularities and begin depositing matrix in and around them to form bone.

TABLE 9.3	Surface Treatments and Various Implant Systems Available Commercially	
Surface Treatment	**Implant System/Surface**	
Blasted and acid washed/etched Implants undergo a blasting process. Afterward, the surface is either washed with nonetching acid or etched with strong acids. RBM-treated implants like the Hahn Tapered Implants have the advantage of resorbable, biocompatible blast media.	Hahn Tapered Implants, DENTSPLY Implants FRI-ALIT and FRIADENT plus, Straumann SLA, Inclusive Tapered Implants	
Anodized This electrochemical process thickens and roughens the titanium oxide layer on the surface of implants.	Nobel Biocare TiUnite	
Acid etched Etching with strong acids increases the surface roughness and the surface area of titanium implants.	BIOMET 3i OSSEOTITE and NanoTite	
Blasted Particles are projected through a nozzle at a high velocity onto the implant. Various materials such as titanium dioxide, aluminum dioxide, and HA are often used.	DENTSPLY Implants ASTRA TECH TiOblast, Zimmer Dental MTX	
HA coated HA is an osteoconductive material that has the ability to form a strong bond between the bone and the implant.	Implant Direct (various), Zimmer Dental MP-1	
Laser ablation High-intensity pulses of a laser beam strike a protective layer that coats the metallic surface. As a result, implants demonstrate a honeycomb pattern with small pores.	BioHorizons Laser-Lok	
Titanium plasma sprayed Powdery forms of titanium are injected into a plasma torch at elevated temperatures.	Straumann ITI titanium plasma-sprayed	

HA, Hydroxyapatite; *RBM*, resorbable blast media.

From Bullis G, Shreya S. Implant surface treatments: a literature review. *Inclusive Mag.* 2014;5(2).

In summary, microroughness on implant surfaces helps in retention of the fibrin clot. This in turn enables the migration of bone progenitor cells that deposit bone in close proximity to the implant improving the BIC. Pits on the implant surface mimic naturally occurring osteoclastic activity and lead osteoblasts to deposit bone on the surface of the implant, leading to improved osseointegration.

Role of Surface Roughness in Peri-implant Disease

Several studies recognized surface roughness as an important factor in the formation of biofilm on implant surfaces.[55,56] By their nature, rougher surfaces encourage more biofilm formation.[57-60]

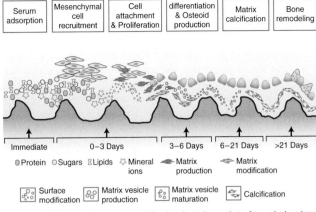

• **Fig. 9.3** Cellular phenomena at the implant–bone interface during healing of implant. (From Anil S, et al. Dental implant surface enhancement and osseointegration. In Turkyilmaz I, ed. *Implant Dentistry: A Rapidly Evolving Practice.* London, UK: InTech; 2011.)

Biofilm formation is directly proportional to surface roughness; the greater the roughness, the higher the rate of biofilm formation is around the implants. The wettability and surface free energy (SFE) of a specific surface also influence the biofilm formation on implants.[57]

Future Directions

Several additional surfaces are being explored as options to improve osseointegration and the rate of bone healing.

Bisphosphonate Surfaces

Bisphosphates are antiresorptive agents known to inhibit osteoclast activity that are used in the treatment of osteoporosis. Bisphosphate-loaded implant surfaces have been reported to improve implant osseointegration.[61,62] It has been shown that bisphosphonate incorporated onto titanium implants increased bone density locally in the peri-implant region[63] with the effect of the antiresorptive drug limited to the vicinity of the implant.[12] An animal study conducted by Peter and colleagues showed a positive effect of zoledronate-coated implants on the peri-implant bone volume fraction in osteoporotic rats.[64]

Abtahi and colleagues conducted a double-blind split-mouth study in which each patient received one bisphosphonate-coated implant and one uncoated implant. After 6 months of osseointegration, resonance frequency analysis indicated better fixation of the coated implants. The implants were coated by using a nanometer-thin fibrinogen coating containing minimal amounts of bisphosphonates that improved early implant fixation with an effect that was maintained at 5 years after prosthetic loading. Reduced marginal bone resorption was also seen. All implants functioned well.[65] At 5 years, the bisphosphonate-coated implants showed only a small amount of resorption (median 0.20 mm). The present data suggest that bisphosphonate-coated implants enable prolonged preservation of the marginal bone.[66] Histologic analysis of test implants removed en bloc at the 6-month follow-up showed mature lamellar bone trabeculae in intimate contact with the implants.[67]

Bisphosphonates inhibit the resorption and renewal of bone mediated by osteoclasts, retaining existing bone, which may increase mineralization under normal function, resulting in an increase in bone mineral density.[68] The prevention of osteoclast-mediated bone resorption and renewal influenced by bisphosphonates results in retention of old bone. Old bone lives out its natural life span and becomes brittle.[69] This may create a nonideal local environment for increased BIC. Bisphosphonates can work as a bony shield to protect the early formed bone, which may explain better fixation seen in some studies.[70]

Statins

Statins are commonly prescribed drugs that decrease cholesterol synthesis by the liver. This reduces serum cholesterol concentrations and lowers the risk of heart attack.[71] Simvastatin induces the expression of bone morphogenetic protein 2 (BMP-2) mRNA that promotes bone formation.[72] Ayukawa and colleagues[73] confirmed that topical application of statins to alveolar bone increased bone formation and concurrently suppressed osteoclast activity at the bone-healing site. In addition, clinical studies reported that statin use is associated with increased bone mineral density.[74-78]

Antibiotic Coating

Antibacterial coatings on the surface of implants that provide antibacterial activity to the implants themselves have been studied as a possible way to prevent surgical site infections associated with implants. Gentamycin, along with the layer of HA, can be coated onto the implant surface, which may act as a local prophylactic agent along with the systemic antibiotics in dental implant surgery.[79] Tetracycline enhances blood clot attachment and retention on the implant surface during the initial phase of the healing process, promoting osseointegration.[12,80]

Functionalization with Biologically Active Substances

The purpose of functionalization of the implant surface with biologically active substances is to diminish the initial inflammatory response after torquing in of the implant and encouraging rapid bone growth. Growth factors and fragments of the organic matrix of bone and other known biologically active peptides are used to coat the surface of implants.[81,82]

There are several growth factors involved in osteogenesis. Four growth factors have potential use in implantology: BMP-2 and BMP-7, fibroblast growth factor (FGF-2), and platelet-derived growth factor (PDGF-B).[83,84]

PDGF-B is a potent mitogen and chemotactic agent for a variety of mesenchymal cells, including osteoblasts.[85] Recently, Chang and colleagues[85] have demonstrated that PDGF stimulates osseointegration of dental implants in vivo. On the other hand, it has been reported that the isolated recombinant PDGF may affect bone formation adversely.[85]

In clinics, the use of platelet-rich plasma or platelet-fibrin clot is the equivalent of pure PDGF usage. This method is gaining popularity because it is safe, and it is possible to use autologous source of growth factors. The method has shown good results in a number of clinical studies.[86-88]

BMPs are a family of growth factors that are present during early stages of bone healing and play an important role in the growth and differentiation of several cell types, including osteoblasts.[89,90] BMP-2 is often used in bone-implant interaction studies because it seems to possess the highest osteoinductive potential among the BMPs.[91] BMPs may be applied to bone sites through various delivery systems such as an absorbable collagen sponge used to augment the bone ridge before implant placement or implants with porous structures coated with rhBMP-2.[92] However, coating an implant is an unreliable way of delivering similar dosages uniformly. The rhBMPs and BMPs are costly, have a high dose requirement (several micrograms up to milligrams), and have a poor distribution profile.[93,94] High doses of BMP-2 have been associated with localized and temporary bone impairment[95] or increased bone resorption caused by stimulation of osteoclast formation.[96] However, once the levels drop, normal bone formation is observed.[70]

Usage of Biologically Active Peptides

Proteins of extracellular bone matrix also have potential use as functional coatings. For example, fibronectin stimulated osteoblastic differentiation and tissue mineralization and contributed to strong osseointegration of implants in experimental models in vivo.[97-99]

Common problems associated with the use of growth factors and biologically active peptides are increase in the cost of implants treated with them, complications with usage, and preservation of the bioactive material before implantation. There are also concerns about the release profile of these components into surrounding tissues (rate of release, area of release, etc.).

Zirconia Implants

In recent years, yttria-stabilized tetragonal zirconia polycrystal (Y-TZP), a high-strength zirconia, has become an attractive new material for dental implants. Zirconia has a tooth-like color and the ability to transmit light, improving the overall esthetic outcome.[100] Moreover, it has a high chemical resistance, high flexural strength (900–1200 MPa), a favorable fracture toughness (KIC; 7–10 MPa/m$^{1/2}$), and a Young's modulus of 210 GPa, which makes it a strong material.[101] Zirconia also has a low affinity for dental plaque, which reduces the risk of inflammatory changes in the peri-implant soft tissues.[102-104]

Zirconia implants are often one-piece implants, which means that both the implant body and the permucosal portion can be digitally designed to fit the local anatomic conditions and individually machined. One-piece implants have the advantage of no implant-abutment movement.[105] Zirconia implants perform well in areas with thin soft tissue biotype and in cases in which soft tissue recession might expose some part of the implant. These advantages make Y-TZP implants a potential alternative to titanium implants in certain clinical situations,[100,105] as well as opening up the possibility for computer-aided design and computer-aided manufacturing (CAD/CAM) of customized zirconia implants.[104]

Surface modifications of zirconia implants such as sandblasting and acid etching trigger tetragonal-to-monoclinic (t → m)phase transformation.[105] This transformation is associated with 3% to 4% phase volume expansion and induces compressive stresses that shield the crack tip from the applied stress.[106] This unique characteristic is known as transformation toughening.[107] However, the surface flaws introduced by sandblasting and acid etching act as stress concentrators and may become potential sites for crack initiation and propagation, causing strength degradation and the possibility of implant fracture.[108,109]

Depprich and colleagues[52] conducted an animal study to compare the osseointegration of acid-etched titanium and zirconia implants of similar macrostructure and found that the BIC during the process of osseointegration was very similar. Langhoff and colleagues[110] conducted a study in sheep using six types of implants with identical implant geometry. All titanium and zirconia implants were sandblasted and partially etched before the surface treatments, similar to the reference. The surfaces of the chemically modified implants were either plasma anodized or coated with CaP. The pharmacologically modified implants were either coated with bisphosphonate or collagen type I. An acid-etched and sandblasted implant made of titanium (grade 4; SPI 1 ELEMENT, Thommen Medical AG, Waldenburg, Switzerland) served as the reference and control for the surface modifications.

The collagen coating was based on an extracellular matrix containing chondroitin sulfate, prepared by fibrillogenesis of the collagen in the presence of chondroitin sulfate, and performed as dip coating in a collagen/chondroitin sulfate solution. The bisphosphonate-coated implants were immobilized with an alendronate solution to a final concentration of 10 mg/cm^2. The zirconia implants were manufactured from yttrium partially stabilized zirconia, medical grade. The zirconia implants were sandblasted and etched in an alkaline bath.

Results of the BIC measurements showed that all titanium implant types were nearly similar at 2 weeks (59%–62% BIC) and increased with time (78%–83%), except the plasma-anodized surface (58%). The two chemical surface modifications performed very differently. The CaP surface showed similar values, with the main increase at 2 to 4 weeks, similar to the reference, and a slight increase toward week 8. In contrast, the plasma-anodized surface lost 2% bone contact initially and did not improve after 4 weeks. Pharmacologically modified surfaces performed close to the reference. The collagen with chondroitin sulfate surface showed slightly higher values than the reference implant at 2 weeks and continued nearly equally, whereas the bisphosphonate-coated surface was higher at 2 and 4 weeks. The zirconia implant presented 20% more bone contact than the titanium implants at 2 weeks, improved toward 4 weeks, then reduced at 8 weeks to below the level of the reference surface. The overall performance of the new surfaces, except the plasma-anodized surface, was better than the reference. Statistically significant differences for BIC were not found.

Biomimetic Formation of Hydroxyapatite on the Implant Surface

The use of coatings with similar composition of the human bone provide an accelerated osseointegration during the earliest healing stages. In particular, CaP apatite has the same chemical composition as the mineral bone phase, which means there is no inflammatory reaction.[111] Many researchers have applied coatings on titanium implants by using techniques like HA plasma spraying.[112] In some clinical studies,[113] this treatment produced a quicker osseointegration at early stages after implant placement, but an accelerated bone loss caused by a bacterial microleakage between the HA layer and the titanium has been observed in the long term.[114] Furthermore, additive techniques such as HA plasma spraying do not allow the formation of crystalline apatite such as in human bone, but amorphous CaP can be caused by high elaboration temperatures.[114] The properties of this layer are not considered appropriate for dental implants because they are extremely soluble, and titanium only achieves mechanical retention and not true adhesion.[115]

Osseointegration of dental implants can be improved by the application of CaP coating by plasma spraying and biomimetic and electrophoretic deposition. Although plasma-sprayed HA-coated dental implants have disadvantages related to coating delamination and heterogeneous dissolution rate of deposited phases, an electrochemical process consisting of depositing CaP crystals from supersaturated solutions releases calcium and phosphate ions from these coatings. This process helps in the precipitation of biological apatite nanocrystals with the incorporation of various proteins, which, in turn, promotes cell adhesion, differentiation into osteoblast, and the synthesis of mineralized collagen (the extracellular matrix of bone tissue).[12,116]

Osteoclast cells are also able to resorb the CaP coatings and activate osteoblast cells to produce bone tissue. Thus these CaP coatings promote a direct bone–implant contact without an intervening connective tissue layer leading to a proper biomechanical fixation of dental implants.[12] Osteoclast cells are also able to resorb the CaP coatings and activate osteoblast cells to produce bone tissue. Thus these CaP coatings promote a direct bone–implant contact without an intervening connective tissue layer, leading to a proper biomechanical fixation of dental implants.[12]

Implants coated with CaP have a better BIC compared with currently available titanium implants. Implants coated with CaP claim to offer a physicochemical matrix for the deposition of new bone by osteoclasts, which could explain the increased BIC. It also leads to an increased attachment of osteogenic cells.[117] Ions released from CaP coating have been reported to control the cellular signals that improve osteoblast differentiation.[118] These ions have a potential to stimulate numerous intracellular signaling pathways in osteoblasts and support the bone formation process.[70,119] Even though it has been suggested that CaP coatings can enhance adhesion/activation of bone cells on the surface of implants,[120] possible delamination of the coating from the surface of the titanium implant and failure at the implant/coating interface may happen when the coating is rather thick.[121]

The hope of developing bioactive implant surfaces is to significantly reduce the time required for osseointegration. The most important mechanisms involved are the protein adsorption capacity, wettability, and an optimized zeta potential, which reduces the electrostatic dispersion between particles. These procedures also aim to increase adhesion, proliferation, and differentiation of osteoblast cells compared with other current surface treatments to facilitate bone formation around the implants.[122]

Alenezi and colleagues investigated the effects of the use of local drug and chemical compound delivery systems on the osseointegration of endosseous implants in animal models. They looked at chemical agents incorporated, coated, or immobilized on implant surfaces and also at chemical agents that were locally delivered at the implant site using carrier materials such as injectable gels, microsphere hydrogel, or collagen sponges. BIC was evaluated for CaP, bisphosphonates, and BMPs. They found that implants coated with CaP and BMPs showed statistically significant bone growth compared with uncoated implants.[70] Well-designed clinical trials will help us better understand the effect of these coatings of implant surfaces and their interaction with bone, as well as the long-term success of these biochemical modifications.

Summary

Our understanding of the role played by dental implant surfaces in the process of osseointegration continues to evolve as research provides additional insights. Research continues in the areas of surface treatments, chemical modifications, and how they both influence the cellular and biological processes. With current reported success rates well above 90%, it is unlikely that new surfaces will provide incremental improvement of these overall rates. However, improvements in outcomes in poor bone quality and in medically compromised patients may well be enhanced by future developments.

References

1. Albrektsson T, Zarb G, Worthington P, Eriksson AR. The long-term efficacy of currently used dental implants: a review and proposed criteria of success. *Int J Oral Maxillofac Implants.* 1986;1:11–25.
2. Smeets R, Stadlinger B, Schwarz F, et al. Impact of dental implant surface modifications on osseointegration. *Biomed Res Int.* 2016;2:1–15.
3. Boyan B, Dean D, Lohmann C. The titanium-bone cell interface in vitro: the role of the surface in promoting osteointegration. In: Brunette D, et al., ed. *Titanium in Medicine.* Springer; 2001.
4. Wennerberg A, Albrektsson T. Suggested guidelines for the topographic evaluation of implant surfaces. *Int J Oral Maxillofac Implants.* 2000;15:331–344.
5. Burger EH, Klein-Nulend J. Mechanotransduction in bone—role of the lacuno-canalicular network. *FASEB J.* 1999;13(suppl):S101–S112. https://doi.org/10.1096/fasebj.13.9001.s101.
6. Mathieu V, Vayron R, Richard G, et al. Biomechanical determinants of the stability of dental implants: influence of the bone-implant interface properties. *J Biomech.* 2014;47:3–13. https://doi.org/10.1016/j.jbiomech.2013.09.021.
7. Dohan Ehrenfest DM, Coelho PG, Kang BS, et al. Classification of osseointegrated implant surfaces: materials, chemistry and topography. *Trends Biotechnol.* 2010;28:198–206. https://doi.org/10.1016/j.tibtech.2009.12.003.
8. Le Guéhennec L, Soueidan A, Layrolle P, Amouriq Y. Surface treatments of titanium dental implants for rapid osseointegration. *Dent Mater.* 2007;23:844–854. https://doi.org/10.1016/j.dental.2006.06.025.
9. Albrektsson T, Wennerberg A. Oral implant surfaces: part 1—review focusing on topographic and chemical properties of different surfaces and in vivo responses to them. *Int J Prosthodont.* 17(5):536–543.
10. Yeo IS. Reality of dental implant surface modification: a short literature review. *Open Biomed Eng J.* 2014;8:114–119. https://doi.org/10.2174/1874120701408010114.
11. Brett PM, Harle J, Salih V, et al. Tonetti, Roughness response genes in osteoblasts. *Bone.* 2004;35:124–133. https://doi.org/10.1016/j.bone.2004.03.009.
12. Anil S, Anand PSS, Alghamdi H, Jansen JA. Dental implant surface enhancement and osseointegration. In: Turkyilmaz I, ed. *Implant Dentistry: A Rapidly Evolving Practice.* InTech; 2011.
13. Rasouli R, Barhoum A, Uludag H. A review of nanostructured surfaces and materials for dental implants: surface coating, patterning and functionalization for improved performance. *Biomater Sci.* 2018;6:1312–1338. https://doi.org/10.1039/c8bm00021b.
14. Gittens RA, Mclachlan T, Cai Y, et al. The effects of combined micron-/submicron-scale surface roughness and nanoscale features on cell proliferation and differentiation. *Biomaterials.* 2011;32:3395–3403. https://doi.org/10.1016/j.biomaterials.2011.01.029.
15. Wennerberg A, Albrektsson T. Effects of titanium surface topography on bone integration: a systematic review. *Clin Oral Implants Res.* 2009;20:172–184. https://doi.org/10.1111/j.1600-0501.2009.01775.x.
16. Fischer K, Stenberg T. Prospective 10-year cohort study based on a Randomized Controlled Trial (RCT) on implant-supported Full-Arch Maxillary Prostheses. Part 1: sandblasted and acid-etched implants and mucosal tissue. *Clin Implant Dent Relat Res.* 2012;14:808–815. https://doi.org/10.1111/j.1708-8208.2011.00389.x.
17. Takeuchi M, Abe Y, Yoshida Y, et al. Acid pretreatment of titanium implants. *Biomaterials.* 2003;24:1821–1827. https://doi.org/10.1016/S0142-9612(02)00576-8.
18. Wennerberg A, Albrektsson T, Johansson C, Andersson B. Experimental study of turned and grit-blasted screws shape implants with special emphasis on effects of blasting in material and surface topoghaphy. *Biomaterials.* 1996;17:15–22.
19. Wennerberg A. The role of surface roughness for implant incorporation in bone. *Cells Materials.* 1999;9(1):1–19.
20. Wennerberg A, Albrektsson T, Andersson B. Bone tissue response to commercially pure titanium implants blasted with fine and coarse particles of aluminum oxide. *Int J Oral Maxillofac Implant.* 1996;11:38–45.
21. Piattelli M, Scarano A, Paolantonio M, et al. Bone response to machined and resorbable blast material titanium implants: an experimental study in rabbits. *J Oral Implantol.* 2002;28:2–8. https://doi.org/10.1563/1548-1336(2002)028<0002:BRTMAR>2.3.CO;2.
22. Oates TW, Arnold AM, Cagna DR, et al. Histomorphometric analysis of the bone-implant contact obtained with 4 different implant surface treatments placed side by side in the dog mandible. *Implant Dent.* 2002;11:394. https://doi.org/10.1097/00008505-200211040-00051.
23. Kang HG, Jeong YS, Huh YH, et al. Impact of surface chemistry modifications on speed and strength of osseointegration. *Int J Oral MaxIllOfac Implant.* 2018;33:780–787. https://doi.org/10.11607/jomi.5871.
24. Wennerberg A, Albrektsson T, Lausmaa J. Torque and histomorphometric evaluation of c.p. titanium screws blasted with 25- and 75-microns-sized particles of Al2O3. *J Biomed Mater Res.* 1996;30:251–260.
25. Pypen CM, Plenk H, Ebel MF, et al. Characterization of microblasted and reactive ion etched surfaces on the commercially pure metals niobium, tantalum and titanium. *J Mater Sci Mater Med.* 1997;8:781–784.
26. Buser D, Schenk RK, Steinemann S, et al. Influence of surface characteristics on bone integration of titanium implants. A histomorphometric study in miniature pigs. *J Biomed Mater Res.* 1991;25:889–902. https://doi.org/10.1002/jbm.820250708.
27. Sittig C, Textor M, Spencer ND, et al. Surface characterization of implant materials c.p. Ti, Ti-6Al-7Nb and Ti-6Al-4V with different pretreatments. *J Mater Sci Mater Med.* 1999;10:35–46. https://doi.org/10.1023/A:1008840026907.
28. Alla RK, Ginjupalli K, Upadhya N, et al. Surface roughness of implants: a review. *Trends Biomater Artif Organs.* 2011;25:112–118.
29. Wieland M, Chehroudi B, Textor M, Brunette DM. Use of Ti-coated replicas to investigate the effects on fibroblast shape of surfaces with varying roughness and constant chemical composition. *J Biomed Mater Res.* 2002;60:434–444.
30. Gaggl A, Schultes G, Mu D, Ka H. Scanning electron microscopical analysis of laser-treated titanium implant surfaces - a comparative study. *Biomaterials.* 2000;21:1067–1073.
31. Hallgren C, Reimers H, Chakarov D, et al. An in vivo study of bone response to implants topographically modified by laser micromachining. *Biomaterials.* 2003;24(5):701–710.
32. Frenkel SR, Simon J, Alexander H, et al. Osseointegration on metallic implant surfaces: effects of microgeometry and growth factor treatment. *J Biomed Mater Res.* 2002;63:706–713. https://doi.org/10.1002/jbm.10408.

33. Clark PA, Rodriguez A, Sumner DR, et al. Biomechanics and mechanotransduction in cells and tissues modulation of bone ingrowth of rabbit femur titanium implants by in vivo axial micro-mechanical loading. *J Appl Physiol.* 2005;98:1922–1929. https://doi.org/10.1152/japplphysiol.01080.2004.-Titanium.

34. Mohseni E, Zalnezhad E, Bushroa AR. Comparative investigation on the adhesion of hydroxyapatite coating on Ti-6Al-4V implant: a review paper. *Int J Adhes Adhes.* 2014;48:238–257. https://doi.org/10.1016/j.ijadhadh.2013.09.030.

35. Rosenberg ES, Torosian JP, Slots J. Microbial differences in 2 clinically distinct types of failures of osseointegrated implants. *Clin Oral Implants Res.* 1991;2(3):135–144.

36. Verheyen CCPM, Dhert WJA, Petit PLC, et al. In vitro study on the integrity of a hydroxylapatite coating when challenged with staphylococci. *J Biomed Mater Res.* 1993;27(6):775–781. https://doi.org/10.1002/jbm.820270610.

37. Ichikawa T, Hirota K, Kanitani H, et al. Rapid bone resorption adjacent to hydroxyapatite-coated implants. *J Oral Implantol.* 1996;22:232–235.

38. Johnson BW. HA-coated dental implants: long-term consequences. *J Calif Dent Assoc.* 1992;20:33–41.

39. Ong JL, Chan D, Chan DCN. Hydroxyapatite and their use as coatings in dental implants: a review. *Artic Crit Rev Biomed Eng.* 2000;28:1–41. https://doi.org/10.1615/CritRevBiomedEng.v28.i56.10.

40. Rams TE, Roberts TW, Feik D, et al. Clinical and microbiological findings on newly inserted hydroxyapatite-coated and pure titanium human dental implants. *Clin Oral Implants Res.* (n.d.);2:121–127.

41. Zablotsky M, Meffert R, Mills O, et al. The macroscopic, microscopic and spectrometric effects of various chemotherapeutic agents on the plasma-sprayed hydroxyapatite-coated implant surface. *Clin Oral Implants Res.* 1992;3:189–198. https://doi.org/10.1034/j.1600-0501.1992.030406.x.

42. Zablotsky MH, Diedrich DL, Meffert RM. Detoxification of endotoxin-contaminated titanium and hydroxyapatite-coated surfaces utilizing various chemotherapeutic and mechanical modalities. *Implant Dent.* 1992;1:154–158.

43. Takeshita F, Kuroki H, Yamasaki A, Suetsugu T. Histopathologic observation of seven removed endosseous dental implants. *Int J Oral Maxillofac Implants.* (n.d.);10:367–372.

44. Takeshita F, Ayukawa Y, Iyama S, et al. A histologic evaluation of retrieved hydroxyapatite-coated blade-form implants using scanning electron, light, and confocal laser scanning microscopies. *J Periodontol.* 1996;67:1034–1040. https://doi.org/10.1902/jop.1996.67.10.1034.

45. Nancollas G, Tucker B. Dissolution kinetics characterization of hydroxyapatite coatings on dental implants. *J Oral Implant.* 1994;20.

46. Choi W, Heo SJ, Koak JY, et al. Biological responses of anodized titanium implants under different current voltages. *J Oral Rehabil.* 2006;33:889–897. https://doi.org/10.1111/j.1365-2842.2006.01669.x.

47. Stanford CM, Schneider GB. Functional behaviour of bone around dental implants. *Gerodontology.* 2004;21:71–77.

48. Davies JE. Understanding peri-implant endosseous healing. *J Dent Educ.* 2003;67(8):932–949.

49. Schliephake H, Scharnweber D, Dard M, et al. Functionalization of dental implant surfaces using adhesion molecules. *J Biomed Mater Res B Appl Biomater.* 2005;73(1):88–96. https://doi.org/10.1002/jbm.b.30183.

50. Mendonça G, Mendonça DBS, Aragão FJL, Cooper LF. Advancing dental implant surface technology - From micron- to nanotopography. *Biomaterials.* 2008;29:3822–3835. https://doi.org/10.1016/j.biomaterials.2008.05.012.

51. Ellingsen JE, Lyngstadaas SP. *Bio-Implant Interface: Improving Biomaterials and Tissue Reactions.* CRC Press; 2003.

52. Depprich R, Zipprich H, Ommerborn M, et al. Osseointegration of zirconia implants: an SEM observation of the bone-implant interface. *Head Face Med.* 2008;4:25. https://doi.org/10.1186/1746-160X-4-25.

53. Rupp F, Liang L, Geis-Gerstorfer J, et al. Surface characteristics of dental implants: a review. *Dent Mater.* 2018;34:40–57. https://doi.org/10.1016/j.dental.2017.09.007.

54. Davies JE, Ajami E, Moineddin R, Mendes VC. *The Roles of Different Scale Ranges of Surface Implant Topography on the Stability of the Bone/Implant Interface*; 2013. https://doi.org/10.1016/j.biomaterials.2013.01.024.

55. Teughels W, Van Assche N, Sliepen I, Quirynen M. Effect of material characteristics and/or surface topography on biofilm development. *Clin Oral Implants Res.* 2006:1768–1781. https://doi.org/10.1111/j.1600-0501.2006.01353.x.

56. Bürgers R, Gerlach T, Hahnel S, et al. In vivo and in vitro biofilm formation on two different titanium implant surfaces. *Clin Oral Implants Res.* 2010;21:156–164. https://doi.org/10.1111/j.1600-0501.2009.01815.x.

57. Han A, Tsoi JKH, Rodrigues FP, et al. Bacterial adhesion mechanisms on dental implant surfaces and the influencing factors. *Int J Adhes Adhes.* 2016;69:58–71. https://doi.org/10.1016/j.ijadhadh.2016.03.022.

58. Quirynen M, Bollen CM. The influence of surface roughness and surface-free energy on supra- and subgingival plaque formation in man. a review of the literature. *J Clin Periodontol.* 1995;22:1–14.

59. Xing R, Lyngstadaas SP, Ellingsen JE, et al. The influence of surface nanoroughness, texture and chemistry of TiZr implant abutment on oral biofilm accumulation. *Clin Oral Implants Res.* 2015;26:649–656. https://doi.org/10.1111/clr.12354.

60. Elter C, Heuer W, Demling A, et al. Supra-and subgingival biofilm formation on implant abutments with different surface characteristics. *Int J Oral Maxillofac Implants.* 2008;23(2):327–334.

61. Kwak HB, Kim JY, Kim KJ, et al. Risedronate directly inhibits osteoclast differentiation and inflammatory bone loss. *Biol Pharm Bull.* 2009;32:1193–1198. https://doi.org/10.1248/bpb.32.1193.

62. Yoshinari M, Oda Y, Inoue T, et al. Bone response to calcium phosphate-coated and bisphosphonate-immobilized titanium implants. *Biomaterials.* 2002;23(14):2879–2885.

63. Josse S, Faucheux C, Soueidan A, et al. Novel biomaterials for bisphosphonate delivery. *Biomaterials.* 2005;26:2073–2080. https://doi.org/10.1016/j.biomaterials.2004.05.019.

64. Peter B, Gauthier O, Laïb S, et al. Local delivery of bisphosphonate from coated orthopedic implants increases implants mechanical stability in osteoporotic rats. *J Biomed Mater Res A.* 2006;76(1):133–143. https://doi.org/10.1002/jbm.a.30456.

65. Abtahi J, Tengvall P, Aspenberg P. A bisphosphonate-coating improves the fixation of metal implants in human bone. A randomized trial of dental implants. *Bone.* 2012;50(5):1148–1151.

66. Abtahi J, Henefalk G, Aspenberg P. Randomised trial of bisphosphonate-coated dental implants: radiographic follow-up after five years of loading. 45:1564–1569. https://doi.org/10.1016/j.ijom.2016.09.001.

67. Guimaraes M, Antes T, Dolacio M, et al. Does local delivery of bisphosphonates influence the osseointegration of titanium implants? A systematic review. *Int J Oral Maxillofac Surg.* 2017;46:1429–1436.

68. Alonso-Coello P, García-Franco AL, Guyatt G, Moynihan R. Drugs for pre-osteoporosis: prevention or disease mongering? *BMJ.* 2008;336:126–129. https://doi.org/10.1136/bmj.39435.656250.AD.

69. Edwards MH, McCrae FC, Young-Min SA. Alendronate-related femoral diaphysis fracture—what should be done to predict and prevent subsequent fracture of the contralateral side? *Osteoporos Int.* 2010;21:701–703. https://doi.org/10.1007/s00198-009-0986-y.

70. Alenezi A, Chrcanovic B, Wennerberg A. Effects of local drug and chemical compound delivery on bone regeneration around dental implants in animal models: a systematic review and meta-analysis. *Int J Oral Maxillofac Implants.* 2018;33:e1–e18. https://doi.org/10.11607/jomi.6333.

71. Goldstein JL, Brown MS. Regulation of the mevalonate pathway. *Nature.* 1990;343:425–430. https://doi.org/10.1038/343425a0.

72. Mundy G, Garrett R, Harris S, et al. Gutierrez, Stimulation of bone formation in vitro and in rodents by statins. *Science.* 1999;286:1946–1949.

73. Ayukawa Y, Yasukawa E, Moriyama Y, et al. Local application of statin promotes bone repair through the suppression of osteoclasts and the enhancement of osteoblasts at bone-healing sites in rats. *Oral Surg Oral Med Oral Pathol Oral Radiol Endod.* 2009;107:336–342. https://doi.org/10.1016/j.tripleo.2008.07.013.

74. Edwards CJ, Hart DJ, Spector TD. Oral statins and increased bone-mineral density in postmenopausal women. *Lancet.* 2000;355:2218–2219.

75. Montagnani A, Gonnelli S, Cepollaro C, et al. Effect of simvastatin treatment on bone mineral density and bone turnover in hypercholesterolemic postmenopausal women: a 1-year longitudinal study. *Bone.* 2003;32:427–433.

76. Du Z, Chen J, Yan F, Xiao Y. Effects of Simvastatin on bone healing around titanium implants in osteoporotic rats. *Clin Oral Implants Res.* 2009;20:145–150. https://doi.org/10.1111/j.1600-0501.2008.01630.x.

77. Ayukawa Y, Okamura A, Koyano K. Simvastatin promotes osteogenesis around titanium implants. A histological and histometrical study in rats. *Clin Oral Implants Res.* 2004;15:346–350. https://doi.org/10.1046/j.1600-0501.2003.01015.x.

78. Yang F, Zhao S, Zhang F, et al. Simvastatin-loaded porous implant surfaces stimulate preosteoblasts differentiation: an in vitro study. *Oral Surg Oral Med Oral Pathol Oral Radiol Endod.* 2011;111:551–556. https://doi.org/10.1016/j.tripleo.2010.06.018.

79. Alt V, Bitschnau A, Osterling J, et al. The effects of combined gentamicin–hydroxyapatite coating for cementless joint prostheses on the reduction of infection rates in a rabbit infection prophylaxis model. *Biomaterials.* 2006;27(26):4627–4634. https://doi.org/10.1016/j.biomaterials.2006.04.035.

80. Persson LG, Ericsson I, Berglundh T, Lindhe J. Osseintegration following treatment of peri-implantitis and replacement of implant components. An experimental study in the dog. *J Clin Periodontol.* 2001;28:258–263.

81. Laurencin CT, Ashe KM, Henry N, et al. Delivery of small molecules for bone regenerative engineering: preclinical studies and potential clinical applications. *Drug Discov Today.* 2014;19:794–800. https://doi.org/10.1016/j.drudis.2014.01.012.

82. King WJ, Krebsbach PH. Growth factor delivery: how surface interactions modulate release in vitro and in vivo. *Adv Drug Deliv Rev.* 2012;64(12):1239–1256. https://doi.org/10.1016/j.addr.2012.03.004.

83. Mukherjee A, Rotwein P. Akt promotes BMP2-mediated osteoblast differentiation and bone development. *J Cell Sci.* 2009;122:716–726. https://doi.org/10.1242/jcs.042770.

84. Bessa PC, Casal M, Reis RL. Bone morphogenetic proteins in tissue engineering: the road from laboratory to clinic, part II (BMP delivery). *J Tissue Eng Regen Med.* 2008;2:81–96. https://doi.org/10.1002/term.74.

85. Hollinger JO, Hart CE, Hirsch SN, et al. Recombinant human platelet-derived growth factor: biology and clinical applications. *J Bone Joint Surg Am.* 2008;90(1):48–54. https://doi.org/10.2106/JBJS.G.01231.

86. Zekiy AO. Molecular approaches to functionalization of dental implant surfaces. *Eur J Mol Biotechnol.* 2015;10:228–240. https://doi.org/10.13187/ejmb.2015.10.228.

87. Inchingolo F, Ballini A, Cagiano R, et al. Immediately loaded dental implants bioactivated with platelet-rich plasma (PRP) placed in maxillary and mandibular region. *Clin Ter.* 2015;166:e146–e152.

88. Kundu R, Rathee M. Effect of Platelet-Rich-Plasma (PRP) and implant surface topography on implant stability and bone. *J Clin Diagnostic Res.* 2014;8:26–30. https://doi.org/10.7860/JCDR/2014/9177.4478.

89. Sakou T. Bone morphogenetic proteins: from basic studies to clinical approaches. *Bone.* 1998;22:591–603.

90. Dimitriou R, Tsiridis E, Giannoudis PV. Current concepts of molecular aspects of bone healing. *Injury.* 2005;36:1392–1404. https://doi.org/10.1016/j.injury.2005.07.019.

91. Laub M, Chatzinikolaidou M, Rumpf H, Jennissen HP. Modelling of protein-protein interactions of bone morphogenetic protein-2 (BMP-2) by 3D-Rapid Prototyping, Materwiss. *Werksttech.* 2002;33:729–737. https://doi.org/10.1002/mawe.200290003.

92. Wikesjö UME, Qahash M, Polimeni G, et al. Alveolar ridge augmentation using implants coated with recombinant human bone morphogenetic protein-2: histologic observations. *J Clin Periodontol.* 2008;35:1001–1010. https://doi.org/10.1111/j.1600-051X.2008.01321.x.

93. Sellers RS, Zhang R, Glasson SS, et al. Repair of articular cartilage defects one year after treatment with recombinant human bone morphogenetic protein-2 (rhBMP-2). *J Bone Joint Surg Am.* 2000;82:151–160.

94. Zhang X, Zhang Z, Shen G, Zhao J. Enhanced osteogenic activity and anti-inflammatory properties of Lenti-BMP-2-loaded TiO2nanotube layers fabricated by lyophilization following trehalose addition. *Int J Nanomedicine.* 2016;11:429–439. https://doi.org/10.2147/IJN.S93177.

95. Guillot R, Pignot-Paintrand I, Lavaud J, et al. *Assessment of a Polyelectrolyte Multilayer Film Coating Loaded with BMP-2 on Titanium and PEEK Implants in the Rabbit Femoral Condyle;* 2016. https://doi.org/10.1016/j.actbio.2016.03.010.

96. Kanatani M, Sugimoto T, Kaji H, et al. Stimulatory effect of bone morphogenetic protein-2 on osteoclast-like cell formation and bone-resorbing activity. *J Bone Miner Res.* 2009;10:1681–1690. https://doi.org/10.1002/jbmr.5650101110.

97. Gao X, Zhang X, Song J, et al. Osteoinductive peptide-functionalized nanofibers with highly ordered structure as biomimetic scaffolds for bone tissue engineering. *Int J Nanomedicine.* 2015;10:7109–7128. https://doi.org/10.2147/IJN.S94045.

98. Albertini M, Fernandez-Yague M, Lázaro P, et al. Advances in surfaces and osseointegration in implantology. Biomimetic surfaces. *Med Oral Patol Oral Cir Bucal.* 2015;20:316–341. https://doi.org/10.4317/medoral.20353.

99. Petrie TA, Reyes CD, Burns KL, García AJ. Simple application of fibronectin-mimetic coating enhances osseointegration of titanium implants. *J Cell Mol Med.* 2009;13:2602–2612. https://doi.org/10.1111/j.1582-4934.2008.00476.x.

100. Oliva J, Oliva X, Oliva JD. Five-year success rate of 831 consecutively placed Zirconia dental implants in humans: a comparison of three different rough surfaces. *Int J Oral Maxillofac Implants.* 2010;25:336–344.

101. Özkurt Z, Kazazoğlu E. Zirconia dental implants: a literature review. *J Oral Implantol.* 2011;37:367–376. https://doi.org/10.1563/AAID-JOI-D-09-00079.

102. Tetè S, Mastrangelo F, Bianchi A, et al. Collagen fiber orientation around machined titanium and zirconia dental implant necks: an animal study. *Int J Oral Maxillofac Implants.* 2009;24(1):5208.

103. Scarano A, Piattelli A, Polimeni A, et al. Bacterial adhesion on commercially pure titanium and anatase-coated titanium healing screws: an in vivo human study. *J Periodontol.* 2010;81:1466–1471. https://doi.org/10.1902/jop.2010.100061.

104. Ding Q, Zhang L, Bao R, et al. Effects of different surface treatments on the cyclic fatigue strength of one-piece CAD/CAM zirconia implants. *J Mech Behav Biomed Mater.* 2018;84:249–257. https://doi.org/10.1016/j.jmbbm.2018.05.002.

105. Assenza B, Tripodi D, Scarano A, et al. Bacterial leakage in implants with different implant–abutment connections: an in vitro study. *J Periodontol.* 2012;83:491–497. https://doi.org/10.1902/jop.2011.110320.

106. Porter DL, Heuer AH. Mechanisms of toughening Partially Stabilized Zirconia (PSZ). *J Am Ceram Soc.* 1977;60:183–184. https://doi.org/10.1111/j.1151-2916.1977.tb15509.x.

107. Piconi C, Maccauro G. Zirconia as a ceramic biomaterial. *Biomaterials*. 1998;20:1–25. https://doi.org/10.1016/B978-0-08-055294-1.00017-9.

108. Gahlert M, Gudehus T, Eichhorn S, et al. Biomechanical and histomorphometric comparison between zirconia implants with varying surface textures and a titanium implant in the maxilla of miniature pigs. *Clin Oral Implants Res*. 2007;18:662–668. https://doi.org/10.1111/j.1600-0501.2007.01401.x.

109. Wang H, Aboushelib MN, Feilzer AJ. Strength influencing variables on CAD/CAM zirconia frameworks. *Dent Mater*. 2008;24:633–638. https://doi.org/10.1016/j.dental.2007.06.030.

110. Langhoff JD, Voelter K, Scharnweber D, et al. Comparison of chemically and pharmaceutically modified titanium and zirconia implant surfaces in dentistry: a study in sheep. *Int J Oral Maxillofac Surg*. 2008;37:1125–1132. https://doi.org/10.1016/j.ijom.2008.09.008.

111. van Oirschot BA, Bronkhorst EM, van den Beucken JJ, et al. A systematic review on the long-term success of calcium phosphate plasma-spray-coated dental implants. *Odontology*. 2016;104:347–356. https://doi.org/10.1007/s10266-015-0230-5.

112. Mertens C, Steveling HG. Early and immediate loading of titanium implants with fluoride-modified surfaces: results of 5-year prospective study. *Clin Oral Implants Res*. 2011;22:1354–1360. https://doi.org/10.1111/j.1600-0501.2010.02123.x.

113. Cannizzaro G, Felice P, Minciarelli AF, et al. Early implant loading in the atrophic posterior maxilla: 1-stage lateral versus crestal sinus lift and 8 mm hydroxyapatite-coated implants. A 5-year randomised controlled trial. *Eur J Oral Implantol*. 2013;6:13–25.

114. Yang Y, Kim KH, Ong JL. A review on calcium phosphate coatings produced using a sputtering process - An alternative to plasma spraying. *Biomaterials*. 2005;26:327–337. https://doi.org/10.1016/j.biomaterials.2004.02.029.

115. Albertini M, Herrero-Climent, Nart J, et al. A biomimetic surface for immediate and early loading of dental implants surface characterization and results from histological studies. *JSM Dent Surg*. 2016;1(1):1008.

116. Lavenus S, Louarn G, Layrolle P. Nanotechnology and dental implants. *Int J Biomater*. 2010:1–9. https://doi.org/10.1155/2010/915327.

117. de Jonge LT, Leeuwenburgh SCG, Wolke JGC, Jansen JA. Organic–inorganic surface modifications for titanium implant surfaces. *Pharm Res*. 2008;25:2357–2369. https://doi.org/10.1007/s11095-008-9617-0.

118. de Jonge LT, Leeuwenburgh SC, van den Beucken JJ, et al. The osteogenic effect of electrosprayed nanoscale collagen/calcium phosphate coatings on titanium. *Biomaterials*. 2010;31:2461–2469. https://doi.org/10.1016/j.biomaterials.2009.11.114.

119. Chai YC, Carlier A, Bolander J, et al. *Current Views on Calcium Phosphate Osteogenicity and the Translation into Effective Bone Regeneration Strategies*; 2012. https://doi.org/10.1016/j.actbio.2012.07.002.

120. Siebers MC, Walboomers XF, Leeuwenburgh SCG, et al. Electrostatic spray deposition (ESD) of calcium phosphate coatings, an in vitro study with osteoblast-like cells. *Biomaterials*. 2004;25. 2019–27.

121. Junker R, Dimakis A, Thoneick M, Jansen JA. Effects of implant surface coatings and composition on bone integration: a systematic review. *Clin Oral Implants Res*. 2009;20:185–206. https://doi.org/10.1111/j.1600-0501.2009.01777.x.

122. Miranda-Rius J, Lahor-Soler E, Brunet-Llobet L, et al. Treatments to optimize dental implant surface topography and enhance cell bioactivity. In: Almasri MA, ed. *Dental Implantology Biomaterial*. IntechOpen; 2016. https://doi.org/10.5772/62682.

PART III

Fundamental Science

10

Medical Evaluation of the Dental Implant Patient

RANDOLPH R. RESNIK AND ROBERT J. RESNIK

The medical evaluation of patients considering dental implant treatment is an important and vital aspect of the treatment planning process. A retrospective analysis of Veterans' Administration Registry data found that the medical status of patients (i.e., medical history, American Society of Anesthesiologists [ASA] category, and medication history) correlated with dental implant failure.[1] It is the primary goal of the clinician to assess the inherent risks associated with the treatment of patients. There exist many factors associated with evaluating the patient's health status and risk including the patients current and past medical and dental history, current and past use of medications, history of allergies, social history, type of treatment, length of treatment, invasiveness of treatment, degree of urgency of treatment, and the past use of sedation (Box 10.1).

Patients presenting for dental implant treatment may apparently appear "healthy"; however, they may actually have serious systemic diseases or taking medications that may increase the morbidity of treatment. Patients today, even those with life-threatening diseases, are more socially active and have a better quality of life because of advances in surgical and medical care. Studies have shown that 30% of dental patients have some type of relevant medical condition.[2] Evaluating patients over the age of 60 years old, 40% have been shown to be on five or more prescription medications, 15% are taking 10 or more prescription medications, and 67% are taking a combination of five or more prescription and over-the-counter (OTC) medications.[3]

Although difficult in many situations, the clinician should do everything possible to identify the medically compromised patient. The goal is for every patient to be treated in a safe and efficient manner. Increased risk to patients may arise from procedures that are too invasive or outside the patient's tolerance in an office setting. Therefore it is imperative for the clinician to make an assessment of risk based on medical and dental history and be conscious of the extent of trauma and stress to the patient with the anticipated procedures.

This chapter is specific for an implant candidate and focuses on the importance of the initial medical evaluation with primary emphasis on the medical history questionnaire and the physical examination. Relevant systemic diseases along with medications that directly affect the dental implant patient are addressed with recommendations on the treatment plan, intraoperative treatment, and postoperative care modifications.

Medical Evaluation

The medical evaluation remains of paramount importance in implant dentistry, perhaps more so than in other disciplines of dentistry. Dental implant treatment is well accepted today as a surgical, prosthetic, and maintenance discipline for patients ranging from adolescence to the elderly population. The need for implant-related treatment increases with the age of the patient; as a result, the implant dentist treats more elderly patients than other specialists in dentistry.

An estimated 12% of the US population is 65 years of age or older; this number is expected to reach 21% (64.6 million) in the year 2030.[4] A 65-year-old person has a life expectancy of another 16.7 years, and an 80-year-old person can expect to live an additional 8 years.[5] These patients often request implant support for their failing fixed restorations or to improve the conditions of their removable prostheses. An increased life span indicates that the number of elderly patients in the dental practice is highly likely to increase in the future. Therefore it is important to design the medical and physical evaluations to accommodate the special conditions of these patients.

• BOX 10.1 Factors Affecting the Risk Assessment of the Implant Patient

- Current and past medical history
- Current and past dental history
- Current and past use of medications
- History of allergies
- Social history and use of recreational drugs
- Type of required treatment
- Length of treatment
- Invasiveness of treatment
- Psychological status
- Degree of urgency of treatment
- Use and type of sedation

Medical History

An extensive written medical history is mandatory for every dental implant candidate. The review of the patient's medical history is the first opportunity for the dentist to speak with the patient. The time and consideration taken at the onset will set the tone for the entire subsequent treatment. This first impression should reflect a warm, caring practitioner who is highly trained to help patients with complex medical and dental histories. A sincere interest and active note-taking process are beneficial. The practitioner should not underestimate the value of the medical history interview. Asking questions that show an understanding of listed medical conditions and related common problems offer several benefits.

The two basic categories of information addressed during the review of the medical history include the medical history and a review of the patient's systemic health. The dental office uses a medical evaluation form to obtain most of this information (Fig. 10.1). Of particular importance is the history of medication usage including OTC medications, herbs and supplements, allergies, and a review of the body systems. The pathophysiology of the systems, the degree of involvement, and the medications being used to treat the conditions are evaluated. It is important to review this form with the patient to ensure that comprehension is adequate to answer all questions accurately and truthfully.

Extraoral and Intraoral Examinations

After the medical history is reviewed, the medical physical examination is initiated because this is the first physical contact the office staff has with the patient. A gentle, caring approach should continue throughout the examination. A complete evaluation of the head and neck is important initially and at all subsequent preventive maintenance (recall) appointments.

The extraoral and intraoral examinations are similar to those addressed in any oral diagnosis textbook. The exposed areas of the patient need to be evaluated (face, neck, arms, and hands) and documented accordingly. Features and facial symmetry are observed, including the ears, nose, and eyes. If the midline, occlusal plane, or smile line of the natural teeth or existing prosthesis is not harmonious, the etiology should be determined. The temporomandibular joint should be evaluated along with maximum occlusal opening because this may complicate or contraindicate surgical and prosthetic procedures. Patients are very receptive to critical evaluation and treatment limitations

About Your Medical History

For the following questions, check YES or NO, whichever applies. Your answers are for our records only, and will be confidential.

THESE FACTS HAVE A DIRECT BEARING ON YOUR DENTAL HEALTH

Sex:_______ Height:_________ Weight:__________ Race:___________

		Date __/__/__	Date __/__/__
General Medical History	1. Are you in good general health?........	❑ Yes ❑ No	❑ Yes ❑ No
	2. Has there been ANY change in your general health in the past year?	❑ Yes ❑ No	❑ Yes ❑ No
	3. My last physical examination was on, approximate date		
	4. Are you PRESENTLY under a physician's care?	❑ Yes ❑ No	❑ Yes ❑ No
	If YES, what condition?........		
	5. The physician's name and address........		
	6. Have you had any serious illness or operation?........	❑ YES ❑ NO	❑ YES ❑ NO
	If YES, please list........		
	7. Have you ever been hospitalized or had a serious illness within the past 5 years?........	❑ Yes ❑ No	❑ Yes ❑ No
	If YES, reason........		
Cardiovascular System	CV1. Do you have or have you ever had any of the following: Please Check ❑ Heart trouble ❑ Heart attack ❑ Coronary insufficiency ❑ Mitral Valve Prolapse ❑ Stroke ❑ Damaged heart valves ❑ Congenital heart disease		
	CV2. Rheumatic heart disease, heart murmur?	❑ Yes ❑ No	❑ Yes ❑ No
	CV3. Chest pain after exertion?........	❑ Yes ❑ No	❑ Yes ❑ No
	CV4. Shortness of breath after mild exercise?........	❑ Yes ❑ No	❑ Yes ❑ No
	CV5. Do your ankles swell?	❑ Yes ❑ No	❑ Yes ❑ No
	CV6. Do you use extra pillows to sleep?........	❑ Yes ❑ No	❑ Yes ❑ No
	CV7. Do you have a cardiac pacemaker?	❑ Yes ❑ No	❑ Yes ❑ No
	CV8. Do you have any blood pressure problems?	❑ Yes ❑ No	❑ Yes ❑ No
	If YES, ...	❑ High ❑ Low	❑ High ❑ Low
Central Nervous System	CN1. Do you have or have you ever had:		
	CN1A. Epilepsy?	❑ Yes ❑ No	❑ Yes ❑ No
	CN1B. Fainting spells?	❑ Yes ❑ No	❑ Yes ❑ No
	CN1C. Seizures?	❑ Yes ❑ No	❑ Yes ❑ No
	CN1D. Emotional disturbances?	❑ Yes ❑ No	❑ Yes ❑ No
	CN2. Do you follow any treatment for a nervous disease?........	❑ Yes ❑ No	❑ Yes ❑ No
Respiratory System	RE1. Do you have a persistent cough or cold?	❑ Yes ❑ No	❑ Yes ❑ No
	RE2. Do you have or have you ever had tuberculosis?........	❑ Yes ❑ No	❑ Yes ❑ No
	RE3. Is there ANY history of tuberculosis in your family?	❑ Yes ❑ No	❑ Yes ❑ No
	RE4. Do you have any sinusitis, sinus trouble?	❑ Yes ❑ No	❑ Yes ❑ No
	RE5. Do you have emphysema, chronic bronchitis, asthma?	❑ Yes ❑ No	❑ Yes ❑ No
Digestive System	GI1. Do you have ANY stomach ulcers?........	❑ Yes ❑ No	❑ Yes ❑ No
	GI2. Do you have or have you ever had:		
	GI2A. Acic Reflux (GERD)?........	❑ Yes ❑ No	❑ Yes ❑ No
	GI2B. Hepatitis?	❑ Yes ❑ No	❑ Yes ❑ No
	GI2C. Jaundice?	❑ Yes ❑ No	❑ Yes ❑ No
	GI2D. Liver disease?	❑ Yes ❑ No	❑ Yes ❑ No
	GI3. Have you ever vomited blood?	❑ Yes ❑ No	❑ Yes ❑ No
	GI4. Do you have ANY diarrhea?	❑ Yes ❑ No	❑ Yes ❑ No

A

• **Fig. 10.1** (A–D) Medical history form.

About Your Medical History

		Date / /	Date / /
Endocrine System	EN1. Do you have diabetes? controlled/uncontrolled	☐ Yes ☐ No	☐ Yes ☐ No
	EN2. Does anyone in your family have diabetes?	☐ Yes ☐ No	☐ Yes ☐ No
	EN3. Do you urinate more than six times a day?	☐ Yes ☐ No	☐ Yes ☐ No
	EN4. Are you thirsty very often or do you have a dry mouth?	☐ Yes ☐ No	☐ Yes ☐ No
	EN5. Do you have hypothyroidism or hyperthyroidism?	☐ Yes ☐ No	☐ Yes ☐ No
Hematogenic System	HB1. Do you have anemia, Sickle Cell disease, blood disorder?	☐ Yes ☐ No	☐ Yes ☐ No
	HB2. Is there ANY family history of blood disorders?	☐ Yes ☐ No	☐ Yes ☐ No
	HB3. Are you hemophilic?	☐ Yes ☐ No	☐ Yes ☐ No
	HB4. Have you had abnormal bleeding after any surgery, extraction, or trauma?	☐ Yes ☐ No	☐ Yes ☐ No
	HB5. Have you ever had a blood transfusion?	☐ Yes ☐ No	☐ Yes ☐ No
	HB6. Immunodeficiency problem?	☐ Yes ☐ No	☐ Yes ☐ No
Allergies	AL1. Are you allergic to or have you reacted adversely to:		
	AL1A. Local anesthetic	☐ Yes ☐ No	☐ Yes ☐ No
	AL1B. Antibiotics, Penicillin, Sulfa Drugs?	☐ Yes ☐ No	☐ Yes ☐ No
	AL1C. Barbiturates, sedatives, or sleeping pills?	☐ Yes ☐ No	☐ Yes ☐ No
	AL1D. Aspirin?	☐ Yes ☐ No	☐ Yes ☐ No
	AL1E. Iodine?	☐ Yes ☐ No	☐ Yes ☐ No
	AL1F. Codeine or other narcotics?	☐ Yes ☐ No	☐ Yes ☐ No
	AL1G. Latex?	☐ Yes ☐ No	☐ Yes ☐ No
	AL1H. Others? Please Specify		
	AL2. Do you have asthma, hay fever or seasonal allergies?	☐ Yes ☐ No	☐ Yes ☐ No
	AL3. Do you have or have you ever had hives or skin rash?	☐ Yes ☐ No	☐ Yes ☐ No
System	UR1. Do you have or have you ever had:		
	UR1A. Kidney trouble?	☐ Yes ☐ No	☐ Yes ☐ No
	UR1B. Dialysis?	☐ Yes ☐ No	☐ Yes ☐ No
	UR1B. Syphilis, gonorrhea?	☐ Yes ☐ No	☐ Yes ☐ No
Bones & Joints	BJ1. Do you have or have you ever had:		
	BJ1A. Arthritis?	☐ Yes ☐ No	☐ Yes ☐ No
	BJ1B. Inflammatory rheumatism?	☐ Yes ☐ No	☐ Yes ☐ No
	BJ1C. Bone infection?	☐ Yes ☐ No	☐ Yes ☐ No
	BJ1D. Osteoporosis?	☐ Yes ☐ No	☐ Yes ☐ No
	BJ1E. Artificial Joint Replacement?	☐ Yes ☐ No	☐ Yes ☐ No
	BJ1F. 1. Have you received or are you currently receiving the intravenous medication known as biphosphonate for example, Zomata (IV) (zoledronic acid) or Aridia (IM) (pamidronate)	☐ Yes ☐ No	☐ Yes ☐ No
	2. Are you taking or have you taken the oral medication known as biphosphonate for osteoporosis or another medical condition for example, Fosamax (alendronate), Actonal (risedronate) or Boniva (ibandronate sodium)	☐ Yes ☐ No	☐ Yes ☐ No
	If yes to 1 or 2		
	3. Have you noticed any changes in your mouth or jaws?	☐ Yes ☐ No	☐ Yes ☐ No
	4. Have you had any jaw pain or toothache(s)?	☐ Yes ☐ No	☐ Yes ☐ No
	5. Have you noticed any foul smell, swelling or discharge in your mouth?	☐ Yes ☐ No	☐ Yes ☐ No
Other	TR1. Do you have or have you ever had:		
	TR1A. Tumor or malignancy?	☐ Yes ☐ No	☐ Yes ☐ No
	TR1B. Chemotherapy or radiation therapy?	☐ Yes ☐ No	☐ Yes ☐ No
	Do you have or have you ever had ANY disease, condition or problem NOT listed above that you think we should know about? If so, please explain		
	TR2. Are you regularly exposed to x-rays or ANY other ionizing radiation or toxic substances?	☐ Yes ☐ No	☐ Yes ☐ No
	TR3. Do you have glaucoma?	☐ Yes ☐ No	☐ Yes ☐ No
	If so,	☐ Wide ☐ Close	☐ Wide ☐ Close
	TR4. Have you ever had any type of radiation treatment? If so, what part of your body was treated and when?		

B

• **Fig. 10.1, cont'd**

About Your Medical History

		Date ___/___/___	Date ___/___/___
TR4.	Are you wearing or do you wear contact lenses?	☐ Yes ☐ No	☐ Yes ☐ No
TR5.	Do you drink alcohol?	☐ Yes ☐ No	☐ Yes ☐ No
	If so, how much and how often?		
TR6.	Do you smoke tobacco?	☐ Yes ☐ No	☐ Yes ☐ No
TR7.	Do you use oral tobacco?	☐ Yes ☐ No	☐ Yes ☐ No
	If so, how much and how often?		

Your Medications

	Date ___/___/___	Date ___/___/___
ME1. Are you taking any of the following medications:	☐ Yes ☐ No	☐ Yes ☐ No
ME1B. Anticoagulants, blood thinning agents?	☐ Yes ☐ No	☐ Yes ☐ No
ME1C. Medicine for high blood pressure?	☐ Yes ☐ No	☐ Yes ☐ No
ME1D. Tranquilizers?	☐ Yes ☐ No	☐ Yes ☐ No
ME1E. Iodine?	☐ Yes ☐ No	☐ Yes ☐ No
ME1F. Aspirin?	☐ Yes ☐ No	☐ Yes ☐ No
ME1G. Codeine or other narcotics?	☐ Yes ☐ No	☐ Yes ☐ No
ME1H. Steroids?	☐ Yes ☐ No	☐ Yes ☐ No
ME1I. Other?	☐ Yes ☐ No	☐ Yes ☐ No
If so, please explain		

MEDICATION LIST

Please provide a list of **any type of medication** you are presently taking as well as the dosage.
(Prescription or Over the Counter)
NEVER DISCONTINUE OR MODIFY ANY MEDICATION THAT WAS PRESCRIBED BY YOUR PHYSICIAN

Name/Type of drugs	Dosage	How many times per day?
_____	_____	_____
_____	_____	_____
_____	_____	_____
_____	_____	_____
_____	_____	_____
_____	_____	_____
_____	_____	_____
_____	_____	_____
_____	_____	_____
_____	_____	_____
_____	_____	_____
_____	_____	_____
_____	_____	_____

C

• **Fig. 10.1, cont'd**

About Your Medical History

		Date __/__/__	Date __/__/__
For Women	Are you pregnant?..	☐ Yes ☐ No	☐ Yes ☐ No
	Are you nursing?...	☐ Yes ☐ No	☐ Yes ☐ No
	Do you have any problems associated with your menstrual period?	☐ Yes ☐ No	☐ Yes ☐ No
	Are you taking oral contraceptives?..	☐ Yes ☐ No	☐ Yes ☐ No
	Are you undergoing hormonal therapy?..	☐ Yes ☐ No	☐ Yes ☐ No

Dental History

What is your chief dental complaint?

	Date	Date
Are you experiencing any discomfort or pain at this time?	☐ Yes ☐ No	☐ Yes ☐ No
Are you satisfied with the appearance of your teeth?....................	☐ Yes ☐ No	☐ Yes ☐ No
Are you able to eat and chew foods satisfactorily?.....................	☐ Yes ☐ No	☐ Yes ☐ No
Do you have headaches, ear aches, or neck pain?.........................	☐ Yes ☐ No	☐ Yes ☐ No
Do you frequently experience sinus problems?...........................	☐ Yes ☐ No	☐ Yes ☐ No
Have you had ANY serious trouble associated with ANY previous dental treatment?...	☐ Yes ☐ No	☐ Yes ☐ No
If YES please explain.........................		

Other Conditions Not Listed

General Dental Responsibility And Consent Statement

I hereby authorize and request the performance of dental services for myself or for:

I also give my consent to ANY advisable and necessary dental procedures, medications or anesthetics to be administered by the attending dentist or his supervised staff for diagnostic purposes or dental treatment. These records may include study models, photographs, x-rays and blood studies. I understand and acknowledge that I am financially responsible for the services provided for myself and or the above named, regardless of insurance coverage. Treatment plans involving extended credit circumstances are subject to a credit check. I also understand that the treatment estimate presented to me is only an estimate. Occasionally, the need may arise to modify treatment. In such a case, I will be informed of the need for additional treatment, and any fee modification.

To the best of my knowledge the information in this form is accurate.

_____   _____
Signature of Patient or Guardian   Date

_____   _____
Signature of Witness   Date

_____   _____
Signature of Doctor   Date

D

• **Fig. 10.1, cont'd**

relating to facial esthetics before reconstruction begins. The high smile should be evaluated, because this may pose esthetic complications related to dental implants. Visible signs of anxiety, abnormal body movements, tremors, lethargy, or difficulty in breathing should be noted along with any abnormalities in the face (e.g., expression, pallor, cyanosis or jaundice, drooping eyelids), neck (e.g., lumps, swelling), arms (e.g., bruising or petechiae), or hands (e.g., finger clubbing, Raynaud phenomenon, rashes, dexterity issues).

The submental, submandibular, parotid, and cervical areas are palpated for lymphadenopathy or unusual swelling. The area between the cricoid notch and the suprasternal notch is palpated for enlargement of the thyroid gland. Thyroid disorders may influence bone metabolism and implant management. Intraoral examination of the lips, labial and buccal mucosa, hard and soft palate, tongue, and oral pharynx is then performed. Any lesions or disease states must be further evaluated before implant procedures commence.

Vital Signs

The recording of vital signs (blood pressure, pulse, temperature, respiration, weight, and height) is also part of the physical examination. Trained dental auxiliary personnel can often gather this information before the patient's history is reviewed by the dentist. If any findings are unusual, the doctor can repeat the evaluation as needed.

Blood Pressure

Blood pressure is a critical component of the medical examination and is often neglected in dental offices. Studies have shown that approximately 10% of dental offices record the patient's blood pressure.[6] The importance of obtaining and recording the blood pressure in every implant patient is twofold. First, the initial recording may serve as a baseline measurement, which, if too high, may indicate an underlying cardiovascular disease that may contraindicate a surgical procedure. Second, when in an acceptable range, the initial blood pressure acts as a baseline measurement specific for that patient. If the patient has a future problem during treatment, the blood pressure difference between baseline and the current situation may alter the medical risk of the patient.

Blood pressure is measured in the arterial system. This makes using a wrist cuff more difficult and less accurate, as the arteries in the wrist are narrower than in the elbow. It is always advisable to use a cuff that measures the blood pressure just above the elbow. Using a cuff that is too small will give you an artificially higher blood pressure, and using a cuff that is too large will give an artificially low blood pressure. Bladder length is a helpful guide in choosing the appropriate cuff size. The American Heart Association (AHA) recommends the cuff to be 80% of the patient's arm circumference and 40% for ideal width.

There are several standard-size cuffs. The small adult size is for an arm circumference of approximately 7 to 9 inches. Regular adult-sized cuffs can be used for arm circumferences that are between 9 and 13 inches. A large adult cuff can be used when the arm circumference exceeds 13 inches but is less than 17 inches.

Blood pressure may be directly influenced by the cardiac output, blood volume, viscosity of the blood, condition of blood vessels (especially the arterioles), and heart rate. The systolic blood pressure is the maximum amount of pressure in your arteries during the contraction of your heart muscle. The diastolic blood pressure is the pressure in the arteries between beats. The difference between the diastolic and systolic blood pressure is the pulse pressure. The pulse pressure is the amount of pressure the heart creates every time is beats. For example, a blood pressure of 120/80 would have a pulse pressure of 40 mm Hg. The average pulse pressure is 30 to 50 mm Hg. A high pulse pressure is greater than 60 mm Hg and is more common in the elderly. Along with age, a high pulse pressure can be indicative of accelerated hypertension or atherosclerosis of the arteries. Blood pressure may be directly influenced by the cardiac output, blood volume, viscosity of the blood, condition of blood vessels (especially the arterioles), and heart rate.

In 2017, the standards for evaluating blood pressure readings were updated with the release of the "Seventh Report of the Joint National Committee on Prevention, Detection, Evaluation and Treatment of High Blood Pressure" (Joint National Committee [JNC] 7).[7] Blood pressure is now divided into four different categories: normal, elevated, stage 1, and stage 2. Normal blood pressure is defined as <120/<80 mm Hg; elevated blood pressure is defined as 120 to 129/<80 mm Hg; stage 1 hypertension is defined as 130 to 139 or 80 to 89 mm Hg; and stage 2 hypertension is defined as >140 or ≥90 mm Hg. A diagnosis of hypertension is not made on a single reading. The diagnosis should be confirmed on at least two or more readings on at least two or more occasions. If the blood pressure reading exceeds a systolic of 140 or diastolic of 90 on two separate readings, then the patient should be referred to their primary care physician.[8]

White-coat hypertension in a medical office can occur with some patients. This is especially true for patients in a dental office, who may be anxious or apprehensive about the pending dental procedure. Before making a diagnosis of hypertension in these individuals, the patient should monitor the blood pressure at home or out of the office. Hypertension tends to have a higher prevalence in African Americans compared with Caucasians. The risk of death from a stroke or heart disease can be doubled for every 20 mm Hg of elevation in systolic blood pressure and every 10 mm Hg in elevation of diastolic blood pressure.

Only personnel that have been trained and retrained on a regular basis in the standardized technique should perform blood pressure monitoring. It is advised to record the blood pressure in both arms and provide at least 2 to 3 minutes between repeating the blood pressure readings. You should always verbally give the patient their blood pressure reading in addition to recording it in their chart. Usually giving the patient at least 5 minutes to rest before checking their blood pressure is advisable. Most dental offices will use an automatic electronic cuff, which will inflate the cuff to the appropriate pressure and automatically measure the blood pressure. It is important that the cuff is in the appropriate position, with the tubes from the cuff running directly over the brachial artery. The patient's feet should be supported on the floor and the arm supported on a table or chair arm at the level of the heart. Do not use one measurement to determine whether a patient has blood pressure issues. Repeat the reading to confirm elevated blood pressure, and refer the patient to their primary care provider when appropriate.

Low blood pressure can also create issues for dental implant surgery. Blood pressure readings of less than 90 mm Hg systolic or less than 60 mm Hg diastolic is considered abnormal, and elective dental implant surgery should be postponed until consultation with the patient's physician. It is always important to recheck the blood pressure to verify the low readings. Low blood pressure can result from dehydration, hypothyroidism, or the patient being over-medicated with antihypertensive medications.

Note: If a female patient presents with a history of a mastectomy, blood pressure should be taken on the arm opposite the side of the mastectomy to avoid possible lymphedema. If a patient relates a history of a double mastectomy, blood pressure should be taken on the ankle (this will usually result in an elevated blood pressure reading).

Pulse

The second vital sign of importance is the pulse. The pulse represents the force of the blood against the aortic walls for each contraction of the left ventricle. The pulse wave travels through the arteries and reaches the wrist 0.1 to 0.2 seconds after each contraction. The actual blood flow takes longer to travel this distance. The usual location to record pulse is the radial artery in the wrist. However, other locations, such as the carotid artery in the neck and the temporal artery in the temporal region, are convenient to use during implant surgery or dental treatment. Pulse monitors are easy to use and are beneficial during surgery or long prosthetic appointments.

Pulse Rate. The normal pulse rate varies from 60 to 90 beats/min in a relaxed, nonanxious patient. Many of the automated blood pressure machines will check the pulse. If there is any significant variation in the blood pressure readings or there is an error on the automated machine, you should check a manual pulse in the brachial or radial artery to ensure the rhythm is regular. The pulse rate can be verified manually for a minimum of 30 seconds to 1 minute.

If you feel any irregularities in the pulse, you should refer the patient back to their primary care provider before proceeding. Sometimes premature ventricular or atrial contractions are normal and can be felt manually with the pulse rate. These extra beats will usually be infrequent. More frequent irregular beats or beat that seem to be just erratically irregular without any particular pattern may indicate a need for primary care provider consultation before proceeding with dental surgery.

Some patients with chronic atrial fibrillation will have an erratically irregular heart rate. These patients are usually on blood thinners (anticoagulants). A rate greater than 100 or less than 60 in these patients can also be problematic and should indicate the need for physician consultation.

The normal cardiac rhythm originates in the sinoatrial node; the pulse reflects the ventricular contractions. The upper limit of normal is considered 100 beats/min; patients in excellent physical condition may have a pulse rate of 40 to 60 beats/min. A pulse rate less than 60 beats/min in a nonathlete or higher than 110 beats/min in a relatively calm patient could be suspect and warrant further medical consultation.

A decreased pulse rate of normal rhythm (less than 60 beats/min) indicates a sinus bradycardia. Naturally, some patients may reach as low as 40 beats/min, although most patients become symptomatic with lightheadedness, dizziness, or can experience syncope with a rate lower than 40 beats/min. An adult pulse rate lower than 60 beats/min in a nonathlete mandates medical evaluation before surgical procedures. Patients receiving beta-blocker medications may have lower than normal pulse rates. These patients may be asymptomatic, but consultation with their physician should be considered. During implant surgery, inappropriate bradycardia may indicate a very serious problem. If the pulse rate of the patient decreases to less than 60 beats/min and is accompanied by sweating, weakness, chest pain, or dyspnea, the implant procedure should be stopped, oxygen administered, and immediate medical assistance obtained. If the resting pulse of the patient is greater than 60 beats/min and drops into the 40s or lower, the dental procedure should be suspended, even if the patient is asymptomatic, until the pulse returns closer to the resting rate.

An increased pulse rate of regular rhythm (more than 100 beats/min) is termed sinus tachycardia. This rate is normal if experienced during exercise or anxiety. However, a medical consultation is suggested when a nonanxious patient has a resting pulse rate higher than 100 beats/min. In patients with anemia or severe hemorrhage, the heart rate increases to compensate for the depletion of oxygen in the tissues. Therefore when increased bleeding during surgery is observed, evaluate the pulse rate and blood pressure.

Pulse rate and temperature are also related, with the pulse rate increasing 5 beats/min for each degree that the body temperature rises. Hyperthyroidism and acute or chronic heart disease also may result in sinus tachycardia. Some patients may be asymptomatic and experience a condition called paroxysmal atrial tachycardia. This condition is characterized by episodes of very fast heartbeats that may last a few minutes or several weeks. All of these conditions affect the surgical procedure and may increase postoperative swelling. The increased swelling favors the occurrence of infections and complications during the first critical weeks after implant placement. This can lead to increased morbidity and failure of the implants.

Pulse Rhythm. As described previously it is critical to not only rely on the automated pulse calculation but also to manually check the pulse for regularity or irregularity for at least 30 seconds in the radial or brachial artery. Extremely anxious patients can have accelerated pulse rates, which can then become irregular with a premature ventricular contraction (PVC) or premature atrial contraction (PAC). Stress reduction protocols can be implemented, and implant procedures may even be contraindicated if the causal conditions are severe.

The presence of an extra pulse beat may indicate a PVC. This condition may be associated with fatigue, stress, or excessive use of tobacco or coffee, but it is also observed during myocardial

infarction (MI). If the PVCs are more frequent over a short period of time, physician consultation should be initiated. If during implant surgery, five or more PVCs are recorded within 1 minute, especially when accompanied by dyspnea or pain, the surgery should be stopped, oxygen administered, the patient placed in a supine position, and immediate medical assistance obtained. If the health history includes cardiovascular disease, including hypertension, the pulse rhythm should be recorded. Sudden death in persons older than 30 years with PVC is six times more frequent than in younger persons.[9]

Pulse Strength. The patient's pulse rate and rhythm may be normal, yet the blood volume can affect the character of the pulse. In anxious patients, the pulse may be bounding as the heart is forced to pump large amounts of blood. If the pulse seems to be strong then weak with some alteration back and forth, this could indicate pulsus alternans, which is frequently observed in left ventricular failure, severe arterial high blood pressure, and advanced coronary disease. Implant surgery is contraindicated, and medical consultation with an electrocardiographic examination is needed to obtain a diagnosis.

Temperature

Technology has altered the way we can now check a patient's temperature. Automated thermometers allow for an accurate temperature by placing a probe under the tongue. Another option is a digital ear thermometer. These devices give quick and reliable temperature measurements of the infrared radiation or heat coming from the tympanic membrane. Axillary and forehead measuring devices are much less sensitive and probably have no utility in a dental implant office. For every degree of fever, the pulse rate raises 5 beats/min and the respiratory rate increases 4 beats/min. If the patient's temperature is greater than 100.5°F, implant surgery should be postponed. If the temperature is greater than 102°F or higher, medical consultation is suggested.

The usual cause of elevated body temperature is bacterial infection and its toxic by-products. Other causes can be exercise, hyperthyroidism, MI, congestive heart failure (CHF), and tissue injury from trauma or surgery. Dental conditions causing an elevated temperature include severe dental abscess, cellulitis, and acute herpetic stomatitis. Elective dental treatment (such as implant surgery or bone grafting) is contraindicated when the patient is febrile (>100.5). The cause of the fever may complicate the postsurgical phase of healing. In addition, because elevated temperature increases the patient's pulse rate, the risks of hemorrhage, edema, infection, and postoperative discomfort are greater. Special attention must be given to a prolonged, sustained fever after surgery because sepsis or possible brain abscess could be present. Very low body temperatures can also be problematic but can also result from inaccurate measurement. If the body temperature is less than 97°F, an alternative method of testing should be used to verify the reading or at a minimum the reading should be repeated. More elderly patients can have normal body temperatures that run just higher than 97°F. Low body temperature can be found in hypothyroidism.

Respiration

Respiration is evaluated while the patient is at rest. The normal rate in the adult varies between 16 and 20 breaths per minute and is regular in rate and rhythm. Patients with advanced respiratory conditions including chronic obstructive pulmonary disease (COPD), CHF, and some forms of asthma may use accessory muscles in the neck or shoulders for inspiration, whether before or during surgery. This is considered a form of dyspnea (difficult or labored breathing). During dental implant surgery, the use of intravenous (IV) drugs including narcotics can cause patients to develop dyspnea.

If dyspnea occurs during surgery, it is important to evaluate the patient's airway for swelling or obstruction. The pulse should immediately be evaluated to rule out the presence of PVCs or irregularity. This could indicate a more serious condition such as a MI.

Hyperventilation is the result of both an increased rate and depth of respiration and may be preceded by frequent sighs, such as is seen in the anxious patient. A respiratory rate greater than 20 breaths per minute requires investigation. Anxiety may increase this rate, in which case sedatives or stress reduction protocols are indicated before implant surgery. Other causes for an increased respiration rate are severe anemia, advanced bronchopulmonary disease, and CHF. All three can affect the surgical procedure or healing response of the implant candidate.

Having a portable pulse oximeter available is always advisable to measure oxygen concentration. It is important to keep the oxygen saturation greater than 90%. This may require supplemental oxygen. There was previous concern regarding oxygen supplementation in patients with chronic COPD depressing the hypoxemic drive. Currently the accepted use of supplemental oxygen in COPD patients is to keep the oxygen level at their baseline or greater than 90%. It is important that every dental office have supplemental oxygen and both a nasal cannula for routine oxygen supplementation and a nonrebreather mask to deliver higher levels of oxygen.

Hypoventilation can also occur from IV sedation. However, the initial evaluation of a patient that is experiencing hypoventilation with or without IV sedation should always be the airway for possible obstruction. If the airway is clear and hypoventilation persists, then pharmaceutical reversal of the sedative agent should be considered.

Height

The height of the patient should be determined, especially in an adolescent patient, to evaluate their growth and development in the determination of when dental implants would be appropriate. Ideally, growth cessation must occur before implant placement is initiated.

Weight

Weight is an important factor when using sedation for implants procedures, because there exists a direct correlation between dosage of sedative drugs and body weight. Additionally, significant changes in weight (gain or loss) should be evaluated to assess malnutrition, obesity, or retention of fluid from either kidney or heart dysfunction. Unintentional loss of weight may be a sign of malignancy, diabetes, or various other systemic diseases. A significant increase in weight may be a sign of cardiovascular disease such as CHF, hypothyroidism, or possible systemic diseases. Of special concern are patients with a history of gastric bypass because absorption rates of certain medications may be affected.

Laboratory Evaluation

Routine laboratory screening of patients in a general dental setting who previously reported a normal health history have found that 12% to 18% have undiagnosed systemic diseases.[10,11] Many of these disorders may influence implant surgery protocol or long-term success rates. The percentage of implant patients with unreported systemic illnesses is most likely higher because the average implant patient is older than those in these general studies. Implant therapy consists of an elective surgery that involves a considerable investment of time and money by the patient.

Although clinical laboratory tests are not a required component of the physical examination in the dental setting, the implant clinician must be well versed in the interpretation of results. In general, the implant clinician should never prescribe laboratory procedures. The reason for this is twofold. First, the patient's physician should be the first to interpret laboratory results because they are more knowledgeable about the specific medical condition of their patients. Second, there exists a medicolegal issue because the implant clinician would be responsible for interpretation of the entire laboratory tests requested.

The most common clinical laboratory evaluation is obtained from urinalysis and venous blood samples and may include a complete blood count (CBC), basic metabolic panel (BMP), comprehensive metabolic panel (CMP), and bleeding disorder tests such as prothrombin time (PT) or partial prothrombin time (PTT). An A1c should also be obtained if the patient relates prediabetic or diabetic conditions because this test gauges how well the patient's diabetes is managed.

Urinalysis

A simple dipstick urinalysis can serve as a valuable screening tool for systemic disease. Urine is a by-product of the kidney and performs several critical functions: filters wastes from the bloodstream; maintains water balance; and reabsorbs or conserves vital proteins and minerals that the body needs. Anything the body does not need is excreted in the urine. For the most part, urine is generally yellow and clear rather than cloudy. However, the color and consistency of urine can change, especially in the presence of systemic disease, infection, or focal urinary tract infection. Glycosuria or sugar spilling in the urine would be one of the most concerning findings for a dentist because this could indicate the presence of diabetes. In normal individuals sugar is absent from the urine. Many individuals with diabetes may not show sugars in the urine; therefore blood screening is the most sensitive way to screen for diabetes.

A urinalysis is not indicated as a routine procedure for dental patients and is rarely used in implant dentistry. The major uses for the urinalysis are a screening for diabetes, renal cancer with the presence of blood, kidney damage evidenced by the presence of protein or microalbumin, issues involving the liver with elevated levels of bilirubin, and infection with the presence of leukocytes or nitrates. Women that are menstruating will frequently have blood in their urine sample.

Complete Blood Cell Count

A CBC is a common screening test that evaluates the cells that circulate in the blood. There are three types of cells suspended in blood plasma: white blood cells (WBCs), red blood cells (RBCs), and platelets. The bone marrow produces these cells and allows them to mature before releasing them into the bloodstream.

The blood sample is read by an automated machine that the cells present and performs a number of other measurements including the physical characteristics of the cells. This would include the size of RBCs; which can be abnormal in cases of anemia (smaller), or vitamin deficiencies like B_{12} or folate (larger). The CBC is a good general screening test, but it may not be required unless major blood loss is anticipated.

However, in implant dentistry, CBCs would be important in patients with a history of anemia or bleeding disorders. CBCs are also useful for patients with chronic renal conditions, which can cause anemia or those that have been on recent (<3 months) steroid or glucocorticoid therapy. Any patient that received chemotherapy for cancer, cured or in remission, or history of WBC disease such as neutropenia (low WBC) or chronic leukemia (markedly elevated WBC) would also require a CBC.[12]

White Blood Cell Count

WBCs are also referred to as leukocytes. The normal total WBC count ranges from 4500 to 11,000 cells/mm^3, and the normal range can vary between laboratories. An increase in WBCs, or leukocytosis, is not specific to one WBC type. Some of the more common issues that create an elevated WBC are acute infection, inflammation, steroid therapy, or abnormal bone marrow production.

There are five different types of WBCs. Neutrophils, which help fight infection, are the most numerous. Lymphocytes, which are usually less than 25 % of the total cell count, help form antibodies and help the body get rid of foreign substances. They can be elevated in viral infections and decreased in immunocompromised patients such as in HIV. One of the first signs of immunodeficiency including HIV may be low lymphocyte count. Basophils are less than 1% of the total count and can increase or decrease based on certain disease states. Infections, severe allergies, and an overactive thyroid can cause abnormally high counts of basophils. Eosinophils, which are usually less than 3% of the total cell count, are elevated in the presence of allergic responses or parasitic infections. Monocytes, making up less than 10% of the count, are responsible for ingesting bacteria or foreign particles. Monocyte counts can be elevated in inflammatory bowel disease (IBD), endocarditis, or bacterial infections of heart, and parasitic or viral infections. A decrease in the number of total WBCs is referred to as leukopenia. Decreased WBC counts usually are the result of a viral infection, immune disorder, or bone marrow disease.

From an implant dentistry perspective, abnormalities in WBC counts can have significant implications. Inflammatory processes can be present with normal WBC counts, but certain types of cells, when increased, can indicate ongoing inflammation or possibly infection. Elevation in band neutrophils or absolute neutrophil counts (ANCs) usually indicates a more serious process like infection or severe inflammation.

When using a WBC count to monitor infection level, it is important to realize that early in the disease process the WBC counts may be normal. It is important to pay attention to shifts in the number of specific WBCs, such as neutrophils, basophils, or monocytes, which is reported as the differential (the breakdown of the five different types of WBCs). WBC counts are critical to dental outpatient care, particularly for patients with immune diseases or undergoing chemotherapy. The counts can indicate infections, leukemic disease (myeloproliferative), immune diseases, and toxicity of drugs (especially chemotherapeutic drugs). The ANC is very important in evaluating a patient's ability to fight infection. This count is calculated by multiplying the WBC count by the percentage of neutrophils. When not using antibiotic prophylaxis, the ANC must be greater than 2000. Counts less than 1500 are considered neutropenia. These individuals should be seen and evaluated by a hematologist or primary care physician and should be given clearance before continuing with implant surgery.

Consideration for antibiotics should begin at an ANC of less than 2500 and most definitely should be used for ANC levels of 1000 to 2000. Dental implant procedures should never be considered in a patient with an ANC of less than 1000.

Red Blood Cell Count

RBCs are responsible for the transport of oxygen and carbon dioxide throughout the body and for control of the blood pH. These cells represent the largest segment of the formed elements of the blood. The normal RBC count is higher in men than in women. Increases may result from polycythemia, smoking, testosterone use, congenital heart disease, or Cushing syndrome. The most common finding is a decreased cell count, which usually indicates anemia.

Hemoglobin

Hemoglobin (Hb) is responsible for carrying oxygen throughout the bloodstream. Each Hb protein carries up to four molecules of oxygen that can be delivered to various cells in the body. The normal level of Hb is 13.5 to 18 g/dL in men and 12 to 16 g/dL in women. The preoperative threshold of 10 g/dL is often used as a minimum baseline for surgery. However, many patients can undergo surgical procedures safely at 8 g/dL as long as their anemia has been chronic and stable.

It is critical for patients with Hb values less than 10 that the history of the rate of decrease be evaluated. Levels that have been consistently decreasing over time could indicate chronic blood loss in the gastrointestinal (GI) tract or through other means including malformation of blood vessels. Patients with a chronic stable anemia can have consistently lower Hb levels as their baseline. Women with heavy periods can develop low Hb counts over time that can sometimes drop below 10 and require supplementation with iron.

It is always a good idea to check with the patient's physician to confirm the chronicity of their anemia and baseline Hb. Significant acute decreases can be just as important at indicating a new process that may need to be addressed before the implant.

Hematocrit

White and red blood cells are suspended in serum and make up the contents of blood. The hematocrit is the percentage of RBCs in a given volume of blood. The hematocrit is a significant indicator of anemia or blood loss. Adult males have a normal value of about 42% to 54% and women 38% to 46%. Values within 75% to 80% of normal are required before sedation or general anesthesia.

Bleeding Tests

Bleeding disorders are the underlying cause of critical bleeding episodes in any type of dental surgery. Blood changes from liquid to solid through the coagulation cascade, which is a complex series of steps that result in a fibrin clot. The body uses platelets to plug the site of injury, and clotting factors then help form the fibrin clot that maintains the platelets in place.

It is important to realize that the platelet count alone does not necessarily provide all the information needed to evaluate a patient for a potential clotting disorder. It is critical to screen the patient for other signs such as easy bruising, heavy menstrual cycles, frequent nosebleeds, and prolonged bleeding after small cuts. The patient's medical history may be a better detector than platelet counts.

Understanding the normal clotting process determines which bleeding test to evaluate. Whenever the integrity of a vessel wall is altered surgically, hemostasis is achieved in three phases: vascular spasm, formation of the platelet plug, and then blood coagulation, which through the formation of fibrin stabilizes the platelet plug. For hemostasis to be maintained or achieved, the blood vessels must be normal, and functional platelets must be present in sufficient number with all clotting factors in the coagulation cascade working properly. In a normal, healthy individual, coagulation is initiated within 20 seconds of blood vessel damage. This is accomplished by two phases of hemostasis: primary and secondary. Primary hemostasis is initiated when platelets adhere to collagen fibers in the vascular endothelium and form the platelet plug. The platelets become inactivated, which results in additional platelet activation and expansion of the platelet plug. The secondary phase consists of a coagulation cascade that has two pathways (Fig. 10.2): contact activation pathway (formerly the intrinsic pathway) and the tissue factor pathway (formerly the extrinsic pathway). These pathways involve a series of enzymatic reactions in which an inactive coagulation factor is converted to an active form, which then activates the next coagulation factors in a series of reactions that result in the formation of fibrin to strengthen the clot. The clotting cascade requires cofactors such as calcium and vitamin K to assist with the synthesis of additional clotting factors.

The tissue factor pathway (extrinsic system) and the contact activation pathway (intrinsic system) lead to completion of hemostasis along a common pathway. Both systems are necessary for normal coagulation. The extrinsic system is activated outside the blood vessels; the intrinsic system is activated within the blood vessels.

Three ways to detect potential bleeding problems are (1) to check the medical history, including any family history of bleeding disorders; (2) to review the physical examination; and (3) to screen the clinical laboratory tests. More than 90% of bleeding disorders can be diagnosed on the basis of the medical history alone.[13]

Bleeding problems in relatives are significant because they indicate inherited coagulation disorders. Hemophilia is a rare inherited condition that can cause minor or major bleeding. It is classified as hemophilia A (lacking clotting factor VIII) and hemophilia B (lacking clotting factor IX, the Christmas factor). Hemophilia B is mostly a hereditary disorder, but 33% of the cases are caused by a spontaneous mutation. The von Willebrand factor is needed to properly carry factor VIII and help blood clot. Without sufficient levels of this factor, blood will not clot properly, resulting in prolonged bleeding after damage to tissue. This hereditary disorder is classified as type 1, 2, or 3 depending on the level of deficiency of the von Willebrand factor. Type 1 is the mildest and type 3 is the most serious. In all of these conditions, WBC, RBC, Hb, and hematocrit most likely will be normal.

It is important to obtain a history of complications from any previous dental or other surgeries. These acquired disorders are present from birth, so uncomplicated previous surgeries most likely indicate there are no inherited disorders. A full personal and family history is still needed, especially in the case of milder forms of the acquired deficiencies. Milder forms of the disease may not cause excessive bleeding in certain conditions but could still create issues during dental implant surgery.

Anticoagulants prevent the production of certain clotting factors and do not break up clots that have already formed. Examples include warfarin, rivaroxiban (Xarelto), apixaban (Eliquis), edoxapan (Savaysa), and dabigatran (Pradaxa). Vitamin K can be used to reverse the effects of Coumadin or warfarin. The newer anticoagulants require more specific reversal medication such as Praxbind for Pradaxa. Currently the Food and Drug Administration (FDA) is evaluating a reversal agent for the other, newer anticoagulant medications like Xarelto and Eliquis. Many times, within 5 days of stopping the medications, the anticoagulant effect of the drug is minimal or eliminated.

Antiplatelet medications decrease platelet aggregation for up to 2 weeks and inhibit the formation of the thrombus. Examples of these medications include aspirin, clopidogrel (Plavix), prasugrel (Effient), ticagrelor (Brilinta), and dipyridamole/aspirin (Aggrenox). Nonsteroidal antiinflammatory drugs (NSAIDs) such as ibuprofen and naproxen may interfere with platelets by blocking platelet aggregation for up to 1 week. This can directly affect clotting during dental surgery.

Any blood dyscrasia history, such as anemia, leukemia, thrombocytopenia (too few platelets), and liver diseases, such as hepatitis or cirrhosis, can be associated with current bleeding disorders. The liver is responsible for synthesizing certain clotting factors and causing defects in both in the quantity and quality of platelet production. Vitamin K is essential for productions of PT, which is required for normal clotting. Therefore it is important that individuals consume daily foods such as green leafy vegetables, such as spinach, lettuce, broccoli, and cabbage, which are high in vitamin K.

Physical Examination

The second method by which the implant dentist can detect a patient with a bleeding disorder is the physical examination. The exposed skin and oral mucosa must be examined for objective signs. Petechiae, ecchymosis, spider angioma, or jaundice may be observed in liver disease patients with bleeding complications. Intraoral petechiae, bleeding gingiva, ecchymosis, hemarthroses, and hematomas may be present in patients with genetic bleeding disorders. Patients with acute or chronic leukemia show signs of oral mucosa ulceration, hyperplasia of the

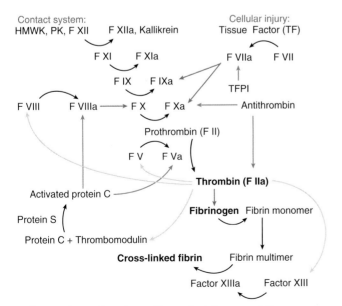

• **Fig. 10.2** Secondary phase of hemostasis is a coagulation cascade.

gingiva, petechiae or ecchymosis of the skin or oral mucosa, or lymphadenopathy. Macular or nodular lesions could be a sign of multiple myeloma.

Clinical Laboratory Testing

The third option for detecting a bleeding disorder is clinical laboratory testing. If a patient's health history and physical examination do not reveal potential bleeding disorders, routine screening with a coagulation profile is not indicated. However, if extensive surgical procedures are expected, a coagulation profile is indicated.

Screening tests for bleeding disorders should include a platelet count, bleeding time, international normalized ratio (INR; formally PT), activated partial thromboplastin time (aPTT), and a thrombin time (TT). In the near future, more sophisticated platelet function analytic studies could replace the bleeding time. NSAIDs (example ibuprofen) and aspirin used within 10 days of this test can affect the results.[14]

International Normalized Ratio and Prothrombin Time. In many cases the most appropriate tests to evaluate patients that are on anticoagulant therapy are the INR and PT. The PT is a test that determines how long it takes blood to clot. Until the early 1990s, the PT was used exclusively to measure the effect of Coumadin on blood clotting. The PT was the test used to measure the effectiveness of the tissue factor pathway (extrinsic system) and common pathways of coagulation. However, because of the variability in laboratory reporting, the World Health Organization (WHO) developed a more standardized system called the INR. In a normal individual, the INR value should be 1.0. The recommended therapeutic range of continuous anticoagulation is an INR between 2.0 and 3.0 for all conditions except artificial heart valves, for which the INR should be between 2.5 and 3.5 (Table 10.1).[15] Each 0.1 increase in the INR means the blood is slightly thinner. An INR > 1.2 in patients not on blood-thinning medication may require additional workup including liver function.

Partial Thromboplastin Time. The PTT is another coagulation test that measures the contact activation pathway (intrinsic system) and common pathways. A more sensitive version of the PTT is the aPTT, which has a normal range of 30 to 40 seconds and is used to monitor heparin therapy. The normal range of the PTT is 25 to 35 seconds and should be used as a routine screening test. Low-dose aspirin only has a minimal effect of INR/PT or PTT.

TABLE 10.1	Target International Normalized Values for Specific Medical Conditions	
Patient Condition	**INR Value**
Normal	1.0
Prevention of myocardial infarction	2.0–3.0
Treatment of pulmonary embolism	2.0–3.0
Treatment of atrial fibrillation	2.0–3.0
Pulmonary embolism	2.0–3.0
Prosthetic heart valves	2.5–3.5
Prevention of venous thrombosis	2.5–3.5

INR, International normalized ratio.

Bleeding Time. The bleeding time test is used to evaluate platelet function The Ivy method is the standardized test usually used. In this test, a blood pressure cuff is placed on the upper arm and inflated to 40 mm Hg. A lancet or scalpel blade is used to make a cut on the underside of the forearm, and the time is measured until bleeding has stopped. Normal values fall between 2 and 9 minutes depending on the method used. The bleeding time measures both coagulation pathways and platelet function and capillary activity. Bleeding time will be elevated in the presence of aspirin for 2 weeks or NSAIDs for up to 10 days. It is important to realize that clotting time is different from bleeding time. Clotting time takes longer because it is the time for blood to actually coagulate or form a clot. Normal values are between 8 and 15 minutes.

Platelet Count. The platelet count is part of the CBC and is usually in range of 150,000 to 450,000 cells/mL of blood. This test identifies the number of platelets (thrombocytes), which is vital to the formation of the blood clot. If the count falls below 150,000 cells/mL, the patient is said to have thrombocytopenia. As platelet counts drop below 100,000, there can be significant bleeding problems in implant patients. Low platelet counts will not affect the PT/INR or PTT tests.

Thrombin Time. The enzymes in thrombin help fibrinogen form fibrin, which help form and strengthen the clot. The TT measures the activity of factor Xa (FXa), which activates prothrombin to thrombin. Thrombin then helps form fibrin and also helps stabilize the clot through cross-linking by activating factor XIII. The reference range for TT is usually less than 20 seconds depending on the test kit used. This test in conjunction with the other coagulation tests can provide valuable information about the patient's ability to form clots.

Additional Oral Anticoagulants. In the United States there are several approved novel oral anticoagulants (NOACs) including rivaroxaban (Xarelto), apixaban (Eliquis), edoxaban (Savaysa), and dabigatran (Pradaxa). These drugs were approved for the treatment of venous thromboembolism, pulmonary embolism, and nonvalvular atrial fibrillation. Because their pharmacokinetics is more predictable than Coumadin/warfarin, they do not require laboratory monitoring. In the studies to approve these drugs they were shown to be as or more effective and safe than Coumadin/warfarin. These drugs are not approved for patients with artificial heart valves or atrial fibrillation related to a defective heart valve.

The previously mentioned coagulation studies do not adequately provide information on the effective inhibition of clotting potential for these drugs. Activity of these NOACs is difficult to measure because of several variables including the reagent and analyzer used. Each NOAC affects the PT/INR test differently, which is more dependent on the time when the blood sample was drawn relative to the time of the most recent dose. In contrast, the INR/PT measurement for Coumadin/warfarin demonstrates activity based on the cumulative effect of several of the most recent doses.

Pradaxa (dabigatran) has almost no effect on coagulation studies and does not correlate to the measurement of INR/PT and PTT until supertherapeutic levels are taken. A normal aPTT usually indicates there are no excess drug levels. The TT is also sensitive to Pradaxa, and a normal TT usually indicates normal blood drug levels.

In contrast, Rivaroxaban (Xarelto) has a sensitivity to INR/PT, and a normal INR/PT usually excludes significant drug levels. Rivaroxaban has no effect on aPTT or TT. Apixaban (Eliquis) cannot be measured by and has no effect on INR/PT, aPTT, or TT. Edoxaban (Savaysa) has almost no effect on INR/PT or TT, but it is sensitive to measurement by aPTT.[16-18]

Dialysis patients pose a number of challenges to the implant dentistry. There are just a few infections that alter drug metabolism and bone lesions. Dialysis patients may be at increased risk for bleeding as well. If the PTT is more than 1.5 times the normal value, surgery should be postponed until physician approval.

Long-term antibiotic therapy can affect the intestinal bacteria that help produce vitamin K, which is necessary for prothrombin production in the liver. Therefore if the implant patient has used long-term administration of antibiotics, then a PT should be obtained to evaluate possible bleeding complications.

It is very important to suspect bleeding disorders in a patient that consumes excessive amounts of alcohol for prolonged periods of time or who has a history of alcohol abuse, because this can lead to liver dysfunction. The liver is the primary site of synthesis of the vitamin K–dependent clotting factors II, VII, IX, and X. Patients with intestinal absorption issues or a diet low in vitamin K can exacerbate this problem.

Alcoholism, independent of liver disease, has been shown to decrease platelet production by megakaryocytes and increased platelet destruction. Most coagulation factors are produced in the liver; 50% of patients with liver disease have hypersplenism resulting from the destruction of platelets. The PT is the single most useful test used to evaluate impaired hepatocyte synthesis of prothrombin complex factors and to assess hemostasis in patients with liver disease. Factor VII has the shortest half-life and is the first to decrease. Factor VIII and the von Willebrand factor tend to increase in chronic hepatic disease patients.

The PT and PTT may be used together to determine coagulation factor defects. A normal PT and abnormal PTT suggest hemophilia. An abnormal PT and a normal PTT suggest factor VII deficiency. If both PT and PTT are longer, then a deficiency of factors II, V, or X or fibrinogen should be considered.

No surgical procedures should be performed on a patient suspected of having a bleeding problem based on history, examination, and clinical laboratory tests without proper preparation, understanding, and concerted management by the dentist and the physician. If the bleeding disorder has been previously undiagnosed, the underlying cause should be addressed before the elective implant surgical procedures begin.

Biochemical Profiles (Serum Chemistry)

The tenets of laboratory diagnosis should be understood, particularly as they relate to implant dentistry. The interpretation of biochemical profiles and the ability to communicate effectively with medical consultants will enhance the treatment of many patients.

The decision to proceed with oral implant treatment may be affected by the results of biochemical profiles by contraindicating the procedure completely, altering the type of implant surgery and reconstruction, postponing the treatment until therapy controls the disease entity, or simply changing the sequence of medications normally used during treatment. Biochemical sanguine profiles are a more necessary part of the medical evaluation for an implant candidate in the presence of systemic diseases or advanced surgical procedures.[19] They are not indicated for every potential implant patient.

The most common metabolic screening assays are the BMP and CMP. The BMP measures the blood levels of the calcium, carbon dioxide (bicarbonate), chloride, creatinine, glucose, potassium, sodium, and blood urea nitrogen (BUN). The CMP measures all of the same tests in the BMP with the addition of albumin, total bilirubin, protein, and the liver enzymes alanine aminotransferase (ALT), aspartate aminotransferase (AST), and alkaline phosphatase (ALP).

It is imperative that dental implant clinicians have a strong understanding of the more common blood chemistry tests. With an understanding of the basic blood profiles such as the BMP and CMP, a dental implant surgeon can have greater insight into the biochemical parameters reflecting the patient's health.

To be comfortable in interpreting the biochemical profile, some time must be spent in learning the BMP/CMP pattern of systemic diseases. This pattern recognition is similar to the tissue patterns a pathologist looks at during a biopsy. The BMP/CMP profile has been described as a "biochemical biopsy" of the blood. These profiles include normal and abnormal values that have interrelationships in the diagnosis of systemic diseases. It is not wise to single out one value to establish a diagnosis. The data should be related with other values obtained in the profile before further determinations are rendered.

Normal Range

The normal values found on the BMP/CMP represent a statistical norm. Any population characteristically shows a bell-shaped curve for a particular measurement. It has been shown that 56% of a sample fall within one standard deviation of the mean and 95% are within two standard deviations. The normal value in the biochemical profile represents two standard deviations. Thus "normal" in the statistical sense does not necessarily mean healthy; instead, the word merely describes the typical range of values expected in any given population. Approximately 1 in 20 results will be outside the two standard deviation ranges. The further from the average value a particular value falls, the more certain its clinical significance. Different laboratories can have different normal results.

As biochemical profiles are compiled for an individual patient over several years, the deviation in a given test may indicate a radical change for that individual, although the result should never deviate from the normal population range. The implant dentist should remember that the healthy patient of today might have a systemic disease in the future. Therefore when evaluating long-term complications, it is of interest to relate a recent biochemical profile to the one first reviewed before the initial surgery.

The patient should fast for at least 6 to 8 hours before the blood is collected to avoid artificial elevations of blood glucose. Most of the other elements of the profile will not be affected. This chapter will limit discussion to the most common tests that are beneficial to the implant dentist (Table 10.2): glucose, calcium, inorganic phosphorus, ALP, lactic dehydrogenase (LDH), creatinine, and bilirubin.

Serum Glucose

The normal range of glucose found in the blood is 70 to 100 mg/mL and is maintained within fairly narrow limits. It is important when evaluating the serum glucose to make sure the specimen has been collected after the patient was fasting for at least 6 to 8 hours. If not, the serum blood level may exceed 120 to 140 depending on the timing of the test from the last meal. Elevated fasting blood sugars are becoming more common as our population ages. Sugars between 100 to 120 fasting can be consistent with the beginning of glucose intolerance, which is a precursor for diabetes (Table 10.3).

TABLE 10.2	Laboratory Evaluation of Disease Indicators
Chemistry	**Disease**
Glucose	Diabetes, steroid dysfunction
Calcium	Renal disease, diet, bone diseases, (carcinoma, parathyroid disease, Paget disease)
Inorganic phosphorus	Renal disease, endocrine (parathyroid, thyroid, steroids), antacids
Alkaline phosphatase	Liver disease, bone diseases (Paget disease, metastases, fractures, hyperparathyroidism)
Lactic dehydrogenase	Hemolytic disorders, liver disorders, myocardial infarction
Creatinine	Renal function
Bilirubin	Liver disease

TABLE 10.3	Hemoglobin A1c Values versus Blood Glucose Levels (Approximate)	
Hemoglobin A1c (%)	**Average Blood Sugar (mg/dL)**	
6	120	
7	150	
8	180	
9	210	
10	240	
11	270	
12	300	

The most common cause of hyperglycemia is diabetes mellitus. If fasting levels of glucose are found to be greater than 120, then a referral to a physician may be warranted. If fasting sugar is greater than 100, then an HbA1c should be added to the blood profile. This test is also referred to as glycosylated Hb and provides average blood sugar concentrations for the past 90 days. For most diabetics the target is less than 7.0%; however, recent studies now show that targets are individualized based on other factors. Patients with longer life expectancy, monotherapy with metformin, and no cardiovascular complications have a target of <6.5%. Patients with frequent hypoglycemic episodes, advanced vascular disease, other comorbidities, and longer history of having diabetes may have a target of <8.0%. An HbA1c greater than 8% should be considered an absolute contraindication to dental implant surgery, and a consultation between the physician and the patient is warranted.

Other causes of hyperglycemia include obesity, insulin resistance, chronic pancreatitis, Cushing syndrome (excess corticosteroid production), polycystic ovary disease, acromegaly, and hemochromatosis (excess iron stores). High fasting blood sugars can be seen in patients that have taken recent or concurrent oral steroids. Hypoglycemia can occur but is much more rare and can be associated with liver damage or excessive insulin production from an insulinoma tumor in the pancreas.

Serum Calcium

Calcium plays a role in several important body functions including nerve impulse transmission, blood coagulation, and muscle contraction. The overwhelming majority of calcium (>99%) is present in the skeleton and teeth. Calcium in the bone provides strength to the skeleton and supplies the intracellular and extracellular calcium. Serum calcium ranges from about 8.8 to 10.4. Bone balance of calcium changes over time. Kids have a positive bone balance (formation > resorption) for skeletal growth. Young adults are usually in neutral bone balance (formation = resorption). Elderly individuals are usually in negative balance during which formation is greater than resorption.

The implant dentist may be the first to detect diseases affecting the bones. Serum calcium levels are influenced by the parathyroid hormone and calcitonin. Serum calcium levels are increased by bone resorption, intestinal absorption, and renal reabsorption of calcium. Vitamin D helps with intestinal reabsorption of calcium and is activated by the parathyroid hormone to allow the intestine to double and even quadruple the absorption of calcium.

Decreased levels of calcium are primarily seen in hypoparathyroidism, decreased dietary or absorptive conditions, hypoproteinemic conditions, and renal disease. Renal disease is much more common, but the diet of the potential implant patient may be severely affected by the lack of denture comfort and stability. The cause and treatment of hypocalcemic serum levels should be addressed before implant reconstruction.

Elevated levels of serum calcium are associated with carcinoma in bones, dietary or absorptive disturbances, and hyperparathyroidism. The osteoporosis that accompanies this disorder has been observed in the mandible. Hyperparathyroidism also causes hypophosphatemia. Hypercalcemia associated with a significant elevation of ALP suggests Paget disease. With all other biochemical values being normal, an elevated calcium value may be the result of laboratory error.[20] If phosphorus or ALP levels are also affected, medical evaluation and treatment are indicated before implant surgery. Calcium levels greater than 11 should be investigated immediately. It is important that lower elevations of calcium also are evaluated, and the patient should be referred back to his or her physician.

Inorganic Phosphorus

Parathyroid hormone also regulates serum levels of phosphorus because of the relationship between calcium and phosphorus in the blood serum. The normal level is between 3 to 4 mg/100 mL. Similar to calcium, it is readily absorbed through the GI tract and can be increased with vitamin D intake. Phosphorus maintains a reciprocal relationship with calcium: as the level of one increases, the other decreases. The most common cause of hyperphosphatemia is renal disease. Low levels of calcium accompany high levels of phosphorus. This results in increased level of parathyroid hormone (PTH), which then increases bone turnover resulting in significant bone mass and density loss.

If an increase in phosphorus is associated with a decrease in calcium and normal renal function, hypoparathyroidism is suspected. If kidney function is abnormal (high BUN/creatinine ratio), the increased phosphorus level is most likely caused by kidney dysfunction. Other endocrine disorders associated with an increased phosphorus level include hyperthyroidism, increased growth hormone secretion, and Cushing syndrome.

Decreased levels of phosphorus may appear in patients with hyperparathyroidism, especially when it is associated with hypercalcemia. The chronic use of antacids containing aluminum hydroxide also may induce hypophosphatemia and warrants investigation for a peptic ulcer.

Alkaline Phosphatase

ALP is an enzyme that is present in the liver, bones, kidneys, and digestive system. The normal ranges are from 44 to 147 IU/mL. There is a rise in ALP levels in all forms of cholestasis (reduction of bile flow), especially in obstructive jaundice. Any damage to the liver can raise the ALP level because damaged cells release ALP into the bloodstream.

In the absence of liver disease, elevations of ALP are often a sign of osteoblastic activity in the skeletal system. Therefore bone metastases, fractures, Paget disease, multiple myeloma, and hyperparathyroidism increase the level of this serum enzyme. Serum ALP is normal in patients with adult osteoporosis. Low levels of ALP are usually not of clinical significance for the dentist.

Lactic Dehydrogenase

LDH is an intracellular enzyme present in all tissues (normal 100–190 U/L) including blood, muscles, brain, kidneys, and pancreas. This enzyme helps convert sugar into energy. If cells become damaged, then LDH is released into the bloodstream. Falsely elevated LDH levels occur as a result of hemolyzed blood specimens. Therefore if all other blood values including liver function tests (LFTs) are normal, LDH testing should be repeated before further investigation.

Because LDH is in many cell types, high levels of LDH can indicate a number of conditions including a cerebrovascular accident (CVA)/stroke, certain cancers, MI, hemolytic anemia, mononucleosis, liver disease (hepatitis), muscle injury, pancreatitis, and sepsis. Elevated levels can be further differentiated to their source as isoenzymes: LDH-1 and LDH-2 are found in the heart and RBCs; LDH-3 is found in lymph tissue, lung, and pancreas; and LDH-4 and LDH-5 are found in the liver and muscle tissue.

When LDH values are elevated, the isoenzyme test should be performed to determine the etiology of the elevation, and the CBC and a blood smear should be evaluated for any abnormalities.

Bilirubin

Bilirubin is a pigment formed by the liver as it breaks down Hb and excretes it into the bile. There are two types of bilirubin: indirect (unconjugated), which is not attached to glucuronic acid; and direct (conjugated), which is attached to glucuronic acid. These values are added together to give the total bilirubin. The level of bilirubin can be an indicator of liver health. Normal serum values of total bilirubin typically are 0.2 to 1 mg/dL. Direct bilirubin should be no more than 0.2 mg/dL.

When evaluating an elevated bilirubin, it is important to differentiate the source of the elevation (indirect, or direct, or both). Some patients are born with a condition called Gilbert syndrome in which the liver does not properly conjugate bilirubin, leading to elevated unconjugated (indirect) bilirubin levels. This condition is present at birth, and most patients will be told some time early in life that they have this harmless condition. Acute elevations of indirect bilirubin are usually a result of hemolytic anemia. The increase in indirect bilirubin in both of these diseases is caused by excess production of bilirubin.

High levels of bilirubin can be associated with jaundice, which can be a result of acute or chronic liver disease or failure, cancer, dysfunction of the bile duct including gallstones, or acute inflammation of the liver such as in hepatitis.

When evaluating liver function, it is important to look at all the tests available in the BMP or CMP because proper liver function is important for healing, drug metabolism, and long-term health.

Aminotransferases

The most sensitive tests to indicate liver damage are liver enzymes referred to as the aminotransferases. The two most common and included in a CMP and LFT profile are the AST (or SGOT) and ALT (or SGPT). An injury to the liver will cause the release of these enzymes into the bloodstream.

AST is less specific for liver damage because it can be found in other tissues outside the liver such as the heart, kidneys, muscles, and brain. Damage to these cells will cause release of AST. ALT or SGPT elevation is more specific for liver disease such as hepatitis or cirrhosis. Some patients have chronic higher than normal levels from conditions like fatty liver, which are usually benign. Some may have mild elevation from medications they take, such as statins. Higher than normal levels should not always be assumed to be from liver damage. The levels are a marker that may or may not demonstrate damage to the liver. Elevation in levels can occur from muscle damage. The level of increase may not be directly proportional to the amount of liver disease or prognosis. Some patients with end-stage liver disease may have only mildly elevated levels. In viral hepatitis A from food these levels can reach the thousands, but recovery is usually full and complete. Patients with chronic hepatitis C infections may have no elevation or only minimal elevation and still develop chronic liver disease or failure.

Creatinine

Creatinine levels are one of the ways to monitor kidney function or kidney disease. If the kidneys become impaired, the blood level of creatinine will rise because the kidneys are unable to excrete enough creatinine into the urine. There is a fairly constant production and excretion of creatinine, which provides a reasonable way to monitor kidney function. The normal creatinine range is 0.6 to 1.1 mg/dL in women and 0.7 to 1.3 mg/dL in men. Diabetics have a high incidence of kidney dysfunction but may have a normal creatinine. In diabetics, a microalbumin screen of the urine can pick up early kidney dysfunction. Microalbumin in the urine is the earliest form of nephropathy or damage from diabetes.

The renal system should not be impaired during implant surgery. Kidney dysfunction may lead to osteoporosis and decreased bone healing. The kidney is required for appropriate activation of Vitamin D to aid in Calcium absorption. Medications can alter pharmacokinetics, and normal healing can also be affected by kidney disease.

Low creatinine levels could be from an issue with the muscles or liver. In older adults reduced muscle mass can cause a low creatine level.

Estimated Glomerular Filtration Rate

The estimated glomerular filtration rate (eGFR) is often included in the BMP or CMP blood panel and can provide more detailed information on kidney function. This test can detect early kidney damage and help with the diagnosis of chronic kidney disease (CKD). More important is a consistent way to monitor kidney status. Normal kidney (stage 1) will have a GFR of 90 or more. Stage 2 kidney disease demonstrates some mild loss of kidney function and has an eGFR between 60 and 89. Stage 3 kidney disease indicates more moderate to severe loss of kidney function and has values of 30 to 59. Stage 4 disease indicates severe loss of kidney function and has values between 15 and 29. Stage 5 indicates kidney failure and has an eGFR of 15 or less. The eGFR will decline with age, even when kidney disease is absent. For example, ages 40 to 49 have an average eGFR of 99, whereas ages 60 to 69 have an average eGFR of 85. A reduced eGFR may require a reduction in dosages of medications metabolized by the kidney.

Blood Urea Nitrogen

Urea is produced mainly in the liver. It enters the bloodstream and is excreted by the kidney in the renal tubules; sweat also can excrete a very small amount of urea. The BUN level can be used as an indicator of kidney and/or liver function. The usual range is 3 to 20 mg/dL. Elevated levels can be seen in a urinary tract obstruction, CHF, a GI bleed, dehydration, use of some medications including some antibiotics, and a high-protein diet.

The BUN can be used in conjunction with the creatinine level and is usually between a ratio of 10 to 1 and 20 to 1. A ratio of greater than 20 can indicate dehydration or GI bleeding. This condition is referred to as prerenal and can also be a result of hypoperfusion of the kidney. When the ratio is less than 10 to 1, it can indicate polyuria such as in diabetes insipidus or Cushing disease and liver disease or failure (Table 10.4).

Systemic Disease and Oral Implants

Systemic diseases play a vital role in treatment planning and implant therapy for patients. There are specific systemic diseases and conditions that undeniably affect bone metabolism, wound

(text continues on p. 19)

TABLE 10.4 **Diagnostic Laboratory Test Summary**

Test Name	Description	Elevated Levels	Decreased Levels
Albumin (blood)	Is produced by liver and most abundant protein in blood; can be used to judge changes in overall health, liver, or kidney function	Dehydration	Inflammation, liver disease, malnutrition, kidney disease, malabsorption
Alkaline phosphatase	Produced by several organs including liver, bone, and kidney	Bone disease such as metastatic cancer, Paget disease, multiple myeloma, liver disease	Malnutrition, hypophosphatemia, hypothyroid, B_{12} deficiency
ALT (SGPT)	Used to access function of the liver	Liver disease (hepatitis, necrosis, cirrhosis, tumor); medications (statins, antibiotics, chemotherapy, narcotics); mononucleosis, obesity (fatty liver)	N/A
Amylase	Enzyme produced by pancreas and used to detect issues with pancreas	Pancreatitis	N/A
ANA	Used as a screen for connective tissue disease; positive test occurs in some individuals without specific disease	Requires further specific tests to confirm lupus, scleroderma, Sjögren syndrome, or myositis	N/A
AST (SGOT)	Used to detect liver disease and provide assessment of liver function	Liver disease, medications, mononucleosis, obesity (similar to AST) AST:ALT >2:1 shows alcoholic liver	Acute renal disease, beriberi, diabetic ketoacidosis, pregnancy, chronic renal dialysis
BMP	Blood panel that measures sodium, potassium, glucose, BUN, creatinine, chloride, CO_2	N/A	Dependent on test (refer to each component)
Bilirubin indirect	Level of bilirubin that is product of liver that is not conjugated (have sugar molecules attached)	Hemolytic anemia, cirrhosis, transfusion reaction, Gilbert disease (lack enzyme to conjugate)	N/A
Bilirubin direct	Level of bilirubin that is conjugated with a sugar molecule but cannot be secreted through blocked bile ducts	Viral hepatitis, drug reactions, alcoholic liver disease, gallstones, tumors, bile duct scarring	N/A
Bleeding time	Measure clot time focused on function of platelets	von Willebrand disease, thrombocytopenia, DIC, medications	N/A
BUN	Measure urea nitrogen formed when protein is broken down; help measure kidney and liver function	Kidney dysfunction, GI bleed, dehydration, shock, medications, CHF, or urinary outlet obstruction	Liver disease, SIADH, malnutrition
BUN/creatinine ratio	Ratio of BUN to creatinine, usually between 10:1 and 20:1	Dehydration, acute kidney failure or injury, diet high in protein (ratio can be normal in chronic kidney disease)	diet low in protein, muscle injury (rhabdomyolysis), pregnancy, cirrhosis, or (SIADH)

TABLE 10.4 Diagnostic Laboratory Test Summary—cont'd

Test Name	Description	Elevated Levels	Decreased Levels
Calcium	Checks blood level calcium not in bones and parathyroid function	Hyperparathyroidism, lung/breast cancer metastasis to bone, Paget disease, excessive intake of vitamin D	Chronic renal failure, vitamin D deficiency, magnesium deficiency, bisphosphonate therapy
Carbon dioxide	Level of carbon dioxide in the blood and important buffer of acid/base regulation	Vomiting, COPD, anorexia, dehydration, hypoventilation	Diarrhea, hyperventilation, kidney or liver disease
Chloride	Important in the monitoring of acid/base disorders	Dehydration, diarrhea, renal tubular acidosis, diuretics, hyperparathyroidism	Overhydration (SIADH), Addison disease, chronic vomiting, heart failure
Creatinine	Important measurement of kidney function	Kidney disease, dehydration, diuresis, medication, radiocontrast induced, hypertensive kidney disease	Decreased muscle mass
Creatinine clearance	Used to estimate glomerular filtration rate and overall kidney function	90+: stage 1 (normal kidney function) 60–89: stage 2 (mildly reduced kidney function) 30–59: stage 3 (moderately reduced kidney function) 15–29: stage 4 (severe kidney disease) <15: end-stage kidney disease	
ESR	Nonspecific marker for inflammation	Collagen vascular disease (lupus, rheumatoid arthritis), vasculitis, infections, malignancy, renal failure, inflammatory bowel disease, anemias	Polycythemia, sickle cell anemia, spherocytosis
Ferritin	Measures amount of iron stored in body	Hemochromatosis, porphyria, liver disease, multiple blood transfusions, liver disease, Hodgkin lymphoma	Hemodialysis, iron deficiency anemia
Glucose	Measurement of blood sugar level that is best interpreted fasting <100	Diabetes, nonfasting level, illness, infection, stress response	Excess insulin secretion, excessive alcohol, Addison's disease (adrenal insufficiency), reactive hypoglycemia
Hematocrit	Ratio of red blood cell volume to the total volume of the blood	Dehydration, diuresis, polycythemia vera, high altitude exposures	Anemia, pregnancy, excessive blood loss
Hemoglobin	Carries oxygen to tissues	Polycythemia, high altitude exposure, extreme exercise program	Anemia, hemolysis, excessive blood loss
Hemoglobin A1c	Measurement of percentage of hemoglobin coated with sugar and provides average of blood sugar over a 3-month period	Poorly controlled diabetes, iron deficiency anemia, vitamin B_{12} deficiency, uremia, alcoholism	Hemolysis, recent blood transfusion, chronic liver disease, excess treatment of diabetes, hypertriglyceridemia
Iron level	Measures amount of iron in blood	Hemochromatosis, hemolysis, liver necrosis, hepatitis, vitamin B_{12} deficiency, excessive blood transfusions	Low dietary intake, heavy menstrual bleeding, GI blood loss, intestinal malabsorption, pregnancy
LPL	Enzyme produced by pancreas to help break down fats and used to help determine disease of the pancreas	Pancreatitis, tumors of pancreas, gallbladder infection, high triglycerides, excessive alcohol, gallstones or infection of gallbladder	May indicate chronic damage to pancreas
LFTs	Measurement of liver functioning (AST, ALT, bilirubin, albumin, alkaline phosphatase)	See Individual Tests	See Individual Tests
MCV	Red blood cell average size	Vitamin B_{12} or folic acid deficiency, ETOH abuse, liver disease, bone marrow dysfunction, hypothyroidism	Anemias, iron deficiency, chronic disease, sideroblastic, chronic renal failure, lead poisoning, thalassemia
PTT	Measures time for blood to clot for intrinsic pathway (factors IX, X, XI, and XII)	Similar to PT	Similar to PT
Platelets	Number of circulating platelets	Acute bleeding, cancer, renal failure, infections, iron deficiency, splenectomy, inflammatory bowel disease, lupus	Hemolytic uremic syndrome, autoimmune disease, pregnancy, ITP, TTP

Continued

TABLE 10.4   Diagnostic Laboratory Test Summary—cont'd

Test Name	Description	Elevated Levels	Decreased Levels
Potassium	Measure level of potassium in blood, essential for proper function of organs and all cells	Acute/chronic kidney disease, Addison's disease (adrenal insufficiency) rhabdomyolysis (breakdown of muscle), HTN medications (ACE/ARB), excessive intake, burn injury	Diabetic ketoacidosis, diarrhea, excessive alcohol or laxative use, hyperhidrosis (excessive sweating), diuretics, folic acid deficiency, primary aldosterone tumor, vomiting
PSA	Measure blood level of PSA released by prostate gland; PSA normally increases with age as prostate enlarges	Prostate cancer, prostatitis, catheter insertion, BPH, UTI, age-related, prolonged bike riding	<0.1 in patients treated for prostate cancer
PT	Measures time for blood to clot by the extrinsic pathway (tissue factor, Xa); INR is standard measure	Liver disease, alcohol abuse, DIC, vitamin K deficiency, clotting factor deficiency, medication induced	Vitamin K supplementation, estrogen therapy, thrombophlebitis
RBC	Measures number of RBCs	Thalassemia trait, altitude exposure, cigarette use, polycythemia	Anemia (including hemolytic), acute blood loss, bone marrow dysfunction
RF	Measures Rheumatoid Factor (RF antibody) level which are proteins that attack healthy tissue	Rheumatoid arthritis, cancer, chronic infections or liver disease, lupus, scleroderma, Sjögren syndrome; also found in individuals with no disease	N/A
Sodium (Na)	Measure level of circulating sodium (important for fluid balance and functioning of nerves and muscles)	Increased dietary intake, Cushing syndrome	Medications (diuretics), CHF, liver disease, SIADH, chronic vomiting, adrenal insufficiency, drinking too much water
TSH	Released by pituitary and causes thyroid gland to release T4 and T3; used to diagnosis thyroid disease	Hypothyroidism, Hashimoto's thyroiditis (antibody attach thyroid), lithium, amiodarone	Hyperthyroidism, subacute thyroiditis (inflammation thyroid), excess thyroid replacement therapy, thyroid cancer (low normal)
T4 free or total	Total T4 measures the amount of T4 in blood released by thyroid and used to diagnose hyper/hypothyroid disease and respond to thyroid replacement; total T4 is protein bound and can be abnormal because of protein levels; free T4 more accurate and not influenced by protein levels	Hyperthyroidism (Graves' disease), pituitary adenoma, excessive thyroid replacement therapy, thyroiditis, birth control pills, pregnancy, excessive iodine intake	Hypothyroidism, pituitary insufficiency, malnutrition, chronic illness, low intake of iodine
T3 free or total	Measure the amount of circulating T3 produced by thyroid; T3 is bound to thyroxine binding globulin; T3 not bound to protein is free T3 and this is thought to be responsible for biologic activities in the body	Hyperthyroidism (Graves' disease), pituitary adenoma, excessive thyroid replacement therapy, thyroiditis, birth control pills, pregnancy, excessive iodine intake; free T3 levels stable in pregnancy and with birth control pills	Hypothyroidism, pituitary insufficiency, malnutrition, illness, medications (amiodarone, phenytoin)
WBC	Measures total number of white blood cells	Bacterial infection, sepsis, steroids very high in CLL	Immunosuppression, viral infections, chemotherapy, antibiotics
Types of WBCs			
Neutrophils	Most abundant type of white blood cell	Bacterial infections, "shift to left," more neutrophils, acute infection	Malignancies, aplastic anemia, severe infections
Lymphocytes	Made up of B cells that produce antibodies and T cells produced in thymus and are part of immune response	Viral infections including mononucleosis and hepatitis	Bone marrow dysfunction, chemotherapy, TB, lupus, rheumatoid arthritis, drug induced
Monocytes	Participate in phagocytosis; produce macrophages to help fight bacteria, fungi, and viruses	TB, chronic inflammatory disorders such as Crohn disease, ulcerative colitis, lupus	Vitamin B_{12} deficiency, bone marrow dysfunction, certain leukemias
Eosinophils	Produced in response to allergens and diseases	Allergic reactions, parasites	Cushing disease, treatment with steroids, stress reactions
Basophils	Least abundant WBC; contain heparin and histamine related to hypersensitivity reactions	Viruses, lymphoma, hypothyroidism, inflammatory bowel disease	Pregnancy, steroid use, hyperthyroidism

ACE, Angiotensin-converting enzyme; *ALT,* alanine transaminase; *ANA;* antinuclear antibody; *ARB,* angiotensin receptor blocker; *AST,* aspartate aminotransferase; *BMP,* basic metabolic profile; *BPH,* benign prostatic hypertension; *BUN,* blood urea nitrogen; *CHF,* congestive heart failure; *COPD,* chronic obstructive pulmonary disease; *DIC,* disseminated intravascular coagulation; *ESR,* erythrocyte sedimentation rate; *ETOH,* alcohol; *GI,* gastrointestinal; *HTN,* hypertension; *INR,* international normalized ratio; *ITP,* idiopathic thrombocytopenic purpura; *LFTs,* liver function tests; *LPL,* lipase; *MCV,* mean corpuscular volume; *PSA,* prostatic-specific antigen; *PT,* prothrombin time; *PTT,* partial thromboplastin time; *RBC,* red blood cell; *RF,* rheumatoid factor; *SIADH,* syndrome of inappropriate antidiuretic hormone secretion; *T3,* triiodothyronine; *T4,* thyroxine; *TB,* tuberculosis; *TSH,* thyroid-stimulating hormone; *TTP,* thrombotic thrombocytopenic purpura; *UTI,* urinary tract infection; *WBC,* white blood cell.

From Resnik RR, Resnik RJ. Medical/medication complications in oral implantology. In Resnik RR, Misch CE, eds. *Misch's Avoiding Complications in Oral Implantology.* St Louis, MO: Elsevier; 2018.

TABLE 10.5 Classifications of Dental Treatment

Classification Type	Treatment
1	Examinations, radiographs, study cast impressions, treatment planning, oral hygiene instruction, stage 2 uncovery with minimum tissue reflection, simple restorative dentistry
2	Extractions, single-tooth implants, multiple implants with minimum tissue reflection, minor augmentation procedures
3	Difficult extractions, multiple implants with more extensive reflection, ridge augmentation, unilateral sinus graft
4	Full-arch implants, autogenous block bone augmentation, large membrane grafts, bilateral sinus graft

healing, and ultimately the success of implant therapy. The implant clinician should use the specific systemic disease information with the planning and management phases of treatment. It is the responsibility of the implant dentist to understand the interrelationship of systemic diseases and implant dentistry. Common conditions that may affect the implant treatment are discussed in three steps. The first section describes the entity in general. The second section discusses dental implant treatment implications. The last section reviews dental implant management.

American Society of Anesthesiologists Physical Status Classification

Systemic diseases have a wide range of effects on a patient, depending on the severity of the disease. There are relatively few systemic diseases that always contraindicate implant surgery or prosthetic rehabilitation. However, several metabolic disorders have contraindications when the conditions are uncontrolled or severe. In 1962, the ASA adopted a classification system for the severity of disease, and the system still is widely used today in medicine. The classification system was designed to estimate the medical risk presented by a patient receiving general anesthesia for a surgical procedure. However, the classification system is valuable for determining any medical risk, regardless of the method of anesthesia or type of surgery (Box 10.2).

The systemic conditions listed in this chapter are those most commonly observed in an implant practice; it is not the intent of this chapter to include all conditions. The diseases discussed are classified as mild, moderate, or severe. A disease entity affects the host with varied intensity. For example, mild diabetes may permit implant treatment, but the same disease in the severe form may contraindicate most implant therapy. As a result, a mild diabetic patient should be treated differently from the severe diabetic patient.

In addition to the range of disease expression, the authors have presented a variety of implant treatments delivered to a patient.[21] In Table 10.5, four levels of surgical and prosthetic dental treatments are established. A systemic condition may contraindicate one class of treatment, yet a more simplified implant procedure can still be performed. The four levels of treatment range from noninvasive procedures with little or no risk of gingival bleeding to those that are most complicated and invasive.

Type 1 procedures can be performed on most patients regardless of systemic condition. Type 2 procedures are more likely to cause gingival bleeding or bacterial invasion of the bony structures. Type 3 procedures are surgical procedures that require more time and technique. Type 4 procedures are advanced surgical procedures with more bleeding and greater risk of postoperative infection and complications.

A relationship can be established between the severity of the disease (mild to severe) and the maximum involvement of the dental implant procedure (Table 10.6). For the more extensive procedure, the patient should be healthier; for a more severe form of the disease, the surgical procedure should be less invasive.

Cardiovascular Diseases

Hypertension

Hypertension is the most common primary diagnosis in the United States and accounts for more than 35 million health care visits per year. In 2018, new statistics from the AHA showed that there is an estimated 103 million adults, or almost half (46%) of the entire adult population, in the United States that have high blood pressure. The death rate from high blood pressure continues to rise each year and still remains the most common cause of cardiovascular deaths.[22]

Untreated, undiagnosed, and uncontrolled hypertension is a serious problem in society today. With increasing age, the prevalence of hypertension increases. More than half of people aged 60 to 69 years and approximately three-quarters of those age 70 and older are affected with hypertension.[2] A recent study showed that the lifetime risk of hypertension is 90% for men and women who were nonhypertensive at age 55 to 65 and live to age 80. Failure to diagnose and detect hypertensive patients can result in life-threatening conditions such as stroke or MI.

Because implant dentists treat a high percentage of elderly patients and there is such a high prevalence in the general population, the incidence of treating dental patients with uncontrolled or undiagnosed hypertension is very high. This places the implant clinician at risk because intraoperative hypertensive episodes may result in cardiac arrhythmias with possible myocardial ischemia issues, which may lead to cardiovascular events such as MI or cerebrovascular events.

TABLE 10.6   Evaluation of Risk in Systemic Diseases

Risk (Disease)	ASA Category	Type 1	Type 2	Type 3	Type 4
Normal (disease)	I	+	+	+	+
Mild	II	+	SRP	Sedation, SRP	Sedation, SRP
Moderate	II	+	Medical consult	Medical consult	Medical consult
Severe	III	Medical consult	Postpone all elective procedures	Postpone all elective procedures	Postpone all elective procedures

+, Procedure may be performed with regular protocol *ASA*, American Society of Anesthesiologists; *SRP*, stress reduction protocol.

Note: ASA IV patients: no treatment.

Classification Guidelines. In late 2017, the American College of Cardiology (ACC) and the AHA released new guidelines for the diagnosis and treatment of high blood pressure. These recommendations show that blood pressure readings greater than 130 mm Hg systolic or 80 mm Hg diastolic should be treated earlier with lifestyle changes and, in some patients that have associated risk factors, with medication. This is a change from the previous guidelines that recommended intervention at blood pressure greater than 140/90. By lowering the definition of high blood pressure, the new guidelines account for complications that can begin with lower readings and now allow for earlier intervention. Although the number of patients now classified as having hypertension will increase, there will be a relatively smaller increase in the need to medicate these patients as opposed to instituting diet, exercise, cholesterol therapy, and other treatment recommendations earlier to prevent future complications from high blood pressure.

The new guidelines define normal blood pressure as less than 120/80 mm Hg. The category of prehypertension has been eliminated; instead these patients are now classified as having elevated blood pressure at 120 to 129/80 mm Hg or stage 1 with a blood pressure between 130 and 139 systolic or 80 and 89 diastolic. In previous guidelines, stage 1 hypertension was classified as 140/90 mm Hg, but in the new classification, this is now stage 2 hypertension. Hypertensive crisis has been redefined as a blood pressure systolic over 180 and/or diastolic over 120 mm Hg. If medically stable, these patients require immediate intervention via consultation with their physician and change of medication. Those patients with chest pain, headache, visual changes, or other somatic complaints may require immediate hospitalization.

Always ensure that proper technique is used to measure blood pressure and use home monitoring with devices that can be validated. White coat hypertension in a medical office is still a concern and should be confirmed by having the patient obtain a blood pressure outside the medical office (i.e., pharmacy, grocery store, home).

Although the definition of Stage 1 hypertension has changed, medication is usually not required for many individuals. The recommendations state that only those individuals that have already had a cardiovascular event like a stroke or heart attack or those at high risk for stroke or heart attack based on factors such as age, presence of diabetes, CKD, or at higher risk for atherosclerotic disease with elevated low-density lipoprotein (LDL) cholesterol or low high-density lipoprotein (HDL) cholesterol should begin medications. Stage 2 hypertension in most cases should be treated with medications.

Hypertension is usually asymptomatic and is the major risk factor for coronary heart disease and CVAs leading to cardiovascular morbidity and mortality for people older than 50 years of age. The medical history should focus on predisposing factors to hypertension such as excessive alcohol intake, history of renal disease, stroke, other cardiovascular diseases, diabetes, increased dietary sodium intake, obesity, and smoking.

Special attention should be given to patients with a history of obstructive sleep apnea (OSA). Sleep apnea has been associated with a number of cardiovascular diseases including dysthymias, MI, and stroke.[23] Greater than 50% of patients with sleep apnea also have hypertension.[24] In contrast to past knowledge that diastolic pressure is more important than systolic pressure, studies have shown that with the aging population, uncontrolled systolic hypertension causes increased rates of cardiovascular and renal diseases.[7]

The side effects of blood pressure medications may alter treatment or require special precautions. For example, orthostatic hypotension affects a patient brought from a supine to an upright position, which can result in syncope and falling, with possible injuries. The patient may feel lightheaded or even faint; these symptoms can be avoided by allowing patients to sit upright for several minutes after the completion of their dental procedure. Patients at high risk include the elderly, those with anxiety, patients taking multiple medications, and those who have undergone lengthy dental procedures.

Patients with difficult-to-control blood pressure may be prescribed multiple classes of antihypertensive medications. Even though these patients are being treated with various antihypertensive medications, they are prone to possible elevation and spikes in blood pressure. With these patients, the clinician should seek medical evaluation and consultation, which may include a postoperative blood pressure–monitoring plan.

Severe hypertension or elevation in blood pressure may lead to angina pectoris, CHF, MI, retinal hemorrhage, or even a cerebrovascular episode. These conditions may be precipitated by a rapid increase in blood pressure during a local anesthetic injection or the inherent stress associated with the surgical procedure. A stress reduction protocol is paramount with hypertensive patients.

Dental Implant Management. Because a high percentage of patients have hypertension, the implant clinician and staff members must be knowledgeable about the measurement, detection, and treatment of hypertension. The accurate measurement of blood pressure, along with a review of all medications including herbal and OTC medications, should be an integral part of the implant consultation and examination (Box 10.3).[25]

An elevated blood pressure is common in the dental office setting because stress associated with treatment (i.e., white coat syndrome) leads to increased levels of catecholamine, which causes an increase in blood pressure and heart rate. Two important steps to decrease the stress in the dental office are a well-monitored stress reduction protocol and proper management of pain and discomfort. Stress reduction protocol may include premedication the night before the appointment with diazepam [Valium] 5 to 10 mg, oral or conscious sedation for the procedure, setting an early morning appointment, minimizing waiting room time, and ensuring the duration of treatment does not exceed the patient's limits. Adequate pain control is also important, including preemptive analgesia, profound anesthesia during the procedure, and sufficient postoperative pain control including long-acting anesthetics. A resting systolic pressure greater than 180 or a diastolic pressure greater than 110 should indicate that all elective procedures be delayed until blood pressure can be reduced to a safer level (Box 10.4).

The use of NSAIDs has been shown to lessen the effectiveness of various antihypertensive medications by inhibiting prostaglandin production, leading to intraoperative hypertensive episodes. Blood pressure regulation is highly prostaglandin dependent, especially as it relates to kidney function through the vasodilatory effects. NSAIDs possess a higher degree of interaction with diuretics angiotensin-converting enzyme (ACE) inhibitors, angiotensin receptor blocker (ARB) inhibitors, and beta-blockers, which may modify prostaglandin-dependent pathways more than drugs that alter non–prostaglandin-sensitive pathways such as calcium channel blockers and central-acting drugs. Therefore the interaction with hypertensive medications and NSAIDs results in a higher propensity to increase blood pressure.[26] Studies have shown that approximately 50 million patients are being treated with antihypertensive therapy, and 12 million use NSAIDs concomitantly. However, the short-term use of NSAIDs has not been shown to have a clinically significant effect.[27]

The implant clinician must take into consideration that beta-blockers may potentiate the cardiovascular effects of epinephrine used in local anesthetics. The nonselective beta-adrenergic drugs, such as propranolol (Inderal) and nadolol, pose the greatest risk of adverse interactions.[10] The cardioselective beta-blockers (Lopressor, Tenormin, and Bystolic) carry less risk of adverse reactions; however, there is competitive clearance through the liver between both classes of beta-blockers and the local anesthetic. This may lead to an increase in serum levels of the local anesthetic.[28] To avoid intraoperative hypertensive episodes, decreasing the dose and increasing the time interval between epinephrine-containing injections is recommended.[29]

Calcium channel blockers (amlodipine, nifedipine, and diltiazem) used to treat hypertension or CHF may lead to gingival hyperplasia around natural teeth or implants (similar to Dilantin). Additionally, this drug classification has been associated with erythema multiforme (a benign rash characterized by patches of red raised skin) and other types of oral ulceration. Gingival overgrowth can result in pain, gingival bleeding, and difficulty in mastication, especially around implant prostheses. The incidence of gingival hyperplasia is approximately 1.7% to 3.8% of patients taking calcium channel blockers[30] (Tables 10.7 and 10.8).

Angina Pectoris

Angina is chest pain that is a result of decreased blood flow to the heart. Atherosclerotic disease of the heart blood vessels is usually responsible for the interruption of blood flow to the heart muscle. There are some other causes of angina including coronary artery spasm and severe aortic valve disease. The classic symptoms are a crushing pain in the substernal area that can radiate across the chest or into the neck or jaw. It can be accompanied by shortness of breath, nausea, diaphoresis, and fatigue. Pain is usually relieved with rest and caused by an imbalance between the amount of oxygen the heart requires and the amount delivered by the coronary arteries, especially with exertion or physical activity.

Men tend to develop coronary disease in the larger vessels and have more classic symptoms. Women tend to develop coronary disease in the smaller vessels, which can lead to variations of the classic symptoms. Women may still experience chest pain but can have the other symptoms of pain into the jaw or neck, fatigue, and shortness of breath.

Angina can be classified as stable, unstable, or Prinzmetal. Stable angina is triggered by exertion such as exercise (i.e., climbing stairs), which results in chest pain that is relieved by resting and/or taking nitroglycerin. Unstable angina is the typical substernal chest pain that is not brought on by exertion or exercise, occurs at rest, can last longer, and sometimes may not be relieved by rest

---

• BOX 10.3 Supplements Associated With Increased Swelling and Increased Blood Pressure

- Celery
- Dandelion
- Elder
- Goldenseal
- Guaiacum
- Juniper

• BOX 10.4 Stress Reduction Protocol

- Premedication the night before a procedure (longer-acting benzodiazepine [diazepam 5–10 mg])
- Early morning appointment
- Explain entire procedure in detail
- Sedation (oral/IV)
- Minimize waiting-room time
- Duration of treatment not to exceed patient's tolerance
- Profound local anesthesia
- Slow/aspiration LA administration
- Sufficient postoperative pain management

IV, Intravenous; LA, local anesthetic.
From Resnik RR, Resnik RJ. Medical/medication complications in oral implantology. In Resnik RR, Misch CE, eds. Misch's Avoiding Complications in Oral Implantology. St Louis, MO: Elsevier; 2018.

TABLE 10.7a Common Antihypertensive Medications

Thiazides Diuretics	Mechanism of Action	Ace Inhibitors	Mechanism of Action	Calcium Channel Blockers Nondihydropyridines	Mechanism of Action
Hydrochlorothiazide	Decrease BP by Decrease Blood Volume	Captopril, Enalapril, Quinapril, Lisinopril, Ramipril	Decrease BP by decreasing peripheral vascular resistance, Blocks Angiotension Converting enzyme in kidney, Results in decrease level of angiotensin which decreases levels of aldosterone, Lower levels of aldosterone result in less sodium and water retention which lowers BP, Can cause dry cough or angioedema	Diltiazem, Verapamil	Acts to vasodilate peripheral vascular system through smooth muscle relaxation Decreases heart rate and stroke volume of heart and can cause blockade of AV node in heart resulting in symptomatic bradycardia
Chlorthalidone	Decrease reabsorption of Sodium in Distal Kidney	Enalapril	Blocks Angiotension Converting enzyme in kidney	Verapamil	Decreases heart rate and stroke volume of heart and can cause blockade of AV node in heart resulting in symptomatic bradycardia
Metolazone	Can cause hypokalemia and hypomagnesemia	Quinapril	Results in decrease level of angiotensin which decreases levels of aldosterone		
		Lisinopril	Lower levels of aldosterone result in less sodium and water retention which lowers BP		
		Ramipril	Can cause dry cough or angioedema	**Calcium Channel Blockers Dihydropyridines**	
Loop Diuretics		**Angiotensin II Receptor Antagonist (ARB)**		Amlodipine (Norvasc)	Block movement of calcium in smooth muscle heart and peripheral smooth muscle
Bumetanide (Bumex)	Inhibits absorbtion of Sodium in Loop of Henle	Candesartan (Atacand), Losartan (Cozaar), Olmesartan (Benicar), Telmisartan (Micardis), Valsartan (Diovan)	lowers BP by vasodilation produced by inhibiting aldosterone production In renal insufficiency can cause worsening renal function and hyperkalemia In renal insufficiency can cause worsening renal function and hyperkalemia Can cause cough or angioedema Decrease Aldosteron decreases sodium absorption and water reabsorption		
Furosemide (Lasix)	Can cause hypokalemia and hypomagnesemia	Losartan (Cozaar)	Decrease Aldosteron decreases sodium absorption and water reabsorption	Felodipine (Plendil)	Lowers BP through smooth muscle relaxation and vasodilation
Torsemide	Increase Prostaglandin synthesis (NSAIDS can interfere and decrease effectiveness of loop diuretics)	Olmesartan (Benicar)	Can cause cough or angioedema	Nifidipine (Procardia)	Can make heart failure worse and cause leg and peripheral edema

Drug	Effect
Demadex	
Telmisartan (Micardis)	In renal insufficiency can cause worsening renal function and hyperkalemia
Valsartan (Diovan)	
Vasodilators	
Hydralazine (Apresoline)	Produce Relaxation of Vascular Smooth Muscle
Minoxidil	Causes decrease in peripheral vascular resistance lowering BP
	Can cause reflex stiumation of heart increasing heart rate, cardiac contractility and O_2 consumption
	Minoxidil reserved for severe hypertension
Central alpha-Agonist in brain	
Clonidine (Catapress)	Stimulate alpha receptors in brain
Methyldopa (Aldomet)	Results in decrease vasoconstriction, heart rate, systemic vascular resistance which then lowers BP

Beta Blocker

Nonselective : Block beta receptor at both B1 (heart) and B2 (lungs) receptors

Propranolol	Decrease Cardiac output which decreases cardiac O_2 consumption by blockade of B1 receptors and lowers BP
Timolol	Causes Peripheral Vasoconstriction and Bronchoconstriction
Nadolol	Blocks effects of epinephrine (adrenaline)
Carvdilol	Decrease Heart Rate and sexual dysfunction
Labetalol	Can cause disturbances in glucose metabolism:

Cardio selective Beta blockers block only B1 (heart) receptors

Acebutolol	
Atenolol	Works specifically on Beta receptors in heart
Esmolol	BP decreases because of lower Heart Rate and Decrease in cardiac contractility and force of blood flow
Metoprolol Succinate	
Cardiovil (Coreg)	
Nebivolol (Bystolic)	Coreg and Bystolyic are 3rd generation beta blockers
	Much more specific for working only on beta receptors in heart

TABLE 10.7b **Common Antihypertensive Medications**

Thiazides Diuretics	Mechanism of Action
Hydrochlorothiazide	Decrease BP by Decrease Blood Volume
Chlorthalidone	Can cause hypokalemia and hypomagnesemia
Metolazone	Decrease reabsorption of Sodium in Distal Kidney

Loop diuretics	Mechanism of Action
Bumetanide (Bumex)	Inhibits absorbtion of Sodium in Loop of Henle
Furosemide (Lasix)	Can cause hypokalemia and hypomagnesemia
Torsemide(Demadex)	Increase Prostaglandin synthesis (NSAIDS can interfere and decrease effectiveness of loop diuretics)

Ace Inhibitors	Mechanism of Action
Captopril	Decrease BP by decreasing peripheral vascular resistance,
Enalapril	Blocks Angiotension Converting enzyme in kidney,
Quinapril	Results in decrease level of angiotensin which decreases levels of aldosterone,
Lisinopril	Lower levels of aldosterone result in less sodium and water retention which lowers BP,
Ramipril	Can cause dry cough or angioedema

Angiotensin II Receptor Antagonist (ARB)	Mechanism of Action
Candesartan (Atacand)	Blocks the binding of of angiotension II on muscle receptors surrounding blood vessels
Losartan (Cozaar)	Results in lowers BP by vasodilation and inhibition of aldosterone production
Olmesartan (Benicar)	In renal insufficiency can cause worsening renal function and hyperkalemia
Telmisartan (Micardis)	In renal insufficiency can cause worsening renal function and hyperkalemia
Valsartan (Diovan)	Can cause cough or angioedema
	Decrease Aldosteron decreases sodium absorption and water reabsorption

Calcium Channel Blockers Nondihydropyridines	Mechanism of Action
Diltiazem (Cardiazem)	Acts to vasodilate peripheral vascular system through smooth muscle relaxation
Verapamil (Calan)	Decreases heart rate and stroke volume of heart
	Can cause blockade of AV node in heart resulting in symptomatic bradycardia

Calcium Channel Blockers Dihydropyridines	Mechanism of Action
Amlodipine (Norvasc)	Block movement of calcium in smooth muscle heart and peripheral smooth muscle
Felodipine (Plendil)	Lowers BP through smooth muscle relaxation and vasodilation
Nifidipine (Procardia)	Can make heart failure worse and cause leg and peripheral edema

Beta blocker Non-Selective Block beta receptor at both B1 (heart) and B2 (lungs) receptors	Mechanism of Action
Cardiovil (Coreg)	Decrease Cardiac output which decreases cardiac O$_2$ consumption by blockade of B1 receptors and lowers BP
Labetalol (Normodyne)	Causes Peripheral Vasoconstriction
Nadolol (Corgard)	Blocks effects of epinephrine (adrenaline)
Pindolol (Visken)	Decrease Heart Rate and can cause sexual dysfunction
Propranolol (Inderol)	Can cause disturbances in glucose metabolism
Sotolol (Betapace)	Can Cause Bronchorestriction as these agents block Beta 2 receptors in lungs
Timolol (Blocardren)	

Cardio selective Beta blockers block only B1 (heart) receptors	Mechanism of Action
Acebutolol (Sectral)	Works specifically on Beta 1 receptors in heart
Atenolol (Tenormin)	BP decreases because of lower Heart Rate and Decrease in cardiac contractility and force of blood flow
Bisoprolol (Zebeta)	Reduce systolic pressure and heart rate
Esmolol (Brevibloc)	Decrease contractility of heart which decrease cardiac output and reduces oxygen demand by the heart
Metoprolol Succinate (Toprol)	
Nebivolol (Bystolic)	Can cause some sexual dysfunction and less likely to cause bronchocontriction

Vasodilators	Mechanism of Action
Hydralazine (Apresoline)	Produce Relaxation of Vascular Smooth Muscle
Minoxidil	Causes decrease in peripheral vascular resistance lowering BP
	Can cause reflex stiumation of heart increasing heart rate, cardiac contractility and O$_2$ consumption
	Minoxidil reserved for severe hypertension

Central alpha-Agonist in brain	Mechanism of Action
Clonidine (Catapress)	Stimulate alpha receptors in brain
Methyldopa (Aldomet)	Results in decrease vasoconstriction, heart rate, systemic vascular resistance which then lowers BP

TABLE 10.8 Blood Pressure Treatment Guidelines

Category	Systolic (mm Hg)	Diastolic (mm Hg)	TREATMENT Preoperative	TREATMENT Intraoperative
Ideal	<120	<80	None	None
Prehypertension	120–139	80–89	Recheck, possible medical consultation	Recheck, stress reduction protocol
Grade 1 hypertension	140–159	90–99	Recheck, possible medical consultation, (relative)	Monitor, stress reduction protocol
Grade 2 hypertension	160–179	100–109	Recheck, medical consultation, (absolute)	Monitor, discontinue procedure, possible emergency room referral
Hypertensive crisis	>180	>110	Recheck, emergency care, (absolute)	Monitor, abort immediately, emergency care

From Resnik RR, Resnik RJ. Medical/medication complications in oral implantology. In Resnik RR, Misch CE, eds. *Misch's Avoiding Complications in Oral Implantology.* St Louis, MO: Elsevier; 2018.

or nitroglycerin. This indicates more advanced coronary disease that requires immediate attention. Prinzmetal angina is caused by coronary artery spasm. Stress and drug use, especially cocaine, are the main causes of this type of angina.

Treatment of angina involves many different medications. Beta-blockers are used to reduce the workload of the heart. Nitroglycerin works to dilate coronary blood vessels, which decrease myocardial oxygen consumption and also reduce the workload of the heart. Aspirin and other antiplatelet agents are critical to prevent thrombus formation. Progressive angina requires cardiac catheterization. If there is significant narrowing, an angioplasty and stent may be used to relieve the blockage and improve symptoms. If the blockage is more severe or not amenable to angioplasty, then bypass surgery may be indicated.

Risk factors for angina pectoris are smoking, hypertension, high cholesterol, obesity, and diabetes. Patients with a history of angina may be taking long-acting nitrates to prevent the occurrence of acute episodes. Sublingual or spray nitroglycerin is recommended for the treatment of acute episodes. It is important to ask any patient with angina about their most recent symptoms including frequency, exacerbating factors, worsening symptoms, how long the chest pain lasts, and what relieves the chest pain. Patients with increased symptoms or more frequent or longer-lasting attacks should be referred to the physician for evaluation. Patients with pain at rest should be immediately referred to their physician.

Dental Implant Management. The major concern for the implant clinician is the precipitation or management of the actual angina attack. Precipitating factors are exertion, cold, heat, large meals, humidity, psychological stress, and dental-related stress. All of these factors cause catecholamine release, which in turn increases the heart rate, blood pressure, and myocardial oxygen demand.[31]

The dental emergency kit should include nitroglycerin tablets (0.3–0.4 mg) or sublingual nitroglycerin spray, which are replaced every 6 months because of their short shelf-life. During an angina attack, all dental treatment should be stopped immediately. Nitroglycerin is then administered sublingually, and 100% oxygen is given at 6 L/min, with the patient in a semisupine or 45-degree position.

Vital signs should be monitored after nitroglycerin is administered because transient hypotension may occur. If the systolic blood pressure falls below 100 mm Hg, then the patient's feet should be elevated. If the pain is not relieved in 8 to 10 minutes with the use of nitroglycerin at 5-minute intervals, emergency medical assistance should be initiated.

Patients with mild angina (up to one attack per month) may undergo most nonsurgical dental procedures performed with the normal protocol (type 1). General cardiac precautions are advised, such as vital signs monitoring, and patients are instructed to bring their own nitroglycerin. Advanced restorative procedures and minor implant surgery (type 2) are performed with nitrous oxide or oral sedation. For more advanced implant procedures (types 3 and 4), appropriate sedation techniques should be used. Appointments should be as short as possible. This may require more than one surgical or restorative appointment. Use of vasoconstrictors should be limited to a maximum of 0.04 to 0.05 mg epinephrine, and concentrations greater than 1/100,000 should be avoided.

Patients with moderate angina (up to one attack per week) tolerate examination and most simple operative procedures (type 1). Prophylactic nitroglycerin (0.3–0.4 mg) or long-acting nitrates are given sublingually just before advanced operative or simple to moderate implant surgery (types 2 and 3). Antianxiety sedation with supplemental oxygen is required. Advanced surgical procedures may require a hospital setting (type 4).

Patients with unstable angina (daily episodes) are limited to examination procedures performed under normal protocol. Medical consultation is recommended for any additional treatment. This form of angina has been represented as an absolute contraindication for elective dental surgery (ASA IV).

The side effects of nitroglycerin are important to recognize because prophylactic administration is in order for the patient with moderate to severe angina because there is a decrease in blood pressure, which causes a decrease of the blood flow to the brain. Fainting is often a possibility; therefore the patient should be sitting or lying down during nitroglycerin administration. The heart attempts to compensate for the decreased blood pressure, and the pulse rate may increase to as much as 160 beats/min. Flushing of the face and shoulders is common after administration of nitroglycerin. If the patient has been taking long-acting nitrates, tolerance to the drug may occur; therefore two tablets may be needed at a time. A headache may occur after administration, which may be treated with OTC analgesics (Table 10.9).

TABLE 10.9	Dental Implant Management in Patients with Angina Pectoris				
Risk	Symptoms	Type 1	Type 2	Type 3	Type 4
Mild	≤1/month; ASA II	+	+	Sedation, supplemental oxygen	Sedation, supplemental oxygen
Moderate	≤1/week; ASA III	+	Sedation, premedication, nitrates, supplemental oxygen	Sedation, premedication, nitrates, supplemental oxygen	Premedication, sedation, outpatient hospitalization
Severe	Daily/more; ASA IV; unstable	+	Physician consultation	Elective procedures contraindicated	Elective procedures contraindicated

+, Procedure may be performed with regular protocol; *ASA*, American Society of Anesthesiologists.

Myocardial Infarction

An MI is a prolonged ischemia or lack of oxygen resulting from a deficiency in the coronary arterial blood supply that causes injury to the myocardium or heart muscle. The end result is cellular death and necrosis of the heart muscle.

About every 40 seconds someone in the United States has a heart attack. Just under 800,000 individuals suffer a heart attack each year in the United States, and three of every four heart attacks are an initial event.[32] One in five heart attacks are silent and there is heart muscle loss, but the individual is unaware of the event.

An acute MI may be precipitated when the patient undergoes unusual stress, either physical (painful stimuli) or emotional (anxiety). The patient usually has severe chest pain in the substernal or left precordial area during an MI episode. The pain may radiate to the left arm or mandible, and is similar to angina pectoris but more severe. Cyanosis, diaphoresis, weakness, nausea or vomiting, and irregular and increased pulse rate are all signs and symptoms of MI.

The complications of MI include arrhythmias and Congestive Heart Failure (CHF), and if a complete occlusion or malignant arrhythmia occurs, then sudden death results. The larger the ischemic area, the greater the risk of heart failure or life-threatening arrhythmias. Any history of MI indicates significant problems in the coronary vessels. Recent infarctions correspond to higher morbidity and death rates with even simple elective surgery.

The risk of MI is less than 1% in the general population in a perioperative setting. Approximately 18% to 20% of patients with a recent history of MI will have an increase of complications, which have a high mortality rate of 40% to 70%. If general anesthesia and surgery are performed within 3 months of MI, the risk of another MI is 30%, and if performed within 3 to 6 months, the risk is 15%. After 12 months, the incidence of recurrent MI stabilizes at about 5%.[33] Acute coronary syndrome consists of three different types of coronary blockages that can result in sudden rupture of plaque inside one of the coronary arteries. When the plaque ruptures, it causes exposure of the soft fatty tissue, which then causes platelets to migrate to the area of rupture and form a clot around the plaque to cover the fatty tissue. When the clot blocks the entire blood supply to the heart muscles, there is coronary occlusion. This can result in one of three scenarios that result in ischemia: unstable angina (as previously described), non-ST segment elevation MI (NSTEMI), or ST elevation MI (STEMI).

There are several variables that determine the type of acute coronary syndrome: length of time blood flow is blocked, and location of the blockage. Unstable angina is a change from stable angina when the pain starts occurring at rest as opposed to occurring with exertion. If the MI does not cause ST-elevation (classic electrocardiogram [ECG] finding of MI) on the ECG but the clinical markers in blood enzymes demonstrate damage has occurred, then this is considered an NSTEMI. The blockage is partial or temporary, so the damage done to heart muscle is usually much smaller. This is still considered a heart attack or MI. Serial troponin and or creatine-kinase (CK)-MB blood levels are drawn and repeated over several hours. Both of these markers indicate damage to the myocardial muscle. Troponin levels may be the earliest indicator of an MI.

If the interruption to the blood supply is more abrupt and prolonged, it will affect a much larger area of the heart and demonstrate ST-segment elevation on the ECG and damage by the serum chemical makers.

Dental Implant Management

Medical Consultation. A medical consultation should precede any extensive restorative or surgical procedure. Even though there are recommendations based solely on the length of time after an MI, the deciding factor on elective dental implant treatment is not only time but also the amount of myocardial damage. The implant clinician should follow the recommendation of the physician concerning treatment options, modifications, or contraindications.

Stress Reduction Protocol. Dental implant surgery after MI may induce arrhythmias or aggravate cardiac ischemia. An increased blood pressure is common in the dental office setting, because stress associated with treatment (i.e., white coat syndrome) leads to increased levels of catecholamine, which cause an increase in blood pressure and heart rate. The most important step in decreasing stress in the dental office is to integrate a comprehensive stress reduction protocol.

Reduction in the Use of Vasoconstrictors. Epinephrine and other vasoconstrictors have several properties that can potentially result in adverse outcomes in patients that have not fully recovered from a recent MI. Epinephrine is chronotropic, which results in an increased heart rate and force of contraction. Both of these result in an increased oxygen demand and could potentiate ischemia. Epinephrine does have some arrhythmogenic properties that could provoke ventricular fibrillation or tachycardia in recovering myocardial muscle. It is best to minimize complications by consulting the patient's treating physician and closely monitoring vital signs when vasoconstrictors are used.

Myocardial Infarction Treatment Summary. The patient's physician should be consulted before elective dental implant treatment to verify the patient's current cardiac status (Table 10.10).

TABLE 10.10 **Dental Implant Management in Patients With Myocardial Infarction**

Risk	Type 1	Type 2	Type 3	Type 4
Mild (>12 months)	+	+	Physician	Physician hospitalization if general anesthesia required
Moderate (6–12 months; ASA III)	+	Postpone all elective procedures	Postpone all elective procedures	Postpone all elective procedures
Severe (<6 months; ASA IV)	Physician consultation	Postpone all elective procedures	Postpone all elective procedures	Postpone all elective procedures

+, Procedure may be performed with regular protocol; *ASA*, American Society of Anesthesiologists.

Absolute (surgical): Recent MI (depending on doctor's recommendation).

Relative (surgical): History of MI (depending on doctor's recommendation).

Congestive Heart Failure

CHF is a pathophysiologic state in which an abnormality in cardiac function is responsible for failure of the heart to pump blood in adequate volume to meet the needs of the metabolizing tissues.[34] Over the past 10 years the number of adults living with heart failure has increased significantly. The most recent data from the AHA's "2017 Heart Disease and Stroke Statistics" update states that about 6.5 million Americans were living with heart failure by the end of 2014. That number may jump to 8 million in the next 10 to 12 years because more people are now surviving heart attacks, leaving the heart weaker and more susceptible to heart failure.[35]

Total direct medical costs for heart failure were over $21 billion in 2012, and it is expected that by 2030 we could see that cost rise to over $53 billion. The overwhelming majority of the cost for health failure is in patients aged 65 years and older; these patients currently account for over 80% of costs related to heart failure and are projected to be responsible for 88% or more of the total costs by 2030.[36]

CHF usually develops over time because the muscles in the heart wall lose their ability to generate appropriate contractile forces and can continue to deteriorate with continuous exposure to volume overload. This results in high levels of pressure in the heart and eventual weakening of the stretched contractile muscles in the heart. Because of the diminished output of the heart, the body responds by increasing vascular resistance (increased blood pressure) throughout the circulatory system, which is initially beneficial to the peripheral tissues. However, this leads to further reductions in cardiac output, because the weakened heart must pump against this increased pressure. The kidney acts to retain sodium and fluid, which continues to exacerbate the problem.

There are many acceptable pharmacologic interventions including diuretics, inotropic drugs, beta-blockers, and ACE/ARB blood pressure medications, among others. Spironolactone has now become the diuretic of choice in treating heart failure. Digoxin was one of the most common drugs used for years to treat heart failure; however, recent CHF treatment algorithms have been updated and digoxin has been replaced by the use of beta-blockers and spironolactone. Digoxin is appropriate for some patients, so implant dentists should be aware of the more common side effects

• **BOX 10.5** **Diagnostic Criteria for Congestive Heart Failure**

- Paroxysmal nocturnal dyspnea or orthopnea
- Neck vein distention
- Rales
- Cardiomegaly
- Acute pulmonary edema
- S3 gallop
- Increased venous pressure >16 cm of water
- Hepatojugular reflux.

Minor Criteria:
- Ankle edema
- Night cough
- Dyspnea on exertion
- Hepatomegaly
- Pleural effusion
- Vital capacity reduced one third from maximum
- Tachycardia (≥120 bpm)

Major or Minor Criteria:
- Weight loss of 4.5 kg or more in 5 days in response to treatment.

of elevated levels like nausea, vomiting, anorexia, headaches, confusion, and visual changes including halos around objects. Patients on digoxin should be questioned about their most recent blood level and stability of blood level over the past several months.

One of newest and most revolutionary treatments for CHF is the medication Entresto. Entresto contains a combination of sacubitril and valsartan. Valsartan (which is classified as an ARB) is used as a single agent to treat hypertension. The drug works in the kidney to block receptors that cause constriction resulting in dilatation of blood vessels, which lowers the resistance against which the heart must pump. Sacubitril is a neprilysin inhibitor that improves blood flow to the kidneys and helps in diuresis and removal of excess volume in the bloodstream.

Symptoms of CHF are listed in Box 10.5, and they include abnormal tiredness or shortness of breath (dyspnea) brought on by slight activity or even occurring at rest (these symptoms are caused by excess fluid in the lungs and partly caused by the excess work required of the heart); wheezing caused by fluid in the lungs (pulmonary edema); peripheral edema or swelling of the ankles (pedal edema) and lower legs; frequent urination at night; jugular venous distension; sounds at auscultation (S₃ gallop); and paroxysmal nocturnal dyspnea (the sensation of being unable to breath), which may interrupt sleep. This symptom is caused by the effect of gravity on fluid that has spent the day down at the feet. As the fluid flows back up, it may pool in the lungs, causing a feeling of suffocation. Excessive weight gain, as much as 20 to 30 pounds, with no change in diet, is also a symptom. This increase, purely from fluid retention, gives some indication of how poorly the heart is pumping. The most common way to make the diagnosis is by using the Framingham criteria. CHF can be diagnosed in patients with two major or one major and two minor criteria.

The most common classification system for heart failure is the New York Heart Association (NYHA). Class 1 is asymptomatic, class II has mild symptoms with moderate exertion, class III has symptoms with minimal activity, and class IV failure has symptoms at rest[37] (Box 10.6).

There are several types of heart failure. Left-sided heart failure involves dysfunction of the left atrium and left ventricle. The left ventricle must function correctly to pump blood to the rest of the body. Left-sided heart failure can be divided into two different subtypes. Systolic failure is when the left ventricle loses its ability to contract fully. This is referred to as heart failure with reduced ejection fraction (HFrEF). Diastolic failure or dysfunction is when the left ventricle cannot relax properly because with the increased pressure and volume the muscle is very stiff. This limits the heart's ability to fill properly between beats, confining the amount of blood that can be pumped out with each beat. Drug treatments are not the same for these two types and are directed at the issue causing the heart failure.

As blood returns to the heart from the venous system in the body, it needs to be reoxygenated. It is collected on the right side of the heart and pumped into the lungs before returning to the left side of the heart. Right-sided heart failure usually occurs as a result of left-sided failure. As the left side increases pressure, the pressure is transferred back through lungs to right side of the heart. Eventually the right side loses contractile power and then backs up into the veins of the body. This results in venous congestion and swelling in the neck or jugular vein distention (JVD). This also causes swelling in the legs, feet, ankles, abdomen, and even in the liver, causing ascites.

In CHF, as the left side of the heart becomes overloaded with fluid, this pressure will be transferred to the lungs, resulting in shortness of breath, dyspnea on exertion, and orthopnea (difficulty breathing when lying down). Heart failure affects the kidney's ability to dispose of sodium and water, leading to edema of the extremities.

An echocardiogram of the heart is the preferred test to gauge the actual output capacity of the heart. Patients with more advanced levels of heart failure such as NYHA class III or class IV may require an implantable defibrillator to prevent sudden death from heart arrhythmias. Most of these patients have heart ejection fractions of less than 30%.

In heart failure there are two proteins, B-brain natriuretic peptide (BNP) and N-terminal-pro-BNP (NT-pro-BNP), which go up when heart failure worsens and down when heart failure improves. BNP (not to be confused with BMP blood panels) levels can be used to monitor the severity of heart failure. Levels <100 are usually not associated with heart failure. In conditions such as sepsis, cirrhosis, and hyperthyroid disorders there is increased or high cardiac output. This can increase levels of BNP and make the test less reliable in gauging the degree of heart failure. Before any dental surgery in a patient with a history of heart failure who is having symptoms, it would be good to review the most recent BNP compared with the patient's baseline. Elevated levels may indicate acute worsening of symptoms and warrant consultation with the patient's physician.

Dental Implant Management. In patients classified as NYHA I and II, no medical consultation is indicated unless there exist additional systemic diseases. In NYHA III and IV, medical consultation is highly recommended for all implant type 3 and 4 procedures. A comprehensive stress reduction protocol is indicated for all patients with CHF. Intraoperatively and postoperatively, pain and anxiety control is important because increased stress can produce an increased myocardial workload with an increase in the degree of heart failure.

Intraoperative Complications. CHF patients are very susceptible to intraoperative cardiovascular morbidity issues. Stress reduction protocol and strict monitoring should be followed. It is advisable to discuss the current condition of the patient with their treating physician. Patients with CHF can be classified as compensated or uncompensated. In uncompensated heart failure, the pulmonary circulation is expanded and congested because the heart is unable to fully compensate. The classic symptoms are seen including shortness of breath, especially with exertion; fatigue; or lying supine. When the CHF patient is treated for heart failure through medical management and the symptoms are controlled, the patient is referred to as compensated.

Patient Positioning. CHF patients should be positioned in the most recumbent position in which they can breathe comfortably and efficiently. This is usually a semireclined or sitting upright position. Usually, the more upright the patient is, the easier it is for the patient to breathe.

Oxygen Supplementation. Oxygen supplementation ($\approx$2 L/min) during implant procedures is highly recommended to minimize the possibility of hypoxia. The use of nitrous oxide in these patients is not advised.

Stress Reduction Protocol. A stress reduction protocol should be implemented prior to the procedure to prevent increased myocardial workload with a damaged heart

Subacute Bacterial Endocarditis and Valvular Heart Disease

Bacterial endocarditis is an infection of the heart valves or the endothelial surfaces of the heart. The infection is the result of the growth of bacteria on damaged or altered cardiac surfaces. The microorganisms most often associated with endocarditis after dental treatment are alpha-hemolytic *Streptococcus viridans* and less frequently staphylococci and anaerobes. The disorder is serious, with a mortality rate of approximately 11%.[38] Dental procedures causing transient bacteremia has been shown to be an etiologic factor of bacterial endocarditis. Patients with gingivitis and certain cardiac conditions are at highest risk. When inflamed gums bleed during dental procedures, bacteria can be introduced into the bloodstream and infect heart valves and the lining of the heart. These bacteria continue to replicate at the infected site. Depending on the type of bacteria infecting the heart tissue, endocarditis can develop quickly or more slowly. Some symptoms include fever, chills, fatigue, muscle aches, night sweats, shortness of breath, edema, and chest pain with inspiration. As a result, the implant dentist should identify the patient at risk for endocarditis and implement prophylactic procedures.

However, endocarditis after a dental procedure is not as common as once believed. New guidelines suggest prophylactic antibiotics for patients only at the highest risk levels. Scientific evidence has shown that the risk of adverse reactions to antibiotics may exceed any benefit for prophylactic treatment based on previous guidelines. This can also increase the likelihood of drug-resistant bacteria.[39]

In 2007, several organizations including the American Dental Association (ADA) and the AHA released updated guidelines for the prevention of infective endocarditis. In 2017, these guidelines were confirmed by a joint review by the AHA and ACC. These groups published a new update to their 2014 guidelines on the management of valvular heart disease.[40]

The updated recommendation states that patients who have routinely taken prophylactic antibiotics in the past are no longer required to do so. The more specific updated infective endocarditis prophylaxis recommendations for dental procedures are only for patients with underlying cardiac conditions that have been linked to the highest risk for developing an adverse outcome. These include patients with prosthetic heart valves, prosthetic material used for cardiac valve repair, a history of endocarditis, a cardiac transplant with abnormal valves, and certain congenital defects of the heart including cyanotic heart disease with shunts and any repaired defects with residual shunts, or other defects that remain at the site of the prosthetic patch.[41]

The risk of bacterial endocarditis increases with the amount of intraoral soft tissue trauma. There is a correlation between the incidence of endocarditis and the number of teeth extracted or the degree of a preexisting inflammatory disease of the mouth.[42] An incidence of bacteremia is six times higher in patients with severe periodontal disease.[43] However, if scaling and root planing are performed before subsequent soft tissue surgery, the risk of endocarditis is greatly reduced. Bacteremia after traumatic tooth brushing, endodontic treatment, and paraffin chewing has also been reported.[44] Endocarditis may even occur in an edentulous patient with denture sores.[45] Chlorhexidine use on isolated gingiva or irrigation of the sulcus 3 to 5 minutes before tooth extraction reduces postextraction bacteremia.

However, these new guidelines suggested that preventative treatment should be initiated in patients with the listed cardiac conditions but not for all dental procedures. The guidelines suggested prophylactic antibiotics only for dental procedures that involve manipulation of gingival tissue and bleeding. Antibiotics are not recommended for routine anesthesia through noninfected tissues or placement or adjustment of removable prosthodontic or orthodontic appliances.

The oral regimen in adults is 2 g amoxicillin orally, 60 minutes before the procedure. A second dose is not necessary because of the prolonged serum levels above the minimal inhibitory concentration of most oral streptococci[46] and the prolonged serum inhibitory activity induced by amoxicillin against such strains (6–14 hours).[47] For patients unable to

---

• BOX 10.7   Endocarditis Prophylaxis Recommendation

The American Dental Association, American Medical Association, and the American Heart Association have recommended antibiotic coverage in patients with the following conditions receiving elective surgery:
- Artificial heart valves
- Past history of infectious endocarditis
- Cardiac transplant that develops a heart valve problem
- Congenital heart disease with shunts or conduits[a] repaired
- Congenital heart defect with residual defect
  - Able to take oral medication: Amoxicillin 2 g (50 mg/kg)
  - Unable to take oral medication: Ampicillin 2 g IM or IV (50 mg/kg IM or IV); cefazolin or ceftriaxone 1 g IM or IV (50 mg/kg IM or IV)
  - Allergic to penicillin or ampicillin: Cephalexin 2 g (50 mg/kg); clindamycin 600 mg (20 mg/kg); azithromycin or clarithromycin 500 mg (15 mg/kg)
  - Allergic to penicillin or ampicillin and unable to take oral medication: Cefazolin or ceftriaxone 1 g IM or IV (50 mg/kg IM or IV); clindamycin 600 mg IM or IV (20 mg/kg IM or IV)

[a]Functional murmurs and organic heart murmurs do not require prophylactic antibiotic.
IM, intramuscular; IV, intravenous.
From Resnik RR, Resnik RJ. Medical/medication complications in oral implantology. In Resnik RR, Misch CE, eds. Misch's Avoiding Complications in Oral Implantology. St Louis, MO: Elsevier; 2018.

---

take oral medications, 2 g ampicillin is administered intramuscularly (IM) or IV 30 minutes before the procedure. If the patient is allergic to penicillin, clindamycin 600 mg or cephalexin (or cefadroxil) 2 g are administered orally 1 hour before the procedure. For patients allergic to penicillin and not able to take oral medications, clindamycin 600 mg IV within 30 minutes of the procedure or cefazolin 1 g IM or IV 30 minutes before the procedure are the recommended regimens for oral procedures.[48] Erythromycin is no longer included because GI upset and complicated pharmacokinetics of various formulations make its use problematic.

In patients who are classified in the high-risk category for development of endocarditis, elective implant therapy may be contraindicated. Edentulous patients restored with implants must contend with transient bacteremia from chewing, brushing, or peri-implant disease. Endosteal implants, with an adequate width of attached gingiva, are the implants of choice for patients in this group who need implant-supported prostheses. Implants may be contraindicated for patients with a limited oral hygiene potential and for those with a history of multiple endocarditis events.

Implant surgery in patients with aortic stenosis is usually contraindicated until after aortic valve replacement. It has been recommended that patients with valve replacements postpone any elective implant surgery until 15 to 18 months after surgical completion because these patients are at high risk for bacterial endocarditis and because of the use of high doses of anticoagulants.[49] Special precautions should always be adhered to in valve replacement patients because their therapeutic bleeding times are usually high (INR 2.5–3.5).

Dental Implant Management. The implant clinician must be familiar with the antibiotic regimens for heart conditions requiring prophylaxis. A similar regimen is suggested for any person requiring antibiotic coverage. There may be future updates, but currently the 2017 AHA and ACC guidelines for endocarditis prophylaxis should be used (Box 10.7).[50]

Cerebrovascular Accident

A stroke is a CVA characterized by a sudden interruption of blood flow to the brain, causing oxygen deprivation. It is most frequently seen in patients with current cardiovascular diseases and is the fourth leading cause of death in the United States and a major cause of adult disability. The majority of strokes are ischemic, resulting from narrowing or blocking of the blood supply to the brain. The etiology of ischemic strokes is embolic and thrombotic. Thrombotic strokes are the result of clots that form inside one of the brain's arteries. The clot blocks blood flow to the brain, causing cell death. Usually, these clots result from plaque or other fatty deposits from atherosclerosis, which break off and become lodged in the blood vessel. Embolic strokes are the results of clots that form in other parts of the body and travel to the brain via the bloodstream. The clot eventually will lodge in a blood vessel and block flow of blood to the brain.

It is important to ask patients if they have ever been diagnosed or treated for "ministrokes" or transient ischemic attacks (TIAs). These attacks are the result of brief (usually less than 24 hours) interruptions in blood flow causing strokelike symptoms. These episodes can be a precursor for a much larger stroke. Unlike a CVA, the blockage is temporary and the clot may dissolve or get dislodged in a very brief time causing the temporary symptoms. TIAs usually cause symptoms for less than 10 minutes and should completely resolve within 24 hours. Unlike a CVA, there is no permanent injury to the brain.

Dental Implant Implications

Bleeding. Although it is important to control blood pressure and treat elevated cholesterol in the management of individuals with a history of strokes, caution should be taken because most patients are on blood-thinning medication. Antiplatelet agents such as aspirin or clopidogrel may be used as single agents or in combination as part of a stroke prevention treatment. Both of these medications irreversibly affect platelets' clotting ability and have been shown to cause increased bleeding. In some cases, warfarin (Coumadin) may also be used, which directly interferes with the body's clotting mechanisms. Evaluation and bleeding control are essential in these types of patients.

Limited Dexterity. Patients who have suffered a compromise in dexterity as the result of a stroke require alternative treatment planning for their final prostheses. A fixed prosthesis is usually the best solution for these patients, because an implant-retained prosthesis may lead to the inability to remove for routine hygiene. Additionally, poor oral hygiene, when combined with xerostomia, causes additional oral problems such as candidiasis, dental caries, periodontal issues, and mucositis lesions, which increase implant prostheses morbidity.

Current Anticoagulant Medications. The goal of anticoagulation medication is to keep the blood thinned so clotting is more difficult. However, it is important to understand these medications work by various pathways and can affect clotting at different points in the clotting cascade or by directly inhibiting platelet function. The antiplatelet agents such as aspirin or clopidogrel have been shown to have a minimal effect on bleeding, both intraoperatively and postoperatively.[19] A number of studies have found no increased risk of bleeding during dental procedures when patients on Coumadin have a therapeutic treatment range INR (below 3.0). In patients with mechanical heart valves, the upper limit of the therapeutic range can reach 3.5 to 4.0. In patients with artificial valves, the INR may be checked 24 hours

TABLE 10.11	Additional Cardiovascular Issues and Treatment Implications	
Positive Response	**Treatment Implications**
Abdominal aneurysm	Rupture leading to high mortality, medical consultation (absolute)
Atrial fibrillation	Thrombin inhibitors, hemostatic measures
Prosthetic heart valve	Maintained at high INR, hemostatic measures
Pacemaker	Cardiovascular issue, stress reduction protocol, no electrosurgery
Fainting/lightheadedness	Orthostatic hypotension
Congenital heart defect	Cardiovascular issue, medical consult to determine extent
Ankle edema	Congestive heart failure, possible varicose veins

INR, International normalized ratio.

From Resnik RR, Resnik RJ. Medical/medication complications in oral implantology. In Resnik RR, Misch CE, eds. *Misch's Avoiding Complications in Oral Implantology.* St Louis, MO: Elsevier; 2018.

before the implant surgery. Under no circumstances should a patient with a mechanical valve on Coumadin be instructed to stop or hold a dose without input from the patient's treating physician.

Hemostatic Agents/Surgical Technique. Ideal surgical technique should be followed, which consists of nontraumatic incision and reflection of tissue. The surgical procedures should be minimized with a decreased surgical duration. The implant clinician must have experience with the use of active and passive hemostatic agents.

Treatment Summary

Absolute (surgical): Recent CVA incident (medical consult)
Relative (surgical): History of CVA + anticoagulants (medical consult)

Additional Cardiovascular Disorders

See Table 10.11.

Endocrine Disorders

Diabetes Mellitus

The most recent Diabetes Statistics Report of 2017 from the Centers for Disease Control and Prevention (CDC) estimated that over 30 million Americans (1 in 10) now have diabetes, with another 84 million (1 in 3) with prediabetes. The majority of new cases of diabetes are in adults 45 to 64 years of age, and there also has been an increase in diabetes in the American youth population. New cases were more prevalent in African Americans. Almost 90% of adults diagnosed were overweight and 40% were not physically active. The diagnosis of diabetes usually involves having an HbA1c (glycosylated Hb) of >6.4%. Glucose tolerance tests have been used previously and still have utility in the diagnosis of gestational diabetes. Using the Hba1c in combination with random fasting an post-prandial sugars has now become the accepted standard of care.[51]

• BOX 10.8   Medication Management of Diabetes

Biguanides: These drugs decrease glucose release from liver and act to block intestinal absorption of glucose. They are in the peripheral system to improve insulin sensitivity by increasing glucose uptake. They are considered euglycemic and should not cause hypoglycemia. Example: Metformin (Glucophage). Many newer medications combine metformin with one of the following categories of medications:

- Sulfonylureas (SFUs). These drugs increase insulin secretion from the pancreas and can cause hypoglycemia. Skipping meals will significantly increase the risk of hypoglycemia. Examples: Amaryl (glimepiride), Glucotrol (glipizide), Micronase (glyburide), Prandin (repaglinide), and Starlix (nateglinide)
- Thiazolidinediones (glitazones or TZDs): These drugs work to decrease insulin resistance in the muscle and fat tissues creating increased utilization of blood glucose. Examples: Actos (pioglitazone), Avandia (rosiglitazone)

GLP-1 Analogs: These drugs work on several systems to increase insulin secretion and inhibit the release of glucose from the liver after eating. They also can delay emptying of food from the stomach, creating a feeling of satiety. They have been shown to also promote weight loss. These medications require injections and are not oral. Examples: Byetta (exenatide), Victoza (liraglutide), and Trulicity (dulaglutide).

DPP-4 Inhibitors: These drugs also increase insulin secretion and limit glucose release from the liver after eating. Examples: Januvia (sitagliptin), Onglyza (saxagliptin), and Trajenta (linagliptin).

SGLT2 inhibitors: These drugs work specifically in the kidney in patients with normal renal function to increase glucose excretion in the urine. Patients on these medications will usually show levels of glucose on a urinalysis. Examples: Invokana (canagliflozin), Farxiga (dapagliflozin), and Jardiance (empagliflozin).

The most current classification of diabetes includes three general clinical categories: type 1 diabetes, type 2 diabetes, and gestational diabetes (pregnancy). In type 1 diabetes, insulin is not produced from the pancreas. This type of diabetes develops most frequently in children or before age 21. However, there is now a form of type 1 diabetes that develops a bit later in life in which the pancreas does not produce insulin. The incidence of type 2 diabetes in the older population is increasing. This type is much more common and accounts for approximately 95% of the diabetic cases and almost always occurs in adults. Initially the defect is coming from the body's inability to respond properly to the action of insulin, which is produced from the pancreas. The incidence of type 2 diabetes is estimated to double by the year 2025 because of aging, unhealthy diets, and obesity.[52] An increased body mass index (BMI) and advanced age can be predictors of undiagnosed diabetes. In patients for whom the clinician has a higher suspicion of diabetes, questions concerning frequent urination (polyuria) or excessively thirst (polydipsia) may be appropriate (Box 10.8).

Diabetes and Dental Implant Healing

Studies have shown that hyperglycemia has a negative effect on bone metabolism, reducing bone mineral density, affecting bone mechanical properties, and impairing bone formation, leading to poor bone microarchitecture.[53] There is a direct correlation between implant osseointegration and glycemic control.[54] Osseointegration is more predictable in anatomic areas with abundant cortical bone, which is why the mandible has shown a greater bone formation than the maxilla.[55]

Implant Failure

Human clinical studies have indicated that no contraindications exist for patients who are well controlled by diet and oral hypoglycemic. However, for insulin-controlled patients, a contraindication for implants may exist depending on the state of control. Researchers have concluded that implants have a high success rate provided the diabetes is controlled (monitor to ensure that glycosylated Hb [HbA1c] < 7.0). An increased failure rate of dental implants has been associated with poor metabolic control.[56] It is imperative that uncontrolled diabetics or patients exhibiting an elevated HbA1c are treated before and during the implant surgery healing period.

Dental Implant Management

Hypoglycemia. The most serious intraoperative complication for diabetic patients is hypoglycemia, which usually occurs as a result of an excessive insulin level, hypoglycemic drugs, or inadequate food intake. Weakness, nervousness, tremor, palpitations, or sweating are all signs of acute hypoglycemia. Mild symptoms can be treated with sugar in the form of orange juice or candy. If the symptoms are not addressed, then they may evolve from minor warning signs to seizure, coma, and, in rare cases, death. In these severe cases, patients may become unconscious or barely arousable. For these symptoms, the emergency administration of 50% IV dextrose should be completed. Additionally, glucagon should be available because this hormone may raise blood sugar through a direct effect on the liver. Glucagon may also be administered IM in a dose of 1 mg for adults over 20 kg. Patients taking sulfonylurea medications for diabetes (including glyburide, glipizide, and glimepiride) who do not have adequate carbohydrate intake before their procedure are at an increased risk of hypoglycemia. It is important that patients on these medications follow their regularly prescribed diet before the dental procedure.

Hyperglycemia. The stress of surgery may provoke the release of counterregulatory hormones that will impair insulin regulation and may result in hyperglycemia and a catabolic state. The cause of hyperglycemia is multifactorial and may include any of several medications such as corticosteroids, beta-blockers, epinephrine, diuretics, and some antipsychotic drugs. Hyperglycemia is usually slower to develop and may not necessarily demonstrate any physical symptoms. Patients should be instructed to monitor their blood sugars in the postsurgical period and contact their physician if their readings remain elevated from their normal baseline. In the acute setting, hyperglycemia can be treated with insulin or by increasing fluids in noncardiac patients. Emergency services should be called for patients who experience erratic breathing and/or fluctuating levels of consciousness associated with high blood sugar levels.

Infection. Diabetic patients are prone to developing infections and vascular complications. The healing process is affected by the impairment of vascular function, chemotaxis, and neutrophil function, as well as an anaerobic milieu. Protein metabolism is decreased, and healing of soft and hard tissue is delayed, which may lead to the susceptibility to infection. Neuropathy and impaired nerve regeneration may be altered as well as angiogenesis.[57]

Determine Glycemic Control. The glycemic control should be evaluated via an HbA1c test (HbA1c, glycated Hb, A1c, or HbA1c) in conjunction with a consultation with the patient's physician. Ideally, the A1c should be maintained at less than 7% when appropriate. The HbA1c test is ideal for evaluation of glycemic control because it will show the glycemic control over the past 3 months. The HbA1c measures the glucose bound to Hb within the RBCs. The test is a weighted average of blood glucose levels during the life of the RBCs (120 days). This test is more accurate in the assessment of diabetic control compared with a fasting blood glucose, which can give a false-positive or false-negative result. It is important to note that target levels for diabetic patients are now individualized rather than generalized. Many times diabetics can be maintained at HbA1c levels greater than 7.0% but less than 8%. The new Medicare quality guidelines consider diabetics less than 9.0% as controlled and greater than 9.0% as uncontrolled. However, it is important to understand studies show that the healing process is much better and complication rate lower in patients with an HbA1c < 7.0%. Because this is an elective procedure, proceeding with surgery in patients with an HbA1c > 7% and ≤8% should be individualized and discussed with their physician and the patient with full disclosure of the increased risks of infection, implant failure, and other complications. Patients with HbA1c > 8% should probably not undergo elective implant surgery because of the higher risk of infection and complications (Table 10.12).

Medication Prophylaxis. Because of the reciprocal relationship between infection and glycemic control, the use of antibiotic prophylaxis is highly recommended. Ideally, a β-lactam antibiotic should be used preoperatively and postoperatively. When antibiotic prophylaxis is administered to diabetic patients, studies have shown a 10.5% reduction in failure rate. Further reduction is achieved by maintaining a strict aseptic technique in combination with good surgical technique. Additionally, it has been reported that the use of a chlorohexidine gluconate (0.12%) rinse at the time of implant placement reduced the failure rate from 13.5% to a remarkable 4.4% in type 2 diabetic patients.[58] A preoperative and postoperative chlorohexidine regimen will decrease morbidity with implants in diabetics. These patients must practice meticulous oral hygiene and be recalled at regular intervals to minimize the possibility of peri-implantitis.

Steroids. Oral steroids like dexamethasone, prednisone, and methylprednisolone will increase blood sugar and should be used with extreme caution in diabetics. A physician consult is recommended for patients under treatment for oral hypoglycemic or insulin-related medications.

Treatment Summary (Diabetes)

Diet-controlled diabetic: Determine/maintain diabetic control.
Hypoglycemic-controlled diabetic: Determine/maintain diabetic, stress reduction protocol; HbA1c < 7%; and individualized treatment recommendations of HbA1c > 7.0% and ≤ 8.0%.
Insulin-controlled diabetic: Determine diabetic control, stress reduction protocol; HbA1c < 7%; individualized treatment recommendations of HbA1c > 7.0% and ≤ 8.0%.

Thyroid Disorders

Thyroid disorders are the second most common endocrine problem, affecting approximately 1% of the general population, principally women. Synthroid (levothyroxine), is one of the most commonly prescribed drugs in the United States.[59,60] Because the majority of patients in implant dentistry are women, a slightly higher prevalence of this disorder is seen in the dental implant practice.

The thyroid gland is one of the larger endocrine glands in the body and is situated at the level of C5 and T1 vertebral bodies, just below the laryngeal prominence. The main function of the thyroid gland is to produce hormones, and the most common are thyroxine (T4) and triiodothyronine (T3). Thyroxine is responsible for the regulation of carbohydrate, protein, and lipid metabolism. In addition, the hormone potentiates the action of other hormones such as catecholamines and growth hormones.

Abnormalities in the anterior pituitary gland or the thyroid can result in disorders of thyroxine production. Excessive production of thyroxine results in hyperthyroidism. Symptoms of this disorder include increased pulse rate, nervousness, intolerance to heat, excessive sweating, weakness of muscles, diarrhea, increased appetite, increased metabolism, and weight loss. Excessive thyroxine may also cause atrial fibrillation, angina, and CHF. Palpation of the patient's neck often reveals an enlarged thyroid gland (goiter) between the cricoid cartilage and the suprasternal notch.

TABLE 10.12	Hemoglobin–Blood Glucose Treatment Regimen		
Risk	**Hemoglobin (A1c)**	**Blood Sugar Level (mg/dL)**	**Treatment Plan**
Low	<6.0	<140	Stress reduction protocol, maintain glycemic control
Low/ medium	6.0–7.0	140–180	Stress reduction protocol, maintain glycemic control Patients with neuropathy, nephropathy, peripheral vascular disease, history of coronary disease, or ophthalmologic manifestation of diabetes (retinopathy) may be at higher risk despite controlled HbA1c. Medical consultation may be appropriate (relative contraindication)
Medium high	7.0–8.0	180–215	Patients without any secondary manifestations of diabetes such as neuropathy, nephropathy, peripheral vascular disease, or ophthalmologic (retinopathy), medical consult may be obtained (relative) Patients with coronary disease or other diabetic related conditions require medical consult (relative/absolute)
High risk	>8.0	>215	Medical referral and better glycemic control (absolute contraindication)

HbA1c, Glycosylated hemoglobin.

From Resnik RR, Resnik RJ. Medical/medication complications in oral implantology. In Resnik RR, Misch CE, eds. *Misch's Avoiding Complications in Oral Implantology.* St Louis, MO: Elsevier; 2018.

The most common form of hypothyroidism is Hashimoto's thyroiditis, which is an autoimmune disease where by the immune system produces antibodies that attack the thyroid gland and create chronic inflammation, which in turn leads to insufficient levels of circulating thyroxine. The related symptoms are a result of a decrease in metabolic rate. The patient complains of cold intolerance, constipation, dry skin, fatigue, and weight gain. In severe cases the patient can develop hoarseness or enter what is termed a myxedema coma. This is a medical emergency with compromised mental activity and hypothermia.

Thyroid function tests are used to confirm the diagnosis of hypothyroidism. The best screening test for thyroid function is to measure the thyroid-stimulating hormone (TSH) level. An increased level indicates underactivity of the thyroid gland, whereas decreased or very low levels indicate over activity of the thyroid. An overactive thyroid gland can cause palpitations, weight loss, tremor, nervousness, and diarrhea. If the TSH level is abnormal, then a free T3 and free T4 can help determine further functioning of the thyroid. T4 and T3 both circulate in the blood, and T4 is converted in the more active form of thyroid hormone T3 in multiple tissues in the body. High levels of T3 and/or T4 indicate an overactive thyroid gland, and low levels indicate an hypofunctioning thyroid gland.

Most people with hypothyroidism are treated with synthetic thyroid replacement medications such as levothyroxine (Synthroid), and the TSH is the best way to monitor this therapy. Some individuals are treated with animal versions of thyroid hormone (Armour Thyroid). The TSH can be artificially low in treatment with Armour Thyroid; therefore a measurement of free T3/T4 is the better way to monitor adequate levels of this treatment.

Dental Implant Management

Hyperthyroidism
Catecholamine Sensitivity. Patients with hyperthyroidism are especially sensitive to catecholamines such as epinephrine in local anesthetics. When exposure to catecholamines is coupled with stress (often related to dental procedures) and tissue damage (dental implant surgery), an exacerbation of the symptoms of hyperthyroidism may occur. This can result in a condition termed thyrotoxicosis or thyroid storm, which is an acute, life-threatening hypermetabolic state clinically presenting with symptoms of fever, tachycardia, hypertension, and neurologic and GI abnormalities. Treatment of thyroid storm in the dental setting includes immediate medical attention. If left untreated, these symptoms may result in CHF and life-threatening cardiac arrhythmias.

Bleeding. The increased blood pressure and heart rate that accompany hyperthyroidism may increase bleeding at the surgical site and require additional hemostatic techniques. It is also important to note that propylthiouracil (PTU) is used to treat hyperthyroidism. This drug is an antagonist of vitamin K, which has an adverse effect on the clotting cascade and may result in significant bleeding or postoperative hemorrhage.

Aspirin/Nonsteroidal Antiinflammatory Drug Use. Use of aspirin or NSAIDs requires extreme caution in the hyperthyroid patient. Aspirin can increase free levels of the T4 hormone because of an interaction with protein binding. Additionally, many hyperthyroid patients are on beta-blockers for heart rate and blood pressure control, and the use of NSAIDs can decrease the efficacy of beta-blockers. Alternative pain medications should be considered in patients with hyperthyroidism (e.g., Ultram).

Hypothyroidism
Central Nervous System Depressants Use. The hypothyroid patient is particularly sensitive to central nervous system (CNS)–depressant drugs, especially narcotics and sedative drugs, such as diazepam or barbiturates. The risk of respiratory depression, cardiovascular depression, or collapse must be considered. Patients with long-standing hypothyroidism may have prolonged bleeding requiring hemostatic control for excessive bleeding. Additionally, hypothyroid patients may exhibit delayed wound healing and predisposition to postoperative infection.

Bone Healing. T4 affects bone metabolism by decreasing recruitment and maturation of bone cells and reducing the bone growth factor of insulin-like growth factor. Studies have shown that medically treated hypothyroid patients exhibit greater bone loss and a less favorable soft tissue response after stage I surgery but with no significant increased risk of failure[59] (Table 10.13).

Adrenal Gland Disorders

The adrenal glands are endocrine organs located just above the kidneys. Epinephrine and norepinephrine are produced by chromaffin cells in the adrenal medulla, which forms the central portion of the gland. These hormones are largely responsible for the control of blood pressure, myocardial contractility and excitability, and general metabolism.[61] The outer portion of the gland or adrenal cortex produces three different types of hormones. Glucocorticoids regulate carbohydrate, fat, and protein metabolism and also help decrease inflammation. Synthetic glucocorticoid medications may be used by the implant dentist to decrease swelling and pain. The mineralocorticoids maintain sodium and potassium balance. A third category of hormones is produced that are

TABLE 10.13 Dental Implant Management in Patients With Thyroid Disorders

Risk		Type 1	Type 2	Type 3	Type 4
Mild	Medical examination <6 months normal Fct last 6 months	+	+	+	+
Moderate	No symptoms No medical examination No Fct test	+	Decrease epinephrine, steroids, CNS depressants	Physician consultation	Physician consultation
Severe	Symptoms	Physician consultation	Postpone all elective procedures	Postpone all elective procedures	Postpone all elective procedures

+, Procedure may be performed with regular protocol; CNS, central nervous system; Fct, function.

mainly sex hormones (testosterone and dehydroepiandrosterone [DHEA]). The hypothalamus stimulated the anterior pituitary gland to produce adrenocorticotropic hormone (ACTH), which then stimulates the adrenal glands to produce cortisol.

Cortisol is one of the most important glucocorticoids secreted by the adrenal cortex. Insufficient production and secretion of cortisol leads to primary adrenocortical insufficiency, also termed Addison's disease. A patient with Addison's disease shows symptoms of weakness, weight loss, orthostatic hypotension, nausea, and vomiting. The physical signs of primary insufficiency do not manifest until 90% of the gland is destroyed. Signs and symptoms develop insidiously over months. When these signs are noted, the implant dentist should require a medical consultation. These patients cannot increase their steroid production in response to stress and in the midst of surgery or long restorative procedures may have cardiovascular collapse. During the physical examination, the dentist can notice hyperpigmented areas on the face, lips, and gingiva.[62] An increase in serum potassium level (hyperkalemia) and decrease in serum glucose level are characteristic of Addison's disease.

When adrenal hypersecretion of cortisol is present, patients will show signs of Cushing syndrome. The characteristic changes associated with this disease are moon facies, truncal obesity or "buffalo hump," muscle wasting, and hirsutism. Patients are hypertensive, and long-term excess function of the cortex decreases collagen production. These patients bruise easily, have poor wound healing, experience osteoporosis, and are also at increased risk for infection. These elements are especially noteworthy to the implant dentist. Laboratory studies show an increase in blood glucose related to an interference with carbohydrate metabolism. The CBC often shows a slight decrease in eosinophil and lymphocyte counts.

Corticosteroids are potent antiinflammatory drugs used to treat a number of systemic diseases and are one of the most prescribed drugs in medicine. Steroids are used for more than 80 conditions such as arthritis, collagen and vascular disorders, kidney diseases, asthma, and dermatologic disorders. However, the continued administration of exogenous steroids suppresses the natural function of the adrenal glands and causes a condition equivalent to Cushing disease. As a result, patients under long-term steroid therapy are placed on the same protocol as patients with hypofunction of the adrenal glands.

Aldosterone is the main mineralocorticoid produced by the adrenal gland and it is essential for sodium conservation by the body. It is regulated by the renin angiotensin system in the kidney. Renin is secreted in response to variations in blood pressure, volume, and sodium and potassium levels by the kidney. Aldosterone works to enhance the reabsorption of sodium and water in the kidneys and secrete potassium, which increases blood pressure. ARB and ACE inhibitor high blood pressure medications block the production of the angiotensin–renin system in the kidneys, thus lowering aldosterone production and sodium retention and leading to the lowering of blood pressure. Overproduction of aldosterone can lead to low levels of potassium and uncontrolled hypertension

Dental Implant Management. Patients with a history of adrenal gland disease, whether hyperfunctioning or hypofunctioning, face similar problems related to dentistry and stress. The body is unable to produce increased levels of steroids during stressful situations, and cardiovascular collapse may occur. As a result, additional steroids are prescribed for the patient just before the stressful situation. These doses are stopped within 3 days. The

healthy patient will accelerate steroid production three to five times higher than regular levels to respond to the stress of surgery or dental procedures. Therefore for patients with known adrenal disorders, the physician should be contacted for consultation. The nature of the disorder and the recommended treatment should be evaluated.

The patient on regular maintenance doses of steroid in excess of prednisone 5 mg/day is at high risk of adrenal suppression. Adrenocortical suppression should be suspected if a patient has received a dose of 20 mg or more of cortisone or equivalent daily via the oral or parenteral route for a continuous period of 2 weeks or longer, within 2 years of dental treatment.[63] Consultation with the patient's physician is indicated, and any modification of medication should only be adjusted by the patient's physician. For simple to advanced operative procedures and simple extractions, and for periodontal or implant surgery (types 1 and 2), the steroid dose should be doubled up to 60 mg of prednisone or equivalent (10 mg dexamethasone). The day after the procedure, the maintenance dose is returned to normal. Oral or IV conscious sedation is used to reduce stress. For moderate to advanced implant surgery or the very anxious patient, general anesthesia may be indicated. The day of the procedure, 60 mg prednisone is administered. This dose is reduced by 50% each day over a 2- to 3-day period to the maintenance dose. Antibiotics are also administered for 3 to 5 days.

Patients at significant or moderate risk for adrenal suppression are those formerly on steroid therapy of 20 mg prednisone or more for longer than 7 days within the preceding year. Simple to complex restorative procedures or simple surgery (types 1 and 2) suggest administration of 20 to 40 mg of prednisone the day of the procedure. Sedation techniques and antibiotics for 3 to 5 days are suggested. The next day the steroid dose is reduced by 50%, and by the third day the dosage is reduced by an additional 50% or returned to normal. For types 3 and 4, moderate to advanced surgical procedures, the protocol is further modified. Prednisone 60 mg or equivalent is administered the day of the surgery. This dose is reduced 50% the next day, and another 50% on the third day. General anesthesia may be used to reduce anxiety in the apprehensive patient.

Patients at low risk for adrenal suppression are those on alternate-day steroid therapy or those whose steroid therapy ended 1 year or more before the implant procedure. For these, dental procedures are scheduled the day steroids are taken or up to 60 mg of prednisone is administered. On the second day the dose is reduced 50%; on the third day, the patient resumes the alternate-day schedule. Sedation and antibiotics are also used.

Steroids act in three different ways that affect implant surgery. They decrease inflammation and are useful in decreasing swelling and related pain. However, steroids also decrease protein synthesis and therefore delay healing. In addition, they decrease leukocytes, reducing the patient's ability to fight infection. Therefore whenever steroids are given to patients for surgery, it may be reasonable to prescribe antibiotics. After a loading dose, amoxicillin or clindamycin are given three times per day for 3 to 5 days (Table 10.14).

Hyperparathyroidism

Hyperparathyroidism is an excess of PTH in the bloodstream caused by overactivity of one or more of the parathyroid glands that maintain calcium balance. The clinical manifestations of this disease vary widely depending on the severity. Mild forms may

TABLE 10.14	Dental Implant Management in Patients With Adrenal Disorders			
Risk	Dosage	Type 1	Type 2	Types 3 and 4
Mild	Equivalent of prednisone on alternate days for >1 year	+	Surgery on day of steroids	Sedation and antibiotics steroids: <60 mg prednisone on day 1 Dose x/2 on day 2 Maintenance dose on day 3
Moderate	Equivalent of prednisone >20 mg or >7 days in past year	+	Sedation and antibiotics: 20–40 mg day 1 Dose x2 on day 2 Dose x4 on day 3	Sedation and antibiotics: 60 mg day 1 Dose x2 on day 2 Dose x4 on day 3
Severe	Equivalent of prednisone 5 mg/day	Physician consultation	Elective procedures contraindicated	Elective procedures contraindicated

+, Procedure may be performed with regular protocol.

be asymptomatic, whereas severe hyperparathyroidism can cause bone, renal, and gastric disturbance. It has been noted that skeletal depletion occurs as a result of stimulation by the parathyroid gland, which results in alveolar bone being affected before bones such as the ribs, vertebrae, or long bones. In the oral and maxillofacial regions, altered trabecular bone patterns may be present that result in mobility of the teeth and compromised bone density. Hyperparathyroidism falls into three categories: primary, secondary, and tertiary. Primary hyperparathyroidism involves one of the parathyroid glands becoming overactive and releasing excess parathyroid hormone. This results in high levels of calcium being released into the bloodstream from the bone, which leads to osteoporotic bones.

Secondary hyperparathyroidism is a chronic condition in which the parathyroid glands release an excess amount of parathyroid hormone because of chronically low blood calcium levels. Secondary hyperparathyroidism is usually caused by conditions such as CKD, vitamin D deficiency, and some GI issues that affect calcium absorption.

Tertiary hyperparathyroidism can occur when the condition causing secondary hyperparathyroidism is treated. This is similar to vitamin D deficiency; however, the parathyroid glands continue to produce excess parathyroid hormone.

Dental Implant Management

Bone Involvement. Dental implants are contraindicated (absolute) in areas of active bony lesions; however, implant placement may be initiated after treatment and healing of the affected areas. Altered trabecular bone pattern with the appearance of ground glass may also occur. In animal studies, secondary hyperparathyroidism affects alveolar bone more than any other bone of the skeleton, and central or peripheral giant cell tumors may be present in active lesion areas.[64]

Parathyroid Control. When the PTH is elevated, a serum calcium level is obtained to determine whether the hyperparathyroidism is primary or secondary, and the condition is usually treated with surgery or medication. In advanced disease, there are certain oral changes that can be present to suggest hyperparathyroidism. These patients have an increased risk for tori, and reduction in the radicular lamina dura is evident on dental radiographs. Many patients with higher levels of PTH develop loose teeth and widening of the periodontal ligament space surrounding the teeth. Additionally, cortical bone loss at the angle of the mandible has been noted in this disorder.

> **• BOX 10.9   Xerostomia Treatment Regimens**

- Drink water frequently: Helps moisten mucosa and loosen mucus.
- Gum/candy: The use of sugarless gum or candy helps stimulate saliva flow.
- Avoid commercial mouth rinses containing alcohol or peroxide: Further desiccates the mucosa.
- Avoid salty foods, dry foods (for example, crackers, toast, cookies, dry breads, dry meats/poultry/fish, dried fruit, bananas), and foods and beverages with high sugar content.
- Avoid drinks containing alcohol or caffeine. Alcohol and caffeine increase urination and desiccate the mucosa.
- Over-the-counter saliva substitutes: Products containing xylitol (e.g., Mouth Kote, Oasis Moisturizing Mouth Spray, or ones containing carboxymethylcellulose).
- Prescription medications, after physician consultation (Evoxac [cevimeline], Salagen [pilocarpine]).

From Resnik RR, Resnik RJ. Medical/medication complications in oral implantology. In Resnik RR, Misch CE, eds, Misch's Avoiding Complications in Oral Implantology. St Louis, MO: Elsevier; 2018.

Xerostomia

Xerostomia (dry mouth) may directly or indirectly have effects on dental implants. A decrease in salivary flow is also accompanied by a change in its composition. An increase in mucin and a decrease in ptyalin result in a more viscous and ropy saliva. Plaque formation is increased, and the reduced antibacterial action of the saliva results in a favorable environment for bacteria growth (Box 10.9).

Dental Implant Management

Oral Complications. Dental implants are not contraindicated in patients suffering from xerostomia. Case reports have been documented with successful implant placement with no increase in failure rate.[65] However, with the lack of saliva, implant patients may be susceptible to more oral lesions and the possibility of irritation from tissue-borne implant prostheses. Additionally, patients are at higher risk for incision line opening.

Oral Bacterial Infections. Patients with xerostomia are at a higher risk for oral infections such as periodontitis, caries, and fungal infections. A comprehensive oral and periodontal examination must be completed with emphasis on a low periodontal pathogen bacterial count to reduce possible postoperative complications.

Increase Saliva Flow. Stimulation of salivary flow may be achieved either by physiologic or pharmacologic means. Mouth rinses, chewing gum, or salivary substitutes may be used.

Final Prosthesis. When planning treatment for patients with xerostomia, a final prosthesis that is not tissue borne is recommended. A fixed-detachable (FP-3) prosthesis is highly recommended because of the lack of soft tissue coverage. If a removable prosthesis is warranted, an RP-4 is recommended because of the lack of soft tissue coverage. Additionally, removable prostheses worn in patients with xerostomia are associated with a high prevalence of fungal infections. If fungal infection is diagnosed, the use of a Nystatin medication is warranted.

Pregnancy

Elective dental implant surgery procedures are contraindicated for the pregnant patient. Not only is the mother the responsibility of the dentist, but so is the fetus. The radiographs or medications that may be needed for implant therapy and the increased stress are all reasons the elective implant surgical procedure should be postponed until after childbirth. However, after implant surgery has occurred, the patient may become pregnant while waiting for the restorative procedures, especially because modalities may require 3 months to 1 year of healing. Periodontal disease is often exacerbated during pregnancy. All elective dental care, with the exception of dental prophylaxis, should be deferred until after the birth. The only exceptions to this are caries control or emergency dental procedures. In these instances, medical clearance should be given for all drugs, including anesthetics, analgesics, and antibiotics to be administered to the patient. In most cases, physicians will approve the use of lidocaine, penicillin, erythromycin, and acetaminophen (Tylenol). Aspirin, vasoconstrictors (epinephrine), and drugs that cause respiratory depression (e.g., narcotic analgesics) are usually contraindicated. Diazepam (Valium), nitrous oxide, and tetracycline are almost always contraindicated.

Dental Implant Management. Elective dental implant therapy should be delayed until after pregnancy. A medical clearance should be obtained before any invasive treatment.

Additional Endocrine Disorders and Treatment Implications

See Table 10.15.

Hematologic System

Erythrocytic (Red Blood Cell) Disorders

In a healthy patient, 4 to 6 million RBCs per milliliter of blood are in circulation. RBCs make up the largest portion of the formed elements in blood. There are two main categories of erythrocyte disorders: polycythemia (increased erythrocyte count) and anemia (decrease in Hb).

Polycythemia. Polycythemia is defined as an increased concentration of Hb in body. It is either the result of increased RBC production or can it be caused by reduction in plasma volume. Most cases of polycythemia are the result of other underlying medical conditions or medications and referred to as secondary polycythemia. Hb levels >16.5 g/dL in women or 18.5 g/dL in men can suggest a diagnosis of polycythemia. Any condition that

TABLE 10.15	Additional Endocrine Issues and Treatment Implications
Positive Response	**Treatment Implications**
Frequent urination	Diabetes (undiagnosed)
Increased thirst	Diabetes (undiagnosed)
Recent weight loss	Anxiety, depression, GI disease, diabetes, hyperthyroidism
Recent weight gain	Heart failure (water retention), corticosteroids, Cushing syndrome, hypothyroidism
Increased appetite	Diabetes, hyperthyroidism
Fatigue	Anxiety, depression, anemia, vitamin B deficiency, hyper/hypothyroidism, chronic pulmonary/cardiovascular disease
Frequent kidney stones	Hypercalciuria from hyperparathyroidism
Increased head/hand shoe size	Paget disease
Nontraumatic bone fractures	Osteoporosis, hyperparathyroidism, myeloma
Slow healing infections/sores	Undiagnosed diabetes, Cushing syndrome, coagulation factor deficiency, vitamin C deficiency, adrenal insufficiency
Pigment changes in skin (dark spots)	Undiagnosed diabetes, Addison disease, melanoma, hemochromatosis

GI, Gastrointestinal.

From Resnik RR, Resnik RJ. Medical/medication complications in oral implantology. In Resnik RR, Misch CE, eds. *Misch's Avoiding Complications in Oral Implantology*. St Louis, MO: Elsevier; 2018.

causes chronic hypoxemia like COPD or even sleep apnea can be a secondary cause of polycythemia. Patients undergoing testosterone replacement can also develop a secondary polycythemia. Complicated implant or reconstruction procedures are usually contraindicated. Very high concentrations of Hb can cause infarcts in tissue such as the heart and stroke. Any patient with an elevated Hb having chest pain or any neurologic symptoms including headache, visuals issues or numbness, and weakness or tingling of extremities should be referred to their physician immediately.

Dental Implant Implications

Thrombus Formation. Because of the higher viscosity of the blood in polycythemic patients, an increased possibility of stroke, MI, or pulmonary embolism may occur.

Bleeding. Excessive bleeding and clotting issues are common with polycythemia patients; good surgical technique and strict hemostatic control measures must be followed to minimize intraoperative and postoperative bleeding episodes.

Treatment Summary

Unless cleared by a physician, polycythemia is an absolute contraindication for dental implant treatment.

Anemia

Anemia is the most common hematologic disorder. Almost all blood dyscrasias may at one time or another be associated with anemia. Anemia is not a disease entity; rather, it is a symptom complex that results from a decreased production of erythrocytes, an increased rate of their destruction, or a deficiency in iron. It is defined as a reduction in the oxygen-carrying capacity of the blood and results from a decrease in the number of erythrocytes or the abnormality of Hb. Hb levels <13.5 g/dL in men or <12.0 g/dL in women can be indicative of anemia. Levels less than 10 g/dL require immediate attention, especially in patients that are symptomatic with shortness of breath, extreme fatigue, or dizziness.

There are a number of different types of anemia, and the most common type is iron-deficiency anemia and relative bone marrow failure. Iron-deficiency anemia may be caused by a decreased intake of iron, a decreased absorption of iron, or an increase in bleeding. Vitamin C increases the absorption of iron. The female patient may normally be anemic in menses or pregnancy. Mild anemia in a man, however, may indicate a serious underlying medical problem. The most common causes of anemia in men are peptic ulcers or carcinoma of the colon. These serious complications warrant medical evaluation of any male patient found to be anemic.

Other forms of anemia include sickle cell anemia (predominant in African Americans), pernicious anemia (low B_{12} or folate levels), and thalassemia (chronic hereditary hemolytic anemia as a result of defective Hb production). These types of anemia are chronic and many patients are well adapted to lower levels of Hb without many symptoms. Sickle cell anemia has different levels of severity, which requires a thorough history and consultation with the patient's physician may be warranted.

The general symptoms and signs are all a consequence of either a reduction of oxygen reaching the tissues or alterations of the RBC. The symptoms of mild anemia include fatigue, anxiety, and sleeplessness. Chronic anemia is characterized by shortness of breath, abdominal pain, bone pain, tingling of extremities, muscular weakness, headaches, fainting, change in heart rhythm, and nausea. The general signs of anemia may include jaundice, pallor, spooning or cracking of the nails, hepatomegaly and splenomegaly, and lymphadenopathy. The oral signs of anemia affect the tongue; symptoms include a sore, painful, smooth tongue; loss of papillae; redness; loss of taste sensation; and paresthesia of the oral tissues.

Complications associated with implant patients with anemia may affect both short-term and long-term prognoses. Bone maturation and development are often impaired in the long-term anemic patient. A faint, large trabecular pattern of bone may even appear radiographically, which indicates a 25% to 40% loss in trabecular pattern. Therefore the initial character of the bone needed to support the implant can be affected significantly. The decreased bone density affects the initial placement and may influence the initial amount of mature lamellar bone forming at the interface of an osteointegrated implant. The time needed for a proper interface formation is longer in poor density bone.[66] However, after the implant is loaded successfully, the local strain environment will improve the bone density at the interface.

Abnormal bleeding is also a common complication of anemia; during extensive surgery, a decreased field vision from the hemorrhage may occur. Increased edema and subsequent increased discomfort postsurgically are common consequences. In addition, the excess edema increases the risk of postoperative infection and its consequences. Not only are anemic patients prone to more immediate infection from surgery; they are also more sensitive to chronic infection throughout their lives. This may affect

the long-term maintenance of the proposed implant or abutment teeth.

Approximately 0.15% of the African American population has sickle cell anemia.[67] Patients with such a disorder usually show marked clinical manifestations and often die before the age of 40. Secondary infections are a common consequence with frequent history of osteomyelitis and bone infection. Because of these complications, implants are contraindicated in patients with sickle cell anemia.

The laboratory tests that diagnose anemia or polycythemia are in the CBC. An accurate test for anemia is the hematocrit, followed by the Hb; the least accurate is the RBC count. The hematocrit indicates the percentage of a given volume of whole blood composed of erythrocytes. The normal values for men range from 40% to 50%, and those for women from 35% to 45%. Hb composes almost 95% of the dry weight of RBCs. Abnormal Hb may result from its combination with substances other than oxygen (e.g., carbon monoxide) or genetic diseases (e.g., sickle cell diseases). Normal values for men are 13.5 to 18 g/dL, and those for women are 12 to 16 g/dL. The minimum baseline recommended for surgery is 10 mg/dL, especially for elective implant surgery. For the majority of anemic patients, implant procedures are not contraindicated. However, preoperative and postoperative antibiotics should be administered, and the risk of bleeding in anemic patients should not be potentiated by the prescription/use of aspirin. Hygiene appointments should be scheduled more frequently for these patients.

Dental Implant Implications

Bleeding. Some anemias are associated with abnormal bleeding. During extensive surgery, the increased bleeding may cause a decreased field of view for the clinician and possible postoperative issues. Most often iron-deficiency anemia and other vitamin-dependent anemias are associated with increased bleeding.

Edema. Increased edema and subsequent increased discomfort postsurgically are common consequences. In addition, the excess edema increases the risk of postoperative infection and morbidity. Anemic patients are prone to more immediate infection from surgery, and they are also more sensitive to chronic infection throughout their lives. This may affect the long-term maintenance of the proposed implant or abutment teeth.

Oral soft tissue issues. The oral signs of anemia affect the tongue. Symptoms include a sore, painful, smooth tongue; loss of papillae; redness; loss of taste sensation; and paresthesia of the oral tissues.

Bone Healing. Bone maturation and development are often impaired in the long-term anemic patient. A faint, large trabecular pattern of bone may even appear radiographically, which indicates a 25% to 40% loss in trabecular pattern. Therefore the initial quality of the bone required to support the implant can be affected significantly. The decreased bone density affects the initial placement and may influence the initial amount of mature lamellar bone forming at the interface of an osseointegrated implant. The time needed for a proper interface formation is longer in poor density bone.[68] However, after the implant is loaded successfully, the local strain environment will improve the bone density at the interface.

Leukocytic Disorders

Leukocyte disorders are an important consideration in hematologic diseases. The WBC count normally ranges from 4500 to 11,000/mm³ in the adult. Leukocytosis is defined as an increase in circulating WBCs in excess of 11,000/mm³. The most common cause of leukocytosis is infection. Leukemia, neoplasms, acute hemorrhage, and diseases associated with acute inflammation or necrosis (e.g., infarction, collagen diseases) are more serious causes of leukocytosis. Physiologic conditions such as exercise, pregnancy, and emotional stress can also lead to leukocytosis. Any patient receiving recent or continuous oral steroids will most likely have an elevated WBC count.

Most oral implant procedures are contraindicated for the patient with acute or chronic leukemia. Acute leukemia can be a fatal disease, but some patients with aggressive therapy including stem cell transplants do have more favorable outcomes. These patients experience serious oral problems, either secondary to the disease process or as complications after chemotherapy. The patient with chronic leukemia will experience anemia and thrombocytopenia. Although the infection is less severe than in acute leukemia, radiolucent lesions of the jaws, oral ulcerations, hyperplastic gingiva, and bleeding complications develop in these patients

Leukopenia is a reduction in the number of circulating WBCs to less than 4500/mm^3. Many times, a low WBC count can be caused by a recent viral infection; however, this should be temporary and past WBC counts should have been normal. Cancer, certain autoimmune diseases (lupus and rheumatoid arthritis [RA]), severe infections, and even some antibiotics can cause a low WBC. There is a subset of patients that have a chronically low WBC count and are otherwise completely healthy. However, these patients require additional testing to confirm that the decrease is in WBCs is benign. These patients should be evaluated by a hematology specialist.

In the potential implant candidate with leukocytosis or leukopenia, many complications can compromise the success of the implants and prosthesis. The most common is infection, not only during the initial healing phase but also long term. Delayed healing is also a consequence of WBC disorders. For most implant procedures, the first few months are critical for long-term success. Delayed healing may increase the risk of secondary infection. Treatment-planning modifications should shift toward a conservative approach when dealing with leukocyte disorders. Complications are more common than in erythrocyte disorders. If the condition is temporary, such as an acute infection, surgical procedures should be delayed until the infection has been controlled and the patient has returned to a normal condition.

Platelet Disorders

A normal platelet count is between 150,000 and 450,000/μL. Thrombocytopenia is a lower than normal platelet count caused by decreased production, increased destruction, or sequestration of platelets in the spleen, which results in potential bleeding complications during surgery. A platelet count should always be obtained in patients with this history, and a value lower than 50,000 U/L contraindicates elective dental surgery because of a significant risk of postoperative bleeding.[69]

It should also be noted that platelet counts can be reduced or normal but bleeding time can be prolonged in the presence of platelet dysfunction. Acquired platelet dysfunction can be the result of a systemic illness like liver or connective tissue disease. Drugs like aspirin or clopidogrel cause an acquired platelet dysfunction that can last 7 days or longer, and concurrent use in the presence of lower than normal platelet counts can prolong

bleeding. Consultation with the patient's physician is indicated in this situation.

Idiopathic thrombocytopenic purpura is a platelet disorder that may present with a number of findings including petechiae, blood in the urine, ecchymosis, and spontaneous prolonged bleeding. Implant dentists need to recognize this condition because it may create prolonged life-threatening bleeding. Oral manifestations include spontaneous gingival bleeding. There may be scattered petechiae on the palate tongue or oral mucosa. There should be consultation with the patient's physician before any dental implant surgery.

Thrombotic thrombocytopenic purpura (TTP) is a rare blood disorder characterized by anemia, neurologic dysfunction, and thrombocytopenia. Neurologically patients will have changes in vision, speech, and mental status as well as fatigue from the anemia and bleeding from the low platelet counts. TTP can be the result of certain medications, including chemotherapy. Any patient with a history of TTP should not undergo any dental implant procedure without clearance from their physician.

Essential thrombocythemia is a condition when the body produces too many platelets. This condition can result in abnormal blood clotting, but because many times the overproduced platelets are dysfunctional, it can also cause abnormal bleeding. Platelet counts can also be elevated from inflammation and caused by several conditions including recent blood loss, infections, pancreatitis, splenectomy, and certain anemias. The platelet counts in these conditions usually resolve as the underlying condition is treated.

It is recommended that patients that have a history of low or high platelet counts be closely evaluated for elective implant surgery.

Dental Implant Management. When treating patients with any hematologic disease, a medical consultation and clearance is warranted, including those with current or past history of reduced or elevated platelet counts because many times there may be an associated platelet dysfunction, which could lead to issues with perioperative and postoperative bleeding. The patient's physician should be presented with a comprehensive summary of the proposed procedure, medications to be prescribed, and the extent of anticipated bleeding.

Additional Hematologic Disorders and Treatment Implications

See Table 10.16.

Pulmonary System

Chronic Obstructive Pulmonary Disease

COPD refers to a group of pulmonary diseases that block airflow, resulting in breathing difficulties. The two most common conditions that make up COPD are chronic bronchitis and emphysema. Chronic bronchitis is an inflammation of the bronchial tubes that produces an increase in mucous production and coughing.

There are close to 15 million American adults that have been diagnosed with COPD and about 10 million of them have chronic bronchitis with about 5 million with emphysema. COPD is now the third most common cause of death behind only cancer and heart disease in the United States. The annual costs to our health care system for COPD-related illness is over $30 billion each year.[70]

TABLE 10.15	Additional Hematologic Issues and Treatment Implications
Positive Response	**Treatment Implications**
Sickle cell anemia	Secondary infections are a common consequence with frequent history of osteomyelitis and bone infection (absolute contraindication)
Leukemia	Experience anemia and thrombocytopenia. Although the infection is less severe than in acute leukemia, radiolucent lesions of the jaws, oral ulcerations, hyperplastic gingiva, and bleeding complications develop in these patients (absolute contraindication)
Thalassemia	Multiple types (alpha, beta) and degrees of severity (major, minor) More severe forms can present some issues such as erythroid mass expansion directly into facial bones causing malocclusions Medical consultation is recommended to determine severity of disease Major (severe forms): absolute contraindication Minor (less severe): relative contraindication
Frequent nosebleeds (epistaxis)	Hypertension, sinus disease, bleeding disorders such as von Willebrand Spontaneous or frequent nosebleeds should have bleeding time and INR
Easy bleeding gums	Gingival disease, bleeding disorder, thrombocytopenia, leukemia, liver disease Further investigation may be warranted with platelet, CBC, bleeding time, PT, PTT
Heavy menstrual periods	Thyroid disease, dysfunctional uterine bleeding (fibroid, polyps, and hormone imbalance), bleeding disorders, platelet dysfunction If no obvious medical reason, check CBC, INR, bleeding time
Family history of bleeding disorder	If family history of bleeding issues, check CBC, INR, PTT, bleeding time to rule out hereditary bleeding disorders such as von Willebrand, hemophilia, and coagulation factor deficiencies
Prolonged bleeding after cuts	Rule out coagulation defect, hereditary bleeding disorder, or platelet dysfunction; check CBC, INR, PTT, bleeding times
Easy bruising or spontaneous bruising	Platelet deficiency, coagulation factor issue, leukemias, vitamin K deficiency, chemotherapy, anticoagulation medication
History of excessive bleeding after dental surgery	If no definitive diagnosis correlates with prolonged bleeding, check CBC, INR, PTT, bleeding time

CBC, Complete blood count; *INR*, international normalized ratio; *PT*, prothrombin time; *PTT*, partial thromboplastin time.

From Resnik RR, Resnik RJ. Medical/medication complications in oral implantology. In Resnik RR, Misch CE, eds. *Misch's Avoiding Complications in Oral Implantology.* St Louis, MO: Elsevier; 2018.

Emphysema occurs when the alveoli in the bronchioles of the lungs become damaged or destroyed, creating symptoms of dyspnea (shortness of breath) that may worsen with mild activity. Patients with COPD may have a combination of both conditions. These patients usually present with fatigue, history of recurrent respiratory infections, wheezing, and shortness of breath. In advanced disease states, patients may become oxygen dependent with tachypnea being present with some audible wheezing and shortness of breath even at rest. The various levels of COPD are classified via the Global Initiative for Chronic Obstructive Lung Disease (GOLD), which classifies patients on their degree of airflow limitation. The airflow limitation is measured during pulmonary function tests (PFTs) and measured as forced expiratory volume (FEV_1).

These guidelines use an ABCD grading system with A being better and D being worse. Treatment involves using long-acting bronchodilators that are beta-agonists (LABA) or muscarinic antagonist (LAMA) and work directly on the lung to improve oxygenation through dilation of the bronchioles. Inhaled corticosteroids (ICS) are not usually used as a single therapy, but many times are used in combination with bronchodilators. More common LABA/IC combinations include Advair, Dulero, Breo, and Symbicort. Common LAMA drugs include Spiriva and Incrusel. Albuterol is a short-acting bronchodilator and is not indicated for continuous monotherapy. It is used as a "rescue" to help treat acute symptoms or exacerbations. Short-acting bronchodilators can have a profound effect on increasing heart rate, especially if used just before an elective dental surgery. Any COPD patient using a long- or short-acting bronchodilator is considered grade A. Patients using a long-acting bronchodilator LABA or LAMA, or both, with persistent symptoms are considered grade B. Grade C is the addition of a LAMA or switching to a LABA and LAMA combination or adding an inhaled corticosteroid to control exacerbations. Grade D patients are the more complex patients requiring more specialized treatment because they do not respond to conventional combinations. Although it is important to get a detailed history of a patient with COPD, there should be specific focus on their current use of medications to control symptoms because they can vary seasonally and under other situations. Patients with grade D symptoms should always get clearance from their physician for elective dental surgery. However, there should be consideration for physician consultation for any grade C or recent worsening of respiratory symptoms in patients with COPD.

Dental Implant Management. Patients with difficulty breathing only on significant exertion and who have normal laboratory blood gases are at minimal risk and may follow all restorative or surgical procedures with normal protocols (types 1–4). Dental management of COPD patients may require repositioning the patient from the normal supine position. Depending on the severity of the disease, orthopnea may result. The patient can be placed in the most recumbent position so that breathing is comfortable. Supplemental oxygen (2–3 L) should be administered throughout the dental procedures.

Patients with difficulty breathing on exertion in general are at moderate risk, as are patients on chronic bronchodilator therapy or who have recently used corticosteroids. These patients may follow examination procedures with normal protocol (type 1). A recent medical examination is recommended for all other procedures. Type 2 procedures should be performed in a hospital setting. If the patient is on bronchodilators, no epinephrine or vasoconstrictors should be added to the anesthetics or gingival retraction cord. Adrenal suppression should be evaluated for any patient on steroid therapy within the past year.

Patients at high risk are those with previously unrecognized COPD, acute exacerbation (e.g., respiratory infection), dyspnea at rest, or a history of carbon dioxide retention. Dental management of patients with COPD is staged according to the severity of the disease. If a patient has been hospitalized for respiratory difficulties, then a medical consultation is warranted. The dentist should inquire regarding the carbon dioxide retention capability of these patients. Patients who retain carbon dioxide have a severe condition and are prone to respiratory failure when given sedatives, oxygen or nitrous oxide, and oxygen analgesia.

Examination procedures may be performed under normal protocol (type 1). Elective moderate procedures or advanced surgical or prosthetic procedures are usually contraindicated. However, if surgery or prosthetic procedures are needed to repair a previously inserted implant, then they should be performed in the hospital. The use of epinephrine should be limited. Drugs that depress respiratory function, such as sedatives (including nitrous oxide), tranquilizers, and narcotics, should be discussed with the physician.

Anesthetic selection. In rare instances, patients with COPD receiving local anesthetics have exhibited adverse reactions. Increased doses of anesthetic solutions that contain sulfites may increase the risk of bronchospasm or allergic reactions. Most local anesthetics that are vasopressor anesthetics (e.g., epinephrine, levonordefrin) will contain the antioxidant sodium (meta) bisulfite. For COPD patients with a known allergy to bisulfites, a local anesthetic without a vasopressor (e.g., mepivacaine HCL 3%, prilocaine HCL 4%) should be used.

Adrenal Suppression. Adrenal suppression may occur with long-term corticosteroid treatment, which is common with more advanced COPD patients.

Cardiovascular Event. For patients who have had a cardiovascular event, the patient's functional capacity should be ascertained (physician consultation) and a stress reduction protocol implemented. The implant clinician should avoid long or extensive surgical procedures.

Oxygen Supplementation. High flow rates of oxygen can result in respiratory depression in patients that are oxygen dependent or have more severe COPD disease. However, there is now supporting evidence that titration of oxygen therapy to maintain saturations between 88% and 92% is the correct approach. Avoid using higher levels of oxygen that would increase pulse oximetry levels to >92%, creating hyperoxia in a COPD patient, which could result in hypercapnia (retention of COPD which can diminish respiratory rate). Nitrous oxide is also contraindicated because of the negative affect on the respiratory drive. Low–flow rate oxygen supplementation (<2 L/min) during implant procedures is highly recommended to minimize the possibility of hypoxia.

Bronchodilators/Inhaled Corticosteroids. Bronchodilators and inhaled corticosteroids are the hallmark of treatment for COPD; however, they have been associated with an adverse effect on oral tissues. β_2-agonists such as albuterol have been associated with a decrease in saliva production and subsequent secretion resulting in xerostomia. Patients should always be instructed to bring their rescue inhaler (usually albuterol) to the procedure or, for more advanced COPD patients, their nebulizer and albuterol solution in case of an emergency.

Use of Sedation. Sedation should be carefully evaluated in patients with COPD, and discussion with their treating physician is recommended. Potent sedatives such as narcotics and barbiturates should be avoided unless approved by the treating physician. These drugs can further depress the respiratory drive in more advanced COPD patients. Antihistamines may desiccate respiratory secretions, which may lead to compromised airflow. Additionally, nitrous oxide should not be used in COPD patients because it can lead to further respiratory depression (Table 10.17).

Additional Pulmonary Disorders and Treatment Implications

See Table 10.18.

Digestive System

Liver Disease (Cirrhosis)

Cirrhosis of the liver is characterized by irreversible scarring and is usually caused by excessive alcohol intake, viral hepatitis B and C, and certain medications. Although patients with advanced disease can present with jaundice and itching, the diagnosis is usually confirmed by liver biopsy and blood tests. Cirrhosis may cause excessive bleeding, mental confusion, kidney failure, and accumulation of fluid in the abdomen (ascites). Cirrhosis is irreversible, and transplantation is becoming the most successful treatment for advanced disease states.

Cirrhosis is the third leading cause of death in young men between the ages of 35 and 54 years. It occurs as a result of injury to the liver with resultant loss of liver cells and progressive scarring. The major cause of cirrhosis is alcoholic liver disease. In 2015, approximately 6.2% of the population met the diagnostic criteria for alcohol abuse and alcohol dependence, but as many as 15 to 20 million may be considered alcoholics. More than 25 million Americans have alcohol-related liver or gallbladder disease, and an estimated 900,000 Americans have cirrhosis.[71,72]

Patients with cirrhosis have several significant issues that can affect dental treatment, including dysfunctional synthesis of clotting factors and the inability to detoxify drugs. Hemostatic defects of liver disease cause not only reduced synthesis of clotting factors but also an abnormal synthesis of fibrinogen and clotting proteins, vitamin K deficiency, enhanced fibrinolytic activity, and quantitative and qualitative platelet defects. Of patients with liver disease,

TABLE 10.17	Dental Implant Management in Patients With Chronic Obstructive Pulmonary Disease			
Risk	**Type 1**	**Type 2**	**Type 3**	**Type 4**
Mild (ASA II)	+	+	+	+
Moderate (ASA III)	+	Physician	Physician/moderate treatment	Physician/moderate treatment
Severe (ASA IV)	Physician consultation	Postpone (hospitalization)	Elective procedures contraindicated	Elective procedures contraindicated

+, Procedure may be performed with regular protocol; *ASA*, American Society of Anesthesiologists.

50% have a prolonged PT and possible significant clinical bleeding. The inability to detoxify drugs may result in oversedation or respiratory depression. The laboratory evaluation of the implant candidate gives much insight into hepatic function. A basic panel of LFTs or a CMP can provide the needed information. In most patients with liver disease, it is recommended that a CBC, LFT, BMP, bleeding time, and an INR/PT test should be performed.

Of special note, patients with normal LFTs can present with constant itching or pruritus. This may be the first symptom of early liver disease, especially primary biliary cirrhosis. This is a progressive disease that causes cholestasis (buildup of bile in the liver) and damages the small bile ducts and over time destroys the ducts, resulting in liver damage. Because this is a progressive disease, it can be fatal, but early diagnosis of the disease can have more favorable outcomes. For baby boomers, hepatitis C has been a significant issue, and until recently many chronic hepatitis C patients were undiagnosed until new screening protocols were instituted. Risk factors include transfusions of blood products (mostly from the 1970s and 1980s), IV drug use, sexual transmission, and tattoos. Because of the opioid and injection drug use epidemic, hepatitis C

infections have increased dramatically since 2005. Many infected individuals can have spontaneous resolution of their infection, but almost 50% of persons with hepatitis C infections are unaware they have or have had the disease. Seventy-five percent of individuals currently with hepatitis C were born between 1945 and 1965 and may be current candidates for elective dental implant surgery. Asking patients at risk, or in this age group, about previous screening through a blood test for hepatitis C is recommended. Newer treatments have now essentially cured this disease for many patients. Individuals affected by hepatitis C can have normal or slightly elevated LFTs, but screening with a hepatitis C antibody blood test should be considered for patients at risk.

Dental Implant Management. Patients with no abnormal laboratory values on CMP, CBC, PTT, and PT are at low risk, and a normal protocol is indicated for all procedures (types 1–4). Patients with an elevated PT of less than 1.5 times the control value, or bilirubin slightly affected, are at moderate risk. These patients should be referred to their physician for evaluation and treatment. The use of sedatives may require physician clearance. Nonsurgical and simple surgical procedures may follow normal protocols (types 1 and 2). However, strict attention to hemostasis is indicated. Bovine collagen such as CollaTape, topical thrombin, or additional sutures may be indicated. Moderate to advanced surgical procedures may require hospitalization (types 3 and 4). Post-surgical close surveillance is indicated. Elective implant therapy is a relative contraindication in the patient with symptoms of active alcoholism.

Patients with a PT greater than 1.5 times the control value, mild to severe thrombocytopenia (platelets lower than 140,000/mL), or several liver-related enzymes or chemicals affected (bilirubin, albumin, ALP, SGOT, and SGPT) are at high risk.

Elective dental procedures such as implants are usually contraindicated. If surgical procedures must be performed on a preexisting implant, hospitalization is recommended. Platelet transfusion may be required for even scaling procedures and administration of mandibular nerve blocks. Fresh frozen plasma may be used to correct PT to under half the control value.

Medications. Many drugs such as local anesthetics (lidocaine, prilocaine, mepivacaine, and bupivacaine), sedatives (lorazepam, valium, and alprazolam), and antibiotics (erythromycin and clindamycin) are metabolized primarily in the liver. Therefore in some patients a dosage reduction may be warranted based on the current liver functioning.

Nonsteroidal Antiinflammatory Drugs. In patients with cirrhosis, NSAIDs have been associated with renal failure and should be avoided. In patients with chronic liver disease, NSAIDs and opioids may be used at reduced doses but only after consultation with the patient's physician. Acetaminophen at a reduced dosage is a possible alternative consideration. New FDA recommendations suggested a maximum dosage of 2 g/day is reasonable. An accepted school of thought is that codeine and opioids should not be used or, if so, used at very infrequent and lower dosages to avoid hepatic encephalopathy.[73] Additionally, tetracycline, erythromycin, and metronidazole should never be used in patients with advanced liver disease.

Stomach Ulcers

Approximately 1 in 10 Americans will suffer from a version of gastritis or ulcer disease during their lifetime. Ulcers form when there is a break or breach of the lining of the stomach or intestine.

Peptic ulcers form in the duodenum of the small intestine from being in contact with stomach acids. Duodenal ulcers are

TABLE 10.18	Additional Pulmonary Issues and Treatment Implications	
Positive Response	**Treatment Implications**
Asthma	Inflammatory process in lung is IgE/allergen mediated Determination of trigger: asthma or bronchospasm, including anxiety Albuterol on hand for surgery Approximation of severity determined by number of medications and frequency of use of albuterol rescue inhaler
Shortness of breath (dyspnea)	Asthma, COPD, heart disease, cardiomyopathy, CHF, arrhythmias, anemia, obesity, heart valve disease
Wheezing	Allergies, asthma, bronchitis, GERD, vocal cord dysfunction
Hemoptysis (blood in sputum)	Bronchitis, pulmonary embolism, CHF, lung cancer, blood thinners, TB
Cough	Postnasal drainage, asthma, GERD, ACE/ARB blood pressure medications, chronic bronchitis in COPD, other respiratory processes like bronchiectasis
Change in exercise tolerance	Any changes walking upstairs or walking more than 50 yards Cardiovascular, pulmonary, poor conditioning
Weight loss	Poorly controlled COPD, malignancy, TB, hyperthyroid, ethyl alcohol abuse
Dysphagia from stroke or other neuromuscular diseases	Risk of aspiration during dental procedure

ACE, Angiotensin-converting enzyme; *ARB,* angiotensin receptor blocker; *CHF,* congestive heart failure; *COPD,* chronic obstructive pulmonary disease; *GERD,* gastroesophageal reflux disease; *IgE,* immunoglobulin E; *TB,* tuberculosis.

From Resnik RR, Resnik RJ. Medical/medication complications in oral implantology. In Resnik RR, Misch CE, eds. *Misch's Avoiding Complications in Oral Implantology.* St Louis, MO: Elsevier; 2018.

the most common type of ulcer. Ulcers that occur in the stomach are referred to as gastric ulcers. In rare cases, esophageal reflux can cause esophageal ulcers. There are several main causes for ulcer disease, including excessive alcohol intake, stress, medications (NSAIDs and aspirin), and a bacterium (*Helicobacter pylori*).

Although there are no direct contraindications to the use of prophylactic antibiotics in patients with ulcer disease (except allergies), some patients may be more sensitive to certain types of antibiotics that may irritate their stomach. Pain management may be hampered by the inability to use NSAIDs or certain narcotics. To prevent bleeding from stomach ulcers, analgesics and antibiotics should be cautiously used (medical clearance) in the treatment of implant surgical patients.

Inflammatory Bowel Disease

IBD is a chronic inflammation of all or part of the digestive tract. The number of people afflicted with this condition continues to increase. The two major forms of IBD are ulcerative colitis and Crohn's disease. Patients will usually have symptoms of chronic or severe diarrhea, fatigue, rectal bleeding, and anemia. Ulcerative colitis is characterized as an inflammatory disease of the rectum and large intestine mainly affecting the mucosal lining. Crohn's disease is an inflammatory disease of the entire digestive tract from mouth to anus, resulting in lesions of healthy tissue in between areas of inflammation. Most cases of Crohn's disease originate within the terminal ileum.

Patients with a history of stomach ulcers are susceptible to infections and healing issues usually associated with the immunosuppressive drugs. Also, their dietary restrictions may affect both of these issues, and postoperative antibiotics are usually indicated.

During dental procedures, stress reduction protocol is essential. Excess stress can affect adrenal function and require additional corticosteroid augmentation. Postoperative pain episodes may increase stress on the adrenal gland, resulting in possible adrenal suppression complications.

Many digestive disorder patients are anemic and, because of malabsorption, may not absorb all the necessary components of clotting factors and certain vitamins. Care should be taken to minimize bleeding.

There are many differences in the oral lesions that manifest in patients with Crohn's disease and those with ulcerative colitis. Many of these patients present with a glossitis, aphthous ulcerations, or a more classic marker of ulcerative colitis, pyostomatitis vegetans. This condition is characterized by pustules with thickened oral mucosa and surrounding erythema with some erosions. Ulcerative colitis has extra GI manifestations that have been associated with erosive temporomandibular joint disease. Crohn's disease has been shown to have oral symptoms such as cobblestoning of the oral mucosa accompanied by ulcerations usually in a linear pattern along with hyperplastic folds of the buccal vestibules (mucosal tags).

A physician consultation is recommended to determine the extent of the patient's digestive disorder along with the current immune status. Most notably, an evaluation of delayed wound healing and postoperative infection susceptibility should be ascertained.

Antibiotics that have a high incidence of antibiotic-associated diarrhea or pseudomembranous colitis should be avoided (e.g., amoxicillin/clavulanic acid, erythromycin, clindamycin). Patients with IBD, especially those with ulcerative colitis, may benefit from the use of probiotics, especially when antibiotics are prescribed. Probiotics are live microorganisms that are added to food to change the intestinal microbial balance. The mechanism of action is controversial; however, theories include strengthening of the gut barrier, pathogen growth inhibition, and enhancement of mucosal and systemic immune responses. Most NSAIDs may precipitate these disease states and should be avoided unless authorized by a physician.

Additional Digestive Disorders and Treatment Implications

See Table 10.19.

Bone Diseases

Diseases of the skeletal system and specifically the jaws often influence decisions regarding treatment in the field of oral implants. Bone and calcium metabolisms are directly related. Approximately 99% of the calcium in the body is held in the bones and teeth. Calcium equilibrium is influenced by several different processes in the body, which then could directly affect bone health. PTH has the most important influence on calcium by impacting the storage of calcium on bones. Even though vitamin D is important for small intestine absorption of calcium, the renal tubules in

TABLE 10.19   Additional Digestive Issues and Treatment Implications

Positive Response	Treatment Implications
Jaundice	Hepatitis, bile duct disorders, sickle cell anemia, autoimmune hemolytic disease pancreatic cancer
Hepatitis	Medical consultation, aseptic technique, preventive measures
Esophageal reflux	Infection, increased tooth decay/erosion
Hiatal hernia	Appointment duration not to exceed patient's tolerance
Nocturnal cough	Gastric reflux disease, chronic sinusitis, allergies
Dark, tar-colored stools	GI bleeding (avoid anticoagulants, NSAIDs; need GI evaluation)
Frequent foul-smelling stools	Crohn disease, pancreatic cancer (gum disease), lactose intolerance (tooth decay, bone demineralization), celiac (gluten intolerance) disease (enamel erosion, aphthous ulcers)
Dysphagia (solid/liquid)	Reflux, esophageal spasm, stricture, esophageal mass, multiple sclerosis, Parkinson disease, stroke, poor oral clearance, high-volume suction, aspiration during treatment, protect airway rubber dam
Persistent pruritus (itching)	Celiac disease, liver disease, biliary disease (sclerosing cholangitis) All can lead to coagulopathy and excessive bleeding

GI, gastrointestinal; *NSAIDs,* nonsteroidal antiinflammatory drugs.

From Resnik RR, Resnik RJ. Medical/medication complications in oral implantology. In Resnik RR, Misch CE, eds. *Misch's Avoiding Complications in Oral Implantology.* St Louis, MO: Elsevier; 2018.

the kidneys reabsorb 95% of the calcium. In the elderly there is increasing evidence to support that lower levels of vitamin D have the most influence on calcium levels.[74]

There exist many diseases that directly affect the dental implant treatment.

Osteoporosis

The most common disease of bone metabolism the implant clinician will encounter is osteoporosis, which is an age-related disorder characterized by a decrease in bone mass, increased microarchitectural deterioration, and susceptibility to fractures. The WHO defines osteoporosis as a bone mineral density level more than 2.5 standard deviations below the mean of normal young women.[75] Forty percent of postmenopausal women in the United States have bone mineral density levels denoting osteopenia, and 7% have scores correlated with osteoporosis.[76] As the population ages, the incidence of osteoporosis will continue to increase in both women and men. Women with osteoporosis are three times more likely to experience tooth loss than those who do not have the disease. It has been shown that dental x-rays may be used as screening for osteoporosis.[77]

After age 60, almost one-third of the population has osteoporosis; it occurs in twice as many women as men. This condition is common in postmenopausal women or those with a history of a premenopausal oophorectomy. The lack of estrogen increases the likelihood of osteoporosis; the addition of estrogen is the single most effective treatment to increase calcium absorption in these women. However, current concerns about the development of breast, ovarian, or endometrial cancer and an increased incidence of stroke, heart attack, and blood clots in these patients have almost eliminated the use of supplemental estrogen.

Many times, if estrogen therapy is initiated, it is at much lower doses and for shorter duration. Half of all women present with bone mineral density below the normal fracture threshold of a 20-year-old woman by the age of 65 years. It is estimated that 1.3 million fractures overall and 133,000 hip fractures occur every year as a result of osteoporosis. Most patients fail to recover normal activity; 24% die of complications related to the fracture within the first year.[78]

The osteoporotic changes in the jaws are similar to other bones in the body. The structure of the bone is normal; however, because of the uncoupling of the bone resorption and formation processes with emphasis on resorption, the cortical plates become thinner, the trabecular bone pattern becomes more discrete, and advanced demineralization occurs. The bone loss related to osteoporosis may be expressed in both the dentate and edentulous patient. In one study of osteoporotic women who had their teeth at age 50, 44% had a complete denture by the age of 60, whereas only 15% of nonosteoporotic women had dentures.[79] A strong correlation was shown between periodontal disease and skeletal osteoporotic changes. In addition, women represent a greater percentage of patients with residual ridge resorption than do men.[80] The loss of trabecular bone is accelerated in the edentulous patient because the factors involved in resorption are already established.

Bone remodeling is a continuous process; however, bone mass increases during youth and diminishes with aging. The peak bone mass is usually reached by the age of 35 to 40 years and is usually 30% higher in men than in women. In the first 3 to 10 years after menopause, bone loss is rapid. Trabecular bone loss in a women 80 years old reaches 40%, but is only 27% in men of the same age. Persons most at risk of osteoporosis are thin, postmenopausal, Caucasian women with a history of poor dietary calcium intake, cigarette smoking, and British or Northern European ancestry.

Estrogen therapy can halt or retard severe bone demineralization caused by osteoporosis and can reduce fractures by about 50% compared with the fracture rate of untreated women. For those patients taking an estrogen supplement, there have been studies to evaluate the effect of estrogen replacement therapy on dental implant failures. Osteoporotic patients not taking estrogen have nearly twice the failure rate of maxillary implants in comparison to patients who were receiving estrogen therapy.[81]

Recent advances in radiology, such as dual-energy x-ray absorptiometry, can measure as little as 1 mg of bone mass change at such sites as the hip, spine, and wrist. Such measurements may accurately predict future fracture risk and identify the patients at risk. The actual diagnosis and treatment of osteoporosis should be attained by the patient's physician. The implant dentist can best assist the patient by noting the loss of trabecular bone and early referral.

Treatment of osteoporosis remains controversial. Its management concentrates on prevention. Regular exercise has shown to help maintain bone mass and increase bone strength. Adequate dietary calcium intake is essential. The advanced demineralization and consequent increase in bone loss of the completely edentulous may become a vicious circle. The denture is less secure, and the patient may not be able to follow the diet needed to maintain proper calcium absorption levels.

The recommended calcium intake is 800 mg/day. The average person in the United States ingests 450 to 550 mg. In postmenopausal women, 1500 mg may be required to maintain a positive calcium balance.[82] Calcium supplements of 1 to 2 g of elemental calcium per day have been shown in several studies to reduce the rate of bone loss. However, there is no evidence that these supplements lead to recovery of bone mass. Plain calcium carbonate tablets contain the greatest fraction of elemental calcium and are relatively inexpensive. It is insoluble and is absorbed after conversion into calcium chloride by gastric hydrochloric acid. Patients with achlorhydria (lack of hydrochloric acid) should be given salts other than calcium carbonate. If the patient has a lactate deficiency, lactate salts are contraindicated. Several food–drug interactions have been reported. Tetracycline and iron do not work effectively with calcium doses. Patients should also avoid phosphate (found in some dairy products or diet soda) or oxalic acid (in spinach and rhubarb) and the phytic acid in bran and whole grains because these decrease calcium absorptions. Patients with a history of renal calculi should avoid calcium supplements. Patients with renal dysfunction need periodic serum and urine calcium level checks, and their serum pH should be monitored to avoid hypercalcemia and metabolic alkalosis.

Vitamin D is also important in treating and preventing osteoporosis because it is required for proper calcium absorption. Without proper levels of vitamin D calcium supplementation may have no effect on bone health; this is especially true in older patients. Calcium and vitamin D supplements may help prevent tooth loss in older adults. Vitamin D is normally made in the skin after exposure to sunlight; however, given the concerns for skin cancer, most individuals are now avoiding direct sun exposure or overexposure. At least 800 IU of vitamin D per day are recommended for postmenopausal women or men over age 70. For more severe cases of vitamin D deficiency higher daily doses of one to several thousand international units of vitamin D may be required. For patients with established osteoporosis, treatment options include bisphosphonates and calcitonin. Bisphosphonates are inhibitors of bone resorption. Calcitonin, which is normally secreted by the thyroid gland, inhibits bone resorption and alters calcium metabolism.

Dental Implant Implications

Surgical Technique. Underpreparation of the osteotomy site (or use of osteotomes) will result in the implant having more bone at the implant interface. Although not contraindicated, immediate stabilization of dental implants is a common concern because of decreased trabecular bone mass. Healing periods and implant surface characteristics should be selected for poorer-quality bone.

Bisphosphonates Use. Oral/IV bisphosphonates are common medications for osteoporosis. (See the section "Bisphosphonates.")

Length of Healing. In osteoporotic patients, there is a decrease in cortical and trabecular bone; the repair process (implant healing) may be compromised. Sufficient time for healing should be adhered to with progressive prosthetic bone loading is highly recommended.

Peri-implantitis. A strong correlation has been shown between periodontal disease and skeletal osteoporotic changes. Strict postoperative recall and periodontal evaluation should be adhered to.

Progressive Bone Loading. Because of poorer bone quality, healing is compromised, necessitating progressive bone loading throughout the prosthetic rehabilitation. The poorer-quality bone is progressively increased to better-quality bone, which results in better bone quality at the implant interface.

Implant Design. Implant design should include greater-width implants. Surface conditions of implant bodies should be designed to increase bone contact and density. Bone stimulation to the healed interface will increase bone density, even in advanced osteoporotic changes (Box 10.10).

Fibrous Dysplasia

Fibrous dysplasia (FD) is a rare, nonheritable, genetic disorder characterized by normal bone being replaced by immature, haphazardly distributed bone and fibrous tissues. The etiology of this bone disease is a gene mutation that prevents the differentiation of cells within the osteoblastic formation. FD can be further classified to involve one site (monostotic FD [MFD]), multiple sites (polyostotic FD [PFD]), or multiple locations (craniofacial FD [CFD]). CFD lesions are usually unilateral and occur twice as often in the maxilla versus mandible. The diagnosis of CFD should be determined from the clinical evidence, histopathologic analysis of the biopsy specimen, and radiologic findings.[55] Most individuals with this disorder are diagnosed early in childhood.

The radiographic appearance is highly variable because of the disproportionately mineralized tissue and fibrous tissue in the lesion. This variability results in radiographic images depicting the typical "ground glass" appearance to early-stage radiolucencies and late-stage radiopacities.[83] Additionally, severe malocclusion, dental abnormalities, and facial asymmetry have been shown to be highly prevalent in CFD patients, which further complicates the prosthetic rehabilitation of these patients.[84]

Dental Implant Implications

Postoperative Healing. Healing after trauma in patients with FD is much different than for those with normal bone. The tissue

---

> ### • BOX 10.10   Common Medications and Implications for Treatment of Osteoporosis
>
> **Bisphosphonates**
> - Alendronate (Fosamax, Fosamax Plus D)
> - Alendronate (Binosto)
> - Denosumab (Prolia)
> - Ibandronate (Boniva)
> - Risedronate (Actonel)
> - Risedronate (Atelvia)
> - Zoledronic acid (Reclast)
>
> **Calcitonin**
> - Calcitonin (Fortical, Miacalcin)
> - Calcitonin (Miacalcin injection)
>
> **Estrogen (Hormone Therapy)**
> - Estrogen (multiple brands)
>
> **Estrogen Agonists/Antagonists (Also Called Selective Estrogen Receptor Modulators)**
> - Raloxifene (Evista)
> - Bazedoxifene (Duavee)
>
> **Anabolic Agents Parathyroid Hormone (Anabolic Agent)**
> - Teriparatide (Forteo)
>
> **Parathyroid Hormone-Related Protein Analog (Anabolic Agent)**
> - Abaloparatide (Tymlos injection)
>
> **Rank Ligand Inhibitor**
> - Denosumab (Prolia injection)

is hypocellular, which leads to slow healing and an increased infection rate. These local infections may spread through the bone and result in more advanced complications.

Informed Consent. Because of the lack of research and studies, patients need to be well informed of possible morbidity and complications.

Treatment Summary

Active lesion areas: Absolute contraindication
Nonlesion areas: Relative contraindication

Vitamin D Disorders (Osteomalacia)

Osteomalacia results in softer than normal bones and is directly related to calcium deficiencies. Lack of vitamin D is the most common cause of osteomalacia. Vitamin D is synthesized by the body in several steps involving the skin, liver, kidney, and intestine. The kidney, in conjunction with PTH, activates vitamin D. With this deficiency, the intestinal uptake and mobilization of calcium from the bone is altered, resulting in hypocalcemia. This will lead to an increased PTH secretion, which increases the clearance of phosphorus from the kidneys. This resultant decrease in the concentration of phosphorus prevents a normal mineralization process. Anticonvulsant drugs, especially diphenylhydantoin and phenobarbital, may cause drug-induced osteomalacia. Many GI disorders also may result in osteomalacia. Osteoporosis is different from osteomalacia. In osteoporosis the bones become more porous and brittle, whereas in osteomalacia the bones are just softer because of demineralization caused by the lower levels of phosphorus and calcium.

The oral findings of osteomalacia are usually not dramatic. A decrease in trabecular bone, indistinct lamina dura, and an increase in chronic periodontal disease have been reported. The treatment for osteomalacia is supplemental oral vitamin D (50,000 IU) usually at weekly doses.

Dental Implant Implications. Treatment for osteomalacia is usually successful, with radiographic changes seen months after treatment. There are no known reports of implant complications in osteomalacia patients; however, there is no contraindication as long as the disease is not active and well controlled.

Hyperparathyroidism

Hyperparathyroidism is caused by overactivity of the parathyroid glands. There are four of these tiny glands located just behind/beside the thyroid gland. Primary hyperparathyroidism results when one or more of the glands become hyperactive, which leads to increased levels of PTH. Surgical intervention is usually required. Vitamin D deficiency, kidney failure, and other disease that results in lower calcium levels will cause a secondary hyperparathyroidism. The treatment for this condition is targeted at the secondary cause. The diagnosis is confirmed with an elevated level of intact PTH.

The clinical manifestations of this disease vary widely, depending on the severity. Mild forms may be asymptomatic. Renal colic disorders often occur with moderate disease. Severe hyperparathyroidism can cause bone, renal, and gastric disturbance. It has been noted that when skeletal depletion occurs as a result of stimulation by the parathyroid gland, alveolar bone may be affected before that of the rib, vertebrae, or long bones.

Oral changes related to this disorder occur only with advanced disease. The loss of lamina dura is the most significant finding. Clinically, patients with this disorder develop loose teeth. Altered trabecular bone pattern with the appearance of ground glass may also occur. In animals, secondary hyperparathyroidism affects alveolar bone loss greater than any other bone of the skeleton.[85] Central or peripheral giant cell tumors may also develop.

Dental Implant Implications. Dental implants are contraindicated in areas of active bony lesions. However, implant placement may be initiated after treatment and healing of the affected areas. Medical consultation is highly recommended.

Osteitis Deformans (Paget Disease)

Osteitis deformans, or Paget disease, is a common metabolic disease characterized by slow, progressive, uncontrolled resorption and deposition of bone. This disease is usually seen in Caucasian men older than 40 years. It is estimated that the rates of Paget disease in the United States are approximately 2% to 3% among patients 55 years and older.[86]

The etiology is unknown and usually affects the maxillary alveolar ridge twice as frequently as the mandibular ridge. Because of the enlargement of the middle one-third of the face, the appearance of a "lionlike" deformity is often noted. Diastemas, tooth mobility, and bone pain are additional characteristics. Radiographically, a decreased radiodensity, large circumscribed radiolucencies, patchy areas of coalesced sclerotic bone (cotton-wool appearance), and marrow spaces that are replaced by fibrous tissue are observed. During the active phases of this disease, bone is highly vascular with the possibility of arteriovenous shunts, which may cause hemorrhagic complications.

Paget disease is marked by high elevations of serum ALP, normal or elevated calcium, and normal phosphate levels. Radionuclear bone scans are used to determine the extent of the disease throughout the body. Edentulous patients are often unable to wear their prostheses without discomfort. There is no specific treatment for Paget disease, and these patients are predisposed to develop osteosarcoma and possibly osteomyelitis.

This disease has a wide spectrum of treatment ranging from no treatment to the use of bisphosphonates. For patients who are symptomatic, IV bisphosphonates are usually the preferred treatments. These drugs help decrease further bone breakdown, formation, and remodeling.

Dental Implant Implications

Bleeding. During the active phases of this disease, bone is highly vascular with the possibility of arteriovenous shunts, which may cause hemorrhagic complications.

Infection. Bone areas that are affected by this disorder are predisposed to develop osteosarcoma and possible osteomyelitis.

Treatment Summary

Oral implants are contraindicated in the regions affected by this disorder or in patients on IV bisphosphonates for the treatment of their Paget symptoms.

Multiple Myeloma

Multiple myeloma is a plasma cell neoplasm that originates in the bone marrow and is characterized by the abnormal proliferation of B cells. Multiple myeloma causes severe hypercalcemia, immune suppression, anemia, and thrombocytopenia because it causes widespread bone destruction. The disease is usually found in patients between 40 and 70 years of age. Usually it affects several bones in the body, with symptoms of skeletal pain. Pathologic fractures may occur. Punched-out lesions appear radiographically. Some patients with early disease may not have any symptoms, but there are increasing examples of the first manifestation of multiple myeloma being an oral gingival or mandibular soft mass.[87]

Secondary oral manifestations of the disease are common (80%) and may affect both the maxilla and the mandible. Paresthesia, swelling, tooth mobility, and tooth movement may occur. Gingival enlargements are also possible. The diagnosis is usually determined through both a urine and serum protein electrophoresis test. The presence of light-chain proteins (Bence-Jones) can also be found. In the past the disease was almost always fatal within a short time after being diagnosed. However, there are now more aggressive treatments including improved chemotherapy and stem cell transplants that have prolonged survival. Although it is rarely curable, the disease is now more manageable.

Dental Implant Implications. Dental implants are usually an absolute contraindication in patients with multiple myeloma because of the severity of this disease; however, a case report has described successful implant placement in a patient with this disease.[88] Although the disease is rarely curable, it is now more manageable, and in just the past few years the 5-year survival rate for these patients has doubled. Given the recent success in treating this disease and the longer survival time, new studies will most likely be done to evaluate the use the of dental implants in patients that have undergone successful treatment for multiple myeloma.

Osteomyelitis

Osteomyelitis is an infection with or without inflammation of the bone. Most always the infection is caused by a bacteria or fungi entering the bone. Open wounds or recent surgery around a bone are the most common sources, but an abscessed tooth is also a potential source for the infection. The radiographic appearance is a poorly defined, radiolucent area with isolated fragments of bone (sequestra) that can exfoliate or become surrounded by bone (involucrum). Osteomyelitis in the oral cavity is usually in the mandible and rarely in the maxilla, most likely because of the increased vascularization. This disorder can also be caused by odontogenic and periodontal infections, trauma, dental implants, immunocompromised states, and hypovascularized bone. The treatment includes aggressive surgical drainage, with possible IV antibiotic intervention.

Dental Implant Implications

Implant Placement. Implant placement in surgical sites that have been previously affected with osteomyelitis leads to an increased morbidity. Because of the lack of vascularity, endosseous implants have a greater chance of bone loss, infection, and failure.

Treatment Summary

Osteomyelitis is usually an absolute contraindication unless the etiologic factors are corrected and adequate blood supply to the affected area is restored. A physician clearance should be obtained along with a comprehensive informed consent on the possible complications that may arise from implant placement into these sites.

Osteogenesis Imperfecta

This is a genetic disorder in which bones break with ease many times with almost no apparent cause. Bone quality is poor, with a thin cortical bone and thin, fine trabeculae. Bones are extremely fragile. Some forms are more severe, but overall the disease is relatively rare. However, osteogenesis imperfecta is the most common inherited bone disease. Bone fractures along with skeletal deformities are common, with very poor healing. Histologically, defective osteoblasts lead to a reduction in bone matrix and abnormal collagen.

Dental Implant Implications. Dental implants are not contraindicated; however, caution should be given to the very poor bone quality and questionable osseous healing.

Cemento-Osseous Dysplasia

This disease usually manifests with lesions in the upper and or lower jaw. Normal bone is replaced with bone that is mixed with connective tissue and abnormal bone. Cemento-osseous dysplasia seems to be more common in middle-aged women, with a higher incidence in African American and Asian women. Most of the time, the lesions are symmetric on both sides of jaw. There is variability in shape, size, and number of lesions. The lesions can expand and may cause some pain, but for the most part the disease is asymptomatic. Many times, the diagnosis is found by accident on a radiograph. There are three types of cemento-osseous dysplasia (i.e., focal, periapical cementoma, florid) that can vary radiographically as radiolucent, radiopaque, or a combination. The lesions are usually associated with the mandibular anterior teeth.

Dental Implant Implications. Dental implants are not contraindicated unless in the sclerotic phase of the disease in which the bone is hypovascular. This bone has the ability to become infected easily, with questionable healing. Special attention must be given so that the disease does not progress to osteomyelitis.

Ectodermal Dysplasia

Ectodermal dysplasia (ED) is a genetically inherited disorder that occurs in 1 per 100,000 live births.[89] Clinically, ED has been divided into two broad categories: an X-linked hypohidrotic form (Christ–Siemens–Touraine syndrome) characterized by the classical triad of hypodontia, hypohidrosis, and hypotrichosis, and by characteristic facial features such as prominent supraorbital ridges and a depressed nasal bridge; and an autosomal inherited hidrotic form (Clouston syndrome), which usually spares the sweat glands but affects teeth, hair, and nails.[90]

In this condition, there is abnormal development of the skin, hair, nails, sweat glands, or teeth. The most common intraoral feature of ED is hypodontia or anodontia. In these patients, conventional prosthodontic procedures often are not successful because of anatomic abnormalities that result in poor retention and stability. Because of this, dental implant therapy aimed at restoring function, esthetics, and psychological rehabilitation is an integral part in the management of adolescent patients with ED. Numerous studies have been completed on dental implants in patients with ED. A 3-year study showed impressive success rates in preadolescents (ages 7–11, 87%), adolescents (ages 12–17, 90%), and adults (older than 17, 97%). Other positive case reports have shown dental implants as a successful adjunct to oral rehabilitation.[91,92]

Dental Implant Implications. Dental implants are not contraindicated in patients with ED. Although not ideal, implants may be placed in preadolescents (i.e., usually anterior mandible), with with functional, esthetic, and psychological advantages. Alveolar bone has been shown to continue to grow after implants have been placed in edentulous ridges of children with ED. Transverse and sagittal growth is not restricted; however, vertical growth may result in submersion of the implants, necessitating prosthetic revision or possible use of longer abutments.

Radiation

Although the survival rate of patients with head and neck cancer has increased over the last 20 years, it still remains one of the deadliest forms of cancer. Aggressive treatment includes surgery, radiation, chemotherapy, or a combination therapy that inevitably leaves the patient with compromised anatomy and physiologic functioning. Patients are left with many deficits including oral mucositis, xerostomia, compromised healing, and reduced angiogenesis. This is a direct result of changes in the vascularity and cellularity of hard and soft tissue, damage to the salivary glands, and increased collagen synthesis that results in fibrosis. Because of these detrimental effects on the bone, wound repair and healing are significantly reduced after surgical procedures. When exposed to high levels of radiation, bone undergoes irreversible physiologic changes that include narrowing of the vascular channels (endarteritis), diminished blood flow, and loss of osteocytes. In time the bone becomes nonvital, which leads to limited remodeling and healing potential.

Dental Implant Implications

Osteoradionecrosis. The most significant risk in placing implants into irradiated bone is osteoradionecrosis (ORN), which is an irreversible devitalization of irradiated bone characterized by necrotic, soft bone that fails to heal properly. The pathophysiologic mechanism is an imbalance in oxygen demand

and oxygen availability, which is caused by endarteritis of the blood vessels. Clinical symptoms include pain, exposed necrotic bone, pathologic fractures, and suppuration. Studies have shown the overall incidence of ORN after radiotherapy to be from 3% to 22%.[93]

Radiotherapy to Previously Placed Implants. There are very few studies on the effects of radiotherapy on preexisting dental implants. Short-term data show very minimal complications and failures. However, in longer-term studies, failure rates seem to be higher.[74] At this time, more studies need to be conducted for conclusive results.

Implant Placement After Radiotherapy. The time between radiotherapy to implant placement seems to affect the prognosis of implants. Most studies have shown that the longer the period for implant placement after radiotherapy, the higher the success rate and the lower the risk of ORN (Box 10.11).[94]

Irradiation Patient Prosthetics. Because of the oral effects of radiotherapy (mucositis and xerostomia), an implant-supported prosthesis (FP-1, FP-2, and FP-3) is recommended over a soft tissue prosthesis (RP-4 and RP-5). This will reduce the possibility of soft tissue irritation associated with postradiotherapy patients wearing removable prostheses.

Past Radiation Treatment. Caution must be emphasized to patients with past radiation therapy because earlier forms of radiation therapy (pre-1980s) were of lower energy, in contrast to current higher energy levels that are less destructive. Because of this lower-energy radiation and associated higher destructive radiotherapy, progressive endarteritis has been shown to take place, which increases over time.[95]

Amount of Radiation Exposure. The presently available literature states that implant placement surgery may be completed on patients who have been irradiated at doses lower than 50 Gy.[96] Unfortunately, very few patients receiving doses greater than 50 Gy have been rehabilitated with implants. Studies have shown that implants placed in patients with a cumulative radiation effect of 18 to 20 (approximately 48–65 Gy standard fractionation) have a rather high success rate. Other reports have shown that doses greater than a cumulative radiation effect of

40 (approximately 120 Gy standard fractionation) exhibit a high degree of failure.[97]

Hyperbaric Oxygen. One treatment proposed to minimize the possibility of ORN is the use of hyperbaric oxygen. Prophylactic hyperbaric oxygen has been advocated to increase oxygen tension in irradiated bone, which will promote capillary angiogenesis and bone formation. Recent data show that oxygen under hyperbaric conditions acts synergistically with growth factors, which stimulates bone growth and turnover and also may act as a growth factor itself. Hyperbaric oxygen also has been shown to act as a stimulator of osseointegration by increasing new bone formation, increasing bone turnover, and increasing the vascular supply to irradiated bone.[98]

Additional Bone Diseases
See Table 10.20.

Systemic Autoimmune Diseases

Autoimmune diseases refer to a group of more than 80 serious, chronic illnesses that can affect almost any organ in the body. Approximately 75% of autoimmune diseases occur in women; these diseases are thought to have a genetic predisposition. However, autoimmune diseases are among the most poorly understood diseases, with symptoms extremely variable among individuals.

Sjögren Syndrome

Sjögren syndrome is an autoimmune disease in which immune cells attack and destroy exocrine glands that produce saliva and tears. This disorder affects an estimated 4 million people in the United States (90% female), with an average age of onset in the late 40s. The classic symptoms of Sjögren syndrome are xerostomia and xerophthalmia (dry eyes). Because of the xerostomia, patients are more susceptible to decay and the mucous membranes become atrophic and friable. Because of the lack of salivary secretions, complications may arise with the use of a tissue-borne prosthesis.

The healing response and integration of implants has been shown to be successful in patients with Sjögren syndrome.[99] These implant-supported prostheses decrease soft tissue–borne prosthetic sore spots and discomfort.

• BOX 10.11   Treatment Protocol for Implant Placement in Radiation Sites

- For sites that have been previously treated with radiotherapy, the authors recommend referral to a dental school, hospital, or clinic that has experience in treating radiotherapy patients.
- If the clinician has experience or can treat the associated complications, the following is recommended.

Ideal Implant Placement
- Preradiation: More than 14 days before radiation
- During radiation: Absolute contraindication[a]
- Postradiation: <6 month or >24 months—relative/absolute contraindication
- 6 to 24 months: Relative contraindication[b]

[a]Radiation therapy medical consultation, possible >20 years ago referral to cancer institution or hospital treatments, for 90 minutes before placement followed by 10 minutes after placement.
[b]Medical consultation, hyperbaric oxygen, informed consent, aseptic technique (<20 Gy cumulative, approximately <50 Gy technique fractionation).
From Resnik RR, Resnik RJ. Medical/medication complications in oral implantology. In Resnik RR, Misch CE, eds. Misch's Avoiding Complications in Oral Implantology. St Louis, MO: Elsevier; 2018.

TABLE 10.20   Additional Bone Disease Responses and Treatment Implications

Positive Response	Treatment Implications
Orthopedic prosthetic device	Antibiotic prophylaxis
Ectodermal dysplasia	Many studies completed showing successful treatment in ectodermal dysplasia patients
Cemento-osseous dysplasia (periapical cemental dysplasia)	Bone quality is questionable because of avascular cementum–like lesions (relative contraindication)
Osteomalacia	Hypomineralized bone, questionable bone quality (relative contraindication)

From Resnik RR, Resnik RJ. Medical/medication complications in oral implantology. In Resnik RR, Misch CE, eds. Misch's Avoiding Complications in Oral Implantology. St Louis, MO: Elsevier; 2018.

Dental Implant Implications

There are no contraindications for dental implants in patients with a history of Sjögren syndrome. However, it is advantageous for the prosthesis to be non–tissue-borne (FP-1, FP-2, FP-3, and RP-4) to minimize soft tissue complications associated with xerostomia.

Systemic Lupus Erythematosus

Systemic lupus erythematosus is a chronic, potentially fatal autoimmune disease in which the immune system attacks cells and tissue in almost any part of the body. There are three main types of lupus in adults. The majority of patients have systemic lupus (eight times higher incidence than other forms) in which the immune system attacks cells and tissue in several areas of the body. In the United States, over 50% of the time, patients with systemic lupus have a major organ such as the heart, lung, kidney, or brain affected. Cutaneous lupus affects only the skin and accounts for a small number of cases (1 of 8). Certain drugs producing symptoms similar to systemic lupus can induce lupus. This category is referred to as drug-induced lupus, and the major contributors are hydralazine, procainamide, and isoniazid. The remaining cases of lupus are neonatal lupus. Lupus occurs in both men and women, but almost 90% of the cases are in women, and most of those cases are women of childbearing age between 14 and 45.[100]

There is no one test to diagnosis lupus. The antinuclear antibody (ANA) test provides some suggestion of lupus; it important to realize that most people with lupus have a positive ANA test, but most people with a positive ANA test do not have lupus. Positive ANA can occur with certain drugs, cancer, and a viral infection. It is interesting to note that those with a positive ANA, but no signs of lupus, may have a false positive test for other diseases like Lyme disease. A positive ANA blood test requires a more sophisticated panel of antibody testing to further differentiate the etiology of the positive ANA and help confirm a diagnosis of lupus. There is no cure for lupus, but symptoms can be controlled in many cases with corticosteroids and immunosuppressive drugs.

Dental Implant Implications

There is no direct contraindication to dental implant treatment in systemic lupus erythematosus patients. However, caution should be taken for possible associated organ damage and the use of high doses of corticosteroids and immunosuppressive drugs, which may contraindicate dental implants in those individuals.

Scleroderma

Scleroderma is a rare, chronic disease characterized by excessive deposits of collagen that causes musculoskeletal, pulmonary, and GI involvement. There are about 75,000 to 100,000 people in the United States that have this disease. The disease is most common in women between the ages of 30 and 50. There are two main types, localized and systemic. Localized scleroderma usually attacks the skin and on occasion the muscle and joints, but it spares the internal organs. These patients usually have discolored patches on the skin (morphea). They can have streaks or bands of thick, hard skin. This is called linear scleroderma and it affects the arms and legs. The more serious type is systemic scleroderma. This form attacks the skin, joints, blood vessels, lungs, kidneys, heart, and other organs and in many cases significantly shortens one's life span. CREST syndrome is a version of systemic scleroderma

that manifests as skin thickening in fingers and toes and as calcified nodules under the skin. Raynaud phenomenon is also associated with CREST, as are esophageal motility issues. A blood test for anticentemere antibodies is usually positive in CREST syndrome. There is no cure for scleroderma. Treatment is aimed at the affected organs, including NSAIDs and immunosuppressant drugs. ACE inhibitors are a mainstay of scleroderma affecting the kidney.[101]

Dental Implant Implications

Numerous reports have discussed the successful treatment of scleroderma patients with dental implants. A fixed prosthesis is recommended because of the inability to retrieve a removable prosthesis due to possible dexterity problems. However, a high percentage of these patients are being treated with immunosuppressive drugs, which may contraindicate the implant therapy.

Rheumatoid Arthritis

RA is a chronic, inflammatory autoimmune disease that causes the patient's immune system to attack the muscles and joints of the body. It is more prominent in the early stages in the fingers, wrist, feet, and ankles rather than the larger joints such as the shoulder, hip, or knee. RA is different from osteoarthritis, which is caused by wear and tear and previous injuries. In RA, the disease affects the lining of the joints, which increases pain and swelling and results in significant bone erosion and deformity of the joints. The inflammation in RA can affect other organs in the body. In most cases the affected joints are symmetric, so if one side of the body is affected, then the other side usually will demonstrate similar manifestations. Life expectancy of patients with RA is shortened by approximately 5 to 10 years.[102]

RA is treated with a wide range of medications including disease-modifying antirheumatic drugs, antiinflammatory drugs, and analgesic medications.

Methotrexate, a drug used to treat cancer, is commonly used to treat RA. Studies have shown the detrimental effect of this medication on bone by delaying bone healing. However, other studies have concluded that that low-dose methotrexate treatment does not affect titanium implant osseointegration.[103]

Dental Implant Implications

There is no direct contraindication for dental implants in patients who have RA. Because of the lack of mobility and dexterity, a fixed-implant restoration is indicated. Special attention should be given to the treatment medications because immunosuppressive, glucocorticoid therapy and biologics may contraindicate implant treatment.

Human Immunodeficiency Virus

Human immunodeficiency virus (HIV) is a retrovirus that is responsible for acquired immunodeficiency syndrome (AIDS), which causes the immune system to be depressed, leading to life-threatening opportunistic infections. According to the US government (https://www.hiv.gov), there are more than 1.1 million in the United States living with HIV and almost 1 in 7 may not be aware they have the disease. Just less than 40,000 individuals were diagnosed with HIV in 2016. The number of new HIV infections did decline between 2008 to 2014, but over the past several years an increase in new cases has been seen. It is most common in homosexual and bisexual men.

Initially, most diagnosed with HIV died from the disease, but a lot has changed in the past 20 years. In 1996, the life expectancy for a 20-year-old with HIV increased to almost 39 years. In 2011, the total life expectancy increased to almost 70 years.[104]

There is no cure for either HIV or AIDS; however, revolutionary new antiretroviral medication and protease inhibitors developed since 1996 have now been able to eliminate active viral load titers from the bloodstream. Many patients demonstrate complete suppression of the virus while taking the medication. Although not a cure, the inactivity improves survival and limits the effect on other organs. These newer medications have slowed or even stopped the damage caused by the HIV infection. They also prevent the virus from developing into more virulent forms and attacking other organs in the body. A postexposure prophylaxis (an antiretroviral) has been shown to reduce the risk of infection after exposure.

Dental Implant Implications

Numerous reports have shown successful dental implant therapy in HIV patients.[105,106]; however, there is insufficient data to determine the association between HIV infection and the success of dental implants. Special care must be taken to evaluate the current status of the patient's immune system and the potentially toxic medications the patient is taking.

Miscellaneous

Sleep Apnea

Obstructive sleep apnea (OSA) occurs when there is partial or complete obstruction of the upper airway during sleep. This in turn causes the chest wall muscles and diaphragm to work harder to clear the obstruction. OSA has both significant medical and dental implications. During the period of obstruction, the oxygen levels in the bloodstream decrease, resulting in diminished delivery of oxygen to vital organs, which can precipitate an MI or stroke.

Patients that are obese, have a larger, thicker neck, deviated septum or smaller nasal canals, enlarged tonsils, large uvula, or large tongue may be at increased risk during surgery, especially if sedation is used. There are many symptoms that can be associated with OSA. Daytime sleepiness, early morning headaches, restless sleep, loud snoring, and waking up feeling like one is choking or gasping are some of the more common ones.

One study demonstrated that "among the associated sleep symptoms and disorders OSA was the highest risk factor for tooth grinding during sleep and was reduced with proper treatment."[107] Untreated patients will most likely have increased morbidity, and implants will be subject to higher related mechanical force issues.

The diagnosis of OSA is made through the use of a sleep study. Sleep studies can be done at home or in a sleep clinic. Home sleep studies are better used as screening tools to confirm the diagnosis. To fully evaluate the potential treatment options, a titration study in a sleep laboratory may be required. The test records the number of slower or apneic (stopped breathing) episodes and oxygen saturation in the bloodstream. The test also monitors arm and leg movements. A sleep specialty physician evaluates the test and makes the diagnosis and recommendations for treatment.

Treatment options include continuous positive airway pressure (CPAP). The CPAP machine uses a hose and mask to deliver constant steady air pressure. Newer devices are much more compact, including Federal Aviation Administration (FAA) travel sizes, and are much quieter. Some individuals find these devices cumbersome and uncomfortable and sometimes give up on this treatment method. It is important to ask patients diagnosed with sleep apnea if they are using their CPAP or other treatment on a regular basis. A variation of the CPAP is bilevel positive airway pressure (BiPAP). This machine supplies BiPAP and coordinates more pressure during inhalation versus exhalation. In less severe cases, oral appliances may be a reasonable option and are much easier to use than CPAP. Most open the airway by bringing the jaw more forward. CPAP machines may place an increased force on the implant-related area. Oral airway devices may not be appropriate for patients with more significant apnea.

It is important to remember that OSA is a medical condition that has a complex pathophysiology. It can be seen as a factor in other medical conditions including CHF and asthma. OSA is not limited to just maxillofacial structural abnormalities. The diagnosis goes beyond just a test on the number of apnea-hypopnea spells. The diagnosis must be considered in conjunction with other of the patient's comorbid conditions. OSA should be diagnosed and treated by a physician, and preferably by a sleep medicine specialist.[108]

OSA has been shown to be a secondary cause of hypertension. Apnea creates significant increases in systolic and diastolic pressure, which creates higher blood pressure levels at night. However, this elevation can continue into the daytime. It has been shown that 50% of patients with hypertension may have OSA (p. 20). More important OSA causes more secondary hypertension than any other source. This same study implies that OSA may be one of the modifiable factors to help prevent hypertension. It is reasonable to consider that patients with resistant hypertension may have untreated sleep apnea.[109]

Elderly (Increased Age)

According to WHO, most developed countries have accepted the chronologic age of 65 years as the definition of an elderly or older person. The treatment of elderly patients is definitely challenging, and because more patients are living longer and are more socially active, they will continue to be a significant part of the implant dentist's practice. Studies have shown that elderly patients are more prone to systemic diseases, more medically compromised, have potentially longer healing periods, more challenging bone conditions (quality and quantity), increased susceptibility to drug interactions, and increased dental implant morbidity.

Dental Implant Implications

Decreased Renal Function. There is an age-related decline in renal functions accelerated by comorbid conditions such as hypertension, heart disease, and diabetes. The age-related decline is more physiologic, whereas the pathologic decline is associated with many medical conditions. In elderly patients, the glomerular filtration rate (GFR) and creatine will give insight into the patient's kidney function. As kidney function declines, especially in stage 3 (GFR 30–59) and above, there is a decreased metabolism and excretion of drugs. Therefore the intervals between drug administration should be longer and dosages should be decreased, except for lipid-soluble drugs and antibiotics, to compensate for the increase in body fat and the reduced immune response. In the presence of significant kidney disease (stage 4 or above), antivirals (acyclovir), β-lactams (amoxicillin), and cephalosporins should be reduced. Nonsteroidal analgesics should not be prescribed in those with stage 3 or greater impairment without consultation with the patient's physician. Caution should be exercised with the use of sedation drugs because they can have more pronounced and longer-lasting effects.

Decreased Gastric Motility. The decreased gastric motility of the elderly patient affects the use of oral analgesics such as hydrocodone and oxycodone. In addition, the use of narcotics in the elderly can cause significant changes in bowel habits, especially constipation. If not contraindicated, a stool softener may be recommended concurrently with use of analgesics. Also, when using antibiotics for any prolonged period, the use of probiotics may help maintain normal gut flora.

Medications. Medications and the number of prescribed drugs usually increase with age, with over 75% of patients 65 years and older taking medications. Many of these drugs are often the cause of adverse or significant drug reactions. Studies have shown more than 70% of drugs taken by elderly patients have potentially adverse effects in the dental practice.[29] Although the incidence of severe drug interactions with commonly prescribed pain medications is relatively low, caution should be used in reviewing the elderly patient's complete medication history before prescribing any analgesics.

Isolated Systemic Hypertension. A major cardiovascular health issue with the elderly is isolated systolic hypertension (ISH). In ISH, systolic blood pressure elevates above 140 mm Hg while the diastolic pressure remains below 90 mm Hg. The difference between the systolic and diastolic is termed the *pulse pressure,* which is a significant risk factor for stroke and heart disease. Recent meta-analysis studies have shown a 10-mm Hg increase in pulse pressure will increase the risk of major cardiovascular events by 20%.[110]

Bone Healing. Clinical studies have shown a direct correlation between delayed bone healing with increasing age. Most likely the etiology results from a reduced number of osteogenic cells and reduced systemic and localized blood flow to the healing site. Therefore longer healing periods along with progressive loading are recommended in older patients.

Bone Quality/Quantity. Both the quality and quantity of bone is affected by aging. Histomorphometric and microradiographic studies have shown that after the age of 50, a marked increase in the cortical porosity leading to decreased bone mass is present. Loss of bone mineral content has been estimated to be approximately 1.5% per year in females and 0.9% in males.[111]

Increased Implant Failure Rate. Studies have shown an increased risk of implant failure as a result of many age-related factors including compromised bone quality and quantity, implant length, treatment protocol, and edentulous locations. Other studies have shown patients older than 60 years were twice as likely to have adverse outcomes.[112]

Prosthetic Treatment. Elderly patients have been shown to have increased difficulty in adapting to the final implant prostheses. Postinsertion issues such as general adaptation, muscle control, hygiene difficulty, tissue inflammation, and overdenture seating were significant in the older population study. Patient education and final expectations should be discussed in detail before initiating treatment.[113]

Treatment Summary. The implant clinician must understand the physical, metabolic, and endocrine changes and the effects associated with the elderly patient before initiating implant treatment. Age is most certainly a prognostic factor in implant failure and morbidity. However, advanced age is not an absolute contraindication to implant therapy. It is imperative that the clinician obtain a detailed medical history and list of medications before devising the dental treatment plan. Patient education along with modification in medication use, surgical technique, soft and hard tissue healing times, and careful assessment of postoperative complications must be strictly enforced.

Adolescent (Decreased Age)

Dental implants are commonly used to correct the congenital absence of teeth in adolescents, and studies have shown this to be a very reliable and predictable treatment option. When a clinician is presented with an adolescent patient, there must be a degree of caution as to the ideal time that implant therapy should be commenced. The concern is that placement of implants too early may lead to the implants interfering with normal growth development and potential esthetic issues. No age-related surgical issues exist unless there are systemic contraindications or psychological issues. If placement of an implant is completed before craniofacial growth is complete, possible interruption of facial growth and esthetic (infraocclusion or labioversion) issues can result.

Dental Implant Implications

Early Consultation. In determining the ideal time for implant placement, the patient/family must be educated on craniofacial growth compared with chronologic age. Chronologic age is a poor indicator of dental development/facial growth; timing of implant placement should coincide with growth cessation.

Determination of Growth Cessation. In the literature, there exist many methods of determining completion of craniofacial/skeletal growth: chronologic age, complete dental development, voice changes, hand–wrist radiographs, cervical vertebral maturation, and superimposition of lateral cephalometric radiographs. The most reliable and safest (no radiation exposure) method has been shown to be when the patient begins to exhibit a lack of growth in stature (0.5 cm/year). When implants are treatment planned in adolescents, clinicians must take into consideration the timing, site development, esthetics, and possible prosthetic limitations including malposition that may develop with age. Most importantly, the determination of growth cessation should be determined by the lack of growth in stature. This method involves no radiographs (decreased radiation exposure) and is the most benign method. The patient's pediatrician should be consulted in the determination of growth cessation (Fig. 10.3).

Smoking

In the United States, an estimated 42.1 million people, or 18.1% of all adults (age 18 years or older), smoke cigarettes. Overall, smoking prevalence has declined from 2005 (20.9%) to 2012 (18.1%); however, tobacco is still the most preventable cause of death and disease in the United States.

Smoking has been directly related to many oral diseases including periodontal disease, malignancies, and dental implant–related complications. Studies have shown that over 7000 different gases and chemicals are found in cigarette smoke (e.g., nitrogen, carbon monoxide, carbon dioxide, ammonia, hydrogen cyanide, benzene, nicotine). In tissues, carbon monoxide displaces oxygen from Hb molecules because of its stronger affinity.[114] Hydrogen cyanide has been shown to cause hypoxia in tissues. The adverse effects that smoking has on successful outcomes in implant surgery are well documented. Multiple retrospective studies have shown that smokers experienced almost twice as many implant failures compared with nonsmokers.[115]

Dental Implant Implications

Increased Incision Opening. Studies have shown that smoking is directly related to increased incision line opening. Possible mechanisms for poor wound healing include the vasoconstrictive nature of nicotine; increased levels of fibrinogen, Hb, and blood viscosity; increased platelet aggregation; and impaired polymorphonuclear neutrophil leukocyte function.[116] Therefore additional sutures along with tension-free closure are recommended.

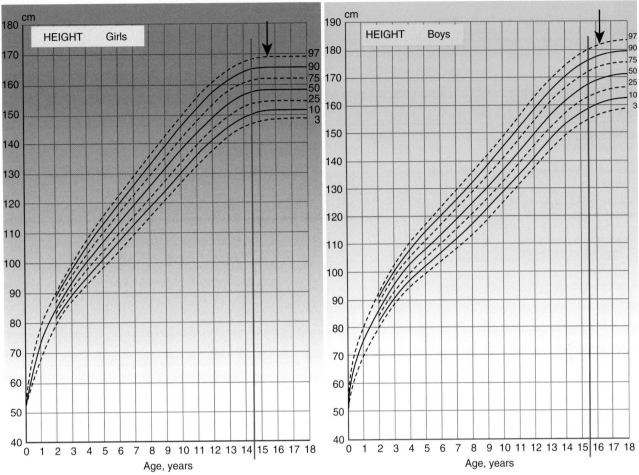

• **Fig. 10.3** Growth cessation chart. Consultation with the patient's pediatrician should be completed to ascertain growth cessation, which usually coincides with <0.5 cm of growth in stature (arrows).

Infection. Tobacco smoke decreases polymorphonuclear leukocyte activity, resulting in lower motility, a lower rate of chemotactic migration, and reduced phagocytic activity. These conditions contribute to a decreased resistance to inflammation and infection.[117]

Implant/Bone Grafting Failure. Meta-analysis studies have shown a definite correlation between smoking and failure rates of implants and bone grafts.

Peri-implantitis. Studies have shown in smokers a strong correlation between peri-implantitis and dental implants.

Informed Consent. With the possible detrimental effects of smoking on implants, it is recommended that patients be informed in detail about the risks of smoking. These possible consequences include increased marginal bone loss after implant placement and the presence of peri-implantitis. Additionally, there is a direct effect on the success rates of bone grafts, with almost double the failure rate in implants placed in grafted maxillary sinuses.

Smoking Cessation. A strong recommendation on smoking cessation before and after implant surgery is recommended because it has been shown to decrease implant morbidity.[118] Ideally, the patient is instructed to cease smoking for 2 weeks before surgery to allow for reversal of increased blood viscosity and platelet adhesion. Smoking cessation is continued for 8 weeks after implant surgery, which coincides with the osteoblastic phase of bone healing.[119] This has been shown to increase wound healing capabilities and reverse subgingival microflora[120] (Table 10.21).

Ideally, smoking cessation should be a gradual process because withdrawal symptoms are less severe in patients who quit slowly. There exists the concept of the "five As" in smoking cessation:
1. Ask: All patients should be asked about possible tobacco use.
2. Assess: Determine whether the patient has ever quit smoking or is interested in smoking cessation.
3. Advise: Every smoking patient should be advised of complications that may arise from continued smoking.
4. Assist: The smoking patient must be instructed on ways to quit smoking or be given a relevant physician referral.
5. Arrange: Make arrangements to evaluate the success of the smoking cessation.[121]

Treatment Summary

Any amount of smoking: Relative contraindication
Excessive smoking (>1.5 packs/day): Absolute contraindication until smoking sessation

Alcohol

Ethyl alcohol is one of the most widely used mood-altering drugs in the world. Approximately 17 million adults aged 18 and older have an alcohol use disorder. This is more common in men than women. Many with alcohol dependence disorders go undiagnosed. Because of the adverse effect of alcohol on dental implants, screening for undiagnosed alcohol-related disorders

TABLE 10.21	Smoking Cessation Techniques	
Technique	**Instructions**	**Possible Side Effects**
Nicotine gum (Nicorette)	Chewing gum that releases nicotine	TMJ, gastric irritation, difficulty for patients wearing removable prostheses
Nicotine inhaler (Nicotrol inhaler)	Puffing for approximately 20 minutes/hour	Dizziness, nausea/vomiting, confusion, blurred vision, palpitations
Nicotine lozenge (Nicorette)	Dissolving	Dizziness, nausea/vomiting, confusion, blurred vision, palpitations
Nicotine nasal spray (Nicotrol)	1–2 doses per hour for 2 months	Nasal mucosa irritation, dizziness, nausea/vomiting, confusion, blurred vision, palpitations
Nicorette microtab sublingual tablets	1–2 tabs hourly	Dizziness, nausea/vomiting, confusion, blurred vision, palpitations
Nicotine patch (Nicoderm CQ)	Worn during day	Skin irritation, dizziness, nausea/vomiting, confusion, blurred vision, palpitations
Rx medication: bupropion SR (Zyban), varenicline tartrate (Chantix)	As directed	Bupropion SR: dry mouth, nausea, headache, dizziness, changes in appetite, weight loss or gain, worsening of anxiety, insomnia. Varenicline tartrate: chest pain, dizziness, severe headache, easy bruising, vivid nightmares, sleep disturbance
Hypnosis	Mixed results supporting effectiveness	N/A
Acupuncture	Mixed results supporting effectiveness	N/A

TMJ, Temporomandibular joint dysfunction.

From Resnik RR, Resnik RJ. Medical/medication complications in oral implantology. In Resnik RR, Misch CE, eds. *Misch's Avoiding Complications in Oral Implantology.* St Louis, MO: Elsevier; 2018.

is beneficial. Excessive alcohol intake has been associated with surgical and dental implant-related issues such as liver and metabolic dysfunction, bone marrow suppression resulting in bleeding complications, predisposition to infection, and delayed soft tissue healing.[122]

Dental Implant Implications

Bleeding Problems. Alcohol interferes with coagulation on multiple levels, leading to decreased platelet production (thrombocytopenia), impaired platelet function (thrombocytopathy), and diminished fibrinolysis. Patients who abuse alcohol are more susceptible to intraoperative and postoperative bleeding complications associated with dental implant surgery.

Infection. Alcohol use leads to significant alterations of cell-mediated immune systems. Alcohol-induced immunosuppression results in a decrease in delayed-type hypersensitivity (DTH), which is a preoperative indicator for postoperative infectious complications.[123] Therefore patients consuming alcohol (especially those who consume it immediately after surgery) are more susceptible to incision line opening and infection.

Increased Bone Loss. Alcohol use also leads to decreased bone formation, increased resorption, and decreased osteoblast function, resulting in decreased bone density and integration issues. The use of alcohol has a direct effect on dental implant healing; studies have shown greater marginal bone loss and implant failure associated with alcohol consumption.

Informed Consent/Decrease Comorbidities. The patient must be well informed of potential consequences of alcohol use, especially immediately after implant surgery.

Cessation Program. Abstinence can reverse many of alcohol's effects on hematopoiesis and blood cell functioning; the patient should be instructed on possible cessation treatments

and programs. Ideally, patients should refrain from using alcohol for a minimum of 2 weeks or after incision line closure occurs.

Psychological

Providing dental implant care to patients with psychological problems is very challenging for clinicians. This group of patients is prone to oral health issues because of poor oral hygiene, poor compliance, and adverse medication effects. Providing comprehensive dental implant care to patients requires good communication skills, perseverance, and flexibility in both the surgical and prosthetic phases of treatment. Additionally, many of the drugs used to treat these patients, including tricyclic antidepressants, selective serotonin reuptake inhibitors (SSRIs), and monoamine oxidase inhibitors, are associated with many drug interactions. Oral manifestations of these diseases and medications include an increase in caries and periodontal disease, increased smoking, xerostomia, chronic facial pain, parafunction (bruxism/clenching), and temporomandibular joint dysfunction.

Dental Implant Implications. Many psychotherapeutic drugs interact with medications that are commonly prescribed in implant dentistry. Clinicians must be aware of drug–drug and drug–disease interactions with respect to the patient's medical history. Most interactions are related to the potentiation of the sedative and anticholinergic actions of the psychotherapeutic drugs. It is important to identify patients taking monoamine oxidase inhibitors or tricyclic antidepressants. Although these are no longer the mainstay of treatment for psychiatric illness, many patients will be placed on these medications to potentiate the effect of other medications. Common examples include amitriptyline, doxepin, nortriptyline, and imipramine. These medications are also being used to treat nonpsychiatric illnesses such as chronic pain and sleep disorders. The main concern is

TABLE 10.22   Medications Linked to Drug-Induced Osteonecrosis of the Jaw

Drug	Classification	Use	Dose	Route
Alendronate (Fosamax)	Bisphosphonate	Osteoporosis	70 mg/week	Oral
Risedronate (Actonel)	Bisphosphonate	Osteoporosis	35 mg/week	Oral
Ibandronate (Boniva)	Bisphosphonate	Osteoporosis	150 mg/month	Oral
Zoledronate acid (Reclast)	Bisphosphonate	Osteoporosis	5 mg/year	IV
Zoledronate acid (Zometa)	Bisphosphonate	Osteoporosis	4 mg/month	IV
Pamidronate (Aredia)	Bisphosphonate	Osteoporosis	90 mg/month	IV
Denosumab (Prolia, Xgeva)	Monoclonal antibody	Osteoporosis, cancer	60 mg/6 months	Subcutaneous
Bevacizumab (Avastin)	Monoclonal antibody	Metastatic cancer	100–400 mg/14 days	IV
Sunitinib (Sutent)	Tyrosine kinase inhibitor	Cancer	5 mg/year	IV
Etidronate (Didronel)	Bisphosphonate	Paget disease	300–750 mg/6 months	Oral
Tiludronate (Skelid)	Bisphosphonate	Paget disease	400 mg daily/3 months	Oral

IV, Intravenous.

From Resnik RR, Resnik RJ. Medical/medication complications in oral implantology. In Resnik RR, Misch CE, eds. *Misch's Avoiding Complications in Oral Implantology.* St Louis, MO: Elsevier; 2018.

the interaction of tricyclic medications and epinephrine because they produce anticholinergic effects on the heart. There is no contraindication to using them together, but patients should be followed more closely for adverse interactions. A physician consult and the implementation of a stress reduction protocol are recommended steps to follow when initiating treatment with these patients.

Medications of Interest to Implant Dentistry

Bisphosphonates

Since the first reported cases of necrotic, exposed bone in patients taking bisphosphonates, there has been much debate over treatment implications regarding dental implants. Bisphosphonates are a group of drugs that are widely used for several bone disorders and have been approved by the FDA for treatment of osteoporosis, metastatic bone cancer, and Paget disease. However, what was once termed bisphosphonate osteonecrosis has now been renamed drug-induced or medication-induced osteonecrosis of the jaws (DIONJ) by the American Medical Association. This has been renamed because of the incidence of osteonecrosis cases involving additional drug classifications such as monoclonal antibody drugs, antiangiogenic drugs, and tyrosine kinase inhibitors (Table 10.22).

Bisphosphonates are mainly used for the treatment of osteoporosis (oral form) and metastatic cancer (IV form) by inducing osteoclastic death or apoptosis at the cellular level. As an osteoporosis drug, bisphosphonates reduce bone resorption via a direct effect on the osteoclast. In osteoporotic patients undergoing bisphosphonate treatment, old bone is retained because bone turnover is suppressed, preventing normal remodeling in this area, which results in the formation of brittle bone. Additionally, bisphosphonates kill functionally resorbing osteoclasts not only at the peripheral sites but also in the bone marrow.

Diagnosis of Drug-Induced Osteonecrosis of the Jaw

Marx has defined characteristics of patients who are diagnosed as having drug-induced osteonecrosis of the jaw (DIONJ). These characteristics include (1) current or previous treatment with a systemic drug that affects bone homeostasis, (2) exposed alveolar bone in the jaws that persists for more than 8 weeks, (3) no history of radiotherapy to the jaws, and (4) no known diagnosis of osteopetrosis or cemento-osseous dysplasia. The definitive symptom of DIONJ is bone exposure in the mandible or maxilla that does not heal. Pain and inflammation are present, with possible secondary infection of the soft tissue. In severe cases, drainage and progressive extension of bone involvement or sequestration result.[124]

Active Lesions

Osteonecrosis may remain asymptomatic for weeks and possibly months. Lesions usually develop around sharp, bony areas and previous surgical sites, including extractions, retrograde apicoectomies, periodontal surgery, and dental implant surgery. Symptoms include pain, soft tissue swelling, infection, loosening of teeth, and drainage. Radiographically, osteolytic changes are seen, and tissue biopsy has shown the presence of actinomyces, which is possibly caused by secondary infection.

Testing

C-Terminal Telopeptide Test (CTx). It has been proposed that assays to monitor markers of bone turnover may help in the diagnosis and risk assessment of developing bisphosphonate-associated osteonecrosis. CTx are fragments of collagen that are released during bone remodeling and turnover. Because bisphosphonates reduce CTx levels, it is believed that serum CTx levels can be a reliable indicator of risk level. The CTx test (also called C-terminal telopeptide and collagen type 1 C telopeptide) is a serum blood test obtained by laboratories or hospitals (ICD-9 diagnostic code 733.40). However, today, the use of the CTx test to determine the possibility of osteonecrosis is controversial.[125,126]

CTx Value	Risk for Drug-Induced Osteonecrosis of the Jaw
300–600 pg/mL (normal)	None
150–299 pg/mL	None to minimal
101–149 pg/mL	Moderate
Less than 100 pg/mL	High

Drug Holiday. Marx has suggested a preoperative protocol for administering possible DIONJ drugs to patients who are undergoing oral surgical procedures. This protocol takes into consideration the type and duration of drug use and radiographic and clinical risk factors. Depending on the laboratory values obtained, a "drug holiday" may be indicated, which includes temporary interruption of bisphosphonate treatment. However, improvement of bisphosphonate levels may not be observed, because measurable levels have been shown to persist in bone for up to 12 years after cessation of therapy.

Drug Holiday Recommendation[125]

Presurgical: Medication stoppage 9 months before surgery
Postsurgical: Medication stoppage 3 months after surgery

Additional Recommendations

Medical History. A comprehensive medical history is essential before any elective treatment is initiated. The most important history of bisphosphonates is the use of IV nitrogen-containing bisphosphonates such as pamidronate (Aredia) and zoledronic acid (Zometa) and new osteoporotic drugs, which have very limited data on the association with DIONJ. In the dental setting, the most common bisphosphonates that implant dentists are exposed to will most likely belong to the family of oral nitrogen-containing bisphosphonates such as risedronate, ibandronate, and alendronate. The latest studies show that oral bisphosphonates have a very low probability of causing osteonecrosis.[127] However, because of the long half-life and short duration of the studies, future long-term complications may become problematic. With this in mind, the implant dentist should be cautioned regarding the possibility of developing osteonecrosis side effects. The risks versus benefits of dental treatment must be discussed with the patient in detail. A well-documented consent form is recommended with possible medical consultation if the patient has been on this medication for more than 3 years.

Reclast. As stated previously, most drugs used to treat osteoporosis are oral, nitrogen-containing bisphosphonate drugs. Reclast (IV: Zoledronate) is given in 5-mg IV doses once a year. Studies have shown that a significant risk occurs after the fourth yearly dose, which is caused by the accumulation of the medication and its 11-year half-life. Elective dental implant surgery or bone graft surgery are best scheduled 9 months after the most recent Reclast dose and 3 months before the next planned dose. However, at this time, very little research has been conducted on the relationship between Reclast and DIONJ. The FDA has placed a warning on the Reclast package inserts that states, "avoid having any type of dental surgery while you are being treated with Reclast." Therefore patients under treatment with Reclast should not be considered for elective dental implant surgery.

Comorbidities. Comorbidities are systemic diseases, medical conditions, medications, gender, and age, all of which can predispose the patient to a greater chance of developing DIONJ. Many chemotherapeutic drugs, diabetes, immune diseases, anemia, smoking, obesity, female gender, and renal dialysis have been noted as comorbidities for DIONJ. Additionally, the use

---

• BOX 10.12 Bisphosphonate Protocol and Suggestions[a]

ORAL BISPHOSPHONATE
Use <3 Years:

1. Proceed with surgery with detailed oral and written informed consent for bisphosphonate-associated osteonecrosis and possible decreased implant healing.
2. Decrease co-morbidities: periodontal disease, infections, smoking, etc.
3. Strict adherence to antibiotic prophylaxis and antimicrobial use (0.12% chlorhexidine)
4. No prophylactic corticosteroids
5. Elective: CTx Test or Drug Holiday
*Early learning curve: Referral

Use >3 Years

1. Proceed with surgery with detailed oral and written informed consent for bisphosphonate-associated osteonecrosis and possible decreased implant healing.
2. Decrease co-morbidities: periodontal disease, infections, smoking, etc.
3. Medical Clearance
4. Strict adherence to antibiotic prophylaxis and antimicrobial use (0.12% chlorhexidine)
5. No prophylactic corticosteroids
6. CTx Test (>150 pg/mL) or Drug Holiday
*Early learning curve: Referral

Drug Holiday (by physician only)
9-month presurgical + 3 month post-surgical

Laboratory Risk Assessment

CTx Value (pg/mL)	Risk for Osteonecrosis
300–600 (normal)	None
150–299	None to minimal
101–149	Moderate
<100	High

IV BISPHOSPHONATE
Absolute Contraindication

[a] Marx RE: Oral and intravenous bisphosphonate-induced osteonecrosis of the jaws: history, etiology, prevention, and treatment. Chicago, IL: Quintessence; 2007.

---

of glucocorticosteroids may be contraindicated in patients taking the DIONJ medications discussed previously because these drugs have been associated with an increased occurrence of osteonecrosis.

Treatment Summary

Oral bisphosphonates: Relative contraindication (informed consent, good surgical technique, CTx test, drug holiday)

IV bisphosphonates: Absolute contraindication (Reclast: absolute/relative contraindication depending on physician clearance) (Box 10.12).

New Therapies for Osteoporosis

Monoclonal Antibodies

Monoclonal antibodies work by inhibiting receptor activator of nuclear factor κ-B (RANK) ligand, which is a type II membrane protein that acts as a primary signal for bone removal. Monoclonal antibodies have a direct effect on the immune system and control bone regeneration and remodeling. These drug molecules irreversibly bind to mineral matrix in bone and have a half-life of approximately 26 days, which is much shorter than bisphosphonates (11 years).

Denosumab (Prolia) is a biyearly subcutaneous injection for the treatment of osteoporosis. This is a human monoclonal antibody that functions as a RANK ligand inhibitor. Inhibition of the RANK ligand results in diminished osteoclast functional and bone resorption. Denosumab recognizes the specific protein that normally activates osteoclasts, inhibiting their activation and preventing them from breaking down bone. Denosumab has also been used to treat metastatic bone disease. These inhibitors do not bind to bone, and their effect on bone remodeling decreases after treatment is stopped. Prolia has a short half-life (26 days) and does not accumulate in the bone like bisphosphonates. It has been shown to be completely inert within 6 months of administration.[128] Osteonecrosis of the jaw has been observed in patients receiving denosumab, and all patients should receive an oral examination before therapy. The risk of developing osteonecrosis of the jaw is less studied compared with the bisphosphonates; however, this has been shown to be a relevant concern.[129]

Immunosuppressive Drugs

Immunosuppressive drugs are medications that are used to inhibit or prevent activity of the immune system. They are usually used to minimize rejection of transplanted organs and tissues and for treatment of autoimmune diseases. These drugs have many side effects, with the majority of them acting nonselectively (acting on normal cells also). There are many classes of immunosuppressive drugs including corticosteroids, calcineurin inhibitors, mTOR inhibitors, IMDH inhibitors, biologics, monoclonal antibodies (Box 10.13).

Glucocorticoids (Long-Term Use)

Glucocorticoids have potent antiinflammatory and immunosuppressive properties. Because these drugs are widely used in the treatment of inflammatory and autoimmune diseases, special attention must be given to patients who are on long-term high doses of glucocorticoids. These drugs impair many healthy anabolic processes in the body and suppress the immune system, which can lead to severe complications in dental implant patients. The long-term use has been shown to have deleterious effects on bone remodeling and repair.

Cytostatics

Cytostatics are common medications in the treatment of malignant disease. These drugs cannot discriminate between malignant and normal tissues and become cytotoxic to normal tissue. Most chemotherapeutic agents are known to have cytotoxic effects on bone, especially on grafted bone in which the blood supply is compromised. Because chemotherapeutic agents have a high affinity for cells that have a high turnover rate, the oral mucosa is often affected. These mucosal ulcerations can become secondarily infected.

Several studies have shown that cyclosporin may negatively influence bone healing around dental implants and may even impair the mechanical retention of dental implants previously integrated in bone.[130]

• **BOX 10.13** Immunosuppressive Drugs

Corticosteroids
- Prednisone (Deltasone, Orasone)
- Budesonide (Entocort EC)
- Prednisolone (Millipred)

Calcineurin Inhibitors
- Cyclosporin (Neoral, Sandimmune, SangCya)
- Tacrolimus (Astagraf XL, Envarsus XR, Prograf)

mTOR Inhibitors
- Sirolimus (Rapamune)
- Everolimus (Afinitor, Zortress)

IMDH Inhibitors
- Azathioprine (Azasan, Imuran)
- Leflunomide (Arava)
- Mycophenolate (CellCept, Myfortic)

Biologics
- Humira (Adalimumab): Rheumatoid arthritis, Crohn's disease, ulcerative colitis, psoriatic arthritis, ankylosing spondylitis
- Remicade (Infliximab): Rheumatoid arthritis, Crohn's disease, ulcerative colitis, psoriatic arthritis, ankylosing spondylitis
- Enbrel (Etanercept): Rheumatoid arthritis, psoriatic arthritis
- Herceptin (Trastuzumab): HER2+ breast cancer
- Lucentis (Ranibizumab): Age-related macular degeneration
- Avonex (Interferon beta-1a): Multiple sclerosis
- Glatiramer acetate (Copaxone): Multiple sclerosis
- Brodalumab (Siliq): Psoriatic arthritis
- Ixekizumab (Taltz): Psoriatic arthritis
- Secukinumab (Cosentyx): Psoriatic arthritis, ankylosing spondylitis
- Ustekinumab (Stelara): Psoriatic arthritis, Crohn's disease

Monoclonal Antibodies
- Basiliximab (Simulect)
- Daclizumab (Zinbryta)
- Muromonab (Orthoclone OKT3)

Tamoxifen

Tamoxifen is a standard treatment for hormone receptor–positive breast cancer in premenopausal women. Because tamoxifen mimics the effects of estrogen, it has a very beneficial side effect that preserves bone mass and prevents bone loss. However, there exist drug-induced osteonecrosis concerns with the administration of this drug, even though there is a very low prevalence.[131]

Aromatase Inhibitors

In postmenopausal women diagnosed with estrogen receptor–positive breast cancer, aromatase inhibitors (AIs) are the mainstay of adjuvant therapy. These medications inhibit the conversion of androgens to estrogens, which results in estrogen deficiency and may accelerate bone loss. There has been an association with an increase in drug-related osteonecrosis of the jaws with this class of medications.[132] However, in patients on AIs, the incidence of osteonecrosis is still significant, and consultation with the treating physician should be considered in these patients.

Treatment Summary of Immunosuppressive Drugs

Most immunosuppressive medications affect the entire immune system, having a higher incidence of adverse effects (e.g., bone marrow suppression leukopenia, thrombocytopenia, anemia). Therefore patients are susceptible to increased infectious episodes, intraoperative bleeding, and compromised bone healing. A medical consult and evaluation are highly recommended before any proposed implant treatment. For most immunosuppressive drugs, concurrent use and the placement of implants are an absolute contraindication. Additionally, patients on long-term corticosteroid use should be evaluated for possible adrenal insufficiency symptoms.

Past immunosuppressive therapy: Relative contraindication after medical consultation

Concurrent immunosuppressive therapy + implant therapy: Absolute contraindication

Biologics

A newer class of therapeutic drugs is termed *biologics*, and it is used to treat an array of medical conditions such as autoimmune diseases and cancers. Biologics use living organisms (genes) and are manufactured by using recombinant DNA technology in the form of vaccines, antitoxins, growth hormones, gene therapy, and recombined proteins and allergens. Biologic medications are advantageous because they specifically target cells that are involved in the pathogenesis of the disease. Some of the most common biologics used today are tumor necrosis factor-α (TNF-α) inhibitors Cimzia (certolizumab pegol), Enbrel (etanercept), Humira (adalimumab), Remicade (infliximab), and Simponi (golimumab). These drugs block the protein TNF-α that stimulates the body to initiate the inflammation process. In conditions such as psoriasis and psoriatic arthritis, TNF-α is produced in excess in the skin and joints, which stimulate accelerated growth of skin cells and may damage joint tissue. Blocking TNF-α stops the inflammatory cycle. Other biologics include the following:

Interleukin (IL)-12 and IL-23 inhibitors Stelara (ustekinumab): These drugs work by specifically targeting IL-12 and IL-23, which create inflammation.
IL-17 inhibitors Cosentyx (secukinumab) and Taltz (ixekizumab): These drugs block IL-17, which is involved in inflammatory and immune responses; Siliq (brodalumab) blocks the receptor for IL-17, which then inhibits the inflammatory process created by IL-17.
T-cell inhibitors Orencia (abatacept): These drugs target T cells, which are involved in the immune and inflammatory response. Blocking T-cell activation leads to reduced inflammation.

Common Disorders Using Biologics for Treatment

Age-Related Macular Degeneration

Age-related macular degeneration (AMD) is an incurable disease that is the most common cause for blindness in the United States. The macula is the central portion of the eye, which is responsible for the central vision in reading, driving, recognizing color, and seeing objects in fine detail. Over 11 million people in the United States have some form of AMD. This number is expected to double to nearly 22 million by 2050. Worldwide the number may exceed 200 million by 2020 and approach 300 million by 2040. Advancing age is the greatest risk factor. In those less than 59, the risk is only about 2%, but the risk is 30% for those over age 75.[133] A newer, more aggressive treatment option to slow the progression of AMD is to inject medications that block vascular endothelial growth factors (VEGFs). With AMD, abnormally high levels of VEGF may be found that can be reduced by injections with anti-VEGF medications such as Lucentis (ranibizumab). These intraocular injections, which may be administered multiple times a month, have been linked to a significant increase in nonocular hemorrhagic events. This may include bruising, GI hemorrhages, formation of hematomas, and subdural hematomas. Despite being injected directly into the eye intravitreally, anti-VEGF agents have demonstrated high levels in the bloodstream. This provides the basis for the potential occurrence of significant systemic adverse events.[134]

Psoriatic Arthritis

Psoriasis is an autoimmune disease that usually affects the skin. Approximately 33% of patients with psoriasis may develop a very painful form of debilitating inflammatory autoimmune arthritis called psoriatic arthritis. The body's immune system attacks healthy tissue mostly in the skin as well as the joints. This defective process creates inflammation that leads to joint pain with swelling and stiffness. Psoriatic arthritis is usually treated very aggressively to avoid permanent joint damage. In most patients, skin symptoms develop before joint problems. This disease most prevalently affects people who have psoriasis and are 30 to 55 years of age. There exist multiple forms including the following:

Symmetric psoriatic arthritis: This makes up about half of the cases of psoriatic arthritis. This creates symptoms in the same joints on both sides of the body simultaneously. This type is very similar to RA.
Asymmetric psoriatic arthritis: A milder form that affects about 35% of patients with psoriatic arthritis but does not appear in the same joints on both sides of body.
Spondylitis: This form creates pain and stiffness in neck and spine.
Distal psoriatic arthritis: The inflammation in this form occurs near distal portion of fingers and toes, and there can be changes in the toenails and fingernails, including lifting from the nail bed and pitting.
Arthritis mutilans: This is only about 5% of the cases and is the most severe. In this form, the inflammation is more aggressive, causing destruction and deformities of the distal joints in the finger and toes.
Ankylosing spondylitis (AS): This is a form of arthritis that primarily creates pain in the lower lumbosacral area of the spine, but it can also affect the ribs, hips, knees, feet, eyes, and bowel. There is a genetic predisposition to development of this disease, and the main gene associated with this condition is *HLA-B27*. Frequently, patients are given steroids and/or methotrexate to treat the symptoms. New treatment options include biologics.

Rheumatoid Arthritis

See "Autoimmune" section.

Polymyalgia Rheumatica

Polymyalgia rheumatica (PMR) is an autoimmune inflammatory disease that directly affects the muscles and joints, mainly in the shoulders and hips. The disease also causes muscle pain and stiffness in the neck, buttocks, and arms. Most of patients diagnosed with PMR are over 50, and the average age is about 70. Onset of symptoms can be abrupt without warning and is usually bilateral. One of the most common complaints is that patients have trouble raising their arms above their shoulders and have aching in joints including the hands and wrists. The stiffness is always worse after prolonged sitting, sleeping, or inactivity. There is no joint swelling. There is no specific test that confirms the diagnosis. Almost all patients with the shoulder and other symptoms have elevated inflammatory markers including elevated sedimentation rate and C-reactive protein. Treatment many times includes steroids, methotrexate, and various biologics.

Eczema (Atopic Dermatitis)

Eczema is a dermatitis that causes dry, itchy, inflamed patches of skin. The etiology of eczema is not fully understood, but it is related to an overactive immune system that many times can be associated with other allergy type symptoms and asthma. There are several types of eczema. (1) Contact dermatitis is caused by contact with chemicals, soaps, plants, or other irritants. (2) Dyshidrotic dermatitis, which is more common in women, affects fingers, the bottom of the feet, and palms. This condition causes itchy, inflamed patches of skin that become erythematous, cracked, and eventually painful. (3) Nummular dermatitis is more prevalent in the winter, with round dry patches mostly on the legs. (4) Seborrheic dermatitis causes scaly, red flaky rashes mostly in the scalp or around the eyes. It can also be seen on the sides of the nose or behind the ears.

For the most part, eczema has been treated with topical steroids, which have very little effect on dental implant surgery. However, recently new biologics have been introduced to treat eczema. Dupixent (dupilumab) is the first biologic medication used to treat eczema. Dupixent works by blocking interleukins from attaching to cell receptors. Interleukins help the immune system combat infection, but when the immune system becomes dysfunctional, the interleukins can cause immune disorders such as eczema. The injection schedule for Dupixent is usually every 2 weeks.

Multiple Sclerosis

Multiple sclerosis (MS) is a chronic disease of the CNS that results in damage to the nerves in the brain, spinal cord, and optic nerves. Symptoms can be mild to severe, from numbness in extremities to complete paralysis or even vision loss. There are over 400,000 people in the United States that have MS. Each year approximately 10,000 new cases are diagnosed. It is over twice as prevalent in women as men, and the diagnosis is usually made after age 20 and before age 50.

Nerves rely on myelin to successfully transmit electrical impulses. MS attacks the myelin sheath, resulting in damage to the nerves and resulting in plaques or lesions that can show up on imaging such as magnetic resonance imaging (MRI). As the nerves lose myelin, impulses from the brain are no longer transmitted to the muscle, causing the symptoms of MS.

Most of the cases of MS are relapse–remitting, which results in new attacks with increasing symptoms, but there are periods of remittance with the periods of relapse. Progressive MS does not have any relapse or remissions; symptoms worsen progressively. These symptoms include muscle weakness, vision problems, coordination and balance issues, memory issues, and numbness in extremities. Difficulty emptying the bladder, constipation, fatigue, dizziness, and muscle spasms are also common symptoms. The exact cause in unknown, but MS is thought to be an autoimmune disorder. There are almost a dozen drugs approved to treat MS, and the most common biologics are Avonex (interferon beta-1a) and glatiramer acetate (Copaxone).

Fibromyalgia

Fibromyalgia causes diffuse musculoskeletal pain accompanied by exhaustion/fatigue, sleep disturbances, mood swings, and sometimes memory issues. Although the etiology of fibromyalgia is unclear, many researchers believe there exists a dysfunctional amplification of pain sensation by the brain, which results in the patient being more sensitive to pain. The disease is much more common in women than men and there is no real cure; however, the symptoms may be treated. Most of the treatment involves relaxation, stress reduction techniques, and exercise. In the United States, fibromyalgia affects about 4 million, or about 2% of the adult population. Although there is no specific test for fibromyalgia, the diagnosis is usually made by combining a detailed history and physical with laboratory and radiologic evaluation.[135] Duloxetine (Cymbalta) and other SSRIs are common treatment options for fibromyalgia. Tricyclic antidepressants like amitriptyline (Elavil) and nortriptyline (Pamelor) are used to help treat fatigue and sleep disturbances. The greatest concern regarding tricyclic antidepressants in implant dentistry is the production of anticholinergic actions on the heart. Epinephrine and levonordefrin are not contraindicated in these patients, but they should be used cautiously. For example, heart rate and blood pressure should be reassessed after each 20- to 40-μg dose of epinephrine administered.[136] Muscle relaxants like cyclobenzaprine, tizanidine, or carisoprodol (Soma) are used to help relieve the muscle pain. These drugs can cause xerostomia. Of greatest concern for dental implant patients is the potential for chronic pain after the implant surgery. There are numerous studies demonstrating chronic persistent pain after dental implant surgery without any neurosensory deficits or evidence of an organic cause. Dental implant surgeons need to take this potential postsurgical complication into consideration when determining whether patients are candidates for implant treatment.[137]

Breast Cancer

The American Cancer Society estimates just over 250,000 new cases of invasive breast cancer will be diagnosed in the United States in 2018. In addition, about 64,000 cases of carcinoma in situ (CIS), which is the earliest form of breast cancer, will be also diagnosed. About 41,000 women will die of breast cancer this same year. The incidence of breast cancer has been stable over the past couple of years, but it remains more common in African American women. Breast cancer remains the second leading cause of cancer death in women, and rates from 1989 to 2015 have dropped almost 40%. Since 2007, deaths from breast cancer have continued to drop in women over age 50. There are currently about 3.1 million breast cancer survivors in the United States, including those that are still being treated.[138]

It is important to recognize that women with breast cancer may be considered cancer free after treatment but, for up to 10 years after the diagnosis, patients may be taking adjuvant therapy (treatment given after chemotherapy and surgery) with medications that could affect dental implant success. This therapy is targeted for hormone receptor–positive breast cancer (the most common type of breast cancer). Approximately 75% of breast cancers express the estrogen and/or progesterone receptors (ERs, PRs).[139] Certain breast cancer cells are stimulated by progesterone and/or estrogen to grow. Medications such as tamoxifen or other similar drugs classified as Aromatase Inhibitors block the hormones from getting to these cells. AIs stop tissues and organs other than the ovaries from making estrogen and are used in postmenopausal women only. In premenopausal women, the AI medications actually stimulate estrogen production from the ovary. Tamoxifen, on the other hand, blocks a cell's ability to use estrogen so it can be used in premenopausal and postmenopausal women. Women that have hormone receptor–positive cancer and are premenopausal will take tamoxifen for 5 years. If they have not entered menopause after 5 years, then they can continue tamoxifen for up to 10 years total. Women that go through menopause while on Tamoxifen can switch to an AI for 5 more years or a total of 10 years of hormone treatment.

The oral cavity can be directly affected by estrogen. Antiestrogen therapies can create issues that can influence dental implant success. There are associated side effects with these types of prolonged hormonal therapies. The complications include oral/pharyngeal mucositis, pain, xerostomia, and dental caries. Of increased concern is the risk for opportunistic bacterial, fungal, and viral infections from the immunosuppressive effect of these drugs as a result of chemotherapy-induced immune suppression.[140] Patients are also at risk for osteonecrosis and the therapies may affect the periodontal tissue, causing gingivitis, gingival bleeding, and periodontal infection.[141]

Treatment Summary for Biologic Medications

Although biologic medications have become very popular in the treatment of many systemic disorders, caution must be exercised in patients that have been treated in the past or are currently being treated. Patients may be susceptible to increased infectious episodes, intraoperative bleeding, and compromised bone healing. A medical consult and evaluation are highly recommended before any proposed implant treatment. For most biologic drugs, concurrent use and the placement of implants is an absolute contraindication. Because of the lack of history and studies with these types of medications, severe caution must be exercised with past biologic use and future implant treatment. Physician consultation and approval is highly recommended.

Past biologic therapy: Relative contraindication after medical consultation
Concurrent biologic therapy + implant therapy: Absolute contraindication

Oral Antithrombotic Medications

Oral antithrombotic medications have been used successfully to treat a variety of thrombotic diseases such as MI, stroke, and deep venous thrombosis, and are frequently used in the prevention of cardiovascular diseases. For decades, clinicians and patients have been conscious of the adverse side effects of these medications, primarily spontaneous bleeding or perioperative bleeding. Many have advocated for years to temporarily discontinue these medications before invasive dental treatments such as dental implant surgery. However, because discontinuation of these drugs may result in serious thrombus complications, a thorough knowledge of the mechanism of action needs to be understood (Table 10.23).

Warfarin Sodium

Warfarin sodium (Coumadin) is used as an anticoagulant in a wide range of conditions such as ischemic heart disease, deep

venous thrombosis, pulmonary emboli, and artificial heart valves. Warfarin sodium has a half-life of 40 hours, which has been known to vary from 20 to 60 hours in some individuals. The mode of action of warfarin sodium is the interference of the synthesis of vitamin K, which is a cofactor in many reactions within the coagulation cascade. Coumadin has been the mainstay of anticoagulant treatment options; however, in the past 3 years there has been a shift to a new class of blood thinners in the treatment of nonvalvular atrial fibrillation and deep venous thrombosis. With an aging population, the number of individuals diagnosed with nonvalvular atrial fibrillation continues to climb, with over 2 million Americans now undergoing treatment. The major concern of atrial fibrillation is the formation of blood clots, so most of these patients will be maintained on blood-thinning medications.

Medication Modification

Until recently, most medical practitioners have believed that anticoagulants should be discontinued before dental surgery to prevent possible bleeding problems. However, there exist many documented cases of embolic complications in patients who discontinue the use of warfarin sodium and develop thrombosis from rebound hypercoagulability. In addition, studies have shown that dental surgery may be performed safely on patients receiving anticoagulant therapy as long as their INR values are within the therapeutic range (2.0–3.5). A brief periprocedural interruption of warfarin therapy is associated with a low risk of thromboembolism (0.7%) and risk of clinically significant bleeding (1.7%); however, the risk versus benefit of interruption is not warranted in most cases.[142]

Medical Consultation

Practitioners should consult with the patient's physician to determine the most recent INR before the surgery (ideally 24–48 hours before surgery). If the INR values are within the therapeutic range (2–3.5) then there is no need to discontinue use of the anticoagulant. If the INR value is higher the therapeutic range (especially higher than 3.5), the physician should take appropriate steps to lower the INR to a safer level or possibly discontinue the warfarin and supplement with heparin therapy or vitamin K. It is important to remember with all anticoagulant patients that special attention should be given to good surgical technique and use of appropriate local measures to control bleeding (hemostatic agents). In addition, many antibiotics can increase the effect of Coumadin thus increasing the chance of bleeding. In general cephalosporins, penicillins, quinolones, and macrolides can increase INR and have a moderate class C rating, which means patient should have their INR checked a bit more frequently while on these antibiotics. Sulfonamides and metronidazole are considered to have more severe interactions and are considered as class D drugs, which usually require reduction in Coumadin dosages. Consultation with a physician for use of any class D drug is absolutely indicated. For class C drugs it is suggested but imperative that the patient also understand the relative increased risk. NSAIDs should not be used in patients on Coumadin.

Aspirin

Aspirin or salicylic acid has been used as an antiinflammatory, analgesic, and antipyretic medication. However, in the 1980s, it

TABLE 10.23   Common Anticoagulant Medications

Drug	ASA (81 mg)	ASA (325 mg)	Clopidogrel (Plavix)	Coumadin (Warfarin)	Dabigatran (Pradaxa)	Rivaroxaban (Xarelto)	Apixaban (Eliquis)
Test to determine coagulation status	Serum thrombin time, bleeding time	Serum thrombin time, bleeding time	Serum thrombin time, bleeding time	INR	No testing needed	No testing needed	No testing needed
Mechanism of action	Inhibiting platelet generation of thromboxane A_2 results in inhibition of thrombus formation	Inhibiting platelet generation of thromboxane A_2 results in inhibition of thrombus formation	Inhibits platelet aggregation and activation	Inhibits production of vitamin K–dependent clotting factors (II, VII, IX, and X)	Direct thrombin inhibitor	Factor Xa inhibitor	Factor Xa inhibitor
Dietary restrictions	None	None	None	Vitamin K	None	None	None
Dosing difficulty	None	None	None	Difficult	Reduce dose CrCl < 30	Reduction CrCl < 50 dosing different for different indications	Reduction CrCl < 50 dosing different for different indications
Need for reduction/interruption	Usually not recommended	Case specific	Case specific, usually not recommended, can precipitate, significant medical clotting issues	Case specific, usually not recommended, can precipitate, significant medical clotting issues	Yes, medical consult, usually 48–72 hours	Yes, medical consult	Yes, medical consult
Days of discontinuation before procedures	Not required in most cases, platelet function inhibited 10–14 days	10 days or more, medical consult	Medical consult, especially if given with ASA	Medical consult, usually 5 days or more	Yes, usually 48–72 hours	Yes, usually 48–72 hours	Yes, usually 48–72 hours
Restarting medication	If discontinued, after hemostasis	If discontinued, after hemostasis	If discontinued, dependent on medical recommendation	If discontinued, dependent on medical recommendation	Usually 24–48 hours and discussion with physician	Usually 24–48 hours and discussion with physician	Usually 24–48 hours and discussion with physician

ASA, American Society of Anesthesiologists; CrCl, creatinine clearance; INR, international normalized ratio.

From Resnik RR, Resnik RJ. Medical/medication complications in oral implantology. In Resnik RR, Misch CE, eds. *Misch's Avoiding Complications in Oral Implantology.* St Louis, MO: Elsevier; 2018.

was discovered that aspirin also had an antiplatelet effect at very low doses (0.5–1 mg/kg) versus higher doses needed for an antipyretic effect (5–10 mg/kg) and antiinflammatory response (30 mg/kg). Because of this research, low-dose aspirin has become a secondary preventive drug for patients who have cardiovascular and peripheral vascular disease. Aspirin works by inhibiting the formation of prostaglandin thromboxane A_2 within the platelet, affecting thrombus formation by irreversibly decreasing platelet aggregation.

Studies

Aspirin inhibits platelet function and can be much more severe in the presence of decreased platelet counts. Studies have shown that this risk is minimal unless a 325-mg aspirin is being used. In a study of tooth extractions, 36 patients were randomized to 325 mg of aspirin or placebo for 2 days before and 2 days after. There

was no significant association between those that took the aspirin and perioperative or postoperative bleeding.[143]

Recommendations

Low-Dose (81 mg) Aspirin. There exists no study supporting the recommendation of low-dose aspirin discontinuation for routine dental implant procedures. In most patients, interruption is not warranted because it may expose the patient to the risk of developing thromboembolism, MI, or CVA.

High-Dose (325 mg) Aspirin. When patients are advised by their physician to take 325 mg of aspirin or doses higher than 100 mg, a physician consultation is recommended. This is especially true of patients on aspirin (any dose) with other anticoagulants such as clopidogrel or dipyridamole. Bleeding times may be appropriate in these patients in combination with physician consultation. Usually aspirin is stopped 7 to 10 days before surgery and can be continued after adequate hemostasis has been confirmed.[144]

Plavix (Clopidogrel)

Clopidogrel is a platelet inhibitor that is approved for the reduction of atherosclerotic events in patients with recent stroke, MI, or peripheral arterial disease. The recent literature has supported longer treatment times for patients with coronary stents and acute coronary syndrome from 3 to 12 months or more in combination with aspirin. The literature does not support the routine discontinuation of this medication in relation to dental implant treatment, but it is important to remember that many patients treated with clopidogrel will be on aspirin or another antiplatelet medication, especially those with cardiac stents.

Recommendation: This regimen should never be discontinued unless under the recommendation of a physician.

Novel Oral Anticoagulants

Pradaxa, Xarelto, and Eliquis are a class of medications termed Novel Oral Anticoagulants (NOAC). NOACs. Orally administered anticoagulants have recently been developed to eliminate the disadvantages associated with warfarin. Dabigatran etexilate (Pradaxa) and rivaroxaban (Xarelto) have been shown to have a more favorable (wider) therapeutic index, fewer drug–drug and drug–food interactions, and a predictable anticoagulant response without the need for anticoagulants. Dabigatran reversibly inhibits thrombin, so the duration of action is predictable and correlates well with plasma drug concentrations. Rivaroxaban is an FXa inhibitor that produces reversible inhibition of FXa activity.[145]

Bleeding

In contrast to the many studies on oral surgery and the use of warfarin, no clinical trials have been completed to offer recommendations on the management of patients on these newer anticoagulants with relation to dental implant surgery. However, there exist several case studies suggesting that, with physician consultation, these drugs can be temporarily discontinued 24 hours before elective oral surgery and restarted the following day, resulting in minimal complications. Because these drugs have a short half-life, brief interruption of usage is usually acceptable. It is imperative that physician consultation be obtained prior to any of these medications being temporarily discontinued. Good surgical technique and the use of hemostatic agents should be adhered to during oral surgery. Currently Praxbind is available to help reverse the effects on Pradaxa and control excessive bleeding. AndrexXA is awaiting final approval to help reverse the excessive or uncontrollable bleeding that may occur from the FXa inhibitors (Xarelto, Eliquis, and Savaysa). Currently there is no approved treatment to control excessive bleeding caused by the FXa inhibitors.

Treatment Summary

Currently there is no accepted reduction protocol for NOACs. Based on the information available, the clinician should consult the patient's physician concerning the proposed implant procedure and the invasiveness of the surgery, anticipated hemostasis complications, and amount of bleeding to be expected. If physician recommendation is for the temporary discontinuation of these drugs, then the typical discontinuation recommendation is for 24 hours before surgery, and the drug should not be restarted until the risk of postoperative bleeding is minimal (usually within 24 hours of surgery).[146] Patients should be closely monitored

postoperatively because bleeding may reoccur after initial hemostasis and continuation of the medication.

Herbal Supplements

OTC herbal and dietary supplements are being consumed at a record pace for general health improvement and treatment of chronic conditions. It is an important part of taking a medical history that you specifically ask about any OTC supplements, herbal medications, or any pills a patient may be taking that are not prescribed by a physician.

Herbs have been known to be associated with unwanted side effects and can cause drug interactions, as well as being associated with surgical complications. Many of these supplements contain active ingredients that exhibit strong biologic effects. The doses are usually unregulated and variable among patients. The *Journal of the American Medical Association* estimates that 15 million adults are at risk for adverse interactions between herbs and prescription medications.[147] The risks of these medications associated with dental implant surgery are increased bleeding, drug interactions, and possible infection.

Recommendation: Patients should discontinue the use of these herbal supplements for at least 2 weeks before implant surgery (Box 10.14).

Selective Serotonin Reuptake Inhibitors

Depression is a prevalent mental illness disorder that is a significant disability with a reduced quality of life. Low levels of serotonin (chemical and neurotransmitter) have been associated with depression. SSRIs have been used to successfully treat depression.

SSRIs have a very low adverse-effect profile because they do not affect blood pressure or heart rate. SSRIs inhibit serotonin reuptake from the synaptic cleft into presynaptic nerve terminals, increasing serotonin neurotransmission. However, SSRIs have been directly associated with lower bone mineral density.[148]

Serotonin found in bone cells (osteocytes, osteoblasts, and osteoclasts) can be activated by SSRIs, which results in altered function. Wu and colleagues stated that SSRIs might have a negative effect on dental implant healing. Their data demonstrate an increased risk of failure with most complications occurring from the anabolic response, which inhibits the bone-remodeling processes triggered by mechanical loading.[149]

Treatment Summary

The concomitant use of SSRIs and dental implants is a relative contraindication. A medical consult and evaluation should ideally be completed before dental implant treatment.

Allergies

Hypersensitivity to titanium is an ever-increasing reportable complication in medicine today that has been associated with a wide range of situations. In orthopedic medicine, there exist many case reports of titanium alloy hypersensitivity. Witt and Swann reported 13 cases of failed total hip prostheses and concluded the tissue reaction in response to metal-wear debris may have been the etiology of the failed implants. This process has been termed *repassivation* and may produce an oxide that surrounds and turns the peri-implant tissues black.[150]

Yamauchi and colleagues reported a titanium-implanted pacemaker developing an allergic reaction. The patient developed a distinct erythema over the implantation site, which

From Resnik RR, Resnik RJ. Medical/medication complications in oral implantology. In Resnik RR, Misch CE, eds. Misch's Avoiding Complications in Oral Implantology. St Louis, MO: Elsevier; 2018.

• BOX 10.14 Herbal Supplement and Adverse Effects

Increased Bleeding
- Arnica
- Barberry
- Bilberry
- Bromelain
- Cat's claw
- Cayenne
- Chamomile
- Chestnut
- Cinnabar root
- Devil's claw
- Dong quai
- Fennel
- Feverfew
- Garlic
- Ginger
- Ginkgo biloba
- Ginseng
- Grape seed
- Green tea
- Kudzu
- Primrose
- Red clover
- Turmeric
- Sweet woodruff
- Vitamin E

Increased Inflammation
- Celery
- Dandelion
- Elder
- Goldenseal
- Juniper

Interactions With Nonsteroidal Antiinflammatory Drugs
- Feverfew
- Gingko
- Ginseng
- St. John's Wort
- Uva-Ursi

Interactions With Anesthesia
- Green tea: Decreases effect of oral atropine
- Dong quai: Increases sedation and lowers seizure threshold
- Kava: Increases sedation
- Valerian: Increases sedation, interacts with opioids
- Vitamin C: In large doses can weaken anesthesia
- Yohimbe: Can interact with some analgesics like morphine

resulted in a generalized eczema. Titanium sensitivity was confirmed by intracutaneous and lymphocyte stimulation testing.[151] In the dental literature, allergic reactions to pure titanium are rare. However, many authors have suggested there is a higher incidence of titanium alloy allergy with respect to dental implants, and it is most likely underreported because of a poor understanding of failure or allergy.[152] du Preez and colleagues have reported a case of implant failure caused by a suspected titanium hypersensitivity reaction around a dental implant. Histologic results showed a chronic inflammatory reaction with concomitant fibrosis.[153] Egusa and colleagues reported

a titanium implant overdenture case that resulted in generalized eczema that fully resolved after implant removal.[154] Sicilia and colleagues, in a clinical study of 1500 consecutive implant patients, reported approximately nine implants with a positive reaction to titanium allergy.[155]

Sensitivity to titanium has been shown to be a result of the presence of macrophages and T-lymphocytes with the presence of B-lymphocytes, which results in a type IV hypersensitivity reaction.[156] All metals, when in a biologic environment, undergo corrosion, which may lead to the formation of metallic ions that trigger the immune system complex with endogenous proteins.[157] Titanium alloy dental implants have been shown to contain many "impurities" that may trigger type IV hypersensitivity reactions. Harloff used spectral analysis to investigate various Ti alloy implants. The results showed that all the Ti alloy samples contained small amounts of other elements such as beryllium (Be), cobalt (Co), chromium (Cr), copper (Cu), iron (Fe), nickel (Ni), and palladium. These impurity elements have been shown to be the etiology of the hypersensitivity reactions.[158]

Treatment Summary

When titanium hypersensitivity is suspected, the implants should be removed and the patient should be referred to their physician for appropriate testing. Case reports have shown that, after complete removal of the implants, complete resolution results.[154] Metal sensitivity is usually diagnosed using a "patch-test," which involves placement of titanium (allergen) to the skin for approximately 3 to 4 days. A positive test would include the appearance of an erythematous reaction. However, there is a possibility of false negatives because the sealing qualities of the skin against direct contact, which may make the test unreliable (Fig. 10.4).

Medical Consultation and Clearance

Oral implantology is a complex specialty with many factors that must be taken into consideration to decrease morbidity and increase the probability of successful treatment. Medical clearance is a necessity with respect to patients who present with complicated systemic conditions, medications, and predisposing factors that may lead to complications. The implant clinician must relay to the physician all necessary information, including
1. A detailed summary of what the patient related as their medical history
2. A list of all current and recent medications
3. A list of all allergies
4. Any medications that will be prescribed by the implant dentist
5. The invasiveness of the intended procedure

The physician will provide with the following:
1. Most recent physical examination: To determine whether the patient is compliant with keeping up with their medical health
2. Documentation of medical health: Very important to determine whether there exists any misinformation or missing health issues that the patient failed to represent on the medical/dental history
3. Medication modification: The physician will recommend any modifications to physician-prescribed medications or dental surgery proposed medications.
4. Acceptable candidate: The physician will clear the patient for dental implant treatment in writing.
5. Contacting the physician: The physician will document whether their recommendation is for the implant dentist to contact them before treatment and, last, to make sure the physician signs and dates the form (Fig. 10.5).

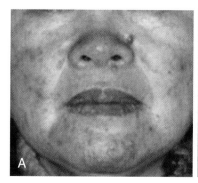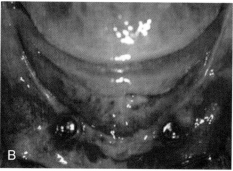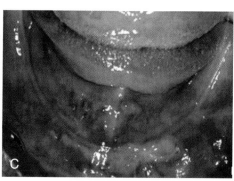

• **Fig. 10.4** Titanium dental implant allergy. (A) Facial eczema after implant placement. (B) Intraoral view of type IV hypersensitivity reaction. (C) Complete resolution after implant removal. (From Egusa H, Ko N, Shimazu T, Yatani H. Suspected association of an allergic reaction with titanium dental implants: a clinical report. *J Prosthet Dent.* 2008;100(5):344–347.)

MEDICAL CONSULTATION FOR DENTAL IMPLANT SURGERY

Patient: _____ Date: _____

The above patient is tentatively scheduled for dental implant surgery. The outpatient surgery will be performed in my office under intravenous conscious sedation. The following information has been provided by the patient.

Medical History: _____

Current Medications: _____

Allergies to Medications: _____

THE FOLLOWING MEDICATIONS ARE PROPOSED FOR THE DENTAL IMPLANT SURGERY:

ANTIMICROBIAL	ANTI-INFLAMMATORY	ANALGESIC	ANESTHESIA	SEDATION
___ Amoxicillin	___ Ibuprofen	___ Hydrocodone	___ 2% Lidocaine 1/100k Epi.	___ Halcion
___ Cephalosporin	___ Dexamethasone	___ Codeine	___ 2% Carbocaine 1/20k Neo.	___ Valium
___ Clindamycin		___ Acetaminophen	___ 3% Carbocaine	___ N20
___ Augmentin		___ Percocet	___ .5% Marcaine 1/200k Epi	___ IV Rx"s
_____		___ Ultram	___ 4% Articaine 1/100k Epi	(Versed,Fentanyl)

PLEASE PROVIDE ANSWERS TO THE FOLLOWING QUESTIONS

1. Date of most recent physical exam: _____

2. Significant medical condition, treatment, disease, injury or comments:

_____

_____

_____

_____

3. Any Recommendations or Modifications of Medications   YES ——— NO ———

   Current Medications _____

   Proposed Medications (Listed Above) _____

4. The above patient is an acceptable candidate for outpatient dental implant surgery   YES ——— NO ———

5. Please contact me prior to treating this patient   YES ——— NO ———

_____

Signature of Physician   **Date**

• **Fig. 10.5** Medical consultation form.

References

1. Weijant RJ. Characteristics associated with the loss and perio implant tissue health of endosseous dental implants. *Int J Oral Maxillofac Implants.* 1992;7:367–372.
2. Scully C. *Scully's Medical Problems in Dentistry.* 7th ed. London: Churchill Livingstone; 2014. 231–231.
3. https://www.wsj.com/articles/when-patients-take-too-many-pills-doctors-deprescribe-1476122784.
4. Dycht K. *Age Wave: The Challenges and Opportunities of an Aging America.* New York: St Martin's Press; 1988.
5. US Bureau of the Census. Population reports. *Population Estimates.* 1988;25:1024.
6. McCarthy FM. Vital signs—the six minute warning. *J Am Dent Assoc.* 1980;100:682–691.
7. Chobanian AV, Bakris GL, Black HR, et al. The seventh report of the joint national committee on prevention, detection, evaluation, and treatment of high blood pressure. *JAMA.* 2003;289(19):2560–2571. https://doi.org/10.1001/jama.289.19.2560.
8. Muntner P, Carey RM, Gidding S, et al. Potential U.S. population impact of the 2017 ACC/AHA high blood pressure guideline. *J Am Coll Cardiol.* 2018;71(2):109–118.
9. Gilbert GH, Minaker KL. Principles of surgical risk assessment of the elderly patient. *J Oral Maxillofac Surg.* 1990;48:972–979.
10. Sabes WR, Green S, Craine C. Value of medical diagnostic screening tests for dental patients. *J Am Dent Assoc.* 1970;80:133–136.
11. Sones ST, Fazio R, Setkowicz A, et al. Comparison of the nature and frequency of medical problems among patients in general specialty and hospital dental practices. *J Oral Med.* 1985;38:58.
12. Misch CE. Medical evaluation of the implant candidate. Part II: complete blood count and bleeding disorders. *Int J Oral Implant.* 1982;10:363–370.
13. Corman L, Bolt RJ, eds. Medical evaluation of the pre-operative patient. *Med Clin North Am.* 1979;63:6.
14. https://www.ncbi.nlm.nih.gov/pmc/articles/PMC4340464/.
15. Hirsch J, Dalan JE, Deykin D, et al. Oral anticoagulants: mechanism of action, clinical effectiveness, and optimal therapeutic range. *Chest.* 1992;102(suppl):312–326.
16. Cuker A, Siegal DM, Crowther MA, Garcia DA. Laboratory measurement of the anticoagulant activity of the non-vitamin K oral anticoagulants. *J Am Coll Cardiol.* 2014;64:1128–1139.
17. Cuker A, Husseinzadeh H. Laboratory measurement of the anticoagulant activity of edoxaban: a systemic review. *J Thromb Thrombolysis.* 2015;39:288–294.
18. Lab Tests Online. *Comprehensive Metabolic Panel*; 2005. Available at: http://www.labtestsonline.org/understanding/analytes/cmp/glance.html.
19. Misch CE. Medical evaluation of the implant candidate. Part III. SMA 12/60. *J Oral Implant.* 1981;9:556–570.
20. Raslavicus PA, Mei Shen E. Laboratory diagnosis by chemical methods. *Dent Clin North Am.* 1974;18:155–170.
21. Misch CE. Medical evaluation. In: Misch CE, ed. *Contemporary Implant Dentistry.* St Louis: Mosby; 1993.
22. Benjamin EJ, Virani SS, Callaway CW, et al. Heart disease and stroke statistics—2018 update: a report from the american heart association. *Circulation.* 2018;137(12):e67–e492.
23. Leung RS, Bradley TD. Sleep apnea and cardiovascular disease. *Am J Respir Crit Care Med.* 2001;164:2147–2167.
24. Lavie P, Herer P, Hoffstein V. Obstructive sleep apnoea syndrome as a risk factor for hypertension: population study. *BMJ.* 2000;320(7233):479–482.
25. Gordy FM, LeJeune RC, Copeland LB. The prevalence of hypertension in a dental school patient population. *Quintessence Int.* 2001;32:691–695.
26. Zamost B, Benumof JL. Anesthesia in geriatric patients. In: Katz J, Benumof JL, Kadis LB, eds. *Anesthesia and Uncommon Diseases: Pathophysiologic and Clinical Correlation.* 2nd ed. Philadelphia: WB Saunders; 1976.
27. Alder M, Kitchen S, Jrion A. *Data Book on the Elderly: A Statistical Portrait.* Washington, DC: US Department of Health and Human Services; 1987.
28. Levy SM, Baker KA, Semla TP, et al. Use of medications with dental significance by a noninstitutionalized elderly population. *Gerodontics.* 1988;4:119–125.
29. Heeling DK, Lemke JH, Semla TP, et al. Medication use characteristics in the elderly. The Iowa 65+ rural health study. *J Am Geriatr Soc.* 1987;35:4–12.
30. Ellis JS, Seymour RA, Steele JG, et al. Prevalence of gingival overgrowth induced by calcium channel blockers: a community-based study. *J Periodontol.* 1999;70:63–67.
31. Herman WW, Konzelman JL. Angina, an update for dentistry. *J Am Dent Assoc.* 1996;127:98–104.
32. Benjamin EJ, Blaha MJ, Chiuve SE, Cushman M, Das SR, Deo R, et al. Heart disease and stroke statistics—2017 update: a report from the American Heart Association. 135:e1–e458. https://doi.org/10.1161/CIR.0000000000000485.
33. Pell S, D'Alonzo CA. Immediate mortality and five year survival of employed men with a first myocardial infarction. *N Engl J Med.* 1964;270:915.
34. Malamed SF. *Sedation: A Guide to Patient Management.* 2nd ed. St Louis: Mosby; 1989.
35. Heart disease and stroke statistics—2018 update. A report from the American heart association. *Circulation.* 2018. [Epub ahead of print].
36. Heidenreich PA, Albert NM, et al. Forecasting the impact of heart failure in the US. A statement policy from the American Heart Association. *Circ Heart Fail.* 2013;6(3):606–619.
37. Yancy CW, Jessup M, Bozkurt B, et al. 2013 ACCF/AHA guideline for the management of heart failure: a report of the American College of Cardiology Foundation/American Heart Association Task Force on Practice Guidelines. *Circulation.* 2013;128:e240–319.
38. Smith MJ, So, RR, Engel AM. Clinical predictors of mortality from infective endocarditis. *IJS.* 2007;5(1):31–34. https://doi.org/10.1016/j.ijsu.2006.06.008.
39. Wilson W, Taubert KA, Gewitz M, et al. Prevention of infective endocarditis: guidelines from the American Heart Association: a guideline from the American Heart Association Rheumatic Fever, Endocarditis, and Kawasaki Disease Committee, Council on Cardiovascular Disease in the Young, and the Council on Clinical Cardiology, Council on Cardiovascular Surgery and Anesthesia, and the Quality of Care and Outcomes Research Interdisciplinary Working Group. *Circulation.* 2007;116(15):1736–1754.
40. Nishimura RA, Otto CM, Bonow RO, et al. 2017 AHA/ACC Focused Update of the 2014 AHA/ACC guideline for the management of patients with valvular heart disease: a report of the American College of Cardiology/American Heart Association Task Force on Clinical Practice Guidelines. *Circulation.* 2017;135:e1159–e1195. Accessed June 19, 2017.
41. Wilson W, Taubert KA, Gewitz M, et al. Prevention of infective endocarditis: guidelines from the American Heart Association: a guideline from the American Heart Association Rheumatic Fever, Endocarditis, and Kawasaki Disease Committee, Council on Cardiovascular Disease in the Young, and the Council on Clinical Cardiology, Council on Cardiovascular Surgery and Anesthesia, and the Quality of Care and Outcomes Research Interdisciplinary Working Group. *Circulation.* 2007;116(15):1736–1754.
42. Burkett LW, Burn CG. Bacteremias following dental extraction: demonstration of source of bacteria by means of a non-pathogen (Serratia marcescens). *J Dent Res.* 1937;16:521.
43. Korn VA, Schaffer EM. A comparison of the postoperative bacteremias induced following different periodontal procedures. *J Periodontol.* 1962;33:226.
44. Grant BF, Harforf TC, Dawson DA, et al. Prevalence of DSM IV alcohol abuse and dependence. United States:1992. *Alcohol Health Res World.* 1994;18:243–248.

45. Cameron IW. SBE in an edentulous patient: a case report. *Br Med J.* 1971;1:821.

46. Dajani AS, Bawdon RE, Berry MC. Oral amoxicillin as prophylaxis for endocarditis: what is the optimal dose? *Clin Inject Dis.* 1994;18:157–160.

47. Fluckiger U, Franciolo P, Blaser J, et al. Role of amoxicillin serum levels for successful prophylaxis of experimental endocarditis due to tolerant streptococci. *J Inject Dis.* 1994;169:397–400.

48. Dajani AS, Taubert KA, Wilson W, et al. Prevention of bacterial endocarditis. Recommendations by the American Heart Association. *J Am Med Assoc.* 1997;277:1794–1801.

49. Chanavaz M. Patient screening and medical evaluation for implant and preprosthetic surgery. *J Oral Implantol.* 1998;24:222–229.

50. Nishimura RA, Otto CM, Bonow RA, et al. 2017 AHA/ACC focused update of the 2014 AHA/ACC guideline for the management of patients with valvular heart disease: a report of the American College of Cardiology/American Heart Association Task Force on Clinical Practice Guidelines. *Circulation.* 2017;135(25): e1159–e1195.

51. https://www.cdc.gov/diabetes/pdfs/data/statistics/national-diabetes-statistics-report.pdf.

52. Gilbert GH, Minaker KL. Principles of surgical risk assessment of the elderly patient. *J Oral Maxillofac Surg.* 1990;48:972–979.

53. Retzepi M, Donos N. The effect of diabetes mellitus on osseous healing. *Clin Oral Implants Res.* 2010;21:673–681.

54. Mellado-Valero A, Ferrer Garcia JC, Herrera Ballester A, et al. Effects of diabetes on the osseo-integration of dental implants. *Med Oral Patol Oral Cir Bucal.* 2007;12:E38–E43.

55. McCracken M, Lemons JE, Rahemtulla F, et al. Bone response to titanium alloy implants placed in diabetic rats. *Int J Oral Maxillofac Implants.* 2000;15:345–354.

56. Javed F, Romanos GE. Impact of diabetes mellitus and glycaemic control on the osseointegration of dental implants: a systematic literature review. *J Periodontol.* 2009;80:1719–1730.

57. Marchand F, Raskin A, Dionnes-Hornes A, et al. Dental implants and diabetes: conditions for success. *Diabetes Metab.* 2012;38:14–19.

58. Jolly DE. Interpreting the clinical laboratory. *Cal Dent Assoc J.* 1995;23:32–40.

59. Attard NJ, Zarb GA. A study of dental implants in medically treated hypothyroid patients. *Clin Implant Dent Relat Res.* 2002;4:220–231.

60. Biron CR. Patients with thyroid dysfunctions require risk management before dental procedures. *RDH.* 1996;16(4):42–44.

61. Liddle GW, Melmon KC. The adrenals. In: Williams RH, ed. *Textbook on Endocrinology.* 5th ed. Philadelphia: WB Saunders; 1974.

62. Dummett CO, Barens C. Oromucosal pigmentation: an updated literary review. *J Periodontol.* 1971;42:726.

63. McCarthy FM. Adrenal insufficiency. In: McCarthy FM, ed. *Essentials of Safe Dentistry for the Medically Compromised Patient.* Philadelphia: WB Saunders; 1989.

64. Henrikson P. Periodontal disease and calcium deficiency: an experimental study in the dog. *Acta Odontol Scand.* 1968;26(suppl 50):1–132.

65. Johnson BS. Altered hemostasis: considerations for dental care. *Cal Dent Assoc J.* 1995;23:41 54.

66. Misch CE. Density of bone: effect on treatment plans, surgical approach, healing and progressive bone loading. *Int J Oral Implant.* 1990;6:23–31.

67. Konotey Ahuke FI. The sickle cell diseases. *Arch Intern Med.* 1974;133:611.

68. Bennett B. Coagulation pathways: inter-relationships and control mechanisms. *Semin Hematol.* 1977;14:301.

69. Marder MZ. Medical conditions affecting the success of dental implants. *Compendium.* 2004;25:739–764.

70. https://www.cdc.gov/copd/data.html.

71. Grant BF, Harforf TC, Dawson DA, et al. Prevalence of DSM IV alcohol abuse and dependence. United States:1992. *Alcohol Health Res World.* 1994;18:243–248.

72. Lieber CS. Medical disorders of alcoholism. *N Engl J Med.* 1995;333:1058–1065.

73. Chandok N, Watt K. Pain management in the cirrhotic patient: the clinical challenge. *Mayo Clin Proc.* 2010;85:451–458.

74. Veldurthy V, Wei R, Oz L, Dhawan P, Jeon YH, Christakos S. Vitamin D, calcium homeostasis and aging. *Bone Res.* 2016;4:16041. Published online 2016 Oct 18 . https://doi.org/10.1038/boneres.2016.41. https://www.ncbi.nlm.nih.gov/pmc/articles/PMC5068478/.

75. *Bone Health and Osteoporosis: a report of the Surgeon General.* Rockville, MD: Department of Health and Human Services; 2004.

76. Chestnut CH. Osteoporosis an undiagnosed disease. *JAMA.* 2001;286:2865–2866.

77. Darcy J, Homer K, Walsh T, et al. Tooth loss and osteoporosis: to assess the association between osteoporosis status and tooth number. *Br Dent J.* 2013;214(4).

78. *National Osteoporosis Foundation: Boning up on Osteoporosis, A Guide to Prevention and Treatment.* Washington, DC: National Osteoporosis Foundation; 1991.

79. Heasman PA. The role of nonsteroidal antiinflammatory drugs in the management of periodontal disease. *J Dent Res.* 1988;16:247–257.

80. Ortman LF, Hausman E, Dunford RG. Skeletal osteopenia and residual ridge resorption. *J Prosthet Dent.* 1989;61:321–325.

81. August M, Chung K, Chang Y, et al. Influence of estrogen status on endosseous implant integration. *J Oral Maxillofac Surg.* 2001;59:1285–1289.

82. Farley JR, Wergedal JE, Baylink DJ. Fluoride directly stimulates proliferation and alkaline phosphatase activity of bone forming cells. *Science.* 1983;222:330.

83. Bajwa MS, Ethunandan M, Flood TR. Oral rehabilitation with endosseous implants in a patient with fibrous dysplasia (McCune-Albright syndrome): a case report. *J Oral Maxillofac Surg.* 2008;66:2605–2608.

84. Ricalde P, Magliocca KR, Lee JS. Craniofacial fibrous dysplasia. *Oral Maxil Surg Clin.* 2012;24:427–441.

85. Padbury Jr AD, Tözüm TF, Taba Jr M, Ealba EL, West BT, Burney RE, et al. The impact of primary hyperparathyroidism on the oral cavity. *J Clin Endocr Metab.* 2006;91(9):3439–3445.

86. Singer FR, Bone 3rd HG, Hosking DJ, et al. Paget's Disease of Bone: an endocrine society clinical practice guideline. *J Clin Endocrinol Metab.* 2014;99(12):4408–4422.

87. https://www.ncbi.nlm.nih.gov/pmc/articles/PMC3244103/.

88. Sager RD, Thesis RM. Dental implants placed in a patient with multiple myeloma. Report of case. *J Am Dent Assoc.* 1990;121:699–701.

89. Clarke A. Hypohidrotic ectodermal dysplasia. *J Med Genet.* 1987;24:659–663.

90. Bergendal B, Bergendal T, Hallonsten AL, et al. A multidisciplinary approach to oral rehabilitation with osseointegrated implants in children and adolescents with multiple aplasia. *Eur J Orthod.* 1996;18:119–129.

91. Smith RA, Vargervik K, Kearns G, et al. Placement of an endosseous implant in a growing child with ectodermal dysplasia. *Oral Surg Oral Med Oral Pathol.* 1993;75:669–673.

92. Davarpanah M, Moon JW, Yang LR, et al. Dental implants in the oral rehabilitation of a teenager with hypohidrotic ectodermal dysplasia: report of a case. *Int J Oral Maxillofac Implants.* 1997;12:252–258.

93. Altasalo K. Bone tissue response to irradiation and treatment model of mandibular irradiation injury. *Acta Otolaryngol.* 1986;428:1–54.

94. Granstrom G. Hyperbaric oxygen as a stimulator of osseointegration. In: Yanagita N, Nakashima T, eds. *Hyperbalic Oxygen Therapy in Otorhinolaryngology.* 54. ; 1998:33–49. Adv Otorhinolaryngol.

95. Jacobsson M. *On Behavior After Irradiation (Master's Thesis).* Goteborg: Sweden: University of Goteborg; 1985.

96. Keller EE. Placement of dental implants in irradiated mandible. A protocol without adjunctive hyperbaric oxygen. *J Oral Maxillofac Surg.* 1997;55:972.

97. Granstrom G. Osseointegration in irradiated tissues. Experience from our first 100 treated patients. *J Oral Maxillofac Surg.* 1996;63:579–585.

98. King MA, Casarett GW, Weber DA. A study of irradiated bone: I. histopathologic and physiologic changes. *J Nucl Med.* 1979;20:1142–1149.

99. Almeida D, Vianna K, Arriaga P, Moraschini V. Dental implants in Sjögren's syndrome patients: a systematic review. *PloS one.* 2017;12(12):e0189507.

100. Pons-Estel GJ, Alarcón GS, Scofield L, et al. Understanding the epidemiology and progression of systemic lupus erythematosus. *Semin Arthritis Rheum.* 2010;39(4):257–268. https://doi.org/10.1016/j.semarthrit.2008.10.007. Epub 2009 Jan 10.

101. https://www.rheumatology.org/I-Am-A/Patient-Caregiver/Diseases-Conditions/Scleroderma.

102. Vital EM, Emery P. Advances in the treatment of early rheumatoid arthritis. *Am Fam Physician.* 2005;72:1002–1004.

103. Friedlander GE, Tross RB, Doganis AC, et al. Effects of chemotherapeutic agents on bone: I. short-term methotrexate and doxorubicin (adriamycin) treatment in a rat model. *J Bone Joint Surg Am.* 1984;66(4):602–607.

104. http://www.natap.org/2016/CROI/croi_25.htm.

105. Shetty K, Achong R. Dental implants in the HIV-positive patient—case report and review of the literature. *Gen Dent.* 2005;53:434–437.

106. Achong RM, Shetty K, Arribas A, et al. Implants in HIV-positive patients: 3 case reports. *J Oral Maxillofac Surg.* 64:1199–1203.

107. Oksenberg A, Aarons E. Reduction of sleep bruxism using a mandibular advancement device: an experimental controlled study. *Sleep Med. Nov.* 2002;3(6):513–515.

108. Jordan AS, McSharry DG, Malhotra A. Adult obstructive sleep apnoea. *Lancet.* 2014;383(9918):736–747.

109. *Hypertension.* 2014;63:203–209. https://doi.org/10.1161/HYPERTENSIONAHA.113.00613.

110. McCracken M, Lemons JE, Rahemtulla F, et al. Bone response to titanium alloy implants placed in diabetic rats. *Int J Oral Maxillofac Implants.* 2000;15:345–354.

111. Peled M, Ardekian L, Tagger-Green N, et al. Dental implants in patients with type 2 diabetes mellitus: a clinical study. *Implant Dent.* 2003;12:116–122.

112. Balshi TJ, Wolfinger GJ. Dental implants in the diabetic patient: a retrospective study. *Implant Dent.* 1999;8:355–359.

113. Jemt T. Implant treatment in elderly patients. *Int J Prosthodont.* 1993;6:456–461.

114. Leow YH, Maibach HI. Cigarette smoking, cutaneous vasculature, and tissue oxygen. *Clin Dermatol.* 1998;16:579–584.

115. Cavalcanti R, Oreglia F, Manfredonia MF, et al. The influence of smoking on the survival of dental implants: a 5-year pragmatic multicenter retrospective cohort study of 1727 patients. *Eur J Oral Implantol.* 2011;4:39–45.

116. van Steenberghe D, Jacobs R, Desnyder M, et al. The relative impact of local and endogenous patient-related factors on implant failure up to the abutment stage. *Clin Oral Implants Res.* 2002;13:617.

117. Jones JK, Triplett RG. The relationship of cigarette smoking to impaired intra-oral wound healing. *J Oral Maxillofac Surg.* 1992;50:237–239.

118. Bain CA. Smoking and implant failure—benefits of a smoking cessation protocol. *Int J Oral Maxillofac Implants.* 1996;11:1667–1674.

119. Bain CA, Moy PK. The association between the failure of dental implants and cigarette smoking. *Int J Oral Maxillofac Impl.* 1993;8:609–615.

120. Grossi SG, Zambon J, Machtei EE. Effects of smoking and smoking cessation on healing after mechanical periodontal therapy. *J Am Dent Assoc.* 1997;128:599–607.

121. Scully C. *Scully's Medical Problems in Dentistry.* 7th ed. London: Churchill Livingstone; 2014.

122. Rees TD. Oral effects of drug abuse. *Crit Rev Oral Biol Med.* 1992;3:163–184.

123. Tonnesen H. Alcohol abuse and postoperative morbidity. *Dan Med Bull.* 2003;50:139–160.

124. Marx RE. *Oral and Intravenous Bisphosphonate-Induced Osteonecrosis of the Jaws.* Hanover Park, IL: Quintessence; 2007.

125. Greenspan SL, Rosen HN, Parker RA. Early changes in serum N-telopeptide and C-telopeptide cross-linked collagen type 1 predict long-term response to alendronate therapy in elderly women. *J Clin Endocrinol Metab.* 2000;85:3537–3540.

126. Marx RE. Bisphosphonates and bisphosphonate-induced osteonecrosis of the jaws. In: Bagheri SC, Bell RB, Kahn HA, eds. *Current Therapy in Oral and Maxillofacial Surgery.* St Louis: Saunders; 2012.

127. Jeffcoat MK. Safety of oral bisphosphonates: controlled studies on alveolar bone. *Int J Oral Maxillofac Implants.* 2006;21:349–353.

128. Damm DD, Jones DM. Bisphosphonate-related osteonecrosis of the jaws: a potential alternative to drug holidays. *Gen Dent.* 2013;61(5):33–38.

129. Aljohani S, Gaudin R, Weiser J, et al. Osteonecrosis of the jaw in patients treated with denosumab: a multicenter case series. *J Craniomaxillofac Surg.* 2018;46(9):1515–1525.

130. Blanchaert RH. Implants in the medically challenged patient. *Dent Clin N Am.* 1998;42:1.

131. Hess LM, Jeter J, Benham-Hutchins M, et al. Factors associated with osteonecrosis of the jaw among bisphosphonate users. *Am J Med.* 2009;121:475–483. e3.

132. Shapiro CL. Bisphosphonate-related osteonecrosis of jaw in the adjuvant breast cancer setting: risks and perspective. *J Clin Oncol.* 2013;31:2648.

133. https://nei.nih.gov/health/maculardegen/armd_facts.

134. Tolentino M. Systemic and ocular safety of intravitreal anti-VEGF therapies for ocular neovascular disease. *Sur Ophthalmol.* 2011;56(2):95–113.

135. https://www.cdc.gov/arthritis/basics/fibromyalgia.htm.

136. Becker DE. Psychotropic drugs: implications for dental practice. *Anesth Prog.* 2008;55(3):89–99.

137. Devine M, Taylor S, Renton T. Chronic post-surgical pain following the placement of dental implants in the maxilla: a case series. *Eur J Oral Implantol.* 2016;9(suppl 2, [1]):179–186.

138. https://www.cancer.org/cancer/breast-cancer/about/how-common-is-breast-cancer.html.

139. Harvey JM, Clark GM, Osborne CK, Allred DC. Estrogen receptor status by immunohistochemistry is superior to the ligand-binding assay for predicting response to adjuvant endocrine therapy in breast cancer. *J Clin Oncol.* 1999;17(5):1474–1481.

140. Sadler GR, Stoudt A, Fullerton JT, et al. Managing the oral sequelae of cancer therapy. *Med surg Nurs.* 2003;12(1):28–36.

141. Watters AL, Epstein JB, Agulnik M. Oral complications of targeted cancer therapies: a narrative literature review. *Oral Oncol.* 2011;47(6):441–448. [PubMed].

142. Garcia DA, Regan S, Henault LE, et al. Risk of thromboembolism with short-term interruption of warfarin therapy. *Arch Intern Med.* 2008;168:63–69.

143. Brennan MT, et al. Aspirin use and post-operative bleeding from dental extractions. *J Dent Res.* 2008;87:740–744.

144. Gulpinar K, Suleyman O, Erpulat O, et al. A preliminary study: aspirin discontinuation before elective operations; when is the optimal timing? *J Korean Surg Soc.* 2013;85(4):185–190.

145. Gomez-Moreno G, Aguilar-Salvaterra A, Martin-Piedra MA, et al. Dabigatran and rivaroxaban, new oral anticoagulants, new approaches in dentistry. *J Clin Exp Dent.* 2010;2:e1–e5.

146. Firriolo JF, Hupp WS. Beyond warfarin: the new generation of oral anticoagulants and their implications for the management of dental patients. *Oral Surg Oral Med Oral Pathol Oral Radiol.* 2012;113(4):431–441.

147. Phillips KA, Veenstra DL. Potential role of pharmacogenics in reducing adverse drug reactions. *JAMA.* 2001;286:2270–2279.

148. Haney EM, Chan BKS, Diem SJ, et al. Association of low bone mineral density with selective serotonin reuptake inhibitor use by older men. *Arch Intern Med.* 2007;167(12):1246–1251.

149. Wu X, Al-Abedalla K, Rastikerdar E, et al. Selective serotonin reuptake inhibitors and the risk of osseointegrated implant failure: a cohort study. *J Dent Res.* 2014;93(11):1054–1061.

150. Witt JD, Swann M. Metal wear and tissue response in failed titanium alloy total hip replacements. *J Bone Joint Surg Br.* 1991;73:559–563.

151. Yamauchi R, Morita A, Tsuji T. Pacemaker dermatitis from titanium. *Contact Dermatitis.* 2000;42:52–53.

152. Siddiqi A, Payne AG, De Silva RK, et al. Titanium allergy: could it affect dental implant integration? *Clin Oral Implants Res.* 2011;22:673–680.

153. du Preez LA, Bütow KW, Swart TJ. Implant failure due to titanium hypersensitivity/allergy? Report of a case. *SADJ.* 2007;62:24–25.

154. Egusa H, Ko N, Shimazu T, Yatani H. Suspected association of an allergic reaction with titanium dental implants: a clinical report. *J Prosthet Dent.* 2008;100:344–347.

155. Sicilia A, Cuesta S, Coma G, et al. Titanium allergy in dental implant patients: a clinical study on 1500 consecutive patients. *Clin Oral Implants Res.* 2008;19:823–835.

156. Holgers KM, Roupe G, Tjellström A, Bjursten LM. Clinical, immunological and bacteriological evaluation of adverse reactions to skin-penetrating titanium implants in the head and neck region. *Contact Dermatitis.* 1992;27:1–7.

157. Hallab N, Merritt K, Jacobs JJ. Metal sensitivity in patients with orthopaedic implants. *J Bone Joint Surg Am.* 2001;83A:428–436.

158. Harloff T, Hönle W, Holzwarth U, et al. Titanium allergy or not? "Impurity" of titanium implant materials. *Health.* 2010;2:306–310.

11

Radiographic Evaluation in Oral Implantology

RANDOLPH R. RESNIK

dvances in radiologic imaging technology have had a significant impact on the surgical and prosthetic phases of
oral implantology. Comprehensive and accurate radiographic assessment is crucial and one of the most important
aspects of dental implant treatment planning. In the past, various imaging techniques have been used to evaluate bone quality,
quantity, and location of anatomic structures in relation to proposed implant sites. Traditionally, implant clinicians have relied
on two-dimensional (2D) conventional radiographic modalities
in implant dentistry that have inherent shortcomings. However, with the advent of computed tomography (CT) and cone
beam computed tomography (CBCT), a new era in all phases
of the radiographic imaging survey of implant patients has
become available to the implant clinician. These technological
advances have significantly increased the level of detailed information available to implant clinicians in the diagnosis, treatment planning, surgical, and prosthetic phases of dental implant
treatment. This chapter will comprehensively review the use of
various radiographic modalities and technology in the presurgical evaluation, treatment planning, and surgical, prosthetic, and
postoperative assessments of implant treatment.

Imaging Objectives in Oral Implantology

The objectives of diagnostic imaging depend on a number of factors, including the amount and type of information required and
the anatomic location of interest. The decision of when to image,
along with which imaging modality to use, depends on the integration of these factors and can be organized into three phases.

Phase 1

Phase 1 is termed presurgical implant imaging assessment and
involves all past radiologic examinations and new radiologic
examinations selected to assist the implant team in determining
the patient's final and comprehensive treatment plan. The objectives of this phase of imaging include all necessary surgical and
prosthetic information to determine the quantity, quality, and
angulations of bone; the relationship of critical structures to the
prospective implant sites; and the presence or absence of disease at
the proposed surgery sites.

Phase 2

Phase 2 consists of surgical and intraoperative implant imaging,
and is focused on assisting in the surgical and prosthetic phases of
intervention of the patient. The objectives of this phase of imaging are to evaluate the surgery sites during and immediately after
surgery, assist in the optimal position and orientation of dental
implants, evaluate the healing and integration phase of implant
surgery, and ensure that abutment position and prosthesis fabrication are correct.

Phase 3

Phase 3 is the final phase comprising the postprosthetic implant
imaging. This phase commences just after the prosthesis placement and continues as long as the implants remain in the jaws.
The objectives of this phase of imaging are to evaluate the long-
term maintenance of implant rigid fixation and function, including the crestal bone levels around each implant, and to evaluate
the implant prosthesis.

Presurgical Imaging (Phase 1)

In the field of oral implantology numerous radiographic imaging
modalities are available for the presurgical assessment of patients
with dental implants. Before cone beam computerized tomography, intraoral radiographs, along with 2D panoramic images, were
used as the sole determinants of implant diagnosis and treatment
planning. With the advancement of radiographic technology, various three-dimensional (3D) imaging systems are now common
place in the dental profession, allowing an unlimited amount of
diagnostic information to be available to the implant team.

The presurgical imaging phase of treatment is one of the most
important in the implant process. The goal of presurgical radiographic evaluation is to assess the available bone quality and
quantity, angulation of bone, and selection of potential implant
sites, and to verify the absence of pathology. With the popular use
of CBCT, the presurgical phase has become more user-friendly
and allows a comprehensive evaluation of the patient. In comparison with CBCT, other types of radiographic modalities (e.g.,
panoramic, periapical, cephalometric, conventional tomography)

have inherent advantages and disadvantages, and have been shown to exhibit false-negative and false-positive results.[1]

In dental and medical radiology a recommended principle when selecting the appropriate radiographic modality is based on radiation dosage. Dental professionals should always adhere to the "as low as reasonably achievable" (ALARA) principle. ALARA basically states that the diagnostic imaging technique selected should include the lowest possible radiation dose to the patient. The American Academy of Oral and Maxillofacial Radiology published guidelines stating that all implant site surveys should be evaluated with a 3D imaging technique such as CBCT or CT.[2] This phase of implant imaging is intended to evaluate the current status of the patient's teeth and bony anatomy, and to develop and refine the patient's treatment plan. Evaluation of the patient by members of the dental implant team is accomplished with a review of the patient's history, a thorough clinical examination, and a review of the patient's radiologic examinations. At this point the clinician should be able to rule out dental or bone disease, and establish a tentative clinical objective that meets the patient's functional and esthetic needs. If the dentist cannot rule out dental or bone disease, then a further clinical or radiologic examination is necessary. The ideal objective of this phase of treatment is to develop and implement a treatment plan for the

patient that enables restoration of the patient's function and esthetics by the accurate and strategic placement of dental implants. The patient's functional and esthetic needs can be transformed physically into a 3D diagnostic template that allows the implant team to identify the specific sites of prospective implant surgery in the imaging examinations. The specific objectives of preprosthetic imaging are listed in Box 11.1.

All of the modalities identified in Box 11.2 have been used in the first diagnostic phase of treatment in oral implantology.[3,4] However, dental implant cases are inherently 3D with respect to the final prosthetics, occlusion, and function of the patient's 3D anatomy. A 3D treatment plan ideally identifies at each prospective implant site the amount of bone width, the ideal position and orientation of each implant, its optimal length and diameter, the presence and amount of cortical bone on the crest, the degree of mineralization of trabecular bone, and the position or relationship of critical structures to the proposed implant sites. Therefore the modalities of choice for presurgical implant treatment planning most commonly utilize CBCT which provides high-resolution and dimensionally accurate 3D information about the patient at the proposed implant sites.

Radiographic Modalities Used in Oral Implantology

Periapical Radiograph

Periapical radiography (digital), one of the most commonly used radiographic modalities in dentistry, has many advantages, such as high resolution, low radiation, convenience, and image modification via digital software capability. However, the implant clinician must understand the inherent disadvantages of this radiologic technique when used in oral implantology.

1. *Image distortion:* Intraoral radiographs are inherently susceptible to image distortion and magnification because the object of interest does not have the same focal spot-to-object distance. When determining the location of anatomic structures the clinician should note that the image may contain distortion, and relying on exact measurements from these images should be cautioned. If the x-ray beam is perpendicular to the image receptor (film or sensor), but the object is not perpendicular to the image receptor and object, then dimensional changes such as foreshortening and elongation will occur (Fig. 11.1). Edentulous sites/quadrants are especially predisposed to these errors because flat maxillary palatal vaults, along with high muscle

---

> **• BOX 11.1** **Objectives of Preprosthetic Imaging**

- Identify normal versus abnormal anatomy.
- Identify anatomic variants.
- Determine bone quality.
- Determine bone quantity.
- Identify ideal implant positioning.
- Use for surgical templates.

> **• BOX 11.2** **Types of Imaging Modalities**

- Periapical
- Panoramic
- Occlusal
- Cephalometric
- Medical computerized technology
- Cone beam computerized technology
- Magnetic resonance imaging

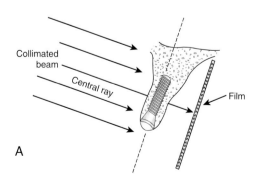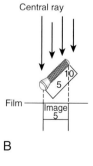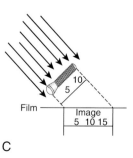

• Fig. 11.1 Film Positioning. (A) Ideally the central ray is perpendicular to the bone, object, and film, which results in minimal distortion. (B) The central ray is perpendicular to the film, but not to the implant, resulting in foreshortening. (C) The central ray is perpendicular to the object, but not the film, resulting in elongation. (*From Resnik RR, Preece JW. Radiographic complications and evaluation. In: Resnik RR, Misch CE, eds. Misch's Avoiding Complications in Oral Implantology. St. Louis, MO: Elsevier; 2018.*)

attachments in the mandible, make accurate positioning of the image receptor difficult.

2. *Two-dimensional radiographic modality:* A true evaluation and determination of the buccal-lingual available bone must be ascertained to evaluate the osseous contours of the existing bone. Because periapical radiography is 2D, vital information on the width of available bone is not obtained. Therefore when attempting to estimate width distances in close approximation to maxillary and mandibular anatomic structures with 2D radiographs, the implant clinician must be conscious of the inherent inaccuracies associated with 2D images.

3. *Poor identification of vital structures:* When evaluating the position of vital structures with intraoral radiographs, extreme caution should be exercised. In the evaluation of the true location of the mental foramen, studies have shown less than 50% of periapical radiographs depict the correct location of the mental foramen.[5] Other studies have concluded that because of insufficient cortical bone around the mandibular canal (MC), only 28% of periapical radiographs will accurately identify the MC.[3] Therefore periapical radiographs exhibit relatively high false-positives and false-negatives with respect to the identification of vital anatomic structures.

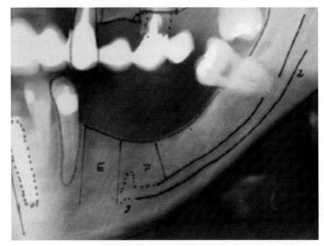

● **Fig. 11.2** All two-dimensional panoramic radiographs exhibit magnification, distortion, overlapping of images, and ghost images, making these images inaccurate as the sole determination for dental implant diagnosis. Therefore panoramic radiographs should not be used for final measurements or determination of vital structures.

Uses in Oral Implantology

Periapical radiographs have many inherent disadvantages, most notably providing only a 2D image of a 3D object. The inability to determine the buccal-lingual bony dimensions is a major shortcoming with respect to implant treatment planning. These radiographs are of little value in determining quantity and quality of bone, identifying vital structures, and depicting the spatial relationship between structures within proposed implant sites. In summary, periapical radiographs should be limited to an initial evaluation of a proposed implant site, intraoperative evaluation, and postoperative assessment.

In terms of the objectives of presurgical imaging, periapical radiography is:

- a useful high-yield modality for ruling out local bone or dental disease;
- limited value in determining quantity because the image is magnified, may be distorted, and does not depict the third dimension (bone width);
- limited value in determining bone density or mineralization (the lateral cortical plates prevent accurate interpretation and cannot differentiate subtle trabecular bone changes); and
- has poor ability in depicting the spatial relationship between the anatomic structures and the proposed implant site.

Panoramic Radiograph

Panoramic radiography is a curved plane tomographic radiographic technique used to depict the body of the mandible, maxilla, and the maxillary sinuses in a single image. Its convenience, speed, and ease have made this type of radiography a popular technique in evaluating the gross anatomy of the jaws. However, the implant clinician must understand the inherent fundamental limitations characteristic of this type of radiograph.

1. *Magnification/Distortion:* All panoramic radiographs exhibit vertical and horizontal magnification, together with a tomographic section thickness that varies according to the anatomic position. Because the x-ray source exposes the jaws using a negative angulation (~8%) to avoid superimposing the occipital bone/base of the skull over the anterior dental region, variable magnification will always be present on panoramic radiographs. Increased magnification stems from variances in patient positioning, focal object distance, the relative location of the rotation center of the x-ray system, and variations in normal anatomic form and size from one patient to the next. Zarch et al.[4] have shown that 83% of panoramic measurements are underestimated, with the greatest magnification being present in the anterior region (Fig. 11.2).

   a. *Horizontal magnification* is determined by the position of the object within the focal trough. The degree of horizontal magnification depends on the distance of the object from the focal trough center and is influenced by the patient's anatomy and positioning within the panoramic machine. In the anterior region the horizontal magnification will increase significantly as the object moves away from the focal trough. This results in anterior magnification being far greater and more variable than posterior magnification.

   b. *Vertical magnification* is determined by the differences between the x-ray source and object. Because the beam angle is directed at a negative [upward] angulation, structures positioned closer to the source are projected higher within the image in relation to structures positioned farther from the x-ray source. Therefore the vertical plane spatial relationships between objects projected on a panoramic radiograph are inaccurate.

2. *Two-dimensional radiographic modality:* The panoramic radiograph is a 2D image depicting 3D structures. Accordingly, it does not demonstrate the buccal-lingual dimension of maxillofacial structures; therefore bone width and vital structures cannot be determined. In addition, it produces a flattened, spread-out image of curved structures, which results in significant distortion of the vital structures and their relationship in space.

3. *Identification of vital structures:* Panoramic radiography does not exhibit an accurate assessment of bone quality/mineralization and the true identification and location of vital structures.

   a. *Visibility of Mental Foramen:* Caution must be exercised in using panoramic images as the definitive diagnostic modality in evaluating the location and visibility of the MC.

Lindh et al.[6] have shown that the MC cortical walls were visible in only 36.7% of panoramic radiographs.

b. *Mental foramen location:* The location of the mental foramen has high patient variability. Yosue and Brooks,[7] in evaluation of the mental foramen, concluded that more than 50% of radiographs will not depict the true location of the mental foramen.

c. *Linear measurements:* Because of the inherent panoramic magnification and distortion disadvantages, calculating linear measurements on panoramic images is inaccurate. Sonic et al.[8] reported in determination of linear measurements for bone assessment with respect to vital structures, an inaccuracy rate of 24% has been shown.

d. *Anterior loops:* The anterior course of the mental nerve in relation to the mental foramen must be identified to prevent neurosensory impairment. Studies completed by Kuzmanovic et al.[9] of anterior loops (mental nerve courses anteriorly to the mental foramen) concluded panoramic radiographs exhibit a high incidence of false-positives and false-negative results, thus being totally inaccurate.

e. *Location of septa:* Septum in the maxillary sinus complicate bone grafting and implant placement. In evaluation of maxillary sinus floor bony septa by Krennmair et al.,[10] correct identification and location have been shown to be approximately 21.3%.

f. *Identification of accessory foramina:* A common anatomic variant in the mandible is the presence of two mental foramen. Accessory (double) foramina have been shown to be identified accurately in less than 50% of panoramic radiographs.[11]

Use in Oral Implantology

Although panoramic radiographs have historically been the gold standard in evaluating potential implant sites, many disadvantages are associated with these types of radiographs. A lower resolution prevents evaluation of the fine detail that is required for the assessment of osseous structures and anatomy. The magnification in the horizontal and vertical planes are nonuniform; thus linear measurements are inaccurate. Often the image has superimposition of real, double, and ghost images, which result in difficulty in visualizing anatomic and pathologic details. The true positions of important vital structures, which are crucial in dental implant treatment, are not easily seen or incorrectly depicted. Therefore panoramic radiographs have value for initial evaluation; however, caution should be exercised when using these types of radiographs for the sole determinant of implant placement because they predispose the implant clinician to many surgical, prosthetic, and medical-legal complications (Fig. 11.3).

Magnetic Resonance Imaging

Magnetic resonance imaging (MRI) is a cross-sectional imaging technique that produces images of thin slices of tissue with excellent spatial resolution. This imaging modality developed by Lauterbur[12] in 1972 uses a combination of magnetic fields that generate images of tissues in the body without the use of ionizing radiation. MRI allows complete flexibility in the positioning and angulation of image sections and can reproduce multiple slices simultaneously. Digital MRI images are characterized by voxels, with an in-plane resolution measured in pixels and millimeters, and a section thickness measured in millimeters (2–3 mm) for high-resolution imaging acquisitions. The image sequences used

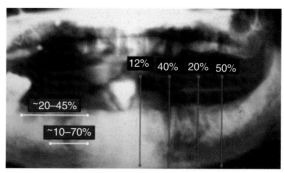

• **Fig. 11.3** Panoramic showing nonuniform magnification in the vertical and horizontal plane depicting inaccurate measurements. Magnification is highly variable, especially in the horizontal plane. (*From Resnik RR, Preece JW. Radiographic complications and evaluation. In: Resnik RR, Misch CE, eds.* Misch's Avoiding Complications in Oral Implantology. *St. Louis, MO: Elsevier; 2018.*)

to obtain magnetic resonance images can be varied to obtain fat, water, or balanced imaging of the patient's anatomy. The images created by MRI are the result of signals generated by hydrogen protons in water or fat such that cortical bone will appear black (radiolucent) or as having no signal. Cancellous bone will generate a signal and will appear white because it contains fatty marrow. Metal restorations will not produce scattering and thus will appear as black images. Therefore MRI has been shown to be less prone to artifacts from dental restorations, prostheses, and dental implants than CT or CBCT scans.[13] As with CT, MRI is a quantitatively accurate technique with exact tomographic sections and no distortion.

Numerous authors have suggested the use of MRI for dental implant evaluation and treatment planning.[14] Vital structures are easily viewed, such as the inferior alveolar canal and the maxillary sinus. In cases where the inferior alveolar canal cannot be differentiated by conventional tomography or CT, MRI would be a viable alternative because the trabecular bone is easily differentiated with the inferior alveolar canal. In cases of nerve impairment or infection (osteomyelitis), MRI may be used because of added advantages including differentiation of soft tissue with respect to CT. Studies have shown that the geometric accuracy of the mandibular nerve with MRI is comparable with CT and is an accurate imaging method for dental implant treatment planning.[15] MRI may be used in implant imaging as a secondary imaging technique when primary imaging techniques such as complex tomography or CBCT fail. Complex tomography fails to differentiate the inferior alveolar canal in 60% of implant cases, and CT fails to differentiate the inferior alveolar canal in about 2% of implant cases. Failure to differentiate the inferior alveolar canal may be caused by osteoporotic trabecular bone and poorly corticated inferior alveolar canal.[16] MRI visualizes the fat in trabecular bone and differentiates the inferior alveolar canal and neurovascular bundle from the adjacent trabecular bone. Double-scout MRI protocols with volume and oriented cross-sectional imaging of the mandible produce orthogonal quantitative contiguous images of the proposed implant sites. Oriented MRI of the posterior mandible is dimensionally quantitative and enables spatial differentiation between critical structures and the proposed implant site. Recent advances in MRI have allowed for higher image resolution, similar to the resolution produced on CBCT scans, with voxel sizes of 300 to 400 μm^3. In addition, technology has allowed for shorter image acquisition times of only 3 to 4 minutes.[17] However, there exist numerous disadvantages for the use of MRI for implant dentistry.

MRI is not useful in characterizing bone mineralization or as a high-yield technique for identifying bone or dental disease. In addition, no commercially available reformatting programs are available to use as reference points.

Use in Oral Implantology

In oral implantology, because of the imaging artifacts associated with CBCT scans, MRI is a possible alternative for the postoperative evaluation of dental implants, especially if associated with a neurosensory impairment (Fig. 11.4).

Cone Beam Tomography (CBCT)

With the advent of cone beam computerized tomography, many of the disadvantages of 2D radiographs and conventional medical CT scanners have been overcome. CBCT has been one of the most significant technological breakthroughs in oral implantology today. Because of the low radiation dose inherent with cone beam technology, the limitations of medical computerized tomography have been overcome. This scanning technology has many advantages, including "in-office" installation and use, which allow the clinician and patient the convenience of on-site scanning capabilities and treatment planning. In addition, the scanning speed (<5 seconds) and integration of interactive software programs have brought an unparalleled advantage to the implant clinician for the evaluation and assessment of potential implant sites.

Today CBCT imaging has become the gold standard for dental implant treatment planning. However, many implant clinicians lack the background and knowledge in evaluating and treatment planning with CBCT, thus predisposing to possible complications. Therefore the implant clinician must have a thorough understanding of inherent disadvantages of CBCT scans, together with knowledge of applied head and neck anatomy, anatomic variants, incidental findings, and pathologic conditions with respect to implant treatment planning.

CBCT images are a result of data collected by numerous detectors and ionizing chambers in the CBCT unit. The data collected by the detectors correspond to a composite of the absorption characteristics of the tissues and structures imaged. This information is transformed into images (raw data) that are reformatted into a voxel (digital) volume for evaluation and analysis. The integration of digital imaging systems in the field of implant dentistry has significantly increased clinicians' diagnostic capabilities. A digital 2D image is described by an image matrix that has individual picture elements called *pixels*. A digital image is described by its width, height, and pixels (i.e., 512 Å~ 512). For larger digital images (i.e., 1.2 M Å~ 1.2 M, where M is megapixels), the image is alternatively described as a 1.5-M image. Each picture element, or pixel, has a discrete digital value that describes the image intensity at that particular point. The value of a pixel element is described by a scale, which may be as low as 8 bits (256 values) or as high as 12 bits (4096 values) for black and white imaging systems, or 36 bits (65 billion values) for color imaging systems. Nine to 11

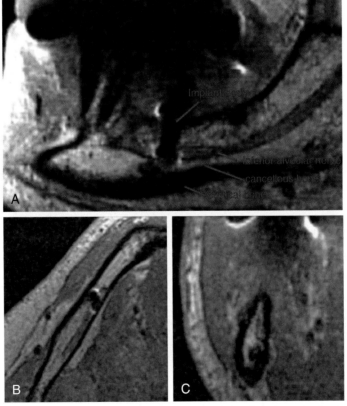

• **Fig. 11.4** Acquired magnetic resonance images—(A) sagittal, (B) axial, and (C) coronal—for three-dimensional assessment of bone after implant placement, with a display of the implant located in the inferior alveolar canal. (*From Wanner L, et al. Magnetic resonance imaging—a diagnostic tool for postoperative evaluation of dental implants: a case report.* Oral Surg Oral Med Oral Pathol Oral Radiol. *2018;125:e103-e107.*)

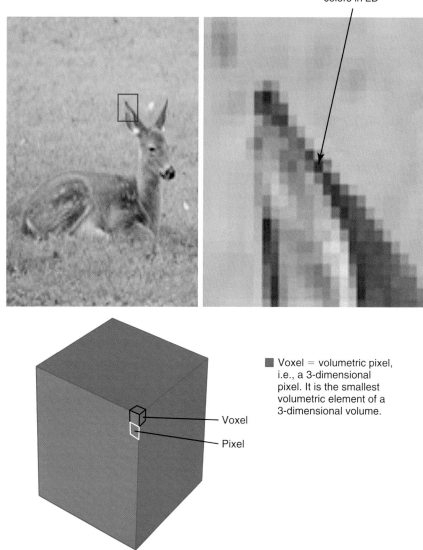

Pixel
The smallest component of an image, which reflects colors in 2D

Voxel = volumetric pixel, i.e., a 3-dimensional pixel. It is the smallest volumetric element of a 3-dimensional volume.

— Voxel

— Pixel

• **Fig. 11.5** The final computed tomography image depends on the pixel (two-dimensional [2D]) and the voxel (three-dimensional) size. (*From Resnik RR, Misch CE. Radiographic imaging in implant dentistry. In: Misch CE, ed.* Dental Implant Prosthetics. *2nd ed. St. Louis, MO: Elsevier; 2015.*)

black and white digital images are displayed optimally on a dedicated black and white monitor. Generally 8 bits, or 256 levels, can be displayed effectively on a monitor. A digital 3D image is described by an image matrix that has individual image or picture elements called *voxels*. A digital 3D image is described not only by its width and height of pixels (i.e., 512 Å~ 512) but also by its depth and thickness. An imaging volume or 3D characterization of the patient is produced by contiguous images, which produce a 3D structure of volume elements (i.e., CT, MRI, and interactive computed tomography [ICT]).

Each volume element has a value that describes its intensity level. Typically 3D modalities have an intensity scale of 12 bits, or 4096 values. The 2D digital images are composed of pixels (2D) and voxels (3D) picture elements. Pixels and voxels possess attributes of size, location, and grayscale value. Each voxel and pixel displayed is characterized by a numerical value that represents the density of the tissues. This is termed the *CT number*. A specific shade of gray or density value is assigned to each CT number that comprises the images (Fig. 11.5).

CT images are inherently 3D images that are typically 512 Å~ 512 pixels with a thickness described by the slice spacing of the imaging technique. Each voxel has a value, referred to in Hounsfield units (HUs), that describes the density of each image. The range of these units is −1000 (air) to +3000 (enamel) HUs (Box 11.3). Most CT scanners are standardized with a Hounsfield value of 0 for water. The CT density scale is quantitative and meaningful in identifying and differentiating structures and tissues (Box 11.4).

Types of Computed Tomography Scanners

Medical

In medical radiology departments the CT scan is the most common diagnostic imaging modality to evaluate hard and soft tissues.

• BOX 11.3 Bone Quality

Density	Hounsfield Units
D1	1250
D2	850–1250
D3	350–850
D4	0–350
D5	<0

• BOX 11.4 Tissue Characterization

Material	Hounsfield Units (HU)
Air	−1000
Water	0
Muscle	35–70
Trabecular bone	150–900
Cortical bone	900–1800
Dentin	1600–2400
Enamel	2500–3000
Extraction Socket	−700
Inferior Alveolar Canal	−700
Mental Foramen	−400
Soft Tissue	300–0

From Patrick, S., Birur, N. P., Gurushanth, K., Raghavan, A. S., & Gurudath, S. (2017). Comparison of gray values of cone-beam computed tomography with hounsfield units of multislice computed tomography: An in vitro study. Indian Journal of Dental Research, 28(1), 66.

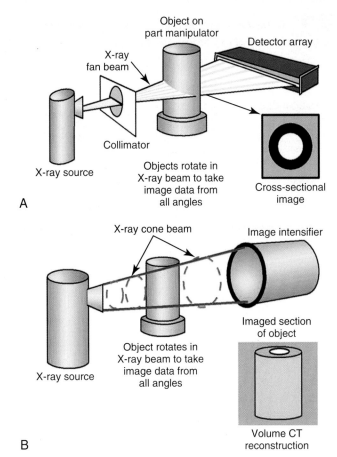

• **Fig. 11.6** (A) A conventional computed tomography (CT) scan uses a very narrow "fan beam" that rotates around the patient, acquiring one thin slice (image) with each revolution. Because of the numerous revolutions needed, the radiation dose is increased. (B) Cone beam volumetric tomography captures all data in one rotation, thus reducing radiation and avoiding distortion and errors in reformatting. (*From Resnik RR, Misch CE. Radiographic imaging in implant dentistry. In: Misch CE, ed. Dental Implant Prosthetics. 2nd ed. St. Louis, MO: Elsevier; 2015.*)

Advances in speed and image quality were apparent in the early 1990s with the advent of spiral and helical CT scanners. However, since its introduction in 1998, multislice (multirow detector CT) has revolutionized the field of medical CT. These CT scanning units are tomographic machines that are classified as 4-, 8-, 12-, 16-, 32-, or 64-slice machines. The number of slices corresponds to the number of times the x-ray beam rotates around the patient's head to acquire the CT data. The CT numbers, or Hounsfield units, are then reconstructed mathematically and formatted into images. However, because these images consist of a series of incremental images grouped together, CT spiral slices produce "average" reconstructed images based on multiple x-rays transversing the scanning area. With this reconstruction of images, a small gap between each slice is present, which contributes to an inherent error within medical scanners.

In the 1980s cross-sectional reconstruction of the CT images dramatically improved the diagnosis and treatment planning in oral implantology. These reformatted images allowed 3D evaluation of vital structures and related oral anatomy. However, even though these advances enhanced diagnostic skills, there were inherent shortcomings to medical scanners used for dental purposes. Because medical scanners were not developed for dental reformatting, there existed inherent errors such as distortion, magnification, and positioning problems that led to inaccuracies when reformatted. In addition, no prosthetic information could be gathered to predict the final prosthetic outcome. This was overcome with the advent of sophisticated scanning appliances, stereolithographic resin bone models, virtual teeth technology, interactive software, computer-generated surgical guides, and CT-based image-guided navigation systems, which allowed for ideal placement and prosthetic outcome to be established.

Although the clinical problems of medical scanners have been remedied, numerous disadvantages remain, including radiation exposure and availability. The amount of radiation exposure of medical scans has been a controversial topic for many years and has been shown to be excessive. The availability has dramatically improved over the years with the advent of cone beam computed technology (Fig. 11.6A).

To overcome some of the disadvantages of conventional medical CT scanners, CBCT has become extremely popular (Table 11.1 and Fig. 11.6B). Because conventional CT is associated with high radiation doses, this medical imaging technique has always been under significant criticism when used for implant treatment planning. However, with the advent of cone beam technology, the limitations of medical CT have been overcome. With cone beam technology, there exists the ability to provide more accurate diagnostic images, along with a fraction of the radiation exposure with conventional CT and adherence to the ALARA principle.[18] Cone beam scanners are made for "in-office" installation and use, allowing the doctor and patient the convenience of on-site scanning capabilities (Fig. 11.7).

CBCT scanners use a rotating x-ray source that generates a conical-shaped beam that can be modified to acquire a desired area of interest. The attenuated x-ray beam data are collected by a

TABLE 11.1	Comparison of Medical Spiral Scanners and Cone Beam Computed Tomography	
Specifications	Medical	Cone Beam
Scanning time	~1–4 minutes	~5–60 seconds
Radiation exposure	More	Less
Scan	Multiple slices	One rotation
Exposed field	One arch at a time	Both arches simultaneously
Scatter	More	Less
Positioning	Very technique sensitive	Much easier

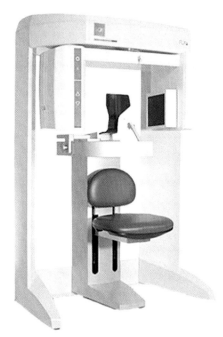

• **Fig. 11.7** Cone beam computed tomography (CBCT) unit: I-Cat Unit with only minimal space requirements (4 × 4 foot footprint).

single collector. These data are then converted to various shades of gray, which are displayed on a computer screen. Reconstruction of these images can be in any plane by simply realigning the image or voxel data. This allows viewing of the data in axial, sagittal, coronal, panoramic, 3D, and soft tissue images (Fig. 11.8).

Focal Spot. The clarity of CT scan images is not dependent on the voxel size. Actually a CBCT unit may have a very small voxel size; however, image quality may be compromised because of a large focal spot. The focal spot is the area of the x-ray tube that emits the x-rays. In general the smaller the focal spot, the sharper the final image quality. Thus a larger source or focal spot will result in projections of shadows of the scanned area, which will result in blurring of the object. This penumbra or blurring of the edges creates a shadow with resultant poor image quality and clarity.

Current CBCT units have focal spots ranging from 0.15 to 0.7 mm (Fig. 11.9).

Field of View. CBCT units vary on the area of interest or what is commonly termed the *field of view* (FOV) in radiology. The FOV describes the scan volume, which is dependent on many factors, including the detector size and shape, beam projection geometry, and beam collimation. Beam collimation is paramount in decreasing radiation exposure to the patient and ensuring only the area of interest to be radiated. Usually smaller scan volumes produce higher resolution images. Currently, CBCT units are classified as small, mid, or large FOVs (Fig. 11.10).

Effective Dose Range of Cone Beam Computed Tomography Scanners. Because of the increasing number of CBCT units being developed and released on the market, it is difficult to generalize radiation dose of CBCT. These units exhibit a wide variation of exposure parameters, such as x-ray spectrum (voltage peak and filtration), x-ray exposure (mA and number of projections), and FOV. Thus the range of units and imaging protocols will result in different absorbed radiation doses.

The effective dose measured in microsieverts is still the most accepted way to determine radiation risk for patients. A number of studies have measured the effective dose on dental CBCT units using thermoluminescent dosimeters with dosimetry phantoms. The phantoms are placed into multiple layers along the axial plane to allow for access to internal anatomy. The thermoluminescent dosimeters are placed on the radiosensitive area to be tested (i.e., ramus, symphysis, thyroid, salivary glands). The operator may control the FOV, kVp, mA, and scanning times to reduce the effective dose. However, these reductions result in a decreased signal and poorer image quality (Fig. 11.11).

Sensor (Detector) Type. The x-ray sensor receives the x-rays and converts them into electrical data, which are then converted to various images via special computer programs. Two types of sensors are used today in CBCT technology: (1) image intensifiers (IIs) with charged coupling devices, and (2) flat panel detectors. Image intensifiers have many disadvantages in comparison with flat panel detectors, including having poorer resolution, being bulkier, and requiring a higher patient radiation dose. Flat panel detectors, although more expensive than image intensifiers, produce images with much higher quality and resolution. Most flat panel detectors used today in CBCT units utilize cesium iodide as the scintillator crystal screen. Cesium iodide scintillators produce the highest spatial resolution possible among various CBCT screens.

Voxel Size. The unit element in the 3D image is termed the *voxel*, which is analogous to the 2D pixel. Images comprised of multiple voxels are stacked in rows or columns that are isotropic. Isotropic correlates to equal dimensions in the x, y, and z planes, and ranges in size from 0.075 to 0.6 mm. Each individual voxel is assigned a grayscale value that corresponds to the attenuation value of the anatomic structure. Thus the smaller the voxel size, the greater the resolution and quality of the image; however, the greater the resultant radiation dose. A voxel size of 0.2 to 0.3 mm is considered ideal because it allows for an equitable trade-off between image quality and absorbed radiation dose (Fig. 11.12).

Spatial Resolution. Spatial resolution is measured in lines per millimeter (lp/mm) and relates to the ability to distinguish two anatomically close objects. On a CBCT image the higher the spatial resolution, the greater the ability to delineate two different objects from one another. Normally, CBCT scanners (voxel size, 0.075–0.6 mm) are most commonly associated with higher spatial resolution than medical-grade scanners (voxel size, 0.6–1 mm). However, decreased spatial resolution on CBCT images may result from: (1) the use of a higher voxel size (>0.4; use of voxel sizes > 0.3 mm for implants is not recommended because of

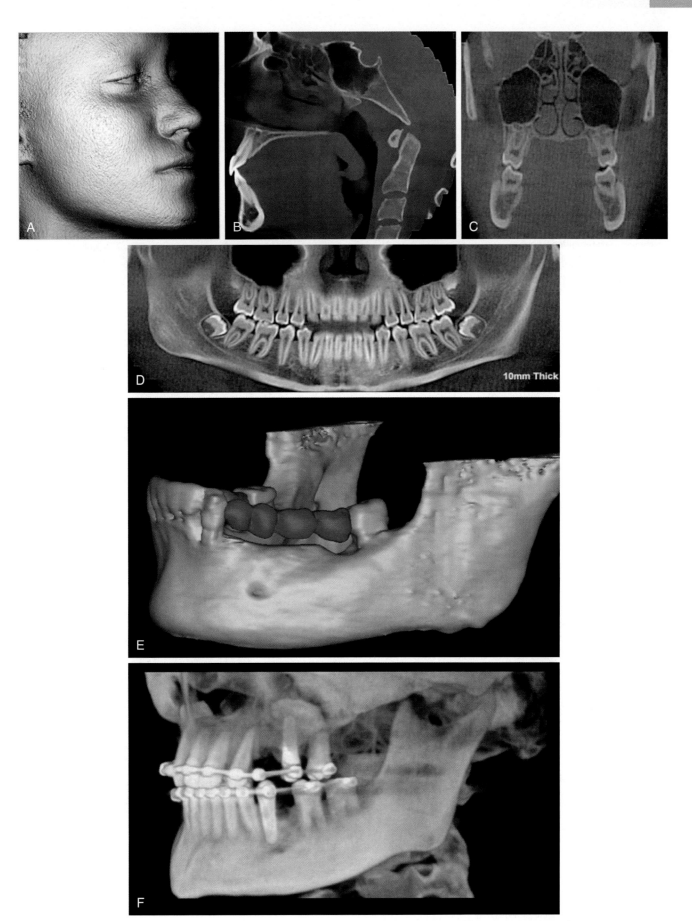

• **FIG. 11.8** Cone Beam Images. (A) Three-dimensional soft tissue image. (B) Lateral cephalometric image. (C) Coronal image. (D) Panoramic image. (E) Lateral osseous image. (F) Maximum intensity projection image (MIP).

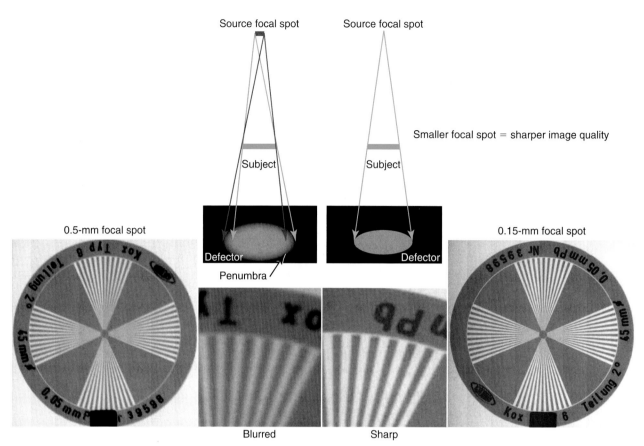

Source focal spot   Source focal spot

Smaller focal spot = sharper image quality

Subject   Subject

0.5-mm focal spot   0.15-mm focal spot

Defector   Defector

Penumbra

Blurred   Sharp

• **Fig. 11.9** Focal Spot. Example showing the difference between a 0.15- and a 0.5-mm focal spot depicting a smaller focal spot is associated with a sharper image. (*From Resnik RR, Misch CE. Radiographic imaging in implant dentistry. In: Misch CE, ed.* Dental Implant Prosthetics. *2nd ed. St. Louis, MO: Elsevier; 2015.*)

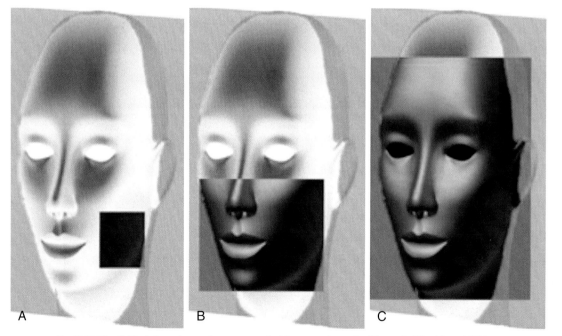

A   B   C

• **Fig. 11.10** The field of view of cone beam computed tomography units: (A) small, (B) mid, and (C) large. (*From Resnik RR, Misch CE. Radiographic imaging in implant dentistry. In: Misch CE, ed.* Dental Implant Prosthetics. *2nd ed. St. Louis, MO: Elsevier; 2015.*)

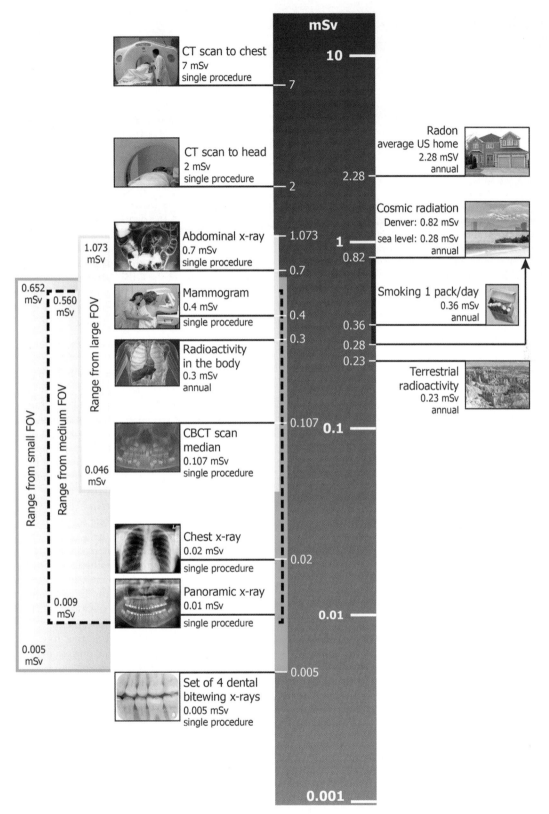

• **Fig. 11.11** Effective dose (microsieverts [mSv]) from cone beam computed tomography (CT) compared with other dose metrics. FOV, field of view. (*From Aanenson JW, Till JE, Grogan HA. Understanding and communicating radiation dose and risk from cone beam computed tomography in dentistry.* J Prosthet Dent. *2018;120:353-360.*)

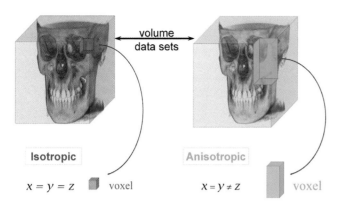

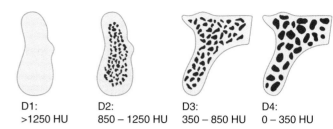

D1:	D2:	D3:	D4:
>1250 HU	850 – 1250 HU	350 – 850 HU	0 – 350 HU

• **Fig. 11.13** Hounsfield unit correlation with the Misch bone density classification (D1–D4).

• **Fig. 11.12** Comparison of volume data sets obtained isotropically (left) and anisotropically (right). Because cone beam computed tomography data acquisition depends on the pixel size of the area detector and not on the acquisition of groups of rows with sequential translational motion, the compositional voxels are equal in all three dimensions, rather than columnar, with height being different from the width and depth dimensions. *(From Scarfe WC, Farman AG. What is cone-beam CT and how does it work? Dent Clin North Am. 2008;52:707-730.)*

the lower spatial resolution); (2) decreased radiation (kVp or mA), which results in increased noise; (3) metallic restorations or dental implants resulting in artifacts; and (4) increased focal spot size.

Contrast Resolution. Contrast resolution is defined as the ability to differentiate tissues of different radiodensities. Ideally, in implant dentistry the ability to produce different shades of gray is important for a clearly diagnostic image. Because CBCT images use less radiation and are produced with lower kVp and mA settings in comparison with MDCT (Multi-Detector Computerized Tomography) units, dental CBCT is associated with slightly higher image contrast, modifiable through software settings. Dental CBCT generally has increased noise and image scatter compared with medical units. A smaller FOV may be used to minimize noise and scatter. However, smaller FOVs are usually associated with slightly higher radiation settings.

Bit Depth. The quality of CBCT images is directly related to the number of shades of gray (bit depth). CBCT units today produce up to 16-bit images, which corresponds to 2^{16} (65,536 shades of gray). However, computer monitors may display up to only 8 bits (2^8; 256 shades of gray). The monitor brightness and contrast may be adjusted to display 8 bits per image, to increase the quality of the image.

Bone Density

MDCT/CBCT. Medical CT data have inherently higher contrast resolution in comparison with dental CBCT images, and medical units permit differentiating between tissues that have a physical density of less than 1%. In contrast, conventional radiography requires a minimum of 10% difference in physical density to be seen.[19] Each medical CT image is composed of pixels and voxels, which are characterized by a given numerical value, which reflects the x-ray beam attenuation. These values are directly affected by the density and thickness of the tissue. These HUs or CT numbers correlate with the density of the medical CT image and range in value from –1000 (air) to +3000 (enamel). A specific shade of gray or density number is assigned to each CT number, which ultimately forms the image. The correlation of these CT numbers has been used to associate the density of the area of interest with various bone densities used for surgical and prosthetic treatment planning. Thus the gray values depicted on medical CT images are considered true attenuation x-ray values (HUs) (Fig. 11.13). When evaluating dental CBCT images in regard to bone density, a direct correlation (accuracy of measurement) does not exist compared with medical CT. Most dental CBCT systems

inherently have an increased variation and inconsistency with density estimates. The density estimates of gray levels (brightness values) are not true attenuation values (HUs), thus inaccuracies in bone density estimates result.[20] This is mainly due to the high level of noise in the acquired images and the slight inconsistencies in the sensitivity of the CBCT detectors. Dental imaging software frequently provides attenuation values (HUs); however, such values should be recognized as approximations lacking the precision of HU values derived from medical CT units.

Scanning Technique

1. *Imaging protocol:* The patient should be positioned within the CBCT unit as per manufacturer's recommendations. When taking the scan, the teeth should be slightly separated so that the different arches may be easily differentiated on re-formation. Cotton rolls, tongue depressors, or a bite registration may be used. In addition, cotton rolls may be placed in the vestibule to separate the lips and cheeks from the buccal mucosa. This will allow for a more accurate representation of the contour and thickness of the gingival tissues.
2. *Position of the scanning template:* The position of the scanning template/radiographic markers in the mouth during CBCT examination is crucial for the accuracy of fabrication of the surgical template. First, it is recommended that an index be used to position and maintain the scanning template in the correct position. This will prevent inaccuracies and help stabilize the template in the mouth. In addition, tissue conditioner or denture adhesive may be used for CBCT templates that are ill fitting or have associated movement.
3. *Mucosal thickness:* When fabricating mucosa-supported surgical guides, the thickness of the mucosa may have a direct effect on the accuracy of the of the planning of the implant sites. Increased mucosa thickness may lead to inaccurate placement of the mucosa-borne guides during the surgical placement procedure. Vasak et al.[21] showed a 1.0-mm buccal mucosa thickness may result in a buccal-lingual deviation larger than 0.41 mm. This will inevitably cause inaccurate measurements and possible misalignment of the surgical guide when placing the implants.

Artifacts

1. *Beam hardening:* Because metallic objects in the oral cavity are associated with higher attenuation coefficients than soft tissue, dental CBCT images inherently are predisposed to these artifacts. One of the most common types of artifacts is termed *beam hardening.* Beam hardening occurs when x-rays travel through the bone/implant, resulting in more low-energy photons being absorbed than high-energy photons. Because of this, the image will have compromised image quality.[22] The titanium alloy

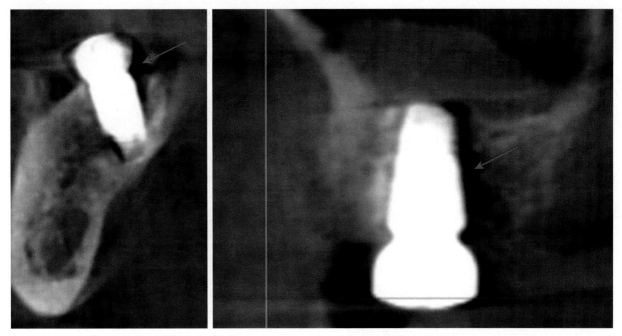

• **Fig. 11.14** Beam Hardening Artifacts. These radiolucent areas next to an implant are caused by the dense nature of titanium implants and the exposure of more low-energy photons (red arrows).

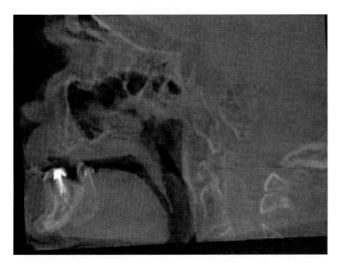

• **Fig. 11.15** Motion artifact due to movement of the patient, leading to overlapping "double images." Usually stand-up CBCT units have a higher incidence of motion-related artifacts. (*From Resnik RR, Preece JW. Radiographic complications and evaluation. In: Resnik RR, Misch CE, eds. Misch's Avoiding Complications in Oral Implantology. St. Louis, MO: Elsevier; 2018.*)

surface is highly susceptible to these types of artifacts because of the high-density nature of the metal. This results in inaccuracies, especially when viewing peri-implant bone levels. Conventional intraoral images will not exhibit these beam hardening artifacts and may appropriately be used to better evaluate the quality and quantity of bone mesial and distal to an implant when beam hardening artifacts may obliterate visualization of interproximal bone, especially when multiple implants are present in the same quadrant. In addition, higher density materials commonly found in the oral cavity (i.e., dental implants, metal based restorations) will lead to complete absorption of the beam and beam hardening artifacts.[23]

Two types of beam hardening artifacts exist that result in linear areas of dark bands or streaks between dense objects and cupping artifacts. Cupping artifacts occur when x-rays pass through the center of a highly dense object and are absorbed more than the peripheral x-rays. This results in an image in which a uniformly dense object appears to be less dense (darker, lower CT numbers) at its center and appears as a "cup" (Fig. 11.14).

2. *Motion-related artifacts:* Motion artifacts are usually the result of patient movement and result in the inaccurate depiction of bony landmarks, measurements, and implants.[24] Patient movements and incorrect patient positioning create blurring problems, double-density line artifacts adjacent to major bony structures, which result in nondiagnostic images. Patients should be instructed to not move and avoid swallowing throughout the scan. The motion blurring causes "double contours" of anatomic structures that result in decreased scan quality and spatial resolution. This may lead to improper implant placement and possible damage to neural structures.[25] Motion-related artifacts may be decreased by using sit-down CBCT units, head restraints, or decreasing scanning times (Fig. 11.15).

3. *Streak (scatter) artifacts:* CBCT images are susceptible to streak artifacts that are caused by x-rays traveling through objects with a high atomic number (metallic restorations). Streak artifacts usually are seen as light and dark lines that arise from the source object, resulting in images with decreased quality and obscuring of anatomic structures. This is caused by photons (x-rays) that are deflected from their original path by metallic objects. When these deflected photons reach the sensor (detector), the intensity of the signal is magnified in a nonuniform magnitude. The end result is an image with decreased resolution and image quality, which ultimately lead to inaccuracies in the reconstructed CT number or voxel density.[26] The FOV of the CBCT is proportional to the amount of scattering, thus smaller FOVs are associated with less scattering. In comparison of scattering with MDCT and CBCT, CBCT images have inherently greater scatter radiation than medical-grade CT images[27] (Figs. 11.16 and 11.17).

4. *Noise:* Two types of noise are associated with CBCT images: additive (results from electrical noise) and photon count (quantum noise). Because CBCT scanners operate at much

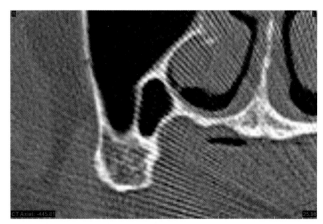

• **Fig. 11.16** Image depicting "streaks" that result from the metal restorations.

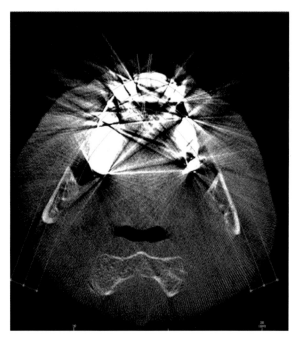

• **Fig. 11.17** Image showing significant streak artifacts that result in total obliteration of the associated anatomy. These artifacts result from full-arch porcelain fused to metal restoration.

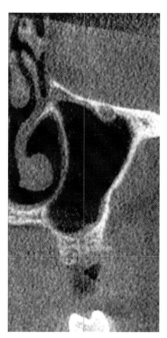

• **Fig. 11.18** Image showing resultant noise (grainy appearance).

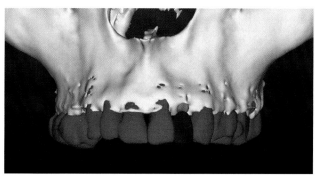

• **Fig. 11.19** Bone dehiscence on three-dimensional images that is caused by reformatting with too high of Hounsfield unit threshold.

lower amperage (mA) settings than MDCT scanners, CBCT images are associated with greater quantum noise. The noise is displayed as a "graining" of the image and is the result of inconsistent distribution of the signal, which results in inconsistent attenuation (gray) values in the projection images (Fig. 11.18).

5. *Bone dehiscence on 3D reformatted images:* MDCT and dental CBCT data have the ability to be reformatted by software algorithms to represent 3D images by projecting only the voxels that represent the surface of the object (surface). The pixels are illuminated on the screen as if a light source is present in the front of the object. The closer the pixels, the brighter they appear. This shading effect allows the object to be projected as a 3D object with depth. However, some 3D images appear to have large voids or no bone present on the surface because of the software averaging volume elements, and the voids appear when the software attempts to reconstruct portions of the image covered by a very thin layer of bone. When evaluating the cross-sectional images, bone will be present. This is a direct result of the reformatting process, which usually selects

a higher HU re-formation, which results in decreased scatter on the 3D image. Therefore the implant clinician should be aware that 3D images *do not accurately* depict the bone in an area; it is only a stylized representation of the facial skeleton (Fig. 11.19).

Incidental Findings

The role of CBCT is rapidly emerging in all aspects of diagnosis and treatment planning with dental implants. Because of varying FOVs, the implant clinician is placed in a position to evaluate maxillofacial areas which he or she may not be familiar. Therefore it is crucial the implant clinician be able to interpret anatomic structures and pathology outside his or her primary area of interest. In radiology an incidental finding is defined as an unexpected discovery found on a radiologic examination performed for an unrelated reason. Unfortunately many normal anatomic variants, developmental anomalies, and imaging artifacts may be misidentified as possible pathologic conditions by inexperienced clinicians.[28] This may lead to unnecessary concern and stress for patients, and embarrassment for the clinician. In addition, possible significant pathologies may exist that go undiagnosed. This problem results in many professional, ethical, clinical, and potential legal issues for the implant clinician.

Complication Prevention

Understanding Incidence of Incidental Findings. Incidental findings on CBCT scans have been well documented in the literature. The exact frequency of incidental findings varies from study to study depending on age, gender, race, and FOV. Price et al.[29] showed a high incidence (3.2 findings/scan) of incidental findings, with approximately 16% requiring intervention or referral. These incidental findings ranged from common benign findings to significant pathologic conditions. Miles[30] reported a minimum of two reportable findings per CBCT and also showed a high incidence of periapical lesions that went undetected on conventional radiographs. Cha et al.[31] determined after evaluation of 500 scans an incidence rate of 24.6% of incidental findings, mostly in the airway region. Arnheiter et al.[32] showed that patients 40 to 49 years old had the largest percentage of reportable incidental findings (70%), with patients aged 20 to 29 years with the lowest percentage (40%).

Obtaining a Radiology Report. Radiology reports immediately after CBCT examinations, before surgery, minimize the liability that may present to the implant clinician. Formal radiology reports may be obtained from many sources, preferably from an appropriately qualified, board-certified maxillofacial radiologist. Unfortunately the geographic distribution of maxillofacial radiologists is not uniform within states or regions within a state, and a careful search will be required. Several, but not all, states require that the report be made by a maxillofacial radiologist licensed in the state, and it is therefore crucial to check with your local dental board or dental practice act to determine whether in-state licensure is required. The implant clinician must be able to recognize and evaluate variations from normal and refer for appropriate medical consultation any significant incidental finding that may be contained in the radiology report.

Use of the Smallest Field of View as Possible. Ideally the smallest FOV should be used for scans when treatment planning for dental implants. A smaller FOV (~mid FOV) will reduce radiation dose to the patient, thus adhering to the ALARA principle. However, caution should be exercised to not take an inadequate FOV that includes insufficient view of the anatomic area of concern. The most common anatomic area for this to occur is the maxillary posterior region, because many practitioners will set the limits of the scan superiorly to exclude the maxillary ostium. When placing implants or bone grafting in the posterior maxilla area, confirming the patency of the ostium is important to minimize complications associated with an obstructed ostiomeatal complex (Fig. 11.20).

Normal Radiographic Anatomy

Due to the complex nature of implant treatment and the potential for complications throughout the surgical and prosthetic phases, the clinician must have a thorough understanding of the normal anatomy of the maxillofacial region. Traditional dental education has focused on the interpretation of conventional 2D radiographic images for diagnosis, but with the introduction and rise of CBCT images, a deeper understanding of anatomy is necessary to examine the patient's structures in three dimensions. This section will address the basic radiographic anatomy as viewed in the three planes (axial, coronal, sagittal) typically shown on a CBCT image.

Mandibular Anatomy

The mandible is the largest, strongest, and lowest bone in the human face area.[33] The mandible is formed by the fusion of the right and left processes, and join in the midline area. It consists of the body (symphysis) and the right rami (ramus). The innervation of the mandible is via the inferior alveolar nerve, which is a branch of the trigeminal nerve. It enters the mandibular foramen on the lingual aspect of the ramus and courses anteriorly, where it divides into two branches: mental nerve and incisive nerve. The mental nerve exits the mental foramen, which gives sensory innervation to the chin, lip, and anterior gingiva. The incisive nerve courses anteriorly to supply the anterior teeth.

Mandibular Canal and Associated Anatomy

The position of the MC as it courses through the mandible from posterior to anterior is highly variable. Although the pathways of the inferior alveolar nerve and the mental nerve have been well described in the literature, it is paramount the implant clinician have a clear understanding of their anatomic features. When evaluating the intraosseous course of the MC buccal-lingually and inferior-superiorly within the mandible, many variations exist based on gender, ethnicity, amount of bone resorption, and age.

The inferior alveolar canal or MC contains the neurovascular bundle, which consists of the inferior alveolar nerve, artery, vein, and lymphatic vessels. The inferior alveolar nerve bundle enters the mandibular foramen, where it transverses anteroinferiorly from lingual to buccal within the body of the mandible. A 3D evaluation of the MC position is recommended when implant placement is going to be positioned in proximity to the nerve. The most accurate assessment of the anatomic position is with CBCT, because images may be enhanced via viewing software

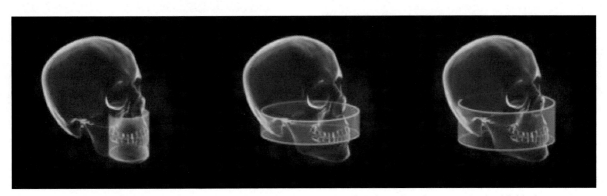

• **Fig. 11.20** Newer cone beam computed tomography units allow for collimation or customized field of views that decrease radiation exposure.

adjustments for contrast, brightness, and grayscale to help depict the anatomic location of the MC.

Image Evaluation. Radiographically the MC appears as a linear, radiolucent shadow, with or without inferior and superior radiopaque borders. Studies have shown the total length to be approximately 62.5 mm, with slightly longer measurements in male individuals (~2.5 mm).[34] The average diameter of the MC is approximately 2.0 to 3.4 mm, with the diameter being the greatest in the posterior near the mandibular foramen.[35] The foramen is triangular in nature near the mandibular foramen, and as it progresses anteriorly, becomes more ovoid in shape.[36] Location is variable depending on the patient's race, gender, and amount of bone resorption. Usually the MC is located on a bony ledge, the lingula, which is located on the medial surface of the ramus. Studies have shown the foramen to be located approximately 19.7 mm from the anterior border of the ramus.[37]

The CBCT data are used with appropriate viewing software to identify and trace the MC. The depiction of the MC enables the implant clinician to assess the position in various multiplanar and 3D re-formations. Initially the MC is most easily drawn on the CBCT reconstructed panoramic view with location confirmation on the cross-sectional images. In most cases the endpoints are first identified (e.g., mandibular foramen, mental foramen), then the location of the MC is extrapolated between these two landmarks.

Buccal-Lingual Path of Mandibular Canal

Radiographic Evaluation. In the posterior region of the mandible the inferior alveolar nerve enters the mandibular foramen on the lingual surface of the mandible and progresses anteriorly in the body of the mandible. In between the MC and the mental foramen, the buccal-lingual position is extremely variable. Studies have shown the buccal-lingual location is dependent on such variables as the amount of bone resorption, age, and ethnicity.[38] The buccal-lingual position of the MC is easily depicted on cross-sectional images after canal location is verified and highlighted (Fig. 11.21).

Clinical Significance. The intraosseous path of the MC is variable in the buccal-lingual position within the mandible, and a comprehensive radiographic survey (CBCT) ideally should be completed before implant osteotomy initiation to determine the anatomic path.

A 2-mm safety zone between the implant and the MC should always be adhered to. Attempting to place an implant buccal or lingual to the neurovascular bundle may result in neurosensory impairment.

Inferior-Superior Path of Mandibular Canal

Evaluation. The vertical position of the MC below the apices of the natural teeth within the mandible is highly variable. Thus generalizations cannot be made because the distance of the canal to the root apices is *not* consistent.[39] An early classification of the vertical positions of the course of the alveolar nerve was reported by Carter and Keen.[40] They described three distinct types: (1) in close approximation to the apices of the teeth, (2) a large nerve approximately in the middle of the mandible with individual nerve fibers supplying the mandibular teeth, and (3) a nerve trunk close to the inferior cortical plate with large plexuses to the mandibular teeth. After the MC is located and drawn on the reconstructed panoramic image using CBCT viewing software, the vertical position of the intraosseous path may be determined by scrolling through the cross-sectional images. The vertical position is then easily seen on individual cross sections or CBCT-generated reconstructed panoramic images (Fig. 11.22).

Clinical Significance. The intraosseous path of the MC is variable in the inferior-superior position within the mandible, and a

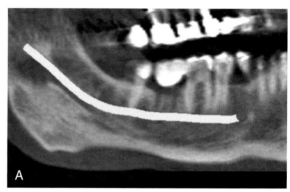
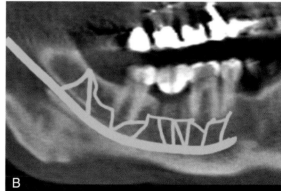
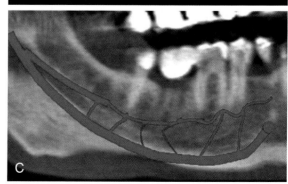

• **Fig. 11.22** Inferior Mandibular Nerves. Type 1 (A), type 2 (B), and type 3 (C) nerves. (*Adapted from Resnik RR, Preece JW. Radiographic complications and evaluation. In: Resnik RR, Misch CE, eds. Misch's Avoiding Complications in Oral Implantology. St. Louis, MO: Elsevier; 2018.*)

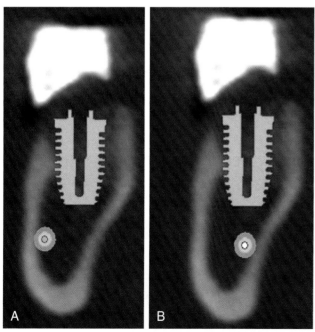

• **Fig. 11.21** Variable Buccal-Lingual Position. (A) Buccal positioned. (B) Lingual positioned. (*From Resnik RR, Preece JW. Radiographic complications and evaluation. In: Resnik RR, Misch CE, eds. Misch's Avoiding Complications in Oral Implantology. St. Louis, MO: Elsevier; 2018.*)

comprehensive radiographic survey (CBCT) ideally should be completed before implant osteotomy. Special care should be exercised in type 1 nerves because their close approximation to the root apexes results in compromised bone height for implant placement. Type 3 nerves are most favorable for implant placement in the posterior mandible because there exists the most ideal amount of bone height. In many instances the MC may not be easily depicted on the CBCT image; thus identification can be extremely challenging. The visibility of the MC varies significantly, even within the same individual.

The MC walls usually are not made up of compact bone, showing only a coalescence of trabecular bone with varying degrees of density.[41] This complicates the determination and location of the true identification of the canal. Studies have shown the unreliability of identifying the entire MC course being a direct result of minimal to no dense cortical plates surrounding the nerve bundle, which has been shown to occur in approximately 30% of cases. The MC has an increased wall density in the posterior (~mandibular foramen > third molar region) in comparison with the anterior region.[42]

With CBCT, images are susceptible to noise and artifacts, with resulting low contrast. Because of these inherent quality issues, distinguishing the MC from other aspects of the internal trabecular components of the mandibular image is difficult. Thresholding, the inability of the software to distinguish between two closely related densities, results in the inability to determine the correct position because of the increased noise. If a highly accurate assessment of the mandibular canal is warranted, the implant clinician may order an MRI survey, which has been shown to depict the soft tissues much better than CBCT.

Mental Foramen

The mental foramen is an opening in the anterolateral aspect of the mandible, commonly in the interproximal space between the first and second premolars; however, individuals may rarely exhibit the position of the foramen as anterior to the cuspid area and as far posteriorly as the bifurcation of the first molar. One of the two terminal branches of the inferior alveolar nerve is the mental nerve, which exits the mental foramen with sensory innervation to the chin, lip, and anterior gingiva. The mental foramen completes after the 12th gestational week, when the mental nerve

separates into several fascicles. If the mental nerve separates before the formation of the mental foramina, the formation of accessory foramen results.[43] The mental foramen location, size, and number are highly variable, with many dependent factors, including gender, ethnic background, age, and skeletal makeup.

Image Evaluation. The mental foramen may be most easily identified on axial, coronal, and cross-sectional images. The relationship between the mental foramen and teeth or vital structures can be evaluated most easily on volumetric 3D images. The location of the mental foramen on 2D periapical and conventional panoramic radiographs has been shown to be inaccurate because they do not show the true location in most cases. In addition, when placing immediate implants in the premolar region, angulation and avoidance of the foramen should be noted because the mental foramen has been shown to be located coronal to the root apex of premolars in 25% to 38% of patients. Thus anytime an implant is to be treatment planned in approximation of the foramen, a CBCT evaluation is recommended.[44] However, the low contrast in CBCT images may make it difficult to do this without obscuring the canal or including too much noise in the process (Fig. 11.23).

Incisive Canal

The mandibular incisive canal is a bony canal within the anterior mandible that is a continuation of the MC. This canal contains the terminal branch of the inferior alveolar nerve, which travels inferiorly to the mandibular anterior teeth and terminates in the midline. In approximately the first molar region, the inferior alveolar nerve bifurcates into the mental and incisive nerves. The mandibular incisive canal terminates as nerve endings within the anterior teeth or bone near the lateral incisor region and will extend only to the midline in 18% of patients and in some cases will anastomosis with the contralateral side.[45]

Radiographic Evaluation. The incisive canal is not always seen radiographically on CBCT. The incisive nerve may be differentiated from the mental nerve by determination of any canal that is anterior to the mental nerve/foramen exit. When present, this radiolucent canal will continue anteriorly from the mental foramen and can be seen as a bifurcation (Fig. 11.24).

Clinical Significance. The incisive canal is often mistaken for an anterior loop of the mental nerve; however, this nerve

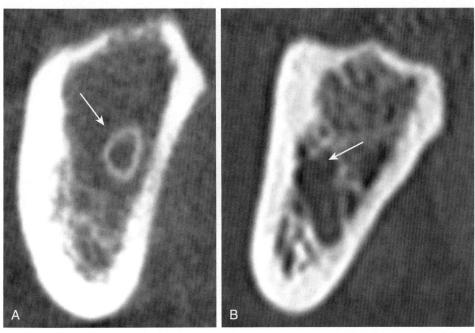

• **Fig. 11.23** (A) The mandibular canal is easily seen when a thick cortical component is present. (B) However, in approximately 30% of patients, the mandibular canal will not have a cortical component.

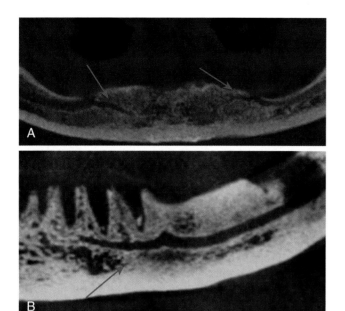

• **Fig. 11.24** Incisive Canal. (A and B) The incisive canal is a continuation of the inferior alveolar canal that contains the incisive nerve, which innervates the mandibular anterior teeth.

innervates the anterior teeth and has no sensory innervation to the soft tissue. However, if the incisive canal is traumatized, cases of excessive bleeding have been reported.

Anterior Loop

As the mental nerve proceeds anteriorly in the mandible, it may on occasion extend beyond the anterior boundary of the mental foramen. This endosteal curved loop is proximal to the mental foramen and exits distally through the mental foramen, and is termed an *anterior loop*. Studies have shown a prevalence rate of approximately 35% to 50%, with a mean distance of 1.16 mm anteriorly to the foramen.[46] Clinically an anterior loop may be determined by probing within the mental foramen in a posterior direction; however, this necessitates full reflection of the mental foramen.

Radiographic Evaluation. The determination of an anterior loop is difficult to identify and cannot be determined accurately with 2D radiography. High false-positive and false-negative results have been noted on conventional panoramic and periapical radiographs. To identify an anterior loop on a reformatted CBCT image, the MC must be highlighted, including the cross-sectional image depicting the mental foramen slice. The anterior part of the mental foramen is marked with a constant perpendicular line (see Fig. 11.25a). In axial images, scrolling from superior to inferior is evaluated for any part of the nerve anterior to the line. If an anterior loop exists, the highlighted nerve will be anterior to the perpendicular line (Fig. 11.25).

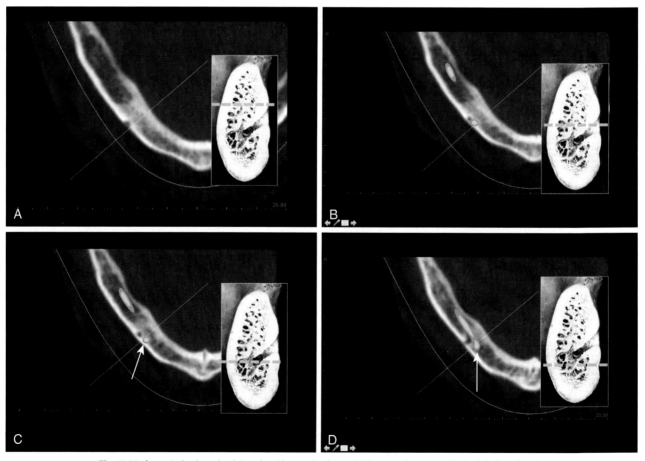

• **Fig. 11.25** An anterior loop is determined by evaluating axial images in a superior to inferior direction. (A) The anterior aspect of the foramen should be marked (line that remains constant in the vertical plane). (B) As the axial images are sequentially evaluated from superior to inferior, if any part of the marked canal extends anterior to the line (C and D, arrows), an anterior loop exists. (*From Resnik RR, Preece JW. Radiographic complications and evaluation. In: Resnik RR, Misch CE, eds.* Misch's Avoiding Complications in Oral Implantology. *St. Louis, MO: Elsevier; 2018.*)

Clinical Significance. The importance of determining the presence of an anterior loop is critical when placing implants anterior to the mental foramen. Inability to establish the existence of an anterior loop may result in implant placement too close to the mental nerve, resulting in possible neurosensory impairment.

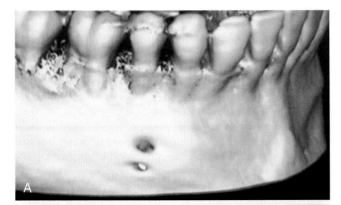

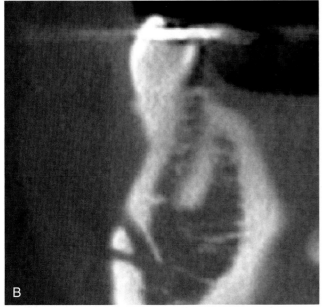

• **Fig. 11.26** (A) 3D CBCT image depicting a small accessory foramen inferior to primary mental foramen. (B) Coronal Image showing large main foramen and smaller accessory foramen.

Accessory and Double Foramina

In approximately 6.6% to 12.4% of patients, an accessory (double) foramen is present, with an average diameter of 1.0 mm.[47-49] Special care should be noted to evaluate for an accessory canal because it may contain components of one of the three branches of the mental nerve. Accessory foramina are believed to be the result of early branching of the inferior alveolar nerve, before exiting the mental foramen during the 12th week of gestation.[50]

Radiographic Evaluation. The ideal technique to determine an accessory foramen is evaluation of coronal images, along with evaluation of the 3D image. In the coronal image the mandibular foramen will be shown bifurcating into two canals, resulting in the presence of two foramina. The evaluation of 3D images will easily depict two canals. Normally, accessory canals are located distal to the mental foramen (Fig. 11.26). In some cases, small openings which represent nutrient vessels may perforate through the buccal plate. These aberrant vessels are of no neural consequence.

Clinical Significance. In the majority of patients, small accessory foramina usually contain a small branch of the mental nerve, which is not problematic because of cross-innervation. However, in some cases a larger branch of the mental nerve (equal or larger size foramen) may exit the mental foramen. If a larger accessory foramen is present and resultant damage to the nerve exists, possible neurosensory impairment is possible. However, usually these accessory foramina are smaller and do not result in any disturbances because of collateral innervation.

Hypomineralization of the Mandibular Canal

When locating the MC, approximately 41% of the time the canal is not seen because of hypomineralization of the bone.[51] Studies have shown that in 20.8% of CBCT scans the MC walls are hypomineralized.[52] This often results in poor localization of the MC and is sometimes an early indication of osteopenia or osteoporosis (Fig. 11.27).

Radiographic Evaluation. The brightness and contrast may be altered using imaging software to more clearly define the canal walls.

Clinical Significance. Lack of identification of the MC may result in the inability to properly locate the MC. This may result in increased morbidity, leading to placement of implants too close to the nerve, with resultant nerve damage. In cases where a CBCT cannot differentiate the canal, an MRI survey is a reasonable alternative.

Mandibular Ramus (Donor Site for Autogenous Grafting)

The mandibular ramus area has become a popular donor site for autogenous onlay and trephine bone grafting. This anatomic area of

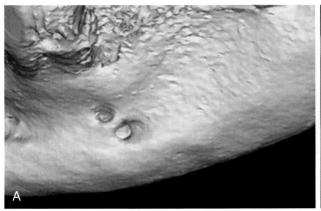

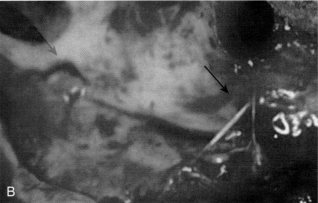

• **Fig. 11.27** (A) Accessory (Double) Foramina which are easily seen on 3D images. (B) Nutrient Canals are small openings which represent nutrient vessels (*green arrow*, mental foramen; *blue arrow*, nutrient canal). (A: From Resnik RR, Preece JW. Radiographic complications and evaluation. In: Resnik RR, Misch CE, eds. Misch's Avoiding Complications in Oral Implantology. St. Louis, MO: Elsevier; 2018.)

the mandible is extremely variable in the amount of bone present, as well as the buccal-lingual and inferior-superior position of the MC. Most commonly the lateral aspect of the ramus is harvested as a block graft, which is used for ridge augmentation procedures.

Image Evaluation. The mandibular ramus is quadrilateral in shape and contains two surfaces, four borders, and two processes. The lateral surface is flat with two oblique ridges, the external and internal. The masseter muscle attaches on the entire lateral ramus surface. The medial surface gives rise to the lingula, which is the entrance of the inferior alveolar nerve and associated vessels. The antegonial notch, anterior to the angle of the mandible, when present, is significant for the presence of parafunction.

The relationship between the lateral cortical plate in the ramus area and the position of the MC is easily seen on cross-sectional images, after nerve location identification. In addition, 3D images and bone models assist in the determination of the osseous morphology in this region to help the clinician select the most appropriate graft site.

Historically, standard 2D radiographs for evaluation of the ramus area as a donor site included conventional panoramic images, in which the location of the external oblique and the MC may be noted. However, 2D evaluation of this area can be difficult to use for determination of the amount of bone present and position of the MC. With this procedure, it is vital that the implant clinician be able to completely determine the exact position of the MC with respect to the external oblique ridge and the lateral cortical bone. Thus overestimation of available bone can result in increased morbidity, so a more accurate representation of this area is with the use of CBCT (Fig. 11.28).

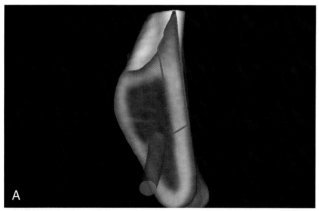

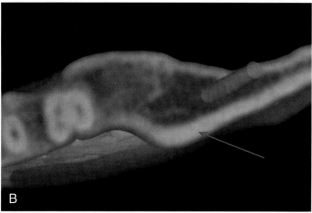

● **Fig. 11.28** The mandibular ramus area can be evaluated. (A and B) Cross-sectional (outline for ramus block graft) (A) and axial 3D image (B) allowing for the evaluation of the proximity of the mandibular nerve to the facial cortical plate. (*A: From Resnik RR, Preece JW. Radiographic complications and evaluation. In: Resnik RR, Misch CE, eds.* Misch's Avoiding Complications in Oral Implantology. *St. Louis, MO: Elsevier; 2018.*)

Lingual Concavities (Posterior)

The trajectory/angulation of the mandible, along with inherent undercuts, poses a significant problem to the implant clinician. Lingual concavities may occur in the anterior region as an hourglass or constriction of the mandibular bone. Butura et al.[53] have shown the incidence to be approximately 4% of patients, which is most likely genetic or developmental in origin.

In the posterior region, concavities are much more common, resulting in undercuts in approximately 35% of patients.[54] Because of these undercuts, implant placement may be difficult, and perforation of the lingual plate may result.

Radiographic Evaluation. Posterior undercuts are most easily seen in cross-sectional and 3D images.

Clinical Significance. In the posterior region, overestimation of available bone is a common complication. If an implant osteotomy is completed in this area, perforation of the lingual plate may result, leading to possible bleeding and possible implant morbidity. Life-threatening lingual bleeding may occur as a result of blood vessel injury, leading to bleeding into the soft tissues. In addition, damage to the lingual nerve may occur on perforation of the lingual cortical plate (Fig. 11.29).

Retromolar Canal/Foramen

The retromolar fossa of the mandible forms a triangular depression, which borders the temporal crest medially and the anterior border of the mandibular ramus laterally. Within this fossa an anatomic variant termed the *retromolar foramen* is present in approximately 14% of patients.[55] The retromolar foramen on the alveolar surface is the terminal end to the retromolar canal, which branches from the MC.

Radiographic Evaluation. The retromolar foramina are not located in a constant position and usually are not bilateral. Most commonly, retromolar foramina should be initially evaluated via CBCT sagittal slices and then verified with cross-sectional images.

Clinical Significance. It is important to confirm the retromolar foramen and canal locations before surgical procedures, because this area is a common donor site for bone grafts. If perforation of the retromolar canal results, excessive bleeding may result (Fig. 11.30).

Mandibular Symphysis (Implant Placement and Bone Donor Site)

The mandibular symphysis area is a common area for implant placement, as well as a donor site for autogenous block grafting. This anatomic region has been shown to be one of the most ideal intraoral donor sites for bone harvesting. However, the mandibular symphysis is susceptible to nonuniform bone resorption and contains various anatomic variations that may lead to surgical complications.

Image Evaluation. The anterior surface of the mandible is termed the mandibular symphysis. A ridge divides the right and left sides, which inferiorly forms the triangular eminence of the mental protuberance. The elevated center of this depressed area forms the mental tubercle, which is the origin of the mentalis muscles. This area should be evaluated on cross-sectional, axial, and 3D images. Two-dimensional imaging of this area should be used only as a preliminary evaluation for bone quantity determination. Poor angulation, bony undercuts, and measurements cannot be determined with 2D radiography. CBCT imaging is highly recommended to prevent implant malposition or overestimation of available bone for harvest procedures, which may lead to increased complications (Fig. 11.31).

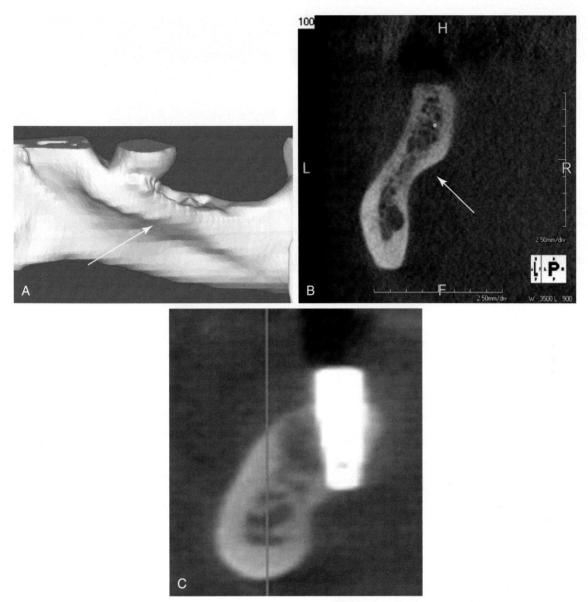

● **Fig. 11.29** (A) Three-dimensional images depicting sublingual undercut. (B) Cross section depicting significant undercut. (C) Nonideal placement of implant perforating the lingual plate that may predispose the patient to possible sublingual bleeding. (*A and B: From Resnik RR, Preece JW. Radiographic complications and evaluation. In: Resnik RR, Misch CE, eds.* Misch's Avoiding Complications in Oral Implantology. *St. Louis, MO: Elsevier; 2018.*)

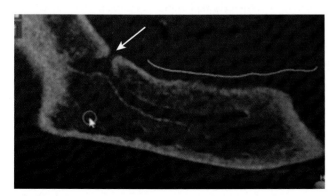

● **Fig. 11.30** Cone beam computed tomography image showing large retromolar canal.

Anterior (Hourglass Shaped)

Radiographic Evaluation. Anterior undercuts are most easily seen in cross-sectional and 3D images.

Clinical Significance. In the anterior region, perforation of the bony plates of the mandible during implant osteotomies may lead to extensive bleeding from sublingual vessels. A significant plexus of sublingual and submental arteries may lead to life-threatening floor of the mouth hematoma formation. Therefore a thorough CBCT examination will determine the exact location and angulation for safe implant placement (Fig. 11.32).

Lingual Foramen/Canal. The interforaminal region in the anterior mandible is usually a relatively safe area for implant placement and bone grafting procedures. However, on the lingual aspect of the mandible, in the midline, lies the lingual foramen or foramina.

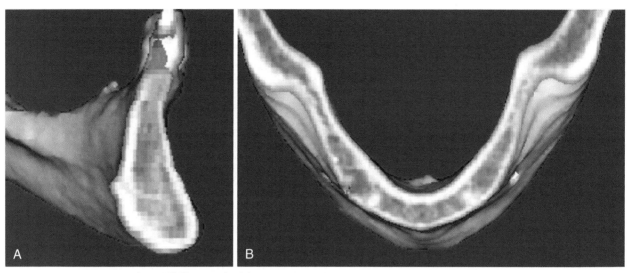

• **Fig. 11.31** (A and B) The symphysial area can be evaluated on cross-sectional images, along with axial slices.

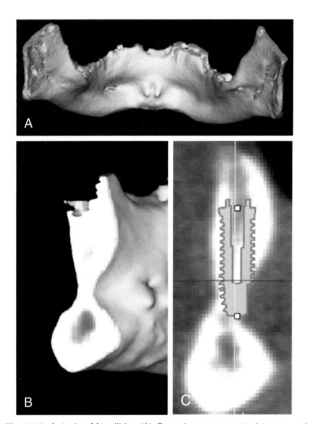

• **Fig. 11.32** Anterior Mandible. (A) Cone beam computed tomography three-dimensional image depicting large undercuts. (B) Cross-sectional image showing hourglass mandibular shape. (C) Interactive treatment plan displaying perforation of an implant if placed in an hourglass mandible. (*A and C: From Resnik RR, Preece JW. Radiographic complications and evaluation. In: Resnik RR, Misch CE, eds.* Misch's Avoiding Complications in Oral Implantology. *St. Louis, MO: Elsevier; 2018.*)

This anatomic structure houses the terminal branches of the lingual artery (sublingual artery), facial artery (submental artery), or the anastomosis of both. As the blood vessels enter within the mandible, they are termed the *mandibular median vascular canal.*

Radiographic Evaluation. Lingual canals and foramina may be seen radiographically as a radiolucent canal in the midline of the mandible and easily depicted on cross-sectional or axial views. Studies have verified the median vascular canal is present in 96% to 100% of patients. The median vascular canal size is proportional to the diameter of the arteries entering the foramen. The average diameter has been shown to be approximately 0.84 mm, with the average distance from the inferior mandibular border to be 11.2 mm. With consideration to the extent of penetration within the mandible, 19.4% of canals end within the lingual third, 52.8% reached the middle third of the mandible, and 27.8% penetrated to the buccal third[56] (Fig. 11.33).

Significance. Potentially, these vessels may cause extensive bleeding in the mandible during endosseous implant placement or symphysial bone grafts. When larger lingual canals exist (>1.0 mm), significant bleeding issues may present with a possible compromised integration because of a potential soft tissue interface with the implant.

Maxillary Anatomy

The maxilla is composed of paired bones, which unite to form the upper jaw, and is composed of four processes: posterolateral (zygomatic, horizontal and medial), palatine (arch and inferior), alveolar, and the superior projecting frontal process. In oral implantology the maxilla presents a difficult and demanding challenge in the treatment and placement of implants with its complex osseous makeup, anatomy, and anatomic variants.

Premaxilla

The anterior premaxilla is one of the most difficult areas for the implant clinician in preoperative assessment, surgical placement, esthetic, and prosthodontic demands. Numerous factors affect the anatomic makeup of the premaxilla that may predispose to surgical complications and result in a decrease in implant survival.

Biomechanics. As a result of the alveolar ridge resorption after tooth loss, the residual available bone migrates to a more palatal position.[57] This leads to difficulties in implant positioning that place the implant clinician at risk because of esthetic issues. Because bone resorption occurs at the result of the buccal plate, implant placement usually occurs in a more palatal position. This

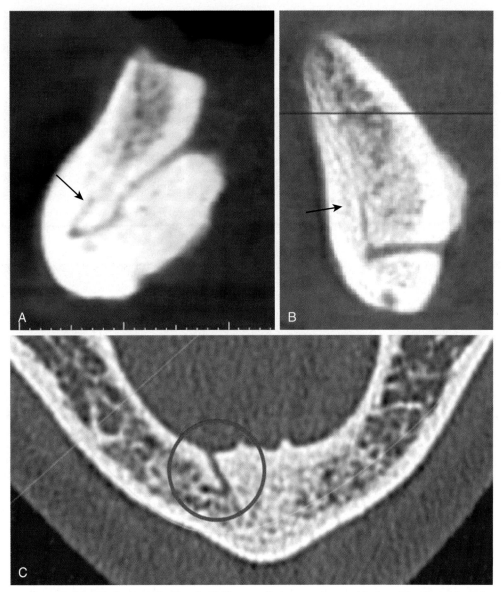

● **Fig. 11.33** Mandibular Vascular Canal. (A) The mandibular vascular canal that contains the sublingual artery anastomosis, which is usually present in the mandibular midline. (B and C) Canal that extends to the facial plate and superiorly (B), and off the midline lingual vascular canal (C).

will create a greater moment force leverage on the bone-implant interface, abutment screws, and implants. Coupled with an angled force in both centric and excursions, more stress is transmitted to premaxillary implants than those in anterior mandibles. Often, more implants and larger-diameter implants are indicated, with bone augmentation by bone spreading or bone graft procedures before or in conjunction with implant placement.

Poor Bone Density. In most patients the bone is less dense in the anterior maxilla than in the anterior mandible. The maxilla most often presents thin porous bone on the labial aspect, very thin porous cortical bone on the floor of the nasal and sinus region, and denser cortical bone on the palatal aspect.[58] The trabecular bone in the premaxilla is usually fine and less dense than the anterior region of the mandible. Due to this poor bone quality, increased difficulty in implant placement and a higher probability of overload implant failures or crestal bone loss may result.

Accelerated Bone Loss. Because of the poor bone quality in the premaxilla, preexisting bone after extractions is predisposed to significant resorption. After tooth loss, the facial cortical plate

rapidly resorbs during initial bone remodeling, and the anterior ridge has been shown to lose up to 25% of its width within the first year, as well as 40% to 50% within the next 3 to 5 years, mostly at the expense of the labial contour (Fig. 11.34).

Nasopalatine Canal/Incisive Foramen

The nasopalatine canal (also termed the incisive canal or anterior palatine canal) is a passageway within the anterior maxilla midline that connects the palate to the floor of the nasal cavity. The entrance of the canal into the oral cavity is via the incisive foramen, which is posterior to the central incisor teeth. The vital structures passing through the canal include the terminal branch of the internal maxillary artery and the nasopalatine nerve, which communicates with the sphenopalatine artery and the greater palatine nerve. The anatomic structures in the nasopalatine canal may present with wide variation in the location, shape, dimensions, and its existence.

Radiographic Evaluation. The location and dimension of the nasopalatine canal is most likely seen on axial and coronal images. Cross-sectional and 3D images may also depict the size, shape,

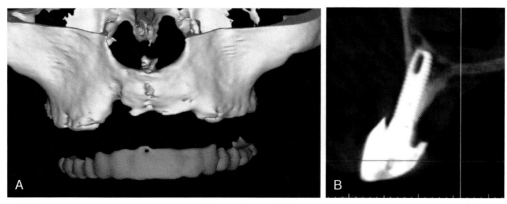

● **Fig. 11.34** The premaxilla presents a challenging area for the implant clinician because of the (A) significant vertical and horizontal bone loss, and (B) minimal bone for implant placement, along with trajectory issues.

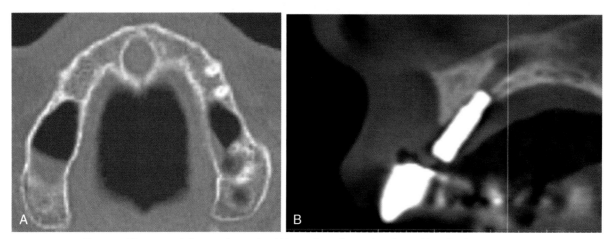

● **Fig. 11.35** The nasopalatine canal area should be evaluated as to the size and location because implant placement in this area may predispose to placement within soft tissue. (A) Very large canal leading to minimal available bone. (B) Implant placement impinging on nasopalatine canal.

and location of the nasopalatine canal, along with evaluation of implant impingement on this space.

Clinical Significance. Determining the morphology of the nasopalatine canal via CBCT images allows the clinician to ascertain whether available bone is present for dental implantation. Placing implants in the anterior maxilla (central incisor area) is the most challenging anatomic location for the implant dentist because of biomechanical, functional, esthetic, and phonetic demands. Especially with immediate implant placement, consideration must be given to the presence of the nasopalatine canal, including a careful evaluation of its morphology and position to minimize implant placement complications.

Implant Placement. The incisive foramen often expands laterally within the palatal bone, and the central incisor implant osteotomy may inadvertently encroach on this structure, resulting in the formation of fibrous tissue at the interface in the mesiopalatal region. If the osteotomy invades the incisive canal, treatment options include tissue removal within the canal and bone graft and/or implant placement. When a large nasopalatine canal exists, a more distally placed implant placement in the central incisor region prevents encroachment on this area. Because most restorations in an edentulous premaxilla are FP-2 or FP-3, the most favorable sites for bone width are selected, even when they are in the interproximal region of central and lateral incisor sites.

Enlarged Incisive Foramen/Canal. When there exists an enlarged canal, the lack of available bone will most likely not

permit ideal implant placement. However, it is important to differentiate enlarged canals from incisive canal cysts. Incisive canal cysts are known to cause localized dilation of the canals, with possible displacement of the teeth. In edentulous patients the nasopalatine canal has been shown to be significantly larger in comparison with dentate patients (Fig. 11.35).

Implant Failure/Bleeding. When implants are positioned in contact with neural tissue, lack of osseointegration and failure of the implant may result. In addition, placement of implants in close approximation to nasopalatine blood vessels may cause excessive bleeding during surgical procedures; however, this is usually self-limiting and controlled by local hemostatic techniques.

Infraorbital Foramen

The infraorbital foramen is located in the anterior aspect of the maxillary bone below the infraorbital margin of the orbit. The infraorbital artery, vein, and nerve exit the foramen. On average the infraorbital foramen to infraorbital margin distance is approximately 6.1 to 10.9 mm.[59]

Radiographic Evaluation. The infraorbital foramen is easily seen on coronal images, along with 3D reformatted images.

Clinical Significance. Anatomic variants have been reported to be as far as 14 mm from the orbital rim in some individuals. In the severely atrophic maxilla the infraorbital neurovascular structures exiting the foramen may be close to the intraoral residual ridge and should be avoided when performing sinus graft procedures, to

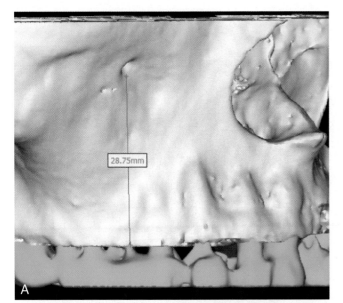

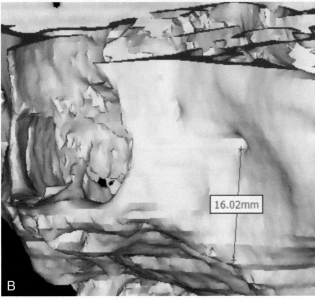

• **Fig. 11.36** (A) Normal location for infraorbital nerve. (B) Variation closer to ridge that may result in neurosensory impairment from retraction or possible transection on reflection of the tissue. (*From Resnik RR, Preece JW. Radiographic complications and evaluation. In: Resnik RR, Misch CE, eds.* Misch's Avoiding Complications in Oral Implantology. *St. Louis, MO: Elsevier; 2018.*)

minimize possible nerve impairment. This is of particular concern on soft tissue reflection and the bone preparation of the superior aspect of the window. Because the infraorbital nerve is responsible for sensory innervations to the skin of the upper cheek; mucosa of the maxillary sinus; maxillary incisors, canines, and premolars; and gingiva, skin and conjunctiva of the eyelid, lateral nose, and mucosa of the upper lip, damage to this nerve may cause significant discomfort to the patient. Most often the nerve is not severed, and a neurotmesis presents that usually resolves within 1 month after the surgery (Fig. 11.36).

Paranasal Sinuses

Frontal. The frontal sinuses are bilateral and funnel-shaped on each side of the midline superior to the orbital bones. The borders of the frontal sinus are inferior, orbital portion of the frontal bone; posterior, separates the dura of the frontal lobe from the lining mucosa; and posterior, separates the dura of the frontal lobe

from the lining mucosa. The frontal sinuses extend to the middle meatus, and drain through the nasofrontal duct and into the frontal recess. The location of the frontal ostia is approximately two-thirds high on the posterior medial wall, which anatomically complicates clearing of the sinus after infection.[60] The frontal recess, which is the drainage pathway of the frontal sinus, drains into the middle meatus or ethmoid infundibulum. On coronal CBCT images, the frontal recess is superior and medial to agger nasi cells.

Ethmoid. The ethmoid sinuses are within the ethmoid bone and divided into two compartments, the anterior and posterior. The anterior ethmoid sinus drains into the middle meatus, and the posterior ethmoids drain into the sphenoethmoidal recess. The borders of the ethmoid sinuses include:

Anterior ethmoid
   Lateral: lamina papyracea of the orbit
   Medial: middle turbinate
   Superior: fovea ethmoidalis, cribriform plate
Posterior ethmoid
   Lateral: lamina papyracea of the orbit
   Medial: superior turbinate
   Superior: fovea ethmoidalis, cribriform plate

The ethmoid sinuses have various radiographic anatomic markers, which are termed *air cells.* The *ethmoid bullae* are the largest and most prominent radiographically in the anterior region. *Agger nasi cells* are usually the most anterior of the anterior air cells and are located in anterior/superior to the middle turbinate. Along the inferior border of the orbits are the *Haller cells,* which may impair mucociliary clearance when they enlarge and impinge on the ethmoid infundibulum. The *Onodi cells* derive from the posterior ethmoid and are located lateral and superior to the sphenoid sinus.[61]

Sphenoid Sinus. The sphenoid sinus is located within the sphenoid bone and contains superiorly the pituitary fossa and olfactory nerves. Inferiorly the pterygoid canal courses beneath the mucosa, with the cavernous portion of the internal carotid artery within the lateral wall. The ostium lies in the superior aspect and drains into the sphenoethmoidal recess.[62]

Maxillary Sinus. The maxillary sinuses are the largest of the paired paranasal sinuses and are often a problematic area for implant clinicians. The posterior maxilla has many inherent disadvantages, including poor bone density, the anatomic minimal interocclusal space, and insufficient bone quantity for ideal implant placement. Thus the implant clinician must have comprehensive knowledge of normal versus abnormal anatomy in association with the maxillary sinus and paranasal sinus anatomy. The maxillary sinus has a high prevalence of anatomic variants and pathology, which predispose the patient to increased morbidity. Thus a comprehensive knowledge and understanding of this area is important for implant clinicians. Radiographically the maxillary sinus has the following borders: Superiorly, the maxillary sinus is bordered by the orbital floor, which houses the infraorbital canal. Inferiorly, the floor of the maxillary sinus approximates the roots of the maxillary teeth. The medial wall coincides with the lateral wall of the nasal cavity and is the location of the maxillary ostium, the area of drainage of the ethmoid infundibulum (Fig. 11.37).

Nasal Cavity

The borders of the nasal cavity are:

Inferior: hard palate
Lateral: medial walls of the right and left maxillary sinus
Superior: nasal, ethmoid, and sphenoid bones
Medial: nasal septum

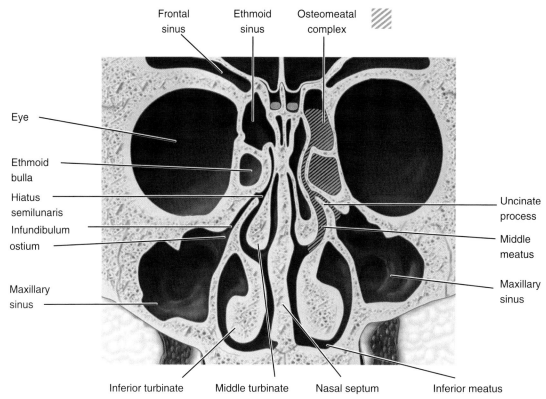

Frontal sinus
Ethmoid sinus
Osteomeatal complex

Eye
Ethmoid bulla
Hiatus semilunaris
Infundibulum ostium
Maxillary sinus

Uncinate process
Middle meatus
Maxillary sinus

Inferior turbinate   Middle turbinate   Nasal septum   Inferior meatus

• **Fig. 11.37** Diagram of Maxillary Sinus Anatomy.

The lateral walls of the nasal cavity are made up of turbinates (concha), which are epithelium-lined bony structures that protrude into the nasal cavity and function to warm/cool and filter inspired air. Below each turbinate are spaces, termed *meatuses*. The middle meatus is most important because this is the area of drainage for the frontal, anterior ethmoid, and maxillary sinuses. The inferior meatus is the drainage site for the nasolacrimal duct. The superior meatus interconnects with the posterior ethmoid and sphenoid sinuses through the sphenoethmoidal recess.[63]

Maxillary Sinus Membrane

The maxillary sinus is lined by the Schneiderian membrane, which is identical to respiratory epithelium. This pseudostratified columnar epithelium is continuous with the nasal epithelium through the maxillary ostium in the middle meatus. The membrane has an average thickness of 0.8 mm and is usually thinner and less vascular than nasal epithelium.[64]

Radiographic Evaluation. A CBCT scan of normal, healthy paranasal sinuses reveals a completely radiolucent (dark) maxillary sinus. Any radiopaque (whitish) area within the sinus cavity is abnormal, and a pathologic condition should be suspected. The normal sinus membrane is radiographically invisible, whereas any inflammation or thickening of this structure will be radiopaque. The density of the diseased tissue or fluid accumulation will be proportional to varying degrees of gray values (Fig. 11.38).

Ostiomeatal Complex

The ostiomeatal unit is composed of the maxillary ostium, ethmoid infundibulum, anterior ethmoid cells, uncinate process, and the frontal recess.

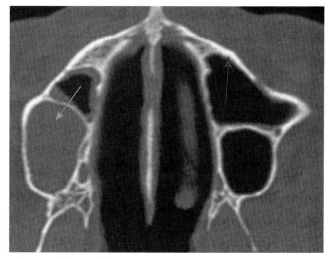

• **Fig. 11.38** The maxillary sinus membrane (Schneiderian membrane) in health should be invisible (red arrow). When inflammation or pathology is present, it will be depicted as an increase in density/radiopacity or a visible increase in thickness (green arrow).

Radiographic Evaluation. The ostiomeatal complex can be evaluated radiographically and most easily seen on a coronal scan that includes the following structures:
1. maxillary sinus ostium
2. infundibulum
3. ethmoid bulla
4. uncinate process
5. hiatus semilunaris

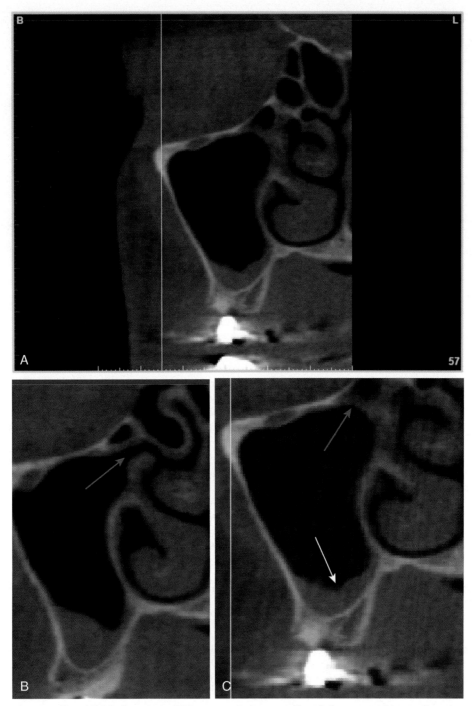

• **Fig. 11.39** (A and B) Maxillary sinus ostium patency is the mucociliary drainage area of the maxillary sinus. (C) Nonpatent ostium (*red arrow*, non-patent ostium; *white arrow*, membrane inflammation).

Maxillary Ostium

The main drainage avenue of the maxillary sinus is through the ostium. The maxillary ostium is bounded superiorly by the ethmoid sinuses and inferiorly by the uncinate process. The maxillary sinus ostium is on the superior aspect of the medial wall of the sinus, approximately halfway between the anterior and posterior walls. The ostium is usually oval shaped and oriented horizontally or obliquely.[65]

Radiographic Evaluation. The maxillary ostium is visualized on coronal images usually in the anterior third of the maxillary sinus. This opening is located in the superior aspect of the maxillary sinus medial (lateral wall of nasal cavity). The patency of the maxillary ostium should always be ascertained when placing implants or bone

grafts into the maxillary sinus. The opening can be verified by scrolling through various coronal images (Fig. 11.39).

Clinical Significance. If the maxillary ostium is nonpatent, the mucociliary clearance of the maxillary sinus may be affected. This can lead to an increased morbidity to implant-related procedures.

Uncinate Process

The uncinate process is an important structure in the lateral wall of the nasal cavity. This finger-like bony projection helps form the boundaries of the hiatus semilunaris and ethmoid bulla, which allow the draining of the frontal and maxillary sinuses.

Radiographic Evaluation. On coronal or cross-sectional CBCT images, the uncinate process is bordered by the medial wall of the maxillary sinus and articulates with the ethmoid process and inferior nasal turbinate. Inferiorly it borders the semilunar hiatus, and posteriorly it has a free margin (Fig. 11.37).

Clinical Significance. A deflected uncinate process (either laterally or medially) can narrow the ethmoid infundibulum, thus affecting the ostiomeatal complex. Perforations may also be present within the uncinate process, leading to communication between the nasal cavity and ethmoid infundibulum. In addition, the uncinate process may be pneumatized. Although this is rare, it may compromise adequate sinus clearance. Uncinate process variations should be evaluated and treated before any procedure in which the physiology of the maxillary sinus is altered (e.g., implant placement or bone grafting).

Hiatus Semilunaris

The hiatus semilunaris is a curved fissure on the lateral wall of the nasal cavity, inferior to the ethmoid bulla. It connects the middle meatus to the anterior ethmoidal air cells and contains the openings for the frontal, maxillary, and anterior ethmoidal sinus (Fig. 11.37).

Radiographic Evaluation. The hiatus semilunaris gains its name from its arched appearance and is best identified in sagittal and cross-sectional images. This anatomic structure is bordered superiorly by the ethmoid bulla and posteriorly by the ethmoid process of the inferior nasal turbinate.

Clinical Significance. Because three different sinuses drain into the hiatus semilunaris, any mechanical blockage in this region may cause inflammation and possible disease into one of the sinuses.

Anatomic Variants

Concha Bullosa

The middle turbinate plays a significant role in proper drainage of the maxillary sinus. Normally the middle turbinate is a thin, bony structure; however, it can be aerated, which is termed a *concha bullosa*. This anatomic variant may be unilateral or bilateral, and it has been shown to have a prevalence rate of up to 53.6% of the population.[66] In addition, there exists a strong association with conchae bullosae and a deviated septum of the contralateral side.[67]

Radiographic Evaluation. Conchae bullosa are easily identified on a CT/CBCT coronal image depicting a radiolucent air space in the center of the middle meatus and surrounded by an ovoid bony rim.

Clinical Significance. In most cases of concha bullosa, no paranasal sinus pathology results. The larger the concha bullosa, the more likely the probability of compromising the drainage of the middle meatus. When enlarged, pressure against the uncinate process may occur, decreasing the infundibulum drainage, and thus affecting the physiology of the maxillary sinus, leading to an increased drainage problem. Caution must be exercised because patients with concha bullosa are more predisposed to postoperative complications from bone grafting and implants in the sinus area (Fig. 11.40).

Paradoxical Middle Turbinate

A paradoxical middle turbinate is an anatomic variant of the middle turbinate, with a prevalence rate of approximately 15% of the population.[68] This anomaly is a reversal of the normal medially directed convexity of the middle turbinate. The inferior edge of the middle turbinate may have various shapes exhibiting excessive curvature, which may predispose the patient to blockage in the nasal cavity, infundibulum, and middle meatus.[69]

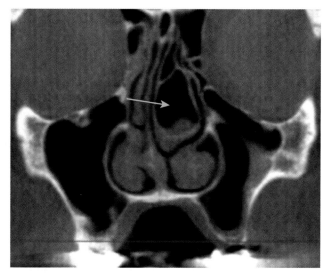

• **Fig. 11.40** An anatomic variant that may predispose the implant patient to postoperative mucociliary impairment is a concha bullosa, which is an aerated middle turbinate.

Radiographic Evaluation. A paradoxical middle turbinate is most easily seen on a coronal CT/CBCT scan image. In certain cross-sectional images, it may also be seen. The convexity of the paradoxical middle turbinate is directed laterally, instead of medially toward the nasal septum.

Clinical Significance. When present, the implant clinician must take into consideration the possibility of postoperative mucociliary complications after bone grafting or implant placement in the maxillary sinus from blockage of the ostium (Fig. 11.41).

Deviated Septum

One of the most common anatomic variants in the oral region is a deviated septum, which may be congenital or traumatic in origin. Studies have shown a prevalence rate of 70%, which increases the possibility of ostiomeatal complex blockage. This occurs when the nasal septum is displaced laterally toward one side of the nasal cavity. When the deviation is severe, the flow of air through the nasal cavity is redirected and may cause nasal obstruction, hypoplasia of the ipsilateral turbinates, or hyperplasia of the contralateral turbinates.

Radiographic Evaluation. A deviated septum can be seen most easily via the coronal and axial image scans. In addition, a 3D image of the midline structure will allow direct evaluation. The nasal septum will be displaced toward one side of the nasal cavity (Fig. 11.42).

Clinical Significance. When the deviation is severe, the airflow through the nasal cavity is compromised, manifesting as nasal congestion. Patients with deviated septums are predisposed to sinus clearance issues, which increase morbidity of bone grafting and implant placement procedures in the maxillary posterior area on the side of deviation. Usually the contralateral side will have normal mucociliary clearance.

Haller Cells

Haller cells are infraorbital ethmoidal air cells that project from the maxillary sinus roof and the most inferior portion of the lamina papyracea. The Haller cells are usually present unilaterally, with a prevalence rate of approximately 6% of the population.[70] The origin of Haller cells is the anterior ethmoid (88%) and posterior ethmoid (12%).[71]

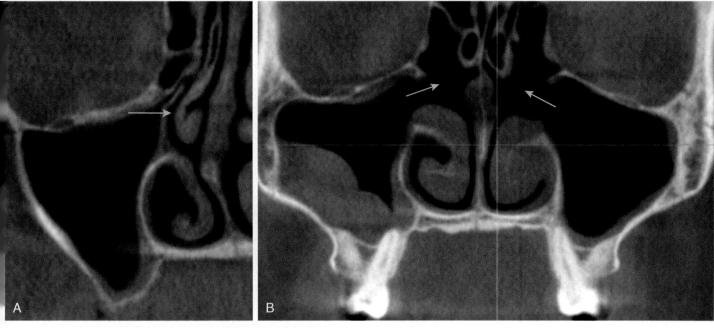

Fig. 11.41 Paradoxical Middle Turbinate (A) An anatomic variant that may predispose the implant patient to postoperative mucociliary impairments is termed a paradoxical middle turbinate. The convex side of the middle turbinate is directed laterally, instead of medially. (B) Image depicting no right or left middle turbinates, which is a recent treatment for patients exhibiting chronic rhinosinusitis to improve mucociliary flow.

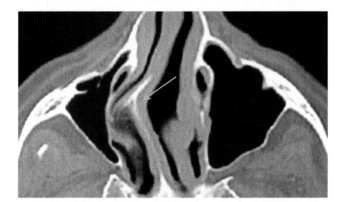

Fig. 11.42 An anatomic variant that may predispose the implant patient to postoperative mucociliary impairments is a deviated septum. The side of deviation may cause blockage of the maxillary ostium.

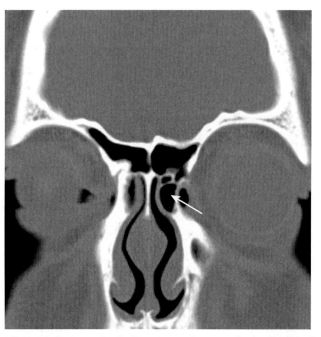

Fig. 11.43 Agger nasi cells that are anterior aerated ethmoid air cells (arrows). (*From Koenig LJ, et al. Diagnostic Imaging: Oral and Maxillofacial. 2nd ed. Philadelphia: Elsevier; 2017.*)

Radiographic Evaluation. Haller cells are identified on coronal images and are located inferior to the ethmoid bulla and adher to the medial roof of the orbit, lateral to the uncinate process.

Clinical Significance. These air cells may expand into the orbit and narrow the ostium of the maxillary sinus, especially in the presence of an infection. Haller cells have been associated with a high incidence of chronic rhinosinusitis because they may impinge on the patency of the maxillary ostium, thus inhibiting ciliary function. Procedures (implants, bone grafts) that may involve the maxillary sinus have an increased morbidity when Haller cells are present.

Agger Nasi Cells

Agger nasi cells are the most anterior ethmoidal air cells that extend anteriorly into the lacrimal bone. They can be identified on CT/CBCT in more than 90% of patients and are associated with a high incidence of frontal sinusitis.[72]

Radiographic Evaluation. Agger nasi cells are most easily seen in CT/CBCT coronal images lateral to the nasal wall (Fig. 11.43).

Clinical Significance. Agger nasi cells may predispose the patient to postoperative sinus complications.

Maxillary Sinus Septa

Antral septa (of buttresses, webs, and struts) are the most common osseous anatomic variant seen in the maxillary sinus. Underwood, an anatomist, first described maxillary sinus septa in 1910. Krennmair et al.[73] further classified these structures into two groups: primary, which are a result of the development of the maxilla; and secondary, which arise from the pneumatization of the sinus floor after tooth loss. The prevalence rate of septa has been reported to be in the range of 33% of the maxillary sinuses in the dentate patient and as high as 22% in the edentulous patient. The most common location of septa in the maxillary sinus has been reported to be in the middle (second bicuspid to first molar) region of the sinus cavity. CT scan studies have shown that 41% of septa are seen in the middle region, followed by the posterior region (35%) and the anterior region (24%). For diagnosis and evaluation of septa, CT scan is the most accurate method of radiographic evaluation.[74] Sinus septa may create added difficulty at the time of surgery.

Radiographic Evaluation. Three-dimensional images depict the anatomic features of septa most easily on CBCT images. They may also be easily seen on reformatted panoramic and axial and sagittal images (Fig. 11.44).

Clinical Significance. Maxillary septa complicate sinus graft surgery and can prevent adequate access and visualization to the sinus floor; therefore inadequate or incomplete sinus grafting is possible. In addition, a higher incidence of membrane perforation results when septa are present.

Maxillary Sinus Hypoplasia

Hypoplasia of the maxillary sinus may be a direct result from trauma, infection, surgical intervention, or irradiation to the maxilla during the development of the maxillary bone. These or other congenital developmental conditions interrupt the maxillary growth center, thus producing a smaller-than-normal maxilla. A malformed and positioned uncinate process is associated with this disorder, leading to chronic sinus drainage problems.

Radiographic Evaluation. Dimensionally smaller than normal maxillary sinus can be seen on panoramic, cross-sectional, coronal, axial, or 3D images.

Clinical Significance. Most often maxillary sinus hypoplasia patients have adequate bone height for endosteal implant placement, and a sinus graft is not required to gain vertical height. If implant placement or bone grafting involves the maxillary sinus,

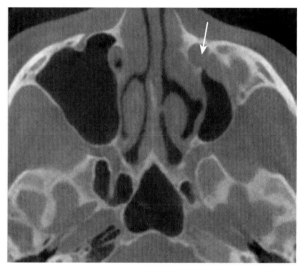

• **Fig. 11.45** Hypoplasia of the maxillary sinus with inflammation (white arrow).

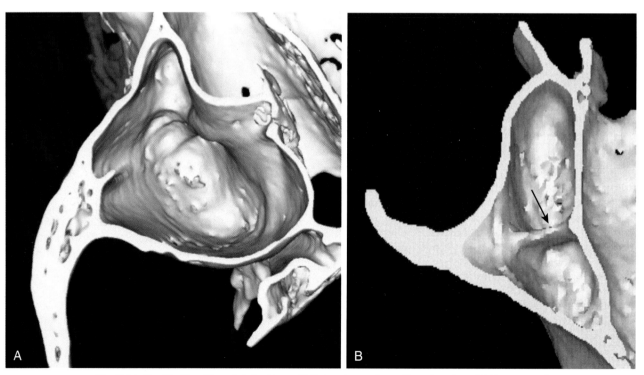

• **Fig. 11.44** The Maxillary Sinus Inferior Floor. (A) Flat and smooth maxillary sinus floor. (B) Narrow maxillary sinus floor with septum separating the sinus cavity.

caution should be exercised, because this condition has been associated with chronic sinus disease (Fig. 11.45).

Inferior Turbinate and Meatus Pneumatization (Big-Nose Variant)

A rather uncommon anatomic variant is when the inferior third of the nasal cavity exhibits pneumatization within the maxilla and resides over the alveolar residual ridge. Studies have shown an incidence rate of approximately 3%. Because the maxillary sinus is lateral to the edentulous ridge, inadequate bone height exists.

Radiographic Evaluation. Big-nose variants may be determined by evaluation on reconstructed CBCT panoramic images, as the nasal cavity will extend distal or posterior to the premolar area.

Clinical Significance. If unaware of this condition, the implant may be placed into the nasal cavity above the residual ridge, often penetrating into the inferior meatus and contacting the inferior turbinate. A sinus graft maybe contraindicated with this patient condition, because the sinus is lateral to the position of the implants. Most likely an onlay graft is required to increase bone height (Fig. 11.46).

Buccal Thickness of Bone in Premaxilla

On average, maxillary buccal cortical plates are less than 1 mm thick, significantly thinner than the mandibular alveolar bones, which are greater than 1 mm. Thin cortical plates (similar to voxel size) tend to become indistinguishable from adjacent cementum or titanium implants on CBCT images.

Radiographic Evaluation. Studies have shown that spatial resolution limitations of CBCT limit bone visibility of thickness less than 0.6 mm, meaning this is the minimum thickness for bone to be measurable. In addition, clinical studies show when bone dehiscence is present, a true dehiscence was present only 50% of the time, and a fenestration was present 25% of the time.[75]

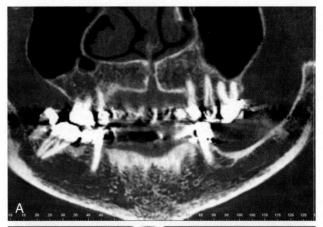
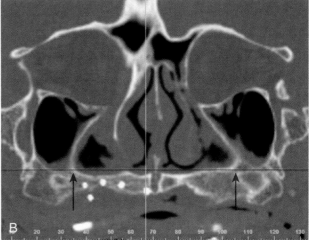

• **Fig. 11.46** (A and B) Big-nose variant, which results in the nasal cavity extending into the first molar region, leaving inadequate bone for implants in the bicuspid region.

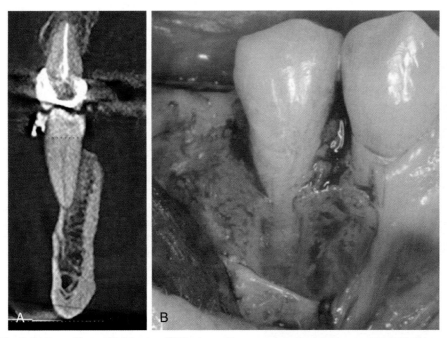

• **Fig. 11.47** Buccal Image Thickness. (A) The buccal bone can be very deceiving as depicted in this cone beam computed tomography cross section showing no buccal bone thickness and (B) photo image after full reflection showing buccal bone is present.

Clinical Significance. Because of the high degree of false-positive results, diagnosis and treatment planning can be problematic. The bone thickness should be correlated with all CBCT images, especially the cross-sectional views (Fig. 11.47).

Intraosseous Anastomosis

Within the lateral wall of the maxilla sinus is the intraosseous anastomosis, which is comprised of the posterior superior alveolar and infraorbital arteries. The vertical component of the lateral access wall for the sinus graft often severs these blood vessels.

Radiographic Evaluation. The intraosseous anastomosis is easily seen on cross-sectional or coronal views of a CBCT scan as a discontinuation of the lateral wall with a radiolucent notch. On average, this structure is approximately 15 to 20 mm from the crest of a dentate ridge.

Clinical Significance. When lateral wall sinus augmentation is indicated, evaluation of the CBCT scans should be completed to determine location and size. If bleeding does occur during the lateral wall osteotomy, this can be addressed by cauterization by the handpiece and diamond bur without water, electrocautery, or pressure on a surgical sponge while the head is elevated (Fig. 11.48).

Canalis Sinuosus

The anterior superior alveolar nerve branches from the infraorbital canal, just lingual to the cuspid area. This radiolucent canal is denoted as the canalis sinuosus. The canal runs forward and inferior to the inferior wall of the orbit and follows the lower margin of the nasal aperture and opens to lateral to the nasal septum.[76] The canalis sinuosus transmits the anterior superior alveolar nerve, artery, and vein.

Radiographic Evaluation. If the clinician is unaware of the canalis sinuosus, this anatomic structure may be misinterpreted as apical pathology on 2D radiographs. Therefore on CBCT scans, this bilateral anatomic structure should be evaluated for its presence. It may be depicted on axial, cross-sectional, or 3D images.

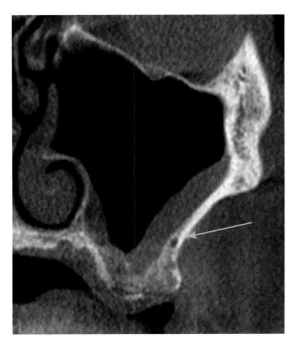

• **Fig. 11.48** Intraosseous anastomosis (arrow) shown on a cross-sectional image seen as discontinuity of the lateral wall and ovoid radiolucency.

Studies have shown the canalis sinuosus to be present on 87.5% of CBCT scans[77] (Fig. 11.49).

Clinical Significance. Because the anterior maxillary region is a common area for dental implant placement, the presence of canalis sinuosus may lead to a high degree of implant morbidity. Impingement into the canal may lead to a soft tissue interface and failure of the implant, and temporary or permanent sensory dysfunction and possible bleeding issues.[78] However, significant sensory impairments are rare because of cross-innervation.

Calcified Carotid Artery Atheroma

Calcified carotid artery atheromas are calcifications located in the common carotid, usually near the bifurcation of the internal and external carotid arteries. These calcifications give radiographic evidence of atherosclerosis, which is an indicator of possible stroke or metabolic disease. It has been shown that approximately 80% of strokes are ischemic and due to atherosclerotic disease in the carotid bifurcation.[79]

Radiographic Evaluation. Carotid artery calcifications are small, multiple radiopacities in the carotid space anterior and lateral to cervical vertebrae C3-C4. These multiple and irregularly shaped calcifications may be vertical in orientation and are usually easily distinguished from the adjacent soft tissue. They can easily be seen on axial and 3D images (Fig. 11.50). An additional common site to evaluate for carotid artery calcifications in large-volume CBCT images is lateral to the pituitary fossa.

Clinical Significance. Because of the significant complications that may arise from the presence of carotid calcifications (ischemic cerebrovascular disease is the second leading cause of death in most developed countries), the patient should be referred to his or her physician for assessment of carotid artery stenosis and possible ultrasound evaluation.

Pathologic Conditions in the Paranasal Sinuses

Pathologic conditions observed on CBCT scans taken for other indications appear to be increasing in prevalence. Signs of inflammation or serious pathologic conditions are a concern when bone augmentation procedures or dental implants are planned for the area. Therefore the implant clinician must have a strong knowledge base for various pathologic conditions in the sinus to understand when proper referral is recommended. In the next part of this chapter, a comprehensive evaluation of maxillary sinus pathology will be discussed, with emphasis on differential diagnosis and clinical relevance.

Odontogenic Rhinosinusitis (Periapical Mucositis)

Odontogenic rhinosinusitis occurs when the sinus membrane is violated by infection of teeth and pathologic lesions of the jaws. The intimate approximation of the roots of the maxillary posterior teeth to the floor of the sinus results in inflammatory changes of the periodontium or surrounding alveolar bone, which promotes the development of pathologic conditions in the maxillary sinus.

Radiographic Appearance. Odontogenic rhinosinusitis will usually produce generalized sinus mucosal hyperplasia, which is seen as a radiopaque band that follows the contours of the sinus floor. A localized periapical mucositis reveals a thickening of the mucous membrane adjacent to the offending tooth and, on occasion, a perforation through to the floor of the sinus. This radiographic appearance has been termed a halo effect (Fig. 11.51).

Differential Diagnosis. Odontogenic rhinosinusitis may be confused with acute rhinosinusitis or mild mucosal thickening.

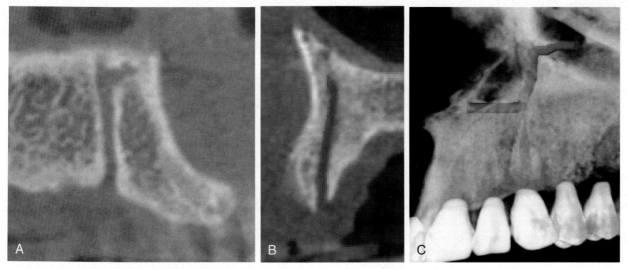

• **Fig. 11.49** Canalis Sinuosus. (A) CBCT panoramic image depicting the canalis sinuosus, which transmits the anterior superior alveolar vessels. (B) Cross-sectional image highlighting in red the nerve. (C) 3D image showing course of the canal.

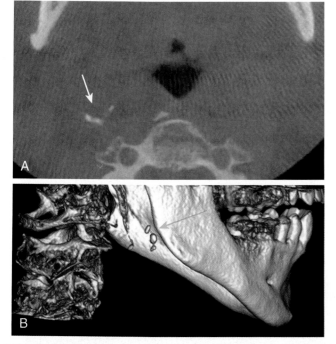

• **Fig. 11.50** (A and B) Carotid calcification atheroma at the level of cervical vertebrae C3-C4 (arrows).

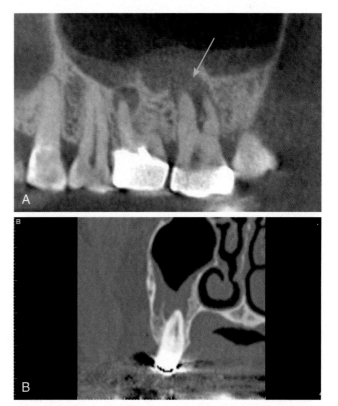

• **Fig. 11.51** Odontogenic rhinosinusitis (A and B) associated with pathologic teeth that extends into the sinus cavity.

However, in odontogenic rhinosinusitis the patient will most likely have pathology associated with an existing tooth (e.g., pain from a posterior tooth or a recent extraction, exudate around the existing natural posterior teeth) and radiographic evidence.

Acute Rhinosinusitis

A nonodontogenic pathologic condition may also result in inflammation in the maxillary sinus in the form of rhinosinusitis. The most common type of rhinosinusitis in the maxillary sinus is acute rhinosinusitis. The signs and symptoms of acute rhinosinusitis are rather nonspecific, making it difficult to differentiate from the common cold, influenza type of symptoms, and allergic rhinitis. However, the most common symptoms include purulent nasal discharge, facial pain and tenderness, nasal congestion, and possible fever. Acute maxillary rhinosinusitis results in 22 to 25 million patient visits to a physician in the United States each year, with a direct or indirect cost of $6 billion dollars. Although four paranasal sinuses exist in the skull, the most common involved in sinusitis are the maxillary and frontal sinuses.[80]

Radiographic Appearance. The radiographic hallmark in acute rhinosinusitis is the appearance of an air-fluid level. A line of demarcation will be present between the fluid and the air within the maxillary sinus. If the patient is supine (CBCT), then the fluid will accumulate in the posterior area; if the patient is upright during the imaging, the fluid will be seen on the floor and horizontal in nature. Additional radiographic signs include smooth, thickened mucosa of the sinus, with possible opacification. In severe cases the sinus may fill completely with supportive exudates, which gives the appearance of a completely opacified sinus. The terms *pyocele* and *empyema* have been applied with these characteristics (Fig. 11.52).

Differential Diagnosis. The differential diagnosis of acute rhinosinusitis and prolonged viral upper respiratory infection are similar. However, a classic air-fluid level in the maxillary sinus will give rise to the confirmation of acute rhinosinusitis. In addition, viral rhinosinusitis will usually improve within 7 to 10 days, whereas acute bacterial rhinosinusitis persists for longer than 10 days.[81]

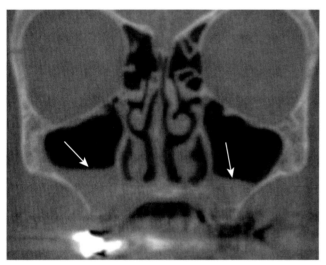

• **Fig. 11.52** Cone beam computed tomography coronal image depicting an air-fluid level that is a classic radiographic sign of acute bacterial rhinosinusitis.

Chronic Rhinosinusitis

If the symptoms of acute rhinosinusitis do not resolve in 12 weeks, it is then termed *chronic rhinosinusitis*. It is the most common chronic disease in the United States, affecting approximately 37 million people. Symptoms of chronic rhinosinusitis are associated with periodic episodes of purulent nasal discharge, nasal congestion, and facial pain.[82]

Radiographic Appearance. Chronic rhinosinusitis has the characteristic feature of sclerotic, thickened cortical bone from long-lasting mucoperiosteal inflammation. In addition, it may appear radiographically as thickened sinus mucosa to complete opacification of the antrum.

Allergic Rhinosinusitis

Allergic rhinosinusitis is a local response within the sinus caused by an irritating allergen in the upper respiratory tract. Therefore the allergen may be the cause of the allergic rhinosinusitis. This category of sinusitis may be the most common form, with 15% to 56% of patients undergoing endoscopy for sinusitis showing evidence of allergy. Allergic rhinosinusitis often leads to chronic rhinosinusitis in 15% to 60% of patients.[83] The sinus mucosa becomes irregular or lobulated, with resultant polyp formation.

Radiographic Appearance. Polyp formation related to allergic rhinosinusitis is usually characterized by multiple, smooth, rounded, radiopaque shadows on the walls of the maxillary sinus. Most commonly, these polyps are located near the ostium and are easily observed on a CBCT scan. In advanced cases, ostium occlusion, along with displacement or destruction of the sinus walls, may be present, with a radiographic image of a completely opacified sinus (Fig. 11.53).

Fungal Rhinosinusitis (Eosinophilic Fungal Rhinosinusitis)

Granulomatous rhinosinusitis is a very serious (and often overlooked) disorder within the maxillary sinus. Patients who have fungal sinusitis are thought to have had an extensive history of antibiotic use, chronic exposure to mold or fungus in the environment, or are immunocompromised.

Differential Diagnosis. Three possible clinical signs may differentiate fungal sinusitis from acute or chronic rhinosinusitis: (1) no response

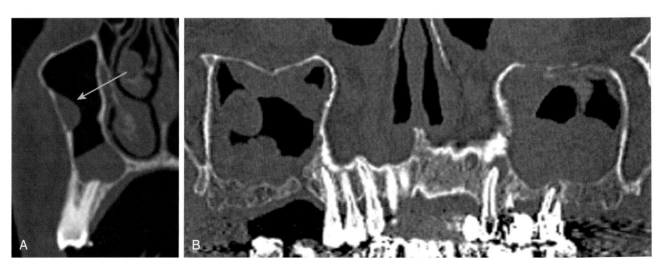

• **Fig. 11.53** (A) Bilateral polyposis, usually associated with allergies, showing the circumferential, polypoid nature of the lesions. (B) Bilateral partially opacified sinuses representing a severe case of allergic rhinosinusitis; severe cases may lead to complete opacification.

to antibiotic therapy; (2) soft tissue changes in sinus associated with thickened reactive bone, with localized areas of osteomyelitis; (3) and association of inflammatory sinus disease that involves the nasal fossa and facial soft tissue. In some cases a positive diagnosis may require mycological and histologic studies.

Radiographic Appearance. Fungal rhinosinusitis is usually unilateral (78% of cases), with bony destruction being rare. Within the sinuses the presence of mild thickening to complete opacification may be present. In most cases varying degrees of density ("double densities") are seen (Fig. 11.54).

Cystic lesions are a common occurrence in the maxillary sinus, and studies have reported a prevalence rate of 2.6% to 20%.[84] They may vary from microscopic lesions to large, destructive, expansile pathologic conditions that include pseudocysts, retention cysts, primary mucoceles, and postoperative maxillary cysts.

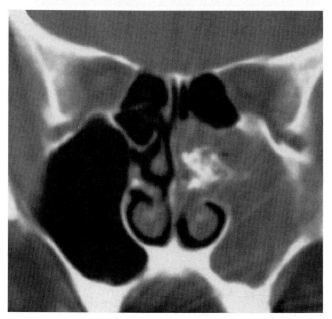

• **Fig. 11.54** Coronal image showing a progressive fungal rhinosinusitis of the left paranasal sinus area. Note the dense radiopacity, which is termed a *fungal ball*.

Pseudocysts (Mucous Retention Cyst)

The most common cysts in the maxillary sinus are mucous retention cysts. After much controversy, in 1984 Gardner[85] distinguished these cysts into two categories: pseudocysts and retention cysts. Pseudocysts are more common and of much greater concern during sinus graft surgery, compared with retention cysts. Pseudocysts reoccur in approximately 30% of patients and are often unassociated with sinus symptoms. As a consequence, many physicians do not treat these lesions. However, when their size becomes large in diameter, pseudocysts may occlude the maxillary ostium during a sinus graft procedure and increase the risk for postoperative infection.

Radiographic Appearance. Pseudocysts are depicted radiographically as smooth, homogenous, dome-shaped, round to ovoid, well-defined homogeneous radiopacities. Pseudocysts do not have a corticated (radiopaque) marginal perimeter and are always on the floor of the sinus cavity (Fig. 11.55).

Retention Cysts

Retention cysts may be located on the sinus floor, near the ostium, or within antral polyps. Because they contain an epithelial lining, researchers consider them to be mucous secretory cysts and "true" cysts. Retention cysts are often microscopic.

Radiographic Appearance. Retention cysts are usually very small and not seen clinically or radiographically. In rare instances they may achieve adequate size to be seen in a CT image and may resemble the appearance of a small pseudocyst.

Primary Maxillary Sinus Mucocele

A primary mucocele is a cystic, expansile, destructive lesion that may include painful swelling of the cheek, displacement of teeth, nasal obstruction, and possible ocular symptoms.[86]

Radiographic Appearance. In the early stages the primary mucocele involves the entire sinus and appears as an opacified sinus. As the cyst enlarges, the walls become thin and eventually perforate. In the late stages, destruction of one or more surrounding sinus walls is evident (Fig. 11.56).

Postoperative Maxillary Cyst

A postoperative maxillary cyst of the maxillary sinus is a cystic lesion that usually develops secondary to a previous trauma or

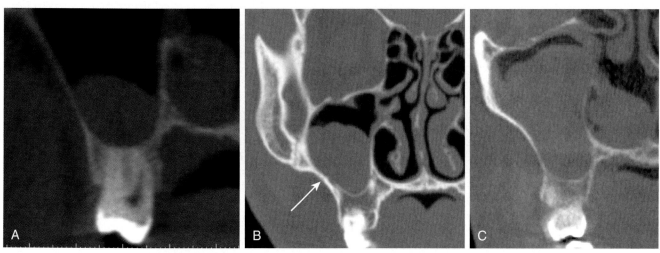

• **Fig. 11.55** Pseudocyst. (A–C) Small pseudocyst (mucous retention cyst) located on the floor of the sinus (A), larger cyst (B), and very large pseudocyst that may lead to obstruction of the sinus (C).

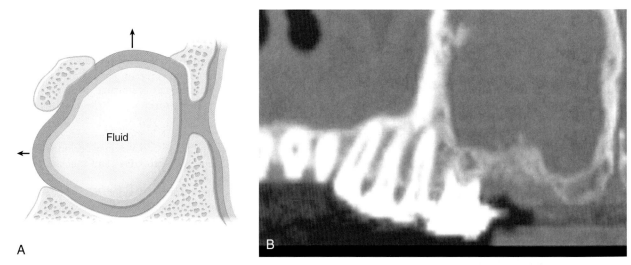

• **Fig. 11.56** Primary Mucocele. (A) Expansile nature of lesion causes destruction of sinus walls. (B) Clinical image depicting right side of a complete radiopaque sinus with expansion of walls.

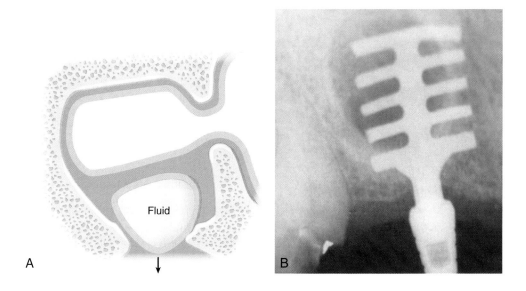

• **Fig. 11.57** (A) Secondary mucocele is a well-defined radiolucent lesion that separates the sinus cavity into two separate compartments, which is usually fluid filled. (B) Radiograph depicting cystic area surrounding the implant.

surgical procedure in the sinus cavity. It has also been termed a surgical ciliated cyst, postoperative maxillary sinus mucocele, or secondary mucocele.[87]

Radiographic Appearance. The cyst radiographically presents as a well-defined radiolucency circumscribed by sclerosis. The lesion is usually spherical in the early stages, with no bone destruction. As it progresses, the sinus wall becomes thin and eventually perforates. In later stages it will appear as two separated anatomic compartments (Fig. 11.57).

Squamous Cell Carcinoma and Adenocarcinoma

Malignant tumors of the paranasal sinuses are rare, with a poorly differentiated squamous cell carcinoma comprising approximately 80% of tumors. Seventy percent of these tumors are found in the maxillary sinus.[88] Symptoms can vary; however, neoplasms of the maxillary sinus usually include nasal obstruction, rhinorrhea, epistaxis, cranial neuropathies, and pain. Advanced cases may include visual disturbances, paresthesias, and possible malocclusion.

Radiographic Appearance. Radiographic signs of neoplasms may include various sized radiopaque masses, complete opacification, or bony wall changes. A lack of a posterior wall on a radiograph should be a sign of possible neoplasm (Fig. 11.58).

Maxillary Sinus Antroliths

Maxillary sinus antroliths are the result of complete or partial encrustation of a foreign body that is present in the sinus. These masses found within the maxillary sinus originate from a central nidus, which can be endogenous or exogenous.[89]

Radiographic Appearance. The radiographic appearance of a maxillary antrolith resembles either the central nidus (retained root) or appears as a radiopaque, calcified mass within the maxillary sinus (Fig. 11.59).

Differential Diagnosis. Because the calcified antrolith is composed of calcium phosphate ($CaPO_4$), calcium carbonate salts, water, and organic material, it will be considerably more radiopaque than an inflammatory or cystic lesion.[90] The central nidus

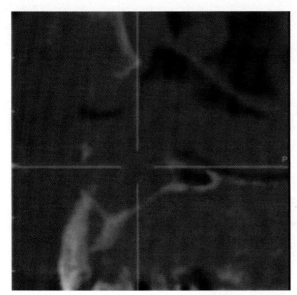

• **Fig. 11.58** Squamous cell carcinoma of the right maxillary sinus showing complete radiopacity with associated expansion and destruction of sinus walls.

of the antrolith is similar to its usual radiographic appearance (Fig. 11.60).

Radiology Reports

A typical radiographic report template will include the following basic information elements.[91]

Patient/Office Identification Section

This section records: date of report, patient name, date of birth, gender, name of the referring doctor, date of the scan, and the name of the scanning center or dental office taking the scan/volume.

Clinical Significance. This section has critical patient record information.

Images Provided

Enter the type of images provided for review. A typical entry would be: "Cone Beam CT images with bone window; Axial, coronal and sagittal planes." Optional information would include the name of the CBCT unit, pixel resolution (e.g., 0.3 mm, size of the volume: small, medium, or large).

Clinical Significance. *Critical/patient record information.* When volume size and pixel resolution are included, patient dose reconstruction is possible when the specific CBCT unit is identified.

Clinical Information

This section would include a brief relevant history and/or clinical note. Entries might include such elements as: "Implant evaluation for edentulous areas of maxilla," "Relationship of endosseous implant to the mandibular canal," etc.

Clinical Significance. This includes critical/patient record information providing the clinician's rationale for taking the diagnostic image.

Diagnostic Objectives

The referring clinician enters his or her specific objectives for the report such as: (1) sinus evaluation; (2) rule out pathology; (3) implant measurements #3,10, 14, 19, 29; (4) rule out osteomyelitis; and (5) mandibular/maxillary pathology.

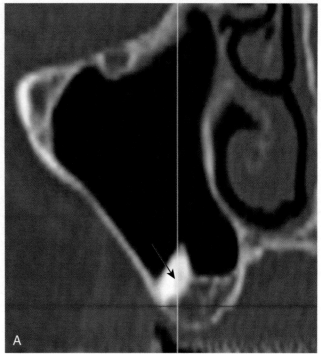

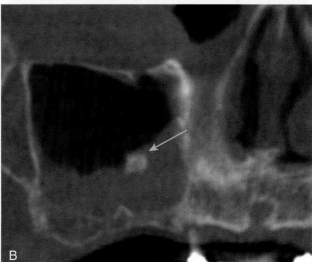

• **Fig. 11.59** Antrolith or calcified masses present in the sinus (arrows). (A) Tooth root, and (B) Restorative material.

Clinical Significance. This includes the clinician's specific request or potential concern for the radiologist to look for as a priority.

Radiographic Findings

This section of the template provides the radiologist/volume interpreter with a list of specific areas within the volume to be evaluated. A standard listing would include:

• maxilla
• paranasal sinuses
• nasal cavity
• air space
• temporomandibular joint (TMJ)

Dental Findings. The radiologist will provide limited comments in this section and typically *will not* report on caries, calculus, and periodontal disease associated with individual teeth. Typically third molar positions will not be reported unless

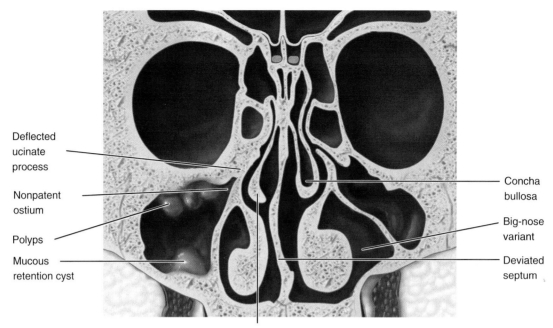

Deflected ucinate process

Nonpatent ostium

Polyps

Mucous retention cyst

Concha bullosa

Big-nose variant

Deviated septum

Paradoxical middle turbinate

• **Fig. 11.60** Summary of the most common pathologic conditions that occur in the paranasal sinuses.

specifically requested by the clinician. The interpretation of these anomalies is within the diagnostic skill set of the dentist.

Clinical Significance. This provides a summary of radiographic findings for the clinician to quickly identify areas of normality and abnormality within the patient volume.

(NOTE: With a digital template for reports, these areas may have a "normal" response listed and subsequently edited as necessary when variations from the normal appearances are identified. For example: "Maxilla: no abnormalities detected; Sinuses: no abnormalities detected, the right and left ostiomeatal complexes were patent; Nasal Cavity: no abnormalities detected, etc." for each area on the list.)

Radiographic Impression

This section of the report template will identify specific variations and deviations from "normal" for each of the areas listed under the radiographic findings and provide the radiologist's impression of the deviation from normal.

Clinical Significance. This gives a summary of radiographic findings providing the clinician with a differential radiographic interpretation of deviations from normal.

Recommendations

This section may be combined with the radiographic impression noted earlier. However, it may be separated to provide general recommendations for clinician guidance related to the findings listed within the radiographic impression section earlier.

The "Recommendations" section would most likely include statements such as: "Physician referral for more thorough evaluation of: ... (Included here would refer any anomaly *not* within the dental scope of practice as defined by your state licensing board.) Other recommendations might include: "Biopsy suggested/recommended for more thorough evaluation of the biological processes involved in ..." (e.g., a large, cystlike lesion in the anterior dental area could represent a cyst of the incisive canal/foramen, large radicular/periapical cyst, ameloblastoma, or central giant cell

tumor, and a biopsy would be helpful in identifying the specific biological nature of the lesion.)

Clinical Significance. This provides the clinician with general guidance related to a specific anomaly and basis for referral.

(NOTE: In general, the radiologist *will not* recommend a specific type of treatment for any finding because this is a consultative report that the clinician must integrate into the patient's overall treatment plan and outcome assessment.)

Radiologist Name and Signature

Level 4: Clinical Significance. This is critical patient record information.

Typical Radiographic Descriptions

Descriptions and entities should be reported as radiographic findings.

Radiographic Findings

Maxilla

Asymmetries between right and left maxillae or sinuses are noted, as well as, changes in bone pattern or texture.

Typical report findings might read:

An asymmetry was noted between the right and left maxillary sinuses; the right maxillary sinus and maxilla exhibit a smaller volume and size than the left, potentially suggestive of maxillary hypoplasia. Correlation of the radiographic observation with the patient's clinical evaluation is suggested.

Clinical Significance. This includes identification of possible hemimaxillary hypoplasia, previous trauma, fibrous dysplasia, etc.

Sinuses

This section will report on findings within all major sinus groups: right and left maxillary, and ethmoid, frontal, and sphenoid sinuses. Under "normal" circumstances the linings of the sinuses are not radiographically visible and are reported as "no abnormalities detected." When the lining becomes visible, sinus pathology is present and reported if the lining is 3 mm or more in thickness.

Common Findings and Sinus Descriptions

Mucositis/sinusitis: "The right maxillary and sphenoid sinuses exhibited an increase in the thickness and density of the sinus lining."

Mucous retention pseudocyst: "A homogeneous ovoid/dome-shaped increase in density was noted within the left maxillary sinus."

Sinusitis: "The right maxillary sinus was partially occupied by homogeneous area of increased density containing bubbles."

Ostiomeatal complex: If the opening is not clearly visible, it should be reported as obstructed/blocked.

Other, less common sinus findings: A thickening, irregularity, and sclerosis of the walls of the sinus may potentially represent a long-standing chronic inflammation of the sinuses. Small, irregular calcifications within the homogeneous density of the tissues of the sinus may be an indication of antrolith formation and an indication of a long-standing chronic sinusitis, small osteomas within the ethmoid sinus.

Typical report findings might read:

The radiographic findings appear consistent with a mild chronic sinusitis of the right and left maxillary sinuses. Review of patient's history for chronic sinusitis/allergy is suggested. Physician referral for more thorough evaluation is suggested if merited by clinical findings and symptoms.

Clinical Significance. This includes identification of potential changes on the sinus region meriting potential physician referral in the presence of symptoms.

Nasal Cavity

This section will include any findings of asymmetry associated with the nasal cavity, including: inferior, middle, and superior turbinates; deviations of the nasal septum; and absence of internal nasal structures potentially associated with previous ear, nose, and throat surgery. A variation in normal anatomy is a dilation within the middle turbinate referred to as a concha bullosa.

Typical report findings might read:

A mild deviation of the nasal septum to the right; enlargement of the middle turbinate consistent with a concha bullosa is considered a variation in normal anatomic form. Deviation of the nasal septum is considered a variation in normal anatomy; referral and treatment are not indicated unless the patient provides a history of difficulty breathing through his nose.

Clinical Significance. This includes identification of possible changes in the nasal cavity potentially influencing breathing patterns.

Air Space

Variations in the size of the airway are noted in the section, as well as potential enlargements of the adenoid and pharyngeal tonsils.

Typical report findings might read:

Narrowing of the airway has been associated with a variety of respiratory disorders, including an increased risk for obstructive sleep apnea. Correlation of the radiographic observation with the patient's clinical history is suggested. Clinical evaluation of the soft tissues of the oral pharynx is suggested.

Clinical Significance. This includes identification of possible airway changes that affect patient breathing patterns.

TMJ

This section reports on variations and deviations in symmetry between the right and left condyles, articular fossae, and joint spaces.

Typical report findings might read:

The right condyle, articular fossa, and joint space exhibited normal bony profiles and contours; the left articular fossa and joint space exhibited normal radiographic contours; the left condyle exhibits a localized discontinuity of the cortical outline, the presence of resorption lacunae, and sclerosis of the underlying bony trabecular pattern consistent with degenerative joint disease (DJD). Correlation of the radiographic observation with the patient's clinical findings and symptoms, if any, is suggested.

Clinical Significance. This includes identification of possible radiographic changes within the bony structures of the TMJ region that affect patient symptoms/occlusion. TMJ-positive findings may predispose the patient to prosthetic rehabilitation complications.

Other Findings

This section is used to report radiographic changes in anatomic structures not associated with the maxilla and mandible but included within the volume, including, but not limited to: calcifications within the carotid artery lateral to the pituitary fossa and within the lower neck, radiographically visible changes within the cervical vertebra, including osteophyte formation, sclerosis, narrowing, and irregularity of intervertebral disc space width with potential bone-to-bone contact; generalized loss or thinning of cortical bone and an absence of internal bony trabeculation suggestive of systemic metabolic disorders of bone/osteoporosis; and increased density noted within one or both mastoid processes. Common incidental radiographic findings included here would be: calcification of the stylohyoid ligament, calcifications of pineal gland and cavernous sinus (middle cranial fossa area), idiopathic soft tissue calcifications within the soft tissues of the skin or soft tissues of the oral pharynx (tonsilloliths), salivary gland/duct calcifications, metallic foreign bodies, ear wax, among others.

Typical report findings might read:

(1) The small areas of increased density noted lateral to the pituitary fossa are anatomically associated with the carotid arteries and are consistent with calcification of the carotid arteries. Vascular calcifications have been associated with an increased risk for cardiovascular disease and stroke. Review of patient's medical history for increased risk factors, such as high blood pressure, elevated cholesterol, stress, and smoking, is suggested. Physician referral is suggested with findings of elevated risk factors or if patient is not currently under the care of a physician. (2) Sclerosis and osteophyte formation within the cervical vertebra may be early indications of DJD of the cervical spine. Correlation of the radiographic observation with the patient's clinical findings and symptoms of chronic neck/muscle pain/headache or other neurologic symptoms is suggested. Physician referral is suggested

for more thorough evaluation if merited by clinical findings and symptoms. (3) Calcification of the pineal gland is considered to be a common incidental radiographic finding that does not require treatment or referral.

Clinical Significance. This provides identification of potential changes indicative of systemic conditions that affect overall patient health and welfare.

Dental Findings

This area provides a summary of radiographic findings that affect dental structures immediately adjacent to the teeth. This area typically reports periapical pathology or other maxillary/mandibular pathology involving the teeth. Evaluation of impacted canines, resorptive changes of adjacent teeth and, dilaceration roots potentially preventing eruption of teeth are noted.

Typical report findings might read:

The maxillary right canine is impacted adjacent to the lingual surface of the apex of the maxillary right lateral incisor; moderate to severe resorptive changes were observed in the root of the lateral incisor.

Clinical Significance. This provides identification of potential changes/conditions that affect treatment planning decisions.

Reporting Implant information

The radiology report template may include separate sections that delineate existing implants or the evaluation of prospective implant sites.

Existing Implants

This section would include a brief notation of the areas that exhibit existing implants and whether the implant exhibits integration with the adjacent bone or the presence of potential changes associated with peri-implantitis.

Implant Measurements

This section typically corresponds to illustrations within the report that exhibit measurements of requested implant sites and will typically state: "Implant measurements have been provided for the requested sites." NOTE: It is important for the clinician to be very specific about the possible sites for which measurements are being requested; it should not be assumed that the radiologist will know the sites for implant placement.

Alternative Report Style for "Incidental Radiographic Findings"

Most incidental findings are unlikely to compromise patient health or dental treatment outcomes, typically do not require referral to a physician, and are found in a high percentage of volumes. They may be provided as a separate list without illustrations depending on the radiologist.

Typical report findings using this format might read:

Incidental findings: deviated nasal septum, concha bullosa, tonsilloliths, ear wax, elongated/calcified stylohyoid ligaments, faint/small calcifications within the pineal gland and cavernous sinuses.

Clinical Significance. This includes identification of potential changes/conditions that will not affect treatment planning decisions or require outside referral.

Styles of Radiology Reports

Each radiologist has her own style and format she uses to construct a report, and it is appropriate for the referring clinician to do his "due diligence" and select the radiologist who will provide the type of report he is comfortable using as a basis for treatment planning decisions (Fig. 11.61). For example, some radiologists specify that their review of the volume is through the assessment of "axial cross sections only," which limits the potential of visualization of radiographic anomalies when CBCT volumes and the software used easily provide axial, coronal, and sagittal cross sections. Our suggestion is to identify a radiologist who provides interpretation based on a complete analysis of the volume using axial, coronal, and sagittal cross sections.

Intraoperative Imaging

The use of surgical imaging has dramatically changed the way that surgical implantology is completed. In the past the disadvantage of periapical radiography perioperatively has been time inefficiency. To verify positioning and location of an osteotomy site or for identification of a vital structure, processing of standard radiograph film can take up to 6 minutes. Because of this, practitioners rarely verified positioning of anatomic structures during surgery. With digital radiography technology, instantaneous images are achieved, allowing for multiple images to be completed in a fraction of the time. Additional advantages of digital intraoperative imaging include manipulation of images, calibration, accurate measurements and positioning, and maintenance of aseptic protocol (Fig. 11.62).

Immediate Postsurgical Imaging

A plain film radiograph (periapical or panoramic) or CBCT should be taken postsurgically so that a baseline image may be used to evaluate against future films. With the ease of image acquisition after surgery, an immediate assessment of positioning and displacement of implants can be evaluated. Because the radiation dose with CBCT has become user-friendly with significantly reduced time and radiation levels (i.e., less than 5 seconds and as low as 15 mSv), immediate postoperative CBCT imaging is a common procedure in implant dentistry today.

Abutment and Prosthetic Component Imaging

When evaluating transfer impressions along with two-piece abutment component placement, radiographs should be taken to verify ideal seating. Intraoral radiographs should be used because of their high geometric resolution to evaluate for any fit discrepancy. However, care must be taken so that the x-ray beam is directed at a right angle to the longitudinal axis of the implant. Even a slight angulation may allow a small opening gap to be unnoticed. When positioning is difficult for intraoral periapical radiographs, bitewing or panoramic radiographs may be used (Figs. 11.63 and 11.64).

Postprosthetic Imaging

In the past, postprosthetic imaging has been limited to intraoral and panoramic radiographs. However, with the advancements in CBCT technology, more accurate CBCT scans with less scattering are available in oral implantology. Therefore CBCT scans are gaining acceptance for use in postprosthetic imaging. There exists no conclusive scientific evidence that low-level ionizing radiation

A. Minimal Information Report:

Patient Name: xxxx   xxxxxxx   DOB: 8/20/1991   Date: xx-xx-xxxx

Scanning Center: or dental office taking volume   Gender: xxxx

Referring Doctor: xxxx xxxxxx   Date of Scan: 5/26/15

Images provided: Cone Beam CT images in the bone window. Axial, coronal and sagittal planes. Closed and open scans provided.

Clinical Info: chronic headaches, jaw pain
Relevant History: not available
Client Notes: implant #3

Diagnostic Objectives:
Rule out pathology

Findings:
Axial, coronal, and sagittal cross-sections of the patient volume were reviewed. Radiographic findings potentially affecting your proposed treatment objectives were not identified.

Radiologist name and signature:
Thank you for the referral of this patient and the opportunity to serve your practice.

B. Medical Style [written only, no illustrations] Report:

Patient Name: xxxx   xxxxxxx   DOB: 8/20/1991   Date: xx-xx-xxxx

Scanning Center: or dental office taking volume   Gender: xxxx

Referring Doctor: xxxx xxxxxx   Date of Scan: 5/26/15

Images provided: Cone Beam CT images in the bone window. Axial, coronal and sagittal planes.

Clinical Info: chronic headaches, jaw pain
Relevant History: not available
Client Notes: implant #3

Diagnostic Objectives:
Rule out pathology

Findings:
Maxilla: no abnormalities detected
Sinuses: a small dome shaped area of increased density was noted within the right maxillary sinus; the right and left osteomeatal complexes were patent.
Nasal Cavity: a deviation the nasal septum to the left was noted.
Mandible: no abnormalities detected
Air Space: no abnormalities detected
TMJs: Both condyles, their articular fossae and eminences exhibit good symmetry and apparently normal bony anatomy; no abnormalities of the bony structures were noted.
Other findings: Sclerosis and osteophyte formation, narrowing and irregularity of intervertebral disc space width with bone to bone contact was noted within the cervical vertebra.
Dental findings: no abnormalities detected

Radiographic Impression:
Sinuses: the radiographic findings appear consistent with a mild chronic mucositis/sinusitis/mucus retention pseudocyst. Review of patient's history for chronic sinusitis/allergy is suggested. Physician referral if merited by clinical findings and symptoms.
Nasal Cavity: deviation of the nasal septum is considered a variation in normal anatomy; referral and treatment is not indicated unless the patient provides a history of difficulty breathing through their nose.
Other Findings: Sclerosis and osteophyte formation, narrowing and irregularity of intervertebral disk space width with bone to bone contact within the cervical vertebra may be indications of DJD of the cervical spine. Correlation of the radiographic observation with the patient's clinical findings and symptoms of chronic neck/muscle pain/headache or other neurological symptoms is suggested. Physician referral is suggested for more thorough evaluation if merited by clinical findings and symptoms.

Radiologist name and signature:
Thank you for the referral of this patient and the opportunity to serve your practice.

Comment: Using the medical model style of radiology report, the radiologist provides a written description of radiographic findings but does not provide illustrations of the various findings or implant measurements.

C. Hybrid Medical with Illustrations

Patient Name: xxxx   xxxxxxx   DOB: 8/20/1991   Date: xx-xx-xxxx

Scanning Center: or dental office taking volume   Gender: xxxx

Referring Doctor: xxxx xxxxxx   Date of Scan: 5/26/15

Images provided: Cone Beam CT images in the bone window. Axial, coronal and sagittal planes.

Clinical Info:
Relevant History:
Client Notes:

Diagnostic Objectives:
1. TMJ Evaluation
2. Rule Out Pathology
etc.

Findings:
Maxilla: no abnormalities detected
Sinuses: no abnormalities detected
Nasal Cavity: no abnormalities detected
Mandible: no abnormalities detected
Air Space: no abnormalities detected
TMJs: no abnormalities detected
Other findings: no abnormalities detected
Dental findings: no abnormalities detected

Radiographic Impression:

Recommendations:

Radiologist name and signature:
Thank you for the referral of this patient and the opportunity to serve your practice.

Comment: Many maxillofacial radiologists provide a hybrid medical model style of report that will include selected images illustrating various radiographic findings. The referring clinician values this kind of report because the illustrations provided allow them to evaluate the severity of the conditions the radiologist has identified and can be used to educate the patient with regard to the radiographic findings.

Patient referral to a physician for additional evaluation based on a radiology report does not have clearly defined guidelines and clearly professional clinical judgment is the key, taking into consideration and integrating clinical findings and patient symptoms. We as healthcare providers have an underlying responsibility to refer patients for additional evaluation when considered appropriate; however, we cannot force our patients to go to physicians if they do not choose to. As a result, documenting in the patient's chart that the radiology report indicated the presence of potential pathology in an area outside of our scope of practice and that the patient was requested to seek a more thorough examination from a physician regarding the condition is prudent and critical.

• **Fig. 11.61** Sample Radiology Report. (A) Minimal information report. (B) Medical style (written only, no illustrations). (C) Hybrid medical style with illustrations. (*From Resnik RR, Preece JW. Radiographic complications and evaluation. In: Resnik RR, Misch CE, eds.* Misch's Avoiding Complications in Oral Implantology. *St. Louis, MO: Elsevier; 2018.*)

has a detrimental effect on bone metabolism and healing. A post-prosthetic radiograph needs to be taken to act as a baseline for future evaluation of component fit verification and also for marginal bone level evaluation.

Recall and Maintenance Imaging

For the evaluation of implant success, immobility and radiographic evidence of bone adjacent to the implant body are the two most accurate diagnostic aids in evaluating success. Follow-up or recall radiographs should be taken after 1 year of functional loading and yearly for the first 3 years.[92] Multiple studies have shown that, in the first year, marginal bone loss and a higher rate of failure are seen.

Evaluation of Alveolar Bone Changes

Radiographically, lack or loss of integration is usually indicated as a radiolucent line around the implant. However, false-negative diagnoses may be made when the soft tissue surrounding an implant is not wide enough to overcome the resolution of

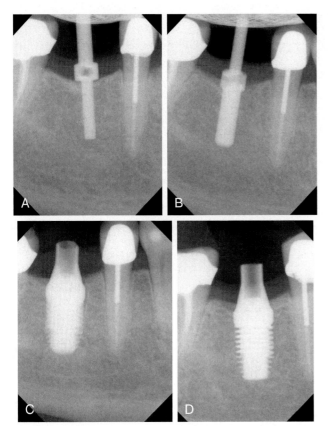

• **Fig. 11.62** Intraoral Radiographs. (A) Initial pilot orientation with slight mesial inclination. (B) Angulation corrected and verified with final depth indicator. (C) Implant placement. Note poor angulation of radiograph leading to distorted measurements. (D) Ideal implant placement radiograph. Note perpendicular orientation of x-ray beam as all threads are seen without distortion. (*From Resnik R, Kircos LT, Misch CE. Diagnostic imaging and techniques. In: Misch CE, ed.* Contemporary Implant Dentistry. *St. Louis, MO: Elsevier; 2008.*)

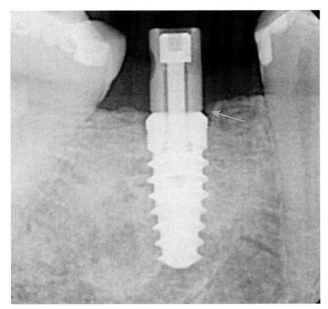

• **Fig. 11.63** Verification of direct transfer coping placement before final impression. Note ideal angulation from thread alignment.

the radiographic modality used (i.e., the implant may not have a direct bone-implant interface). Also, false-positive diagnoses may be made when a "Mach band effect" results from an area of lower radiographic density adjacent to an area of high density (implant), which results in a more radiolucent area than is actually present.[93] However, studies have shown that the possibility of the Mach band effect is significantly reduced with digital image processing. In addition, digital radiography has been shown to have the advantage over conventional radiography with respect to "edge enhancement," which is the ability to detect space between the implant and the surrounding bone. Because of the variability of operator-controlled problems, a strict quality-assurance protocol should be used to maintain ideal image quality over time. Proper positioning, along with kVp and mA settings, should be documented for future reference.

Periapical Radiographs. In recall radiographic examinations the marginal bone level is compared with the immediate postprosthetic films. Therefore radiographs similar in geometry, density, and contrast are paramount. Standardized periapical radiographs are essential to ensure accuracy. However, reproducing positioning is difficult. Numerous film-holding devices have been documented that attach to the implant, abutment, or prosthesis to standardize image geometry. When proper projections are achieved, implant threads on both sides of the implant are clearly seen. If the threads are not clearly seen in the radiographs, modification of the beam angle needs to be made. If diffuse threads are present on the right side of the implant, then the beam angle was positioned too much in the superior direction. If the threads are diffuse on the left side, then the beam angle was from an inferior angulation (Fig. 11.65). With digital enhanced radiographs, numerous techniques have been postulated to measure bone levels around implants. Computer-assisted measurements, rulers, calipers, and suprabony thread evaluation have been shown to have highly reproducible results.[94]

Bitewing Radiographs. In cases where the x-ray source cannot be positioned perpendicular to the implant because of oral anatomy or existing prosthesis, horizontal or vertical bitewings may be taken to evaluate the crestal bone area. With this projection the central beam is perpendicular to the implant and alveolus, the object-film distance is relatively small, and very minor distortions are present. The only limitation of bitewing radiographs is that the apical portion cannot be seen.

Panoramic Radiographs. Panoramic radiographs usually are not used routinely for evaluation of osseous bone levels and recall examinations. Because panoramic radiographs use intensifying screens, resolution is not as good as with intraoral radiographs. However, when film positioning or when multiple implants need to be evaluated, panoramic radiography is the imaging technique of choice.

Computed Tomography. Two-dimensional radiographs (periapical, panoramic) have limitations in that they relay no buccolingual information about the present condition of alveolar bone. CBCT does allow 3D information about the osseous status around an implant. Resolution and scattering have always been a problem in evaluation of implants; however, with the advent of cone beam technology, this is greatly improved. CBCT can be of great benefit in the evaluation of sinus augmentation graft prognosis. With the advantage of bone density evaluation using Hounsfield units, important information on bone maturation may be determined. Also, this radiographic modality is the image

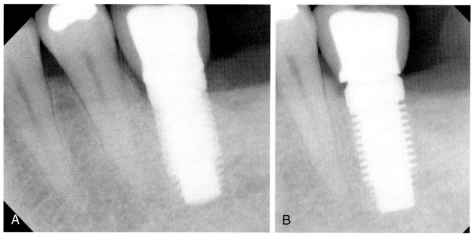

• **Fig. 11.64** Seating of Final Prosthesis. (A) Poor x-ray angulation showing a false-negative or complete seating of the prosthesis. Note the diffuse threads. (B) A corrected angulation image exposes the seating problem.

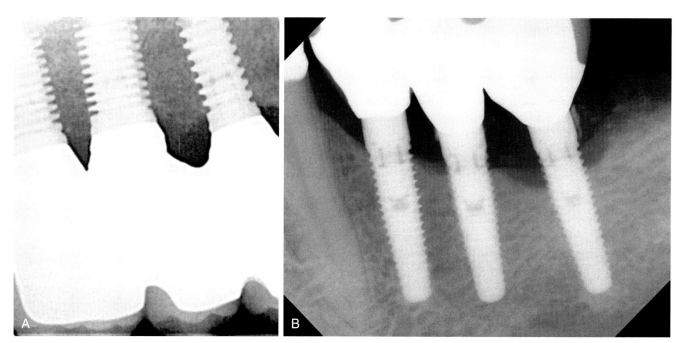

• **Fig. 11.65** Alveolar Bone Level Evaluation. (A) Ideal positioning showing ideal thread orientation. (B) Improper angulation showing diffuse thread orientation.

of choice for evaluation of sinus infection or postsurgical sinusitis complications (Figs. 11.66 and 11.67).

Legal Issues and Cone Beam Computed Tomography

With CBCT becoming more prevalent in diagnosis and treatment planning for dental implants, many legal issues are coming to light. The implant clinician, as a medical professional, is liable for nondiagnosis of any abnormality on the CBCT scan. Dentists are held to a standard when diagnosing and treating patients. To

help meet this standard, the implant clinician must use the CBCT survey in a proper and ideal manner, thus maximizing diagnostic accuracy. Therefore it is imperative for the practitioner to stay current with some of the many potential legal issues associated with CBCT.

To Take a Scan or Not

In medicine, radiographic equipment is usually not approved for a particular purpose or indication. Nor is there any actual standard of care or universally accepted guidelines for the use of CBCT technologies. Instead, any applicable standard of care is mandated by the legislature, a court, or dental board.[95] On

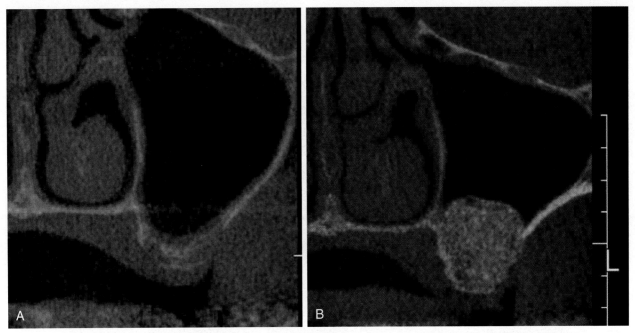

• **Fig. 11.66** Maxillary sinus evaluation. (A) Preoperative cone beam computed tomography (CBCT). (B) Postoperative CBCT depicting maxillary rhinosinusitis after sinus augmentation.

the other hand, even in the absence of an express guideline, an implant clinician is more likely to be questioned for failing to use available CBCT technologies preoperatively if a complication arises.

Technical Parameters

The doctor ordering the scan must be careful to select the correct parameters of the scan. Inadequate or improper CBCT settings and settings may lead to liability. Examples include ordering a scan with low resolution when a high resolution is indicated (e.g., tooth fracture).

Field of View

The FOV (anatomic limits of the scan) is crucial in the preoperative assessment of an implant patient. Ideally the FOV should be the smallest possible to reduce the patient x-ray dosage and improve spatial resolution. However, if the FOV is too small, inadequate sufficient evaluation of the anatomic area will result. This is most commonly seen in the posterior maxillary augmentation when too small a field of view is used. If there is any type of pathology in the sinus and the scan is not taken high enough to determine the patency of the ostium, the doctor is at risk of causing serious sinus issues because of the inability to determine the patency of the ostium and the nature of the pathology.

Interpreting the Scan

There is no current consensus on the legal ramifications of interpreting CBCT scans. However, as a general proposition the implant dentist remains responsible for interpreting the entire scan.[96] The implant clinician has three options. The implant clinician may: (1) interpret the scan themselves; (2) send the CBCT data to a licensed radiologist, or (3) have the CBCT data evaluated by the hospital or imaging center radiologist.

Referral to Radiologist

Ideally, most clinicians will decrease their liability by referring their CBCT scans to a radiologist for evaluation. However, if the doctor sends the scan to a radiologist who is unqualified to interpret the scan, the dentist may have liability for the negligent referral.[97] In addition, the CBCT scan must be read by a radiologist licensed in the same state as the implant clinician. Otherwise, the dentist may be subject to disciplinary action by the state dental board for aiding and abetting the radiologist's unlicensed practice of medicine and for negligent referral of the patient's scan to the unlicensed provider.[98] The implant clinician also should confirm that the radiologist's malpractice insurance covers the reading of CBCT scans.

Waiver of Liability

Many implant clinicians who are untrained in CBCT interpretation request their patients sign a waiver of liability regarding the interpretation of the CBCT scans or a waiver of the right to have the scan read by a radiologist. In general, a patient cannot consent to the negligence of their dentist or other health care provider.[99] Waivers of liability typically have no legal effect and are inadmissible.

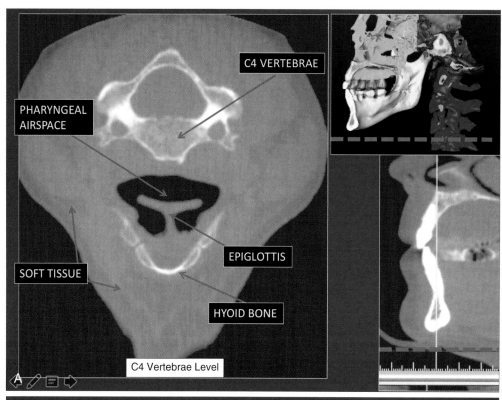

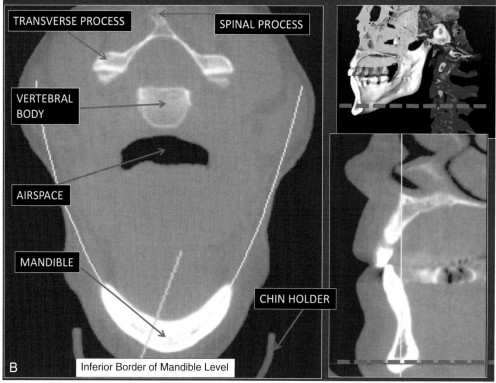

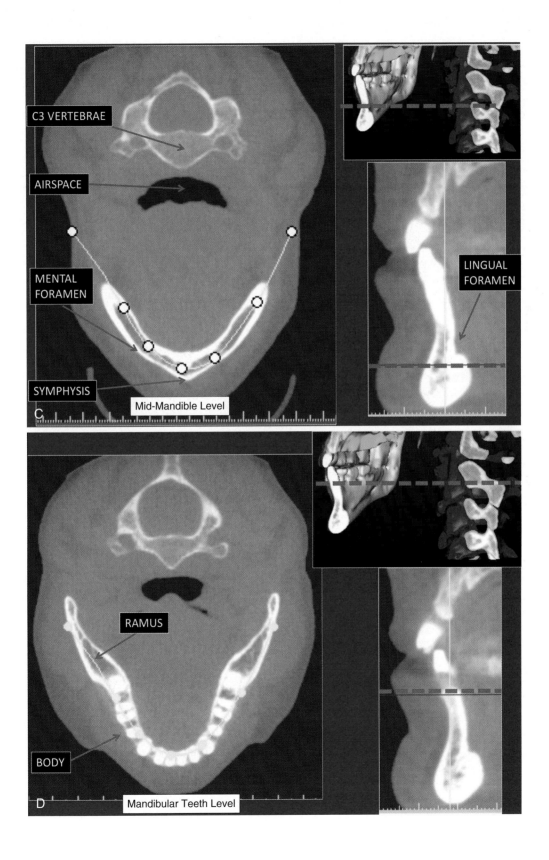

C3 VERTEBRAE

AIRSPACE

MENTAL FORAMEN

SYMPHYSIS

Mid-Mandible Level

C

LINGUAL FORAMEN

RAMUS

BODY

Mandibular Teeth Level

D

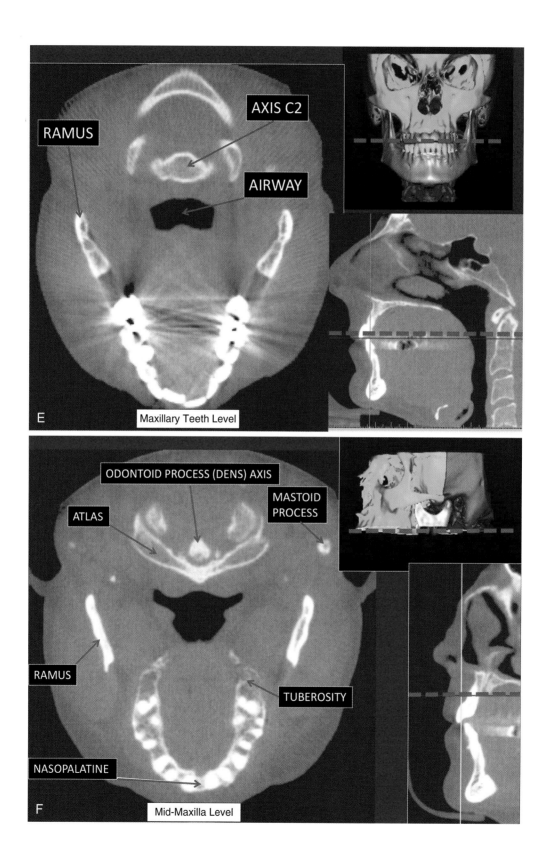

E Maxillary Teeth Level

RAMUS

AXIS C2

AIRWAY

F Mid-Maxilla Level

ODONTOID PROCESS (DENS) AXIS

ATLAS

MASTOID PROCESS

RAMUS

TUBEROSITY

NASOPALATINE

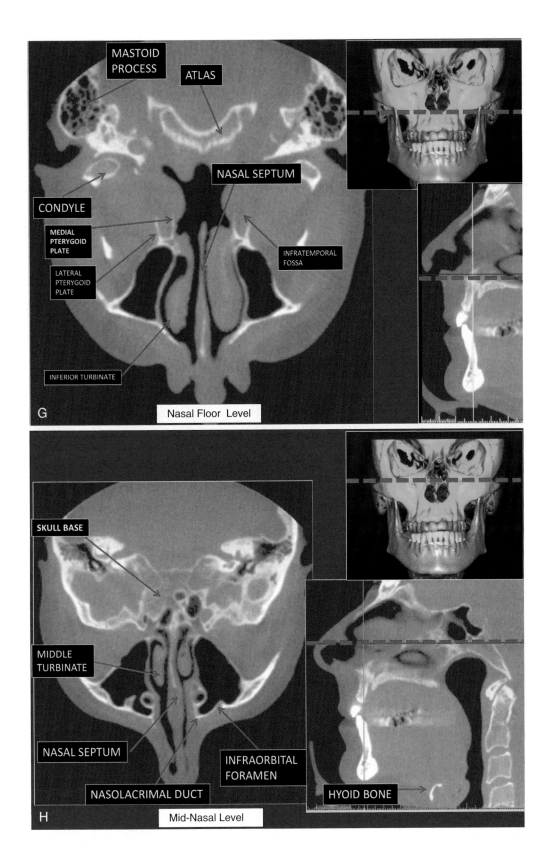

G   Nasal Floor Level

H   Mid-Nasal Level

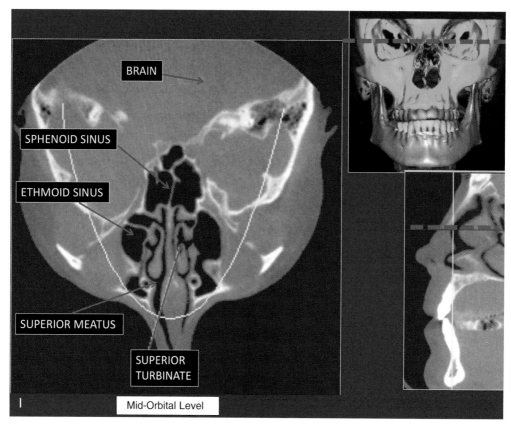

BRAIN

SPHENOID SINUS

ETHMOID SINUS

SUPERIOR MEATUS

SUPERIOR TURBINATE

I — Mid-Orbital Level

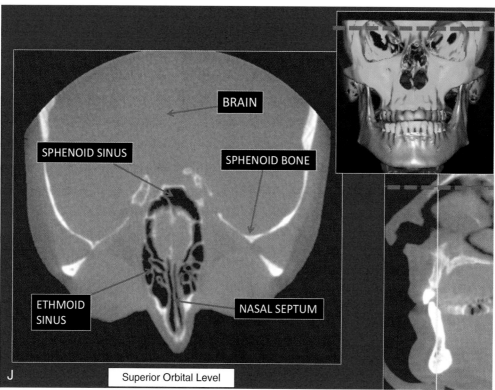

BRAIN

SPHENOID SINUS

SPHENOID BONE

ETHMOID SINUS

NASAL SEPTUM

J — Superior Orbital Level

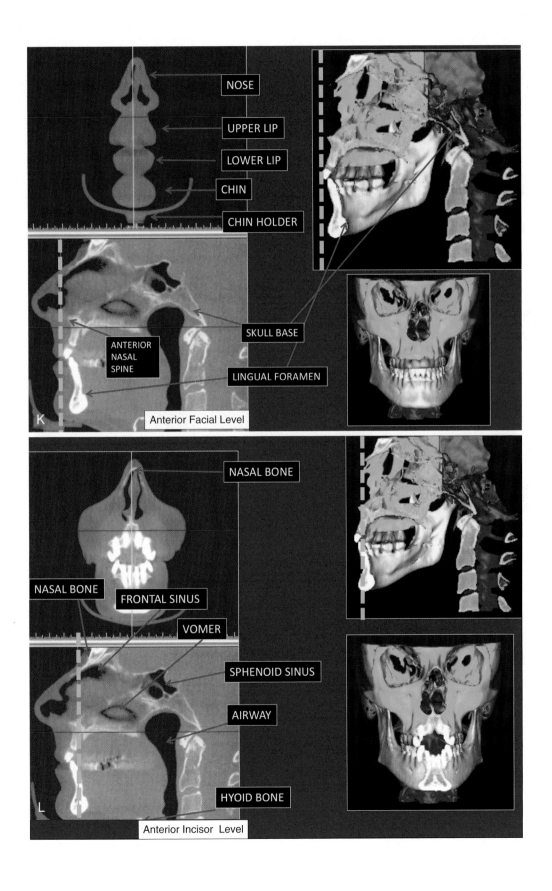

NOSE

UPPER LIP

LOWER LIP

CHIN

CHIN HOLDER

SKULL BASE

ANTERIOR NASAL SPINE

LINGUAL FORAMEN

K   Anterior Facial Level

NASAL BONE

NASAL BONE

FRONTAL SINUS

VOMER

SPHENOID SINUS

AIRWAY

HYOID BONE

L   Anterior Incisor Level

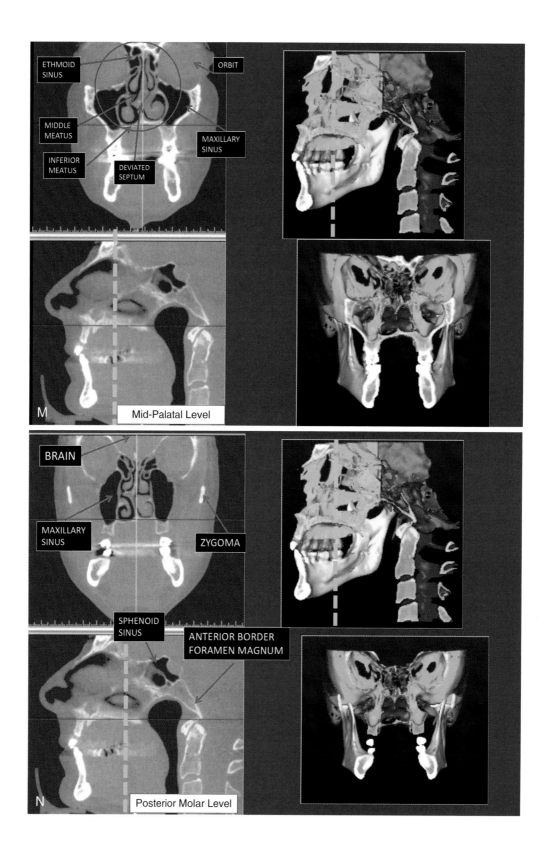

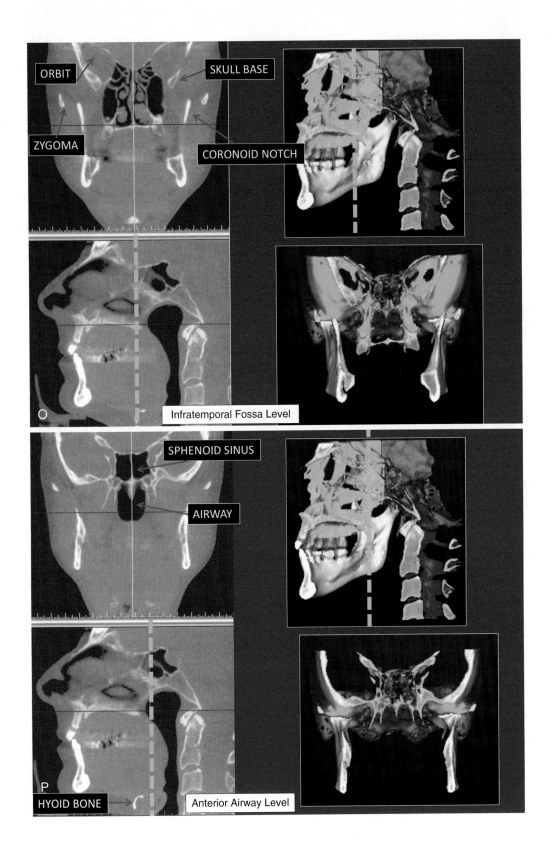

ORBIT

SKULL BASE

ZYGOMA

CORONOID NOTCH

O   Infratemporal Fossa Level

SPHENOID SINUS

AIRWAY

P

HYOID BONE   Anterior Airway Level

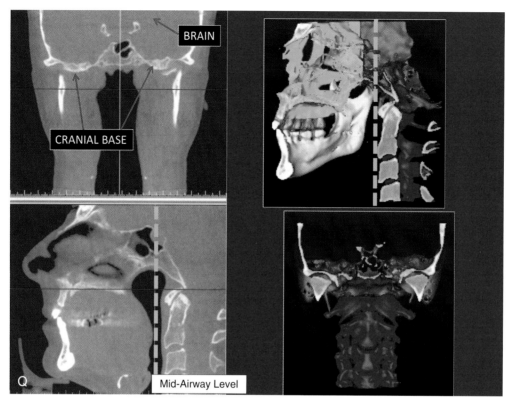

• **Fig. 11.67** Cone Beam Computed Tomography (CBCT) Images. (A) Axial view at the C3 level below the mandible. (B) Axial view at the inferior border of the mandible. (C) Axial view at the midmandible level of the mandible. (D) Axial view at the CEJ of the mandibular teeth. (E) Axial view at the incisal edges of the maxillary and mandibular teeth. (F) Axial view at the midmandible level of the mandible. (G) Axial view at the inferior border of the nasal cavity. (H) Axial view at the midnasal cavity level. (I) Axial view at the midorbit level. (J) Axial view at the superior orbit level. (K) Coronal view at the soft tissue anterior to the maxillary and mandibular teeth. (L) Coronal view at the maxillary and mandibular anterior teeth. (M) Coronal view at the midpalate level. (N) Coronal view at the molar level. (O) Coronal view at the third molar region. (P) Coronal view just anterior to the airway. (Q) Coronal view within the airway region. CEJ, Cementoenamel Junction.

Summary

One of the keys to preventing potential complications during the surgical and prosthetic phases of implant treatment is to have as clear a picture of the patient's current anatomic makeup as possible. Identifying deficiencies of bone allows the clinician to modify the bony architecture to achieve optimal implant location for prosthetic success. Knowing the exact locations of vital structures allows us to plan safe zones during treatment to avoid potentially catastrophic complications. Proper planning is absolutely paramount to success in any endeavor, and having a strong plan in place before the initiation of implant treatment is no exception.

Cone beam technology has ushered in a new era of accuracy in treatment planning. Clinicians are no longer having to rely on "guesswork" by extrapolating anatomic measurements from a distorted 2D image. Templates may be made based on these new 3D images to assist clinicians during tough surgical cases, especially early on respective learning curves. There are just so many benefits to using CBT technology that it is hard to distinguish a reason not to possess one before the initiation of implant treatment. The present legal climate is beginning to echo this sentiment, as CBT is closer to becoming the standard of care across the board.

With the combination of 3D imaging and a thorough knowledge of the anatomic areas that are focused on in this chapter, a clinician can acquire a further degree of confidence that the likelihood of complications has been reduced, which makes the implant treatment process less stressful for both patient and provider.

References

1. Beason RC, Brooks SL. Preoperative implant site assessment in southeast Michigan. *J Dent Res.* 2001;80:137.
2. Tyndall DA, Brooks SL. Selection criteria for dental implant site imaging: a position paper of the American Academy of Oral and Maxillofacial Radiology. *Oral Surg Oral Med Oral Pathol Oral Radiol Endod.* 2000;89(5):630–637.
3. Denio D, Torabinejad M, Bakland LK. Anatomical relationship of the mandibular canal to its surrounding structures in mature mandibles. *J Endod.* 1992;18(4):161–165.
4. Zarch SH Hoseini, et al. Evaluation of the accuracy of panoramic radiography in linear measurements of the jaws. *Iran J Radiol.* 2011;8(2):97.
5. Yosue T, Brooks SL. The appearance of mental foramina on panoramic radiographs. I. Evaluation of patients. *Oral Surg Oral Med Oral Pathol.* 1989;68(3):360–364.

6. Lindh C, Petersson A, Klinge B. Measurements of distances related to the mandibular canal in radiographs. *Clin Oral Implants Res.* 1995;6(2):96–103.

7. Yosue T, Brooks SL. The appearance of mental foramina on panoramic radiographs. I. Evaluation of patients. *Oral Surg Oral Med Oral Pathol.* 1989;68(3):360–364.

8. Sonick M, Abrahams J, Faiella RA. A comparison of the accuracy of periapical, panoramic, and computerized tomographic radiographs in locating the mandibular canal. *Int J Oral Maxillofac Implants.* 1994;9:455–460.

9. Kuzmanovic DV, Payne AG, Kieser JA, Dias GJ. Anterior loop of the mental nerve: a morphological and radiographic study. *Clin Oral Implants Res.* 2003;14(4):464–471.

10. Krennmair G, Ulm GW, Lugmayr H, et al. The incidence, location, and height of maxillary sinus septa in the edentulous and dentate maxilla. *J Oral Maxillofac Surg.* 1999;57:667–671.

11. Naitoh M, Yoshida K, Nakahara K, et al. Demonstration of the accessory mental foramen using rotational panoramic radiography compared with cone-beam computed tomography. *Clin Oral Implants Res.* 2011;22:1415–1419.

12. Lauterbur PC. *Image Formation by Induced Local Interactions: Examples Employing Nuclear Magnetic Resonance*; 1973.

13. Gray CF, Redpath TW, Smith FW, Staff RT. Advanced imaging: magnetic resonance imaging in implant dentistry. *Clin Oral Implants Res.* 2003;14(1):18–27.

14. Zabalegui J, Gil JA, Zabalegui B. Magnetic resonance imaging as an adjunctive diagnostic aid in patient selection for endosseous implants: preliminary study. *Int J Oral Maxillofac.* 1990;5(3).

15. Eggers G, Rieker M, Fiebach J, Kress B, Dickhaus H, Hassfeld S. Geometric accuracy of magnetic resonance imaging of the mandibular nerve. *Dentomaxillofac Radiol.* 2005;34(5):285–291.

16. Kircos LT. Magnetic resonance imaging of the mandible utilizing a double scout technique for preprosthetic imaging. *J Magn Reson Med.* 1993;7:190–194.

17. Wanner Laura, et al. Magnetic resonance imaging—a diagnostic tool for postoperative evaluation of dental implants: a case report. *Oral Surg Oral Med Oral Pathol Oral Radiol Endod.* 2018;125(4):e103–e107.

18. Engstrom H, Svendsen P. Computed tomography of the maxilla in edentulous patients: Normal Anatomy. *Oral Surg Oral Med Oral Pathol Oral Radiol Endod.* 1981;52(5):557–560.

19. Gulsahi Ayse. In: Turkyilmaz Ilser, ed. *Bone Quality Assessment for Dental Implants, Implant Dentistry - The Most Promising Discipline of Dentistry, Prof.* ; 2011. ISBN: 978-953-307-481-8.

20. Angelopoulos Christos, Aghaloo Tara. Imaging technology in implant diagnosis. *Dental clinics of North America.* 2011;55(1):141–158.

21. Vasak C, Watzak G, Gahleitner A, Strbac G, Schemper M, Zechner W. Computed tomography-based evaluation of Guided surgery template (NobelGuide)-guided implant positions: a prospective radiological study. *Clin Oral Implants Res.* 2011;22:1157–1163.

22. Schulze RK, Berndt D, d'Hoedt B. On cone-beam computed tomography artifacts induced by titanium implants. *Clin Oral Implants Res.* 2010;21(1):100–107.

23. Haramati N, Staron RB, Mazel-Sperling K, et al. CT scans through metal scanning technique versus hardware composition. *Comput Med Imaging Graph.* 1994;18(6):429–434.

24. Pettersson A, Komiyama A, Hultin M, Nasstrom K, Klinge B. Accuracy of virtually planned and template guided implant surgery on edentate patients. *Clin Implant Dent Relat Res.* 2012;14:527–537.

25. Visconti MA,PG, et al. Influence of maxillomandibular positioning in cone beam computed tomography for implant planning. *Int J Oral Maxillofac Surg.* 2013;42(7):880–886.

26. Wang Jing, Mao Weihua, Solberg Timothy. "Scatter correction for cone-beam computed tomography using moving blocker strips." SPIE Medical Imaging. *International Society for Optics and Photonics.* 2011.

27. *Specialty Imaging: Dental Implants Tamimi.*

28. Scarfe William C. Incidental findings on cone beam computed tomographic images: a Pandora's box? *Oral surgery, oral medicine, oral pathology and oral radiology.* 2014;117(5):537–540.

29. Price JB, Thaw KL, Tyndall DA, Ludlow JB, Padilla RJ. Incidental findings from cone beam computed tomography of the maxillofacial region: a descriptive retrospective study. *Clin. Oral Impl. Res.* 2012;23:1261–1268.

30. Miles DA, BA, DDS MS, FRCD(C). Clinical experience with cone-beam volumetric imaging—report of findings in 381 cases. Available from: http://www.learndigital.net/articles/2007/CBCT_Touch_Briefings.pdf.

31. Cha JY, Mah J, Sinclair P. Incidental findings in the maxillofacial area with 3- dimensional cone-beam imaging. *Am J Orthod Dentofacial Orthop.* 2007;132:7–14.

32. Arnheiter C, Scarfe WC, Farman AG. Trends in maxillofacial cone-beam computed tomography usage. *Oral Radiol.* 2006;22:80–85.

33. Standring Susan, Ellis H, Healy J, et al. Gray's anatomy: the anatomical basis of clinical practice. *Am J Neuroradiol.* 2005;26(10):2703.

34. Liu T, Xia B, Gu Z. Inferior alveolar canal course: a radiographic study. *Clin Oral Impl Res.* 2009;20:1212–1218.

35. Ikeda K, Ho KC, Nowicki BH, Haughton VM. Multiplanar MR and anatomic study of the mandibular canal. *Am J Neuroradiol.* 1996;17:579–584.

36. Lopes PT, Pereira GA, Santos AM. Morphological analysis of the lingula in dry mandibles of individuals in Southern Brazil. *J Morphol Sci.* 2010;27(3-4):136–138.

37. Hayward J, Richardson ER, Malhotra SK. The mandibular foramen: its anteroposterior position. *Oral Surg Oral Med Oral Pathol.* 1997;44:837–843.

38. Kim ST, Hu KS, Song WC, et al. Location of the mandibular canal and the topography of its neurovascular structures. *J Craniofac Surg.* 2009;20:936–939.

39. Anderson LC, Kosinski TF, Mentag PJ. A review of the intraosseous course of the nerves of the mandible. *J Oral Implantol.* 1991;17:394–403.

40. Carter RB, Keen EN. The intramandibular course of the inferior alveolar nerve. *J Anat.* 1971;108(pt 3):433–440.

41. Denio D, Torabinejad M, Bakland LK. Anatomical relationship of the mandibular canal to its surrounding structures in mature mandibles. *J endod.* 1992;18:161–165.

42. 5 Gowgiel JM. The position and course of the mandibular canal. *J Oral Implantol.* 1992;18:383–385.

43. Naitoh M, Hiraiwa Y, Aimiya H, Gotoh K, Ariji E. Accessory mental foramen assessment using cone-beam computed tomography. *Oral Surg Oral Med Oral Pathol Oral Radiol Endod.* 2009;107:289–294.

44. Fishel D, Buchner A, Hershkowith A, Kaffe I. Roentgenologic study of the mental foramen. *Oral Surg Oral Med Oral Pathol.* 1976;41(5):682–686.

45. Jacobs R, Mraiwa N, Van Steenberghe D, Sanderink G, Quirynen M. Appearance of the mandibular incisive canal on panoramic radiographs. *Surg Radiol Anat.* 2004;26(4):329–333. Epub 2004 Jun 10.

46. Filo K, Schneider T, Locher MC, et al. The inferior alveolar nerve's loop at the mental foramen and its implications for surgery. *J Am Dent Assoc.* 2014;145:260–269.

47. Hanihara T, Ishida H. Frequency variations of discrete cranial traits in major human populations IV. Vessel and nerve related variations. *J Anat.* 2001;199:273–287.

48. Singh Rajani, Srivastav AK. Study of position, shape, size and incidence of mental foramen and accessory mental foramen in Indian adult human skulls. *Int J Morphol.* 2010;28(4):1141–1146.

49. Juodzbalys G, Wang HL, Sabalys G. Anatomy of mandibular vital structures. Part II: Mandibular incisive canal, mental foramen and associated neurovascular bundles in relation with dental implantology. *J Oral Maxillofac Res.* 2010;1:e3.

50. Serman NJ. The mandibular incisive foramen. *Anat.* 1989;167:195–198.
51. De Oliveira-Santos C, Souza PH, de Azambuja Berti-Couto S, et al. Assessment of variations of the mandibular canal through cone beam computed tomography. *Clin Oral Investig.* 2012;16:387–393.
52. Leite Guilherme Mariano Fiuza, et al. Anatomic variations and lesions of the mandibular canal detected by cone beam computed tomography. *Surg Radiol Anat.* 2014;36(8):795–804.
53. Butura Caesar C, et al. Hourglass mandibular anatomic variant incidence and treatment considerations for all-on-four implant therapy: report of 10 cases. *J Oral Maxillofac Surg.* 2011;69(8):2135–2143.
54. Watanabe H, Mohammad Abdul M, Kurabayashi T, Aoki H. Mandible size and morphology determined with CT on a premise of dental implant operation. *Surg Radiol Anat.* 2010;32:343e349.
55. Athavale SA, et al. Bony and cadaveric study of retromolar region. *People's Journal of Scientific Research.* 2013;7 6(2). July 2013.
56. Babiuc IULIANA, Tarlungeanu Ioana, Pauna Mihaela. Cone beam computed tomography observations of the lingual foramina and their bony canals in the median region of the mandible. *Rom J Morphol Embryol.* 2011;52(3):827–829.
57. Atwood DA, Coy WA. Clinical cephalometric and densitometric study of reduction of residual ridges. *J Prosthet Dent.* 1971;26:200–295.
58. Misch CE. Density of bone: effect on treatment plans, surgical approach, healing and progressive bone loading. *Int J Oral Implantol.* 1991;6:23–31.
59. Macedo VC, Cabrini RR, Faig-Leite H. Infraorbital foramen location in dry human skulls. *Braz. J. Morphol. Sci.* 2009;26(1):35–38.
60. DelBalso AM. *Maxillofacial Imaging.* Philadelphia: W.B. Saunders CO; 1990:72.
61. Kantarci M, Karasen R, Alper F, et al. Remarkable anatomic variations in paranasal sinus region and their clinical importance. *Eur J Radiol.* 2004;50:296–302.
62. Seiden A, Tami T, Pensak M, et al. *Otolaryngology the Essentials.* New York: Thieme Medical Publishers; 2002:77–118.
63. Parks Edwin T. Cone Beam Computed Tomography for the Nasal Cavity and Paranasal Sinuses. *Dent Clin North Am.* 2014;58(3):627–651.
64. Van den Bergh JPA, ten Bruggenkate CM, et al. Anatomical aspects of sinus floor elevations. *Clin Oral Implants Res.* 2000;11:256–265.
65. Prasanna LC, Mamatha H. The location of maxillary sinus ostium and its clinical application. *Indian J Otolaryngol Head Neck Surg.* 2010;62(4):335–337.
66. Zinreich S, Albayram S, Benson M, Oliverio P. The ostiomeatal complex and functional endoscopic surgery. In: Som P, ed. *Head and Neck Imaging.* 4th ed. St Louis: Mosby; 2003:149–173.
67. Stallman Jamie S, Joao Lobo N, Som Peter M. The incidence of concha bullosa and its relationship to nasal septal deviation and paranasal sinus disease. *Am J Neuroradiol.* 2004;25(9):1613–1618.
68. Llyod GA. CT scan of the paransal sinuses: study of a control series in relation to endoscopic sinus surgery. *Laryngo Rhino Otol.* 1990;104:477–481.
69. Wani Asif A, et al. CT scan evaluation of the anatomical variations of the ostiomeatal complex. *Indian J Otolaryngol Head Neck Surg.* 2009;61(3):163–168.
70. Arslan Halil, et al. Anatomic variations of the paranasal sinuses: CT examination for endoscopic sinus surgery. *Auris Nasus Larynx.* 1999;26(1):39–48.
71. Kainz J, Braun H, Genser P. [Haller's cells: morphologic evaluation and clinico-surgical relevance]. *Laryngo-rhino-otologie.* 1993;72(12):599–604.
72. Brunner E, Jacobs JB, Shpizner BA, et al. Role of the agger nasi cell in chronic frontal sinusitis. *Ann. Otol. Rhinol. Laryngol.* 1996;105(9):694–700.
73. Krennmair G, Ulm CW, Lugmayr H, et al. The incidence, location and height of maxillary sinus septa in the edentulous and dentate maxilla. *J Oral Maxillofac Surg.* 1999;57:667–671.
74. Kim MJ, Jung UW, Kim CS, et al. Maxillary sinus septa: prevalence, height, location and morphology: a reformatted computed tomography scan analysis. *J Periodontol.* 2006;77:903–908.
75. Leung Cynthia C, et al. Accuracy and reliability of cone-beam computed tomography for measuring alveolar bone height and detecting bony dehiscences and fenestrations. *Am J Orthod Dentofacial Orthop.* 2010;137(4):S109–S119.
76. Neves FS, Souza MC, Franco LCS, Caria PHF, Almeida PB, Rebello IC. Canalis sinuosus: a rare anatomical variation. *Surg Radiol Anat.* 2012;34:563–566.
77. Wanzeler Ana Márcia Viana, et al. Anatomical study of the canalis sinuosus in 100 cone beam computed tomography examinations. *J Oral Maxillofac Surg.* 2014;19(1):49–53.
78. Jacobs RL, Martens W, Mraiwa N, Adriaenses P, Gelan J. Neurovascularization of the anterior jaw bones revisited using high resolution magnetic resonance imaging. *Oral Surg Oral Med Pathol Oral Radiol Endod.* 2007;103:683–693.
79. Almog DM, Tsimidis K, Moss ME, Gottlieb RH, Carter LC. Evaluation of a training program for detection of carotid artery calcifications on panoramic radiographs. *Oral Surg Oral Med Oral Pathol Oral Radiol Endod.* 2000;90:111–117.
80. American Academy of Otolaryngology—Head and Neck Surgery. Fact sheet: 20 questions about your sinuses. Available at http://www.entnet.org/healthinfo/ sinus/sinus_questions.cfm.
81. Rosenfeld RM, Andes D, Bhattacharyya N, et al. Clinical practice guideline: adult sinusitis. *Otolaryngol Head Neck Surg.* 2007;137(suppl 3):S1–S31.
82. Beule A. Epidemiology of chronic rhinosinusitis, selected risk factors, comorbidities, and economic burden. *GMS Curr Top Otorhinolaryngol Head Neck Surg.* 2015;14(11):1–31.
83. Beninger MS, Mickleson SA. Functional endoscopic sinus surgery, morbidity and early results. *Henry Ford Hosp Med J.* 1990;38:5.
84. Yoshiura K, Ban S, Hijiya K, et al. Analysis of maxillary sinusitis using computed tomography. *Dentomaxillofac Radiol.* 1993;22:86.
85. Gardner DG. Pseudocysts and retention cysts of the maxillary sinus. *Oral Surg Oral Med Oral Pathol.* 1984;58:561–567.
86. Kudo K, et al. Clinicopathological study of postoperative maxillary cysts. *J Jpn Stomatol Soc.* 1972;21:250–257.
87. Misch CM, Misch CE, Resnik RR, et al. Postoperative maxillary cyst associated with sinus elevation procedure: a case report. *J Oral Implantol.* 1991;18:432–437.
88. Tiwari R, Hardillo JA, Mehta D, et al. Squamous cell carcinoma of maxillary sinus. *Head Neck. Mar.* 2000;22(2):164–169.
89. Blaschke FF, Brady FA. The maxillary antrolith. *Oral Surg Oral Med Oral Pathol.* 1979;48:187–191.
90. Karges MA, Eversol LR, Poindexter BJ. Report of case and review of literature. *J Oral Surg.* 1971;29:812–814.
91. Resnik RR, Misch CE, eds. *Misch's Avoiding Complications in Oral Implantology.* St. Louis, MO: Elsevier; 2018.
92. Gröndahl K, Lekholm U. The predictive value of radiographic diagnosis of implant instability. *Int J Oral Maxillofac Implants.* 1997;12(1).
93. Sunden S, Gröndahl K, Gröndahl HG. Accuracy and precision in the radiographic diagnosis of clinical instability in Brånemark dental implants. *Clin Oral Implants Res.* 1995;6(4):220–226.
94. Wouters FR, Lavstedt S, Frithiof L, Söder PÖ, Hellden L, Salonen L. A computerized system to measure interproximal alveolar bone levels in epidemiologic, radiographic investigations: II. Intra-and inter-examiner variation study. *Acta Odontol Scand.* 1988;46(1):33–39.
95. Friedland B, Miles DA. Liabilities and risks of using cone beam computed tomography. *Dental Clinics.* 2014;58(3):671–685.
96. Friedland B. Clinical radiological issues in orthodontic practice. In: *Seminars in orthodontics* . WB Saunders; 1998, June;4(2):64–78
97. *Estate of Tranor v Bloomsburg Hosp.* 60 F. Supp. 2d 412, 416 (M.D. Pa. 1999) .
98. Texas Occupations Code, Title 3, Subtitle D, Chapter 251; California Business and Professions Code x2264.
99. Dahl D. *Doctors' 'no sue' contracts spark debate,* Lawyers USA May 21, 2007.

12

Applied Anatomy for Dental Implants

MOHAMED SHARAWY

The surgical anatomy of the maxilla and mandible provide the foundation required to safely insert dental implants. The anatomy is also a requisite to the understanding of complications that may inadvertently occur during surgery, such as injury to blood vessels or nerves, as well as postoperative complications such as infection. This information also provides the operator with the confidence needed to deal with these complications. This chapter addresses those issues important in the field of oral implantology.

Surgical Anatomy of the Maxilla as an Organ

The maxilla is pyramidal in shape, with the root of the zygoma as its apex (Figs. 12.1 and 12.2). The latter can be palpated in the buccal vestibule of the oral cavity. The root of the zygoma divides the facial surface of the maxilla into anterolateral and posterolateral surfaces of the pyramid. The third surface of the pyramid is the orbital plate of the maxilla. The base of the pyramid is the lateral wall of the nose or the medial wall of the maxillary sinus. The alveolar process of the maxilla related to the anterolateral surface carries the incisors, the canines, and the premolars, whereas that of the posterolateral surface carries the molars and ends as the maxillary tuberosity. The intraoral part of the maxilla is limited by the mucobuccal fold and the orbicularis oris muscle anteriorly and by the buccinator muscle posteriorly. The posterolateral surface of the maxilla above the mucobuccal fold forms the anterior wall of the infratemporal fossa and is difficult to palpate. However, the anterolateral surface of the maxilla beyond the mucobuccal fold can be palpated easily under the skin along with the anterior nasal spine, the anterior nasal aperture, and the frontal process of the maxilla. Intraorally, it is possible to palpate the canine eminence, the canine fossa (distal to the canine eminence and a common site for facial access to the maxillary sinus), the maxillary tuberosity, and the hamular notch. The maxilla extends as a horizontal plate medially to form the anterior two-thirds of the hard palate. The horizontal plate of the palatine bone forms the posterior one-third of the hard palate. The palatine bone has a vertical plate that articulates with the base of the maxilla; it also has a pyramidal process that interposes between the maxillary tuberosity and the pterygoid processes of the sphenoid bone. Mucosal incision

at the maxillary tuberosity that extends into the hamular notch may expose the pyramidal process of the palatine bone. Distal to this point, one may expose the medial pterygoid muscle, which takes origin from the tuberosity and the lateral pterygoid plate of the sphenoid. The medial wall of the maxilla begins at the sharp edge of the anterior nasal aperture and extends posteriorly, with a concavity that bounds the nasal fossa and continues distal to the canine. Once there, it forms the medial wall of the maxillary sinus and continues all the way back to the maxillary tuberosity. The medial wall of the maxilla provides attachment to the inferior nasal concha and to the vertical plate of the palatine bone. The opening of the maxillary sinus is found in the medial wall of the maxilla, close to the floor of the orbit. The opening is reduced in diameter by the uncinate process of the ethmoid bone. The latter provides the superior and middle conchae of the lateral nasal wall. The orbital plate of the maxilla forms the floor of the orbit and also the roof of the maxillary sinus. The infraorbital canal carries the infraorbital nerve and vessels, and it forms a ridge that can be seen in the sinus cavity.

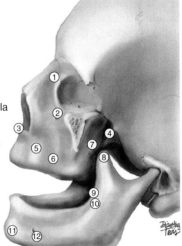

1. Frontal process of maxilla
2. Infraorbital foramen
3. Anterior nasal spine
4. Pterygomaxillary fissure
5. Canine eminence
6. Canine fossa
7. Posterolateral surface of maxilla
8. Coronoid process
9. Retromolar triangle
10. External oblique ridge
11. Mental eminence
12. Mental foramen

• **Fig. 12.1** Anatomical features of the maxilla and mandible that are of clinical importance.

The authors thank Francis T. Lake for contributing to the section on blood supply of edentulous jaws and Lewis Hinley for skillful medical illustration.

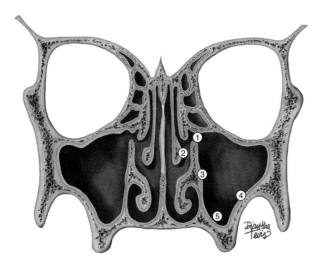

1. Maxillary sinus opening
2. Middle meatus
3. Medial wall of sinus
4. Lateral wall of sinus
5. Floor of sinus and alveolar recess

• **Fig. 12.2** Anatomical features of the maxillary sinus.

Muscles Attached to the Maxilla

As the maxillary alveolar bone resorbs, the crest of the residual ridge migrates toward the muscles that take their origin from the basal bone of the maxilla. Descriptions of muscles of surgical importance to oral implantologists follow (Figs. 12.3–12.5).

Orbicularis Oris Muscle

The orbicularis oris muscle originates from the modiolus at each corner of the mouth. The muscle fibers fan out into the upper and lower lips, in which they form upper and lower peripheral portions under the skin and marginal portions under the vermilion zone of the lips. Some of the orbicularis oris fibers attach to the ala of the nose and to the nasal septum. In the midline of the upper lip, the peripheral portions from both sides interdigitate to create the philtrum. The marginal portions interdigitate and create the labial tubercle. Although unattached to the bone of the maxilla, the muscle limits the depth of the upper and lower facial vestibule. The orbicularis oris receives innervation from the buccal and mandibular branches of the facial nerve.

Incisivus Labii Superioris Muscle

The incisivus labii superioris muscle originates from the floor of the incisive fossa of the maxilla above the eminence of the lateral incisor and deep to the orbicularis oris. To expose the bone of the premaxilla between the canines, a mucoperiosteal flap reflection may detach the incisivus labii superioris. It may also detach the septalis and oblique fibers of the nasalis muscle. The first fiber is attached to the skin of the nasal septum and the latter fiber to the ala of the nose. These small muscles will reattach after placement of the flap. However, if the muscles were damaged, then drooping of the septum and flaring of the ala of the nose may result.

Buccinator Muscle

The buccinator muscle originates from the base of the alveolar process opposite to the first, second, and third molar of both jaws. This muscle also takes origin from the pterygoid hamulus of the medial pterygoid plate of the sphenoid bone, bridging the gap

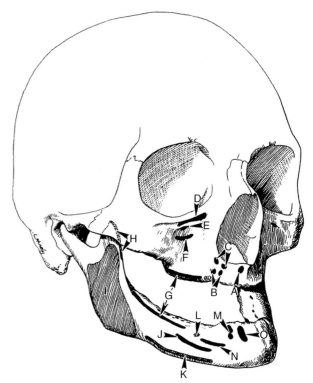

• **Fig. 12.3** *A,* Origin of depressor septi muscle; *B,* origin of superior incisivus muscle; *C,* origin of nasalis muscle; *D,* origin of levator labii superioris muscle; *E,* infraorbital foramen; *F,* origin of levator anguli oris (caninus) muscle; *G,* origin of buccinator muscle; *H,* insertion of lateral tendon of temporalis muscle; *I,* insertion of masseter muscle; *J,* origin of depressor anguli oris (triangularis) muscle; *K,* insertion of platysma muscle; *L,* mental foramen; *M,* origin of inferior incisivus muscle; *N,* origin of depressor labii inferioris muscle; and *O,* origin of mentalis muscle.

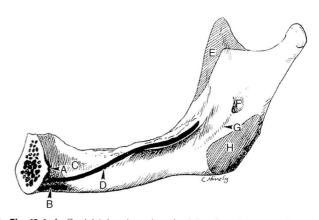

• **Fig. 12.4** *A,* Genial tubercles, site of origin of genioglossus (superior tubercle) and geniohyoid (inferior tubercle) muscles; *B,* digastric fossa, site of origin of anterior belly of digastric muscle; *C,* sublingual fossa, location of sublingual gland; *D,* mylohyoid line, site of origin of mylohyoid muscle; *E,* insertion of medial tendon of temporalis muscle; *F,* mandibular foramen; *G,* mylohyoid groove, formed by mylohyoid nerve; and *H,* site of insertion of medial pterygoid muscle.

between the maxillary tuberosity anteriorly and the hamulus posteriorly. Extension of a subperiosteal frame design into the pterygoid plates may interfere with the fibers of these muscles without adding too much to the retention of the implant. When incising and reflecting the mucosa overlying the areas of the maxillary tuberosity and hamular notch before taking impressions for maxillary subperiosteal implants, avoid injuring the tendon of the

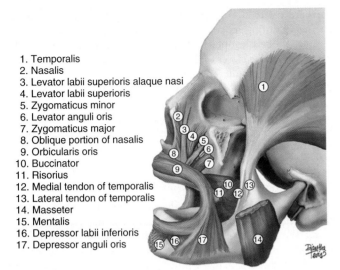

1. Temporalis
2. Nasalis
3. Levator labii superioris alaque nasi
4. Levator labii superioris
5. Zygomaticus minor
6. Levator anguli oris
7. Zygomaticus major
8. Oblique portion of nasalis
9. Orbicularis oris
10. Buccinator
11. Risorius
12. Medial tendon of temporalis
13. Lateral tendon of temporalis
14. Masseter
15. Mentalis
16. Depressor labii inferioris
17. Depressor anguli oris

• **Fig. 12.5** Muscles attached to the maxilla and mandible.

1. Maxillary n.
2. Pterygopalatine ganglion
3. Infraorbital n.
4. Posterior superior alveolar n.
5. Middle superior alveolar n.
6. Anterior superior alveolar n.
7. Buccal n.
8. Mandibular n.
9. Lingual n.
10. Inferior alveolar n.
11. Nerve to mylohyoid
12. Auriculotemporal n.
13. Mental branch of inferior alveolar n.

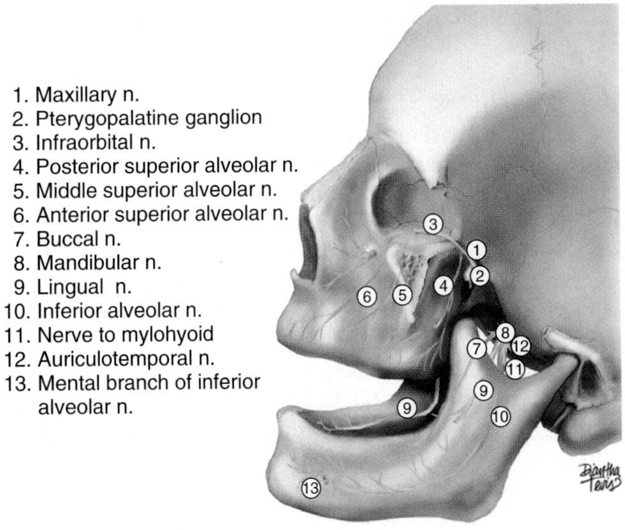

• **Fig. 12.6** Sensory innervation of the maxilla and mandible.

tensor veli transact muscle, which passes around the pterygoid hamulus. The tendon moves on an underlying bursa whenever the soft palate moves; therefore it may become irritated by the subperiosteal frame and result in inflammation and pain. Fibers of the buccinator and medial pterygoid muscles are also found in the area of reflection. The majority of the fibers of the medial pterygoid muscle originate from the medial surface of the lateral pterygoid plate of the sphenoid bone, whereas the rest of the fibers form the tuberal head, which takes origin from the maxillary tuberosity. Near the pterygoid hamulus, a fibrous tissue raphe or, in some cases, a broad fascialike structure is found between the transaction and the superior pharyngeal constrictor muscles. In some cases, no raphe or fascia is found. Injury to the latter muscle should be avoided during reflection of the mucosa, particularly on the palatal aspect of the area of the hamulus.

Levator Labii Superioris Muscle

The levator labii superioris muscle takes origin from the infraorbital margin above the infraorbital foramen; therefore it is rarely of concern to the implant surgeon. The zygomatic branch of the facial nerve innervates this muscle.

Levator Anguli Oris (Caninus) Muscle

The levator anguli oris muscle originates in the maxilla below the infraorbital foramen. The infraorbital nerve and vessels arise between this muscle and the levator labii superioris. In the severe atrophic division D maxilla, the infraorbital foramen is relatively close to the crest of the ridge. Reflection of the tissues for autogenous grafts and implant placement into sinus grafts may approximate this region and cause paresthesia. In subperiosteal implant cases that require extensive framework extension for retention, the operator should be aware of the location of the infraorbital neurovascular bundle in relation to the caninus and levator labii superioris muscles. The zygomatic branch of the facial nerve innervates the caninus muscle.

Sensory Innervation of the Maxilla

The maxillary nerve (V2) innervates the maxilla (Fig. 12.6). The nerve leaves the middle cranial fossa by passing through the foramen rotundum and appears in the pterygopalatine fossa. It exits the fossa

and passes briefly into the infratemporal fossa; from there it enters the floor of the orbit or the roof of the maxillary sinus by passing through the infraorbital fissure. The nerve then exits the orbit via the infraorbital foramen. The pterygopalatine portion of the maxillary nerve provides the descending palatine and sphenopalatine branches. The sphenopalatine nerve enters the nasal cavity from the pterygopalatine fossa by passing through the sphenopalatine foramen. The nerve supplies the nasal cavity and becomes the incisive nerve that supplies the palatine mucosa opposite to the upper six anterior teeth. The descending palatine nerve terminates as the great palatine nerve, which supplies the mucosa of the hard palate, and the lesser palatine nerves, which supply the mucosa of soft palate. These sensory nerves also carry parasympathetic fibers from the sphenopalatine ganglion that innervate the mucous glands of the palate. The infratemporal portion of V2 branches into the posterior alveolar nerve and zygomatic nerve. The latter divides into the zygomaticofacial and zygomaticotemporal cutaneous nerves. The posterior superior alveolar nerve supplies the buccal gingiva, buccal alveolar bone, second and third molars, and two roots of the first molar. The infraorbital portion of V2 gives rise to anterior superior alveolar and occasionally middle superior alveolar nerves. These nerves run in bony grooves in the facial wall of the maxillary sinus under the Schneiderian membrane. The nerves supply the sinus wall and the premolars; the canine, lateral, and central incisor on the same side; and the central incisor at the contralateral side. The infraorbital nerve exits the maxilla at the infraorbital foramen and supplies cutaneous branches to the lower eyelid, side of the nose, and upper lip. Implantologists often need to block V2 or several of its branches. Luckily this can be achieved by an intraoral route. V2 can be reached via the great palatine foramen and descending palatine canal, or via the pterygomaxillary fissure by following the slope of the posterolateral surface of the maxilla into the pterygopalatine fossa.

Posterior Superior Alveolar (Dental) Nerve

The nerve arises within the pterygopalatine fossa, courses downward and forward, passing through the pterygomaxillary fissure, and enters the posterior aspect of the maxilla. It runs between the bone and the lining of the maxillary sinus. This nerve supplies the sinus, the molars, the buccal gingiva, and the adjoining portion of the cheek; it may be injured during a sinus augmentation with a lateral approach. Clinically this does not appear to be of major consequence.

Infraorbital Nerve

This nerve is a continuation of the main trunk of the maxillary division. It leaves the pterygopalatine fossa by passing through the inferior orbital fissure to enter the floor of the orbit. It runs in the infraorbital groove and then in the infraorbital canal. The nerve exits the orbit through the infraorbital foramen to give cutaneous branches to the lower eyelid, the ala of the nose and the skin, and the mucous membrane of the lip and cheek. The infraorbital foramen is located between the levator labii superioris muscle, which takes origin above the foramen, and the levator anguli oris (caninus) muscle, which takes origin below the foramen. The foramen and neurovascular contents are within 5 to 10 mm of an extremely resorbed maxilla. When applying onlay grafts, which expose the entire maxilla, the implant dentist must be very aware of this situation. Fixation screws or implants may cause paresthesia when inserted through the graft and into this structure. Subperiosteal implants designed for an atrophied maxilla should not extend into the site of the infraorbital nerve and vessels. In some cases of maxillary sinus disorder, the site of the infraorbital foramen becomes tender, probably as a result of inflammation of the infraorbital nerve. This is an important diagnostic test for possible postoperative involvement after sinus augmentation procedures.

Middle Superior Alveolar (Dental) Nerve

This branch of the infraorbital nerve is given off as the infraorbital nerve passes through the infraorbital groove. The middle superior alveolar nerve runs downward and forward in the lateral wall of the sinus to supply the maxillary premolars. This region is routinely violated in the lateral approach to sinus grafts, with apparently no consequence.

Anterior Superior Alveolar (Dental) Nerve

This branch of the infraorbital nerve arises within the infraorbital canal. It initially runs laterally within the sinus wall and then curves medially to pass beneath the infraorbital foramen. The branch turns downward to supply the maxillary anterior teeth. A nasal branch passes into the nasal cavity to supply the mucosal lining of a portion of the nasal cavity. Before elevation of nasal mucosa and placement of grafts, this nerve must be anesthetized. The infraorbital nerve block or V2 block anesthesia is suggested. Implant dentists must also anesthetize this branch before placement of implants in the incisor region. The anterior, middle, and posterior superior alveolar nerves intermingle to form the superior dental plexus. The posterior, middle, and anterior superior alveolar nerves run in the facial wall of the maxillary sinus between its lining membrane and the bone. During antrostomy procedures to augment the floor of the sinus, the operator should be aware of these structures, which are present even in the absence of teeth.

Palatine Nerve

The greater (anterior) and lesser (posterior) palatine nerves supply the hard and soft palate, respectively. They exit the pterygopalatine fossa through the superior opening of the descending palatine canal, travel downward, and enter the oral cavity by way of the greater and lesser palatine foramina. The greater palatine nerve runs forward in a groove on the inferior surface of the hard palate to supply the palatal mucosa as far forward as the incisor teeth. Here the nerve communicates with the nasopalatine nerve. The nerve supplies the gingiva, mucous membrane, and glands of

the hard palate. The greater palatine artery and vein accompany the nerve during its course in the hard palate. As the maxillary alveolar process atrophies, it shifts to the palate and brings the crest of the ridge closer to the groove in which the greater palatine neurovascular bundle is found. The restoring dentist should be aware that an incision too palatal to the crest of the ridge in the atrophied maxilla might injure these vital structures. This foramen is entered for a V2 block anesthesia. One may find it by taking a blunt instrument and pressing firmly along the alveolar palatal bone angle. The instrument will depress over the foramen when in the correct position.

Nasopalatine (Sphenopalatine) Nerve

The nasopalatine nerve leaves the pterygopalatine fossa through the sphenopalatine foramen located in the medial wall of the fossa. The nerve enters the nasal cavity and supplies portions of the lateral and superior aspects of the nasal cavity. The longest branch reaches the nasal septum, in which it turns downward and forward, traveling on the surface of the septum. While on the septum it forms a groove on the vomer bone. The nerve supplies the nasal mucosa, descends to the floor of the nose near the septum, passes through the nasopalatine canal, and then exits onto the hard palate through the incisive foramen. The latter opening is deep in the incisive papilla. The nerve communicates with the greater palatine nerve. The incisive nerve should be anesthetized before elevation of the mucosa of the floor of the nose for subnasal grafts or implants that engage the nasal floor in the incisor region.

Arterial Supply to the Maxilla

The majority of arterial blood supply (Fig. 12.7) comes from the maxillary artery, which is one of the terminal branches of the external carotid artery. The artery starts deep in the neck of the mandibular condyle (mandibular portion) and then proceeds either superficial or deep to the lateral pterygoid muscle (pterygoid portion). It then branches close to the pterygomaxillary fissure, in which one branch enters the fossa (pterygopalatine portion). The other branch, called the *infraorbital artery*, enters the floor of the orbit via the infraorbital fissure; it proceeds in the infraorbital canal and exits on the face by passing through the infraorbital foramen. Branches of the maxillary artery are as follows:

1. Ophthalmic a.
2. Infraorbital a.
3. Deep temporal a.
4. Posterior superior alveolar a.
5. Middle superior alveolar a.
6. Anterior superior alveolar a.
7. Buccal a.
8. Inferior alveolar a.
9. Middle meningeal a.
10. Maxillary a.
11. Superior temporal a.
12. External carotid a.
13. Mental branch of inferior alveolar a.
14. Facial a.

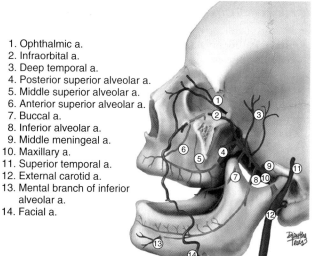

• **Fig. 12.7** Arterial supply of the maxilla and mandible.

1. Mandibular portion: deep auricular, tympanic, middle meningeal, and inferior alveolar arteries
2. Pterygoid portion: deep temporal, lateral pterygoid, medial pterygoid, and masseteric arteries
3. Pterygopalatine portion: posterior superior alveolar, descending palatine, and sphenopalatine arteries
4. Infraorbital portion: anterior and middle superior alveolar, palpebral, nasal, and labial arteries

Supplemental arterial blood supply reaches the maxilla via two branches from the cervical portion of the facial artery (ascending palatine and tonsillar arteries), two dorsolingual arteries from the lingual artery, and the ascending pharyngeal branch of the external carotid artery. All the collateral circulation reaches the maxilla from the area of the soft palate. During orthognathic surgery to correct maxillary prognathism, the surgeon often cuts the posterior, middle, and anterior superior alveolar arteries, as well as the descending palatine arteries, without compromising the blood supply to the maxilla because of the presence of supplemental blood supply from the branches mentioned previously. It is important to note that the maxillary artery supplies blood to the bone of the mandible via its inferior alveolar artery and its branches to the muscles of mastication. Detaching the masseter and medial pterygoid muscles without reattaching it could result in necrosis of the ramus of the mandible. In addition, all the arterial branches mentioned previously arise from the external carotid; therefore bilateral arteriosclerosis of the carotids, which is common in old age and in uncontrolled diabetic patients, may compromise the blood supply to the maxilla and could result in delay of healing after insertion of implants or bone grafting to the area. More detailed consideration of applied anatomy of the arterial supply to both the maxilla and mandible is presented at the end of this chapter.

Venous Drainage of the Maxilla

The veins follow the arteries and carry the same names. The maxilla drains into the maxillary vein. The latter communicates freely with the pterygoid plexus of veins and then joins the superficial temporal vein to form the posterior facial vein within the parotid gland. Infection from the maxilla may follow the maxillary vein to the pterygoid plexus veins and then to the cavernous sinuses via emissary veins, causing infected cavernous sinus thrombosis. Adequate arterial supply and healthy venous drainage are essential for bone regeneration and remodeling of bone grafts.

Lymphatic Drainage

The maxilla, including the maxillary sinuses, drains its lymphatics into the submandibular lymph nodes. In addition, the posterior portion of the maxilla and soft palate drain into the deep facial lymph nodes, which are part of the deep cervical nodes. Palpation of lymph nodes is an essential part of the physical examination of the head and neck.

Surgical Anatomy of the Mandible

The clinician should be familiar with the anatomical features of dentulous and edentulous mandibles, not only from radiographs but also from physical examination (see Figs. 12.1–12.4). The symphysis, inferior border, premasseteric notch, gonial angle, lateral pole of condyle, and coronoid process are all palpable under the skin. Intraoral palpable features of the mandible from the facial surface include the external oblique ridge and retromolar triangle, with the coronoid process at its tip, the external oblique ridge bordering it laterally, and the internal oblique ridge bordering it medially. The latter is called the *temporal crest* because this is the site for insertion of the medial tendon of the temporalis muscle. The mental foramen can be located at the midpupillary line at the apices of the premolars. From the lingual aspect, palpate the internal oblique ridge and torus mandibularis at the premolar region. Reflection of the mucoperiosteal flap beyond the mucobuccal fold facially exposes the mentalis muscles lateral to the midline, the mental foramen with the mental neurovascular bundle, the depressor labii inferiori, and the triangularis close to the inferior border in the premolar region, the transaction at the base of the alveolar process opposite to the molars, and the temporalis tendons at the anterior border of the ramus. An atrophied edentulous mandible loosens the alveolar process, and the crest of the ridge may be found at the same level as the external and internal oblique ridge. It is possible to palpate the superior genial tubercle with its genioglossus muscle attachment. Reflection of the mucoperiosteal flap after a midcrest incision may expose the mental neurovascular bundle, which is abnormally located at or occasionally lingual to the crest of the ridge. The transact muscle may loosen its attachment to the external oblique ridge, whereas the mylohyoid may rise above the level of the ridge. The lingual nerve, which has a close relationship to the alveolar bone of the third molar in the dentulous mandible, may run close to the crest of the edentulous ridge; in some cases it may be found under the retromolar pad.

Muscle Attachment to the Mandible

The loss of teeth begins a cascade of events that leads to alveolar bone loss in width and height. As the mandibular alveolar bone resorbs, the residual ridge migrates toward many of the muscles that originate or insert on the mandible (see Figs. 12.3–12.5). The origin, insertion, innervation, and function of the muscles of surgical importance to the implant dentist are discussed.[1-7]

Lingual or Medial Attachments

Mylohyoid Muscle. The mylohyoid muscle is the main muscle of the floor of the mouth. It takes origin from the entire length of the mylohyoid lines on the medial aspect of the mandible bilaterally. The most posterior fibers of the mylohyoid insert into the body of the hyoid bone, whereas the other fibers meet in the midline to form a median raphe that extends from the mandible to the hyoid bone. The structures above the mylohyoid muscle are sublingual or intraoral in location, and the structures below the mylohyoid muscle are extraoral or subcutaneous. With a severely resorbed residual ridge, the origin of the mylohyoid muscle approximates the crest of the ridge, especially in the posterior mandible. In these cases surgical manipulation at the crest of the ridge may injure the mylohyoid muscle. A mandibular periosteal reflection for subperiosteal implant often reflects this muscle to the second molar region. The substructure of the implant then has a permucosal site in the first molar area and a lingual primary strut above and below the mylohyoid muscle. Surgical manipulation of the tissue of the floor of the mouth may lead to edematous swelling of the sublingual space (above the mylohyoid muscle), swelling of the submandibular space (below the mylohyoid muscle), or both. Ecchymosis resulting from blood accumulation may occur subcutaneously and/or submucosally. In some cases, infection may start and spread lingually and lead to an abscess or cellulitis either sublingually (intraoral) or submandibularly (extraoral), depending on the site of origin of the infection in relation to the origin of the mylohyoid muscle. Extensive bilateral cellulitis of the sublingual spaces may push the tongue backward or compress the pharynx, which may result in airway obstruction and necessitate a tracheotomy or cricothyroidotomy to maintain the airway. Functionally, the mylohyoid muscle raises the hyoid bone and floor of the mouth, or it can depress the mandible if the hyoid bone is fixed. The mylohyoid nerve that innervates the muscle is a motor branch of the inferior alveolar nerve. The latter is a branch of the mandibular nerve (V3).

Genioglossus Muscle. The genioglossus muscle forms the bulk of the tongue. It takes origin from the superior genial tubercle. The anterior fibers insert into the dorsal surface of the tongue from the root to its tip, and the posterior fibers insert into the body of the hyoid bone. The genioglossus muscle is the main protruder of the tongue. The genial tubercles, particularly the superior pair, may be located near the crest of the alveolar ridge in divisions C to D of the atrophic mandible. During the elevation of the lingual mucosa and before making an impression for a subperiosteal implant, one should be aware of the origin of this structure to avoid causing injury during the procedure. A portion of this muscle may be reflected from the genial tubercle. However, the muscle should not be completely detached from the tubercle because this may result in retrusion of the tongue and possible airway obstruction. A branch of the hypoglossal nerve (cranial nerve XII) supplies the genioglossus.

Medial Pterygoid Muscle. The majority of the fibers of the medial pterygoid muscle take origin from the medial surface of the lateral pterygoid plate of the sphenoid bone. A small slip of muscle originates from the tuberosity of the maxilla. The muscle inserts on the medial surface of the angle of the mandible. The medial pterygoid muscle bounds the pterygomandibular space medially. This space is entered when an inferior dental nerve block is administered. Furthermore, during surgical procedures medial to the medial tendon of the temporalis muscle, such as in preparation for the insertion of a unilateral subperiosteal implant, the pterygomandibular space is usually involved. Infection of this space is dangerous because of its proximity to the parapharyngeal space and the potential for spread of the infection to the mediastinum. Surgical exposure of tissue posterior to the maxillary tuberosity may also involve the medial pterygoid muscle because a portion of the muscle takes origin from the maxillary tuberosity. However, the numbers of fibers originating from the tuberosity are few compared with the fibers from the medial surface of the lateral pterygoid plate. A branch of the mandibular division (V3) of the trigeminal nerve innervates the muscle.

Lateral Pterygoid Muscle. Although the lateral pterygoid muscles rarely are involved in surgery for implants, their possible action in mandibular flexure or adduction during opening, as well as the effect of this phenomenon on subperiosteal implants or prosthetic full-arch splitting of mandibular implants in the molar region, warrants their consideration. The lateral pterygoid muscle consists of superior and inferior heads. The superior head takes origin from the infratemporal surface and crest of the greater wing of the sphenoid bone (roof of the infratemporal fossa), whereas the inferior head takes origin from the lateral surface of the lateral plate of the pterygoid process of the sphenoid bone. The fibers of the superior head run downward to insert on the anterior band of the temporomandibular joint (TMJ) disk (about 15% of its fibers)

and the pterygoid fovea on the neck of the mandible. The fibers of the inferior head run upward to insert on the pterygoid fovea and also on the medial pole of the condyle, median capsule, and median collateral ligament of the TMJ disk. Because of the angulation of the lateral pterygoid muscles, many authors believe that the mandibular flexure causing alteration in the mandibular arch width, and sometimes pain in patients with a full-arch subperiosteal implant or prosthetic splint, may be caused by contraction of the lateral pterygoid muscles. The muscles normally function in protraction of the mandible and are innervated by a branch of the mandibular nerve (V3).

Temporalis Muscle. The temporalis is a fan-shaped muscle of mastication. It takes origin from the temporal fossa and inserts into the coronoid process of the mandible and the anterior border of the ramus as far inferiorly as the last molar at the site of the retromolar fossa. The muscle has two tendons that insert into the mandible. The superficial tendon is located laterally, and the deep tendon is inserted medially. The temporalis tendons and their associated fascia project anteromedially and inferiorly and serve as a common point for attachment for the temporalis, masseter, and medial pterygoid muscles, as well as for the transaction and superior pharyngeal constrictor muscles. The long buccal nerve and vessels are also located in this area. This temporalis tendon–fascial complex extends into what is traditionally called the *retromolar triangle.* Surgical exposure of the mandibular ramus medially would involve this tendon–fascial complex, with its contents of muscle fibers, nerves, and vessels, and may lead to transaction and postoperative pain. Incisions placed on the anterior ascending ramus for subperiosteal implants or harvesting bone from the external oblique and ramus should be inferior to the insertion of the two tendons of the temporalis muscle. The temporalis muscle is a powerful elevator and retractor of the mandible and, like all the major muscles of mastication, is innervated by a branch of V3.

Buccal or Facial Muscle Attachments

Mentalis Muscle. The external surface of the mandible in the midline presents a ridge indicative of the location of the symphysis menti (see Fig. 12.5). The ridge leads inferiorly to a triangular elevation known as the *mental protuberance.* The base of the triangle is raised on either side into the mental tubercles. The mentalis muscles take origin from the periosteum of the mental tubercles and the sides of the mental eminence and insert into the skin of the chin and superiorly interdigitate with the orbicularis oris of the lower lip. Above the mentalis origin, the incisivus muscles take origin from small fossae called the *incisivus fossae.* Complete reflection of the mentalis muscles for the purpose of extension of a subperiosteal implant or symphyseal intraoral graft may result in "witch's chin," probably caused by the failure of muscle reattachment. If the muscle is completely detached to expose the symphysis, then an elastic bandage is applied externally to the chin for 4 days to help in the reattachment of the muscle. Another approach is to incise the muscle and leave a proximal portion attached to bone and reflect the distal portion. The distal and proximal portions should be approximated with resorbable sutures before suturing the mucosa. The mentalis muscle receives its nerve supply from the marginal (mandibular) branch of the facial nerve.

Buccinator Muscle. The fibers of the transaction muscle (cheek muscle) take origin from the lateral surfaces of the alveolar processes of the maxilla and the mandible in the area of the molars, the maxillary tuberosity, the pterygoid hamulus, the pterygomandibular raphe, and the retromolar fossa of the mandible. The insertion of the muscle is complex. The upper and lower fibers of the transaction blend with the fibers of the orbicularis oris at the upper and lower lips. The central fibers decussate at the modiolus before they insert into the orbicularis oris. The modiolus is the site of crossing and intermingling of fibers from the transaction muscle with fibers from the elevator and depressor muscles of the angle of the mouth. The modiolus forms a palpable node inside the angle of the mouth opposite the upper first premolar tooth. The parotid duct opposite the maxillary second molar pierces the transaction muscle. The buccopharyngeal fascia, which is a part of the visceral fascia of the neck, covers the muscle. Lateral to the fascia is the buccal pad of fat.

Some patients wearing lower subperiosteal implants complain of episodic swelling and pain at the site of origin of the transaction muscle, particularly after periods of heavy mastication or bruxism. Incision of these swellings does not usually yield exudate or purulence. The condition responds well to heat application, transactionary drugs, and rest. Although the cause for this condition is not known, one may speculate that myositis of a detached transaction muscle may cause it. The process of muscle reattachment to the implant surface or to a new site should be investigated. The buccal branch of the facial nerve innervates the muscle.

Masseter Muscle. This strong muscle of mastication covers the lateral surface of the ramus and angle of the mandible. The masseter has a dual origin from superficial and deep heads. The superficial head takes origin from the anterior two-thirds of the lower border of the zygomatic arch. The deep head originates from the posterior one-third of the zygomatic arch and the entire deep surface of the arch. The muscle inserts into the outer surface of the ramus of the mandible from the sigmoid notch to the angle. However, the muscle can be deflected easily during surgery to expose the bone for the ramus extension needed for lateral support of a subperiosteal implant. The space between the masseteric fascia and the muscle is a potential surgical space, known as the *masseteric space,* into which an infection may spread, causing myositis and trismus. The masseter is one of the main elevators of the jaw. The masseteric nerve provides the innervation of the muscle and is a branch of the mandibular division (V3) of the trigeminal nerve.

Innervation of the Lower Jaw and Associated Structures

Inferior Alveolar (Dental) Nerve

This nerve arises as a branch of the mandibular nerve (V3) in the infratemporal fossa (see Fig. 12.6). It appears at the inferior border of the inferior head of the lateral pterygoid muscle, courses downward, and enters the mandibular foramen on the medial aspect of the ramus. Before the nerve enters the mandibular foramen, it gives numerous sensory branches that innervate the mandibular bone. These small nerves are in association with small vessels in neurovascular channels. The inferior dental nerve can run as one unit through the mandibular canal until it reaches the premolar region, in which it divides into the mental and the incisive nerves. The mental nerve exits the canal through the mental foramen. In an excessively resorbed ridge, the mental foramen, with its contents of mental nerve and vessels, can be found on the crest of the ridge. When making an incision or reflection of the mucosa in this area, avoid injury to these vital structures. Knowledge of the position of the inferior dental canal in vertical and buccolingual dimensions is of paramount importance during site preparation for implants. The potential use of reconstruction techniques on

computed tomographic scans and magnetic resonance imaging may increase clinicians' ability to locate the inferior dental canal precisely within the jawbone. Much less expensive techniques using panoramic cross-sectional tomographic imaging are also available. In some cases the inferior dental nerve may divide into two or three rami that occupy separate canals as the nerve travels in the mandible to supply the bone. These variations can be determined by conventional radiographic techniques, and the operator should modify the surgical approach and type of implant to avoid injury to the portion of the nerve that exits the foramen. Injury to the portion of the inferior alveolar nerve that remains in the atrophied bone and does not innervate soft tissues is of far less consequence. The nerves in the bone, when in contact with an implant, may account for the rare but occasional observation of tenderness, even though the implant is rigid and appears healthy. In addition, the fibrous tissue around these nerves may cause an increase in the amount of fibrous tissue around an implant that is inserted in contact with these structures.

Lingual Nerve

The lingual nerve is a branch of the mandibular nerve that is given off in the infratemporal fossa. It appears at the inferior border of the inferior head of the lateral pterygoid muscle anterior to the inferior alveolar nerve. It passes downward and forward between the ramus of the mandible and the medial pterygoid muscle. The nerve enters the oral cavity above the posterior edge of the mylohyoid muscle close to its origin at the third molar region. Because the nerve lies just medial to the retromolar pad, incisions in this region should remain lateral to the pad, and the mucosal reflection should be done with the periosteal elevator in constant contact with bone to prevent injury to the nerve. The nerve proceeds on the surface of the hyoglossus muscle and then crosses the duct of the submandibular gland medially to enter the floor of the mouth and the tongue. While in the infratemporal fossa, the nerve is joined by the chorda tympani nerve, which is a branch of cranial nerve VII. The chorda tympani nerve carries taste fibers from the anterior two-thirds of the tongue and parasympathetic preganglionic fibers to the submandibular autonomic ganglion. The ganglion is connected to the lingual nerve on the surface of the hyoglossus muscle. The postganglionic neurons from the submandibular ganglion supply the submandibular and sublingual salivary glands. The branches of the lingual nerve in the oral cavity carry sensory information from the lingual mucosa, the mucosa of the floor of the mouth, and the anterior two-thirds of the tongue. Improper reflection of a lingual mucoperiosteal flap may injure the lingual nerve and produce ipsilateral paresthesia or anesthesia of the innervated mucosa, loss of taste, and reduction of salivary secretion. The extent of involvement depends on the degree of injury to the nerve.

Nerve to the Mylohyoid

The mylohyoid motor branch of the inferior dental nerve is given off just before the nerve enters the mandibular foramen. This branch descends in a groove on the medial surface of the mandibular ramus and then appears in the submandibular triangle at the posterior border of the mylohyoid muscle. The nerve supplies the mylohyoid muscle and then proceeds on its surface with the submental artery (branch of the facial artery) until it reaches the anterior belly of the digastric muscle, which it also supplies. Because the nerve is so closely related to the ramus of the mandible, surgical intervention in this area may lead to injury of this important motor nerve.

Long Buccal Nerve

This nerve is a sensory branch of the mandibular division of the trigeminal nerve and is distributed to the skin and mucous membrane of the cheek and the buccal transact opposite the mandibular molar region. The nerve courses between the two heads of the lateral pterygoid muscle, then precedes medial to, or sometimes within, the medial temporalis tendon to gain access to the surface of the buccinator muscle. The nerve supplies the skin of the cheek and runs down to the level of the external oblique ridge, penetrates the buccinator, and spreads its branches under the cheek mucosa, alveolar mucosa, and attached gingivae opposite to molar teeth. The implantologist who is planning to access the ramus for the purpose of excising a block graft should be aware of the buccal nerve and avoid injuring it. In addition, surgical manipulation in this area (e.g., during insertion of a subperiosteal implant) may injure this nerve.

Blood Supply to the Maxilla and Mandible

The head and neck region has an abundant blood supply, with many anastomoses (see Fig. 12.7). The upper and lower jaws are no exception. The blood supply to both the mandible and maxilla is derived from a common source, the external carotid artery. The external carotid artery is a branch of the common carotid artery, which is a direct branch off the arch of the aorta on the left side and a branch of the brachiocephalic artery on the right side of the body.

The main artery supplying the mandible is the inferior alveolar (dental) artery, which serves as the nutrient artery to the bone and other tissues within the lower jaw. The bone tissue of the maxillae is supplied by branches of two major vessels, the posterior superior alveolar (dental) artery, and the infraorbital artery. The major branch of the infraorbital artery that supplies the maxilla is the anterior superior alveolar (dental) artery. The posterior superior alveolar and infraorbital arteries are branches of the maxillary artery, which is one of the two terminal branches of the external carotid artery.

General Concepts

The circulation of blood within long bones is centrifugal; that is, the blood circulates from the marrow (medullary) region outward through the cortical bone to end in vessels located in the periosteum and soft tissues associated with the bone.[8,9] The blood supply to the medullary region is by way of nutrient arteries, which are relatively large vessels that pass through the bone by way of nutrient canals to enter the marrow spaces. Within the marrow spaces, the nutrient artery forms a network of vessels called the *endosteal* or *medullary plexus.* Vessels from this plexus enter the cortical bone through Volkmann canals and eventually reach the surface of the bone. While blood is passing through the cortical bone, numerous vessels are given off at right angles to these intraosseous vessels within Volkmann canals. These branches are the vessels that are found within the haversian canals of the osteons.[8,9] Osteonal bone is the major type of bone found in the cortical bone of the jaws. Once the intraosseous vessels reach the outer surface of the bone, they anastomose with vessels within the fibrous layer of the periosteum or with arteries supplying the soft tissues. The network of vessels associated with the periosteum is called the *periosteal plexus.* The periosteal plexus in turn communicates with vessels that are supplying arterial blood to muscles and other soft tissues in the area.

The mandible and maxilla are membrane bones and as such do not develop in the same manner as long bones. Most researchers agree that the circulation of blood within the body of the mandible[10] and in the maxilla[11,12] is centrifugal under normal conditions. As in the long bones, endosteal and periosteal plexuses exist that are connected with one another.[12,13] In addition to these vascular networks, a periodontal plexus is found associated with the teeth.[12,13] When teeth are present, intraosseous vessels send branches into the alveolar processes (intraalveolar arteries), to the teeth (apical arteries), and to branches of the periodontal plexus. The intraalveolar arteries and periodontal plexus in turn connect with vessels of the periosteal plexus, as well as with vessels within the soft tissues surrounding the bone. Once a tooth is removed, its periodontal plexus is lost. When abnormal circulatory conditions exist within the mandible or maxilla, such as occlusion of the nutrient artery, the blood supply to the bone is reversed so that the direction of flow is from the outside to the inside of the bone.[10,11,14] This is called *centripetal circulation.*

Maxilla

The vessels that supply the maxilla are branches of the third part of the maxillary artery. The posterior superior alveolar artery leaves the maxillary artery and travels on the infratemporal portion of the maxilla, in which it divides into several branches. Some of the branches enter alveolar canals within the posterior aspect of the maxilla to become intraosseous arteries, which supply the molar and premolar teeth and the lining of the maxillary sinus. Other branches of the posterior superior alveolar artery travel on the surface of the maxilla to supply the transact of the posterior maxillary teeth. Injury to this artery within the bone during lateral-approach sinus elevation procedures may cause hemorrhage, which requires coagulation or the use of bone wax to control the bone bleeding.

The infraorbital artery leaves the maxillary artery and enters the orbital cavity by way of the inferior orbital fissure. The artery runs in the infraorbital groove and later in the infraorbital canal. Both of these structures are located in the floor of the orbit. The infraorbital canal opens on the face as the infraorbital foramen. Within the canal the artery gives off the anterior superior alveolar artery, which descends through anterior alveolar canals to supply the maxillary anterior teeth and the mucous membrane of the maxillary sinus. The anterior and posterior superior alveolar arteries join together to form an arterial loop. The middle superior alveolar artery is rarely a separate branch.[15] The infraorbital artery also supplies branches to the maxillary sinus.[16]

Gingival, buccal, labial, palatal, nasal, and maxillary sinus blood vessels anastomose with the arterial networks associated with the maxilla. These vessels not only join with the periosteal plexus, but they also penetrate the bone to connect with vessels of the endosteal and periodontal plexuses. In addition, abundant midline crossover is possible in the soft tissues of the palate and face.[13]

The mucoperiosteum of the anterior maxilla is supplied by branches of the infraorbital artery and the branches of the superior labial artery, which is a major branch of the facial artery.[13] The buccal mucoperiosteum of the maxilla is supplied by vessels of the posterior superior alveolar, anterior superior alveolar, and buccal arteries. Branches from the greater (anterior) palatine and the nasopalatine arteries supply the mucoperiosteum of the hard palate. The lesser (posterior) palatine artery supplies the soft palate. Communications of the lesser palatine arteries with the ascending pharyngeal branch of the external carotid artery and the ascending palatine branch of the facial artery are critical in many of the surgical orthognathic procedures that are performed on the maxilla.[12] In these surgical procedures, the major nutrient arteries to the maxilla are sometimes severed, but the blood supply is maintained by means of the anastomoses present in the soft palate. The vessels of the soft palate unite with vessels of the hard palate, which in turn communicate with the periosteal, periodontal, and endosteal plexuses of the upper jaw. Thus the vitality of the tissues of the maxilla is maintained through an arterial supply derived entirely from vessels that normally supply the soft palate.

Mandible

The major artery supplying the blood of the mandible is the inferior alveolar artery. The artery enters the medial aspect of the ramus of the mandible and courses downward and forward within the mandibular canal to enter the body of the mandible. The artery branches in the premolar region to give rise to two terminal branches: the mental and incisive arteries. The incisive artery continues medially within the body to anastomose with the artery of the opposite side. This artery is often severed during the harvest of a monocortical symphyseal block of bone for grafting resorbed ridges. Crushing bone around the vessel or using bone wax easily controls the bleeding. The mental artery exits the body of the mandible through the mental foramen and supplies the region of the chin and anastomoses with the submental and inferior labial arteries. Near its origin the inferior alveolar artery gives off a lingual branch, which supplies blood to the oral mucosa.[16]

Studies in animals have demonstrated that the coronoid process, the condylar process, and the angle of the mandible are supplied by arteries that provide blood to the muscles that attach to these sites.[16] Studies of human cadaver material show that the condylar process is supplied by the vascular network of the TMJ joint capsule and the lateral pterygoid muscle. In addition, researchers found that vessels from the temporalis muscle supplied the coronoid process exclusively, and the inferior alveolar artery supplied the angle of the mandible, as well as the muscles attached to the area. The same researchers found that the vessels that supply the pterygomasseteric sling (i.e., the medial pterygoid and masseter muscles) also supply the anterior portion of the ramus.[17] Empirical findings from mandibular osteotomy procedures in humans support many of these findings.[18] Thus the repositioning of the inferior alveolar artery laterally, which is a procedure that may be needed in some cases before implant insertion, should not eliminate the blood supply to the bone in this region (see the discussion that follows).

Changes in Blood Supply to the Mandible with Age. Although the normal circulation within the body of the mandible is centrifugal in young individuals, the direction of blood flow may reverse with aging. It has been shown that the inferior alveolar artery is susceptible to arteriosclerotic changes and tends to become tortuous and narrow with age.[19,20] Blockage of the inferior alveolar artery occurs years before any clinical evidence of blockage in the carotid vessels is found. Angiographic studies of living human subjects of all ages demonstrated blockage of the inferior alveolar in 79% of all individuals studied, and in 33% of the patients arterial flow was absent.[20] The incidence of absence of flow in the inferior alveolar artery increased with age. The reduction or absence in flow within the inferior alveolar artery may be associated with tooth extraction.[20] Studies in completely edentulous humans indicated that the inferior alveolar artery degenerates to such an extent as to be negligible in the supply of blood to the mandible.[19] In these cases the blood supply to the bone and internal structures was dependent on the connections with the external

blood supply located within the periosteum and soft tissues associated with the mandible.[19,20] Major arteries that probably supply blood to the mandible after the interruption of the inferior alveolar artery blood flow include the mental artery,[14] the mandibular branch of the sublingual artery,[14] the facial artery,[10] and muscular branches of the maxillary artery. These anastomoses are critical in surgical procedures in which mucoperiosteal flaps are created in the mandible. The changes in pattern of blood flow to the atrophic mandible are of special importance to implant dentistry. Mucoperiosteal flap reflection for subperiosteal implant usually exposes 75% of the body of the mandible and approximately 50% of the inferior one-third of the rami. Dehiscence of the mucosa at the incision lines has been reported. The reduction in atrophied bone blood supply may be a contributing factor. Onlay grafts from the iliac crest to severely atrophied mandibles are also associated with occasional incision line opening postoperatively. Limitation of surgical reflection of muscles that attach to the bone improves blood supply but may complicate primary closure without tension. However, muscle attachments at the basal bone of the mandible, which are not in the way of the graft placement, should not be reflected. In addition, endosteal implants placed in an atrophied anterior mandible may have less blood supply to the interface and may require longer time for load-bearing bone to develop. Misch has suggested 5 months of healing in very dense bone when found in an atrophied anterior mandible.[21] These speculations, of course, require experimental verification. Similar blood flow reversal with age has not been reported in the maxilla, but final comment concerning blood flow in the aged edentulous maxilla awaits further investigation.

Implantologists may encounter neurovascular bundles such as the infraorbital, incisal, greater palatine, anterior, middle, and posterior superior alveolar nerves in the maxilla (e.g., during antral augmentation procedures or mucoperiosteal flap reflection) and the mental nerve, inferior dental nerve, and the lingual nerve in the mandible (e.g., during placement of root or blade implants or reflection of microperiosteal flaps). Stretching, compression, partial resection, or total transaction can mechanically injure the nerve.

Factors that affect nerve response to mechanical injury include the following:
1. Size and number of funiculi (nerve bundles) within the nerve trunk.
2. Funicular pattern: The branching within the nerve trunk will lead to an increase in density or number of nerve fibers per cross section of the nerve. Therefore injury to the nerve at one spot may cause damage to more fibers than to the adjacent area of the nerve that has less funicular branching.
3. The amount of epineural tissue: The connective tissue that surrounds the nerve is called the *epineurium*. The thinner the epineurium is, the greater the possibility is that partial injury to the nerve could damage the nerve fibers.
4. Position of the nerve fibers in the nerve trunk: The peripheral fibers leave the nerve first, whereas the central fibers innervate the most distal tissue. If a patient develops paresthesia of the lower lip after surgical placement of implants in the molar region, then it means that the nerve damage went through the center of the nerve to affect the mental nerve fibers.
5. Physiologic susceptibility: For an unknown reason, the motor fibers respond differently when subjected to mechanical deformation compared with sensory fibers.

Nerve fibers of the peripheral nervous system (PNS) show greater capacity for regeneration than nerves of the central nervous system (CNS). The axons of both myelinated and unmyelinated fibers in the PNS are surrounded by Schwann cells, which are covered by basal lamina. They later provide a continuous tube, even after the nerve fiber is cut into distal and proximal segments. The proximal segment is still connected to a living nerve cell body, whereas the distal segment gradually degenerates and eventually disappears. This is known as *Wallerian degeneration.* The Schwann cells of the distal segment proliferate and form a cell strand known as a *Schwann cell column* or *band of Büngner* within the basal lamina tube.[22] The Schwann cells also become phagocytic, and along with macrophages they clean the distal segment from degenerating axons. Sprouting of new axons takes place approximately 4 weeks after injury, and it takes 5 weeks for a sizeable number of axons to occupy the distal segment. The excess sprouts degenerate, and one fiber finds its way into the distal segments. If regenerating axons evade the Schwann cell column and enter the connective tissue, then they cease to grow after elongation of a few millimeters. The Schwann cells and the basal lamina are indispensable for axonal regeneration because they retain growth factors. The Schwann cells also provide new myelin for the regenerating fibers, although the conduction property is less efficient and the functional recovery may never be complete. The sprouting stage may cause pain to the patient, and the area may be sensitive to touch. The rate of recovery will depend on the type of injury (e.g., a crushed nerve regenerates faster than a severed nerve).

References

1. Sharawy M. *Companion of Applied Anatomy.* 4th ed. Augusta, Ga: Medical College of Georgia Printing Service; 1999.
2. Hickey JC, Zarb GA, Bolender CL. *Boucher's Prosthetic Treatment for Edentulous Patients.* 9th ed. St Louis: Mosby; 1982.
3. Atwood DA, Coy WA. Clinical cephalometric and densitometric study of reduction of residual ridges. *J Prosthet Dent.* 1977;26:280–299.
4. DuBrul EL. *Sicher's Oral Anatomy.* St Louis: Mosby; 1982.
5. Atwood DA. Some clinical factors related to rate of resorption of residual ridges. *J Prosthet Dent.* 1962;12:441–450.
6. Atwood DA. Reduction of residual ridges: a major oral disease entity. *J Prosthet Dent.* 1971;29:266–279.
7. Bays RA. The pathophysiology and anatomy of edentulous bone loss. In: Fonseca RJ, Davis WH, eds. *Reconstructive Pre-Prosthetic Oral and Maxillofacial Surgery.* Philadelphia: WB Saunders; 1986.
8. Brookes M. *The Blood Supply of Bone.* London: Butterworths; 1971.
9. Rhinelander FW. Circulation of bone. In: Bourne GH, ed. *The Biochemistry and Physiology of Bone.* New York: Academic Press; 1972:10.
10. Hellem S, Ostrup LT. Normal and retrograde blood supply to the body of the mandible in the dog. II. The role played by periosteo-medullary and symphyseal anastomoses. *Int J Oral Surg.* 1981;10:31–42.
11. Bell WH, Levy BM. Revascularization and bone healing after anterior mandibular osteotomy. *J Oral Surg.* 1970;28:196–203.
12. Bell WH. Biologic basis for maxillary osteotomies. *Am J Phys Anthropol.* 1973;38:279–290.
13. Bell WH. Revascularization and bone healing after anterior maxillary osteotomy: a study using adult rhesus monkeys. *J Oral Surg.* 1969;27:249–255.
14. Castelli WA, Nasjleti CE, Diaz-Perez R. Interruption of the arterial inferior alveolar flow and its effects on mandibular collateral circulation and dental tissues. *J Dent Res.* 1975;54:708–715.
15. Perint J. Surgical anatomy and physiology: detailed roentgenologic examination of the blood supply in the jaws and teeth by applying radiopaque solutions. *J Oral Surg.* 1949;2:2–20.
16. Williams PL, Warwick R. *Gray's Anatomy.* 36th ed. Philadelphia: WB Saunders; 1980.
17. Castelli W. Vascular architecture of the human adult mandible. *J Dent Res.* 1963;42:786–792.
18. Bell WH. Biologic basis for modification of the sagittal ramus split operation. *J Oral Surg.* 1977;35:362–369.
19. Bradley JC. Age changes in the vascular supply of the mandible. *Br Dent J.* 1972;132:142–144.
20. Bradley JC. A radiological investigation into the age changes of the inferior dental artery. *Br J Oral Surg.* 1975;13:82–90.
21. Misch CE. Density of bone, its effect on treatment planning, surgery, healing, and progressive bone loading. *Int J Oral Implantol.* 1990;6:23–31.
22. Ide C. Peripheral nerve regeneration. *Neurosci Res.* 1996;25:101–121.

13

Dental Implant Infections

JOSEPH E. CILLO, JR.

Introduction

Dental implants are a contemporary solution to tooth loss and oral reconstruction with a known high success rate of osseointegration. It is estimated that between 100,000 and 300,000 dental implants are placed per year.[1] Although the success rate is high, dental implant infections may occur that lead to lack or loss of osseointegration and may result in subsequent implant failure. These failures may be divided into either early or late based on the time of their occurrence during a dental implant's life span. Early dental implant failure occurs before osseointegration and prosthetic loading, whereas late failures occur after loading and may occur years to decades later. Early dental implant failure may be attributed to bacterial contamination, such as pellicle or biofilm formation, and inflammation that prevents or prolongs osseointegration. Similarly, long-term survival of dental implants depends, in part, on control of bacterial infection in the peri-implant region. Peri-implant disease may contribute to increased bone loss and eventual dental implant failure. The capability to diminish the potential early deleterious effects of bacterial contamination during both the surgical and prosthetic aspects of dental implant therapy and later effects of bacterial involvement in the peri-implant tissues begins with the understanding of the microenvironment and its denizens. This understanding of the oral microenvironment and its influence on dental implant surgery and prosthetics may allow for strategies to decrease the occurrence and spread of dental implant infections.

Overview of Oral, Head, and Neck Infection and Spread

Dental implants are uniquely engineered biomaterials ubiquitously used to replace teeth for restoration of oral function. The most common form of dental implant is the screw-type, or endosseous, implant comprised of a single implant unit that is inserted within a dentoalveolar or basal bone osteotomy. An implant's presence in the bacteria-laden milieu of the oral cavity would indicate the high likelihood of an increase in infection risk. However, the failure rate because of infection for dental implants (0.0%–1.1%) placed in this contaminated environment is similar to that of orthopedic joint arthroplasties performed in a near-sterile environment (0.1%–1.3%).[2] Conversely, orthopedic device placement that breaches the immune barrier of the epidermis and exposes the underlying sterile tissue to an unsterile external environment results in much higher infection-associated failure rates of up to 23.0%.[2]

The success of dental implant resistance to infection-associated failure may be caused by the ability of oral tissues to heal rapidly in the continuous presence of commensal bacteria and opportunistic pathogens, and the tolerance of the oral immune system. The main cause of infection-associated dental implant failure is when local tissue is unable to adhere, spread, and heal in the presence of microbial contaminants and an intolerant immune system. The role of saliva in the development of dental implant infection is complicated. Saliva has been shown to have antimicrobial[3,4] and antifungal[5] properties that may be a contributing factor to infection prevention. However, saliva is responsible for pellicle formation to which viable bacteria may adhere and mature to hinder healing and yield infection.

Signs and Symptoms of Oral Infection

The signs and symptoms of surgical site infections (SSI) have remained consistent and are generally similar throughout the human body. Diagnosis is based on the clinical signs of infection such as hyperplastic soft tissues, suppuration, color changes of the marginal peri-implant tissues, and gradual bone loss. The four fundamental signs of infection are pain or tenderness (*dolor*), localized swelling (*tumor*), redness (*rubor*), and heat or fever (>38°C) (*calor*) are the hallmark signs of infection.[6] This may or may not be associated with purulent drainage (pus) or fistula formation.

The occurrence of hematologic bacterial seeding with dental implant surgery is common and may occur as soon as 30 minutes after placement. Hematologic spread of oral microorganisms caused by this transient bacteremia may result in bacterial colonization in extraoral sites and is a proposed mechanism for systemic injury by free toxins and systemic inflammation caused by soluble antigens of oral pathogens. Some of the numerous species involved include *Staphylococcus epidermidis*, *Eubacterium* spp., *Corynebacterium* spp., and *Streptococcus viridans*, *Fusobacterium nucleatum*, *Porphyromonas gingivalis*, *S. mutans*, and *Campylobacter rectus*.[7,8] Systemic hematologic spread of oral commensals and pathogens to distant body sites may cause extraoral infections and inflammation, leading to cardiovascular disease, such as infective endocarditis with early colonizers *S. gordonii*, *S. sanguinis*, and *S. oligofermentans*,[9-11] adverse pregnancy outcomes, rheumatoid arthritis, inflammatory bowel disease, and colorectal cancer (direct and specific carcinogenesis of colonic adenomas from *F. nucleatum* induces tumor growth,[12] respiratory tract infections, organ inflammation, and abscesses by virulent oral species). Development of dangerous and life-threatening conditions, such as Ludwig angina, airway compromise, or carotid cavernous sinus fistula may also occur.[13]

Spread of Head and Neck Infection

Regardless of their pathogenic potentials in the oral cavity, once colonized in the extraoral sites, oral bacteria often become bona fide pathogens, especially in immunocompromised individuals, causing disease manifestation (Figs. 13.1–13.4).[7] Spread of infection from a dental implant, or any oral source, will travel through the path of least resistance, which is generally fascial spaces. Fascial spaces are potential spaces that exist without the presence of pathology or infection and lay between loose fibrous connective tissue fasciae and underlying organs and other tissues. The loose fibrous connective tissue that makes up the fascia of the head and neck is found in varying degrees of density with a tensile strength somewhat less than dense fibrous connective tissue located elsewhere in the body. In the head and neck, fascia may be divided into the superficial and deep layers with 16 fascial spaces divided into four subtypes. These four subtypes are the fascial spaces of the face, suprahyoid fascial spaces, infrahyoid fascial spaces, and the fascial spaces of the neck.

The superficial fascia of the head and neck lies just under the skin (as it does in the entire body), invests the superficially situated mimetic muscles (platysma, orbicularis oculi, and zygomaticus major and minor), and, located in distinct anatomic areas, is composed of two layers, an outer fatty layer and a thin inner membrane.[14] The deep fascia is absent in the face and scalp and begins at the anterior border of the masseter muscle and invests the muscles of mastication

The fascial spaces of the face are subdivided into five spaces: canine, buccal, masticatory (further divided into the masseteric, pterygomandibular, and temporal spaces), parotid, and infratemporal. The canine space is located between the levator anguli oris and the levator labii superioris muscles. Infection may spread to this space from dental abscess or dental implant–related procedures performed in the anterior maxillary region. Direct surgical access is achieved by incision through the maxillary vestibular mucosa above the mucogingival junction. The buccal space is bounded anterior to the masticator space and lateral to the buccinator muscle with no true superior or inferior boundary and consists of adipose tissue (the buccal fat pad that fills the greater part of the space), Stensen duct, the facial artery and vein, lymphatic vessels, minor salivary glands, and branches of cranial nerves VII and IX.[15] The buccal space frequently communicates posteriorly with the masticator space where it joins the buccopharyngeal fascia.[16]

When infection is involved in the buccal space, the buccal space can serve as a conduit for spreading disease between the mouth and the parotid gland. The lack of fascial compartmentalization in the superior, inferior, and posterior directions permits the spread of pathology both to and from the buccal space.[17] Surgical access to the buccal space infections may be easily accomplished through the intraoral approach. However, more complicated infections, directed by location within the buccal space and suspicion of malignancy, may require a preauricular and/or submandibular approach. The masticator space is a well-defined fibrous tissue that surrounds the muscles of mastication and contains the internal maxillary artery and the inferior alveolar nerve. Most masseteric space infections result from spread in the mandibular molar region,[18] with trismus being the most pronounced clinical feature, and often precludes intraoral examination. Computed tomography (CT) and/or magnetic resonance imaging (MRI) may be an invaluable resource in the assessment of masseteric space infections because they can often influence the surgical approach and distinguish abscess from cellulitis.[18] Abscess formation in this area is easily reached by intraoral surgical access for simple, isolated abscesses for incision and drainage, but with extension into adjacent spaces, an external approach may be required. The pterygomandibular space is bounded by the mandible laterally and by the medial pterygoid muscle medially and inferiorly. The posterior border is formed by parotid glandular tissue, which curves medially around the posterior mandibular ramus and anteriorly by the pterygomandibular raphe, the fibrous junction of the buccinator, and superior constrictor muscles. Other structures in this space are important in the administration of local anesthesia, including the inferior alveolar vessels, the sphenomandibular ligament, and the interpterygoid fascia.[19] Surgical access to this space for incision and drainage may be achieved intraoral in the case of simple infections, but it may require extraoral access when multiple adjacent spaces are involved.[20] The temporal fascia surrounds the temporalis muscle in a strong fibrous sheet that is divided into clearly distinguishable superficial and deep layers that originate from the same region, with the muscle fibers of the two layers intermingled in the superior part of the muscle.[21]

The sublingual space is bounded between the mylohyoid muscle and the geniohyoid and genioglossus muscles. This space contains the lingual artery and nerve, the hypoglossal nerve, the glossopharyngeal nerve, Wharton duct, and the sublingual salivary gland, which drains into the oral cavity through several small

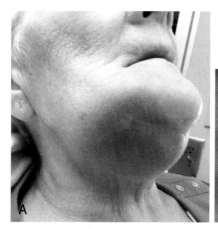
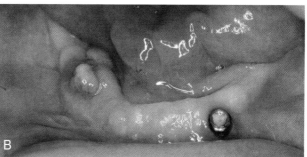

• **Fig. 13.1** (A) Extraoral and intraoral edema and fluctuance involving the floor of mouth and (B) submental and submandibular spaces from dental implant infection.

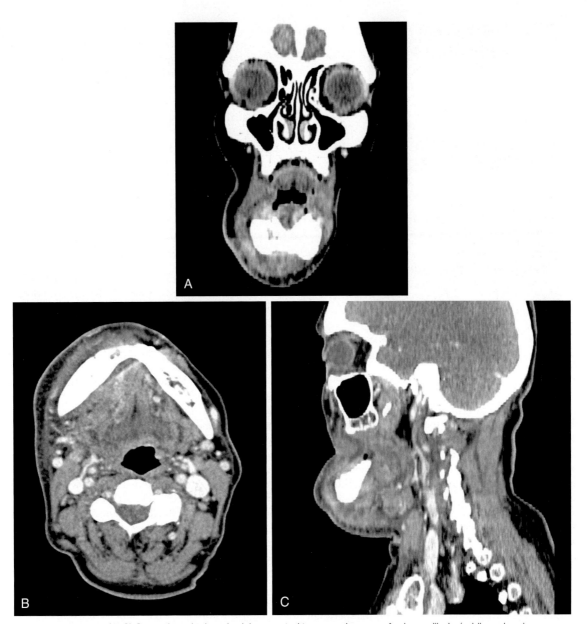

• **Fig. 13.2** (A–C) Coronal, sagittal, and axial computed tomography scan of submandibular/sublingual and submental spaces of dental implant infection.

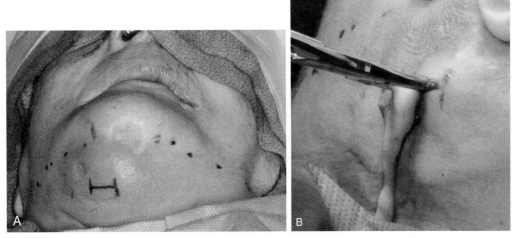

• **Fig. 13.3** Intraoperative images of (A) extraoral incision and (B) drainage of submental and submandibular space abscess.

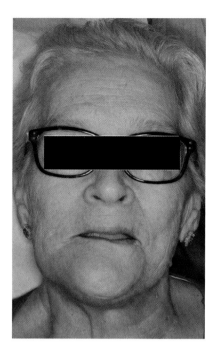

• **Fig. 13.4** Postoperative recovery from extraoral incision and drainage of dental infection.

excretory ducts in the floor of the mouth and a major duct known as the Bartholin duct. The submental space is bounded anteriorly by the symphysis of the mandible, laterally by the anterior bellies of digastric muscles, superiorly by the mylohyoid muscle, and inferiorly by the superficial fascia of the platysma muscle. There are no vital structures that traverse the submental space. This space is usually involved in odontogenic infections from the anterior mandibular teeth with surgical access for drainage of infection generally through an extraoral incision below the chin.[22] The submandibular space extends from the hyoid bone to the mucosa of the floor of the mouth and is bound anteriorly and laterally by the mandible and inferiorly by the superficial layer of the deep cervical fascia. The mylohyoid muscle separates it superiorly from the sublingual space, which communicates with it freely around the posterior border of the mylohyoid. Most oral infections that perforate the lingual mandible above the mylohyoid line will involve the sublingual space. When infection has spread to the bilateral submandibular, sublingual, and submental spaces, it represents Ludwig angina, a potentially life-threatening condition that requires immediate surgical drainage and intravenous antibiotic therapy.

The lateral pharyngeal space (also called the parapharyngeal space) is an inverted cone with its base at the base of skull and apex at the hyoid bone and is bounded posteriorly by the prevertebral fascia, anteriorly by the raphe of the buccinator and superior constrictors muscles, and laterally by the mandible and parotid fascia. The lateral pharyngeal space can be divided into anterior (prestyloid) and posterior (retrostyloid) compartments by the styloid process. The anterior compartment contains only fat, lymph nodes, and muscle, whereas the posterior compartment contains the carotid artery, the internal jugular vein, and cranial nerves IX through XII. Infections in the anterior space may present with pain, fever, and neck swelling below the angle of the mandible and trismus. Rotation of the neck away from the side of the swelling causes severe pain from tension on the ipsilateral sternocleidomastoid muscle. Because this space communicates with the other fascia spaces, spread of infection may also arise from numerous sources,

including the tonsils, parotid, and submandibular, peritonsillar, masticator, or retropharyngeal spaces. Airway impingement caused by medial bulging of the pharyngeal wall and supraglottic edema may occasionally occur, which may require the procurement of a stable airway by either tracheotomy or intubation.[23] The treatment of lateral pharyngeal space infections requires surgical drainage through either a transoral or extraoral approach.[24]

Fascial Spaces of the Neck

The fascial spaces of the neck all lie between the deep cervical fascia surrounding the pharynx anteriorly and the spine posteriorly. The retrovisceral space is divided into the retropharyngeal and danger spaces by the alar fascia and serves as the main route for oropharyngeal infections to descend into the mediastinum. The other fascial spaces of the neck include the prevertebral and carotid sheath spaces.

The retropharyngeal space is bounded anteriorly by the constrictor muscles and posteriorly by the alar layer of the deep cervical fascia and connects posteriorly to the danger space. Infections in this space may present with symptoms of fever, stiff neck, drooling, dysphagia, and bulging of the posterior pharyngeal wall. They may be complicated by the development of supraglottic edema with airway obstruction, aspiration pneumonia caused by rupture of the abscess, and acute mediastinitis that may lead to empyema or pericardial effusions. Proximity to the danger space may allow infection to spread to the mediastinum to the level of the diaphragm and possibly posteriorly to the prevertebral space. Surgical drainage should be performed in the operating room via a transoral approach with the head down to prevent rupture during intubation and septic aspiration.

The danger space is bounded superiorly by the skull base, anteriorly by the alar fascia, and posteriorly by the prevertebral fascia, ending at the level of the diaphragm. Danger space infections may track from the anteriorly located retropharyngeal space between the buccopharyngeal fascia and alar fascia and pass inferiorly to the mediastinum and the pericardium and may result in conditions such as purulent pericarditis.[25]

Microbiology of Dental Implant Infection

The oral cavity is awash in a milieu of different microbial species and colonies. More than 19,000 types of eukaryotic and prokaryotic bacteria, fungal, protozoan, and viral species coexist in the oral microenvironment.[26-28] This diverse microbiome consists of beneficial, pathologic, and opportunistic organisms, and when in balance may produce a benign or even beneficial result to the individual. When development of dysbiotic polymicrobial communities ensue with a misrepresentation between normally dominating species and normally outcompeted or contained species, more deleterious microbial species may increase in number to fill the void. Longitudinal studies have shown that successful implants are colonized by a predominantly gram-positive, facultative flora, which is established shortly after implantation, with no change in composition in patients with clinically stable implants over 5 years.[29] The transition from a gram-positive, facultative flora in health to a gram-negative, anaerobic flora in disease is the hallmark of impending dental implant infection and failure. In patients with bone loss and pocket formation around implants, significantly different flora develops consisting of gram-negative anaerobic bacteria, particularly fusobacteria, spirochetes, and black-pigmenting organisms such as high proportions of *Prevotella intermedia*. Although there may be nonmicrobial primary causes for implant failure, gram-negative anaerobes play a role in peri-implant infections, and their elimination may lead to improvement of the clinical condition. The introduction and growth of deleterious microorganisms may also occur within the implant and on the prosthesis because the dental implant/abutment interface cannot totally seal the passage of microorganisms. Therefore the implant interior may become a reservoir of pathogenic microorganisms that produce and maintain chronic inflammation in the tissues around implants.

The numerically predominant species in the oral microbiota is the streptococci species. Most of the oral streptococci are commensal, nonperiodontopathogenic bacteria, but some are known to cause local and distant disease. Oral streptococci are divided into five different groups: (1) Mutans group (prominent members are *S. mutans* and *S. sobrinus*), (2) Salivarius group (*S. salivarius*), (3) Anginosus group (*S. anginosus* and *S. intermedius*), (4) Sanguinis group (*S. sanguinis* and *S. gordonii*), and (5) Mitis group (*S. mitis* and *S. oralis*).[30-32] These oral streptococci species are known to be the early colonizers for oral biofilm formation and heavily influence the development of further infection and biofilm formation. As an early colonizer, oral streptococci have been found to have metabolic interactions between other members of the oral biofilm, which may develop either a corporative or disobliging relationship. Symbiotic relationships exist between oral streptococci and the genus *Veillonella*, *V. atypica*, and *V. parvula* most prominently[33,34]; *Actinomyces naeslundii*[35,36]; *F. nucleatum*[37]; and the periodontal pathogen *Aggregatibacter actinomycetemcomitans*.[38] These symbiotic relationships include such events as coaggregation between *S. cristatus* and *F. nucleatum* and lactic acid–based cross-feeding between *S. gordonii* and the late colonizer and periodontal pathogen *A. actinomycetemcomitans*.

Anaerobic bacteria genera in the oral cavity include *Actinomyces, Arachnia, Bacteroides, Bifidobacterium, Eubacterium, Fusobacterium, Lactobacillus, Leptotrichia, Peptococcus, Peptostreptococcus, Propionibacterium, Selenomonas, Treponema,* and *Veillonella*. In adults, anaerobes are always present with greatest proportions found in the gingival sulcus rather than in the gingival margin, tooth surfaces, buccal mucosa, tongue, or saliva.[39] Proportions of anaerobic bacteria from the healthy gingival sulcus consist of gram-positive bacilli (5%–14%), gram-negative bacilli (13%–29%), *Veillonella* (2%–8%), and gram-positive cocci (1%–15%) of the cultivable flora.[39] Marginal plaque and tooth surface plaque consist mainly of gram-positive bacilli and gram-positive cocci, whereas *Veillonella* is the most numerous anaerobe in saliva.

Spirochetes are distinctive double-membrane bacteria that generally have characteristic helically coiled or spiraled cells and are known to be an abundant phylum in periodontitis.[40] *Treponema denticola*, a gram-negative, obligate anaerobic, motile, and highly proteolytic bacterium, is the most common spirochete in both periodontitis and peri-implantitis. Once spirochetes have developed in the dental implant site, they are responsible for bone loss and may be extremely difficult to eradicate. Spirochetes have developed a defense mechanism against antibiotic administration by transformation into spherical dense granular bodies, which make them highly resistant to antibiotics.[41] This phenomenon is seen with serial infections treated by multiple rounds of oral antibiotics that seem to resolve and then recur repeatedly.

Genera of fungi frequently found in the mouth include *Candida, Cladosporium, Aspergillus, Fusarium, Glomus, Alternaria, Penicillium,* and *Cryptococcus*.[42] Interactions between the mycobiome and the bacterial microbiome may play a role in health

and disease. In some cases, the occurrence of bacteria correlates positively with the presence of fungi, such as when *Mycobacterium* superinfection occurs occasionally with aspergillosis[43] or when bacteria compete with fungi, such as when the growth of *Candida* species and possibly other fungi is suppressed when *Pseudomonas aeruginosa* dominates.[44] These microorganisms are known to colonize dental implants, dental implant prostheses surfaces, and internal components that may lead to peri-implant mucositis and peri-implantitis.[45,46]

Archaea are prokaryotic organisms (which means they do not possess nuclei) that have been isolated in the oral cavity as a source of disease. The presence or increase in level of methanogenic Archaea alters the composition of the polymicrobial community, resulting in changes in virulence and composition of microflora at diseased sites. Antagonistic interactions of methanogenic Archaea and treponemes,[47] and *Synergistes* spp. have been suggested to be possible syntrophic partners of the methanogens.[48] *Methanobrevibacter oralis* is a species of coccobacillary, nonmotile, gram-positive, methane-producing archaeon considered to be the major methanogenic archaea found in the oral cavity and associated with severe periodontitis.[49] It has a high prevalence in subgingival plaque of chronic periodontitis patients while being undetectable in healthy subjects.[50] An increase in the inoculum of methanogenic Archaea and sulfate-reducing bacteria have been reported to be associated with the severity of periodontitis[51,52] and has a significant increased prevalence in peri-implantitis sites.[53] *Methanobacterium congelense/curvum* is also an archaeon that is found in peri-implantitis sites but at a significantly lower volume.

Periodontal pathogens such as *Porphyromonas gingivalis, Tannerella forsythia, Prevotella intermedia,* and *Capnocytophaga ochracea* have been shown clustered together in peri-mucositis sites, suggesting that periodontal pathogens may play important roles in the pathogenesis of peri-implant diseases. Progression to peri-implantitis reveals a relative abundance of *Eubacterium minutum, Prevotella intermedia,* and *Propionibacterium acnes* in peri-implantitis.[54,55] Various microorganisms have been identified as possible pathogenic determinants in the multispecies infection of peri-implantitis. Some, such as *Enterococcus faecalis,* are persistent and may vegetate in bone after tooth extraction and colonize a dental implant after placement in the healed site that may cause fixture loss, marginal bone loss, or progression to osteomyelitis.[56]

Recent evidence has suggested that the peri-implant crevice may be immunologically, histologically, and microbiologically distinct from the subgingival sulcus.[57-59] Certain periodontal pathogens (such as *P. gingivalis* and *T. denticola*) may be shared between tooth and implants in certain individuals.[60-64] However, most of the flora, especially the abundant species, remain distinct between the two ecosystems, which may indicate that proximity is not sufficient to fully determine the local environmental microbiology. The diverse anatomy of the oral cavity has allowed unique microenvironments that shape the evolution of a diverse bacterial flora. The buccal epithelium, subgingival crevice, maxillary anterior vestibule, tongue, soft and hard palate, tonsils, and the tooth surface are all colonized by different combinations of bacterial species or phylotypes.[27] As such, the periodontal microbiome tends to be more diverse than the peri-implant microbiome, particularly in health. The disease process appears to shape the microbial populations through increased diversity in the diseased microenvironments in both periodontal and peri-implant healthy and diseased individuals.[58] Not all species present in the subgingival sulcus are capable of surviving and thriving in the peri-implant sulcus, and evidence to support that bacteria can translocate from diseased teeth to healthy teeth and do not necessarily colonize the niche[65] and the architecture, surface energy, and surface characteristics of abiotic structures such as dental implants dictates the composition of the ecosystem around them.[66,67]

Causes and Risks of Dental Implant Infection

Infection is one of the most important causes of early dental implant failure and may be an indication of a much more critical result than if the same complications occur later because of disturbance of the primary bone healing process. Several authors have defined the criteria for implant failure and postoperative infection. Esposito and colleagues[68,69] defined dental implant failure and infection as implant mobility measured manually and/or any infection directing implant removal with any biologic complications such as wound dehiscence, suppuration, fistula, abscess, and osteomyelitis. Similarly, Abu-Ta'a and colleagues[70] defined dental implant failures caused by infection as the presence of signs of infection and/or radiographic peri-implant radiolucencies that could not respond to antibiotics and/or judged a failure after performing explorative flap surgery by an experienced surgeon. Quirynen and colleagues classified dental implant infection failures into one of four groups: infection before the implant placement, perisurgical infection, severe postsurgical infection, and peri-implant disease.[71]

Infection Before the Implant Placement

Active Infection Site

Immediate dental implant placement and function after tooth extraction has become a widely accepted practice in contemporary dental implantology (Fig. 13.5).[72] Whether completed with or without immediate function, comparative clinical studies have found that implant survival rates (SRs) after immediate dental implant placement are similar to rates seen with delayed dental implant placement. Immediate dental implant placement has several advantages, such as reduction in the number of surgical

treatments, reduction of the time between tooth extraction, and placement of a definitive prosthesis and maintenance of alveolar ridge dimensions. However, there are certain situations that may endanger the success of the immediate dental implant placement, including periodontal disease or periapical lesions. Active infection in a fresh extraction site may be considered a harbinger for immediate dental implant placement failure. Placement of a dental implant in the presence of an active infection has traditionally been considered a contraindication because of the possibility of septic embolism that may cause immediate or late postsurgical infection, such as osteomyelitis or peri-implant abscess, and may increase the risk of implant nonintegration. This remains a controversial subject in dental implantology because of a lack of high-level prospective research to substantiate these claims[73] and a body of literature that consists mainly of retrospective case reports and series.[74]

Clinical case series have shown favorable results in immediate dental implant placement into chronically infected sites.[75-83] High implant SRs have been reported even when implants were placed immediately in infected extraction sockets and provisionalized within 36 hours. Early or immediate loading of dental implants placed into periodontally or endodontically infected sites produced no statistically significant difference in failure rates between chronically infected or noninfected sites.[82] In immediately placed and loaded dental implants into chronically infected sites in the esthetic zone of the anterior maxilla, Anitua and colleagues[75] found no failures and a success rate of 93%, leading them to conclude that immediate loading of implants inserted into fresh and infected extraction sockets is not a risk factor for implant survival. Systematic reviews of the literature reveal a high SR and support the hypothesis that implants may be successfully osseointegrated when placed immediately after extraction of teeth that present with endodontic[76,81] or periodontal lesions.[77] This was contingent on appropriate clinical decontamination procedures being performed before dental implant placement, such as meticulous cleaning, socket curettage/debridement, and chlorhexidine (0.12%) rinse/irrigation.[78,80,83] Nonocclusal loading on implants placed in cleaned periodontically or endodontically infected

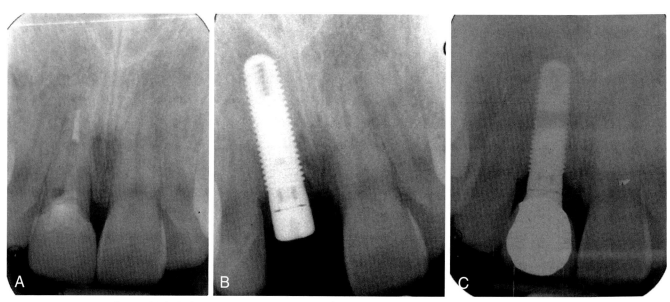

• **Fig. 13.5** Periapical radiographs of (A) nonrestorable tooth #9 with periapical radiolucency, (B) extraction of tooth #9 with immediate implant placement, and (C) 1-year postprosthesis loading.

extraction sites has shown complete initial primary stability (100%) and a 98.7% success rate on postoperative reverse torque testing of osseointegration at 3 and 4 months.[84] Similarly, Bell and colleagues[79] found high, comparable, and statistically insignificant success rates, defined as successful osseointegration and restoration, and absence of evidence of bone loss or peri-implantitis at last follow-up, between implants placed in fresh extraction sockets with chronic periapical pathology (97.5%) and healed sites (98.7%). A statistically significant higher failure rate is seen for dental implants placed adjacent to retained teeth with periapical pathology. Placement of dental implants in sockets affected by chronic periapical pathology can be considered a safe and viable treatment option, but placement adjacent to teeth with periapical radiolucencies carries a high risk of failure.

A metaanalysis of dental implant failure and marginal bone loss after immediate placement into infected versus noninfected sites found that immediate placement into an infected site showed 116% increase in the risk of implant failure, with no statistically significant difference in marginal bone loss.[85] However, the reviews and analyses used have been found to be of low or moderate methodological quality[86] and with the presence of uncontrolled confounders, respectively, and should also be interpreted with caution.[85] It would be recommended that sound clinical judgment be used in determining whether immediate dental implant placement into an actively infected site is prudent, despite decontamination procedures, and whether a delayed protocol until proper site healing has been achieved should be followed.

Periodontal Disease

Periodontal disease is a chronic infectious and inflammatory response to pathologic changes in periodontium to an anaerobic microenvironment. These changes generally result in an imbalance and aggregation of deleterious microorganisms that may lead to the development of peri-mucositis, peri-implantitis, and bone loss. Comparisons of clinical, microbiologic, and host response characteristics between healthy dental implants and healthy teeth and between infected implants and periodontally diseased teeth have been found to be similar, respectively, with subjects at risk for periodontal disease also at risk for peri-implantitis.[87] The bacteria associated with periodontal diseases are predominantly gram-negative anaerobic bacteria and may include *A. actinomycetemcomitans, P. gingivalis, P. intermedia, B. forsythus, C. rectus, E. nodatum, P. micros, S. intermedius,* and *Treponema* sp., with bacterial numbers associated with disease up to 100,000 times larger than those associated with healthy teeth. The frequency of four periodontopathogenic bacteria in tooth sulci (*A. actinomycetemcomitans, P. gingivalis, T. forsythia,* and *T denticola*) are significantly higher around natural teeth with deeper periodontal pockets but not in peri-implant sulci in partially edentulous subgroups or in the peri-implant sulci or the alveolar gingiva of completely edentulous patients. Cytokine and interleukin creation from periodontal pathogens stimulate the production of inflammatory mediators secreted in peri-implant sulcus fluid, leading to peri-implant tissue destruction.[88]

A systematic review of implant failure rates, postoperative infection, and marginal bone loss from dental implant placement in periodontally compromised patients compared with periodontally healthy patients found some evidence that patients treated for periodontitis may experience more implant loss and complications around implants, including higher bone loss and peri-implantitis, than patients without periodontitis.[89] Similarly, individuals with both aggressive or chronic periodontal disease have a greater significant risk for implant loss, peri-implant bone loss, and peri-implantitis compared with patients without periodontal disease. The risk is greater for patients with aggressive periodontitis compared with patients with chronic periodontitis.[90]

There are different types of periodontal disease, including gingivitis, which is the mildest form, and aggressive periodontitis, which is a form of periodontitis that occurs in patients who are otherwise clinically healthy and may include rapid attachment loss, bone destruction, and familial aggregation. Another type is chronic periodontitis, which results in inflammation within the supporting tissues of the teeth, progressive attachment and bone loss, and is characterized by pocket formation and/or gingival recession (Fig. 13.6). Necrotizing periodontal diseases are another type and are characterized by necrosis of gingival tissues, periodontal ligament, and alveolar bone. General and local periodontitis have been implicated as "microbial reservoirs" in the etiology of peri-implant diseases.

Gingivitis is a reversible inflammatory process in the soft tissue surrounding teeth. When this phenomenon surrounds an osseointegrated dental implant without the loss of marginal bone beyond normal resorption it is known as peri-implant mucositis. Gingivitis is ubiquitous in the adult population and if left untreated may progress to periodontal disease and bone loss. Gingivitis is generally very treatable and, regarding dental implants, rarely leads to implant loss or infection; it is not a contraindication for implant surgery or prosthetics when an appropriate oral hygiene regimen is established.

Dental implant placement in patients with a history of generalized aggressive periodontal disease might be considered a viable option to restore oral function despite the aggressive nature of this

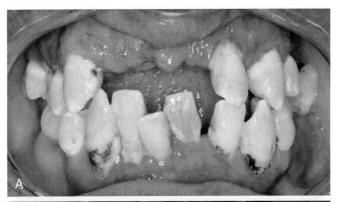
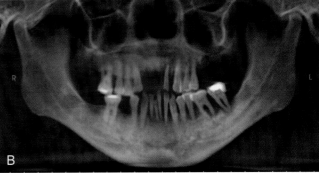

• **Fig. 13.6** Aggressive periodontal disease consisting of (A) generalized pathologic migration, calculi deposits, purulent exudate, gingival inflammation, grades II and III mobility, greater than 5-mm probing depths, and (B) radiographic signs of severe bone resorption with multiple bone defects.

disease and its assault on local bone levels. Outcomes similar to those seen in chronic periodontal disease and healthy periodontium[91] with high SRs and low marginal bone loss[92] have been found in generalized aggressive periodontal disease subjects. A systematic review of the literature revealed that the 3-year SR was high but statistically significantly lower in generalized aggressive periodontal disease subjects (SR 97.98% versus 100%) compared with healthy periodontal and chronic periodontitis subjects.[93] The only significant difference seen at the 3-year time point between these groups was an increased probing depth and attachment loss in the generalized aggressive periodontal disease subjects.[91] At 10-year follow-up, bone and attachment loss were higher with a lower SR, 83% compared with 100% in generalized aggressive periodontal disease subjects compared with healthy individuals.[94] Similarly, the probability of a dental implant infection failure in individuals with a history of aggressive periodontal disease is significantly higher (almost four times as great) compared with individuals with either healthy or chronic periodontal disease.[95] Long-term dental implant success may be achievable with postperiodontal treatment long-term stability with excellent patient cooperation and strict periodontal maintenance protocol.[96] Several case reports have detailed medium-term dental implant reconstruction success in aggressive periodontal management, involving scaling and root planning and periodontal surgery, in the treatment and implant maintenance.[96-98] The functioning SRs of fixtures and superstructures of osseointegrated implants also tend to be generally high in subjects with aggressive periodontal disease (between 95.9% and 100%) over short- and long-term follow-up.[99]

Immediate dental implant placement into fresh extraction sockets with periodontal infection has been evaluated at single- and multiple-tooth reconstruction and shown to be a valid option with predictable results. Single dental implants placed into periodontally infected extraction sites have shown, at 12-month follow-up, to be asymptomatic with no signs of infection or bleeding on probing, no decrease in radiographic bone–implant contact, and no loss of clinical attachment level or keratinized mucosa width at the midbuccal location per implant.[100]

Chronic Periodontitis

There is conflicting evidence over medium- and long-term success between dental implants placed to restore periodontitis- and nonperiodontitis-associated tooth loss. Over a 10-year period, dental implants have lower SRs and more biologic complications between periodontitis- and nonperiodontitis-associated tooth loss.[101] However, although this difference was significant between these two groups, the success rate was still high between the chronic periodontitis group (90.5%) and nonperiodontitis group (96.5%). Similarly, dental implant suprastructures and dental implant survival are not significantly different over a 10-year period, but they have significantly increased incidences of peri-implantitis at 10 years and peri-implant marginal bone loss at 5 years with periodontitis-associated tooth loss.[102] The important aspect of dental implant treatment associated with existing periodontitis or a history of chronic periodontitis is proper periodontal therapy. Implant reconstruction can be successfully accomplished in patients with periodontitis when appropriate regular periodontal therapy and maintenance are achieved. Residual pockets, nonattendance to a periodontal maintenance program, and smoking are negative factors for long-term dental implant outcomes in periodontitis-associated tooth loss.[103]

Immediate Loading in Periodontal Disease

Immediately placed and immediately loaded dental implants have been shown to be predictable and successful.[104] Immediate implant loading of complete mandibular implant–retained prostheses may be a viable treatment option for edentulous individuals with a history of chronic periodontal infection. Dental implants immediately placed in chronically infected sockets and immediately loaded with a fixed full-arch maxillary and mandibular prosthesis have been shown to have excellent short-term success[105] and a 3-year cumulative surgical and prosthetic SR.[106] Crestal bone height is also an indicator of dental implant success because increased bone loss may lead to a change in the microenvironment and microorganism composition. This will eventually lead to dental implant failure and need for removal. Immediately restored dental implants in patients with periodontal disease, after 1 year, exhibit crestal bone loss rates similar to those seen for conventionally restored implants.[107] Immediate dental implant rehabilitation in subjects with untreated periodontitis may also be feasible when appropriate periodontal therapy is provided and regularly maintained.[108] This shows that immediate dental implant placement and restoration is possible in individuals with periodontal disease as long as periodontal maintenance is regularly and consistently sustained.

Perisurgical Infection

Intraoral surgery, in general, and dental implant surgery, specifically, are classified as clean-contaminated surgery because the surgical field may be contaminated by many sources of microorganisms that can easily infiltrate the surgical site. There are numerous sources of potential perisurgical-site infections. Several specific potential sources of perisurgical contamination are mostly derived from surgical instrumentation, such as air, aspiration, instrumentation, and saliva in the surgical field, and its relationship with the skin of the face, lips, and nose.[109] Several techniques have been used to avoid perisurgical cross-contamination of the surgical field, including saliva secretion reduction with atropine,[110] double aspiration to avoid salivary contamination of surgery, and chlorhexidine rinses to reduce oral microbial load.[71] Chlorhexidine has been shown to have effective antibacterial activity on the salivary flora and development of oral biofilms[111-113] but not on developed and mature biofilms.[114] Additionally, chlorhexidine has been shown to be affected by its local salivary environment, such as pH. Chlorhexidine is more effective in alkaline than in acidic environments,[115] and the presence of organic substances and food compounds will reduce antimicrobial activity.[116] However, the effect of saliva on the antimicrobial activity of chlorhexidine has been shown to be weak but statistically significant.[117] Extraoral microbial organism presentation has been suggested in perisurgical contamination, such as from the nose. A meshed nose guard to prevent contact with the highly contaminated nasal skin is highly recommended for field isolation to prevent infection; otherwise, covering the nostrils by a mask and sterile adhesive plastic film is not essential in avoiding airborne microbial contamination during dental implant surgery.[118] Clinical manifestations of the infections caused by perioperative contamination are usually in the form of peri-implant abscesses, periapical radiolucency, marginal bone loss, orocutaneous fistulas, and/or osteomyelitis.

Severe Postsurgical Infection

Postoperative infections are rare complications that usually occur within the first month after dental implant placement, with an incidence as high as 11.5%. These infections generally occur during the osseointegration period. Dental implant placement in the mandible and submerged healing are more prone to postoperative infections.[119] Signs and symptoms of postoperative dental implant infection are similar to other oral infections and include pain, swelling, heat, and redness. If the infected implant is not removed and the area debrided and decontaminated, an orocutaneous fistula[120,121] and/or osteomyelitis may develop.

Osteomyelitis

Dental implant–related osteomyelitis of the jaws is a rare complication that has been reported in the literature (Figs. 13.7 and 13.8).[122-130] The incidence of dental implant–related

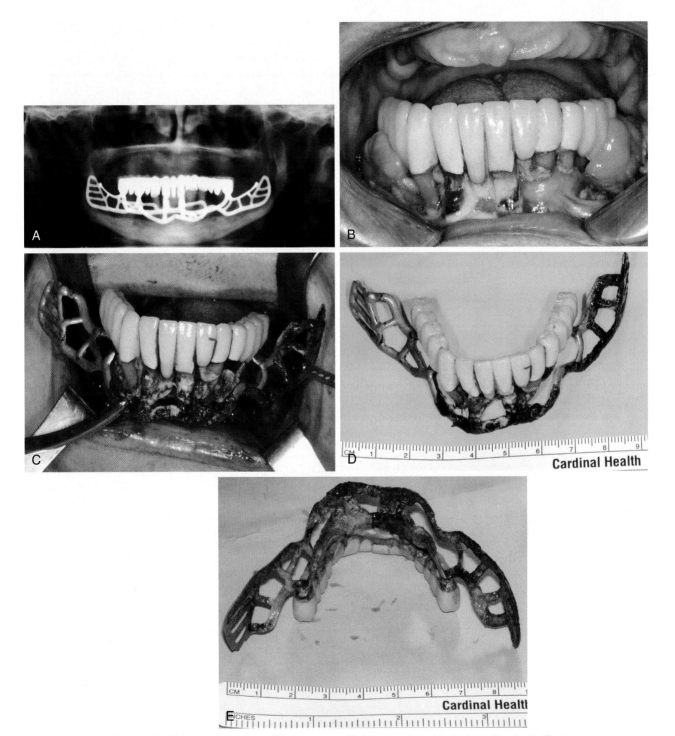

• **Fig. 13.7** (A–E) Advanced osteomyelitis from a mandibular subperiosteal implant resulting in significant bone loss, implant mobility, chronic infection, and pain. After removal, note the amount of calculus and slime layer as evidence of suspected developed biofilm.

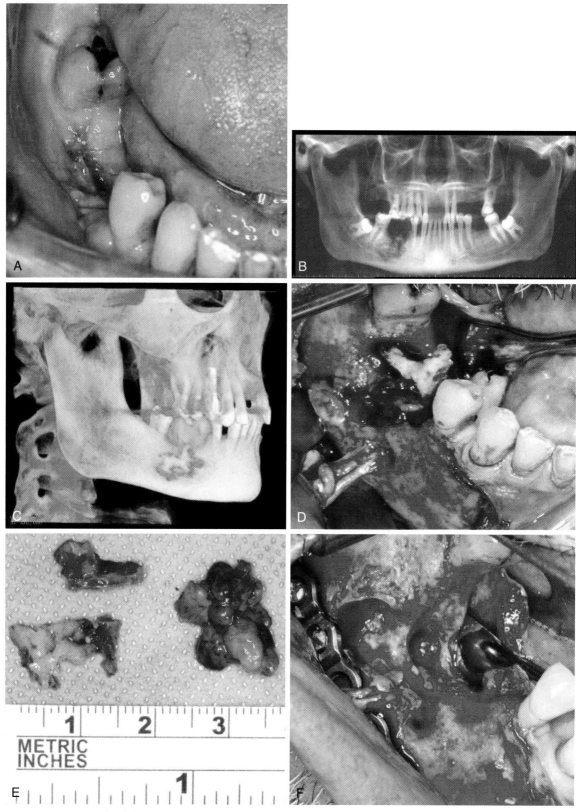

• **Fig. 13.8** (A–F) Clinical and radiographic presentation of dental implant–related mandibular osteomyelitis. Extension of osteomyelitis necessitated placement of a mandibular fracture plate to prevent pathologic fracture during debridement.

osteomyelitis of the jaws has ranged from 5%[131] to 26%[130] of all cases. Osteomyelitis of the jaws is an acute and chronic inflammatory process in the medullary spaces or cortical surfaces of bone that extends away from the initial site of involvement. Several local and systemic factors are generally involved in the development and spread of osteomyelitis of the jaws. Local factors, such as trauma from tooth extraction or dental implant placement, can decrease vascularity and vitality of bone in the area. Systemic factors, such as immunosuppression or diabetes mellitus, can impair host defense mechanisms.

The mandible is a much more prevalent location for osteomyelitis than the maxilla because of the latter's rich vascularity.[124,130,132-135] Introduction of bacterial pathogens into the bone, such as in the surgical placement of a dental implant, allows the bacteria access into the jaw bone to initiate a local infection and inflammatory response. The inflammatory response developed toward these pathogens leads to a compromise of local blood flow. Medullary infection then spreads throughout the marrow spaces and vessel thrombosis leads to extensive bone necrosis. Lacunae in the bone then empty the osteocytes, fill with purulence, and proliferate in the necrotic tissue. Suppurative inflammation may then extend through cortical bone to the periosteum, which further compromises vascular supply. This predisposes the bone to further become necrotic, which leads to sequestrum that separates from the surrounding vital bone.

Local and systemic host factors may increase the patient susceptibility. Comorbidities such as chronic systemic diseases, alcoholism, immunosuppression, malnutrition, diabetes mellitus, intravenous drug abuse, malignancy, and diseases can result in hypovascularized bone (such as osteopetrosis, Paget disease, florid cemento-osseous dysplasia, and radiation therapy), or, more recently, medication-related osteonecrosis of the jaw (MRONJ) caused by antiresorptive and antiangiogenic therapies has also been associated with an increased frequency of osteomyelitis.

The classic presentation of osteomyelitis of the jaws indicates an acute phase that can present either as a suppurative or nonsuppurative infection causing vascular compromise, which results in local tissue ischemia and necrosis with bony sequestrum. The two major groups of osteomyelitis (acute and chronic) are differentiated by the clinical course of the disease after onset, relative to surgical and antimicrobial therapy with an arbitrary time limit of 1 month used to differentiate the two groups.[135-138]

Chronic osteomyelitis of the jaws is classified into various types based on clinical characteristics by the Zurich classification system, which is primarily based on the clinical course and appearance of the disease and on imaging studies.[134] Chronic osteomyelitis of the jaws can be divided into primary and secondary chronic osteomyelitis, with secondary types further subclassified into three major clinical types: suppurative chronic osteomyelitis, osteoradionecrosis of the jaw, and MRONJ. Suppurative chronic osteomyelitis has major symptoms of abscess/purulence formation, sequestration, and exposed bone.[134] This is in contrast to primary chronic osteomyelitis, which may present with nonsuppurative chronic inflammation of the jawbone, the absence of causative dental infection, pus formation, fistula formation, or sequestration.

Radiologic features of mandibular dental implant–related osteomyelitis are generally similar to other types of osteomyelitis of the jaws. Early stages may initially appear normal radiographically and may not manifest itself until at least 10 days after initiation of the inflammatory process. Progression of the infection may include radiolucent or mixed radiolucent-radiopaque lesions with poorly defined borders that may be limited to the area of the failed implant or may extend to a large part of the mandible.[123] After sufficient bone resorption has occurred, an irregular moth-eaten area of radiolucency may appear, which is generally pathognomonic for osteomyelitis.

Histopathologic findings may range from acute osteomyelitis and chronic osteomyelitis with features of a fibroosseous-like lesion and occasional rimming of atypical osteoblasts.[123] Routine histology will show loss of osteocytes from lacunae in addition to peripheral resorption, bacterial colonization, and acute inflammatory infiltrate consisting of polymorphonuclear leukocytes in haversian canals and peripheral bone. Furthermore, inflamed connective tissue in the intertrabecular bone, scattered sequestrum, and pockets of abscess are generally seen.

Progression of dental implant–related osteomyelitis involves a host of virulent causative organisms. These may include *Streptococcus, Peptococcus,* and *Peptostreptococcus* species in general[128] and *S. anginosus*[130] and *S. intermedius,*[134,139] specifically. Osteomyelitis of the jaw may also exhibit large areas of bone occluded with well-developed biofilms that comprise microbial organisms embedded in an extracellular polymeric substance with a predominance of the *Actinomyces* genus.[140]

Conservative treatment alone is often insufficient to provide a cure for chronic osteomyelitis.[141,142] Progression of an incorrectly diagnosed or treated osteomyelitis of the jaws can result in serious complications such as pathologic fracture and/or osteolytic extension to the inferior border of the mandible. This generally will require an aggressive surgical intervention to include debridement of the infected area until bleeding bone is visualized. The condition may progress to the point in which it will require either marginal mandibulectomy or segmental mandibular resection. The resultant continuity defect from mandibular resection may also require titanium reconstruction plate stabilization with or without hard- and soft-tissue reconstructive procedures.[125]

Medication-Related Osteonecrosis of the Jaws

Although the reason remains unknown, current literature reveals a low rate of MRONJ in dental implant patients taking antiresorptive medication compared with other invasive procedures, such as tooth extraction.[143-145] Although the mechanism in the development of dental implant–related MRONJ is believed to be mainly mechanical, such as in dental implant placement,[146] a microbial biofilm component has been identified.[147] These cases have shown large areas of necrotic bone occluded with biofilms that compromise many bacterial morphotypes and species, such as *Fusobacterium,* bacillus, *Actinomyces,* staphylococcus, streptococcus, *Selenomonas,* and treponemes and yeast (*Candida* species), all with observed coaggregation.[147] This represents some more diverse bacterial organisms in addition to fungal organisms not generally seen in osteomyelitis of the jaws,[140] which may provide an important therapeutic implication because microorganisms present in biofilm represent a clinical antibiofilm target for prevention and treatment efforts.

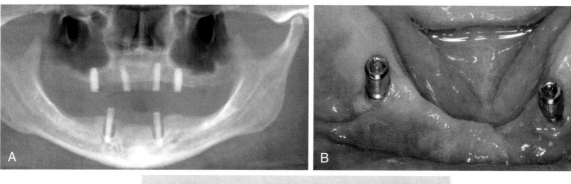

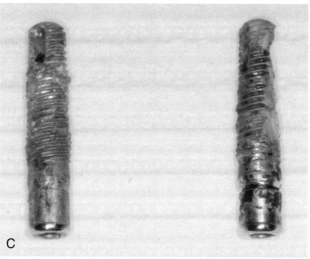

• **Fig. 13.9** (A and B) Advanced peri-implantitis involving two mandibular overdenture dental implants. Note the excessive amount of peri-implant bone loss. (C) Although stable, the implants required removal because of chronic infection.

Biologics

"Biologics" are monoclonal antibodies used against specific targets in the treatment of autoimmune diseases such as rheumatoid arthritis, psoriatic arthritis, and ulcerative colitis. Commonly prescribed medications include adalimumab (Humira), infliximab (Remicade), and certolizumab (Cimzia). Serious postoperative infections may occur when biologic drugs that suppress the immune system have been used and are more likely when combined with other drugs that also suppress the immune system. Individuals that are to undergo any oral or dental implant surgical procedures should have prior consultation with their prescribing physician to evaluate infection risks and the possible need for discontinuation of the medication in question.

Peri-implant Disease

Peri-mucositis and Peri-implantitis

Peri-implant mucositis is characterized by biofilm-induced inflammation localized on the soft peri-implant mucosa but with no evidence of destruction of the supporting bone (Fig. 13.9). Progression of the inflammation may lead to gradual destruction of the bone, manifesting as peri-implantitis. Peri-implant mucositis and peri-implantitis are analogous to gingivitis and periodontitis of natural teeth.[148] Mucositis occurs in approximately 80% of patients with dental implants and in 50% of the implants. The prevalence of peri-implantitis has varied reportedly from 28% to 56% among patients, and 12% to 43% among implants.[149] Evidence indicates that peri-implant mucositis occurs in 50% to 90% of implants, whereas 20% of implants with an average function time of 5 to 11 years develop peri-implantitis.[149] Putative pathogens associated with peri-implantitis are present at a moderate relative abundance in peri-implant mucositis, suggesting that peri-implant mucositis is an important early transitional phase during the development of peri-implantitis.[54] Peri-implant mucositis and peri-implantitis are analogous to gingivitis and periodontitis of natural teeth.[148] The current literature does not warrant development of a correlation of potential bacterial initiators or promoters of peri-implantitis.

Peri-implantitis is an irreversible inflammatory reaction in the soft and hard peri-implant tissues. Plaque accumulation around dental implants has been shown to result in the development of peri-implant inflammation. Contributing factors for the development of peri-implantitis include periodontal disease, smoking, excess cement, and lack of supportive therapy.[150] Periodontopathogenic bacteria that have been implicated in peri-implantitis include *P. gingivalis, P. intermedia, Prevotella nigrescens,* and *A. actinomycetemcomitans.*[151,152] Peri-implantitis has more floral clinical symptoms because in the initial phase it may present the same signs as peri-implant mucositis, but these are later accompanied by the symptoms of bone loss itself.

The most common signs of peri-implantitis are the presence of bacterial plaque and calculus, edema and redness of peri-implant tissues, peri-implant mucosal hyperplasia with a lack of keratinized gingiva, increased probing depths that may reach the apex of the implant, bleeding and purulence on probing and/or palpation, vertical bone destruction in relation to a peri-implant pocket, radiologic presence of bone reabsorption, implant mobility, and possibly pain.[153]

Lack of treatment of peri-implantitis will progress to marginal bone loss. A continuously moving implant and peri-implant radiolucency indicate that the disease is reaching its outcome, characterized by total loss of the bone–implant interface. Radiologic examination is very important because although radiographs only show bone on mesial and distal implant surfaces, the bone defects have a circular or funnel-shaped form; therefore they are larger than those observed on radiographs.

Biofilm

Most infections of the oral cavity are caused by bacteria, fungi, and yeast organized into biofilms. Oral microbial flora comprises one of the most diverse human-associated biofilms that is heavily influenced by oral streptococci as the main group of early colonizers. Oral streptococci species are believed to make up over 80% of the early biofilm constituents.[154] Their initial attachment determines the composition of later colonizers in the oral biofilm. Biofilms are a complex, multispecies, highly communicative community of multilayered accumulations of bacteria or fungi, immersed in an extracellular polymeric matrix.[155,156] Biofilms form in a rapid sequence of events and mature into a complex, interacting community of microorganisms that have different properties than when present in isolation, resulting in a community that is more resistant to antimicrobial agents, stress, and host defenses. This makes the treatment of biofilm infections with traditional antibiotics alone ineffective, and surgical removal of diseased tissue is required.

The earliest stage of biofilm formation is adhesion of microbial cells to a surface, such as dental implant or prostheses, with an acquired salivary pellicle. The salivary pellicle is a thin acellular organic film that forms on any type of surface on exposure to saliva. The role of the pellicle is diverse, with functions known to be highly influenced by the physicochemical properties of both substrata and ambient media, which include protection, lubrication, remineralization, hydration, and acting as a diffusion barrier and buffer.[157] The next stage involves development of an irreversible bond between bacterial adhesins and the acquired salivary pellicle surface with the degree of adherence dependent on the microbial species, the number of cells, and the physicochemical properties of a given surface. Secretory IgA, α-amylase, and cystatins have been identified as dominant proteins in the salivary pellicle that strengthen adherence to smooth titanium surfaces and cause an upregulation of metabolic activity in early oral microbial colonizers, such as S. oralis.[158] Once colonized, the involved microorganisms begin to produce an extracellular polysaccharide matrix.[156] Within this matrix, the subsequent growth in layers of biofilm depend on many factors such as salivary flow, nutrient content, iron availability, pH, osmolarity, oxygen content, concentration of antibacterial agents, and ambient temperature.[159] As microcolonies form, maturation of the biofilm ensues such that the structure and function of microorganisms within the biofilm

may resemble multicellular organisms caused by interactions and communication between cells, even of different species, which function as a consortium, cooperating in a relatively complicated and coordinated manner.[156] Once established, biofilm may cause a pathogenic process even in anatomically distant sites because of dislodged fragments that contain aggregates of bacterial cells, production of endotoxin, evasion of the immunologic response of the host, and formation of a niche for replication of bacterial cells resistant to antimicrobials.

Microbial samples obtained by traditional methods tend to destroy the three-dimensional structure of biofilm, resulting in mixtures of bacteria from unspecified districts of biofilm associated with peri-implant diseases. Advances in microbial analyses methods indicate that peri-implant disease may be viewed as a mixed anaerobic infection, and in most cases the composition of the flora is comparable to subgingival flora of chronic periodontitis dominated by gram-negative bacteria, such as P. gingivalis, P. intermedia, B. forsythus, and gram-positive bacteria, such as peptostreptococci or staphylococci.[61]

The presence of biofilm also effects dental implant restorative materials. Biofilm may lead to a friction coefficient and threaten the biomechanical behavior of a single implant-supported restoration and lead to infection-related failure.[160] Effects of dental implant restorative material/surface properties (such as surface charge, hydrophobicity, roughness, topography, and chemistry) on bacterial adhesion and biofilm formation have shown that negatively charged surfaces, super-hydrophobic surfaces, super-hydrophilic surfaces, and nanometer-scale surface roughness reduce bacterial adhesion. The presence of an acquired pellicle-containing host and bacterially derived proteins poses a great challenge to the control of bacterial adhesion and biofilm formation based on surface modifications. Factors other than surface properties, such as dietary intake and complex oral microbiome, also affect biofilm formation.

Biofilms may act as directors or promoters of cell-mediated (osteoclast) bone resorption or induce bone resorption via various microbial mechanisms. Once established, local host defenses and repair mechanisms act to wall off and eradicate the dead bone via sequestration.[161] Therefore biofilms play an important role in the pathogenesis of osteonecrosis of the jaw (ONJ) in addition to explicating the septic nature of this condition.

Prophylactic Antibiotics

Administration of preoperative, perioperative, or postoperative systemic antibiotics is generally undertaken to prevent dental implant infection. Although numerous prophylactic systemic antibiotic regimens have been suggested to minimize failure, the role of antibiotics in implant dentistry remains contentious. There appears to be no consensus regarding antibiotics in association with routine dental implant placement, the type of regimen to use, or effectiveness in preventing early implant loss. Furthermore, most of the antibiotic regimens used are not in accordance with the recommendations current in the published data.[162,163] Systematic antibiotic administration in patients that receive dental implants significantly reduces implant failure, but there are no apparent significant effects of prophylactic antibiotics on the occurrence of postoperative infections in healthy patients receiving implants.[164,165]

References

1. Gupta A, Dhanraj M, Sivagami G. Status of surface treatment in endosseous implant: a literary overview. *Indian J Dent Res.* 2010;21(3):433–438. https://doi.org/10.4103/0970-9290.70805.

2. Yue C, Zhao B, Ren Y, et al. The implant infection paradox: why do some succeed when others fail? Opinion and discussion paper. *Eur Cell Mater.* 2015;29:303–310.

3. Farnaud SJ, Kosti O, Getting SJ, Renshaw D. Saliva: physiology and diagnostic potential in health and disease. *Sci World J.* 2010;10:434–456. https://doi.org/10.1100/tsw.2010.38.

4. Malamud D, Abrams WR, Barber CA, Weissman D, Rehtanz M, Golub E. Antiviral activities in human saliva. *Adv Dent Res.* 2011;23(1):34–37. https://doi.org/10.1177/0022034511399282.

5. Hanasab H, Jammal D, Oppenheim FG, Helmerhorst EJ. The antifungal activity of human parotid secretion is species-specific. *Med Mycol.* 2011;49(2):218–221. https://doi.org/10.3109/13693786.2010.512299.

6. Young PY, Khadaroo RG. Surgical site infections. *Surg Clin North Am.* 2014;94(6):1245–1264. https://doi.org/10.1016/j.suc.2014.08.008.

7. Han YW, Wang X. Mobile microbiome: oral bacteria in extra-oral infections and inflammation. *J Dent Res.* 2013;92(6):485–491. https://doi.org/10.1177/0022034513487559.

8. Bölükbaşı N, Özdemir T, Öksüz L, Gürler N. Bacteremia following dental implant surgery: preliminary results. *Med Oral Patol Oral Cir Bucal.* 2012;17(1):e69–e75.

9. Herzberg MC. Platelet-streptococcal interactions in endocarditis. *Crit Rev Oral Biol Med.* 1996;7:222–236.

10. Herzberg MC, Meyer MW, Kilic A, Tao L. Host-pathogen interactions in bacterial endocarditis: streptococcal virulence in the host. *Adv Dent Res.* 1997;11:69–74.

11. Matta M, Gousseff M, Monsel F, et al. First case of Streptococcus oligofermentans endocarditis based on sodA gene sequences determined after amplification directly from valvular samples. *J Clin Microbiol.* 2009;47:855–856.

12. Kostic AD, Chun E, Robertson L, et al. Fusobacterium nucleatum potentiates intestinal tumorigenesis and modulates the tumor-immune microenvironment. *Cell Host Microbe.* 2013;14(2):207–215. https://doi.org/10.1016/j.chom.2013.07.007.

13. Shimizu Y, Tsutsumi S, Yasumoto Y, Ito M. Carotid cavernous sinus fistula caused by dental implant-associated infection. *Am J Otolaryngol.* 2012;33(3):352–355. https://doi.org/10.1016/j.amjoto.2011.08.002.

14. Stuzin JM, Baker TJ, Gordon HL. The relationship of the superficial and deep facial fascias: relevance to rhytidectomy and aging. *Plast Reconstr Surg.* 1992;89(3):441–449.

15. Kim HC, Han MH, Moon MH, Kim JH, Kim IO, Chang KH. CT and MR imaging of the buccal space: normal anatomy and abnormalities. *Korean J Radiol.* 2005;6(1):22–30.

16. Tart RP, Kotzur IM, Mancuso AA, Glantz MS, Mukherji SK. CT and MR imaging of the buccal space and buccal space masses. *RadioGraphics.* 1995;15:531–550.

17. Smoker WRK. Oral cavity. In: Som PM, Curtin HD, eds. *Head and Neck Imaging.* 3rd ed. St. Louis: Mosby; 1996:488–544.

18. Schuknecht B, Stergiou G, Graetz K. Masticator space abscess derived from odontogenic infection: imaging manifestation and pathways of extension depicted by CT and MR in 30 patients. *Eur Radiol.* 2008;18(9):1972–1979. https://doi.org/10.1007/s00330-008-0946-5.

19. Khoury JN, Mihailidis S, Ghabriel M, Townsend G. Applied anatomy of the pterygomandibular space: improving the success of inferior alveolar nerve blocks. *Aust Dent J.* 2011;56(2):112–121.

20. Bratton TA, Jackson DC, Nkungula-Howlett T, Williams CW, Bennett CR. Management of complex multi-space odontogenic infections. *J Tenn Dent Assoc.* 2002;82(3):39–47.

21. Lee JY, Kim JN, Kim SH, et al. Anatomical verification and designation of the superficial layer of the temporalis muscle. *Clin Anat.* 2012;25(2):176.

22. Ural A, Imamoğlu M, Umit Işık A., et al. Neck masses confined to the submental space: our experience with 24 cases. *Ear Nose Throat J.* 2011;90(11):538.

23. Potter JK, Herford AS, Ellis 3rd E. Tracheotomy versus endotracheal intubation for airway management in deep neck space infections. *J Oral Maxillofac Surg.* 2002;60(4):349–354.

24. Dzyak WR, Zide MF. Diagnosis and treatment of lateral pharyngeal space infections. *J Oral Maxillofac Surg.* 1984;42(4):243–249.

25. Goodman LJ. Purulent pericarditis. *Curr Treat Options Cardiovasc Med.* 2000;2(4):343–350.

26. Kulik EM, Sandmeier H, Hinni K, Meyer J. Identification of archaeal rDNA from subgingival dental plaque by PCR amplification and sequence analysis. *FEMS Microbiol Lett.* 2001;196:129–133.

27. Aas JA, Paster BJ, Stokes LN, Olsen I, Dewhirst FE. Defining the normal bacterial flora of the oral cavity. *J Clin Microbiol.* 2005;43:5721–5732.

28. Keijser BJ, Zaura E, Huse SM, et al. Pyrosequencing analysis of the oral microflora of healthy adults. *J Dent Res.* 2008;87:1016–1020.

29. Mombelli A. Microbiology of the dental implant. *Adv Dent Res.* 1993;7(2):202–206.

30. Whiley RA, Beighton D. Current classification of the oral streptococci. *Oral Microbiol Immunol.* 1998;13(4):195–216.

31. Facklam R. What happened to the streptococci: overview of taxonomic and nomenclature changes. *Clin Microbiol Rev.* 2002;15:613–630.

32. Burton JP, Wescombe PA, Cadieux PA, Tagg JR. Beneficial microbes for the oral cavity: time to harness the oral streptococci? *Benef Microbes.* 2011;2(2):93–101. https://doi.org/10.3920/BM2011.0002.

33. Delwiche EA, Pestka JJ, Tortorello ML. The veillonellae: gram-negative cocci with a unique physiology. *Annu Rev Microbiol.* 1985;39:175–193.

34. Distler W, Kroncke A. The lactate metabolism of the oral bacterium *Veillonella* from human saliva. *Arch Oral Biol.* 1981;26:657–661.

35. McNab R, Ford SK, El-Sabaeny A, Barbieri B, Cook GS, Lamont RJ. LuxS-based signaling in *Streptococcus gordonii:* autoinducer 2 controls carbohydrate metabolism and biofilm formation with *Porphyromonas gingivalis. J Bacteriol.* 2003;185:274–284.

36. Rickard AH, Palmer Jr RJ, Blehert DS, et al. Autoinducer 2: a concentration-dependent signal for mutualistic bacterial biofilm growth. *Mol Microbiol.* 2006;60:1446–1456.

37. Edwards AM, Grossman TJ, Rudney JD. *Fusobacterium nucleatum* transports noninvasive *Streptococcus cristatus* into human epithelial cells. *Infect Immun.* 2006;74:654–662.

38. Brown SA, Whiteley M. A novel exclusion mechanism for carbon resource partitioning in *Aggregatibacter actinomycetemcomitans. J Bacteriol.* 2007;189:6407–6414.

39. Sutter VL. Anaerobes as normal oral flora. *Rev Infect Dis.* 1984;6(suppl 1):S62–S66.

40. Park OJ, Yi H, Jeon JH, et al. Pyrosequencing analysis of subgingival microbiota in distinct periodontal conditions. *J Dent Res.* 2015;94(7):921–927. https://doi.org/10.1177/0022034515583531.

41. Nordquist WD. Oral spirochetosis associated with dental implants: important clues to systemic disease. *Int J Clin Implant Dent.* 2009;1(1):32–39.

42. Cui L, Morris A, Ghedin E. The human mycobiome in health and disease. *Genome Med.* 2013;5(7):63. https://doi.org/10.1186/gm467.

43. Darling WM. Co-cultivation of mycobacteria and fungus. *Lancet.* 1976;2:740. 40.

44. Kerr J. Inhibition of fungal growth by *Pseudomonas aeruginosa* and *Pseudomonas cepacia* isolated from patients with cystic fibrosis. *J Infect.* 1994;28:305–310.

45. Matsubara VH, Igai F, Tamaki R, Tortamano Neto P, Nakamae AE, Mori M. Use of silver nanoparticles reduces internal contamination of external hexagon implants by candida albicans. *Braz Dent J.* 2015;26(5):458–462. https://doi.org/10.1590/0103-644020130087.

46. Trindade LA, de Araújo Oliveira J, de Castro RD, de Oliveira Lima E. Inhibition of adherence of C. albicans to dental implants and cover screws by Cymbopogon nardus essential oil and citronellal. *Clin Oral Investig.* 2015;19(9):2223–2231. https://doi.org/10.1007/s00784-015-1450-3.

47. Lepp PW, Brinig MM, Ouverney CC, Palm K, Armitage GC, Relman DA. Methanogenic Archaea and human periodontal disease. *Proc Natl Acad Sci U S A.* 2004;101(16):6176–6181.

48. Vianna ME, Conrads G, Gomes BP, Horz HP. T-RFLP-based mcrA gene analysis of methanogenic archaea in association with oral infections and evidence of a novel Methanobrevibacter phylotype. *Oral Microbiol Immunol.* 2009;24(5):417–422. https://doi.org/10.1111/j.1399-302X.2009.00539. x.

49. Huynh HT, Nkamga VD, Drancourt M, Aboudharam G. Genetic variants of dental plaque Methanobrevibacter oralis. *Eur J Clin Microbiol Infect Dis.* 2015;34(6):1097–1101. https://doi.org/10.1007/s10096-015-2325-x.

50. Li CL, Liu DL, Jiang YT, et al. Prevalence and molecular diversity of Archaea in subgingival pockets of periodontitis patients. *Oral Microbiol Immunol.* 2009;24(4):343–346. https://doi.org/10.1111/j.1399-302X.2009.00514.x.

51. Bringuier A, Khelaifia S, Richet H, Aboudharam G, Drancourt M. Real-time PCR quantification of Methanobrevibacter oralis in periodontitis. *J Clin Microbiol.* 2013;51(3):993–994. https://doi.org/10.1128/JCM.02863-12.

52. Vianna ME, Holtgraewe S, Seyfarth I, Conrads G, Horz HP. Quantitative analysis of three hydrogenotrophic microbial groups, methanogenic archaea, sulfate-reducing bacteria, and acetogenic bacteria, within plaque biofilms associated with human periodontal disease. *J Bacteriol.* 2008;190(10):3779–3785. https://doi.org/10.1128/JB.01861-07.

53. Faveri M, Gonçalves LF, Feres M, et al. Prevalence and microbiological diversity of Archaea in peri-implantitis subjects by 16S ribosomal RNA clonal analysis. *J Periodontal Res.* 2011;46(3):338–344. https://doi.org/10.1111/j.1600-0765.2011.01347.x.

54. Zheng H, Xu L, Wang Z, et al. Subgingival microbiome in patients with healthy and ailing dental implants. *Sci Rep.* 2015;5:10948. https://doi.org/10.1038/srep10948.

55. Shiono Y, Ishii K, Nagai S, et al. Delayed *Propionibacterium acnes* surgical site infections occur only in the presence of an implant. *Sci Rep.* 2016;6:32758. https://doi.org/10.1038/srep32758.

56. Flanagan D. *Enterococcus faecalis* and dental implants. *J Oral Implantol.* 2017;43(1):8–11. https://doi.org/10.1563/aaid-joi-D-16-00069.

57. Berglundh T, Zitzmann NU, Donati M. Are peri-implantitis lesions different from periodontitis lesions? *J Clin Periodontol.* 2011;38(suppl 11):188–202.

58. Kumar PS, Mason MR, Brooker MR, O'Brien K. Pyrosequencing reveals unique microbial signatures associated with healthy and failing dental implants. *J Clin Periodontol.* 2012;39:425–433.

59. Salvi GE, Aglietta M, Eick S, Sculean A, Lang NP, Ramseier CA. Reversibility of experimental peri-implant mucositis compared with experimental gingivitis in humans. *Clin Oral Implants Res.* 2012;23:182–190.

60. Leonhardt A, Adolfsson B, Lekholm U, Wikstrom M, Dahlen G. A longitudinal microbiological study on osseointegrated titanium implants in partially edentulous patients. *Clin Oral Implants Res.* 1993;4:113–120.

61. Mombelli A, Décaillet F. The characteristics of biofilms in peri-implant disease. *J Clin Periodontol.* 2011;38(suppl 11):203–213. https://doi.org/10.1111/j.1600-051X.2010.01666.x.

62. Rutar A, Lang NP, Buser D, Burgin W, Mombelli A. Retrospective assessment of clinical and microbiological factors affecting peri-implant tissue conditions. *Clin Oral Implants Res.* 2001;12:189–195.

63. Tabanella G, Nowzari H, Slots J. Clinical and microbiological determinants of ailing dental implants. *Clin Implant Dent Relat Res.* 2009;11:24–36.

64. Takanashi K, Kishi M, Okuda K, Ishihara K. Colonization by *Porphyromonas gingivalis* and *Prevotella intermedia* from teeth to osseointegrated implant regions. *Bull Tokyo Dent Coll.* 2004;45:77–85.

65. Christersson LA, Slots J, Rosling BG, Genco RJ. Microbiological and clinical effects of surgical treatment of localized juvenile periodontitis. *J Clin Periodontol.* 1985;12:465–476.

66. Größner-Schreiber B, Teichmann J, Hannig M, Dörfer C, Wenderoth DF, Ott SJ. Modified implant surfaces show different biofilm compositions under in vivo conditions. *Clin Oral Implants Res.* 2009;20(8):817–826. https://doi.org/10.1111/j.1600-0501.2009.01729.x.

67. Yoshinari M, Oda Y, Kato T, Okuda K, Hirayama A. Influence of surface modifications to titanium on oral bacterial adhesion in vitro. *J Biomed Mater Res.* 2000;52(2):388–394.

68. Esposito M, Cannizzaro G, Bozzoli P, Chec-chi L, Ferri V, Landriani S, et al. Effectiveness of prophylactic antibiotics at placement of dental implants: a pragmatic multicentre placebo-controlled randomised clinical trial. *Eur J Oral Implantol.* 2010;3:135–143.

69. Esposito M, Cannizzaro G, Bozzoli P, et al. Efficacy of prophylactic antibiotics for dental implants: a multicentre placebo-controlled randomised clinical trial. *Eur J Oral Implantol.* 2008;1:23–31.

70. Abu-Ta'a M, Quirynen M, Teughels W, van Steenberghe D. Asepsis during periodontal surgery involving oral implants and the usefulness of peri-operative antibiotics: a prospective, randomized, controlled clinical trial. *J Clin Periodontol.* 2008;35:58–63. 25.

71. Quirynen M, De Soete M, van Steenberghe D. Infectious risks for oral implants: a review of the literature. *Clin Oral Impl Res.* 2002;13:1–19.

72. Jensen OT. Dental extraction, immediate placement of dental implants, and immediate function. *Oral Maxillofac Surg Clin North Am.* 2015;27(2):273–282. https://doi.org/10.1016/j.coms.2015.01.008.

73. Aghaloo TL, Mardirosian M, Delgado B. Controversies in implant surgery. *Oral Maxillofac Surg Clin North Am.* 2017;29(4):525–535. https://doi.org/10.1016/j.coms.2017.07.007.

74. Hegde R, Krishna Prasad D, Shetty DV, Shetty M. Immediate placement and restoration of implant in periapical infected site in the maxillary esthetic zone: a case report. *J Indian Prosthodont Soc.* 2014;14(suppl 1):299–302. https://doi.org/10.1007/s13191-014-0357-z.

75. Anitua E, Piñas L, Alkhraisat MH. Long-term outcomes of immediate implant placement into infected sockets in association with immediate loading: a retrospective cohort study. *J Periodontol.* 2016;87(10):1135–1140. https://doi.org/10.1902/jop.2016.160104.

76. Corbella S, Taschieri S, Tsesis I, Del Fabbro M. Postextraction implant in sites with endodontic infection as an alternative to endodontic retreatment: a review of literature. *J Oral Implantol.* 2013;39(3):399–405. https://doi.org/10.1563/AAID-JOI-D-11-00229.

77. Crespi R, Capparé P, Crespi G, Lo Giudice G, Gastaldi G, Gherlone E. Dental implants placed in periodontally infected sites in humans. *Clin Implant Dent Relat Res.* 2017;19(1):131–139. https://doi.org/10.1111/cid.12425.

78. Chrcanovic BR, Martins MD, Wennerberg A. Immediate placement of implants into infected sites: a systematic review. *Clin Implant Dent Relat Res.* 2015;17(suppl 1):e1–e16. https://doi.org/10.1111/cid.12098.

79. Bell CL, Diehl D, Bell BM, Bell RE. The immediate placement of dental implants into extraction sites with periapical lesions: a retrospective chart review. *J Oral Maxillofac Surg.* 2011;69(6):1623–1627. https://doi.org/10.1016/j.joms.2011.01.022.

80. Blus C, Szmukler-Moncler S, Khoury P, Orrù G. Immediate implants placed in infected and noninfected sites after atraumatic tooth extraction and placement with ultrasonic bone surgery. *Clin Implant Dent Relat Res.* 2015;17(suppl 1):e287–e297. https://doi.org/10.1111/cid.12126.

81. Montoya-Salazar V, Castillo-Oyag R, Torres-Sanchez C, Lynch CD, Gutirrez-Perez JL, Torres-Lagares D. Outcome of single immediate implants placed in post-extraction infected and non-infected sites, restored with cemented crowns: a 3-year prospective study. *J Dent.* 2014;42(6):645–652.

82. Zuffetti F, Capelli M, Galli F, Del Fabbro M, Testori T. Post-extraction implant placement into infected versus non-infected sites: a multicenter retrospective clinical study. *Clin Implant Dent Relat Res.* 2017;19(5):833–840. https://doi.org/10.1111/cid.12523.

83. Waasdorp JA, Evian CI, Mandracchia M. Immediate placement of implants into infected sites: a systematic review of the literature. *J Periodontol.* 2010;81(6):801–808. https://doi.org/10.1902/jop.2010.090706.

84. Meltzer AM. Immediate implant placement and restoration in infected sites. *Int J Periodontics Restorative Dent.* 2012;32(5):e169–e173.

85. Zhao D, Wu Y, Xu C, Zhang F. Immediate dental implant placement into infected vs. non-infected sockets: a meta-analysis. *Clin Oral Implants Res.* 2016;27(10):1290–1296. https://doi.org/10.1111/clr.12739.

86. de Oliveira-Neto OB, Barbosa FT, de Sousa-Rodrigues CF, de Lima FJC. Quality assessment of systematic reviews regarding immediate placement of dental implants into infected sites: an overview. *J Prosthet Dent.* 2017;117(5):601–605. https://doi.org/10.1016/j.prosdent.2016.09.007.

87. Ata-Ali J, Ata-Ali F, Ata-Ali F. Do antibiotics decrease implant failure and postoperative infections? a systematic review and meta-analysis. *Int J Oral Maxillofac Surg.* 2014;43(1):68–74. https://doi.org/10.1016/j.ijom.2013.05.019.

88. Melo RF, Lopes BM, Shibli JA, Marcantonio Junior E, Marcantonio RA, Galli GM. Interleukin-1β and interleukin-6 expression and gene polymorphisms in subjects with peri-implant disease. *Clin Implant Dent Relat Res.* 2012;14:905–914.

89. Chrcanovic BR, Albrektsson T, Wennerberg A. Periodontally compromised vs. periodontally healthy patients and dental implants: a systematic review and meta-analysis. *J Dent.* 2014;42(12):1509–1527. https://doi.org/10.1016/j.jdent.2014.09.013.

90. Lee DW. Periodontitis and dental implant loss. *Evid Based Dent.* 2014;15(2):59–60. https://doi.org/10.1038/sj.ebd.6401031.

91. Mengel R, Schroeder T, Flores-de-Jacoby L. Osseointegrated implants in patients treated for generalized chronic periodontitis and generalized aggressive periodontitis: 3- and 5-year results of a prospective long-term study. *J Periodontol.* 2001;72(8):977–989.

92. Brignardello-Petersen R. Implants placed in patients with a history of aggressive periodontitis had high survival rates and low marginal bone loss. *J Am Dent Assoc.* 2017;148(4):e37. https://doi.org/10.1016/j.adaj.2017.02.023.

93. Theodoridis C, Grigoriadis A, Menexes G, Vouros I. Outcomes of implant therapy in patients with a history of aggressive periodontitis. A systematic review and meta-analysis. *Clin Oral Investig.* 2017;21(2):485–503. https://doi.org/10.1007/s00784-016-2026-6.

94. Mengel R, Behle M, Flores-de-Jacoby L. Osseointegrated implants in subjects treated for generalized aggressive periodontitis: 10-year results of a prospective, long-term cohort study. *J Periodontol.* 2007;78(12):2229–2237.

95. Monje A, Alcoforado G, Padial-Molina M, Suarez F, Lin GH, Wang HL. Generalized aggressive periodontitis as a risk factor for dental implant failure: a systematic review and meta-analysis. *J Periodontol.* 2014;85(10):1398–1407. https://doi.org/10.1902/jop.2014.140135.

96. Ramesh A, Ravi S, Kaarthikeyan G. Comprehensive rehabilitation using dental implants in generalized aggressive periodontitis. *J Indian Soc Periodontol.* 2017;21(2):160–163. https://doi.org/10.4103/jisp.jisp_213_17.

97. Rajan G, Natarajarathinam G, Kumar S, Parthasarathy H. Full mouth rehabilitation with zygomatic implants in patients with generalized aggressive periodontitis: 2-year follow-up of two cases. *J Indian Soc Periodontol.* 2014;18(1):107–111. https://doi.org/10.4103/0972-124X.128262.

98. Rasaeipour S, Siadat H, Rasouli A, Sajedinejadd N, Ghodsi S. Implant rehabilitation in advanced generalized aggressive periodontitis: a case report and literature review. *J Dent (Tehran).* 2015;12(8):614–620.

99. Kim KK, Sung HM. Outcomes of dental implant treatment in patients with generalized aggressive periodontitis: a systematic review. *J Adv Prosthodont.* 2012;4(4):210–217. https://doi.org/10.4047/jap.2012.4.4.210.

100. Marconcini S, Barone A, Gelpi F, Briguglio F, Covani U. Immediate implant placement in infected sites: a case series. *J Periodontol.* 2013;84(2):196–202. https://doi.org/10.1902/jop.2012.110279.

101. Karoussis IK, Salvi GE, Heitz-Mayfield LJ, Brägger U, Hämmerle CH, Lang NP. Long-term implant prognosis in patients with and without a history of chronic periodontitis: a 10-year prospective cohort study of the ITI dental implant system. *Clin Oral Implants Res.* 2003;14(3):329–339.

102. Schou S, Holmstrup P, Worthington HV, Esposito M. Outcome of implant therapy in patients with previous tooth loss due to periodontitis. *Clin Oral Implants Res.* 2006;17(suppl 2):104–123.

103. Zangrando MS, Damante CA, Sant'Ana AC, Rubo de Rezende ML, Greghi SL, Chambrone L. Long-term evaluation of periodontal parameters and implant outcomes in periodontally compromised patients: a systematic review. *J Periodontol.* 2015;86(2):201–221. https://doi.org/10.1902/jop.2014.140390.

104. Del Fabbro M, Testori T, Francetti L, Taschieri S, Weinstein R. Systematic review of survival rates for immediately loaded dental implants. *Int J Periodontics Restorative Dent.* 2006;26(3):249–263.

105. Gomes JA, Sartori IAM, Able FB, de Oliveira Silva TS, do Nascimento C. Microbiological and clinical outcomes of fixed complete-arch mandibular prostheses supported by immediate implants in individuals with history of chronic periodontitis. *Clin Oral Implants Res.* 2017;28(6):734–741. https://doi.org/10.1111/clr.12871.

106. Alves CC, Correia AR, Neves M. Immediate implants and immediate loading in periodontally compromised patients-a 3-year prospective clinical study. *Int J Periodontics Restorative Dent.* 2010;30(5):447–455.

107. Horwitz J, Machtei EE. Immediate and delayed restoration of dental implants in patients with a history of periodontitis: a prospective evaluation up to 5 years. *Int J Oral Maxillofac Implants.* 2012;27(5):1137–1143.

108. Malo P, Nobre Mde A, Lopes A, Ferro A, Gravito I. Immediate loading of implants placed in patients with untreated periodontal disease: a 5-year prospective cohort study. *Eur J Oral Implantol.* 2014;7(3):295–304.

109. Lang NP, Wet AC. Histologic probe penetration in healthy and inflamed peri-implant tissues. In: Brånemark PI, Zarb GA, Albrektsson T, eds. *Tissue-Integrated Prostheses: Osseointegration in Clinical Dentistry.* Chicago: Quintessence; 1985:211–232.

110. Haanaes HR. Implants and infections with special reference to oral bacteria. *J Clin Periodontol.* 1990;17:516–524.

111. Ribeiro LG, Hashizume LN, Maltz M. The effect of different formulations of chlorhexidine in reducing levels of mutans streptococci in the oral cavity: a systematic review of the literature. *J Dent.* 2007;35:359–370. https://doi.org/10.1016/j.jdent.2007.01.007.

112. Roldan S, Herrera D, Santa-Cruz I, O'Connor A, Gonzalez I, Sanz M. Comparative effects of different chlorhexidine mouth-rinse formulations on volatile sulphur compounds and salivary bacterial counts. *J Clin Periodontol.* 2004;31:1128–1134. https://doi.org/10.1111/j.1600-051X.2004.00621.x.

113. van der Mei HC, White DJ, Atema-Smit J, van de Belt-Gritter E, Busscher HJ. A method to study sustained antimicrobial activity of rinse and dentifrice components on biofilm viability *in vivo*. *J Clin Periodontol*. 2006;33:14–20. https://doi.org/10.1111/j.1600-051X.2005.00859.x.

114. Vitkov L, Hermann A, Krautgartner WD, et al. Chlorhexidine-induced ultrastructural alterations in oral biofilm. *Microsc Res Tech*. 2005;68:85–89. https://doi.org/10.1002/jemt.20238.

115. Gilbert P, Moore LE. Cationic antiseptics: diversity of action under a common epithet. *J Appl Microbiol*. 2005;99:703–715. https://doi.org/10.1111/j.1365-2672.2005.02664.x.

116. Spijkervet FK, van Saene JJ, van Saene HK, Panders AK, Vermey A, Fidler V. Chlorhexidine inactivation by saliva. *Oral Surg Oral Med Oral Pathol*. 1990;69:444–449. https://doi.org/10.1016/0030-4220(90)90377-5.

117. Abouassi T, Hannig C, Mahncke K, et al. Does human saliva decrease the antimicrobial activity of chlorhexidine against oral bacteria? *BMC Research Notes*. 2014;7:711. https://doi.org/10.1186/1756-0500-7-711.

118. Van Steenberghe D. Complete nose coverage to prevent airborne contamination. *Clinical Oral Implants Research*. 1997;8:512–516.

119. Figueiredo R, Camps-Font O, Valmaseda-Castellón E, Gay-Escoda C. Risk factors for postoperative infections after dental implant placement: a case-control study. *J Oral Maxillofac Surg*. 2015;73(12):2312–2318. https://doi.org/10.1016/j.joms.2015.07.025.

120. Mahmood R, Puthussery FJ, Flood T, Shekhar K. Dental implant complications –extra-oral cutaneous fistula. *Br Dent J*. 2013;215(2):69–70. https://doi.org/10.1038/sj.bdj.2013.683.

121. Fujioka M, Oka K, Kitamura R, Yakabe A, Endoh H. Extra-oral fistula caused by a dental implant. *J Oral Implantol*. 2011;37(4):477–479. https://doi.org/10.1563/AAID-JOI-D-09-00008.1.

122. Schlund M, Raoul G, Ferri J, Nicot R. Mandibular osteomyelitis following implant placement. *J Oral Maxillofac Surg*. 2017;75(12):2560.e1–2560.e7. https://doi.org/10.1016/j.joms.2017.07.169.

123. Shnaiderman-Shapiro A, Dayan D, Buchner A, Schwartz I, Yahalom R, Vered M. Histopathological spectrum of bone lesions associated with dental implant failure: osteomyelitis and beyond. *Head Neck Pathol*. 2015;9(1):140–146. https://doi.org/10.1007/s12105-014-0538-4.

124. Semel G, Wolff A, Shilo D, Akrish S, Emodi O, Rachmiel A. Mandibular osteomyelitis associated with dental implants. A case series. *Eur J Oral Implantol*. 2016;9(4):435–442.

125. Yahalom R, Ghantous Y, Peretz A, Abu-Elnaaj I. The possible role of dental implants in the etiology and prognosis of osteomyelitis: a retrospective study. *Int J Oral Maxillofac Implants*. 2016;31(5):1100–1109. https://doi.org/10.11607/jomi.4527.

126. Naval L, Molini MS, Herrera G, Naval B. Dental implants and osteomyelitis in a patient with osteopetrosis. *Quintessence Int*. 2014;45(9):765–768. https://doi.org/10.3290/j.qi.a32443.

127. Pigrau C, Almirante B, Rodriguez D, et al. Osteomyelitis of the jaw: resistance to clindamycin in patients with prior antibiotics exposure. *Eur J Clin Microbiol Infect Dis*. 2009;28(4):317–323. https://doi.org/10.1007/s10096-008-0626-z.

128. Kesting MR, Thurmuller P, Ebsen M, Wolff KD. Severe osteomyelitis following immediate placement of a dental implant. *Int J Oral Maxillofac Implants*. 2008;23:137.

129. O'Sullivan D, King P, Jagger D. Osteomyelitis and pathological mandibular fracture related to a late implant failure: a clinical report. *J Prosthet Dent*. 2006;95(2):106–110.

130. Chatelain S, Lombardi T, Scolozzi P. Streptococcus anginosus dental implant-related osteomyelitis of the jaws: an insidious and calamitous entity. *J Oral Maxillofac Surg*. 2018;S0278–2391 (18):30032–30036. https://doi.org/10.1016/j.joms.2018.01.010.

131. Baltensperger M. *A Retrospective Analysis of 290 Osteomyelitis Cases Treated in the Past 30 Years at the Department of Cranio-Maxillofacial Surgery Zurich with Special Recognition of the Classification*. Zurich: Med Dissertation; 2003.

132. Hudson JW. Osteomyelitis of the jaws: a 50-year perspective. *J Oral Maxillofac Surg*. 1993;51:1294.

133. Topazian RG. Osteomyelitis of the jaws. In: Topazian RG, Goldberg MH, Hupp JR, eds. *Oral and Maxillofacial Infections*. 4th ed. Philadelphia, PA: WB Saunders; 2002:214–242.

134. Baltensperger M, Eyrich GK. Osteomyelitis of the jaws: Definition and classification. In: Baltensperger M, Eyrich GK, eds. *Osteomyelitis of the Jaws*. Berlin: Springer-Verlag; 2009:5–47.

135. Koorbusch GF, Deatherage JR, Curé JK. How can we diagnose and treat osteomyelitis of the jaws as early as possible? *Oral Maxillofac Surg Clin North Am*. 2011;23(4):557–567. https://doi.org/10.1016/j.coms.2011.07.011.

136. Marx RE. Chronic osteomyelitis of the jaws. *Oral Maxillofac Surg Clin North Am*. 1991;3(2):367–381.

137. Mercuri LG. Acute osteomyelitis of the jaws. *Oral Maxillofac Surg Clin North Am*. 1991;3(2):355–365.

138. Koorbusch GF, Fotos P, Goll KT. Retrospective assessment of osteomyelitis. Etiology, demographics, risk factors, and management in 35 cases. *Oral Surg Oral Med Oral Pathol*. 1992;74(2):149–154.

139. Doll C, Hartwig S, Nack C, Nahles S, Nelson K, Raguse JD. Dramatic course of osteomyelitis in a patient treated with immediately placed dental implants suffering from uncontrolled diabetes: a case report. *Eur J Oral Implantol*. 2015;8(4):405–410.

140. Sedghizadeh PP, Kumar SK, Gorur A, Schaudinn C, Shuler CF, Costerton JW. Microbial biofilms in osteomyelitis of the jaw and osteonecrosis of the jaw secondary to bisphosphonate therapy. *J Am Dent Assoc*. 2009;140(10):1259–1265.

141. Coviello V, Stevens MR. Contemporary concepts in the treatment of chronic osteomyelitis. *Oral Maxillofac Surg Clin North Am*. 2007;19:523.

142. Baur DA, Altay MA, Flores-Hidalgo A, et al. Chronic osteomyelitis of the mandible: Diagnosis and management—an institution's experience over 7 years. *J Oral Maxillofac Surg*. 2015;73:6559.

143. Chadha GK, Ahmadieh A, Kumar S, Sedghizadeh PP. Osseointegration of dental implants and osteonecrosis of the jaw in patients treated with bisphosphonate therapy: a systematic review. *J Oral Implantol*. 2013;39(4):510–520. https://doi.org/10.1563/AAID-JOI-D-11-00234.

144. Kwon TG, Lee CO, Park JW, Choi SY, Rijal G, Shin HI. Osteonecrosis associated with dental implants in patients undergoing bisphosphonate treatment. *Clin Oral Implants Res*. 2014;25(5):632–640. https://doi.org/10.1111/clr.12088.

145. Yuan K, Chen KC, Chan YJ, Tsai CC, Chen HH, Shih CC. Dental implant failure associated with bacterial infection and long-term bisphosphonate usage: a case report. *Implant Dent*. 2012;21(1):3–7. https://doi.org/10.1097/ID.0b013e3182425c62.

146. Pichardo SE, van Merkesteyn JP. Bisphosphonate related osteonecrosis of the jaws: spontaneous or dental origin? *Oral Surg Oral Med Oral Pathol Oral Radiol*. 2013;116(3):287–292. https://doi.org/10.1016/j.oooo.2013.05.005.

147. Sedghizadeh PP, Kumar SK, Gorur A, Schaudinn C, Shuler CF, Costerton JW. Identification of microbial biofilms in osteonecrosis of the jaws secondary to bisphosphonate therapy. *J Oral Maxillofac Surg*. 2008;66(4):767–775. https://doi.org/10.1016/j.joms.2007.11.035.

148. Heitz-Mayfield LJ, Lang NP. Comparative biology of chronic and aggressive periodontitis vs. periimplantitis. *Periodontol 2000*. 2010;53:167–181.

149. Zitzmann NU, Berglundh T. Definition and prevalence of peri-implant diseases. *J Clin Periodontol*. 2008;35(suppl 8):286–291.

150. Renvert S, Quirynen M. Risk indicators for peri-implantitis. A narrative review. *Clin Oral Implants Res*. 2015;26(suppl 11):15–44. https://doi.org/10.1111/clr.12636.

151. Botero JE, González AM, Mercado RA, Olave G, Contreras A. Subgingival microbiota in peri-implant mucosa lesions and adjacent teeth in partially edentulous patients. *J Periodontol*. 2005;76(9):1490–1495.

152. Renvert S, Roos-Jansåker AM, Lindahl C, Renvert H, Rutger Persson G. Infection at titanium implants with or without a clinical diagnosis of inflammation. *Clin Oral Implants Res.* 2007;18(4):509–516.
153. Bowen-Antolín A, Pascua-García MT, Nasimi A. Infections in implantology: from prophylaxis to treatment. *Med Oral Patol Oral Cir Bucal.* 2007;12:e323–e330.
154. Rosan B, Lamont RJ. Dental plaque formation. *Microbes Infect.* 2000;2:1599–1607.
155. Donlan RM, Costerton JW. Biofilms: survival mechanisms of clinically relevant microorganisms. *Clin Microbiol Rev.* 2002;15:167–193.
156. Dufour D, Leung V, Levesque C. Bacterial biofilm: structure, function, and antimicrobial resistance. *Endodontic Topics.* 2010;22(1):2–16. 03.
157. Lindh L, Aroonsang W, Sotres J, Arnebrant T. Salivary pellicles. *Monogr Oral Sci.* 2014;24:30–39. https://doi.org/10.1159/000358782.
158. Dorkhan M, Svensäter G, Davies JR. Salivary pellicles on titanium and their effect on metabolic activity in Streptococcus oralis. *BMC Oral Health.* 2013;13:32. https://doi.org/10.1186/1472-6831-13-32.
159. Davey ME, O'Toole GA. Microbial biofilms: from ecology to molecular genetics. *Microbiol Mol Biol Rev.* 2000;64:847–867.
160. Bordin D, Cavalcanti IM, Jardim Pimentel M, et al. Biofilm and saliva affect the biomechanical behavior of dental implants. *J Biomech.* 2015;48(6):997–1002. https://doi.org/10.1016/j.jbiomech.2015.02.004.
161. Nelson CL, McLaren AC, McLaren SG, et al. Is aseptic loosening truly aseptic? *Clin Orthop Rel Res.* 2005;437:25.
162. Camps-Font O, Viaplana-Gutiérrez M, Mir-Mari J, Figueiredo R, Gay-Escoda C, Valmaseda-Castellón E. Antibiotic prescription for the prevention and treatment of postoperative complications after routine dental implant placement. A cross-sectional study performed in Spain. *J Clin Exp Dent.* 2018;10(3):e264–e270. https://doi.org/10.4317/jced.54637.
163. Deeb GR, Soung GY, Best AM, Laskin DM. Antibiotic prescribing habits of oral and maxillofacial surgeons in conjunction with routine dental implant placement. *J Oral Maxillofac Surg.* 2015;73(10):1926–1931. https://doi.org/10.1016/j.joms.2015.05.024.
164. Chrcanovic BR, Albrektsson T, Wennerberg A. Prophylactic antibiotic regimen and dental implant failure: a meta-analysis. *J Oral Rehabil.* 2014;41(12):941–956. https://doi.org/10.1111/joor.12211.
165. Keenan JR, Veitz-Keenan A. Antibiotic prophylaxis for dental implant placement? *Evid Based Dent.* 2015;16(2):52–53. https://doi.org/10.1038/sj.ebd.6401097.
166. Esposito M, Grusovin MG, Worthington HV. Interventions for replacing missing teeth: antibiotics at dental implant placement to prevent complications. *Cochrane Database Syst Rev.* 2013;(7):CD004152. https://doi.org/10.1002/14651858.CD004152.pub4.

14

Pharmacology in Implant Dentistry

RANDOLPH R. RESNIK

Because of the increase in demand and use of dental implants in dentistry today, a thorough understanding of the indications and protocol for the use of pharmacologic agents in implant dentistry is essential for the implant clinician. The morbidity of implant-related complications may on occasion be significant; therefore ideal medication selection and sufficient dosage levels of medications are preoperatively and postoperatively indicated. In addition, the scope of implant treatment often encompasses an older population with more complex cases and medical histories. As a result, treatment requires a greater understanding of the use of pharmacologic agents to decrease implant morbidity and possible complications.

Currently in implant dentistry, no consensus exists on the pharmacologic protocol based on both the patient's health status and procedure type. Many practitioners use medications empirically or generically with respect to all procedures with little basis on scientific facts and studies. The author has developed a pharmacologic protocol with the goal of decreasing complications and increasing the success rate of implants with an emphasis on the patient's health status and the invasiveness of the procedure. Therefore this chapter will provide the implant dentist with an overview of the pharmacokinetics and pharmacodynamics of various classifications of medications, together with an understanding of the proper prescribing protocol used in implant dentistry today with respect to different patient and procedure characteristics.

Antimicrobials

An important complication to prevent after implant surgery is infection. Infectious episodes may lead to a multitude of problems, including pain, swelling, loss of bone, and possible failure of the implant. Because of the risk for morbidity resulting from infections, antimicrobial therapy is an essential component of the surgical protocol. Although adverse effects are associated with antibiotic therapy, these are usually mild and infrequent. The most common antimicrobials used in implant dentistry today consist of antibiotics (local and systemic) and antimicrobial rinses (0.12% chlorhexidine gluconate).

Antibiotics

The use and understanding of the various antibiotic regimens available in implant dentistry are beneficial for the initial success and long-term maintenance of implant therapy. Antibiotic therapy in implant dentistry may be classified as either prophylactic (prevent infection) or therapeutic (treat infection). The field of dentistry has been shown to prescribe a considerable amount of antibiotics administered in the United States (7%–11%).[1]

Prophylactic Antibiotics

In general surgery, including its subspecialties, principles of antibiotic prophylaxis are well established. Guidelines are specifically related to the procedure, the type of antibiotic, and the dosage regimen.[2,3] The use of prophylactic antibiotics in dentistry has also been documented in the prevention of complications for patients at risk for development of infectious endocarditis and immunocompromised patients. However, in oral implantology, there exists no consensus on the use and indications for prophylactic antibiotics. Disadvantages with the use of antibiotics include cost, development of resistant bacteria, adverse reactions, and possible resultant lax surgical technique.[4-6] As a result the need for prophylactic antibiotics in healthy patients, type of antibiotic, dosage, and duration of coverage is controversial. On the other hand, postoperative surgical wound infections can have a significant impact on the well-being of the patient and the survival of the implant or bone graft. Documented cases of potential consequences of infection range from increased pain and edema to even patient death. According to Esposito and Hirsch,[7] one of the main causes of dental implant failure is due to bacterial contamination at implant insertion.

A local inoculum must be present for a surgical wound infection to occur, to overcome the host's defenses and allow growth of the bacteria. This process has many variables, including various host, local tissue, systemic and microbial virulence factors. Antibiotic prophylaxis is only one component of this complex cascade; however, the efficacy and impact of antimicrobial prophylaxis has been proven to be significant.[4]

Several studies have concluded there is a benefit of preoperative antibiotics for dental implantology.[8-10] In the most comprehensive and controlled study to date, 33 hospitals formed the Dental Implant Clinical Research Group and concluded the use of preoperative antibiotics significantly improved dental implant survival, both in early and later stages. In the evaluation of 2973 implants, a significant difference was found with the use of preoperative antibiotics (4.6% failure) compared with no antibiotics (10% failure).[8,9]

The main goal of the use of prophylactic antibiotics is to prevent infection during the initial healing period from the surgical wound site, thus decreasing the risk for infectious complications of the soft and hard tissues. Although there is no conclusive evidence on the mechanism of preoperative antibiotics, most likely a greater aseptic local environment is achieved. A landmark study by Burke[11] defined the scientific basis for the perioperative use of antibiotics to prevent surgical wound infection. From this work, several accepted principles have been established in the perioperative use of prophylactic antibiotics.[12]

Principle 1: The Procedure Should Have a Significant Risk for and Incidence of Postoperative Infection. To evaluate the risk for postoperative wound infection, the American College of Surgeons (Committee on Control of Surgical Wound Infections) developed a classification of operative wounds and risk for infection. All surgical procedures were classified according to four levels of contamination and infection rates (Box 14.1). Within these classifications, it is generally accepted that all class 2, 3, and 4 procedures warrant the use of prophylactic antibiotics.[13] By definition, elective dental implant surgery falls within the class 2 (clean-contaminated) category. Class 2 medical and dental surgical procedures have been shown to have an infection rate of approximately 10% to 15%. However, with proper surgical technique and prophylactic antibiotics, the incidence rate of infection may be reduced to less than 1%.[14,15] In a healthy patient, risk for infection after dental implant surgery is influenced by numerous factors, such as type and location of surgery, skill of the surgeon, methods of intraoperative management, patient factors, and aseptic technique.[14,16] Moreover, additional patient-related (systemic and local) risk factors that are not addressed in these classifications have also been correlated with increased susceptibility to infection. These factors must be addressed in reference to evaluation for the use and duration of antibiotic prophylaxis (Box 14.2).

One of the most significant surgical factors that may contribute to infection is poor aseptic technique. Various routes of transmission of virulent bacteria include: (1) direct contact with the patient's blood or other body fluids; (2) indirect contact with contaminated objects; (3) contact of infected nasal, sinus, or oral mucosa; and (4) inhalation of airborne microorganisms. To prevent these conditions, a controlled, well-monitored aseptic setting should be achieved for the surgical procedures that are at high risk of infection. The aseptic surgical site includes proper disinfection and draping procedures of the patient, hand scrubbing, sterile gowns worn by all surgical members, and maintenance of complete sterility of the instrumentation.

Another important surgical factor related to postoperative infection is the duration of the surgical procedure. This factor has been shown to be the second most critical risk factor (after wound contamination) affecting postoperative infection rates.[17] In general, surgical operations lasting less than 1 hour have an infection rate of 1.3%, whereas those lasting 3 hours increase the rate to more than 4%.[18-20] It is postulated that the rate of infection doubles with every hour of the procedure.[21] The skill and the experience of the surgeon with the placement of implants has been shown to be significant in postoperative infections and implant failures. A recent study has shown that less-experienced surgeons (<50 implants placed) have a 7.3% increase in failure rates in comparison with experienced surgeons.[9]

In the medical literature it is well documented that the insertion of any prosthetic implant or device increases the chance of infection at the surgical site. A dental implant can act as a foreign body, and the host's defenses may therefore be compromised. The surface of the implant has been shown to facilitate bacterial adherence, and the presence of an implant can compromise the host's defenses. This may result in normal flora with low virulence potential to cause infections at the implant-host interface, which has been shown to be very difficult to treat.[22-24]

The probability of risk for infection for a given procedure is related to local, systemic, and surgical factors. The patient's American Society of Anesthesiologists (ASA) score may be used as the systemic factor and then correlated with various local and surgical factors. A risk index may then be modified from the literature to correlate these factors to dental implant surgeries (Table 14.1). The probability of wound infection may then be correlated with the type of wound contamination (class 1–4) and the risk index. Therefore a class 2 wound with a risk index 2 has a greater risk for complications, and a class 1 wound with risk index 0 has the least risk for postoperative infection.[18,25]

TABLE 14.1 Probability of Wound Infection by Type of Wound, Risk Index, and American Society of Anesthesiologists Status

Operation Classification	RISK INDEX		
	0	1	2
Clean	1.0%	2.3%	5.4%
Clean-contaminated	2.1%	4.0%	9.5%

Risk index classification: 0: ASA 1 or ASA 2, and no local or surgical factors; 1: ASA ≥2, at least one of the local or surgical factors is present; 2: ASA ≥2, both local and surgical factors are present.

ASA, American Society of Anesthesiologists.

Data are from Cruse PJ, Foord R. A 5-year prospective study of 23,649 surgical wounds. *Arch Surg.* 1973;107:206-210.

• BOX 14.3 Microorganisms Most Commonly Associated with Peri-implant Complications

- *Staphylococcus* spp.
- *Actinomyces* spp.
- Surface translocating bacteria
- *Wolinella* spp.
- *Capnocytophaga* spp.
- *Fusobacterium* spp.
- *Entamoeba gingivalis*
- Motile rods
- Fusiforms
- Spirochetes
- Enteric gram-negative bacteria
- *Candida albicans*

Principle 2: The Appropriate Antibiotic for the Surgical Procedure Must Be Selected. The prophylactic antibiotic should be effective against the bacteria that are most likely to cause an infection. In the majority of cases, infections after surgery are from organisms that originate from the site of surgery.[12] Most postoperative infections are caused by endogenous bacteria, including aerobic gram-positive cocci (streptococci), anaerobic gram-positive cocci (peptococci), and anaerobic gram-negative rods (bacteroides)[14] (Box 14.3).

Although oral infections are usually mixed infections in which anaerobes outnumber aerobes 2:1, it has been shown that anaerobes need the aerobes to provide an environment to proliferate.[26] Subsequent studies have shown that the early phase of intraoral infections involves streptococci that prepare the environment for subsequent anaerobic invasion.[27,28] With that in mind, the ideal antibiotic must be effective against these pathogens.

The second factor in selecting the correct antibiotic is to use the antibiotic with the least amount of adverse effects. These effects may vary from mild nausea to the extreme allergic reaction.

The final selection factor is that the antibiotic should ideally be bactericidal. The goal of antibiotic prophylaxis is to kill and destroy the bacteria. Bacteriostatic antibiotics work by inhibiting growth and reproduction of bacteria, thus allowing the host defenses to eliminate the resultant bacteria. However, if the host's defenses are compromised in any way, the bacteria and infection may flourish. Bactericidal antibiotics are advantageous over bacteriostatic antibiotics in that: (1) there is less reliance on host resistance, (2) the bacteria may be destroyed by the antibiotic alone, (3) results are faster than with bacteriostatic medications, and (4) there is greater flexibility with dosage intervals.[14]

Principle 3: An Appropriate Tissue Concentration of the Antibiotic Must Be Present at the Time of Surgery. For an antibiotic to be effective, a sufficient tissue concentration must be present at the time of bacterial invasion. To accomplish this goal, the antibiotic should be given in a dose that will reach plasma levels that are three to four times the minimum inhibitory concentration of the expected bacteria.[29] The minimum inhibitory concentration is defined as the lowest antibiotic concentration to destroy the specific bacteria. Usually the antibiotic must be given at twice the therapeutic dose and at least 1 hour before surgery to achieve this cellular level.[16] It has been shown that normal therapeutic blood levels are ineffective to counteract bacterial invasion. If antibiotic administration occurs after bacterial contamination, no preventive influence has been seen compared with taking no preoperative antibiotic.

Principle 4: Use of the Shortest Effective Antibiotic. In a healthy patient, continuing antibiotics after surgery often does not decrease the incidence of surgical wound infections.[3,30,31] Therefore, depending on the procedure and infection risk, in some patients a single dose of antibiotics is usually sufficient. However, for patients or procedures with increased risk factors (see Box 14.2), a longer dose of antibiotics is warranted.[12] With the high degree of morbidity associated with dental implant infections, one must weigh the benefits versus risk involved for the extended use of antibiotics.

Complications of Antibiotic Prophylaxis

With the use of prophylactic antibiotics for dental implant procedures, many side effects may develop. It is estimated that approximately 6% to 7% of patients who are taking antibiotics will have some type of adverse event.[32] Incidence of significant complications with the use of prophylactic antibiotics are minimal; however, a small percentage can be life-threatening. The risks associated with antibiotics include gastrointestinal (GI) tract complications, colonization of resistant or fungal strains, cross-reactions with other medications, and allergic reactions.

Allergic reactions have a wide range of complications, ranging from mild urticaria to an anaphylaxis and death. Studies have shown that 1% to 3% of the population receiving penicillin will exhibit the urticaria type of reactions, with 0.04% to 0.011% having true anaphylactic episodes. Of this small percentage of anaphylactic reactions, 10% will be fatal.[33]

An unusual but increasing complication in the general population after antibiotic use is pseudomembranous colitis (PMC). This condition is caused by the intestinal flora being altered and colonized by *Clostridium difficile.* Penicillin and clindamycin use have been significantly associated with PMC; however, all antibiotics have been shown as potential causative agents. The risk levels of colitis related to antibiotics are outlined in Table 14.2. The most common treatment for antibiotic-induced colitis is vancomycin or metronidazole.

The most recent concern of antibiotic use is the development of resistant bacteria. It has been observed that the overgrowth of resistant bacteria begins only after the host's susceptible bacteria are killed, which usually takes at least 3 days of antibiotic use. Therefore short-term (1 day) use of antibiotics has been shown to have little influence on the growth of resistant bacteria.[14]

TABLE 14.2	Risks for Antibiotic-Induced Pseudomembranous Colitis	
High	**Medium**	**Low**
• Ampicillin	• Penicillin	• Tetracyclines
• Amoxicillin	• Erythromycin	• Metronidazole
• Cephalosporin	• Quinolones	• Vancomycin
• Clindamycin		

Antibiotics Used in Implant Dentistry

Beta-Lactam Antibiotics. The most common beta-lactam antibiotics used in implant dentistry are the penicillins and cephalosporins. These antibiotics have similar chemical structures, and the mechanism of action is by inhibiting bacterial cell wall synthesis (bacteriocidal) via the interruption of the cross-linking between peptidoglycan molecules.

Penicillin V. Penicillin V is one of the more common antibiotics currently used in dentistry. It is well absorbed and will achieve peak serum levels within 30 minutes of administration with detectable blood levels for 4 hours. Penicillin V is effective against most *Streptococcus* species and oral anaerobes. The main disadvantages of penicillin are four times per day dosing and susceptibility to resistant bacteria.

Amoxicillin. Amoxicillin is a derivative of ampicillin, with the advantage of superior absorption and a bioavailability of 70% to 80% with a very low toxicity. It has excellent diffusion in infected tissues, and adequate tissue concentrations are easily achieved. Amoxicillin is considered broad spectrum and is effective against gram-negative cocci and gram-negative bacilli. This antibiotic also has greater activity than penicillin V against streptococci and oral anaerobes.

Amoxicillin/Clavulanic Acid (Augmentin). A combination of two antibiotics was synthesized to counteract the activity of beta-lactamase destruction of penicillins by resistant bacteria such as *Streptococcus aureus*. Clavulanic acid, a beta-lactam antibiotic, was added to amoxicillin to form Augmentin. This combination antibiotic has an affinity for penicillinase-producing bacteria. It functions as a "suicide molecule" that inactivates the resistant bacteria. As a result of an increase in the prevalence of these specific bacteria (especially in the sinus), Augmentin is becoming more popular in oral implantology. This antibiotic is used mainly in cases in which penicillinase bacteria are suspected (or known by culture) and is practical as a perioperative antibiotic for sinus augmentation procedures (Fig. 14.1 and Box 14.4).

Cephalosporins. The cephalosporin family is designated according to their generation (generations 1–5), with increasing generation equaling increasing spectrum activity. The first generation (cephalexin) has coverage similar to amoxicillin (i.e., gram-positive cocci with a limited activity against gram-negative pathogens). The second-generation cephalosporins have greater gram-negative pathogen and anaerobic coverage. Third-generation cephalosporins exhibit even greater gram-negative activity, with the fourth generation demonstrating efficacy against most gram-positive and -negative activity. Fifth-generation cephalosporins have activity against methicillin-resistant *Staphylococcus aureus*.

A disadvantage that is often discussed is the cross-reactivity with patients who are allergic to penicillin. They are often used in dentistry as an alternative for the patient who is allergic to penicillin, although cross-reactivity between these two drugs may

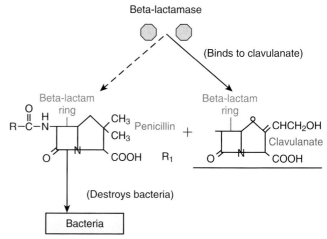

• **Fig. 14.1** Beta-lactamase inactivation by the addition of clavulanic acid to amoxicillin (Augmentin). Because of the high binding affinity of clavulanic acid, beta-lactamase will be inactivated, allowing penicillin to destroy the bacteria.

• BOX 14.4   Common Penicillin Antibiotics

Generic	Brand Name
Amoxicillin	Amoxil, Polymox, Trimox, Wymox
Ampicillin	Omnipen, Polycillin, Polycillin-N
Bacampicillin	Spectrobid
Carbenicillin	Geocillin, Geopen
Cloxacillin	Cloxapen
Dicloxacillin	Dynapen, Dycill, Pathocil
Flucloxacillin	Flopen, Floxapen, Staphcillin
Mezlocillin	Mezlin
Nafcillin	Nafcil, Nallpen, Unipen
Oxacillin	Bactocill, Prostaphlin
Penicillin G	Bicillin L-A
Penicillin V	Beepen-VK, Betapen-VK, V-Cillin K
Ticarcillin	Ticar

occur. Rates of cross-reactivity to first-generation cephalosporins with patients who are allergic to penicillin have been cited to be approximately 8% to 18%. The most recent gram-positive and -negative bacteria studies have shown that only patients who have had type I (immunoglobulin E: immediate hypersensitivity reactions) should not be administered a cephalosporin. If the patient has a previous history of a reaction that was not immunoglobulin E mediated (types II, III, or IV, or idiopathic reactions), a first-generation cephalosporin may be administered. Newer second- and third-generation cephalosporins exhibit a broader spectrum, less cross-reactivity, and a greater resistance to beta-lactamase destruction (Box 14.5).[34]

Macrolides

For years the most common macrolide used in dentistry was erythromycin. It is active against most streptococci, staphylococci, and some anaerobes, and it is an alternative for patients who are allergic to penicillin. Erythromycin has the advantage of excellent absorption and, unlike many drugs, is affected by the presence of food. It is administered primarily by the oral route and has a relatively low toxicity. However, this antibiotic has a high incidence

---

• BOX 14.5 | Common Cephalosporin Antibiotics

Generic	Brand Name
First Generation	
• Cefadroxil (cefadroxyl)	Duricef, Ultracef
• Cefalexin (cephalexin)	Keflex, Keftab
• Cefalotin (cephalothin)	Keflin
• Cefapirin (cephapirin)	Cefadyl
• Cefazolin (cephazolin)	Ancef, Kefzol
Second Generation	
• Cefaclor	Ceclor, Ceclor-CD, Keflor
• Cefprozil (cefproxil)	Cefzil
• Cefuroxime	Ceftin, Kefurox
Third Generation	
• Cefdinir	Omnicef, Cefdiel
• Cefixime	Suprax
• Cefmenoxime	Cefmax
• Cefotaxime	Claforan
• Cefpodoxime	Vantin
• Ceftizoxime	Cefizox
• Cefoperazone	Cefobid
• Ceftazidime	Ceptaz, Fortum, Fortaz
Fourth Generation	
• Cefepime (parenteral)	Maxipime
• Cefpirome (parenteral)	Cefrom
Fifth Generation	
• Ceftobiprole (parenteral)	Zeftera
• Ceftaroline (parenteral)	Teflaro

• BOX 14.6 | Common Macrolides Antibiotics

Generic	Brand Name
• Azithromycin	Zithromax
• Erythromycin	
• Clarithromycin	Biaxin

---

of nausea and is bacteriostatic rather than bacteriocidal, and it is therefore not an ideal first-line choice for infections in the oral cavity.

Erythromycin has questionable use when a severe infection exists or when the patient is immunocompromised and requires bacteriocidal activity. Even more disturbing is its implication in numerous drug interactions, including its proclivity for elevating serum levels of digoxin, theophylline, and carbamazepine. Erythromycin has also been found to retard conversion of terfenadine (Seldane), a nonsedating antihistamine, to its active metabolite. As a result, elevated serum concentrations of the predrug may result and lead to cardiotoxicity, presenting a particular form of ventricular tachycardia called *torsades de pointes*.

Therefore two novel macrolides have shown to be advantageous over erythromycin (i.e., clarithromycin [Biaxin] and azithromycin [Zithromax]). Unlike other macrolides, they do not appear to inhibit hepatic cytochrome P450 isozymes, which account for most drug interactions inherent with erythromycin. Biaxin has been shown to produce less nausea and has better gram activity; Zithromax appears to be more effective against *Haemophilus influenzae* (Box 14.6).

Clindamycin

The use of clindamycin is popular for the treatment of dental infections primarily because of its activity against anaerobic bacteria. It also is active against aerobic bacteria, such as streptococci and staphylococci, and it has superior effects against Bacteroides fragilis. Clindamycin (Cleocin phosphate) is supplied as an aqueous

(300 mg/2 mL) solution that is sometimes used in the incorporation of graft material for sinus augmentation procedures. However, it is bacteriostatic in normal concentrations and has a rather high toxicity in larger concentrations. As a result the main disadvantage of clindamycin is the occurrence of diarrhea in 20% to 30% of patients treated. This antibiotic also has a higher incidence of antibiotic-associated PMC caused by *C. difficile* when administrated for extended periods. PMC has been reported to occur with most long-term antibiotics.

The toxicity of antibiotics related to PMC is elevated with ampicillin, amoxicillin, cephalosporin, and clindamycin. Penicillin, erythromycin, and quinolones are moderate risk, and the lowest occurrence is with tetracycline, metronidazole, and vancomycin. The latter group is often used even to treat PMC conditions.

The patient should be informed that if either diarrhea or abdominal cramping occurs during or shortly after antibiotic therapy, the drug should be discontinued and the physician should be notified. Antidiarrheal medications should be avoided in these cases because they hinder the fecal elimination of the pathogen. If it is necessary to continue management of the dental infection, consultation with the patient's physician is warranted.

Tetracyclines

Tetracycline is a bacteriostatic antibiotic that inhibits protein synthesis. Tetracycline has been available since the 1950s and has a wide spectrum of activity against streptococci, staphylococci, oral anaerobes, and gram-negative aerobic rods. Because this antibiotic has been so extensively used in the past, there exists a high degree of bacterial resistance. Tetracycline is an attractive adjunct for the treatment of gingival and periodontal disease with a high bioavailability in the gingival sulcus. For these reasons tetracyclines are primary agents for treating implant disease and infections around implant posts. Their efficacy for managing infrabony infections is questionable, considering their inactivity when chelated with calcium complexes. The disadvantages of this antibiotic include a high incidence of promoting *Candida* spp. infections, and it may be associated with photosensitivity reactions. Tetracycline has been shown to be advantageous in allowing for reosseointegration resulting from peri-implant disease. Case reports have shown that application of 50 mg/mL tetracycline for 5 minutes and then bone grafting resulted in bone growth fill in the peri-implant defects.[35]

Fluoroquinolones

Fluoroquinolones are bactericidal antibiotics and have a broad antibacterial spectrum, which may be used either orally or parenterally. Ciprofloxacin is one of the first-generation quinolones and is the prototype antibiotic for this antibiotic classification. Newer third-generation (Levaquin, Avelox) quinolones have been developed with great activity against resistant bacteria and anaerobic bacteria. However, the U.S. Food and Drug Administration has placed warnings on this antibiotic class because of the potential for disabling and potentially permanent side effects related to tendon damage. Therefore these antibiotics are no longer used to

• BOX 14.7 Common Fluoroquinolones Antibiotics

Generic	Brand Name
First Generation	
• Nalidixic acid	NegGam, Wintomylon
• Oxolinic acid	Uroxin
Second Generation	
• Ciprofloxacin	Cipro, Cipro XR, Ciprobay, Ciproxin
• Norfloxacin	Lexinor, Noroxin, Quinabic,
• Ofloxacin	Janacin
	Floxin, Oxaldin, Tarivid
Third Generation	
• Gatifloxacin	Tequin
• Levofloxacin	Levaquin
• Moxifloxacin	Avelox
• Temafloxacin	Omniflox
Fourth Generation	
• Trovafloxacin	Trovan

treat dental implant–related issues unless no other options exist. Physician consultation and approval are recommended in these situations (Box 14.7).

Metronidazole

Metronidazole is a bacteriocidal antibiotic that is most often used for anaerobic infections. Because metronidazole has no activity against aerobic bacteria, it is seldom used for mixed infections unless it is combined with another antibiotic. However, it may be combined with penicillin when managing severe infections. Patients should be cautioned against drinking alcoholic beverages while taking this medication, because disulfiram-like reactions have been reported. These consist of severe nausea and abdominal cramping caused by the formation of a toxic compound resembling formaldehyde. Metronidazole should not be prescribed for patients who are taking the oral anticoagulant warfarin (Coumadin).

The more common antibiotics and dosages used in oral implantology for prophylaxis, grafting and implant insertion, postoperative infection, and long-term complications are listed in Table 14.3

TABLE 14.3 Commonly Used Antibiotics in Oral Implantology

Generic Name	Brand Name	Bactericidal/Bacteriostatic	THERAPEUTIC Usual Adult Dosage	Maximum Adult Dosage	Prophylactic Dosages
Amoxicillin	Amoxil, Polymox, Trimox	Bactericidal	250–500 mg TID	4 g/day	SBE: 2 g 1 hr before; Surgical: 1 g 1 hr before
Amoxicillin/Clavulanic acid	Augmentin	Bactericidal	250–500 mg TID or 825 mg BID	4 g/day	Surgical: 825 mg
Cephalexin	Biocef, Cefanex, Keftab, Keflex	Bactericidal	250 mg QID or 500 mg BID	4 g/day	SBE: 2 g 1 hr before; Surgical: 1 g 1 hr before
Cefadroxil	Duricef, Ultracef	Bactericidal	500 mg BID	4 g/day	SBE: 2 g 1 hr before; Surgical: 1 g 1 hr before
Azithromycin	Zithromax	Bacteriostatic	500 mg immediately, 1000 mg/day	—	SBE: 500 mg 1 hr before
Clarithromycin	Biaxin	Bacteriostatic	250 mg	—	SBE: 500 mg 1 hr before
Erythromycin	E-mycin, E-tab	Bacteriostatic	250 mg QID	4 g/day	—
Tetracycline	Achromycin, Sumycin	Bacteriostatic	250 mg QID	4 g/day	—
Clindamycin hydrochloride	Cleocin HCl	Bacteriostatic	150–300 mg TID or QID	1.8 mg/day	SBE: 600 mg 1 hr before; Surgical: 600 mg 1 hr before
Metronidazole	Flagyl	Bactericidal	250 mg TID or QID	4 g/day	
Levofloxacin	Levaquin	Bactericidal	500 mg/day	500 mg/day	Surgical: 500 mg
Moxifloxacin	Avelox	Bactericidal	400 mg/day	400 mg/day	—
Trimethoprim/sulfa-methoxazole	Bactrim Septra	Bacteriostatic	160 mg (DS) BID 80 mg BID	—	—

DS, Double strength; SBE, subacute bacterial endocarditis.

Levofloxacin and Moxifloxacin: *Physician approval prior to prescribing.*

Prophylactic Antibiotics in Oral Implantology

Postoperative wound infections can have a significant effect on the success of dental implants and bone-grafting procedures. The occurrence of surgical host defenses allows an environment conducive to bacterial growth. This process is complex, with interactions of host, local, systemic and microbial virulence factors. Various measures attempt to minimize infection by modifying the host and local tissue factors. The use of antimicrobials has been shown to be significant in reducing postoperative infections and decreases failure rate in implant dentistry.[36-38]

The antibiotic chosen for prophylaxis should encompass the bacteria most known to be responsible for the type of infection related to the surgical procedure. Therefore the following antibiotics are suggested against pathogens known to cause postoperative surgical wound infections in bone grafting or implant surgery:

1. **Amoxicillin** is the usual drug of choice; however, if the patient is allergic to amoxicillin, use
2. **Cephalexin** (nonanaphylactic allergy to penicillin) or
3. **Clindamycin** (anaphylactic allergy to penicillin).

For sinus involvement procedures (e.g., sinus grafts) the following antibiotics are suggested:

1. **Augmentin**
2. **Ceftin** (if history of recent use of antibiotics [within 4 weeks]) or doxycycline

Therapeutic Use of Antibiotics: Postoperative Infections

Acute postoperative infections have been shown to most commonly occur on the third to fourth day after surgery. The most common microorganisms associated with peri-implant, postoperative complications have been previously listed in Box 14.3.

Local signs of infection are pain, inflammation, bleeding, and exudate at the site of surgery. Systemic signs include fever, headache, nausea, muscle aches, vomiting, and weakness. When surgical wound infections arise, a specific diagnosis is advantageous to treat the complication. When evaluating the various antibiotics that are possibly effective against the bacteria in question, a broad-spectrum beta-lactam antibiotic is most often the first-line medication. The duration of treatment should include antibiotic administration for 3 days beyond the occurrence of significant clinical improvement (i.e. usually the fourth day), and therefore for a minimum of 7 days.[39]

Therapeutic Antibiotics in Implant Dentistry

The recommended treatment for intraoral infections associated with grafting or implant therapy includes:

1. **Surgical drainage**
2. **Systemic antibiotics**:

    Amoxicillin (500 mg): two immediately, then one tablet three times daily for 1 week or if penicillin allergy exists

    Clindamycin (300 mg): two immediately, then one tablet three times daily for 1 week

    NOTE: If no improvement is seen after 4 days, a culture and sensitivity test may be obtained to select the antibiotic that is most effective against the responsible organisms.

3. **0.12% chlorhexidine gluconate rinse** (½ oz twice daily for 2 weeks)

Prescription: 0.12% chlorhexidine gluconate (16 oz)
1. Patient presurgical rinse: used in the aseptic protocol before surgery for reduction of bacterial load
2. Surface antiseptic: intraoral and extraoral scrub of patient, scrubbing of hands before gowns and gloves
3. Postsurgical rinse: rinse twice a day until incision line closure
4. Peri-implant maintenance on daily basis
5. Treatment of postoperative infections

Chlorhexidine

Another medication used for antimicrobial prophylaxis for implant surgery is the use of an oral rinse, 0.12% chlorhexidine digluconate (Peridex; Procter & Gamble, Cincinnati, OH). Chlorhexidine gluconate is a potent antibacterial that causes lysis by binding to bacterial cell membranes. It has high substantivity that allows it, at high concentrations, to exhibit bacteriocidal qualities by causing bacterial cytoplasm precipitation and cell death.[40,41] In the oral cavity, chlorhexidine has been shown to have a slow release from tissue surfaces over a 12-hour period.[42,43]

In vitro studies have shown an inhibitory effect of chlorhexidine on cultured epithelium and cell growth; however, clinical studies have not shown this effect.[44-46] To the contrary, the use of chlorhexidine has been shown to be an effective adjuvant in reducing plaque accumulation, enhancing mucosal health,[46-48] improving soft tissue healing,[49,50] treating periodontal disease, preventing alveolar osteitis,[51,52] improving tissue healing after extractions,[53] and reversing peri-implantitis,[54] and has been shown to have no adverse effect on implant surfaces.[55]

When evaluating the effect of preoperative chlorhexidine before dental implant surgery, a significant reduction in the number of infectious complications (2 to 1) and a sixfold difference in implant failures in comparison with no use of chlorhexidine have been shown.[56]

Use of Chlorhexidine in Oral Implantology

As a consequence of many reported benefits of chlorhexidine, this antiseptic has been advocated for many uses in oral implantology (Box 14.8).

Miscellaneous

Citric Acid

Citric acid has been reported in the literature for the detoxification of exposed implant surfaces resulting from bone loss. Citric acid is stated to remove the smear layer, lipopolysaccharides, and exposure of collagen fibrils. The detoxification results in the improvement of the blood clot formation with a greater fibrin retention fibrin.[57,58] Numerous articles have evaluated the in vitro and in vivo effectiveness of citric acid; however, there is no agreement on the ideal concentration and duration for application. In a rhesus monkey study, implants were decontaminated with citric acid with a 40% concentration and developing reosseointegration 40 months after surgery.[59] In most detoxification protocols, citric acid is used in different concentrations (10%, 20%, or 40%) with a cotton pellet to burnish the exposed surfaces (Fig. 14.2).

Management of Postoperative Inflammation

The management of postsurgical swelling is crucial to pain management, control of edema, and incidence of postoperative

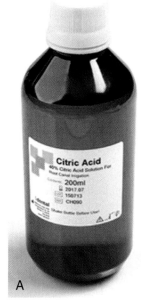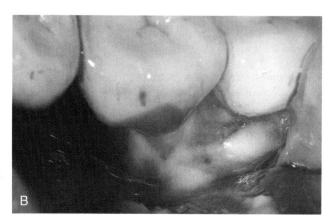

• **Fig. 14.2** Citric Acid. (A) 40% citric acid solution. (B) Citric acid is used to detoxify implant surface before bone grafting in the treatment of peri-implantitis.

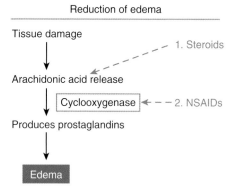

• **Fig. 14.3** Mechanism of action for nonsteroidal antiinflammatory drugs (NSAIDs) and steroids in the reduction of inflammation.

infection. In most dental implant surgeries, tissue is traumatized, which results in some degree of an inflammatory reaction. By controlling the extent of inflammation associated with surgical procedures, edema, trismus, pain, and infection may be reduced.

The mediators of the inflammatory process include cyclooxygenase (COX) and prostaglandins, which play a significant role in the development of postoperative inflammation and pain (Fig. 14.3). When tissue manipulation or damage occurs, phospholipids are converted into arachidonic acid by way of phospholipase A_2. Arachidonic acid, which is an amino acid, is released into the tissue, which produces prostaglandins by enzymatic breakdown by COXs. The end result is the formation of leukotrienes, prostacyclins, prostaglandins, and thromboxane A_2, which are the mediators for inflammation and pain. For postoperative treatment, medications such as ibuprofen (nonsteroidal antiinflammatory drugs [NSAIDs]) and glucocorticosteroids (steroids) are used, which play an integral part in counteracting the negative effects of this cascade.

Nonsteroidal Antiinflammatory Drugs

NSAIDs have an analgesic effect, as well as an antiinflammatory effect. This drug class reduces inflammation by inhibiting the synthesis of prostaglandins from arachidonic acid. Therefore the use of the popular analgesic drug ibuprofen has a secondary beneficial antiinflammatory effect. NSAIDs do not have a ceiling effect for inflammation; however, higher doses to achieve antiinflammatory qualities are accompanied by serious side effects. In implant dentistry the use of ibuprofen is suggested as a preemptive analgesic agent, because it has antiinflammatory properties in type 1 to 5 procedures.

Glucocorticosteroids

The adrenal cortex, which uses cholesterol as a substrate, synthesizes and secretes two types of steroid hormones—androgens and corticosteroids. The corticosteroids are classified by their actions: (1) glucocorticoids, which have effects on carbohydrate metabolism and have potent antiinflammatory actions; and (2) mineralocorticoids, which have sodium-retaining qualities. The use of synthetic glucocorticosteroids has become popular in the postoperative management of pain and inflammation after oral surgical procedures. These synthetic glucocorticoids have greater antiinflammatory potency in comparison with natural steroids with very little sodium and water retention. Most of these steroids have similar chemical structures; however, they differ in their milligram potency.[60] Their antiinflammatory effects are achieved by altering the connective tissue response to injury, thus causing a decrease in hyperemia, which results in less exudation and cellular migration, along with infiltration at the site of injury.[61,62]

A wide range of glucocorticoid preparations are available for local, oral, and parenteral administration. In relation to the naturally occurring cortisol (hydrocortisone), synthetic glucocorticoids are longer acting and more potent. The main differences are based on the classification as short-acting (<12 hours),

TABLE 14.4	Synthetic Glucocorticoids		
Glucocorticoids	Antiinflammatory Potency	Equivalent Dose (mg)	Duration (hr)
Short-acting			
Hydrocortisone	1.0	20	<12
Cortisone	0.8	25	<12
Intermediate-acting			
Prednisone	4.0	5	24–36
Prednisolone	4.0	5	24–36
Long-acting			
Dexamethasone	25	0.75	>48

intermediate-acting (12–36 hours), and long-acting (>36 hours). A summary of the most common glucocorticosteroids is shown in Table 14.4.[60]

Mechanism of Action

Glucocorticoids bind to glucocorticoid receptors within cells and form a glucocorticoid-GR complex. This complex alters the synthesis of messenger RNA from the DNA molecule, thus affecting the production of different proteins. By suppressing the production of proteins that are involved in inflammation, glucocorticoids also activate lipocortins, which have been shown to inhibit the action of phospholipase A_2. Phospholipase A_2 is a key enzyme involved in the release of arachidonic acid from cell membranes.

Arachidonic acid is an omega-6 fatty acid that is incorporated into cell membranes. When a cell is damaged, arachidonic acid is released from cell membranes and is converted into inflammatory and pain prostaglandins by cyclooxygenase-2 (COX-2) enzymes. The release of arachidonic acid requires the activation of the enzyme phospholipase A_2. However, lipocortins, which cause the inhibition of phospholipase A_2, prevent the release of arachidonic acid, thereby reducing the amounts of inflammatory prostaglandins.

Adrenal Suppression

Glucocorticoids are essential for the body to adapt to stressful situations. Adrenal insufficiency may predispose a person to an inability to respond to stress. Adrenal suppression has been shown to occur after 7 to 10 days of steroid administration. In stressful situations, cardiovascular collapse may occur and, if not treated appropriately, may be life-threatening. Because most dental implant procedures maintain a high level of stress, the implant dentist must be able to assess the level of adrenal suppression on patients taking glucocorticoid replacement therapy.

Prolonged, long-term steroid therapy causing adrenal suppression is a well-known phenomenon. The amount of suppression is a function of both the duration of treatment and the dose administered. Studies have shown that short-term use of corticosteroids does not significantly affect the hypothalamus-pituitary-adrenal (HPA) axis, and normal levels of cortisol, which are initially suppressed, recover to normal levels after 7 days.[63] The conclusion is that the HPA axis, although altered by the initial dexamethasone therapy, is restored completely. In addition, the amount of surgical stress involved with oral surgical procedures appears to be of insufficient magnitude to overcome the HPA suppression of the negative feedback mechanism caused by the steroid administration. Therapeutic levels of steroid are present at a cellular level to prevent any manifestations of adrenal insufficiency.[64]

Timing

The use of synthetic steroids should be based on the production of the natural steroid cortisol (hydrocortisone) in the body. Normally, cortisol is produced from plasma cholesterol at a rate of 15 to 30 mg/day.[65] Under stressful situations (e.g., infection, illness, trauma), as much as 300 mg of cortisol can be secreted. Plasma concentrations of cortisol are several-fold higher in the morning compared with the afternoon. Studies have shown that a dose of dexamethasone given in the morning (8:00 a.m.) does not significantly alter the level of endogenous circulating cortisol. However, the same dose in the late afternoon (4:00 p.m.) can cause complete suppression of the HPA cycle.[66] This secretion rate is dictated by the pituitary-adrenal axis with a feedback-inhibition cycle.[67] Therefore administration of glucocorticoids should ideally be given in the early morning so that simulation of normal diurnal rhythm is achieved, thus minimizing the possibility of HPA suppression.[68]

Glucocorticoid Use in Implant Dentistry

Since the advent of glucocorticoids in 1942, these medications have been used clinically in two ways: (1) therapeutic treatments in various inflammatory diseases and autoimmune diseases, and (2) prophylactic treatment of inflammation and associated pain. They are still used for an array of autoimmune diseases. Glucocorticoids have been well documented in the dental literature as being advantageous in the prevention of postoperative complications after traumatic oral surgery,[69] intraoral sagittal osteotomy,[70] vestibuloplasty with palatal mucosal grafts, and reduction of edema and pain after oral surgical procedures.[61,62,71,72] In addition, they have been shown to be associated with less need of pain medication after oral surgical procedures.[73,74] These drugs have been shown to have the ability to be long-lasting in duration and cause minimal effects on wound healing, infection, and adrenal suppression, with minimal central nervous system (CNS) alteration.[66]

Antiinflammatory/Analgesic. The use of glucocorticoids is an integral part in the treatment of postsurgical edema after dental implant procedures. The selection of the ideal synthetic glucocorticoid for dental implant surgery should maintain high antiinflammatory potency with minimal mineralocorticoid effects. The glucocorticoid that best suits the requirements is the long-acting glucocorticoid dexamethasone (Decadron). It is imperative that this drug be administered before surgery so that adequate blood levels are obtained. Also, it should be given in the morning in conjunction with the natural release of cortisol. This timing will interfere the least with the adrenocortical system. Because inflammation usually peaks between 48 and 72 hours, the postoperative regimen of dexamethasone should not exceed 3 days after implant surgery unless a nerve impairment is present. The dose should not exceed the equivalence of 300 mg cortisol and with high doses, a decreasing dose the second and third day to reduce possible side effects. This high-dose, short-term glucocorticoid therapy has been shown not to significantly affect the HPA axis.[64,75,76] Studies evaluating the efficacy of dexamethasone have shown positive results with preventing and controlling postoperative pain and discomfort after implant placement surgery (Box 14.9).[77]

Prescription:

- Dexamethasone (Decadron Tablets 0.5 mg, 0.75 mg, 4 mg, and 6 mg)
- Dexamethasone Injectable (4 mg/mL—30-mL vial)
1. Antiinflammatory/Analgesic: administer 4 mg according to pharmacologic protocol
2. Neurosensory impairment: 8 mg for days 1–3, 4 mg for days 4–6

NOTE: Also may use injectable form to be placed locally at site of nerve injury (1–2 mL of 4 mg/mL)

3. Postoperative nausea and vomiting: 8 mg to be administered in two 4 mg doses intravenously

^aMethylprednisolone (Medrol) is an alternative to dexamethasone but has significantly less antiinflammatory potency.

Neurosensory Impairment. The use of dexamethasone has been shown to decrease the morbidity of neurosensory impairments. Not only does dexamethasone reduce the inflammation at the site of nerve injury, it has been shown to improve the regeneration of severed and compressed inferior alveolar nerves.[78]

Postoperative Nausea and Vomiting. A significant additional benefit of the administration of dexamethasone is the potent antiemetic effects for the prophylactic treatment of postoperative nausea and vomiting. This is now an accepted medication for hospital-based outpatient surgery, usually given in doses of 8 to 10 mg intravenously.[79-81] When using intravenous (conscious) sedation for dental implant procedures, it is highly effective in reducing pain and inflammation, along with preventing postoperative nausea and vomiting. Usually an 8-mg dose is recommended split into two administrations to reduce the possibility of perineal pain and itching.

Contraindication to Glucocorticosteroids

Contraindications to the use of corticosteroids include active infections (viral, bacterial, fungal), tuberculosis, ocular herpes simplex, primary glaucoma, acute psychosis, and diabetes mellitus. Special attention must be given to patients with diabetes, because glucocorticoids have an antiinsulin action that results in increased serum glucose and glycosuria.[82] Dexamethasone has been reported to induce immunosuppression when prescribed for long periods, which could be a concern with implant therapy.[83] However, the recommended use in our pharmacologic protocol involves only short-term use, thus minimizing the risks for these unwanted complications.

Cryotherapy

An additional therapeutic regimen to help reduce the amount and duration of postoperative inflammation is the application of cold dressings. It is reported that cold dressings in the form of ice bags or premanufactured ice packs applied extraorally to the surgical site will minimize edema.[84] The application of cold dressings is believed to cause vasoconstriction of the capillary vessels, thus reducing the flow of blood and lymph in this region, resulting in less inflammation.[85] Also, with the lower temperature at the surgical site, cell metabolism is reduced. As a result the cells in the region of trauma consume less oxygen, which allows them to survive a longer period of ischemia. Localized hypothermia will induce vasoconstriction and lowers microcirculation by more than 60%, and these effects may last for up to 30 minutes after cessation. In addition, there exists a reduction in pain as a result of less edema as well as restoration of motor and sensory nerve conduction.[86]

Prescription: Ice Packs^a

1. Ice packs (cold dressings) should be applied extraorally over the surgical site for 20 minutes on/20 minutes off for first 24 to 36 hours.

^aCaution must be taken to limit the application of ice for no longer than 36 hours, because prolonged use may cause rebound swelling and cell destruction.

When applying ice to the surgical site, caution should be exercised to not cause a thermal necrosis of the tissue from too long of an application. Ideally cryotherapy should be applied for 20 minutes, followed by 20 minutes of rest. The rationale for this protocol includes possible vasodilation (reactive hyperemia) after the initial cryotherapy-induced vasoconstriction. The vasodilation is a compensatory reaction also termed a "hunting response," which results from the blood flow through the arteriovenous anastomoses.[87] Therefore to prevent the possibility of increased edema, the 20 minutes on/20 minutes off protocol is recommended (Box 14.10).

Postsurgical Pain Management

Pain has been documented to be inadequately treated in 50% of all surgical procedures.[88] These painful experiences predispose the patient to amplification of noxious stimuli (hyperalgesia) and cause typically painless sensations to be experienced as pain (allodynia).[89,90] Therefore patients who have had painful experiences may have increased pain and the need for additional analgesic use in future surgeries. The goal for pain control in oral implantology is to obtain analgesic levels before the cessation of local anesthesia and a well-administered postoperative analgesic regimen for patient comfort.

Mechanism of Pain

The mechanism of painful stimuli is modulated by the peripheral nervous system and CNS. Noxious stimuli (tissue damage) cause peripheral nociceptors to transmit signals along nerve fibers lying in the dorsal root ganglion. Their axons synapse in the dorsal horn of the spinal cord and then travel along the spinothalamic tract of the spinal cord to the thalamus and the cortex. Within the cortex and thalamus, the signals originating from tissue damage form the subjective interpretation of pain.

With repeated noxious stimuli, peripheral nociceptors become more responsive. The sensitivity to these receptors is further enhanced by tissue factors and inflammatory mediators released in the course of tissue damage. Numerous inflammatory mediators are present that include prostaglandins, kinins, leukotrienes, substance P, and histamine. These mediators initiate and magnify the nociceptive impulses that are transmitted to the CNS for the perception of pain.

The most important mediators, prostaglandins, are extremely important in sensitizing peripheral neurons to the local stimuli. Prostaglandins are also synthesized in the spinal cord and brain, and enhance pain sensitivity by recruiting secondary neurons to respond to the primary stimulus.[91]

One of most commonly used analgesics, NSAIDs, works at the site of tissue damage and the spinal cord and brain to prevent prostaglandin formation by inhibiting COX. COX is an enzyme

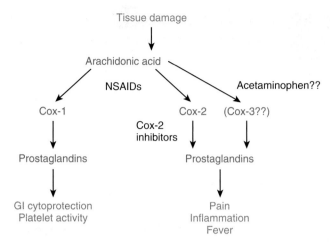

• **Fig. 14.4** Mechanism of action of the various cyclooxygenase enzymes. *COX*, Cyclooxygenase; *GI*, gastrointestinal; *NSAIDs*, nonsteroidal antiinflammatory drugs.

• **BOX 14.11** Analgesic Classifications in Dentistry

Nonopioids
- Nonsteroidal antiinflammatory drugs
- Acetaminophen
- Tramadol
- Cyclooxygenase-2 inhibitors

Opioids
- Codeine
- Hydrocodone
- Oxycodone
- Meperidine

Adjuvants
- Glucocorticoids
- Long-acting anesthetics
- Tricyclic antidepressants

TABLE 14.5 Common Analgesic Medications in Oral Implantology

Medication	Advantages	Disadvantages
NSAIDs Nonselective	Inexpensive Over the counter Excellent pain relief Excellent antiinflammatory effects	Many drug interactions Limited use in patients with gastrointestinal issues
Acetaminophen	Inexpensive Over the counter Good pain relief	No antiinflammatory effects
Opioids	Good to excellent pain relief	Addiction potential Drug interactions No antiinflammatory effects
Corticosteroids	Excellent antiinflammatory action	Use in patients with diabetes is restricted Alteration of the hypothalamus-pituitary-adrenal axis

NSAID, Nonsteroidal antiinflammatory drug.

that breaks down arachidonic acid to prostaglandin synthesis. In the tissue, two well-identified COXs exist, COX-1 and COX-2. COX-1 enzymes support hemostasis (platelet degranulation and adhesion), stomach mucosal integrity, and regulation of kidney function. COX-2 enzymes are an inducible form whose synthesis is activated in damaged tissue, which leads to the formation of proinflammatory prostaglandins that play a major role in inflammation, pain, and fever. A relatively new COX has been described (COX-3) that is found in the brain and is thought to be the site of action of acetaminophen.[92]

In contrast with NSAIDs, opioids have a different mechanism of action to reduce pain. Opioids act on the CNS by binding to specific receptors (μ-opioid), thus preventing transmission of nociceptive pathways, while also activating inhibitory pathways that descend to the spinal cord. By binding to these μ-opioid receptors, substance P is barred from being released, thus preventing painful stimuli.[93]

Protocols Postoperative Pain

In implant dentistry different classifications and mechanisms of pain suppression may be used. The most effective technique to decrease pain is a combination of preemptive analgesia and a multimodal pain management protocol. By using a multimodal therapy protocol, lower dosages of medication can be used, which results in fewer side effects and advantageous outcomes. Therefore the author has developed a pain control protocol that simplifies and standardizes the various aspects of pain relief (Fig. 14.4, Box 14.11, and Table 14.5).

Prophylactic Analgesics
1. Preemptive Analgesia

Postoperative Analgesics
1. Nonopioid Analgesics (Nonnarcotics)
2. Opioid Analgesics (Narcotics)
3. Adjuvants

Preemptive Analgesia

Preemptive analgesia is defined as the introduction of an analgesic regimen before the onset of noxious stimuli. In relation to dental implant surgery, it is advantageous to have adequate analgesic blood levels present before the initiation of surgery. The concept of preemptive analgesia is based on advances in evidence-based clinical research. It has recently been refined and evolved to a broader concept that surgical incision alone is not the trigger for central sensitization. The goal is to prevent sensitization of the nervous system to subsequent stimuli that could possibly amplify pain. Dental implant surgery is ideal for this type of treatment because it is usually elective, and the timing of noxious stimuli is known.

Manipulation of hard and soft tissues during implant and bone grafting procedures predisposes the patient to postoperative pain. The extent of tissue reflection, amount of bone preparation, inherent patient factors, and duration of the surgical procedure have an effect on the intensity and duration of postoperative pain. Hyperalgesia is characterized by enhanced sensations of pain, a pain threshold reduction, and an increase in the suprathreshold noxious stimuli. With administration of analgesics before tissue

---

• BOX 14.12   Preemptive Analgesics

Prescriptions

- Ibuprofen (400 mg)
- Acetaminophen (1000 mg)
- Celecoxib (200mg)

Given 1 hour before the procedure.

• BOX 14.13   Nonopioid Analgesics

Prescriptions

- Ibuprofen (400–600 mg): 400 mg every 4 hours; not to exceed 1200 mg/day
- Acetaminophen (500 mg): 1 g every 6 hours; not to exceed 4 g/day
- Celecoxib (50, 100, 200, 400 mg): 200 mg twice daily as needed
- Tramadol: 50–100 mg oral dose every 4–6 hours as needed; not to exceed 400 mg/day
- Ultram: 50 mg tramadol
- Ultracet: 37.5 mg tramadol/1000 mg acetaminophen
- Ultram ER: 100 mg tramadol–extended release once daily

TABLE 14.6	Relative Risks of Nonsteroidal Antiinflammatory Drugs for Gastrointestinal Complications	

NSAID	Relative Risk
None	1
Ibuprofen	2.1
Ketoprofen	3.2
Naproxen	4.3
Indomethacin	5.5
Aspirin	8–11
Ketorolac	24.7

NSAID, Nonsteroidal antiinflammatory drug.

---

damage, the sensitivity of these receptors is dramatically reduced and may be eliminated.[94] Many studies on the ideal medication to use for preemptive analgesia with ibuprofen (400 mg), acetaminophen (1000 mg), or celecoxib (200 mg) show positive results for the reduction of postoperative pain[95] (Box 14.12).

Postoperative Medications

Nonopioid Medications

The nonopioid analgesics used in implant dentistry include acetaminophen, NSAIDs, COX-2 inhibitors, and tramadol (Box 14.13).

Acetaminophen (Paracetamol). The mode of action of acetaminophen is not known; however, it is believed to involve the prostaglandin pathways within the CNS, with little influence on peripheral prostaglandin synthesis. The COX-3 enzyme has been described that is fully expressed in the brain, spinal cord, and heart. The primary function of this enzyme is to regulate pain responses and fever, and it has been postulated to be the site of action of acetaminophen.[96]

Acetaminophen is indicated for mild-to-moderate pain and is a safe alternative to NSAIDs. It has excellent analgesic and antipyretic properties, and is void of side effects that are associated with NSAIDs. Like NSAIDs, acetaminophen also has a ceiling dose (4 g/day) for analgesic effects. However, unlike NSAIDs, acetaminophen is limited in that it has minimal antiinflammatory qualities. The main side effect is liver damage, which is associated with long-term use of this drug.

Nonsteroidal Antiinflammatory Drugs. NSAIDs are one of the most commonly used analgesics in implant dentistry today. Clinical trials have shown that NSAIDs are effective in all levels of pain (mild, moderate, severe).[97,98] The mechanism of action of NSAIDs is thought to arise from the inhibition of the synthesis of prostaglandins from arachidonic acid. With the inhibition of COX, conversion of arachidonic acid to the immediate precursors of prostaglandins is prevented. Thus with the lack of prostaglandins in the tissue, the hyperanalgesia and edema associated with the acute inflammation are minimized.[99]

The main reasons that NSAIDs are so widely used is the fact that they work very well as analgesics and have variable effects on inflammation (drug and dose dependent). Inflammation and pain are two separate entities, with analgesic doses having a ceiling effect[100] and antiinflammatory doses not having a ceiling effect. In regard to the analgesic effect, there exists no reason to exceed the analgesic ceiling for the treatment of acute pain, because higher doses give no additional pain relief while increasing the likelihood of side effects.

There are two classes of NSAIDs: "nonselective" (e.g., ibuprofen) and "selective" (e.g., celecoxib). The COX enzyme is actually present in two different forms, COX-1 and COX-2. COX-1 enzymes protect the gastric mucosa from the acid that the stomach naturally produces and also is involved with platelet aggregation. COX-2 enzymes are responsible for producing prostaglandins that mediate pain and inflammation. The selective NSAIDs target only the COX-2 enzymes, which decrease pain and inflammation while maintaining the protective factors of the stomach, along with not interrupting platelet function. The side effects of NSAIDs are numerous, including GI disturbances (dyspepsia, erosions, ulcerations) and liver, renal, and cardiac effects.[101] This group of medications is responsible for the largest number of serious drug-related complications, surpassing all other drugs by a wide margin.[102] The various types of NSAIDs and their associated risks are listed in Table 14.6.[103] NSAIDs have very little effect on platelet aggregation because bleeding times are not prolonged. With prolonged use of NSAIDs, interference with most classes of antihypertensives has been noted. Therefore if patients take NSAIDs for more than 5 days postoperatively, blood pressure should be monitored. Although NSAIDs have numerous advantages, they may have a potential detrimental effect on bone metabolism. Numerous animal studies have been inconclusive. Some have shown that NSAIDs may impair angiogenesis and osteoblast/osteoclast precursor differentiation, especially in the first month after implant placement. However, other studies have shown no differences in long-term healing outcomes.[104]

Ibuprofen. Ibuprofen was first introduced in 1969 as a new NSAID and has since been the most popular prescribed NSAID.[105] Ibuprofen is a nonselective COX inhibitor because it inhibits two isoforms of COX, COX-1 and COX-2. It is available under a number of different trade names, including Advil and Motrin (200 mg). Ibuprofen is used to treat mild-to-moderate pain and has been proven to significantly reduce postoperative dental pain in clinical studies.[106,107] The analgesic ceiling dose is 400 mg/dose and 1200 mg/day[108]; at these doses it has been shown to be as safe as acetaminophen, while achieving better analgesia with less nausea and cramping.[109]

Aspirin. Acetylsalicylic acid was the first prototypical NSAID. It has analgesic, antiinflammatory, and antipyretic properties. However, at analgesic doses its relative risk for GI complications is high. Acetylsalicylic acid is not a drug of choice in the management of dental implant surgical patients because of its very significant antiplatelet effects.

COX-2 Inhibitors. An additional type of NSAID specifically targets the COX-2. Because this class of medications is selective for COX-2, the risk for GI side effects is reduced. These drugs do not block COX-1 enzymes, which produce prostaglandins that protect the stomach and promote blood clotting. Because COX-1 is not altered, the possibility of ulcers or increase in bleeding is reduced. Recently rofecoxib (Vioxx) and valdecoxib (Bextra) have been taken off the market because of a possible increase in heart attacks and strokes. Currently celecoxib (Celebrex) 200 mg is available in the United States.

Acetaminophen + Nonsteroidal Antiinflammatory Drugs (Ibuprofen). Prescribing acetaminophen and NSAIDs together has become popular in clinical practice with positive results.[110] Although NSAIDs have few regulatory restrictions, many significant adverse effects may be present at high doses or with longer courses of treatment. Acetaminophen is safe and widely accepted; however, it has minimal pain relief by itself. Combining an NSAID and acetaminophen allows for the benefits of both medications without increasing dose or risk. Typically acetaminophen is given in a dosage regimen of 1 g every 6 hours, and ibuprofen in a dosage of 400 mg every 8 hours. This dosage regimen is advantageous because asynchronous dosing has been shown to be less effective.[111]

Tramadol. Tramadol represents a unique classification of analgesic because it is a synthetic analog of codeine; however, it has a reduced affinity for opioid receptors while having an action on 5-hydroxytryptamine-noradrenaline reuptake inhibitors. Therefore it is a centrally acting analgesic with two complementary characteristics: opioid and antidepressant. It works by inhibition of norepinephrine and serotonin reuptake within pain pathways of the CNS and also by its relative weak affinity for the μ-opioid receptor.[109] Tramadol is a nonscheduled drug and is associated with fewer opioid-like side effects, such as dependence, sedation, respiratory depression, and constipation.[112,113] The analgesic efficacy of tramadol is similar to codeine (60 mg) and is indicated for moderate to moderately severe pain management. This drug is an appropriate analgesic alternative for the treatment of postoperative pain in patients who have NSAID-related GI and opioid intolerance. Tramadol has been shown to be effective in the reduction of pain when used in combination with acetaminophen. Ultracet (tramadol/acetaminophen) has demonstrated excellent efficacy in pain studies and is supplied as a combination analgesic containing 37.5 mg tramadol and 325 mg acetaminophen.[114,115]

Narcotics (Opioids)

Narcotics (opioids) are the primary medications for analgesia of moderate-to-severe pain from dental origin. They are centrally acting analgesics that act as agonists at μ- and κ-opioid receptors. Morphine, which is a naturally occurring opioid, is generally accepted as the prototypical narcotic. All other narcotics are compared in potency to morphine.

Unlike nonopioids, opioids do not have a ceiling effect for analgesia. As the dose increases, the analgesic effect increases. However, in addition to relieving pain by μ-receptor binding, euphoria, nausea, vomiting, and constipation may occur. With

high doses, sedation and respiratory depression are possible. With chronic use, physical and psychological dependence are common.

The following section discusses the most commonly used narcotics in oral implantology. Structurally these narcotics are similar to morphine and provide the same degree of pain relief and unlimited efficacy at equipotent doses.

Codeine. Codeine is a naturally occurring alkaloid that is classified as a mild analgesic. Codeine has excellent antitussive properties; however, it is associated with high degrees of nausea and constipation. Orally administered codeine is only 60% bioavailable, which results in only 10% being demethylated to morphine. This 10% is the only part responsible for analgesic properties, thus allowing 90% to have no analgesic efficacy. Because of the side effects and low potency compared with other opioids, codeine is usually not the first choice of narcotics used in oral implantology.

Hydrocodone. Hydrocodone bitartrate is a semisynthetic narcotic analgesic and antitussive with multiple actions qualitatively similar to codeine. It is usually used as a combination analgesic, being combined with either acetaminophen or ibuprofen. For several years this narcotic has been the most frequently dispensed prescription medication in the United States. Hydrocodone is habit forming, and the most frequent adverse reactions are dizziness, sedation, nausea, and vomiting.

Oxycodone. Oxycodone is a semisynthetic opioid with analgesic action similar to morphine. It is recommended for moderate-to-severe pain, with its principal actions being analgesia and sedation. It has excellent oral bioavailability because it retains half of its analgesic activity when administered orally. Oxycodone has the same adverse effects as most other opioids, with an increased potential for abuse and drug dependence. Oxycodone is marketed as a combination narcotic, combined with either acetaminophen (Percocet) or aspirin (Percodan). A slow-release oxycodone (Oxycontin) has recently been released, which has a high abuse potential.

Meperidine. Meperidine is mostly used in hospital settings via intramuscular administration. A majority of meperidine is converted to normeperidine, which is a metabolite that has no analgesic property; however, it is a strong CNS stimulant. Because meperidine in oral form has a poor oral bioavailability (25%), a greater risk evolves with the accumulation of normeperidine. As a result, meperidine is a poor choice for an orally administered opioid.

Combination Analgesic Therapy for Postoperative Pain

A pain management strategy using multiple analgesics with different mechanisms of action is termed *combination analgesic therapy*. The goal of combining different types of analgesics is to increase the analgesic effect while decreasing possible side effects. When multiple drugs are used in combination, synergistic and additive effects allow for the use of lower doses of each individual drug.

With combination therapy, acetaminophen or NSAIDs are used with an opioid. Because of the ceiling effects of acetaminophen and NSAIDs, further increases in dosage will not provide any additional analgesia; however, they will increase side effects (Table 14.7).

Analgesic Agents in Oral Implantology

The selection of an analgesic or analgesic regimen for management of postsurgical pain is ideally related to the expected pain intensity. This may be based on the patient's medical history, past pain threshold, type of procedure, extent of tissue reflection, and

TABLE 14.7	Combination Analgesics		
Generic Name	Brand Name	Average Adult Dosage	Schedule
5 mg codeine/300 mg acetaminophen	Tylenol #1	1–2 tablets every 4 hr	III
15 mg codeine/300 mg acetaminophen	Tylenol #2	1–2 tablets every 4 hr	III
30 mg codeine/300 mg acetaminophen	Tylenol #3	1–2 tablets every 4 hr	III
60 mg codeine/300 mg acetaminophen	Tylenol #4	1 tablet every 4 hr	III
5 mg hydrocodone/500 mg acetaminophen	Vicodin/Lortab 5/500	1–2 tablets every 4–6 hr (maximum: 8 tablets/24 hr)	III
7.5 mg hydrocodone/750 mg acetaminophen	Vicodin ES	1 tablet every 4–6 hr	III
7.5 mg hydrocodone/650 mg acetaminophen	Lorcet	1 tablet every 4–6 hr	III
10 mg hydrocodone/660 mg acetaminophen	Vicodin	1 tablet every 4–6 hr	III
10 mg hydrocodone/650 mg acetaminophen	Lorcet 10/650	1 tablet every 4–6 hr	III
7.5 mg hydrocodone/200 mg ibuprofen	Vicoprofen	1–2 tablets every 6 hr	III
5 mg oxycodone/325 mg acetaminophen	Percocet 5/325	1–2 tablets every 4–6 hr	II
7.5 mg oxycodone/500 mg acetaminophen	Percocet 7.5/500	1–2 tablets every 4–6 hr (maximum: 8 per day)	II
10 mg oxycodone/650 mg acetaminophen	Percocet 10/650	1 tablet every 4–6 hr	II
5 mg oxycodone/400 mg ibuprofen	Combunox	1 tablet every 6 hr (maximum: 4 per day)	II

duration of procedure. Because of the various agents and numerous options for the treatment of postsurgical pain after dental implant surgery, a pain control protocol was formulated to aid in the proper administration of these agents. According to the World Health Organization guidelines, the procedure and patient must be evaluated and classified as mild, moderate, or severe.

Mild Pain

Mild pain is self-limited and usually will be resolved with regular recommended doses of NSAIDs.

Moderate Pain

Moderate pain involves more intense pain than mild and usually will not be resolved totally by NSAIDs. The expected pain will interfere with function and disrupt the activities of daily living.

Severe Pain

Severe pain is defined as pain that interferes with some or all of the activities of daily living. The patient may be confined to bed, and strong opioid treatment will need to be continued for days. Adjuvant drug therapies may be needed for supplementation.

Control of Postoperative Surgical Pain

Currently in the United States an alarming increase in prescription opioid deaths has been reported. A source of a substantial number of opioids are from leftover postoperative medications that are later shared among friends and family members. Among health care providers who prescribe opioids, dentists have been shown to be the most prevalent providers of these medications.[116] Therefore the dental profession has an obligation to counsel patients on the misuse of opioids and to use caution in the prescribing practices of opioids.

The implant dentist is placed in a challenging position with respect to the management of postoperative pain. Many of the procedures performed are rather invasive, which may lead to

intense pain postoperatively. Identifying patients who may be susceptible to poor pain management or uncontrolled acute pain is difficult. Therefore it is advantageous for implant clinicians to be able to assess patients and propose pain management plans that will minimize the risk and maximize inherent benefits. Thus good practice involves a comprehensive initial assessment, individualized pain management strategy, and reassessment if necessary.

The goal of postsurgical pain management is to optimize patient comfort through pharmacologic and behavioral strategies. The World Health Organization formulated an analgesic "ladder" for the treatment of pain management. The following protocol describes three steps in the treatment of acute pain (Box 14.14)[103]:

1. The first step is to maximize the use of NSAIDs (acetaminophen, ibuprofen) for mild-to-moderate pain.
2. When moderate pain is expected or persists, an opioid (hydrocodone, codeine) should be added to the NSAID. The fixed dose of opioids with the NSAIDs provides additive analgesia. Adjuvant medications such as glucocorticoids and cryotherapy are often suggested.
3. Moderate-to-severe pain that is expected or persists should be treated by increasing the dosage of the opioid. Adjuvant medications such as glucocorticoids and cryotherapy are often suggested.

With the guidelines from the World Health Organization, a pain control protocol was formulated for treatment of procedures based on the expected postoperative pain.

Pain Control Protocol

Preoperative Evaluation

1. A thorough evaluation that includes a comprehensive medical and dental history: This should include screening for past or current use of opioids, benzodiazepines, sedative-hypnotics, antidepressants, or anxiolytics.

2. Access and check the Prescription Monitoring Program for the past and current use of the earlier drug categories. This information can be compared with the patient's medical and dental history, along with determining the extent of a patient's history of chronic opioid or sedative medications. In some cases a physician consultation and clearance may be recommended.

Development of a Pain Control Protocol

After obtaining this information, the following prescribing protocol may be followed:

Step 1: Preemptive analgesics—the use of ibuprofen (400 mg), acetaminophen (1000 mg), or celecoxib (200 mg)—should be taken 1 hour before the procedure.

Step 2: Nonopioid analgesics should be used as the first line of pain control.
   a. NSAIDs are ideally used because they exhibit great pain control together with antiinflammatory effects. Avoid NSAIDs if there exists a known hypersensitivity, GI bleeding, or history of aspirin allergy. For patients at risk for bleeding, a selective COX–2 inhibitor (e.g., celecoxib) may be considered.
   b. If an increased analgesic effect is required, the combination of an NSAID with acetaminophen may be used. Avoid acetaminophen if there is a history of liver disease or hypersensitivity to the medication.
   c. Adjuvant multimodal pain strategies should be integrated into the management of acute postoperative pain (e.g., cryotherapy, long-acting anesthetics, glucocorticosteroids).

Step 3: If an opioid is warranted, the following protocols should be adhered to:
   a. The lowest effective opioid dose of immediate-release opioids should be prescribed.

   b. Quantity should be proportional to the expected duration of pain; usually this will cover 3 days, and a quantity exceeding 7 days is rare.
   c. Obtain medical clearance before prescribing opioid medication to any patient with a history of chronic use.

Local Anesthetics

Local anesthetics are an integral component of all dental implant surgical procedures. They are necessary to perform surgery without pain and are effective for decreasing onset and duration of pain. The dental surgeon must have significant knowledge of the pharmacokinetics of the different local anesthetics used in implant dentistry. The most commonly used dental anesthetics are amides, which are known for their low toxicity and relative lack of allergenicity.

Local anesthetics prevent postoperative pain by blocking the generation and conduction of action potentials in sensory neurons. This will prevent surgically induced nociceptive impulses from reaching the CNS and causing centrally mediated postoperative hyperalgesia. Table 14.8 provides local anesthetic dosage information.

Lidocaine

The compound with which most other local anesthetics are compared is 2% lidocaine-1/100,000 epinephrine. This solution is most commonly used in infiltration or block anesthesia, and is considered a medium-duration anesthetic. Lidocaine is supplied in two other forms: a higher-concentration vasoconstrictor (1/50,000 epinephrine) and with no vasoconstrictor (plain).

Mepivacaine

Mepivacaine is an anesthetic that is very similar to lidocaine in onset of action, duration, and toxicity. The usual dosage used in dentistry is a 2% solution with the addition of 1/20,000 levonordefrin (Neo-Cobefrin) as the vasoconstrictor. This local anesthetic is also made in a 3% (plain) solution, which is used for short procedures or when a vasoconstrictor is contraindicated.

Articaine

Articaine is a newer amide type of anesthetic that was approved in 2000 by the U.S. Food and Drug Administration for use in the United States. Articaine differs structurally from other amide anesthetics, allowing it to have a better lipid solubility, which improves permeability of the lipid barriers in nerve membranes. Articaine

• BOX 14.14 World Health Organization Analgesic Ladder

Three-Step Conceptual Model
1. Nonopioid + adjuvant
2. Nonopioid + adjuvant + opioid (moderate)
3. Nonopioid + adjuvant + opioid (severe)

TABLE 14.8 Local Anesthetic Dosage Information

Anesthetic Solution	Maximum Dose	pKa	Onset (min)	DURATION (MIN) Maxilla	Mandible	Elimination Half-Life (min)
2% lidocaine (1:100,000 epinephrine)	7 mg/kg	7.9	2–4	170	190	90
2% mepivacaine (1:20,000 Neo-Cobefrin)	6.6 mg/kg	7.6	2–4	130	185	115
4% articaine (1:100,000 epinephrine)	7 mg/kg	7.8	2–4	140	270	20
0.5% bupivacaine (1:200,000 epinephrine)	1.3 mg/kg	8.1	5–8	340	440	210
3% mepivacaine, no epinephrine	6.6 mg/kg	7.6	2–4	90	165	115

Data are from Haas DA. An update on local anesthetics in dentistry. *J Can Dent Assoc.* 2002;68:546-551.

TABLE 14.9 Maximum Manufacturer-Recommended Number of Anesthetic Capsules

Weight of Patient (lb)	2% Lidocaine 1/100,000 Epinephrine	2% Mepivacaine 1/20,000 Neo-Cobefrin	4% Articaine 1/100,000 Epinephrine	5% Bupivacaine 1/200,000 Epinephrine
80	6.5	6.5	3.5	5
100	8	8	4.5	6.5
120	10	10	5.5	8
140	11.5	11	6	9
160	13	11	7	10
180	13.5	11	7	10
200	13.5	11	7	10

Data are from Malamed SF. *Handbook of Local Anesthesia.* 4th ed. St. Louis, MO: Mosby; 1997.

also has a very short half-life (20 minutes) in comparison with the other amide anesthetics. This shorter half-life results because it is hydrolyzed over 90% by plasma esterases and not by the liver as with the other amides. As a result, articaine is of less concern in liver-impaired individuals and is a safer drug for reinjections in longer-duration procedures.

Long-Acting Anesthetics

Postoperative dental pain has been shown to reach its maximum intensity during the first 12 hours postoperatively.[117] When comparing analgesia (reduction in the sensation of pain) with anesthesia (complete elimination of feeling and sensation of pain), complete elimination of pain can be beneficial throughout the immediate postoperative period. Local anesthetics play a key role in the postoperative pain experience for the patients. If the implant surgeon can keep the patient comfortable during the initial period, pain and discomfort in the short term will also be minimized. The greater duration of anesthesia and decreased postoperative pain is effective in reducing the amount of analgesics required after surgery.[118]

The most common long-acting amide anesthetic is bupivacaine (Marcaine). This local anesthetic can play a vital role in pain management. Because of its unique pharmacokinetics, bupivacaine has been studied extensively and has been proven to be safe and far superior to other long-acting local anesthetics. Bupivacaine is an amide local anesthetic that is structurally similar to lidocaine and mepivacaine. It is more potent and less toxic than other types of amide anesthetics. Because of its high pKa (8.1), bupivacaine lasts two to three times longer than lidocaine or mepivacaine. The epinephrine concentration of bupivacaine is much lower (1/200,000 epinephrine) than standard anesthetics, thus limiting its ability to affect hemostasis.

Local Anesthetic Overdosage

A serious complication, local anesthetic overdosage, is of great concern in implant dentistry. Because many implant-related surgeries are of longer duration, a greater amount of anesthetic is often administered. Special attention must be taken during implant surgery as to the number of cartridges and type of anesthetic used during a procedure. Table 14.9 lists anesthetics and the manufacturers' maximum recommended dose by weight of patient to carpules. However, the maximum number of cartridges is time

• BOX 14.15 Signs and Symptoms of Local Anesthetic Toxicity

Mild Symptoms
- Talkativeness
- Slurred speech
- Apprehension
- Localized muscle twitching
- Light-headedness/dizziness
- Tinnitus
- Disorientation

Progressive Symptoms
- Lethargy
- Unresponsiveness
- Drowsiness/sedation
- Lack of muscle tone
- Mild drop in blood pressure, heart, and respiratory rate

dependent. The elimination half-life is not indicative of anesthetic duration; however, it may be used as a guide for repeated anesthetic administration during a lengthy procedure. After one half-life, as much as 50% of the permissible dose can be administered with reasonable safety if liver function is normal.

Special care must be given to the use of combination local anesthetics. In implant dentistry, it is common to use two amide anesthetics together—lidocaine and bupivacaine. Although acceptable, total doses should not exceed combined maximum recommended doses. Calculations should factor in the total dose of the combination and whether sufficient time has elapsed for elimination of the initial dose.[81] If local anesthetic toxicity reactions occur,[119] CNS excitation, convulsions, respiratory depression, and cardiac arrest may occur (Box 14.15).

Most amide anesthetics (except for articaine) are metabolized by the liver by a microsomal enzyme system. Therefore special attention should be given to patients with decreased liver function, especially in elderly patients (e.g., chronic alcoholism, hepatitis). The half-life of lidocaine has been shown to be greater than 2.5 times the normal values in patients with hepatic disease.[120] Special attention must be given to the amount of anesthetic used, and concern for reinjection must be strictly evaluated in these

TABLE 14.10 Most Commonly Used Oral and Intravenous Sedative Agents

Sedative Agent	Class	Administration	Onset (min)	Duration	Half-Life (hr)	Active Metabolites	Oral Dose	IV Dose	Amnesia	Analgesia
Triazolam	Benzodiazepine	PO	60	1–2 hr	2–3	No	0.125–0.25 mg	—	Yes	No
Diazepam	Benzodiazepine	PO/IV	PO: 60 IV: 1–2	0.25–0.5 hr	21–37	Yes	0.2–0.5 mg/kg (maximum: 15 mg)	0.1 mg/kg	Yes	No
Lorazepam	Benzodiazepine	PO/IV	PO: 120–240	IV: 1–2 hr	10–20	No	0.053 mg/kg (maximum: 4 mg)	0.03–0.04 mg/kg	Yes	No
Brevital	Barbiturate	IV	0.5	0.3 hr	4	No	—	0.2–0.4 mg/kg	Yes	No
Fentanyl	Narcotic	IV	0.5	0.75–1 hr	3–4	No	—	1–2 mg/kg	No	Yes
Propofol	Sedative hypnotic	IV	0.2–0.5	3–8 min	0.5–1.5	No	—	25–100 mg/kg/min	Yes	No
Midazolam	Benzodiazepine	PO/IV	0.5–1	0.25–1.25 hr	1–4	No	0.5 mg/kg	0.01–0.1 mg/kg	Yes	No

IV, Intravenous; *PO*, by mouth.

patients. In addition to liver dysfunction, the kidneys are the primary organs responsible for excretion of the local anesthetics and its metabolites. Patients with significant renal impairment will also have difficulty in removing the anesthetics from the blood, resulting in an increased chance of toxicity.

Patients with cardiovascular disease should be well evaluated before the use of epinephrine-containing anesthetics, and care should be taken as to the amount of epinephrine administered. Recommendations on the maximum safe dose for a healthy patient are 0.2 versus 0.04 mg epinephrine for the patient with cardiac impairment. It should be noted that when epinephrine is not included in the anesthetic, the systemic uptake of the drug is more rapid and the maximum number of carpules given is significantly less in comparison with anesthetics with vasoconstrictors.

Post-Surgical Anesthetic Use

To keep the patient as comfortable as possible, the use of long-acting anesthetics is highly recommended both in the beginning and at the end of the procedure. By administering a long-acting anesthetic at the end, the patient will remain "pain free" longer and will have a decrease in the initiation of noxious stimuli. However, care must be given to the number and amount of local anesthetic to avoid overdosage.

Sedative Agents

The use of conscious sedation is a valuable adjunct to dental implant procedures. The American Dental Association defines conscious sedation as a minimally depressed level of consciousness that retains the patient's ability to independently and continuously maintain an airway and respond appropriately to physical stimulation or verbal command, and that is produced by a pharmacologic or nonpharmacologic method or combination thereof.[121] Several sedative agents are currently available for oral and intravenous

sedation. Table 14.10 provides the most commonly used oral and intravenous sedative agents.

Benzodiazepines

The benzodiazepines are the most effective drugs available for dental-related anxiety. These drugs have depressant effects on the subcortical levels of the CNS. Benzodiazepines produce anxiolysis and anterograde amnesia, which are extremely useful for patients undergoing conscious sedation for dental procedures. The exact mechanism is not known, but benzodiazepines are thought to have an effect on the limbic system and the thalamus, which are involved with emotions and behavior.[122]

Diazepam (Valium)

Diazepam is usually not an effective agent for highly apprehensive patients unless administered intravenously. However, it is extremely effective if given orally the night before the procedure with a dose of 5 to 10 mg. Advantages of diazepam for dental procedures are that it reduces salivary flow and relaxes skeletal muscles.

The main disadvantage of diazepam is the 24-hour half-life for adults and an 85-hour half-life for elderly patients. The active metabolites (desmethyldiazepam and oxazepam) are responsible for the prolonged sedation and recovery, along with impaired psychomotor impairment.[122,123]

Midazolam (Versed)

Midazolam is a fast-acting benzodiazepine that is twice as potent as diazepam. It is available as a syrup and also as a formulated injectable solution. Midazolam possesses anticonvulsant properties and also is an excellent muscle relaxant, sedative, and amnesic. The inhibitory effects in the CNS are intensified; therefore midazolam should not be combined with other CNS depressant drugs.

Triazolam (Halcion)

Triazolam is an orally administered benzodiazepine and short-term hypnotic drug. When given orally, this drug is fast acting and has been shown to be safe and effective for dental procedures. Studies have shown that triazolam given in doses of 0.25 to 0.5 mg does not produce adverse effects in respiration, heart rate, or arterial pressure. This drug is also ideal for patients with hypertension, because blood pressure has been shown to decrease by five points.[122,123]

Additional Sedative Anxiolytics

Fentanyl

Fentanyl is a synthetic opioid agonist narcotic that produces analgesia, drowsiness, sedation, and euphoria, but no amnesia. All opioid agonists produce dose-dependent depression of ventilation. Respiratory depression is a result of a decreased response of the ventilatory centers to carbon dioxide. For this reason, care should be taken when administering opioid agonists, especially in combination with other sedatives. Nausea and vomiting are another undesirable effect of opioid agonists. Opioid-induced nausea and vomiting are caused by direct stimulation of dopamine receptors in the chemoreceptor trigger zone in the fourth floor of the fourth ventricle.[122]

Propofol (Diprivan)

Propofol is an intravenous sedative-hypnotic agent commercially introduced in the United States in 1989 by Zeneca Pharmaceuticals. It was the first of a new class of intravenous anesthetic agents: the alkylphenols. Propofol is an ideal sedative anesthetic for dentistry because it is fast-acting and possesses a short half-life. The elimination half-life of propofol has been estimated to be between 2 and 24 hours. However, its duration of clinical effect is much shorter because propofol is rapidly distributed into peripheral tissues. Because of its pronounced respiratory depressant effect and its narrow therapeutic range, propofol should be administered only by individuals trained in airway management.[122,123]

Reversal Agents

Flumazenil (Anexate, Lanexat, Mazicon, Romazicon) is a benzodiazepine antagonist used as a reversal agent for the treatment of benzodiazepine overdose. It reverses the effects of benzodiazepines by competitive inhibition at the benzodiazepine binding site on the $GABA_A$ receptor. It was introduced in 1987 by Hoffman-LaRoche under the name Anexate.

The onset of action is rapid, and usually effects are seen within 1 to 2 minutes. The peak effect is seen at 6 to 10 minutes. The recommended dose for adults is 200 mg every 1 to 2 minutes until the effect is seen, to a maximum of 3 mg per hour. It is available as a clear, colorless solution for intravenous injection, containing 500 mg in 5 mL. It is hepatically metabolized to inactive compounds, which are excreted in the urine.[122,123]

NOTE: Many benzodiazepines have longer half-lives than flumazenil. Therefore repeated doses of flumazenil may be required to prevent recurrent symptoms of overdosage after the initial dose of flumazenil wears off. It is hepatically metabolized to inactive compounds that are excreted in the urine.

Naloxone (Narcan) is a drug used as a reversal for narcotic toxicity. Naloxone is injected intravenously for fastest action. The drug acts after about 2 minutes, and its effects may last about 45 minutes.

Many opioids have a longer half-life than naloxone. Therefore patients who are receiving naloxone should be monitored for resedation and may require repeated doses of naloxone if resedation or respiratory depress occurs.[122,123]

Comprehensive Pharmacologic Protocol

Because of the many variables (e.g., local, systemic, surgical) that need to be considered with the use of pharmacologic agents in implant dentistry, a protocol has been developed to standardize the prophylactic use of these agents. A five-category classification is proposed based on the patient's ASA status and procedure type (Table 14.11).

a. **Patient selection:** Patients are evaluated according to their ASA status: ASA1—normal, healthy patient; ASA2—mild systemic disease; ASA3—severe systemic disease; and ASA4—patient with severe systemic disease that is a threat to life.

b. **Procedures:** The specific procedures are categorized into the protocol according to the extent, invasiveness, surgery duration, and expected bleeding.

c. **Antimicrobials:** The type of antibiotic is selected that is most specific to combat the type of bacteria present in the surgical area. The duration of antibiotic administration can be either a single preoperative dose or extended postoperatively. The duration of antibiotic use is dictated by the patient's health status and invasiveness of the procedure. The first-line antibiotic is amoxicillin for type 1 to 4 categories and Augmentin for type 5 category. Second-line antibiotics include clindamycin (types 1–4) and Ceftin or doxycycline for type 5. The use of chlorhexidine is recommended with all implant procedures before and after surgery.

d. **Glucocorticoid:** Dexamethasone (4 mg) is recommended for type 2 to 5 surgeries, with an increase dose and duration in relation to the extent and invasiveness of surgery.

e. **Analgesic:** Ibuprofen is the ideal preemptive analgesic to be used in all surgeries. Alternatives to ibuprofen would include acetaminophen. See earlier Pain Control Protocol section consisting of maximizing nonopioid medications first and adding narcotics only if warranted.

Possible Drug Interactions in Oral Implantology

See Table 14.12 for possible drug interactions.

TABLE 14.11   Pharmacologic Protocol for Oral Implantology

	Patient Selection	Procedures	Antibiotic	Glucocorticoid	Antimicrobial	Analgesic
CATEGORY 1	ASA1/ASA2 >ASA2 = Category 2	• Single implants with minimal reflection	**Amoxicillin 1 g:** 1 hr before surgery	None	**Chlorhexidine:** ½ oz BID for 2 weeks	Pain control protocol **PCP 1–2**
CATEGORY 2	ASA1/ASA2 >ASA2 = Category 4	• Traumatic extractions with pathology • Socket grafting • Single-tooth implants with extensive reflection • Multiple implants with minimal tissue reflection • SA-1 sinus procedures • Immediate implants without pathology	**Amoxicillin 1 g:** 1 hr before surgery, then 500 mg 6 hours after	**Decadron 4 mg** • 1 tablet a.m. day of surgery	**Chlorhexidine:** ½ oz BID for 2 weeks	Pain control protocol **PCP 1–2**
CATEGORY 3	ASA1/ASA2 >ASA2 = Category 4	• Single implants with bone grafting and excessive tissue reflection • Multiple implants with extensive reflection • Bone grafting (allograft/autograft)	**Amoxicillin 1 g:** 1 hr before surgery, then 500 mg TID for 3 days	**Decadron 4 mg** • 1 tablet a.m. day of surgery • 1 tablet a.m. day after surgery • 1 tablet a.m. 2 days after surgery	**Chlorhexidine:** ½ oz BID for 2 weeks	Pain control protocol **PCP 2–3**
CATEGORY 4	**Any of the following:** • >ASA2 • Long-duration surgery • Less experienced surgeon • Immunocompromised • Active periodontal disease	• Any category 3 procedures with surgical or patient factors • Immediate implants with pathology • Autogenous onlay grafting	**Amoxicillin 1 g:** 1 hr before surgery, then 500 mg TID for 5 days	**Decadron 4 mg** • 2 tablets a.m. day of surgery • 2 tablets a.m. day after surgery • 1 tablet a.m. 2 days after surgery	**Chlorhexidine:** ½ oz BID for 2 weeks	Pain control protocol **PCP 3–4**
CATEGORY 5	All SA-3/SA-4 sinus patients	All SA-2, SA-3, and SA-4 sinus procedures	**Augmentin** (875 mg/125 mg): 1 tablet BID starting 1 day before, then 1 tablet BID for 5 days	**Decadron 4 mg** • 2 tablets a.m. day before surgery • 2 tablets a.m. day of surgery • 1 tablet a.m. day after surgery • 1 tablet a.m. 2 days after surgery	**Chlorhexidine:** ½ oz BID for 2 weeks	Pain control protocol **PCP 2–3**

ASA, American Society of Anesthesiologists; *PCP*, pain control protocol; *SA*, subantral; *SBE*, subacute bacterial endocarditis.

Alternative Medications

Amoxicillin (1 g) = cephalexin (1 g), clindamycin (600 mg)

Augmentin (875/125) = Ceftin (500 mg) = doxycycline (100 mg)

SBE prophylaxis: change preoperative antibiotic dose to amoxicillin (2 g), cephalexin (2 g), or clindamycin

Continued

TABLE 14.11	Pharmacologic Protocol for Oral Implantology—cont'd

Pain control protocol:

PCP 1: ibuprofen 400 mg 1 hour before surgery

PCP 2: ibuprofen 400 mg + 5 mg/300 mg hydrocodone PRN

PCP 3: ibuprofen 400 mg + 7.5 mg/300 mg hydrocodone

PR PCP 4: ibuprofen 400 mg + 10 mg/300 mg hydrocodone PRN

Recommended Pain Control Protocol:

PCP 1: mild pain expected

Ibuprofen: 400 mg 1 hour before surgery

PCP 2: mild-to-moderate pain expected

Ibuprofen: 400 mg 1 hour before surgery (continue QID for 2 days)

+Hydrocodone (Vicodin): 5 mg/300 mg as needed

PCP 3: moderate pain expected

Ibuprofen: 400 mg 1 hour before surgery (continue QID for 2 days, then PRN)

+Hydrocodone (Vicodin ES): 7.5 mg/350 mg (QID) for 2 days, then PRN

PCP 4: severe pain expected

Ibuprofen: 400 mg 1 hour before surgery (continue qid for 4 days, then PRN)

+Hydrocodone (Vicodin HP): 10 mg/300 mg (QID) for 2 days, then PRN

Alternative Medications:

Ibuprofen (400 mg) > acetaminophen (500 mg) or naproxen sodium (375 mg)

Hydrocodone (5 mg/500 mg) > Tylenol #2/tramadol (50 mg)

Hydrocodone (7.5 mg/750 mg) > Tylenol #3/tramadol (100 mg)/Nucynta (50, 75, 100 mg)

Hydrocodone (10 mg/660 mg) > oxycodone (Percocet) 7.5/500 mg

If the patient cannot take medication by mouth:

1. Ibuprofen oral suspension (over the counter)

2. Lortab Elixir (7.5 mg hydrocodone/500 mg APAP/15 mL)

From Misch International Implant Institute.

APAP, acetyl-para-aminophenol.

TABLE 14.12 Drug Interactions

Medication	Interacting Medication	Adverse Effects
All penicillins	Bacteriostatic antibiotics	Static drug will impair action of penicillin
	Methotrexate (Rheumatrex)	Decreases secretion of methotrexate
All cephalosporins	Bacteriostatic antibiotics	Static drug will impair action of penicillin
	Anticoagulants	Risk for bleeding disorders might be increased in anticoagulated patients
Lincomycins Clindamycin (Cleocin)	Erythromycin	Possibility of antagonism AVOID CONCURRENT USE
Macrolides: Dirithromycin (Dynabac) Clarithromycin (Biaxin) Erythromycin	Anticoagulants	Risk for bleeding disorders is increased in anticoagulated patients—monitor patient
	Benzodiazepines	Possible increased benzodiazepine levels resulting in CNS depression, avoid in elderly
	CCBs diltiazem (Cardizem) and verapamil (Isoptin, Calan, Verelan)	QT interval prolongation, could cause sudden death
	Cyclosporine (Sandimmune, Neoral)	Increased cyclosporine renal toxicity
	"Statins" (Lipitor, Zocor, Mevacor)	Increased statin levels with possible muscle toxicity
Metronidazole (Flagyl)	Anticoagulants (Coumadin)	Risk for bleeding disorders is increased in anticoagulated patients
	Ethanol	Severe disulfiram-like reactions
	Tacrolimus (Prograf)	Metronidazole doubles Prograf levels
Quinolones: Ciprofloxacin (Cipro) Gatifloxacin (Tequin) Levofloxacin (Levaquin) Moxifloxacin (Avelox)	Antacids	Decreased quinolone absorption
	Anticoagulants (Coumadin)	Increased risk for bleeding disorders Monitor international normalized ratio
	Antineoplastics	Quinolone serum levels may be decreased
	Cyclosporine (Sandimmune, Neoral)	Cyclosporine renal toxicity may be enhanced
	NSAIDs	Enhanced CNS stimulation
	Caffeine	Increased caffeine effects
		Muscle weakness—tendon damage
NSAIDs and aspirin	Anticoagulants (warfarin [Coumadin])	Increase risk for bleeding disorders in anticoagulated patient, possible GI hemorrhage
	Antihypertensives (all but CCBs) (angiotensin-converting enzyme inhibitor, beta blockers, diuretics)	Decreased antihypertensive effect Monitor blood pressure
	Bisphosphonates	GI toxicity
	Cyclosporine (Neoral, Sandimmune)	Nephrotoxicity of both agents may be increased
	Methotrexate (Rheumatrex, Mexate)	Toxicity of methotrexate may be increased, and increased possibility of stomatitis
	SSRIs	GI bleeding, depletion of platelet serotonin required for aggregation
	NSAID + salicylates	Blockage of antiplatelet action with increased GI effects
Acetaminophen	Barbiturates, carbamazepine, phenytoin, rifampin, sulfinpyrazone	The hepatotoxicity of APAP may be increased by high-dose or long-term administration of these drugs
	Sedatives/anxiolytics	Increased sedation and respiratory depression
	Ethanol	Increased hepatotoxicity of APAP with chronic ethanol ingestion
Tramadol (Ultram, Ultracet)	Any drug that enhances serotonin activity (SSRI antidepressants, "triptans" for acute migraine	Possible serotonin syndrome
	MAOIs (Marplan, Nardil, Parnate)	MAOI toxicity enhanced
	Quinidine	Tramadol increased/metabolite decreased
All opioids	Alcohol, CNS depressants, local anesthetics, antidepressants, antipsychotics, antihistamines, cimetidine	Increased CNS and respiratory depression may occur Use with caution
Hydrocodone/Codeine	2D6 inhibitors, amiodarone, cimetidine, desipramine, fluoxetine, paroxetine, propafenone, quinidine, ritonavir	Inhibition of biotransformation of codeine to active analgesic form Use different narcotic on patients taking 2D6 inhibitor
	SSRI antidepressants and bupropion	Analgesic effect reduced

Continued

TABLE 14.12 Drug Interactions—cont'd		
Medication	**Interacting Medication**	**Adverse Effects**
Amides (e.g., lidocaine)	Alcohol, CNS depressants, opioids, antidepressants, antipsychotics, antihistamines	Increased CNS and respiratory depression may occur
	Antiarrhythmic drugs	Increased cardiac depression
	Beta blockers, cimetidine	Metabolism of lidocaine is reduced
	Bupivacaine	Toxicity is additive, total dose should not exceed the combined maximum dosages
Vasoconstrictors (epinephrine, levonordefrin)	TCAs—high dose (amitriptyline, desipramine, imipramine, nortriptyline, etc.)	Increased sympathomimetic effects possible Limit epinephrine to 0.04 mg with high-dose TCAs
	Beta blockers (nonselective) (e.g., propranolol, nadolol)	Hypertensive and/or cardiac prescription possible Limit epinephrine to 0.04 mg/2 hour visit
	Phenothiazines (e.g., chlorpromazine)	Vasoconstrictor action inhibited, leading to possible hypotensive responses Use with caution
Antihistamines: Diphenhydramine (Benadryl) Hydroxyzine (Atarax, Vistaril) Promethazine (Phenergan)	Anticholinergics	Increased dry mouth, tachycardia, urinary retention
	CNS depressants (alcohol, narcotics)	Enhanced duration and intensity of sedation Reduce dosages
Benzodiazepines (Triazolam)	Rifampin, carbamazepine	Increased metabolism leading to decreased sedative response

APAP, Acetyl-para-aminophenol; *CCB,* calcium channel blocker; *CNS,* central nervous system; *GI,* gastrointestinal; *MAOI,* monoamine oxidase inhibitor; *NSAID,* nonsteroidal antiinflammatory drug; *SSRI,* selective serotonin reuptake inhibitor; *TCA,* tricyclic antidepressant.

From Resnik RR, Resnik RJ. Medical/medication complications in oral implantology. In: *Misch's Avoiding Complications in Oral Implantology.* Philadelphia: Elsevier; 2018.

References

1. Dana R, Azarpazhooh A, Laghapour N, et al. Role of dentists in prescribing opioid analgesics and antibiotics: an overview. *Dent Clin North Am.* 2018;62(2):279–294.
2. Munckhof W. Antibiotics for surgical prophylaxis. *Aust Prescr.* 2005;28(2):38–40.
3. Stone HH, Haney BB, Kolb LD, et al. Prophylactic and preventative antibiotic therapy. *Ann Surg.* 1979;189:691–699.
4. Peterson LJ, Booth DF. Efficacy of antibiotic prophylaxis in intraoral orthognathic surgery. *J Oral Surg.* 1976;34:1088.
5. Peterson JA, Cardo VA, Stratigos GT. An examination of antibiotic prophylaxis in oral and maxillofacial surgery. *J Oral Surg.* 1970;28:753.
6. Gynther GW, Kondell PA, Moberg LE, et al. Dental implant installation without antibiotic prophylaxis. *Oral Surg Oral Med Oral Pathol Oral Radiol Endod.* 1998;85:509–511.
7. Esposito M, Hirsch JM. Biological factors contributing to failure of osseointegrated oral implants. *Eur J Oral Sci.* 1998;106:721–764.
8. Laskin D, Dent C, Morris H. The influence of preoperative antibiotics on success of endosseous implants at 36 months. *Annu Periodontol.* 2000;5:166–174.
9. Dent CD, Olson JW, Farish SE, et al. Influence of preoperative antibiotics on success of endosseous implants up to and including stage 2 surgery. *J Oral Maxillofac Surg.* 1997;55:19–24.
10. Larsen P, McGlumphy E. Antibiotic prophylaxis for placement of dental implants. *J Oral Maxillofac Surg.* 1993;51:194.
11. Burke JF. The effective period of preventive antibiotic action in experimental incisions and dermal lesions. *Surgery.* 1961;50:161.
12. Peterson LJ. Antibiotics: their use in therapy and prophylaxis. In: Kruger GO, ed. *Oral and Maxillofacial Surgery.* St Louis: Mosby; 1984.
13. Woods RK, Dellinger MD. Current guidelines for antibiotic prophylaxis surgical wounds. *Am Fam Physician.* 1998;57:2731–2740.
14. Peterson LJ. Antibiotic prophylaxis against wound infections in oral and maxillofacial surgery. *J Oral Maxillofac Surg.* 1990;48:617.
15. Olson M, O'Connor M, Schwartz ML. Surgical wound infection: a 5-year prospective study of 10,193 wounds at the Minneapolis VA Medical Center. *Ann Surg.* 1984;199:253.
16. Page CP, Bohnen JMA. Antimicrobial prophylaxis for surgical wounds: guidelines for clinical care. *Arch Surg.* 1993;128:79.
17. Haley RW, Culver DH, Morgan WM, et al. Identifying patients at risk of surgical wound infection: a simple multivariate index of patient susceptibility and wound contamination. *Am J Epidemiol.* 1985;121:206–215.
18. Garibaldi RA, Cushing D. Risk factors for post-operative infection. *Am J Med.* 1991;91(suppl 3B). 158S–157S.
19. Cruse PJ, Foord R. A five-year prospective study of 23,649 surgical wounds. *Arch Surg.* 1973;107:206–210.
20. Cruse PJ, Foord R. The epidemiology of wound infection: a 10-year prospective study of 62,939 wounds. *Surg Clin North Am.* 1980;60:27–40.
21. Rider CA. Infection control within the oral surgeon's office. *Compend Contin Educ Dent.* 2004;25:529–534.
22. Gristina AG, Costerton JW. Bacterial adherence and the glycocalyx and their role in musculoskeletal infections. *Orthop Clin North Am.* 1984;15:517–535.
23. Lee KH, Maiden MF. Microbiata of successful osseointegrated dental implants. *J Periodontol.* 1999;70:131.
24. Drake DR, Paul J. Primary bacterial colonization of implant surfaces. *Int J Oral Maxillofac Implants.* 1999;14:226.
25. Culver DH, Horan TC, Gaynes RP, et al. Surgical wound infection rates by wound class, operative procedure and patient risk index: National Nosocomial Infections Surveillance System. *Am J Med.* 1991;91:152–157.
26. Greenberg RN, James RB, Marier RL, et al. Microbiologic and antibiotic aspects of infections in the oral and maxillofacial region. *J Oral Surg.* 1979;37:873–884.

27. Aderhold L, Knothe H, Frenkel G. The bacteriology of dentogenous pyogenic infections. *Oral Surg Oral Med Oral Pathol.* 1981;52:583–587.
28. Lewis MA, MacFarlane TW, McGowan DA. Quantitative bacteriology of acute dento-alveolar abscesses. *J Med Microbiol.* 1986;21:101–104.
29. Norris LH, Doku HC. Antimicrobial prophylaxis in oral surgery. *Oral Maxillofacial Surg Infect.* 1992;2:85–92.
30. Hossein K, Dahlin C. Influence of different prophylactic antibiotic regimens on implant survival rate: a retrospective clinical study. *Clin Dent Res Relat Res.* 2005;7:32–35.
31. Binhamed A, Stowkeych A. Single preoperative dose versus long-term prophylactic regimens in dental implant surgery. *Int J Oral Max Implants.* 2005;20:115–117.
32. Alanis A, Weinstein AJ. Adverse reactions associated with the use of oral penicillins and cephalosporins. *Med Clin North Am.* 1983;67:113.
33. Parker CW. Allergic reactions in man. *Pharmacol Rev.* 1982;34:85–104.
34. Pichichero ME. Prescribing cephalosporins to penicillin-allergic patients. *North Am Pharmacother.* 2006;54:1–4.
35. Tinti C, Parma-Benfenati S. Treatment of peri-implant defects with the vertical ridge augmentation procedure: a patient report. *Int J Oral Maxillofac Implants.* 2001;16(4):572–577.
36. Esposito M, Grusovin MG, Worthington HV. Interventions for replacing missing teeth: antibiotics at dental implant placement to prevent complications. *Cochrane Database Syst Rev.* 2013;7:CD004152.
37. Ata-Ali J, Ata-Ali F, Ata-Ali F. Do antibiotics decrease implant failure and postoperative infections? A systematic review and meta-analysis. *Int J Oral Maxillofac Surg.* 2014;43:68–74.
38. Chrcanovic BR, Albrektsson T, Wennerberg A. Prophylactic antibiotic regimen and dental implant failure: a meta-analysis. *J Oral Rehabil.* 2014;41:941–956.
39. Newman MG, Van Winkehoff AJ. *Antibiotic and Antimicrobial use in Dental Practice.* 2nd ed. Chicago: Quintessence; 2001.
40. Hugo WB, Longworth AR. The effects of chlorhexidine on the electrophoretic mobility, cytoplasmic constituents, dehydrogenase activity and cell walls of E. coli and S. aureus. *J Pharmacy Pharmacol.* 2001;18:569–578.
41. Ciancio SG, Bourgault PC. *Clinical Pharmacology for Dental Professionals.* 3rd ed. Chicago: Year Book Medical Publishers; 1989.
42. Schiott C, Loe H. The effect of chlorhexidine mouthrinses on the human oral flora. *J Periodont Res.* 1970;5:84–89.
43. Bonesvoll P, Lokken P. Influence of concentration, time, temperature and pH on the retention of chlorhexidine in the oral cavity after mouth rinses. *Arch Oral Biol.* 1974;19:1025–1029.
44. Helgeland K, Heyden G. Effect of chlorhexidine on animal cells in vitro. *Scand J Dent Res.* 1971;79:209–215.
45. Goldschmidt P, Cogen R. Cytopathologic effects of chlorhexidine on human cells. *J Periodontol.* 1977;48:212–215.
46. Sanz M, Newman MG. Clinical enhancement of post-periodontal surgical therapy by a 0.12% chlorhexidine gluconate mouthrinse. *J Periodontol.* 1989;60:570–576.
47. Langeback J, Bay L. The effect of chlorhexidine mouthrinse on healing after gingivectomy. *Scand J Dent Res.* 1976;84:224–228.
48. Newman MG, Sanz M. Effect of 0.12% chlorhexidine on bacterial recolonization following periodontal surgery. *J Periodontol.* 1989;60:577–581.
49. Brownstein CN, Briggs SD. Irrigation with chlorhexidine to resolve naturally occurring gingivitis: a methodologic study. *J Clin Periodontol.* 1990;17:558.
50. Beiswanger DD, Mallat ME. Clinical effects of a 0.12% chlorhexidine rinse as an adjunct to scaling and root planning. *J Clin Dent.* 1992;3:33.
51. Larson PE. The effect of a chlorhexidine rinse on the incidence of alveolar osteitis following the surgical removal of impacted third molars. *J Oral Maxillofac Surg.* 1991;49:932.
52. Ragano JR, Szkutnik AJ. Evaluation of 0.12% chlorhexidine rinse on the prevention of alveolar osteitis. *Oral Surg Oral Med Oral Pathol.* 1991;72:524.
53. Lang NP, Schild U. Effect of chlorhexidine (0.12%) rinses on periodontal tissue healing after tooth extraction. I. Clinical parameters. *J Clin Periodontol.* 1994;21:422.
54. Hammerle CHF, Fourmousis I. Successful bone fill in late peri-implant defects using guided tissue regeneration: a short communication. *J Periodontol.* 1995;66:303.
55. Thomson-Neal D, Evans GH. Effects of various prophylactic treatments on titanium, sapphire and hydroxyapatite-coated implants: an SEM study. *Int J Periodont Restorative Dent.* 1989;9:300.
56. Lambert PM, Morris HF. The influence of 0.12% chlorhexidine digluconate rinses on the incidence of infectious complications and implant success. *J Oral Maxillofac Surg.* 1997;55:25–30.
57. Leite FR, Sampaio JE, Zandim DL, et al. Influence of root-surface conditioning with acid and chelating agents on clot stabilization. *Quintessence Int.* 2010;41(4):341–349.
58. Valderrama P, Wilson Jr TG. Detoxification of implant surfaces affected by peri-implant disease: an overview of surgical methods. *Int J Dent.* 2013:740680.
59. Hanisch O, Tatakis DN, Boskovic MM, et al. Bone formation and reosseointegration in peri-implantitis defects following surgical implantation of rhBMP-2. *Int J Oral Maxillofac Implants.* 1997;12(5):604–610.
60. *Accepted Dental Therapeutics.* 40th ed. Chicago: American Dental Association; 1984.
61. Esen E, Tasar F. Determination of the anti-inflammatory effects of methylprednisolone on the sequelae of third molar surgery. *J Oral Maxillofac Surg.* 1999;57:1201–1206.
62. Messer EJ, Keller JJ. The use of intraoral dexamethasone after extraction of mandibular third molars. *Oral Surg.* 1975;40:594–597.
63. Hooley JR, Hohl TH. Use of steroids in the prevention of some complications after traumatic surgery. *J Oral Surg.* 1974;32:8634–8866.
64. Williamson LW, Lorson EL, Osborn DB. Hypothalamic-pituitary-adrenal suppression after short-term dexamethasone therapy for oral surgical procedures. *J Oral Surg.* 1980;38:20–28.
65. Misch CE, Moore P. Steroids and the reduction of pain, edema and dysfunction in implant dentistry. *Int J Oral Implant.* 1989;6:27–31.
66. Nichols T, Nugent CA, Tyle FH. Diurnal variation in suppression of adrenal function by glucocorticoids. *J Clin Endocrinol Metab.* 1965;25:343.
67. Bahn SL. Glucocorticosteroids in dentistry. *J Am Dent Assoc.* 1982;105:476–481.
68. Messer EJ, Keller JJ. The use of intraoral dexamethasone after extraction of mandibular third molars. *Oral Surg.* 1975;40:594–597.
69. Ross R, White CP. Evaluation of hydrocortisone in prevention of postoperative complications after oral surgery: a preliminary report. *J Oral Surg.* 1958;16:220.
70. Guernsey LH, DeChamplain RW. Sequelae and complications of the intraoral sagittal osteotomy in the mandibular. *Oral Surg Oral Med Oral Pathol.* 1971;32:176–192.
71. Neuper EA, Lee JW, Philput CB, et al. Evaluation of dexamethasone for reduction of postsurgical sequelae of third molar removal. *J Oral Maxillofac Surg.* 1992;50:1177–1182.
72. Moore PA, Barr P, Smiga ER, et al. Preemptive rofecoxib and dexamethasone for prevention of pain and trismus following third molar surgery. *Oral Surg Oral Med Oral Pathol Oral Radiol Endod.* 2005;99:E1–E7.
73. Hooley JR, Francis FH. Betamethasone in traumatic oral surgery. *J Oral Surg.* 1969;27:398–403.
74. Baxendale BR, Vater M, Lavery KM. Dexamethasone reduces pain and swelling following extraction of third molar teeth. *Anaesthesia.* 1993;48:961–964.

75. Sisk A, Bonnington GJ. Evaluation of methylprednisolone and flurbiprofen for inhibition of postoperative inflammatory response. *Oral Surg Oral Med Oral Pathol*. 1985;60:137–145.

76. Montgomery MT, Hogg JP, Roberts DL, et al. The use of glucocorticosteroids to lessen the inflammatory sequelae following third molar surgery. *J Oral Maxillofac Surg*. 1990;48:179–187.

77. Bahammam MA, Kayal RA, Alasmari DS, et al. Comparison between dexamethasone and ibuprofen for postoperative pain prevention and control after surgical implant placement: a double–masked, parallel–group, placebo–controlled randomized clinical trial. *J Periodontol*. 2017;88(1):69–77.

78. Gao W, Tong D, Li Q, et al. Dexamethasone promotes regeneration of crushed inferior alveolar nerve by inhibiting NF-κB activation in adult rats. *Arch Oral Biol*. 2017;80:101–109.

79. Wang JJ, Ho ST, Lee SC, et al. The prophylactic effect of dexamethasone on postoperative nausea and vomiting in women undergoing thyroidectomy: a comparison of droperidol with saline. *Anesth Analg*. 1999;89:200–203.

80. Liu K, Hsu CC, Chia YY. Effect of dexamethasone on post-operative emesis and pain. *Br J Anaesth*. 1998;80:85–86.

81. Moore PA. Adverse drug interactions in dental practice: interactions associated with local anesthetics, sedatives and anxiolytics. *J Am Dent Assoc*. 1999;130:541–554.

82. Beaver WT. Combination analgesics. *Am J Med*. 1984;77:38–53.

83. Coutinho AE, Chapman KE. The anti-inflammatory and immunosuppressive effects of glucocorticoids, recent developments and mechanistic insights. *Mol Cell Endocrinol*. 2011;335:2–13.

84. Filho JRL, Silva EDO. The influence of cryotherapy of reduction of swelling, pain, trismus after third molar extraction. *J Am Dent Assoc*. 2005;136:774–778.

85. Forsgren H, Heimdahl A. Effect of application of cold dressings on postoperative course in oral surgery. *Int J Oral Surg*. 1985;14:223–228.

86. Meeusen R, Lievens P. The use of cryotherapy in sports injuries. *Sports Med*. 1986;3:398–414.

87. Laureano Filo JR, de Oliveira e Silva ED, Batista CI, et al. The influence of cryotherapy on reduction of swelling, pain and trismus after third-molar extraction: a preliminary study. *J Am Dent Assoc*. 2005;136(6):774–778.

88. Carr DB, Jacox AK. *Clinical Practice Guidelines for Acute Pain Management: Operative or Medical Procedures and Trauma*. Washington, DC: Agency for Health Care Policy and Research, DHHS publication no. 95-0034; 1992.

89. Bachiocco V, Scesi M. Individual pain history and familial pain tolerance models: relationships to post-surgical pain. *Clin J Pain*. 1993;9:266–271.

90. Taenzer P, Melzack R. Influence of psychological factors on postoperative pain, mood and analgesic requirements. *Pain*. 1986;24:331–342.

91. Huynh MP, Yagiela JA. Current concepts in acute pain management. *J Calif Dent Assoc*. 2003:1–13.

92. Chandraasekharan NV, Dai H. COX-3, a cyclooxygenase-1 variant inhibited by acetaminophen and other analgesic/antipyretic drugs: cloning, structure, and expression. *Proc Natl Acad Sci U S A*. 2002;99:13926–13931.

93. Basbaum AL, Leveine JD. Opiate analgesia. How central is a peripheral target? *N Engl J Med*. 1991;325:1168–1169.

94. Gottschalk A, Smith DS. New concepts in acute pain therapy: preemptive analgesia. *Am Fam Physician*. 2001;63:1979–1984.

95. Al-Sukhun J, Al-Sukhun S, Penttila H, et al. Preemptive analgesic effect of low doses of celecoxib is superior to low doses of traditional nonsteroidal anti-inflammatory drugs. *J Craniofac Surg*. 2012;23(2):526–529.

96. Schwab JM, Schluesener HJ. COX-3: just another COX or the solitary elusive target of paracetamol? *Lancet*. 2003;361:981–982.

97. Ahmad N, Grad HA. The efficacy of non-opioid analgesics for postoperative dental pain: a meta-analysis. *Anesth Prog*. 1997;44:119–126.

98. Dionne RA, Gordon SM. Nonsteroidal anti-inflammatory drugs for acute pain control. *Dent Clin North Am*. 1994;38:645–667.

99. Jackson DL, Moore PA. Preoperative nonsteroidal anti-inflammatory medication for the prevention of postoperative dental pain. *J Am Dent Assoc*. 1989;119:641–647.

100. Ruffalo RL, Jackson RL, Ofman JJ, et al. The impact of NSAID selection on gastrointestinal injury risk for cardiovascular events: identifying and treating patients at risk. *Therapy*. 2002;20:570–576.

101. Hernández-Diaz S, García-Rodríguez LA. Epidemiologic assessment of the safety of conventional nonsteroidal anti-inflammatory drugs. *Am J Med*. 2001;110(suppl 3A):20S–27S.

102. Smalley WE, Griffin MR. The risks and costs of upper gastrointestinal complications attributable to NSAIDS. *Gastroenterol Clin North Am*. 1996;25:373–379.

103. United States Department of Health and Human Services. *Agency for Health Care Policy and Research Clinical Practice Guidelines, Number 9*. Washington, DC: U.S. Government Printing Office; 1994.

104. Bryce G, Bomfim DI, Bassi GS. Pre- and post-operative management of dental implant placement. Part 1: management of postoperative pain. *Br Dent J*. 2014;217(3):123–127.

105. Busson M. Update on ibuprofen: review article. *J Int Med Res*. 1986;14:53–62.

106. Cooper SA. Five studies on ibuprofen for post-surgical dental pain. *Am J Med*. 1984;77:70–77.

107. Winter L, Bass W. Analgesic activity of ibuprofen (Motrin) in post-operative oral surgical pain. *Oral Surg Oral Med Oral Pathol*. 1978;45:159–166.

108. Seymour RA, Ward-Booth P. Evaluation of different doses of ibuprofen and ibuprofen tablets in postoperative dental pain. *Br J Oral Maxillofac Surg*. 1996;34:110–114.

109. Driessen B, Reimann W. Interaction of the central analgesic, tramadol, with the uptake and release of 5-hydroxytryptamine in the rat brain in vitro. *Br J Pharmacol*. 1992;105:147–151.

110. Bailey E, Worthington HV, van Wijk A, et al. Ibuprofen and/or paracetamol (acetaminophen) for pain relief after surgical removal of lower wisdom teeth. *Cochrane Database Syst Rev*. 2013;(12): CD004624.

111. TGA Medicines Evaluation Committee, 2003. Australia: Therapeutic Goods Administration; 2003. Review of Non-Prescription Analgesics: Multiple Strength of Oral Liquids.

112. Moore PA. Pain management in dental practice: tramadol vs. codeine combinations. *J Am Dent Assoc*. 1999;130:1075–1079.

113. Vickers MD, O'Flaherty D. Tramadol: pain relief by an opioid without depression of respiration. *Anaesthesia*. 1992;47:291–296.

114. Mullican WS, Lacy JR. Tramadol/acetaminophen combination tablets and codeine/acetaminophen combination capsules for the treatment of pain: a comparative trial. *Clin Ther*. 2001;23:1429–1445.

115. Medve RA, Wang A. Tramadol and acetaminophen tablets for dental pain. *Anesth Prog*. 2001;48:79–81.

116. Volkow ND, McLellan TA, Cotto JH, Karithanom M, Weiss SR. Characteristics of opioid prescriptions in 2009. *JAMA*. 2011;305:1299–1301.

117. Seymour RA, Blair GS. Postoperative dental pain and analgesic efficacy. *Br J Oral Surg*. 1983;21:290–297.

118. Kaurich MJ, Otomo-Corgel J. Comparison of postoperative bupivacaine with lidocaine on pain and analgesic use following periodontal surgery. *J West Soc Periodontol Periodontal Abstr*. 1997;45:5–8.

119. Moore PA. Prevention of local anesthesia toxicity. *J Am Dent Assoc*. 1992;123:60–64.

120. Thomson PD, Melmo KL. Lidocaine pharmacokinetics in advanced heart failure, liver disease, and renal failure in humans. *Ann Intern*. 1973;78:499–513.

121. American Dental Association. *American Dental Association guidelines for the use of conscious sedation, deep sedation and general anesthesia for dentists*. http://www.ada.org/prof/resources/positions/statements/anesthesia_guidelines.pdf. Accessed July 16, 2007.

122. Stoelting RK. *Pharmacology and Physiology in Anesthetic Practice*. 4th ed. Philadelphia: Lippincott Williams & Wilkins; 2006.

123. *Mosby's Dental Drug Reference*. 8th ed. St Louis: Elsevier; 2008.

PART IV

Treatment Planning Principles

15

Interactive Computed Tomography and Dental Implant Treatment Planning

RANDOLPH R. RESNIK

One of the most significant advances in cone beam computed tomography (CBCT) technology is interactive computed tomography (ICT). ICT describes a technique that was developed to bridge the gap between the CBCT radiographic survey and the surgical placement of implants or bone grafts. With this technology, the implant clinician's computer becomes a diagnostic radiologic workstation with unlimited tools to measure the length and the width of the alveolus, determine bone quality, evaluate vital structures, diagnosis pathology, place type and specific sized implants, and evaluate and preplan the final prosthesis. When viewing the data via the interactive software, various views may be obtained that include axial, cross-sectional, panoramic, sagittal, coronal, and three-dimensional (3D). Specific areas or regions of the patient's anatomy can be selected for display, which may be manipulated via magnification or grayscale modifications to facilitate the evaluation of anatomic structures, anatomic variants, or disease processes.

An important feature of ICT is the implant clinician may perform electronic surgery (ES) by selecting and placing various sized implants into specific anatomic areas. With an appropriately designed diagnostic template, ES can be performed to develop the patient's treatment plan electronically in three dimensions. Electronic implants can be placed at arbitrary positions and orientations with respect to each other, the alveolus, vital anatomic structures, and the final prosthesis. ES and ICT enable the development of a 3D treatment plan that can be integrated with the patient's anatomy and visualized before surgery by the implant team and the patient for approval or modification. With the number and size of implants accurately determined, along with the density of bone at the proposed implant sites, the implant clinician can determine the exact specifications of the implants or bone grafting needed before surgery. Recent advances have allowed this technology to go one step further, with the advent of navigational surgery. Navigational surgery allows the clinician to place implants precisely in "real time" with specialized computer software and global positioning system (GPS)–like technology.

Therefore this chapter will discuss an overview of the basic concepts and use of ICT technology in implant dentistry, including:

(1) evaluating and determining the ideal implant position prior to obtaining an CBCT, (2) obtaining a CBCT scan, (3) obtaining a dataset, (4) integrating the dataset into interactive computer software programs (5) developing various treatment plans with the CBCT data (6) designing a surgical template from the treatment plan, and (7) integrating the surgical plan/template into the actual surgical procedure.

Evaluation and Determination of the Ideal Implant Position Prior To Obtaining a CBCT

The ideal location of the final tooth position or prosthesis must be determined to correlate the positioning of the implant in relation to the available bone. Without a known prosthetically driven location, the implant may be surgically placed in an incorrect position, leading to biomechanical issues and future complications. Therefore a relationship between the implant and final prosthesis location must exist in combination with the radiographic survey to achieve this information. If no correlation exists, the ideal implant positioning may be in error and lead to final placement complications (Fig. 15.1). Various methods of radiographic visualization in determination of the ideal location of the planned implants exist in two categories: radiographic templates and virtual restorations.

Fabrication of Radiographic Template (Scanning Template)

In the literature, there exists significant confusion in the use of prosthodontic terminology and nomenclature when describing radiographic and surgical templates. The terms *stent*, *guides*, *model*, and *appliances* have been used interchangeably in the description of these prostheses. Additional terms sometimes used in identifying these prostheses include scan appliance, scan stent, radiographic or surgical appliance, and radiopaque appliance. However, according to the *Journal of Prosthetic Dentistry*'s "Glossary of Prosthodontic Terms," the definition of *template* best describes the purpose of the prosthesis (Box 15.1).

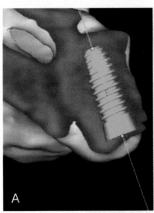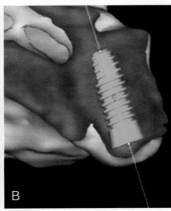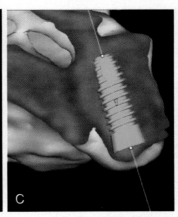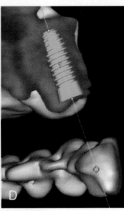

• **Fig. 15.1** (A–C) If no correlation exists between the implant and final prosthesis, the implant may not be planned in the ideal position. (D) With a radiopaque template, the ideal implant position may be correctly transferred to the surgical treatment plan, thereby allowing for implant placement to be directly related to the final prosthesis.

• BOX 15.1 Prosthodontic Glossary of Terms

Template: A thin, transparent form duplicating the tissue surface of a dental prosthesis and used as a guide for surgically shaping the alveolar process; a guide used to assist in proper surgical placement and angulation of dental implants

Stent: Named for the dentist who first described their use, Charles R. Stent, such ancillary prostheses are used to apply pressure to soft tissues to facilitate healing (i.e., periodontal stent, skin graft stent)

Appliance: A device or restoration; something developed by the application of ideas or principles that are designed to serve a special purpose or perform a special function; a broad term applied to any material or prosthesis that restores or replaces lost tooth structure, teeth, or oral tissues

Model: A facsimile used for display purposes; a miniature representation of something

Guide: No definition exists in the "Prosthodontic Glossary of Terms"

Many different types of radiographic templates have been used in implant dentistry. A radiopaque template describes a prosthesis that is fabricated to wear during the CBCT survey that relates the ideal prosthesis position in reference to the bone. Radiopaque templates are usually fabricated through the process of diagnostic tooth positioning via diagnostic waxing, denture teeth arrangement, or duplication of the existing prosthesis. This information is then transferred to the template and used in the radiographic survey (i.e., patient wears radiopaque template during the CBCT survey). In some instances the radiopaque template can be transformed into a surgical placement template for use during implant placement (Fig. 15.2).

Radiopaque Material

A radiopaque material must be used to correlate tooth position and tissue in relation to available bone and vital structures. Many different materials have been described in the literature and may be used in the fabrication of a radiopaque template. The most common material used today in implant dentistry is barium sulfate ($BaSO_4$), which is an inorganic compound that has been used for years as a radiocontrast material in medical diagnostic imaging (Fig. 15.3). This material is ideal for maxillofacial imaging because it may accurately depict the existing contours of the teeth or soft tissue without scattering artifacts. Various techniques to incorporate $BaSO_4$ into the radiographic template include: (1) filling the edentulous area with $BaSO_4$, (2) painting the outside aspects of the buccal and lingual surfaces of the template, and (3) use of preformed $BaSO_4$ teeth. When using $BaSO_4$, care must be made not to use too high of a concentration of $BaSO_4$ because it may cause excessive scatter in the scan. Therefore commercially available monomer and polymer kits are available that include ideal concentrations (i.e., Salvin Dental Inc.). Other radiopaque materials that have been used include gutta percha, amalgam, lead foil, and metal sleeves. However, these materials are useful for delineating the position of the final tooth position but give little information regarding the contours of the restoration.[1,2]

In the literature the radiopaque prosthesis worn during the CBCT scan has been termed many different names (radiopaque template, barium sulfate template or appliance, scanning template, and scanning appliance). The radiopaque prosthesis may be fabricated by various techniques:

1. *Clear vacuum formed:* One of the simplest methods to fabricate a radiopaque template is with the use of a clear vacuum-formed prosthesis from a study cast. After fabrication of a diagnostic wax-up, a duplicate study cast is made. A clear vacuum-formed matrix is created. With the use of $BaSO_4$, the material is added to the edentulous site and allowed to cure. The patient then wears the prosthesis during the scanning process. This prosthesis may be fabricated by a laboratory or with an in-office technique (Box 15.2).

2. *Prosthesis duplication:* If the patient's current prosthesis needs no modification because of esthetics or function, the prosthesis is duplicated via a denture duplicator. The patient wears the fully edentulous radiopaque template during the scanning process. Care must be made so that the prosthesis is stable during the scanning procedure. It is highly recommended to place denture adhesive on the prosthesis before the scan to avoid inaccuracies in the location of the teeth on the scan. Another option would be to make a clear vacuum-form matrix over the existing denture. The matrix is trimmed and barium sulfate is painted over the buccal surfaces of the matrix. The patient wears the denture (with matrix) during

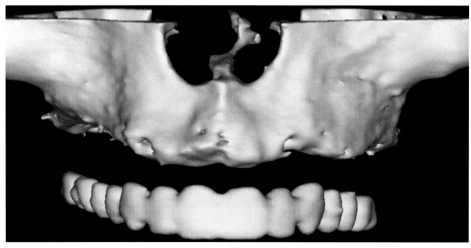

• **Fig. 15.2** Radiopaque template made from a diagnostic wax-up with the correct tooth position and vertical dimension. Note the amount of bone loss (space between the radiopaque template and residual ridge.

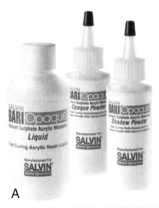

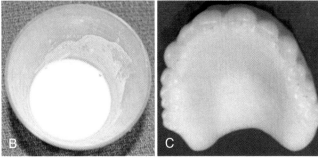

• **Fig. 15.3** (A) Barium sulfate monomer and polymer (Salvin Dental Specialties, Inc., Charlotte, N.C.). (B) Homogenous mixture that may be added to the radiographic template before the cone beam computed tomography (CBCT) scan. (C) Barium sulfate complete denture (i.e., scanning appliance), which is worn by patient for the CBCT scan.

the CBCT survey. Once the scan is obtained, the matrix is removed. (Fig. 15.4; Box 15.3).

3. *Virtual teeth:* Most software programs today allow for an alternative to a radiographic template. This technique has been generically termed the "virtual teeth" function. The benefit of this technique is the clinician may design the replacement teeth via the specialized computer program without the fabrication of a radiopaque template. This specialized tool may be used for single tooth replacement and short edentulous spans. However, caution must be exercised because the use of this modality should be limited to ideal cases in which no maxillomandibular changes are required (Fig. 15.5; Box 15.4).

Flapless Template Techniques

1. *Flapless full arch technique (single scan):* Barium sulfate is used to identify the teeth from the diagnostic wax-up in a 20% $BaSO_4$ solution. If a soft tissue (flapless surgery) template is to be made, teeth are ideally identified with a 20% $BaSO_4$ solution, and the base (soft tissue) uses a 10% mix. This allows for differentiation of the teeth from the soft tissue. Poor mixing will result in a nonhomogeneous mixture that exhibits areas of high radiolucency.

2. *Flapless full arch technique (double scan):* The drawbacks of single scan CBCT-generated surgical techniques are associated with increased costs, more time consuming, and a technique sensitive process. To combat these disadvantages, a new scanning technique, referred to as the *dual-scan technique*, has been introduced to the profession for flapless procedures on fully edentulous patients. This scanning technique allows for fast, easy, and accurate scanning data to be obtained at a significantly reduced cost. With the dual-scan technique, the scan can be obtained at the initial appointment, without the need for a duplicate prosthesis or irreversible modification of the existing prosthesis.

The dual-scan technique utilizes two scans to obtain the data to fabricate a fully guides tissue supported template. The first scan is obtained with the patients current prosthesis with added

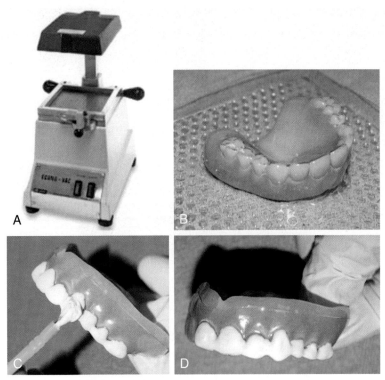

• **Fig. 15.4** Alternative technique for immediate fabrication of a radiopaque template for a fully edentulous patient. (A) Thermoform machine. (B) Fabricate thermoform template over existing denture. (C) Paint on buccal and lingual contours. (D) Patient wears the radiopaque template during scan. *(From Resnik RR, Misch CE. Diagnostic casts, surgical templates, and provisionalization. In: Misch CE, ed.* Dental Implant Prosthetics. *2nd ed. St. Louis, MO: Mosby; 2015.)*

• BOX 15.3 Laboratory Steps for Radiopaque (Full Edentulism) Denture Template

Option 1: Laboratory-Fabricated Template

1. With the use of a denture duplicator flask (Lang Dental Manufacturing, Chicago, Ill.), mix and fill half of the flask with alginate.
2. Place the denture (teeth first) into alginate with the teeth perpendicular to the bottom of the flask.
3. After alginate is set, trim excess that covers the denture flange.
4. Lubricate the alginate and exposed denture with separating material.
5. Fill the other half of the flask, along with the ridge part of the denture, with alginate.
6. Close the flask, ensuring complete closure. After the alginate is set, open and remove the denture.
7. Pour acrylic clear acrylic resin (Clear Surgical Template) or radiopaque acrylic resin (Radiopaque Template) into the incisal and occlusal surfaces, ensuring no bubbles. Pour the remainder of the mixture into the palate or vestibule area.
8. Cure for a minimum of 20 minutes on the laboratory bench or in a pressure pot at 30 psi.
9. Trim excess and polish.

NOTE: If modifications need to be made to the existing prosthesis, the try-in denture should be duplicated after all necessary changes are made.

Option 2: Immediate Template

1. With the patient's existing complete denture, fabricate a vacuum-formed clear template with clear thermoforming material (~0.060 inch, 5 x 5 inches).
2. Using barium sulfate monomer and polymer, paint the facial and lingual surfaces of the template. Allow it to dry.
3. Administer the cone beam computed tomography scan with the radiopaque template.
4. After scan is completed, the vacuum form matrix is removed from the denture. (Figure 15.4)

---

radiopaque markers along with a bite registration (centric relation). The second scan is obtained only with the current prosthesis with added radiopaque markers. After the scans are obtained, the raw data (Digital Imaging and Communications in Medicine [DICOM] datasets) are reformatted with any of the third-party software programs available today. By superimposing the spherical markers over each other, a 3-D bone model is fabricated along with the radiographic template.

Scanning Process

First Scan: The patients existing prosthesis is modified by adding self-stick radiopaque markers Suremark Clearmarkers (3D Diagnostix) over the flange and palatal areas. A bite registration material is then obtained and is worn during the first scan to allow for stability of the prosthesis. Ideally, specifications of the scan should include a 512-x-512 matrix, thickness of less than 1.0 mm, a high resolution reconstruction computer algorithm, and exported in DICOM format.

Second Scan: For the second scan, the prosthesis (with the markers attached) is removed from the patient's mouth and placed onto a holder (attached to the chin cup holder) that allows the prosthesis to be positioned parallel to the floor. The prosthesis should be placed in relatively the same position as the first scan.

Merging of the Two Datasets

Most software programs today will allow for the merging of the two dataset files. The CBCT dataset files are merged by aligning the radiopaque markers so that the prosthesis will be visible over the available bony anatomy, thereby allowing the radiographic template and patient's anatomy to be viewed together or separately. The virtual planning is then completed on the bone and/or prosthetic

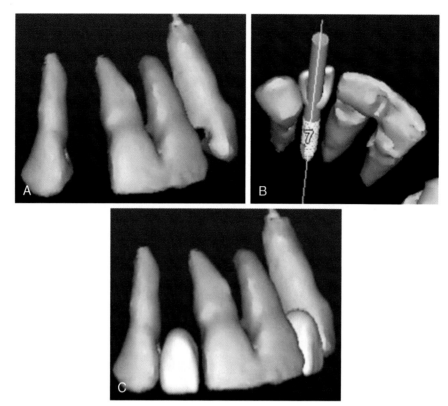

• **Fig. 15.5** Virtual Teeth. (A) Missing maxillary right lateral incisor. (B and C) Virtual tooth #7 moved into ideal position.

model, which allowing for fabrication of the final treatment plan and surgical template.[3] (Fig. 15.6; Box 15.5).

Obtaining a Cone Beam Computed Tomography Scan

Medical Scan vs. Cone Beam Computed Tomography

The second step in the interactive treatment planning technique is obtaining a CT scan (CBCT or medical). Today medical scans are becoming less popular, mainly because of the availability and benefits of the CBCT units in the office setting. Today a wide range of CBCT machines are available in implant dentistry. With most CBCT units, there are two components of CBCT production: acquisition configuration and image detection.

1. *Acquisition configuration:* The first step in the CBCT process is the acquisition of the data via the x-ray source. With most units a partial or rotational scan originates from the x-ray source, whereas a reciprocating area detector moves around the area of interest via a fixed fulcrum. During this rotation, each projection image x-ray beam is captured by the detector. The dimensions of the data acquisition are dependent on the field of view (FOV), which is dictated by inherent detector size and shape. Most CBCT imaging machines use a 360-degree complete circular arch scan to acquire the data.

2. *Image detection:* Current CBCT units have two types of image detectors: an image intensifier tube/charge-coupled device or a flat panel imager. The resolution of the images is mainly determined by the voxel (individual volume elements) size specified within the CBCT unit. The voxel dimension is dependent on the pixel size of the detector and is displayed in submillimeters (range 0.07 to 0.04 mm). The voxel resolution on CBCT units is isotropic or equal in the x, y, and z dimensions.[4]

For interactive treatment planning, it is imperative to reduce artifacts and increase resolution and accuracy of the scan. Therefore to maximize accuracy, the following should be adhered to:

- Use the smallest FOV that encompasses the area of interest. The FOV are usually classified as either small, mid, or large.
- Patients should wear a radiopaque template when indicated. If there is a lack of retention of the radiographic prosthesis, the patient should wear the prosthesis with denture adhesive to ensure stability. The prosthesis may also be relined with tissue conditioner or soft reline material to improve retention. Any movement or improper seating will result in errors, leading to incorrect implant position.
- Always separate the arches (i.e., cotton roll), so the ideal contours of the teeth can be ascertained and the maxilla and mandible can be differentiated in the reformatting process (Fig. 15.7).

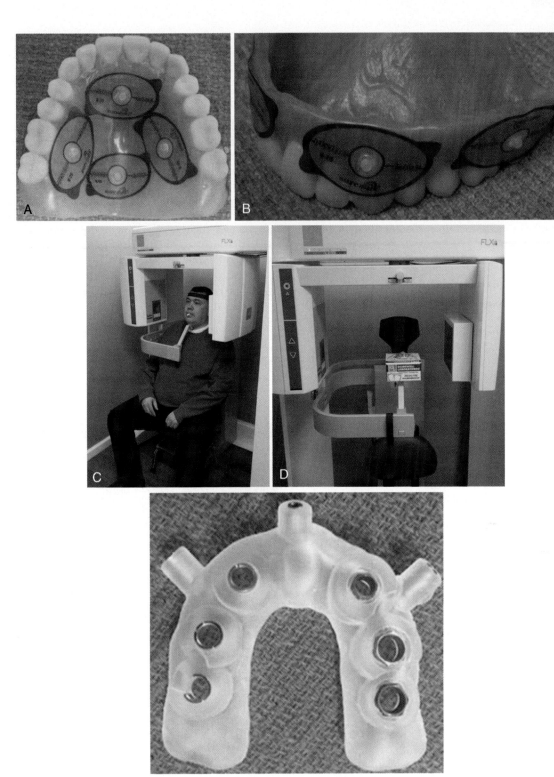

• **Fig. 15.6** Double Scan. (A) Markers are placed on the palate (SureMark Markers). (B) Markers placed on right and left flanges. (C) Cone beam computed tomography (CBCT) scan acquired with patient wearing the existing prosthesis + markers. (D) CBCT scan acquired prosthesis + markers. (E) Final CBCT surgical template fabricated.

Obtain Dataset

The data generated from the CBCT scan include multiple slices with varying thickness (i.e., 1 to 5 mm), which is dependent on the type of scanner. The number of individual projection frames may number from 100 to more than 600, each with greater than a million pixels, with each pixel containing 12 to 16 bits of data per pixel. All of the images are stored in a file termed a *dataset*. To create the volumetric dataset, the acquisition computer will reconstruct the data in a format that will allow transfer to other computers for evaluation and manipulation of the information.

Ideally the dataset should be saved in the Digital Imaging and Communication in Medicine (DICOM) format. This format was developed to create a generalized system for digital image acquisition, storage, and display in medical radiography. If the dataset is saved in a ".dcm" format, the data are easily transferred into the various available CBCT software programs for data evaluation (Fig. 15.8).

Integrate Dataset Into Specialized Software

Most treatment planning software have their own specific protocol; however, all are compatible with DICOM files. These files may be directly generated and downloaded from the scanner. If the dataset is saved in a "viewer" format, in most cases the data will not be able to be extracted for reformation purposes in other third-party software programs.

Reconstruction (Manipulation of Data to Formulate a Treatment Plan)

With the use of CBCT-generated software programs (e.g., SimPlant, Co-Diagnostix), the anatomic relationship can be predictably determined before surgery for ideal treatment planning

purposes. After successful integration of the dataset into the software program, there exist several different methods to evaluate the images.

Determination of Panoramic Curve

The initial viewing window of most CBCT software programs will consist of any of the following images: axial, coronal, sagittal, panoramic, and cross-sectional views, along with 3D representations. In many programs a spline is present that allows the clinician to represent the area or depth of the image in a buccal-lingual orientation. These sagittal cuts allow for anatomic structures to be seen clearly (e.g., mandibular canal [MC]). The clinician can then scroll through the various cross-sectional images that may aid in the visualization of the dimensions of bone (buccal to lingual).

Mandibular Canal Identification

Methods for Identifying the Mandibular Canal

The identification of the MC is manually performed and estimated on multiple endpoints that cross reference in all available image types of the dataset (Fig. 15.9; Box 15.6).[5]

• BOX 15.5 Double Scan

1. The first scan is taken with the patient wearing the radiolucent prosthesis with Dual Scan Markers 3D Diagostix and bite registration. The bite registration is used to stabilize the prosthesis during the scanning procedure.
2. Positioning of the patient is comparable with a standard dental computed tomography scan. The transaxial slice plane must be parallel to the floor.
3. The maxilla and mandible, including the scan template, must be within the FOV.
4. The second scan is taken of the prosthesis alone, applying the same general settings that were used to obtain the first scan.
5. It is important that the position of the prosthesis is in the same position as the mouth position. The materials to hold the prosthesis must be more radiolucent than the prosthesis itself. Polyethylene and polyurethane foam materials may be used. Alternatively, a cardboard box can be used to secure the prosthesis in a vertical position.

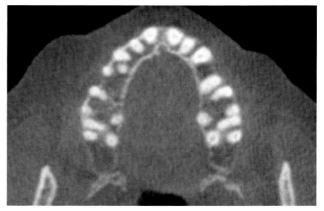

• **Fig. 15.8** Individual image stored in Digital Imaging and Communication in Medicine (DICOM) format. A dataset is made of many dicom images.

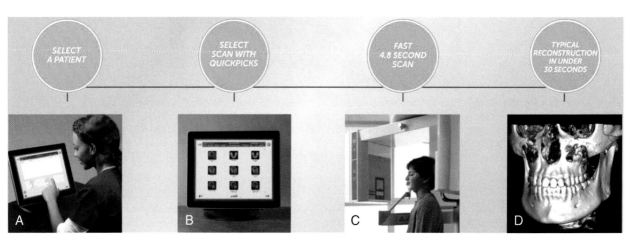

• **Fig. 15.7** Cone Beam Computed Tomography (CBCT) Scan Acquisition (I-cat). (A) Patient information added. (B) Field of view selected. (C) CBCT scan taken (~< 5 seconds). (D) Reconstruction of scan data (~<30 seconds).

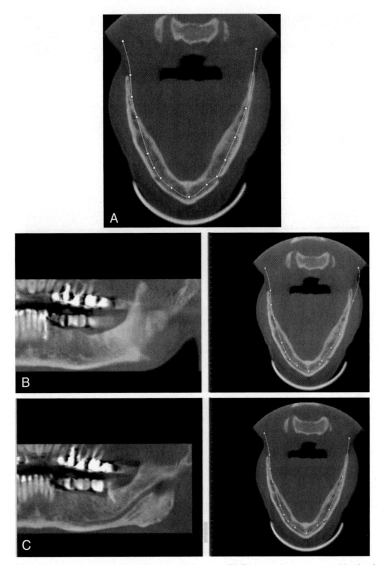

• **Fig. 15.9** (A) Panoramic curve outlined in an axial image. (B) Panoramic curve outside the focal trough of the mandibular canal (MC) resulting in no visualization of MC. (C) Panoramic curve changed within the MC allowing for evaluation of MC.

• BOX 15.6　Identification of Mandibular Canal

Manipulation of Images

1. Select the reconstructed panoramic view using the CBCT software to access the MC.
2. If the MC is not seen clearly, manipulate the mandibular curve in the axial view buccal-lingually
3. When the MC can be seen clearly, the nerve is drawn (main nerve canal) from the posterior to the mental foramen.
4. In the cross-sectional views, scroll until the mental canal/foramen is seen. Draw the first nerve (green) from the MC to the exit of the mental foramen. Draw the second nerve (orange) from anterior to posterior.
5. If the MC cannot be seen clearly, mark the posterior and anterior limits of the MC and extrapolate via cross-sectional images. The MC can then be drawn, connecting the extrapolating points on the panoramic image.

Additional Techniques

If the CBCT examination does not depict the MC clearly, an MRI examination may be completed to more easily see the cortical and cancellous bone, nerve, and blood vessels. Studies have shown that MRI images provide less variability in determining the locations of the mandibular nerve, the mental foramen, and the mandibular foramen than CBCT images. Even though there exists no ionizing radiation, MRI technology is limited in dentistry because of cost, availability, and no cross referencing.

The accurate identification of the MC is crucial for preoperative treatment planning for implant placement in the posterior mandible. Because the amount of available bone height present between the alveolar ridge and the MC dictates the positioning and size of the dental implant, any inaccuracies may lead to an increased morbidity. Because of the varying inability to ascertain cortical borders in the MC and with different trabecular patterns, in some cases it may be difficult to determine the exact location. Studies have shown the visibility of the MC decreases toward the mental foramen. This unreliability of visualization of the MC near the mental foramen is due to the lack of definite walls in the anterior portion of the canal. Even with the wide variation of CBCT images, the identification of this structure is directly proportional to the density of the bone and the thickness of the cortical bone surrounding the MC.

Lofthag-Hansen et al.[6] determined that the MC is visible on only one-third of cross-sectional images. However, when other images (sagittal and axial) were evaluated, the visibility of the MC increased significantly to approximately 87%. Therefore assessing multiple sequential images increases the localization of the MC[6] (Fig. 15.10).

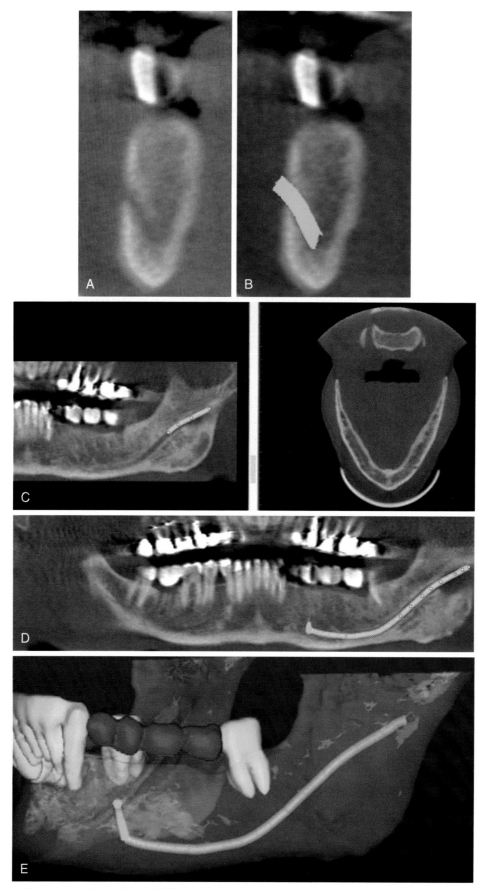

• **Fig. 15.10 Mandibular Canal (MC) Identification.** (A) Mental foramen and canal are identified in the cross-section view. (B) Foramen and canal are marked by using the nerve marking module within the software. (C) In the CBCT panoramic view the MC is marked from the posterior in small segments. (D and E) The canal is marked anteriorly until the MC marking connects with the mental canal.

Evaluation of Bone Density

The determination of the bone density values allows for modification of the surgical (drilling protocol, insertion torque, implant size determination, number of implants) and prosthetic (healing time, progressive bone loading) protocols. The bone density is a relative measurement on CBCT units because it is based on many factors, including gray values, machine calibration and settings, and software interpretation, whereas on medical-grade CT scanners, it is directly related to the Hounsfield units (Fig 15.11; Box 15.7).

Virtual Implant Placement

Manual implant placement may be performed in most of the associated views after reformatting the DICOM images. The digital software will allow the user to place a "virtual implant" in the proposed position according to anatomic factors. Analysis may be made for ideal positioning, and modifications are easily completed. Most software programs have implant libraries that consist of various implant types and allow for the determination of the exact implant dimensions (i.e., the diameter, length, and thread size). The implant position may be evaluated and adjusted accordingly with respect to bony anatomy, prosthesis type, and location of vital structures (Figs. 15.12 and 15.13).

Safety Zone

Most software programs contain safety zone features that prevent implant placement too close to a vital structure (i.e., implant in approximation to the MC). Usually a 2-mm safety zone will be preset within the program that will prevent implant placement too close to the MC (Fig. 15.14).

Bone Graft Simulation

When advanced cases of ridge resorption are present, bone grafting defects may need to be addressed and evaluated. Bone grafting procedures (e.g., sinus augmentation, ridge augmentation) may be simulated and completed via the interactive software programs (Fig. 15.15). With some software programs, actual bone graft volume may be determined.

Treatment Plan to Surgical Placement

The implant profession has seen a major shift and demand from traditional freehand implant placement to computer-guided surgical intervention. This can be accomplished by facilitating the accurate translation from the interactive treatment plan to reality with the use of surgical guides (templates). The three-dimensional computer-assisted interactive implant treatment planning software tools have facilitated an accurate and precise clinical method to ensure proper placement. This computerized transfer process can be accomplished via the use of fabricated stereolithographic drill guides or direct navigation. The use of surgical templates has been shown to be a reliable and proven method to transfer the surgical plan to the surgical field through guided drilling templates.

Surgical Template Fabrication

Commercial

After the treatment plan is verified the clinician can easily upload the saved plan to a third-party site for template fabrication. In most software programs the patient data, type of template, drilling sequence, and drill diameters may be manually inserted into the program (Fig. 15.16).

In-Office

New techniques have allowed for the integration of the following; (1) CBCT, (2) digital scan, and (3) surgical template from a computer-aided design/computer-aided manufacturing (CAD/CAM). This type of template is usually milled or 3D printed (3D additive manufactured). Although the milled guides are the most dimensionally stable and less brittle, cost and the time-consuming nature are disadvantages. Affordable,

---

• BOX 15.7   Bone Density Relationship to Hounsfield Numbers[29]

D1: >1250
D2: 850–1250
D3: 350–850
D4: 0–350

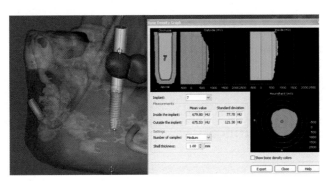

• Fig. 15.11 Bone Density Determination. The bone density may be determined "inside" the implant (i.e., provides the clinician with information when drilling the osteotomy) and "outside" the implant (i.e., provides the clinician with information on the healing of the implant).

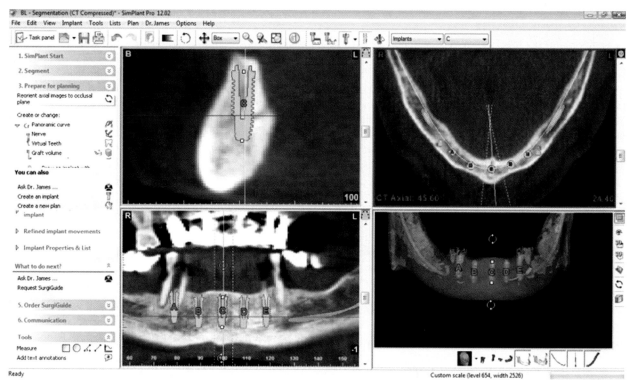

• **Fig. 15.12** Virtual Implant Placement. Mesial-distal space evaluated and measured.

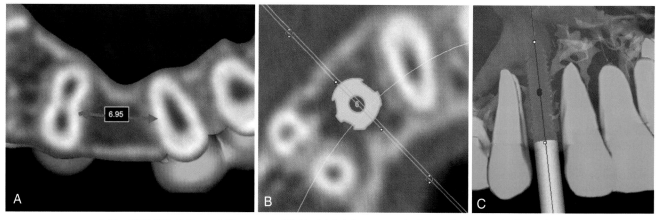

• **Fig. 15.13** Virtual Implant Placement. (A) Mesial-distal space evaluated and measured. (B) Implant placement and evaluation between adjacent roots. (C) Final positioning verified in cross section.

high-quality, in-office 3D printers are now available that produce guides with limited waste and minimal polymerization shrinkage, to combat these drawbacks. These 3D printers are highly accurate and produce precise anatomic models and surgical templates (Figs. 15.17 and 15.18).

Surgical Implant Placement With Surgical Template

A surgical template (guide) is defined as a prosthesis used to assist in the surgical placement of implants. In the literature, three different surgical template designs are based on surgical restriction: nonlimiting, partial-limiting, and complete-limiting design.

Surgical Restriction Templates

Non-limiting Design

A non-limiting surgical template is a template that allows for a generalized location of the ideal implant site. No actual directional guide is built into this type of template other than possibly the buccal or lingual contours of the ideal positioning of the teeth. A simple and inexpensive method to fabricate this type of template is duplication of an existing prosthesis or modification of Preston's clear splint for the diagnosis of tooth contours, tooth position, and occlusal form.[7]

The diagnostic wax-up is completed to evaluate the tooth size, position, contour, and occlusion in the edentulous regions where implants will be inserted. A full arch, irreversible hydrocolloid or polyvinyl siloxane impression is made of the diagnostic wax-up and poured in dental stone. On the duplicate cast of the wax-up teeth a vacuum acrylic shell (0.060 to 0.080 inch) is vacuum formed to fit over the teeth and gingival contours of the buccal aspect of the ridge. If no natural teeth are present in the posterior, then the posterior portion of the template should be maintained to cover the retromolar pads or tuberosities and palate to aid in positioning.

The occlusal surface is trimmed over the ideal and optional implant sites, maintaining the facial and facial-occlusal line angle of the surgical template. A black line then is drawn on the template with a marker to indicate the center of each implant and the desired angulation. This provides latitude for the implant dentist for implant placement, yet communicates the ideal tooth position and angulation during surgery.

The surgical template should relate to the ideal facial contour. Many edentulous ridges have lost facial bone, and the template can assist in determining the amount of augmentation required for implant placement or support of the lips and face. The surgical template may be used for a bone graft, and later the same template may be used for insertion of implants and again for implant uncovery.

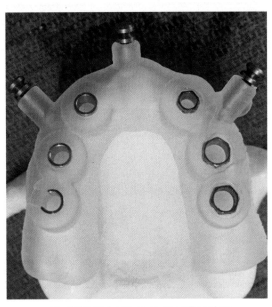

• **Fig. 15.14** Safety Zone. Most software programs have safety zones that prevent placement of implants too close to a vital structure. In this example a 2.0-mm safety zone is present around the implant in the prevention of placement too close to the mandibular nerve.

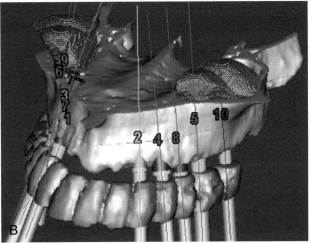

• **Fig. 15.16** Third-Party Surgical Template.

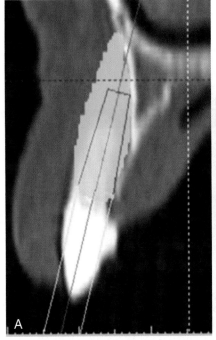

• **Fig. 15.15** Bone Graft Simulation. (A) Buccal bone graft required. (B) Sinus grafting simulation.

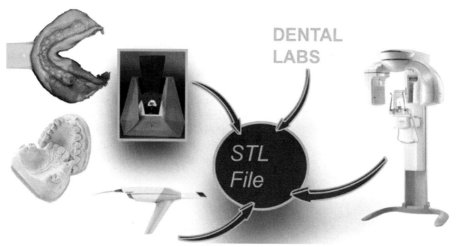

• **Fig. 15.17** STL File. STL file is obtained from study casts, digital impression, or CBCT scans.

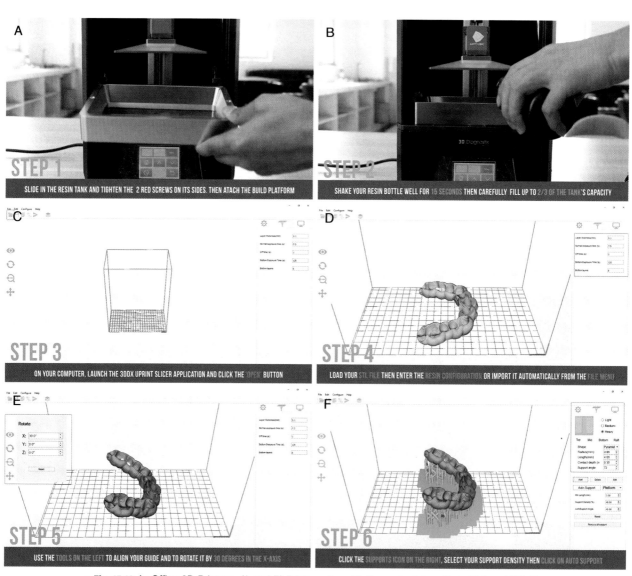

• **Fig. 15.18** In-Office 3D Printers. (A and B) Printer setup. (C) Computer integration. (D) Load STL file. (E–G) Design of Template. (H and I) Printing. (J and K) Printing complete. (L) Metal sleeves placed into template.

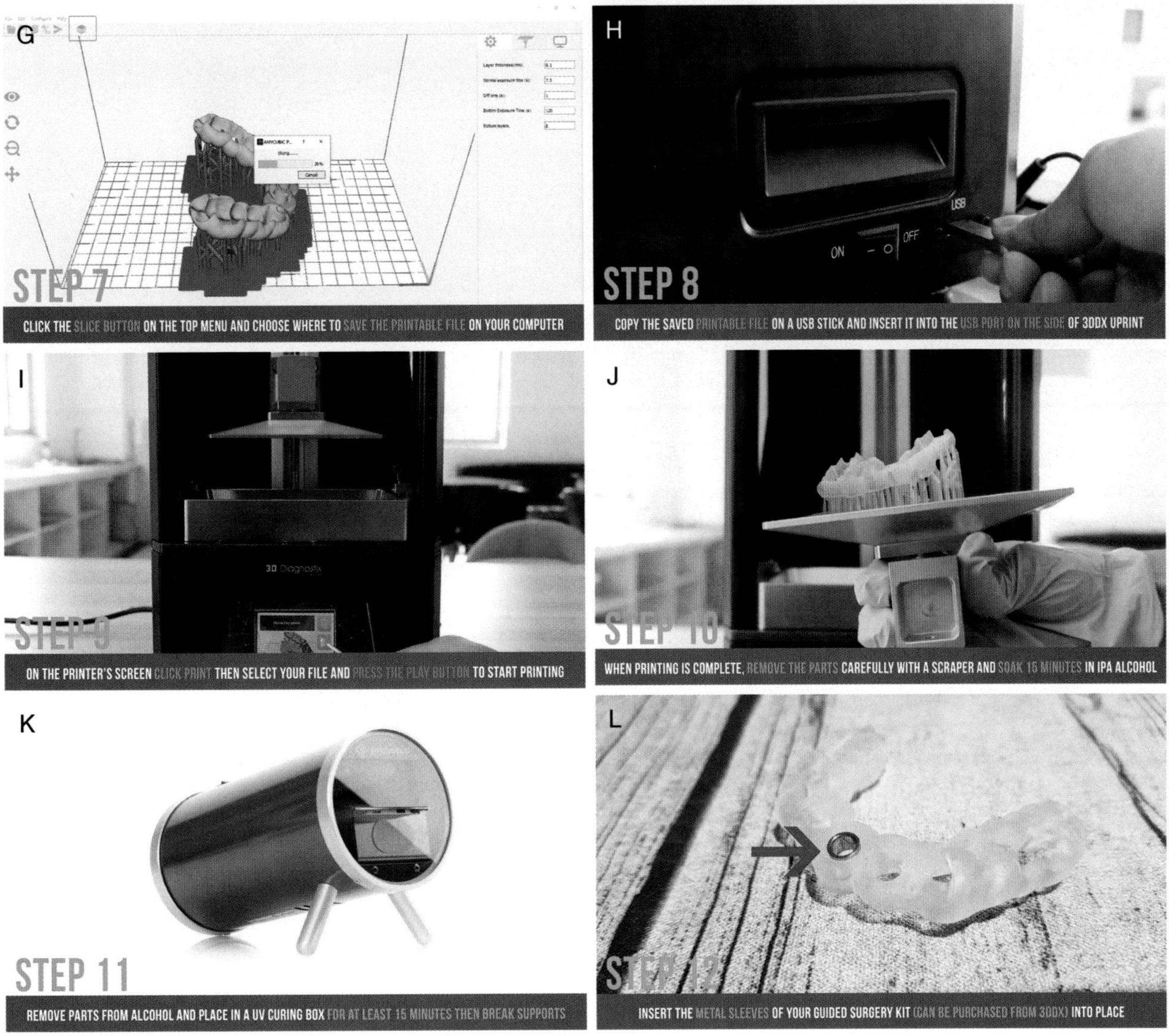

• **Fig. 15.18, cont'd**

Partial-Limiting Design

The partial-limiting design incorporates a guided sleeve or a slot that allows for angulation of one drill size, usually the pilot drill. Therefore after the first drill is used, the remainder of the osteotomy sites are completed freehand. Various techniques can be used, including manual laboratory-fabricated templates or templates fabricated from a radiographic template, which is then converted into a surgical guide template.

Complete-Limiting Design

With the complete-limiting design, the position, angulation, and depth of the osteotomy are dictated by the guided tubes or sleeves, thus restricting any variation by the implant surgeon.

This type of template prevents any osteotomy error in the buccolingual and mesiodistal planes (i.e., complete-limiting). In addition, drill stops can be incorporated to prevent from over-preparing the site. With the complete-limiting design, the final position of the implant is known before the actual surgery. The complete-limiting design is ideal because the prosthetic final abutment or provisional restoration can be prefabricated for immediate provisionalization after implant placement (Fig. 15.19).

CBCT Templates by Support

When using a CBCT-generated treatment plan, the complete-limited design is the most common. There are three types of CBCT supported guides: tooth, bone, or tissue.

Tooth-Supported Guides

Tooth-supported guides are the most accurate and easiest guide to use.[8,9] These guides are mainly used in partially edentulous patients and are highly dependent on the accuracy of the impression and study cast. These guides typically are translucent, thus allowing visualization of the complete seating of the guide. No gaps should be present between the guide and teeth on the study cast or in the mouth. In addition, the guide must be stable and have no movement when lightly manipulated (Fig. 15.20).

Indications

1. Partially edentulous patients
2. Sufficient number of teeth for guide support

Requirements (one of the following)

1. Study cast + CBCT
2. Stereolithography (STL) STL file of study cast + CBCT
3. Digital impression + CBCT

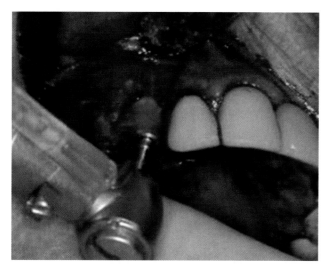

● **Fig. 15.19** Complete-Limiting Template. Accurate template fabricated from cone beam computed tomography data.

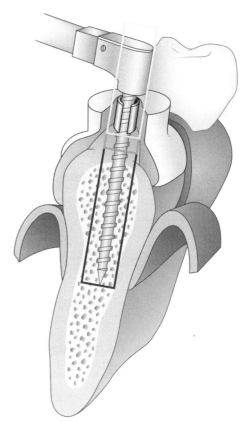

● **Fig. 15.21** Bone-Supported Guide. Surgical template that is completely supported by the existing bone. This type of template is often used when existing bone modification is indicated.

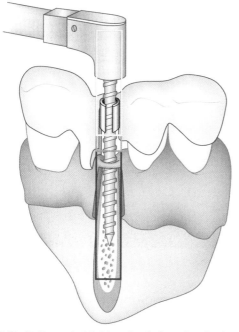

● **Fig. 15.20** Tooth-Supported Guides. Surgical template that is completely supported by adjacent teeth and is the most accurate type of template.

Bone-Supported Guides

Bone-supported guides may be used in partially or fully edentulous patients. These guides require extensive full-thickness reflection to expose the bony ridges to allow proper seating of the guide. If bone modification is indicated, proper seating of the guide may be difficult, resulting in errors in implant placement. In some cases a bone reduction guide may be used before seating the bone-supported guide. It should be noted that small bone protuberances may exist that are below the resolution of the scan. Therefore meticulous evaluation of the bony contours should be evaluated before osteotomy site preparation (Fig. 15.21).

Indications
1. Edentulous patients
2. Partially edentulous patients (minimum of three teeth missing)

Soft Tissue–Supported Guides

Soft tissue–supported guides are usually indicated for completely edentulous patients, and these surgeries are usually termed *flapless.* In some cases the guides are difficult to seat correctly, especially if there exists overextension beyond the vestibule or floor of the mouth. Bite registrations are sometimes used to ensure ideal placement and positioning. In many cases, stabilizing pins or screws are placed to improve stability during osteotomy and implant placement. The most challenging cases for the use of soft tissue guides are the maxilla with flat palatal vaults and mandibles with high floor of the mouth with very little vestibule. Most full arch soft tissue–supported guides are fabricated via the "dual scan" technique (Fig. 15.22).

Indications
1. Only edentulous patients
2. Must have sufficient support
   a. Maxilla (palate)
   b. Mandible: sufficient vestibular or lingual support of prosthesis

Requirements
Dual Scan technique.

Studies: Accuracy studies comparing the three types of guides have shown tooth-supported guides being the most accurate, followed by bone-supported guides. Soft tissue guides are the least accurate, mainly because of the consistency and changes of the soft tissue.[8,10]

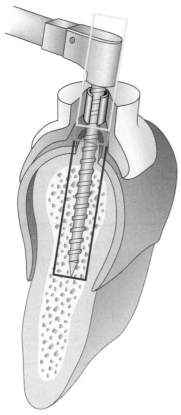

• **Fig. 15.22 Soft Tissue–Supported Guide.** Surgical template that is completely supported by the soft tissue and is used mainly in flapless surgery.

CBCT by Drill Guidance (Fig. 15.23)

Pilot Guide (Fig. 15.24)

- Ideal for initial position (buccal-lingual, mesial-distal)
- Only first drill used
- Must freehand final drills and implant placement
- May have depth control (guided drills with stop)
  Uses: position and angulation of the implant

Universal Guide (Fig. 15.25)

- Compatible with all implant systems
- Drill guidance
- Depth control
- Finalize osteotomy with surgical system
- Must place implant freehand
  Uses: depth, position and angulation

Fully Guided (Fig. 15.26)

- Brand-specific surgical kits
- Drill guidance with depth control (full sequence)
- Implant guidance with depth control
- Immediate smile possible
  Uses: depth, position, angulation, and implant placement

Requirements of a Surgical Template

1. The template should allow the clinician to place the implant in the ideal position according to the x, y, and

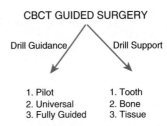

CBCT GUIDED SURGERY

Drill Guidance | Drill Support

1. Pilot   1. Tooth
2. Universal   2. Bone
3. Fully Guided   3. Tissue

• **Fig. 15.23** Summary of Cone Beam Computed Tomography (CBCT) Surgical Templates.

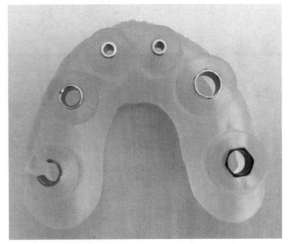

• **Fig. 15.24 Pilot Guide.** Surgical template depicting pilot guide placement in the anterior (# 8, # 9). After the first drill the clinician must complete the osteotomies freehand. The premolar implants are for universal guide placement and the molar sites are for fully guided implant placement.

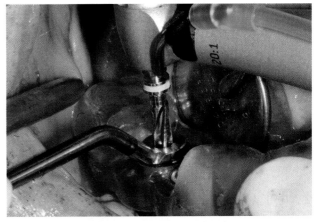

• **Fig. 15.25 Universal Guide.** Surgical template that can be used with any implant surgical system. All drills except the last drill are used from a universal surgical kit and special keys that fit directly into the surgical tubes.

z axes (i.e., buccolingual, mesiodistal, and apicocoronal dimensions).
2. The template must be stable and rigid when placed in the correct position. There should exist no "rocking" or incomplete seating of the template.
3. If the arch being treated has remaining natural teeth, the template should encompass as many teeth as possible to stabilize the template in position. When no remaining teeth

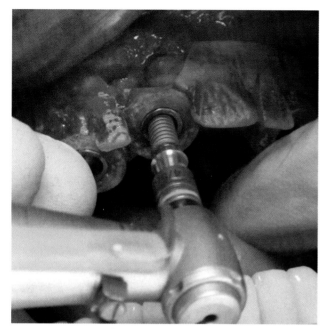

• **Fig. 15.26** **Fully Guided.** Surgical template that allows for all osteotomy drills to be used along with implant placement through the guide.

are present, the template should extend onto nonreflected soft tissue regions (i.e., the palate and tuberosities in the maxilla or the retromolar pads in the mandible) for tissue-borne templates.
4. Access for irrigation must be present because osteotomy drilling without irrigation will result in overheating the bone (necrosis) and lack of implant integration. The surgical guide tube diameter is approximately 0.2 mm larger; therefore adequate irrigation is difficult to achieve.
5. The template must be able to be sterilized to ensure surgical asepsis. Templates should be able to be disinfected with 3.2% glutaraldehyde and immersed in 0.12% chlorhexidine during the surgery.

Surgical Template Fabrication

Surgical guides are computer-generated drilling guides that are fabricated through the process of stereolithography. The surgical guide concept is based on the presurgical treatment plan, using specialized dental implant software for ideal implant positioning. The surgical osteotomy drill guides may be either bone-, teeth-, or mucosa-borne. Surgical templates have metal cylindrical tubes that correspond to the number of desired osteotomy preparations and specific drill diameters. The diameter of the drilling tube is approximately 0.2 mm larger than the corresponding drill, thus making angle deviation highly unlikely.

Clinical data and studies of computer-aided stereolithographic surgical guides have shown that implant placement is improved, and allow precise translation of a predetermined treatment plan directly to the surgical field. Nickenig et al.[9] evaluated the margin of error with freehand vs. guided implant placement and showed an apical deviation of 0.6 to 0.9 mm (guided) and 2.0 to 2.5 mm (freehand).

There are two types of surgical guide fabrication techniques from the treatment planning software: (1) laser photopolymerization of liquid resin, and (2) CAD/CAM.

Additional Types of Templates (Guides)
Stereolithographic Models
The fabrication of stereolithographic models is a laser-dependent rapid polymerization technique using sequential layers of special polymers that can duplicate the exact shape of the osseous anatomy.[10-13] These types of models include:
1. Surgical guide models used in the fabrication of surgical guides
2. Presurgical models used in the preoperative evaluation for implant placement, bone grafting, and orthognathic surgery (Fig. 15.27); and
3. Bone reduction guides: similar to reduction copings in conventional crown and bridge, and used to reduce osseous height before implant placement (Fig. 15.28).

Surgical Guidance Templates and Navigation Systems
Navigational systems, originally developed in neurosurgery, are now available to facilitate dental implant placement procedures during surgery. The navigational implant systems are based on CBCT imaging in combination with optical positioning, which assists in the accurate placement of dental implants.[15] Using preoperative planning software and real-time display, the depth and trajectory of the drilling sequence can be made to the specifics of preplanned position. Navigational systems have been shown to prevent damage to adjacent teeth and vital structures such as the inferior alveolar nerve.[16,17]

Dental implant surgical navigation is comparable with a GPS that is composed of three components: (1) localizer (Satellite in Space), (2) instrument or surgical probe (Tracking waves emitted by the GPS Unit), and (3) CBCT dataset (Road Map).[18]

Two different types of navigational systems are currently available: optical and electromagnetic. With an optical system, also referred to as an infrared system, infrared sensors along with light reflectors are fixed to the patient's head and a handheld probe to track the position of the instruments within the surgical field. Electromagnetic systems use an electromagnetic field and reference points on a device that is attached to the patient's head and a wired surgical instrument.

When placing implants with navigational surgery, a generalized protocol includes:
1. Stent (template) fabrication
   • A thermoplastic stent is fabricated directly on the patient's teeth.
2. CBCT imaging
   • The patient is scanned wearing the prefabricated stent, along with fiducial markers for cross-referencing jaw positions with the CBCT scan.
3. Implant treatment planning
   • The implant and prosthesis are treatment planned using CBCT software.
4. Implant surgery
   • Using the dynamic guidance process, implant placement is completed in real time. The surgical handpiece is equipped with a 3D positioning device, such as electromagnetic digitizers[19] or light-emitting diodes.[20] Extraoral markers attached to the surgical guide are also necessary so that the computer can analyze the positions of the jaw and the handpiece relative to each other. Continuous reevaluation of locations and matching to the CT scan data during surgery allow for visualization of osteotomies and comparison of planning and drilling. Some computer systems are equipped with audible or visual warnings when osteotomies deviate from pre-planned positions or when a vital structure is about to be entered.

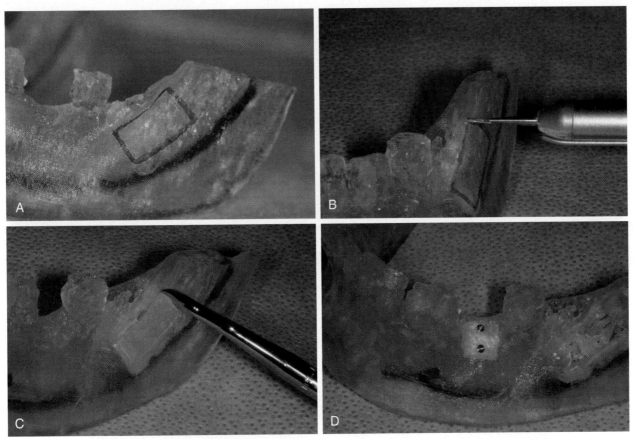

• **Fig. 15.27** Bone Grafting Model. (A) Ramus bone graft model. (B) Bone cuts in model. (C) Donor graft removed. (D) Graft placed into recipient site.

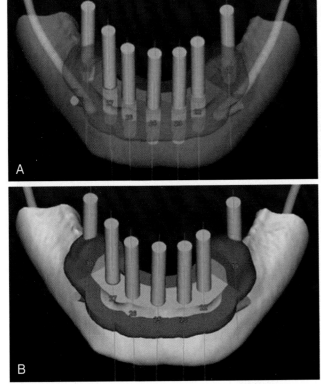

• **Fig. 15.28** Bone Reduction Guide. (A) The amount of bone reduction is determined via the prosthetic treatment plan. (B) Outline of bone reduction showing the relationship between implants and bone height.

Studies

Research studies have shown this approach, although complex, can yield favorable results in the vicinity of 0.5 mm.[21,22] Other studies have shown guided surgery with CAD/CAM guides can achieve precision consistently within 1 mm of the planned implant location at the entrance and 5 degrees of the desired angulation[23] (Fig. 15.29).

Stackable Templates for Provisional Restorations (Immediate Smiles)

Taking the CT-generated technology to the next level involves fabricating provisional restorations before implant insertion. First, the virtual treatment plan is created by the implant dentist, followed by the manufacturer developing the computer-generated stereolithographic surgical guides. A dental laboratory uses the surgical guide and articulated diagnostic casts to fabricate provisional and (in some cases, final) prostheses. The implant dentist then uses the surgical guide to place the implants and abutments. The provisional (or final) prosthesis is then inserted immediately after the placement (Fig. 15.30).

Digital Technology

The use of dental CAD/CAM technology has become overwhelming popular today in all phases of dentistry. Chairside CAD/CAM systems for dental offices have allowed clinicians the opportunity to design, mill, and place ceramic restorations in a single appointment, along with treatment planning and fabricating implant restorations. The ability to fabricate various prosthetic restorations without using traditional dental laboratory methods has proved to be rewarding in many ways.

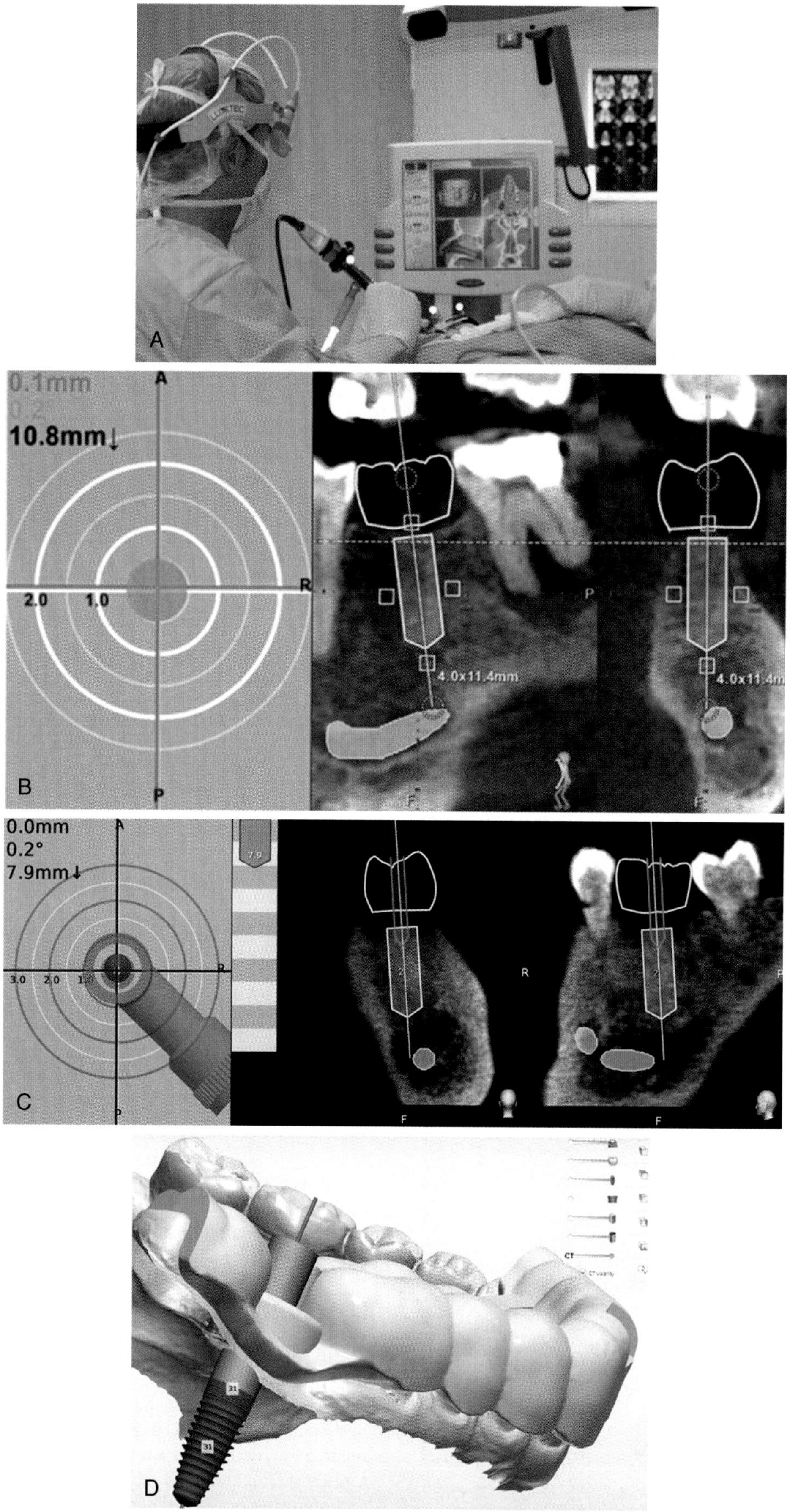

• **Fig. 15.29 Navigational Surgery.** (A) Setup for navigational surgery. (B and C) Implant treatment plan. (D) Final implant placement.

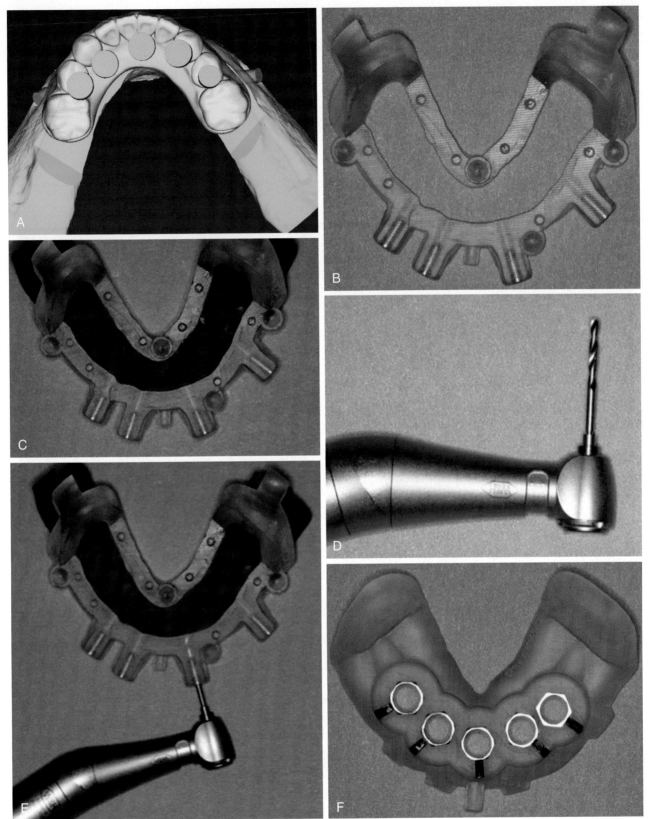

• **Fig. 15.30** Stackable Guides. (A) Interactive treatment plan. (B and C) Stackable reduction guide. (D and E) Fixation screws. (F) Implant placement guide. (G) Implant placement. (H) Abutments inserted. (I) Nonengaging abutment. (J) Gasket placement. (K and L) Polymethylmethacrylate temporary.

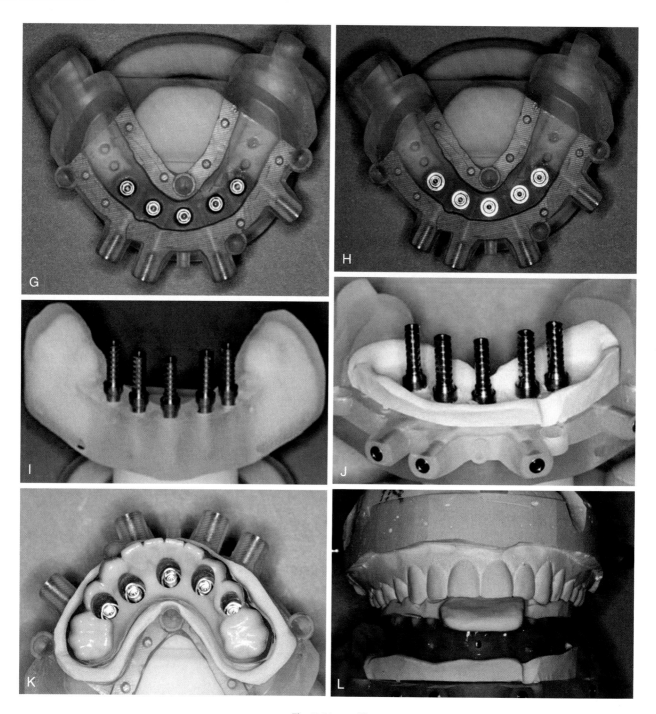

• **Fig. 15.30, cont'd**

The prototypic workflow for CAD/CAM typically begins with the accumulation of data either intraorally or from model-based scanners. The acquired digital data are processed using various specialized computer programs that build 3D-specific information via modeling algorithms. The information then can be analyzed and the acquired data altered via dental-specific CAD software to design a full array of restorations (Box 15.8).

Optical Impressions

Digital optical impressions are becoming the ideal and most accurate technique to be integrated into the clinical practice workflow. This technology is user friendly and requires a minimal learning curve. Digital impressions are advantageous over

---

• **BOX 15.8** Definitions

CAD/CAM: computer-aided design/computer-aided manufacturing
Stereolithographic guide: Surgical guides that assist placement of implants to coincide with the planned position using stereolithography (3D layering/printing) to create solid plastic 3D objects from CAD drawings by selectively solidifying an ultraviolet-sensitive liquid resin (photopolymer) using a laser beam
STL file: file for stereolithographic CAD systems
Computer-guided surgery (static): use of a static surgical template that reproduces the virtual implant position directly from CBCT data and does not allow intraoperative modification of the position of the implant
Computer-navigated surgery (dynamic): use of a surgical navigation system that directly reproduces the virtual implant position from the CBCT data and allows for intraoperative implant position changes

- Eliminates the need for traditional impressions
- Eliminates the need for bite registrations
- Increases marginal accuracy
- Decreases the number of appointments
- Improves workflow efficiency

traditional techniques in that they are more efficient, less time consuming, give greater patient comfort, and increase the profitability of the dental practice. The optical scan produces a positive replica of the teeth and tissues, not a negative replica such as a conventional impression. The position of teeth, soft tissue contours, existing restorations, edentulous spaces, and occlusal contacts can be evaluated easily using the high-resolution 3D images.

Studies have shown the accuracy of optical impressions to be far greater than conventional techniques. Because no dimensional discrepancies exist, such as with conventional impressions, the accuracy is far superior. In addition, instantaneous diagnosis and treatment planning can be accomplished, along with user-friendly patient educational resources (Box 15.9).

Digital Systems

Two types of digital systems are used today for clinical dentistry: (1) digital impression systems, and (2) CAD/CAM systems with clinical oriented software. For the dental laboratory, there exists a full spectrum of technology, including scanners, milling machines, and rapid prototype units. The dental laboratory has available greater sophisticated technology that is based on the CAD/CAM workflow of digital data, which are sent by the dental office. The data is usually transmitted electronically to the dental laboratory for use in multiple applications, which may include study cast fabrication, prosthetic design, implant treatment planning, and restoration fabrication. After obtaining the digital impression data, the laboratory may convert the digital impression into an analog model through the milling or rapid prototyping techniques.

Most CAD/CAM systems today require a direct method of data input for capture of intraoral conditions into the CAD software. These systems use a digital intraoral camera or scanner for image acquisition directly in the oral cavity. Some chairside CAD/CAM systems use intraoral camera systems to scan stone master casts produced by the clinician via the traditional technique. However, the goal of the digital impression system is to replace the traditional analog method of recording a patient's intraoral condition through the traditional impression technique.

Most of these digital chairside impression systems include both the hardware for scanning and the software for management of patient data. The learning curves with the various systems differ slightly, with the understanding of the specific imaging modality of the individual scanner (static images versus video streaming) being paramount.[24]

Digital Scanner Process

The digital scanner software will capture and store the digital data from the intraoral scan and also record all of the necessary medical and prescription information. The accumulated data are archived within the computer and then transmitted digitally to the laboratory via the Internet. Once transmitted, the data may be used by the dental laboratory for evaluation, design, or milling for the particular case. The laboratory may convert the digital impression into an analog model through the process of milling or rapid prototyping such as stereolithography.[25] After model fabrication, the laboratory may initiate a direct restoration or use the model as a reference or evaluation of the final CAD/CAM restoration (Fig. 15.31).

For chairside CAD/CAM systems the intraoral camera or scanner is capable of both designing and milling within the office setting; however, greater skill set is required.

Studies have shown that digital systems are more accurate than traditional techniques; however, meticulous care must be exercised in proper setup, consistent protocols, and calibration of milling parameters to ensure accuracy.[26]

Implant Treatment Planning

Significant improvements in CAD/CAM systems have allowed chairside and laboratory workflows to be integrated into implant therapy. CAD x-ray software has led to advancements in implant treatment planning and guided implant surgery. With the use of CBCT data, special implant software has allowed the integration of CAD data from digital impression systems to aid in restorative implant planning and placement. The specialized software may virtually wax-up teeth that is based on a functional and esthetic position, and export the virtual restoration into a CBCT software environment that aids in ideal implant positioning by use of a surgical template.

Restorative Implant Applications

CAD/CAM restorative applications have expanded into implant-level digital impressions, design and milling of custom healing abutments, custom prosthetic abutments, interim restorations, single-tooth prostheses, multiple and full arch prostheses, overdenture bar substructures, and telescopic implant prosthetics (Figs. 15.32–15.34).

Laboratory Implant Applications

Laboratories now have the capability to transition traditional clinical impressions and master casts to CAD/CAM implant prostheses. There exists a full array of laboratory-based benchtop scanners that vary from small scanners for simple impression, die, and model scanning, to large scanners that allow for scanning of fully articulated models.

Materials

Major advancements have been made in CAD/CAM technology, including material type, strength, chemistry, biocompatibility, and esthetics. Glass ceramic materials may be used for chairside fabrication of single-tooth restorations that can be adhesively bonded, with the future allowing for multiple teeth restorations. Materials such as zirconium oxide, commercially pure titanium, titanium alloy, noble metals and alloys, composite resins, wax, and fiber-reinforced acrylics are primarily the mainstay of laboratory-processed restorations. Laboratory-based CAD/CAM materials are supplied in a form where multiple restorations may be milled within one large blank of material (monolithic) to reduce material waste and costs.

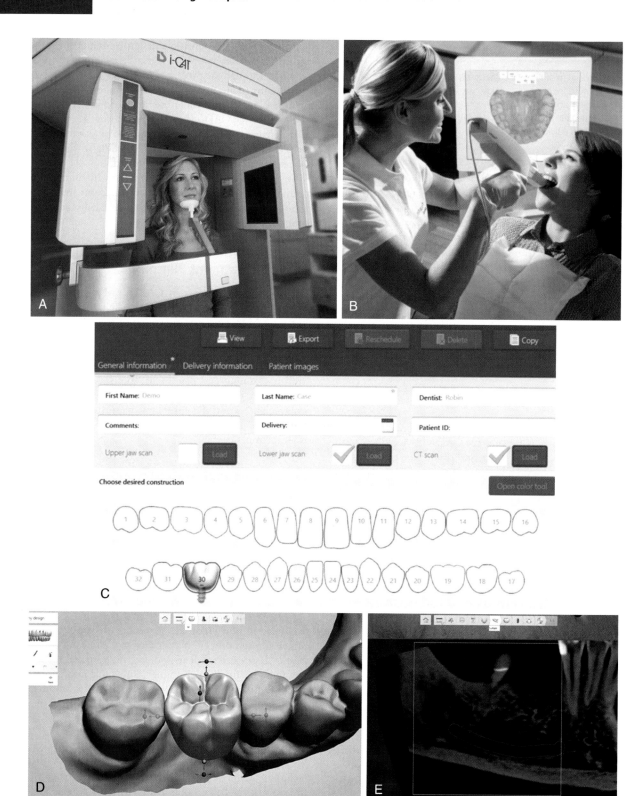

• **Fig. 15.31** Integration of cone beam computed tomography (CBCT), digital scanning, and specialized software to fabricate an in-office surgical template: (A and B) step 1: upload CBCT scan + surface scan into implant studio, (C) implant treatment planning, (D) prosthesis development, (E) nerve position verified, (F) final implant position, (G–I) guide development, (J–L) final plan, and (M) final template.

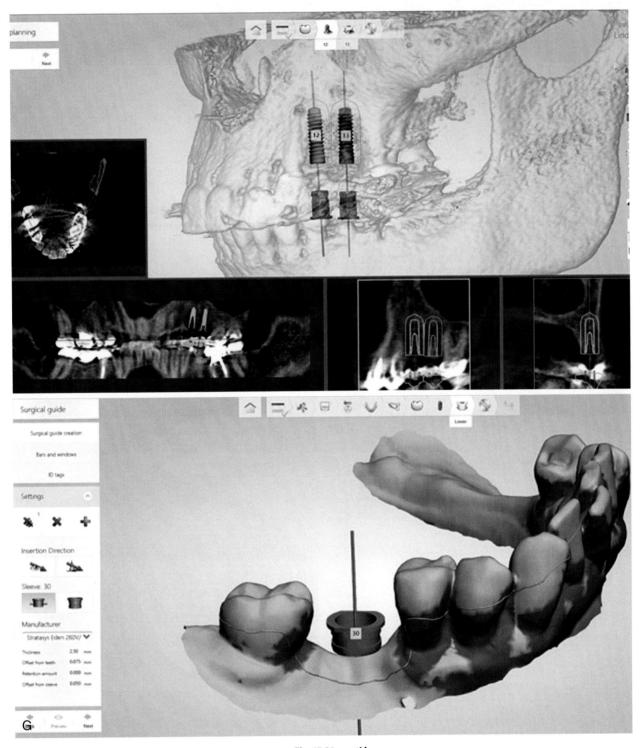

• Fig. 15.31, cont'd

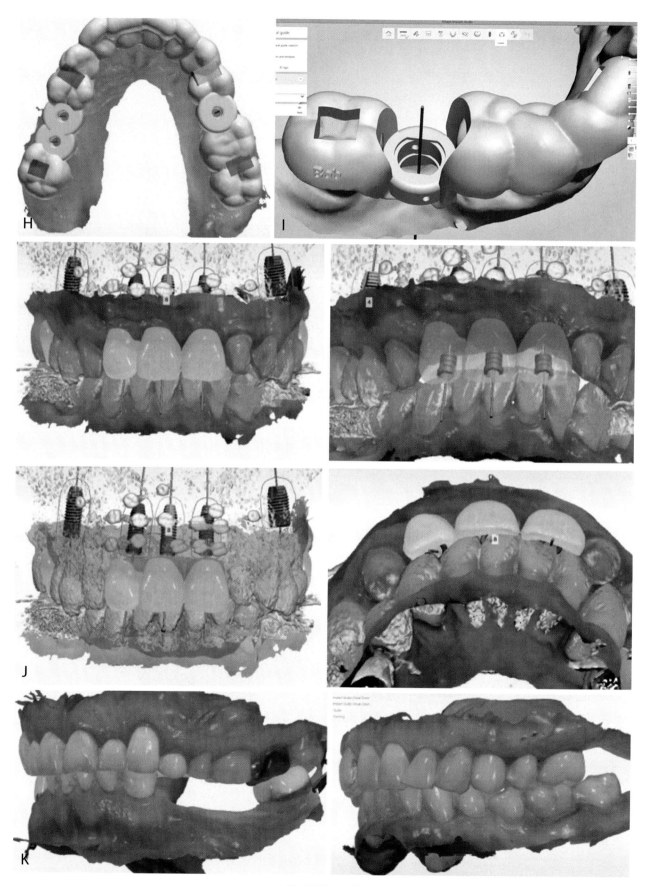

• Fig. 15.31, cont'd

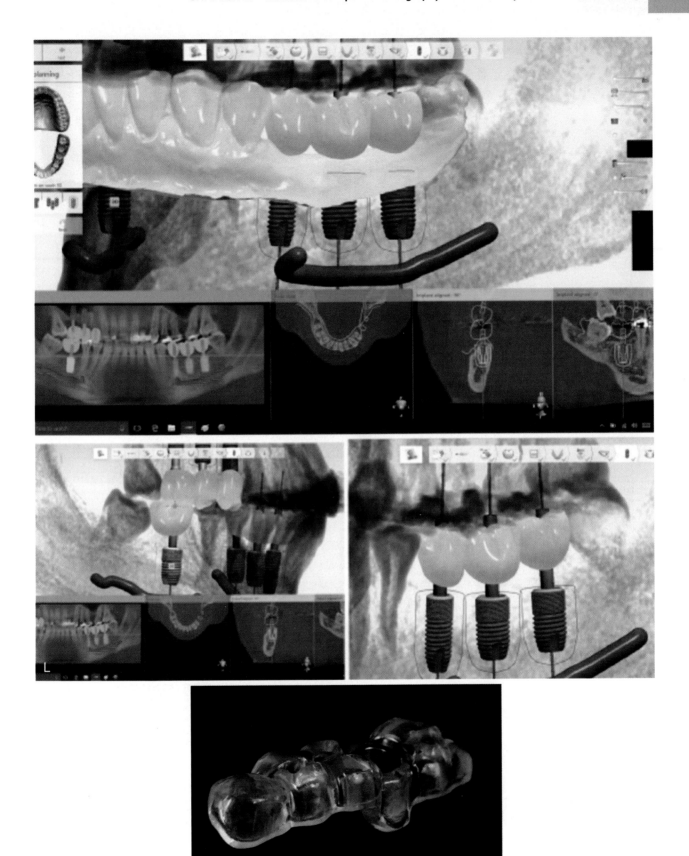

• Fig. 15.31, cont'd

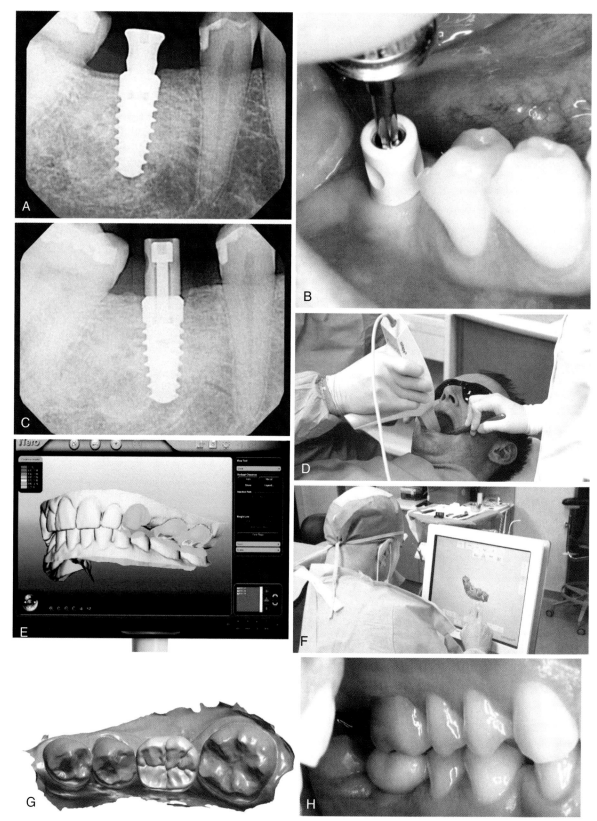

• **Fig. 15.32** Digital Impression Technique. (A) Implant placement. (B) Scanning abutment placed. (C) Verification of complete seating of abutment. (D) Digital impression. (E and F) Design of crown with specialized software. (G) In-office crown milling. (H) Final restoration.

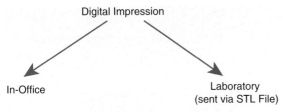

Digital Impression

In-Office

Laboratory
(sent via STL File)

• **Fig. 15.33** Types of Digital Impressions.

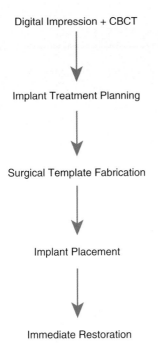

Digital Impression + CBCT

Implant Treatment Planning

Surgical Template Fabrication

Implant Placement

Immediate Restoration

• **Fig. 15.34** Immediate Placement/Restoration Protocol.

Surgical Template Complications

Overheating the Bone

Because of the tolerances between the drill size and the surgical template tubes (i.e., usually less than 0.2 mm), inadequate irrigation often results. It is imperative to use as much irrigation as possible to prevent this complication.

1. This may involve the use of supplemental irrigation in the form of external irrigation (i.e., monoject curved syringe). In most templates the facial aspect may be altered, which allows for the delivery of additional saline solution (Fig. 15.35).
2. "Bone dance" preparation is most important in better quality bone (D1 or D2 bone). Bone dancing includes preparing the osteotomy in a "pumping" motion, which allows irrigation to enter into the template tube and osteotomy.[27]
3. Refrigerate irrigation: Barrak et al.[28] showed that cooling the irrigation fluid to 10°C is a safe method for implant site preparation and drilling through a drilling guide in terms of temperature control. The results showed no mean increase in temperature resulted. Therefore the sterile saline irrigation fluid may be stored in a refrigerator before surgical procedures.[28]

Inadequate Access

A common complication with surgical templates may exist with posterior implant placement. Because most guided drills are longer than standard surgical drills, in many cases the clinician may not have sufficient interarch space to drill the osteotomies (Fig. 15.36). In addition, most tubes used in surgical templates are approximately 5 mm in height, which further increases the difficulty in drill access. Many surgical template manufacturers may fabricate "buccal" or "lingual" accesses within the guides, which allows the clinician greater access (Fig. 15.37).

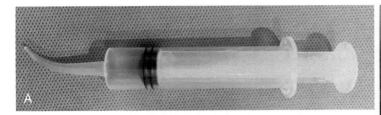

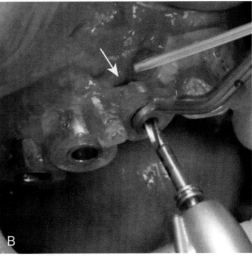

• **Fig. 15.35** (A) Monoject Curved Syringe, (B) Facial aspect of template altered to allow for external irrigation.

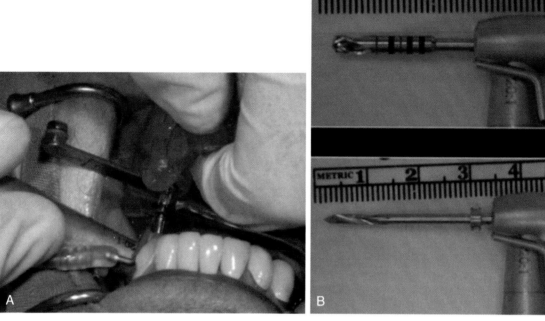

• **Fig. 15.36** (A) Posterior implant placement with cone beam computed tomography (CBCT) template limits available room for access. (B) Standard surgical drill versus guided drill with depth stopper is approximately 10 mm longer.

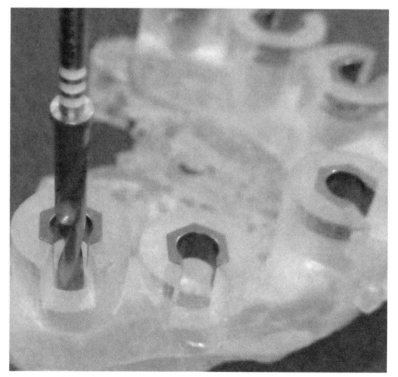

• **Fig. 15.37** Lateral Access Drilling Tube. Surgical drill is inserted from the lateral access, thereby decreasing amount of interocclusal space by approximately 5 mm. This allows for easier posterior guided implant placement in compromised interocclusal space cases.

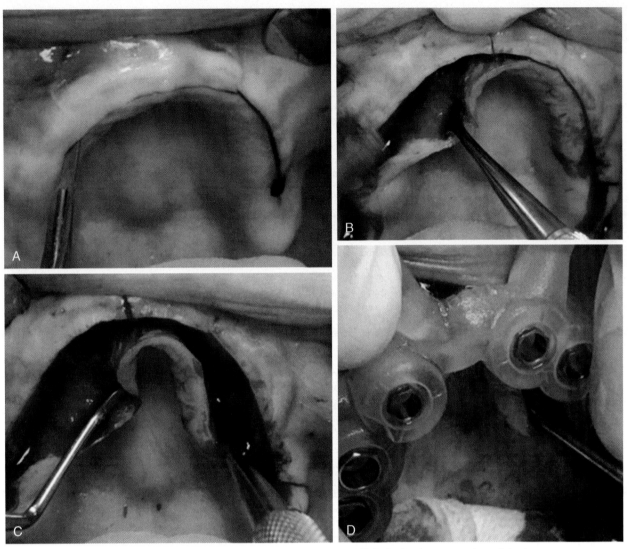

• **Fig. 15.38** Difficulty in Seating Template. (A) Incision. (B and C) Reflection for access of template placement. (D) Seating template underneath soft tissue flap.

Difficulty in Template Seating

With bone-supported guides, many clinicians may have difficulty in seating the template because of the extent of required reflection. It is imperative that the template seats completely on bone, and no soft tissue prevents the seating. Therefore the incision and reflection should be preplanned to accommodate the size and peripheral extent of the surgical template (Fig. 15.38).

Summary

Digital technology is responsible for the most innovative advancement that dentistry has ever seen. Being able to obtain a digital replica of the oral-facial structures to enhance diagnosis and treatment planning, along with the use in surgical and prosthetic treatments, has changed implant dentistry forever. Optical scans of the teeth and soft tissue can be combined with 3D CBCT images to even further enhance the scope of implant dentistry. These advances in both CAD/CAM technology and dental material science are paving the future for applications of digital implant dentistry. The digital systems for CAD/CAM dentistry have allowed for the clinical workflow and final clinical outcomes for patient therapy in implant dentistry. As the CAD/CAM systems continue to evolve, the research and clinical evidence of the effectiveness of CAD/CAM dentistry will take implant dentistry to the next level.

References

1. Basten CHJ, Kois JC. The use of barium sulfate for implant templates. *J Prosthet Dent.* 1996;76(4):451–454.
2. Plemons JM, Watkins P, et al. Barium-coated surgical stent and computer-assisted tomography in the preoperative assessment of dental implant patients. *Int J Periodontics Restorative Dent.* 1992;12:52–61.
3. Resnik, R. "Dual CBCT Scanning Technique for Completely Edentulous Arches." *Dentistry today* 35, no. 12 (2016): 50-52.
4. Scarfe William C, Farman Allan G. What is cone-beam CT and how does it work? *Dental Clinics.* 2008;52(4):707–730.
5. Chau A. Comparison between the use of magnetic resonance imaging and conebeam computed tomography for mandibular nerve identification. *Clin Oral Implant Res.* 2012;23:253–256.

6. Lofthag-Hansen S, Gröndahl K, Ekestubbe A. Cone-beam CT for preoperative implant planning in the posterior mandible: visibility of anatomic landmarks. *Clin Implant Dent Relat Res.* 2009;11:246.

7. Hebel MKS, Gajjar R. Anatomic basis for implant selection and positioning. In: Babbush C, ed. *Dental Implants: the Art and Science.* Philadelphia: WB Saunders; 2001:85–103.

8. Ozan O, Turkyilmaz I, Ersoy AE, et al. Clinical accuracy of 3 different types of computed tomography-derived stereolithographic surgical guides in implant placement. *J Oral Maxillofac Surg.* 2009;67(2):394–401.

9. Nickenig HJ, Wichmann M, Hamel J, et al. Evaluation of the difference in accuracy between implant placement by virtual planning data and surgical guide templates versus the conventional free-hand method–a combined in vivo–in vitro technique using cone-beam CT (Part II). *J Oral Maxillofac Surg.* 2010;38(7):488–493.

10. Turbush SK, Turkyilmaz I. Accuracy of three different types of stereolithographic surgical guide in implant placement: an in vitro study. *J Prosthet Dent.* 2012;108(3):181–188.

11. Lal K, White GS, Morea DN, Wright RF. Use of stereolithographic templates for surgical and prosthodontic implant planning and placement. Part I. The concept. *J Prosthodont.* 2006;15:51–58.

12. Lal K, White GS, Morea DN, Wright RF. Use of stereolithographic templates for surgical and prosthodontic implant planning and placement. Part II. A clinical report. *J Prosthodont.* 2006;15:117–122.

13. Molé C, Gérard H, Mallet JL, et al. A new three-dimensional treatment algorithm for complex surfaces: applications in surgery. *J Oral Maxillofac Surg.* 1995;53:158–162.

14. Nikzad S, Azari A. A novel stereolithographic surgical guide template for planning treatment involving a mandibular dental implant. *J Oral Maxillofac Surg.* 2008;66(7):1446–1454.

15. Ewers R, Schicho K, Truppe M, et al. Computer-aided navigation in dental implantology: 7 years of clinical experience. *J Oral Maxillofac Surg.* 2004;62:329e34.

16. Birkfellner W, Solar P, Gahleitner A, et al. In-vitro assessment of a registration protocol for image guided implant dentistry. *Clin Oral Implants Res.* 2001;12:69e78.

17. Siessegger M, Schneider BT, Mischkowski RA, et al. Use of an image-guided navigation system in dental implant surgery in anatomically complex operation sites. *J Craniomaxillofac Surg.* 2001;29:276e81.

18. Sukegawa S, Kanno T, Furuki Y. Application of computer-assisted navigation systems in oral and maxillofacial surgery. *Japanese Dental Science Review.*

19. Solar P, Grampp S, Gsellmann B. A computer-assisted navigation for oral implant surgery using 3D-CT reconstruction and real time video-projection. In: Farman AG, ed. *Computer Assisted Radiology—CAR.* Amsterdam: Elsevier; 1996.

20. Shapira L. Image-guided implantology: real-time guidance of dental implant surgery in the operative field using CT-scan image. In: Vannier MW, Inamura K, Farman AG, et al., eds. *Proceedings of the 16th International Congress, Computer-Assisted Radiology and Surgery.* Paris: France; 2002.

21. Gaggl A, Schultes G. Assessment of accuracy of navigated implant placement in the maxilla. *Int J Oral Maxillofac Implants.* 2002;17:263–270.

22. Casap N, Wexler A, Persky N, et al. Navigation surgery for dental implants: assessment of accuracy of the image guided implantology system. *Oral Maxillofac Surg.* 2004;62:116–119.

23. Nickenig HJ, Eitner S, Rothamel D, Wichmann M, Zoller JE. Possibilities and limitations of implant placement by virtual planning data and surgical guide templates. *Int J Comput Dent.* 2012;15(1):9–21.

24. Seelbach P, Brueckel C, Wöstmann B. Accuracy of digital and conventional impression techniques and workflow. *Clin Oral Investig.* 2013;17(7):1759–1764.

25. Dunne P. Digital dentistry and SLA technology. *Lab Management Today.* 2008;Nov/Dec:44-45.

26. Fasbinder DJ, Neiva GF, Dennison JB, et al. Evaluation of zirconia crowns made from conventional and digital impressions [abstract]. *J Dent Res.* 2012;91 (speciss A). Abstract 644.

27. Jeong SM, Yoo JH, Fang Y, Choi BH, Son JS, Oh JH. The effect of guided flapless implant procedure on heat generation from implant drilling. *J Craniomaxillofac Surg.* 2014;42(6):725–729.

28. Barrak I, Joób-Fancsaly A, Varga E, Boa K, Piffko J. Effect of the combination of low-speed drilling and cooled irrigation fluid on intraosseous heat generation during guided surgical implant site preparation: an in vitro study. *Implant dentistry.* 2017;26(4):541–546.

29. Misch CE. *Contemporary Implant Dentistry.* 3rd ed. St Louis: Mosby; 2008.

16

Available Bone and Dental Implant Treatment Plans

CARL E. MISCH AND RANDOLPH R. RESNIK

Long-term success in implant dentistry requires the evaluation of more than 50 dental criteria, many of which are unique to this discipline.[1] However, the doctor's training and experience, and the amount and density of available bone in the edentulous site of the patient, are arguably the primary determining factors in predicting individual patient success. Today the prosthodontic requirements and desires of the patient should be determined first; then an array of factors that include patient force factors, bone density, key implant positions, implant number, and size evaluated. In the past the available bone was not modified and was the primary intraoral factor influencing the treatment plan. Greenfield,[2] as early as 1913, documented the importance of the amount of available bone. However, with the predictability of bone augmentation today, patients with even large osseous defects are becoming candidates for dental implants. Therefore this chapter will describe the three-dimensional concept of available bone and the implant treatment options (Misch classification) for each type of bone anatomy.

Literature Review

The process of bone volume atrophy after tooth loss and loss of alveolus has been fully documented in the literature (Fig. 16.1).[3-19] Characteristic bone volume changes after tooth loss were evaluated in the anterior mandible by Atwood (Fig. 16.2).[4-6] The six described residual ridge stages are beneficial to appreciate the shapes and range of bone loss. Tallgren[7] reported the amount of bone loss occurring the first year after tooth loss is almost 10 times greater than the following years. The posterior edentulous mandible resorbs at a rate approximately four times faster than the anterior edentulous mandible.[8]

It has been suggested that, in the mandibular symphysis, females present higher total reduction and more rapid bone loss during the first 2 years.[9] More recent studies in complete denture wearers have confirmed the higher rate of resorption in the first year of edentulouness.[10,11] The anterior maxilla resorbs in height slower than the anterior mandible. However, the original height of available bone in the anterior mandible is twice as much as the anterior maxilla. Therefore the resultant maxillary atrophy, although slower, affects the potential available bone for an implant patient with equal frequency.[7] The changes in the edentulous anterior maxillary ridge dimension can be dramatic in height and width (up to 70%),

especially when multiple extractions are performed.[12] In addition, many patients lose additional bone by simultaneous alveolectomy procedures after tooth extraction before the delivery of a maxillary denture.[13] Although slight differences exist between different alveolectomy techniques, all are detrimental to the ridge volume.[14]

The residual ridge shifts palatally in the maxilla and lingually in the mandible as related to tooth position, at the expense of the buccal cortical plate in all areas of the jaws, regardless of the number of teeth missing.[15-19] However, after the initial bone loss, the maxilla continues to resorb toward the midline, whereas the mandibular basal bone is wider than the original alveolar bone position and results in the late mandible resorption progressing facially. This, in addition to a marked change in mandibular position, leads to the classical appearance of the denture wearer with a protruding chin and a mandibular lip.[20] The posterior maxilla loses bone volume faster than any other region. Not only can periodontal disease cause initial bone loss before the loss of teeth, the crestal bone loss is substantial after tooth extraction. In addition, the maxillary sinus after tooth loss expands toward the crest of the edentulous ridge. As a result the posterior maxilla is more often indicated for bone augmentation compared with any other intraoral location. In 1974, Weiss and Judy[21] developed a classification of mandibular atrophy and its influence on subperiosteal implant therapy. In 1982, Kent[22] presented a classification of alveolar ridge deficiency designed for alloplastic bone augmentation. Another bone volume classification was proposed by Lekholm and Zarb[23] in 1985 for residual jaw morphology related to the insertion of Brånemark fixtures. They described five stages of jaw resorption, ranging from minimal to extreme (Fig. 16.3). The mandibular resorption was described only in loss of height. All of the five stages of resorption in either arch used the same implant modality, surgical approach, and type of final prosthesis. In addition, as the bone volume decreased, the number of implants decreased.

A maxillary alveolar process of resorption after tooth loss after Atwood's description for the mandible was presented by Fallschüssel[24] in 1986. The six resorption categories of this arch ranged from fully preserved to moderately wide and high, narrow and high, sharp and high, wide and reduced in height, and severely atrophic. The classifications of Atwood, Zarb and Lekholm, and Fallschüssel do not describe the actual resorption process in chronologic order and are more descriptive of the residual bone.[25] Another bone resorption classification, which included the expansion of the maxillary sinuses, was also proposed by Cawood and Howell[26] in 1988. Although similar to other categories, the bone volume changes are not reflective of the changes required for implant placement or bone-grafting procedures.

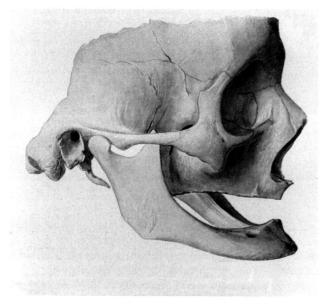

• **Fig. 16.1** Maxillary and mandibular atrophy after tooth loss was documented by J. Misch in 1922.

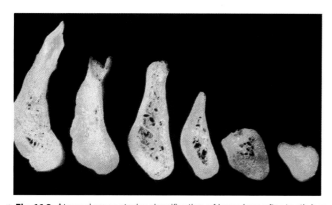

• **Fig. 16.2** Atwood presented a classification of bone loss after tooth loss in the anterior mandible in 1963.

In 1985, Misch and Judy established four basic divisions of available bone for implant dentistry in the edentulous maxilla and mandible, which follow the natural resorption phenomena of each region, and determined a different implant approach to each category.[1,27-33] The angulation of bone and crown height were also included for each bone volume, because they affect the prosthetic treatment. These original four divisions of bone were further expanded with two subcategories to provide an organized approach to implant treatment options for surgery, bone grafting, and prosthodontics (Fig. 16.4). The ability to organize the available bone of the potential implant site into specific related categories of common treatment options and conditions is of benefit to both the beginning and experienced clinician alike. Improved communication among health professionals and the collection of relevant specific data for each category are also beneficial. The Misch-Judy bone classification has facilitated these processes during the past three decades within the profession, universities, implant programs, and international implant societies. To understand the available bone classification, the clinician must first have a knowledge of dental implant size (i.e., width or diameter and height or length).

Implant Size

The category and design of the final prosthesis and key implant positions are first determined after a patient interview and evaluation of existing medical and dental conditions. The patient force factors and bone density are of particular note. The abutments necessary to support the restoration are then established in implant number and size, and without initial regard to the available bone conditions.

Implant Width (Diameter)

Manufacturers describe the root form implant in dimensions of width and length (e.g., Hahn 4.3 mm × 16.0 mm). The implant length corresponds to the height of available bone. Therefore this text refers to root form implant height or length. The width of a root form implant is most often related to the diameter and mesiodistal length of available bone. Most root form implants have a round cross-sectional design to aid in surgical placement; therefore the diameter of the implant corresponds to the implant width. Many manufacturers propose implants with a crest module wider than

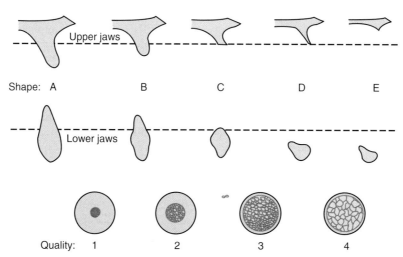

• **Fig. 16.3** Lekholm and Zarb presented a classification of bone loss in the edentulous jaws in 1985.

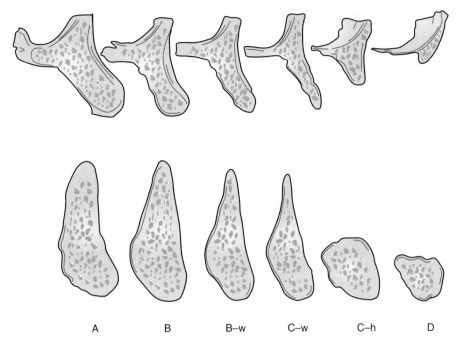

A   B   B–w   C–w   C–h   D

• **Fig. 16.4** In 1985, Misch and Judy presented a classification of available bone (Divisions A, B, C, and D), which is similar in both arches. Implant, bone grafting methods, and prosthodontic-related treatment were suggested for each category of bone. *h*, Inadequate height; *w*, inadequate width.

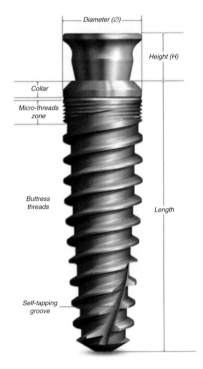

Diameter (∅)

Height (H)

Collar

Micro-threads zone

Buttress threads

Length

Self-tapping groove

• **Fig. 16.5** Tapered dental implant showing width and length along with distinct difference between crest diameter and body. (*From Glidewell Dental, Newport Beach, California.*)

the implant body dimension. Yet the often-stated dimension of the manufacturer is the smaller body width. For example, the Nobel Biocare 3.75-mm-diameter implant has a 4.1-mm crest module. The clinician should be knowledgeable of all implant dimensions, especially because the crestal dimension of bone (where the wider crest module dimension is placed) is usually the narrowest region of the available bone and where the implant is closest to an adjacent tooth (Fig. 16.5).

All teeth are not equal when considered as abutments for a prosthesis. The restoring dentist knows how to evaluate the surface area of the natural abutment roots. A healthy maxillary first molar with more than 450 mm² of root surface area constitutes a better abutment for a fixed prosthesis than a mandibular lateral incisor with 150 mm² of root support. The larger-diameter teeth correspond to the regions of the mouth with greater bite force. It is interesting to note the increase in surface area for natural teeth is most dependent on diameter and a change in design, more so than length.

All sizes and designs of implants do not have the same surface area and should not be considered as equals for prosthetic abutments. With a greater surface area of implant–bone contact, less stress is transmitted to the bone, and the implant prognosis improved. For a generic cylinder root form implant design, each 0.25-mm increase in diameter corresponds to a surface area increase of approximately 5% to 8%. Therefore a cylinder root form implant 1 mm greater in diameter will have a total surface area increase of approximately 20% to 30%. Because stress (S) equals force (F) divided by the functional area (A) over which it is applied (S = F/A), the greater diameter decreases the amount of stress at the crestal bone–implant interface. Because early bone loss relates to the crestal bone regions and prosthetic complications may be related to the crest module size of an implant, the width of the implant is much more critical than its height, after a minimum height has been obtained.

Implant Height (Length)

The height of the implant also affects its total surface area. A cylinder root form implant 3 mm longer provides a 20% to 30% increase in surface area. The advantage of increased height does not express itself at the crestal bone interface, but rather in initial stability of the implant, the overall amount of bone–implant interface, and a greater resistance to rotational torque during abutment screw tightening. The increased height of an implant in an

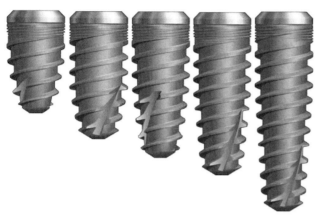

• **Fig. 16.6** Implant Length. Most implant systems include various implant sizes varying in length, with "long" implants being approximately 16 mm and "short" implants being approximately ~8 mm in length. *(From Glidewell Dental, Newport Beach, California.)*

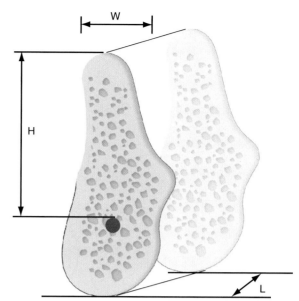

• **Fig. 16.7** Available bone is measured in height (H), width (W), and length (L). Also considered are crown height space and angulation of bone (direction of force to the implant body).

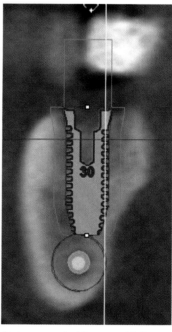

• **Fig. 16.8** Cone beam computed tomographic image of implant placement with 2 mm safety zone to prevent neurosensory impairment.

immediate extraction site larger in diameter than the implant also increases the initial bone contact percent, which can decrease the initial risk for movement at the interface. In addition, the crestal bone and opposing anatomic landmark are often composed of cortical bone, which is denser and stronger than trabecular bone. As a result, it may help stabilize the implant while the trabecular woven bone forms. In this way a direct bone–implant interface is encouraged. This may be of particular advantage when an immediate-loading protocol of implants is used for a transitional prosthesis. However, after the implant has healed, the crestal region is the zone that receives the majority of the stress. As a result, implant length is not as effective as the width to decrease crestal loads around an implant (i.e., prevent future bone loss).

The minimum height for long-term survival of endosteal implants is in part related to the density of bone. The denser bone may accommodate a shorter implant (i.e., 8 mm), and the least dense, weaker bone requires a longer implant (i.e., 12 mm). After the minimum implant height is established for each implant design and bone density, the width is more important than additional length. This chapter primarily presents the volume of bone requirements for ideal bone density situations or D2, which is coarse trabecular bone surrounded by porous to dense cortical bone.

Before 1981 the Brånemark screw–type implant body and osteointegrated approach was provided as a single diameter (3.75 mm) and was used only in the completely edentulous anterior maxilla and mandible.[34] The implant drills cut 10 mm deep, and the "10-mm" implant was 9 mm in length. By 1990 this philosophy had been expanded to all jaw regions and many implant sizes. However, failure rates reported in the literature for implants shorter than 9 mm tended to be higher independently from the manufacturer design, surface characteristic, and type of application.[35-50] For many years there existed a 12-mm height minimum that applied to most screw-shape endosteal implant designs in good-density (D2) bone.[51-53] However, with newer implant designs and implant coatings, this has been disproved. Currently many studies are available that discuss the high success of short dental implants (~8 mm). With newer implant designs and implant coatings, shorter length implants are gaining acceptance (Fig. 16.6).

Measurement of Available Bone

Available bone describes the amount of bone in the edentulous area considered for implantation. It is measured in width, height, length, angulation, and crown height space (CHS; Fig. 16.7).

Historically the available bone was never modified, and it dictated the implant position and size (or contraindicated implant treatment). Today if the bone is inadequate to support an ideal abutment for the intended prosthesis or bone grafting, the ideal site is often indicated, or an alternative site may be considered. As a general guideline, 2 mm of surgical error is maintained between the implant and a vital structure. Unfortunately, today many implants are placed in violation of this principle, leading to complications and morbidity of the patient. For example, implants placed too close to the mandibular canal may result in neurosensory impairment (Fig. 16.8). Implants placed into the nasal cavity or maxillary sinus may result in infection. Therefore, when evaluating an edentulous site, bone may be evaluated in four parameters: (1) height, (2) width, (3) length, and (4) angulation.

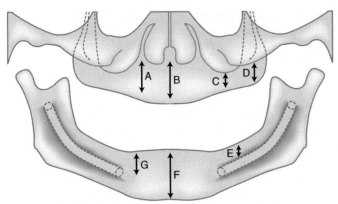

• **Fig. 16.9** The height of available bone is measured from the crest of the edentulous ridge to the opposing landmark. The opposing landmark may be in the maxillary canine region (*A*), floor of the nares (*B*), maxillary sinus (*C*), tuberosity (*D*), bone above the inferior mandibular canal (*E*), anterior mandible (*F*), or mandibular canine region (*G*).

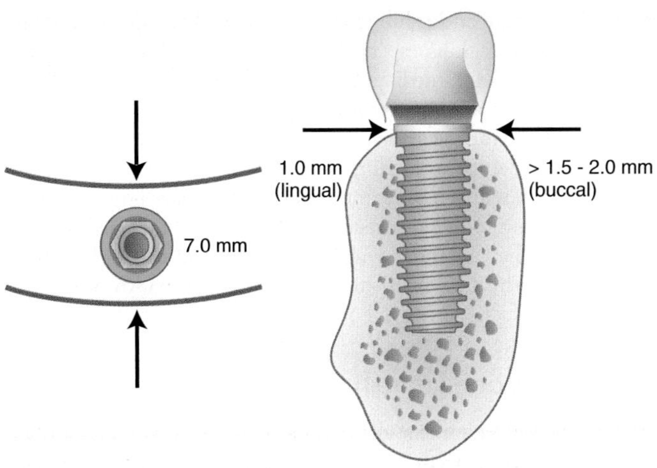

• **Fig. 16.10** Minimum bone width for a 4-mm-diameter root form is 7 mm to allow for greater than 1.5 mm on the buccal and a minimum of 1.0 mm on the lingual.

Available Bone Height

The available bone height is first estimated by radiographic evaluation in the edentulous ideal and optional regions, where implant abutments are required for the intended prosthesis. A cone beam computed tomography (CBCT) survey is the most common method for the determination of the available bone height.

The height of available bone is measured from the crest of the edentulous ridge to the opposing landmark. The anterior regions are limited by the maxillary nares or the inferior border of the mandible. Usually the anterior regions of the jaws have the greatest height, because the maxillary sinus and inferior alveolar nerve limit this dimension in the posterior regions. The maxillary canine eminence region often offers the greatest height of available bone in the maxillary anterior.[54] In the posterior jaw region, there is usually greater bone height in the maxillary first premolar than in the second premolar, which has greater height than the molar sites because of the concave morphology of the maxillary sinus floor. Likewise the mandibular first premolar region is commonly anterior to the mental foramen and provides the most vertical column of bone in the posterior mandible. However, on occasion, this premolar site may present a reduced height compared with the anterior region, because of the mental foramen position or the anterior loop of the mandibular canal (when present) as it passes below the foramen and proceeds superiorly, then distally, before its exit through the mental foramen (Fig. 16.9).

The dilemma of available bone in implant dentistry involves the existing anatomy of the edentulous mandible and maxilla. The initial mandibular bone height is influenced by skeletal anatomy, with angle Class II patients having shorter mandibular height, and angle Class III patients exhibiting the greatest height. The initial edentulous anterior maxillary available bone height is less than the mandibular available bone height. The opposing landmarks for the initial available bone height are more limiting in the posterior regions. The posterior mandibular region is reduced because of the presence of the mandibular canal, approximately situated 12 mm above the inferior border of the mandible. As a result, in the areas where greater forces are generated and the natural dentition has wider teeth with two or three roots, shorter implants, if any, are often used and in insufficient number because of the anatomic limiting factors. A study of 431 patients revealed that in the partially edentulous maxilla and mandible, the placement of posterior implants at least 6 mm in length was possible in only 38% and 50%, respectively. The anterior regions of edentulous arches could receive implants 55% and 61% of the time, respectively.[55] The existing bone anatomy of the implant patient often

requires modification to enhance long-term implant success. For example, sinus grafts in the posterior maxilla permit the placement of posterior endosteal implants into restored bone height.

The available bone height in an edentulous site is a crucial dimension for implant consideration, because it affects both implant length and crown height. Crown height affects force factors and esthetics. In addition, bone augmentation is more predictable in width than height, so even when the width is inadequate for implant placement, bone grafting may be used to create a site ideal for restorative and implant insertion requirements.

Available Bone Width

The width of available bone is measured between the facial and lingual plates at the crest of the potential implant site. The crest of the edentulous ridge is most often supported by a wider base. In most areas, because of this triangular-shaped cross section, an osteoplasty can be performed that results in a greater width of bone, although of reduced height. However, the anterior maxilla often does not follow this rule, because most edentulous ridges exhibit a labial concavity in the incisor area, with an hourglass configuration. Crest reduction affects the location of the opposing landmark, with possible consequences for surgery, implant height selection, appearance, and the design of the final prosthesis. This is particularly important when a type 1 fixed prosthesis (FP-1) is planned, with the goal of obtaining a normal contour and proper soft tissue drape around a single tooth replacement.

After adequate height is available, the next most significant criterion affecting long-term survival of endosteal implants is the width of the available bone. Root form implants of 4-mm crestal diameter usually require a minimum of 7 mm of bone width (4.0 mm + 2.0 mm buccal + 1.0 mm lingual) to ensure sufficient bone thickness and blood supply around the implant for predictable survival. These dimensions provide more than 1.5 mm of bone on the buccal side and at least 1.0 mm on the lingual side. When measuring necessary bone width, always determine the true diameter of the implant at the crest module, because many implant systems base the diameter on the root area of the implant, not the neck area. Because the bone usually widens apically, this minimum dimension rapidly increases. For root form implants the minimum bone thickness is located in the midfacial and midlingual contour of the crestal region exclusively (Fig. 16.10). The crestal aspect of the residual ridge is often cortical in nature and exhibits greater density than the underlying trabecular bone regions, especially in the mandible. This mechanical advantage permits immediate fixation of the implant, provided this cortical layer has not been removed by osteoplasty.

The initial width of available bone is related to the initial crestal bone loss after implant loading. Edentulous ridges that are greater than 6 mm in width have demonstrated less crestal bone loss than when minimum bone dimensions are available. In general, extraction sockets having more width at the crest also lose less bone during initial healing than sites with minimum width of cortical plates on the facial or lingual of the extraction site.

Available Bone Length

The mesiodistal length of available bone in an edentulous area is often limited by adjacent teeth or implants. As a general rule the implant should be at least 1.5 mm from an adjacent tooth and 3 mm from an adjacent implant. This dimension not only allows surgical error but also compensates for the width of an implant or tooth crestal defect, which is usually less than 1.4 mm. As a result, if bone loss occurs at the crest module of an implant or from periodontal disease with a tooth, the vertical bone defect will not spread to a horizontal defect and cause bone loss on the adjacent structure.[56] Therefore in the case of a single-tooth replacement, the minimum length of available bone necessary for an endosteal implant depends on the width of the implant. For example, a 5-mm-diameter implant should have at least 8 mm of mesiodistal bone, so a minimum of 1.5 mm is present on the buccal and 1.0 mm on the lingual. A minimum mesiodistal length of 7 mm is usually sufficient for a 4-mm-diameter implant. Of course the diameter of the implant is also related to the width of available bone and, in multiple adjacent sites, is primarily limited in this dimension. For example, a width of bone of 5.0 mm without augmentation requires a 3.5-mm or smaller implant, with inherent compromises (such as minimal surface area and greater crestal stress concentration under occlusal loads). Therefore in the narrower ridge, it is often indicated to place two or more narrow-diameter implants when possible to obtain sufficient implant–bone surface area to compensate for the deficiency in width of the implant. Because the implants should be 3 mm apart and 1.5 mm from each tooth, 13 mm or more (3.5 mm + 3.5 mm + 3.0 mm between implants + 1.5 mm + 1.5 mm from adjacent teeth) in available bone mesiodistal length may be required when the narrower implant dimensions are used to replace a posterior tooth.

The ideal implant width for single-tooth replacement or multiple adjacent implants is often related to the natural tooth being replaced in the site. The tooth has its greatest width at the interproximal contacts, is narrower at the cement-enamel junction (CEJ), and is even narrower at the initial crestal bone contact, which is ideally 2 to 3 mm below the CEJ (or 3 mm below the free gingival margin).[57] The ideal implant diameter corresponds to the width of the natural tooth 2 mm below the CEJ, if it also is 1.5 mm from the adjacent tooth. In this way, the implant crown emergence through the soft tissue may be similar to a natural tooth. For example, a maxillary first premolar is approximately 8 mm at the interproximal contact, 5 mm at the CEJ, and 4 mm at a point 2 mm below the CEJ. Therefore a 4-mm-diameter implant (at the crest module) would be the ideal implant diameter, if it also is at least 1.5 mm from the adjacent roots (2 mm below the CEJ) (Fig. 16.11).

Available Bone Angulation

Bone angulation is the fourth determinant for available bone. The initial alveolar bone angulation represents the natural tooth root trajectory in relation to the occlusal plane. Ideally it is perpendicular to the plane of occlusion, which is aligned with the forces of occlusion and is parallel to the long axis of the prosthodontic restoration. The incisal and occlusal surfaces of the teeth follow the curve of Wilson and curve of Spee. As such the roots of the maxillary teeth are angled toward a common point approximately 4 inches away. The mandibular roots flare, so the anatomic crowns are more lingually inclined in the posterior regions and labially inclined in the anterior area compared with the underlying roots. The first premolar cusp tip is usually vertical to its root apex.

The maxillary anterior teeth are the only segment in either arch that does not receive a long axis load to the tooth roots, but instead are usually loaded at a 12-degree angle. As such, their root diameter is greater than the mandibular anterior teeth. In all other regions of the mouth the teeth are loaded perpendicular to the curve of Wilson or curve of Spee. Rarely does the bone angulation remain ideal after the loss of teeth, especially in the anterior edentulous arch (Fig. 16.12). In this region, labial undercuts and resorption after tooth loss[12,15,16] often mandate greater angulation of the implants or correction of the site before insertion. In the posterior mandible the submandibular fossa mandates implant placement with increasing angulation as it progresses distally. Therefore in the mandibular second premolar region the angulation may be 10 degrees to a horizontal plane; in the first molar areas, 15 degrees; and in the second molar region, 20 to 25 degrees.

The limiting factor of angulation of force between the body and the abutment of an implant is correlated to the width of bone. In edentulous areas with a wide ridge, wider root form implants may be selected. Such implants may allow up to 25 degrees of divergence with the adjacent implants, natural teeth, or axial forces of occlusion with moderate compromise. The angled load to an implant body increases the crestal stresses, but the greater diameter implant decreases the amount of stress transmitted to the crestal bone. In addition, the greater width of bone offers some latitude in angulation at implant placement. The implant body may often be inserted so as to reduce the divergence of the abutments without compromising the permucosal site.

The narrow yet adequate width ridge often requires a narrower design root form implant. Compared with larger diameters, smaller-diameter designs cause greater crestal stress and may not offer the same range of custom abutments. In addition, the narrower width of bone does not permit as much latitude in placement regarding angulation within the bone. This limits the acceptable angulation of bone in the narrow ridge to 20 degrees from the axis of the adjacent clinical crowns or a line perpendicular to the occlusal plane.

Divisions of Available Bone

Division A (Abundant Bone)

Division A abundant bone often forms soon after the tooth is extracted. The abundant bone volume remains for a varied amount of time that is dependent on many factors. Studies have shown the original crestal width may be reduced by more than 30% within 2 years.[12] Division A bone corresponds to abundant available bone in all dimensions (Box 16.1 and Fig. 16.13). It should be emphasized that the available bone height may be greater than 20 mm for Division A, but this does not mean the implant length must be equal to the bone height. Because the stresses to the implant interface are dependent on bone density, the ideal implant length is bone-density and force-factor driven.

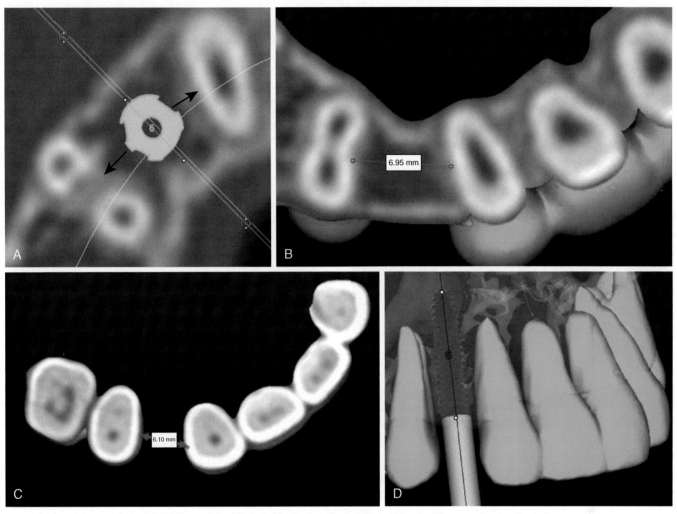

• **Fig. 16.11** (A) Determining ideal position between adjacent tooth roots, (B) measuring spacing between roots, (C) measuring clinical crown space, and (D) verifying ideal position in third dimension.

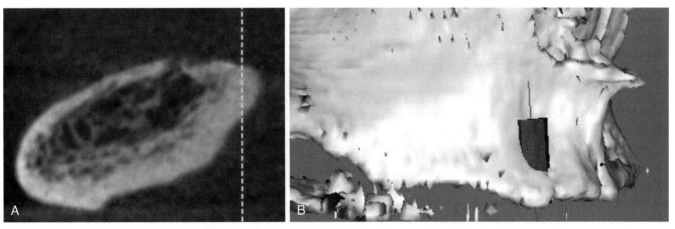

• **Fig. 16.12** Bone Angulation. (A) Mandibular anterior angulation contraindicating dental implants. (B) Maxillary anterior depicting nonideal bone trajectory issues because of extensive atrophy.

The Division A width of more than 6.5 mm (1.5 mm on buccal, 1.0 mm on lingual) is predicated on an implant diameter of at least 4 mm at the crest module, because abundant long-term data have been published regarding this implant size.[35,43] In abundant bone width (A+ bone) of greater than 7 mm a wider (5-mm-diameter) implant may be inserted, provided that 1.5 mm of bone remains around the buccal and 0.5 mm on the lingual aspects of the implant. Osteoplasty may often be performed to obtain additional bone width.

The implant choice in Division A bone is a root form of 4 mm or greater in diameter. A larger-diameter implant is suggested in the molar regions (5–6 mm in diameter). The length of the implant (8–16 mm) is primarily dependent on the bone density and secondarily dependent on the force factors. Longer implants

- Width > 7 mm
- Height > 10 mm
- Mesiodistal length > 7 mm
- Angulation of occlusal load (between occlusal plane and implant body) < 25 degrees
- CHS ≤ 15 mm
- Prosthesis:
  - Fixed: FP-1 likely, possible FP-2
  - Removable: RP-4 or RP-5

- The larger the diameter of an implant, the greater the surface area and the less stress distributed through the crestal bone region.
- The larger-diameter implants are closer to the lateral cortical plates of bone, which have greater density and therefore increased strength, modulus of elasticity, and bone-implant contact percentages.
- The larger-diameter implants are less likely to fracture, because the strength of the material is increased by a power of four related to the radius of the implant. (A 4-mm-diameter implant is 16 times stronger than a 2-mm-diameter implant.)
- The smaller-diameter implants (~ 3.0 mm) are often one piece to decrease the risk for fracture. The one-piece implants require an immediate restoration, rather than a submerged or one-stage approach. As such, likely loading and micromovement may occur at the bone–implant interface, with an increased risk for crestal bone loss and/or implant failure.
- The emergence profile angle of the crown is related to the implant diameter. The larger-diameter teeth can be most esthetically restored with a wider-diameter implant.
- The larger the implant diameter, the less stress applied to the abutment screw, and therefore complications such as screw loosening or fracture are less likely.
- The larger-diameter abutment provides greater cement retention for the final restoration crown.
- Oral hygiene procedures are more compromised around smaller-diameter implants restored with greater emergence profile angles and over contoured restorations.
- The crest module and crestal portion of many two-piece, small-diameter implants are smooth metal to increase the interbody wall thickness, thus creating shear loads to the crestal bone and an increased risk for bone loss.
- Implant costs to the patient are related to implant number, not diameter. Therefore increases in implant numbers for smaller-diameter implants increase the cost to the patient (and the doctor).
- Division A root form implants are designed for variable bone density and can provide the greatest range of prosthetic options.

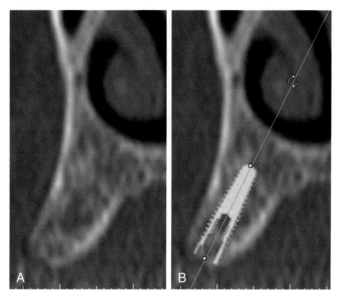

• **Fig. 16.13** Division A Bone. (A) Cone beam computed tomographic image depicting adequate bone width and length. (B) Because of adequate bone, Division A implant inserted ideally in the bone.

are usually suggested in immediate placement and loading treatment options. Division A bone ideally should not be treated with smaller-diameter implants for the final prosthesis. There are several advantages to the use of implants equal to or greater than 4 mm in diameter, compared with smaller-diameter implants (Box 16.2).

A patient with Division A bone should be educated that this is the most ideal time to restore his or her edentulous condition with implants. All too often the doctor fails to inform the patient about the rapid decrease in bone volume width and the consequences of delaying treatment. When the bone volume is Division A, there is a decrease in treatment costs, with a reduction in the number and complexity of surgeries to the edentulous area with significant benefits to the patient. Unfortunately, these patients may not have significant problems with their existing restoration and therefore may not be motivated to address the situation. As the bone resorbs and the problems arise, a greater appreciation for the benefits of implant-supported restorations are realized. Just as the restoring dentist explains the need to replace a single tooth before tipping and extrusion of adjacent teeth and the risk for additional tooth loss, the patient should be educated as to the benefit of implant treatment while the area presents abundant bone.

The prosthetic options for Division A can be all fixed and removable options. An FP-1 prosthesis definitely will require a Division A ridge. An FP-2 prosthesis most often also requires a

Division A bone. The FP-2 restoration is the most common posterior restoration supported by multiple adjacent implants in partially edentulous patients, because of either bone loss or osteoplasty before implant placement. An FP-3 prosthesis is most frequently the option selected in the anterior Division A bone when the maxillary smiling lip position is high or a mandibular low lip line during speech exposes regions beyond the natural anatomic crown position.

For removable implant overdentures in Division A bone the final position of the tooth and superstructure bar must be evaluated before surgery. A limited CHS may be present with Division A bone, and a final type 4 removable prosthesis (RP-4) or RP-5 result may require a significant osteoplasty before implant placement. Division A bone may represent a contraindication for high-profile O-ring attachments or superstructures placed several millimeters above the tissue for hygiene considerations, because of a compromised CHS to accommodate prosthetic components (Fig. 16.14). In cases of inadequate CHS, prosthesis complication failure in the form of tooth debonding, fractured prosthesis, or attachment problems may occur.

Division B (Barely Sufficient Bone)

As the bone resorbs, the width of available bone first decreases at the expense of the facial cortical plate, because the cortical bone is usually thicker on the lingual aspect of the alveolar bone,

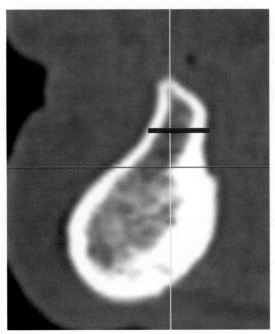

• **Fig. 16.14** Osteoplasty indicated (only if the crown height space is not compromised) to change a Division B ridge to a Division A.

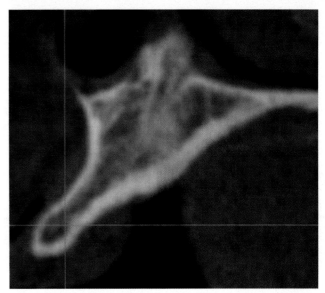

• **Fig. 16.15** Osteoplasty contraindicated because bone augmentation is required. If osteoplasty is performed, a compromised crown height space will result.

• BOX 16.3   Division B Dimensions

- 2.5 to 7 mm wide
  - B+: 4 to 7 mm
  - B–w: 2.5 to 4 mm
- Height > 10 mm
- Mesiodistal length > 6 mm
- Angulation < 20 degrees
- CHS < 15 mm
- Prosthesis:
  - Fixed: most likely FP-2 or FP-3
  - Removable: RP-4 or RP-5

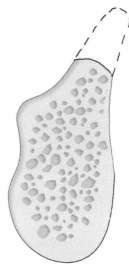

• **Fig. 16.16** Division B bone ridge may be modified by osteoplasty to increase the width of bone. The osteoplasty increases the crown height space for the prosthesis.

especially in the anterior regions of the jaws. Studies have shown a possible 25% decrease in bone width the first year and a 40% decrease in bone width within the first 1 to 3 years after tooth extraction.[12,15,16] The resulting narrower ridge is often inadequate for many 4-mm-diameter root form implants. Slight-to-mild osseous atrophy is often used to describe this clinical condition. After Division B bone volume is reached, it may remain for more than 15 years in the anterior mandible.[5] However, the posterior mandibular height resorbs four times faster than the anterior region. The posterior maxillary regions exhibit less available bone height (i.e., as a consequence of sinus expansion) and have the fastest decrease of bone height of any intraoral region. As a result the posterior regions of the jaws may become inadequate in height (C–h) earlier than the anterior regions.

Division B bone offers sufficient available bone height with compromised width (Box 16.3). The Division B available bone width may be further classified into ridges 4 to 7 mm wide and B minus width (B–w) 2.5 to 4 mm wide, where bone grafting techniques are usually indicated (Fig. 16.15). The minimum mesiodistal width of a Division B ridge is less than that of Division A; a smaller-diameter implant (i.e., 3 mm) may be used depending on the area of concern and force factors. Because the ridge width and implant diameter are narrower and forces

increase as the angle of load increases, the angulation of occlusal load is also less. A CHS of 15 mm or less (similar to Division A) is necessary in Division B to decrease the moment of forces with lateral or offset loads, especially because of the narrower width dimension.

Three treatment options are available for the Division B edentulous ridge:
1. Modify the existing Division B ridge to Division A by osteoplasty to permit the placement of root form implants 4 mm or greater in width (Fig. 16.16). When more than 10 mm of bone height results, the bone converts to Division A. When less than 10 mm of bone height results, the bone converts to Division C–h.
2. Insert a narrow Division B root form implant (e.g., 3.0-mm implant for maxillary lateral incisors or mandibular anteriors).
3. Modify the existing Division B bone into Division A by bone augmentation.

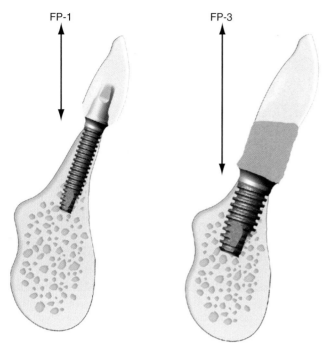

FP-1   FP-3

• **Fig. 16.17** Options to treat a Division B ridge in the anterior mandible include a narrow implant with a final prosthesis closer to anatomic dimensions (FP-1) (left) or osteoplasty with Division A root forms and extended crown heights (FP-2 or FP-3) (right).

The final prosthesis must first be considered to select the ideal approach to this bone category. When a Division B ridge is changed to a Division A by osteoplasty procedures, the final prosthesis design has to compensate for the increased CHS. For example, before surgery the available bone height may be compatible with an FP-1 prosthetic design. If at the time of surgery the ridge is found deficient in width for implant placement, it is not unusual to remove 1 to 3 mm of crestal bone before reaching a Division A width. This will result in the final restoration, requiring an additional 3 mm in height and prosthesis type changing to an FP-2 or FP-3 (Fig. 16.17).

The osteoplasty option is less likely the treatment of choice for an FP-1 prosthesis with a B–w ridge, because even greater bone height reduction is required. Therefore changing a Division B to an A will most likely always result in the fixed prosthesis being a FP-2 or FP-3.

The most common approach is to modify the narrower Division B ridge into another bone division by osteoplasty when the final prosthesis is an implant overdenture (Figs. 16.18 to 16.20). The edentulous ridge crest may be reduced, thereby increasing the width of the ridge. If the CHS is less than 15 mm, the ridge division becomes Division A with a greater width than 6 mm, ideal for a RP-4 or RP-5. If the ridge height is reduced so that the CHS is greater than 15 mm, the bone division may be changed to Division A. However, caution should be exercised to not decrease the height to a Division C–h bone volume, where vertical cantilevers or lateral forces may be present on the prosthesis. An RP-4 or RP-5 restoration most often requires option 1—osteoplasty—where adequate CHS is created to permit the fabrication of the overdenture and superstructure bar with attachments without prosthetic compromise.

The second main treatment option for the narrow available bone Division B is the small-diameter root form implant. Smaller-diameter root form implants (~3.0 mm, not "mini-implants") are designed primarily for Division B available bone. The Division B bone is narrower, so the implant body of the implant must bisect

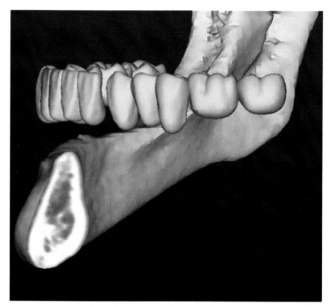

• **Fig. 16.18** Evaluation of necessary amount of osteoplasty is determined by evaluating the position of the final prosthesis.

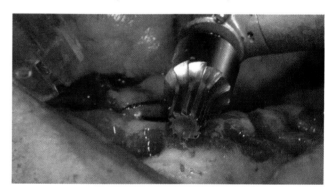

• **Fig. 16.19** Osteoplasty completion with ridge reduction bur.

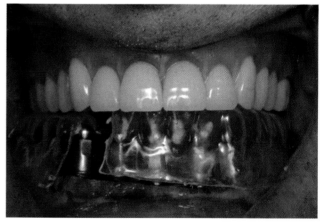

• **Fig. 16.20** Evaluation of necessary interocclusal space for final prosthesis via a diagnostic template fabricated from the patients existing prosthesis or diagnostic wax-up.

the bone and implant angulation becomes less flexible. The Division B root form implants present several inherent disadvantages compared with the larger-diameter implants (Box 16.4).[56-61] As a result of these concerns for the Division B root form, this option is mostly used for single-tooth replacement of a maxillary lateral incisor or mandibular incisors where the restricted available bone is in mesiodistal width and buccal-lingual length.[62,63]

• BOX **16.4** Disadvantages of Division B Root Forms

1. Almost twice the stress is concentrated at the top crestal region around the implant.
2. Less overall surface area means that lateral loads on the implant result in almost three times greater stress than Division A root forms.
3. Fatigue fractures of the abutment post are increased, especially under lateral loads.
4. The crown emergence profile is less esthetic (except for maxillary lateral or mandibular incisors).
5. Conditions for daily care are compromised around the cervical aspect of the crown.
6. The implant design is often poor in the crestal region. To increase implant body wall thickness to reduce fracture, no threads or compressive force design are present, but this further increases stress and the amount of shear loads to bone.
7. The angle of load must be reduced to less than 20 degrees to compensate for the small diameter.
8. Two implants are often required for proper prosthetic support, unless anterior single-tooth replacement for maxillary laterals or mandibular incisors, so surface area ends up being greater because of implant number, *not* size.
9. Implant costs are not related to diameter, so an increase in implant number results in greater cost to the doctor and patient.

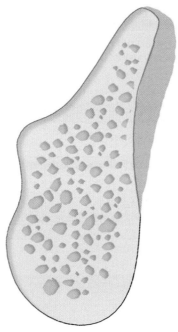

• **Fig. 16.21** Division B ridge anatomy may be modified to Division A by augmentation procedures.

The third alternative treatment for Division B bone is to change the Division B ridge into a Division A by grafting the edentulous ridge with autogenous or a combination of autograft and allograft with or without guided bone regeneration techniques (Fig. 16.21). If this graft is intended for implant placement, a healing period of at least 4 to 6 months is needed for maturation of the graft and before endosteal implants should be placed. An FP-1 restoration most often mandates the augmentation option. The emergence profile angle of the final crown, which does not compromise hygiene, requires a Division A root form implant with the exception of maxillary lateral incisors or mandibular incisors.

Stress factors may also dictate the surgical approach to Division B bone. In the presence of unfavorable stress factors, the number and width of abutments should be increased without increasing the CHS to provide a greater surface area of resistance to the magnified forces. Augmentation is indicated in Division B bone to accomplish this goal.

The success of regenerative materials for augmentation correlates with the number of osseous walls in contact with the graft material.[64] Therefore a five-wall bony defect as a tooth socket forms bone more predictable with an allograft versus a one-wall defect as an onlay graft. The distinction between B and B–w is especially important when augmentation is the method of choice. Bone augmentation is most predictable when the volume to augment is minimal and is for width, and least predictable when height is desired. For example, usually a width increase of 1 to 3 mm may be obtained with an allograft and a guided bone regeneration, whereas greater than 3 mm of width is more predictable with an autologous block graft. Some regions of the mouth are better suited than others for height augmentation (e.g., the floor of the maxillary sinus versus the posterior mandible).

Bone Spreading

An alternative for the augmentation approach for Division B bone is bone spreading. A narrow osteotomy may be made between the bony plates, and bone spreaders are sequentially tapped into the edentulous site. The Division B ridge may be expanded to a Division A with this technique and allow a Division A implant or an allograft to be inserted.[65]

The Division B–w ridge requires greater than 2 mm of width increase, and therefore autologous bone is beneficial to predictably grow bone width. If the Division B–w ridge contour should be altered for improved prosthodontic relationships, a block graft of autogenous bone is usually indicated. The autograft may be harvested from an intraoral region (such as the symphysis or ramus) and placed along the lateral aspect of the ridge that corresponds to ideal arch form (Fig. 16.22). The implant placement should be delayed until after the augmentation process to permit ideal implant placement and to ensure complete bone formation before placing the implant. In most cases, Division A root form implants may be placed 4 to 6 months after the autologous bone graft.[64-66]

The patient delaying treatment with a Division B bone condition should be notified of future bone volume resorption. The augmentation of bone in height is much less predictable and requires more advanced techniques than the augmentation of width alone. For example, the patient may not be experiencing problems with a maxillary denture, but the Division B bone will resorb in height and decrease the stability and retention of the removable soft tissue–supported prosthesis over time. When treatment is delayed, until patient problems begin, the overall result may be more difficult to achieve and more costly to the patient.

The final prosthesis type for Division B ridges is dependent on the surgical option selected. Grafted ridges will more often be used when a fixed prosthesis is desired, whereas ridges treated with osteoplasty before implant placement are likely to be supporting removable prostheses. The most common osteoplasty driven treatment for a Division B ridge is the anterior mandible. The treatment option may be influenced by the region to be restored. For example, in the partially edentulous anterior maxilla, augmentation is most often selected because of esthetics. In the edentulous anterior mandible, osteoplasty is common because esthetics are less of a concern (Fig. 16.23).

Division C (Compromised Bone)

The Division C ridge is deficient in one or more dimensions (width, length, height, or angulation) (Box 16.5) regardless of the position of the implant body into the edentulous site. The resorption pattern occurs first in width and then in height. As a result the Division B ridge continues to resorb in width, although height of bone is still present, until it becomes inadequate for any design of endosteal implant. This bone category is called Division C minus width (C–w) (Fig. 16.24). The resorption process continues, and the available bone is then reduced in height (C–h).

Moderate-to-advanced atrophy may be used to describe the clinical conditions of Division C. The posterior maxilla or mandible result with Division C–h more rapidly than the anterior regions because the maxillary sinus or mandibular canal limit vertical height sooner than the opposing cortical plates in the anterior regions. When the anterior mandible is C–h, the floor of the mouth is often level or below the residual mandibular crest of the ridge. During swallowing, it may prolapse over the residual crest and implant sites, causing constant irritation of the permucosal implant posts and impairing proper design of the prosthetic superstructures.

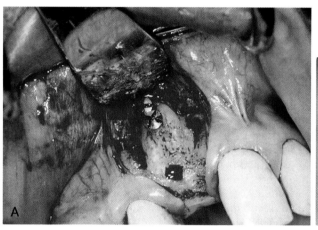
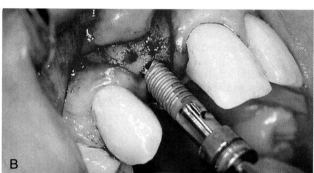

• **Fig. 16.22** (A) Reentry of an onlay ramus bone graft to a Division B–w ridge. The ridge is now converted to Division A. (B) Root form implant may now be inserted without compromise to implant position or existing width of bone.

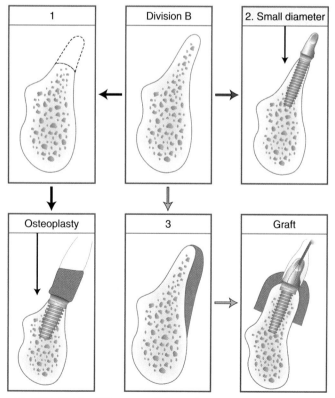

• **Fig. 16.23** Division B Summary; (1) Osteoplasty may compromise crown-height space, (2) Small diameter implant may be biomechanically non-ideal, (3) Augmentation is the most ideal treatment as it restores implant to pre-existing conditions.

• **BOX 16.5** **Division C Bone**

- Width (C–w bone): 0 to 2.5 mm
- Height (C–h bone):
- Angulation of occlusal load (C–a bone): >30 degrees
- CHS: >15 mm
- Prosthesis:
  - Fixed: most likely FP-2 or FP-3
  - Removable: ideally RP-5 because of increased CHS

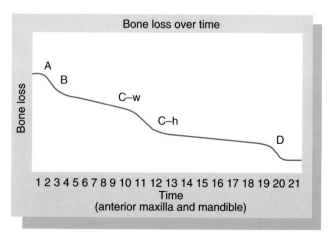

• **Fig. 16.24** Bone resorbs from Division A to Division B rapidly and from Division C–w to C–h to Division D slowly. There exists a long plateau from Division B to Division D. This is why it is important to prevent bone loss immediately after an extraction to resorb.

The doctor must appreciate that the C–w bone will resorb to a C–h ridge as fast as the A resorbs to B and faster than B resorbs to C–w. In addition, without implant or bone graft intervention, the C–h available bone will eventually evolve into Division D (severe atrophy). Many completely edentulous patients are treated with implants in the mandible and conventional dentures in the maxilla, primarily because the mandibular C–h arch is more often the cause of patient complaint (Fig. 16.25). However, the patient should be educated about the future maxillary bone loss that will render maxillary implant treatment almost impossible without advanced bone graft procedures before placement.

The Division C edentulous ridge does not offer as many elements for predictable endosteal implant survival or prosthodontic management compared with Divisions A or B. Anatomic landmarks to determine implant angulations or positions in relation to

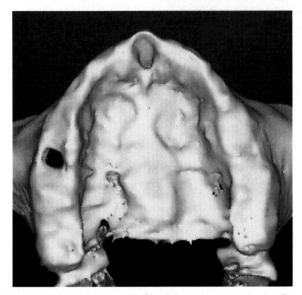

• **Fig. 16.25** Division C Premaxilla: Significant ridge resorption leading to a C–w and then a C–h ridge.

the incisal edge are usually not present; therefore greater surgical skill is required. The doctor and patient should realize that Division C ridge implant-supported prostheses are more complex and have slightly more complications in healing, prosthetic design, or long-term maintenance. On the other hand, the patients usually have greater need for increased prosthodontic support. In spite of the reduced bone volume, altered treatment plans that decrease stress can provide predictable, long-term treatment.

There is one uncommon subcategory of Division C, namely, C–a. In this category, available bone is adequate in height and width, but angulation is greater than 30 degrees regardless of implant placement (Fig. 16.26). When present, this condition is most often found in the anterior mandible; other less-observed regions include the maxilla with severe facial undercut regions or the mandibular second molar with a severe lingual undercut. Root form implants placed in this bone category may be positioned within the floor of the mouth and compromise prosthetic reconstruction, speech, and comfort (Fig. 16.27).

Implant treatment planning for the completely edentulous C–h arch is more complex than in Division A or B. There are seven implant treatment options for Division C bone (Box 16.6); all of these options require greater clinician skill than similar treatment modalities in Division A or B.

Treatment Options

A C–w ridge may be treated by osteoplasty, which most likely will change the ridge to a C–h, not Division A (i.e., because of the lack of height after osteoplasty). This most often occurs in the mandibular anterior region to allow for root form implants. On occasion the C–w osteoplasty may convert the ridge to Division D, especially in the posterior mandible or maxilla. Care should be taken not to let this occur, because bone grafting procedures will be contraindicated or more challenging after the height has been reduced.

Another treatment option is to alter the Division C by grafting. After the ridge is augmented, it is treated with the options available in the acquired bone division. The patient who desires a fixed prosthesis often requires an autogenous graft before implant placement to acquire proper lip support and ideal crown height.

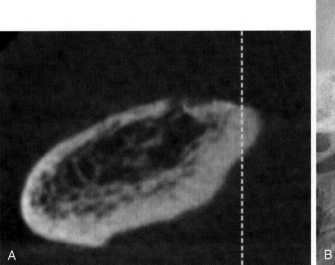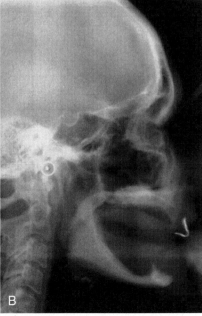

• **Fig. 16.26** (A) Cone beam computed tomography cross section depicting a C–a anterior mandible; the resultant angulation contraindicates dental implant placement. (B) Lateral cephalogram of an anterior mandible with a 45-degree trajectory to the occlusal plane.

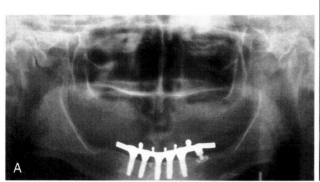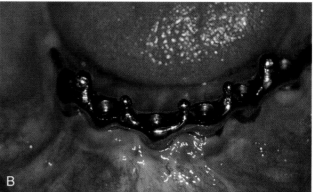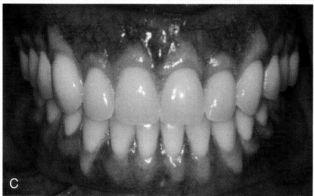

• **Fig. 16.27** (A) A panoramic radiograph of an edentulous C–h mandible with a disk implant in the posterior left connected to five anterior root form implants with an overdenture bar. (B) An intraoral view of the overdenture bar for a RP-4 prosthesis in a C–h mandible. (C) The five root forms and disk implant support a bar for a mandibular RP-4 overdenture opposing a conventional maxillary denture. *(From Misch DE. Available bone and dental implant treatment plans. In: Misch CE, ed.* Dental Implant Prosthetics. *2nd ed. St. Louis, MO: Mosby; 2015.)*

• **BOX 16.6** **Division C Treatment Options**

- Osteoplasty (C–w)
- Root form implants (C–h)
- Augmentation procedures before implant insertion
- Subperiosteal implant (C–h, C–a partial, or completely edentulous mandible)
- Disk Implants

Augmentation of C–w is most often used when prosthetic guidelines require a fixed restoration or excess force factors require greater surface area implants and improved biomechanics for the prosthesis. The C–w augmentation is more difficult than for Division B bone, because the need for bone volume is greater, yet the recipient bed is more deficient. Therefore block bone grafts are usually indicated.[66-68] Soft tissue complications, such as incision line opening and lack of papilla, are more common in C–w augmentations compared with Division B.

The C–h posterior maxilla is a common and unique edentulous condition. The residual ridge resorbs in width and height after tooth loss, similar to other regions. However, because of the initial extensive ridge width dimension, a decrease of 60% in dimension still is adequate for 4-mm-diameter implants. In addition to the residual alveolar bone resorption, the maxillary sinus expands after tooth loss (pneumatization). As a result the available bone height is decreased from both the crestal and apical regions. Sinus grafts,

which elevate the maxillary sinus floor membrane and then graft the previous sinus floor region, were developed by Tatum[65] in the mid-1970s. This area is the most predictable intraoral region to augment in excess of 10 mm of vertical bone. Therefore sinus grafting (either lateral wall or transcrestal) is often prescribed before placing endosteal implants in the C–h posterior maxilla (Fig. 16.28).

Various implant approaches are used in the Division C–h available bone. Shorter endosteal implants are the most common options.[52,53] A C–h root form implant is usually 4 mm or greater in width at the crest module and 10 mm or less in height. Many previous studies indicated implant survival is decreased once an implant is 10 mm or less in height.[35,69,70] For example, a large multicenter study of 31 different sites and 6 different implant designs observed 13% failure with 10-mm implants, 16% failure with 8-mm implants, and 25% failure with 7-mm-long implants.[35] The implant failure does not occur after surgery but rather after prosthetic delivery. However, many recent studies have shown high success rates for short implants in comparison with longer implants.

When endosteal root form implants are used in Division C–h bone with greater crown heights, additional implants should be placed to increase the overall implant-bone surface area, and the prosthesis should load the implants in an axial direction. Because the CHS is greater than 15 mm, the design of a removable prosthesis should often reduce cantilever length and incorporate a stress relief mechanism. In these cases, reduced long-term predictability

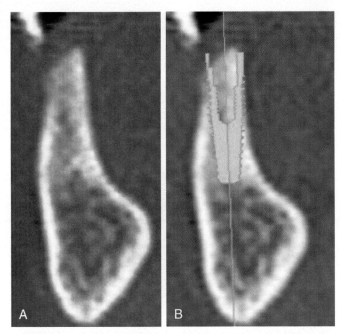

• **Fig. 16.28** Division C–w Implant Placement. (A) Cone beam computed tomography cross section showing compromised width of bone, ideally requiring bone augmentation. (B) Small-diameter implant placement showing inadequate available bone that would most likely result in crestal bone loss.

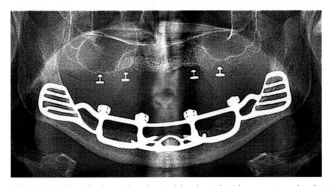

• **Fig. 16.29** Mandibular subperiosteal implant that is a custom implant placed on top of the bone, which retains an RP-4 prosthesis.

is usually expected if additional implants or less stressful prostheses are not used, because a greater moment force is transmitted to the implants. The most efficient way to reduce stress is by maintaining the overdenture prosthesis as an RP-5, not an RP-4 prosthesis. With an RP-5 prosthesis the soft tissue will absorb most of the primary force because the implants or attachments are used only for secondary support.

An alternative design to endosteal implants in the posterior mandibular edentulous Division C–h arch is subperiosteal and disk design implants (Fig. 16.29).[71-73] Subperiosteal implants are more predictable in the mandibular arch than in the maxilla; however, they have fallen out of favor recently. The limitations of anatomy for root form implants may be bone angulation, a square arch form, or inadequate bone height. When the anterior bone angulation is unfavorable, root form implants may be positioned too far lingually for prosthodontic support, speech, or hygiene. The superstructure and abutment posts for the subperiosteal implant are designed and cast before implant placement. The permucosal posts may be designed with greater latitude than endosteal implants. When anterior root forms are placed in an edentulous mandible with a square arch form, the superstructure

may not be cantilevered distally because of the poor anteroposterior distance. As a result a fixed restoration or RP-4 overdenture prosthesis is contraindicated with anterior root forms in a square arch form. A subperiosteal implant may provide anterior and posterior bone support, and the square arch form does not contraindicate an RP-4 prosthesis. Autogenous grafts or nerve repositioning may be necessary to place endosteal implants in the posterior Division C–h mandible. The increase in treatment time, surgical risks, and postoperative complications (such as paresthesia) are to be thoroughly discussed with the patient. Circumferential or unilateral subperiosteal implants permit the placement of posterior prosthodontic units without risk for paresthesia from nerve repositioning or lengthened treatment time associated with autogenous bone grafts and endosteal implants.[73]

Another alternative for the posterior mandible or premaxilla with Division C–h bone is a disk design implant that engages the lateral aspect of the cortical bone and may be used in available bone height of 3 mm or more. As a general rule, these implants are used in addition to other root form implants. Their inclusion in the treatment plan for C–h posterior sections of edentulous mandibles eliminates cantilevers in full-arch restorations.[71,74]

The prosthetic options for Division C ridges more often consist of removable prosthesis in the completely edentulous maxillary arch. A maxillary overdenture in a Division C ridge allows for support of the upper lip without hygiene compromise. In a Division C mandible the greater CHS often mandates an overdenture design with soft tissue support (RP-5). A fixed restoration in the Division C mandible often requires both anterior and posterior implant support. The fixed prosthesis in Division C bone with greater than 15 mm CHS is most often a hybrid prosthesis, with denture teeth attached to a precious metal substructure with acrylic resin. In this way the complications and costs of a porcelain-metal fixed restoration may be reduced.

In general, Division C–h presents less favorable biomechanical factors to the implant support. Therefore additional implants or teeth, cross-arch stabilization, soft tissue support, or an opposing removable prosthesis often need to be considered in the prosthetic design to improve the long-term prognosis. Treating the Division C ridge requires greater experience, caution, and training than does the previous two bone divisions; however, excellent results may be achieved.

The completely edentulous patient who does not have implant treatment should be well educated that the bone resorption process will continue, with significantly increased risk for the conventional removable restoration. Waiting to treat the patient until irreparable problems develop is a poor treatment alternative that results in the need for more advanced procedures such as iliac crest grafts and significant risk for associated complications.

In conclusion, as in all other bone divisions, the final prosthesis determines the treatment option. For mandibular RP-4 restorations, five root forms in the anterior mandible may be used (if the other dental criteria permit). However, the greater CHS or a square arch form may mandate an RP-5 prosthesis with anterior root form implants. The combination of anterior root forms and posterior subperiosteal implants (or disk implants) is an uncommon treatment option for RP-4 or fixed prosthesis in the mandibular arch. These types of treatment options require an advanced skill set not only surgically, but also prosthetically. Augmentation is often required for a fixed prosthesis in either of the Division C complete edentulous arches if stress factors are high and cannot be reduced.

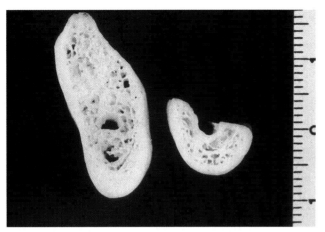

• **Fig. 16.30** The left posterior mandible is Division A, with abundant bone in height and width (left). The residual ridge on the right is a Division D with a dehiscent mandibular canal.

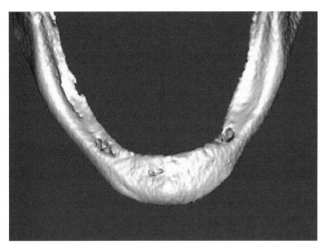

• **Fig. 16.31** Division D mandible with mainly basal bone in the anterior mandible and dehiscence nerves in the posterior.

Division D (Deficient Bone)

Long-term bone resorption may result in the complete loss of the residual ridge, accompanied by basal bone atrophy (Fig. 16.30). Severe atrophy describes the clinical condition of the Division D ridge. At one time, it was believed that only the alveolar process would resorb after tooth loss and the basal bone would remain. However, bone loss may continue beyond the previous roots of teeth and even include the bone over the inferior mandibular nerve or the nasal spine of the maxilla. Basal bone loss eventually results in a completely flat maxilla. In the mandible the superior genial tubercles become the most superior aspect of the ridge. The mentalis muscle will lose much of its attachment, even though the superior portion of the muscle attaches near the crest of the resorbed ridge. The buccinator muscle may approach the mylohyoid muscle and form an aponeurosis above the body of the mandible. The mandibular arch also presents with mental foramina and portions of the mandibular canal dehiscent. Therefore it is not infrequent that these patients report neurosensory deficits of the lower lip, especially during mastication. The CHS is greater than 20 mm, which is a significant force multiplier and can rarely be reduced enough to render long-term success (Fig. 16.31 and Box 16.7).

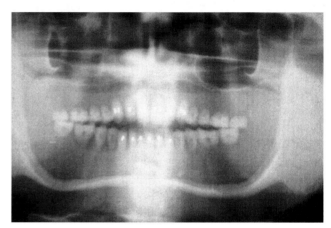

• **Fig. 16.32** Division D mandible with extensive atrophy leading to possible pathologic fracture of mandible.

The prosthetic result for Division D without augmentation is the poorest treatment outcome of all the divisions of bone. Fixed restorations are nearly always contraindicated, because the CHS is so significant. Completely implant-supported overdentures are indicated whenever possible to decrease the soft tissue and nerve complications, but require anterior and posterior implant support, which almost always requires bone augmentation before implant placement. Bone augmentation for Division D is difficult to improve the CHS enough to warrant a fixed restoration unless there are favorable force factors. An RP-5 restoration is not suggested, because bone loss will continue in the soft tissue–supported region of the overdenture, and usually the buccal shelf (primary stress bearing area) is not present.

The completely edentulous Division D patient is the most difficult to treat in implant dentistry. Benefits must be carefully weighed against the risks and complications. Although the practitioner and patient often regard this condition as the most desperate, these patients do not usually understand the possible chronic complications that may result (e.g., oral antral fistulae, deviated facial). If implant failure occurs, the patient may become a dental cripple—unable to wear any prosthesis and worse off than before treatment (Fig. 16.32).

Autogenous iliac crest bone grafts to improve the Division D are strongly recommended before any implant treatment is attempted.[74] After autogenous grafts are in place and allowed to heal for 5 or more months, the bone division is usually Division C–h or Division A, and endosteal implants may be inserted (Figs. 16.33 and 16.34).

Autogenous bone grafts should always be indicated for the placement of implants, never to increase support for a denture. The autogenous bone grafts are not intended for improved denture support. If soft tissue–borne prostheses are fabricated on autogenous grafts, studies have shown 90% of the grafted bone resorbs within

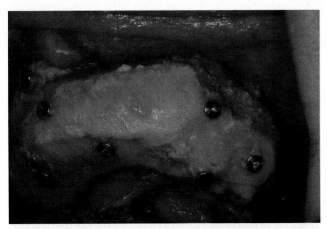

• **Fig. 16.33** Autogenous Iliac Crest Graft: An autologous iliac crest bone graft in situ. The block is fixated with screws to the host bone.

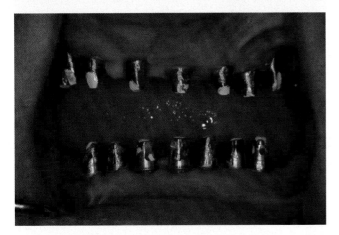

• **Fig. 16.34** Post–Graft Implant Placement.

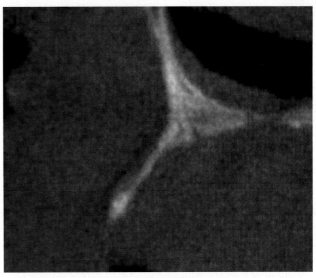

• **Fig. 16.35** Division D premaxilla revealing no host bone present.

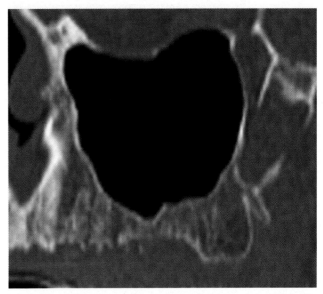

• **Fig. 16.36** Division D posterior maxilla showing bone posterior to the edenulous area, however insufficient bone where implants are indicated.

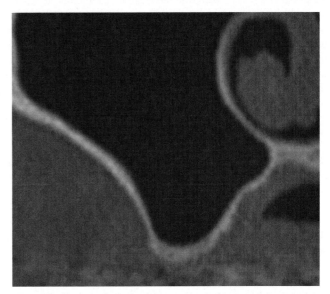

• **Fig. 16.37** Preoperative cone beam computed tomography cross section showing no bone present.

5 years as a result of accelerated resorption.[75] Additional augmentation to compensate for this resorption is not indicated. Repeated relines, highly mobile tissue, sore spots, and patient frustration are all postoperative consequences. On the other hand, autogenous bone grafts are maintained long term in conjunction with implant placement because of the stress to the bone. Another option with a low success rate is the addition of dense hydroxyapatite to improve denture support. Migration of the graft at the time of surgery or in the future after soft tissue loading is a frequent sequel.

The partially or completely edentulous patient with a posterior Division D maxilla may undergo sinus graft procedures with a combination of autograft and allograft regenerative materials.[65] The CHS may be insufficient for onlay grafts in the posterior maxilla, despite a lack of available bone height, because the sinus expands faster than the crest of the ridge resorbs. Endosteal implants of adequate height can rarely be positioned without a sinus graft. After the Division D posterior maxilla is restored to Division A or C–h, root form implants may be inserted for posterior prosthodontic support. In most cases, greater surface area is required in the form of increasing implant number or implant diameter (Figs. 16.35 to 16.39).

Endosteal root form implants without autogenous grafts may be used on rare occasions in the anterior Division D mandible when the remaining bone is dense and the opposing arch is edentulous. Care must be taken during placement, because mandibular fracture at insertion or during postoperative healing is a possible complication.[76,77] Under these conditions the CHS is very great, and the number of implants often four or fewer. Implant failure

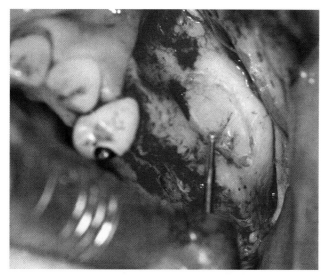

• **Fig. 16.38** Lateral wall sinus augmentation window preparation.

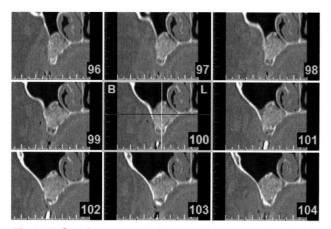

• **Fig. 16.39** Cone beam computed tomography cross sections depicting post–sinus graft.

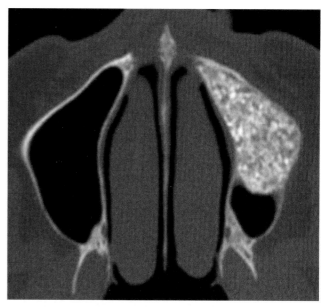

• **Fig. 16.40** Axial View of Post–Sinus Augmentation.

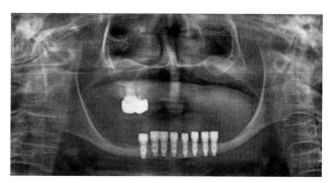

• **Fig. 16.41** Anterior root form implants were placed in a Division D mandible. As a result of the failure of one implant, the mandible has fractured and has a continuity defect.

after loading is a greater risk. Implant failure results with circumferential bone loss, which may be associated with mandibular fracture through the implant site. An RP-5 removable restoration is usually indicated for Division D with only anterior implants. However, the RP-5 restoration allows for continued bone resorption and atrophy to continue in the posterior regions. Therefore the prudent therapy is to educate the patient as to the risks of his or her current condition and offer an autologous bone graft and implants to support an RP-4 restoration. The choice to render treatment is the doctor's, not the patient's. The implant support should not be compromised when implant failure may result in significantly greater risks.

The Division D arch requires greater doctor training and results in more frequent complications related to grafting, early implant failure, and soft tissue management; therefore treatment options include a more guarded prognosis. It should be the goal of every implant clinician to educate and treat the patient before a Division D bone condition develops. In contrast, the profession treats periodontal diseases before pain in the region occurs, and carious lesions are removed before abscess formation. The profession monitors bone loss around teeth in fractions of a millimeter and offers continued care to reduce the risks for future tooth and bone loss. Likewise the prudent practitioner should monitor bone loss in edentulous sites, and offer education and treatment before deleterious effects (Figs. 16.40 to 16.42).

Summary

In implant dentistry the prosthesis is designed at the onset of treatment to satisfy the patient's needs and desires, and obtain optimal results. This may range from a completely fixed prosthesis to one with primarily soft tissue support. After the final prosthesis type has been established, the key implant positions, patient force factors, bone density in the implant sites, and implant number, size, and design are determined. The primary criterion for proper implant support is the amount of available bone. Four divisions of available bone, based on the width, height, length, angulation, and CHS in the edentulous site, have been presented. Consistent implant treatment plan procedures elaborated for each category of bone may be followed.

The Division A edentulous ridge offers abundant bone in all dimensions. Division A root form implants are optimally used and most often as independent support for the prosthesis. Division B bone may provide adequate width for narrower, small-diameter root from endosteal implants. The decreased width and surface area usually require additional implants to be included in the final prosthesis design. Division B may be changed in condition to a Division A by augmentation or osteoplasty. The treatment options may be selected in light of the area to be treated. For example, in the anterior maxilla, augmentation is most often selected because of esthetics. In the anterior mandible,

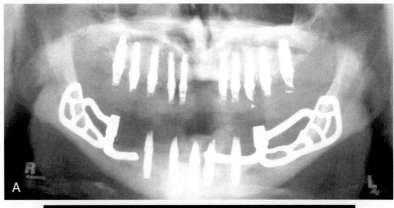

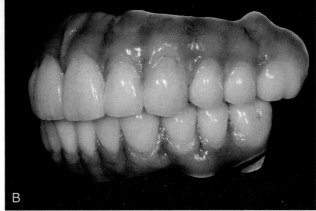

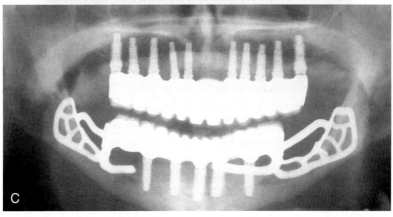

● **Fig. 16.42** (A) A panoramic radiograph of 10 implants inserted into an edentulous maxilla after bilateral sinus grafting. The mandible has five endosteal implants in a C–h anterior mandible. The posterior mandible has bilateral subperiosteal implants inserted for posterior prosthetic support. (B) The maxillary and mandibular FP-3 restoration. (C) A panoramic radiograph of the FP-3 prostheses in situ. *(From Misch DE. Available bone and dental implant treatment plans. In: Misch CE, ed. Dental Implant Prosthetics. 2nd ed. St. Louis, MO: Mosby; 2015.)*

osteoplasty is common because of the available bone height and low esthetic concerns. In the posterior mandible, multiple Division B implants may be used, because the bone density is good, the available bone height is limited, and esthetics are not a primary factor. When stress factors are greater, bone augmentation precedes Division A root form implants, regardless of the anatomic location.

The Division C edentulous ridge exhibits moderate resorption and presents more limiting factors for predictable endosteal implants. The decision to restore with endosteal implants or to upgrade the bone division by augmentation before implant placement is influenced by the prosthesis, patient force factors, and

patient's desires. The Division D edentulous ridge corresponds to basal bone loss and severe atrophy, resulting in dehiscent mandibular canals or a completely flat maxilla. The patient often requires augmentation with autogenous bone before implant and prosthodontic reconstruction.

If the existing conditions do not qualify for a predictable end result, the patient's mind or mouth must be modified. For example, the expectations of the patient must be reduced so the prosthesis may be changed from FP-1 to RP-4, or the bone must be augmented to improve the height and width and to change the division so that long-term implant support and prosthetic design will be compatible.

References

1. Misch CE, Judy KWM. Patient dental-medical implant evaluation form. *Int Cong Oral Implant.* 1987.
2. Greenfield EJ. Implantation of artificial crown and bridge abutments. *Dent Cosmos.* 1913;55:364–369.
3. Misch J. In: *Lehrbuch der Grenzgebiete der Medizin und Zahnheilkunde.* Vol. 1. 2nd ed. Leipzig, Germany: FCW Vogal; 1922.
4. Atwood DA. Postextraction changes in the adult mandible as illustrated by microradiographs of midsagittal sections and serial cephalometric roentgenograms. *J Prosthet Dent.* 1963;13:810–824.
5. Atwood DA. Reduction of residual ridges: a major oral disease entity. *J Prosthet Dent.* 1971;26:266–279.
6. Atwood DA, Coy WA. Clinical, cephalometric and densitometric study of reduction of residual ridges. *J Prosthet Dent.* 1971;26:280–295.
7. Tallgren A. The continuing reduction of the residual alveolar ridges in complete denture wearers. A mixed longitudinal study covering 25 years. *J Prosthet Dent.* 1972;27:120–132.
8. Atwood DA. Some clinical factors related to the rate of resorption of residual ridges. *J Prosthet Dent.* 1962;12:441–450.
9. Karkazis HC, Lambadakis J, Tsichlakis K. Cephalometric evaluation of the changes in mandibular symphysis after 7 years of denture wearing. *Gerodontology.* 1997;14:10–15.
10. Karagaclioglu L, Ozkan P. Changes in mandibular ridge height in relation to aging and length of edentulism period. *Int J Prosthodont.* 1994;7:368–371.
11. Kovacic I, Celebic A, Knezovic Zlataric D, et al. Influence of body mass index and the time of edentulousness on the residual alveolar ridge resorption in complete denture wearers. *Coll Antropol Suppl.* 2003;2:69–74.
12. Lam RV. Contour changes of the alveolar process following extraction. *J Prosthet Dent.* 1960;10:25–32.
13. Berg H, Carlsson GE, Helkimo M. Changes in shape of posterior parts of upper jaws after extraction of teeth and prosthetic treatment. *J Prosthet Dent.* 1975;34:262–268.
14. Gazabatt C, Parra N, Meissner C. A comparison of bone resorption following intraseptal alveolectomy and labial alveolectomy. *J Prosthet Dent.* 1965;15:435–443.
15. Pietrokovski J, Sorin S, Hirschfeld Z. The residual ridge in partially edentulous patients. *J Prosthet Dent.* 1976;36:150–157.
16. Pietrokovski J, Massler M. Alveolar ridge resorption following tooth extraction. *J Prosthet Dent.* 1967;17:21–27.
17. Pietrokowski J. The bony residual ridge in man. *J Prosthet Dent.* 1975;34:456–462.
18. Parkinson CF. Similarities in resorption patterns of maxillary and mandibular ridges. *J Prosthet Dent.* 1978;39:598–602.
19. Wical KE, Swoope CC. Studies of residual ridge resorption. Part I: use of panoramic radiographs for evaluation and classification of mandibular resorption. *J Prosthet Dent.* 1974;32:7–12.
20. Tallgren A, Lang BR, Miller RL. Longitudinal study of soft-tissue profile changes in patients receiving immediate complete dentures. *Int J Prosthodont.* 1991;4:9–16.
21. Weiss CM, Judy KWM. Severe mandibular atrophy: biological considerations of routine treatment with complete subperiosteal implants. *J Oral Implant.* 1974;4:431–469.
22. Kent JN. Correction of alveolar ridge deficiencies with non-resorbable hydroxyapatite. *J Am Dent Assoc.* 1982;105:99–100.
23. Lekholm U, Zarb G. Patient selection and preparation. In: Brånemark PI, ed. *Tissue Integrated Prostheses: Osseo-Integration in Clinical Dentistry.* Chicago: Quintessence; 1985.
24. Fallschüssel GKH. Untersuchungen zur Anatomie des zahnlosen Oberkiefers. *Z Zahnarztl Implantol.* 1986;2:64–72.
25. Gruber H, Solar P, Ulm C. Maxillomandibular anatomy and patterns of resorption during atrophy. In: Watzek G, ed. *Endosseous Implants: Scientific and Clinical Aspects.* Chicago: Quintessence; 1996.
26. Cawood JJ, Howell RA. A classification of the edentulous jaws classes I to VI. *Int J Oral Maxillofac Surg.* 1988;17:232–279.
27. Misch CE. *Treatment Planning and Implant Dentistry [Abstract].* Dearborn, Mich: Misch Implant Institute Manual; 1985.
28. Misch CE, Judy KWM. Classification of partially edentulous arches for implant dentistry. *Int J Oral Implant.* 1987;4:7–12.
29. Misch CE. Available bone influences prosthodontic treatment. *Dent Today.* Feb. 1988:44–75.
30. Misch CE. Bone classification, training keys to implant success. *Dent Today.* May. 1989:39–44.
31. Misch CE. Classifications and treatment options of the completely edentulous arch in implant dentistry. *Dent Today.* Oct. 1990:26–30.
32. Misch CE. Divisions of available bone in implant dentistry. *Int J Oral Implant.* 1990;7:9–17.
33. Misch CE. Classification de l'os disponible en implantologie [in French]. *Implantodontie.* 1992;6/7:6–11.
34. Brånemark PI. Osseointegration and its experimental background. *J Prosthet Dent.* 1983;50:399–410.
35. Minsk L, Polson A, Weisgold A, et al. Outcome failures of endosseous implants from a clinical training center. *Compend Contin Educ Dent.* 1996;17:848–859.
36. Stultz RE, Lofland R, Sendax VI, et al. A multicenter 5-year retrospective survival analysis of 6,200 integral implants. *Compend Contin Educ Dent.* 1993;14:478–486.
37. Saadoun A, LeGall MG. An 8-year compilation of clinical results obtained with Steri-Oss endosseous implants. *Compend Contin Educ Dent.* 1996;17:669–688.
38. van Steenberghe D, DeMars G, Quirynen M, et al. A prospective split mouth comparative study of two screw-shaped self-tapping pure titanium implant system. *Clin Oral Impl Res.* 2000;11:202–209.
39. Naert I, Koutsikakis G, Duyck J, et al. Biologic outcome of implant-supported restorations in the treatment of partial edentulism, part I: a longitudinal clinical evaluation. *Clin Oral Implants Res.* 2002;13:381–389.
40. Pylant T, Triplett RG, Key MC, et al. A retrospective evaluation of endosseous titanium implants in the partially edentulous patient. *Int J Oral Maxillofac Implants.* 1992;7:195–202.
41. Naert I, Quirynen M, van Steenberghe D, et al. A six-year prosthodontic study of 509 consecutively inserted implants for the treatment of partial edentulism. *J Prosthet Dent.* 1992;67:236–245.
42. Jemt T, Lekholm U. Oral implant treatment in posterior partially edentulous jaws: a 5-year follow-up report. *Int J Oral Maxillofac Implants.* 1993;8:635–640.
43. Lekholm U, van Steenberghe D, Herrmann I, et al. Osseointegrated implants in the treatment of partially edentulous jaws: a prospective 5-year multicenter study. *Int J Oral Maxillofac Implants.* 1994;9:627–635.
44. Higuchi KW, Folmer T, Kultje C. Implant survival rates in partially edentulous patients: a 3-year prospective multicenter study. *J Oral Maxillofac Surg.* 1995;53:264–268.
45. Gunne J, Jemt T, Linden B. Implant treatment in partially edentulous patients: a report on prostheses after 3 years. *Int J Prosthodont.* 1994;7:142–146.
46. Friberg B, Jemt T, Lekholm U. Early failures in 4,641 consecutively placed Brånemark dental implants: a study from stage 1 surgery to the connection of completed prostheses. *Int J Oral Maxillofac Implants.* 1991;6:142–146.
47. Jemt T, Lekholm U. Implant treatment in edentulous maxillae: a 5-year follow-up report on patients with different degrees of jaw resorption. *Int J Oral Maxillofac Implants.* 1995;10:303–311.
48. Testori T, Younan R. Clinical evaluation of short, machined-surface implants followed for 12 to 92 months. *Int J Oral Maxillofac Implants.* 2003;16:894–901.
49. Testori T, Wisemen L, Wolfe S, et al. A prospective multicenter clinical study of the Osseotite implant: four-year interim report. *Int J Oral Maxillofac Implants.* 2001;16:193–200.

50. Weng D, Jacobson Z, Tarnow D, et al. A prospective multicenter clinical trial of 3i machined-surface implants: results after 6 years of follow-up. *Int J Oral Maxillofac Implants*. 2003;16:417–423.

51. Misch CE. Density of bone: effect on treatment plans, surgical approach, healing and progressive bone loading. *Int J Oral Implant*. 1990;6:23–31.

52. Misch CE. Short dental implants: a literature review and rationale for use. *Dent Today*. 2005;24:64–68.

53. Misch CE, Steigenga K, Barboza E, et al. Short dental implants in posterior partial edentulism: a multicenter retrospective 5 year case study. *J Periodontol*. 2006;77:1470–1477.

54. Razavi R, Zena RB, Khan Z, et al. Anatomic site evaluation of edentulous maxillae for dental implant placement. *J Prosthet Dent*. 1995;4:90–94.

55. Oikarinen K, Raustia AM, Hartikainen M. General and local contraindications for endosseal implants—an epidemiological panoramic radiographic study in 65 year old subjects. *Community Dent Oral Epidemiol*. 1995;23:114–116.

56. Tarnow DP, Cho SC, Wallace SS. The effect of interimplant distance on the height of inter-implant bone crest. *Periodontology*. 2000;71:546–549.

57. Hebel KS, Gajjar R. Achieving superior aesthetic results: parameters for implant and abutment selection. *Int J Dent Symp*. 1997;4:42–47.

58. Rangert B, Krogh P, Langer B, et al. Bending overload and implant fracture: a retrospective clinical analysis. *Int J Oral Maxillofac Impl*. 1995;10:326–334.

59. Misch CE, Bidez MW. Occlusion and crestal bone resorption: etiology and treatment planning strategies for implants. In: McNeill C, ed. *Science and Practice of Occlusion*. Chicago: Quintessence; 1997.

60. Misch CE, Wang HL. The procedures, limitations and indications for small diameter implants and a case report. *Oral Health*. 2004;94:16–26.

61. Misch CE, Bidez MW. Implant protected occlusion, a biomechanical rationale. *Compend Contin Educ Dent*. 1994;15:1330–1342.

62. Misch CE. Maxillary anterior single tooth implant health esthetic compromise. *Int J Dent Symp*. 1995;3:4–9.

63. Misch CE, D'Alessio R, Misch-Dietsh F. Maxillary partial anodontia and implant dentistry—maxillary anterior partial anodontia in 255 adolescent patients: a 15 year retrospective study of 276 implant site replacements. *Oral Health*. 2005;95:45–57.

64. Misch CE, Dietsh F. Bone grafting materials in implant dentistry. *Impl Dent*. 1993;2:158–167.

65. Tatum HO. Maxillary and sinus implant reconstructions. *Dent Clin North Am*. 1980;30:207–229.

66. Misch CM, Misch CE, Resnik RR, et al. Reconstruction of maxillary alveolar defects with mandibular symphysis grafts for dental implants: a preliminary procedural report. *Int J Oral Maxillofac Impl*. 1992;3:360–366.

67. Misch CM, Misch CE. The repair of localized severe ridge defects for implant placement using mandibular bone grafts. *Impl Dent*. 1995;4:261–267.

68. Misch CM. Ridge augmentation using mandibular ramus bone grafts for the placement of dental implants: presentation of a technique. *Pract Perio Aesth Dent*. 1996;8:127–135.

69. Ivanoff CJ, Grondahl K, Sennerby L, et al. Influence of variations in implant diameters: a 3-to 5-year retrospective clinical report. *Int J Oral Maxillofac Implants*. 1999;14. 173-160.

70. Scurria MS, Morgan ZV, Guckes AD, et al. Prognostic variables associated with implant failure: a retrospective effectiveness study. *Int J Oral Maxillofac Implants*. 1998;13:400–406.

71. Scortecci GM. Immediate function of cortically anchored disk design implants without bone augmentation in moderately to severely resorbed completely edentulous maxillae. *J Oral Implant*. 1999;25:70–79.

72. Judy KW, Misch CE. Evolution of the mandibular subperiosteal implant. *N Y Dent J*. 1983;53:9–11.

73. Misch CE, Dietsh F. The unilateral mandibular subperiosteal implant: indications and technique. *Int J Oral Implant*. 1992;8:21–29.

74. Misch CE, Dietsh F. Endosteal implants and iliac crest grafts to restore severely resorbed totally edentulous maxillae: a retrospective study. *J Oral Implantol*. 1994;20:110.

75. Curtis TA, Ware WH, Beirne OR, et al. Autogenous bone grafts for atrophic edentulous mandibles: a final report. *J Prosthet Dent*. 1987;57:73–78.

76. Albrektsson T. A multicenter report on osseointegrated oral implants. *J Prosthet Dent*. 1988;60:75–84.

77. Mason ME, Triplett RG, van Sickels JE, et al. Mandibular fractures through endosseous cylinder implants: report of cases and review. *J Oral Maxillofac Surg*. 1990;48:311–317.

17

Prosthetic Options in Implant Dentistry

RANDOLPH R. RESNIK AND CARL E. MISCH

Implant dentistry is similar to all aspects of medicine in that treatment begins with a diagnosis of the patient's condition. Most treatment options are derived from the obtained diagnostic information. Traditional dentistry provides limited treatment options for the edentulous patient. Because the dentist cannot add abutments, the restoration design is directly related to the existing oral condition. In contrast, implant dentistry can provide a range of additional abutment locations, thus allowing for a wide spectrum of treatment options. Bone augmentation may further modify the existing edentulous condition in both the partial and total edentulous arch, and therefore also affects the final prosthetic design. As a result, a number of treatment options are available to most partially and completely edentulous patients. Therefore once the diagnosis is complete, the implant treatment plan of choice at a particular moment is patient and problem based. Not all patients should be treated with the same restoration type or design.

Almost all human-made creations, whether art, buildings, or prostheses, require the end result to be visualized and precisely planned for optimal results. Blueprints indicate the finest details for buildings. The final structure should be clearly identified before the project begins, yet implant dentists often forget this simple but fundamental axiom. Historically in implant dentistry, bone available for implant insertion dictated the number and locations of dental implants. The prosthesis then was often determined after the position and number of implants were selected. The goals of implant dentistry are to replace a patient's missing teeth to normal contour, comfort, function, esthetics, speech, and health, regardless of the previous atrophy, disease, or injury of the stomatognathic system. It is the final prosthesis, not the implants, that accomplishes these goals. In other words, patients are missing teeth, not implants. The prosthesis should be designed first, to satisfy predictably a patient's needs and desires. In the stress treatment theorem[1] the final restoration is planned first, similar to the architect designing a building before making the foundation. Only after this is accomplished can the abutments necessary to support the specific predetermined prosthesis be designed (Fig. 17.1).

Completely Edentulous Prosthesis Design

The completely edentulous patient is too often treated as though cost was the primary factor in establishing a treatment plan. However, the clinician and staff should specifically ask about the patient's desires. Some patients have a strong psychological need to have a fixed prosthesis (FP) as similar to natural teeth as possible. In contrast, some patients do not express serious concerns whether the restoration is fixed or removable as long as specific problems are addressed. In general a patient with existing teeth that are to be extracted are more likely to have interest in a fixed-implant prosthesis. However, a patient with a removable prosthesis (RPs) is most commonly interested in an overdenture prosthesis. The existing anatomy is evaluated after it has been determined whether a fixed or removable restoration is desired, to assess the ideal final prosthetic design.

An axiom of implant treatment is to provide the most *predictable*, most *cost-effective* treatment that will satisfy the patient's anatomic needs and personal desires. In the completely edentulous patient a removable implant-supported prosthesis offers several advantages over a fixed-implant restoration (Box 17.1). However, some completely edentulous patients require a fixed restoration because of personal choice or because their oral condition makes the fabrication of teeth difficult if a removable prosthesis is planned. For example, when the patient has abundant bone and implants have already been placed, the lack of crown height space may not permit an RP.[2]

Too often treatment plans for completely edentulous patients consist of a maxillary denture and a mandibular overdenture with two implants. However, in the long term, this treatment option may prove a disservice to the patient. The arches will continue to lose bone, and the bone loss may even be accelerated in the premaxilla.[3,4] Once this dimension is lost, the patient will have much more difficulty with retention and stability of the restoration. In addition, the lack of posterior implant support in the mandible will allow posterior bone loss to continue.[5] Facial changes and reduced posterior occlusion with the maxillary prosthesis is to be expected. The clinician should diagnose the amount of bone loss and its consequences on facial esthetics, function, and psychological and overall health. Patients should be made aware of future compromises in bone loss and the associated problems with minimal treatment options, which do not address the continued loss of bone in regions where implants are not inserted.

It is even more important to visualize the final prosthesis at the onset with a fixed-implant restoration. After this first important step, the individual areas of ideal or key abutment support are determined to assess whether it is possible to place the implants to support the intended prosthesis. The patient's force factors and

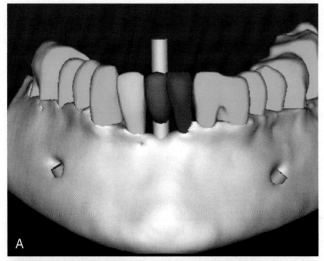

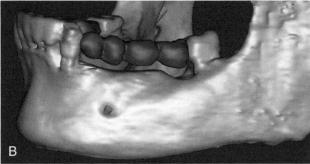

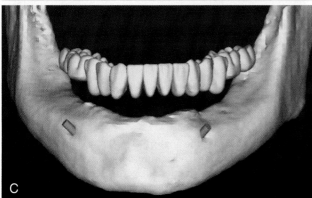

• **Fig. 17.1** When evaluating edentulous sites for implant treatment plans, CBCT images should be used to determine the most ideal prosthesis. (A) 3D CBCT image of implant placed in the missing # 25 area. The position of the implant to the adjacent teeth can easily be determined along with the crown height space. The final prosthesis will most likely be a FP-2. (B) CBCT image showing the osseous contour in relation to the clinical crown of the prosthesis. Note the vertical defect on the second molar which will most likely change the prosthesis type, (c) 3D CBCT image of an edentulous arch depicting the discrepancy between the bone level and prosthesis. In this situation, the prosthesis will most likely be a FP-3.

bone density in the region of implant support are evaluated. The additional implants to support the expected forces on the prosthesis designed may then be determined, with implant size and design selected to match force and area conditions. Only then is the available bone evaluated to assess whether it is possible to place the implants to support the intended prosthesis. In inadequate natural or implant abutment situations, the existing oral conditions or the needs and desires of the patient must be altered. In

other words, either the mouth must be modified by augmentation to place implants in the correct anatomic positions, or the mind of the patient must be modified to accept a different prosthesis type and its limitations. A fixed-implant restoration may be indicated for either the partially or the completely edentulous patient. The psychological advantage of fixed teeth is a major benefit, and edentulous patients often feel the implant teeth are better than their own. The improvement over their removable restoration is significant.

The completely implant-supported overdenture (RP-4) usually will require the same number of implants as a fixed-implant restoration. Thus the cost of implant surgery may be similar for fixed or removable prostheses. FPs often last longer than overdentures, because attachments are not present which require replacement, and acrylic denture teeth wear faster than porcelain to metal or zirconia.[6] The chance of food entrapment under a removable overdenture is often greater than for a fixed restoration, because soft tissue extensions and support are often required in the latter. The laboratory fees for a FP may be similar to a bar, coping attachments, and overdenture. Because the denture or partial denture fees are much less than FPs, many clinicians charge the patient a much lower fee for removable overdentures on implants. However, chair time and laboratory fees are often similar for fixed or removable restorations that are completely implant supported. Therefore, implant overdentrues (e.g. RP-4) should often parallel the cost of a fixed prosthesis. or clinicians to undercharge for overdenture implant-supported prostheses.

Partially Edentulous Prosthesis Design

A common axiom in traditional prosthodontics for partial edentulism is to provide a fixed partial denture whenever applicable.[7,8] The fewer natural teeth missing, the better the indication for a fixed partial denture. This axiom also applies to implant prostheses in the partially edentulous patient. Ideally the fixed partial denture is completely implant supported rather than joining implants to teeth. This concept leads to the use of more implants in the treatment plan. Although this may be a cost disadvantage, it is outweighed by significant intraoral health benefits. The added implants in the edentulous site result in fewer pontics, more retentive units in the restoration, and less stress to the supporting bone. As a result, complications are minimized, and implant and prosthesis longevity are increased (Box 17.2).

- Greater masticatory force
- Greater patient satisfaction
- Psychological (feels more like natural teeth)
- Less food entrapment
- Less maintenance (no attachments to change or adjust)
- Longevity (less prosthesis failure)
- Possible overhead cost as completely implant-supported overdentures

TABLE 17.1   Prosthodontic Classification

Type	Definition
FP-1	Fixed prosthesis; replaces only the clinical crown; looks like a natural tooth.
FP-2	Fixed prosthesis; replaces the crown and a portion of the root; crown contour appears normal in the occlusal half but is elongated or hypercontoured in the gingival half.
FP-3	Fixed prosthesis; replaces missing crowns and gingival color and portion of the edentulous site; prosthesis most often uses denture teeth and acrylic gingiva, but may be porcelain to metal, or zirconia.
RP-4	Removable prosthesis; overdenture that is completely implant supported, no soft tissue support.
RP-5	Removable prosthesis; overdenture supported by both soft tissue (primary) and implant (secondary). The primary stress bearing areas are maintained in the prosthesis (maxilla—residual ridge and horizontal palate; mandible—the line should not begin with a dash. Please move the elements on the last two lines to ensure this doesn't happen. buccal shelf).

From Misch CE. Bone classification training keys. *Dent Today.* 1989;8:39-44.

Prosthetic Options

In 1989, Misch[9,10] proposed five prosthetic options for implant dentistry (Table 17.1). The first three options are FPs (FP-1, FP-2, and FP3). These three options may replace partial (one tooth or several) or total dentitions and may be cemented or screw retained. They are used to communicate the appearance of the final prosthesis to all of the implant team members and the patient. These options depend on the amount of hard and soft tissue structures replaced and the aspects of the prosthesis in the esthetic zone. Common to all fixed options is the inability of the patient to remove the prosthesis. Two types of final removable implant restorations are RPs (RP-4 and RP-5); they depend on the amount of implant and soft tissue support, not the appearance of the prosthesis.

Fixed Prostheses

FP-1

An FP-1 is a fixed restoration and appears to the patient to replace only the anatomic crowns of the missing natural teeth. There must be minimal loss of hard and soft tissues to fabricate this prosthesis type. The volume and position of the residual bone must permit *ideal placement* of the implant in a location similar to the root of a natural tooth.

The final restoration appears similar in size and contour to most traditional FPs used to restore or replace natural crowns of teeth (Fig. 17.2).

The FP-1 prosthesis is most often desired in the maxillary anterior region, especially in the esthetic zone during smiling or speaking and patients with a high smile line. The final FP-1 prosthesis appears to the patient to be similar to a crown on a natural tooth. However, the implant abutment can rarely be treated exactly as a natural tooth prepared for a full crown. For example, the cervical diameter of a maxillary central incisor is ~6.5 mm with an oval to triangular cross-section. However, the implant abutment is usually 4 mm in diameter and round in cross-section. Therefore inherent discrepancies are present between natural teeth and implants.

In addition, the placement of the implant rarely corresponds exactly to the crown-root position of the original tooth. The thin labial bone lying over the facial aspect of a maxillary anterior root remodels after tooth loss and the crest width shifts to the palate, decreasing up to 40% within the first 2 years.[11] The occlusal table is also usually modified in unesthetic regions to conform to the implant size and position, and to direct vertical forces to the implant body. For example, posterior mandibular implant-supported prostheses have narrower occlusal tables at the expense of the buccal contour, because the implant is smaller in diameter and placed in the central fossa region of the tooth.[12]

Because the width or height of the crestal bone is frequently lacking after the loss of multiple adjacent natural teeth, bone augmentation is often required before implant placement to achieve natural-looking crowns in the cervical region (Fig. 17.3). There are rarely interdental papillae in edentulous ridges; therefore soft tissue augmentation also is often required to improve the interproximal gingival contour. Ignoring this step in the process causes open "black" triangular spaces (i.e., where papillae should usually be present) when the patient smiles. FP-1 prostheses are especially difficult to achieve when more than two adjacent teeth are missing. The bone loss and lack of interdental soft tissue complicate the final esthetic result, especially in the cervical region of the crowns (Fig. 17.4). The restorative material of choice for an FP-1 prosthesis is zirconia or lithium disilicate.

FP-2

FP-2 appears to restore the anatomic crown and a portion of the root of the natural tooth. The volume and topography of the available bone is more apical compared with the ideal bone position of a natural root (1 to 2 mm below the cement-enamel junction) and dictate a more apical implant placement compared with the FP-1 prosthesis. As a result, although the incisal edge is in the correct position, the gingival third of the crown is overextended or hypercontoured, usually apical and lingual to the position of the original tooth. These restorations are similar to teeth exhibiting periodontal bone loss and gingival recession (Fig. 17.5).

The patient and the clinician should be aware from the onset of treatment that the final prosthetic teeth will appear longer than healthy natural teeth (without bone loss). The esthetic zone of a patient is established during smiling in the maxillary arch and during speech of sibilant sounds for the mandibular arch (Figs. 17.6 and 17.7). If the high lip line during smiling or the low lip line during speech do not display the cervical regions, the longer teeth are usually of no esthetic consequence, provided that the patient has been informed before treatment.

As the patient becomes older, the maxillary esthetic zone is altered. Only 10% of younger patients do not show any soft tissue during smiling, whereas 30% of 60-year-olds and 50% of 80-year-olds do not display gingival regions during smiling (Fig. 17.8). The low lip position during speech is not affected as much as the high smile line. Only 10% of older patients show the mandibular soft tissue during speech.[13,14]

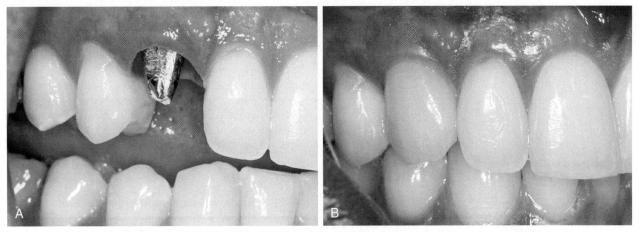

• Fig. 17.2 (A) An implant is positioned in the maxillary right canine position. The hard and soft tissue conditions are ideal for a crown of normal contour and size. (B) The maxillary right canine implant crown in position. The soft tissue drape is similar to a natural tooth, and the crown contour is similar to the clinical crown contour of a natural tooth. This is the goal of an FP-1 prosthesis.

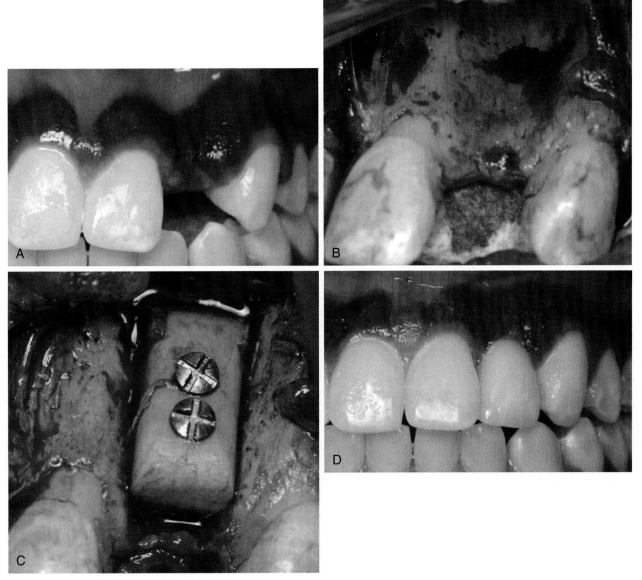

• Fig. 17.3 FP-1 (A) congenitally missing left lateral incisor, (B) large osseous defect resulting in inadequate amount of bone for implant placement, (C) autogenous block graft, and (D) final FP-1 zirconia restoration.

A multiple-unit FP-2 restoration does not require as specific an implant position in the mesial or distal position because the cervical contour is not displayed during function. The implant position may be chosen in relation to ideal bone width, angulation, or hygienic considerations rather than purely esthetic

demands (compared with the FP-1 prosthesis). On occasion the implant may even be placed in an embrasure between two teeth. This often occurs for mandibular anterior teeth for full-arch fixed restorations. If this occurs, the most esthetic area usually requires the incisal two-thirds of the two crowns to be ideal in width, as though the implant were not present. Only the cervical region is compromised. Although the implant is not positioned in an ideal mesiodistal position, it should be placed in the correct facial-lingual position to ensure that contour, hygiene, and direction of forces are not compromised. The material of choice for an FP-2 prosthesis is zirconia or lithium disilicate.

FP-3

The FP-3 fixed restoration appears to replace the natural teeth crowns and has pink-colored restorative materials to replace a portion of the soft tissue. As with the FP-2 prosthesis, the original available bone height has decreased by natural resorption or osteoplasty at the time of implant placement. To place the incisal edge of the teeth in proper position for esthetics, function, lip support, and speech, the excessive vertical dimension to be restored requires teeth that are unnatural in length. However, unlike the FP-2 prosthesis, the patient may have a normal-to-high maxillary lip line during smiling or a low mandibular lip line during speech. The ideal high smile line displays the interdental papilla of the maxillary anterior teeth but not the soft tissue above the midcervical regions. Approximately 7% of males and 14% of females have a high smile, or "gummy" smile, and display more than 2 mm of gingival above the free gingival margin of the teeth[13] (Fig. 17.9).

The patient may also have greater esthetic demands even when the teeth are out of the esthetic smile and speech zones. Patients report that the display of longer teeth appears unnatural even though they must lift or move their lips in unnatural positions to see the covered regions of the teeth. As a result of the restored gingival color of the FP-3, the teeth have a more natural appearance in size and shape, and the pink restorative material mimics the interdental papillae and cervical emergence region. The addition of gingival-tone acrylic, porcelain, or zirconia for a more natural FP appearance is often indicated with multiple implant abutments because bone loss is common with these conditions. There are basically three approaches for an FP-3 prosthesis: (1) a hybrid restoration of denture teeth and acrylic and metal

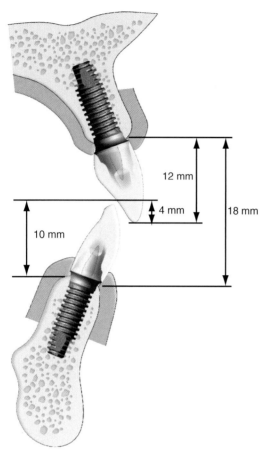

Fig. 17.4 The hard and soft tissue must be ideal in volume and position to obtain an FP-1 appearance for the final restoration. When multiple teeth are replaced, bone and tissue augmentation is usually required to obtain an FP-1 prosthesis.

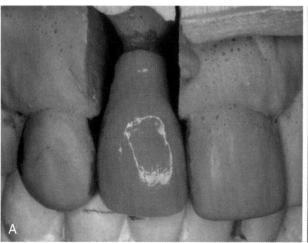
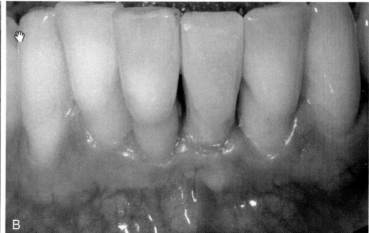

Fig. 17.5 (A) FP-2 prosthesis resulting from implant placement too far apically. Ideally the implant neck should be 2 to 3 mm below the free gingival margin of the adjacent teeth. (B) Because the FP-2 prosthesis is hypercontoured, it is often not esthetically pleasant. However, in this example, because of the bone and tissue loss of the adjacent teeth, the FP-2 prosthesis blends in very well.

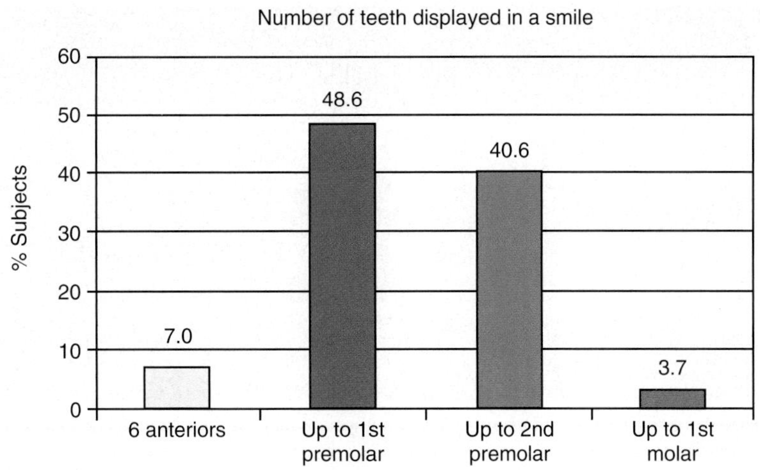

Number of teeth displayed in a smile

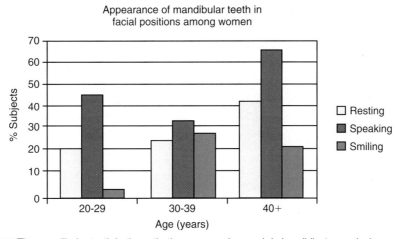

• **Fig. 17.6** The number of teeth observed during a high smile line is variable. Almost 50% of patients display the teeth up to a first premolar. Only 3.7% of patients display the maxillary teeth to the first molar. (*Adapted from Tjan AHL, Miller GD. Some esthetic factors in a smile.* J Prosthet Dent. *1984;51:24-28.*)

Appearance of mandibular teeth in facial positions among women

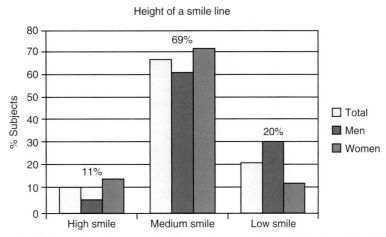

• **Fig. 17.7** The mandibular teeth in the esthetic zone are observed during sibilant sounds, because more teeth show during speech than at rest or smiling. (*Adapted from Cade RE. The role of the mandibular anterior teeth in complete denture esthetics.* J Prosthet Dent. *1979;42:368-370.*)

Height of a smile line

• **Fig. 17.8** A smile that shows interdental papillae but no cervical tissue is ideal and found in 70% of patients. A low smile line shows no soft tissue during smiling and is seen in 20% of patients (more men than women). A high smile line displays interdental papillae and the cervical regions above the teeth, and is observed in 11% of patients (more women than men). (*Adapted from Tjan AHL, Miller GD. Some esthetic factors in a smile.* J Prosthet Dent. *1984;51:24-28.*)

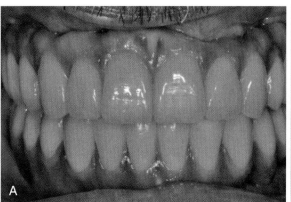
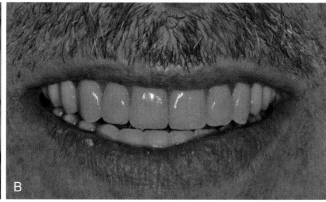

• **Fig. 17.9** (A) A full-arch FP-3 maxillary implant prosthesis. Note the maxillary placement of implants in embrasure areas and irregular tissue level. (B) The high smile line of the same patient. The low lip position during smiling permitted the fabrication of an FP-2 prosthesis.

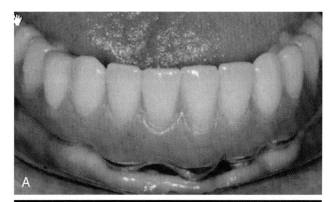
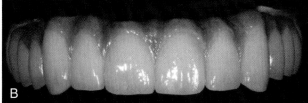
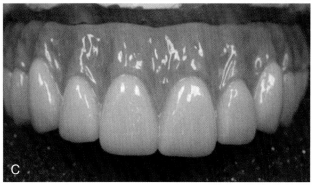

• **Fig. 17.10** FP-3 Restorative Materials. (A) The hybrid FP-3 consisting of acrylic and denture teeth on a metal substructure; (B) porcelain fused to metal FP-3 consisting of a metal substructure and porcelain; and (C) monolithic zirconia, which is fabricated from a solid block of zirconia and stained to the teeth and tissue colors.

substructure,[15] (2) a porcelain-metal restoration, or (3) a monolithic zirconia prosthesis. The most important factor involved in selecting the prosthetic material is esthetics, longevity, and durability. Today the material that is advantageous and fulfills these requirements is monolithic zirconia (Figs. 17.10 and 17.11; Table 17.2).

Another factor that determines the restoration material is the amount of crown height space.[2,16] An excessive crown height space means a traditional porcelain-metal restoration will have a large amount of metal in the substructure, so the porcelain thickness will not be greater than 2 mm. Otherwise there is an increase in porcelain fracture. Precious metals are indicated for implant restorations to decrease the risk for corrosion and improve the accuracy of the casting, because nonprecious metals shrink more during the casing process. However, the large amount of metal in the substructure acts as a heat sink and complicates the application of porcelain during the fabrication of the prosthesis. In addition, as the metal cools after casting, the thinner regions of metal cool first and create porosities in the structure. This may lead to fracture of the framework after loading. Furthermore, when the casting is reinserted into the oven to bake the porcelain, the heat is maintained within the casting at different rates; thus the porcelain cool-down rate is variable, which increases the risk for porcelain fracture. In addition, the amount of precious metal in the casting adds to the weight and cost of the restoration. An FP-3 porcelain-to-metal restoration is more difficult to fabricate for the laboratory technician than an FP-2 prosthesis. The pink porcelain is more difficult to make appear as soft tissue and usually requires more baking cycles. This increases the risk for porosity or porcelain fracture (Figs. 17.12 and 17.13).

An alternative to the traditional porcelain-metal FP is a hybrid prosthesis (see Table 17.2). This restoration design uses a smaller metal framework, with denture teeth and acrylic to join these elements together. This prosthesis is less expensive to fabricate and is highly esthetic because of the premade denture teeth and acrylic pink soft tissue replacements. In addition, the intermediary acrylic between the denture teeth and framework may reduce the impact force of dynamic occlusal loads. The hybrid prosthesis is easier to repair in comparison to porcelain, because the denture tooth may be replaced with less risk than adding porcelain to a traditional porcelain-metal restoration. However, the fatigue of acrylic is greater than the traditional prosthesis; therefore repair of the restoration is more commonly needed.

Monolithic zirconia has been able to curtail all of the complications from the hybrid and porcelain fused to metal restorations. Monolithic zirconia has been shown to have a high flexural and compressive strength, which approximates 1465 MPa. Because of its monolithic nature, minimal interocclusal space (~8 mm) is needed for the fabrication of the prosthesis and can be fabricated with ~0.5-mm interocclusal space. A high 5-year success rate has

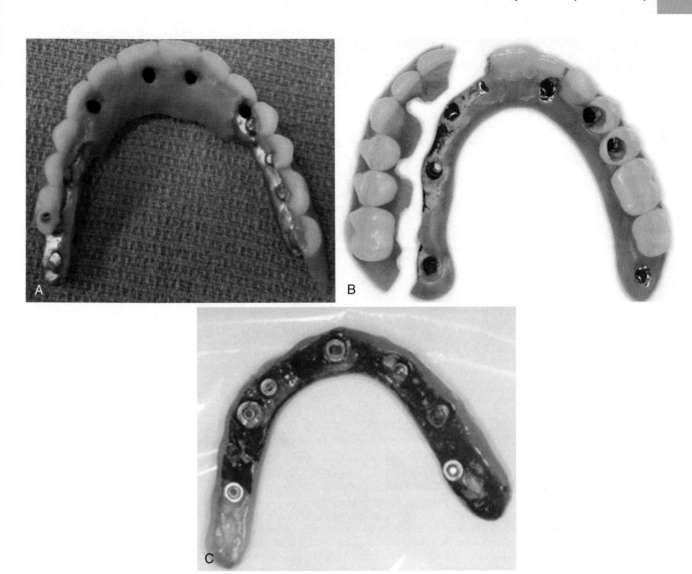

• Fig. 17.11 Complications of FP-3 Hybrid Prostheses. (A) Attrition and wear of the denture teeth, especially if opposing natural teeth or porcelain; (B) delamination is common, which is usually caused by excess force on the prosthesis; and (C) the acrylic and denture teeth tend to harbor bacteria, leading to difficulty in hygiene and often causing peri-implant disease.

TABLE 17.2   Comparison of Porcelain-to-Metal Versus Hybrid Prostheses Versus Zirconia (FP-3)

Consideration	Porcelain	Hybrid	Monolithic Zirconia-Metal
Occlusal vertical	>12 mm	≥15 mm	≥10 mm
Technique	Same	Same	Same
Retention	Cement or screw	Cement or screw	Cement or screw
Precision of fit	Fair	Fair/Good	Good
Esthetics	Same	Same	Same
Soft tissue	Difficult	Easier	Easier
Time/appointments	Same	Less	Same
Weight	More	Less	More
Cost	More	Less	More
Impact forces	More	Less	Excellent
Volume (bulk)	Same	Same	Same
Long term	Same	Same	Excellent
Occlusion	Stable	Variable	Stable
Speech	Same	Same	Same
Biofilm accumulation	Medium	High	Low
Hygiene	Same	Same	Same
Complications	Medium	High	Low
Aging of materials	Less	More	Less

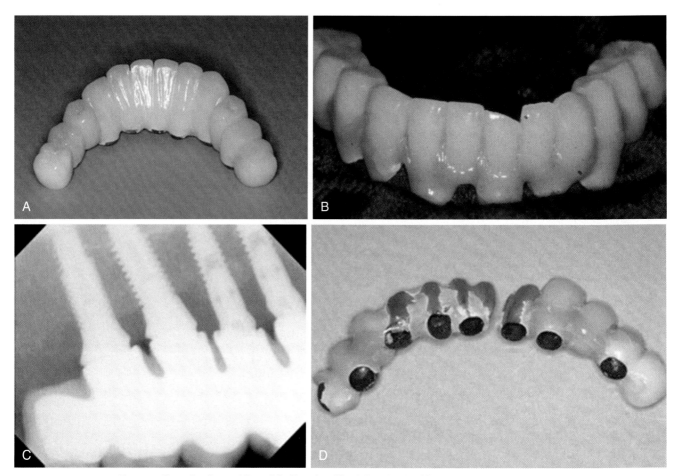

• **Fig. 17.12** Complications of Porcelain Fused to Metal Prosthesis. (A) Porcelain fused to metal prostheses tends to be very heavy, especially if there are increased amounts of tissue loss (i.e., more metal substructure needed). This often results in patients reporting compromised opening or temporomandibular joint symptoms. (B) Porcelain fracture is the most common complication, often requiring the refabrication of the prosthesis. (C) Marginal integrity is a significant problem because of the difficulty in obtaining a passive casting, and (D) to increase the marginal integrity, the metal framework is often soldered; however, this results in an increased possibility of prosthesis fracture.

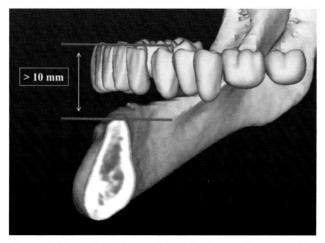

• **Fig. 17.13** Interocclusal Space. Interocclusal space is measured from the incisal edge to the alveolar crest. An FP-3 prosthesis requires a minimum of 10 mm for a monolithic zirconia, ~12 mm for a porcelain fused to metal prosthesis, and >15 mm for a hybrid prosthesis. The amount of space can be easily determined from the cone beam computed tomography images.

been shown with minimal complications.[17] Antagonistic wear is minimal and is advantageous to porcelain and natural teeth enamel. Lastly, there is less peri-implant disease, as lower thickness of biofilm accumulates in comparison with a porcelain product.

The crown height space determination for a hybrid prosthesis is approximately 15 mm from the bone to the occlusal plane. When less than this space is available, a porcelain-to-metal restoration is suggested. When a greater crown height space is present, a hybrid prosthesis is often fabricated. Implants placed too facial, lingual, or in embrasures are easier to restore when vertical bone has been lost and an FP-2 or FP-3 prosthesis is fabricated, because even extremely high smile lip lines do not expose the implant abutments. The greater crown heights allow the correction of incisal edge positions. However, the FP-2 or FP-3 restoration has greater crown height compared with the FP-1 fixed types of prostheses; therefore a greater moment of force is placed on the implant cervical regions, especially during lateral forces (e.g., mandibular excursions or with cantilevered restorations). As a result, additional implant abutments or shorter cantilever lengths should be considered with these restorations (Figs. 17.14 and 17.15).

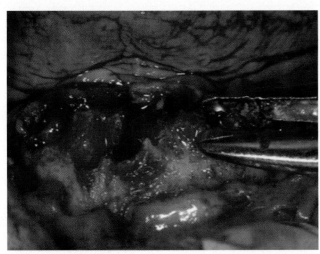

Fig. 17.14 Techniques to Increase Interocclusal Space. Ideally the amount of interocclusal space is determined before the placement of implants. An osteoplasty is usually required before placement for an increased interocclusal space.

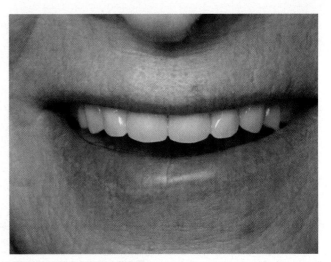

Fig. 17.16 The soft tissue profile may be changed or modified very easily with an RP-4 and RP-5 prosthesis. This can be completed by adding bulk to the flange areas of the prosthesis.

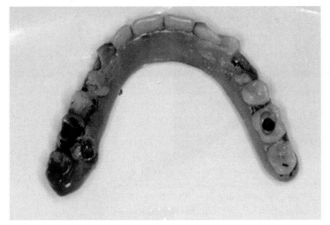

Fig. 17.15 FP-3 Hybrid Complication. When there exists insufficient interocclusal space, it is common for denture teeth to fracture or debond.

An FP-2 or FP-3 prosthesis rarely has the patient's interdental papillae or ideal soft tissue contours around the emergence of the crowns, because these restorations are used when there is more crown height space and the lip does not expose the soft tissue regions of the patient. In the maxillary arch, wide open embrasures between the implants may cause food impaction or speech problems. These complications may be solved by using a removable soft tissue replacement device or making overcontoured cervical restorations. The maxillary FP-2 or the FP-3 prosthesis is often extended or juxtaposed to the maxillary soft tissue so that speech is not impaired. Hygiene is more difficult to control, although access next to each implant abutment is provided.

The mandibular restoration may be left above the tissue, similar to a sanitary pontic. This facilitates oral hygiene in the mandible, especially when the implant permucosal site is level with the floor of the mouth and the depth of the vestibule. However, if the space below the restoration is too great, the lower lip may lack support in the labiomental region. Rarely can this space be left in the maxilla, because this will usually impact esthetics or affect the speech (e.g., the patient may exhibit "whistling" sounds or saliva extrusion through the spaces).

Removable Prostheses

There are two types of removable prostheses RPs (RP-4 and RP-5), based on support of the restoration (see Table 17.1). Patients are able to remove the prosthesis but not the implant-supported superstructure attached to the abutments. The difference in the two categories of removable restorations is not in appearance (as it is in the fixed categories). Instead, the two removable categories are determined by the amount of implant and soft tissue support.[18] The most common removable implant prostheses are overdentures for completely edentulous patients, which have been reported with high predictability.[6,19-23] One of the most significant benefits of a removable implant prosthesis (RP-4 and RP-5) is the ability to enhance the soft tissue profile. With an FP (FP-1, FP-2, or FP-3) in an edentulous patient, it is often difficult to increase the fullness of the soft tissue without overcontouring the prosthesis and making hygiene difficult (Fig. 17.16).

RP-4

RP-4 is an RP that is completely supported by the implants, teeth, or both with no soft tissue support. The prosthesis is rigid when inserted: Overdenture attachments usually connect the RP to a low-profile tissue bar or superstructure that splints the implant abutments. Usually five or six implants in the mandible and six to eight implants in the maxilla are required to fabricate completely implant-supported RP-4 prostheses in patients with favorable dental criteria.

The implant placement criteria for an RP-4 prosthesis are different from that for an FP. More interocclusal space is required to allow for sufficient space for acrylic and denture teeth. In addition, a superstructure and overdenture attachments must be added to the implant abutments. This requires a more lingual and apical implant placement in comparison with the implant position for an FP. If implant placement is not more lingually or apically positioned, insufficient space will be present to retain the denture teeth. The implants in an RP-4 prosthesis (and an FP-2 or FP-3 restoration) should be placed in the mesiodistal position for the best biomechanical and hygienic situation. On occasion the position of an attachment on the superstructure or prosthesis may also affect the amount of spacing between the implants. For example, a Hader clip requires the implant spacing to be greater than 6 mm from edge to edge, and as a consequence reduces the number

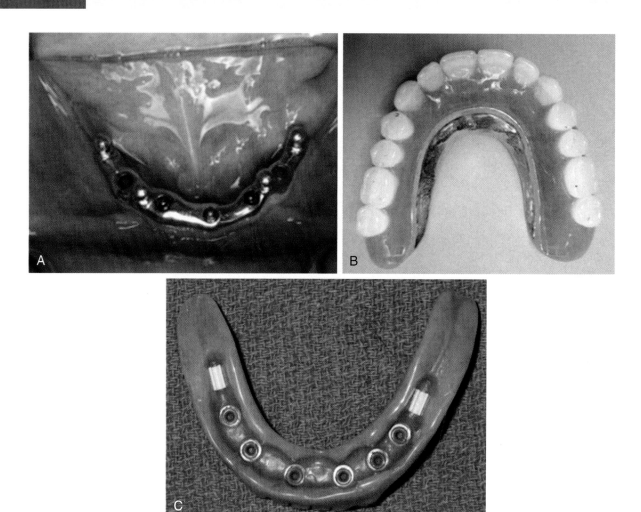

• **Fig. 17.17** RP-4 Prosthesis. An RP-4 prosthesis is a totally implant-supported prosthesis with no soft tissue support. (A) Usually this type of prosthesis is retained with a splinted bar. (B) A maxillary RP-4 is a palateless prosthesis that usually is reinforced with metal or fiber to increase strength. (C) The mandibular RP-4 prosthesis is totally implant supported with no soft tissue support (e.g., no buccal shelf extension).

of implants that may be placed between the mental foramina. The RP-4 prosthesis may have the same appearance as an FP-1, FP-2, or FP-3 restoration. A porcelain-to-metal prosthesis with attachments in selected abutment crowns can be fabricated for patients with the cosmetic desire of an FP. The overdenture attachments permit improved oral hygiene or allow the patient to sleep without the excess forces of nocturnal bruxism on the prosthesis (Fig. 17.17).

RP-5

RP-5 is an RP with soft tissue (primary) and implant (secondary) support. There exist many options with an RP-5 prosthesis. For example, the completely edentulous mandibular overdenture may have: (1) two anterior implants independent of each other, (2) splinted implants in the canine region to enhance retention, (3) three splinted implants in the premolar and central incisor areas to provide lateral stability, or (4) implants splinted with a cantilevered bar to reduce soft tissue abrasions and to limit the amount of soft tissue coverage needed for prosthesis support. The primary advantage of an RP-5 restoration is the reduced cost. The prosthesis is similar to traditional overdentures supported by natural teeth (Fig. 17.18). In the maxilla, depending on the arch form, four, five, or six implants are indicated. The final prosthesis is a full-arch conventional denture that receives the primary support from the soft tissue and secondarily from the implants.

A preimplant treatment denture may be fabricated to ensure the patient's satisfaction. This technique is especially indicated for patients with demanding needs and desires regarding the final esthetic result. The implant clinician can also use the treatment denture as a guide for implant placement. The patient can wear the prosthesis during the healing stage. After the implants are uncovered, the superstructure is fabricated within the guidelines of the existing treatment restoration. Once this is achieved, the preimplant treatment prosthesis may be converted to the RP-4 or RP-5 restoration. The clinician and the patient should realize that the bone will continue to resorb in the soft tissue–borne regions of the prosthesis. Relines and occlusal adjustments every few years are common maintenance requirements of an RP-5 restoration. Bone resorption with RP-5 prostheses may occur two to three times faster than the resorption found with full dentures.[5] This can be a factor when considering this type of treatment in young patients, despite the lesser cost and low failure rate.

Summary

In traditional dentistry, the restoration reflects the existing condition of the patient. Existing natural abutments are first evaluated, and a removable or fixed restoration is fabricated accordingly.

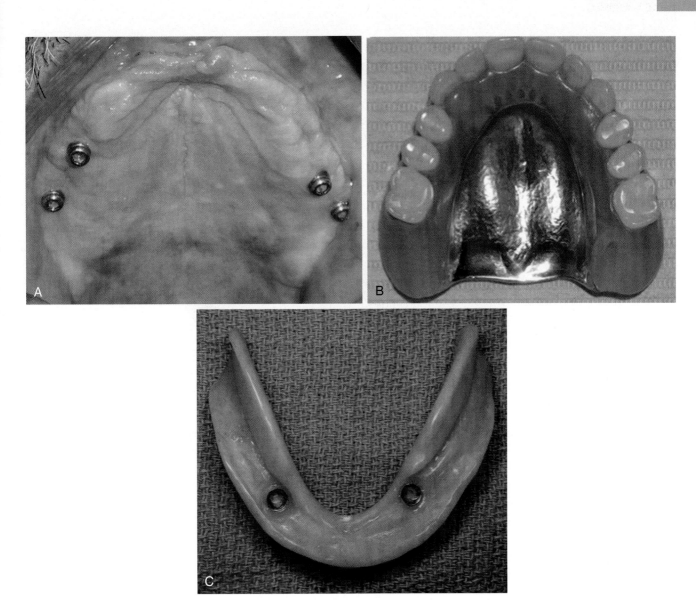

• **Fig. 17.18** RP-5 Prosthesis. An RP-5 prosthesis is a soft tissue–supported prosthesis with secondary implant support. (A) Usually an RP-5 prosthesis is retained with nonsplinted attachments (e.g., no substructure bar). (B) A maxillary RP-5 prosthesis is a complete palate (e.g., must have full palatal support). (C) The mandibular RP-5 prosthesis is soft tissue supported with buccal shelf flange extension.

Implant dentistry is unique because an additional foundation base may be created for a desired prosthodontic result. Therefore both the psychological and anatomic needs and desires of the patient should be evaluated and determined. The prosthesis that satisfies these goals and eliminates the existing problems may then be designed. The prosthesis may be fixed or removable for the completely edentulous patient, whereas fixed restorations are planned for most partially edentulous patients.

If only one implant approach is used for all patients, the same surgical and prosthetic scenarios and flaws are invariably repeated. For example, if all edentulous mandibles are treated with two implants, not only are the implant and surgery similar regardless of intraoral or extraoral conditions, but an RP-5 prosthesis will usually result despite the patient's needs and desires. Many patients will accept an RP-5 prosthesis; however, many will not.

Therefore patients need to be educated on the advantages and disadvantages of the various types of prostheses.

The benefits of implant dentistry can be realized only when the prosthesis is first discussed and determined. An organized treatment approach based on the prosthesis permits predictable therapy results. Five prosthetic options postulated by Misch are available in implant dentistry. Three restorations are fixed and vary in the amount of hard and soft tissue replaced; two are removable and are based on the amount and type of support for the restoration (Figs. 17.19 and 17.20). The amount of support required for an implant prosthesis should initially be designed similar to traditional tooth-supported restorations. Once the intended prosthesis is designed, the implants and treatment surrounding this specific result can be established.

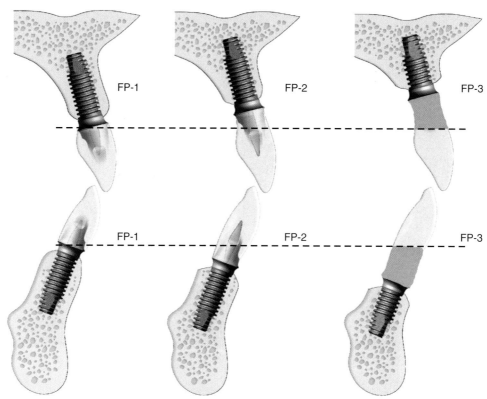

• **Fig. 17.19** Fixed restorations have three categories: FP-1, FP-2, and FP-3. The restoration type is related to the contour of the restoration. (FP-1 is ideal, FP-2 is hypercontoured, and FP-3 replaces the gingiva drape with pink porcelain or acrylic.) The difference between FP-2 and FP-3 most often is related to the high maxillary lip position during smiling or the mandibular lip position during sibilant sounds of speech. FP-2 and FP-3 restorations often require more implant surface area support by increasing implant number or size, or by adjusting design considerations.

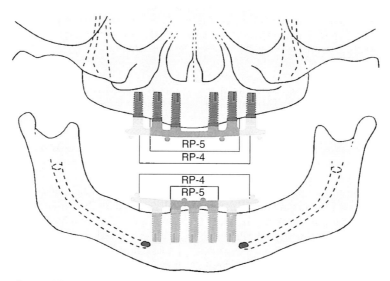

• **Fig. 17.20** Removable prostheses have two categories based on implant support. RP-4 prostheses have complete implant support anteriorly and posteriorly. In the mandible the superstructure bar often is cantilevered from implants positioned between the foramina. The maxillary RP-4 prosthesis usually has more implants and little to no cantilever. An RP-5 restoration has primarily anterior implant support and posterior soft tissue support in the maxilla or mandible. Often fewer implants are required, and bone grafting is less likely indicated.

References

1. Misch CE. Consideration of biomechanical stress in treatment with dental implants. *Dent Today*. 2006;25(80). 82,84,85; quiz 85.
2. Misch CE, Goodacre CJ, Finley M, et al. Consensus conference panel reports: crown-height space guidelines for implant dentistry—part 1. *Implant Dent*. 2005;14:312–318.
3. Jacobs R, van Steenberghe D, Nys M, et al. Maxillary bone resorption in patients with mandibular implant-supported overdentures: a survey. *Int J Prosthodont*. 1996;9:58–64.
4. Barber HD, Scott RF, Maxon BB, et al. Evaluation of anterior maxillary alveolar ridge resorption when opposed by the transmandibular implant. *J Oral Maxillofac Surg*. 1990;48:1283–1287.
5. Jacobs R, Schotte A, van Steenberghe D, et al. Posterior jaw bone resorption in osseointegrated implant overdentures. *Clin Oral Implants Res*. 1992;2:63–70.
6. Goodacre CJ, Bernal G, Rungcharassaeng K, et al. Clinical complications with implants and implant prosthodontics. *J Prosthet Dent*. 2003;90:121–132.
7. Dykema RW, Goodacre CJ, Phillips RW. *Johnston's Modern Practice on Fixed Prosthodontics*. 4th ed. Philadelphia: WB Saunders; 1986.
8. Tylman SD, Malone WFD. *Tylman's Theory and Practice of Fixed Prosthodontics*. 7th ed. St Louis: Mosby; 1978.
9. Misch CE. Bone classification, training keys. *Dent Today*. 1989;8:39–44.
10. Misch CE. Prosthetic options in implant dentistry. *Int J Oral Implantol*. 1991;7:17–21.
11. Misch CE. Early maxillary bone loss after tooth extraction: a clinical observation. In: *Misch Implant Institute Manual*. Dearborn, MI: Misch Implant Institute; 1991.
12. Misch CE. Posterior single tooth replacement. In: Misch CE, ed. *Dental Implant Prosthetics*. St Louis: Mosby; 2005.
13. Tjan AH, Miller GD, The JG. Some esthetic factors in a smile. *J Prosthet Dent*. 1984;51:24–28.
14. Cade RE. The role of the mandibular anterior teeth in complete denture esthetics. *J Prosthet Dent*. 1979;42:368–370.
15. Brånemark PI, Zarb GA, Albrektsson T. *Tissue Integrated Prostheses*. Chicago: Quintessence; 1985.
16. Misch CE, Misch-Dietsh F. Preimplant prosthodontics. In: Misch CE, ed. *Dental Implant Prosthetics*. St Louis: Mosby; 2005.
17. Sulaiman TA, Abdulmajeed AA, Donovan TE, et al. Fracture rate of monolithic zirconia restorations up to 5 years: a dental laboratory survey. *J Prosthet Dent*. 2016;113(3):436–439.
18. Misch CE. Implant overdentures relieve discomfort for the edentulous. *Dentist*. 1989;67:37–38.
19. Naert I, Quirynen M, Theuniers G, et al. Prosthetic aspects of osseointegrated fixtures supported by overdentures: a 4-year report. *J Prosthet Dent*. 1991;65:671–680.
20. Spiekermann H, Jansen VK, Richter J. A 10-year follow-up of IMZ and TPS implants in the edentulous mandible using bar-retained overdentures. *Int J Oral Maxillofac Implants*. 1995;10:231–243.
21. Chan MFW, Johnston C, Howell RA, et al. Prosthetic management of the atrophic mandible using endosseous implants and overdentures: a 6-year review. *Br Dent J*. 1995;179:329–337.
22. Johns RB, Jemt T, Heath MR, et al. A multicenter study of overdentures, supported by Brånemark implants. *Int J Oral Maxillofac Implants*. 1992;7:513–522.
23. Zarb GA, Schmitt A. The edentulous predicament. I. The longitudinal effectiveness of implant-supported overdentures. *J Am Dent Assoc*. 1996;127:66–72.

18

Bone Density: A Key Determinant for Treatment Planning

RANDOLPH R. RESNIK AND CARL E. MISCH†

Available bone is a crucial part of implant dentistry and describes the external architecture or volume of the edentulous area considered for implants. In the early days of oral implantology, the available bone was not modified in the implant candidate. Instead the existing bone volume was the primary factor used to develop a treatment plan. Short implants and fewer implants were used in less-available bone, and long implants in greater numbers were inserted in larger bone volumes. Today, the treatment plan should start with the determination of the final prosthesis first, then evaluate patient force factors followed by the bone density.

The internal structure of bone is described in terms of quality or density, which reflects a number of biomechanical properties, such as strength and modulus of elasticity. The external and internal architecture of bone controls virtually every facet of the practice of implant dentistry. The density of available bone in an edentulous site is a determining factor in treatment planning, implant design, surgical approach, healing time, and initial progressive bone loading during prosthetic reconstruction.[1,2] This chapter presents the aspects of bone density related to overall planning of an implant prosthesis.

Influence of Bone Density on Implant Success Rates

The quality of bone is often dependent on the arch position.[3-7] The densest bone is usually observed in the anterior mandible, followed by the anterior maxilla and posterior mandible, and the least-dense bone is typically found in the posterior maxilla. Following a standard surgical and prosthetic protocol, Adell et al.[8] reported an approximately 10% greater success rate in the anterior mandible compared with the anterior maxilla. Schnitman et al.[9] also noted lower success rates in the posterior mandible compared with the anterior mandible when the same protocol was followed. The highest clinical failure rates have been reported in the posterior maxilla, where the force magnitude is greater and the bone density is poorer.[5-7,9-13] Therefore, the literature is quite abundant on implant survival relative to the arch position.

In addition to arch location, several independent groups have reported different failure rates related to the quality of the bone.[3-21]

Engquist et al.[16] observed that 78% of all reported implant failures were in soft bone types. Friberg et al.[3] observed that 66% of their group's implant failures occurred in the resorbed maxilla with soft bone. Jaffin and Berman,[15] in a 5-year study, reported a 44% implant failure rate when poor-density bone was observed in the maxilla. The article documented a 35% implant loss in any region of the mouth when bone density was poor. Fifty-five percent of all implant failures within their study sample occurred in the soft bone type. Johns et al.[17] reported a 3% failure rate of implants in moderate bone densities but a 28% implant failure rate in the poorest bone type. Smedberg et al. reported a 36% failure rate in the poorest bone density.[18] The reduced implant survival most often is more related to bone density than arch location. In a 15-year follow-up study, Snauwaert et al.[12] reported early annual and late failures were more frequently found in the maxilla. Herrmann et al.[13] found implant failures were strongly correlated to patient factors, including bone quality, especially when coupled with poor bone volume (65% of these patients experienced failure). These reported failures are not primarily related to surgery healing but instead occur after prosthetic loading. Therefore over the years, many independent clinical groups, following a standardized surgical protocol, documented the indisputable influence of bone density on clinical success (Fig. 18.1). However, a protocol established by Misch, which adapts the treatment plan, implant selection, surgical approach, healing regimen, and initial prosthetic loading, has resulted in similar implant success rates in all bone densities and all arch positions.[22-25] This chapter proposes a scientific rationale for the modification of a treatment plan in function of implant density to achieve comparable success rates in all bone types.

Etiology of Variable Bone Density

Bone is an organ that is able to change in relation to a number of factors, including hormones, vitamins, and mechanical influences. However, biomechanical parameters, such as duration of edentulous state, are predominant.[26-30] Awareness of this adaptability has been reported for more than a century. In 1887 Meier[31] qualitatively described the architecture of trabecular bone in the femur. In 1888 Kulmann[32] noticed the similarity between the pattern of trabecular bone in the femur and tension trajectories in construction beams.

†Deceased.

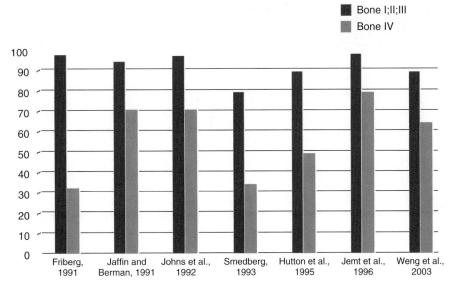

● **Fig. 18.1** Over the years, several clinical reports observed higher success rates in better bone quality (bone I to III) and lower survival rates in poor bone quality (bone IV).

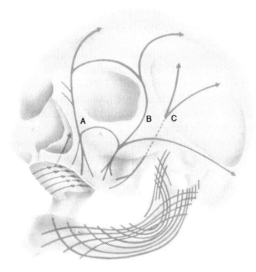

● **Fig. 18.2** The maxilla is a force distribution unit, which allows for force to be redirected away from the brain and orbit (A,B,and C). The mandible is designed to absorb force, thereby forming denser and thick cortical bone and courser trabecular bone.

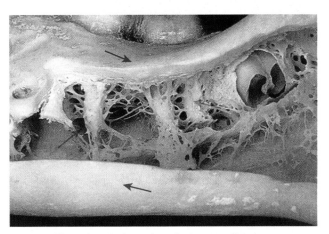

● **Fig. 18.3** The trabecular bone in a dentate mandible is coarser compared with the maxilla (*green arrows*). The mandible, as an independent structure, is a force-absorbing element. In addition, the cortical bone is thicker and more dense (*red arrows*).

Wolff,[33] in 1892, further elaborated on these concepts and published, "Every change in the form and function of bone or of its function alone is followed by certain definite changes in the internal architecture, and equally definite alteration in its external conformation, in accordance with mathematical laws." The modified function of bone and the definite changes in the internal and external formation of the vertebral skeleton as influenced by mechanical load were reported by Murry.[34] Therefore the external architecture of bone changes in relation to function, and the internal bony structure is also modified.

MacMillan[35] and Parfitt[36] have reported on the structural characteristics and variation of trabeculae in the alveolar regions of the jaws. For example, the maxilla and mandible have different biomechanical functions (Fig. 18.2). The mandible, as an independent structure, is designed as a force absorption unit. Therefore, when teeth are present, the outer cortical bone is denser and thicker, and the trabecular bone is coarser and denser (Fig. 18.3). In contrast, the maxilla is a force distribution unit. Any strain to the maxilla is transferred by the zygomatic arch and palate away from the brain and orbit. As a consequence the maxilla has a thin cortical plate and fine trabecular bone supporting the teeth (Fig. 18.4). They also noted that the bone is densest around the teeth (cribriform plate) and denser around the teeth at the crest compared with the regions around the apices (Fig. 18.5). Alveolar bone resorption associated with orthodontic therapy also illustrates the biomechanical sensitivity of the alveolar processes.[37] Generalized trabecular bone loss in the jaws occurs in regions around a tooth from a decrease in mechanical strain.[38] Orban[39] demonstrated a decrease in the trabecular bone pattern around a maxillary molar with no opposing occlusion compared with a tooth with occlusal contacts on the contralateral side (Fig. 18.6). Bone density in the jaws also decreases after tooth loss. This loss is primarily related to the length of time the region has been edentulous and not loaded appropriately, the initial density of the bone, flexure and torsion in the mandible, and parafunction before and after tooth loss. In general, the density change after tooth loss is greatest in the posterior maxilla and least in the anterior mandible.

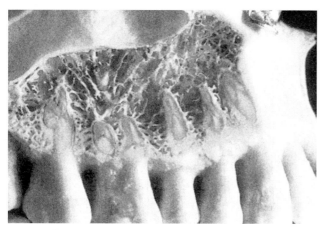

• **Fig. 18.4** The dentate maxilla has a finer trabecular pattern compared with the mandible. The maxilla is a force distribution unit and is designed to protect the orbit and brain.

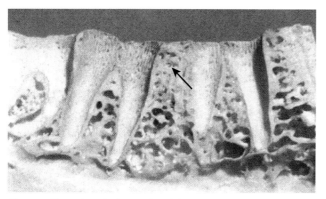

• **Fig. 18.5** The trabecular bone of each jaw has structural variations. The trabecular bone is densest next to the teeth, where it forms the cribriform plate. Between the teeth the bone is usually densest near the crest and least dense at the apex.

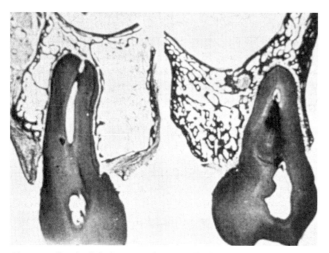

• **Fig. 18.6** On the left the opposing mandibular tooth was removed. A lack of occlusal contact resulted in loss of trabecular bone around the maxillary tooth. The tooth on the right is from the same monkey, with the opposing mandibular tooth in place. The trabecular bone is much denser around the tooth. The disuse atrophy observed on the left is from inadequate microstrain conditions to maintain the bone. (*From Orban B*. Oral Histology and Embryology. *3rd ed. St. Louis, MO: Mosby; 1953.*)

Cortical and trabecular bone throughout the body are constantly modified by either modeling or remodeling.[40] Modeling has independent sites of formation and resorption, and results in the change of the shape or size of bone. Remodeling is a process of resorption and formation at the same site that replaces previously existing bone and primarily affects the internal turnover of bone, including that region where teeth are lost or the bone next to an endosteal implant.[41,42] These adaptive phenomena have been associated with the alteration of the mechanical stress and strain environment within the host bone.[43,44] Stress is determined by the magnitude of force divided by the functional area over which it is applied. Strain is defined as the change in length of a material divided by the original length. The greater the magnitude of stress applied to the bone, the greater the strain observed in the bone.[45] Bone modeling and remodeling are primarily controlled, in part or whole, by the mechanical environment of strain. Overall the density of alveolar bone evolves as a result of mechanical deformation from microstrain.

Frost[46] proposed a model of four histologic patterns for compact bone as it relates to mechanical adaptation to strain. The pathologic overload zone, mild overload zone, adapted window, and acute disuse window were described for bone in relation to the amount of the microstrain experienced (Fig. 18.7). These four categories also may be used to describe the trabecular bone response in the jaws. The bone in the acute disuse window loses mineral density, and disuse atrophy occurs because modeling for new bone is inhibited and remodeling is stimulated, with a gradual net loss of bone. The microstrain of bone for trivial loading is reported to be 0 to 50 microstrain. This phenomenon may occur throughout the skeletal system, as evidenced by a 15% decrease in the cortical plate and extensive trabecular bone loss consequent to immobilized limbs for 3 months.[47] A cortical bone density decrease of 40% and a trabecular bone density decrease of 12% also have been reported with disuse of bone.[48,49] Interestingly, bone loss similar to disuse atrophy has been associated with microgravity environments in outer space, because the microstrain in bone resulting from the Earth's gravity is not present in the "weightless" environment of space.[50] In fact, an astronaut aboard the Russian Mir space station for 111 days lost nearly 12% of his bone minerals.[51,52]

The *adapted window* (50–1500 microstrain) represents an equilibrium of modeling and remodeling, and bone conditions are maintained at this level. Bone in this strain environment remains in a steady state, and this may be considered the homeostatic window of health. The histologic description of this bone is primarily lamellar or load-bearing bone. Approximately 18% of trabecular bone and 2% to 5% of cortical bone are remodeled each year[26] in the physiologic loading zone, which corresponds to the adapted window. This is the range of strain ideally desired around an endosteal implant, once a stress equilibrium has been established (Fig. 18.8). Bone turnover is required in the adapted window, as Mori and Burr[53] provide evidence of remodeling in regions of bone microfracture from fatigue damage within the physiologic range.

The *mild overload zone* (1500–3000 microstrain) causes a greater rate of fatigue microfracture and increase in the cellular turnover rate of bone. As a result the bone strength and density may eventually decrease. The histologic description of bone in this range is usually woven or repaired bone. This may be the state for bone when an endosteal implant is overloaded and the bone interface attempts to change the strain environment. During the repair process the woven bone is weaker than the more mature, mineralized lamellar bone.[41] Therefore while bone is loaded in the mild overload zone, care must be taken because the "safety range" for bone strength is reduced during the repair.[42]

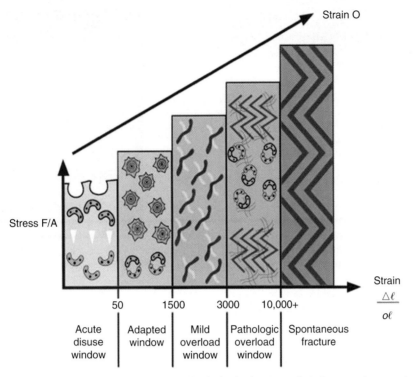

• **Fig. 18.7** Four zones for bone related to mechanical adaption to strain before spontaneous fracture. The acute disuse window is the lowest microstrain amount. The adapted window is an ideal physiologic loading zone. The mild overload zone causes microfracture and triggers an increase in bone remodeling, which produces more woven bone. The pathologic overload zone causes increase in fatigue fractures, remodeling, and bone resorption.

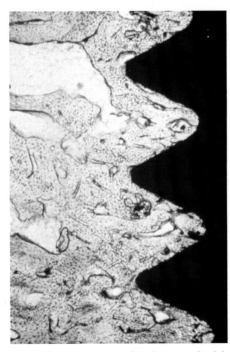

• **Fig. 18.8** An ideal bone–implant interface has organized: lamellar bone next to the implant. The adapted window zone of microstrain balances remodeling and allows the bone to maintain this condition.

Pathologic overload zones are reached when microstrains are greater than 3000 units.[46] Cortical bone fractures occur at 10,000 to 18,000 microstrain (1%–2% deformation). Therefore pathologic overload may begin at microstrain levels of only 18% to 40% of the ultimate strength or physical fracture of cortical bone. The

bone may resorb and form fibrous tissue, or when present, repair woven bone in this zone, because a sustained turnover rate is necessary. The marginal bone loss evidenced during implant overloading may be a result of the bone in the pathologic overload zone. Implant failure from overload may also be a result of bone in the pathologic overload zone.

Bone Classification Schemes Related to Implant Dentistry

An appreciation of bone density and its relation to oral implantology has existed for almost 50 years. Linkow and Chercheve,[54] in 1970, classified bone density into three categories:

Class I bone structure: This ideal bone type consists of evenly spaced trabeculae with small cancellated spaces.
Class II bone structure: The bone has slightly larger cancellated spaces with less uniformity of the osseous pattern.
Class III bone structure: Large, marrow-filled spaces exist between bone trabeculae.

Linkow stated that Class III bone results in a loose-fitting implant; Class II bone was satisfactory for implants; and Class I bone was the most ideal foundation for implant prostheses. In 1985 Lekholm and Zarb[55] listed four bone qualities found in the anterior regions of the jawbone (Fig. 18.9). Quality 1 was composed of homogeneous compact bone. Quality 2 had a thick layer of compact bone surrounding a core of dense trabecular bone. Quality 3 had a thin layer of cortical bone surrounding dense trabecular bone of favorable strength. Quality 4 had a thin layer of cortical bone surrounding a core of low-density trabecular bone. Irrespective of the different bone qualities, all bone was treated

1   2   3   4

• **Fig. 18.9** Four bone qualities for the anterior region of the jaws. Quality 1 is composed of homogenous compact bone. Quality 2 has a thick layer of cortical bone surrounding dense trabecular bone. Quality 3 has a thin layer of cortical bone surrounded by dense trabecular bone of favorable strength. Quality 4 has a thin layer of cortical bone surrounding a core of low-density trabecular bone. *(From Lekholm U, Zarb GA. Patient selection and preparation. In: Brånemark PI, Zarb GA, Albrektsson T, eds.* Tissue Integrated Protheses: Osseointegration in Clinical Dentistry. *Chicago: Quintessence; 1985.)*

with the same implant design and standard surgical and prosthetic protocol.[8] Following this protocol, Schnitman and others[3,9,16] observed a 10% difference in implant survival between Quality 2 and Quality 3 bone, and 22% lower survival in the poorest bone density. Johns et al.[17] reported 3% failure in type III bone, but 28% in type IV bone. Smedberg et al.[18] reported a 36% failure rate in type IV bone. Higuchi and others also experienced a greater failure in the soft bone of the maxilla.[19] It is obvious that a standardized surgical, prosthetic, and implant design protocol does not yield similar results in all bone densities. In addition, these reports are for implant survival, not the quality of health of surviving implants. The amount of crestal bone loss also has been related to bone density[56-60] and further supports a different protocol for soft bone.

In 1988 Misch[1,2] proposed four bone density groups independent of the regions of the jaws based on macroscopic cortical and trabecular bone characteristics. The regions of the jaws with similar densities were often consistent. Suggested treatment plans, implant design, surgical protocol, healing, and progressive loading time spans have been described for each bone density type.[24,60,61] Following this regimen, similar implant survival rates have been observed for all bone densities.[22-24]

Misch Bone Density Classification

Dense or porous cortical bone is found on the outer surfaces of bone and includes the crest of an edentulous ridge. Coarse and fine trabecular bone types are found within the outer shell of cortical bone and occasionally on the crestal surface of an edentulous residual ridge. These four macroscopic structures of bone may be arranged from the least dense to the most dense, as first described by Frost[25,46] (Fig. 18.10).

In combination, these four increasing macroscopic densities constitute four bone categories described by Misch (D1, D2, D3, and D4) located in the edentulous areas of the maxilla and mandible (Fig. 18.11). The regional locations of the different densities of cortical bone are more consistent than the highly variable trabecular bone.

D1 bone is primarily dense cortical bone. D2 bone has dense-to-porous cortical bone on the crest and, within the bone, has coarse trabecular bone. D3 bone types have a thinner porous cortical crest and fine trabecular bone in the region next to the implant. D4 bone has very little to no crestal cortical bone. The fine trabecular bone composes almost all of the total volume of bone next to the implant (Table 18.1 and Fig. 18.12). A very soft bone, with incomplete mineralization and large intertrabecular spaces, may be addressed as D5 bone. This bone type is most often immature bone in a developing sinus graft.

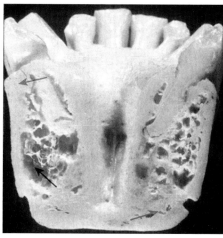

• **Fig. 18.10** The macroscopic structure of bone may be described, from the least dense to the most dense, as (1) fine trabecular (*red arrow*), (2) coarse becular (*yellow arrow*), (3) porous cortical (*green arrow*), and (4) dense cortical *(orange arrow).*

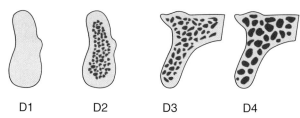

D1   D2   D3   D4

• **Fig. 18.11** Four bone densities found in the edentulous regions of the maxilla and mandible. D1 bone is primarily dense cortical bone; D2 bone has dense-to-thick porous cortical bone on the crest and coarse trabecular bone underneath; D3 bone has a thinner porous cortical crest and fine trabecular bone within; and D4 bone has almost no crestal cortical bone. The fine trabecular bone composes almost all of the total volume of bone.

TABLE 18.1 **Misch Bone Density Classification Scheme**

Bone Density	Description	Tactile Analog	Typical Anatomic Location
D1	Dense cortical	Oak or maple wood	Anterior mandible
D2	Porous cortical and coarse trabecular	White pine or spruce wood	Anterior mandible Posterior mandible Anterior maxilla
D3	Porous cortical and fine trabecular	Balsa wood	Anterior maxilla Posterior maxilla Posterior mandible
D4	Fine trabecular	Styrofoam	Posterior maxilla Anterior maxilla
D5	Osteoid	Soft Styrofoam	Poorly mineralized bone graft

Determining Bone Density

The bone density may be determined by various techniques including tactile sensation, during surgery, the general location, or radiographic evaluation (CBCT).

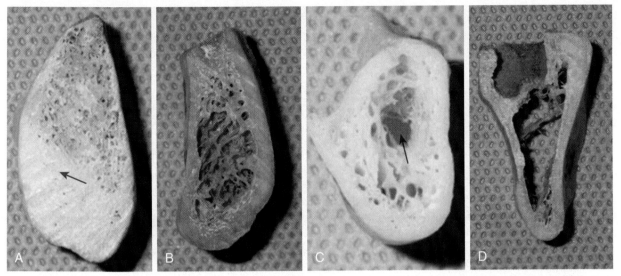

• **Fig. 18.12** The four macroscopic bone qualities are (A) D1 (*arrow*), (B) D2, (C) D3 (*arrow*), and (D) D4. The bone-density variance is dependent on anatomic location and the local strain history of the bone after tooth loss.

TABLE 18.2	Usual Anatomic Location of Bone Density Types (% Occurrence)			
Bone	Anterior Maxilla	Posterior Maxilla	Anterior Mandible	Posterior Mandible
D1	0	0	92	8
D2	8	0	66	26
D3	75	22	0	3
D4	38	40	0	22
D5	Immature, poorly mineralized bone graft			

Location

A review of the literature and a survey of completely and partially edentulous patients postsurgery indicated that the location of different bone densities often may be superimposed on the different regions of the mouth[3-7,11-13,15-18,62-66] (see Tables 18.1 and 18.2). D1 bone is almost never observed in the maxilla and is rarely observed in most mandibles (Fig. 18.13). In the mandible, D1 bone is observed approximately 6% of the time in the Division A anterior mandible and 3% of the time in the posterior mandible, primarily when the implant is engaging the lingual cortical plate of bone. In a C–h bone volume (moderate atrophy) in the anterior mandible the prevalence of D1 bone approaches 25% in male individuals. The C–h mandible often exhibits an increase in torsion, flexure, or both in the anterior segment between the foramina during function. This increased strain may cause the bone to increase in density. D1 bone also may be encountered in the anterior Division A mandible of a Kennedy Class IV partially edentulous patient with a history of parafunction and recent extractions. In addition, D1 bone has been observed in the anterior or posterior mandible when the angulation of the implant may require the engagement of the lingual cortical plate.

The bone density D2 is the most common bone density observed in the mandible (Figs. 18.14 and 18.15). The anterior mandible consists of D2 bone approximately two-thirds of the time. Almost half of patients have D2 bone in the posterior mandible. The maxilla presents D2 bone less often than the mandible. Approximately one-fourth of patients have D2 bone, and this is more likely in the partially edentulous patient's anterior and premolar region, rather than the completely edentulous posterior molar areas. Single-tooth or two-tooth, partially edentulous spans in either arch almost always have D2 bone.

Bone density D3 is common in the maxilla (Fig. 18.16). More than half of patients have D3 bone in the upper arch. The anterior edentulous maxilla has D3 bone approximately 75% of the time, whereas almost half of the patients have posterior maxillae with D3 bone (more often in the premolar region). Almost half of the posterior mandibles also present with D3 bone, whereas approximately 25% of the anterior edentulous mandibles have D3 bone.

The softest bone, D4, is most often found in the posterior maxilla (approximately 40%), especially in the molar regions or after a sinus graft augmentation (where almost two-thirds of the patients have D4 bone) (Fig. 18.17). The anterior maxilla has D4 bone less than 10% of the time—more often after an onlay iliac crest bone graft. The mandible presents with D4 bone in less than 3% of the patients. When observed, it is usually Division A bone in a long-term, completely edentulous patient after an osteoplasty to remove the crestal bone.

Generalizations for treatment planning can be made prudently based on location. The bone density by location method is the first way the clinician can estimate the bone density in the implant sites to develop an initial treatment plan. It is safer to err on the side of less-dense bone during treatment planning, so the prosthesis will be designed with slightly more, rather than less, support. Therefore the initial treatment plan before computed tomography (CBCT) radiographic scans or surgery suggests the anterior maxilla is treated as D3 bone, the posterior maxilla as D4 bone, the anterior mandible as D2 bone, and the posterior mandible as D3

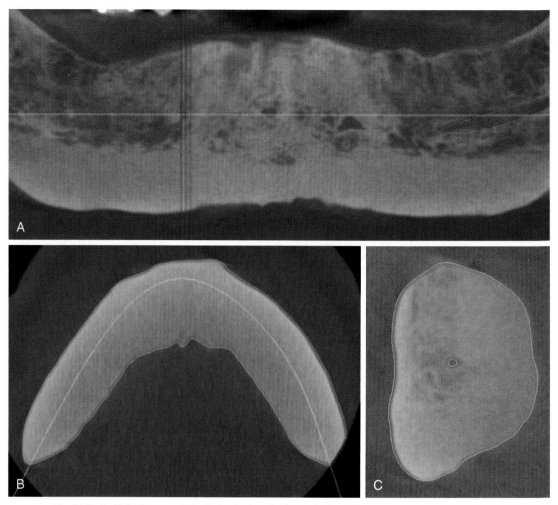

• **Fig. 18.13** (A–C) D1 bone: note the lack of trabecular bone. D1 bone has almost all cortical bone, leading to a tendency to overheat during preparation and compromised blood supply during healing.

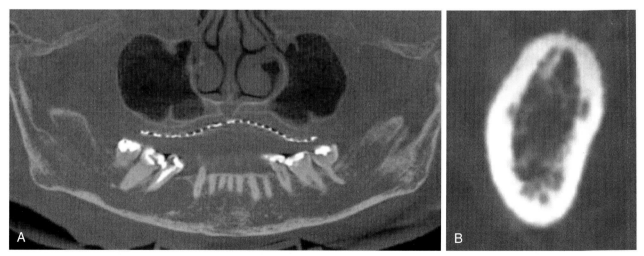

• **Fig. 18.14** D4 Bone. (A) Cone beam computed tomography panoramic exhibiting very poor bone quality (minimal trabecular bone) in a patient with osteoporosis. (B) Cortical bone will be mottled in a patient with osteoporosis.

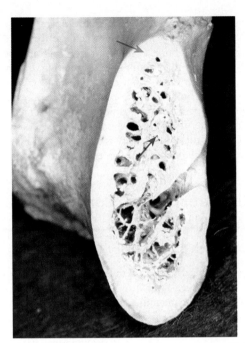

• **Fig. 18.15** A cross section of a D2 mandible in the region of the mental foramen. A thick cortical plate (*green arrow*) exists on the crest, and a coarse trabecular bone (*red arrow*) pattern exists within.

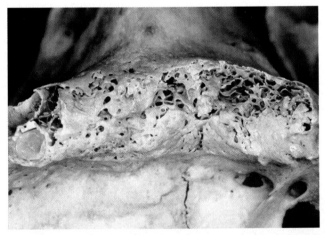

• **Fig. 18.16** A posterior maxilla demonstrating D3 bone with a thin porous cortical plate on the crest with fine trabecular bone underneath.

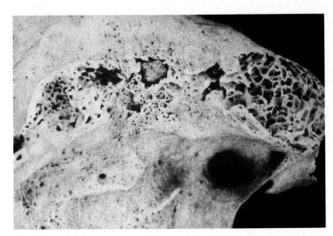

• **Fig. 18.17** In a D4 posterior maxilla the posterior crestal region has little to no cortical bone on the crest and is composed primarily of fine trabecular bone.

bone. A more accurate determination of bone density is made with CBCT images before surgery or tactilely during implant surgery.

Radiographic Evaluation

Periapical or panoramic radiographs are minimally beneficial in determining bone density, because of their two-dimensional nature and the lateral cortical plates often obscure the trabecular bone density. In addition, the more subtle changes of D2 to D3 cannot be quantified by these radiographs. Therefore the initial treatment plan, which often begins with these radiographs, follows the bone density by location method. Bone density may be more precisely determinedusing cone beam computerized tomography (CBCT).[67-70] With conventional computerized tomography (CT), each image is comprised of pixels. Each pixel in the CT image is assigned a number, also referred to as a Hounsfield or CT number. The CT Hounsfield scale is calibrated such that the Hounsfield unit values are based on water (0 HU) and air (–1000 HU). In general the higher the CT number, the denser the tissue. The HU is a quantitative measurement used in CT scanning to express CT numbers in a standardized form. The HU was created by Sir Godfrey Hounsfield and obtained from a linear transformation of the measured attenuation coefficients of water (0 HU) and air(-1000 HU).

When evaluating dental cone beam computed tomography (CBCT) images in regard to bone density, there does not exist a direct correlation (accuracy of measurement) compared with medical CT. Most dental CBCT systems inherently have an increased variation and inconsistency with density estimates.

The density estimates of gray levels (brightness values) are not true attenuation values (HU); thus inaccuracies in bone density estimates may result.[71] This is mainly due to the high level of noise in the acquired images and the slight inconsistencies in the sensitivity of the CBCT detectors. Dental imaging software frequently provides attenuation values (HU); however, such values should be recognized as approximations lacking the precision of HU values derived from medical CT units.

HUs have been correlated with bone density and treatment planning for dental implants.[72-74] In a retrospective study of CT scan images from implant patients, Kircos and Misch[69] established a correlation between CT HUs and density at the time of surgery. The Misch bone density classification may be evaluated on the CT images by correlation to a range of HUs (Box 18.1).[69] The very soft bone observed after some immaterialized bone grafts may be 50 to 180 units.[69] Even negative numbers, suggestive of fat tissue, have been observed with the cortical plates of some jaws, including the anterior mandible. Norton and Gamble[72] also found an overall correlation between subjective bone density scores of Lekholm and Zarb and the CT values. Several studies correlating torque forces at implant insertion with preoperative bone density values from CTs have reported similar conclusions.[75-77] Preoperative CT scan data of areas that lead to successful and unsuccessful implant placement have been reported. In the mandible, failed sites exhibited higher HUs than usual. This was correlated with failure in dense bone, possibly because of the lack of vascularization or overheating during surgery. By contrast, in the maxilla the bone density was low for the failed sites.[68] The bone density may be different near the crest, compared with the apical region where the implant placement is planned.[74] The most critical region of bone density is the crestal 7 to 10 mm of bone, because this is where most stresses are applied to an osteointegrated bone–implant interface. Therefore when the bone density varies from the most crestal to apical region around the implant, the crestal 7 to 10 mm determines the treatment-plan protocol (Figs. 18.18 and 18.19).

Many CBCT software programs are now available that allow for preoperative determination of bone density in the implant site area. Fig. 18.18 displays an implant ideally positioned in the bone within a CT scan image. An average HU is given inside the implant, which correlates to the bone density that the implant surgeon will be drilling into. The HU outside of the implant relays the average bone density around the periphery of the implant, which gives the clinician information on the bone–implant contact (BIC). This is especially important to determine the prosthetic protocol or progressive bone loading.

Tactile Sense

There is a great difference in the tactile sensation during osteotomy preparation in different bone densities, because the density is directly related to its strength.[1,2,77,78] To communicate more broadly to the profession relative to the tactile sense of different bone densities, Misch[1,2] proposed the different densities of his classification be compared with materials of varying densities. Site preparation and implant placement in D1 bone is similar to the resistance on a drill preparing an osteotomy in oak or maple wood (e.g., hard wood). D2 bone is similar to the tactile sensation of drilling into white pine or spruce (e.g. soft wood). D3 bone is similar to drilling into a compressed balsa wood. D4 bone is similar to drilling into a compressed Styrofoam. This clinical observation may be correlated to different histomorphometric

bone density determinations.[62] When an implant drill can operate at 1500 to 2500 rpm, it may be difficult to feel the difference between D3 and D4 bone. In D4 bone the drill may be inserted to the full desired depth without the drill rotating. In other words, a bone compression rather than extraction process may be used with the drill. D3 bone is easy to prepare but requires the drill to rotate while it is pressed into position. When this tactile method is the primary site, the surgeon should know how to modify the treatment plan if this bone density is different from first estimated when developing the treatment plan (Fig. 18.20).

Scientific Rationale of a Bone Density–Based Treatment Plan

Bone Strength and Density

Bone density is directly related to the strength of bone before microfracture.[79,80] Misch et al.[78] reported on the mechanical properties of trabecular bone in the mandible, using the Misch density classification. A tenfold difference in bone strength may be observed from D1 to D4 bone. D2 bone exhibited a 47% to 68% greater ultimate compressive strength, compared with D3 bone (Fig. 18.21). In other words, on a scale of 1 to 10, D1 bone is a 9 to 10 relative to strength. D2 bone is a 7 to 8 on this scale. D3 bone is 50% weaker than D2 bone and is a 3 or 4 on the strength scale. D4 bone is a 1 to 2 and up to 10 times weaker than D1 bone (Fig. 18.22). Misch and Bidez[81] performed three-dimensional, finite stress analyses on bone volumes of Division A, B, and C–w patients. Each model reproduced the cortical and trabecular bone material properties of the four densities described. Clinical failure was mathematically predicted in D4 bone and some D3 densities under occlusal loads (Fig. 18.23). The bone densities that originally relied on clinical impression are now fully correlated to quantitative objective values obtained from CT scans and bone strength measurements. These values can help prevent failure in specific situations of weak densities.

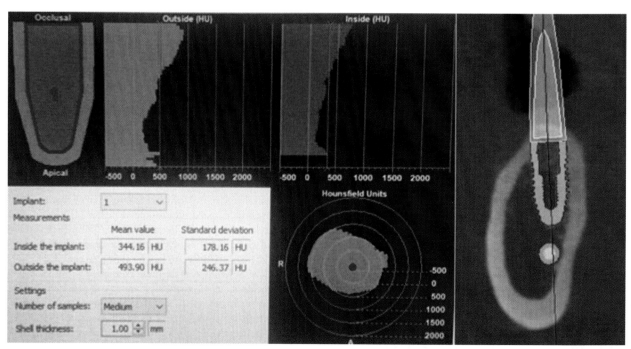

• **Fig. 18.18** Cone beam computed tomography determination of bone density inside and outside of implant. The inside density would correlate to the osteotomy preparation bone density. The outside density will correlate to the bone density that will encompass the implant after insertion.

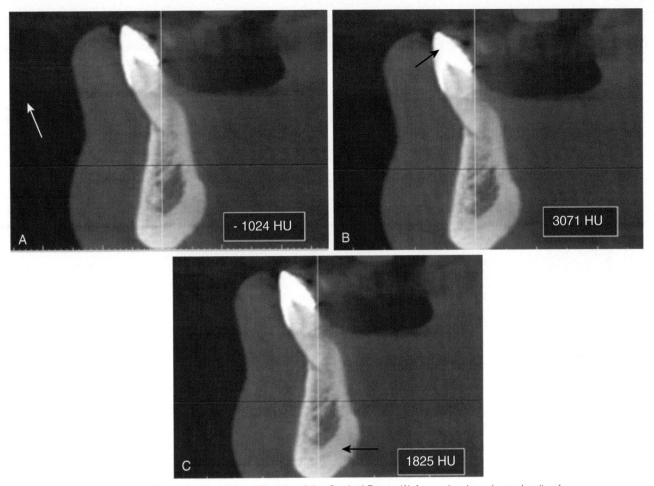

• **Fig. 18.19** Determination of Bone Density of the Cortical Bone. (A) Arrow showing a bone density of –1024 HU, which denotes air. (B) Bone density measurement on the crown, which correlates to 3071 HU. (C) Bone density measurement on cortical bone, which corresponds to a bone density of 1071 HU.

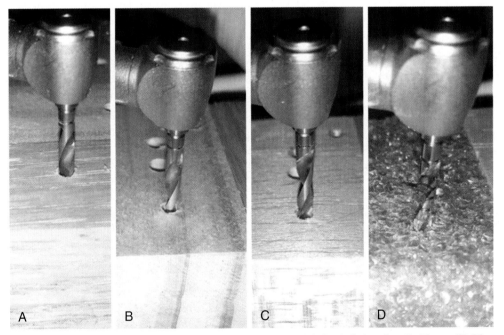

• **Fig. 18.20** Tactile Sensation. (A) D1 bone (hard wood), which is basically basal cortical bone. (B) D2 bone (soft wood), the ideal bone for preparation and healing. (C) D3 bone (balsa wood), minimal cortical bone and course trabeculae. (D) D4 bone (Styrofoam), which has no cortical bone with minimal trabeculae.

Elastic Modulus and Density

The elastic modulus describes the amount of strain (changes in length divided by the original length) as a result of a particular amount of stress. It is directly related to the apparent density of bone.[80] The elastic modulus of a material is a value that relates to the stiffness of the material. The elastic modulus of bone is more flexible than titanium. When higher stresses are applied to an implant prosthesis, the titanium has lower strain (change in shape) compared with the bone. The difference between the two

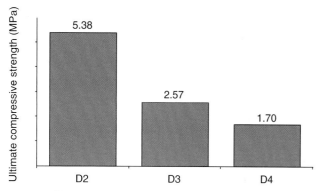

• **Fig. 18.21** The ultimate compressive strength of D2 trabecular bone is greater than D3 trabecular bone. D4 trabecular bone is the weakest.

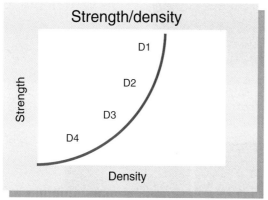

• **Fig. 18.22** The strength of bone is related directly to the density of bone.

materials may create microstrain conditions of pathologic overload and cause implant failure (Fig. 18.24A). When the stresses applied to the implant are low, the microstrain difference between titanium and bone is minimized and remains in the adapted window zone, maintaining load-bearing lamellar bone at the interface (Fig. 18.24B).

Misch et al.[78] found the elastic modulus in the human jaw to be different for each bone density (Fig. 18.25). As a result, when a stress is applied to an implant prosthesis in D1 bone, the titanium–D1 bone interface exhibits a very small microstrain difference. In comparison, when the same amount of stress is applied to an implant in D4 bone, the microstrain difference between titanium and D4 bone is greater and may be in the pathologic overload zone (Fig. 18.26). As a result, D4 bone is more likely to cause implant mobility and failure.[81] Several studies using finite element analysis models with various implant designs and bone qualities have evaluated the stress/strain distribution in the bone around the implants. Conclusions agree with the prior study to show the importance of bone quality in the treatment planning phase for long-term prognosis.[82-87]

Bone Density and Bone–Implant Contact Percentage

The initial bone density not only provides mechanical immobilization of the implant during healing but after healing also permits distribution and transmission of stresses from the prosthesis to the implant–bone interface. The mechanical distribution of stress occurs primarily where bone is in contact with the implant. Open marrow spaces or zones of unorganized fibrous tissue do not permit controlled force dissipation or microstrain conditions to the local bone cells. Because stress equals force divided by the area over which the force is applied, the less the area of bone contacting the implant body, the greater the overall stress, all other factors being equal. Therefore the BIC percent may influence the amount of stress/strain at the interface.

Misch[2] noted in 1990 that the bone density influences the amount of bone in contact with the implant surface, not only at first stage surgery but also at the second stage uncovery and early prosthetic loading. The BIC percentage is significantly greater in cortical bone than in trabecular bone. The very dense D1 bone of a C–h resorbed anterior mandible or of the lingual cortical plate of a Division A anterior or posterior mandible provides the highest

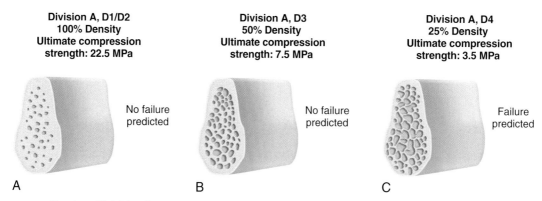

• **Fig. 18.23** (A) A finite element analysis study of D1 bone with a Division A, B, or C bone volume predicted no implant failure. (B) In a finite element analysis study of D3 bone of one-third the strength, no failure was predicted in Division A bone. (C) In a finite element analysis study, D4 bone was inadequate in strength for implant success, even in Division A bone volume.

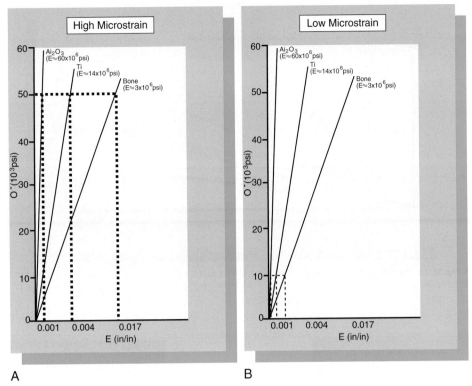

• **Fig. 18.24** (A) When the microstrain is high (50 × 10³ psi in this example), the change in shape difference of titanium and bone is large and may result in a pathologic overload zone. As a result, fibrous tissue at the interface and implant mobility is expected. (B) When the microstrain is low (10 × 10³ psi in this example), the change in shape difference between titanium and bone is small and may result in the ideal adapted window zone. As a result, organized, lamellar bone may remain at the implant interface.

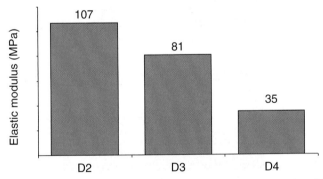

• **Fig. 18.25** The elastic modulus for D2 trabecular bone is greater than D3 trabecular bone, and D4 trabecular bone has the lowest elastic modulus.

percentage of bone in contact with an endosteal implant and may approximate more than 85% BIC (Fig. 18.27). D2 bone, after initial healing, usually has 65% to 75% BIC (Fig. 18.28). D3 bone typically has 40% to 50% BIC after initial healing (Fig. 18.29). The sparse trabeculae of the bone often found in the posterior maxilla (D4) offer fewer areas of contact with the body of the implant. With a machined-surface implant, this may approximate less than 30% BIC and is most related to the implant design and surface condition (Fig. 18.30). Consequently, greater implant surface area is required to obtain a similar amount of BIC in soft bone compared with a denser bone quality found around an anterior mandibular implant.

Bone Density and Stress Transfer

Crestal bone loss and early implant failure after loading results may occur from excess stress at the implant–bone interface.[49-52,56-59,82-86]

A range of bone loss has been observed in implants with similar load conditions.[59] Misch[2] noted in 1990 that part of this phenomenon may be explained by the evaluation of finite element analysis stress contours in the bone for each bone density. As a result of the correlation of bone density, elastic modulus bone strength, and BIC percent, when a load is placed on an implant, the stress contours in the bone are different for each bone density. In D1 bone, highest strains are concentrated around the implant near the crest, and the stress in the region is of lesser magnitude. D2 bone, with the same load, sustains a slightly greater crestal strain, and the intensity of the stress extends farther apically along the implant body (Fig. 18.31). D4 bone exhibits the greatest crestal strains, and the magnitude of the stress on the implant proceeds farthest apically along the implant body (Fig. 18.32). As a result the magnitude of a prosthetic load may remain similar and yet give one of the following three different clinical situations at the bone–implant interface, based on bone density: (1) physiologic bone loads in the adapted window zone and no marginal bone loss, (2) mild overload to pathologic overload bone loads and crestal bone loss, or (3) generalized pathologic overload and implant failure. Therefore to obtain a similar clinical result in each implant prosthesis, the variables in each patient must be either eliminated or accounted for in the treatment plan. Because the myriad of variables cannot be eliminated relative to bone density, the treatment plans (including implant number, size, and design) should be modified.

Treatment Planning

In oral implantology today, it is becoming more common for the initial radiographic survey to be with a CBCT scan. Therefore the implant clinician may use the location and radiographic survey

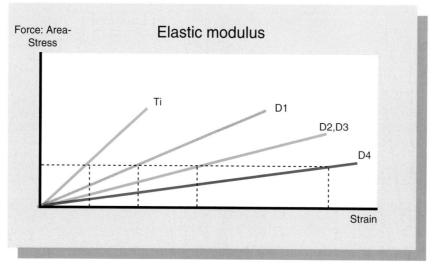

• **Fig. 18.26** The microstrain difference between titanium and D4 bone is great and may be in the pathologic overload zone, whereas at the same stress level, the microstrain difference between titanium and D2 bone may be within the ideal adapted window zone.

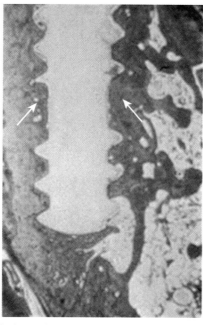

• **Fig. 18.27** D1 bone density has the greatest amount of bone–implant contact. Because stress equals force divided by area, the increase in the area of contact results in a decreased amount of stress.

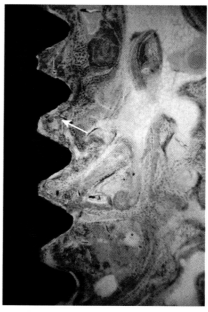

• **Fig. 18.28** In D2 bone density, one finds primarily coarse trabecular bone next to the implant. The bone–implant contact is greater than D3 bone but less than D1 bone.

as indicators on the bone density qualitative evaluation of the patient. After the initial assessment of the bone density is determined, additional factors such as implant key position and number, implant size and design, and available bone are evaluated.

There exist four key principles that help form the basis for treatment-plan modification in function of the bone quality: (1) each bone density has a different strength, (2) bone density affects the elastic modulus, (3) bone density differences result in different amounts of BIC percent, and (4) bone density differences result in a different stress/strain distribution at the implant–bone interface when implants are loaded. Therefore bone density is an implant treatment-plan modifier in several ways—prosthetic factors, implant size, implant design, implant surface condition, implant number, and the need or method of prosthetic progressive bone loading.

As the bone density decreases, the strength of the bone also decreases. To decrease the incidence of microfracture of bone, the strain to the bone must be reduced. Strain is directly related to stress. Consequently, the stress to the implant system should also be reduced as the bone density decreases (Box 18.2). One way to reduce the biomechanical loads on implants is by prosthesis design to decrease force. The most ideal technique is the splinting of multiple implants. Additional techniques include the cantilever length being shortened or eliminated, narrower occlusal tables designed, and offset loads minimized, all of which reduce the amount of load.[45] RP-4 restorations, rather than fixed prostheses, permit the patient to remove the prosthesis at night and reduce nocturnal parafunctional forces. RP-5 prostheses permit the soft tissue to share the occlusal

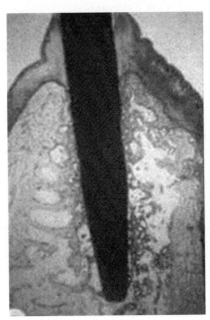

• **Fig. 18.29** The fine trabecular bone of D3 initially heals next to the implant with 40% to 50% bone–implant contact.

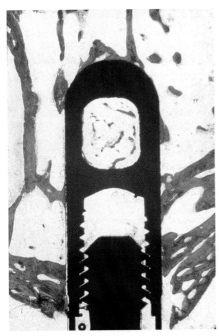

• **Fig. 18.30** D4 bone has the least bone–implant contact. As a result the stress is greatest for the D4 bone-implant interface. Trabecular bone is fine, the strength is poor, and the modulus of elasticity microstrain difference is greatest. The microstrain difference for each bone density is not the same. D4 bone is most at risk, whereas D1 bone is least at risk.

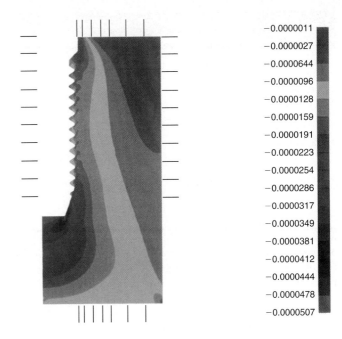

−0.0000011
−0.0000027
−0.0000644
−0.0000096
−0.0000128
−0.0000159
−0.0000191
−0.0000223
−0.0000254
−0.0000286
−0.0000317
−0.0000349
−0.0000381
−0.0000412
−0.0000444
−0.0000478
−0.0000507

• **Fig. 18.31** Stress transfer around the implant interface is different for each bone density. In this two-dimensional finite element analysis, D2 bone has an intermediate stress intensity around the implant (green). Very little of the high intensity stress (red) reaches the implant interface

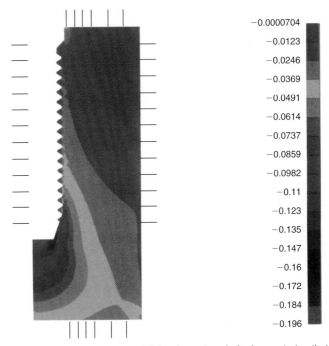

−0.0000704
−0.0123
−0.0246
−0.0369
−0.0491
−0.0614
−0.0737
−0.0859
−0.0982
−0.11
−0.123
−0.135
−0.147
−0.16
−0.172
−0.184
−0.196

• **Fig. 18.32** A two-dimensional finite element analysis demonstrates that D4 bone has a higher stress intensity around the implant, and the higher intensity even extends to the zone around the apical threads (red).

force and reduce the stress on the implants. The use of occlusal guards help dissipate parafunctional forces on an implant system. As the bone density decreases, these prosthetic factors become more important.

The load on the implant may also be influenced by the direction of force to the implant body.[81] A load directed along the long axis of the implant body decreases the amount of stress in the crestal bone region compared with an angled load. Therefore as the bone density decreases, axial loads on the implant body become more critical. Bone grafting or bone spreading to increase the width of bone and to better position the implant relative to the intended load is considered for soft bone types.

Stress may also be reduced by increasing the functional area over which the force is applied. Increasing implant number is an excellent way to reduce stress by increasing functional loading area. Three implants rather than two may decrease applied implant moments in half and bone reaction forces by two-thirds, depending on implant position and size.[45] An implant prosthesis with normal patient forces in the bone should ideally have at least one implant per tooth. In the molar region, two implants for each missing molar may be appropriate. In D2 bone with normal patient forces a pontic may replace a tooth between two implants. In D3 bone, one implant per tooth is often appropriate.

The surface area of the implant macrogeometry may be increased to decrease stress to the implant–bone interface.[60,88] The width of the implant may decrease stress by increasing the surface area.[60,89] This may also reduce the length requirement. For every 0.5-mm increase in width, there is an increased surface area between 10% and 15% for a cylinder implant, and even greater difference is found with threaded-implant body designs. Because the greatest stresses are concentrated at the crestal region of the implant, width is more significant than length for an implant design, once adequate length has been established. D4 bone should often require wider implants compared with D1 or D2 bone. This may require onlay grafts or bone spreading to increase the width of bone when other stress factors are high. This implant length requirement may require sinus grafts in the posterior maxilla. However, because the crestal region is where pathologic overload of bone most often occurs after prosthetic loading, once initial healing is complete the length of the implant is not as effective to decrease crestal bone loss (and the quality of implant health) as other factors (e.g., implant design, implant width).

The macro design affects the magnitude of stresses and their impact on the bone–implant interface[10,82,90,91] and can dramatically change the amount and contour of the bone strains concentrated at the interface. Different implant design criteria respond to different bone densities. Bone densities exhibit a tenfold difference in strength, and the elastic modulus is significantly different between D1 and D4.

Coatings or the surface condition on an implant body can increase the BIC percentage and therefore the functional surface area. A rougher surface is strongly suggested in soft bone and has resulted in improved short-term survival rates compared with machined titanium.[11] After 1 to 2 years, the mechanical load on the overall implant design is more critical to the amount and type of bone contact compared with the surface condition on the implant body. Rough surface conditions also may have some disadvantages. Plaque retention when exposed above the bone, contamination, and increased cost are a few of the concerns with roughened surfaces. The benefit and risk of surface conditions suggest the roughest surfaces are most often used in only softer bone types.

Progressive bone loading provides for a gradual increase in occlusal loads, separated by a time interval to allow the bone to mature and accommodate to the local strain environment.[2] Over time, progressive loading changes the amount and density of

the implant–bone contact. The increased density of bone at the implant interface improves the overall support system mechanism. The softer the bone, the more important the need for progressive loading.[1,2]

Summary

A key determinant for clinical success is the diagnosis of the bone density in a potential implant site. The strength of bone is directly related to bone density. The modulus of elasticity is related to bone density. The percentage of BIC is related to bone density, and the axial stress contours around an implant are affected by the density of bone. As a consequence, past clinical reports that did not alter the protocol of treatment related to bone density had variable survival rates. To the contrary, altering the treatment plan to compensate for soft bone types has provided similar survival rates in all bone densities. Once the prosthetic option, key implant position, and patient force factors have been determined, the bone density in the implant sites should be evaluated to modify the treatment plan. The treatment plan may be modified by reducing the force on the prosthesis or increasing the area of load by increasing implant number, implant position, implant size, implant design, or implant body surface condition.

References

1. Misch CE. Bone character: second vital implant criterion. *Dent Today*. 1988;7:39–40.
2. Misch CE. Density of bone: effect on treatment plans, surgical approach, healing, and progressive loading. *Int J Oral Implant*. 1990;6:23–31.
3. Friberg B, Jemt T, Lekholm U. Early failures in 4,641 consecutively placed Brånemark dental implants: a study from stage I surgery to the connection of completed prostheses. *Int J Oral Maxillofac Implants*. 1991;6:142–146.
4. van Steenberghe D, Lekholm U, Bolender C, et al. Applicability of osseointegrated oral implants in the rehabilitation of partial edentulism: a prospective multicenter study on 558 fixtures. *Int J Oral Maxillofac Implants*. 1990;5:272–281.
5. Hutton JE, Heath MR, Chai JY, et al. Factors related to success and failure rates at 3 year follow up in a multicenter study of overdentures supported by Brånemark implants. *Int J Oral Maxillofac Implants*. 1995;10:33–42.
6. Esposito M, Hirsch JM, Lekholm U, et al. Biological factors contributing to failures of osseointegrated oral implants. (II) Etiopathogenesis. *Eur J Oral Sci*. 1998;106:721–764.
7. Morris HF, Ochi S, Crum P, et al. AICRG, Part I: a 6-year multicentered, multidisciplinary clinical study of a new and innovative implant design. *J Oral Implantol*. 1804;30:125–133.
8. Adell R, Lekholm U, Rockler B, et al. A 15-year study of osseointegrated implants in the treatment of the edentulous jaw. *Int J Oral Surg*. 1981;6:38/–416.
9. Schnitman PA, Rubenstein JE, Whorle PS, et al. Implants for partial edentulism. *J Dent Educ*. 1988;52:725–736.
10. Minsk L, Polson A, Weisgold A, et al. Outcome failures of endosseous implants from a clinical training center. *Compend Contin Educ Dent*. 1996;17:848–859.
11. Fugazzotto PA, Wheeler SL, Lindsay JA. Success and failure rates of cylinder implants in type IV bone. *J Periodontol*. 1993;64:1085–1087.
12. Snauwaert K, Duyck D, van Steenberghe D, et al. Time dependent failure rate and marginal bone loss of implant supported prostheses: a 15-year follow-up study. *Clin Oral Investig*. 1800;4:13–18.
13. Herrmann I, Lekholm U, Holm S, et al. Evaluation of patient and implant characteristics as potential prognostic factors for oral implant failures. *Int J Oral Maxillofac Implants*. 1805;18:218–230.

14. Brånemark PI, Hansson BO, Adell R, et al. *Osseointegrated Implants in the Treatment of the Edentulous Jaw—Experience from a 10-Year Period.* Stockholm: Almquist and Wiksell International; 1977.
15. Jaffin RA, Berman CL. The excessive loss of Brånemark fixtures in the Type IV bone: a 5-year analysis. *J Periodontol.* 1991;62:2–4.
16. Engquist B, Bergendal T, Kallus T, et al. A retrospective multicenter evaluation of osseointegrated implants supporting overdentures. *Int J Oral Maxillofac Implants.* 1988;3:129–134.
17. Johns Jr B, Jemt T, Heath MR, et al. A multicenter study of overdentures supported by Brånemark implants. *Int J Oral Maxillofac Implants.* 1992;7:513–522.
18. Smedberg JI, Lothigius E, Bodin L, et al. A clinical and radiological two-year follow-up study of maxillary overdentures on osseointegrated implants. *Oral Clin Implants Res.* 1993;4:39–46.
19. Higuchi KW, Folmer T, Kultje C. Implant survival rates in partially edentulous patients: a 3-year prospective multicenter study. *J Oral Maxillofac Surg.* 1995;53:264–268.
20. Weng D, Jacobson Z, Tarnow D, et al. A prospective multicenter clinical trial of 3i machined surface implants: results after 6 years of follow up. *Int J Oral Maxillofac Implants.* 1803;18:417–423.
21. Jemt T, Chai J, Harnett J. A 5-year prospective multicenter follow-up report on overdentures supported by osseointegrated implants. *Int J Oral Maxillofac Implants.* 1996;11:291–298.
22. Misch CE, Hoar JE, Hazen R, et al. Bone quality based implant system: a prospective study of the first two years of prosthetic loading. *J Oral Implantol.* 1999;25:185–197.
23. Kline R, Hoar JE, Beck GH. A prospective multicenter clinical investigation of a bone quality based dental implant system. *Implant Dent.* 2002;11:224–234.
24. Misch CE, Poitras Y, Dietsh-Misch F. Endosteal implants in the edentulous posterior maxilla—rationale and clinical results. *Oral Health.* 2000;90:7–16.
25. Misch CE, Steigenga J, Cianciola LJ, et al. Short dental implants in posterior partial edentulism: a multicenter retrospective 5-year case series study. *J Periodontol.* 1800;77:1340–1347.
26. Roberts EW, Turley PK, Brezniak N, et al. Bone physiology and metabolism. *J Calif Dent Assoc.* 1987;15:54–61.
27. Klemetti E, Vaino P, Lassila V, et al. Trabecular bone mineral density and alveolar height in postmenopausal women. *Scand J Dent Res.* 1993;101:166–170.
28. Mercier P, Inoue S. Bone density and serum minerals in cases of residual alveolar ridge atrophy. *J Prosthet Dent.* 1981;46:250–255.
29. Atwood DA, Coy WA. Clinical cephalometric and densitometric study of reduction of residual ridges. *J Prosthet Dent.* 1971;26:280–295.
30. Lavelle CLB. Biomechanical considerations of prosthodontic therapy: the urgency of research into alveolar bone responses. *Int J Oral Maxillofac Implants.* 1993;8:179–184.
31. Meier GH. Die architektur der spongiosa. *Arch Anat Physiol Wess Med.* 1993;34:615–628.
32. Kulmann C. *Die graphische Statik 1.* Aufl, Zurich: Meyer and Zeller; 1888.
33. Wolff J. *Das Gesetz der Transformation der Knochen.* Berlin: A Hirshwald; 1892.
34. Murry PDF. *Bones: A Study of Development and Structure of the Vertebral Skeleton.* Cambridge: Cambridge University Press; 1936.
35. MacMillan HA. Structural characteristics of the alveolar process. *Int J Ortho.* 1926;12:722–730.
36. Parfitt AM. Investigation of the normal variations in the alveolar bone trabeculation. *Oral Surg Oral Med Oral Pathol.* 1962;15:1453–1463.
37. Harris EF, Baker WC. Loss of root length and crestal bone height before and during treatment in adult and adolescent orthodontic patients. *Ann J Orthod Dentofac Orthop.* 1990;98:463–469.
38. Neufeld JO. Changes in the trabecular pattern of the mandible following the loss of teeth. *J Prosthet Dent.* 1958:685–697.
39. Orban B. *Oral Histology and Embryology.* 3rd ed. St Louis: Mosby; 1953.
40. Enlow DH. *Principles of Bone Remodeling: an Account of Post-Natal Growth and Remodeling Processes in Long Bones and the Mandible.* Springfield, Ill: Thomas; 1963.
41. Roberts WE, Smith RK, Zilberman Y, et al. Osseous adaptation to continuous loading of rigid endosseous implants. *Am J Orthod.* 1984;86:96–111.
42. Garretto LP, Chen J, Parr JA, et al. Remodeling dynamics of bone supporting rigidly fixed titanium implants. A histomorphometric comparison in four species including human. *Implant Dent.* 1995;4:235–243.
43. Rhinelander FW. The normal circulation of bone and its response to surgical intervention. *J Biomed Mater Res.* 1974;8:87–90.
44. Currey JD. Effects of differences in mineralization on the mechanical properties of bone. *Philos Trans R Soc Lond B Biol Sci.* 1984;1121:509–518.
45. Bidez MW, Misch CE. Force transfer in implant dentistry: basic concepts and principles. *J Oral Implantol.* 1992;18:264–274.
46. Frost HM. Mechanical adaptation. Frost's mechanostat theory. In: Martin RB, Burr DB, eds. *Structure, Function, and Adaptation of Compact Bone.* New York: Raven Press; 1989.
47. Kazarian LE, Von Gierke HE. Bone loss as a result of immobilization and chelation: preliminary results in Macaca mulatta. *Chin Orthop Relat Res.* 1969;65:67–75.
48. Minaire MC, Neunier P, Edouard C, et al. Quantitative histological data on disuse osteoporosis: comparison with biological data. *Calcif Tissue Res.* 1974;17:57–73.
49. Uhthoff HK, Jaworski ZF. Bone loss in response to long-term immobilisation. *J Bone Joint Surg Br.* 1978;60-B:418–429.
50. Simmons DJ, Russell JE, Winter F. Space flight and the non-weight bearing bones of the rat skeleton. *Trans Orthop Res Sco.* 1981;4:65.
51. Ingebretsen M. Out of this world workouts. *World Traveler Feb.* 1997:10–14.
52. Oganov VS. Modern analysis of bone loss mechanisms in microgravity. *J Gravit Physiol.* 1804;11:143–146.
53. Mori S, Burr DB. Increased intracortical remodeling following fatigue damage. *Bone.* 1993;14:103–109.
54. Linkow LI, Chercheve R. *Theories and Techniques of Oral Implantology.* Vol. 1. St Louis: Mosby; 1970.
55. Lekholm U, Zarb GA. Patient selection and preparation. In: Brånemark PI, Zarb GA, Albrektsson T, eds. *Tissue Integrated Prostheses: Osseointegration in Clinical Dentistry.* Chicago: Quintessence; 1985.
56. Misch CE. Early crestal bone loss etiology and its effect on treatment planning for implants. *Postgraduate Dentistry.* 1995;2:3–17.
57. Oh T, Yoon J, Misch CE, et al. The cause of early implant bone loss: myth or science? *J Periodontol.* 2002;73:322–333.
58. Misch CE, Suzuki JB, Misch-Dietsh FD, et al. A positive correlation between occlusal trauma and peri-implant bone loss—literature support. *Implant Dent.* 2005;14:108–116.
59. Manz MC. Radiographic assessment of peri-implant vertical bone loss: DICRG interim report no. 9. *J Oral Maxillofac Surg.* 1997;55:62–71.
60. Misch CE, Bidez MW, Sharawy M. A bioengineered implant for a predetermined bone cellular response to loading forces: a literature review and case report. *J Periodontol.* 2001;72:1276–1286.
61. Misch C. Progressive bone loading. *Dent Today.* 1995;12:80–83.
62. Trisi P, Rao W. Bone classification: clinical-histomorphometric comparison. *Clin Oral Implants Res.* 1990;10:1–7.
63. Orenstein IH, Synan WJ, Truhlar RS, et al. Bone quality in patients receiving endosseous dental implants: DICRG interim report no. 1. *Implant Dent.* 1994;3:90–94.
64. Quirynen M, Naert I, van Steenberghe D, et al. A study of 589 consecutive implants supporting complete fixed prostheses. Part I: periodontal aspects. *J Prosthet Dent.* 1992;8:655–663.
65. Rothman SLG. Interactive implant surgical planning with Sim/Plan. In: Rothman SLG, ed. *Dental Applications of Computerized Tomography: Surgical Planning for Implant Placement.* Chicago: Quintessence; 1998.

66. Genant HK. Quantitative computed tomography: update. *Calcif Tissue Int.* 1987;41:179–186.

67. Cann CE. Quantitative CT for determination of bone mineral density: a review. *Radiology.* 1988;166:509–522.

68. Rothman SLG. Computerized tomography of the mandible. In: Rothman SLG, ed. *Dental Applications of Computerized Tomography: Surgical Planning for Implant Placement.* Chicago: Quintessence; 1998.

69. Kircos LT, Misch CE. Diagnostic imaging and techniques. In: Misch CE, ed. *Contemporary Implant Dentistry.* 2nd ed. St Louis: Mosby; 1999.

70. Todisco M, Trisi P. Bone mineral density and bone histomorphometry are statistically related. *Int J Oral Maxillofac Implants.* 2005;20:898–904.

71. Angelopoulos C, Aghaloo T. Imaging technology in implant diagnosis. *Dent Clin North Am.* 2011;55:141–158.

72. Norton MR, Gamble C. Bone classification: an objective scale of bone density using the computerized tomography scan. *Clin Oral Implants Res.* 2001;12:79–84.

73. Turkyilmaz I, Tözüm TF, Tumer C, Bone density assessments of oral implant sites using computerized tomography. *J Oral Rehabil.* 2007; 34(4):267–272.

74. Shahlaie M, Gantes B, Schulz E, et al. Bone density assessments of dental implant sites: 1. Quantitative computed tomography. *Int J Oral Maxillofac Implants.* 2003;18:224–231.

75. Homolka P, Beer A, Birkfellner W, et al. Bone mineral density measurement with dental quantitative CT prior to dental implant placement in cadaver mandibles: pilot study. *Radiology.* 2002;224:247–252.

76. Aranyarachkul P, Caruso J, Gantes B, et al. Bone density assessments of dental implant sites: 2. Quantitative cone-beam computerized tomography. *Int J Oral Maxillofac Implants.* 2005;20:416–424.

77. Ikumi N, Tsutsumi S. Assessment of correlation between computerized tomography values of the bone and cutting torque values at implant placement: a clinical study. *Int J Oral Maxillofac Implants.* 2005;20:253–260.

78. Misch CE, Qu Z, Bidez MW. Mechanical properties of trabecular bone in the human mandible implications of dental implant treatment planning and surgical placement. *J Oral Maxillofac Surg.* 1999;57:700–706.

79. Carter DR, Hayes WC. Bone compressive strength: the influence of density and strain rate. *Science.* 1976;194:1174–1176.

80. Rice JC, Cowin SC, Bowman JA. On the dependence of the elasticity and strength of cancellous bone on apparent density. *J Biomech.* 1988;21:155–168.

81. Misch CE, Bidez MW. Implant protected occlusion. *Pract Periodontics Aesthet Dent.* 1995;7:25–29.

82. Kitagawa T, Tanimoto Y, Nemoto K, et al. Influence of cortical bone quality on stress distribution in bone around dental implants. *Dent Mater J.* 1805;24:219–224.

83. Sevimay M, Turhan F, Kilicarsian MA, et al. Three-dimensional finite element analysis of the effect of different bone quality on stress distribution in an implant-supported crown. *J Prosthet Dent.* 1805;93:227–234.

84. Tada S, Stegaroiu R, Kitamura E, et al. Influence of implant design and bone quality on stress/strain distribution in bone around implants: a 3-dimensional finite element analysis. *Int J Oral Maxillofac Implants.* 1803;18:357–368.

85. Crupi B, Guglielmino E, LaRosa G, et al. Numerical analysis of bone adaptation around an oral implant due to overload stress. *Proc Inst Mech Eng [H].* 2004;218(6):407–415.

86. Ichikawa T, Kanitani H, Wigianto R, et al. Influence of bone quality in the stress distribution—an in vitro experiment. *Clin Oral Implants Res.* 1997;8:18–22.

87. Bassi F, Procchio M, Fava C, et al. Bone density in human dentate and edentulous mandibles using computed tomography. *Clin Oral Implants Res.* 1999;10:356–361.

88. Steigenga JT, Alshammari KF, Nociti FH, et al. Dental implant design and its relationship to long term implant success. *Implant Dent.* 1803;12:306–317.

89. Petrie CS, Williams JL. Comparative evaluation of implant designs: influence of diameter, length and taper on strains in the alveolar crest: a three-dimensional finite element analysis. *Clin Oral Implants Res.* 1805;16:486–494.

90. Rieger MR, Adams WK, Kinzel GL, et al. Finite element analysis of bone-adapted and bone-bonded endosseous implants. *J Prosthet Dent.* 1989;62:436–440.

91. Schenk RK, Buser D. Osseointegration: a reality. *Periodontology.* 1998;1800(17):22–35.

19

Treatment Plans Related to Key Implant Positions and Implant Number

CARL E. MISCH[†] AND RANDOLPH R. RESNIK

In the past, treatment planning for implant dentistry was primarily driven by the existing bone volume in the edentulous sites (i.e., bone-driven treatment planning). As a result, implants were placed in areas where bone was present, however not necessarily in the best position for prosthetic rehabilitation. Because of the nonideal positioning, atypical prostheses resulted that led to significant biomechanical issues. A second historical phase of treatment planning has since developed based on esthetics and ideal biomechanics. In this scheme, implant positions are primarily dictated and controlled by the teeth (prosthesis) being replaced. If the available bone is insufficient or in a nonideal position, bone augmentation is completed to increase the bone volume to position the implants more ideally.

It is generally accepted that when implants are inserted into abundant bone volume and allowed sufficient time to integrate before loading, the surgical success rate is greater than 98%. In most studies this success rate is not related to implant position, number, size, or design and, more importantly, prosthesis success.[1] Research has shown that when the implant is occlusally loaded with the prosthesis for a period, the failure rate may be greater than three to six times the surgical failure rate. For example, a metaanalysis reveals 15% failure rates (with several reports >30% failure) when the implant prosthesis is occlusally loaded in softer bone.[1] This failure most often occurs during the first 18 months of loading and is termed *early loading failure*. The primary cause of this complication in implant dentistry is related to biomechanical factors, with excessive biomechanical stress applied to the implant support system or bone too weak to support the load.[2]

Therefore it is imperative for the implant clinician to reduce the biomechanical stress to the implant prosthesis. This may be accomplished by several methods (e.g., eliminating cantilevers, ideal implant positioning, adequate implant number and splinting implants whenever possible).[1] Mechanical complications of the implant components or prosthesis far outnumber surgical failures, which may include abutment screw loosening, uncemented prostheses, and restorative material failure. These potential complications may be exacerbated by parafunctional habits, nonfavorable opposing dentitions, and improper occlusal schemes. Because mechanical complications are related to biomechanical factors,

Misch[2] developed a treatment plan sequence to decrease the risk for biomechanical overload, consisting of the following:
1. development of the prosthesis design
2. evaluation of patient force factors
3. determination of bone density in the edentulous sites
4. determination of key implant positions and implant number
5. determination of implant size
6. determination of available bone in the edentulous sites

This chapter will discuss the key implant positions and related treatment planning principles for an implant prosthesis to reduce the biomechanical stress to the system.

Key Implant Positions Rules for a Fixed Implant Prosthesis

The position of dental implants within the arch is crucial to long-term success. Some implant positions are more critical than others in regard to force reduction. For a fixed prosthesis, four general guidelines have been postulated to assist the clinician in treatment planning (Box 19.1):
1. Cantilevers on the prosthesis should be reduced and preferably eliminated (especially in the maxilla); therefore the terminal abutments in the prosthesis are key positions.
2. More than three adjacent pontics should not be designed in the prosthesis.
3. The canine and first molar sites are key positions, especially when adjacent teeth are missing.
4. The arch is divided into five segments. When more than one segment of an arch is being replaced, a key implant position is at least one implant in each segment.

> **• BOX 19.1 Guidelines for Key Implant Positions**
>
> - No cantilevers
> - Maximum of three adjacent pontics
> - Canine
> - Molar rule
> - Arch dynamics

[†]Deceased.

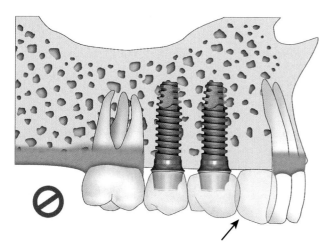

• **Fig. 19.1** Ideal key implant positions include the terminal abutment positions when adjacent teeth are missing. Without a terminal abutment, a cantilever situation will exist on the restoration, which increases biomechanical complications. This is particularly important when excessive forces are present.

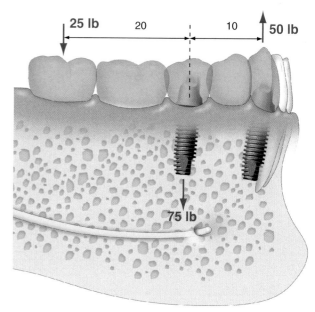

• **Fig. 19.2** A cantilever on two implants may be considered a class 1 lever. For example, when the center of each implant is 10 mm apart, with a 20-mm cantilever, a mechanical advantage of 2 is created. Therefore the load on the cantilever will be multiplied by 2 on the posterior implant, and the implant close to the cantilever receives the majority of the stress of the two loads.

Rule # 1: Minimize Cantilevers

The first rule for ideal key implant positions dictates that the use of cantilevers should be reduced and minimized in the design of the prosthesis (Fig. 19.1). Cantilevers are force magnifiers to the implants, abutment screws, cement or prosthesis screws, and implant–bone interface. Force magnifiers are variables that increase or potentiate force to the system. It is well accepted that cantilevers on fixed partial dentures supported by natural teeth have a higher complication rate than prostheses with terminal abutments, including unretained restorations. This is especially noted with parafunction or reduced crown height spaces.[3] Therefore the ideal key implant positions include the terminal abutment positions when adjacent teeth are missing.

The length of the cantilever is directly related to the amount of the additional force placed on the abutments of the prosthesis. For example, when a 25-lb force is placed along the long axis of an implant, the implant system (i.e., crown, cement, abutment, abutment screw, implant body, implant marginal bone, and implant–bone interface) receives a 25-lb load. When a force of the same magnitude (25 lb) is applied on a 10-mm cantilever, the moment force on the abutment is increased to a 250-lb millimeter force. As a result, any part of the implant system is at an increased risk for biomechanical failure (e.g., porcelain fracture, uncemented prosthesis, abutment screw loosening, crestal bone loss, implant failure, implant component or body fracture) (Fig. 19.2).

A cantilevered restoration on multiple implants may be compared with a class I lever. The extension of the prosthesis from the last abutment is the *effort arm* of the lever. The last abutment next to the cantilever acts as a fulcrum when a load is applied to the lever. The distance between the last abutment and the farthest abutment from the end of the cantilever represents the *resistance arm* and may be called the *anteroposterior distance* or *A-P spread* of the implants. The length (usually in millimeters) of the cantilever (effort arm) divided by the resistance arm represents the *mechanical advantage*. Therefore when two implants are 10 mm apart with a cantilever or extension of 20 mm, the mechanical advantage is two (20 mm/10 mm). In this example a 25-lb force on the cantilever results with a 50-lb force on the farthest abutment from the cantilever (25 lb × 2 = 50 lb). The abutment closest to the

cantilever (fulcrum) receives a force equal to the sum of the other two forces, or in this example, 75 lb (25 lb + 50 lb). Therefore cantilevers magnify forces to all of the abutments that support the prosthesis.

Therefore the ideal treatment plan should minimize the use of cantilevers. However, in some clinical conditions a cantilever is the most prudent treatment option. For example, in an edentulous mandible, available bone in the posterior regions may be insufficient for root form implant placement, without advanced procedures (e.g., nerve repositioning, iliac crest bone grafts). An alternative treatment plan may be to cantilever pontics from anterior implants. However, when terminal abutments are not designed in the treatment plan and a cantilever is planned, other force and surface area factors should compensate for the increase in force (Fig. 19.3). When this option is considered, the force factors of parafunction, bone density, crown height, masticatory dynamics, implant location, and opposing arch are closely scrutinized. In addition to force modifiers, the A-P distance (A-P spread) of the distal and anterior implants is also a factor. When the implants are in one plane, the cantilever should rarely extend farther than the A-P distance, regardless of how low the patient force factors. When the force factors are unfavorable, the cantilever length should be reduced or eliminated, the implant number increased, the implant size increased, or the implant design surface areas increased. The square arch form is the least desirable because this equates to a short, minimal A-P spread. The tapered arch form is the most ideal because the distance between the anterior and posterior implants is the greatest. The ovoid arch form is associated with an arch form between the square and tapered (Fig. 19.4).

Rule # 2: Limit the Number of Adjacent Pontics

In most prostheses designs, greater than three adjacent pontics are contraindicated on implants, just as they are contraindicated on natural tooth abutments.[4] The exception to this rule is when very

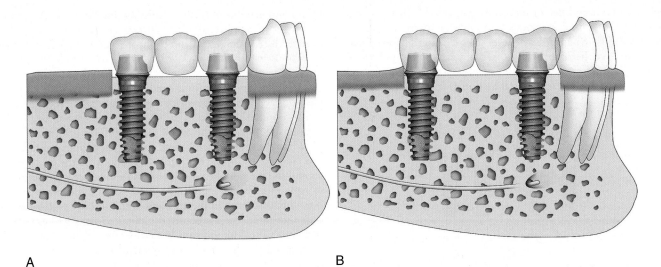

A   B

• **Fig. 19.3** (A) When three adjacent teeth are being replaced, the terminal abutments are key implant positions. When all patient force factors are low and bone density is good, two implants may be adequate
to replace the three missing teeth. However, when force factors are high, an implant for each missing
tooth is recommended. (B) When four adjacent teeth are missing, the terminal abutments are key implant
positions. Rarely are these two implants sufficient to replace four posterior teeth (i.e., exception would
be opposing a complete denture). More commonly, three implants are placed with the additional implant
being placed ideally in the most available position because of higher occlusal forces.

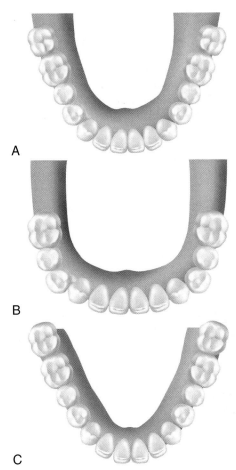

A

B

C

• **Fig. 19.4** The anteroposterior distance (A-P spread) of five implants in the
mandible is measured from the distal of the last two implants to the mid
position of the most anterior implant. Because these splinted implants form
an arch, the cantilever may extend up to 2.5 times the A-P distance (when
patient force factors are low and bone density is good). Arch shape affects
the A-P distance. The ovoid arch form (A) often has an A-P distance of 6
to 8 mm. A square arch form (B) often has an A-P dimension of 2 to 5 mm.
A tapered arch form (C) has the greatest A-P distance, larger than 8 mm.

low force factors are present along with favorable implant conditions (i.e., bone density, available bone, minimal force factors). The
complication resulting from multiple adjacent abutments is the
additional force that is applied, especially in the posterior regions.

The adjacent abutments are subjected to considerable additional force when they must support three missing teeth, especially in the posterior regions of the mouth. In addition, all pontic
spans between abutments flex under load. The greater the span
between abutments, the greater the flexibility in the prosthesis.
The greater the load, the greater the flexure. This resultant flexure
places shear and tensile loads on the abutments.[5] In addition, the
greater the flexure, the increased risk for porcelain/zirconia fracture, uncemented prostheses, and abutment screw loosening.

The flexure of restorative materials in a long span is more of a
problem for implants than natural teeth. Because natural tooth
roots have associated mobility both apically and laterally, the
tooth acts as a stress absorber, and the amount of material flexure
may be reduced. An implant is more rigid than a tooth (and also
has a greater modulus of elasticity than a natural tooth), so the
complications of increased load and material flexure are greater
for an implant prosthesis. This is especially crucial with maxillary
anterior prostheses, where angled forces magnify the amount of
the force to the implant system.

The span of the pontics in the ideal treatment plan should be limited in size by reducing the occlusal table and cusp height. If replacing a molar-size space (mesiodistal), the size of two premolar-sized
teeth may be used. By narrowing the occlusal table, the amount of
damaging forces (i.e., shear, off-axis) will reduce the amount of force
to the system. By decreasing the cusp height, the potential of shear
forces is reduced significantly (Fig. 19.5).

Rule # 3: Implant Positioned in Canine Site

A fixed restoration replacing a canine is at greater risk than nearly
any other restoration in the mouth. The maxillary or mandibular
adjacent incisor is one of the weakest teeth in the mouth, and
the first premolar is often one of the weakest posterior teeth. A
traditional fixed prosthetic axiom indicates it is contraindicated to

replace a canine and two or more adjacent teeth.[4,6] Therefore if a patient desires a fixed prosthesis, and force factors are not favorable, implants are required whenever the following adjacent teeth are missing in either arch: (1) the first premolar, canine, and lateral incisor; (2) the second premolar, first premolar, and canine; and (3) the canine, lateral, and central incisors (Fig. 19.6). Whenever

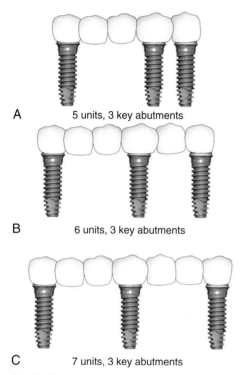

A   5 units, 3 key abutments

B   6 units, 3 key abutments

C   7 units, 3 key abutments

• **Fig. 19.5** (A–C) A five- to seven-unit fixed prosthesis has three key positions for the abutments. The terminal abutment follows rule 1 (no cantilever), and a one-pier abutment is positioned following rule 2 (no three adjacent pontics). Rarely are these three abutments sufficient to support the prosthesis in the long term. Additional abutments are required when force factors are moderate to severe or bone density is poor around the implant.

these combinations of teeth are missing, implants are required to restore the patient because: (1) the length of the span is three adjacent teeth, (2) the lateral direction of force during mandibular excursions increase the stress, and (3) the magnitude of the bite force is increased in the canine region compared with the anterior region. Therefore under these conditions, at least two key implant positions are required to replace these three adjacent teeth, usually in the terminal positions of the span (especially when one of the terminal abutments is the canine position) (Figs. 19.7 and 19.8).

When the three adjacent teeth are the first premolar and canine and lateral incisors, the key implant positions are the first premolar and the canine. These positions result in an anterior cantilever to replace the lateral incisor. However, because the lateral incisor is the smallest tooth in the arch and in the anterior region has the least bite force, the cantilever is of limited negative impact. In addition, the canine implant is usually larger than a lateral incisor implant for the esthetic requirements of the restoration. This further reduces the effect of the cantilever (Fig. 19.9). In addition, the occlusion is modified so that no occlusal contact is present on the lateral incisor pontic in centric occlusion or excursions of the mandible. When force factors are greater than usual, a small-diameter implant may also be used to support the lateral incisor, and three implants with no cantilever reduce the increased force factor risks.

When there are multiple missing teeth and the canine edentulous site is a pier abutment position, the canine position is a key implant position to help disocclude the posterior teeth in mandibular excursions. As a result, when four or more adjacent teeth are missing, including a canine and at least one adjacent posterior premolar tooth, the key implant positions are the terminal abutments, the canine position, and additional pier abutments, which limit the pontics spans to no more than two teeth (Fig. 19.10).

The canine site is also crucial for the ideal occlusion. In most fixed-implant treatment plans an implant-protected occlusion is recommended. This occlusal scheme allows for disocclusion off of the canine (i.e., canine guidance), thereby protecting the teeth from harmful forces. Williamson and Lundquist[7] showed in electromyographic studies that when a mutually protected occlusion is present, two-thirds of the temporalis/masseter muscle fibers do

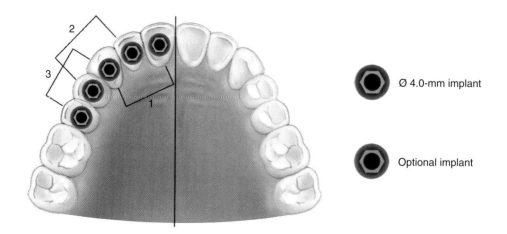

Ø 4.0-mm implant

Optional implant

• **Fig. 19.6** Whenever the canine and three adjacent teeth are missing, implants are required to support a fixed prosthesis. Therefore when (*1*) the canine, lateral, and central; (*2*) the lateral, canine, and first premolar; or (*3*) the canine, first, and second premolar teeth are missing, an implant should always be placed in the canine position.

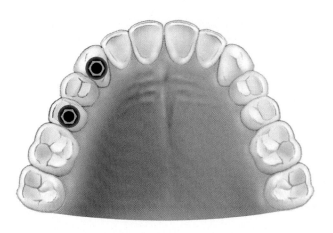

• **Fig. 19.7** When the canine, first premolar, and second premolar teeth are missing, key implant positions are in the canine and second premolar positions to support these three teeth.

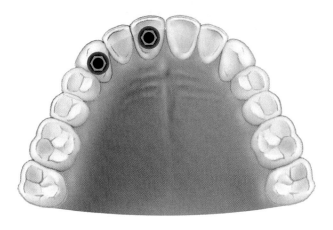

• **Fig. 19.8** When the canine, lateral, and central incisor teeth are missing, key implant positions are in the central and canine positions to support these three teeth.

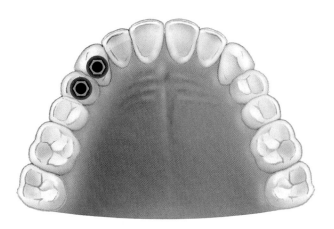

• **Fig. 19.9** When the first premolar, canine, and lateral incisors are missing, the key implant positions are the first premolar and canine position. Although this may result in a cantilever on the restoration, the lateral incisor is the smallest tooth, the anterior region has less bite force, and the canine implant may be larger than the lateral incisor implant for esthetic requirements.

not contract. Therefore by positioning an implant in the cuspid position, the resultant muscle activity from the temporalis and masseter muscles is greatly reduced.[7]

Rule # 4: Implant Positioned in Molar Site

The first molar is also a key implant position when three adjacent posterior teeth are missing. The bite force doubles in the molar position compared with the premolar position in both the maxilla and mandible. In addition, the edentulous span of a missing first molar is 10 to 12 mm, compared with a 7-mm span for a premolar. As a result, when three or more adjacent teeth are missing, including a first molar, the key implant positions include the terminal abutments and the first molar position (Fig. 19.11). For example, in a patient missing the second premolar, first molar, and second molars, three key implant positions are needed to restore the full contour of the missing molar teeth: the second premolar and second molar terminal abutments and the first molar pier abutment (Fig. 19.12). When one implant replaces a molar (for a span of less than 13 mm), the implant should be at least 5 mm in diameter. When a smaller-diameter implant is selected, the molar may be considered the size of two premolars.

Rule # 5: Implant Positioned in Each Arch Segment

An arch (maxilla or mandible) may be divided into five segments, similar to an open pentagon (see Fig. 8.15). The two central and two lateral incisors are one segment, the canines are independent segments, and the premolars and molars on each side form a segment. In other words, each segment is essentially a straight line, with little inherent biomechanical advantage to a lateral force. However, when two or more segments of an arch are connected, the tripod effect is greater, and as a benefit, an A-P distance (A-P spread) is created from the most distal terminal abutments to the most anterior pier abutment (Fig. 19.13).

When multiple adjacent missing teeth extend beyond one of the open pentagon segments, a key implant position needs to be situated within each segment. Therefore if the patient is edentulous from first premolar to first premolar, the key implant positions include the terminal abutments (the two first premolars), the two canines, and either of the central incisor positions (Fig. 19.14). These implant positions follow the rules of (1) no cantilever, (2) no three adjacent pontics, (3) the canine position, and (4) at least one implant in each edentulous segment of an arch.

Implant Number

In the past the number of implants most often was determined by the amount of available bone in the mesiodistal dimension. For example, in an edentulous arch, five to six implants were often used in abundant bone between the mental foramina for a full-arch fixed prosthesis, whereas four implants were used in moderate-to-severe resorption for a fixed full-arch prosthesis (Fig. 19.15).[8] However, this treatment option does not consider the force magnifiers of crown or height space, or the A-P distance (A-P spread) of the implants in relation to the bilateral posterior cantilevers replacing the posterior teeth.

Usually a completely edentulous arch is supported by a 12-unit fixed prosthesis, extending from first molar to first molar. Rarely are second molars replaced in the prosthesis, unless the opposing arch has a second molar present. In this scenario the position of the implants cannot follow the four key implant position rules,

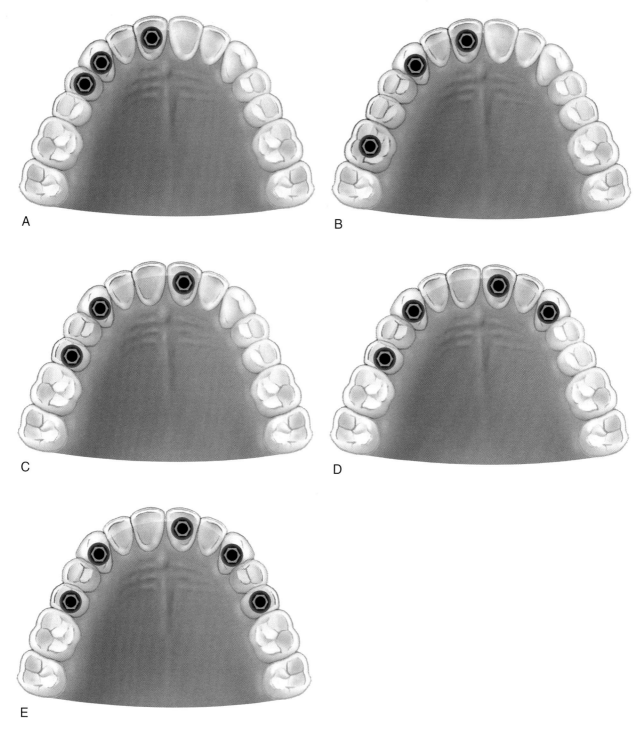

• **Fig. 19.10** (A) When the central, lateral, canine, and first premolar are missing, the ideal key implant positions are the central and first premolar (rule 1, no cantilever) and the canine position (rule 3, the canine and first molar position). (B) When the central, lateral, canine, first premolar, second premolar, and first molar are missing, the three key implants positions are the central and first molar sites (rule 1) and the canine site (rules 2 and 3, no three adjacent pontic and canine and first molar position). (C) When the central, central, lateral, canine, first premolar, and second premolar are missing, there are three key implant positions: the central and second premolar (rule 1, no cantilever) and the canine position (rule 3, the canine and first molar position). (D) When eight adjacent teeth are missing from second premolar to the opposite canine, there are four key implant positions: the canine and second premolar position (rule 1), the opposite canine (rule 3), and one of the central incisor positions (rule 2). (E) When 10 adjacent teeth are missing from second premolar to second premolar, there are five key implant positions: the two second premolar sites (rule 1), the two canine sites (rule 3), and one of the central incisor positions (rule 2).

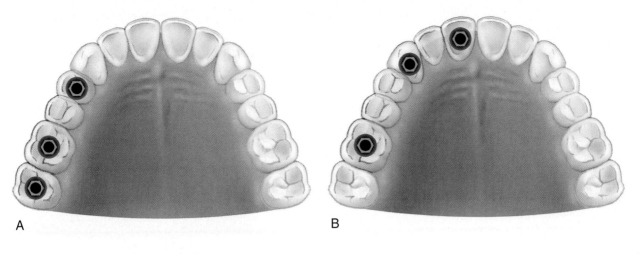

A

B

C

• **Fig. 19.11** (A) When the patient is missing four teeth from the first premolar to second molar, there are three key implant positions to replace the four teeth: the first premolar and second molar sites (rule 1) and the first molar position (rule 3). (B) When the patient is missing six adjacent teeth from the central incisors to the first molar, there are three key implant positions: the central and first molar position (rule 1) and the canine position (rule 3). When a larger implant cannot be inserted into the molar site, an additional implant is required to follow rule 2. (C) When the patient is missing teeth from first molar to first molar, there are five key implant positions: the two first molars (rule 1), the two canines (rule 3), and a central incisor (rule 2). Additional implants in the posterior region are indicated when a larger-diameter implant is not positioned in the first molar sites (rule 2). Implants in the second premolar site are also usually indicated when force factors are moderate or bone density is D3. Even more implant support is suggested when force factors are severe or bone density is D4.

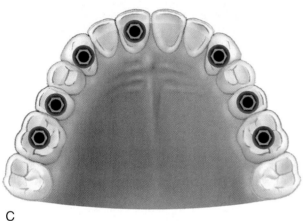

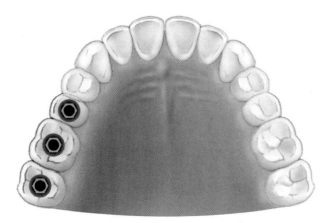

• **Fig. 19.12** In a patient missing the second premolar and first molar and second molars, three key implant positions are needed to restore the full contour of the missing molars: the second premolar and second molar terminal abutments and the first molar pier abutment.

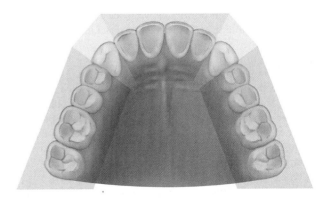

• **Fig. 19.13** An arch may be considered as an open pentagon: the two premolar and molar sites, the two canine sites, and the central and lateral incisors represent the five sides.

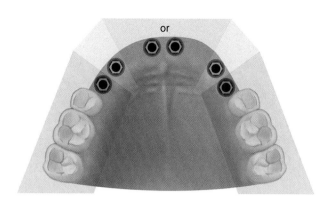

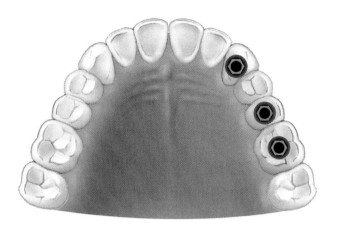

• **Fig. 19.14** When a patient is missing eight teeth from first premolar to first premolar, there are five key positions: the first premolar sites (rule 1: no cantilever; and rule 4: one implant in each open pentagon segment), the two canines (rule 3: the canine and first molar rule; and rule 4: an implant in each pentagon segment), and an implant in one of the central incisor positions (rule 2: no three adjacent pontics; and rule 4: an implant in each open pentagon segment).

• **Fig. 19.16** When four adjacent teeth are missing from the canine to first molar, the two terminal key implant positions are usually inadequate to support the prosthesis. One or two additional implants are required in most clinical situations (depending on patient force factors and bone density). The additional implant of choice is in the second premolar site, especially when a larger-diameter implant is not placed in the molar site.

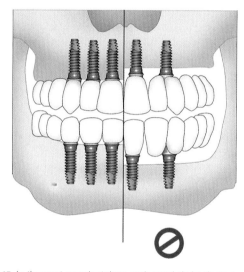

• **Fig. 19.15** In the past an edentulous arch used six implants to support a fixed prosthesis in abundant bone situations and four implants to support a complete full arch prosthesis when minimal bone volumes were present.

and include either four pontics between the anterior implants or three pontics cantilevered from the most distal implants. In addition, the number of implants in a treatment plan should rarely use a minimum number. There is no safety factor if an implant fails. For example, if 25 patients receive four implants to support a fixed prosthesis, there would be 25 fixed prostheses and 100 implants. If each patient lost one implant, there would remain only three implants and, as a result, nearly all 25 fixed prostheses would be at risk for overload failure. If 20% of the implants fail (with one failure per patient), only 5 of the 25 patients would have four implants to support the restoration (20% prosthesis success). This type of treatment planning may initially be less expensive for the patient, but an implant failure anytime after implant surgery places the patient's prosthesis at considerable risk.

The key implant positions are often not enough support for the implant restoration, unless all patient force factors are low

(e.g., parafunction, masticatory dynamics, crown height) and the bone density is good (D1, D2). Therefore most often additional implants (besides the key implants) are added to the treatment plan.

One of the most efficient methods to increase surface area and decrease stress is to increase the implant number. For example, only two implant key positions as terminal abutments for a four-unit implant prosthesis in the canine and posterior region represent inadequate implant support, unless patient force factors are low, bone density is ideal, and implant size is not compromised. In most situations three implants to replace four missing teeth is an ideal implant number. When force factors are high and bone density is poor (i.e., posterior maxilla), four implants to replace four teeth is often appropriate (Fig. 19.16).

Previous studies have shown that three abutments for a five-tooth span distribute stress more favorably than do two abutments for the same span. The one additional implant may decrease the implant reaction force by two times and reduce metal flexure fivefold. In addition, in the three-abutment scenario, moment forces are reduced.[9,10] In full-arch prostheses, studies comparing six implants and four implant abutments show better distribution and reduced stress on the six-implant system components (crown, cement, abutment, abutment screw, marginal bone, implant–bone interface, and implant components).[11]

The decision on the number of implants in the treatment plan begins with the implants in the ideal key positions. Additional numbers are most often required and are primarily related to the patient force factors and to bone density in the edentulous sites. Therefore in a young, large man with severe bruxism with greater-than-normal crown height space in the posterior regions of the mouth, opposing an implant restoration will require one implant for each missing root (two implants for each molar). Likewise, patients with moderate force factors and poor bone density (D4 bone) in the implant sites may also require this many implants.

As a general observation the number of implants to replace all of the mandibular teeth range from five to nine, with at least four between the mental foramina. When fewer than six implants are used, a cantilever must be designed in a fixed prosthesis as a result of the mandibular flexure. Cantilevers in the mandible should

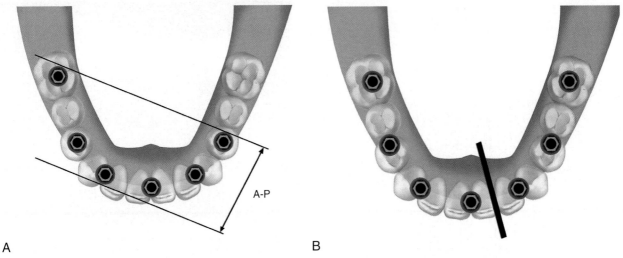

• **Fig. 19.17** (A) When six or more implants are positioned in the mandible (first molar, two first premolar, two canine, and one central incisor), a cantilever may be designed in the mandible because of the dynamics of an arch, with four of the five sections of an open pentagon joined, the large anteroposterior distance (A-P), and the favorable mandibular bone density. (B) When seven or more implants are placed in an edentulous mandible, two separate prostheses with no posterior cantilever may be designed. The mandible flexure and torsion are free to occur when the separation between the two prostheses is between the mental foramina.

ideally be projected in only one posterior quadrant to increase the A-P distance and reduce the force to the implants (Fig. 19.17). When implants are positioned in four of the five open pentagon positions in the mandible, a cantilever is at a reduced risk for overload because of favorable dynamics of an arch, increased large A-P distance, and favorable bone density. When seven or more implants are used, two separate restorations may be fabricated with no posterior cantilever to permit mandibular flexure and torsion (see Fig. 8.19B). Usually the second molar is not replaced in the edentulous mandible. A greater number of implants is generally required in the maxilla to compensate for the less-dense bone and more unfavorable biomechanics of the premaxilla, and range from 7 to 10 implants, with at least 3 implants from canine to canine (Fig. 19.18).

In most situations an implant should be positioned at least 1.5 mm from an adjacent natural tooth and 3 mm from an adjacent implant.[12-18] Using these guidelines, each 4-mm-diameter implant requires 7 mm of mesiodistal space (Fig. 19.19). Therefore the maximum number of implants between adjacent teeth can be calculated by taking the crest module of an implant (e.g., 4.0 mm) and adding these dimensions (Fig. 19.20). For example, an edentulous span of 21 mm is required for three adjacent implants 4 mm in diameter, and 28 mm for four adjacent implants between two teeth. As a general rule, it is better to err on the side of safety in numbers than on the side of too few implants. Therefore when in doubt, add an additional implant to the treatment plan.

Commonly, implant-supported crowns in the posterior regions of the mouth are the size of premolars. This concept often permits the placement of two implants to replace an intratooth molar, when the span is at least 14 mm for 4-mm-diameter implants (3 mm between each implant and 1.5 mm from the adjacent teeth). When the missing molar is the most distal in the arch, a 12.5-mm span is required for two 4-mm-diameter implants (3 mm between each implant and 1.5 mm from the anterior tooth), because the 1.5-mm distance from the last tooth is no longer required.

There are several advantages of a 7- to 8-mm-wide premolar and a molar-sized crown. More implants may be used to restore

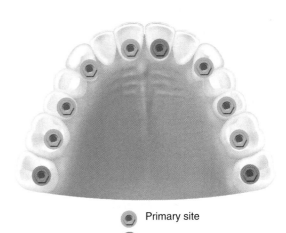

   Primary site

   Secondary site

• **Fig. 19.18** The ideal seven-implant positioning for a maxillary edentulous arch includes at least one central incisor position, bilateral canine positions, bilateral second premolar sites, and bilateral sites in the distal half of the first molars. In the case of heavy stress factors, an additional anterior implant and bilateral second molar positions (to increase the anteroposterior distance) may be of benefit.

the missing teeth. Implants may range from 4 to 5 mm in diameter, which are the most common sizes, and often the available bone has adequate buccolingual bone dimension in this region. The emergence of the crown contours on implants of this dimension permit sulcular probing. In addition, the occlusal table width decreases mesial and distal moment forces compared with a molar-sized crown.[19]

Additional Treatment Planning Principles

Independent Prosthesis

As a general rule an implant-supported prosthesis should be independent from the natural adjacent teeth. This concept will

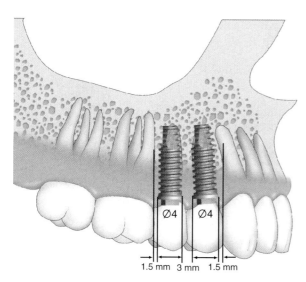

• **Fig. 19.19** The minimum mesiodistal dimension for two standard 4-mm diameter implants is 1.5 mm + 4 mm + 3 mm + 4 mm + 1.5 mm = 14 mm.

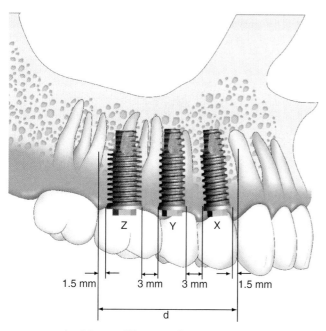

d = 1.5 mm +ØZ + 3mm+ØY + 3mm+ØX + 1.5mm

• **Fig. 19.20** When three adjacent teeth are missing (two premolars and first molar), the mesiodistal dimension averages 7.1 mm + 6.6 mm + 10.4 mm = 24.1 mm. In this situation, planning 4-mm-diameter implants to fabricate two premolars of 7 mm each (1.5 mm + 4 mm + 1.5 mm) and one 5-mm-diameter implant for the first molar allows more bone around each implant.

reduce the risk for marginal decay on the natural teeth next to the adjacent pontic or abutment. The incidence of decay on a tooth splinted in a fixed partial denture accounts for 22% of the complications within 10 years, whereas individual crowns have less than 1% risk for decay within this time frame.[20] Unrestored natural teeth exhibit less risk for decay, and implants do not decay at all. A second common complication of teeth-supported fixed prosthetic restorations is endodontic-related factors that occur in approximately 15% of cases within 10 years.[21] Implant abutments

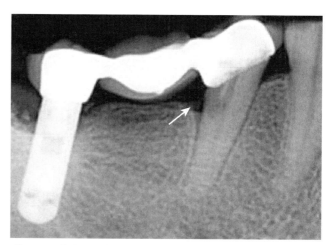

• **Fig. 19.21** Independent Implant Prosthesis. Ideally implants should always be kept independent from natural teeth because of numerous biomechanical differences. One of the most common complications is recurrent decay on the natural tooth abutment.

do not require endodontic procedures, and unsplinted natural tooth crowns have less endodontic procedures. Independent implant prostheses may also reduce or eliminate pontics, whereas simultaneously increasing the number of abutments and distributing forces more effectively. The increase in abutment number decreases the risk for an unretained restoration, which is the third most common fixed prosthesis complication supported by natural teeth. Therefore independent implant prostheses cause fewer complications and exhibit greater long-term success rates of the prosthesis and greater survival rates of the adjacent teeth.[22] However, when an implant restoration is joined to a natural tooth, an increased risk for abutment screw loosening, implant marginal bone loss, tooth decay, and unretained restoration occurs. In addition, the distribution of occlusal forces is optimized when independent implant prostheses are designed. As a result the ideal treatment plan for a partially edentulous patient includes an independent implant restoration (Fig. 19.21).

Splinted Implants

The splinting of dental implants is controversial. Many clinicians use the same existing treatment planning principles from natural teeth as they do for dental implants. However, implants and teeth are much different biomechanically. The fact that teeth adapt to forces much differently from implants is significant when deciding to splint versus nonsplint.

There exist many advantages to splinting implants. Splinted implants increase the functional surface area of support, increase the A-P distance (A-P spread) to resist lateral loads, distribute force over a larger area, increase cement retention of the prosthesis, decrease the risk for abutment screw loosening, decrease the risk for marginal bone loss, and decrease the risk for implant component fracture. In other words, the entire system benefits.[23-26]

In addition to biomechanical reasons, if an independent implant fails over time, the implant is removed, the site is grafted, the site is reimplanted, and a new crown is fabricated. When multiple splinted implants have an implant that fails, the affected implant may often be sectioned below the crown, and the implant or crown site converted to a pontic using the same prosthesis. As a result, rather than several surgical and prosthetic procedures over an extended period when independent units are restored, the complication may be solved in one relatively short appointment when the crowns are splinted together.

The splinted implants distribute less force to the implant bodies, which decreases the risk for marginal bone loss and implant body fracture. In a report by Sullivan,[27] a 4-mm single implant replacing a molar had implant body fracture in 14% of the cases. In comparison, multiple implants splinted together had a 1% implant body fracture.[1]

Splinted implants reduce the risk for screw loosening. The highest prosthetic complication with single-tooth implants is abutment screw loosening. In a report by Balshi and Wolfinger,[28] single-tooth implants replacing a molar had 48% screw loosening over a 3-year period. When two implants were splinted together to replace a molar, the incidence rate of screw loosening was reduced to 8% over the same period.

The exception to the splinted implant rule is a full-arch mandibular implant prosthesis. The body of the mandible flexes distal to the foramen on opening and has torsion during heavy biting with potential clinical significance for full-arch implant prostheses.[29,30] As a result a full-arch mandibular implant prosthesis replacing the first or second molars should not be splinted to molars on the opposite side. Therefore full-arch mandibular restorations should have a cantilever or be made in two or three sections to accommodate the mandibular dynamics during function. The concept of flexure and torsion does not affect the maxilla, where all implants often are splinted together, regardless of their positions in the arch.

When implant crowns are splinted, they provide greater prosthesis retention and transfer less force to the cement interface. As a result a cemented implant restoration is less likely to become uncemented. This is especially significant when the abutments are short or lateral forces are present.

Many implant clinicians do not like to splint implants because of the associated technical complexities. The prosthesis path of insertion, the need for nonengaging abutments, and prosthetic insertion difficulties may deter many practitioners. However, with advancements in prosthetic and laboratory techniques and materials, this is becoming less of a concern in implant dentistry today.

When splinting implants, many clinicians and patients complain about the ability to perform interproximal hygiene. However, this concept is not as significant with implants for two reasons. First, a very low percentage of the population flosses regularly, especially if floss threaders are indicated.[31] Because the implants are usually 3 mm or more apart, if a patient does wish to perform interproximal hygiene, most aids (e.g., floss threader, proxy brush, water-pik) can easily clean this region.

A second reason that splinted units are not popular is the inability to repair restorative material fracture. However, when dental implants are splinted together, the crown marginal ridges between the implants are supported by metal/zirconia connectors; therefore the porcelain/zirconia is placed under compression. As independent units the margins of porcelain-to-metal crowns are most often placed under shear loads, which increase the risk for fracture. However, the increased use of monolithic zirconia has decreased material fracture significantly. Also, screw-retained prosthetic restorations are becoming more popular; therefore the prosthesis may be removed and repaired much easier.

And lastly, clinicians have the mindset of natural teeth and recurrent decay. A single crown on a natural tooth has a caries risk of less than 1% within 10 years. However, when natural teeth are splinted together, decay at the interproximal margin often occurs

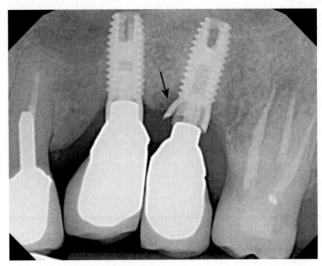

• **Fig. 19.22** Splinted Prosthesis. Implants should be splinted together whenever possible, as the force (i.e., occlusal load) is distributed over a greater area. Note the fracture of the most posterior implant, which is likely due to occlusal force issues.

at a rate of approximately 22%.[32] In addition, the endodontic risk is increased when crowns are splinted. A single crown has an endodontic risk of 3% to 5.6%. Splinted teeth have an endodontic risk of 18%.[20] Therefore independent units reduce the incidence of complications and allow the practitioner to more readily treat these complications. However, implants do not decay or need endodontic therapy. As a result, independent units would not be required to address these complications (Fig. 19.22).

Treatment Planning Should Not Be Dictated by Finances

Many patients have unrealistic expectations with regard to treatment duration and implant treatment. It is not uncommon for a patient to demand that the treatment be "completed faster," especially when bone augmentation is ideally indicated. For example, a percentage of clinicians may not be comfortable with such procedures and may proceed with placing implants without bone grafting because the cost is greater and the procedure is more complex. Manufacturers have even further complicated the situation with questionable treatments of ultrashort implants, "mini-implants", excessive angled implants, or shortcut procedures.

Therefore because most biomechanical-related complications often occur within the first few years of function, the clinician may place themselves at significant risk when a nonideal or shortcut procedure is recommended. As a result, when failure occurs and remediation treatment is required, often the patient expects the clinician to repeat the treatment for no charge. Further, if the patient seeks care from another provider, this is often associated with a greater cost. As a result the patient is more likely to seek litigation-related remedies.

Summary

A biomechanical-based treatment plan reduces complications after implant loading with the prosthesis. To reduce stress conditions, there are key implant positions for a prosthesis replacing missing teeth: (1) minimize cantilevers in the design of the prosthesis, (2) greater than three adjacent pontics should be avoided, (3) the canine and first molar sites are vitally important positions in an arch, and (4) the maxillary arch is divided into five segments. When more than one segment of an arch is being replaced, a key implant position is at least one implant in each missing segment.

Increasing the number of implants is the most efficient method to increase surface area and reduce overall stress. Therefore after the key implant positions are selected, additional implants are indicated to reduce the risks for overload from patient force factors or implant sites with reduced bone density. When in doubt of the number of implants required, adding an additional implant is advantageous.

References

1. Goodacre CJ, Bernal G, Rungcharassaeng K, et al. Clinical complications with implant and implant prostheses. *J Prosthet Dent.* 2003;90:121–132.
2. Misch CE. Consideration of biomechanical stress in treatment with dental implants. *Dent Today.* 2006;25:80–85.
3. Rosenstiel SF, Land MF, Fujimoto J. *Contemporary Fixed Prosthodontics.* 4th ed. St Louis: Mosby; 2006.
4. Shillinburg HT, Hobo S, Lowell D, et al. Treatment planning for the replacement of missing teeth. In: Shillinburg HI, Hobo S, eds. *Fundamentals of Fixed Prosthodontics.* 3rd ed. Chicago: Quintessence; 1997.
5. Smyd ES. Mechanics of dental structures: guide to teaching dental engineering at undergraduate level. *J Prosthet Dent.* 1952;2:668–692.
6. Tylman SD. *Theory and Practice of Crown and Fixed Partial Prosthodontics.* St Louis: Mosby; 1965.
7. Williamson EH, Lundquist DO. Anterior guidance: its effect one electromyographic activity of the temporal and masseter muscles. *J Prosthet Dent.* 1983;49:816–823.
8. Adell R, Lekholm U, Rockler B, et al. A 15-year study of osseointegrated implants in the treatment of the edentulous jaw. *Int J Oral Surg.* 1981;6:387–416.
9. Bidez MW, Misch CE. *The Biomechanics of Interimplant Spacing.* Charleston, SC: Proceedings of the 4th International Congress of Implants and Biomaterials in Stomatology; 1990.
10. Rangert B, Renouard F. *Risk Factors in Implant Dentistry.* Chicago: Quintessence; 1999.
11. McAlarney ME, Stavropoulos DN. Theoretical cantilever lengths versus clinical variables in fifty-five clinical cases. *J Prosthet Dent.* 2000;83:332–342.
12. Tarnow DP, Cho SC, Wallace SS. The effect of interimplant distance on the height of interimplant bone crest. *J Periodontol.* 2000;71:546–569.
13. Hatley CL, Cameron SM, Cuenin MF, et al. The effect of dental implant spacing peri-implant bone using the rabbit (Oryctolagus cuniculus) tibia model. *J Prosthodont.* 2001;10:154–159.
14. Gastaldo JF, Cury PR, Sendyk WR. Effect of the vertical and horizontal distances between adjacent implants and between a tooth and an implant on the incidence of interproximal papilla. *J Periodontol.* 2004;75:1242–1246.
15. Novaes Jr AB, Papalexiou V, Muglia V, et al. Influence of interimplant distance on gingival papilla formation and bone resorption: clinical-radiographic study in dogs. *Int J Oral Maxillofac Implants.* 2006;21:45–51.
16. Papalexiou V, Novaes Jr AB, Ribeiro RF, et al. Influence of the interimplant distance on crestal bone resorption and bone density: a histomorphometric study in dogs. *J Periodontol.* 2006;77:614–621.
17. Desjardins RP. Tissue-integrated prostheses for edentulous patients with normal and abnormal jaw relationships. *J Prosthet Dent.* 1988;59:180–187.
18. Hobo S, Ichida E, Garcia LT. *Osseointegration and Occlusal Rehabilitation.* Chicago: Quintessence; 1989.
19. Allahyar G, Morgano SM. Finite element analysis of three designs of an implant-supported molar crown. *J Prosthet Dent.* 2004;5:434.
20. Goodacre CJ, Bernal G, Rungcharassaeng K, et al. Clinical complications in fixed prosthodontics. *J Prosthet Dent.* 2003;90:31–41.
21. Bergenholtz G, Nyman S. Endodontic complications following periodontal and prosthetic treatment of patients with advanced periodontal disease. *J Periodontol.* 1984;55(2):63–68.
22. Priest GE, Priest J. The economics of implants for single missing teeth. *Dent Econ.* 2004:130–138.
23. Skalak R. Biomechanical considerations in osseointegrated prostheses. *J Prosthet Dent.* 1983;49:843.
24. Rangert B, Jemt T, Jorneus L. Forces and moments on Brånemark implants. *Int J Oral Maxillofac Implants.* 1998;4:241.
25. Wang TM, Leu IJ, Wang J, et al. Effects of prosthesis materials and prosthesis splinting on peri-implant bone stress around implants in poor quality bone: a numeric analysis. *Int J Oral Maxillofac Implants.* 2002;17:231.
26. Guichet DL, Yoshinobu D, Caputo AA. Effects of splinting and interproximal contact tightness on load transfer by implants restorations. *J Prosthet Dent.* 2002;87:528.
27. Sullivan D, Siddiqui A. Wide-diameter implants: overcoming problems. *Dent Today.* 1994;13:50–57.
28. Balshi TJ, Wolfinger GJ. Two-implant-supported single molar replacement: interdental space requirements and comparison to alternative options. *Int J Perio Rest Dent.* 1997;17:426–435.
29. Abdel-Latif H, Hobkirk J, Kelleway J. Functional mandibular deformation in edentulous subjects treated with dental implants. *Int J Prosthodont.* 2000;13:513–519.
30. Hobkirk JA, Havthoulas TK. The influence of mandibular deformation, implant numbers, and loading position on detected forces in abutments supporting fixed implant superstructures. *J Prosthet Dent.* 1998;80:169–174.
31. Segelnick S. A survey of floss frequency, habit and technique in a hospital dental clinic and private periodontal practice. *NY State Dent J.* 2004;70:28–33.
32. Scurria MS, Bader JD, Shugars DA. Meta-analysis of fixed partial denture survival: prostheses and abutments. *J Prosthet Dent.* 1998;79:459–464.

PART V

Edentulous Site Treatment Planning

20

Treatment Plans for Partially and Completely Edentulous Arches in Implant Dentistry

CARL E. MISCH[†] AND RANDOLPH R. RESNIK

Partially Edentulous Arches

A classification of patient conditions is necessary to organize treatment plans in a consistent approach. Because more than 65,000 possible combinations of teeth and edentulous spaces exist in a single arch, no universal agreement exists regarding the use of any one classification system. Numerous classifications have been proposed for partially edentulous arches. Their use allows the profession to visualize and communicate the relationship of hard and soft structures. This chapter reviews a classification for diagnosis and treatment planning for patients who are partially or completely edentulous and require implant prostheses. By using this classification, which Misch[1] first presented in 1985, the doctor is able to convey the dimensions of the bone available in the edentulous area and also indicate the strategic position of the area to be restored.

History

Cummer,[2] Kennedy,[3] and Bailyn[4] originally proposed the classifications of partially edentulous arches that are most familiar to the profession. These classifications were developed to organize removable partial denture (RPD) designs and concepts. Other classifications have also been proposed[5-12] (including one by the American College of Prosthodontists), none of which has been universally accepted. The Kennedy classification, however, has been most accepted in most American dental schools.

The Kennedy classification divides partially edentulous arches into four classes: Class I has bilateral posterior edentulous spaces, Class II has a unilateral posterior edentulous space, Class III has an intradental edentulous area, and Class IV has an anterior edentulous area that crosses the midline.

The Kennedy classification is difficult to use in many situations without certain qualifying rules. The eight Applegate rules are used to help clarify the system. They may be summarized in three general principles.

1. The first principle is that the classification should include only natural teeth involved in the final prosthesis and follow rather than precede any extractions of teeth that might alter the original classification. This concept, for example, considers whether second or third molars are to be replaced in the final restoration.
2. The second principles is that the most posterior edentulous area always determines the classification.
3. The third principle is that edentulous areas, other than those determining the classification, are referred to as modifications and are designated only by their number. The extent of the modification is not considered.

Classification of Partially Edentulous Arches

The implant dentistry bone volume classification developed by Misch and Judy[13] in 1985 may be used to build on the four classes of partial edentulism described in the Kennedy-Applegate system. This facilitates communication of teeth positions and the primary edentulous sites among the large segment of practitioners already familiar with this classification, and it enables the use of common treatment methods and principles established for each class. The implant dentistry classification for partially edentulous patients by Misch and Judy[13] also includes the same four available bone volume divisions previously presented for edentulous areas. Other intradental edentulous regions that are not responsible for the Kennedy-Applegate class determination are not specified within the available bone section, should implants not be considered in the modification region. However, if the modification segment is also included in the treatment plan, then it is listed, followed by the available bone division it characterizes.

Treatment Planning: Class I

In Class I patients, distal edentulous segments are bilateral, and natural anterior teeth are present (Fig. 20.1). The majority of these arches are missing only molars, and almost all have retained at least the anterior incisors and canines. Therefore once restored to proper occlusal vertical dimension, the natural anterior teeth contribute to the distribution of forces throughout the mouth in centric relation occlusion. More importantly, when opposing natural teeth or in fixed implant prosthesis, they also permit excursions

---

[†]Deceased.

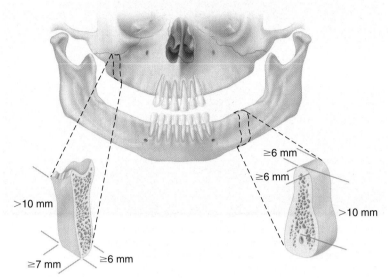

• **Fig. 20.1** A Class I, Division A dental arch has bilateral posterior missing teeth and abundant bone volume in the edentulous sites. (*From Misch CE. Treatment plans for partially and completely edentulous arches in implant dentistry. In: Misch CE, ed.* Dental Implants Prosthetics. *2nd ed. St. Louis, MO: Mosby; 2015.*)

during mandibular movement to disclude the posterior implant-supported prostheses and protect them from lateral forces. However, many of these mandibular Class I patients oppose a maxillary denture, in which case bilateral balance is more appropriate.

The Class I patient is more likely to wear an RPD than Class II or III patients because mastication and/or support of an opposing removable prosthesis is more difficult when not wearing a mandibular prosthesis. The posterior soft tissue–supported Class I partial dentures are designed to primary load either the edentulous regions or the natural anterior teeth. The clasp design, which places less force on the tooth (e.g., bar clasp), will ultimately place more force on the bone. The RPDs, which place more force on the abutment teeth (e.g., precision partial dentures), will place less force on the bone. In either case the removable prosthesis often accelerates the posterior bone loss. In addition, a partial denture that is not well designed or maintained distributes additional loads to abutment teeth and may even contribute to poor periodontal health. The combinations of these conditions lead to bone loss in the edentulous regions and poorer adjacent natural abutments.[14] As a result, it has been observed by authors that long-term Class I patients who have been wearing an RPD often exhibit Division C ridges and mobile abutment teeth.

Class I patients often have mobile anterior teeth, because long-term lack of bilateral posterior support caused by the wearing of a poorly fitting RPD, or none at all, has resulted in an overload to the remaining dentition. Therefore these patients often require a posterior implant prosthesis to be independent from the mobile natural teeth. In addition, the occlusal scheme must accommodate the specific conditions of mobile anterior teeth. This requires increased implant support in the posterior segments compared with most Class II or III patients, as well as greater attention and frequency for occlusal adjustments.

The treatment plan must consider the factors of force previously identified and relate them to the existing bilateral edentulous condition. Osteoplasty cannot be as aggressive in the Class I patient to increase bone width, compared with the Class IV or fully edentulous patient with implants primarily in the anterior regions, because of the opposing anatomic landmarks (maxillary

sinus or mandibular canal). Augmentation procedures are often required to improve posterior bone volume, increase the implant surface area, and permit the fabrication of an independent implant restoration.

Financial concerns may require the staging of treatment over years. The posterior region with the greatest volume of bone usually is restored first, if no bone grafting is required. In this manner, implants of greater size and surface area can resist the unilateral posterior forces while the patient awaits future treatment. If many years pass before implants are to be inserted in the lesser available bone, then continued resorption may require augmentation before reconstruction. If both posterior segments require bone grafting, the patient is encouraged to have both posterior segments augmented at the same time. In this way the autologous portion of the graft may be harvested and distributed to both posterior regions, decreasing the number of surgical episodes for the patient.

Division A Treatment Plans

When patients are placed in a Class I, Division A category, an independent implant-supported fixed prosthesis is usually indicated. Two or more endosteal root form implants are required to replace molars with independent prostheses (Fig. 20.2). The greater the number of teeth missing, the larger the size and/or number of implants required. Posterior available bone is limited in height by the mandibular canal in the mandible or the maxillary sinus in the maxilla. The first premolar-positioned implants must avoid encroachment on the apex of the canine root and yet avoid the anterior loop of the mandibular canal or maxillary sinus (Fig. 20.3).

Division B Treatment Plans

Class I, Division B patients have narrow bone in posterior edentulous spaces and anterior natural teeth. A fixed prosthesis is also indicated in these categories. Available bone height is restricted by the mandibular canal or maxillary sinus. Therefore osteoplasty to increase bone width has limited applications. Endosteal small-diameter root form implants may be placed in the mandibular

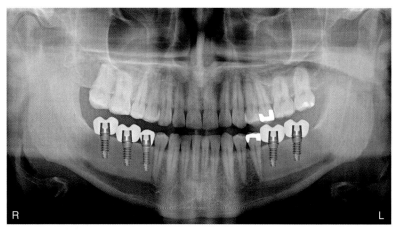

• **Fig. 20.2** A Mandible with a Class I, Division A Classification. The key implant positions are determined, and the implant sizes are ideal (4 mm × 10 mm in premolars and 5 mm × 10 mm in the molars). (*From Misch CE. Treatment plans for partially and completely edentulous arches in implant dentistry. In: Misch CE, ed.* Dental Implants Prosthetics. *2nd ed. St. Louis, MO: Mosby; 2015.*)

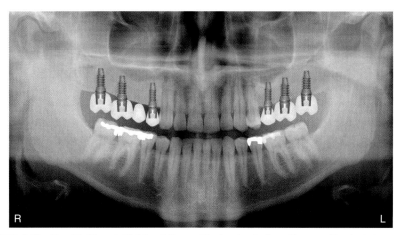

• **Fig. 20.3** A Maxilla with Class I, Division A Bone. The key implant positions and implant sizes are positioned without limitation. (*From Misch CE. Treatment plans for partially and completely edentulous arches in implant dentistry. In: Misch CE, ed.* Dental Implants Prosthetics. *2nd ed. St. Louis, MO: Mosby; 2015.*)

posterior Division B edentulous ridge. If narrow-diameter root forms are used, then a greater number than for the Division A ridge is indicated, and the use of one implant for every missing tooth root with no cantilever is recommended.

The patient who is missing molars and both premolars requires additional implant support. Four Division B root forms may be the foundation of an independent fixed partial denture (FPD) in the mandible, depending on the other stress factors. If stress factors are too great (as a result of parafunction) or bone density is poor (as in the maxilla), then the Division B bone should be augmented to Division A before larger-diameter implant insertion. The anterior teeth in Class I patients should provide disclusion of the posterior implants during all excursions when opposing natural teeth or a fixed prosthesis. Molar endosteal implants should not be rigidly cross-splinted to each other in the Class I patient. Flexure of the mandible during opening may cause a rigid splint to exert lateral forces on the posterior implants. Therefore independent restorations are indicated (Fig. 20.4).

Division C Treatment Plans

When inadequate bone exists in height, width, length, or angulation, or if crown/implant ratios are equal to or greater than 1, the practitioner must consider several options. The first treatment option is not to use implant support but rather to orient the patient toward a conventional removable partial prosthesis. However, although this condition is easiest to treat with a traditional soft tissue–borne restoration, bone loss will continue and can eventually compromise any restorative modality.

The second option is to use bone augmentation procedures. If the intent of the bone graft is to change a Division C to a Division A or B for endosteal implants, then at least some autogenous bone is indicated. Augmentation is used most often in the Class I maxilla, where sinus grafts with a combination of allografts and autogenous bone are a predictable modality. Implants may be placed after the graft has created a Division A ridge, and the treatment plan follows the options previously addressed.

In the mandible the third option is nerve repositioning and endosteal implants in Class I patients who are poor candidates for bone augmentation. Risks of long-term paresthesia exist that may include hyperesthesia and pain. Reports in the literature concern dysesthesia and fracture of the severely atrophic mandible.[15] In addition, the gain of height in the C–h mandible may permit the placement of only implants 10 mm in height, still insufficient to compensate for the increased crown height and resultant unfavorable crown/implant ratio. It is recommended that nerve repositioning be attempted only by clinicians with prior extensive training and experience with the procedures.

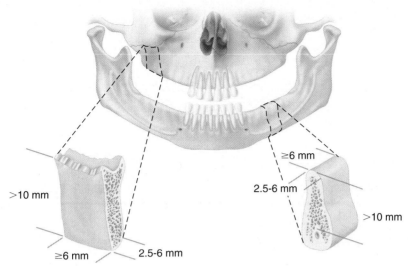

• **Fig. 20.4** A Class I, Division B dental arch has adequate height of bone but is barely sufficient in width. (*From Misch CE. Treatment plans for partially and completely edentulous arches in implant dentistry. In: Misch CE, ed.* Dental Implants Prosthetics. *2nd ed. St. Louis, MO: Mosby; 2015.*)

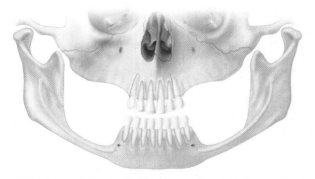

• **Fig. 20.5** A Class I, Division D patient is usually seen in the maxilla when the maxillary sinus has expanded and less than 5 mm of bone is present in height under sinus. (*From Misch CE. Treatment plans for partially and completely edentulous arches in implant dentistry. In: Misch CE, ed.* Dental Implants Prosthetics. *2nd ed. St. Louis, MO: Mosby; 2015.*)

In the fourth option the mandibular anterior teeth are extracted and root form implants are placed between the mental foramens. This is especially a predictable treatment because the patient will benefit from increased masticatory efficiency and force along with improved esthetics.

Division D Treatment Plans

Class I, Division D usually occurs most often in the long-term edentulous maxilla. A sinus graft is usually performed before implant placement. Class I, Division D ridges are rarely found in the mandibular partially edentulous patient. When observed, the most common causes are from trauma or surgical excision of neoplasms. These patients often need autogenous bone onlay grafts to improve implant success and prevent pathologic fracture before prosthodontic reconstruction. After the bone graft is mature and the available bone improved, the patient is evaluated and treated in a manner similar to other patients with favorable bone volume (Fig. 20.5).

Treatment Planning: Class II

Kennedy-Applegate Class II partially edentulous patients are missing teeth in one posterior segment. These patients are often able to function without a removable restoration and are less likely to tolerate or overcome the minor complications of wearing the prosthesis. As a result, they are not as likely to wear a removable restoration. The available bone is therefore often adequate for endosteal implants, even when long-term edentulism has been present. However, the local bone density may be decreased. Endosteal implants with minimum osteoplasty are a common modality in these patients, who are more often Class II, Division A or B types.

Because the patient is less likely to wear the RPD, the opposing natural teeth have often extruded into the posterior edentulous region. The occlusal plane and tipped or extruded teeth should be closely evaluated and restored as indicated to provide a favorable environment in terms of occlusion and forces distribution. It is not unusual to require extraction of the second molar, endodontics, crown lengthening and a crown of the first molar, and enameloplasty for the second premolar (Fig. 20.6).

Division A Treatment Plans

When patients are placed in a Class II, Division A category, an independent implant-supported fixed prosthesis is usually indicated. Two or more endosteal root form implants are required to replace molars with independent prostheses. The greater the number of teeth missing, the larger the size and/or number of implants required. Posterior available bone is limited in height by the mandibular canal in the mandible or the maxillary sinus in the maxilla. The first premolar-positioned implants must not encroach on the apex of the canine root while still avoiding the anterior loop of the mandibular canal or maxillary sinus (Fig. 20.7).

Division B Treatment Plans

Class II, Division B patients have narrow bone in posterior edentulous spaces and anterior natural teeth. A fixed prosthesis is also indicated in these categories. Available bone height is restricted

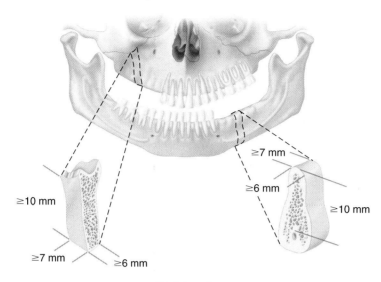

Division A

• **Fig. 20.6** A Class II patient has posterior missing teeth in one quadrant. When the available bone is abundant, it is Division A. (*From Misch CE. Treatment plans for partially and completely edentulous arches in implant dentistry. In: Misch CE, ed.* Dental Implants Prosthetics. *2nd ed. St. Louis, MO: Mosby; 2015.*)

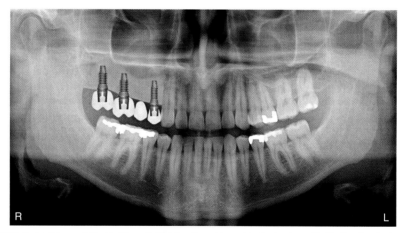

• **Fig. 20.7** A maxillary arch that is Class II, Division A may have implants placed in the key implant positions and are of ideal sizes. (*From Misch CE. Treatment plans for partially and completely edentulous arches in implant dentistry. In: Misch CE, ed.* Dental Implants Prosthetics. *2nd ed. St. Louis, MO: Mosby; 2015.*)

by the mandibular canal or maxillary sinus. Therefore osteoplasty to increase bone width has limited applications. Endosteal small-diameter root form implants may be placed in the mandibular posterior Division B edentulous ridge. If narrow-diameter root forms are used, then a greater number than for the Division A ridge is indicated, and the use of one implant for every missing tooth root with no cantilever is recommended.

The patient who is missing molars and both premolars requires additional implant support. Four Division B root forms may be the foundation of an independent FPD in the mandible, depending on the other stress factors. If stress factors are too great (as a result of parafunction) or bone density is poor (as in the maxilla), then the Division B bone should be augmented to Division A before larger-diameter implant insertion. The anterior teeth in Class II patients should provide disclusion of the posterior implants during all excursions (Fig. 20.8).

Division C Treatment Plans

When inadequate bone exists in height, width, length, or angulation, or if crown/implant ratios are equal to or greater than 1, then the practitioner must consider several options. In the mandible the first treatment option is not to use implant support but to consider a posterior cantilevered FPD replacing one premolar-sized crown, using two or three anterior teeth as abutment support. This is the easiest option and is strongly recommended when only molars are missing.

The second option is to use bone augmentation procedures. If the intent of the bone graft is to change a Division C to a Division A or B for endosteal implants in the mandible, then autogenous bone is indicated. Augmentation is used most often in the Class II maxilla as the first choice, where sinus grafts with a combination of allografts and autogenous bone are a predictable modality. Implants may be placed after the graft has created a Division

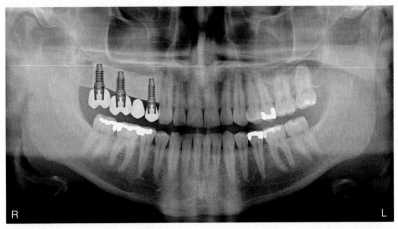

• **Fig. 20.8** A maxillary Class II, Division B patient often has a membrane bone augmentation to increase width (pink) followed by implants in the key implant positions and of ideal sizes.

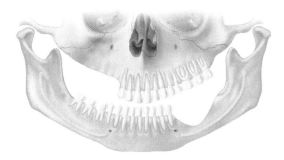

Division C

• **Fig. 20.9** A Class I, Division C–h arch has 7 to 9 mm of bone in height in the edentulous site. (*From Misch CE. Treatment plans for partially and completely edentulous arches in implant dentistry. In: Misch CE, ed. Dental Implants Prosthetics. 2nd ed. St. Louis, MO: Mosby; 2015.*)

A ridge, and the treatment plan follows the options previously addressed.

The third option for the Division C mandibular patient is to place a Class II unilateral subperiosteal implant or a disc implant above the canal.

The fourth treatment option in the mandible is nerve repositioning and endosteal implants in Class II patients who are poor candidates for bone augmentation. Risks of long-term paresthesia exist that may include hyperesthesia and pain. In addition, the gain of height in the C–h mandible may permit the placement of only implants 10 mm high, which is still insufficient to compensate for the increased crown height and resultant unfavorable crown/implant ratio (Fig. 20.9).

Division D Treatment Plans

Class II, Division D usually occurs most often in the long-term edentulous maxilla. A sinus graft is usually performed before implant placement. Class II, Division D ridges are rarely found in the mandibular partially edentulous patient. When observed, the most common causes are from trauma or surgical excision of neoplasms. These patients often need autogenous bone onlay grafts to improve implant success and prevent pathologic fracture before prosthodontic reconstruction. After the graft is mature and the available bone improved, the patient is evaluated and treated in a manner similar to other patients with favorable bone volume (Fig. 20.10).

Treatment Planning: Class III

Typically the two most common Class III patients consulting for implants are either missing a single tooth or have a long posterior edentulous span. A multitooth posterior edentulous region most often can be restored as an independent prosthesis. A review of the literature demonstrates that joining implants in teeth in the same prosthesis under those conditions is possible.

A single-tooth implant is the treatment of choice when the bone and soft tissues are within normal range before or during implant treatment. Fixed prostheses increase the risk for decay, pulpal involvement, and periodontal disease on the natural abutment teeth.[16] Both the traditional prosthesis and the abutment teeth have a poorer survival rate than implant prostheses. As a result, single-tooth implants are often indicated (Fig. 20.11).

Division A Treatment Plans

Class III, Division A patients are usually excellent candidates for endosteal root form implant placement in the edentulous space. This will allow for the restoration of natural teeth to be independent and allow the fabrication of shorter span restorations. It is easier to obtain maximum available height of bone for implant placement anterior to the mandibular foramen or maxillary sinus. As a general rule the final prosthesis should be completely implant supported, and two implants should support each section of three missing tooth roots (not three missing crowns). Mobile natural teeth adjacent to the edentulous span cause greater loads on the implants; therefore one implant for each missing root may be indicated. If the adjacent teeth are mobile, then the implant must support both the missing teeth and mobile teeth during occlusion.

Division B Treatment Plans

In Class III, Division B patients, narrow-diameter endosteal implants may be placed in the mandibular long-span edentulous space. This treatment plan is primarily used for a fixed prosthesis when the span is too long or occlusal forces are too great for the natural abutments to act as sole support for the final prosthesis. The final implant prosthesis should be independent of these teeth (Figs. 20.12 and 20.13).

Division C or Division D Treatment Plans

When Division C is found in Class III patients the most common treatment plan in the maxilla is bone augmentation before implant insertion and an independent implant prosthesis. Sinus grafting in the posterior Division C ridge is predictable.

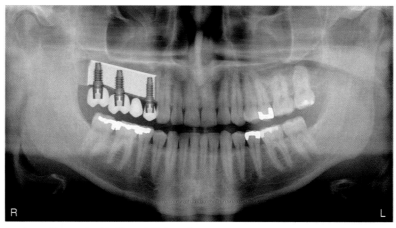

• **Fig. 20.10** A maxillary arch with Class II, Division C–h most often has a sinus bone graft (white) and then implants in the key implant positions and of ideal implant sizes. (*From Misch CE. Treatment plans for partially and completely edentulous arches in implant dentistry. In: Misch CE, ed.* Dental Implants Prosthetics. *2nd ed. St. Louis, MO: Mosby; 2015.*)

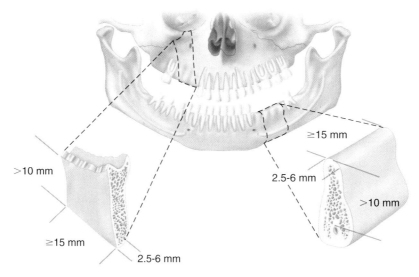

Division B

• **Fig. 20.11** A Class III patient has an intratooth edentulous space. When it is adequate in height but barely sufficient in width, it is Division B bone. (*From Misch CE. Treatment plans for partially and completely edentulous arches in implant dentistry. In: Misch CE, ed.* Dental Implants Prosthetics. *2nd ed. St. Louis, MO: Mosby; 2015.*)

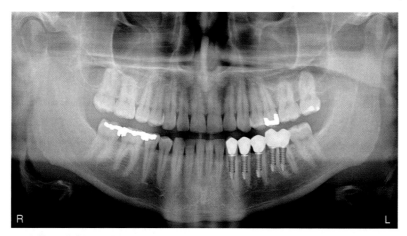

• **Fig. 20.12** A Class III, Division B mandible may use smaller-diameter implants. When this option is used, one implant for each tooth root missing is often indicated. (*From Misch CE. Treatment plans for partially and completely edentulous arches in implant dentistry. In: Misch CE, ed.* Dental Implants Prosthetics. *2nd ed. St. Louis, MO: Mosby; 2015.*)

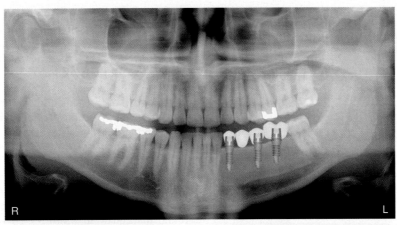

• **Fig. 20.13** A Class III, Division B mandible may have a membrane bone graft to gain abutment width (gray) followed by ideal implant sizes in the key implant positions. (*From Misch CE. Treatment plans for partially and completely edentulous arches in implant dentistry. In: Misch CE, ed. Dental Implants Prosthetics. 2nd ed. St. Louis, MO: Mosby; 2015.*)

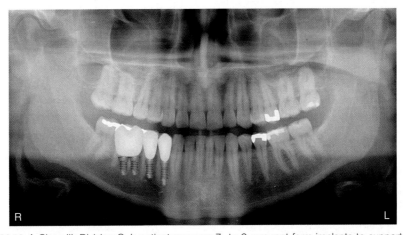

• **Fig. 20.14** A Class III, Division C–h patient may use 7- to 9-mm root form implants to support a fixed prosthesis. Incisal guidance on the anterior teeth during all mandibular excursions is indicated to eliminate greater forces on the extended crown heights. (*From Misch CE. Treatment plans for partially and completely edentulous arches in implant dentistry. In: Misch CE, ed. Dental Implants Prosthetics. 2nd ed. St. Louis, MO: Mosby; 2015.*)

In the mandible, a traditional fixed prosthesis for Division C bone volume for Class III patients should often be considered, because bone grafting for height is difficult, requires an additional skill set, and is less predictable than in the maxilla (Figs. 20.14 and 20.15).

Treatment Planning: Class IV

In the Class IV patient the anterior edentulous space crosses the midline. In the past, traditional FPDs were often the treatment of choice when the canines were present. Today an independent implant prosthesis is often warranted. However, a lack of anterior bone volume in the maxilla is common, and bone grafts before implant placement are typically necessary to prevent the implants from being placed palatally in relation to the natural roots. A cantilever is often created off the implant bodies to place the maxillary incisor edge in proper position for esthetics and speech. The moment force generated is greater than when found in the mandibular counterpart. This, in addition to other factors, makes the premaxilla one of the more difficult regions of the mouth to treat successfully. As a general rule, one implant for each tooth is considered in the premaxilla unless facial bone

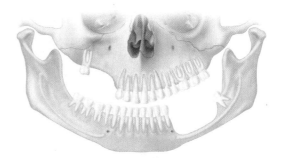

Division D

• **Fig. 20.15** A Class III, Division D patient is more often observed in the maxillary arch. (*From Misch CE. Treatment plans for partially and completely edentulous arches in implant dentistry. In: Misch CE, ed. Dental Implants Prosthetics. 2nd ed. St. Louis, MO: Mosby; 2015.*)

loss has been significant that decreases the available length. In the mandible, usually one implant can replace two teeth, with the implants placed in the embrasure areas with a screw-retained prosthesis (Fig. 20.16).

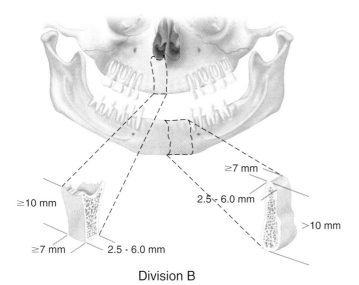

≥7 mm

2.5 6.0 mm

>10 mm

≥10 mm

≥7 mm   2.5 - 6.0 mm

Division B

• **Fig. 20.16** A Class IV patient has missing teeth that cross the midline. When the bone is adequate in height but barely sufficient in width, it is Division B. (*From Misch CE. Treatment plans for partially and completely edentulous arches in implant dentistry. In: Misch CE, ed.* Dental Implants Prosthetics. *2nd ed. St. Louis, MO: Mosby; 2015.*)

Division A Treatment Plans

Division A patients are good candidates for endosteal root form implant placement in the edentulous space. Ideally the prosthesis should be restored independently of the natural teeth. As a general rule the final prosthesis should be completely implant supported, and two implants should support each section of three missing tooth roots (not three missing crowns), as long as there are favorable force factors. Mobile natural teeth adjacent to the edentulous span cause greater loads on the implants. Therefore one implant for each missing root may be indicated (Figs. 20.17 and 20.18).

Division B Treatment Plans

The Class IV, Division B patient is most often treated with augmentation before implant placement. If the ridge is Division B and inadequate in width for Division A root form implants, then the narrow-diameter root forms compromise esthetics and oral hygiene procedures. Bone augmentation is more often used in anterior edentulous regions with narrow bone, and Division A implants are indicated to improve the final crown contour, esthetic appearance, and daily maintenance. Implant and tooth replacement should remain independent. The canine is an important natural abutment. When the canine and two adjacent teeth are missing, a fixed prosthesis is contraindicated (according to

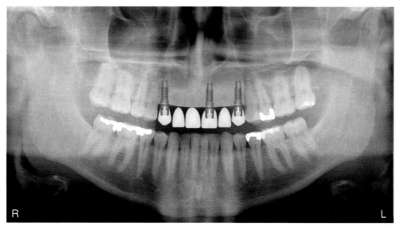

• **Fig. 20.17** A Class IV, Division A patient has implants positioned in the key implant positions of ideal width and length. (*From Misch CE. Treatment plans for partially and completely edentulous arches in implant dentistry. In: Misch CE, ed.* Dental Implants Prosthetics. *2nd ed. St. Louis, MO: Mosby; 2015.*)

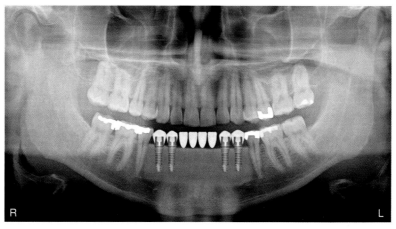

• **Fig. 20.18** A Class IV, Division A mandible has implants positioned in the key implant positions. When force factors are low to moderate and bone density is good, the implant between the canine positions may be eliminated when posterior implants are connected to the canine implants. (*From Misch CE. Treatment plans for partially and completely edentulous arches in implant dentistry. In: Misch CE, ed.* Dental Implants Prosthetics. *2nd ed. St. Louis, MO: Mosby; 2015.*)

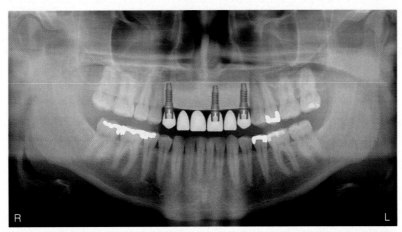

• **Fig. 20.19** A maxillary Class IV, Division B patient usually has bone augmentation (pink) to increase the bone volume width. After augmentation the key implant positions and ideal implant sizes may be used to support a fixed prosthesis. (*From Misch CE. Treatment plans for partially and completely edentulous arches in implant dentistry. In: Misch CE, ed.* Dental Implants Prosthetics. *2nd ed. St. Louis, MO: Mosby; 2015.*)

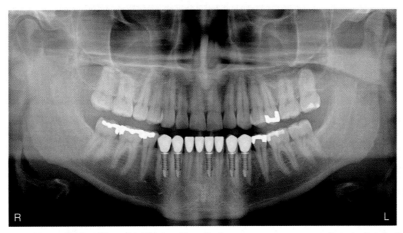

• **Fig. 20.20** A mandibular Class IV, Division B patient may use a narrower-diameter implant (3.0 to 3.5 mm) of ideal implant length (≥12 mm). The key implant positions should be selected, including an implant between the canine positions. (*From Misch CE. Treatment plans for partially and completely edentulous arches in implant dentistry. In: Misch CE, ed.* Dental Implants Prosthetics. *2nd ed. St. Louis, MO: Mosby; 2015.*)

basic prosthodontic principles). In other words an implant should replace a canine whenever multiple teeth are missing, which includes the canine (Figs. 20.19 and 20.20).

Division C and D Treatment Plans

The first option for a Class IV patient is to use bone augmentation procedures. If the intent of the bone graft is to change a Division C or D to a Division A or B for endosteal implants, then autogenous bone is indicated. Implants may be placed after the graft has created a Division A ridge, and the treatment plan follows the options previously addressed (Figs. 20.21 to 20.23).

Classification of Completely Edentulous Arches

Completely edentulous classifications in the literature include the classification of Kent and the Louisiana Dental School.[17] The classification was originally for ridge augmentation with

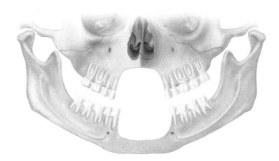

Division C

• **Fig. 20.21** A Class IV, Division C–h dental arch has compromised bone in height. If the bone is compromised in width, it is C–w. (*From Misch CE. Treatment plans for partially and completely edentulous arches in implant dentistry. In: Misch CE, ed.* Dental Implants Prosthetics. *2nd ed. St. Louis, MO: Mosby; 2015.*)

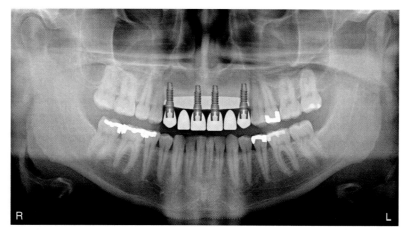

• **Fig. 20.22** A maxillary Class IV, Division C–w patient should have block bone graft procedures to increase the width of bone followed by implants in the key implant positions. An additional implant may be necessary if bone density is poor or force factors are greater than normal. (*From Misch CE. Treatment plans for partially and completely edentulous arches in implant dentistry. In: Misch CE, ed.* Dental Implants Prosthetics. *2nd ed. St. Louis, MO: Mosby; 2015.*)

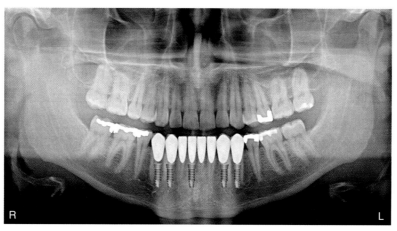

• **Fig. 20.23** A mandibular Class IV, Division C–h mandible often may have implants positioned in key implant positions. Bone density is usually good, and in centric occlusion the implants may be loaded in their long axis. (*From Misch CE. Treatment plans for partially and completely edentulous arches in implant dentistry. In: Misch CE, ed.* Dental Implants Prosthetics. *2nd ed. St. Louis, MO: Mosby; 2015.*)

HYDROXYAPatite and a conventional denture. This classification treats all regions of an edentulous arch in similar fashion and does not address regional variation. Likewise the classification of Lekholm and Zarb[18] addressed only the anterior maxilla and mandible, always resulted in root form implants without regard for bone grafting, and always used a fixed prosthesis, regardless of biomechanical considerations. The divisions of bone previously presented by Misch and Judy[13] are the basis of the classification of the completely edentulous patient presented in this chapter. Its purpose is to allow communication of not only the volume of bone but also its location. It organizes the most common implant options of prosthodontic support for the completely edentulous patient.

The edentulous jaw is divided into three regions (one anterior and two posterior) and described according to the Misch-Judy classification.[19] In the mandible the right and left posterior sections extend from the mental foramen to the retromolar pad, and the anterior area is located between the mental foramina. The anterior section usually extends from first premolar (mesial) to first premolar (mesial) because of the foramen's most common

location (i.e., between the two premolar teeth). The right and left posterior regions of the edentulous maxilla also start from the first premolar (mesial) sites, where the maxillary sinus most often determines the height of available bone. The anterior section of the maxilla consists of the region between the first premolars and is usually anterior to the maxillary sinus (Fig. 20.24). The division of bone in each section of the edentulous arch then determines the classification of the edentulous jaw. The three areas of bone are evaluated independently from each other. Therefore one, two, or three different divisions of bone may exist. The term type is used in the completely edentulous classification, rather than class, as in the partially edentulous classification.

Type 1

In the Type 1 edentulous arch the division of bone is similar in all three anatomic segments. Therefore four different categories of Type 1 edentulous arches are present.

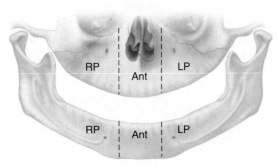

• **Fig. 20.24** A completely edentulous jaw is divided into three segments. The anterior component (Ant) is between the mental foramina or in front of the maxillary sinus. Right (RP) and left (LP) posterior segments correspond to the patient's right and left sides. (*From Misch CE. Treatment plans for partially and completely edentulous arches in implant dentistry. In: Misch CE, ed. Dental Implants Prosthetics. 2nd ed. St. Louis, MO: Mosby; 2015.*)

Division A

In the Type 1, Division A ridge, with abundant bone in all three sections, as many root forms as needed may be placed to support the final prosthesis. As a general rule the range of 5 to 9 implants may be used in the mandible and 6 to 10 implants in the maxilla for a fixed prosthesis.

Division B

The Type 1, Division B edentulous ridge presents adequate bone in all three sections in which to place narrow-diameter root form implants. It is common practice to modify the anterior section of bone in the mandible by osteoplasty to a Division A and to place ideal size root form implants in this region. It is less common to have sufficient height in either the posterior maxilla or mandible to permit osteoplasty to improve the division. Therefore several narrower implants are often indicated in the mandible if posterior implants are inserted without grafting. One implant is used for every tooth root to compensate for the decrease in surface area of implant support. Augmentation by bone spreading may be indicated in the maxilla, if the patient desires a fixed prosthesis, especially when opposing natural teeth. If stress factors are great, then lateral augmentation may also be necessary in the posterior regions to increase implant diameter.

Division C

Type 1, Division C–w edentulous arches present adequate height of available bone but have inadequate width. If the patient desires an implant-supported removable prosthesis, then an osteoplasty may be used to convert the ridge to C–h. The treatment plan then follows a Type 1, Division C–h formula. When a fixed restoration is desired, an autogenous onlay graft in the C–w arch is usually warranted to restore the ridge to Division A before implant insertion.

Type 1, Division C–h edentulous arches often do not present all the essential requirements for predictable long-term implant support for fixed prostheses. An implant-supported RP-4 or RP-5 removable prosthesis is often indicated to reduce occlusal loads. The prosthesis should be completely implant supported (RP-4) to halt the continued bone loss in the posterior regions of the mouth. When only Division C anterior root form implants are inserted, posterior soft-tissue support (RP-5) may be required.

The edentulous maxilla is often treated with a conventional removable prosthesis until the mandible is completely restored. If

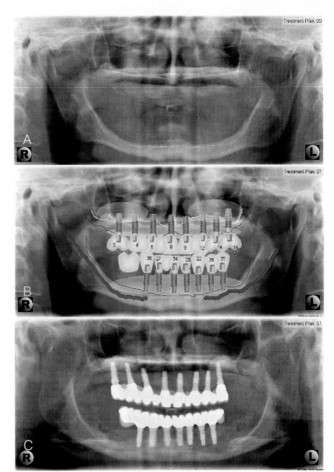

• **Fig. 20.25** (A) A Type I, Division C–h mandible and maxilla should be restored to Division A with autogenous grafts when a fixed prosthesis is desired. (B) Computer-assisted treatment plans with five to nine implants placed in the grafted bone volumes can be developed before treatment (XCPT, Naples, FL). (C) Panoramic radiograph of a patient with division C–h maxilla and mandible restored to division A arches with iliac crest grafts, endosteal implants, and fixed maxillary and mandibular prostheses. (*From Misch CE. Treatment plans for partially and completely edentulous arches in implant dentistry. In: Misch CE, ed. Dental Implants Prosthetics. 2nd ed. St. Louis, MO: Mosby; 2015.*)

this denture needs additional retention or stability, then HA can be used to augment the premaxilla. This squares the ridge shape and provides resistance to occlusal excursions during function. Intramucosal inserts may also be used to increase the retention of the removable complete denture. However, the patient and doctor should realize that bone loss will continue and will make future implant placement even more difficult.

The C–h maxilla should often consider subnasal augmentation combined with root form implants in the canine eminence region and sinus graft with root form implants with an RP-4 prosthesis. Additional surgical training is required for these last two alternatives, and they have a greater incidence of complication.

Fixed prostheses may need autogenous iliac crest grafts to change the anterior division of bone and improve long-term success and esthetics. Sinus grafts are also indicated in these situations (Fig. 20.25).

The edentulous arches classified as Type 1, Division D are the most challenging to traditional and implant dentistry. If an implant fails in a Type 1, Division D patient, then pathologic fractures or almost unrestorable conditions may result; yet these are

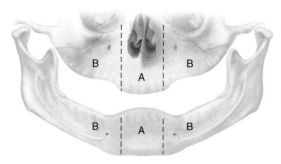

• **Fig. 20.26** A Type 2, Division A, B arch has an anterior section classified as Division A (*A*) and posterior sections classified as Division B (*B*). The anterior region dominates the overall treatment plan in all edentulous arches and usually has a greater volume of bone than the posterior. (*From Misch CE. Treatment plans for partially and completely edentulous arches in implant dentistry. In: Misch CE, ed.* Dental Implants Prosthetics. *2nd ed. St. Louis, MO: Mosby; 2015.*)

the patients who need the most help for support of their prostheses. The benefits versus risks must be weighed carefully for each patient. Endosteal implants may be placed in the anterior mandible. However, the unfavorable crown height of greater than 20 mm and mandibular fracture during implant placement or after implant failure may result in significant complications.[20]

Often the best solution is to change the division with autogenous grafts, then reevaluate the improved conditions and appropriately alter the treatment plan. The Type 1, Division D ridges most often use autogenous iliac crest grafts. After 6 months a total of five to nine implants may be placed in the anterior and posterior regions.

Type 2

In the Type 2 completely edentulous arch the posterior sections of bone are similar but differ from the anterior segment. The most common arches in this category present less bone in the posterior regions, under the maxillary sinus, or over the mandibular canal than in the anterior segment. These edentulous ridges are described in the completely edentulous classification with two division letters following Type 2, with the anterior segment being listed first because it often determines the overall treatment plan. Therefore a mandible with Division A between the foramina and Division C distal to the mandibular foramen is a Type 2, Division A, C arch. This condition is common in the mandible, because the posterior regions resorb four times faster than the anterior regions. Because onlay grafts in the posterior mandible are more difficult to perform predictably, the anterior region is often the only segment used for implant support.

In the Type 2, Division A, B arch the posterior segments may be treated with narrow-diameter implants, whereas the anterior section is adequate for larger-diameter root form implants to support the prosthesis (Fig. 20.26). When possible, the posterior Division B section is changed into Division A. Autogenous grafts are more debilitating and require extended healing periods but may be indicated for the benefit of increased posterior bone width when stress factors and patient desires are high. Smaller segments can be augmented with intraorally harvested block grafts. In the posterior maxilla, bone spreading and Division A root forms should be considered. The softer the bone is, the easier it is to spread.

Two primary modules exist to restore the Type 2, Division A, C edentulous ridge. In the mandible the most common option is the

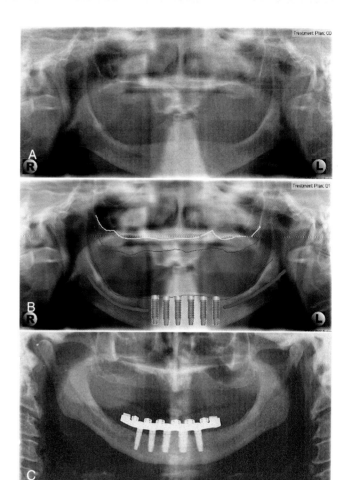

• **Fig. 20.27** (A) A treatment option for Type 2, Division A, C. (B) A computer-generated treatment plan with favorable biomechanics places implants in the anterior section of the mandible and restores the arch with cantilevered posterior sections (XCPT, Naples, FL). (C) In a situation with higher masticatory dynamics or nocturnal parafunction, this type of arch may mandate the fabrication of a RP-4 prosthesis rather than a fixed restoration. (*From Misch CE. Treatment plans for partially and completely edentulous arches in implant dentistry. In: Misch CE, ed.* Dental Implants Prosthetics. *2nd ed. St. Louis, MO: Mosby; 2015.*)

use of the anterior section only for implant-supported root form implants (Fig. 20.27). The maxillary arch may be treated with a combination of sinus graft and endosteal implants if additional posterior support is required for the prosthesis. Because the bone density of the mandible is usually superior to that of the maxilla, and the moment forces remain directed within the arch form, rarely does the mandible require additional posterior support with grafts or circumferential subperiosteal implants. However, for a patient with a square arch form or high masticatory dynamics such as opposing natural teeth, posterior support may be required for an RP-4 or fixed prosthesis.

An edentulous ridge with severe posterior bone loss and abundant bone in the anterior region is uncommon and occurs more frequently in the maxilla. The Type 2, Division A, D patient is treated in a similar manner to the patient with a Type 2, Division A, C arch. Sinus grafts and endosteal implants in the maxilla or only anterior implants with or without an autogenous graft in the mandible are most often the treatment of choice.

The Type 2, Division B, C edentulous arch can be treated with two main treatment options. The anterior section may be changed

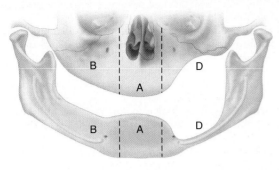

• **Fig. 20.28** This Type 3, Division A, B, D arch has abundant anterior bone (A), moderate atrophy of bone in the posterior right (B), and severe atrophy in the left posterior segment (D). Sinus grafting is a common treatment if posterior implants are required in the maxilla. However, bone augmentation in the posterior mandible for Division D is more unusual, and additional anterior implants in the Division A with a cantilever are more typical. Another option is to use narrower implants in the right posterior, splinted to the anterior implants. *(From Misch CE. Treatment plans for partially and completely edentulous arches in implant dentistry. In: Misch CE, ed. Dental Implants Prosthetics. 2nd ed. St. Louis, MO: Mosby; 2015.)*

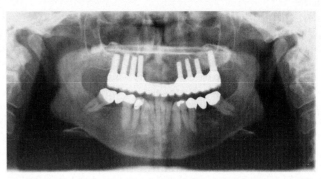

• **Fig. 20.29** The square dentate maxilla with Type 3, Division C, D, E may require bilateral sinus grafts and implants in the canine with nasal elevation to support a fixed prosthesis. *(From Misch CE. Treatment plans for partially and completely edentulous arches in implant dentistry. In: Misch CE, ed. Dental Implants Prosthetics. 2nd ed. St. Louis, MO: Mosby; 2015.)*

to Division A by osteoplasty if anatomic conditions permit. These patients are then treated exactly as the previously described Type 2, Division A, C. When the ridge does not present sufficient height after osteoplasty to upgrade the division, the posterior segments may be improved by sinus grafts and the whole arch treated in the same manner as Type 1, Division B or Type 2, Division B, A. Onlay grafts are less predictable than sinus grafts; therefore the anterior mandible may be changed to a Division C by osteoplasty, and a mandibular complete subperiosteal implant and RP-4 restoration or anterior root forms and RP-5 prosthesis may be selected for Type 1, Division C mandibular patients.

Patients who have advanced atrophy in the posterior segments and adequate ridge width and height in the anterior may be described as Type 2, Division B, D. This condition almost never occurs in the mandible, but it can be found on occasion in the maxilla. These patients are treated in a manner similar to patients with Type 2, Division B, C, as previously described. The primary difference is that the posterior graft is more extensive and requires additional months for healing before implant insertion and prosthodontic reconstruction. In the mandible, Type 2, Division C, D patients may be treated similar to a Type 1, Division D mandible with autogenous bone grafts before implant placement.

Type 3

In Type 3 edentulous arches the posterior sections of the maxilla or mandible differ from each other. This condition is less common than the other two types and is found more frequently in the maxilla than the mandible. The anterior bone volume is listed first, then the right posterior, followed by the left posterior segment. Therefore the edentulous maxilla with no bone available for implants in the left posterior section, abundant bone in the anterior section, and adequate bone in the right posterior segment is a Type 3, Division A, B, D edentulous arch (Fig. 20.28).

The patient with a mandible that has adequate bone in the right posterior segment and inadequate bone on the other side, but abundant bone in the anterior, is a Type 3, Division A, B, C edentulous ridge. A narrow-diameter implant may be placed in the right posterior segment, as well as root forms in the anterior section as indicated by the prosthesis. If additional prosthetic

support is needed in the left mandibular region, then in most cases additional anterior root forms are placed and splinted to the posterior implants and the teeth or bar cantilevered without implant support on the left posterior region. The Type 3, Division A, C, B patient is treated as a mirror image of Type 3, Division A, B, C.

The Type 3, Division A, D, C (or Type 3, Division A, C, D) patient receives a treatment plan similar to the plans discussed under Type 2, Division A, C. Endosteal root form implants are placed in the anterior section; if the prosthesis needs additional posterior support, then grafts are considered, especially in the posterior maxilla. Patients with Type 3 arches with anterior Division B or C are treated similar to the corresponding Type 2 patients with an anterior Division B or C. In the maxilla, it is not unusual that the premaxilla presents insufficient bone volume, and one posterior quadrant requires a sinus graft (Type 3, Division C, A, D). In that case and if appropriate bone volume is present in the cuspid area with favorable force factors, then a full-arch fixed prosthesis can be fabricated after sinus graft and implant placement in the posterior regions, bypassing the premaxilla (Fig. 20.29).

The arch is Type 3, even when the anterior region is similar to one of the posterior sections. For example, the Type 3, Division C, D, C ridge has Division C in the anterior, severe atrophy on the right section, and moderate atrophy in the left section. In a mandibular arch of this type, implant placement in the anterior section only may be sufficient to restore the patient, although a subperiosteal implant may be indicated. The maxilla usually requires sinus grafts and subnasal elevation because of the poor biomechanics and bone quality.

The anterior section usually determines the treatment plan. Rarely are posterior implants inserted without any anterior implant support. In traditional prosthetics, Kennedy-Applegate Class I, modification I patients with anterior missing teeth are often restored with an anterior FPD and posterior RPD. This limits rocking of the prosthesis and decreases the forces transmitted to the abutments. Conventional prosthetics also dictate that an FPD is not indicated when the canine and two adjacent teeth are missing. This applies also when the anterior six teeth are missing and implants cannot be inserted. These time-tested, traditional prosthodontic axioms indicate that posterior implants alone should not be placed without any anterior implant or natural tooth support. However, this concept is often ignored in the maxilla, where practitioners often rely solely on sinus grafts and implants in the posterior segments. If no canine implants are inserted, then the lack of anterior support can cause rotation of the prosthesis and accelerate posterior implant loss. The two posterior sections are not connected because the span between the first premolars is too great, and the posterior implants are placed almost in a straight line with little biomechanical advantage. Anterior rocking and posterior lateral forces on these straight-line implants increase implant failure. The patient's condition is then often worse than before any implant therapy. It is usually far more prudent to convince the patient to be treated with an anterior onlay graft and anterior implants so that a full-arch restoration (RP-4 or fixed) may be fabricated.

Summary

An implant dentistry classification has been postulated that permits visualization of teeth and bone in partially edentulous arches. The foundation of this classification is the Kennedy-Applegate system, which is the most-used classification in prosthodontics. In addition, a classification for the completely edentulous arch is discussed, which is based on the quantity of available bone.

References

1. Misch CE. *Available Bone Improved Surgical Concept in Implant Dentistry*. Congress XI, Birmingham, AL: Paper presented at the Alabama Implant Study Group; 1985.
2. Cummer WE. Possible combinations of teeth present and missing in partial restorations. *Oral Health*. 1920;10:421.
3. Kennedy E. *Partial Denture Construction*. Brooklyn, NY: Dental Items of Interest; 1928.
4. Bailyn M. Tissue support in partial denture construction. *Dent Cosmos*. 1928;70:988.
5. Neurohr F. *Partial Dentures: a System of Functional Restoration*. Philadelphia: Lea & Febiger; 1939.
6. Mauk EH. Classification of mutilated dental arches requiring treatment by removable partial dentures. *J Am Dent Assoc*. 1942;29:2121.
7. Godfrey RJ. Classification of removable partial dentures. *J Am Coll Dent*. 1951;18:5.
8. Beckett LS. The influence of saddle classifications on the design of partial removable restoration. *J Prosthet Dent*. 1953;3:506.
9. Friedman J. The ABC classification of partial denture segments. *J Prosthet Dent*. 1953;3:517.
10. Austin KP, Lidge EF. *Partial Dentures: A Practical Textbook*. St. Louis: Mosby; 1957.
11. Skinner CNA. Classification of removable partial dentures based upon the principles of anatomy and physiology. *J Prosthet Dent*. 1959;9:240–246.
12. Applegate OC. *Essentials of Removable Partial Denture Prosthesis*. 3rd ed. Philadelphia: WB Saunders; 1965.
13. Misch CE, Judy WMK. Classifications of the partially edentulous arches for implant dentistry. *Int J Oral Implantol*. 1987;4:7–12.
14. Laney WR, Gibilisco JA. *Diagnosis and Treatment in Prosthodontics*. Philadelphia: Lea & Febiger; 1983.
15. Davis WH. Neurologic complications in implant surgery. In the American Association of Oral and Maxillofacial Surgeons Congress. *Clin Study Guide*. 1992.
16. Walton JN, Gardner MF, Agar JR, et al. A survey of crown and fixed partial denture failures: length of service and reasons for replacement. *J Prosthet Dent*. 1986;56:416–420.
17. Kent JN. Correction of alveolar ridge deficiencies with nonresorbable hydroxylapatite. *J Am Dent Assoc*. 1982;105:99–100.
18. Lekholm U, Zarb GA. Patient selection and preparation. In: Brånemark PI, Zarb GA, Albrektsson T, eds. *Tissue Integrated Prostheses: Osseointegration in Clinical Dentistry*. Chicago: Quintessence; 1985.
19. Misch CE. Classification of partially and completely edentulous arches in implant dentistry. In: Misch CE, ed. *Contemporary Implant Dentistry*. St. Louis: Mosby; 1993.
20. Tolman DE, Keller EE. Management of mandibular fractures in patients with endosseous implants. *Int J Oral Maxillofac Implants*. 1991;6:427–436.

21

Preimplant Prosthodontic Factors Related to Surgical Treatment Planning

CARL E. MISCH[†], RANDOLPH R. RESNIK, AND FRANCINE MISCH-DIETSH

Implants serve as a foundation for the prosthetic support of missing teeth. However, in the partially edentulous patient, the existing teeth may often require restorations or treatment. The existing conditions of the stomatognathic system should be evaluated and treated, when indicated. As such, preimplant prosthodontic considerations are a vital phase of the overall treatment before implant surgery. For example, the surgical decision to augment or perform an osteoplasty before implant surgery is primarily dependent on the desired prosthetic result. Most all conventional forms of construction, from buildings to art form, require a detailed plan and a clear vision of the end result before the project is initiated.

Overall Evaluation

The preimplant prosthodontic evaluation of the patient's overall condition closely resembles traditional dentistry. When a restoring dentist first evaluates the prosthetic needs of a patient, an orderly process is required, regardless of the current state of the dentition. In other words, regardless of whether the patient has all teeth or is missing all teeth, after the dentist accepts the responsibility of long-term professional guidance and treatment as necessary, a consistent approach to care is beneficial. There are five initial elements that should be assessed in sequence and treated when indicated. These elements include maxillary anterior tooth position, the existing occlusal vertical dimension (OVD), the mandibular incisor edge position, the maxillary occlusal plane, and the mandibular occlusal plane (Box 21.1). These elements are evaluated in a partially edentulous patient during the initial clinical examination and on mounted diagnostic casts (which may also serve as diagnostic wax-up procedures).

Maxillary Anterior Tooth Position

The position of the existing maxillary anterior teeth is first assessed. Most often these natural teeth are adequate in location and incisal edge position. However, if their position is undesirable for any

reason, orthodontics or conventional prosthetic intervention may be indicated. If the maxillary incisor edge is modified in either the horizontal or vertical plane, this may lead to changes in the other four elements of the stomatognathic system.

The labial position of the maxillary anterior teeth is first determined with the lip in repose (i.e., resting position). This is primarily evaluated by overall support of the maxillary lip and its relationship to the balance of the face, especially in relation to the nose and presence or absence of a philtrum in the midline (Fig. 21.1).[1-7] When the teeth are positioned more labial, the vertical position of the lip is elevated. Likewise, a more palatal position of the maxillary anterior teeth results in a more inferior or extended position of the lip. If the labial or horizontal position is going to be altered, then orthodontic therapy is ideally the treatment of choice. On occasion, a prosthetic or surgical approach may be indicated, with or without orthodontic treatment.

The next step in the evaluation process (when the labial position is acceptable) is the vertical position of the maxillary anterior teeth related to the lip in repose. The maxillary canine is the key for this position. Misch has suggested the canine tip be located approximately 1 mm level with the lip in repose, regardless of the age or sex of the patient (Fig. 21.2).[8] A horizontal line drawn from one canine tip to the contralateral side should be level to the horizon. Normally, the central incisors are 1 to 2 mm longer in a horizontal plane to the canines. If the patient is wearing a maxillary complete denture, then the maxillary anterior tooth position is often incorrect, compared with the natural tooth position. As a result of resorption of the premaxilla, the denture shifts apically and posteriorly after the bone loss pattern. No other region of the mouth should be restored until this position is corrected because it negatively influences the proper position of every other segment (e.g., OVD, mandibular anterior tooth position, posterior planes of occlusion).

The maxillary anterior horizontal and vertical tooth positions are evaluated before any other segment of the arches, including the OVD. If the maxillary anterior teeth are significantly malpositioned, the clinician should obtain further diagnostic studies, such as a cone beam radiograph, to determine the relationship of the maxilla to the cranial base. The patient may have unfavorable

[†]Deceased.

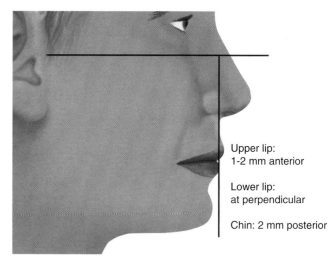

• **Fig. 21.1** Ideal soft tissue position. The labial position of the teeth is first evaluated relative to the support of the maxillary lip. A vertical line drawn through the subnasal point and perpendicular to the Frankfort plane can be used as a baseline. Ideally, the maxillary lip should be 1 to 2 mm anterior to this line, the lower lip even with the line, and the chin 2 mm behind the line.

Upper lip: 1-2 mm anterior

Lower lip: at perpendicular

Chin: 2 mm posterior

skeletal relationships (vertical maxillary excess or deficiency). If the position of the natural maxillary anterior teeth is undesirable for any reason, then orthodontics, orthognathic surgery, or prosthetic intervention may be indicated. After the position of the maxillary anterior teeth is acceptable, the next prosthetic step is the evaluation of the OVD.

Existing Occlusal Vertical Dimension

To determine the crown height space (CHS), the overall issue of OVD must be addressed. The patient's existing OVD should be evaluated early in an implant prosthetic treatment plan because any modification will significantly modify the overall treatment. Not only will a change in OVD require at least one full arch to be reconstructed, it will also affect the CHS and therefore the potential number, size, position, and angulation requirements of the implants. The OVD is defined as the distance between two points (one in the maxilla and the other directly below in the mandible) when the occluding members are in contact.[9] This dimension requires clinical evaluation of the patient and cannot be based solely on the diagnostic casts.

The determination of the OVD is not a precise process because a range of dimensions is possible without clinical symptoms.[10-23] At one time, it was believed OVD was very specific and remained stable throughout a patient's life. However, this position is not necessarily stable when the teeth are present or after the teeth are lost. Long-term studies have shown this is not a constant dimension and often decreases over time without clinical consequence in the dentate or partially or completely edentulous patient.

The OVD may be altered without the symptoms of pain or dysfunction however is case specific. However, this is not to say that altering the OVD has no consequence. A change in OVD affects the CHS. As such, it may affect the biomechanics of the support system of an implant prosthesis. In addition, any change in the OVD will also modify the horizontal dimensional relationship of the maxilla to the mandible; therefore a change in OVD will modify the anterior guidance, range of function, and esthetics.

The most important effect of OVD on tooth (implant) loading may be the effect on the biomechanics of anterior guidance. The more closed (decreased) the OVD, the farther forward the mandible rotates and the more class III the chin appears (Figs.

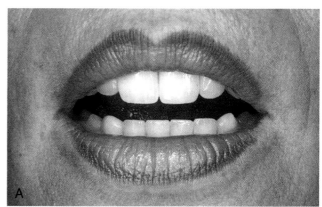
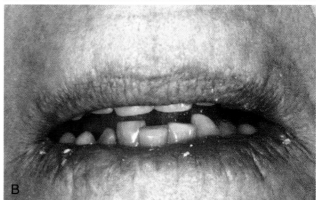

• **Fig. 21.2** (A) Vertical position of the maxillary anterior teeth is assessed by evaluating the position of the canines. The ideal position is determined by the canine to lip in repose position: a horizontal line is drawn from canine tip to canine tip, and the central incisors are 1 to 2 mm longer. (B) This position is consistent (within 1 mm) regardless of the age or sex of the patient.

21.3 and 21.4). In a class II, division 2 patient, the more closed the OVD, the steeper is the anterior guidance and the greater the vertical overlap of the anterior teeth. Anterior guidance is necessary to maintain incisal guidance during mandibular excursions to decrease the risk of posterior interferences. In completely edentulous patients restored with fixed implant prosthodontics, a change

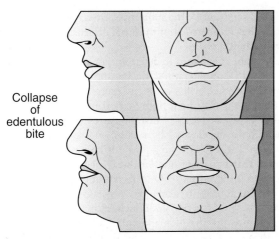

• **Fig. 21.3** Decreased vertical dimension. As the edentulous bite collapses, a closed occlusal vertical dimension results that rotates the chin farther forward. This gives a class III appearance.

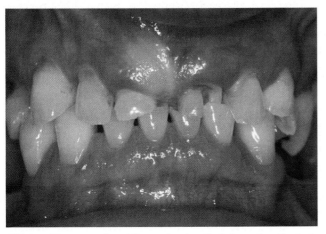

• **Fig. 21.4** The more closed the occlusal vertical dimension, the farther forward the mandibular teeth occlude.

in OVD in either direction may affect biomechanics. Opening the OVD and decreasing the incisal guidance, with a resulting bilaterally balanced occlusion, may increase forces placed on posterior implants during mandibular excursion. Closing the OVD may increase the forces to anterior implants during any excursion. On occasion, a change in the OVD may also affect the sibilant sounds by altering the horizontal position of the mandible. According to Kois and Phillips, three situations primarily mandated the modification of the OVD: (1) esthetics, (2) function, and (3) structural needs of the dentition.[12] Esthetics is related to OVD for incisal edge positions, facial measurements, and the occlusal plane. Function is related to the canine positions, incisal guidance, and angle of load to teeth or implants. Structural requirements are related to dimensions of teeth for restoration, while maintaining a biological width.

Methods to Evaluate Occlusal Vertical Dimension

In traditional prosthodontics, a range of techniques has been described to establish the OVD. Objective methods use facial dimension measurements, whereas subjective methods rely on esthetics, resting arch position, and closest speaking space. There is no consensus on the ideal method to obtain the OVD; therefore this dimension is part art form and part science. However, it is a

crucial component of the rehabilitation process, so OVD should be determined before completion of a final treatment plan.

Subjective Methods

The subjective methods to determine OVD include the use of resting interocclusal distance and speech-based techniques using sibilant sounds. Niswonger proposed the use of the interocclusal distance ("freeway space"), which assumes that the patient relaxes the mandible into the same constant physiologic rest position.[13] The practitioner then subtracts 3 mm from the measurement to determine the OVD. Two observations conflict with this approach. First, the amount of freeway space is highly variable in the same patient, depending on factors such as head posture, emotional state, presence or absence of teeth, parafunction, and time of recording (greater in the morning). Second, interocclusal distance at rest varies 3 to 10 mm from one patient to another. As a result, the distance to subtract from the freeway space is unknown for a specific patient; therefore the physiologic rest position should not be the primary method to evaluate OVD. However, the distance should be evaluated once the OVD is established, to ensure a freeway space exists when the mandible is at rest.

Silverman stated that approximately 1 mm should exist between the teeth when making an S sound.[14]

Pound further developed this concept for the establishment of centric and vertical jaw relationship records for complete dentures.[15,16] Although this concept is acceptable, it does not correlate to the original OVD of the patient; therefore the speaking space should not be used as the only method to establish OVD. After the OVD has been determined, the speaking space should be observed, and the teeth should not touch during sibilant sounds. On occasion, a short adjustment period of a few weeks may be required to establish this criterion. Therefore a transitional prosthesis should be used to evaluate this position in case it must be modified before the final restoration.

Kois[12] has noted that the subjective method of esthetics to establish an OVD is the most difficult to teach inexperienced dental students and therefore is least likely to be initially addressed when teaching the concepts of determining OVD. However, experienced clinicians often value this method more than any other to assess OVD. After the position of the maxillary incisor edge is determined, the OVD influences esthetics of the face in general.

Objective Methods

Facial dimensions are directly related to the ideal facial esthetics of an individual and can be easily assessed regardless of the clinician's experience.[17-25] This objective evaluation is usually the method of choice to evaluate the existing OVD or establish a different OVD during prosthetic reconstruction. In addition, it may be performed without the need of additional diagnostic tests.

Facial measurements can be traced back to antiquity when sculptors and mathematicians followed the golden ratio for body and facial proportions, as described by Pythagoras. The golden ratio relates to the length and width of a golden rectangle as 1 to 0.618. Many human body proportions follow the golden ratio because it is considered the most esthetically appealing to the human eye.[18-20,25] Leonardo da Vinci later contributed several observations and drawings on facial proportions, which he called divine proportions.[21] He observed the distance between the chin and the bottom of the nose (i.e., OVD) was a similar dimension as

(1) the hairline to the eyebrows, (2) the height of the ear, and (3) the eyebrows to the bottom of the nose. Each of these dimensions equaled one-third of the face.

Many professionals, including plastic surgeons, oral surgeons, artists, orthodontists, and morticians, use facial measurements to determine OVD. A review of the literature found that many different sources reveal many correlations of features that may correspond to the OVD (Box 21.2; Fig. 21.5).

All these measurements do not correspond exactly to each other, but they usually do not vary by more than a few millimeters (with the exception of the vertical height of the ear) when facial features appear in balance. An average of several of these measurements may be used to assess the existing OVD. In a clinical study by Misch, the OVD was often slightly larger than the facial measurements listed (more in men than women), but it was rarely a smaller dimension.[22] The subjective criteria of pleasing esthetics may then be considered after the facial dimensions are within balance to each other.

Radiographic methods to determine an objective OVD are also documented in the literature. Tracings on a cephalometric radiograph are suggested when gross jaw excess or deficiency is noted. Such conditions may stem from vertical maxillary excess, vertical maxillary deficiency, vertical mandibular excess (long chin), vertical mandibular deficiency (short chin), and apertognathia or class II, division 2 (deep bite) situations. Orthodontic treatment planning of a dentate patient often includes a lateral cephalogram and may be used to evaluate OVD (glabella-subnasale, subnasale-menton). The same measurements may be performed on the edentulous patient.[26,27] Esthetics are influenced by OVD because of the relationship to the maxillomandibular positions. The smaller the OVD, the greater the class III jaw relationship becomes; the greater the OVD, the more class II the relationship becomes. The maxillary anterior tooth position is determined first and is most important for the esthetic criteria of the reconstruction. Alteration of the OVD for esthetics rarely includes the maxillary tooth position. For example, the OVD position may be influenced by the need to soften the chin for a patient with a large mental protuberance. After the OVD satisfies the esthetic requirement of the prosthetic reconstruction, it may still be slightly refined. For example, the OVD may be modified to improve the direction of force on the anterior implants.

In addition, anterior mandibular implants on occasion are too facial to the incisal edge position, and increasing the OVD makes them much easier to restore. Therefore because the OVD is not an exact measurement, the ability to alter this dimension within limits may often be beneficial. The evaluation of the pretreatment OVD is also very important for the patient wearing a complete maxillary denture opposing a partially edentulous mandible, especially in the case of edentulous posterior segments that are not compensated by a removable partial denture (Kennedy-Applegate class I). Under these conditions, a combination (Kelly) syndrome may be present and is especially noteworthy if the OVD is within normal limits.[28]

• BOX 21.2 Occlusal Vertical Dimension Correlations

1. The horizontal distance between the pupils
2. The horizontal distance from the outer canthus of one eye to the inner canthus of the other eye
3. Twice the horizontal length of one eye
4. Twice the horizontal distance from the inner canthus of one eye to the inner canthus of the other eye
5. The horizontal distance from the outer canthus of the eye to the ear
6. The horizontal distance from one corner of the lip to the other, following the curvature of the mouth (cheilion to cheilion)
7. The vertical distance from the external corner of the eye (outer canthus) to the corner of the mouth
8. The vertical height of the eyebrow to the ala of the nose
9. The vertical length of the nose at the midline (from the nasal spine [subnasion] to the glabella point)
10. The vertical distance from the hair line to the eyebrow line
11. The vertical height of the ear
12. The distance between the tip of the thumb and the tip of the index finger when the hand lays flat, with the fingers next to each other

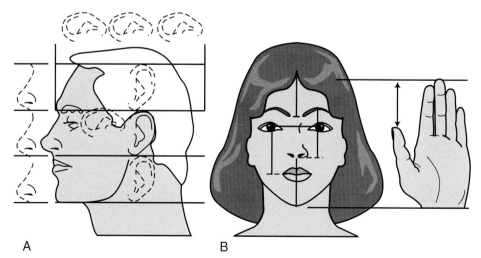

A   B

• Fig. 21.5 Occlusal vertical dimension (OVD) may initially be evaluated by objective measurements, comparing facial dimensions to the existing OVD. Leonardo da Vinci described divine proportions in the following way: (A) "The distance between the chin and the nose and the hairline and the eyebrows are equal to the height of the ear and a third of the face. From the outer canthus of the eye to the ear, the distance is equal to the height of the ear and to one-third of the face height." (B), In addition, facial height (from chin to hairline) is equal to the height of the hand, and the nose is the same length as the distance between the tip of the thumb and the tip of the index finger.

The clinical symptoms include (1) maxillary incisor denture position up and rotated back from ideal, (2) lower natural anterior teeth overerupted and beyond the mandibular occlusal plane, (3) horizontal occlusal plane tilted apically in the anterior and occlusally in the posterior regions, (4) enlarged tuberosities encroaching on the mandibular interarch space, (5) maxillary palatal hyperplasia, and (6) highly mobile tissue in the premaxilla. In addition, because the mandibular posterior teeth have been missing many years for this syndrome to develop, there is a lack of posterior bone in the mandible to place endosteal implants (Fig. 21.6).

The proper maxillary incisal edge position and OVD are especially critical for these patients because of the incidence of mandibular incisor extrusion beyond the maxillary occlusal plane. The extrusion is usually accompanied by the alveolar process. To position the maxillary incisors properly, the mandibular anterior teeth must be repositioned at the proper incisal plane. Endodontic therapy and crown lengthening procedures usually precede the restorations on the lower arch to obtain a retentive and esthetic restoration.

On occasion, the remaining roots of the mandibular anterior teeth are too short to consider for long-term prognosis after the crown lengthening is performed. Under these conditions, extraction of the mandibular anterior teeth, alveoloplasty, and implant placement may be indicated. When the arch shape is ovoid to tapered, five anterior implants may be adequate to serve as support for a full arch implant–supported restoration. Therefore the implants replace the teeth extracted from overeruption, and they can also replace the posterior missing teeth. This is usually very helpful because long-term edentulous posterior segments are usually deficient in bone volume. Thus this approach eliminates the need for posterior bone grafts to restore the lower arch with a fixed implant–supported restoration.

Mandibular Incisor Edge Position

After the maxillary incisal edge and the OVD are deemed clinically acceptable, the position of the lower anterior teeth is evaluated. When natural teeth are present, or when a fixed prosthesis is planned in the anterior region, the mandibular teeth incisal edge should contact the lingual aspect of the maxillary anterior natural teeth at the desired OVD position. A vertical overlap with the maxillary anterior teeth is usually in the range of 3 to 5 mm. The incisal guidance is defined as the influence of contacting surfaces of the mandibular and maxillary anterior teeth on mandibular movements.[9] The incisal guide angle is formed by the intersection of the plane of occlusion and a line within the sagittal plane, determined by the incisal edge of the maxillary and mandibular central incisors when in maximal intercuspation (MI). The incisal guide angle is responsible for the amount of posterior tooth separation during mandibular excursions, and to do so, it should be steeper than the condylar disc assembly (Christensen phenomenon). Therefore any planned prosthesis and associated compensating curves should be developed within these confines. If they are not, then the maxillomandibular arch position may be improper (i.e., in the skeletal class II patient) and the posterior teeth may exhibit lateral contacts during mandibular excursions. Under these conditions, the masseter and temporalis muscles do not reduce their contraction force during these movements (as they do when only anterior teeth occlude in excursions), and the strong muscles of mastication continue to contract and place an increased force on the entire stomatognathic system.

The incisal guidance can be evaluated on the mounted diagnostic models. A steep incisal guidance helps in avoiding posterior interferences in protrusive movement. However, the steeper the incisal guide angle is, the greater force applied to anterior crowns. This may present a significant problem for an anterior single-tooth implant

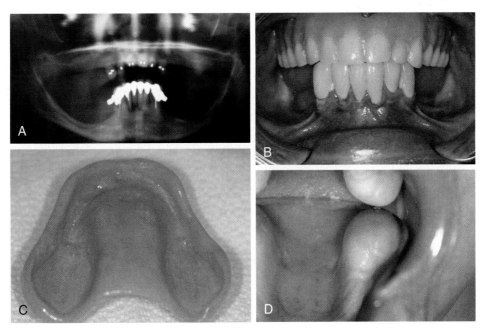

• **Fig. 21.6** (A) Combination syndrome describes the clinical conditions occurring when a maxillary denture opposes mandibular anterior teeth and no partial denture. The mandibular teeth overerupt as the maxillary denture seats up in the anterior and down in the posterior. (B) Clinical view of retained maxillary anterior teeth with passive eruption of the mandibular alveolar bone with no posterior support, (C) Maxillary prosthesis showing extensive premaxilla atrophy and enlarged tuberosities, (D) In most cases of combination syndrome, tuberosity reduction is indicated prior to prosthetic treatment.

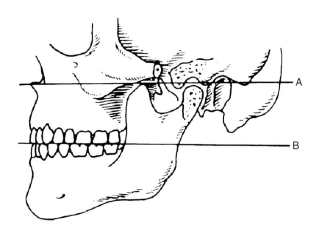

• **Fig. 21.7** Ala–tragus line (Camper plane) *(Line A)* is parallel to the occlusal plane of the maxillary teeth *(Line B)*.

replacement. On occasion, the tooth is lost as a result of severe parafunction from a steep incisal guidance (usually from fracture after endodontic therapy). On the other hand, if the existing incisal guidance is shallow, it may be necessary to plan recontouring or prosthetic restoration of posterior teeth that exhibit contact during excursions.

Existing Occlusal Planes (Posterior Maxillary and Mandibular Planes of Occlusion)

After the maxillary anterior teeth position, OVD, and mandibular anterior teeth position are deemed acceptable, the horizontal occlusal planes are evaluated in the posterior regions of the mouth. Their position related to the curves of Wilson (mediolateral) and Spee (anteroposterior [A-P]) and to each other should allow harmonious occlusion, with maximum occlusal interdigitation and canine or mutually protected occlusion. Ideally, the maxillary posterior occlusal plane should be parallel to the Camper plane (i.e., to the midtragus position) (Fig. 21.7). The occlusal plane of existing teeth is critical in evaluating partially edentulous patients in relationship to the final implant prosthesis. Occlusal modification, endodontic therapy, or crowns are indicated to remedy tipping or extrusions of adjacent or opposing natural teeth. A pretreatment diagnostic wax-up is strongly suggested to evaluate the needed changes before implant placement. A proper curve of Spee and curve of Wilson are also indicated for proper esthetics and are reproduced in the compensating curves for complete denture fabrication (Fig. 21.8).

The occlusal plane seems like an obvious step in the patient dental evaluation; however, the existing occlusal plane is not routinely evaluated before the fabrication of the prosthesis. The restoring clinician should explain to the patient the existence of extrusion or exfoliation of the surrounding teeth, which is often obvious on radiographs or diagnostic casts. The need to restore the missing tooth sooner rather than later is apparent to the patient because the teeth are already shifting as a result of the arch collapse. If the patient cannot afford the complete treatment plan related to the missing teeth then the opposing arch with the poor occlusal plane should be treated first, and not the arch with the missing tooth. In this way, opposing quadrants will ultimately be restored to a proper relationship. An occlusal plane analyzer may be used on diagnostic casts to evaluate pretreatment conditions and assist in intraoral occlusal plane correction. Occlusal analyzers are fabricated in several sizes. The average size corresponds to a 4-inch sphere and provides a starting point for ideal curves of Wilson and Spee. Any discrepancy observed on the cast may be

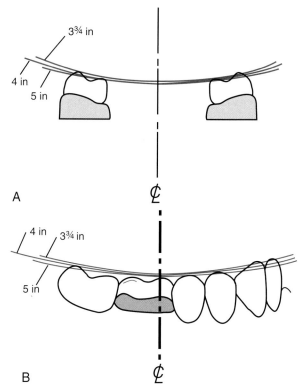

• **Fig. 21.8** Occlusal planes. (A) The curve of Spee is also similar to the radius of a 4-inch sphere and is related to skull size. (B) The curve of Wilson is evaluated before reconstruction in the region. The radius of the average curve corresponds to the radius of a 4-inch sphere.

corrected in the mouth. A laboratory-assisted template may be fabricated with this intent. In the laboratory, a vacuum or press fit of an acrylic shell is prepared over the cast. The occlusal plane analyzer is then used to evaluate and correct an improper occlusal plane. A handpiece is used to grind the acrylic shell and protruding occlusal cusps on the duplicate diagnostic cast. The clear acrylic shell is then taken intraorally and inserted over the teeth. Any cusp extending through the acrylic shell is recontoured to the level of the surrounding acrylic. As such, the occlusal plane is rapidly corrected to an ideal condition (Fig. 21.9).

The natural dentition opposing a partially edentulous ridge also must be carefully examined, and often regions before surgical placement of the implants, especially in the posterior regions of the mouth. The opposing teeth have often drifted or tipped into the opposing edentulous site as a result of improper or missing opposing occlusal contacts.

The CHS in the edentulous site may be significantly reduced as a result of posterior extrusion or exfoliation. The implant drills and implant body insertion often require a posterior CHS of more than 8 mm from the ideal plane of occlusion so the handpiece, drill, or implant may be inserted at the correct position and angulation. This problem is increased when a guided surgical template is used.

The partially edentulous posterior ridge with facial resorption may require implant insertion more medial in relation to the original central fossa of the natural dentition. Enameloplasty of the stamp cusps of the opposing teeth is often indicated to redirect occlusal forces over the long axis of the implant body and may be determined with the diagnostic casts and modified in the mouth before the opposing arch impression and bite registration at the final impression appointment. Then, at the final prosthesis delivery, the final modifications of the opposing dentition are made. The goal of preprosthetic evaluation is to identify and restore the prosthetic parameters within normal limits. The correct tooth positions

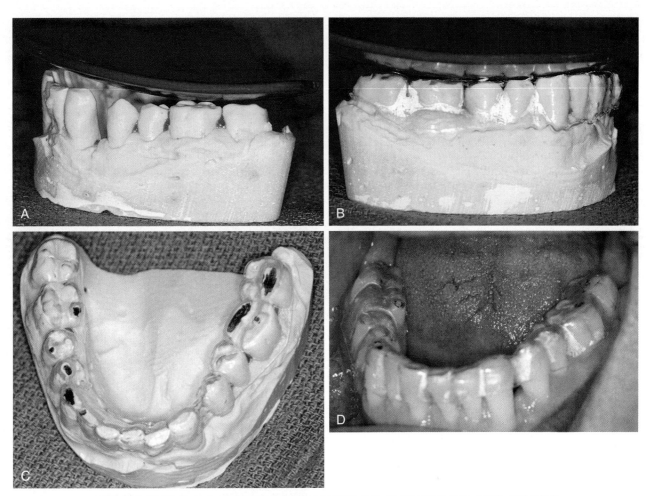

• **Fig. 21.9** (A) Misch occlusal analyzer fabricated in three sizes as follows: ¾-inch, 4-inch, and 5-inch sphere. The occlusal plane of the patient is evaluated before the restoration of the opposing arch. (B) A press-form (vacuum) shell is placed over a duplicate study cast of the patient. The template and teeth are adjusted so the casts follow the Misch occlusal analyzer more accurately. (C) The areas on the cast are marked to indicate the areas to modify intraorally. The modified template is inserted in the mouth, and the dental regions above the template are recontoured. (D) Intraorally, the correction is performed using the template.

should be first determined so that, even if the total treatment time is extended over several years, at least each segment will aim toward a consistent goal. Too often the restoring dentist assumes the patient wants the cheapest or fastest treatment related to each treatment session. As a consequence, the mouth is restored one tooth at a time, fitting the restoration into the patient's present occlusal condition, which usually worsens over time and never improves on its own. As a result, after the patient has been in the same practice for several decades, the mouth is in poorer condition than when the patient started. Although it is easier to restore an entire mouth to the correct occlusal relationships at one time, it is also possible to obtain a similar result one tooth at a time, as long as each step proceeds along the predetermined course of treatment.

Specific Criteria

After the five elements of the existing teeth (restorations) have been evaluated and modified where necessary, several other conditions may modify and hinder the course of implant treatment if overlooked. These conditions should be considered before the final treatment plan is presented to the patient (Box 21.3) and include the following.

• **BOX 21.3**   **Specific Criteria to Evaluate**

1. Lip lines
2. Maxillomandibular arch relationship
3. Existing occlusion
4. Crown height space
5. Temporomandibular joint status
6. Extraction of hopeless or guarded-prognosis existing teeth
7. Existing prostheses
8. Arch form (ovoid, tapering, and square)
9. Natural tooth adjacent to implant site
10. Soft tissue evaluation of edentulous sites

Lip Lines

Lip positions are evaluated, including resting lip line, maxillary high lip line (smile), and mandibular low lip line (speech) in relation to the vertical position of the teeth. The lip line positions are especially noted if anterior teeth are to be replaced. The resting lip positions are highly variable, but in general they are related to the patient's age. In general, older patients show less maxillary teeth at rest and during smiling, but they demonstrate more mandibular teeth during sibilant sounds.[4] Prosthetic guidelines for incisal edge position established relative to esthetics, phonetics, and occlusion are applied.[1-8,29-35]

A common removable prosthetic guideline is a 1- to 2-mm incisal edge display with the lip at rest, regardless of the patient's age. Instead, the goal should be to position the prosthetic teeth in the most likely location for the patient's natural teeth. Males tend to show fewer teeth than a female of the same age. In a 50-year-old male, the maxillary incisal edge is often level with the upper lip at rest. This is a similar position for a 60-year-old female. The average upper lip is 20 to 22 mm for women and 22 to 26 mm for men. The maxillary incisal edge is usually at an average of 22 to 24 mm from the floor of the nose depending on the length and contour of the lip. For a short upper lip, the standard guideline for incisal edge of the central incisor would not be acceptable because this would decrease the height of the maxillary arch.

The position of the maxillary incisor in relation to the maxillary lip and the age of the patient is much more variable than the position of the canine. The lip bow in the center of the upper lip rises several millimeters on some females and is barely obvious on others. The higher the lip bow, the more central incisor surface is seen on the patient, regardless of age. Men rarely exhibit an exaggerated lip bow and therefore have a more consistent incisor edge to lip position. The canine position at the corner of the lip is not affected by the lip bow effect. As such, it is a more consistent position and usually corresponds to the length of the resting lip position from 30 to 60 years of age in both males and females.[8]

In the natural dentition, the maxillary lip is most often longer than the incisal edge after the patient turns 65 years old. However, most patients desire the maxillary teeth to be at least slightly visible. It is risky to extend the maxillary tooth position to decrease the age of the smile without considering the consequences of an increased crown height on moment forces (biomechanics). If pontics rather than implants support the anterior crowns, the poor biomechanical condition is magnified.

An alternative to increasing the length of the anterior teeth may be to increase the thickness of the alveolar ridge. This extra support brings out the lip and also raises the vermilion border. As a result, the teeth are not longer, but the border of the lip is higher. In addition, if the added width to the ridge is with autologous bone, replacing teeth with implants rather than pontics further improves the situation. The fuller maxillary lip may also look younger because vertical age lines may also be reduced.

High Lip Line

The maxillary high lip line is determined while the patient displays a natural, broad smile.[36,37] There are three categories of maxillary lip lines: low, average (ideal), and high ("gummy"). The low lip line displays no interdental papilla or gingiva above the teeth during smiling. The high lip demonstrates all of the interdental papilla and more than 2 mm of tissue above the cervices of the teeth. The clinical characteristics of the average or ideal esthetic smile include a full length of crown exposure (crowns of normal height), a normal tooth position and alignment (lateral incisors may not be completely straight), a normal tooth form, the interdental papilla, and minimal gingival exposure over the cervicals of the teeth (lip at the free gingival margin of the centrals and canines) (Fig. 21.10). Approximately 70% of the adult population has a smile line within a few millimeters of the free gingival margin.

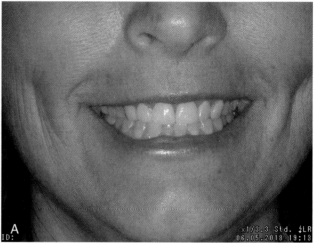

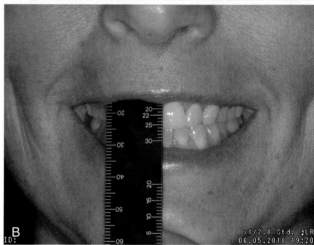

• **Fig. 21.10** (A) An ideal high smile line, although this patient shows ideal clinical crown and the interdental papillae in the anterior, the right posterior shows less teeth than the posterior left. (B) Measuring the height of the exposed clinical crown.

The FP-1 prosthesis in implant dentistry attempts to reproduce a normal crown contour. However, with a high lip position during smiling, this goal must also include the soft tissue drape around the crown. As a consequence, the esthetic requirements are much more demanding and often mandate additional surgical steps to enhance the soft and hard tissues before the crown restoration. The selection of an FP-2 and an FP-3 fixed prosthesis is often based solely on the evaluation of the high lip line. An FP-2 prosthesis is easier to fabricate because it requires fewer porcelain bake cycles.

Approximately 15% to 20% of adults have a low lip line and do not show the interdental papilla when smiling (more males than females) (Fig. 21.11). In these patients, the soft tissue drape does not require a primary focus and can often be compromised with an FP-2 restoration, when the patient is notified before treatment. However, an average to high lip position during smiling contraindicates this restoration type because of poor cervical esthetics. The pink porcelain or zirconia restoration (FP-3) to replace the soft tissue may be esthetic, but it is rarely the treatment of choice for single- tooth replacement. On the other hand, in multiple missing adjacent anterior teeth, the pink porcelain or zirconia is often the treatment of choice because the soft tissue drape is usually unable to be ideal, even with bone and tissue grafts.

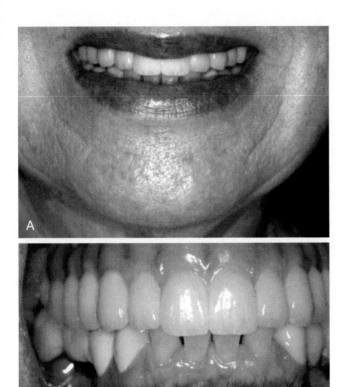

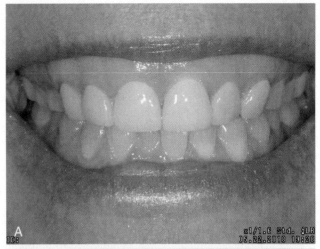

• **Fig. 21.11** (A) A low, high smile line shows no interdental papillae during smiling. (B) The patient in (A) has a full arch implant–supported FP-3 prosthesis.

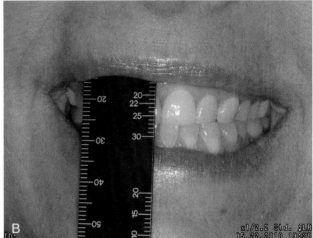

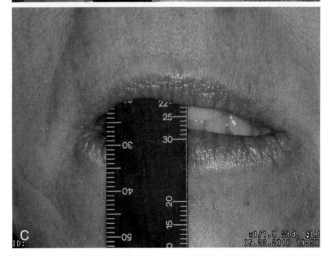

• **Fig. 21.12** (A) A high smile line exposes all of the clinical crown, the interdental papillae, and the full gingival margin above the teeth. (B) Measurement of the high smile line. (C). Measurement of the low smile line.

In a completely edentulous patient, the labial flange of the patient's existing denture may be removed and the lip position evaluated before the completed treatment plan of a fixed restoration. When the lip needs the support of the labial flange for esthetics, yet a fixed restoration is planned, autogenous, allografts or hydroxyapatite (HA) may be indicated to increase labial tissue thickness for proper lip support.

A gummy or high smile line occurs in 14% of the young female patients and 7% of young male patients (Fig. 21.12).[36] The normal clinical crown width/height ratio is 0.86 for the central incisor, 0.76 to 0.79 for the lateral incisor, and 0.77 to 0.81 for the canine. If the patient demonstrates a band of gingiva over the cervical areas of the teeth, then the height of the clinical crowns are evaluated, relative to their width. Esthetic crown lengthening is often a good option when the height of the central clinical crown is less than 10 mm (and the width is greater than 8 mm). Often the effect of crown lengthening is a dramatic improvement and may be accomplished at the same time as the implant surgery.

In patients with a high lip line who are missing all their anterior teeth, the prosthetic teeth can be made longer (up to 12 mm) instead of the average 10 mm height to reduce the gingival display and result in a more esthetic restoration. Therefore the height of the maxillary anterior teeth is determined by first establishing the incisal edge by the lip in repose. Second, the high smile line determines the height of the tooth (from 9–12 mm). Third, the width of the anterior teeth is determined by the height/width ratios.

The cervical third of the maxillary premolars is also observed during a high smile line. It is not unusual to reveal the cervical third and gingiva of the premolar with a high lip line. These teeth should not appear too long or unnatural in height. Resorption may also cause the implants to be inserted more palatally in this area. The position of these crowns may then be too palatal and therefore affect the esthetic result. Bone grafts are the primary method to eliminate the need for ridge laps or the addition of pink porcelain at the gingiva. They are also indicated to reduce crown height.

Mandibular Lip Line

The mandibular low lip position is often neglected, with disastrous esthetic results. The mandibular incisors are more visible in middle age and older patients during speaking than maxillary teeth. In addition, lower central incisors are often visible in their incisal two-thirds during exaggerated smiles.[37,38] Although the maxillary high lip line is evaluated during smiling, the mandibular low lip position should be assessed during speech. In pronunciation of the S sound, or sibilants, some patients may expose the entire anterior mandibular teeth and gingival contour. Patients are often unaware of this preexisting lip position and blame the final restoration for the display of the mandibular gingiva, or complain that the teeth look too long. Therefore it is recommended to make the patient aware of these existing lip lines before treatment and emphasize that these lip positions will be similar after treatment. An FP-3 mandibular restoration may be indicated to restore the patient with a low mandibular lip position.

Maxillomandibular Arch Relationship

After the maxillary anterior teeth positions, OVD, and mandibular anterior teeth positions are evaluated, the maxillomandibular relationships are assessed in the vertical, horizontal, and lateral planes. An improper skeletal position may be modified by orthodontics or surgery. It is far better to discuss these options with the patient before implant surgery because the implant placement may compromise the final prosthetic result if the arch positions are altered after implant insertion. Specific compromises of the final result should be discussed with patients when orthognathic surgery or orthodontic therapy is declined by patients with skeletal discrepancies.

Arch relationships are often affected in edentulous ridges. The anterior and posterior edentulous maxilla resorbs toward the palate after tooth loss.[39] The width of the alveolar ridge may decrease 40% within a few years, primarily at the expense of the labial plate. Consequently, implants are often placed lingual to the original incisal tooth position. The final restoration is then overcontoured facially to restore the incisal two-thirds in the ideal tooth position for esthetics. This results in a cantilevered force on the implant body. The maxilla is affected more often than the mandible because the incisal edge position in the esthetic zones cannot be modified and is dictated by esthetics, speech, lip position, and occlusion. Anterior cantilevered crowns from maxillary anterior implants often require additional implants splinted together and an increase in the A-P distance between the most distal to most anterior implant positions to compensate for the increased lateral loads and moment forces, especially during mandibular excursions.

An anterior cantilever on implants in the mandibular arch may correct an Angle's skeletal class II jaw relationship. The maxillary anterior teeth support the lower lip at rest in both Angle's skeletal class I and II relationships. A traditional complete mandibular denture cannot extend beyond the anatomic support or neutral zone of the lips without decreasing stability of the prosthesis. However, with implants, the denture teeth may be set in a more ideal esthetic and functional position. The anterior cantilever in the mandible is also dependent on adequate implant number and A-P distance between the splinted implants. To counteract the anterior cantilever effect, the treatment plan should provide increased implant support by increasing the surface area by number, size, design, or A-P implant position. In these cases, an RP-4,

designed to prevent food impaction, may facilitate daily care and help control the occlusal forces, compared with an FP-3 prosthesis.

The palatal resorption pattern of the maxilla, paired with the anterior rotation of the mandible in long-term, complete denture patients, may mimic a class III relationship on a lateral cephalometric radiograph. However, in this condition, class III mandibular mechanics do not apply (primarily vertical chewers with little to no anterior excursions during mastication or parafunction). In contrast, these patients exhibit a full range of mandibular excursions and can contribute significant lateral forces on the maxillary restoration, which is cantilevered off the implant base to obtain a class I esthetic restoration. Therefore additional splinted implants are suggested in the maxilla, with the widest A-P distance available. This usually requires sinus grafts and posterior implants in the first or second molar position splinted to the anterior implant support.

Transversal arch relationships include the existence of posterior crossbites, which occur frequently in implant dentistry. Edentulous maxillary posterior arches resorb palatally and medially after tooth loss. Sinus grafts can restore available bone height, but the ridge still remains medial to the opposing mandibular tooth central fossa. This is especially pronounced when opposing a division C–h or moderate atrophic mandible because the mandible widens after the residual alveolar ridge resorbs. For example, when mandibular implants are used in C–h bone volume for implant support opposing a complete denture, the posterior teeth may be set in crossbite (especially when out of an esthetic zone) to decrease the moment forces developing on the maxillary posterior teeth, causing denture instability.

Existing Occlusion

MI is defined as the complete intercuspation of the opposing teeth independent of condylar position, which is sometimes described as the best fit of teeth regardless of the condylar position.[9] *Centric occlusion* is defined as the occlusion of opposing teeth when the mandible is in centric relation (CR).[9] This may or may not coincide with the tooth position of MI. Its relationship to CR (a neuromuscular position independent of tooth contact with the condyles in an anterior, superior position) is noteworthy to the restoring dentist because of the potential need for occlusal adjustments to eliminate deflective tooth contacts and the evaluation of their potential noxious effects on the existing dentition and for the planned restoration. Correction of the problems before treatment presents many advantages and may follow a variety of approaches, depending on the severity of the incorrect tooth position: selective odontoplasty (a subtractive technique), restoration with a crown (with or without endodontic therapy), or extraction of the offending tooth. The existing occlusion is best evaluated with facebow-mounted diagnostic casts and open-mouth bite registration in CR.

Controversy exists as to the necessity for MI to be harmonious with CR occlusion. A vast majority of patients do not have such a relationship, yet they do not exhibit clinical pathology or accelerated tooth loss. Therefore it is difficult to state that these two positions must be similar. What is important is to evaluate the existing occlusion and the mandibular excursions to consciously decide whether the existing situation should be modified or be maintained. In other words, dentists should determine whether they are going to ignore or control the occlusion of the patient (Fig. 21.13). As a general rule, the more teeth replaced or restored, the more likely the patient is restored to CR occlusion. For example, if a completely edentulous mandible is to be restored with an implant-supported fixed prosthesis, then the CR occlusion position provides consistency and reproducibility between the articulator and the intraoral condition. Slight changes in OVD to position anterior implant abutments in a more favorable restoration position may be studied and implemented on the articulator without the need to record the new occlusal vertical position on the patient.

On the other hand, when one anterior tooth is being replaced, the existing MI position is often satisfactory to restore the patient, even though a posterior interference and anterior slide into full interdigitation may be present. The underlying question that helps determine the need for occlusal correction before restoration of the implant patient is the observation of negative symptoms related to the existing condition. This may include temporal mandibular joint conditions, tooth sensitivity, mobility, tooth fractures or abfraction, or porcelain fracture. The fewer and less significant the findings, the less likely an overall occlusal modification is required before restoration of the patient. However, to properly assess these conditions, the dentist must not ignore them before treatment.

Crown Height Space

The interarch distance is defined as the vertical distance between the maxillary and mandibular dentate or edentate arches under specific conditions (e.g., the mandible is at rest or in occlusion).[9] A dimension of only one arch does not have a defined term in prosthetics; therefore Misch proposed the term *crown height space*.[40] The CHS for implant dentistry is measured from the crest of the bone to the plane of occlusion in the posterior region and the incisal edge of the arch in question in the anterior region (Fig. 21.14). The ideal CHS for an FP-1 fixed implant prosthesis should range between 8 and 12 mm. This space accounts for the biological width, abutment height for cement retention or prosthesis screw fixation, occlusal material strength, esthetics, and hygiene considerations

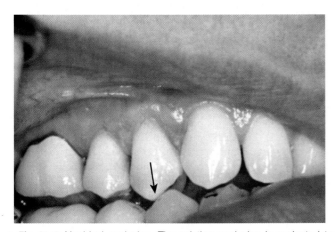

• **Fig. 21.13** Nonideal occlusion. The existing occlusion is evaluated to determine whether the maximal intercuspation is similar to centric relation. The mandibular excursions are also evaluated. The lack of canine contact and premature first premolar contact and the uneven occlusal plane indicated correction of the occlusion before final reconstruction.

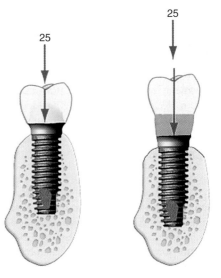

• **Fig. 21.15** Crown height is not a multiplier of force when the load is in the long axis of the implant. However, any angled force or cantilever increases the force and the crown height magnifies the effect.

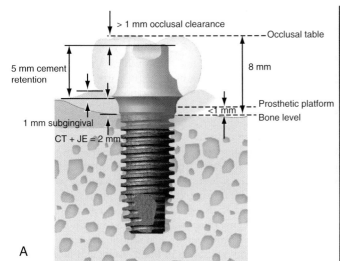

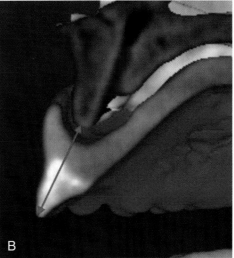

• **Fig. 21.14** (A) Crown Height Space The crown height space (CHS) is measured from the occlusal plane to the level of the bone. *CT,* Connective tissue; *JE,* junctional epithelium. Ideally a minimum of 8 mm is required between the bone level and the occlusal table, however id dependent on the type of prosthesis material. (B) CBCT cross-section depicting the available crown height space.

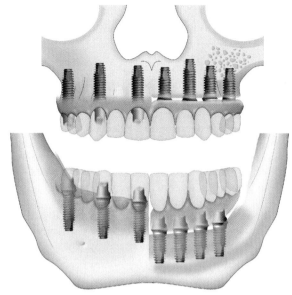

• **Fig. 21.16** The greater the crown height space (CHS), the more implants are required to restore the patient *(right)*. The less the CHS (left side), fewer implants are required to restore the patient.

around the abutment crowns. Removable prostheses often require more than 12 mm of CHS for denture teeth and acrylic resin base strength, attachments, bars, and oral hygiene considerations.[41,42]

Excessive Crown Height Space

Mechanical complication rates for implant prostheses are often the highest of all complications reported in the literature [43,44] and are often caused by excessive stress applied to the implant-prosthetic system. Implant body or component failure may occur from overload and result in prosthesis failure and bone loss around the failed implants.[43] Crestal bone loss may also be related to excessive forces and often occurs before implant body fracture.

The biomechanics of CHS are related to lever mechanics. The issues of cantilevers and implants were demonstrated in the edentulous mandible in which the length of the posterior cantilever directly related to complications or failure of the prosthesis.[44] Rather than being a posterior cantilever, the CHS is a vertical cantilever and therefore is also a force magnifier. When the direction of a force is in the long axis of the implant, the stresses to the bone are not magnified in relation to the CHS (Fig. 21.15). However, when the forces to the implant are on a cantilever or a lateral force is applied to the crown, the forces are magnified in direct relationship to the crown height. Bidez and Misch have evaluated the effect of a cantilever on an implant and its relation to crown height.[45,46] When the crown height is increased from 10 to 20 mm, two of six of these moments are increased 200%. When the available bone height is decreased, the CHS is increased. An angled load to a crown also magnifies the force to the implant. Maxillary anterior teeth are usually at an angle of 12 degrees or more to the occlusal planes. Therefore even implants placed in an ideal position are usually loaded at an angle. In addition, maxillary anterior crowns are often longer than any other teeth in the arch, so the effects of crown height cause greater risk. The angled force to the implant may also occur during protrusive or lateral excursions because the incisal guide angle may be 20 degrees or more. Anterior implant crowns will therefore be loaded at a considerable angle during excursions, compared with the long axis of the

implant. As a result, an increase in the force to maxillary anterior implants should be compensated for in the treatment plan.

Most forces applied to the osteointegrated implant body are concentrated in the crestal 7- to 9-mm bone, regardless of implant design and bone density. Therefore implant body height is not an effective method to counter the effect of crown height. Moderate bone loss before implant placement may result in a crown height–bone height ratio greater than 1, with greater lateral forces applied to the crestal bone than in abundant bone (in which the crown height is less). A linear relationship exists between the applied load and internal stresses.[47,48] Therefore the greater the load applied, the greater is the tensile and compressive stresses transmitted at the bone interface and to the prosthetic components. The greater the CHS, the greater number of implants are usually required for the prosthesis, especially in the presence of other force factors. This is a complete paradigm shift to the concepts advocated originally with many implants in greater available bone and small crown heights and fewer implants with greater crown heights in atrophied bone (Fig. 21.16). Because an increase in the biomechanical forces are in direct relationship to the increase in CHS, the treatment plan of the implant restoration should consider stress-reducing options whenever the CHS is increased. Methods to decrease stress are presented in Box 21.4.[40,41]

CHS is defined as excessive when it is greater than 15 mm. Treatment of excessive CHS as a result of vertical resorption of bone before implant placement includes surgical methods to increase bone height or stress reduction methods to the prosthesis. Several surgical techniques may be considered to increase bone height, including block onlay bone grafts, particulate bone grafts with titanium mesh or barrier membranes, interpositional bone grafts, and distraction osteogenesis.[41,42,49]

Bone augmentation may be preferred to prosthetic replacement. Surgical augmentation of the residual ridge height will reduce the CHS, improve implant biomechanics, and often permit the placement of wider body implants with the associated benefit of increased surface area. Although prosthetics is the most commonly used option to address excess CHS, it should be the last option used. Gingiva-colored prosthetic materials (pink porcelain or acrylic resin) on fixed restorations or changing the prosthetic design to a removable restoration should often be considered when restoring excessive CHS.

In the maxilla, a vertical loss of bone results in a more palatal ridge position. As a result, implants are often inserted more palatal than the natural tooth position. Removable restorations have several advantages under these clinical circumstances. The removable

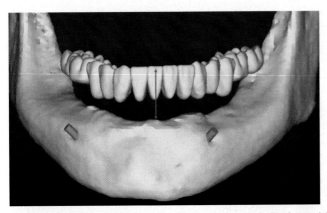

• **Fig. 21.17** Large crown height space requires a greater bulk of material (i.e., porcelain-metal prosthesis or zirconia), which increases the risk of possible prosthetic complications.

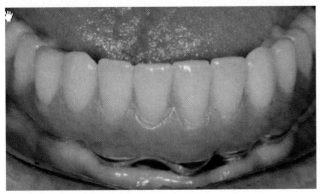

• **Fig. 21.18** Excessive crown height space. For an edentulous full arch prosthesis, a hybrid prosthesis (titanium milled bar + acrylic) may be used to decrease the thickness and weight associated with restoring a large space. Another prosthesis option is zirconia which is much lighter than conventional metal fused to porcelain.

prosthesis does not require embrasures for hygiene and may be removed during sleep to decrease the effects of an increase in CHS on nocturnal parafunction. The prosthesis may also improve the deficient lip facial support. The overdenture may have sufficient bulk of acrylic resin to permit denture tooth placement without infringement of the substructure and to decrease the risk of prosthesis fracture. However, it has identical requirements to a fixed prosthesis because it is rigid during function (hidden cantilever situation).

In the case of removable prostheses with mobility and soft tissue support, two prosthetic levers of height should be considered. The first is the height of the attachment system to the crest of the bone. The greater the height distance, the greater are the forces applied to the bar, screws, and implants. The second CHS to consider is the distance from the attachment to the occlusal plane. This distance represents the increase in prosthetic forces applied to the attachment. Therefore in a CHS of 15 mm, an O-ring may be 7 mm from the crest of bone, resulting in a lever action of 7 mm applied to the implants. The distance from the rotation point of the O-ring to the occlusal plane may be an additional 8 mm. Under these conditions, a greater lever action is applied to the prosthesis than to the implant interface. This results in increased instability of the restoration under lateral forces.[42]

A larger CHS results in the substructure requiring a greater bulk of material. This often may predispose the patient to fractured

restorative material (Fig. 21.17). With metal based casted substructure, control of surface porosities after casting becomes increasingly difficult because their different parts cool at different rates.[50] If not controlled properly, both of these factors increase the risk of porcelain fracture after loading.[51] For excessive CHS, considerable weight of the prosthesis (approaching 3 ounces of alloy) may affect maxillary trial placement appointments because the restoration does not remain in place without the use of adhesive. Because noble metals must be used to control the alloy's heat expansion or corrosion, the cost of such implant restorations is dramatically increased. Proposed methods to produce hollow frames to alleviate these problems include using special custom trays to achieve a passive fit, which can double or triple the labor costs.[52]

An alternative method to fabricate fixed prostheses in situations of a CHS 15 mm or greater is the fixed complete denture or hybrid prosthesis, which has a smaller metal framework, denture teeth, and acrylic resin to join the materials together (Fig. 21.18). Unfortunately, this type of prosthesis has a high incidence of fracture/delamination. On occasion, undercontoured interproximal areas are designed by the laboratory in restorations of large CHS to assist oral hygiene, and they have been referred to as high-water restorations. This is an excellent method in the mandible; however, it results in food entrapment, affects air flow patterns, and may contribute to speech problems in the anterior maxilla.

Because crown height is a considerable force magnifier, the greater the crown height, the shorter the prosthetic cantilever should extend from the implant support system. In crown heights of more than 15 mm, no cantilever should be considered unless all other force factors are minimal. The occlusal contact intensity should be reduced on any offset load from the implant support system. Occlusal contacts in CR occlusion may even be eliminated on the most posterior aspect of a cantilever. In this way, a parafunction load may be reduced because the most cantilevered portion of the prosthesis is only loaded during functional activity while eating food.

Reduced Crown Height Space

Issues related to CHS are accentuated by an excessive CHS that places more forces on the implant and prosthetic system, and reduced CHS makes the prosthetic components weaker. A reduced CHS has biomechanical issues related to a reduced strength of implant material or prosthetic components, an increased flexibility of the material, and a reduction of retention requirement of the restoration. The fatigue strength and flexure of a material is related to its radius to the power of 4. In fixed restorations,

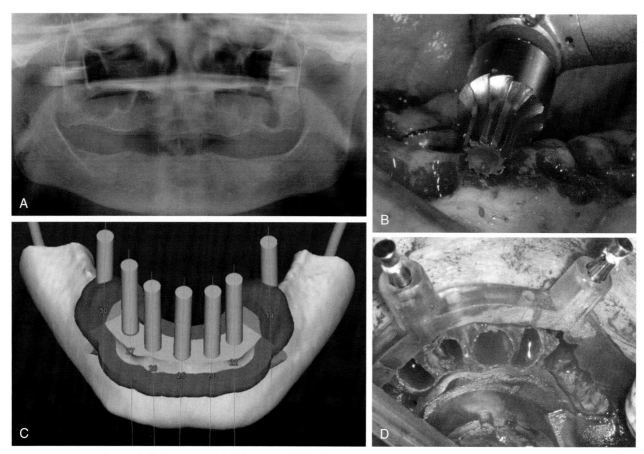

• **Fig. 21.19** Reduced crown height space (CHS). (A) Panoramic radiograph depicting a compromised CHS (red arrows). (B) An osteoplasty using a ridge reduction bur is indicated to increase the CHS before implant insertion. (C) A cone beam computerized tomography reduction guide may be fabricated via interactive treatment planning software to simulate the amount of bone to be removed. (D) Stackable reduction surgical guide fixated onto host bone for preparation of ridge reduction.

the flexure of the reduced-diameter material may cause porcelain fracture, screw loosening, or uncemented restorations. Therefore in the situation of reduced CHS, material failures are more likely (Box 21.5).

Skeletal discrepancies (deep bite), reduced OVD from attrition or abrasion, minimal bone atrophy after tooth loss, and supraeruption of unopposed teeth may all result in less than ideal space for prosthetic replacement of the dentition. Traditional prosthetic and restorative procedures are indicated to restore the proper OVD and plane of occlusion. However, on occasion, even when the opposing arch is corrected, the CHS may still be less than ideal (<8 mm). The 8-mm minimum requirement for CHS consists of 2-mm occlusal material space, 4-mm minimum abutment height for retention, and 2 mm above the bone for the biological width dimension (which does not include the sulcus because a crown margin may be 1 mm subgingival for retention or esthetics). When the reduced OVD is in partially edentulous patients, the OVD may be restored by orthodontics, which is the preferred method. This correction may also require a surgical orthognathic surgery, such as a LeFort I osteotomy and superior repositioning. However, prosthetics is a common approach and may involve an entire arch.

When the opposing teeth are in the correct position and the CHS is insufficient, additional space may be gained surgically with osteoplasty and soft tissue reduction of one arch, provided adequate bone height remains after the procedure for predictable implant placement and prosthetic support (Fig. 21.19). If a removable implant-supported prosthesis is planned, an aggressive alveoloplasty should often be performed after tooth extraction to provide adequate prosthetic space.

Additional prosthetic space can also be obtained in many clinical situations by soft tissue reduction, especially in the maxilla. Soft tissue reduction should be performed in conjunction with second-stage surgery if the implants heal in a submerged location. This allows the thicker tissue to protect the implants from uncontrolled loading by a soft tissue–supported prosthesis during healing. If the implants heal permucosally, then the reduction procedures should be done during implant placement. Soft tissue reduction procedures may include gingivectomy, removal of connective tissue, or apical repositioning of flaps. Efforts should be made to maintain adequate keratinized tissue around the implants. Soft tissue reduction also has the benefit of decreased probing depths around the implants. However, the definition of

CHS is from the bone to the occlusal plane; therefore although the prosthetic space is improved, the CHS remains similar when only soft tissue reduction is performed. Too little CHS can be further complicated when the surgeon places the implant above the bone. When the CHS is less than ideal, the following prosthetic parameters should be identified[42]:

1. Available space
2. Abutment taper
3. Surface area of abutment
4. Cement type
5. Surface finish
6. Occlusal topography and material
7. Load on final restoration
8. Fit of restoration to abutment
9. Retention of prosthesis
10. Implant manufacturer
11. Implant platform to occlusal plane dimension

The consequences of insufficient CHS include a decrease in abutment height (which may lead to inadequate retention of the restoration), inadequate bulk of restorative material for strength or esthetics, and poor hygiene conditions compromising long-term maintenance.[53] In addition, the final restoration flexes inversely to the cube of the thickness of material. A fixed prosthesis half as thick will flex eight times as much and will further result in loss of cement retention, loosening/fracture of fixation screws, or porcelain fracture.[54] Inadequate thickness of occlusal porcelain or acrylic, or unsupported occlusal material caused by inadequate metal substructure design, may also result in complications such as component fracture.

Minimum restorative requirements vary in function of the implant system. The minimum restoration space may be determined by limiting the occlusal material to 1 mm and reducing the abutment height to the top of the retaining screw.

When fabricating a cemented restoration, the restoration technique (indirect versus direct) may be influenced by the CHS. Because additional abutment height for retention may be gained by a subgingival margin, the indirect technique (making an implant body level impression) may have an advantage over a direct intraoral impression. An implant body level impression permits the subgingival restoration to be placed more than 1 mm subgingival, with greater accuracy, representing benefit in a reduced CHS situation, especially when the soft tissue is several millimeters thick. The indirect technique is also used for custom abutments, which can be designed with increased diameter to increase the overall surface area for retention. A custom abutment may also be fabricated to decrease the total occlusal convergence angle to increase retention for cemented prostheses.

The retention and resistance difference between a 3-mm high and a 5-mm high implant abutment may be as great as 40% for a 4.5-mm-diameter abutment. Less than 3 mm of abutment height indicates a screw retained crown, 3 to 4 mm requires a screw retained or resin-cemented restoration, and greater than 4 mm of abutment height allows for clinician's preference. Splinting implants together, regardless of whether they are screw retained or cement retained, can also increase retention.

Conditions such as cement hardness, surface condition of the abutment, and occlusal material (zirconia vs. porcelain vs. metal) are also to be considered in limited CHS situations. The occlusal material is important to consider in reduced CHS for two primary reasons. When zirconia or metal is used as the occluding surface, it is possible to provide greater retention for the prosthesis as a result of an increase in abutment height. The abutment height may be

greater because the occlusal space required above the abutment is only 1 mm, whereas porcelain requires 2 mm of occlusal space and acrylic resin requires 3 mm or more. When a screw is used to retain the crown, the strength of occlusal porcelain is reduced by 40%. Acrylic resin requires the most dimension for strength and is much more likely to fracture when the CHS is limited. This is why acrylic resin overdentures require more CHS than a porcelain-metal fixed prosthesis.

The surgeon may magnify the prosthetic problem of limited CHS by placing the implant at an angle to the ideal position. Angled abutments lose surface area of retention from the abutment screw hole and further compromise the limited space conditions. In addition, a 30-degree taper on an abutment to correct parallelism loses more than 30% of the abutment surface area and dramatically decreases the retention for the abutment.

Overdentures also exhibit greater complications in situations of reduced CHS. Removable prostheses have space requirements for elements such as a connecting bar and the type and position of attachments and restorative material (metal versus resin). According to English, the minimum CHS for individual attachments is 4.5-mm CHS for locator-type attachments and between 12 and 15 mm for a bar and O-rings.[55] Marinbach reported the ideal CHS for removable prostheses is >14 mm and the minimum height is 10.5 mm (i.e., nonbar overdenture).[42] The lowest possible profile attachment should be used in situations of reduced CHS to fit within the contours of the restoration, provide greater bulk of acrylic resin to decrease fracture, and allow proper denture tooth position without the need to weaken the retention and strength of the resin base.

Overdenture bars may be screw retained or cement retained. The most common current method of retention for a fixed prosthesis is screw retained. The most common method of bar retention by almost the same percentage for overdentures is screw retention; yet the advantages of cement retention for a fixed prosthesis also apply to an overdenture bar. Therefore in minimum CHS situations, the screw-retained bar has a clear advantage.

Temporomandibular Joint

The temporomandibular joint (TMJ) may exhibit signs and symptoms of dysfunction. Symptoms include pain and muscular tenderness experienced by the patient. Noises or clicking in the joint during opening, deviation of the mandible during jaw opening, and limited jaw movements are signs of potential dysfunction observed during the patient examination. Patient complaints or signs gathered during this phase should be carefully evaluated before further reconstructive treatment.

Palpation of the temporalis, masseter, and internal and external pterygoid muscles is part of the TMJ examination. The muscles should not be tender during this process. Parafunction may contribute to TMJ disorders and is a direct source of muscle tenderness. Under these conditions, the muscles are usually hypertrophied as a result of the excess occlusal forces. The masseter and temporalis muscles are easily palpated. The lateral pterygoid muscle is often overused in this patient profile, yet is difficult to palpate. The ipsilateral medial pterygoid muscles can be as diagnostic and are easier to evaluate in the hamular notch region. They act as the antagonist to the lateral pterygoid muscle in hyperfunction and, when tender, they are a good indicator of overuse of either muscle. Deviation to one side on opening indicates muscle imbalance on the same side as the deviation and possible degenerative joint disease.[56,57] The patient should also be able to perform unrestricted mandibular excursions. Maximal

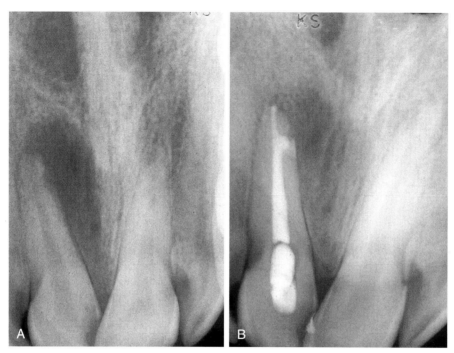

• **Fig. 21.20** (A) A nonvital tooth with an endodontic lesion of more than 5 mm has less than an 88% treatment success rate. (B) The postoperative follow-up of the tooth indicates endodontic success. It may now be restored with less risk of failure. If not successful, extraction rather than retreatment is considered because the retreatment success rate is 65%.

opening is noted during this examination and is normally greater than 40 mm from the maxillary incisal edge to the mandibular incisal edge in an Angle's skeletal class I patient. If any horizontal overjet or vertical overbite exists, it is subtracted from the 40-mm minimum opening measurement.[58] The range of opening without regard to overlap or overbite ranges from 38 to 65 mm in men and 36 to 60 mm in women, from one incisal edge to the other. The practitioner is encouraged to carefully evaluate the TMJ status. It is beyond the scope of this text to address the methods of treatment of TMJ dysfunction. However, many patients with soft tissue–borne prostheses and TMJ dysfunction benefit from the stability and exacting occlusal aspects that implant therapy provides. As such, these patients may benefit from implant support to improve their condition.

Extraction of Teeth with Hopeless or Guarded Prognosis

Maintaining natural teeth in health, function, and esthetics is a primary goal of all dentists. In the past, the maintenance of a natural tooth was paramount because tooth replacement techniques were costly and not as predictable as repairing the natural tooth. However, advanced repair procedures such as apicoectomy, furcation treatment, or functional crown lengthening, may have a lower success rate than an implant to replace the tooth. Therefore on occasion, the natural tooth is significantly compromised and extraction with replacement of an implant is indicated. A tooth may be considered for extraction because of prosthetic, endodontic, or periodontal considerations. On rare occasions, extraction is considered rather than orthodontics to restore the teeth in a more esthetic or functional position.

Caries

Caries on a natural tooth is most often able to be removed and the tooth restored. However, on occasion, the tooth is unrestorable after the decay is removed. A prosthetic axiom is to have at least 1.5 to 2 mm of tooth structure for a crown with a cervical ferule effect. In addition, adequate retention and resistance from the tooth preparation should exist. As a result of the caries, endodontic therapy, post and core, and functional crown lengthening may be required. Thus the procedures to save the tooth are costly and not predictable. On occasion, the end result may not be predictable or esthetically pleasing. For example, when a central incisor requires considerable functional crown lengthening, the gingival margin may be compromised and have a poor esthetic result.

Endodontic Therapy

A patient with a history of an increased decay rate with recurrent caries under a crown, requiring endodontics with a post and core before restoration, may also be better served with an extraction and implant insertion. The repeated recurrent decay can be eliminated, at least for that tooth, with an implant. When caries extend within the root canal, the outer structural walls of the natural root may be too thin for a predictable post or restoration. As a result, extraction and implant insertion has a better prognosis.

Endodontic considerations may also consider tooth extraction rather than traditional treatment. When the root canal cannot be accessed because of abnormal root anatomy, an extraction and implant insertion may be considered. On occasion, the endodontic procedure is compromised or an apicoectomy has a moderate to high risk of paresthesia. An implant after extraction may be less invasive and have less risk of paresthesia. A tooth with "split root" syndrome may have undergone root canal therapy, with pain still present during function. Rather than an apicoectomy, an extraction and implant insertion is usually a definitive treatment that eliminates more predictably pain during function.

A vital tooth has endodontic success rates above 93%, whereas a nonvital tooth has an 89% rate. A large periapical lesion (larger than 5 mm) compromises the success rate of traditional

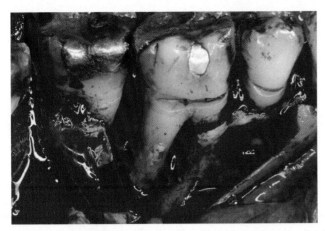

● **Fig. 21.21** Root resection prognosis. A mandibular first molar with a distal root resection generally has a success rate of 75%. Even when successful, the mesial root requires endodontic treatment, core, and crown and the distal root needs replacement. Therefore an implant or three-unit fixed partial denture is indicated. It is more cost-effective to extract, implant, and fabricate one crown, even when bone grafting is indicated.

TABLE 21.1	Extract or Maintain Natural Tooth: 0-, 5-, and 10-Year Rule	
Prognosis	**Protocol**
>10 years	Keep the tooth and restore as indicated
5–10 years	Ideally maintain the teeth and implants as independent prostheses
<5 years	Extract the tooth and graft or immediately place implant in site

endodontics. A nonvital tooth with large periapical pathology has a success rate of 78% (Fig. 21.20).[59,60] Therefore endodontic therapy should be performed and evaluated over several months before post, core, and crown treatment. A retreatment of an endodontic tooth with a periapical lesion has a reported success rate of 65%. As a result, consideration for extraction and implant replacement may be considered for nonvital teeth with more than 5-mm apical radiolucencies that do not resolve or endodontic retreatment when periapical lesions are present. The existing teeth in a partially edentulous patient should be evaluated for longevity and existing disease. Implant dentistry has modified the treatment plan philosophy in these patients.

Periodontal Disease

Advanced periodontal disease may be addressed with extraction of questionable abutments more frequently than in the past, provided the resulting edentulous area offers sufficient bone for predictable endosteal implant placement and a predictable prognosis.[61] Herodontics are discouraged when the prognosis is poor or failure of treatment may result in inadequate bone for implant placement. The cost of the questionable periodontal treatment may result in the patient's inability to afford the more predictable implant therapy later. This is especially noted when the existing available bone around the tooth roots is compromised in height, especially in the posterior mandible. Unsuccessful periodontal treatment and continual bone loss may render the remaining bone inadequate for extraction and placement of implants.

The etiology of furcation involvements includes bacteria and plaque in the furca, with extension of inflammation in the region with loss of interradicular bone. This leads to a progressive and site-specific loss of attachment in most individuals. A first molar furcation entrance cannot be accessed with hand instruments 58% of the time.[62] In addition, pulpal pathoses with accessory canals in the furca may cause problems. Vertical root fracture after endodontic therapy may also occur.

Furcation treatment of molars may include root amputation. The lowest success rate for root resection was found on mandibular distal root resection (75%) (Fig. 21.21). Even when successful, the missing root indicates endodontics, core and crown, and the replacement of the distal root. An implant replaces the entire

tooth, with a higher success rate and often lower cost. A maxillary molar that has lost bone to the furcation has lost almost 30% of the root surface area of support. Therefore when a tooth has a short root or is multirooted, a considerable functional crown lengthening may compromise the remaining support or result in a furcation involvement. The endodontics, post and core, and functional crown lengthening may not be as predictable as extraction and implant insertion. In addition, the cost of conventional treatment may be twice the cost of an implant. Traditional methods to save a tooth have increased in cost over the years. Multirooted endodontic therapy now approaches the cost of an implant surgery. When functional crown lengthening and endodontic post treatment is also required, the fees are usually greater than extraction and implant insertion. Therefore part of the equation of whether to extract or treat a tooth may also relate to the cost of the service provided. The natural molar tooth that requires endodontics, root amputation, post and core placement, and nevertheless a compromised root with poor root surface area may be cost prohibitive for the service provided.

An implant in the site after tooth extraction is often less expensive and more predictable long term. However, the recent trend to extract teeth with a good prognosis after endodontic or periodontal treatment is discouraged. Implants are not yet 100% predictable, and implants should not be substituted for natural teeth presenting a good or even fair prognosis. Table 21.1 summarizes the decision-making protocol involving a natural tooth abutment. The dentist evaluates the natural teeth for their quality of health with widely used prosthetic, periodontal, and endodontic indexes. After this is accomplished, the dentist obtains an estimate of longevity and decides whether to extract or to treat and maintain the tooth, following a 0-year, 5-year, or 10-year rule. If the natural tooth has a favorable prognosis for more than 10 years, it is included in the treatment plan. The decision to use it or not as an abutment requires additional information, but few reasons support removal of the tooth to restore the partially edentulous patient.

If the natural tooth prognosis (after periodontal, endodontic, or restorative therapy when necessary) is in the 5- to 10-year range, independent implant-supported prostheses are indicated. If the edentulous region does not provide sufficient implant support for an independent restoration, then placement of as many implants as possible around the tooth, with treatment alternatives that will permit removal of the tooth without sacrificing the restoration, is indicated. For example, a coping may be placed on the tooth with a 5- to 10-year prognosis, and the tooth may act as "living pontic" in the final restoration, surrounded by sufficient implant support. Whether the tooth is missing or present does not matter. In this way, the prosthesis may be removed in the future and the tooth may be removed (if indicated). The prosthesis essentially is maintained without compromise.[63-65]

The copings on the teeth should be designed with a different path of insertion than fixed partial dentures (FPDs) and should be cemented with permanent cement, whereas the fixed implant prosthesis usually is cemented with a weaker (soft access) or temporary cement. Thus the FPD path of removal differs from that of the natural tooth coping and, along with the weaker cement, allows the prosthesis to be removed while the coping remains permanently cemented on the tooth. The preparation of copings on natural teeth often requires additional removal of tooth structure to prevent overcontoured restorations and, consequently, may mandate endodontic therapy. If hygiene is poor with patients with a high caries index or with grade II or grade III furca involvement in molars, the tooth most often is considered in the 0- to 5-year category and is considered for extraction, especially when other teeth in the same quadrant are missing or hopeless, or only 8 to 10 mm of bone remains between the crest of bone and the opposing landmark. A less than 5-year prognosis for a natural tooth adjacent to an edentulous site, despite restorative or periodontal therapy, warrants extraction of the tooth, with grafting and planning for additional implant abutment support as part of the initial treatment plan. This treatment scenario may often be faster, easier, and less costly over a 5- to 10-year period compared with maintaining a questionable adjacent tooth. Mandibular molars with grade I furcation involvement often are placed in the 5- to 10-year prognosis category. However, maxillary molars are at higher risk of furca complications and are lost 33% of the time within 5 years. Mandibular molars have a 20% failure at this same reference time. After the molar has a grade II or higher furca, it has a greater risk of failure and may be placed in the 0- to 5-year category.[66-69] The dentist should evaluate teeth especially next to multiple edentulous sites. A natural tooth distant from the future implant restoration site is less likely to affect the implant reconstruction and alter the treatment sequences in this site. However, failure of a natural tooth adjacent to an implant site may cause failure of the adjacent implant and almost always (whether failure occurs or not) causes the restoration to be delayed and compromised. Therefore if the practitioner is not sure whether the tooth is in the 0- to 5-year or 5- to 10-year category, the tooth more often should be considered to have the poorer prognosis.

Existing Prostheses

When present, existing prostheses are evaluated for proper design and function. A removable partial soft tissue–supported restoration opposing the proposed implant-supported prosthesis is of particular interest. The occlusal forces vary widely as the underlying bone remodels. The patient may not even wear the opposing removable partial denture in the future, which will dramatically modify the occlusal conditions. Therefore continued maintenance and follow-up evaluations are indicated, including relines and occlusal evaluation.

The patient should be asked whether esthetic desires are met with the current restorations. It is not unusual that the prosthesis is completely acceptable, yet the patient wishes a different shade or contour for the teeth. If unacceptable to the patient, the reasons for dissatisfaction are noted. In addition, the existing restorations are evaluated throughout the mouth for clinical harmony. It is better to leave a poor esthetic restoration that is in occlusal harmony than to provide one that is esthetic but improper in position because the latter may influence all future restorations. Pontic regions of existing prostheses may often be improved with the addition of connective tissue grafts.

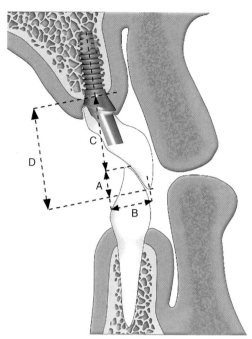

• **Fig. 21.22** Dental arch form may be different than the arch form of the residual arch. A tapered dentate arch form on a square residual bone form is the worst combination because the anterior teeth are cantilevered from the implant abutments. (A) Amount of vertical overbite, (B) Amount of maxillary anterior cantilever, (C) Vertical crown height space minus overbite, (D) Maxillary bone level to incisal edge.

An acceptable preexisting maxillary removable prosthesis, which will be replaced with a fixed implant prosthesis, may be used as a template for implant reconstruction when fabricating an implant-supported fixed or removable implant prosthesis. The thickness of the labial flange of the existing denture is evaluated and is often removed to evaluate the difference in lip position and support. If implants may be correctly inserted, yet additional lip support is needed once the labial flange is eliminated, an HA, connective tissue, or acellular dermal onlay graft is usually indicated. This graft is not intended for implant support or placement; rather, it is intended to enhance the support of the labial alveolar mucosa to improve maxillary lip support.

Arch Form

The edentulous arch form in the horizontal plane is described as ovoid, tapering, or square. In the edentulous patient, the ovoid arch form is the most common, followed by the square, then the tapered form. The square arch form may result from the initial formation of the basal skeletal bone. However, the presence of a square arch form is more common in maxillary implant patients as the result of labial bone resorption of the premaxilla region when anterior teeth are lost earlier than the canine. The tapering arch form is often found in skeletal class II patients as a result of parafunctional habits during growth and development. It is common to find different arch forms in the upper and the lower arches.

Two different arch forms are to be considered for implant prostheses. The first arch form is of the residual edentulous bone and determines the A-P distance for implant support. The second arch form is of the replacement teeth position. The dentate and edentulous arch form are not necessarily related, and the worst situation in the maxilla corresponds to a square residual arch form that supports a tapered dental restoration. The cantilever off the available bone is greatest in this combination (Fig. 21.22).

The most ideal biomechanical arch form depends on the restorative situation. The tapering residual ridge arch form is favorable for anterior implants supporting posterior cantilevers. The square dental arch form is preferred when canine and posterior implants are used to support anterior teeth in either arch. The ovoid arch form has qualities of both tapered and square arches.

The arch form is a critical element when anterior implants are splinted together and support a posterior cantilever restoration. For these conditions, a square arch form provides a poorer prognosis than a tapered arch form. The A-P distance or A-P spread is the distance from the center of the most anterior implant to a line joining the distal aspect of the two most distal implants.[55,70] The distance provides an indication as to the amount of cantilever that can be reasonably planned. When five anterior implants in the mandible are used for prosthesis support, the cantilevered posterior section of the restoration should not exceed 2.5 times the A-P spread, when all patient force and stress factors are low. The actual length of the cantilever depends on implant position and on other stress factors, including parafunction, crown height, implant width, and number. In other words, the predominant factors to determine the cantilever length are related to stress and not the A-P distance.[45,46] For example, the distance between two implants supporting a cantilever (C) form a class I lever. For implants 10 mm apart and a 10-mm posterior cantilever, the following forces are applied: a 25-pound force on cantilever C results in a 25-pound force on the most anterior implant from the cantilever (A) and 50 pounds for the nearest implant to the cantilever (B), which acts as a fulcrum. An interimplant distance of 5 mm with the same 10-mm cantilever and a 25-pound force applied on C results in a 50-pound force on A and a 75-pound force on B. The diminution in the distance between implants significantly increases the forces to both implants, but in the first example if a patient with parafunction bites with a 250-pound force on C, the force on implant A is 250 pounds and the force on implant B is 500 pounds. In other words, parafunction is much more meaningful in terms of force than the interimplant distance when designing a cantilever. Therefore A-P distance is only one stress factor to evaluate for cantilever length. Parafunction, crown height, masticatory dynamics, arch position, opposing arch, direction of force, bone density, implant number, implant width, implant design, and A-P distance are all factors to be considered. When the force factors are low and the area factors (implant number, width, and design) are high, the cantilever length may be as much as 2.5 times the A-P distance.

As mentioned previously, anterior endosteal implants often may not be inserted in their ideal location in the maxilla as a result of labial plate resorption and inadequate bone width at the implant site. This not only requires implant placement more palatally compared with the original natural teeth, but it may also negate the lateral and central positions and require the use of the canine regions in more advanced atrophic arches. The resulting restoration is a fixed, anteriorly cantilevered prosthesis to restore the original arch form. Under these conditions, greater stresses are placed on the dentate tapered arch forms compared with dentate square arch forms, with all other factors identical. The maxillary anterior cantilever to replace teeth in a dentate-tapered arch form requires the support of additional implants of greater width and number to counteract the increase in lateral load and moment force. For example, not only are the canine implants necessary, but two more anterior additional implants are suggested, even if bone grafting is required before their placement. In addition, additional posterior implants in the first

BOX 21.6 Teeth Adjacent to Implant Site

1. Abutment options
2. Extract or maintain
3. Adjacent bone anatomy
4. Cantilevers
5. Attaching Implants to teeth
6. Natural and implant pier abutments

BOX 21.7 Natural Abutment Evaluation

1. Abutment size
2. Crown/root (implant) ratio
3. Endodontic status
4. Root configuration
5. Tooth position (in the arch)
6. Parallelism
7. Root surface area
8. Caries: restorability
9. Periodontal status
10. Opposing arch contacts

to second molar region splinted to the most anterior implants are highly suggested. Therefore if a maxillary arch form requires this treatment approach, at least eight implants (four on each side) and an increased A-P distance from molar implants splinted to incisor implants is suggested. In the maxilla, the recommended anterior cantilever dimension is less than for the posterior cantilever in the mandible because of poor bone density and forces directed outside the arch during excursions.

Natural Teeth Adjacent to Implant Site

A common prosthetic axiom is to provide the partially edentulous patient with a fixed prosthesis whenever possible. Implant dentistry often may provide the additional abutments necessary to fulfill this goal, regardless of the number of teeth missing. The ability to add abutments in specific locations, rather than being limited to a particular remaining natural abutment that may not always be in optimum health, enables the dentist to expand this prosthetic axiom to most patients. The dentist may use implants as independent support for the restoration or rarely, along with natural teeth in the same prosthesis. In either situation, the treatment plan is strongly influenced by the dental evaluation of the remaining natural abutments adjacent to the edentulous site. Natural teeth may require additional therapy before the final prosthesis can be completed. It is best to communicate with the patient regarding all required treatment involved in the rehabilitation process before the surgical placement of the implants. Otherwise, treatment outcome sequences and cost may conflict with the originally projected result and lead to dissatisfaction, the need to modify the original treatment plan, or a poorer prognosis.

Whether considered for abutment support or not, teeth adjacent to a partially edentulous site are evaluated thoroughly and from a different perspective than the rest of the dentition. Often the adjacent tooth exhibits bone loss next to the edentulous site and presents a less than optimal quality of health. In addition, the available bone characteristics immediately adjacent to the tooth are highly influenced by its presence. Often this is a determining factor in the choice between an independent implant prosthesis, a traditional FPD, or a removable restoration. When multiple teeth are missing, the treatment becomes even more complex with additional restorative options, such as whether implants and natural teeth may serve as abutments in the same prosthesis.

The dental criteria of the adjacent tooth to an edentulous space addressed in this section are outlined in Box 21.6, as well as important parameters to evaluate in considering implants and teeth in the same restoration. Additional considerations to help assess the restorability of teeth adjacent to potential implant sites appear in Box 21.7.

Abutment Options

Several options are available for the restoration of an edentulous segment. Under ideal conditions, placing implant abutments in sufficient number to fabricate a completely implant-supported prosthesis has several advantages. The most common cause of failure of tooth-supported fixed prostheses is caries of the abutment teeth.[71-73] Unrestored natural teeth do not decay as often as restored teeth, and implant abutments do not decay. The second most common cause of fixed prosthesis failure is endodontic failure or complications of a natural tooth abutment. Implant abutments do not need endodontic therapy. As a result, the 10-year survival rates indicate a greater than 25% improved survival rate for implant prosthesis compared with FPDs supported by natural teeth.[74,75] Natural teeth abutments compared with unrestored natural teeth are more difficult to clean, collect and retain more plaque, are often more temperature or contact sensitive, and are more subject to future prosthetic periodontal or endodontic treatment. Caries, endodontic problems, or both may cause not only a loss of the fixed prosthesis more than 25% of the time within 10 years, but they almost as often lead to the failure and extraction of at least one of the natural tooth abutments. As a result, an independent implant restoration is the treatment of choice for almost every multiple-tooth edentulous site in a partially edentulous patient.[76]

Natural teeth respond to occlusal forces differently than implants. A light force produces most of the recorded movement of a tooth, whereas the amplitude of implant movement is related directly to the force applied.[77-79] In arches with implant and natural abutments, it is easier to adjust two independent prostheses. When planning an independent implant prosthesis, instead of using a natural tooth as one of the terminal abutments, the dentist usually requires the addition of at least one more implant. An increase in implant abutment number enhances the implant–bone interface and therefore reduces the stress to the support system and improves the ability of the fixed restoration to withstand additional forces, when necessary. In addition, because of the additional retentive units, uncemented or unretained restorations occur with less frequency. Unretained restorations are the third most common complication reported in fixed prosthodontics.[73,74] Abutment screw loosening is a common complication reported for implant prostheses, especially during the first year.[43,80-86]

The increase in implant number also decreases the amount of forces on the abutment screws, thus the risk of abutment screw loosening; as a result, many reasons justify the use of a sufficient number of implants for an independent prosthesis. So many advantages exist for an independent implant-supported fixed prosthesis with multiple units that such a treatment is always the first choice when possible. Unfortunately, completely implant-supported fixed prostheses in partially edentulous patients are not always feasible and carry a higher surgical risk. Thus the natural tooth occasionally may be considered a potential abutment. However, the dentist

should consider splinting of implants and natural teeth within the same prosthesis only when the surface area of the implant support does not permit replacement of the total number of missing teeth and additional implant placement is not a possibility.

Adjacent Bone Anatomy

The edentulous bony structure adjacent to a natural tooth varies in height, width, length, and angulation and is a reflection of the history of the former tooth. If the ridge topography is not ideal for endosteal implant placement in the site immediately adjacent to the natural abutment, then the dentist should consider a bone graft or a pontic. An osteoplasty needed to obtain adequate bone width in the area adjacent to a natural tooth may compromise the adjacent natural root support, increase the crown height of the final restoration, and affect the esthetic outcome. Therefore osteoplasty to gain additional width is rarely indicated in this situation.

If an ideal prosthodontic abutment position is adjacent to a natural tooth and inadequate bone width is available, augmentation of the edentulous site before implant insertion may improve the bone anatomy without compromising the natural abutment. However, inadequate bone height adjacent to a tooth offers a poorer prognosis for augmentation than in other situations. In general, to grow bone in height is more difficult than to grow it in width. However, when the inadequate bone height of the edentulous site includes the region adjacent to a natural root, the ability to grow additional bone height becomes even more unpredictable and usually unsuccessful. Bone height augmentation is not predictable on a natural tooth root with a horizontal defect. If the natural tooth root has lost bone adjacent to the site, then the bone augmentation in height usually will not occur above the position of bone on the root. An alternative for inadequate bone height next to a natural tooth is orthodontic extrusion, along with the bone graft. The orthodontic movement will increase bone height next to the tooth and improve the bone graft prognosis. However, the tooth usually requires endodontics and restoration after the orthodontic process. An implant apically positioned more than 3 to 4 mm below the cement-enamel junction (CEJ) and interproximal bone level of the natural tooth root presents potential soft tissue contour problems (Fig. 21.23). The soft tissue between the tooth and implant creates a more shallow slope, unlike the steep drop of the level of the bony crest between the elements. Under these conditions, a soft tissue pocket greater than 6 mm may result in the implant crown adjacent to the natural tooth. Therefore when a bone graft for height in a multitooth edentulous site is required to place an implant adequately adjacent to a natural root, the dentist should consider a pontic to replace the missing element next to the natural tooth. The pontic may be supported by a cantilever from implants or teeth or using dual support from teeth and implants. In case of inadequate bone volume adjacent to a tooth, the dentist considers treatment options in this order: (1) graft the site if inadequate in width to permit division A or division B implant placement, (2) cantilever a pontic from two or more natural teeth or two or more division A implants, and (3) fabricate a fixed prosthesis with one pontic connecting an implant with one or two teeth, depending on the adjacent tooth status (Fig. 21.24).

Cantilevers

Cantilevers in fixed prostheses result in moment loads or torque on the abutments.[87-91] They are used more frequently for implant-supported prostheses than natural teeth abutments, and several widely diverging guidelines have been recommended for their use,

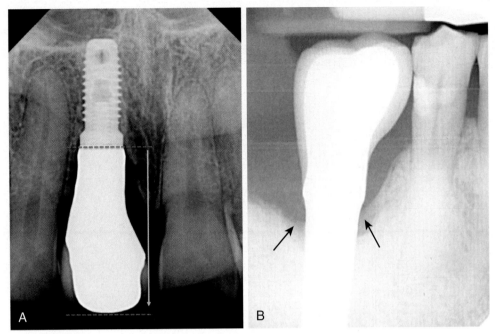

• **Fig. 21.23** Apically positioned implant. (A) Maxillary implant insertion well below the ideal position (i.e., 3 mm below the free gingival margin). (B) Implant positioned too apical leading to crestal bone loss and peri-implant disease.

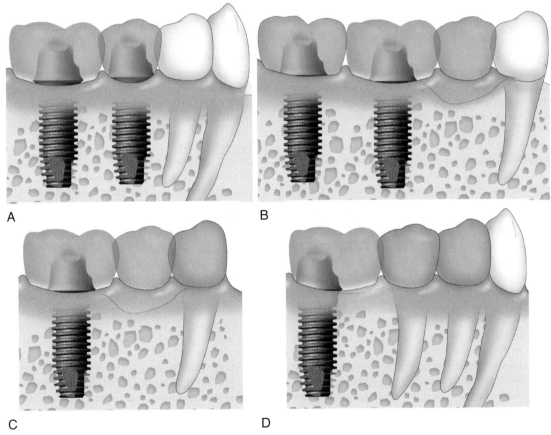

• **Fig. 21.24** (A) When inadequate bone adjacent to a tooth can be grafted for implant placement and an independent prosthesis, this is the ideal treatment of choice. (B) When inadequate bone adjacent to a tooth cannot be grafted, one option is to cantilever the missing tooth from the anterior teeth or from posterior implants. The posterior implants permit the replacement of more than one tooth but require at least two implants in most situations. (C) When the inadequate bone adjacent to a tooth cannot be grafted, another option is to insert an implant more distal and make a three-unit fixed partial denture by connecting the implant to the nonmobile tooth. (D) When the inadequate bone adjacent to a tooth cannot be grafted and the tooth is slightly mobile, one option is to insert an implant more distal and make a four-unit fixed partial denture by connecting the implant to two anterior teeth (when the most anterior tooth is nonmobile).

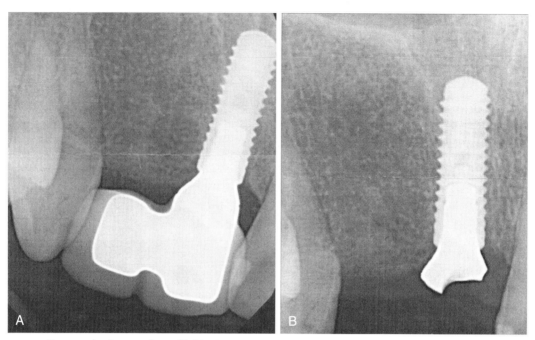

• **Fig. 21.25** Implant cantilever. (A) Maxillary central incisor implant with cantilevered lateral incisor. (B) Because of excessive horizontal forces, the implant prosthesis fractured at the abutment level.

ranging from no extension at all to several teeth.[87-93] The force on the cantilever may be compared with a class I lever. The distance between the most anterior and most distal abutments is divided into the length of the cantilever to determine the mechanical advantage to the farthest abutment from the cantilever. For example, if the implants are 10 mm apart and a distal cantilever of 15 mm is present, then the mechanical advantage is 1.5 times. A 25-pound compressive load (chewing force) is magnified to a tensile load of 37.5 pounds on the most anterior abutment. The abutment closest to the cantilever acts as a fulcrum and receives the sum of the two loads, or a compressive load of 62.5 pounds.

The most common complication for a cantilevered restoration is uncementation of the abutment farthest from the cantilever. This occurs because cement is about 20 times weaker in tension compared with compression forces. For example, the compressive strength of zinc phosphate cement is 12,000 pounds per square inch (psi), but its tensile strength before fracture is only 500 psi. Takayama has suggested that the cantilever should not extend beyond the distance between the implants to keep the mechanical advantage less than one times this distance.[94] The most common distance between two implant centers is 7 to 8 mm (i.e., for a 4-mm diameter implant) so that the outer dimensions of the implants may be 3 mm apart and the crowns on the implants are similar in size to a premolar. Thus the size of the cantilever should not be greater than a premolar of similar size when two implants support the prosthesis. Ideally, if present, a cantilever should extend mesially, rather than distally, to reduce the amount of occlusal force on the lever.[95] The most important factor in determining the length of the cantilever is the amount of force the patient places on the cantilever. In other words, the amount of force generated against the cantilever is more critical than the other factors, including the cantilever length and mechanical advantage. In addition, an angled force is more detrimental than a force in the long axis of the abutments.

The crown height also influences the amount of the force on the cement and bone interface. As such, the cantilever magnifies

any other force factor presented; therefore it should be used with caution. When cantilevers are used in the final restoration, the occlusion on the cantilevered pontics should be reduced, with no contact on the pontic during mandibular excursions. Cantilevers on two implants should not be used when force factors are moderate to severe or when other force factors are present (Fig. 21.25). Instead, additional implants or grafting and implants positioned without cantilevers typically reduce complications.

Attaching Implants to Teeth

Before 1988, many practitioners connected an implant to one or two natural teeth. These implants were designed to have either a fibrous tissue or a direct bone interface. When the root form osseointegration concept of Brånemark for full arch edentulous fixed prostheses became more dominant in the mid-1980s, these implants came to be used in partially edentulous arches. It was hypothesized at the time that joining a rigid implant to a natural tooth would cause biomechanical complications on the implant, implant prosthesis, or both. Since that time, several reports have indicated that a rigid implant may be joined to a natural tooth in the same prosthesis.[96,97] In fact, implant-cantilevered prostheses in partial edentulous patients have more reported complications than when implants are joined to teeth. There are more partially edentulous patients missing posterior teeth than anterior teeth. As a result, the most common scenario for which a root form implant may be joined to a natural tooth is in the posterior regions. Of these cases, the most common scenario is as a terminal abutment in a patient missing the molars. For example, if a patient is missing the first and second molars in a quadrant (with no third molar present), then the segment requires at least two implants of proper size and design to independently restore these two teeth. If adequate bone exists in the second molar and distal half of the first molar but inadequate bone exists in the mesial half of the first molar, then a premolar-size pontic is required. The pontic may be cantilevered from the anterior natural teeth or the posterior implants. Either of

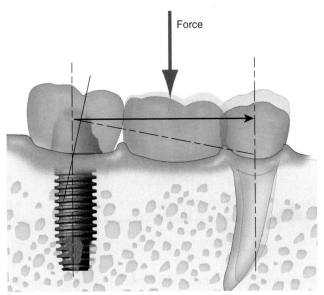

• **Fig. 21.26** Splinting a rigid implant to a natural tooth has caused concerns relative to the biomechanical differential in movement between the implant and tooth. Because the tooth moves more than the implant, the implant may receive a moment force created by the "cantilever" of the prosthesis.

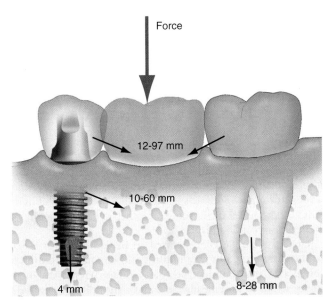

• **Fig. 21.27** Three- or four-unit precious metal prosthesis with an implant and a posterior tooth rigidly splinted has some inherent movement. The implant moves apically 0 to 5 mm, and the tooth moves apically 8 to 28 mm but can rotate up to 75 mm toward the implant because of a moment force. The metal in the prosthesis can flex from 12 to 97 mm, depending on the length of the span and the width of the connecting joints. The abutment-to-implant component movement may be up to 60 mm because of abutment prosthetic screw flexure. As a result, a vertical load on the prosthesis creates little biomechanical risk when joined to a nonmobile tooth because of the design.

these options may result in complications because of tensile forces on the cement seal of the abutment farthest from the pontic.

The connection of natural teeth and osseointegrated implants within a single rigid prosthesis has generated concern in publications, with studies and guidelines for both extremes.

In other words, some articles report complications, but others state that no problem exists. To be more applicable to a particular

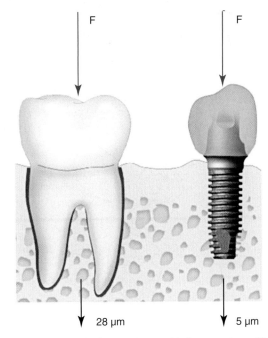

• **Fig. 21.28** Tooth and implant movement. Under normal conditions, the same force applied to a tooth and an implant results in the tooth moving significantly more (28 µm) compared with an implant (5 µm).

situation, more information is required to design a successful treatment plan. Two prosthetic designs are available for the connection of implants and teeth within the same prosthesis: a conventional FPD or an FPD with a nonrigid connector. To address this issue, the mobility of the natural abutment should be assessed (Figs. 21.26 and 21.27).

Etiology

The mobility of potential natural abutments influences the decision to join implants and teeth more than any other factor. In the implant-tooth rigid fixed prosthesis, five components may contribute movement to the system: the implant, the bone, the tooth, the prosthesis, and implant and prosthetic components.

Existing Tooth Mobility

The tooth exhibits normal physiologic movements in vertical, horizontal, and rotational directions. The amount of movement of a natural tooth is related to its surface area and root design. The number and length of the roots; their diameter, shape, and positions; and the health of the periodontal ligament primarily influence tooth mobility. A healthy tooth exhibits no clinical mobility in a vertical direction. Actual initial vertical tooth movement is about 28 µm and is the same for anterior and posterior teeth.[98] The immediate rebound of the tooth is about 7 µm and requires almost 4 hours for full recovery, so additional forces applied within 4 hours depress the tooth less than the original force.[78] The vertical movement of a rigid implant has been measured as 2 to 5 µm under a 10-pound force and is mostly attributable to the viscoelastic properties of the underlying bone (Fig. 21.28).[79] The implant movement is not as rapid as the tooth movement because the tooth movement is a consequence of the periodontal ligament, not the surrounding bone elasticity.

Horizontal tooth mobility is greater than vertical movement. A very light force (500 g) moves the tooth horizontally 56 to 108 µm (Fig. 21.29). The initial horizontal mobility of a healthy, nonmobile

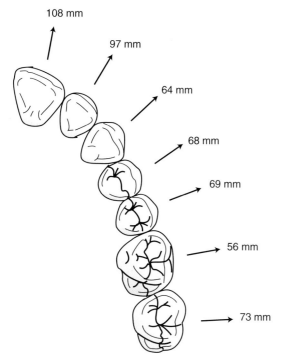

• **Fig. 21.29** Horizontal movement of teeth. A healthy natural tooth may move laterally from 56 to 108 mm, with anterior teeth moving significantly more than posterior teeth.

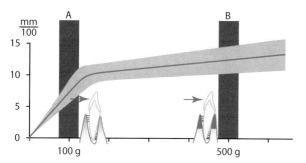

• **Fig. 21.30** Teeth have a primary tooth movement related to a periodontal ligament. This accounts for the 28-µm apical and 56- to 108-µm lateral movement. They also have a delayed secondary mobility related to the viscoelastic nature of bone.

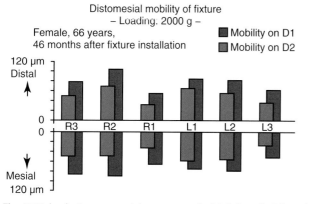

• **Fig. 21.31** Implant movement is more mesiodistal than faciolingual, reaching values between 40 and 115 µm.

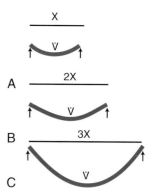

• **Fig. 21.32** Bridge flexure is related to the cube of the span between abutments. (A) Whereas a one-pontic prosthesis may flex 12 µm, (B) a two-pontic prosthesis flexes up to 97 µm. (C) Therefore the flexure will further increase the biomechanical mismatch between the teeth and implants.

posterior tooth is less than that of an anterior tooth and ranges from 56 to 75 µm, which is two to nine times the vertical movement of the tooth. Initial horizontal mobility is even greater in anterior teeth and ranges from 90 to 108 µm in healthy teeth.

Muhlemann found that tooth movement may be divided into initial mobility and secondary movement.[77] The initial mobility is observed with a light force, occurs immediately, and is a consequence of the periodontal ligament. If an additional force is applied to the tooth, then a secondary movement is observed, which is related directly to the amount of force. The secondary tooth movement is related to the viscoelasticity of the bone and measures up to 40 µm under considerably greater force (Fig. 21.30). The secondary tooth movement is similar to implant movement.

Prosthesis Movement

A fixed prosthesis that connects a tooth and implant also illustrates movement. Studies have shown that with a 25-pound vertical force, a prosthesis with a 2-mm connector fabricated in noble metal results in a 12-µm movement for one pontic and 97-µm movement for a two pontic span (Fig. 21.31).[99] The FPD movement helps compensate for some difference in vertical mobility of a healthy tooth and implant.

Rangert and colleagues reported an in vitro study of a fixed prosthesis supported by one implant and one natural tooth and showed that the abutment or gold cylinder screw joint of the system also acts as a flexible element. The inherent flexibility matched the vertical mobility of the natural tooth. The minimal movement of the tooth and the fact that implant, prosthesis, and abutment components have some mobility indicate that the risk is small in the vertical direction, with the biomechanical difference of an implant and a tooth in the same prosthesis when one or two pontics separate these units.[100]

Implant Mobility

The implant–bone interface also exhibits lateral movement. Sekine and colleagues evaluated the movement of endosteal implants with rigid fixation and found a range of 12 to 66 µm of movement in the labiolingual direction.[79] Komiyama measured 40 to 115 µm of implant movement in the mesiodistal direction under a force of 2000 g (≈4.5 psi) and a labiolingual range of 11 to 66 mm (Fig. 21.32).[101] The greater implant movement in the mesiodistal dimension corresponds to the lack of cortical bone around the implants in this direction, compared with the thicker lateral cortical plates present in the labiolingual dimension. The mobility

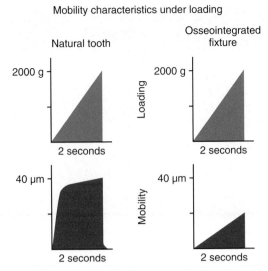

Mobility characteristics under loading

• **Fig. 21.33** Sekine compared tooth movement with a gradual load over 2 seconds *(left)* with implant movement. The secondary tooth movement was similar to implant movement.

of implants varies in direct proportion to the load applied and the bone density, which reflects the elastic deformation of bone tissue.

Although the implant has a range of mobility, the mobility is related to the viscoelastic component of bone, not the physiologic aspect of a periodontal membrane. As such, when the implant and tooth are loaded in the same prosthesis, the tooth immediately moves (primary tooth movement), and then the tooth and implant move together. In other words, secondary tooth movement is similar to implant movement because they both depend on the viscoelasticity of the bone. In a study by Sekine and colleagues[79] when a tooth was gradually loaded over a 2-second period, the tooth immediately moved 36 μm and then gradually moved an additional 6 μm. The implant gradually loaded had movement directly related to the amount of load and eventually moved as much as 22 μm. The secondary tooth movement was similar to the implant movement (Fig. 21.33).

In summary, when all factors are considered, an implant moves vertically and horizontally, the abutments and prosthesis flex, and the tooth has apical and lateral movements. However, the major difference in movement between implants and teeth is more related to the direction of movement (the horizontal dimension is more compared with much less difference in the vertical dimension).

Guidelines for Joining Implants to Teeth

No Lateral Force on Prosthesis. To decrease biomechanical conditions, which increase the risk of complications, a requisite to join an implant to a natural tooth is that no lateral force should be designed on a unilateral prosthesis. Lateral forces increase the amount of tooth movement and decrease the amount of implant movement (faciolingual versus mesiodistal). Horizontal forces placed on an implant also magnify the amount of stress at the crestal bone region.

Natural Tooth with No Clinical Mobility

A vertical movement or force placed on a posterior implant joined to a healthy posterior tooth causes mesial tension on the implant.

The implant can move vertically 3 to 5 μm and mesially 40 to 115 μm, and a noble metal–fixed prosthesis with one pontic allows mesiodistal movement of 6 μm. A natural tooth with

no clinical mobility could be connected rigidly to an osseointegrated implant with no lateral forces because the implant, bone, and prosthesis compensate for the slight tooth movement. Finite element, photoelastic, and clinical documentation confirm that implants can be connected rigidly to stable teeth.[102] However, the occlusion should be modified to allow the initial occlusal contacts on the natural tooth so that the implant does not bear the major portion of the initial load.[103]

The lateral mobility of healthy anterior incisor teeth often is recorded as (+) with a range of movement from 90 to 108 μm. Visual clinical evaluation by the human eye can detect movement greater than 90 μm. When the horizontal mobility of a natural tooth (anterior or posterior) can be observed, mobility is greater than 90 μm and too great to be compensated by the implant, bone, and prosthesis movement.

When the vertical posterior tooth movement, vertical implant movement, mesiodistal implant movement, and prosthesis movement are compared with the same conditions of a "mobile" tooth with lateral loads, the biomechanical risk factors are not the same. One of the primary conditions for joining an implant to natural teeth is the lack of observable clinical movement of the natural abutment during functional movement. Nonmobile posterior teeth with no lateral forces on the prosthesis may join rigid implants. However, implants rarely should be connected to an individual anterior tooth because (1) anterior teeth exhibit more than 10-fold greater clinical mobility than the implant, and (2) the lateral forces applied to the restoration during mandibular excursions are transmitted to the natural tooth and implant abutments.

When the natural abutment exhibits clinical horizontal movement or conditions promote horizontal forces against the abutment tooth, two options can be selected for the final prosthesis. The first, and the option of choice, is to place additional implants and to avoid the inclusion of natural abutments in the final prosthesis. This may include the extraction of the mobile tooth and replacement with an implant. The other option is to improve stress distribution by splinting additional natural abutments until no clinical mobility of the splinted units is observed.

Rigid Connectors Are Contraindicated

Implants should not be joined to mobile teeth with rigid attachments, which basically adds a cantilever on the implant (the tooth acting as a living pontic). If the natural teeth are mobile in relation to the implant in the same prosthesis, several complications may occur that may be detrimental to the tooth and implant.

If the prosthesis is cemented, movement may break the cement–implant abutment seal. Cement does not adhere as well to titanium as to dentin. In addition, the mobile tooth will move (which decreases the impact force) rather than break the cement seal on the tooth. However, the rigid implant will have greater stresses applied to the cement (or screw)-retained crown. After the prosthesis is loose from the implant, greater stress is applied to the natural mobile tooth. The tooth may increase in mobility as a result or fracture as a consequence (especially when endodontic procedures were performed) (Fig. 21.34).

Nonrigid Connectors Are Contraindicated

A mobile attachment between the implant and natural tooth is usually not a benefit. A mobile attachment moves more than an implant or a tooth; therefore it is not an "attachment." The pontic is cantilevered from the implant with little to no support from the tooth. It is usually better to have a rigid connector between implants and teeth than a mobile attachment.

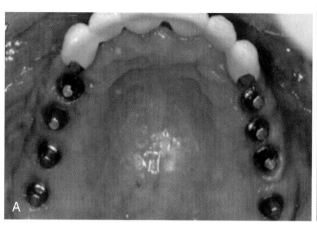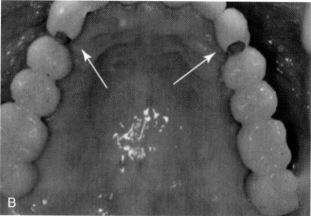

• **Fig. 21.34** Rigid connection implant. (A and B) Treatment plan involving connecting posterior implant-supported crowns to natural teeth. Ideally, the implants should be independent from the teeth.

Although nonrigid connectors have been advocated in the literature, a nonrigid connector in a unilateral prosthesis rarely is indicated for implant-fixed prostheses and may be detrimental.[104] Nonrigid connection does not improve the stress distribution between the different abutments and has been reported to have caused migration of the natural teeth.[105,106]

If the nonrigid connector exhibits any clinically observed mobility, it moves more than the implant. As such, the implant-supported part of the restoration is cantilevered to the attachment. In addition, the nonrigid (or mobile) attachment adds cost, creates over contoured abutments, impairs daily hygiene, and does not decrease the clinical tooth movement.

Prevent Tooth Intrusion. When implants are joined to teeth that act as a terminal abutment, a definitive cement should be used for the natural tooth. The tooth cannot intrude unless it becomes unretained from the abutment (or has a nonrigid connector between the units).

Reports of intrusion of the natural tooth connected to an implant usually include the use of temporary cement to lute a coping to the natural abutment, leaving the final restoration uncemented on the coping, or the use of a nonrigid connector.[107]

A possible explanation for tooth intrusion may be that the tooth is pushed vertically 28 μm but wants to rebound only 8 μm. The fixed prosthesis rebounds immediately and pulls on the tooth. The cement seal eventually breaks, causing a space to develop, which is first occupied by air. The prosthesis then acts as an orthodontic appliance and continually pushes the tooth in a vertical direction. Eventually, the space is occupied by saliva, and hydraulics continue the downward force during mastication. The tooth eventually submerges or intrudes from the prosthesis.

Ideal, Favorable Conditions. An alternative may be to join the implant(s) to a natural tooth if all other factors are favorable. This treatment option is more likely in the presence of a division C–h ridge in the pontic region when inadequate bone height adjacent to the natural tooth decreases the prognosis of a vertical bone graft. This option is also available when a posterior implant is positioned too distal to restore with a single crown. It is almost always better to splint the implant to the adjacent tooth rather than fabricating a cantilevered crown from one implant, especially when parafunction is present.

Pier (Intermediary) Abutments

A pier abutment is one between two other abutments, sometimes referred to as intermediate abutment. The intermediate abutment may be an implant or a natural tooth, and each type plays a different

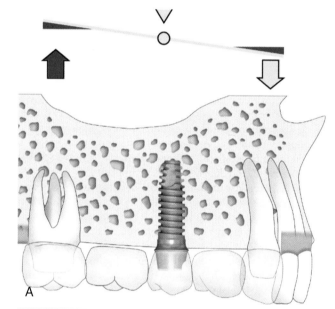
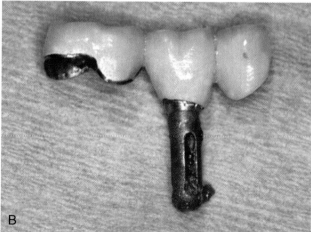

• **Fig. 21.35** (A) When an implant acts as a pier abutment, the biomechanical risk of uncemented restorations is increased, especially under lateral loads. The more rigid implant may act as the fulcrum of a class I lever. The cement seal breaks on the more rigid tooth or the least retentive abutment. (B) This implant was overloaded and failed because the cement seal broke on the natural tooth. The compressive force on the pontic led to a tensile force on the tooth, and the implant acted as a fulcrum. Cement is 10 times weaker under tension. After the cement seal broke from the tooth, all the loads were applied to the implant only, which then failed from overload.

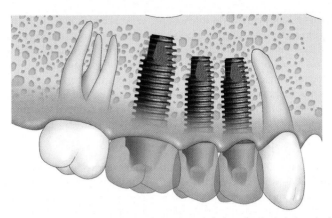

• **Fig. 21.36** Ideal option is to graft the sites and place implants in terminal abutment locations and to fabricate an independent prosthesis.

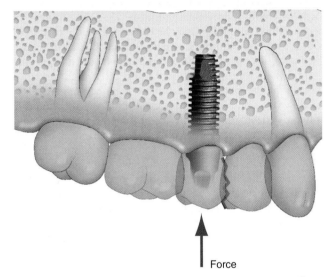

Force

• **Fig. 21.37** When grafting and additional implants are not an option, an attachment should not be used to simulate the movement of the tooth.

role in the overall treatment. When an implant serves as a pier abutment between two natural teeth, the difference in movement between implant and tooth may increase the complication rate compared with one tooth joined to two implants. The pier implant exhibits less movement than a terminal abutment and acts as the fulcrum of a class I lever (Fig. 21.35). This problem is magnified by a longer lever arm such as a pontic between the implant and tooth. A pier implant abutment may cause complications even when joined to nonmobile teeth as terminal abutments. The cement tensile strength is often 20 or more times less than the compressive strength. Therefore when the implant acts as a fulcrum, an uncemented abutment (usually the least mobile tooth or least retentive crown) is a common consequence, with decay being the next most common occurrence. Uncemented restorations are a common complication in FPDs, even when all aspects of treatment are within acceptable limits. Any condition that may increase this problem, such as the one presently addressed, should be carefully avoided. For most clinical situations, an additional implant can be placed in at least one of the sites next to a tooth to provide the support needed to fabricate an independent, cantilevered, implant-supported prosthesis. The better option is to perform bone grafting, place implants in both terminal abutment locations next to the natural teeth, and avoid connecting implants to teeth (Fig. 21.36).When bone grafting is not an option and additional implants cannot be inserted, a mobile attachment can be used to restore the

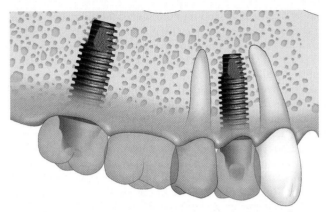

• **Fig. 21.38** When a natural tooth serves as a pier abutment between two or more implants, the tooth may act as a living pontic. No stress breaker is needed in this situation.

implant pier abutment between two natural nonmobile teeth (Fig. 21.37). The nonrigid attachment may connect the implant and the least retentive crown to prevent the implant pier abutment from acting as a fulcrum. In conventional fixed prostheses, the "male" portion of a nonrigid attachment usually is located on the mesial aspect of the posterior pontic, whereas the "female" portion is in the distal aspect of the natural pier abutment tooth. This prevents mesial drift from unseating the attachment.[108] However, an implant does not undergo mesial drifting, and the nonrigid connector location is more flexible. When a natural tooth rather than an implant serves as a pier abutment between two or more implants, the situation is completely different from the previous scenario. When the two or more implants may support the load of the prosthesis alone, the natural tooth becomes a living pontic. In other words, in absence of the tooth, the dental unit would be a pontic. Because the tooth has greater mobility than the implant and does little to contribute to the support of the prosthetic load, it is referred to as a pontic with a root, or a living pontic (no more than one adjacent site should be a pontic) (Fig. 21.38). This scenario is best when no additional pontics are between the implants and the tooth. On occasion, multiple implants are splinted together to cantilever one or two pontics, yet a healthy, natural tooth is positioned among the implants. The tooth essentially is ignored in the development of the treatment plan, other than the dentist having to fabricate a crown rather than a pontic in the splinted prosthesis. For a natural pier abutment between two implants, a stress breaker is not indicated. One advantage of keeping the natural tooth, even though it does not contribute to the support of the prosthesis, is the proprioceptive aspect of the periodontal complex.[97-109] Implant prostheses have higher bite forces during mastication than natural tooth restorations because of the decrease in occlusal awareness. A living pontic may decrease the interaction of the forces found during function.

Natural Abutment Evaluation

The evaluation of a potential abutment adjacent to an edentulous site includes the following: (1) abutment size, (2) crown/root (implant) ratio, (3) tooth position, (4) parallelism, (5) caries, (6) root configuration, (7) root surface area, (8) endodontic status, and (9) periodontal status.

Abutment Size

Uncemented restorations are one of the most common complication of fixed prostheses.[71-73] After the crown on the natural abutment becomes uncemented, a significant concern is caries. Decay may proceed rapidly and result in loss of the abutment, creating a need for endodontic treatment, post and core, a new prosthesis, or an abutment with even poorer retention. These same conditions exist if the natural retainer becomes uncemented from an implant-tooth restoration. In addition, the implant is at greater risk. The fixed prosthesis then acts as a cantilever with a dramatic increase in moment force on the implant. Crestal bone loss, prosthesis or abutment screw fracture, implant fracture, or mobility and failure of the implant are likely complications. When natural and implant abutments are combined in the same prosthesis, uncementation occurs more frequently on the implant. Tooth mobility fatigues the cement seal and increases the forces on the implant. The parameters of retention are similar for a tooth or implant and mainly are influenced by the diameter and height of the abutment.[110-112] Molars are more retentive than premolars because of their increased surface area, with all other factors being equal. Wider implant abutments are more retentive than narrower ones. Limited crown height because of limited interarch space also decreases retention. Splinting of teeth with limited crown height to improve retention often compromises access for hygiene in the interproximal areas. Instead, crown lengthening is often indicated in case of limited interarch space to improve the retention of the prosthesis and the esthetic result without compromising home care. A customized abutment of larger diameter can be used on an implant abutment of reduced height. Crowns of reduced size require minimal tapering and additional retentive elements, such as grooves or boxes to limit the path of insertion and direction of dislodgment.[111-113]

Crown/Root Ratio

The crown/root ratio represents the height of the crown from the most incisal or occlusal position to the crest of the alveolar ridge around the tooth compared with the height of the root within the bone. This criterion is most important when lateral forces are expected against the crown, as in mandibular excursions. The lateral forces act as a class I lever on the tooth, with the fulcrum at the crest of the bone. As the crown height increases, the root height decreases, creating a force multiplier.

The crown/root ratio is indicative of the risk of mobility and amount of additional stress the tooth may sustain when used as an FPD abutment. A patient with a history of periodontal disease may show an increased crown/root ratio, yet no abutment mobility. However, the long-term risk of mobility is increased if the tooth is used as an abutment for a prosthesis. Lateral forces are most detrimental in this situation because of the increased moment force. Splinting may be indicated to distribute stress, and occlusal schemes must be modified to protect these abutments from horizontal stresses.[114] The most ideal crown/root ratio for a fixed prosthetic abutment is 1:2, but this is rarely observed. A more common condition is 1:1.5, and a 1:1 ratio is the minimum requirement when opposing natural teeth or implants and when serving as an abutment for an implant-tooth prosthesis.[115] In addition, the doctor and patient must realize that teeth with an increased crown/root ratio often are restored with an FP-2 or an FP-3 prosthesis. A high lip line during smiling and low lip line during speech should be evaluated carefully to determine the prosthetic design. Crown/implant ratio is not considered in a similar way as a crown/root ratio. The implant does not rotate around a center located two thirds down the endosteal/root portion, as does a tooth. Instead, it captures the force at the crest of the ridge. The implant length does not affect its mobility and does not affect its resistance to a lateral force. Although a minimum

height requirement does exist and approaches 9 mm, implants greater than 12 mm in healed bone sites do not demonstrate clinical benefit. This is not to say crown height is not important. Crown height is a vertical cantilever on a tooth or implant and will magnify angled, lateral, or cantilever forces. However, the effect of crown height cannot be reduced by increasing the length of the implant. Instead, the dentist should consider reduced cantilever lengths or reduction of angled forces on the prosthesis.

Tooth Position

The dentist considers tooth position next to the edentulous site, including whether the tooth is in the anterior region of the mouth, the intermediate position, or the posterior region. Regardless of arch position, some considerations remain similar. When the natural tooth adjacent to the implant site is in the anterior region, greater mobility and often lateral directions of force are present. Therefore under these conditions the implant is rarely connected to a natural tooth as a terminal abutment. The most common situation in which an implant may be connected rigidly to a natural tooth as a terminal abutment is in a posterior edentulous site with a second or first premolar adjacent to the potential implant site.

The bone adjacent to a natural tooth often is compromised, especially in the long-term edentulous Kennedy-Applegate class I or class II patient. Under these conditions, the edentulous site is often deficient in width and height. As previously mentioned, bone grafting in width is much more predictable than height, especially in the posterior mandibular regions. A sinus graft may provide adequate height of bone for endosteal implants in the posterior maxilla, but onlay grafts on the posterior mandible are much less predictable, and nerve repositioning before implant placement is fraught with potential complications. Bone width augmentation is an usual treatment plan, and bone grafting for height in the posterior maxilla has become a routine procedure, but the posterior mandible is less often a candidate for height augmentation, unless block grafts or more advanced grafting techniques are selected.

When adjacent teeth have been missing for a long time period, the remaining natural abutment often has drifted from its ideal position and frequently exhibits tipping, tilting, rotation, or extrusion. The dentist should consider correction of the natural abutment position in the original treatment plan for the partially edentulous patient, whether or not the natural abutment is joined to the implant. A good habit to utilize is to evaluate and correct any dental unit that will contact the new restoration. Enameloplasty to improve the occlusion or change the contact shape and position next to the implant prosthesis is not unusual. The path of insertion of the implant prosthesis and the size and shape of the interproximal space also may require modification. Treatment also may consist of a crown when beyond the ability merely to reshape the tooth. Orthodontic movement to correct interarch or gross occlusal correction, especially when skeletal patterns require improvement, may be indicated. One can plan orthodontic treatment along with the healing phase for rigid fixated implants. One also may use orthodontic treatment to develop available bone for an implant next to a natural tooth. Moving the tooth slowly through the bone to a more remote position generates bone growth and an improved implant site.

Parallelism

As previously discussed, clinical movement can be eliminated by splinting natural abutments. As such, splinting mandibular incisors is more common in implant dentistry than traditional prosthodontics. These teeth often are crowded or rotated. In addition, the path of insertion of a prosthesis that includes anterior and posterior dental units often requires more extensive tooth preparation. Some of the indications for attachments in a fixed or removable partial denture include joining nonparallel teeth or splinting anterior and posterior teeth in the same prosthesis. The attachment should usually be rigid in design, size, and fabrication. All of these factors limit the path of insertion of the final prosthesis. Several abutments may need endodontic therapy to achieve this goal. If this is not explained to the patient before treatment begins and endodontic therapy is required, the patient often feels that inadequate treatment has been rendered.

Endodontic therapy or posts and crowns for overlapping anteriors still may provide inadequate embrasures for hygiene. This condition not only compromises esthetics but also may result in the loss of more than one tooth because of periodontal disease. Selective extraction of incisors may even be indicated if rotations or overlapping of teeth create an unfavorable environment for daily maintenance.[116]

Caries

The dentist should eliminate all carious lesions before implant placement, even when the teeth will be restored with crowns after implant healing for the final prosthesis. Rigidly fixated implants usually require several months of healing after initial placement. The progression of the decay may alter the final treatment plan, with a decrease in crown retention and increased risk for endodontic therapy, posts, cores, or even loss of a desired abutment. Should endodontic therapy be indicated, the obturation of the canals ideally should be completed before implant surgery to avoid possible confusion in the differential diagnosis, if both treatments were overlapping in time and location. If caries are eliminated at the same time as implant surgery, then elimination of caries should be performed before reflection of any tissue.

Root Configuration

The natural root configuration may affect the amount of additional stress the tooth may withstand without potential complications.[116] Tapered or fused roots and blunted apexes are examples of decreased ability to withstand the additional occlusal loads required for a fixed prosthesis. The maxillary second molar often presents these varied root configurations. Additional implants and independent implant-supported restorations usually are indicated in the presence of these conditions, rather than the use of these teeth as terminal abutments. Root dilaceration or curvatures improve the support quality of an abutment tooth. However, such root morphology also is likely to encroach on the adjacent available bone volume and increase the risk of implant placement. This is exemplified best in the maxillary canine and first premolar region. The canine presents a distal angulation of 11 degrees and has a distal root curvature in 60% of the cases. As such, the first premolar edentulous site is limited. An implant inserted into this site usually should be shorter and should follow the angulation of the canine rather than that of the second premolar. The dentist must evaluate carefully any adjacent natural tooth with curved roots at the apex before implant placement.

Roots with a circular cross section do not represent as good a prosthodontic abutment as those with an ovoid cross section. Therefore the maxillary premolar is a better abutment than the maxillary central incisor, although their root surface areas are similar.[111] The maxillary lateral incisor may exhibit less lateral mobility than the central incisor as a result of its cross-sectional anatomy.[78]

All these factors from traditional prosthodontics are also part of the implant candidate's dental evaluation.

Root Surface Area

In general, the greater the root surface area of a proposed abutment tooth, the greater is the prosthetic support. Posterior teeth provide greater periodontal surface area and greater support than anterior teeth. Teeth affected by periodontal disease lose surface area and represent poorer support elements for a prosthesis. For a maxillary first molar, bone loss to the beginning of the root furcation corresponds to a root surface area loss of 30%.[117] Ante's law requires the root surface area of the abutment teeth to be equal to or greater than that of the teeth replaced by the pontics of the fixed restoration.[118] Although empirical at its inception, Ante's law has withstood the test of time and still serves as a clinical guideline.

Endodontic Evaluation

The natural abutment adjacent to or included in a combined tooth and implant-supported prosthesis should present a healthy pulpal status or successful endodontic treatment. If the pulpal or endodontic status of an abutment is questionable, then the prudent treatment is endodontic therapy. In this way, the abutment crown may be evaluated for retention, for need for post and core, and for any other related criteria before final prosthodontic treatment. Potential lesions of endodontic origin are evaluated best before implant surgery because an exacerbation of the lesion during early implant healing may result in a pathway of destruction to the adjacent implant site, implant failure, and extensive bone loss.

In the literature, success has been reported as low as 47% to as high as 98%. However, most studies report success in the range of 85% to 90% at 5 or more years.[117,119,120] As such, when endodontic treatment has a good prognosis and the tooth may be restored adequately, root canal treatment is in order. However, a number of implant failures each year are attributed to adjacent tooth endodontic failure. At first, this may seem contradictory. Implant healing failures are rare in most practices and account for less than 2% of implants inserted, when using a classic two-step approach. However, when these 2% failures are evaluated, a large number of failures occur next to natural teeth that had an endodontic complication during early implant healing.

Assessment of endodontic success before implant surgery often is difficult.[121-123] The patient may be symptom free, yet a low-grade infection is present at the apex. The healing implant interface is more prone to complications with such a tooth having this condition because the healing interface is weaker than the previous bone condition and a pathway may exist to the developing implant interface. If a tooth is asymptomatic, but has a past endodontic treatment and periapical radiolucency, consideration should be given to retreatment or extraction. When the periapical lesion is 5 mm or greater, the success of endodontic retreatment is not predictable. During the treatment planning phase, teeth adjacent to the edentulous segment should be scrutinized for potential endodontic problems, keeping in mind that the preparation of a tooth for a crown has a 3% to 6% risk of pulpal death as a consequence of the procedure. In addition, past periodontally involved teeth are at greater risk of pulpal disease after tooth preparation.

Periodontal Status

The periodontal evaluation of natural abutments to be connected to implants is identical to the evaluation of other FPD abutments. Special attention may be directed to the adjacent implant site, which may be contaminated by bacteria during periodontal

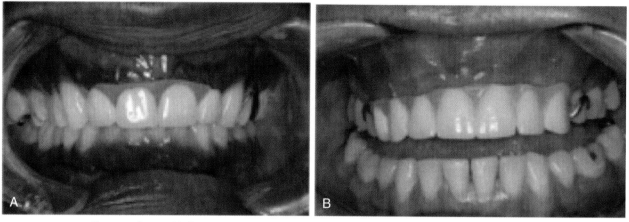

• **Fig. 21.39** Removable "treatment" prosthesis (A and B) To determine the ideal soft tissue profile, esthetics and jaw relationship, a temporary removable prosthesis may be used. Note how the facial flanges have been modified to reduced facial soft tissue profile.

surgery. The incision line and flap design for implant placement often includes the abutment teeth. The implant surgeon should decide whether periodontal therapy is indicated on the abutment teeth before or at the same time as implant placement. A reduction in the number of surgical procedures is a noteworthy benefit to the patient; however, active infection should be minimized during implant placement. Therefore the pathologic condition of the abutment teeth most often is addressed before the soft tissue reflection in the region of the implant osteotomy. Dental prophylaxis and oral hygiene considerations are usually scheduled before implant surgery. The use of 0.12% chlorhexidine to reduce the bacterial count is most beneficial.

In summary, a completely implant-supported prosthesis is desirable, independent of the natural teeth. Grafting the edentulous site or the use of additional implants is the usually treatment of choice. However, when insufficient implant support is available, the natural teeth may be considered as potential abutments. The most important natural tooth criterion for implant-tooth–supported restorations is tooth mobility. A clinical assessment of zero mobility often allows a rigid connection between the tooth and implant. However, if mobility is present, the practitioner should design the prosthesis to include more natural abutments and return the dental elements to zero mobility or consider an independent implant restoration. Splinting natural teeth is the usual method to reduce mobility.

Several additional factors are critical for dual implant-tooth support of a fixed prosthesis: crown size, crown/root ratio, tooth position, parallelism, caries, root configuration, root surface area, endodontics, and periodontal status. Although these same criteria are important for any fixed restoration, each presents unique aspects in implant- and tooth-supported prostheses.

Soft Tissue Support

The evaluation of the soft tissue support is a primary concern when evaluating potential implant sites. Of utmost importance is the soft tissue support when planning an RP-5 overdenture prostheses (i.e., gains primary support from the soft tissue and secondary support from the implants). The following factors need to be evaluated: ridge shape, size, parallelism, and palate shape. Large ridge forms with minimal resorption provide a better support than smaller ridge forms with greater atrophy, in either the maxilla or mandible (Fig. 21.39).

Prosthesis support depends on the shape of the residual ridge and, in the maxilla, the palatal vault. A square ridge form yields optimal resistance and stability. A relatively flat one represents a compromised factor for retention and stability, although support is still adequate. Tapering ridges on the palatal vault usually equate with poor stability.[124-126] Ridge parallelism is also evaluated. The edentulous ridge parallel to the occlusal plane is most favorable for soft tissue support. If ridges are divergent, stability of the denture will be greatly affected.

The lateral throat form in patients with a maxillary denture or RP-5 restoration should be evaluated. A soft palate slope is favorable when it has a long, gradual slope from the junction of the hard and soft palate,[127] which allows a greater extension of the posterior palatal seal and enhances retention. On the other hand, a soft palate class III, which drops abruptly, may lead to soreness, loss of valve seal, and gagging. These elements are of great diagnostic value in the evaluation of the maxillary fully edentulous patient who may consider an implant-supported overdenture. A greater number of unfavorable anatomic structures may direct the treatment plan toward an RP-4 prosthesis with greater implant support and no soft tissue support to address all the needs of the patient. It must be emphasized to the patient that a partial or total soft tissue–borne prosthesis will not stabilize bone loss. In contrast, bone loss will continue and may even be accelerated because the prosthesis is more often worn and bite forces are increased. As a result, all soft tissue–borne prostheses should be considered transitional dentures. Most of these prostheses require repeated relines, rebasing, and refabrication to replace the missing bone. A totally implant-supported prosthesis (fixed or removable) does not require soft tissue support and may be considered a definitive restoration.

Many soft tissue–supported restorations are fabricated because the patient cannot afford a totally implant-supported prosthesis especially in the completely edentulous patient. However, the clinician often forgets that if a patient cannot afford the ideal treatment today, it does not mean the patient cannot afford any further treatment later. For example, if a patient requires four first molars replaced, but cannot afford all restorations at this time, the doctor most often can still restore one of the molars. Then a few years later the next tooth may be restored. Eventually, the four molars are treated and the arch form and occlusion restored. In similar fashion, a patient who can afford only two implants to retain a

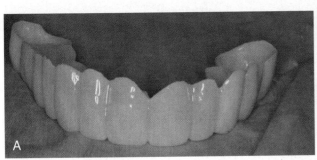
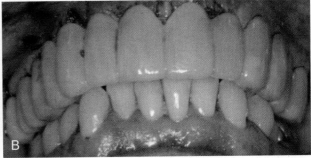

● **Fig. 21.40** Smile transition (Glidewell Laboratories, Newport Beach, California). (A) Interim prosthesis used to restore function, evaluate jaw relations ("treatment prosthesis"). (B) The interim prosthesis is inserted over the remaining abutment teeth which allows for evaluation of esthetics, function, jaw relations, as well as decreases force to the future implant sites.

● **BOX 21.8** Implant Treatment Prostheses

1. Assist with diagnosis
   a. Crown lengthening indications
   b. Occlusal plane evaluation
   c. Hopeless teeth determination
2. Evaluate the psychological profile of the patient
   a. Denture before implant surgery
3. Improve soft tissues before final impression for implant overdentures
4. Maintain soft tissue profile during postoperative healing period
5. Evaluate occlusal vertical dimension
6. Evaluate temporomandibular joint status
7. Improve implant position related to final tooth position
8. Evaluate esthetics before surgery
9. Evaluate hygienic contours of fixed restorations
10. Determine whether removable restoration is required for maxillary lip support (RP versus FP)
11. Protect bone graft or implants during healing
12. Patient's financial and compliance management
13. Progressive bone loading procedures
14. Phonetics and esthetics for full arch implant–FPs on complete edentulous patients

FP, Fixed prosthesis; *RP*, removable prosthesis.

mandibular denture could possibly afford further treatment later. Therefore a lifetime strategy for health should be established, which may include the addition of more implants in the future to reduce and eventually halt the continued bone loss and consequences on esthetics and function.

Pretreatment Prostheses

Fixed Treatment Prostheses

Pretreatment prostheses in implant dentistry are often indicated to obtain a diagnosis, improve soft tissue health before fabricating soft tissue–borne restorations, reestablish or confirm the vertical dimension, evaluate esthetic considerations, or treat TMJ dysfunction (Fig. 21.40). In addition, the pretreatment prosthesis may be used to select a prosthetic option, to progressively load bone to improve its strength, and as a transitional restoration to protect a healing bone graft or implant. Immediate loading of an implant system often uses a transitional prosthesis out of occlusion in a partial edentulous situation. In the completely edentulous immediate load restoration, the transitional prosthesis has no cantilevers in nonesthetic areas.

Treatment prostheses may also help evaluate the psychological attitude of a patient before irreversible implant procedures (Box 21.8).

Diagnosis in medicine is the first step to establishing a treatment for a disease or disorder. Likewise, to establish a treatment plan for a partially or completely edentulous patient, a proper diagnosis should be established. A treatment prosthesis may be required to help in this process. For example, questionable teeth may require initial restoration to assess their prognosis related to whether or not the extraction of the tooth and implant replacement therapy is required. A treatment prosthesis may correct the existing occlusal plane, identify extruded teeth, and indicate whether endodontic therapy, crown lengthening, or extraction is required to complete the final treatment plan. Remember, after prosthetic crown lengthening is performed, usually at least 4 mm of tooth structure is supracrestal (2 mm for connective tissue and junctional epithelial attachment and 2 mm to create a ferrule effect with the crown to reduce the risk of root fracture). Also, the crown/root ratio is increased and the mobility of the tooth should be evaluated. Excessive mobility may require additional implants, splinting teeth, or even extraction and additional implant insertion. A long-span partially edentulous patient often wears a fixed-treatment prosthesis, which also acts as an interim prosthesis. Metal-reinforced transitional prostheses may be used when four or five pontics are present. These fixed, transitional treatment prostheses may be used during bone grafts or healing of implants to decrease forces on the soft tissues and on the graft or healing implants.

Removable Treatment Prostheses

Treatment prostheses may be used to improve the soft tissues used for support, stability, or retention before RP-5 overdenture or complete denture restorative procedures. The first evidence of residual ridge destruction by an ill-fitting denture is often deformed and traumatized overlying soft tissue.[128] The soft tissue bed may exhibit different degrees of redundant hyperplasia, epulis, hypertrophy, or abrasions.[129,130] A tissue conditioning treatment is usually indicated to restore soft tissue health before making the final impression for the soft tissue bone prosthesis. The soft tissue conditioner may need to be replaced every 2 to 3 days, although 10 to 14 days are usually sufficient to return the soft tissue to normal condition. The existing denture can often be used as the treatment prosthesis. Additional treatment such as surgical removal of excessive hypermobile tissues is often warranted before soft tissue conditioning.

It should be noted that soft tissue conditioners are different from soft liners used in soft tissue support areas of removable prostheses. Tissue conditioners usually change dimensions during the first 18 to 24 hours. As such, as the tissues return to a more normal condition,

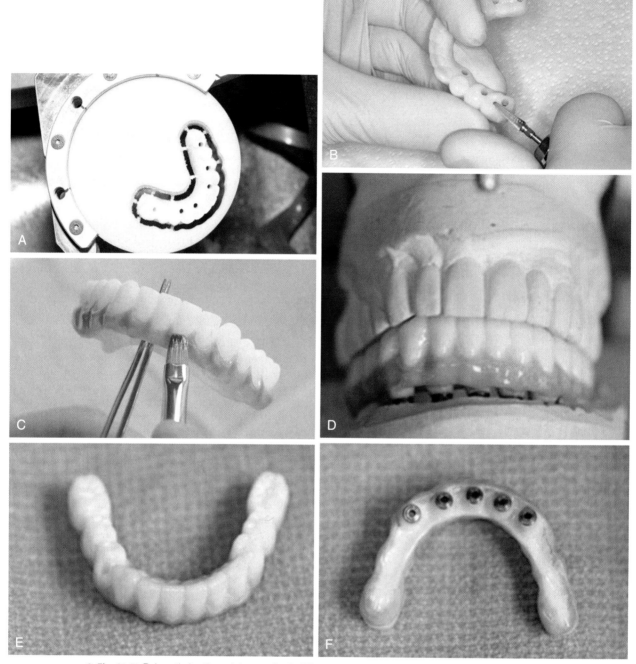

• **Fig. 21.41** Polymethylmethacrylate prosthesis (PMMA). (A) From a diagnostic wax-up or scan of an interim prosthesis, a PMMA prosthesis is milled. (B) Prosthesis polishing. (C) Staining of the prosthesis. (D–F) Final interim PMMA prosthesis.

the material changes dimension to allow and encourage these changes. However, many tissue conditioners contain modifiers required for this reaction leach out of the material, halt the process within a day, and result in a stiff material. Soft liners, on the other hand, stay soft longer than tissue conditioners, especially when coated with a sealer. However, the material does not change dimension during the first day and therefore will not accommodate a changing tissue condition.

Most often, tissue conditioners are used to improve abused tissues before a final soft tissue impression for a removable prosthesis. In addition, these materials are used after implant surgery in regions under a removable prosthesis, while the implant–bone interface heals. The tissue conditioner may respond to the swelling and tissue changes immediately after soft tissue reflection. In

addition, it is relieved over the implant site. At the suture removal appointment, the tissue conditioner is removed and replaced with a sealed soft liner. This material remains soft during extended periods and is less likely to load the implant through the soft tissue.

Postimplant Placement Transitional Prosthesis

Usually for full arch prostheses, a transitional prosthesis maybe fabricated to function as a long-term provisional prosthesis. The most common transitional prosthesis is made of polymethylmethacrylate (PMMA). Because of advanced innovations in dental computer-aided design (CAD)/computer-aided manufacturing (CAM) technology, these prostheses can now be milled from a single block of

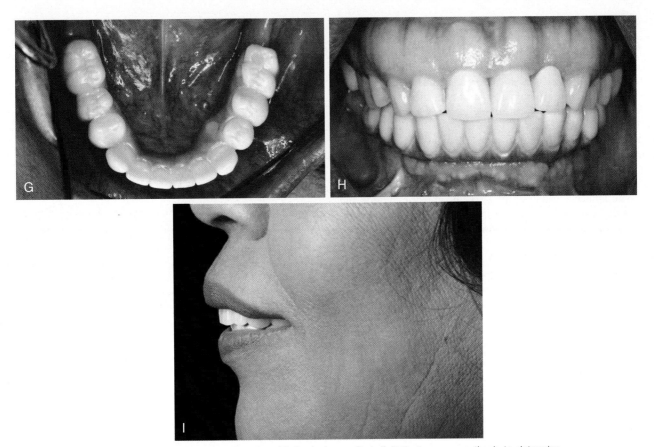

Fig. 21.41, cont'd (G) Intraoral insertion. (H) Occlusion verified. (I) Patient wears prosthesis to determine ideal esthetics, occlusion, and vertical dimension.

• BOX 21.9 Advantages of a Polymethylmethacrylate Interim Prosthesis

- CAD/CAM milled from a single block of polymethylmethacrylate
- Avoids traditional wax try-in procedures
- Patient is able to evaluate function, esthetics, and contours of the prosthesis
- Ease of final prosthesis after patient approval
- Maintains vertical dimensions and prevent soft tissue collapse.

CAD/CAM, Computer-aided design/computer-aided manufacturing.

---

material, resulting in a strong, durable, and esthetic provisional that is resistant to wear, fracture, and staining. The patient may then adapt to the prosthesis with emphasis on the esthetics, occlusion, and vertical dimension before the completion of the final prosthesis (Fig. 21.41; Box 21.9). In addition, these type of prostheses allow the patient and clinician the latitude to determine if any changes such as vertical dimension, occlusion, esthetics, and soft tissue profile require changes to be made in final prosthesis.

Occlusal Vertical Dimension

Long-term edentulous patients who have been wearing the same denture may require a treatment prosthesis to restore the OVD and ridge relationship before implant treatment.[131] The OVD may gradually collapse, especially in the completely edentulous patient, as a result of continued bone loss and prosthesis occlusal wear. TMJ and myofascial dysfunction may be the further consequence of this condition. A treatment prosthesis to reestablish the

proper OVD or assess a symptomatic joint helps determine the patient's specific needs regarding the dysfunction.

As the OVD decreases, the mandibular jaw rotates forward and closes in a more prognathic pseudo–class III relationship. To place the implants in the correct angulation, the OVD should be reestablished before implant surgery so the correct position of the teeth relative to the arch is established. In the case of immediate implant loading, a treatment prosthesis is delivered at or soon after the implant surgery. The design of the prosthetic superstructure concomitant with the implant substructure is necessary for immediate loading in implant overdentures. Therefore a treatment prosthesis is indicated to establish the proper OVD and tooth position before the placement of the implants and fabrication of the superstructure bar.

As the OVD increases, the maxillomandibular relationship evolves toward a class II relationship. This influences the position or angulation of the implant. In addition, the location of an overdenture bar may be equally influenced by variations of the OVD. The treatment prosthesis may be used to establish prosthetic position of teeth.

If a PMMA was prosthesis cannot be utilized, an alternative if for the placement of a conventional removable prosthesis. This type of prosthesis is most likely fabricated with acrylic teeth to facilitate recontouring and the addition of cold-cured acrylic for repairs or to change the OVD or lip support.

Esthetic Assessment

On occasion, a patient's desire for esthetic improvement may be very demanding or unrealistic. In the completely edentulous patient, a treatment denture (partial or complete) may be used to satisfy those esthetic concerns before implant surgery. Tooth shape, surface quality, size and position, tooth color, lip and soft tissue contour, tooth position, gingival color, soft tissue contour, and papilla support may all be evaluated. If the patient cannot be satisfied with the pretreatment prosthesis, it is far better to realize this before implant placement or final prosthesis insertion. Although demanding patients may not be satisfied with the pretreatment prosthesis, they can decide to lower expectations and continue with treatment or be referred to another dentist. If the latter is chosen, it is prudent to contact the next practitioner and inform them that another pretreatment prosthesis is indicated before implant placement.

A high lip line in the maxilla or low lip line position in the mandible may influence the need for a specific gingival contour and color in the restoration, yet the maintenance needs of the restoration may compromise the final esthetic result. A fixed restoration must be designed to allow access for proper hygiene procedures around the teeth and implants. A pretreatment prosthesis may help determine whether an implant-supported removable prosthesis rather than a fixed restoration is required to satisfy the patient's esthetic goals and desires for the restoration, yet may be removed to allow proper daily maintenance. The maxillary vermilion border of this lip is usually altered by the loss of the maxillary anterior teeth. After bone is also lost, the natural support of the entire lip is often deficient and is dependent on the labial flange of the prosthesis. An FPD may require an anterior cantilever away from the soft tissue in a horizontal and vertical dimension to provide this support. A pretreatment prosthesis can provide the information required to determine whether a fixed prosthesis will compromise esthetics, support, or hygiene in this region above the teeth.

Another advantage of a transitional prosthesis is the ability to progressively load the implants. A prosthesis to improve the quality of bone is most always used in D3 or D4 bone-supporting implants before the fabrication of the final restoration. Interim (provisional) acrylic restorations that gradually load bone for progressive loading may be considered pretreatment prostheses. A decrease in crestal bone loss and decrease in implant failure, especially in soft bone types, are particular advantages with progressively loaded treatment prostheses. Pretreatment prostheses also assist in the determination of the final form and function of the final prosthesis, especially for completely edentulous patients. "Pretreatment" prosthesis may be the first full arch–fixed restoration they have worn after several years of wearing a complete denture, thereby allowing an easier transition period.

Summary

Preimplant prosthodontics for partial or fully edentulous patients include overall evaluation of five intraoral segments: (1) the maxillary incisal edge, (2) the OVD, (3) the mandibular incisor edge, (4) the maxillary occlusal plane, and the (5) mandibular occlusal plane.

In addition, there are 10 specific criteria that affect a treatment plan: (1) lip lines, (2) maxillomandibular relationships, (3) existing occlusion, (4) CHS, (5) TMJ status, (6) extraction of hopeless or guarded-prognosis teeth, (7) existing prosthesis, (8) arch form, (9) natural tooth adjacent to an edentulous space, and (10) soft tissue evaluation. Pretreatment prostheses are also used in an implant prosthetic evaluation process.

The prosthodontic evaluation of the implant candidate borrows several conventional criteria from the evaluation of natural abutments. In addition, many of these situations require a unique approach for implant prosthodontics and may influence the implant treatment plan. The goal of the implant surgeon is to achieve

predictable, rigid fixation of endosteal implants. The restoring dentist's responsibility is to maintain the implant–bone interface in an environment that satisfies all the traditional prosthodontic criteria.

References

1. Rufenacht CR. *Fundamentals of Esthetics*. Chicago: Quintessence; 1990.
2. Lynn BD. The significance of anatomic landmarks in complete denture service. *J Prosthet Dent*. 1964;14:456.
3. Harper RN. The incisive papilla: the basis of a technique to reproduce the positions of key teeth in prosthodontics. *J Dent Res*. 1948;27:661.
4. Vig RG, Brundo GC. The kinetics of anterior tooth display. *J Prosthet Dent*. 1978;39:502–504.
5. Hulsey CM. An esthetic evaluation of lip-teeth relationships present in smile. *Am J Orthod*. 1970;57:132.
6. Matthews TG. The anatomy of smile. *J Prosthet Dent*. 1978;39:128.
7. Robinson SC. Physiological placement of artificial anterior teeth. *Can Dent J*. 1969;35:260–266.
8. Misch CE. Incisal edge position, the canine is the guide. *J Prosth-Odontics*. (in press).
9. The glossary of prosthodontic terms. *J Prosthet Dent*. 1999;81: 39–110.
10. Sharry JJ. *Complete Denture Prosthodontics*. New York: McGraw-Hill; 1968.
11. Shannon TEJ. Physiologic vertical dimension and centric relation. *J Prosthet Dent*. 1956;6:741–747.
12. Kois JC, Phillips KM. Occlusal vertical dimension: alteration concerns. *Compend Contin Educ Dent*. 1997;18:1169–1180.
13. Niswonger ME. The rest position of the mandible and centric relation. *J Am Dent Assoc*. 1934;21:1572–1582.
14. Silverman MM. Accurate measurement of vertical dimension by phonetics and the speaking centric space, part I. *Dent Dig*. 1951;57:265.
15. Pound E. Let /S/ be your guide. *J Prosthet Dent*. 1977;38:482–489.
16. Pound E. Utilizing speech to simplify a personalized denture service. *J Prosthet Dent*. 1970;24:586–600.
17. McGee GF. Use of facial measurements in determining vertical dimension. *J Am Dent Assoc*. 1947;35:342–350.
18. Danikas D, Panagopoulos G. The golden ratio and proportions of beauty. *Plast Reconstr Surg*. 2004;114:1009.
19. Amoric M. The golden number: applications to cranio-facial evaluation. *Funct Orthod*. 1995;12:18.
20. Haralabakis NB, Lagoudakis M, Spanodakis E. A study of esthetic harmony and balance of the facial soft tissue [in Greek (modern)]. *Orthod Epitheor*. 1989;1:175.
21. da Vinci L. *The Anatomy of Man*. Drawings from the collection of Her Majesty Queen Elizabeth II, Windsor, United Kingdom, ca 1488.
22. Misch CE. Vertical Occlusal Dimension by Facial Measurement, *Continuum: Misch Implant Institute Newsletter*, summer, 1997.
23. Misch CE. Objectives subjective methods for determining vertical dimensions of occlusion. *Quintessence Int*. 2000;31:280–281.
24. Mach MR. Facially generated occlusal vertical dimension. *Compendium*. 1997;18:1183–1194.
25. Ricketts RM. The biologic significance of the divine proportion and Fibonacci series. *Am J Orthod*. 1982;1:357–370.
26. Brzoza D, Barrera N, Contasti G, et al. Predicting vertical dimension with cephalograms, for edentulous patients. *Gerodontology*. 2005;22:98–103.
27. Ciftci Y, Kocadereli I, Canay S, et al. Cephalometric evaluation of maxillomandibular relationships in patients wearing complete dentures: a pilot study. *Angle Orthod*. 2005;75:821–825.
28. Kelly E. Changes caused by a mandibular removable partial denture opposing a maxillary complete denture. *J Prosthet Dent*. 1978;27:140–150.
29. Renner RP, Boucher LJ. *Removable Partial Dentures*. Chicago: Quintessence; 1987.

30. Laney WR, Gibilisco JA. *Diagnosis and Treatment in Prosthodontics.* Philadelphia: Lea & Febiger; 1983:164–165.

31. Kokich VO, Kiyak Hl, Shapiro PA. Comparing the perception of dentists and lay people to altered dental esthetics. *J Esthetic Dent.* 1999;11:311–324.

32. Kokich VG, Spear FM, Kokich VO. Maximizing anterior esthetics: an interdisciplinary approach: esthetics and orthodontics. In: McNamara JA, ed. *Craniofacial Growth Series.* Ann Arbor, Mich: Center for Human Growth and Development, University of Michigan; 2001.

33. Levin EI. Dental esthetics and the golden proportion. *J Prosthet Dent.* 1978;40:244.

34. Pound E. *Personalized Denture Procedures: Dentist's Manual.* Anaheim, Calif: Denar Corp; 1973.

35. Robbins WJ. *The Incisal Edge Position in Complex Restorative Dentistry.* Texas GP: spring; 2000:12–13.

36. Tjan AHL, Miller GD, Josephine GP. Some esthetic factors in a smile. *J Prosthet Dent.* 1984;51:24–28.

37. Crispin BJ, Watson JF. Margin placement of esthetic veneer crowns. Part 1: anterior tooth visibility. *J Prosthet Dent.* 1981;45:278–282.

38. Cade RE. The role of the mandibular anterior teeth in complete denture esthetics. *J Prosthet Dent.* 1979;42:368–370.

39. Pietrokovski J, Masseler M. Alveolar ridge resorption following tooth extraction. *J Prosthet Dent.* 1967;17:21–27.

40. Misch CE. Natural teeth adjacent to multiple implant sites: effect on diagnosis and treatment plan. In: Misch CE, ed. *Dental Implant Prosthetics.* St Louis: Mosby; 2005.

41. Misch CE, Goodacre CJ, Finley JM, et al. Consensus Conference Panel Report: crown-height space guidelines for implant dentistry—part 1. *Implant Dent.* 2005;14:312–318.

42. Misch CE, Goodacre CJ, Finley JM, et al. Consensus Conference Panel Report: crown-height space guidelines for implant dentistry—part 2. *Implant Dent.* 2006;15:113–121.

43. Goodacre CJ, Bernal G, Rungcharassaeng K, et al. Clinical complications with implants and implant prostheses. *J Prosthet Dent.* 2003;90:121–132.

44. Bragger U, Aeschlimann S, Burgin W, et al. Biological and technical complications and failures with fixed partial dentures (FPD) on implants and teeth after four to five years of function. *Clin Oral Impl Res.* 2001;12:26–43.

45. Bidez MW, Misch CE. Issues in bone mechanics related to oral implants. *Impl Dent.* 1992;1:289–294.

46. Bidez MW, Misch CE. Force transfer in implant dentistry: basic concepts and principles. *J Oral Implant.* 1992;18:264–274.

47. Kakudo Y, Amano N. Dynamic changes in jaw bones of rabbit and dogs during occlusion, mastication and swallowing. *J Osaka Univ Dent Soc.* 1972;6:126–136.

48. Kakudo Y, Ishida A. Mechanism of dynamic responses of canine and human skull due to occlusal masticatory and orthodontic forces. *J Osaka Univ Dent Soc.* 1972;6:137–144.

49. Jensen OT, Cockrell R, Kuheke L, et al. Anterior maxillary alveolar distraction osteogenesis—a prospective 5-year clinical study. *Int J Oral Maxillofac Implants.* 2002;17:507–516.

50. Bidger DV, Nicholls JI. Distortion of ceramometal fixed partial dentures during the firing cycle. *J Prosthet Dent.* 1981;45:507–514.

51. Bertolotti RL, Moffa JP. Creep rate of porcelain-bonding alloys as a function of temperature. *J Dent Res.* 1980;59:2061–2065.

52. Bryant RA, Nicholls JI. Measurement of distortion in fixed partial dentures resulting from degassing. *J Prosthet Dent.* 1979;42:515–520.

53. Finley JM. *Personal Communication;* 2005.

54. Smyd E. Mechanics of dental structures. Guide to teaching dental engineering at undergraduate level. *J Prosthet Dent.* 1952;2:668–692.

55. English CE. The mandibular overdenture supported by implants in the anterior symphysis: a prescription for implant placement and bar prosthesis design. *Dent Implantol Update.* 1993;4:9–14.

56. Dawson PE. *Evaluation, Diagnosis and Treatment of Occlusal Problems.* 2nd ed. St Louis: Mosby; 1989.

57. Dawson PE. Determining the determinants of occlusion. *Int Periodont Rest Dent.* 1983;6:9.

58. Tanaka TT. Recognition of the pain formula for head, neck and TMJ disorders. The general physical examination. *Calif Dent Assoc J.* 1984;12:43–49.

59. Farzaneh M, Abitbol S, Friedman S. Treatment outcome in endodontics: the Toronto study. Phases I and II: orthograde retreatment. *J Endod.* 2004;30:627–633.

60. Farzaneh M, Abitbol S, Lawrence HP, et al. Treatment outcome in endodontics—the Toronto study. Phase II: initial treatment. *J Endod.* 2004;30:302–309.

61. Klokkevold PR, Newman MG. Current status of dental implants: a periodontal perspective. *Int J Oral Maxillofac Implants.* 2000;15:56–65.

62. Bower RC. Furcation morphology relative to periodontal treatment: furcation entrance architecture. *J Periodontol.* 1979;50:23–27.

63. Linkow LI, Chercheve R. *Theories and Techniques in Oral Implants.* St Louis: Mosby; 1970.

64. Balshi TJ. Osseointegration for the periodontally compromised patient. *Int J Prosthodont.* 1988;1:51–58.

65. Reider CE. Copings on tooth and implant abutments for superstructure prostheses. *Int J Periodontics Restorative Dent.* 1990;10:437–454.

66. Langer B, Sullivan DY. Osseointegration: its impact on the interrelationship of periodontics and implant dentistry, part II. *Int J Periodontics Rest Dent.* 1989;9:165–183.

67. Hamp SE, Ravald N, Teiwik A, et al. Modes of furcation treatment in a long-term prospective study. *J Parodontol.* 1992;11:11–23.

68. Muller HP, Eger T, Lange DE. Management of furcation-involved teeth: a retrospective analysis. *J Clin Periodontol.* 1995;22:911–917.

69. Wang HL, Burgett FG, Shyr Y, et al. The influence of molar furcation involvement and mobility on future clinical periodontal attachment loss. *J Periodontol.* 1994;65:25–29.

70. English CE. Prosthodontic prescriptions for mandibular implant overdentures—part 1. *Dent Implantol Update.* 1996;7:25–28.

71. Holm C, Tidehaq P, Tillberg A, et al. Longevity and quality of FPDs: a retrospective study of restorations 30, 20, and 10 years after insertion. *Int J Prosth.* 2003;16:283–289.

72. Goodacre CJ, Bernal G, Rungcharassaeng K, et al. Clinical complications in fixed prosthodontics. *J Prosthet Dent.* 2003;90:31–41.

73. Tan K, Pjetursson BE, Lang NP, et al. A systematic review of the survival and complication rates of fixed partial dentures (FPDs) after an observation period of at least 5 years. III. Conventional FPDs. *Clin Oral Impl Res.* 2004;15:654–666.

74. Priest G. Failure rates of restorations for single tooth replacement. *Int J Prosthodont.* 1996;9:38–45.

75. Pjetursson BE, Tan K, Lang NP, et al. A systematic review of the survival and complication rates of fixed partial dentures (FPDs) after an observation period of at least 5 years. I. Implant-supported FPDs. *Clin Oral Impl Res.* 2004;15:625–642.

76. Priest G, Priest J. The economics of implants for single missing teeth. *Dental Econ.* 2004:130–138.

77. Muhlemann HR. Tooth mobility: a review of clinical aspects and research findings. *J Periodontol.* 1967;38:686–708.

78. Parfitt GS. Measurement of the physiologic mobility of individual teeth in an axial direction. *J Dent Res.* 1960;39:608–612.

79. Sekine H, Komiyama Y, Hotta H, et al. Mobility characteristics and tactile sensitivity of osseointegrated fixture-supporting systems. In: van Steenberghe D, ed. *Tissue Integration in Oral Maxillofacial Reconstruction.* Amsterdam: Elsevier; 1986.

80. Dixon DI, Breeding LC, Sadler JB, et al. Comparison of screw loosening, rotation, and deflection among three implant designs. *J Prosthet Dent.* 1995;74:270–278.

81. US Food and Drug Administration. *MDR Data Device Experience Network Database.* Rockville, MD: Center for Devices and Radiological Health CDRH/FDA; 1995.

82. Balshi TJ, Hernandez RE, Pryszlak MC, et al. A comparative study of one implant versus two replacing a single molar. *Int J Maxillofac Implants*. 1996;11:372–378.

83. Gunne J, Astrand P, Ahlen K, et al. Implants in partially edentulous patients. *Clin Oral Implants Res*. 1992;3:49–56.

84. Naert I, Quirynen M, van Steenberghe D, et al. A six year prosthodontic study of 509 consecutively inserted implants for the treatment of partial edentulism. *J Prosthet Dent*. 1992;67:236–245.

85. Hemmings KW, Schmitt A, Zarb GA. Complications and maintenance requirements for fixed prostheses and overdentures in the edentulous mandible: a 5-year report. *Int J Oral Maxillofac Implants*. 1994;9:191–196.

86. Gunne J, Jemt T, Linden B. Implant treatment in partially edentulous patients: a report on prostheses after 3 years. *Int J Prosthodont*. 1994;7:143–148.

87. English CE. The critical A-P spread. *Implant Soc*. 1990;1:2–3.

88. Falk H, Laurell L, Lundgren D. Occlusal force pattern in dentitions with mandibular implant-supported fixed cantilever prostheses occluded with complete dentures. *Int J Oral Maxillofac Implants*. 1989;4:55–62.

89. Falk H, Laurell L, Lundgren D. Occlusal interferences and cantilever joint stress in implant-supported prostheses occluding with complete dentures. *Int J Oral Maxillofac Implants*. 1990;5:70–77.

90. White SN, Caputo AA, Anderkvist T. Effect of cantilever length on stress transfer by implant-supported prostheses. *J Prosthet Dent*. 1994;71:493–499.

91. Wang S, Hobkirk JA. Load distribution on implants with a cantilevered superstructure: an in vitro pilot study. *Implant Dent*. 1996;5:36–42.

92. McAlarney ME, Stavropoulos DN. Determination of cantilever length-anterior-posterior spread ratio assuming failure criteria to be the compromise of the prosthesis retaining screw-prosthesis joint. *Int J Oral Maxillofac Implants*. 1996;11:331–339.

93. Schackleton JL, Carr L, Slabbert JC, et al. Survival of fixed implant supported prostheses related to cantilever lengths. *J Prosthet Dent*. 1994;71:23–26.

94. Takayama H. Biomechanical considerations on osseointegrated implants. In: Hobo S, Ichida E, Garcia CT, eds. *Osseointegration and Occlusal Rehabilitation*. Chicago: Quintessence; 1989.

95. English CE. Biomechanical concerns with fixed partial dentures involving implants. *Implant Dent*. 1993;2:221–242.

96. Astrand P, Borg K, Gunne J, et al. Combination of natural teeth and osseointegrated implants as prosthesis abutments: a 2-year longitudinal study. *Int J Oral Maxillofac Implants*. 1991;6:305–312.

97. Cavicchia, Fabrizio, Bravi F. Free-standing vs tooth-connected implant supported fixed partial restorations: a comparative retrospective clinical study of the prosthetic results. *Int J Oral Maxillofac Implants*. 1994;9(6).

98. Adell R, Lekholm U, Rockler B, et al. A 15-year study of osseointegrated implant in the treatment of the edentulous jaw. *Int J Oral Surg*. 1981;6:387.

99. Bidez MW, Lemons JE, Isenberg BF. Displacements of precious and nonprecious dental bridges utilizing endosseous implants as distal abutments. *J Biomed Mater Res*. 1986;20:785–797.

100. Rangert B, Gunne J, Sullivan DY. Mechanical aspects of a Brånemark implant connected to a natural tooth: an in vitro study. *Int J Oral Maxillofac Implants*. 1991;6:177–186.

101. Komiyama Y. Clinical and research experience with osseointegrated implants in Japan. In: Albrektsson T, Zarb G, eds. *The Brånemark Osseointegrated Implant*. Chicago: Quintessence; 1989.

102. Ismail YH, Misch CM, Pipko DJ, et al. Stress analysis of a natural tooth connected to an osseointegrated implant in a fixed prosthesis. *J Dent Res*. 1991;70:460.

103. Misch CE, Bidez MW. Implant protected occlusion, a biomechanical rationale. *Compendium*. 1994;15:1330–1342.

104. Shillingburg HT, Fisher DW. Nonrigid connectors for fixed partial dentures. *J Am Dent Assoc*. 1973;87:1195–1199.

105. Misch CM, Ismail YH. Finite element analysis of tooth to implant fixed partial denture designs. *J Prosthodont*. 1993;2:83–92.

106. Pesun IJ. Intrusion of teeth in the combination implant-to-natural-tooth fixed partial denture: a review of the theories. *J Prosthodont*. 1997;6:268–277.

107. Cho GC, Chee WL. Apparent intrusion of natural teeth under an implant supported prosthesis: a clinical report. *J Prosthet Dent*. 1992;68:3–5.

108. Shillingburg HT, Fisher DW. Nonrigid connectors for fixed partial dentures. *J Am Dent Assoc*. 1973;87:1195–1199.

109. Kay HB. Free standing implant-tooth interconnected restorations: understanding the prosthodontic perspective. *Int J Periodontics Restorative Dent*. 1993;13:47–69.

110. DeClercq M, Naert I, Theuniers G, et al. Damages at implant parts and prosthetical superstructures supported by osseointegrated implants. *J Dent Res*. 1989;68:901.

111. Shillinburg HT, Hobo S, Whitsett LD, et al. *Fundamentals of Fixed Prosthodontics*. 3rd ed. Chicago: Quintessence; 1997.

112. Kaufmann EG, Coelho AB, Colin L. Factors influencing the retention of cemented gold castings. *J Prosthet Dent*. 1961;11:487–502.

113. Jorgensen KD. The relationship between retention and convergence angle in cemented veneer crowns. *Acta Odontol Scand*. 1955;13:35–40.

114. Reynolds JM. Abutment selection for fixed prosthodontics. *J Prosthet Dent*. 1968;19:483.

115. Penny RE, Kraal JH. Crown to root ratio: its significance in restorative dentistry. *J Prosthet Dent*. 1979;42:34–38.

116. Laney WR, Gibilisco JA. *Diagnosis and Treatment in Prosthodontics*. Philadelphia: Lea & Febiger; 1983.

117. Rapp EL, Brown Jr CE, Newton CW. An analysis of success and failure of apicoectomies. *J Endod*. 1991;17:508–512.

118. Ante IH. The fundamental principles of abutments. *Mich Dent Soc Bull*. 1926;8:14.

119. Sjogren U, Hagglund B, Sundquist G, et al. Factors affecting the long-term results of endodontic treatment. *J Endod*. 1990;16:498–504.

120. Peak JD. The success of endodontic treatment in general dental practice: a restrospective clinical and radiographic study. *Prim Dent Care*. 1994;1:9–13.

121. Esposito M, Hirsch J, Lekholm U, et al. Differential diagnosis and treatment strategies for biologic complications and failing oral implants: a review of the literature. *Int J Oral Maxillofac Implants*. 1999;14:472–490.

122. Brisman DL, Brisman AS, Moses MS. Implant failures associated with asymptomatic endodontically treated teeth. *J Am Dent Assoc*. 2001;132:191–195.

123. Shaffer M, Juruaz D, Haggerty P. The effect of periradicular endodontic pathosis on the apical region of adjacent implants. *Oral Surg Oral Med Oral Pathol Oral Radiol Endod*. 1998;86:578–581.

124. Laney WR, Desjardins RP. Surgical preparation of the partially edentulous patient. *Dent Clin North Am*. 1973;17:611–630.

125. Zarb GA, Bolender CL, Hickey JC, et al. Diagnosis and treatment planning for the patient with no teeth remaining. In: Zaeb GA, Bolender CL, eds. *Boucher's Prosthodontic Treatment for Edentulous Patients*. 10th ed. St Louis: Mosby; 1990.

126. House MM. *Full Denture Technique*. Notes from study club; 1950.

127. House MM. The relationship of oral examination to dental diagnosis. *J Prosthet Dent*. 1958;8:208–219.

128. Lytle RB. Soft tissue displacement beneath removable partial and complete dentures. *J Prosthet Dent*. 1962;12:34–43.

129. Lambson GO. Papillary hyperplasia of the palate. *J Prosthet Dent*. 1966;16:636–645.

130. Lytle RB. The management of abused oral tissue in complete denture construction. *J Prosthet Dent*. 1957;7:27–42.

131. Turbyfill WF. The successful mandibular denture implant. Part two. *Dent Econ*. 1996:104–106.

22

Single and Multiple Tooth Replacement: Treatment Options

RANDOLPH R. RESNIK AND NEIL I. PARK

The introduction of the dental implant has greatly expanded the scope of services that clinicians can provide to restore dental patients to optimal form, function, and esthetics. Patients with missing teeth or pathology that necessitate tooth extraction now have numerous treatment options beyond fixed bridges or removable prosthetics. The progressive loss of bone as a consequence of tooth extraction can now be minimized. Implant technology has allowed practitioners to come much closer to the ideal goal of assisting patients with attaining or retaining dental health.

Clinicians are often confronted with patients with either an edentulous condition or a pathology that necessitates tooth removal. The clinician has an ethical and legal obligation to educate the patient as to the advantages and disadvantages of every therapeutic option available to restore the patient back to dental health.

The goal of this chapter is to provide clinicians with a comprehensive treatment protocol for common edentulous conditions, including advantages and disadvantages of each. By informing the patient of each option available (including no treatment), the dental professional can aid the patient in forming an educated choice for treatment that meets his or her needs and values.

Tooth Replacement

In the United States, 70% of the dentate population is missing at least one tooth. Single-tooth replacement will most likely comprise a larger percentage of prosthetic dentistry in the future, compared with past generations. In 1960 the average American older than 55 years had just seven original teeth. Currently, the average 65-year-old has 18 natural teeth, and baby boomers (those born between 1946 and 1964) can expect to have at least 24 natural teeth when they reach 65 years of age[1] (Fig. 22.1).

When evaluating options for tooth replacements, it is prudent of the clinician to use evidence-based medicine, which consists of conscientious, explicit, and judicious use of the best literature and research in making decisions concerning the care of individual patients. Over the years researchers have observed that external clinical evidence would both invalidate previously accepted treatment and allow replacement with new modalities that are more

efficacious and safer. Therefore an evidence-based approach should be applied to treatment planning for the replacement of teeth.[2]

When discussing a treatment plan with a patient, it is quite easy to get mentally focused on a certain treatment option, based on the actual needs and perceived values of the patient. Implant clinicians sometimes favor certain treatments (i.e., overdenture versus fixed prosthesis) according to their learning curve, training, or personal preferences. It is imperative from an ethical and legal perspective that the clinician discuss all treatment options, including a conversation concerning each option's advantages and disadvantages. Most state dental boards in the United States require as part of their dental law code that all patients be given all possible and viable options, including advantages and disadvantages.

In the treatment planning of a single edentulous site, five possible treatment options exist for the replacement of the missing tooth (Box 22.1). When evaluating single edentulous spaces, many factors must be taken into consideration when determining treatment options. One of the most important is the interocclusal space, which must be assessed carefully regardless of the treatment selected. Patients with insufficient vertical space may be contraindicated for any prosthesis without the prior correction of the occlusal plane and maxillomandibular relationships. In addition,

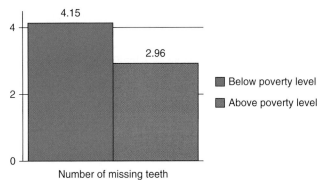

• **Fig. 22.1** The average number of missing teeth in a 20- to 64-year-old population is similar, regardless of income.

the condition, prognosis, and angulation of the adjacent teeth need to be evaluated to determine whether there are any factors that would contraindicate treatment.

Single Missing Tooth

No Treatment

Even though in most cases the option of no treatment is not ideal, the patient should always be informed of the possible ramifications that may occur if no treatment is rendered. Proposing this treatment option may seem counterintuitive to clinicians, because the goal of dentistry is to restore a patient to optimal function; however, the presentation of this option does allow the clinician to enter into a discussion as to the various consequences of tooth loss.

Advantages

The only advantages of no treatment are: (1) the patient will not have to undergo further procedures to address the situation; and (2) there will be no financial demands for the patient.

Disadvantages

However, with no treatment, many disadvantages result.

Movement of Adjacent Teeth. When a patient loses a single tooth, numerous consequences may result that will create an occlusal disharmony and the potential for further dental complications. If a tooth is extracted in any position anterior to the second molars, the patient can expect for the tooth distal to it to begin tilting mesially into the edentulous space. This will most likely result in a change of the occlusal plane on that side. As the teeth experience this mesial tilt, the direction of load changes, which may cause excessive stress to the periodontal ligament. The contacting teeth in the opposing arch will begin to supraerupt in relation to the changes in the occlusal plane. The correction of future supraerupted teeth may require orthodontic or endodontic/crown therapy. In some situations extraction may be necessary.

Occlusal Force Issues. Another consequence of the single missing tooth is the patient will typically favor the fully dentate side to chew with, because of a decreased masticatory efficiency on the partially edentulous side. This situation results in the overuse of the fully dentate side, leading to fatigue-related issues with the teeth. Examples of these complications include fracture of crowns (porcelain, zirconia), fractures of enamel/existing restorations, significant occlusal wear, or myofascial pain syndrome (Fig. 22.2).

Removable Partial Denture

Advantages

The main advantages of the removable partial denture (RPD) in restoring a single missing tooth is based on convenience. The patient can receive a tooth-borne RPD after a few appointments, and there is a lack of invasive treatment in this modality. Most

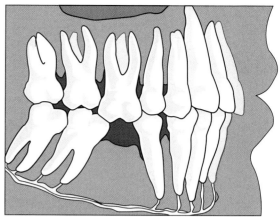

• **Fig. 22.2** Consequences of No Treatment. Complications that may arise from not restoring a single edentulous site such as supraeruption of teeth, tipping of adjacent teeth, eventual loss of adjacent teeth from caries, and food impaction.

often there is a lower associated cost in comparison with most other treatment options.

Disadvantages

Decreased Acceptance. Removable partials dentures, even those that are primarily tooth borne, have a low patient acceptance rate compared with other treatment options. Patients experience difficulty in eating, because food debris may become trapped under the prosthesis. Speech patterns are often disrupted, because the patient must acclimate to the partial framework in the mouth. The prosthesis is often bulky, covering part of the palatal tissue on the maxilla or the lingual tissue on the mandible.

Increased Morbidity to Abutment Teeth. Reports of RPDs indicate that the health of the remaining dentition and surrounding oral tissues often deteriorates. In a study that evaluated the need for repair of an abutment tooth as the indicator of failure, the "success" rates of conventional RPDs were 40% at 5 years and 20% at 10 years.[3] Patients wearing partial dentures often exhibit greater mobility of the abutment teeth, greater plaque retention, increased bleeding on probing, higher incidence of caries, speech inhibition, taste inhibition, and noncompliance of use. A report by Shugars et al.[4] found abutment tooth loss for a RPD may be as high as 23% within 5 years and 38% within 8 years.

Increased Bone Loss. The natural abutment teeth, on which direct and indirect retainers are designed, must submit to additional lateral forces. Because abutment teeth are often compromised by deficient periodontal support, many partial dentures are designed to minimize the forces applied to them. The result is an increase in mobility of the removable prosthesis and greater soft tissue support. These conditions protect the remaining teeth but accelerate the bone loss in the edentulous regions.[5] Notably, bone loss is accelerated in the soft tissue support regions in patients wearing the removable prosthesis compared with patients not wearing the partial.

Accidental Swallowing of Prosthesis. Another drawback of the fabrication of a one-tooth RPD (Nesbit) is that no cross-arch stabilization exists; therefore accidental swallowing or aspiration may occur if it becomes dislodged. Numerous case reports have discussed the inadvertent swallowing of the prosthesis, which necessitated medical treatment, including removal from the esophagus.[6,7]

In conclusion, the evidence-based evaluation for the replacement of a single edentulous site with an RPD is not ideally

Removable Partial Denture Treatment

Advantages
1. Ease of hygiene
2. Soft tissue replacement in esthetic areas
3. Soft tissue support
4. Minimal tooth preparation
5. Reduced cost
6. Reversible Treatment

Disadvantages
1. Material bulkiness—often requires cross-arch stabilization
2. Greater food debris and plaque accumulation
3. Inherent movement
4. Speech and function compromised
5. Accelerates bone loss in edentulous site
6. Abutment teeth loss
7. Possible aspiration

Resin-Bonded Prosthesis

Advantages
1. Minimal preparation of teeth
2. Conservative (reversible) treatment
3. Esthetics

Disadvantages
1. High debond rates (~50% within 3 years)
2. Risk for decay on abutment teeth when partially debonded
3. Movement of abutment teeth if dislodgement occurs

methods. Therefore even if preparation is required, it is usually restricted to the enamel.

Reversible Treatment. The prosthesis usually can be removed without damaging the abutment teeth. This is helpful especially if used as an interim treatment (i.e., future implant placement in a growing patient).

Conventional, Fast Treatment. Minimal appointments are required. Usually involves a conventional or digital impression followed by a second appointment insertion.

Inexpensive. Overhead costs, laboratory bills, and chair time are greatly reduced.

Disadvantages

Higher Failure Rate. There is a higher debond of the prosthesis in comparison with conventional bridges. Failure rates reported in the literature are greatly disparate, but the majority of reports indicate a failure rate of at least 30% within 10 years and as high as 54% within 11 months. Most failures occur from cement (bonding) failure during function.[8]

Higher Recurrent Caries. This type of prosthesis is highly susceptible to partial or total dislodgement, which may result in decay.[9]

Nonideal Space. In many cases diastemas are present or the pontic space is too large or small (nonideal space). This will result in difficulty in space distribution between pontic and abutment teeth. Often esthetic issues may result.

Relapse of Abutment Teeth. If the prosthesis is partially dislodged, it may result in one of the abutment teeth moving, especially if prior procedures have included orthodontic treatment (Box 22.3 and Fig. 22.3B).

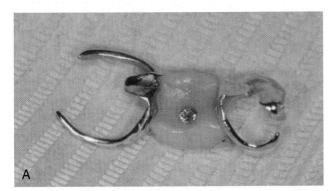

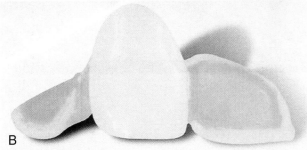

• **Fig. 22.3** Nonideal Single-Tooth Replacement Options. (A) Removable partial denture. (B) Resin-bonded prosthesis.

indicated. Partial dentures may accelerate the loss of adjacent teeth and allow for continued bone loss, along with predisposing the patient to increased morbidity (Box 22.2 and Fig. 22.3A).

Resin-Bonded Fixed Partial Denture

Another option to replace a missing tooth is with a resin-bonded prosthesis (i.e., Maryland bridge). Resin-retained bridges have been used clinically since the 1960s and have undergone many transformations over the years. This prosthesis type is used to replace a single missing tooth by cementing or bonding a pontic tooth to the adjacent teeth. This conservative treatment is usually not used as a first line of treatment because of an unpredictable longevity.

Advantages

Conservative Treatment. Almost no tooth preparation is indicated because retention does not rely on conventional retentive

Fixed Partial Denture

In the past the most common treatment for a single tooth was a fixed partial denture (FPD), which includes the preparation of the adjacent teeth. Because of the high success rates of this type of treatment, FPDs have been the treatment of choice since the 1950's.[10,11]

Advantages

Common Type of Treatment. A fixed prosthesis is a conventional and common type of procedure that most clinicians are comfortable performing. The prosthesis can be fabricated rather quickly, because a laboratory can generate a complete restoration in 1 to 2 weeks, and satisfies the criteria of normal contour, comfort, function, esthetics, speech, and health. Most patients have an increased compliance with this type of treatment, especially because no surgical intervention is needed.

Minimal Need for Soft and Hard Tissue Augmentation. With an FPD, augmentation of the edentulous area is uncommon. Because the pontic may be modified to encompass any defect, surgical augmentation procedures are usually not needed. In some instances lack of attached tissue will be present on abutment teeth; however, this is rare.

Disadvantages

Increased Caries Rate. Despite the many advantages that an FPD has over its removable counterpart, the treatment modality does have inherent disadvantages. Caries and endodontic failure of the abutment teeth are the most common causes of FPD prosthesis failure.[12] Caries occurs more than 20% of the time, and endodontic complications to the abutments of an FPD 15% of the time. Caries on the abutment crown primarily occur on the margin next to the pontic. Fewer than 10% of patients floss on a regular basis, and those using a floss threader are even less.[13] As a result the pontic will act as a large overhang next to the crown and a reservoir for plaque. The long-term periodontal health of the abutment teeth may also be at greater risk as a result of the plaque increase, including bone loss.

Increased Endodontic Treatment. When a vital tooth is prepared for a crown, studies have shown that the patient has up to a 6% chance of experiencing an irreversible pulpal injury and subsequent need for endodontic treatment.[14] Not only does tooth preparation present a risk for endodontics on each of the vital abutment teeth, but the crown margin next to the pontic is also more at risk for decay and the need for endodontics as a result. Up to 15% of abutment teeth for a fixed restoration require endodontic therapy, compared with 6% of nonabutment teeth with crown preparations.[15]

Unfavorable Outcomes of Fixed Partial Denture Failure. Many issues may result when an FPD fails. This may include not only the need to replace the failed prosthesis but also the loss of an abutment tooth and the need for additional pontics and abutment teeth in the replacement bridge. Endodontic therapy is not 100% successful, and metaanalysis reports show a 90% success rate at the 8-year mark. Because approximately 15% of FPD abutment teeth require endodontics, many abutment teeth may be lost. In addition, an endodontic posterior tooth abutment is at a greater risk for fracture. Reports indicate that abutment teeth for an FPD fail because of endodontic complications (e.g., fracture) four times more often than those with vital pulps.[16] The fracture of the tooth may result in failure of the prosthesis and abutment tooth.

The abutment teeth of an FPD may be lost from caries, endodontic complications, or root fracture at rates up to 30% for 8 to 14 years.[17] Recent reports indicate 8% to 18% of the abutment teeth retaining an FPD are lost within 10 years. This is most alarming because 80% of abutments have no previous decay or are minimally restored before the fabrication of the FPD[18] (Box 22.4 and Fig. 22.4A).

Single-Tooth Implant

The last treatment option to replace a missing tooth is a single-tooth implant. In the past, patients were advised to set their desires aside and accept the limitations of an FPD. The primary reasons for suggesting the FPD were its clinical ease and reduced treatment time.

Ideally the primary reason to suggest or perform a treatment should not only be related to treatment time, cost, or difficulty to perform the procedure but also should reflect the best possible long-term solution for each individual.

Advantages

Higher Success Rate. Prior to the 1990's, few long-term studies focusing on single-tooth implant replacement with osseointegrated implants in any region of the mouth had been published. Early reports indicated that single-tooth implant results were less

---

> **• BOX 22.4** **Fixed Partial Denture**

Advantages
1. Fast treatment
2. Restores function, esthetics, and intraarch health
3. Proven long-term survival
4. Reduced cost
5. Requires minimal crown height space for retention

Disadvantages
1. Increased rate of caries and endodontic failure of abutment teeth
2. Increased plaque
3. Irreversible preparation of abutment teeth
4. Fracture complications (porcelain, tooth)
5. Esthetics complications (crowns less esthetic than natural teeth)

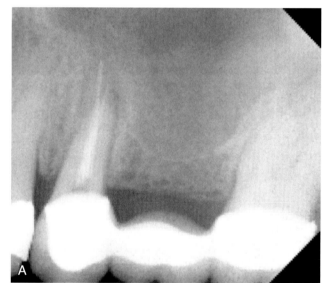

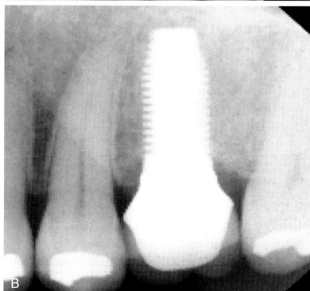

> **• Fig. 22.4** Common Single-Tooth Replacement Options. (A) Fixed partial denture. (B) Dental implant.

predictable than they have become in the "since the late 2000s". For example, in 1990 Jemt et al.[19] reported a 9% implant failure within 3 years of prosthesis completion on 23 implants (21 in the maxilla, 2 in the mandible). In 1992 Andersson et al.[20] published a preliminary report of a prospective study of 37 implants restored with single-tooth crowns in 34 patients. A 3-year follow-up included this "developmental group" and an additional 23 patients with 28 crowns. The cumulative success rate recorded was 93.7%, with 89% of the developmental group in function 3 to 4 years.[20] From approximately 1993 to present, single-tooth implants have become the most predictable method of tooth replacement, with success rates that exceed 95%.[21]

Hygiene. The dental implant treatment plan allows for easier hygiene because the proximal surfaces are able to be easily accessed for flossing. This acts as a preventative measure against periodontal and carious pathologies.

No Alteration of Adjacent Teeth. Adjacent teeth do not have to be altered with the implant option, which decreases the risk for recurrent caries or endodontic issues in these teeth. Because of these advantages, the patient is at a much lower risk for losing further teeth in the future.

Better Cost Comparison. Cost comparison studies conclude that the implant restoration demonstrates a more favorable cost-effectiveness ratio.[22] Even when the adjacent teeth are not lost, the conventional FPD often needs to be replaced every 10 to 20 years on average because of decay, endodontic complications, porcelain fracture, or unretained restoration (which may decay and require endodontics).

Higher Success Rate. The single-tooth implant exhibits the highest survival rates of the five treatment options presented for single-tooth replacement. In addition, the adjacent teeth have the highest survival rate and the lowest complication rate, which is a considerable advantage.

Disadvantages

Increased Treatment Time. The single-tooth implant procedure does take considerably longer for treatment than does the RPD or FPD. From the initial surgical placement the average implant requires 3 to 6 months for osseointegration to occur. This time frame is dependent on the patient's bone density in that area, as well as the volume of bone that was present at placement. In an effort to accelerate the process, immediate placement and loaded implants are a popular technique in implant dentistry today; however, limitations do exist.

Possible Need for Additional Treatment. Especially in esthetic areas, modifications to the soft tissue may be necessary in an effort to change the soft tissue drape or to enhance the patient's tissue biotype. In addition, in some cases the hard tissue (bone) may require augmentation for ideal implant placement and long-term success.

Esthetics. Based on available bone and crown height space (CHS), the final prosthesis may feature a traditional tooth contour (FP1), a longer crown form (FP2), or may require the addition of pink porcelain/zirconia to mimic normal soft tissue contours (FP3). The patient must be aware of these possible prosthetic outcomes because their esthetic values may dictate the need for adjunctive bone grafting procedures.

In conclusion, the single-tooth implant exhibits the highest survival rates of all treatment options presented for single-tooth replacement. The adjacent teeth have the highest survival rate and the lowest complication rate, which is a considerable advantage (Fig. 22.4B and Box 22.5).

• BOX 22.5 Implant

Advantages
1. Less risk for caries, endodontics, restoration and tooth fracture, unretained prosthesis
2. No preparation of adjacent teeth
3. Improved hygiene conditions
4. Improved esthetics: in most cases
5. Maintains hard and soft tissue bone at site
6. Decreases adjacent tooth loss

Disadvantages
1. Increased treatment time
2. Possible hard and soft tissue grafting

Specific Single-Tooth Implant Indications

Anodontia

The absence of one or more teeth is known as anodontia and may be complete (rare) or partial (also called *hypodontia*). It is many times more common than supernumerary teeth.[23] The primary cause of partial anodontia (third molars excluded) is familial heredity, and the incidence rate ranges from 1.5% to as high as 10% in the U.S. population.[24] Congenital absence appears to occur less often in Asians and African Americans (2.5%) than in whites (5.15%). The highest average has been reported in Scandinavian countries (10.1% in Norway and 17.5% in Finnish Skolt-Lapps). In addition, a number of syndromes exist in the literature that include multiple missing teeth, of which ectodermal dysplasia is the most common. A high correlation is found between primary tooth absence and a permanent missing tooth; however, a missing tooth occurs more frequently in the permanent dentition. Caprioglio et al.[25] evaluated the records of almost 10,000 patients between the ages of 5 and 15 years. Of all the missing single teeth, the mandibular second premolar was most often missing (38.6%), followed by the maxillary lateral incisor (29.3%), the maxillary second premolar (16.5%), and the mandibular central incisor (4.0%). The remaining teeth were absent at a rate of only 0.5% to 1.8%, with the maxillary first molar being the least affected. The missing mandibular second premolar primarily occurred in male patients, and the missing maxillary lateral incisor primarily occurred in female patients.[25] The most common multiple teeth lost (other than third molars) are the maxillary lateral incisors followed by the mandibular second premolars and maxillary second premolars (Figs. 22.5 and 22.6).

Congenitally missing teeth are therefore a common scenario in a general practice. Fortunately, fewer than 1% of those individuals who are missing teeth are missing more than two teeth, and fewer than 0.5% of this group is missing more than five permanent teeth. In the majority of children with more than five teeth missing, it is related to ectodermal dysplasia.[26]

A congenital missing mandibular second premolar most often has a deciduous second molar. In some cases, the deciduous second molar may be extracted at the approximate age of 5–6 years old. This may allow the permanent molar to then erupt in a more mesial position. When the first deciduous molar is lost naturally (around the age of 9–11 years), the first permanent premolar and first molar may be orthodontically positioned adjacent to each other. This approach eliminates the need for a second premolar replacement. Because the second premolar space is eliminated

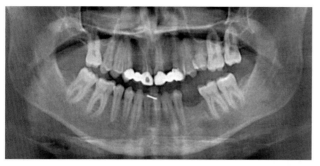

• **Fig. 22.5** Congenitally missing mandibular left second premolar: the most common missing tooth. Note the increased mesial-distal distance due to retaining the primary molar.

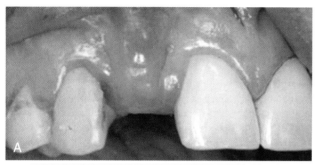

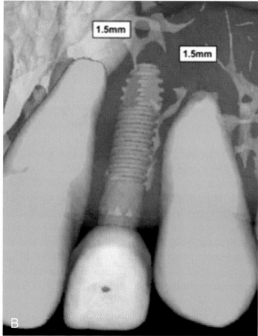

• **Fig. 22.6** Congenitally missing maxillary lateral incisor: the most difficult missing tooth to be replaced by an implant. (A) Clinical image of missing lateral incisor. (B) Ideal implant placement being approximately 1.5 mm from roots.

with orthodontics, no bone graft, implant surgery, or crown (or combination of these treatments) is required to replace the tooth. Few disadvantages exist to the use of orthodontics to eliminate this posterior missing tooth space.

A common scenario is to maintain the deciduous second molar for as long as possible. Often the deciduous tooth will break down and need to be extracted. When the deciduous second molar is maintained, it may become ankylotic approximately 10% of the time. As a result the opposing maxillary second premolar extrudes, and the adjacent teeth often tip over the deciduous tooth. In addition, because the deciduous molar is 1.9 mm larger than a premolar, the mesiodistal space is larger than the usual premolar space after the deciduous molar is lost at a later date in the adult patient's life.

An implant is usually the treatment of choice to replace the second premolar. However, the deciduous tooth does not have a buccolingual width of bone that is adequate for a larger-diameter implant. The crown for this larger tooth dimension is supported by a regular-size implant, which increases forces on the abutment screw and increases the risk for screw-loosening complications. However, this is most often the treatment of choice in adult patients rather than preparing the adjacent teeth for a traditional FPD. An alternative in an adult implant patient is to augment the site for width and place a larger-diameter implant (5 mm). This improves the emergence profile and decreases the risk for abutment screw loosening.

Another option in an adult patient missing a permanent premolar is orthodontic closure of the space. However, care is taken so the anterior component of teeth does not shift distally and open the centric occlusal bite relationship. To prevent this occurrence, an orthodontic implant (transitional anchorage device) may be inserted distal to the canine root and used as anchorage to pull the molars forward to close the space (Fig. 22.7). This approach may also negate the need to extract a third molar in that quadrant when performed on adolescents.

Single-Tooth Implant Size Specifics

When an edentulous site is evaluated, the clinician must use specific parameters in determination if the site is an acceptable implant site. The ideal diameter of a single-tooth implant directly is dependent on the mesiodistal dimension of the missing tooth and the buccolingual dimension of the implant site. When evaluating the size of the dental implant, specific guideline measurements should be adhered to:

- 1.5–2.0 mm from an adjacent tooth
- 3.0 mm between implants
- 2 mm from a vital structure
- 1.5–2.0 mm mm of buccal bone (after implant placement)
- 1.0 mm of lingual bone (after implant placement)

Caution should be exercised in placing implants with compromised facial bone. When an implant has a facial bone thickness less than 1.0 mm of cortical bone, an increased risk for bone loss and implant failures may occur.[27] As a consequence the ideal implant diameter is 1.5 mm or more from each adjacent tooth, 1.5 mm or more from the facial plate, and 1.0 mm from the lingual plate (i.e., the lingual plate is always thicker and more resistant to bone loss in comparison with the facial plate).

Anterior Teeth Replacement

Mandible

One of the more difficult edentulous areas in the oral cavity to treatment plan is the mandibular anterior. Because of the compromised mesial-distal length, placing one implant for each missing tooth is difficult, if not impossible. When missing two mandibular incisors (~#24–#25), usually one implant may be placed interproximally, slightly lingual with a screw-retained prosthesis. If all four lower incisors are missing, two implants may be placed interproximally, distributing the cantilever amount equally. This

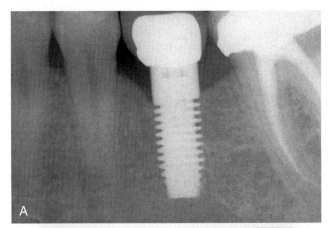

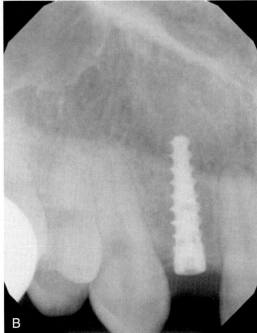

• **Fig. 22.7** (A and B) Postorthodontic treatment of the most common congenitally missing sites.

area involves lower force factors. When all of the lower incisors are missing (~#23–#26), then usually two implants are placed in the interproximal areas (#23–#24 and #25–#26), and a four-unit prosthesis is fabricated. This allows the implants to be far enough away from the mesial aspect of the cuspids, and therefore not causing a peri-implant problem. When mandibular cuspid to cuspid are missing, then usually four implants are placed, with the distal implants being in the #22 to #23 and #26 to #27 embrasure areas (Fig. 22.8). This prevents developing an osseous defect on the mesial of the cuspids.

Maxillary

The maxillary anterior edentulous spaces are one of the most difficult treatment areas. Contrary to missing posterior teeth, nearly all patients have an emotional response regarding a maxillary anterior missing tooth. No question exists regarding the need to replace the tooth, and financial considerations are less important. When posterior teeth are extracted, little resistance to the preparation of adjacent teeth may be given to the dentist. However, when anterior, normal-looking teeth must be prepared to serve as FPD abutments, the patient is more anxious and often looks for

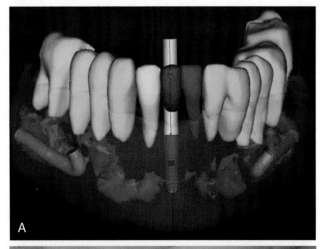

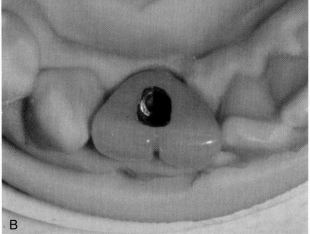

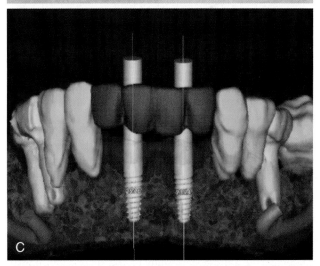

• **Fig. 22.8** Treatment Plans for Mandibular Anterior. (a) Missing # 24 or # 25 - implant placement as long as ideal space is available. (b) Missing # 24 and # 25 - implant placed in the embrasure area with a screw retained prosthesis, (c) Missing # 23 - # 26 - two implants placed in the embrasure area.

an alternative. In the patient's perspective, anterior FPD restorations are never as esthetic as natural teeth. In part, this is because patients are able to distinguish between good and poor esthetic results. Because patients are able to notice only the restorations that are not natural in appearance, they believe anterior FPDs are not esthetic. In younger patients with congenitally missing maxillary lateral incisors or with trauma to the maxillary central incisor (which resulted in its failure, often after endodontic therapy), parents are eager to provide the best possible replacement option. They often perceive this option to be a single-tooth implant. As a consequence of these psychological factors, a common site for a single-tooth implant in a restorative practice is the maxillary central or lateral incisor.

The highly esthetic zone of the premaxilla often requires both hard (bone and teeth) and soft tissue restoration. The soft tissue drape is often the most difficult aspect of treatment. As a consequence, maxillary anterior single-tooth replacement is often a challenge, regardless of the experience and skill of the dentist. Endodontic failure is less likely in the maxillary anterior region compared with posterior teeth, but the cause of pulp necrosis may more often lead to root resorption, compared with the posterior regions.

Before 1990 few long-term studies of anterior single-tooth implant replacement with osteointegrated implants were conducted. However, recently studies are becoming more prevalent. Misch et al.[28] reported on 276 anterior maxillary single implants to restore missing teeth from agenesis. In 255 adolescent patients the implants were monitored for a range of 2 to 16 years, with a 98.6% implant and prosthesis survival rate. In the same year, Wennstrom et al.[29] reported on a 5-year prospective study with 45 single-tooth implants, with a 97.7% implant survival rate with minimal bone loss. Zarone et al.[30] reported on lateral maxillary agenesis replacement with 34 implants, with a 97% survival rate at 39 months.

More clinical studies have been conducted for a maxillary anterior single-tooth replacement with an implant than any other treatment option. Retrospective reports are available, as with other modalities; however, of more importance is the fact that many prospective clinical studies confirm the data of previous reports. The maxillary anterior single-tooth implant has a very high success rate compared with any other treatment option to replace missing teeth with an implant restoration (i.e., overdentures, short-span FPD, full-arch FPD, or single-tooth implant).[31] In a systematic review of single-implant restorations in all regions of the mouth, Creugers et al.[32] reported a cumulative rate of 97% success at 4 years, with 83% reporting uncomplicated maintenance. Lindhe et al.[33] published a metaanalysis of implants with nine studies on single implants, with a total of 570 single crowns with a follow-up range of 1 to 8 years and a 97.5% survival rate. A review of the literature by Goodacre et al.[34] found single-tooth implant studies had the highest survival rate of any prosthesis type and averaged 97%.

More recently a trend toward single-stage and immediate-extraction implants has emerged. This appears especially attractive in the maxillary anterior region, where the soft tissue drape is ideal before the extraction and patients are more anxious to have a fixed replacement. In a prospective study of 102 single-tooth implants in the anterior maxilla, Kemppainen et al.[35] reported a 99% success rate using one-stage and two-stage implants. Other studies have recommended one stage and immediate load with some success in specific situations.

As important as implant versus prosthesis survival rates is the fact that the adjacent teeth prognosis is improved with single-tooth implants compared with any other option. In a 10-year report, Priest[36] indicated adjacent teeth next to implants have less decay, endodontic risk, sensitivity, plaque retention, and evidence of adjacent tooth loss over 10 years. Studies by Misch et al.[37] also resulted in similar conclusions. As such, the maxillary anterior

single-tooth implant has become the treatment of choice when bone and space parameters are sufficient or may be created.

One of the most common procedures performed in implant dentistry is a single-tooth replacement. Although implant success rates are high in the maxillary regions, high patient expectations, high esthetic requirements, and sensitive soft and hard tissue management compound the complexity of the anterior teeth restoration. A single maxillary central crown on a natural tooth is often a difficult challenge for the restoring dentist. This challenge is significantly compounded when an implant serves as the prosthetic support. As a consequence, implants to replace a maxillary anterior single tooth remain one of the more difficult treatments to perform in implant dentistry.

Posterior Teeth Replacement

Premolar Replacement

The most ideal and easiest posterior tooth to replace with an implant is the first premolar in the maxillary arch (Fig. 22.9). When used as an abutment for a three-unit FPD, the canine is at an increased risk for material fracture or uncementation (because of the lateral forces applied) and is often more difficult to restore

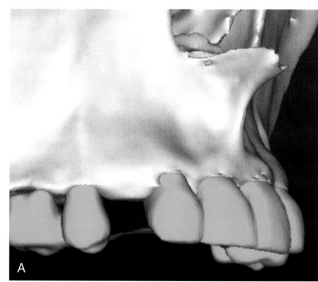
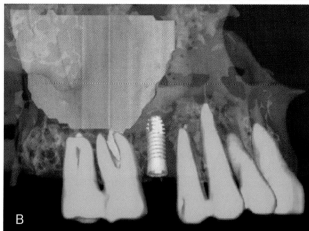

• **Fig. 22.9** Premolar Replacement. (A) The maxillary first premolar is the safest and easiest position to place an implant. (B) In most cases an implant can be positioned anterior to the maxillary sinus in the second premolar position.

to its original appearance than are other anterior or posterior teeth. The vertical available bone is usually greater in the first premolar locations than in any other posterior tooth positions. In the maxilla, it is almost always anterior or below the maxillary sinus, and is the perfect site for a clinician initially learning implant placement. In the mandible the first premolar is almost always anterior to the mental foramen and associated mandibular neurovascular complex. The bone trajectory for implant insertion is more favorable in the mandibular first premolar than for any other tooth in the arch.

The maxillary premolars are often in the esthetic zone of patients with a high smile line. The need for bone grafting before maxillary first premolar implant placement is common because the extraction process of the thin buccal root often results in facial bone loss during or after the extraction. Implant placement without bone grafting may result in a recessed emergence profile, which in the past was corrected with a facial ridge lap to the crown. However, the crown with a ridge lap contour does not allow proper hygiene or probing of the facial sulcular region of the crown and should be used as a last resort.

To ensure a proper esthetic result and to avoid the need for a crown with a ridge lap, the implant body is often positioned similar to an anterior implant, under the buccal cusp tip (one-third buccal, two-thirds lingual) rather than midcrest (which is under the central fossa). The slight buccal implant placement improves the cervical emergence profile of the maxillary premolar crown.

The natural premolar tooth is 7 mm wide in the mandible and 6.5 to 7 mm in the maxilla. The premolar root is usually 4.2 mm in diameter on average at a distance of 2 mm below the cement-enamel junction (CEJ), which is the ideal position of the bone. As a consequence the most common implant diameter is usually 4 mm at the crest module. This also provides approximately 1.5 mm of bone on the proximal surfaces adjacent to the natural teeth when the mesiodistal space is 7 mm or greater. However, when the mesiodistal dimension is only 6.5 mm, a 3.5-mm implant is suggested.

The maxillary canine root is often angled 11 degrees distally and presents a distal curve 32% of the time, which may extend over the shorter root of the maxillary first premolar. With posterior implant insertion, the implant body is often longer than the natural tooth root. The surgeon may inadvertently place the implant parallel to the second premolar and, consequently, into the natural canine root. This may not only result in endodontic therapy of the canine but also may cause root fracture and loss of the tooth. Therefore in the maxillary first premolar region, care must be taken to evaluate the canine angulation and vertical height limitation. The first premolar implant may need to be placed parallel to the canine root, and a shorter implant than is considered ideal may be required (Fig. 22.10). A tapered implant body at the apical third may also be of benefit to avoid encroachment on the apical region of the canine.

The second premolar root apices may be located over the mandibular neurovascular canal (or foramen) or maxillary sinus. The foramen is often 2 mm or more above the neurovascular canal. Hence the second premolar available bone height may be less than the first molar region. This also results in a reduced height of bone compared with the anterior region of the jaws. As a result a shorter implant than ideal is a common consequence in the second premolar site.

First Molar Implant Replacement. The first molar is one of the most common teeth to be extracted. The natural molars receive twice the load of the premolars and have 200% more root surface area; therefore it is logical that the implant support in a molar region should be greater than in the premolar position. Its mesiodistal dimension usually ranges from 8 to 12 mm, depending on the original tooth size and the amount of mesial drift of the second molar before implant placement. It should be noted that the ideal size of the implant should be measured by the intratooth distance from the adjacent CEJ of each tooth, not the interproximal distance at the marginal ridges. A tipped adjacent tooth should be recontoured to a more ideal condition, so that food impaction does not occur under the interproximal contacts in the enlarged triangular interdental papilla space, which is formed after the implant crown is inserted.

When one 4-mm-diameter implant is placed to support a crown with a mesiodistal dimension of 12 mm, this may create a

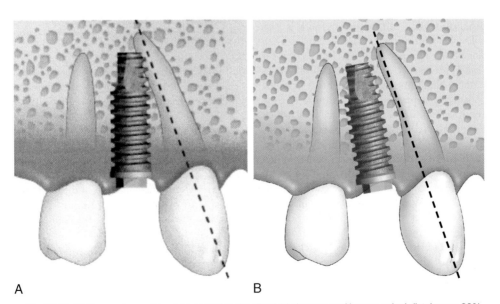

A   B

• **Fig. 22.10** (A) The canine root is often angled to the distal 11 degrees and has an apical distal curve 32% of the time. As a consequence the first premolar implant may contact the canine root. (B) The first premolar implant may need to be angled so it is parallel to the canine rather than the second premolar.

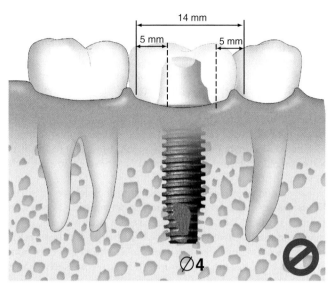

• **Fig. 22.11** When a 4-mm-diameter implant replaces a molar, a mesial and distal cantilever is created on the crown, which is nonideal. In addition, if a large occlusal table exists (buccal-lingually), shear forces may result because of the mesial,distal, buccal, and lingual cantilevers.

4- to 5-mm cantilever on the marginal ridges of the implant crown (Fig. 22.11). The magnified occlusal forces (especially important in parafunction) may cause bone loss (which may complicate home care), increase abutment screw loosening, and increase abutment or implant failure because of overload.

Sullivan[38] reported a 14% implant fracture rate for single molars fabricated on 4.0-mm implants composed of grade 1 titanium and concluded that this is not a viable treatment. Rangert et al.[39] reported that overload-induced bone resorption appeared to precede implant fracture in a significant number of 4.0-mm-diameter single-molar implant restorations. Therefore a larger-diameter implant should be inserted to enhance the mechanical properties of the implant system through increased surface area, stronger resistance to component fracture, increased abutment screw stability, and enhanced emergence profile for the crown.

When the mesiodistal dimension of the missing tooth is 8 to 12 mm with a buccolingual width greater than 7 mm, a 5- to 6-mm-diameter implant body is suggested (Fig. 22.12). Langer et al.[40] also recommended the use of wide-diameter implants in bone of poor quality or for the immediate replacement of failed implants. The larger-diameter implant does not require as long an implant body to result in a similar loading surface area, which is also a benefit because of the reduced posterior available vertical bone height because of anatomic limitations and landmarks present, such as the maxillary sinus or mandibular canal. When the mesiodistal dimension of the missing tooth site is 14 to 20 mm, two 4- to 5-mm-diameter implants should be considered to restore the region (Fig. 22.13). When two implants replace the molar region, the mesiodistal offset loads to the prosthesis can be eliminated because each implant may be placed 1.5 mm from the adjacent tooth. The total surface area of support is greater for the two implants, compared with the surface area provided by one larger-diameter implant (two 4-mm-diameter implants > one 5- or 6-mm-diameter implant). In addition, the two regular-size implants provide more stress reduction than just one larger-diameter implant, which in turn reduces the incidence of abutment screw loosening.

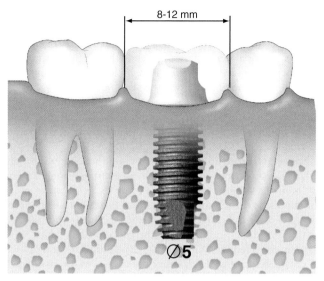

• **Fig. 22.12** When the mesiodistal space in the posterior regions is 8 to 12 mm, a 5- to 6-mm-diameter implant is suggested.

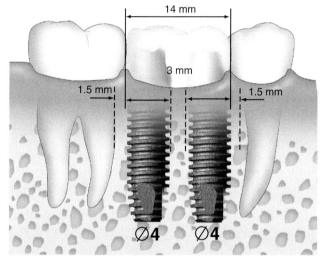

• **Fig. 22.13** When the mesiodistal space is 14 to 20 mm, two implants should be used to support the crowns.

In 1996 Bahat et al.[41] reported on the results of various implant numbers and size selection. The overall failure rate was 1.2%, with the two 5-mm implants having 100% success. In 1997, Balshi et al.[42] compared the use of one implant and two implants to replace a single molar. The 3-year cumulative success rate was 99%. Prosthesis mobility and screw loosening were the most common complications for the one-implant group (48%); this complication rate was reduced to 8% in the two-implant group.

In a finite element analysis of three different implant-supported molar crown designs, Geramy and Morgano[43] showed a 50% decrease in mesiodistal and buccolingual stress between 5-mm and standard-diameter implants. The double-implant design had the least stress of all. Therefore, whenever possible, two implants should be used to replace a larger single-molar space to reduce cantilever loads and abutment screw loosening.

When the posterior space is 14 to 20 mm, the largest implant diameter for the two implants may be calculated by subtracting 6 mm (1.5 mm from each tooth for soft tissue and surgical risk and 3 mm between the implants) from the intratooth distance and

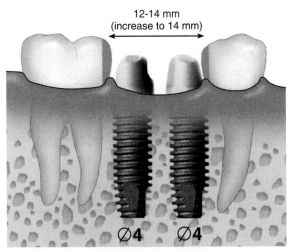

● **Fig. 22.14** When the space between natural teeth is 12 to 14 mm, the choice of implant size and number is less obvious.

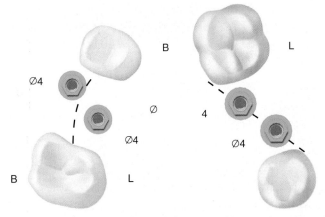

● **Fig. 22.15** On the left (in the maxilla) the mesial implant is positioned more facial and the distal implant more palatal. On the right (mandible) the mesial implant is placed more lingual and the distal implant more buccal.

dividing by 2 to determine the size of each implant (16 mm – 6 mm = 10 mm ÷ 2 = 5-mm implants). Remember, when two adjacent molars are missing, it is advantageous to place each implant 1.5 to 2 mm from the adjacent teeth (or under the mesial of the first molar and distal of the second molar crown) and splint the implants together, rather than placing the implant in the center of each tooth. This eliminates the cantilever to the mesial and distal from the implants.

Ideally two implants should be 3 mm apart because crestal bone loss around each implant may occur. The width of the crestal defect is usually less than 1.5 mm. Therefore the two adjacent implants 3 mm or more apart will not convert an angular defect next to an implant to be a horizontal defect that may increase sulcus depths and cause loss of papilla height.[44] Although this region is often out of the esthetic zone, the loss of papilla height increases food impaction.

When the mesiodistal space is 12 to 14 mm from adjacent CEJs, the treatment plan of choice is less obvious. A 5-mm-diameter implant may result in cantilevers up to 5 mm on each marginal ridge of the crown. However, two implants present a greater surgical, prosthetic, and hygiene risk. Unfortunately the 12- to 14-mm space is not unusual. The primary goal is to obtain at least 14 mm of space instead of 12 to 14 mm (Fig. 22.14). Additional space may be gained in several ways. Orthodontics may be the treatment of choice to upright a tilted second molar or increase the intratooth space. One anterior implant may be placed and an orthodontic spring incorporated in the transitional crown; the spring pushes and uprights the distal tooth and moves it more distal. After orthodontic movement the second implant may be inserted with less risk and improved hygiene between each implant. Another option is to use orthodontics to reduce the space and place only one implant and crown.

The implants may not be centered in the crestal width of bone. Instead, one implant is placed buccal and the other on a diagonal toward the lingual (Fig. 22.15). The diagonal dimension increases the mesiodistal space by 0.5 to 1.0 mm. When implants are placed in such a way, consideration is given to oral hygiene and occlusion. In the mandible the most anterior implant is placed to the lingual aspect of the midcrest, and the more distal implant is placed to the facial aspect to facilitate access of a floss threader from the vestibule into the intraimplant space. The occlusal contacts are also slightly modified on the buccal aspect of the mesial implant to

occlude over the central fossa. In the maxilla the anterior implant is placed to the buccal aspect and the distal implant to the palatal region to improve the esthetics of the more visible half of the tooth. The distal occlusal contact is placed over the lingual cusp, and the mesial occlusal contact is located in the central fossa position. The cervical esthetics of the maxillary molar is compromised on the distal half of the tooth to the benefit of greater intratooth distance and easier access for home care. This maxillary implant placement requires the intraimplant furcation to be approached from the palate rather than the buccal approach as in the mandible.

Second Molar Implant Replacement. In general, when third molars are missing, the second mandibular molar is usually not restored. The mandibular second molar is not in the esthetic zone of the patient. Ninety percent of the masticatory efficiency is generated anterior to the mesial half of the mandibular first molar, so function is rarely a primary reason to replace the second molar. A 10% greater occlusal force is measured on the second molar compared with the first. As a result, biomechanical stress–related complications are more of a risk, including abutment screw loosening. This tooth is more likely to exhibit working or nonworking interfaces during mandibular excursions. As a result of the increased forces and occlusal interferences, a greater incidence of porcelain or zirconia fracture occurs.

The CHS decreases as it proceeds posteriorly, and represents limited access for implant placement, along with abutment screw and abutment insertion, especially when opposing natural dentition. A reduced CHS results in the abutment height being reduced, so the retention of the crown may be compromised. Cheek biting is more common in this region because of the proximity of the buccinator muscle.

The course of the mandibular canal anterior to the mid-first molar most commonly corresponds to the level of the mental foramen. However, in the region of the second molar, its course becomes highly variable, with less available bone height and an elevated risk for paresthesia and neurovascular bundle damage during implant surgery and insertion. The bone quality in the second mandibular molar region is often inferior to other regions of the mandible, with an increased risk for bone loss or implant failure as a consequence. The submandibular fossa topography is deeper in the second molar regions compared with the premolar or first molar sites, and mandates greater implant body angulation, with associated increased stresses at the crestal region of the implant, thereby increasing the risk for bone loss and abutment screw loosening. In addition, the

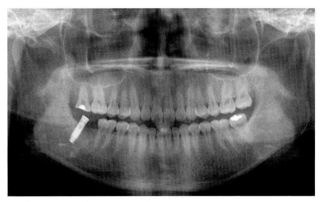

• **Fig. 22.16** Second Molar Replacement. Replacing second molar teeth is usually not recommended because of the compromised crown height space.

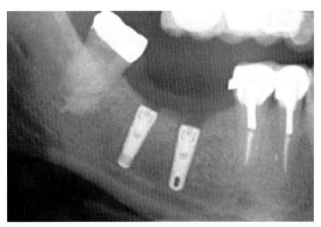

• **Fig. 22.17** Complications that may occur from the placement of second molars that result in neurosensory impairment.

TABLE 22.1	Disadvantages of Replacing Second Molars

1. Not in esthetic zone
2. Extruded maxillary second molar not esthetic or occlusal consequence
3. Less than 5% of total chewing efficiency in this region
4. A 10% higher bite force (increased bone loss risk, porcelain/zirconia fracture risk, and abutment screw–loosening risk)
5. More often exhibits occlusal interferences during excursions
6. Higher and less predictable location of mandibular canal in that site
7. Less dense bone
8. Submandibular fossa depth greater
9. Angulation of bone to occlusal plane greater
10. Limited to unfavorable crown height space for cement retention (increased risk for uncementation)
11. Limited access for occlusal screw placement
12. Limited access for correct implant body placement
13. Crossbite position—implant placed more buccal than maxillary tooth
14. Hygiene access more difficult
15. Cheek biting more common
16. More incision line opening after surgery
17. Greater mandibular flexure during parafunction
18. Greater cost to patient

facial artery is located in the submandibular fossa before it crosses the mandibular notch and crosses over the face. Perforation of the lingual plate in the region of the second molar may violate the facial artery and cause life-threatening bleeding. The mandible exhibits increased flexure and torsion in this area during opening or heavy biting on one side, and masticatory dynamics are less favorable. As a result the implant may not integrate in a patient with moderate-to-severe bruxism or clenching. Finally, the cost of an implant or fixed prosthesis to replace the second molar often does not warrant the benefits achieved. As a consequence the mandibular second molar is usually not replaced when the third molar and second molar are the only posterior mandibular teeth missing.

The primary disadvantage of electing not to replace a mandibular second molar tooth is the potential extrusion and loss of the maxillary second molar, or a loss of proper interproximal contact with the adjacent tooth, with increased risk for caries, periodontal disease, or both. The extrusion of the maxillary second molar is usually not an esthetic or occlusal concern. When the mandible moves into an excursion, the maxillary second molar is behind the mandibular first molar and does not alter the mandibular pathway of movement even if the maxillary second molar extrudes. If extrusion of the maxillary second molar is a concern for the patient or doctor, then a crown on the mandibular first molar may include an occlusal contact with the mesial marginal ridge of the maxillary second molar, or the maxillary second molar may be bonded to the maxillary first molar.

On the other hand, a missing maxillary second molar opposing a mandibular second molar with extrusion may result in occlusal concern when the mandible moves into an excursion. The extrusion of a mandibular second molar results in an occlusal interference when the mandible moves into protrusive or lateral excursion. Hence, as a general rule, maxillary second molars are usually replaced with an implant when opposing a natural tooth (Fig. 22.16).

The mandibular second molar is usually replaced when the third molar is in function and will remain present. In addition, some patients desire an intact dentition and wish to have the tooth replaced, regardless of whether they have a third molar. If the bone is abundant and no paresthesia or surgical risk is apparent, then the second molar may be replaced. However, this is usually the exception rather than the rule of treatment and usually replaces only a premolar-sized tooth (Fig. 22.17 and Table 22.1).

Multiple Missing Teeth

No Treatment

Advantages

There are no advantages to no treatment for multiple teeth other than finances and time. When a patient is missing multiple teeth, the education and communication to the patient is even more important. Although there is no financial or time commitment for the patient, the disadvantages are more significant in comparison with a single missing tooth.

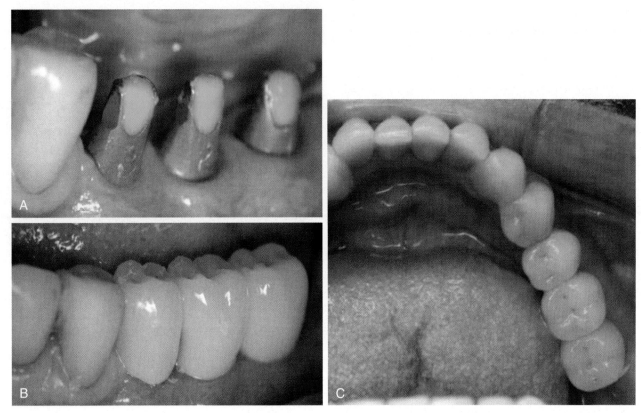

• **Fig. 22.18** Multiple Implant Prosthesis: (a) Three cementable abutments for cement-retained prosthesis, (b) Buccal clinical view, (c) Occlusal view.

Disadvantages

Decreased Masticatory Function. The main disadvantage of not replacing multiple teeth is the decreased masticatory function. Patients will place more force and stress on their remaining teeth, which leads to an increased morbidity. The forces of mastication are transmitted to the remaining teeth, which results in a greater possibility of decay, mobility, periodontal issues, and loss of teeth. The longer the edentulous ridge remains without stimulation, the greater the chance that bone loss will occur. This may lead to the future need for hard and soft tissue augmentation procedures to increase hard and soft tissue volume for implant placement.

Tooth Movement. The remaining teeth may continue to shift in relation to the stresses of mastication, causing movement and tilting. Teeth in the opposing arch will supraerupt because of the lack of stimulation by an opposing tooth, causing root exposure and occlusal disharmony. These phenomena combine to drastically complicate the implant restoration.

Esthetics. If no treatment is rendered for the edentulous area, obvious esthetic issues will result. In most cases, patient acceptance of the edentulous areas is not well accepted, and esthetics is usually a motivating factor in seeking rehabilitation.

Removable Partial Denture

See Box 22.2 for the advantages and disadvantages of RPD treatment.

Implant-Supported Multiple Crowns (Fig. 22.18)

Advantages

Ideal Prosthesis. The implant-supported fixed prosthesis is the closest available treatment option for an edentulous patient to return to optimal form, function, and esthetics. Most patients who receive a fixed prosthesis will state that it "feels like normal teeth," which carries a profound psychological impact. The prosthesis does not require removal and is less likely to impact food in comparison with a removable prosthesis.

Less Bone Loss in Cantilevered Areas. Wright et al.[45] have evaluated posterior mandibular bone loss in implant overdentures (overdenture removable prosthesis [RP-5]) compared with cantilevered fixed prostheses from anterior implants. The annual bone loss index observed in the RP-5 overdentures ranged from +0.02 to –0.05, with 14 of 20 patients losing bone in the posterior regions. The fixed prostheses group had a range from +0.07 to –0.015, with 18 of 22 patients gaining posterior bone area. Reddy et al.[46] also found a similar clinical observation in 60 consecutively treated cantilevered fixed prostheses supported by five to six implants placed between the foramina. The mandibular body height was measured 5, 10, 15, and 20 mm distal to the last implant. The baseline measurements up to 4 years after function increased from 7.25 ± 0.25 to 8.18 ± 0.18 mm. Nearly all of the bone growth occurred during the first year of function. Therefore an important role for the complete implant-supported restoration is the maintenance and even regeneration of posterior bone in the mandible.

Decreased Maintenance. Because no attachments are used with a fixed implant prosthesis, far less maintenance is needed. This will also decrease the financial outlay the patient must commit to in comparison with an overdenture treatment.

Disadvantages

Cost. The cost of a fixed prosthesis is usually higher than other treatment plans, which may serve as a barrier to acceptance. In patients with severe parafunction the argument does arise for fabrication of a removable overdenture as opposed to the porcelain fixed restoration.

Esthetics. The esthetics for a fixed detachable prosthesis may be inferior to an removable prosthesis. Because soft tissue support for facial appearance often is required for an implant patient with advanced bone loss, a fixed prosthesis will usually not be as soft tissue supportive as an overdenture. Because there is no labial flange with a fixed prosthesis, compromises in the soft tissue may result. If overcontouring of the prosthesis is completed by the laboratory, this will often result in difficulty for hygiene access.

Food Impaction. With a fixed prosthesis a common complaint exists with an increase in food impaction. This will most likely result when custom abutments are used to offset nonideal implant positioning.

Types of Prostheses

The clinician should have a strong understanding of the various prosthetic options that may be used for single- or multiple-implant restoration in partially edentulous arches. The primary methods used for retention of these prostheses are cement and screw retention. Although other options exist, including friction-fit component systems, these methods find their greatest utility with the retention of removable prostheses.

Screw-Retained Restorations

Screw-retained restorations can be secured to the implant body directly (Fig. 22.19) or attached through the use of a standardized abutment, which is in turn held in place to the implant with a retaining screw (Fig. 22.20). The early work by Brånemark et al., which focused on rehabilitation of the fully edentulous arch, featured screw-retained restorations exclusively (Fig. 22.21). The updated version of that type of restoration (Fig. 22.22) features a much lower profile for the abutment and provides the patient with a restoration that provides improved esthetics and function (Box 22.6).

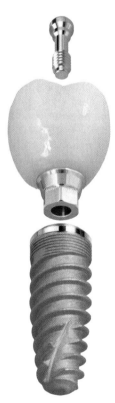

● **Fig. 22.19** Screw-retained crown.

Advantages

Retrievability. Screw-retained restorations are easily removed by the clinician at any time after delivery should there be a complication, such as prosthesis fracture or chipping, that requires intervention with the prosthesis outside the mouth. Although a

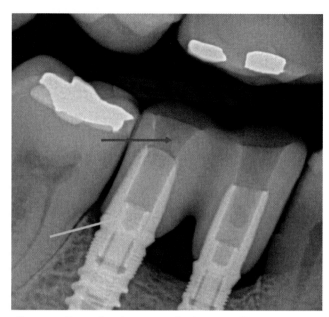

● **Fig. 22.20** Two splinted screw retained crowns. Note screw access channel (green arrows) and retaining screw (red arrows).

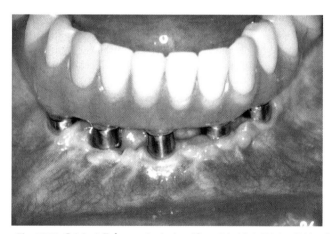

● **Fig. 22.21** Original Brånemark design "Swedish High-Water Bridge." *(From Misch CE. The completely edentulous mandible: treatment plans for fixed restorations. In: Dental Implant Prosthetics. 2nd ed. St. Louis, MO: Elsevier; 2015.)*

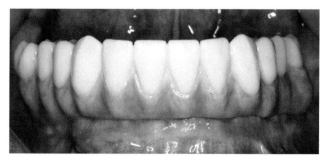

● **Fig. 22.22** Contemporary design of full-arch screw-retained bridge.

cement-retained prosthesis can also be removed by the clinician, it is a less predictable procedure and risks damage to the patient's restoration and implants. For this reason, screw retention is often recommended for long-span, full-arch, and cantilevered restorations, or in cases where the prosthesis may require removal in the future.

Lack of Cement. The absence of the cement interface between the restoration and the implant abutment is another important advantage of a screw-retained prosthesis. Excess cement at the margin has been shown to be an important iatrogenic contributing factor to implant complications, such as implant peri-mucositis and peri-implantitis. Although there are established techniques for mitigating that risk, it remains an important consideration. For example, in clinical situations where the soft tissue interface is part of the patient's smile, and it is necessary to place the margin of the restoration subgingivally, a screw-retained restoration is recommended.

Lack of Crown Height Space. In areas where there is minimal interocclusal space (i.e., CHS), a screw-retained restoration will provide better retention for the prosthesis. Cementation on short implant abutments provides the same risk for debonding as with restorations on natural teeth.

Disadvantages

Esthetics Is Dependent on Implant Positioning. For a screw-retained prosthesis, the esthetics of the prosthesis is highly dependent on the implant positioning in the x, y, and z axes. The most common area in the oral cavity that presents a problem is the maxillary anterior. Because of the inherent trajectory of the alveolus in this area, it is not uncommon for the implant to be facially positioned. Therefore the access hole would be required to be in the buccal aspect of the crown, which leads to an obvious esthetic issue.

• BOX 22.6   Screw-Retained Crowns

Advantages
- Retrievable
- Known retention
- No risk for leaving residual cement
- Limited interocclusal space

Disadvantages
- Highly dependent on implant position (unesthetic)
- Access hole
- More expensive
- Occlusion (access hole wearing)
- Multiple splinted units—passivity
- Porcelain fracture—unsupported porcelain

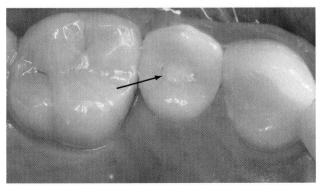

• Fig. 22.23 Screw-retained prosthesis (bicuspid) with access hole filled with composite.

Access Hole. The greatest disadvantage to screw-retained restorations involves the screw access hole in the restoration. Particularly on ceramic or metal-ceramic restorations, the patient can often see the vestiges of this access and, without proper preoperative explanation, may be concerned. Fortunately this result can be largely mitigated by clinicians using newer composites that offer a remarkably good match to the restorative material used (e.g., opaque composite material) (Fig. 22.23).

Difficulty in Obtaining a Passive Fit. Some authors have reported increased difficulty in obtaining a passive fit for multiimplant screw-retained restorations compared with cement retained. The reasoning is that because there is some degree of spatial relief provided around each cement-over abutment, the overall restoration should be more forgiving of a minor misfit. Although there is some logic to this argument, it is fortunate that improved clinical and laboratory techniques, specifically the use of the implant verification jig and computer-aided design/computer-aided manufacturing (CAD/CAM) techniques, have made such challenges to passive fit increasingly rare.

Cement-Retained Restorations

Cement-retained restorations consist of a conventional crown or bridge prosthesis cemented over one or more abutments, which have been secured to the implant with an abutment screw (Fig. 22.24). The abutment for a cement-retained restoration can be either a

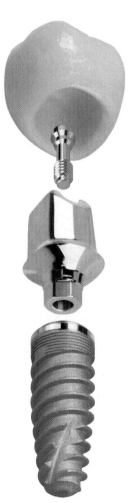

• Fig. 22.24 Cement-retained crown, shown in position over a screw-retained custom abutment.

standardized abutment or a custom abutment. Standardized abutments have pre-prepared margins that attempt to mimic the soft tissue contours of the implant interface. Custom abutments, although originally fabricated with a waxing and casting technique, are now largely milled from precision titanium components using CAD/CAM methodology (Box 22.7).

Advantages

More Traditional Prosthetic Technique. Many clinicians prefer a cement-retained prosthesis because the prosthetic and laboratory procedures parallel traditional prosthetics. The preparation, impression, laboratory, and insertion techniques are similar to procedures completed on natural teeth. Therefore many clinicians and their office staff are comfortable completing cement-retained prostheses.

Passive Fit. A cement-retained prosthesis has been shown to be advantageous because a more passive fit is obtained. Because a cementable prosthesis contains a "cement space," the prosthesis will be more passive in comparison with a screw-retained prosthesis. The cement space is ideally approximately 40 μm and will compensate for any fit variation. When a screw-retained prosthesis is fixated to implants, permanent strain conditions develop as the force is transmitted from the prosthetic screws to the implant body. Therefore studies have concluded that most screw-retained prostheses exhibit some degree of nonpassiveness.[47]

No Access Hole. Another key advantage of cement-retained restorations is the lack of a screw access hole in the restoration. Although an occlusal access hole in a posterior crown can predictably be filled in a reasonably esthetic manner, angled implants where the screw access is from the facial or incisal can create esthetic challenges. Even though specially designed screw-retained components have been fabricated to correct these angles, many clinicians find the cemented restoration to be a more viable solution.

The screw access hole, even when correctly placed on the occlusal surface of the crown, may still present clinical difficulties. When using ceramic and metal-ceramic restorations, there may exist unsupported ceramic material around the screw channel that is susceptible to chipping. Although this complication rarely occurs in the now commonly used stronger monolithic materials like BruxZir zirconia (Glidewell Dental), it is still a risk when using layered ceramic materials. In addition, the occlusal contacts may fall in the area of a screw access hole, resulting in an occlusal scheme that varies from the original restorative plan.

Disadvantages

Retrievability Difficulty. Retrievability Cement-retained restorations are more difficult for the clinician to remove from the

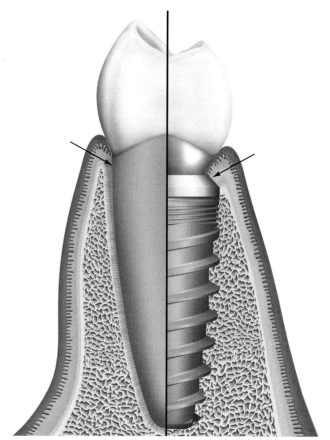

• **Fig. 22.25** Natural tooth versus implant soft tissue attachments. There exists no attachment of the tissue to the implant surface as seen with a natural tooth (arrows).

patient after delivery. Even when a provisional cement is used, the clinician risks damage to the restoration or implant in the removal process. When using a cement-retained restoration, the clinician must follow the same retentive principles established for crowns on natural teeth. The preparation must be sufficiently retentive or there will be a significant risk for debonding. A cemented restoration also requires greater interocclusal distance than does a screw-retained restoration.

Requires Increased Crown-Height Space. A cement-retained restoration requires a minimum of 7 to 8 mm of CHS, whereas a screw-retained restoration can be successfully delivered with a space of 5 to 7 mm. (Internal data, Glidewell Dental).

Cement Retention. Perhaps the most significant disadvantage for the use of cement-retained implant restorations is the risk for excess retained cement and the peri-implant complications that could result. Because of the absence of strong fibrous attachments between the implant and the soft tissue, the peri-implant tissues are more easily displaced and retain cement easier in comparison with a natural tooth with its stronger fibrous connections (Fig. 22.25).

Miscellaneous Restorations

Angulated screw channel

In some clinical situations the angulation of the implant requires an access hole through the facial aspect of the implant restoration. New technology has led to the development of the angulated screw channel (ASC). The ASC allows a screw-retained prosthesis to be fabricated when angulations of the implant are less than 25 degrees. This is accomplished by using a lingual access to fixate the prosthesis.

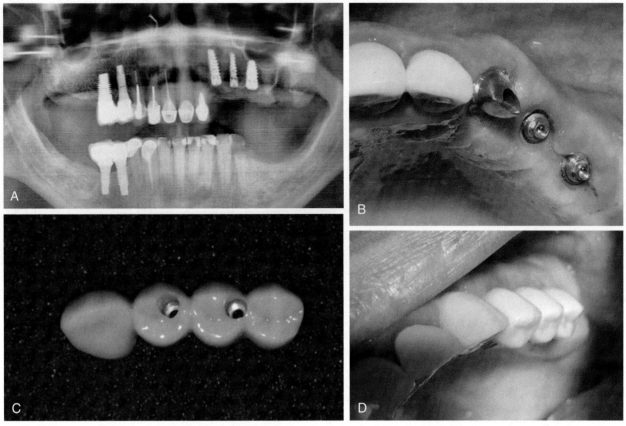

• **Fig. 22.26** Combination Prosthesis. (A) Radiograph depicting #11/#12/#13 implant placement. (B) Intraoral view of # 11 custom abutment and #12 to #13 screw-retained abutments. (C) Combination screw-cement prosthesis with #11 (cementable) and #12 to #13 (screw-retained). (D) Final insertion of screw-cementable prosthesis.

Screw-cementable (combination) prosthesis

In clinical cases in which multiple implants are splinted together, and one or more of the implants are positioned with the screw access within the buccal aspect of the prosthesis, a combination prosthesis may be fabricated. This technique combines the advantages of cement and screw-retained prostheses into the same prosthesis. The combined prosthesis allows for the use of a temporary cement over the telescoped abutment (cement-retained) and fixation screws on the screw-retained part of the prosthesis. This allows for retrievability, along with ease of seating and enhanced esthetics (Fig. 22.26).

Ideal Positioning for Screw and Cement-Retained Prosthesis

Ideal implant positioning must be completed to optimize the esthetics of the implant restoration. The following are recommendations for ideal implant positioning (implant body long axis) for screw and cement-retained prostheses (Fig. 22.27):

Anterior

Cement retained: slightly lingual to incisal edge
Screw retained: cingulum area

Posterior

Cement retained: central fossa
Screw retained: central fossa

Abutment Options

Abutments for Cement-Retained Restorations

Standardized (Stock) Abutments

Standardized (stock) abutments are prefabricated components that are screw retained and intended to be connected directly to the endosseous implant platform. These abutments are used for the retention of a cemented prosthesis and are indicated for a single- or multiple-implant prostheses. Each stock abutment is specific for the restorative platform and the implant type. There are several common designs (e.g., straight, angled, esthetic), which vary based on the position and contours of the margins (Fig. 22.28).

Standardized abutments are advantageous in that they are inexpensive and often can be modified by the clinician or laboratory for the specific case. The disadvantages of these abutments are that they are more likely to allow tissue show-through (i.e., darkness because of tissue translucency) and have been associated with poorer tissue health.[48]

Custom Abutments

Custom abutments may be fabricated by using a castable abutment or through a CAD/CAM process. They may be produced from titanium, gold alloy, or milled zirconia with a titanium base (Fig. 22.29). These abutments can be designed with the margin in the ideal position with respect to the soft tissue drape around the implant.

Custom abutments allow for better soft tissue health, along with correction of nonideal implant placement. The disadvantage of custom abutments includes an increased laboratory cost.

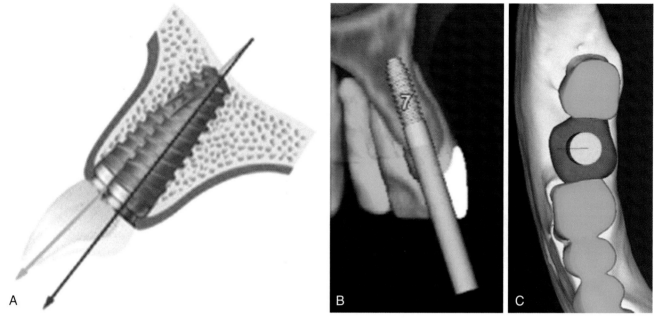

• **Fig. 22.27** Ideal Positioning: (a) Cement-Retained - slightly lingual to incisor edge (green arrow) and Screw-retained - cingulum area (red arrow), (b) CBCT cross section depicting ideal placement for cement-retained prosthesis. and (C) posterior screw and cement retained.

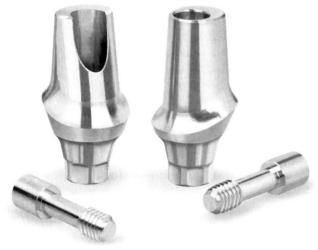

• **Fig. 22.28** Standardized abutments for cemented restorations.

Abutments for Screw-Retained Restorations

With few exceptions, most abutments for screw-retained restorations are standardized components (e.g., multiunit abutments). The contemporary design of today's multiunit abutment differs markedly from the component introduced in the original Brånemark protocol. Although the Standard Abutment once marketed by Nobelpharma (Fig. 22.30) provided the advantages of screw retention, the cylindrical design placed the restoration well above the soft tissue emergence of the implant, resulting in the Swedish high water design (Fig. 22.31). With the development of the multiunit abutments (Fig. 22.32), it is now possible to design prostheses that mimic a natural emergence profile from the soft tissue (Fig. 22.33).

Restorative Materials

There are few, if any, areas of restorative dentistry that have advanced as far in recent years as the choices of restorative materials that are

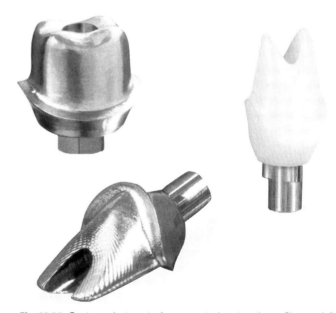

• **Fig. 22.29** Custom abutments for cemented restorations. Shown, left to right, are posterior titanium abutment, anterior titanium abutment, and anterior ceramic-titanium hybrid abutment.

offered to the clinician providing implant restorations. Use of these materials is made possible by concomitant advances in CAD/CAM. In addition to the advanced computer-guided milling machines that enable the fabrication of these designs, there is rapid development in additive manufacturing, or three-dimensional printing, in providing implant restorations. In implant dentistry today the state-of-the-art esthetic restorative crown and bridge materials consist of monolithic ceramics such as zirconia (ceramic) and lithium disilicate (glass-ceramic), as well as porcelain fused to metal.

Zirconia

The use of zirconia is increasingly more popular than the traditional porcelain fused-to-metal prostheses. Most monolithic zirconia

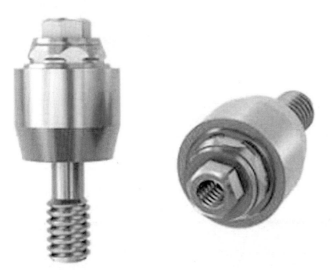

• **Fig. 22.30** "Standard Abutment," which is no longer in production.

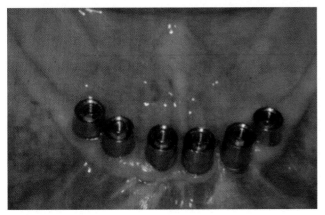

• **Fig. 22.31** Swedish High Water Design: Standard abutments which attach to the implant place the prosthesis above tissue level.

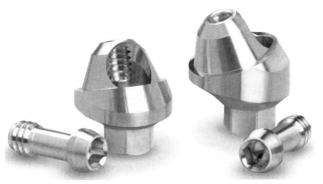

• **Fig. 22.32** Multiunit Abutment (Glidewell Dental).

restorations are made of a partially stabilized zirconia (i.e., 3% yttria, 97% zirconia). Compared with other all-ceramic crown and bridge materials, monolithic zirconia exhibits a unique combination of high flexural strength, fracture toughness, and exceptional esthetics. Originally these restorations were specifically fabricated for posterior prostheses; however, with improved zirconia formulations and manufacturing processes, enhanced translucency and shading are present, which make them an anterior esthetic option as well.

The posterior monolithic zirconia (e.g., BruxZir Full Strength Solid Zirconia) can be used for screw-retained crowns in the

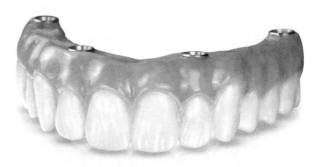

• **Fig. 22.33** Monolithic full-arch prosthesis, secured by multiunit abutments (BruxZir).

posterior, posterior bridges, and full-arch restorations (Fig. 22.34). Advanced staining techniques have enabled technicians to create a one-piece restoration with strength far exceeding hybrid restorations or layered restorations, while offering excellent esthetics. In the anterior regions of the mouth a third-generation material (e.g., BruxZir Esthetic) exhibits excellent translucency and shading and tensile strength that far exceeds other esthetic restorative materials. It can be used for anterior crowns, veneers, anterior screw-retained crowns, and short span bridges in the anterior (Fig. 22.35).

Lithium Disilicate and Lithium Silicate

Lithium disilicate, introduced by Ivoclar Vivadent as IPS e.max, and lithium silicate, manufactured by Glidewell Dental as Obsidian, are highly esthetic and versatile glass ceramic monolithic materials that can be milled or pressed to create veneers, crowns, and short span bridges. Although not providing the same flexural strength or fracture toughness shown by zirconia materials, they exhibit higher levels of translucency than the full-strength versions of these materials (Fig. 22.36).

Metal-Ceramic

Metal-ceramic restorations were developed in the 1970s to provide a higher-strength alternative to the feldspathic porcelains that were then available. By creating a cast metal framework that was layered with feldspathic porcelain, dental laboratories were able to significantly increase the strength of the restoration, and still maintain high esthetics. Two major technological advances have enabled the development of a new generation of metal-ceramic restorations that exhibit even greater strength, esthetics, and accuracy of fit. The advent of direct metal laser sintering, or three-dimensional printing of dental frameworks, provided a new level of fit and consistency for the metal underlying the metal-ceramic restoration. In addition, a pressable lithium silicate material, Obsidian, was developed that is significantly stronger than the feldspathic porcelains previously used for veneering. The combination created a strong and highly esthetic restoration that provides a better fit than a cast metal veneered restoration. Obsidian pressed to metal restorations can be used in the anterior or posterior for single crowns, short or long span bridges, and screw-retained implant crowns (Fig. 22.37).

Gold Alloy

For more than 100 years, gold alloy restorations have been a predictable and highly useful dental material. No dental material has more long-term documentation than gold alloy. This material has declined in popularity because of the increasing cost of noble metals, as well as patients' demand for more esthetic restorations. Gold alloy is primarily used for crowns, bridges, and screw-retained implant crowns in the posterior (Fig. 22.38).

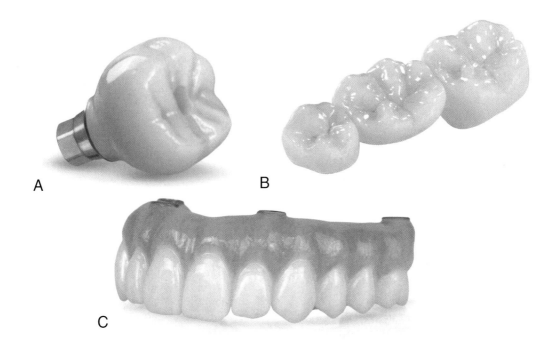

• **Fig. 22.34** Monolithic Zirconia. (A) BruxZir SRC (screw-retained crown), (B) BruxZir bridge, and (C) BruxZir full-arch screw-retained bridge.

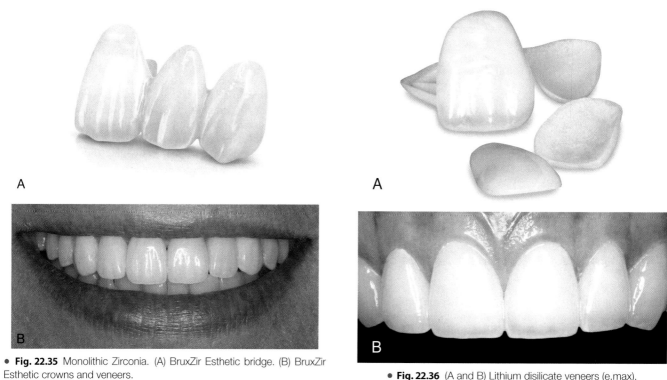

• **Fig. 22.35** Monolithic Zirconia. (A) BruxZir Esthetic bridge. (B) BruxZir Esthetic crowns and veneers.

• **Fig. 22.36** (A and B) Lithium disilicate veneers (e.max).

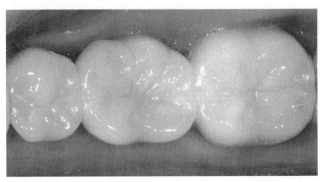

• **Fig. 22.37** Lithium disilicate (Obsidian pressed to metal restorations).

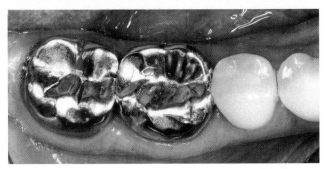

• **Fig. 22.38** Gold alloy crowns.

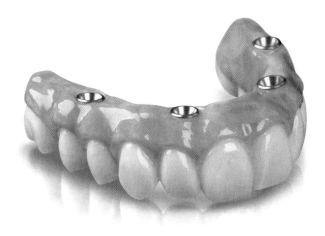

• **Fig. 22.39** Polymethylmethacrylate provisional full-arch bridge on implants.

Polymethylmethacrylate

Polymethylmethacrylate (PMMA) is a stable resin that demonstrates strength and translucency when milled using CAD/CAM technology. It is commonly used to create short- and medium-term provisionals for implant restorations to evaluate esthetics and phonetics, and to enable progressive loading treatment plans. It is also used for patient prototyping in the production of full-arch zirconia implant bridges, enabling the patient to wear a PMMA replica of his or her final zirconia bridge to provide a meaningful final approval for the design (Fig. 22.39 and Table 22.2).

TABLE 22.2	Current Recommendations for Single- and Multiple-Implant Crowns

Single-Implant Crowns

Anterior

1. Monolithic zirconia (BruxZir Esthetic)
2. Monolithic glass-ceramic (IPS e.max, Obsidian)
3. Metal-ceramic (Obsidian pressed to metal)
4. Metal-ceramic (porcelain fused to metal)

Posterior

1. Monolithic zirconia (BruxZir Full-Strength)
2. Metal-ceramic (Obsidian pressed to metal)
3. Metal-ceramic (porcelain fused to metal)

Multiple-Implant Crowns

Anterior

1. Monolithic zirconia (BruxZir Esthetic)
2. Monolithic glass-ceramic (IPS e.max, Obsidian)
3. Metal-ceramic (Obsidian pressed to metal: laser-sintered in non-, semi-, or precious)

Posterior

1. Monolithic zirconia (BruxZir Full-Strength)
2. Metal-ceramic (Obsidian pressed to metal: laser-sintered in non-, semi-, or precious)
3. Metal-ceramic (porcelain fused to metal)

References

1. Misch CE. *Dental Implant Prosthetics*. 2nd ed. St Louis: Mosby; 2015.
2. Chalmers I. The Cochrane Collaboration: preparing, maintaining, and disseminating systematic reviews of the effects of health care. *Ann N Y Acad Sci*. 1993;703:156–165.
3. Wetherell J, Smales R. Partial dentures failure: a long-term clinical survey. *J Dent*. 1980;8:333–340.
4. Shugars DA, Bader JD, White BA, et al. Survival rates of teeth adjacent to treated and untreated posterior bounded edentulous spaces. *J Am Dent Assoc*. 129:1085.
5. Rissin L, House JE, Conway C, et al. Effect of age and removable partial dentures on gingivitis and periodontal disease. *J Prosthet Dent*. 1979;42:217–223.
6. Krišto B, Krželj I. Foreign body in the esophagus: chronically impacted partial denture without serious complication. *Otolaryngology Case Reports*. 2016;1(1):5–7.
7. Hashmi S, Walter J, Smith W, Latis S. Swallowed partial dentures. *J Royal Society Med*. 2004;97(2):72–75.
8. Priest GF. Failure rates of restorations for single tooth replacements. *Int J Prosthodont*. 1996;9:38–45.
9. Wood M, Kern M, Thomson VP, et al. Ten year clinical and microscopic evaluation of resin bonded restorations. *Quintessence Int*. 1996;27:803–807.
10. Johnston JE, Phillips RN, Dykema RW, eds. *Modern Practice in Crown and Bridge Prosthodontics*. Philadelphia: WB Saunders; 1971.
11. Creugers NH, Kayser HF, Van 't Hof MA. A meta-analysis of durability data on conventional fixed bridges. *Community Dent Oral Epidemiol*. 1994;22:448–452.

12. Walton JN, Gardner FM, Agar JR. A survey of crown and fixed partial denture failures, length of service and reasons for replacement. *J Prosthet Dent.* 1986;56:416–421.

13. Payne BJ, Locker D. Oral self-care behaviours in older dentate adults. *Community Dent Oral Epidemiol.* 1992;20:376–380.

14. Jackson CR, Skidmore AE, Rice RT. Pulpal evaluation of teeth restored with fixed prostheses. *J Prosthet Dent.* 1992;67:323–325.

15. Bergenholtg G, Nyman S. Endodontic complications following periodontal and prosthetic treatment of patients with advanced periodontal disease. *J Peridontol.* 1984;55:63–68.

16. Randow K, Glantz PO, Zoger B. Technical failures and some related clinical complications in extensive fixed prosthodontics: an epidemiological study of long-term clinical quality. *Acta Odontol Scand.* 1986;44:241–255.

17. Bell B, Rose CL, Damon A. The Normative Aging Study: an interdisciplinary and longitudinal study of health and aging. *Int J Aging Hum Dev.* 1972;3:5–17.

18. Misch CE, Misch-Dietsh F, Silc J, et al. Posterior implant single tooth replacement and status of abutment teeth: multicenter 10 year retrospective report. *J Periodontol.* 2008;79(12):2378–2382.

19. Jemt T, Lekholm U, Grondahl K. Three year follow up study of early single implant restoration ad modum Brånemark. *Int J Periodontics Restorative Dent.* 1990;10:340–349.

20. Andersson B, Odman P, Lidvall AM, et al. Single tooth restoration supported by osseointegrated implants: results and experience from a prospective study after 2 to 3 years. *Int J Oral Maxillofac Implants.* 1995;10:702–711.

21. Schmitt A, Zarb GA. The longitudinal clinical effectiveness of osseointegrated dental implants for single tooth replacement. *Int J Prosthodont.* 1993;6:187–202.

22. Goodacre CJ, Bernal G, Rungcharassaeng K, et al. Clinical complications with implants and implant prostheses. *J Prosthet Dent.* 2003;90:121–132.

23. Graber TM. Anomalies in number of teeth. In: Graber TM, ed. *Orthodontics: Principles and Practice.* 2nd ed. Philadelphia: WB Saunders; 1966.

24. Maklin M, Dummett Jr CO, Weinberg R. A study of oligodontia in a sample of New Orleans children. *J Dent Child.* 1979;46:478–482.

25. Caprioglio D, Vernole B, Aru G, et al. *Le Agenesie Dentali.* Milan, Italy: Masson; 1988:1–14.

26. Oosterle LJ. Implant considerations in the growing child. In: Higuchi KW, ed. *Orthodontic Applications of Osseointegrated Implants.* Chicago: Quintessence; 2000.

27. Spray JR, Black CG, Morris HF, et al. The influence of bone thickness on facial marginal bone response: stage 1 placement through stage 2 uncovering. *Ann Periodontol.* 2000;5:119–128.

28. Misch CE, D'Alessio R, Misch-Dietsh F. Maxillary partial anodontia and implant dentistry-maxillary anterior partial anodontia in 255 adolescent patients: a 15-year retrospective study of 276 implant site replacement. *Oral Health.* 2005;95:4557.

29. Wennstrom JL, Ekestubbe A, Grondahl K, et al. Implant-supported single-tooth restorations: a 5-year prospective study. *J Clin Periodontol.* 2005;32:567–574.

30. Zarone F, Sorrentino R, Vaccaro F. Prosthetic treatment of maxillary lateral incisor agenesis with osseointegrated implants: a 24-39 month prospective clinical study. *Clin Oral Implants Res.* 2006;17:94–101.

31. Lindhe T, Gunne J, Tillberg A. A meta-analysis of implants in partial edentulism. *Clin Oral Implants Res.* 1998;9:80–90.

32. Creugers NH, Kreuler PA, Snoek RJ, et al. A systematic review of single tooth restorations supported by implants. *J Dent.* 2000;28:209–217.

33. Lindhe T, Gunne J, Tillberg A. A meta-analysis of implants in partial edentulism. *Clin Oral Implants Res.* 1998;9:80–90.

34. Goodacre CJ, Bernal G, Rungcharassaeng K, et al. Clinical complications with implants and implant prostheses. *J Prosthet Dent.* 2003;90:121–132.

35. Kemppainen P, Eskola S, Ylipaavalniemi A. Comparative prospective clinical study of two single tooth implants: a preliminary report of 102 implants. *J Prosthet Dent.* 1997;77:382–387.

36. Priest GF. Failure rates of restorations for single tooth replacements. *Int J Prosthodont.* 1996;9:38–45.

37. Misch CE, D'Alessio R, Misch-Dietsh F. Maxillary partial anodontia and implant dentistry-maxillary anterior partial anodontia in 255 adolescent patients: a 15-year retrospective study of 276 implant site replacement. *Oral Health.* 2005;95:45–57.

38. Sullivan DY. Wide implants for wide teeth. *Dent Econ.* 1994;84:82–83.

39. Rangert B, Krogh PH, Langer B, et al. Bending overload and fixture fracture: a retrospective clinical analysis. *Int J Oral Maxillofac Implants.* 1995;10:326–334.

40. Langer B, Langer L, Herrman I, et al. The wide fixture: a solution of special bone situations and a rescue for the compromised implant. *Int J Oral Maxillofac Implants.* 1993;8:400–408.

41. Bahat O, Handelsman M. Use of wide implants and double implants in the posterior jaw, a clinical report. *Int J Oral Maxillofac Implants.* 1996;11:379–386.

42. Balshi TJ, Wolfinger GJ. Two-implant-supported single molar replacement: interdental space requirements and comparison to alternative options. *Int J Periodontics Restorative Dent.* 1997;17:426–435.

43. Geramy A, Morgano SM. Finite element analysis of three designs of an implant-supported molar crown. *J Prosthet Dent.* 2004;92:434–440.

44. Tarnow DR, Cho SC, Wallace SS. The effect of inter-implant distance on the height of inter-implant bone crest. *J Periodontol.* 2000;71:546–549.

45. Wright PS, Glastz PO, Randow K, et al. The effects of fixed and removable implant-stabilized prostheses on posterior mandibular residual ridge resorption. *Clin Oral Implants Res.* 2002;13:169–174.

46. Reddy MS, Geurs NC, Wang IC, et al. Mandibular growth following implant restoration: does Wolff's Law apply to residual ridge resorption? *Int J Periodontics Restorative Dent.* 2002;22:315–321.

47. Carr AB, Stewart RB. Full–arch implant framework casting accuracy: preliminary in vitro observation for in vivo testing. *J Prosthodontics.* 1993;2(1):2–8.

48. Broggini N, et al. Persistent acute inflammation at the implant-abutment interface. *J Dental Res.* 2003;82(3):232–237.

23

Treatment Planning for the Edentulous Posterior Maxilla

RANDOLPH R. RESNIK AND CARL E. MISCH[†]

Historically the maxillary posterior region has been one of the most difficult regions in the oral cavity to treat. Maxillary posterior partial or complete edentulism is one of the more common treatment areas in implant dentistry. However, the maxillary posterior edentulous region presents many unique and challenging conditions in implant dentistry that many years ago led to an area with the highest implant failure rate. Over the years many new surgical protocols and technological advances have led to this region being as predictable as any other region in the oral cavity. Most noteworthy of these surgical methods includes sinus augmentation to increase available bone height, ridge augmentation to increase bone width, better-designed shorter implants, and modified surgical approaches to insert implants in poorer bone density.[1] Grafting of the maxillary sinus to overcome the problem of reduced vertical available bone has become a very popular and predictable procedure since the 1990's. After the initial introduction by Tatum in the mid-1970s and the initial publication of Boyne and James in 1980, many studies have been published about sinus grafting with results higher than 90%.[2-38] This chapter will address the various disadvantages inherent with the posterior maxilla, along with the treatment planning factors and concepts specific to the maxillary posterior partial or complete edentulous regions.

Inherent Disadvantages of Posterior Maxilla Treatment

Poor Bone Density

In general the bone quality is poorest in the edentulous posterior maxilla compared with any other intraoral region.[30] A literature review of clinical studies reveal poorer bone density may result in decreased implant loading survival by an average of 16% and has been reported to be as low as 40%.[31] The cause of the poorer success rate is related to several factors. Bone strength is directly related to its density, and the poor density bone of this region is often 5 to 10 times weaker in comparison with bone found in the anterior mandible (~ D2 Bone Quality).[32] Bone densities directly influence the percent of implant–bone surface contact (bone–implant contact or

BIC), which accounts for the force transmission to the bone. The bone–implant contact (~<30%) is the lowest in D4 (Type 4) bone compared with other bone densities. The stress patterns distributed within poor bone density migrate farther toward the apex of the implant. As a result, bone loss is more pronounced and occurs also deeper along the implant body, rather than only crestally as in other denser bone conditions. D4 bone also has been shown to exhibit the greatest biomechanical elastic modulus difference compared with titanium under load.[32] This biomechanical mismatch develops a higher strain condition to the bone, which may be in the pathologic overload range. As such, modified surgical protocols are warranted to increase bone-implant contact.

In the posterior maxilla the poorer deficient osseous structures and the minimal cortical plate on the crest of the ridge will compromise the initial implant stability (insertion torque) at the time of placement (Fig. 23.1). The labial cortical plate is usually thin, and the ridge is often wide. As a result the lateral cortical bone–implant contact to stabilize the implant is often insignificant because implant placement rarely engages the buccal plate. Therefore initial healing of an implant in D4 bone is often compromised, and clinical reports indicate a lower initial healing success than with D2 or D3 bone.

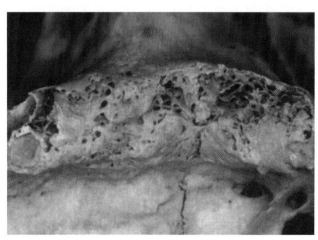

• **Fig. 23.1** D4 bone density, which is usually found in the posterior maxilla. This type of bone usually exhibits minimal cortical bone and has very fine trabeculae.

[†] Deceased

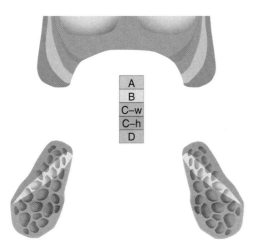

• **Fig. 23.2** As bone resorbs in the maxilla, the ridge shifts toward the lingual and encroaches on the maxillary sinus. This also will result in a change in the relationship of the maxilla and mandible.

Decreased Available Bone

In the posterior maxilla the implant clinician is often confronted with a decreased bone quantity, thereby compromising implant placement. The dentate maxilla is usually associated with a thinner cortical plate on the facial compared with the mandible. Because the trabecular bone of the posterior maxilla is finer than other dentate regions, the loss of maxillary posterior teeth usually results in an initial decrease in bone width at the expense of the labial bony plate. The width of the posterior maxilla will decrease at a more rapid rate than in any other region of the jaws.[25] The resorption phenomenon is accelerated by the loss of vascularization of the alveolar bone and the existing fine trabecular bone type. However, because the initial residual ridge is so wide in the posterior maxilla, even with a significant decrease in the width of the ridge, ideal size root form implants usually can be placed (Fig. 23.2).

Increased Pneumatization of the Maxillary Sinus

Pneumatization is a normal physiologic process that occurs in all paranasal sinuses during the growth period, which results in an increased volume. Histologic studies have shown that the pneumatization process occurs by osteoclastic resorption of the cortical walls of the sinus. However, the etiology of maxillary sinus pneumatization is poorly understood and has been associated with heredity, pneumatization drive of the nasal mucous membrane, craniofacial configuration, bone density, growth hormones, and intra-sinus air pressure.[39]

The pneumatization process has been shown to increase in size after tooth extraction. Most likely this is a result of a decrease in functional forces that are transferred to the bone after tooth loss and the remodeling process involving disuse atrophy according to Wolff's law.[40] Because of the proximity and possible protrusion of the maxillary sinus roots into the sinus, the lack of cortical bone lining after extraction will allow the sinus to expand. Studies have also shown that pneumatization is greater after molar extraction in comparison with premolar extractions, mainly because of the greater resultant defect.[41] Sharan and Madjar[39] in pneumatization studies showed that a preextraction curving sinus floor resulted in greater expansion. In addition, when two or more adjacent posterior teeth were extracted or when a second molar was extracted (in comparison with the first molar), greater expansion was reported (Fig. 23.3).

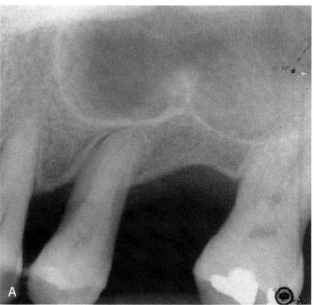

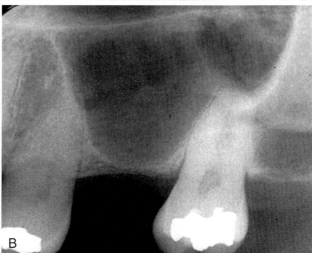

• **Fig. 23.3** Maxillary Sinus Pneumatization. (A and B) After tooth loss the maxillary sinus expands (non-uniformly) and approaches the maxillary sinus floor, which decreases available bone for implant placement.

Resultant Increased Crown Height Space

As the vertical bone loss increases, the crown height space increases. This most likely will result in implant placement inferior to the adjacent interproximal bone (if present) and inferior to the ideal apical-coronal position (i.e., 2–3 mm below the free gingival margin). The inferior positioning results in an increased crown height space, thereby increasing morbidity to the long-term prognosis of the implant prosthesis. Sevimay et al.,[42] in a three-dimensional finite element analysis, showed that when increasing the crown height from 10 to 20 mm, the strain values placed on the implant prosthesis increased 72% for tensile stress and 41% for compressive stress (Fig. 23.4). Therefore, implant prostheses in this area are at an increased risk in comparison to other areas of the oral cavity.

Lingual Oriented Ridge Position

As a result of the horizontal bone resorption process the ridge will progressively shift toward the palate until the ridge is resorbed into a medially positioned narrower bone volume.[29] The posterior maxilla continues to remodel toward the midline as the bone resorption

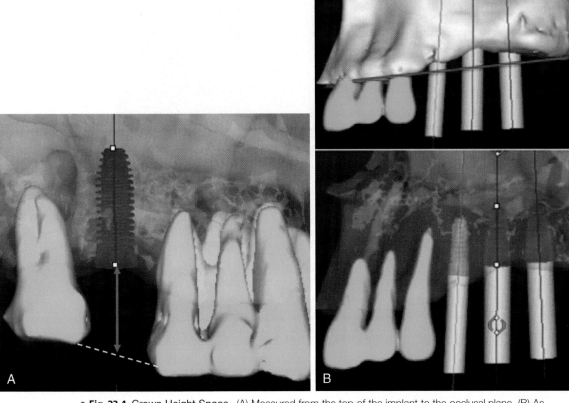

• **Fig. 23.4** Crown Height Space. (A) Measured from the top of the implant to the occlusal plane. (B) As bone resorbs from Division A to Division D, the vertical height position becomes more apical. This results in an increased crown height, even if vertical grafting is completed within the sinus.

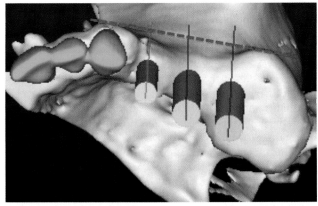

• **Fig. 23.5** Another component of the maxillary posterior resorption process is the shifting of the ridge to the lingual. Because of the lingual positioning, implants are often placed in a nonideal buccal-lingual position.

process continues. Because of this resorption pattern, the buccal cusp of the final prosthesis will usually be cantilevered facially to satisfy the esthetic requirements at the expense of biomechanics in the moderate-to-severe atrophic ridges (Fig. 23.5).

Anatomic Location

Because of the maxillary posterior's anatomic location, access is a common problem. Especially when lack of opening is present,

surgical placement of implants in the posterior is sometimes difficult because of the lack of interocclusal space. Most commonly, maximum mouth opening is measured in the anterior by using the interincisal distance. Studies vary on the definition of a restricted opening; however, it is usually within the 35- to 40-mm distance.[43] Because the posterior opening is far less than the anterior, obtaining sufficient space for implant placement or prosthetic procedures is usually difficult. Insufficient space also becomes increasingly problematic when using a cone beam computed tomography (CBCT) surgical template for implant placement. In addition, the lack of space will increase the risk for swallowed or aspirated objects (Fig. 23.6).

Increased Biting Force

The occlusal forces in the posterior region are greater than in the anterior regions of the mouth. Studies have shown that the maximum bite force in the anterior region ranges from 35 to 50 lb/in^2. The bite force in the molar region of a dentate person ranges from 200 to 250 lb/in^2. Therefore, a 5:1 ratio exists between the maxilla and mandible. Parafunctional forces may increase the resultant force as much as threefold, which leads to greater implant and prosthetic morbidity.[44-46] As a consequence the maxillary molars of the natural teeth have 200% more surface area than the premolars and are significantly wider in diameter (Fig. 23.6).[1] Both of these features will reduce the stress to bone, which also decreases

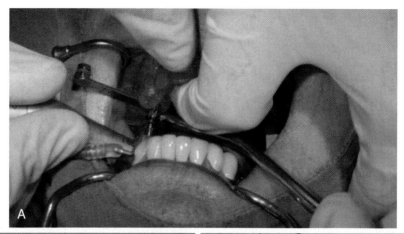

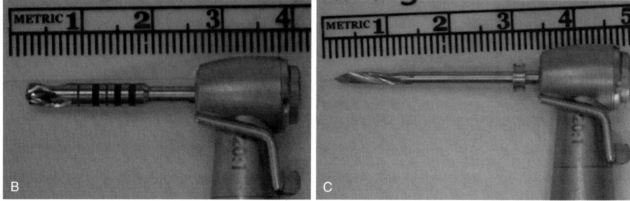

• **Fig. 23.6** (A) It is often difficult to have adequate space for implant placement, especially in the posterior maxilla. With the popularity of guided surgery, it becomes even more difficult because greater space is required for implant placement. (B) Standard surgical drill, (C) Guided drill kits contain drills that are usually longer (~10 mm) than regular-size drills.

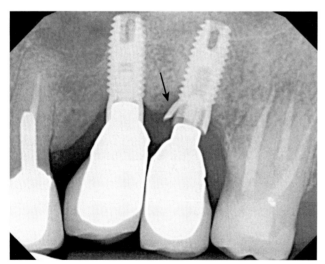

• **Fig. 23.7** Increased biting force may lead to accelerated crestal bone loss, along with mechanical stress complications such as fractured prostheses, screw loosening, and fractured implants.

the strain of the bone. Following this natural selection, implant support should be greater in the posterior molar region than any other area of the mouth.[1] Therefore the decrease in bone quantity and quality and increased forces should be considered in the treatment plan of this region of the mouth (Fig. 23.7).[47]

Requirement of Greater Surface Area Diameter Implants and Minimized Occlusal Forces

When treatment planning in the posterior maxilla to combat biomechanical forces, ideally conditions should be simulated as those found with natural teeth. Because stresses occur primarily at the crestal region, biomechanical designs of implants to minimize their noxious effects should be implemented.[47] Implant diameter is an effective method to increase surface area at the crestal region and combat the forces.[47,48] Ideally Division B implants are not used in the posterior maxilla. A 12-year retrospective study of 653 sinus grafts performed by Misch revealed 14 implant failures.[49] Eight implant failures were caused by implant fracture at the neck of smaller-diameter implants. Therefore implants of at least 5 mm in diameter are suggested, or multiple splinted 4-mm implants in the molar area.

Over the years the concept of implant length has become less important to long-term implant success. Because the majority of force is transmitted only to the middle-crestal area of the implant, less emphasis is now placed on the need for longer implants. In general the better the bone quality, the less critical the implant length. However, with poorer bone quality, or extensive graft areas, greater length increases the surface area, allowing for better initial fixation or primary stability.

In certain cases, increasing implant number is an excellent method to decrease associated stresses. Normally one implant is indicated for each missing tooth. However, if narrower implants are indicated, then more implants should be placed and splinted

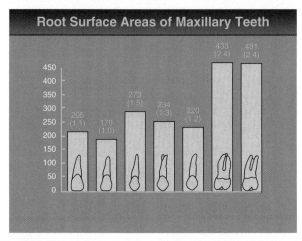

• **Fig. 23.8** Root surface areas are significantly greater in the posterior versus the anterior.

together to reduce stresses to the bone. If excessive force factors are present, two implants for each molar are then recommended.

And lastly, posterior cantilevers on implant prostheses should be minimized. Narrow occlusal tables with centered implant contact points prevent shear type of forces, which are detrimental to the implant interface (Fig. 23.8).

Maxillary Sinus Has High Incidence of Pathology

The maxillary sinus has the highest incidence of pathology in comparison with any of the other paranasal sinuses. Most studies report 30% to 40% of asymptomatic patients have some type of pathology present in their sinuses (i.e., inflammation, cysts, mucoceles, rhinosinusitis, fungal infections, carcinomas, antroliths). Therefore because many posterior maxillas require grafting, the presence of pathology results in complications and delayed treatment (Fig. 23.9).[51,52]

Treatment History

Treatment of the Posterior Maxilla—Literature Review

Over the years several strategies have been advocated to restore the posterior maxilla and address the deficiency of bone volume and poor bone quality. The various approaches can be categorized as follows:
• Avoid the maxillary sinus and place implants anteriorly, posteriorly, or medially.[52-54]
• Place implants and perforate the sinus floor.[55,56]
• Perform sinus augmentation procedures with simultaneous or delayed implant placement.[2-6,13,57-62]
• Elevate sinus floor during implant placement.[2,3,5,57-66]
• Use alternative types of implants.
• Use subperiosteal implants.[67,68]
• Perform horizontal osteotomy, interpositional bone grafting, and endosteal implants.[69,70]

In the early days of oral implantology, implants were inserted in the posterior maxilla without modifying the maxillary sinus topography. Shorter-length implants were often placed below the antrum. The decreased surface area, compounded by poor bone quality, resulted in poor implant stability and increased failure rates. Attempts to place larger endosteal implants posterior to the

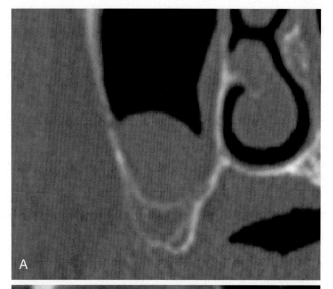

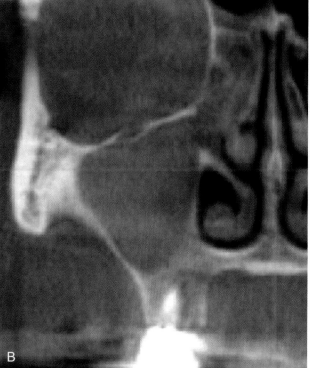

• **Fig. 23.9** The maxillary sinus has a high incidence of pathology, which can range from (A) cystic lesions and (B) completely opacified sinus cavities.

antrum and into the tuberosity and pterygoid plates also resulted in compromised situations. Although feasible from a surgical standpoint, rarely are third- or fourth-molar abutments indicated for proper prosthodontic support. This approach often requires a greater pontic space (i.e., three or more pontics between the anterior and posterior implants). The resultant prosthesis span will result in excessive flexibility of the prosthesis, unretained restorations, excess stresses, and implant failure.

In the late 1960s Linkow reported that the blade-vent implant could be blunted and the maxillary sinus membrane slightly elevated to allow implant placement "into" the sinus in the posterior maxilla.[71] This technique required the presence of at least 7 mm of vertical bone height below the antrum.

Geiger and Pesch[55] reported that ceramic implants placed through the maxillary sinus floor could heal and stabilize without complication. Brånemark et al.[56] have shown that implants may be placed into the maxillary sinus without consequence if integration occurs between the implants and the bone below the sinus. Yet they also report a higher failure rate (70% success rate for 5–10 years) for this technique. Ashkinazy[54] and others have reported on using tomographic radiographs to determine whether adequate bone exists on the palatal aspect of the maxillary sinus for blade implants. However, Stoler[72] stated that after 25 consecutive computed tomographic scans of maxillae, adequate bone for implant support was not found on the medial aspect of the sinus. Thus it seems that if sufficient bone is present medial to the sinus, it is the rare exception.

In the early 1970s Tatum[2,3,58,63] began to augment the posterior maxilla with onlay autogenous rib bone to produce adequate vertical bone for implant support. He found that onlay grafts below the existing alveolar crest would decrease the posterior intradental height significantly, yet very little bone for endosteal implants would be gained. Therefore in 1974 Tatum developed a modified Caldwell-Luc procedure for elevation of the sinus membrane and subantral (SA) augmentation.[2,3] The Caldwell-Luc procedure was established by the American George Caldwell and the Frenchman Henry Luc, who in 1893 described a new technique and procedure to access the maxillary sinus using a lateral window.[73] The crestal ridge of the maxilla was infractured and used to elevate the maxillary sinus membrane. Autogenous bone was then added in the area previously occupied by the inferior third of the sinus. Endosteal implants were inserted in the grafted bone after approximately 6 months. Implants were then loaded with a final prosthesis after an additional 6 months.[2,3]

In 1975 Tatum developed a lateral approach surgical technique that allowed the elevation of the sinus membrane and implant placement in the same surgical appointment. The implant system used was a one-piece ceramic implant, and a permucosal post was required during the healing period. Early ceramic implants were not designed adequately for this procedure, and results with the technique were unpredictable. In 1981 Tatum[58] developed a submerged titanium implant for use in the posterior maxilla.[3] The advantages of submerged healing, the use of titanium instead of aluminum oxide as a biomaterial, improved biomechanics, and improved surgical technique made this implant modality more predictable.

From 1974 to 1979 the primary graft material for the sinus graft procedure was autologous bone. In 1980 the application of the SA augmentation technique with a lateral maxillary approach was further expanded by Tatum with the use of synthetic bone. That same year, Boyne and James[4] reported on the use of autogenous bone for SA grafts. Most of the data published in the 1980s were anecdotal or based on very small sample sizes. In 1987 Misch[5] organized a treatment approach to the posterior maxilla based on the amount of bone below the antrum, and in 1989 he expanded the treatment approach to include the available bone width related to the surgical approach and implant design (Fig. 23.10).[61,62] Since then, minor modifications regarding the graft materials or surgical approach have been proposed.

In the 1990s the profession developed a much greater interest in the sinus graft technique.[13] Several reports flourished in the literature, reporting on minor changes in the technique, different materials used in the graft, different origins for the autogenous portion of the graft, histomorphometric data relative to the graft healing, and other retrospective studies relative to the survival rates of implants placed in grafted sinuses with a simultaneous or delayed approach.[60-62,74-87]

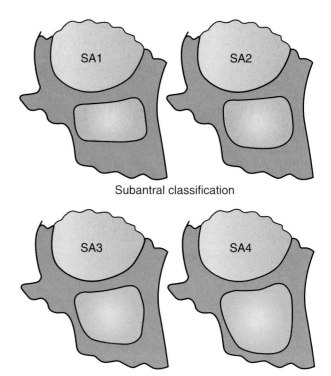

• **Fig. 23.10** In 1987 Misch presented four subantral treatment options based on the amount of bone below the maxillary sinus. Subantral augmentation category 1 (SA-1) sinus used traditional implant approaches. SA-2 used a sinus lift procedure within the osteotomy. For SA-3 and SA-4 a Tatum sinus graft procedure is performed before implant insertion.

Long-term results have been reported by Tatum et al.[60] to be greater than 95% in more than 1500 SA augmentations performed. The sinus graft procedure has been the most predictable method to grow bone height from 5 to 20 mm compared with any other intraoral bone-grafting technique, with a graft success rate and an implant survival rate greater than 95%.

An alternative technique, which was a less invasive technique using osteotomes, was introduced in 1994 by Summers.[88] And more recently, newer techniques include the use of shorter implants, placement of implants to avoid the sinus, elongated zygomatic implants, and pterygoid plate implants.

Sinus Graft Options for the Posterior Maxilla

A classification based on the amount of available bone height between the floor of the antrum and the crest of the residual ridge in the region of the ideal implant locations was presented by Misch[5] in 1987 and later modified by Resnik in 2017 (Table 23.1). This protocol detailed a surgical approach, bone graft material, and timetable for healing before prosthetic reconstruction. In 1988 Cawood and Howell also classified the edentulous posterior maxilla, which included the loss of bone and pneumatization of the maxillary sinus.[89] In 1995 Misch modified his 1987 classification to include the lateral dimension of the sinus cavity, and this dimension was used to modify the healing period protocol, because smaller-width sinuses (0–10 mm) tend to form bone faster than larger-width (>15 mm) sinuses. Other classifications of the sinus graft procedure have been proposed by Jensen[90] in 1998 and Chiapasco[80,91] in 2003. In 2017 Resnik further modified the Misch classification to include different augmentation techniques and the use of short implants with regard to existing force factors.

TABLE 23.1	Healing Times for Treatment Categories			
Procedure	Height (mm): Favorable/ Unfavorable Conditions	Procedure	Healing Time (Months): Graft	Healing Time (Months): Implant
SA-1	≥ 8 / ≥ 10	Division A root form placement	No Graft	4–6 (no bone grafting)
SA-2	≥ 6 / ≥ 8	Sinus "bump"; simultaneous Division A root form placement	No Graft	6–8 (no bone grafting)
SA-3	≥ 5 / ≥ 8	Sinus graft (transcrestal or lateral wall + implant placement)	6–8	6–8[a]
SA-4	< 5 / < 5	Lateral wall approach sinus graft; delayed Division A root form placement	6–8	6–10[a]

[a]Evaluate at implant insertion.

SA, Subantral augmentation option.

Misch-Resnik Maxillary Posterior Classification

There exist four treatment classifications based on the amount of bone available below the maxillary sinus (i.e., SA-1, SA-2, SA-3, and SA-4). Because implants in the posterior maxilla are susceptible to biomechanical stress, each category has been further divided into two divisions: favorable and unfavorable force factors.

Favorable Conditions
- Good quality of bone (D2/D3 bone) with the presence of cortical bone
- Minimal occlusal force factors
- No parafunction
- Ideal crown/implant ratio

Unfavorable Conditions
- Parafunction, high force factors
- Poor quality of bone (D3/D4 bone) with no cortical bone
- Increased occlusal force factors
- Parafunctional forces present
- Poor crown/implant ratio

Subantral Option 1: Conventional Implant Placement

The first SA treatment option, SA-1, is applied when there exists sufficient available bone height to permit the placement of endosteal implants without entry into the sinus proper. The minimum "ideal" bone height is related to force factors and the bone density. For posterior maxillae with favorable force factors, a small-length implant (~ 8 mm) may be used as long as there exists sufficient bone for a minimum width to accommodate a 5-mm-diameter implant. For unfavorable force factors a minimum of 10 mm of height is required.

Patients with narrower bone volume (Division B) may be treated with osteoplasty or augmentation to increase the width of bone. The insertion of smaller surface area implants is not suggested because the forces are greater in the posterior regions of the mouth, and the bone density is less than in most regions. In addition, the narrow ridge is often more medial than the central fossa of the mandibular teeth and will result in an offset load on the restoration, which will increase the strain to the bone. Osteoplasty in the SA-1 posterior maxilla may change the SA category if the height of the remaining bone is less than 8/10 mm after the bone modification is completed. Augmentation for width may be accomplished with membrane grafting, bone spreading, and autogenous onlay or appositional grafts. Larger-diameter implants are often required in the molar region, and bone spreading to

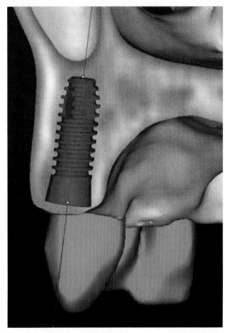

• **Fig. 23.11** Subantral option 1 (SA-1) technique that includes implant placement that does not enter the sinus proper.

place wider implants is the most common approach when the bone density is poor. If less than 2.5 mm of width is available in the posterior edentulous region (Division C–w), the most predictable treatment option is to increase width with onlay autogenous bone grafts.[92] After graft maturation the area is then reevaluated to determine the proper treatment plan classification. However, Division C–w posterior maxillas are unpredictable and require an increased skill set.

Although a common axiom in implant dentistry is to remain 2 mm or more from an opposing landmark, this is not indicated in the SA region (i.e., inferior floor of the sinus). As long as pathology is not present in the maxillary sinus, there exist no contraindications for placement of implants at the level of or engaging the cortical plate of the sinus floor. Healing of implants in the SA-1 category is allowed to continue uneventfully for a minimum of 4 to 6 months, depending on the bone density. Usually progressive loading is recommended during the prosthetic phases of the treatment when D3 or D4 bone is present (Figs. 23.11 and 23.12; Box 23.1).

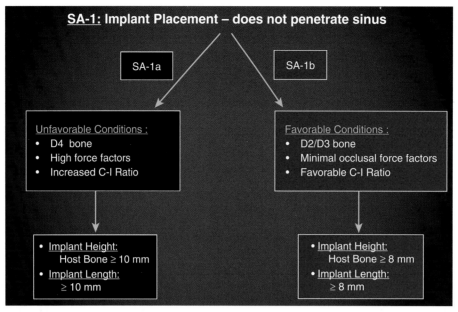

● **Fig. 23.12** Subantral option 1 (SA-1) protocol decision tree related to favorable versus unfavorable factors. *C-I,* Crown/implant.

● **BOX 23.1** SA-1: Implant Placement—Does Not Penetrate Sinus

Indications

Favorable conditions: >8 mm host bone (implant ≥8 mm in length)
Unfavorable conditions: >10 mm host bone (implant ≥10 mm in length)

See Surgical Protocol (Chapter 37)

Subantral Option 2: Sinus Lift and Simultaneous Implant Placement

The second SA option, SA-2, is selected when there is a minimum of 6/8 mm of vertical bone present (Fig. 23.11). In the SA-2 technique the sinus floor is elevated via the implant osteotomy 1 to 2 mm (Figs. 23.12 and 23.13). This technique was originally developed by Tatum[2,3] in 1970 and published by Misch[5] in 1987 and many years later by Summers[93] in 1994. The endosteal implant osteotomy is prepared as determined by the density of bone protocol. The depth of the osteotomy is approximately 1 to 2 mm short of the floor of the antrum. A cupped-shape osteotome of the same diameter (or slightly smaller) as the final osteotomy is selected.[94] It is of a different end shape than osteotomes used for bone spreading.[93] The osteotome is inserted and tapped firmly in 0.5- to 1-mm increments beyond the osteotomy until its final position up to 2 mm beyond the prepared implant osteotomy. This surgical approach causes a greenstick-type fracture in the antral floor and slowly elevates the unprepared bone and sinus membrane over the broad-based osteotome. The implant may be inserted into the osteotomy after the sinus membrane elevation and extend up to 2 mm above the floor of the sinus. The implant is slowly threaded into position so that the membrane is less likely to tear as it is elevated. The apical portion of the implant engages the denser bone on the cortical floor, with bone over the apex, and an intact sinus membrane. The implant may ideally extend up to 2 mm beyond the sinus floor, and the 1- to 2-mm bony covering over the apex may result in as much as a 3-mm elevation of the sinus mucosa (Fig. 23.14).

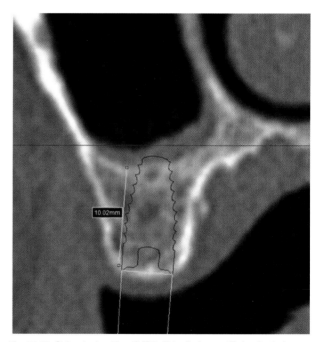

● **Fig. 23.13** Subantral option 2 (SA-2) technique with implant placement that includes a small bump into the sinus (~1 mm).

Because of the autologous bone present above the apical portion of the implant, along with the osteoprogenitor cell–rich sinus membrane, new bone formation is accelerated. The success of the intact sinus membrane elevation cannot be confirmed before or at the time of implant placement. Attempts to feel the elevation of the membrane from within an 8-mm-deep implant osteotomy that is approximately 3 mm in diameter may easily cause separation of the sinus lining.

The patient's prosthodontic treatment may proceed similar to that in the SA-1 category. If inadequate bone is formed around the apical portion of an implant after initial healing, the progressive loading protocol for D4 bone is suggested.

Some authors have reported the attempted SA-2 sinus lift procedure to gain more than 3 mm of implant vertical height.

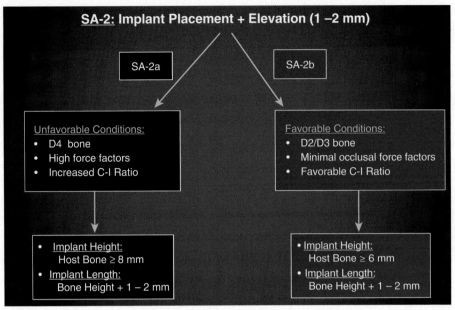

● **Fig. 23.14** Subantral option 2 (SA-2) protocol decision tree related to favorable versus unfavorable factors.

SA-2: Implant Placement: Membrane Bump 1-2mm No Graft (Osteotome Technique)

Indications

<u>Favorable conditions:</u> > 6 mm host bone (Implant length= Bone height + 1-2)
<u>Unfavorable conditions:</u> > 8 mm host bone (Implant length= Bone height + 1-2)

See Surgical Protocol (Chapter 37)

Blind surgical techniques such as the SA-2 technique increase the risk for sinus membrane perforation. When the sinus mucosa is perforated, the risk for postoperative infection increases. Membrane perforation is the primary reason why the SA-2 technique is restricted to elevating the membrane only 1 to 2 mm. In addition, the presence of a septum in the area of elevation increases the possibility of a perforation. If a sinus infection occurs, a bacterial smear layer may accumulate on the implant apex, which may precipitate mucociliary clearance issues and possible sinus infections.

Worth and Stoneman[95] have reported a comparable phenomenon of bone growth under an elevated sinus membrane, called *halo formation*. They observed the natural elevation of the sinus membrane around teeth with periapical disease. The elevation of the membrane resulted in new bone formation once the tooth infection was eliminated (Figs. 23.13 and 23.14; Box 23.2).

Subantral Option 3: Sinus Graft with Immediate Endosteal Implant Placement

The third approach to the maxillary posterior edentulous region, SA-3, is indicated when at least 5 mm of vertical bone height and sufficient width are present between the antral floor and the crest of the residual ridge in the area of the required prosthodontic abutment (Fig. 23.15). The 5-mm minimum is necessary because this is the amount of bone needed to achieve rigid fixation for implant placement.

There exist two different options for the grafting of the sinus area in the SA-3 protocol. In the first technique the bone graft is performed transcrestally. The osteotomy is performed, and the floor is fractured similar to the SA-2 technique. Before the implant placement, the layering technique is used consisting of a collagen membrane (first layer) and allograft (second layer). Autogenous bone may be placed in SA-3 cases when poor bone quality is present.

The second technique is the Tatum lateral maxillary wall approach. With this procedure an osteotomy of the lateral maxillary wall is performed to allow for bone graft placement before dental implant insertion. This results in a lateral access window, which exposes the sinus membrane and allows for the lateral window to be rotated in and upward in a superior position. As long as there is sufficient width, the implant may be placed at the same time after the grafting is complete. The graft material selected is usually allograft, unless there is easy access to autogenous bone. Autogenous bone is of less importance because of the existing host bone (minimum 5 mm of height) (Boxes 23.1 and 23.2). When the original ridge width is Division B or C–w, membrane grafting or onlay graft in conjunction with the sinus augmentation is a possible treatment option, and usually the case is classified as SA-4 because implant placement will be delayed.

The 5-mm minimum of initial bone height in an SA-3 posterior maxilla may have cortical bone on the residual crest, and cortical-like bone on the original antral floor may stabilize an implant that is inserted at the time of the graft and permit its primary stability. Therefore an endosteal implant may be inserted at this appointment and has been advocated for many years by Misch[5] and others (Figs. 23.15 and 23.16; Box 23.3).[12,15,59]

Subantral Option 4: Sinus Graft Healing and Extended Delay of Implant Insertion

In the fourth option for implant treatment of the posterior maxilla, SA-4, the maxillary sinus region for future endosteal implant insertion is first augmented. This option is indicated when less than 5 mm remains between the residual crest of bone and the floor of the maxillary sinus. There is inadequate vertical bone in

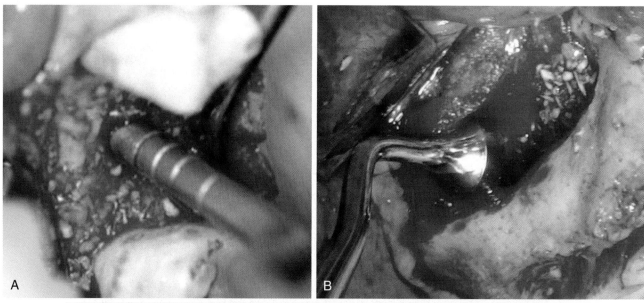

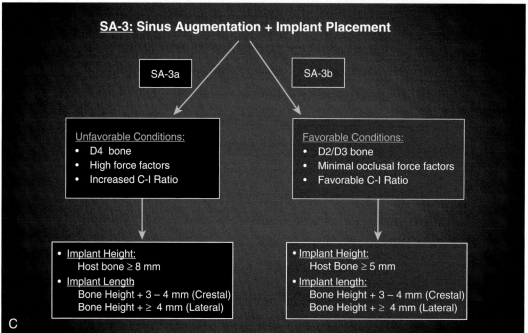

SA-3: Sinus Augmentation + Implant Placement

SA-3a

SA-3b

Unfavorable Conditions:
- D4 bone
- High force factors
- Increased C-I Ratio

Favorable Conditions:
- D2/D3 bone
- Minimal occlusal force factors
- Favorable C-I Ratio

- Implant Height:
  Host bone ≥ 8 mm
- Implant Length:
  Bone Height + 3 – 4 mm (Crestal)
  Bone Height + ≥ 4 mm (Lateral)

- Implant Height:
  Host Bone ≥ 5 mm
- Implant length:
  Bone Height + 3 – 4 mm (Crestal)
  Bone Height + ≥ 4 mm (Lateral)

C

• **Fig. 23.15** Subantral Option 3 (SA-3) Technique. (A) Implant placement with bone graft (crestal). (B) Implant placement with bone graft (lateral wall). (C) Decision tree related to favorable versus unfavorable factors and crestal versus lateral wall technique.

these conditions to predictably place an implant at the same time as the sinus graft and less recipient bone to act as a vascular bed for the graft and for primary stability (Fig. 23.17). The SA-4 protocol corresponds to a larger antrum and minimal host bone on the lateral, anterior, and distal regions of the graft, because the antrum generally has expanded more aggressively into these regions.

Unfortunately, in SA-4 posterior maxillas there is less autologous bone to harvest in the tuberosity, which further delays the bone regeneration in the site. In addition, there are usually fewer septa or webs in the sinus, which decreases complications, and it typically exhibits longer mediodistal and lateromedial dimensions. Therefore the fewer bony walls, less favorable vascular bed, minimal local autologous bone, and larger graft volume all mandate a longer healing period and slightly altered surgical approach.

The Tatum lateral wall approach for sinus graft is performed as in the previous SA-3 procedure (lateral wall). Most SA-4 regions provide better surgical access than the SA-3 counterparts because the antrum floor is closer to the crest compared with the SA-3 maxilla. The medial wall of the sinus membrane is elevated to the level of the height of the lateral window so that adequate height is available for future endosteal implant placement.

The combination of graft materials used and their placement are similar to those for the SA-3 technique. However, less autogenous bone is often harvested from the tuberosity, so in some cases an additional harvest site may be required, most often from the mandible (i.e., from the ascending ramus). Because of the compromised host bone present, more autogenous bone is required.

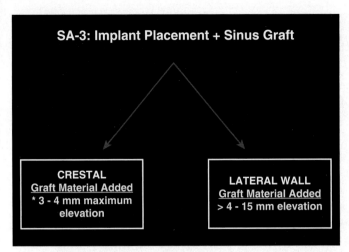

• **Fig. 23.16** Subantral option 3 (SA-3) technique that includes crestal versus lateral wall techniques.

• **BOX 23.3**   **SA-3: Subantral Option 3 Requirements Graft + Implant Placement: Sinus Grafted with Implant Placement (Lateral Wall or Osteotome)**

Indications

Favorable conditions: > 5 mm host bone (Implant length = Bone height + 3-4 mm (crestal), > 4-15 mm (lateral)
Unfavorable conditions: > 8 mm host bone (Implant length= Bone height + 3-4 mm (crestal), > 4-15 mm (lateral)

See Surgical Protocol (Chapter 37)

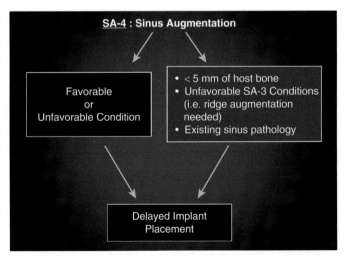

• **Fig. 23.17** Subantral Option 4 (SA-4) Bone-Grafting Indications.

The augmented region is left to mature for 6 to 10 months before reentry for placement of endosteal implants. The amount of initial healing is related to the antral size (including small, medium, or large lateral-medial size) and the amount of autologous bone used in the inferior third of the antrum. Typically the width of crestal bone is wide enough in SA-4 regions for the placement of root form implants after the graft matures.

The implant placement surgery at reentry for the SA-4 technique is similar to SA-1 with one exception. The previous access

window may appear completely healed with bone; soft and filled with loose graft material, or with cone-shaped fibrous tissue ingrowth (with the base of the cone toward the lateral wall); or in any variation states. If the graft site appears clinically as bone, the implant osteotomy and placement follow the surgical approach designated by the bone density. Usually with the SA-4 technique, implant placement is completed under a stage II process.

The time interval for stage II uncovery and prosthetic procedures after implant insertion is dependent on the density of bone at the reentry implant placement. The crest of the ridge and the original antral floor may be the only cortical bone in the region for implant fixation. The most common bone density observed is D4, and often it is softer than the region in general. Progressive loading after uncovery is most important when the bone is particularly soft and less dense.

The width of the host site for sinus grafts is most often Division A; however, when Division C–w to B exists, guided bone regeneration or an onlay graft for width is indicated. When the graft cannot be secured to the host bone, it is often ideal to perform the sinus graft 6 to 9 months before the bone graft for width. After graft maturation the implants may be inserted.

There are many advantages of the SA-4 technique over the SA-3 technique:

1. The healing of the graft may be assessed before the implant placement surgery via a CBCT scan. Because of the advances in CBCT technology, radiation exposure is not a significant disadvantage. In addition, the bone quality may be evaluated during the implant osteotomy before implant insertion. The healing time for the implant is no longer arbitrary but more patient specific.

2. Postoperative sinus graft infection occurs in approximately 3% to 5% of patients, which is much higher than the percentage for implant placement surgery. If the sinus graft becomes infected with an implant in place, a bacterial smear layer may develop on the implant and make future bone contact with the implant less predictable. The infection is also more difficult to treat when the implants are in place, and may result in greater resorption of the graft as a consequence. If the infection cannot be adequately treated, the graft and implant must be removed. Therefore there is also a decreased risk for losing the graft and implant if a postoperative infection occurs with a delayed implant insertion. Reports in the literature indeed indicate a higher failure rate of implants when inserted simultaneously compared with a delayed approach.[60,80,91,92]

3. Blood vessels are required to form and remodel bone. A titanium implant in the center of the sinus graft does not provide a source of blood vessels; therefore obtaining a vascular supply is more difficult and usually requires an increased healing time.

4. Bone width augmentation may be indicated in conjunction with sinus grafts to restore proper maxillomandibular ridge relationships or increase the implant diameter in the molar region. Augmentation may be performed simultaneously with the sinus graft. As a result, larger-diameter implants may be placed with the SA-4 technique.

5. The bone in the sinus graft will be much denser after ideal healing with the SA-4 approach. As such, implant angulation and position may be improved because it is not dictated by existing anatomic limitations at the time of the sinus graft.

The primary disadvantage of the SA-4 approach is the delayed implant placement, thereby requiring an additional surgery (Figs. 23.17 and 23.18; Box 23.4).

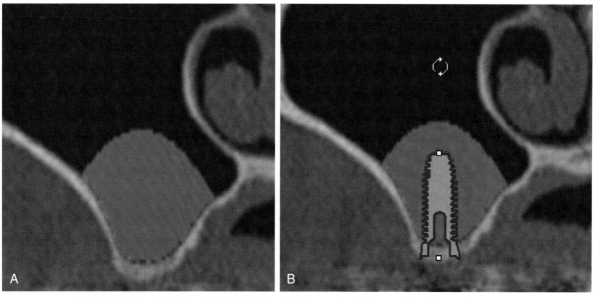

• **Fig. 23.18** Subantral Option 4 (SA-4) Protocol. (A) Lateral wall sinus grafting (Phase 1). (B) Delayed implant placement after sufficient healing (Phase 2).

• BOX 23.4 **Subantral Option 4 Requirements Graft: Sinus Grafted (Lateral Wall) with Delayed Implant Placement**

Indications

Favorable or unfavorable conditions: <5 mm host bone

See Surgical Protocol (Chapter 37)

• BOX 23.5 **Summary of Treatment Protocol with Respect to Available Bone**

<5 mm	SA-4 Lateral wall
5 mm	SA-3 or SA-4
6 mm	SA-2, SA-3, or SA-4
7 mm	SA-2, SA-3, or SA-4
8 mm	SA-1, SA-2, or SA-3
9 mm	SA-1, SA-2
10 mm	SA-1 or SA-2
>10 mm	SA-1

SA, Subantral option.

Summary

In the past the posterior maxilla has been reported as the least predictable area for implant survival. Causes cited include inadequate bone quantity, poor bone density, difficult access, and high occlusal forces. Previous implant modalities attempted to avoid this region, with approaches such as excessive cantilevers when posterior implants are not inserted or an increased number of pontics when implants are placed posterior to the antrum.

The maxillary sinus may be elevated and SA bone regenerated to improve implant height. Tatum began to develop these

techniques as early as the mid-1970s. Misch developed four options for treatment of the posterior maxilla in 1987 based on the height of bone between the floor of the antrum and the crest of the residual bone. These options were further modified by Resnik to include specific bony dimensions dependent on favorable versus unfavorable conditions as well as the transcrestal augmentation technique and short length implants. Although management of the posterior maxilla presents many challenges for the implant practitioner, progress on a number of fronts has made it increasingly possible to create successful bone-supported prostheses in this region by adhering to the classifications described earlier in this chapter (Box 23.5).

References

1. Misch CE. Treatment planning for edentulous maxillary posterior region. In: Misch CE, ed. *Contemporary Implant Dentistry.* St Louis: Mosby; 1993.
2. Tatum OH. *Maxillary Subantral Grafting.* Lecture presented at Alabama Implant Study Group. 1977.
3. Tatum OH. Maxillary and sinus implant reconstruction. *Dent Clin North Am.* 1986;30:207–229.
4. Boyne PJ, James RA. Grafting of the maxillary sinus floor with autogenous marrow and bone. *J Oral Surg.* 1980;38:613–616.
5. Misch CE. Maxillary sinus augmentation for endosteal implants: organized alternative treatment plans. *Int J Oral Implant.* 1987;4:49–58.
6. Smiler DG, Holmes RE. Sinus lift procedure using porous hydroxylapatite: a preliminary clinical report. *J Oral Implantol.* 1987;13:2–14.
7. Chanavaz M. Maxillary sinus: anatomy, physiology, surgery and bone grafting relating to implantology—eleven years of clinical experience. *J Oral Implantol.* 1990;16:199–209.
8. Tidwell JK, Blijdorp PA, Stoelinga PJW, et al. Composite grafting of the maxillary sinus for placement of endosteal implants. *Int J Oral Maxillofac Surg.* 1992;21:204–209.
9. Smiler DG, Johnson PW, Lozada JL, et al. Sinus lift grafts and endosseous implants: treatment of the atrophic posterior maxilla. *Dental Clin North Am.* 1992;36:151–186.
10. Jensen J, Sindet-Petersen S, Oliver AJ. Varying treatment strategies for reconstruction of maxillary atrophy with implants: results in 98 patients. *J Oral Maxillofac Surg.* 1994;52:210–216.

11. Chiapasco M, Ronchi P. Sinus lift and endosseous implants: preliminary surgical and prosthetic results. *Eur J Prosthodont Rest Dent.* 1994;3:15–21.

12. Blomqvist JE, Alberius P, Isaksson S. Retrospective analysis of one-stage maxillary sinus augmentation with endosseous implants. *Int J Oral Maxillofac Implants.* 1996;11:512–521.

13. Jensen OT, Shulman LB, Block MS, et al. Report of the sinus consensus conference of 1996. *Int J Oral Maxillofac Implants.* 1998;13(suppl):11–45.

14. Valentini P, Abensur DJ. Maxillary sinus grafting with anorganic bovine bone: a clinical report of long-term results. *Int J Oral Maxillofac Impl.* 2003;18:556–560.

15. Lozada JL, Emanuelli S, James RA, et al. Root form implants in subantral grafted sites. *J Cal Dent Assoc.* 1993;21:31–35.

16. Wallace SS, Froum SJ. Effect of maxillary sinus augmentation on the survival of endosseous dental implants. A systematic review. *Ann Periodontol.* 2003;8:328–343.

17. Del Fabbro M, Testori T, Francetti L, et al. Systematic review of survival rates for implants placed in grafted maxillary sinus. *Int J Periodont Restorative Dent.* 2004;24:565–577.

18. Peleg M, Garg AK, Mazor Z. Predictability of simultaneous implant placement in the severely atrophic posterior maxilla: a 9-year longitudinal experience study of 2132 implants placed into 731 human sinus grafts. *Int J Oral Maxillofac Implants.* 2006;21:94–102.

19. Hising P, Bolin A, Branting C. Reconstruction of severely resorbed alveolar ridge crests with dental implants using a bovine bone mineral for augmentation. *Int J Oral Maxillofac Implants.* 2001;16:90–97.

20. Piattelli M, Favero GA, Scarano A, et al. Bone reactions to anorganic bovine bone (Bio-Oss) used in sinus augmentation procedures: a histologic long-term report of 20 cases in humans. *Int J Oral Maxillofac Implants.* 1999;14:835–840.

21. Valentini P, Abensur D, Wenz B, et al. Sinus grafting with porous bone mineral (Bio-Oss) for implant placement: a 5-year study on 15 patients. *Int J Periodontics Restorative Dent.* 2000;20:245–253.

22. Velich N, Nemeth Z, Toth C, et al. Long-term results with different bone substitutes used for sinus floor elevation. *J Craniofac Surg.* 2004;15:38–41.

23. Fugazzotto PA, Vlassis J. Long-term success of sinus augmentation using various surgical approaches and grafting materials. *Int J Oral Maxillofac Implant.* 1998;13:52–58.

24. Hallman M, Sennerby L, Lundgren S. A clinical and histologic evaluation of implant integration in the posterior maxilla after sinus floor augmentation with autogenous bone, bovine hydroxyapatite, or a 20:80 mixture. *Int J Oral Maxillo Implants.* 2002;17:635–643.

25. Rodoni LR, Glauser R, Feloutzis A, et al. Implants in the posterior maxilla: a comparative clinical and radiologic study. *Int J Oral Maxillofac Implants.* 2005;20:231–237.

26. Maiorana C, Sigurta D, Mirandola A, et al. Bone resorption around dental implants placed in grafted sinuses: clinical and radiologic follow-up to 4 years. *Int J Oral Maxillofac Implants.* 2005;20:261–266.

27. Chanavaz M. Sinus grafting related to implantology statistical analysis of 15 years of surgical experience, 1979-1994. *Oral Implantol.* 1996;22:119–130.

28. Aghaloo TL, Moy PK. Which hard tissue augmentation techniques are the most succesful in furnishing bony support for implant placement? *Int J Maxillofac Implants.* 2007;22(suppl):49.

29. Pietrokovski J. The bony residual ridge in man. *J Prosthet Dent.* 1975;34:456–462.

30. Misch CE. Bone character: second vital implant criterion. *Dent Today.* 1988;7:39–40.

31. Goodacre JC, Bernal G, Rungcharassaeng K, et al. Clinical complications with implants and implant prostheses. *J Prosthet Dent.* 2003;2:121–132.

32. Misch CE, Qu Z, Bidez MW. Mechanical properties of trabecular bone in the human mandible: implications for dental implant treatment planning and surgical placement. *J Oral Maxillofac Surg.* 1999;57:700–706.

33. Blitzer A, Lawson W, Friedman WH, eds. *Surgery of the Paranasal Sinuses.* Philadelphia: WB Saunders; 1985.

34. Lang J, ed. *Clinical Anatomy of the Nose, Nasal Cavity and Paranasal Sinuses.* New York: Thieme; 1989.

35. Anon JB, Rontal M, Zinreich SJ. *Anatomy of the Paranasal Sinuses.* New York: Thieme; 1996.

36. Stammberger H. History of rhinology: anatomy of the paranasal sinuses. *Rhinology.* 1989;27:197–210.

37. Takahashi R. The formation of the human paranasal sinuses. *Acta Otolaryngol.* 1984;408:1–28.

38. Karmody CS, Carter B, Vincent ME. Developmental anomalies of the maxillary sinus. *Trans Am Acad Ophthalmol Otol.* 1977;84:723–728.

39. Sharan A, Madjar D. Maxillary sinus pneumatization following extractions: a radiographic study. *Int J Oral Maxillofac Implants.* 2008;23(1).

40. Weinmann JP, Sicher H. *Bone and Bones. Fundamentals of Bone Biology.* 2nd ed. St Louis: Mosby; 1955:123–126.

41. Wehrbein H, Diedrich P. Progressive pneumatization of the basal maxillary sinus after extraction and space closure [in German]. *Fortschr Kieferorthop.* 1992;53:77–83.

42. Sevimay M, et al. Three-dimensional finite element analysis of the effect of different bone quality on stress distribution in an implant-supported crown. *J Dent Res.* 2005;93(3):227–234.

43. Dworkin SF, LeResche L. Research diagnostic criteria for temporomandibular disorders: review, criteria, examinations and specifications, critique. *J Craniomandib Disord.* 1992;6:301–355.

44. Gibbs C, Mahan P, Mauderli A. Limits of human bite strength. *J Prosthet Dent.* 1986;56:226–237.

45. Hagberg C. Assessment of bite force: a review. *J Craniomandib Disord Facial Oral Pain.* 1987;1:162–169.

46. Brunski JB. Forces on dental implants and interfacial stress transfer. In: Laney WR, Tolman DE, eds. *Tissue Integration in Oral, Orthopedic and Maxillofacial Reconstruction.* Chicago: Quintessence; 1990:108–124.

47. Fanuscu MI, Iida K, Caputo AA, et al. Load transfer by an implant in a sinus-grafted maxillary model. *Int J Oral Maxillofac Implants.* 2003;18:667–674.

48. Herzberg R, Doley E, Schwartz-Arad D. Implant marginal bone loss in maxillary sinus grafts. *Int J Oral Maxillofac Implants.* 2006;21:103–110.

49. Misch CE. *Contemporary Implant Dentistry-E-Book: Arabic Bilingual Edition.* St Louis: Elsevier; 2007.

50. Hsiao YJ, Yang J, Resnik RR, Suzuki JB. Prevalence of maxillary sinus pathology based on cone-beam computed tomography evaluation of multiethnicity dental school population. *Implant Dent.* 2019;28(4):356–366.

51. Manji A, Faucher J, Resnik RR, Suzuki JB. Prevalence of maxillary sinus pathology in patients considered for sinus augmentation procedures for dental implants. *Implant Dent.* 2013;22(4):428–435.

52. Linkow LI. Tuber blades. *J Oral Implant.* 1980;9:190–216.

53. Tulasne JF. Implant treatment of missing posterior dentition. In: Albrektsson T, Zarb G, eds. *The Brånemark Osseointegrated Implant.* Chicago: Quintessence; 1989.

54. Ashkinazy LR. Tomography in implantology. *J Oral Implant.* 1982;10:100–118.

55. Geiger S, Pesch HJ. Animal experimental studies of the healing around ceramic implants in bone lesions in the maxillary sinus region. *Deutsche Zahnarztl Z.* 1977;32:396–399.

56. Brånemark PI, Adell R, Albrektsson T, et al. An experimental and clinical study of osseointegrated implants penetrating the nasal cavity. *J Oral Maxillofac Surg.* 1984;42:497–505.

57. Linkow LI. *Maxillary Implants: A Dynamic Approach to Oral Implantology.* North Haven, Conn: Glarus; 1977.

58. Tatum OH. *Omni Implant Systems, S Series Implants.* St Petersburg, Fla: Omni; 1981.

59. Raghoebar GM, Brouwer TJ, Reintsema H, et al. Augmentation of the maxillary sinus floor with autogenous bone for the placement of endosseous implants: a preliminary report. *J Oral Maxillofac Surg.* 1993;51:1198–1203.

60. Tatum OH, Lebowitz MS, Tatum CA, et al. Sinus augmentation: rationale, development, long term results. *N Y St Dent J.* 1993;59:43–48.

61. Misch CE. Treatment plans for implant dentistry. *Dent Today.* 1993;12:56–61.

62. Misch CE. Maxillary posterior treatment plans for implant dentistry. *Implantodontie.* 1995;19:7–24.

63. Tatum OH. The Omni implant system. In: Hardin JF, ed. *Clarke's Clinical Dentistry.* Philadelphia: Lippincott; 1984.

64. Feigel A, Maker M. The significance of sinus elevation for blade implantology: report of an autopsy case. *J Oral Implant.* 1989;15:232–247.

65. Jensen J, Simonsen EK, Sindet Pedersen S. Reconstruction of the severely resorbed maxilla with bone grafting and osseointegrated implants: a preliminary report. *J Oral Maxillofac Surg.* 1990;48:27–32.

66. Wood RM, Moore DL. Grafting of the maxillary sinus with intraorally harvested autogenous bone prior to implant placement. *Int J Oral Maxillofac Impl.* 1988;3:209–214.

67. Linkow LI. Maxillary pterygoid extension implants: the state of the art. *Dent Clin North Am.* 1980;24:535–551.

68. Cranin AN, Satler N, Shpuntoff R. The unilateral pterygo-hamular subperiosteal implant evolution of a technique. *J Am Dent Assoc.* 1985;110:496–500.

69. Keller EE, van Roekel NB, Desjardins RR, et al. Prosthetic surgical reconstruction of severely resorbed maxilla with iliac bone grafting and tissue integrated prostheses. *Int J Oral Maxillofac Impl.* 1987;2:155.

70. Sailer HF. A new method of inserting endosseous implants in totally atrophic maxillae. *J Cranio Maxillofac Surg.* 1989;17:299–305.

71. Linkow LI. Clinical evaluation of the various designed endoosseus implants. *J Oral Implant Transplant Surg.* 1966;12:35–46.

72. Stoler A. *The CAT-Scan Subperiosteal Implant.* Hong Kong: International Congress of Oral Implantologist World Meeting; 1986.

73. Fonseca RJ, Marciani RD, Turvey TA. *Oral and Maxillofacial Surgery.* 2nd ed. St Louis: Saunders; 2008.

74. Boyne PT. Analysis of performance of root form endosseous implants placed in the maxillary sinus. *J Long Term Effects Med Implants.* 1993;3:143–159.

75. Small SA, Zinner ID, Panno FV, et al. Augmenting the maxillary sinus for implants, report of 27 patients. *Int J Oral Maxillofac Impl.* 1993;8:523.

76. Gonzalez-Garcia R, Naval-Gias L, Munoz-Guerra MF, et al. Preprosthetic and implantological surgery in patients with severe maxillary atrophy. *Med Oral Patol Oral Cir Bucal.* 2005;10:343–354.

77. Merkx MA, Maltha JC, Steolinga PJ. Assessment of the value of anorganic bone additives in sinus floor augmentation: a review of clinical reports. *Int J Oral Maxillofac Surg.* 2003;32:1–6.

78. Tong DC, Rioux K, Drangsholt M, et al. A review of survival rates for implants placed in grafted maxillary sinuses using meta analysis. *Int J Oral Maxillofac Implants.* 1998;13:175–182.

79. Hallman M, Sennerby I, Zetterqvist L, et al. A 3-year prospective follow-up study of implant-supported fixed prostheses in patients subjected to maxillary sinus floor augmentation with a 80:20 mixture of deproteinized bovine bone and autogenous bone: clinical, radiographic and resonance frequence analysis. *Int J Oral Maxillofac Surg.* 2005;34:273–280.

80. Chiapasco M. Tecniche ricostruttive con innesti e/o osteo-tomie. In: Chiapasco M, Romeo E, eds. *Riabilitazione Implanto-Protesica Dei Casi Complessi.* Torino, Italy: UTET ed; 2003.

81. Loukota RA, Isaksson SG, Linner EL, et al. A technique for inserting endosseous implants in the atrophic maxilla in a single stage procedure. *Br J Oral Maxillofac Surg.* 1992;30:46–49.

82. Jensen OT, Greer R. Immediate placement of osseo-integrated implants into the maxillary sinus augmented with mineralized cancellous allograft and Gore-Tex, 2nd stage surgical and histological findings. In: Laney WR, Tolman DE, eds. *Oral Orthopedic and Maxillofacial Reconstruction.* Chicago: Quintessence; 1992.

83. Hirsch JM, Ericsson I. Maxillary sinus augmentation using mandibular bone grafts and simultaneous installation of implants—a surgical technique. *Clin Oral Impl Res.* 1991;2:91–96.

84. Hurzeler MB, Kirsch A, Ackermann KL, et al. Reconstruction of the severely resorbed maxilla with dental implants in the augmented maxillary sinus—a 5 year clinical investigation. *Int J Oral Maxillofac Impl.* 1996;11:466–475.

85. Chiapasco M, Romeo E, Vogel G. Tridimensional reconstruction of knife-edge edentulous maxillae by sinus elevation, onlay grafts, and sagittal osteotomy of the anterior maxilla: preliminary surgical and prosthetic results. *Int J Oral Maxillofac Implants.* 1998;13:394–399.

86. Widmark G, Andersson B, Andrup B, et al. Rehabilitation of patients with severely resorbed maxillae by means of implants with or without bone grafts: a 1-year follow-up study. *Int J Oral Maxillofac Implants.* 1998;13:474–482.

87. Yildirin M, Spiekermann H, Biesterfeld S, et al. Maxillary sinus augmentation using xenogenic bone substitute material Bio-Oss in combination with venous blood. A histologic and histomorphometric study in humans. *Clin Oral Implants Res.* 2000;11:217–229.

88. Summers RB. A new concept in maxillary implant surgery: the osteotome technique. *Compend Contin Educ Dent.* 1994;15:152.

89. Cawood JL, Howell RA. A classification of the edentulous jaws. *Int J Oral Maxillofac Surg.* 1988;17:232–236.

90. Jensen O. *The Sinus Bone Graft.* Carol Stream, Ill: Quintessence; 1999.

91. Misch CE, Chiapasco M. Identification for and classification of sinus bone grafts. In: Jensen O, ed. *The Sinus Bone Graft.* 2nd ed. Carol Stream, Ill: Quintessence; 2006.

92. Misch CE, Dietsh F. Bone grafting materials in implant dentistry. *Impl Dent.* 1993;2:158–167.

93. Summers RB. Maxillary implant surgery: the osteotome technique. *Compend Cont Educ Dent.* 1994;15:152–162.

94. Zaninari A. Rialzo del Seno Mascellare Prima parte. *Tam Tam Dentale.* 1990;2:8–12.

95. Worth HM, Stoneman DW. Radiographic interpretation of antral mucosal changes due to localized dental infection. *J Can Dent Assoc.* 1972;38:111.

24

The Edentulous Mandible: Fixed Versus Removable Prosthesis Treatment Planning

RANDOLPH R. RESNIK AND CARL E. MISCH[†]

Historically, the edentulous mandibular patient has been one of the most common patients to be treated with dental implants. The placement of dental implants in this area has been shown to be very successful in obtaining the support, retention, and stability of a mandibular prosthesis, whether it is fixed or removable. From a bone volume conservation standpoint, complete edentulous patients should be treated with sufficient implants to support a prosthesis in the maxilla or mandible. The continued bone loss after tooth loss and associated compromises in esthetics, function, and health make all edentulous patients possible implant candidates. The bone loss that occurs during the first year after tooth loss is 10 times greater than in the following years. In the case of multiple extractions, this often means an approximate 4-mm vertical bone loss within the first 6 months. As the bony ridge resorbs, the muscle attachments become level with the edentulous ridge, thereby compromising the fit of a mandibular prosthesis. Rather than waiting until the patient has lost most of the residual bone, the clinician should inform and emphasize to the patient the benefits of implants and why they should be inserted before the bone is lost. Therefore the profession should treat bone loss from extractions in a similar fashion as bone loss from periodontal disease. Rather than waiting until the bone is resorbed or the patient complains, the dental professional should educate the patient about the bone loss process caused not only by periodontal disease but also by the lack of stimulation and its consequences of bone resorption, and explain how implants are available to treat the condition. Therefore most completely edentulous patients should be informed of the necessity of dental implants to maintain bone volume, function, masticatory muscle activity, esthetics, and psychological health. Ideally patients who have non-restorable teeth should be given the option to include implants to support the future prosthesis. The traditional complete denture may be presented as a temporary measure to provide cosmetic and oral function during implant treatment. For an edentulous patient, two treatment options exist: (1) fixed (FP-1, FP-2, or FP-3) or (2) removable (RP-4 or RP-5) prosthesis (Fig. 24.1).

† Deceased

Mandibular Treatment Planning Principles

Anteroposterior Spread

The distance from the center of the most anterior implant to a line joining the distal aspect of the two most distal implants on each side is called the *anteroposterior* (A-P) *distance* or the *A-P spread*[1] (Fig. 24.2). In theory, the greater the A-P spread, the farther the distal cantilever may be extended to replace the missing posterior teeth. As a general rule, when five to six anterior implants are placed in the anterior mandible between the foramina to support a fixed prosthesis, the cantilever should not exceed two times the A-P spread, with all other stress factors being low.

The range of implant and prosthesis survival may be because of the broad application of the same implant position, regardless of crown height, opposing dentition, implant length, A-P position of implants, and parafunction. The arch form, the position of the mental foramina, force factors, and bone density are important criteria when four to six implants are placed only in the anterior segment to replace the entire mandibular arch. The anterior arch form and foramina position affect the position of the distalmost implants. Therefore a cantilever distance is variable for different patients.

The A-P distance is affected by the arch form. The types of arch forms may be separated into square, ovoid, and tapering. A square arch form in the anterior mandible has a 0- to 6-mm A-P spread between the most distal and most anterior implants (Fig. 24.3). An ovoid arch form has an A-P distance of 7 to 9 mm and is the most common type (Fig. 24.4). A tapering arch form has an A-P distance greater than 9 mm (Fig. 24.5).

Hence whereas a tapering arch form may support a 20-mm cantilever, a square arch form requires the cantilever to be reduced to 12 mm or less, however is directly dependent upon force factors. The position of the mental foramen can affect the A-P spread. The mental foramen is most often found between the root apices of the premolars. However, it may be located as far anterior as just distal to the canine and as far distal as the mesial of the first molar apex.[2] The farther forward the foramen, the shorter the cantilever length

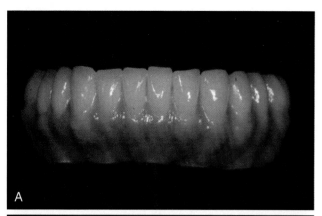

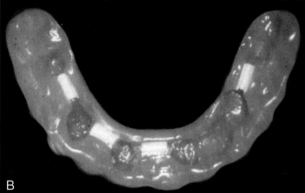

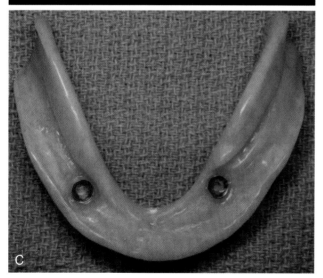

• **Fig. 24.1** Mandibular Edentulous Prostheses. (A) Fixed prothesis (FP-3), which is commonly fabricated from zirconia, porcelain fused to metal, or acrylic/denture teeth. (B) Removable prosthesis (RP-4), which is totally implant supported; note the flangeless nature of the prosthesis. (C) Removable prosthesis (RP-5), which is primarily supported by the soft tissue.

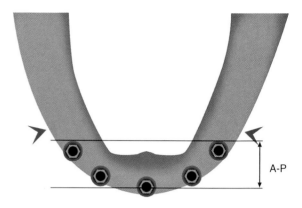

• **Fig. 24.2** The anteroposterior (A-P) distance is determined by a line drawn from the distal portion of the distalmost implant on each side of the arch and another parallel line drawn through the center of the anteriormost implant from the cantilever.

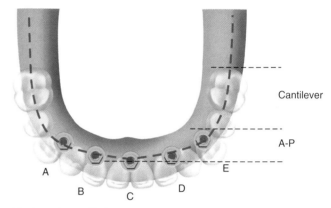

• **Fig. 24.3** A mandibular square arch form has an anteroposterior (A-P) distance of 0 to 6 mm. As a result a cantilever is limited. (*From Misch CE. The completely edentulous mandible: treatment plans for fixed restorations. In:* Dental Implant Prosthetics. *2nd ed. St. Louis, MO: Mosby; 2015.*)

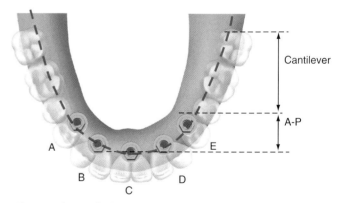

• **Fig. 24.4** A mandibular ovoid arch form has an anteroposterior (A-P) distance of 7 to 9 mm and is the most common type. A cantilever may extend to 18 mm with the ovoid-type arch. (*From Misch CE. The completely edentulous mandible: treatment plans for fixed restorations. In:* Dental Implant Prosthetics. *2nd ed. St. Louis, MO: Mosby; 2015.*)

because the A-P spread is reduced. The A-P spread is only one of the force factors to be considered for the extent of the distal cantilever. If the stress factors are high (e.g., parafunction, crown height, masticatory musculature dynamics, opposing arch), the cantilever length of a prosthesis should be reduced and may even be contraindicated. The density of bone is also an important criterion. The softest bone types (D3 and D4) should not have as great of a cantilever than the denser types (D1 and D2).

Therefore, the length of the posterior cantilever depends on the specific force factors of the patient, of which A-P spread is

only one. The number and size of implants may also affect the cantilever length. Stress equals force divided by the area over which force is applied. The area over which the forces are applied from the prosthesis to the implants can be modified through the number, size, and design of the implants. A cantilever rarely is indicated on three implants even with a similar A-P spread as five implants.

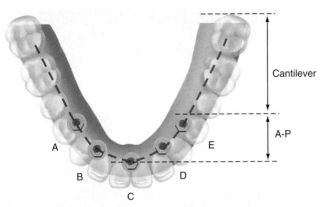

• **Fig. 24.5** A mandibular tapered arch form has an anteroposterior (A-P) distance of greater than 9 mm and is the type least observed. A cantilever is least at risk for this arch form. (*From Misch CE. The completely edentulous mandible: treatment plans for fixed restorations. In: Dental Implant Prosthetics. 2nd ed. St. Louis, MO: Mosby; 2015.*)

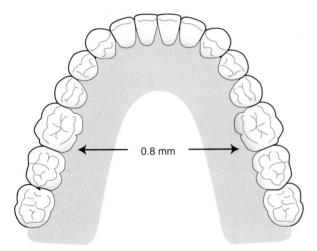

• **Fig. 24.6** The flexure of the mandible during opening and protrusive movements occurs distal to the mental foramina. The amount of flexure depends on the amount of the bone volume and the sites in question. The medial movement from the first molar to the first molar region may be 800 mm.

Mandibular Flexure

Medial Movement

Many reports have addressed the dimensional changes of the mandible during jaw activity as a result of masticatory muscle action.[3-6] Five different movements have been postulated.

Medial convergence is the one most commonly addressed.[7] The mandible between the mental foramina is stable relative to flexure and torsion. However, distal to the foramina, the mandible exhibits considerable movement toward the midline on opening.[8,9] This movement is caused primarily by the attachment of internal pterygoid muscles on the medial ramus of the mandible.

The distortion of the mandible occurs early in the opening cycle, and the maximum changes may occur with as little as 28% opening (or about 12 mm). This flexure has also been observed during protrusive jaw movements.[10] The greater the active opening and protrusive movements, the greater the amplitude of mandibular flexion. The amount of movement varies among individuals and depends on the density and volume of bone, and the location of the site in question. In general the more distal the sites, the more medial flexure. The amplitude of the mandibular body flexure toward the

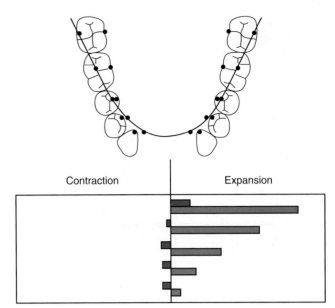

• **Fig. 24.7** Unilateral molar biting causes the mandible to undergo torsion, with the bottom of the mandible expanding outward and the crest of the mandible rotating medially. (*From Misch CE. The completely edentulous mandible: treatment plans for fixed restorations. In: Dental Implant Prosthetics. 2nd ed. St. Louis, MO: Mosby; 2015.*)

midline has been measured to be as much as 800 μm in the first molar-to-first molar region to as much as 1500 μm in the ramus-to-ramus sites (Fig. 24.6). In a study by Hobkirk and Havthoulas[11] on deformation of the mandible in subjects with fixed dental implant prostheses, medial convergence up to 41 mm was observed.

Torsion

Torsion of the mandibular body distal to the foramina has also been documented in both animal and human studies.[12,13] Hylander[14] evaluated larger members of the rhesus monkey family (macaque) and found the mandible twisted on the working side and bent in the parasagittal plane on the balancing side during the power stroke of mastication and unilateral molar biting (Fig. 24.7). Parasagittal bending of the human jaw during unilateral biting was confirmed by Marx,[15] who measured localized mandibular distortion in vivo in humans by using strain gauges on screws attached to cortical bone in the symphyseal and gonial regions. Abdel-Latif et al.[12] confirmed that the mandibles of patients with implant prostheses measured up to 19 degrees of dorsoventral shear. The torsion during parafunction is caused primarily by forceful contraction of the masseter muscle attachments (Fig. 24.8). Therefore parafunctional bruxism and clenching may cause torsion-related problems in the implant support system and prosthesis when the mandibular teeth are splinted from the molar-to-molar regions.

The posterior bone gain in edentulous patients restored with cantilevered prostheses from anterior implants may be a consequence of the mandibular flexure and torsion, which stimulate the bone cells in the region. Because the bite force may increase 300% with an implant prosthesis compared with a denture, the increased torsion may stimulate the posterior mandibular body to increase in size, as reported by Wright et al.[16] and Reddy et al.[17]

Misch[18] has observed the increase in flexure in the posterior mandible is a result of the mental foramen weakening of the facial cortical plate. As such, the mandible flexes and has torsion distal to the foramen. The most common position of the mental foramen is between the first and second premolar teeth. Therefore, when bilaterally

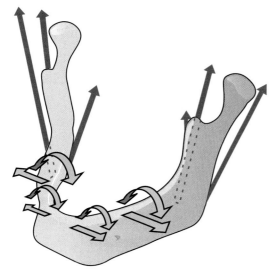

• **Fig. 24.8** The mandible flexes toward the midline on opening or during protrusive movements as a result of the internal pterygoid muscle attachments on the ramus (blue arrows). The mandible also torques, with the inferior border rotating out and up, and the crestal region rotating lingually. The movement is caused by the masseter muscles during forceful biting or parafunction (red arrows).

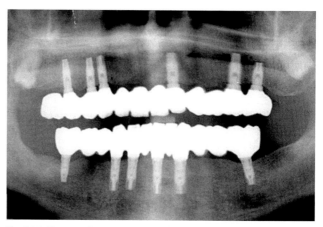

• **Fig. 24.9** Some authors propose that the ideal implant positions to support a mandibular full-arch prosthesis are the bilateral molars and bilateral canines, splinted together with a rigid structure. These positions are not ideal because of the mandibular dynamics (flexure and torsion) during opening and function.

<table>
<tr><td>• BOX 24.1</td><td>Advantages of Mandibular Implant Overdentures</td></tr>
</table>

1. Enhanced soft tissue support
2. Increased chewing efficiency compared with conventional dentures
3. Less expense/implants
4. Esthetics
5. Ease of hygiene
6. Parafunctional habits
7. Less food impaction

splinting teeth distal to the premolar positions, mandibular dynamics should be considered. Posterior rigid, fixated implants splinted to each other in a full-arch restoration are subject to a considerable buccolingual force on opening and during parafunction.[19,20]

A study by Miyamoto et al.[21] identified jaw flexure as the primary cause of posterior implant loss in full-arch splinted mandibular prostheses. The more distal the rigid splint from one side to the other, the greater the risk that mandibular dynamics may influence the implants or prosthesis prognosis. In addition, the body of the mandible flexes more when the size of the bone decreases. As a result the division C minus height (C–h) or division D mandible flexes or exhibits torsion more than the division A mandible, all other factors being similar.

The difference in movement between an implant and a tooth has been addressed as a concern for dentists when splinting these objects together. The natural tooth movement ranges from 28 μm apically and 56 to 108 μm laterally. In contrast, the rigid implant has movement up to 5 μm apically and 10 to 60 μm laterally. Yet the mandibular flexure and torsion may be more than 10 to 20 times the movement of a healthy tooth. Therefore the flexure and torsion of the mandibular body are more critical in the patient evaluation compared with whether an implant should be joined to the natural dentition.

Some authors have suggested four implants in the mandible with a full-arch splinted fixed restoration—two in the first molars and two in the canine regions (Fig. 24.9).[22] Additional implants have been used with this full-arch splinted restorative option, with up to four other implants in the premolar and the incisor regions.[23] However, complete cross-arch splinting of posterior molar implants with a rigid, fixated prosthesis should be reconsidered in the mandible. The flexure of the mandible is thwarted by the prosthesis, but this introduces lateral stresses to the implant system (cement, screw, crestal bone, and implant–bone interface).[24-26] These lateral stresses place the molar implants, screws, and bone at increased risk because of the mandibular flexure and torsion previously addressed.

In complete mandibular subperiosteal implants, pain on opening was noted in 25% of the patients at the suture removal appointment when a rigid bar connected molar-to-molar regions. When the connecting bar was cut into two sections between the foramina, the pain on opening was immediately eliminated. This clinical observation

does not mean that the other 75% of patients did not have flexure of the mandibular arch on opening. The observation does demonstrate, however, that flexure may be relevant to postoperative complications.

Implant Overdentures Advantages (RP-4 and RP-5)

For an implant-supported overdenture the implants ideally should be placed in planned, specific sites, and their number should be predetermined by the clinician and patient. The primary indications for a mandibular implant overdenture (IOD) are problems often found with lower dentures, such as lack of retention or stability, decrease in function, difficulties in speech, tissue sensitivity, and soft tissue abrasions. If an edentulous patient is willing to remain with a removable prosthesis, an overdenture is often the treatment of choice. In addition, if cost is a concern for the patient, the overdenture may serve as a transitional prosthesis until additional implants may be inserted and restored. When evaluating mandibular IODs, many advantages exist (Box 24.1).

Enhanced Soft Tissue Support

Bone loss dictates the appearance of the inferior third of the face. A maxillary overdenture often provides improved support for the lips and soft tissues of the face compared with a fixed prosthesis because the prosthesis contour does not have to accommodate daily hygiene requirements. Denture teeth also provide an esthetic replacement for the natural dentition, which is more challenging for the technician to re-create with porcelain fused to metal restorations. For the laboratory to create pink

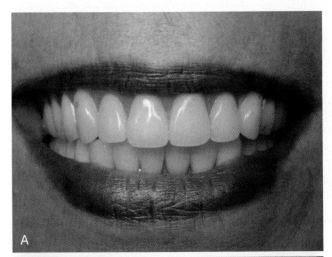

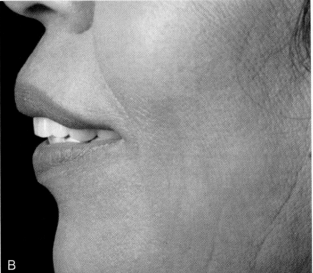

• **Fig. 24.10** (A and B) Soft tissue support: because of the ability to modify the flange of the prosthesis, ideal soft tissue support can be obtained.

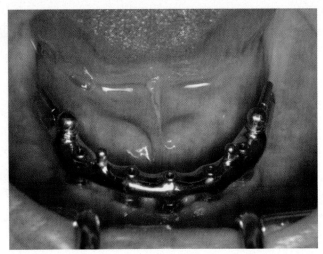

• **Fig. 24.11** Hygiene: because of the removable nature of the overdenture, hygiene access is much easier to complete in comparison with a fixed prosthesis.

interdental papilla, as well as replace the soft tissue drape, is easier with an overdenture compared with porcelain-metal fixed restorations or zirconia prosthesis. In addition, the teeth can be positioned in the most esthetic position, without any restriction as to the relationship to the atrophied crest, because stability now is provided by the implant and does not depend on tooth position on the crest of the ridge (Fig. 24.10).

Increased Chewing Efficiency Compared with Conventional Dentures

A study of chewing efficiency compared wearers of complete dentures with patients with implant-supported overdentures. The complete-denture group required 1.5 to 3.6 times the number of chewing strokes compared with the overdenture group.[27] The chewing efficiency with an IOD is improved by 20% compared with a traditional complete denture.[28,29]

Less Expense/Implants

When cost is a factor, two implant-retained IODs may improve the patient's condition at a significantly lower overall treatment cost than a fixed implant–supported prosthesis. A survey

by Carlsson et al.[30] in 10 countries indicated a wide range of treatment options. The proportion of IODs selected versus fixed implant dentures was highest in the Netherlands (93%) and lowest in Sweden and Greece (12%). Cost was cited as the number one determining factor in the choice. However, in general, overdenture treatment is less expensive than a fixed implant prosthesis, mainly because of the decreased number of implants required.

Esthetics

The esthetics for many edentulous patients with moderate-to-advanced bone loss is improved with an overdenture compared with a fixed restoration. Soft tissue support for facial appearance often is required for an implant patient because of advanced bone loss, especially in the maxilla. Interdental papilla and tooth size are easier to reproduce or control with an overdenture. Denture teeth easily reproduce contours and esthetics compared with time-consuming and technician-sensitive porcelain-metal or zirconia fixed restorations. The labial flange may be designed for optimal appearance, not daily hygiene.

Ease of Hygiene

Hygiene conditions and home and professional care are improved with an overdenture compared with a fixed prosthesis. Peri-implant probing is diagnostic and easier around a bar than a fixed prosthesis because the crown often prevents straight-line access along the abutment to the crest of the bone. The overdenture may be extended over the abutments to prevent food entrapment during function. Speech is not compromised because the denture may extend onto the soft tissues in the mandible and prevent air and saliva from escaping (Fig. 24.11).

Parafunctional Habits

An overdenture may be removed at bedtime to reduce the noxious effect of nocturnal parafunction, which increases stresses on the implant support system. The overdenture also may provide stress relief between the superstructure and prosthesis, and the soft tissue may share a portion of the occlusal load. The prosthesis

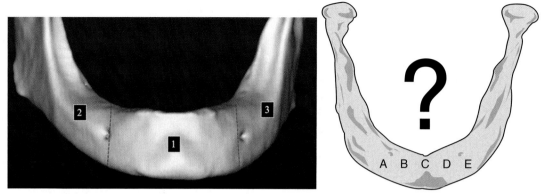

• **Fig. 24.12** (A) The mandible is divided into three regions for treatment planning. (B) The anterior mandible is positionally documented via *A*, *B*, *C*, *D*, and *E* positions.

is usually easier to repair than a fixed restoration. In most cases, there exists a reduced cost of overdenture treatment in comparison to a fixed prosthesis. In addition, long-term denture patients do not appear to have a psychological problem associated with the ability to remove their implant prostheses.[31,32] Therefore, denture patients usually adapt very well into an overdenture treatment.

Less Food Impaction

Especially with an RP-5 prosthesis, there is less food impaction with an overdenture in comparison with a fixed prosthesis. The flanges of the prosthesis (RP-5) usually extend to form a peripheral seal that minimizes food impaction. Because of the nature of the fixed mandibular prosthesis, it often is overextended for esthetic reasons. In comparison with a conventional denture, food particles migrate and become impacted under the prosthesis during swallowing. Because a lower denture "floats" and moves during function, the food more readily goes under and out, whereas the IOD traps the food debris against the implants, bars, and attachments.

Review of the Overdenture Literature

In 1986 a multicenter study reported on 1739 implants placed in the mandibular symphysis of 484 patients. The implants were loaded immediately and restored with bars and overdentures with clips as retention. The overall success rate was 94%.[33] Engquist et al.[34] reported a 6% to 7% implant failure for mandibular implant–supported overdentures and a 19% to 35% failure rate for maxillary IODs. Hyperplasia below the bar occurred in 25% of the patients. Jemt et al.[35] reported on a 5-year prospective, multicenter study on 30 maxillae (117 Brånemark implants) and 103 mandibles with 393 implants. Survival rates in the mandible were 94.5% for implants and 100% for prostheses; in the maxilla the survival rates were 72.4% for implants and 77.9% for prostheses. Higher failure rates in the maxilla were related directly to poor density and quantity of bone with a characteristic cluster failure pattern.[35]

Wismeijer et al.[36] reported on 64 patients with 218 titanium plasma-sprayed implants, with a 97% survival rate with overdentures in a 6.5-year evaluation. Naert et al. found 100% implant success at 5 years for overdentures with different anchorage systems. In Belgium, Naert at al. reported on 207 consecutively treated patients with 449 Brånemark implants and Dolder-bar

overdentures. In this report the cumulative implant failure rate was 3% at the 10-year benchmark.[37]

Misch[38] reported a less than 1% implant failure rate and no prosthesis failure over a 7-year period with 147 patients when using the organized treatment options and prosthetic guidelines presented in this chapter. Kline et al.[39] reported on 266 implant-supported overdentures for 51 patients, with an implant survival rate of 99.6% and a prosthesis survival rate of 100%. Mericke-Stern[40] reported a 95% implant survival rate with two IODs.

In a randomized clinical report Awad et al. compared satisfaction and function in complete dentures (48 patients) versus two IODs in 56 patients. There was significantly higher satisfaction, comfort, and chewing ability in the IOD group.[41]

Thomason et al.,[42] in the United Kingdom, reported a 36% higher satisfaction for the IOD patients than the complete denture wearers in the criteria of comfort, stability, and chewing.

In a 10-year study of IODs in Israel, with 285 implants and 69 IODs, Schwartz-Arad et al.[43] reported the implant survival rate was 96.1% with higher success rates in the mandible. Many reports have been published over the last two decades that conclude that implant-supported overdentures represent a valid beneficial option for denture wearers. It should be noted that the majority of reports are for IODs supported by only two implants.[44,45]

Mandibular Overdenture Treatment Planning (RP-4 and RP-5)

Anatomy of the Mandible

In treatment planning the mandible for a fixed or removable prosthesis, the mandible is divided into three regions: (1) anterior mandible, (2) posterior right, and (3) posterior left. The available bone in the anterior mandible is divided into five equal columns of bone serving as potential implant sites, labeled A, B, C, D, and E, starting from the patient's right side.[46,47] Regardless of the treatment option being used, all five implant sites are mapped out at the time of treatment planning and surgery (Fig. 24.12).

Mandibular Implant Site Selection

Anterior retention and stability for an overdenture offer several advantages. The greatest available height of bone is located in the anterior mandible, between the mental foramina. This region also usually presents a favorable bone density (e.g., D2) for implant support. In addition, overdentures with posterior movement (RP-5) gain better acceptance than removable prostheses with anterior movement. An axiom in removable partial denture design is to gain rigid prosthetic support in the anterior region. When the prosthesis has poor anterior and poor posterior support, it rocks back and forth. This rocking action applies torque to the abutments and increases stresses on the overdenture components and bone–implant interface. Therefore anterior forces should be resisted by implants or bars, whereas posterior forces may be directed on a soft tissue area such as the mandibular buccal shelf (i.e., primary stress-bearing area). In addition, the IOD treatment options presented are designed for anterior implant placement with adequate bone quantity.

In this way the patient always has the option to obtain additional implant support in the future. For example, a patient may receive adequate support for an IOD with four implants. However, if the patient desires a fixed prosthesis in the future, these four implants may fall short of the new requirements. If the clinician did not plan an additional implant site at the initial surgery but instead placed the four implants an equal distance apart, the additional space may not be available without removing one of the present implants. In addition, a patient may desire a completely implant-supported restoration as an RP-4 or fixed prosthesis but cannot afford the treatment all at once. Three implants in the A, C, and E positions and an overdenture may be provided currently, two implants may be added in the B and D locations later, and a completely implant-supported overdenture or fixed restoration may be fabricated.

In addition, if an implant complication occurs that results in an implant failure, corrective procedures may be completed. If implants were placed in the A, B, D, and E positions, and an implant fails to achieve rigid fixation, the failed implant may be removed and an additional implant placed in the C position at the same time. This saves time as additional surgery is not required which eliminates the additional bone healing time before another implant can be reinserted.

Overdenture Treatment Options

In 1985 Misch[39,48] presented organized treatment options for implant-supported mandibular overdentures in the completely edentulous patient. The treatment options range from primarily soft tissue support with secondary implant retention (RP-5) to a completely implant-supported prosthesis (RP-4) with rigid stability (i.e., no soft tissue support) (Table 24.1). The initial treatment options are presented for completely edentulous patients with Division A (abundant) or B (sufficient) anterior bone, treated with Division A anterior root form implants of 4 mm or greater in diameter.

When evaluating the patient for an overdenture, the clinician should evaluate the patient's existing dentures concerning support, retention, and stability. Support is related to the resistance to occlusal load. Retention describes the resistance of the prosthesis to movement away from the tissues. Stability is the lateral resistance criterion. The patient's complaints, anatomy, desires, and financial commitment determine the amount of implant support, retention, and stability required to address these conditions predictably. The amount of resistance provided in IODs is related to the number and position of the implants.

TABLE 24.1 Mandibular Overdenture Treatment Options

Option	Description	Removable Prosthesis Type
OD-1	2 implants (B and D positions) independent of each other	RP-5 Ideal posterior ridge form Ideal anterior and posterior ridge form Cost is a major factor (two-legged chair)
OD-2	3 implants (A, C, and E positions)	RP-5 Ideal posterior ridge form (three-legged chair)
OD-3	4 implants (A, B, D, and E positions)	RP-4 (favorable force factors) RP-5 (unfavorable force factors) Patient desires greater retention, major stability, and support (four-legged chair)
OD-4	5 implants (A, B, C, D, and E positions)	Patient has high demands or desires Retention, stability, and support (four-legged chair)

OD, Overdenture option.

Overdenture Option 1

The first treatment option for mandibular overdentures (OD-1) is indicated primarily when cost is the most significant patient factor and minimal retention is required. The patient should be educated about the amount of retention that may be obtained. Most two implant overdentures can be correlated with a two-legged chair (i.e. rotation and hinging will occur). Bone volume should be abundant (Division A or B) in the anterior, and the posterior ridge form should be an inverted U shape, with high parallel walls for good-to-excellent anatomic conditions for conventional denture, support, and stability. The buccal shelf (primary stress bearing area) should be prominent to withstand the forces. Under these conditions, two implants may be inserted in the B and D positions. The implants usually remain independent of each other and are not connected with a superstructure. The most common type of attachment used in OD-1 is a Locator or an O-ring design, because there will be associated prosthesis movement.

Positioning of the implants in the B and D positions is a much better prosthetic option in OD-1 than positioning in the A and E regions (Fig. 24.13). Independent implants in the A and E positions allow a greater amplitude of rocking of the prosthesis compared with implants in the B and D regions (Fig. 24.14). When using B and D implants, the anterior movement of the prosthesis is reduced, and the prosthesis even may act as a splint for the two implants during anterior biting forces, thereby decreasing the stress to each implant. However, most situations do not allow the prosthesis to act as a true splint because a stress relief attachment permits movement in any plane. As a result, only one implant is loaded at a time in most situations. The stability and support of the prosthesis are gained primarily from the anatomy of the mandible and prosthesis design, which is similar to a complete denture. The implant support mechanism is poor because stress relief is permitted in any plane.

The primary patient advantage with OD-1 is cost. The existing restoration often may be adapted with an intraoral rebase and pickup procedure around the implants and attachments. Additional indications are when arch shape is considerably tapered such that a connecting bar would be cantilevered too far to the facial or would interfere with speech and mastication if too lingual. Hygiene procedures also are facilitated with independent attachments.

The disadvantages of the OD-1 relate to its relatively poor implant support and stability, compared with the other options, because of the independent nature of the two implants. The other disadvantages of OD-1 relate to an increase in prosthetic maintenance appointments. For the prosthesis to be inserted and function ideally, the two implants should be parallel to each other, perpendicular to the occlusal plane, at the same horizontal height (parallel to the occlusal plane), and equal distance off the midline. If one implant is not parallel to the other, the prosthesis will wear one attachment faster because of the greater displacement during insertion and removal than the other. If the angulation difference is severe, the prosthesis may not engage one attachment at all. The implants also should be perpendicular to the occlusal plane. Because the goal is to allow the posterior regions of the overdenture to rock downward and load the soft tissue over the mandibular buccal shelves for support, the hinge rotation should be at 90 degrees to the rotation path. In addition, because only two implants sustain the occlusal load during function or parafunction, minimization of the forces to the implant components and crestal bone by placing them in the long axis of the implant body and perpendicular to the occlusal plane is ideal (Fig. 24.15).

The two independent implants should be positioned at the same occlusal height, parallel to the occlusal plane. If one implant is higher than the other, the prosthesis will disengage from the lower implant during function and rotate primarily on the higher implant. This situation will accelerate the wear of the attachment on the lower implant. In addition, because the higher implant receives the majority of the occlusal load, an increased risk for complications may occur, including abutment screw loosening, crestal bone loss, and implant failure.

The implants should be equal distance off the midline. If one implant is more distal (farther from the midline), it will serve as the primary rotation point or fulcrum when the patient occludes in the posterior segments. As such, the more medial implant attachment will wear faster, and the more distal implant will receive a greater occlusal load (Box 24.2 and Fig. 24.16).

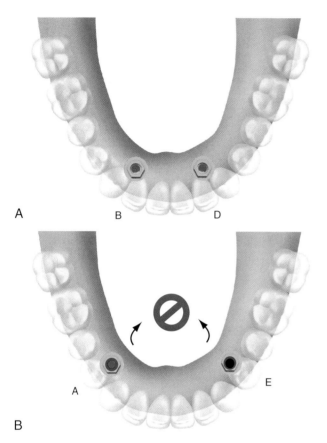

• **Fig. 24.13** Overdenture option 1 consists of two independent implants. These are best placed in the *B* and *D* positions (A) to limit the forward rocking of the restoration during function. Independent implants in the *A* and *E* positions (B) allow a greater rocking of the restoration and place greater leverage forces against the implants.

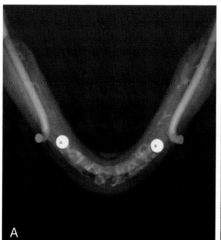
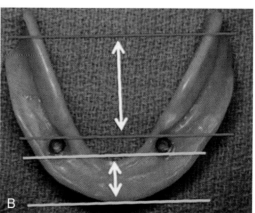

• **Fig. 24.14** Two-Implant Overdenture. (A) *A* and *E* position. (B) This position often results in an anterior and posterior "rocking" of the prosthesis. In addition, the attachment may impinge on the next phase tongue space requiring overcontouring of acrylic.

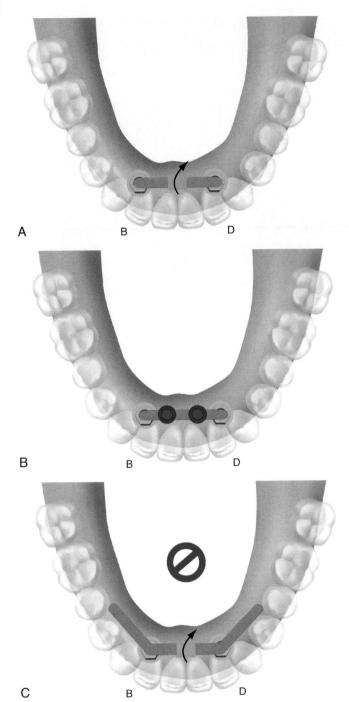

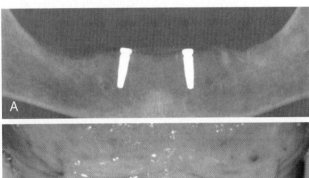
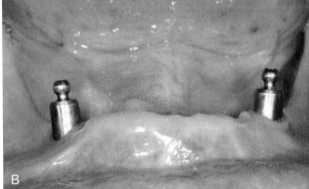

• **Fig. 24.16** (A) When two implants are used in the treatment plan, the implants should be as parallel as possible. (B) Two implants that are not parallel and at different heights, which most likely will lead to prosthetic complications.

• **Fig. 24.15** (A) Treatment option 2 has implants in the *B* and *D* positions, and a bar joins the implants. The bar should not be cantilevered off the distal side of the implants. The prosthesis movement will be reduced, and too much force on the bar and implants will increase complications. Attachments such as an O-ring (B) or a Hader clip (C), which allow movement of the prosthesis, can be added to the bar. The attachments are placed at the same height at equal distance off the midline and parallel to each other.

Overdenture Option 2

Three root form implants are placed in the A, C, and E positions for the second overdenture treatment option (OD-2). The advantages of splinting A, C, and E implants compared with implants in the B and D positions are many. The additional implant provides a sixfold reduction in superstructure flexure

(i.e. if splinted bar is used) and limits the consequences previously discussed.[49] In addition, screw loosening occurs less frequently because three coping screws retain the superstructure rather than two. Implant reaction forces are reduced with a third implant compared with two implants. The greater surface area of implant to bone allows better distribution of forces. The risk for abutment or coping screw loosening is reduced further because force factors are decreased. Three permucosal sites distribute stresses more efficiently and minimize crestal bone loss. Because the crestal bone is the first region of the bone to be affected, this represents a major advantage. The reduction in the maximum moment of force is twofold with a three-implant system compared with two implants in the A and E regions (Fig. 24.17).[50] A three implant overdenture (RP-5) can be correlated to a 3-legged chair for patient educational purposes.

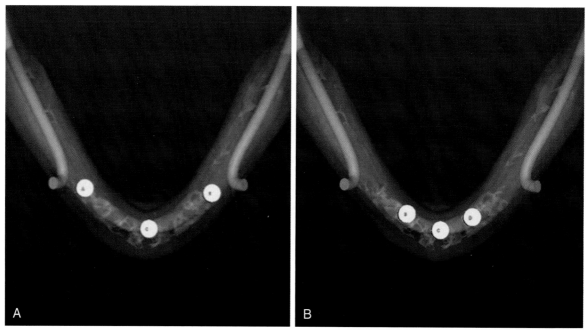

• **Fig. 24.17** Three-Implant Overdenture. (A) A-C-E positions. (B) B-C-D positions.

Ideally, the implants in the A, C, and E positions should not form a straight line. The C implant is anterior to the more distal A and E implants and directly under the cingulum position of the denture teeth. The prosthesis benefits from direct occlusal load to the implant support in the anterior arch. When more than two implants are in the anterior mandible, a tripod support system may be established. The greater the A-P spread of the A, C, and E implants, the greater the biomechanical advantage to reduce stress on the implant and the better the lateral stability of the implant bar and overdenture system. Rotation of the prosthesis may also be more limited compared with OD-1. Therefore the third implant for OD-2 is a considerable advantage for the mandibular edentulous patient. This is usually the first treatment option for a patient with minimal complaints who is concerned primarily with retention and anterior stability when cost is a moderate factor. The posterior ridge form determines the posterior lingual flange extension of the denture, which limits lateral movement of the restoration. If the anterior and posterior ridge form is favorable (Divisions A or B), the implants are placed in the A, C, and E areas, and a wide range of attachments is available (Fig. 24.18).[50]

If the posterior ridge form is poor (Division C–h), the lack of lateral stability places additional forces on the anterior implants. Implants then are best placed in the B-C-D position to allow greater freedom of movement of the prosthesis. The greater the stress to the system, the greater prosthesis movement/stress relief indicated. This increases the posterior movement of the prosthesis but decreases the amount of stress placed on the implants and screw-retained bar.

The prosthesis movement for three implants with C–h posterior bone should be greater to minimize forces on the implants and bar or individual attachment system. If the patient with poor posterior ridge form requires more stability, more than three implants are indicated. In Division D posterior mandibles, five anterior implants are indicated to support the prosthesis (Box 24.3).

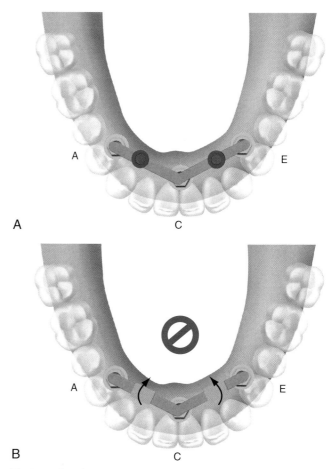

• **Fig. 24.18** Overdenture option 3 corresponds to implants in the A, C, and E positions connected with a bar. The attachments should be positioned to allow movement of the distal section of the prosthesis (A). Two non-aligned Hader clips will not allow movement (B).

Overdenture Option 3

In the third mandibular overdenture option (OD-3), four implants are placed in the A, B, D, and E positions. These implants usually provide sufficient support to include a distal cantilever up to 10 mm on each side if the stress factors are low. The cantilevered superstructure is a feature of the four or more implant treatment option for three reasons: The first relates to the increase in implant support compared with OD-1 to OD-3. The second is that the biomechanical position of the implants is improved in an ovoid or tapering arch form compared with OD-1 or OD-2. The third is related to the additional retention provided for the superstructure bar, which limits the risk for screw loosening and other related complications of cantilevered restorations (Fig. 24.19).

In considering a distal cantilever for a mandibular overdenture bar, the implant position is the primary local determinant. Cantilevers may be compared with a class 1 lever in mechanics. The distalmost implant on each side acts as a fulcrum when occlusal forces are applied to the distal cantilever. Therefore the amount of the occlusal force is magnified by the length of the cantilever, which acts as a lever. For example, a 25-lb load to a 10-mm cantilever results in a 250-lb moment force.

This moment force is resisted by the length of the bar anterior to the fulcrum. Therefore if the two anterior implants are 10 mm from the fulcrum (distal implants), the effect of the posterior cantilever is countered. If the implants are 5 mm apart, the mechanical advantage of the lever is the 10-mm cantilever divided by the 5-mm A-P spread, which equals 2. A 25-lb distal force is magnified to 50 lb to the anterior implant and 75 lb (50 + 25 = 75) to the distal (fulcrum) implant.

The mandibular arch form may be square, tapering, or ovoid. Square arch forms limit the A-P spread between implants and may not be able to counter the effect of a distal cantilever. Therefore rarely are distal cantilevers designed for square arch forms. In a tapering arch form the A-P spread between implants in the A-E and B-D positions is greater and therefore permits a longer distal cantilever. This A-P spread is often at least 10 mm, and therefore often permits a cantilever up to 10 mm from the A and E positions. In an ovoid arch, which is most common, the A-P spread between AE and BD is usually 8 mm. Therefore the cantilever may be up to 8 mm long distally from the A and E implants.

The A-P spread is only one factor to determine the length of the cantilever. When stress factors such as occluding forces are greater, the cantilever is decreased. When the crown height is doubled, the moment forces are doubled. Therefore under ideal, low-force conditions (crown height less than 15 mm, no parafunction, older females, opposing maxillary denture), the cantilever may be up to 1.5 times the A-P spread for OD-3 overdentures.

The patient's indications for this OD-3 include moderate-to-poor posterior anatomy that causes a lack of retention and stability, soft tissue abrasions, and difficulty with speech. The edentulous posterior mandible resorbs four times faster than the anterior mandible. In the C–h posterior mandible the external oblique and mylohyoid ridges are high and often correspond to the crest of the residual ridge. The muscle attachments therefore are at the crest of the ridge. The patient's complaints and desires are more demanding than for the previous treatment options.

The OD-3 prosthesis is indicated to obtain greater stability and a more limited range of prosthesis motion. The overdenture attachments often are placed in the distal cantilevers. The prosthesis is still RP-5, but with the least soft tissue support of all RP-5 designs. The anterior attachment must allow vertical movement for the distal aspect of the prosthesis to

---

• BOX 24.3 Overdenture Treatment Option 2: Three Implants (A-C-E)

Advantages
- Increased retention
- Less invasive surgery and prosthetics
- Increased A-P spread from options 1

Disadvantages
- May not meet patient expectations (RP-5 prosthesis)
- Increased maintenance appointments
- Continuous cost associated with attachment replacement
- Prosthesis reline must be completed more often
- Relies on soft tissue for primary support

Indications
- Relatively low cost
- Less-complicated surgery and prosthetics
- Patient who needs minimal increased retention (RP-5)

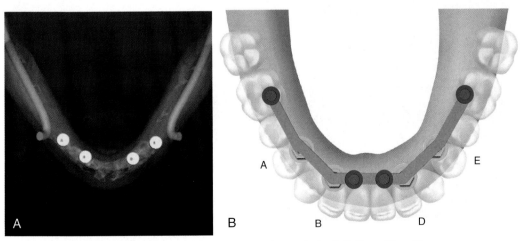

• **Fig. 24.19** (A and B) Four-implant overdenture in the A, B, D, and E position.

rotate toward the tissue. Clips, which permit rotation, are difficult to use on cantilevered superstructures. The clip must be placed perpendicular to the path of rotation to allow movement, not along the cantilevered bar, where its only function then is retention.

The patient benefits from the three implants because of greater occlusal load support and lateral prosthesis stability. The prosthesis loads the soft tissue over only the first and second molars and retromolar pad regions. Therefore the amount of occlusal force is reduced because the bar does not extend to the molar position, where the forces are greater. The amount of distal cantilever is related primarily to the force factors and to the arch form, which corresponds to the A-P spread from the center of the most anterior implants to the distal portions of the A and E implants. However, without the "C" implant position, the A-P spread is not as great (Box 24.4).

Overdenture Option 4

The fourth mandibular overdenture option (OD-4) is designed for three types of patients. This is a minimum treatment option for patients with moderate-to-severe problems related to a

traditional restoration. The needs and desires of the patient are often most demanding and may include limiting the bulk or amount of the prosthesis, major concerns regarding function or stability, posterior sore spots, and the inability to wear a mandibular denture.

The second patient condition is for the treatment of continued bone loss in the posterior mandible. If no prosthetic load is on the posterior bone, the resorption process is delayed considerably and usually is reversed. The third patient condition is a patient who suffers from severe soft tissue sore spots or a history of xerostomia. Because of the completely supported nature of this implant treatment plan, no resultant force will be applied to the soft tissue.

Therefore even when no posterior implants are inserted, the attachments, cantilevered bar, and overdenture avoid load to the residual ridge and often halt its resorption process. Studies have shown that completely implant-supported prostheses may increase the amount of posterior bone height, even when no posterior implants are inserted.[17,51] A better option to prevent this bone loss is the insertion of posterior implants before bone atrophy begins. This treatment option is more likely when the patient desires a fixed restoration or the arch form is square (Fig. 24.20 and Box 24.5).

Division C–h Anterior Mandibles

The four treatment options proposed for mandibular implant–supported overdentures provide an organized approach to solving a patient's complaints or anatomic limitations. The prosthesis support and range of motion should be part of the initial diagnosis. The treatment options initially proposed are designed for completely edentulous patients with Division A anterior bone in desire of an overdenture. These options are modified if the anterior bone is Division C–h. The increase in crown/implant ratio and decrease in implant surface area mandate modification of these initial options.

In the C–h anterior bone volume patient, one more implant is added to each option and OD-1 is eliminated completely. Ideally an RP-5 with good buccal shelf support is recommended.

• **BOX 24.4** **Treatment Option 3: Four Implants (A-B-D-E)**

Advantages
- Increased anteroposterior spread from options 1 and 2
- May cantilever with bar
- May be used as an RP-4 or RP-5 according to force factors
- Possible no soft tissue support (RP-4)

Disadvantages
- More implants required
- More expensive treatment
- Surgical and prosthetic procedures more complicated

Indications
- Increased retention
- Decreased prosthesis movement
- More range of prosthetic options

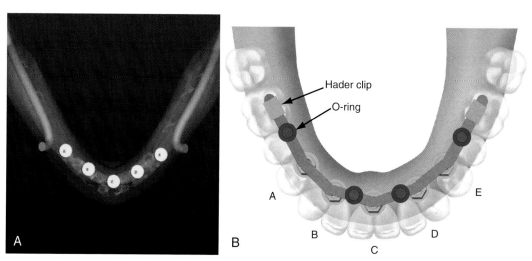

• **Fig. 24.20** (A and B) Five-implant overdenture and a removable RP-4 prosthesis with implants in the A, B, C, D, and E positions.

Patient Education on Various Mandibular Overdenture Options

The clinician and staff can explain the amount of support each treatment option can provide by comparing them with the support system of a chair. Treatment option OD-1 is related to a two-legged chair. The prosthesis provides some vertical support but can rock back and forth. Option OD-2 with three implants is compared with a three-legged chair. This system provides further support but can be rocked one way or the other under lateral forces. A four-legged chair provides the greatest support and is similar to OD-3 and OD-4, which are stable, retentive prostheses.

Fixed Prosthesis

Fixed Prosthesis Advantages

Psychological

A fixed prosthesis provides the psychological advantage of acting and feeling similar to natural teeth, whereas an overdenture, even if fully implant supported, remains a removable prosthesis. In today's society, most patients do not want to be able to remove the prosthesis. A fixed prosthesis often is perceived as an actual body part of the patient, and if a patient's primary request is not to remove the prosthesis, an implant-supported overdenture would not satisfy the psychological need of this patient (Box 24.6).

Improved Speech

The complete mandibular denture, and overdentures to an extent, often move during mandibular jaw movements during function and speech. The contraction of the mentalis, buccinator, or mylohyoid muscles may lift the prosthesis off the soft tissue. As a consequence the teeth may touch during speech and elicit clicking noises. The retentive nature of a fixed prosthesis allows it to remain in place during mandibular movement. The tongue and perioral musculature may resume a more normal position because they are not required to limit the denture or overdenture movement.

Decreased Soft Tissue Irritation

Soft tissue abrasions and accelerated bone loss are more symptomatic of horizontal movement of the prosthesis under lateral forces.

A mandibular denture may move up to 10 mm during function. An implant-supported overdenture may limit lateral movements and direct more longitudinal forces. Under these conditions, specific occlusal contacts and the control of masticatory forces are nearly impossible. An implant fixed prosthesis provides ideal stability of the prosthesis, and the patient is able consistently to reproduce a determined centric occlusion.[52] A fixed prosthesis is especially beneficial in patients with xerostomia (i.e., dry mouth) because there is no tissue contact, which minimizes any possible soft tissue irritation (Fig. 24.21).

Increased Biting Force

Higher bite forces have been documented for mandibular fixed prosthesis on implants. The maximum occlusal force of a patient with dentures may improve 300% with an implant-supported prosthesis.[53] Jemt et al.[54] showed a decrease in occlusal force when the bar connecting implants was removed, which they attributed to the loss of support, stability, and retention. If enough implant support is provided, the resulting prosthesis may be completely supported, retained, and stabilized by the implant prosthesis (i.e., RP-4). Müller et al.[55] reported a greater masseter thickness, chewing efficiency, and bite force in edentulous patients with fixed implant–supported prostheses in a cross-sectional multicenter study.

Less Bone Resorption

When implants are placed in the anterior mandible, the resorption of bone is decreased. Studies have confirmed that after the extraction of mandibular teeth, an average of 4-mm vertical bone loss occurs during the first year after treatment. This bone loss will continue indefinitely, with the mandible experiencing a fourfold greater vertical bone loss than the maxilla.[56] The bone underneath an overdenture may resorb as little as 0.6 mm vertically over 5 years, and long-term resorption may remain at less than 0.05 mm per year.[57,58]

A more recent clinical study by Wright et al.[17] has evaluated the posterior mandibular bone loss in IODs (RP-5) compared with cantilevered fixed prostheses from anterior implants. The annual bone loss index observed in the RP-5 overdentures ranged from +0.02 to +0.05, with 14 of 20 patients losing bone in the posterior regions. On the other hand, the fixed prostheses group had a range from +0.07 to +0.015, with 18 of 22 patients gaining posterior bone area. Reddy et al.[18] also found a similar clinical observation in 60 consecutively treated cantilevered fixed prostheses supported by five to six implants placed between the foramina. The mandibular body height was measured 5, 10, 15, and 20 mm distal to the last implant. The baseline measurements up to 4 years after function increased from 7.25 ± 0.25 to 8.18 ± 0.18 mm. Nearly all of the bone growth occurred during the first year of function. Therefore

---

• BOX 24.5 Treatment Option 4: Five Implants (A-B-C-D-E)

Advantages
- Increased anteroposterior spread from options 1, 2, and 3
- Usually bar-retained cantilever can be used
- RP-4 prosthesis
- No soft tissue support

Disadvantages
- More implants required
- More expensive treatment
- Surgical and prosthetic procedures more complicated

Indications
- Highest amount of retention for an overdenture
- Decreased prosthesis movement
- More range of prosthetic options

• BOX 24.6 Advantages of Mandibular Fixed Implant Prosthesis

1. Psychological
2. Improved speech
3. Decreased soft tissue irritation
4. Increased biting force
5. Less bone resorption
6. Less soft tissue extension
7. Less long-term expenses
8. Less interocclusal space requirement
9. Patients with limited dexterity
10. Increased chewing efficiency

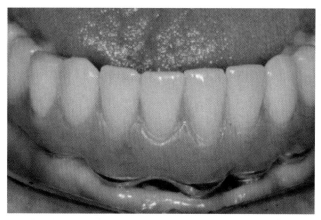

• **Fig. 24.21 Soft Tissue Irritation.** Because there is no contact with the soft tissue for a fixed prosthesis, patients who have a history of soft tissue irritation or xerostomia benefit greatly from a fixed prosthesis.

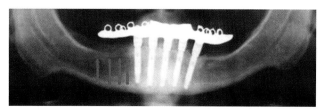

• **Fig. 24.22 Fixed Implant Prosthesis.** A net increase in bone is seen with an FP-3 prosthesis (red arrows). With a removable overdenture prosthesis, bone loss is seen and is continuous.

an important advantage for a complete implant-supported prosthesis is the maintenance and possible regeneration of posterior bone in the mandible. This is especially important because posterior bone loss in this region may lead to neurosensory changes and even mandibular body fracture (Figs. 24.22 and 24.23).

Less Soft Tissue Extension

The implant fixed prosthesis reduces the soft tissue coverage and extension of the prosthesis. This is especially important for new denture wearers, patients with tori or exostoses, or patients with low gagging thresholds. Also, the existence of a labial flange in a conventional denture may result in exaggerated facial contours for the patient with recent extractions. Implant-supported prostheses do not require labial extensions or extended soft tissue coverage. Fixed prosthesis should ideally be convex on the intaglio surface, not concave which leads to hygiene difficulty.

Less Long-Term Expenses

Mandibular overdenture wearers often incur greater long-term expenses than those with fixed restorations. Attachments such as Locator, O-rings, or clips wear and must be replaced regularly. Replacements appear more frequent during the first year, but remain a necessary maintenance step. Denture teeth wear faster on an IOD than with a traditional denture because bite force and masticatory dynamics are improved.

Walton and McEntee[59] noted that there were three times more maintenance and adjustments for removable prostheses compared with fixed restorations. IODs often require attachments to be changed on a regular basis, and denture teeth often wear, requiring a new prosthesis to be fabricated more often. In a review of literature by Goodacre et al., IODs have retention and adjustment problems 30% of the time, relines 19%, clip or attachment fracture 17%, and fracture of

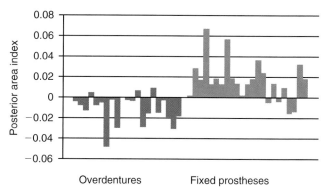

• **Fig. 24.23** Implant overdentures with posterior soft tissue support lose bone in the posterior regions almost 75% of the time. Fixed prostheses cantilevered from anterior implants gain bone in the posterior regions more than 80% of the time (right side of graph).

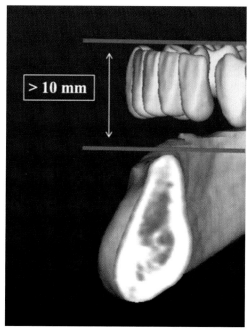

• **Fig. 24.24 Crown/Implant Ratio.** It is imperative that sufficient space is present to fabricate a fixed prosthesis, which is approximately 10 mm for a porcelain fused-to-metal prosthesis (i.e., 8 mm for a zirconia prosthesis).

the prosthesis 12%. A fixed prosthesis (FP-3) requires less repair and less maintenance. Patient education of the long-term maintenance requirement should be outlined at the onset of implant therapy.[60]

Less Interocclusal Space Requirement

The mandibular overdenture treatment plan may require up to 15 mm of space between crestal bone and the occlusal plane. When sufficient crown height space is lacking, the prosthesis is more prone to component fatigue and fracture. The required crown height space (i.e., 15 mm for a bar-retained overdenture and 9 mm for independent attachments) provides adequate bulk of acrylic to resist fracture, space to set denture teeth without modification, and room for attachments, bars, soft tissue, and hygiene. However, with a fixed prosthesis, only 8mm is required for a zirconia prosthesis and 10 mm for a porcelain fused to metal prosthesis. An osteoplasty to increase crown height space before implant placement or a fixed restoration is often indicated when abundant bone height and width are present (Fig. 24.24).

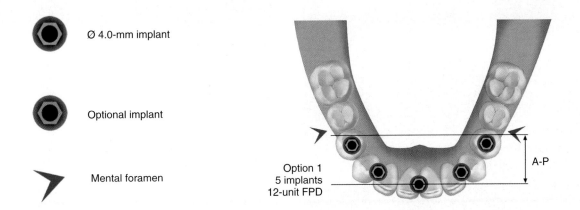

Ø 4.0-mm implant

Optional implant

Mental foramen

Option 1
5 implants
12-unit FPD

A-P

• **Fig. 24.25** The most common number of implants between the foramina for option 1 is five. These implants provide as great an anteroposterior (A-P) distance as possible between the foramina, with sufficient interimplant spacing for treatment of complications. *FPD,* Fixed partial denture.

Patients with Limited Dexterity

A fixed implant prosthesis is ideal for patients with limited dexterity, such as patients with autoimmune disorders (e.g., rheumatoid arthritis, scleroderma). With a removable prosthesis, it may be difficult or impossible to remove a prosthesis because of the attachment fixation. Today, numerous hygiene devices are available to assist patients with daily hygiene.

Increased Chewing Efficiency

Gonçalves et al.[61] showed in studies that a fixed implant prosthesis results in significantly increased chewing efficiency in comparison with an IOD. In the fixed implant prosthesis group the masseter and temporalis muscle showed greater thickness and patient satisfaction was much greater than with a removable prosthesis.[61]

Mandibular Fixed Prosthesis (FP-1, FP-2, and FP-3)

In the past the functional and esthetic rehabilitation of edentulous patients have always been areas of frustration and challenge in the dental profession. However, with the use of dental implants, patients are now able to obtain clinically successful rehabilitation through the use of a fixed prosthesis. Currently, edentulous patients have a full array of treatment options for a fixed prosthesis in the mandibular arch.

Implant Treatment Options for Fixed Restorations

Treatment Option 1: The Brånemark Approach

Among the fixed implant–supported options, the prosthesis following the Brånemark protocol has been shown to have excellent longevity and clinical efficacy.[62] This classical treatment plan involves four to six implants between the mental foramina, and bilateral distal cantilevers replace the mandibular posterior teeth, usually to the first molar region. The mandible does not flex or exhibit significant torsion between the mental foramina. Therefore anterior implants may be splinted together without risk or compromise. The placement of four to six anterior root forms between the mental foramina and a distal cantilever posterior of the most distal implant to replace the posterior teeth was the treatment of choice for clinical reports from 1967 to 1981 with the Brånemark system.[62] This treatment approach resulted in an 80% to 90%

implant survival rate for 5 to 12 years after the first year of loading. In a long-term, 18- to 23-year study, Attard and Zarb[63] reported an 84% success rate using this treatment option (Fig. 24.25).

Treatment option 1 depends greatly on patient force factors; arch form; and implant number, size, and design. As a result, this option should be reserved for patients with low force factors, opposing a removable prosthesis, lower biting force, favorable bone density, and available bone for ideal implant dimensions (Box 24.7 and Fig. 24.26).

Treatment Option 2: Modified Brånemark Technique

A second mandibular fixed treatment plan involves a modified Brånemark technique. Bidez and Misch[19] have evaluated dentate and edentulous mandibles, and developed a three-dimensional bone-strain model of flexure and torsion. Studies were performed to evaluate different splinted implant options that would not compromise the prosthetic foundation. As a consequence a number of implant site options have become available.[64]

A slight variation of the ad modum Brånemark protocol is to place additional implants above the mental foramina because the mandible flexes distal to the foramen. An implant above one or both foramina presents several advantages. First, the number of implants may be increased to as many as seven, which increases the implant surface area. Second, the A-P spread for implant placement is greatly increased. The more distal implant positions will reduce the class 1 lever forces generated from the distal cantilever prosthesis (Fig. 24.27). Third, the

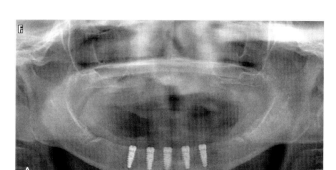

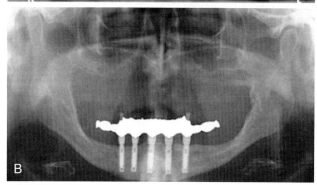

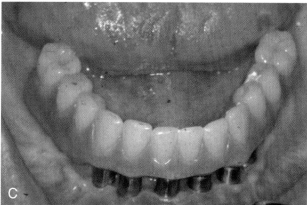

• **Fig. 24.26** Treatment Option 1. (A) Clinical image of traditional Bråne-mark mandibular technique. (B) Five-implant FP-3 prosthesis. (C) Hybrid Brånemark fixed prosthesis.

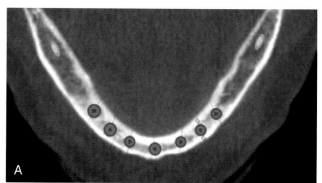

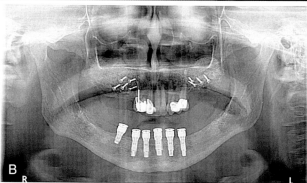

• **Fig. 24.28** Treatment Option 2. (A) Cone beam computed tomography treatment plan for implants over the foramen area. (B) Clinical image of adding an implant over the right foramen to increase the anteroposterior spread.

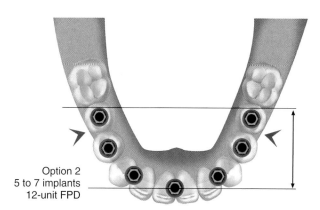

Option 2
5 to 7 implants
12-unit FPD

• **Fig. 24.27** Treatment option 2 has five key implant positions: two implants placed over the mental foramina, two implants in the canine positions, and one implant in the midline. Secondary implants may be positioned in the first premolar sites. *FPD,* Fixed partial denture.

length of the cantilever is reduced dramatically because the distalmost implants are positioned at least one tooth more posterior.

A prerequisite for treatment option 2 is the presence of available bone in height and width over one or both foramina. When available bone is present, the foramen often requires implants of reduced height compared with the anterior implants. The most distal implant bears the greatest load when loads are placed on the cantilever (acts as fulcrum); therefore the greatest forces are generated on the shortest implants. A minimum recommended implant height of 8 mm and a greater diameter or an enhanced surface area design are recommended to compensate for the reduced implant length.

The key implant positions in treatment option 2 are the second premolar positions, the canine positions, and the central incisor or midline position. The two optional implant sites are the first premolar sites and are more often indicated when the patient force factors are greater than usual (Box 24.8 and Fig. 24.28).

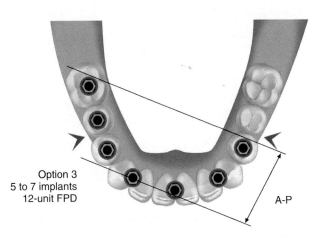

• Fig. 24.29 Treatment option 3 has key implant positions in one first molar site, bilateral first premolar positions, and two canine sites. Secondary implants may be used in the bilateral second premolar and midline position. The anteroposterior (A-P) distance is measured from the two distal-most implants to the anteriormost implant from the cantilever. *FPD*, Fixed partial denture.

Treatment Option 3: Anterior Implants and Unilateral Posterior Implant

The third fixed treatment option is used when inadequate bone is present over the foramina and support is required more posteriorly. The Bidez and Misch[65] strain model of an edentulous mandible indicated that implants in one posterior section may be splinted to anterior implants without compromise. Misch evaluated full-arch fixed prostheses on implants with one posterior segment connected to the anterior region over 20 years and found no additional complications experienced during this time frame compared with those with independent segments.[65]

Therefore an improved treatment plan option to support a fixed mandibular prosthesis consists of additional implants in the first molar or second premolar position (or both) connected to four or five implants between the mental foramina. Hence five to seven implants usually are placed in this treatment option (Fig. 24.29).

The key implant positions for treatment option 3 are the first molar (on one side only), the bilateral first premolar positions, and the bilateral canine sites. The secondary implant positions include the second premolar position on the same side as the molar implant and the central incisor (midline) position. On occasion an additional site may include the position over the mental foramen on the side of the cantilever. Although mandibular movement during function occurs, it has not been observed to cause complications, because the side opposite to the molar implant has no splinted implant(s).

Treatment option 3 is a better option than anterior implants with bilateral cantilevers (option 1 or 2) for several reasons. When one or two implants are placed distal to the foramina on one side and are joined to anterior implants between the foramina, a considerable biomechanical advantage is gained. Although the number of implants may be the same as option 1 or 2, the A-P spread is 1.5 to 2 times greater because, on one side, the distal aspect of the last implant now corresponds to the distal aspect of the first molar. In addition, only one cantilever is present rather than bilateral cantilevers. When force factors are greater, six to seven implants may be used for this option. Five implants between the foramina and one or two implants distal on one side encompass the most common placement.[66] This approach is superior to treatment option 1 or 2 with bilateral cantilevers because: (1) the A-P

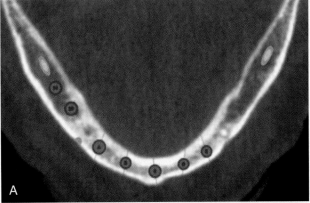
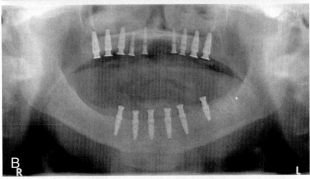
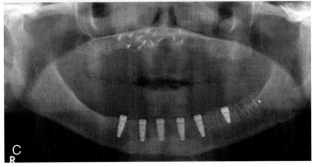

• Fig. 24.30 Treatment Plan 3 Options. (A) Two unilateral posterior implants. (B and C) Clinical images of one unilateral implant that increases the anteroposterior spread and reduces the bilateral cantilever effect.

spread is dramatically increased, (2) more implants may be used if desired, and (3) only one side has a cantilever. However, this option requires available bone in at least one posterior region of the mandible (Fig. 24.30 and Box 24.9).

Treatment Option 4: Anterior Implants and Bilateral Posterior Implants

Treatment plan options for fixed full-arch prostheses also may include bilateral posterior implants as long as they are not splinted together in one prosthesis. This option is selected when force factors are great or the bone density is poor. Poor bone quality most often is observed in the posterior maxilla, but on occasion it is also found in the mandible. Several options for fixed restorations are available when bilateral posterior implants are included; however, the prosthesis needs to be in more than one piece.[67]

In treatment option 4, implants are placed in all three segments of the mandible. Key implant positions for this treatment option include the two first molars, two first premolars, and two canine sites. Secondary implants may be added in the second premolars or the incisor (midline) position (or both) (Fig. 24.31).

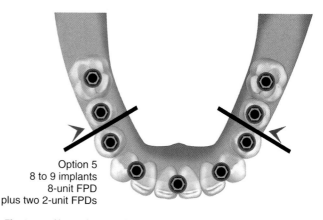

Option 5
8 to 9 implants
8-unit FPD
plus two 2-unit FPDs

• **Fig. 24.32** Alternative prosthetic design is for three separate prostheses, first premolar to first premolar supported by four or five implants, and two posterior segments. *FPD,* Fixed partial denture.

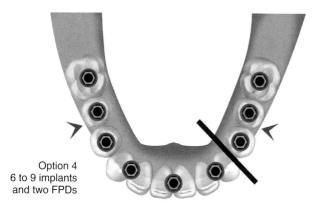

Option 4
6 to 9 implants
and two FPDs

• **Fig. 24.31** Treatment option 4 has implants in both molar sites. Other key positions include the two first premolar positions and the two canine sites. Secondary implants may also be positioned into second premolar locations and the midline. *FPD,* Fixed partial denture.

Prosthetically, all implants in the anterior and one posterior side may be splinted together for a fixed prosthesis. The other posterior segment is restored independently with an independent three-unit, fixed prosthesis supported by implants in the first premolar and first molar region.

Three implants (first premolar, second premolar, and molar) are used most often for the smaller segment to compensate for force factors and the alignment of the implants (because they are almost in a straight line). At least six implants typically are used in this option, but seven are more often used, so the smaller segment has three implants (Fig. 24.32).

The primary advantage of this treatment option is the elimination of cantilevers. As a result, risks for occlusal overload are reduced. Another advantage is that the prosthesis has two segments rather than one. The larger segment (molar to contralateral canine) has an improved advantage because it has implants in three to four different horizontal planes. Because no cantilever is present, less damaging forces are applied to the prosthesis. If the prosthesis requires repair, the affected segment may be removed more easily because only the segment requiring repair needs to be removed. The prosthesis should exhibit posterior disclusion in excursions to limit lateral loads, especially to the prosthesis supported by fewer implants.

Disadvantages for treatment option 4 include the need for abundant bone in both mandibular posterior regions and the additional costs incurred for one to four additional implants.

Another modification for the completely edentulous mandible is to fabricate three independent prostheses rather than two. The anterior region of the mandible may have four to five implants. The key implants are in the two first molar sites, the two first premolar sites, and two canine regions. Secondary positions are the two second premolar and central incisor (midline) sites. With this protocol, the posterior restorations extend from first molar to first premolar, and an anterior restoration replaces the six anterior teeth.

The advantages of this option are smaller segments for individual restorations in case one should fracture or become uncemented. In addition, if greater mandibular body movement is expected because of parafunction or a decrease in size of the body of the mandible, the independent restorations allow the most flexibility and torsion of the mandible.

The primary disadvantage of option 4 is the greater number of implants required. In addition, the available bone needs are greatest with this treatment option. Nine implants are rarely required to replace the lower teeth, regardless of the bone density or force factors present. Option 4 is the treatment of choice when force factors are severe (Box 24.10 and Fig. 24.33).

Treatment Option 5: All-on-Four Protocol

The treatment option 5 includes the "all-on-four" concept, which was developed to avoid regenerative procedures that potentially increase the treatment costs and patient morbidity. This protocol, developed

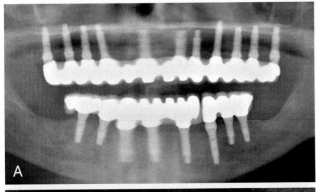

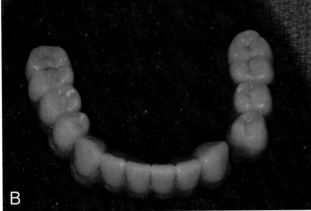

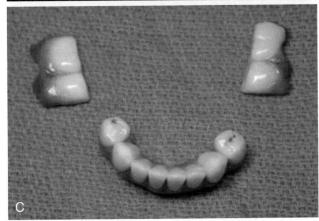

• **Fig. 24.33** Treatment Plan 4. (A and B) Clinical image of eight implant mandibular implants with two independent prostheses. (C) An additional prosthetic option is three independent prostheses with one anterior and two posterior.

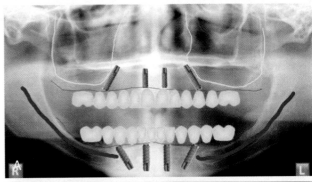

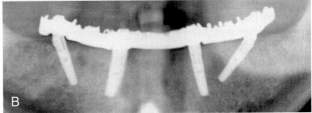

• **Fig. 24.34** All-on-Four Protocol. (A) Two implants are positioned in the anterior and two implants in the posterior at an angle to increase the anteroposterior spread and avoid the mental foramen. (B) Clinical image of mandibular all-on-four.

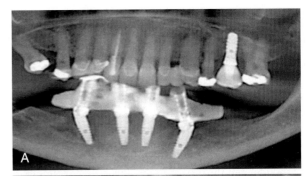

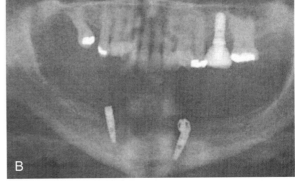

• **Fig. 24.35** All-on-Four Complication. (A and B) If one or more of the implants fail, the prosthesis is lost, and new implants and bone augmentation may need to be completed to redo the prosthesis.

by Malo, uses four implants in the anterior part of a completely edentulous jaw to support a provisional, fixed, and immediately loaded prosthesis. Most commonly, the two most anterior implants are placed axially, whereas the two posterior implants are placed at an angle (i.e., usually at an approximately 45-degree angle) to increase A-P spread along with decreasing the cantilever length (Fig. 24.34).[68,69]

Tilted implants have been shown to generate favorable biomechanical outcomes[70] and in a metaanalysis, there was no significant difference in either failure rate compared with axially placed implants[71] or marginal bone loss.[72] The tilted implants offer several advantages, which include the use of longer implants (i.e., greater surface area and primary stability), reduced or eliminated cantilever length, and avoidance of vital structures such as the inferior alveolar canal.[73] This procedure has become popular among clinicians and patients because of the decreased treatment costs and treatment duration.[74] The literature has shown high survival rates and a low incidence of complications with this procedure (Fig. 24.35).[75,76] Most dental implant and prosthetic survival rates approach 98% (Box 24.11).[47,48,77,78] However, all-on-four protocols require the clinician to have additional surgical and prosthetic skills. Because of the increased skill level required, clinicians early on their learning curve should exercise caution in these cases.

• BOX 24.11 Fixed Treatment Option 5: All-on-Four

Advantages
- Fixed immediate protocol
- Accepted surgical and prosthetic protocol
- Fewer implants, lower costs
- Faster treatment

Disadvantages
- Technically difficult (surgical and prosthetic)
- Complications are difficult to remedy

Indications
- Immediate placement implants
- Immediate loading

Summary

The treatment of the edentulous mandible is a common procedure that implant clinicians see on a regular basis. There exists a full array of options for patients which include 5 fixed treatment plans and 4 removable overdenture treatment options. IODs borrow several principles from tooth-supported overdentures. The advantages of IODs relate to the ability to place rigid, healthy abutments in the positions of choice. The number, location, superstructure design, and prosthetic range of motion can be predetermined and based on a patient's expressed needs and desires. Two implants placed just anterior to the mental foramina rarely should be used. The overdenture should be designed to satisfy the patient's desires and anatomic limitations predictably.

Many completely edentulous patients desire a fixed restoration rather than a removable prosthesis. The financial cost for a fixed implant prosthesis often have been a deterrent but should be more similar to a completely implant-supported overdenture. The number and position of implants should be related to the amount of stress transmitted to the bone during occlusion and parafunction, and the density of the bone. Other considerations include mandibular flexure and torsion. Five treatment options generally are available for this fixed complete mandibular implant-supported restoration. These treatment options accommodate the stronger mandibular bone dynamics without affecting the prosthesis.

References

1. English CE. The mandibular overdenture supported by implants in the anterior symphysis: a prescription for implant placement and bar prosthesis design. *Dent Implantol Update.* 1993;4:9–14.
2. Cutright B, Quillopa N, Shupert W, et al. An anthropometric analysis of key foramina for maxillofacial surgery. *J Oral Maxillofac Surg.* 2003;61:354–357.
3. De Marco TJ, Paine S. Mandibular dimensional change. *J Prosthet Dent.* 1974;31:482–485.
4. Fischman B. The rotational aspect of mandibular flexure. *J Prosthet Dent.* 1990;64:483–485.
5. Goodkind RJ, Heringlake CB. Mandibular flexure in opening and closing movement. *J Prosthet Dent.* 1973;30:134–138.
6. Grant AA. Some aspects of mandibular movement: acceleration and horizontal distortion. *Ann Acad Med Singapore.* 1986;15:305–310.
7. Hylander WL. The human mandible: lever or link? *Am J Phys Anthropol.* 1975;43:227–242.
8. Osborne J, Tomlin HR. Medial convergence of the mandible. *Br Dent J.* 1964;117:112–114.
9. Regli CP, Kelly EK. The phenomenon of decreased mandibular arch width in opening movement. *J Prosthet Dent.* 1967;17:49–53.
10. McDowell JA, Regli CP. A quantitative analysis of the decrease in width of the mandibular arch during forced movements of the mandible. *J Dent Res.* 1961;40:1183–1185.
11. Hobkirk JA, Havthoulas TK. The influence of mandibular deformation, implant numbers, and loading position on detected forces in abutments supporting fixed implant superstructures. *J Prosthet Dent.* 1998;80:169–174.
12. Abdel-Latif HH, Hobkirk JA, Kelleway JP. Functional mandibular deformation in edentulous subjects treated with dental implants. *Int J Prosthodont.* 2000;13:513–519.
13. Omar R, Wise MD. Mandibular flexure associated with muscle force applied in the retruded axis position. *J Oral Rehabil.* 1981;8:209–221.
14. Hylander WL. Mandibular function in Galago crassicaudatus and Macaca fascicularis: an in vivo approach to stress analysis of the mandible. *J Morphol.* 1979;159:253–296.
15. Marx H. Untersuchungen des funktionsbedingten elastis-chen Deformierung der menschlichen Mandibula. *Dtsch Zahnarztl Z.* 1966;21:937–938.
16. Wright PS, Glastz PO, Randow K, et al. The effects of fixed and removable implant-stabilized prostheses on posterior mandibular residual ridge resorption. *Clin Oral Implants Res.* 2002;13:169–174.
17. Reddy MS, Geurs NC, Wang IC, et al. Mandibular growth following implant restoration: does Wolff's Law apply to residual ridge resorption? *Int J Periodontics Restorative Dent.* 2002;22:315–321.
18. Misch CE. Treatment options for mandibular full arch implant-supported fixed prostheses. *Dent Today.* 2001;20:68–73.
19. Miyamoto Y, Fujisawa K, Takechi M, et al. Effect of the additional installation of implants in the posterior region on the prognosis of treatment in the edentulous mandibular jaw. *Clin Oral Implants Res.* 2003;14:727–733.
20. Zarone F, Apicella A, Nicolais L, et al. Mandibular flexure and stress build-up in mandibular full-arch fixed prostheses supported by osseointegrated implants. *Clin Oral Implants Res.* 2003;14:103–114.
21. Miyamoto Y, Fujisawa K, Takechi M, et al. Effect of the additional installation of implants in the posterior region on the prognosis of treatment in the edentulous mandibular jaw. *Clin Oral Implants Res.* 2003;14:727–733.
22. Parel SM, Sullivan D. Full arch edentulous ceramometal restoration. In: Parel SM, Sullivan D, eds. *Esthetics and Osseointegration.* Dallas: Osseointegration Seminars; 1989.
23. Balshi TJ. Opportunity to prevent or resolve implant complications. *Implant Soc.* 1990;1:6–9.
24. Fishman BM. The influence of fixed splints on mandibular flexure. *J Prosthet Dent.* 1976;35:643–667.
25. de Oliveria RM, Emtiaz S. Mandibular flexure and dental implants: a case report. *Implant Dent.* 2000;9:90–95.
26. Paez CY, Barco T, Roushdy S, et al. Split-frame implant prosthesis designed to compensate for mandibular flexure: a clinical report. *J Prosthet Dent.* 2003;89:341–343.
27. Geertman ME, Slagter AP, van Waas MA, et al. Comminution of food with mandibular implant retained overdentures. *J Dent Res.* 1994;73:1858–1864.
28. Rissin L, House JE, Manly RS, et al. Clinical comparison of masticatory performance and electromyographic activity of patients with complete dentures, overdentures and natural teeth. *J Prosthet Dent.* 1978;39:508–511.
29. Sposetti VJ, Gibbs CH, Alderson TH, et al. Bite force and muscle activity in overdenture wearers before and after attachment placement. *J Prosthet Dent.* 1986;55:265–273.
30. Carlsson GE, Kronstrom M, de Baat C, et al. A survey of the use of mandibular implant overdentures in 10 countries. *Int J Prosthodont.* 2004;17:211–217.

31. Feine JS, de Grandmont P, Boudrias P, et al. Within subject comparisons of implant-supported mandibular prostheses: choice of prosthesis. *J Dent Res*. 1994;73:1105–1111.
32. de Grandmont P, Feine JS, Tache R, et al. Within subject comparisons of implant-supported mandibular prostheses: psychometric evaluation. *J Dent Res*. 1994;73:1096–1104.
33. Babbush CA, Kent JN, Misiek DJ. Titanium plasma spray (TPS) Swiss screw implants for the reconstruction of the edentulous mandible. *J Oral Maxillofac Surg*. 1986;44:247–282.
34. Engquist B, Bergendal T, Kallus T, et al. A retrospective multicenter evaluation of osseointegrated implants supporting overdentures. *Int J Oral Maxillofac Implants*. 1988;3:129–134.
35. Jemt T, Chai J, Harnett J. A 5-year prospective multicenter follow-up report on overdentures supported by osseointegrated implants. *Int J Oral Maxillofac Implants*. 1996;11:291–298.
36. Wismeijer D, Van Waas MAJ, Vermeeren J. Overdenture supported by implants: a 6.5 year evaluation of patient satisfaction and prosthetic after care. *Int J Oral Maxillofac Implants*. 1995;10:744–749.
37. Naert I, Alsaadi G, Quirynen M. Prosthetic aspects and patient satisfaction with two-implant-retained mandibular overdentures: a 10-year randomized clinical study. *Int J Prosthodont*. 2004;17(4).
38. Misch CE. Treatment options for mandibular implant overdentures: an organized approach. In: Misch CE, ed. *Contemporary Implant Dentistry*. St Louis: Mosby; 1993.
39. Kline R, Hoar J, Beck GH, et al. A prospective multicenter clinical investigation of a bone quality based dental implant system. *Implant Dent*. 2002;11:224–234.
40. Mericke-Stern R. Clinical evaluation of overdenture restorations supported by osseointegrated titanium implants: a retrospective study. *Int J Oral Maxillofac Implants*. 1990;5:375–383.
41. Awad MA, Lund JP, Dufresne E, Feine JS. Comparing the efficacy of mandibular implant-retained overdentures and conventional dentures among middle-aged edentulous patients: satisfaction and functional assessment. *Int J Prosthodont*. 2003;16(2).
42. Thomason JM, Lund JP, Chehade A, et al. Patient satisfaction with mandibular implant overdentures and conventional dentures 6 months after delivery. *Int J Prosthodont*. 2003;16:467–473.
43. Schwartz-Arad D, Kidron N, Dolev E. A long-term study of implants supporting overdentures as a model for implant success. *J Periodontol*. 2005;76:1431–1435.
44. Takanashi Y, Penrod JR, Lund JP, et al. A cost comparison of mandibular two-implant overdenture and conventional denture treatment. *Int J Prosthodont*. 2004;17:181–618.
45. Attard NJ, Zarb GA. Long-term treatment outcomes in edentulous patients with implant overdentures: the Toronto study. *Int J Prosthodont*. 2004;17:425–433.
46. Malo P, de Araujo Nobre M, Lopes A, et al. A longitudinal study of the survival of all-on-4 implants in the mandible with up to 10 years of follow-up. *J Am Dent Assoc*. 2011;142(3):310–320.
47. Agliardi E, Panigatti S, Clerico M, et al. Immediate rehabilitation of the edentulous jaws with full fixed prostheses supported by four implants: interim results of a single cohort prospective study. *Clin Oral Implants Res*. 2010;21(5):459–465.
48. Misch CE. Implant overdentures relieve discomfort for the edentulous patient. *Dentist*. 1989;67:37–38.
49. Jager K, Wirz EJ. In: *Vitro Spannung Analysen on Implantaten fur Zahnartzt und Zahntechniker*. Berlin: Quintessenz; 1992.
50. Bidez MW, Misch CE. The biomechanics of interimplant spacing. In: *Proceedings of the Fourth International Congress of Implants and Biomaterials in Stomatology*. Charleston, SC; 1990:24–25.
51. Davis WH, Lam PS, Marshall MW, et al. Using restorations borne totally by anterior implants to preserve the edentulous mandible. *J Am Dent Assoc*. 1999;130:1183–1189.
52. Jemt T, Stalblad PA. The effect of chewing movements on changing mandibular complete dentures to osseointegrated overdentures. *J Prosthet Dent*. 1986;55:357–361.
53. Haraldson T, Jemt T, Stalblad PA, et al. Oral function in subjects with overdentures supported by osseointegrated implants. *Scand J Dent Res*. 1988;96:235–242.
54. Jemt T, Book K, Karlsson S. Occlusal force and mandibular movements in patients with removable overdentures and fixed prostheses supported by implants in the maxilla. *Int J Oral Maxillofac Implants*. 1993;8:301–308.
55. Müller Frauke, et al. Masseter muscle thickness, chewing efficiency and bite force in edentulous patients with fixed and removable implant-supported prostheses: a cross-sectional multicenter study. *Clin Oral Implants Res*. 2012;23:2.
56. Tallgren A. The reduction in face height of edentulous and partially edentulous subjects during long-term denture wear: a longitudinal roentgenographic cephalometric study. *Acta Odontol Scand*. 1966;24:195–239.
57. Naert I, Gizani S, Vuylsteke M, et al. A 5-year randomized clinical trial on the influence of splinted and unsplinted oral implants in the mandibular overdenture therapy. 1. Peri-implant outcome. *Clin Oral Implants Res*. 1998;9:70–177.
58. Adell R, Lekholm U, Rockler B, et al. A 15-year study of osseointegrated implants in the treatment of the edentulous jaw. *Int J Oral Surg*. 1981;10:387–416.
59. Walton JN, McEntee MI. Problems with prostheses on implants: a retrospective study. *J Prosthet Dent*. 1994;71:283–288.
60. Goodacre CJ, Bernal G, Rungcharassaeng K, Kan JY. Clinical complications with implants and implant prostheses. *J Prosthet Dent*. 2003;90(2):121–132.
61. Gonçalves TMSV, et al. Mastication improvement after partial implant-supported prosthesis use. *J Dent Res*. 2013;92(suppl 12):189S–194S.
62. Smith DE, Zarb GA. Criteria for success of osseointegrated endosseous implants. *J Prosthet Dent*. 1989;62(5):567–572.
63. Attard NJ, Zarb GA. Long-term treatment outcomes in edentulous patients with implant-fixed prostheses: the Toronto study. *Int J Prosthodont*. 2004;17:417–424.
64. Misch CE, Bidez MW. Implant-protected occlusion: a biomechanical rationale. *Compendium (Newtown, Pa.)*. 1994;15(11):1330–1332.
65. Bidez M, Misch C. *Clinical Biomechanics in Implant Dentistry*; 2005.
66. Misch Carl E, Resnik R. Misch's avoiding complications in oral implantology-e-book. *Elsevier Health Sci*. 2017.
67. Bidez MW, Misch CE. Force transfer in implant dentistry: basic concepts and principles. *J Oral Implantol*. 1992;18(3):264–274.
68. Paulo Maló, Bo Rangert, Nobre Miguel. All-on-four immediate-function concept with Brånemark system implants for completely edentulous mandibles: a retrospective clinical study. *Clin Implant Dent Relat Res*. 2003;5:2–9.
69. Paulo Malo, Bo Rangert, Nobre Miguel. All-on-4 immediate-function concept with brånemark system implants for completely edentulous maxillae: a 1-year retrospective clinical study. *Clin Implant Dent Relat Res*. 2005.
70. Rossetti PH, Bonachela WC, Rossetti LM. Relevant anatomic and biomechanical studies for implant possibilities on the atrophic maxilla: critical appraisal and literature review. *J Prosthodont*. 2010;19:449–457.
71. Menini M, Signori A, Tealdo T, et al. Tilted implants in the immediate loading rehabilitation of the maxilla: a systematic review. *J Dent Res*. 2012;91:821–827.
72. Francetti L, Romeo D, Corbella S, Taschieri S, Del Fabbro M. Bone level changes around axial and tilted implants in full-arch fixed immediate restorations. Interim results of a prospective study. *Clin Implant Dent Relat Res*. 2012;14:646–654.
73. Bevilacqua M, Tealdo T, Menini M, et al. The influence of can- tilever length and implant inclination on stress distribution in maxillary implant-supported fixed dentures. *J Prosthet Dent*. 2011;105:5–13.
74. Malo P, Nobre M, Lopes A. The rehabilitation of completely edentulous maxillae with different degrees of resorption with four or

more immediately loaded implants: a 5-year retrospective study and a new classification. *Eur J Oral Implantol.* 2011;4(3):227–243.

75. Babbush CA, Kanawati A, Kotsakis GA, Hinrichs JE. Patient-related and financial outcomes analysis of conventional full-arch rehabilitation versus the All-on-4 concept: a cohort study. *Implant Dent.* 2014;23(2):218–224.

76. Maló P, Lopes A, de Araújo Nobre M, Ferro A. Immediate function dental implants inserted with less than 30 N· cm of torque in full-arch maxillary rehabilitations using the All-on-4 concept: retrospective study. *Int J Oral Maxillofac Surg.* 2018.

77. Butura CC, Galindo DF, Jensen OT. Mandibular all-on-four therapy using angled implants: a three-year clinical study of 857 implants in 219 jaws. *Dent Clin North Am.* 2011;55(4):795–811.

78. Babbush CA, Kutsko GT, Brokloff J. The all-on-four immediate function treatment concept with NobelActive implants: a retrospective study. *J Oral Implantol.* 2011;37(4):431–445.

25

The Edentulous Maxilla: Fixed versus Removable Treatment Planning

RANDOLPH R. RESNIK AND CARL E. MISCH[†]

In all phases of implant dentistry the treatment planning of the edentulous maxilla is the most complicated for the long-term success of implants and the prosthesis. The maxillary arch is predisposed to inherent anatomic disadvantages, which has led to many studies verifying a much lower success rate in comparison with the mandible. Historically, most research studies on edentulous arches were completed on the mandible because most patients often described the instability of the mandibular denture in comparison with the maxillary. In general, patients are more likely to wear a maxillary denture in comparison with the mandibular edentulous prosthesis. Many patients often waited longer periods before seeking treatment in the edentulous maxilla, which resulted in extensive resorption.

The maxillary arch has a lower success rate mainly because in the past the maxillary arch principles followed the same principles that are used in the mandibular arch. The long-term prognosis for implants in the maxilla has been shown to be less predictable in comparison with the mandible. Because of the resorption pattern of the maxilla (i.e., horizontal bone loss twice as much as vertical

resorption soon after extraction), anatomic structures such as the nasal cavity and the maxillary sinus play an important role in treatment planning. Because of the high prevalence of reduced quantity and quality of bone, along with increased esthetic demand, the maxillary arch requires more detailed approaches to treatment planning with respect to a fixed or removable prosthesis (Fig. 25.1).

Treatment Planning Factors

When evaluating a patient for maxillary implants, one of the most important diagnostic tools is the patient's existing denture. From the patient's denture, the smile line, amount of lip support, size and shape of the teeth, interocclusal space (crown height space), and the relative retention of the prosthesis can be determined.

Smile Line

The smile line is an important variable when evaluating the amount of teeth the patient should show with movement of the upper lip during

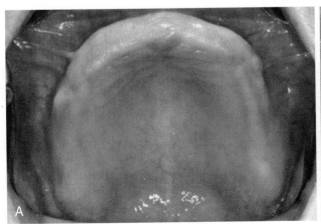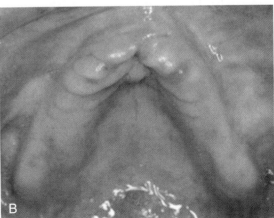

• **Fig. 25.1** The maxilla varies greatly, from abundant bone with attached tissue (A) to a severely resorbed maxilla with compromised hard and soft tissue (B).

[†] Deceased

speech and smiling. Tjan et al.[1] reported that the average smile allows approximately 75% to 100% of the maxillary incisors and interproximal gingiva to be visible. With an edentulous arch the clinician should evaluate the amount of ridge showing when smiling without the denture. If the residual ridge does show during smiling, the treatment planning for an implant prosthesis may be very challenging (Fig. 25.2).

Lip Support

The lip and soft tissue support is derived from the maxillary anterior teeth contours and also the position of the residual ridge. The lip and soft tissue support should be evaluated with the existing denture in place and not in place. This will give crucial information on whether a fixed or removable prosthesis would be more ideal. If the existing denture greatly supports the lip, then a fixed prosthesis may not be the most ideal because it is often difficult to obtain lip support from a fixed maxillary prosthesis. The soft tissue support is mainly from the buccal flange of the maxillary prosthesis as resorption in the maxilla proceeds in a cranially and medially direction.

In addition, a patient with a short upper lip will most likely show the maxillary teeth on repose. Therefore short upper lips are far more challenging than long upper lips. With a long upper lip, very little to none of the maxillary teeth will be visible (Fig. 25.3).

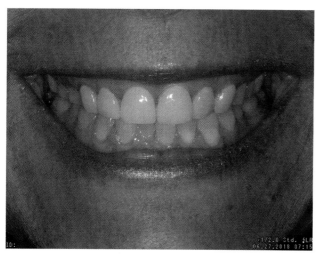

• **Fig. 25.2** Smile Line. When patients exhibit a high smile line, caution should be exercised in the treatment planning of the edentulous arch because the final esthetics may be problematic.

Ridge Position

Depending on the amount of bone resorption, the residual ridge is usually significantly lingual to the ideal position of the teeth in the maxillary anterior and posterior. This discrepancy must be taken into consideration when evaluating the ideal position of the implants so that a prosthesis may be fabricated that fulfills adequate lip support, phonetics, and patient approval, and allows for sufficient tongue space. When the difference between the ridge and the tooth position (i.e., square arch form and tapered tooth position) is present, significant prosthetic difficulties such as anterior force factors (i.e. from the cantilevered discrepancy between the ridge and tooth position) may predispose to complications.

Soft Tissue

The thickness and quality of the soft tissue should be evaluated both clinically and via a cone beam computed tomography examination. As the maxillary ridge resorbs, the tissue thins and is less dense with loss of keratinized tissue. In severely resorbed premaxillary regions, the tissue will become hypermobile, which leads to very little support for the prosthesis. Often maxillary edentulous patients seek an esthetic fixed prosthesis similar to natural teeth. Therefore it is imperative the patient understand the difficulty in achieving a papillary architecture similar to preextraction condition. Regenerating papilla, which would result in a FP-1 (fixed prosthesis with normal size clinical crown) prosthesis, is usually difficult and in some cases impossible to achieve.[2]

Crown Height Space (Interocclusal Space)

The amount of space between the residual ridge and the incisal edge is an important factor in the treatment planning of a maxillary prosthesis. For a fixed versus a removable implant prosthesis, there exist different dimensional tolerances to accommodate the prosthesis. Therefore a preoperative evaluation and determination of the amount of crown height space needs to be completed before any surgical placement of dental implants. In general this may be accomplished with an articulated setup of maxillary and mandibular arches. However, a study cast will not relate an accurate assessment of the thickness of the soft tissue. Therefore newer software programs that allow for the three-dimensional evaluation of the teeth in maximum intercuspation can easily be accomplished with a cone beam computed tomography survey.

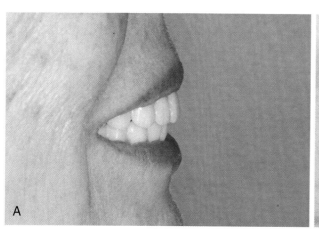
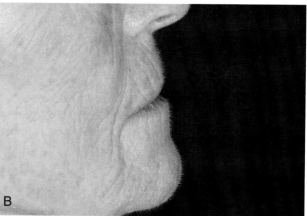

• **Fig. 25.3** Lip Support. (A) The lip support should be evaluated with the denture in and the denture out to determine the future prosthetic demands (B).

Conventional screw-retained implant prostheses (i.e., zirconia or porcelain-fused prostheses) can be fabricated with 8-10 mm (zirconia) between the edentulous ridges and the opposing occlusal plane. For a hybrid prosthesis, approximately 15 mm of interocclusal room is required, as increased space is required to prevent acrylic material fracture.[3] Sufficient crown height space will allow for adequate bulk of material and permits for more ideal esthetics and hygiene ability. If space is compromised, an increase in prosthetic complications may occur.[4,5]

For a removable prosthesis in the maxillary arch, compromised space can be more problematic in comparison with the mandibular arch. When inadequate space is available for a removable prosthesis, fracture of the prosthesis or compromised esthetics may result. A significant variable is whether the implants would be independent or bar retained. For an independent attachment implant-supported overdenture (IOD), a minimum of 9 mm of space is required (i.e., Locator Attachment). If a bar-retained prosthesis is to be fabricated, a minimum of 12 to 14 mm of space is needed, depending on the attachment system.[6] To prevent fracture of the denture base or attachments, 2 to 3 mm is needed to provide adequate strength as a denture base material (Fig. 25.4) and prevent denture teeth dislodgement.[7]

Literature Review

In general, studies have shown the maxillary overdenture and maxillary fixed prosthesis to be less predictable and associated with a higher morbidity and failure rate in comparison with the mandibular arch prostheses. Jemt[8] evaluated maxillary fixed prostheses with 449 implants for a 5-year period and found a cumulative implant and prosthesis survival rate to be 92.1% and 95.9% for 5 years, respectively. The mean marginal bone loss was approximately 1.2 mm at the 5-year evaluation. In this study, speech problems were the most common patient complaints, followed by resin prosthesis fractures as the most common prosthetic complication.

Maxillary overdentures have been reported to have the highest failure rate in comparison with any other type of prosthesis. When evaluating maxillary overdenture success, Hutton et al.[9] showed a nine-times

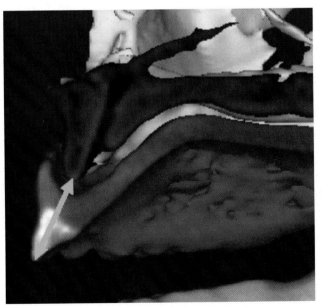

• **Fig. 25.4 Maxillary Crown Height Space.** Measured from the residual ridge to the incisal edge, the minimum space requirement is 8 to 10 mm for a fixed prosthesis, 9 mm for an independent attachment overdenture, and 12-14 mm for a bar-retained prosthesis.

greater failure in the maxilla compared with the mandible. Numerous studies have shown implant failure rates of 2% to 5% before loading, and up to 30% after loading.[10-13] For late failure, maxillary overdenture studies have shown failure rates up to 5% to 15%.[14-17]

Wilbom et al. evaluated maxillary fixed versus overdenture prostheses for a 5-year period. Interestingly, the survival rate was 77% in the overdenture group and 46% in the group originally treatment planned for a fixed prosthesis; however, it was then changed to an overdenture. With this study a very high failure rate was seen, especially with patients in whom the prosthesis was changed from a fixed to a removable prosthesis.[18]

Maxillary dentures have also been associated with various inherent disadvantages in comparison with a fixed prosthesis. Most of the issues stem from the increased palatal coverage that a conventional denture or RP-5 overdenture in comparison to a RP-4 overdenture. Shannon et al.[19] showed compromised parotid flow when palatal coverage was present, thereby decreasing salivary flow when wearing an RP-5 overdenture. Patients often report a lack of taste sensation when wearing a maxillary overdenture with palatal coverage. This has been shown with multiple studies.[20,21]

In addition, longitudinal studies on implant-supported maxillary overdentures have shown an increased frequency rate of maxillary hyperplasia of up to 30%.[22] In retrospective follow-up studies, hyperplasia was observed in more than 64% of the subjects originally planned for a fixed maxillary prosthesis but who had an overdenture treatment because of implant failure.[23] Most commonly, hyperplastic tissue is seen around the retaining bars.

Fixed Maxillary Treatment Plans

A review of the literature found many articles that indicate that full maxillary fixed implant–supported prostheses are fabricated on an average of six standard-diameter implants with posterior molar cantilevers. More recently, numerous articles have shown the success of a fixed prosthesis on four implants. However, the edentulous maxilla has been shown to have the lowest implant survival for either fixed or removable implant restorations, compared with mandibular prostheses.[24-27] All reports concur with the finding that maxillary bone tends to be of poorer quality and volume, and presents several biomechanical disadvantages. To compensate for the poor local conditions, a greater number of implants should be planned, along with a greater anteroposterior (A-P) distance. Therefore a number of core principles are used when treatment planning an edentulous maxillary arch for a fixed prosthesis; following these principles increases the success rate.

1. The number of implants is related to the dental arch form.
2. The arch form is dictated by the final dentition or prosthesis, not the edentulous ridge arch form.
3. Key implant positions exist: anterior, canine, premolar, and molar.
4. An RP-4 (totally implant supported removable prosthesis) prosthesis is treatment planned the same as a fixed prosthesis.

Three common dental arch forms for the maxilla exist: square, ovoid, and tapering. As a consequence of bone resorption the edentulous ridge arch form usually will differ from the dentate arch form. The dental arch form of the patient is determined by the final teeth position in the premaxilla and not the arch shape of the residual ridge. A residual ridge may appear square because of resorption or trauma. However, the final teeth position may need to be cantilevered facially with the final prosthesis. In other words, a dental ovoid arch form may be needed to restore a residual edentulous square arch form. The number and position of implants are related to the arch form of the final dentition (prosthesis), not the existing edentulous arch form (Table 25.1).

TABLE 25.1	Treatment Plan for Edentulous Premaxilla		
Arch Form	Anterior Cantilever (mm)	Number of Anterior Implants	Implant Position
Square	< 8	2	Canines
Ovoid	8–12	3	Two canines and one incisor
Tapering	>12	4	Two canines and two incisors

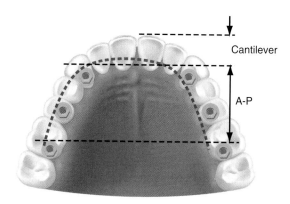

• **Fig. 25.6** Fixed Treatment Plan 1: When force factors are low, a square dentate arch form may use six implants for a fixed or RP-4 (totally implant supported removable prosthesis) prosthesis. *A-P,* Anteroposterior distance.

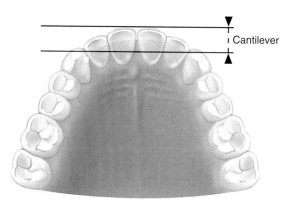

• **Fig. 25.5** Dental Arch Form Determination: Two horizontal lines are drawn. The first line bisects the incisal papilla and connects the tips of the canines. The second line is parallel and along the facial position of the central incisor. The distance between these lines determines whether the dentate arch form is square, ovoid, or tapering.

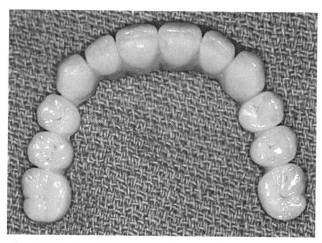

• **Fig. 25.7** Maxillary FP-3 (type 3 fixed prosthesis) Prosthesis. This prosthesis follows a square dentate arch form, and therefore is supported by six implants (canines, second premolars, and first molars). Because of the square arch form a minimal cantilever results.

• **BOX 25.1** Maxillary Fixed Prosthesis (FP-1,2,or 3) Treatment Plan 1

Indications: Square arch form
Implants: 6
Positions (bilateral):
  Canine
  Second bicuspid
  First molar

The dental arch form in the anterior maxilla is determined by the distance from two horizontal lines. The first line is drawn from one canine (i.e., in a diagnostic wax-up or existing prosthesis if no teeth are present) incisal edge tip to the other. This line most often bisects the incisive papilla. The second line is drawn parallel to the first line, along the facial position of the anterior teeth (Fig. 25.5). When the distance between these two lines is less than 8 mm, a square dental arch form is present. When the distance between these two lines is 8 to 12 mm, an ovoid dentate arch form is present—the most commonly observed. When the distance between the two lines is greater than 12 mm, the dentate arch form is tapering.

Therefore with respect to dental arch form, the authors have postulated four different options for the maxillary fixed prosthesis.

Maxillary Fixed Prosthesis Treatment Option 1 (Box 25.1)

In a dental square arch form, lateral and central incisors are minimally cantilevered facially from the canine position, resulting in a

lesser requirement of an implant in the central or lateral position. When maxillary fixed prosthesis treatment option 1 is used, mandibular excursions and occlusal forces exert less stress on the canine implants. As a result, implants in the canine position to replace the six anterior teeth may suffice when the force factors are low and if they are splinted to additional posterior implants (Figs. 25.6 and 25.7).

Maxillary Fixed Prosthesis Treatment Option 2

If the final teeth position is an ovoid arch form, at least three implants should be inserted into the premaxilla: one in each canine and preferably one in a central incisor position (Fig. 25.8). The central incisor position increases the A-P distance from the canine to central and provides improved biomechanical support to the prosthesis. In long-term edentulous maxillae with significant atrophy, treatment option 2 will most likely require bone augmentation before implant insertion (Box 25.2). When patient force factors are low to moderate, the anterior implant may be positioned in a lateral incisor site if the central site in nonideal. The three implant positions in the premaxilla will resist the additional forces created in this arch form, enhance prosthesis retention, and reduce the risk for abutment screw loosening.

The suggested locations for this treatment option are at least one central (or lateral) incisor position, bilateral canine positions,

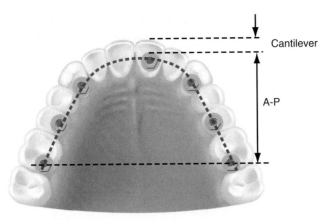

• **Fig. 25.8** Fixed Treatment Plan 2: In an ovoid dentate arch form, three implants should be planned in the premaxilla: one in each canine position and one additional implant. In addition, at least four posterior implants should be splinted to form an arch. *A-P*, Anteroposterior distance.

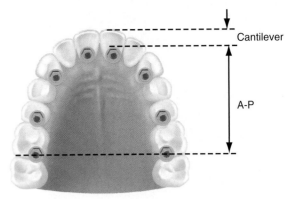

• **Fig. 25.9** Fixed Treatment Plan 3: In a tapered arch form the anterior cantilever is greater and should be supported by implants in the premaxilla. At least four posterior implants should be added to restore the completely edentulous arch. *A-P*, Anteroposterior distance.

> • **BOX 25.2** | **Maxillary Fixed Prosthesis (FP-1,2,or 3) Treatment Plan 2**

Indications: Ovoid arch form
Implants: 7
Positions (bilateral):
 Central incisor (unilateral)
 Canine
 Second bicuspid
 First molar

---

bilateral second premolar sites, and the bilateral distal half of the maxillary first molar sites. The seven implants should be splinted together to function as an arch. These implant positions create sufficient space between each implant to allow for greater implant diameters (i.e., when required for force or bone density factors). Implants should ideally be at least 3 mm apart after placement.

Maxillary Fixed Prosthesis Treatment Option 3

The prosthesis treatment planned in a tapered dental arch form places the greatest forces on the anterior implants, especially during mandibular excursions when the residual bone is an ovoid or square ridge form. The anterior teeth create a significant facial cantilever from the canine position, and anterior biting forces often lead to a shear type of forces. As such, four implants should be considered to replace the six anterior teeth (Figs. 25.9 and 25.10).

The bilateral canine and central incisor positions represent the best option. These positions are preferred when other force factors are greater, such as crown height, parafunction, and masticatory muscular dynamics. The worst-case scenario is a patient who requires restoration of a dental tapered arch form with a square residual ridge form. Not only are four implants then ideally required to compensate for the cantilevered tooth position, but these implants should be connected to additional posterior implants, which can extend to the second molar sites. Therefore in treatment plan 3, when force factors are moderate or the dental arch form is tapered, the minimum implant number should increase to eight implants (Box 25.3). When force factors are greater than usual or bone density is poorer, additional implants may be used in any of the arch forms. In the square and ovoid arch form, at least one additional implant is positioned in the premaxilla. For patients with higher force factors

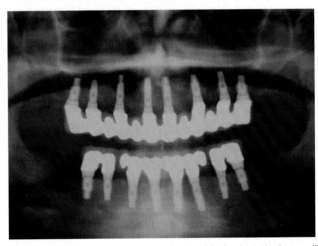

• **Fig. 25.10** Tapered arch form treated with eight implants in the maxilla and splinted prosthesis.

> • **BOX 25.3** | **Maxillary Fixed Prosthesis (FP-1,2,or 3) Treatment Plan 3**

Indications: Tapered arch form
Implants: 8
Positions (bilateral):
 Central incisor
 Canine
 Second bicuspid
 First molar

---

or poor bone density, two additional implants are planned in the distal half of the second molar position to improve the arch form. This will result in an increased A-P distance compared with the first molar site, which will compensate for the increased force factors or poor bone density (Fig. 25.11). The implant number and position guidelines also may counter the effect of an incisal cantilever off the residual anterior bone for an esthetic tooth position and is indicated for patients with chronic parafunction (such as bruxism).

The disadvantage of second-molar implants for an ideal treatment plan is the additional cost of the second molar implant, possible bone grafting, and the prosthesis. In addition, many patients do not have an existing second molar in the mandibular arch. However, the reason for this implant position is for force transfer, not necessarily esthetics or functional purposes.

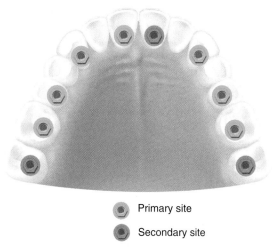

Primary site

Secondary site

• **Fig. 25.11** The ideal seven-implant positioning for a maxillary edentulous arch includes at least one central incisor position, bilateral canine positions, bilateral second premolar sites, and bilateral sites in the distal half of the first molars. In case of heavy stress factors, an additional anterior implant and bilateral second molar positions (to increase the anteroposterior distance) may be of benefit.

• BOX 25.4 Maxillary Fixed Prosthesis (FP-1,2,or 3) Treatment Plan 4

Indications:
    Shorter treatment time required
    Contraindication to bone grafting
    Low force factors
Implants: 4
Positions (bilateral):
    Anterior
    Posterior (angled at 30–45 degrees), anterior to sinus

Maxillary Fixed Treatment Option 4: All-on-Four

In implant dentistry today a shift in treatment options has become popular to minimize treatment time, treatment costs, and decrease patient morbidity. The all-on-four treatment concept has been reported by Maló et al.[28] in many reports in an attempt to address these objectives in implant dentistry today. In general the all-on-four technique includes placing four implants in the maxillary arch, with two axially placed implants in the anterior and two posterior implants positioned angulated at 30 to 45 degrees.[28] Even though the placement of four implants is far less than what has been accepted for years (i.e., usually six to eight implants required for a fixed prosthesis in the maxilla) in implant dentistry, high success rates of 93% to 98% have been shown[29-32] (Box 25.4).

Maló et al.[28] state that the all-on-four technique in the maxilla uses a more favorable bone density in the anterior, along with longer implants in the posterior that are angulated, which increases the A-P spread. Zampelis et al.[33] concluded in a finite element analysis model that the tilted posterior implants have a biomechanical advantage in comparison with cantilevering axial placed implants. The all-on-four technique is most commonly used for immediate load situations (see Chapter 33).

In conclusion, the all-on-four technique has shown very promising results in the literature. However, careful patient selection, along with an experienced surgical and prosthetic clinician with an increased skill set, is essential for successful treatment results. Because of the pneumatization of the maxillary sinuses and the requirement of bone grafting in many cases, the all-on-four technique allows for the avoidance of the sinus anatomy by tilting the implants, which ultimately increases the A-P spread (Fig. 25.12).

Removable Maxillary Treatment Plans

The primary advantage of a maxillary Implant Overdenture (IOD) compared with a fixed prosthesis is the ability to provide a flange for maxillary lip support and the reduced fee compared with a fixed restoration. As a consequence, before the selection of a specific prosthesis type and to facilitate the diagnosis, the labial flange above the maxillary teeth of the existing denture (or wax try-in of a new prosthesis) may be removed and the facial appearance of the maxillary lip without labial support assessed.

Maxillary IOD complications, such as attachment wear and prosthesis or component fracture, are more frequent than with a fixed restoration and primarily occur as a result of inadequate bulk of acrylic and minimal strength of the framework, compared with a fixed restoration (Table 25.2).

Fewer reports have been published for maxillary IOD compared with the mandible. Most of these reports discuss RP-5 restorations with posterior soft tissue support and anterior implant retention. According to Goodacre et al.,[34] the restoration with the highest implant failure rate is a maxillary overdenture (19% failure rate). In 1994 Palmqvist et al.[35] reported similar poor results in a 5-year prospective, multicenter study on 30 maxillae and 103 mandibles. Jemt and Lekholm[36] reported that the survival rate of mandibular implants was 94.5% versus 100% for mandibular prostheses. In the maxillae the implant survival rate was 72.4%, and the prosthesis survival rate was 77.9%. The authors suggested that the treatment outcome may be predicted by bone volume and quantity. A prospective study by Johns et al.[11] reported on maxillary IODs at 1, 3, and 5 years.[9,37] Sixteen patients were followed throughout the whole study with a cumulative success rate of 78% for prostheses and 72% for implants. A pooled implant survival rate of maxillary removable designs was reported at 76.6% at 5 years.[11,37-39]

Alternatively, Misch followed 75 maxillary IODs (RP-4) and 615 implants for 10 years with 97% implant survival rate and 100% prosthesis survival rate.[40] The primary differences in these treatment modalities have been a completely implant-supported, retained, and stabilized maxillary IOD (RP-4); a greater implant number; and key implant positions following the guidelines of treatment planning based on basic biomechanical concepts to reduce failure and decrease risks.

Maxillary Removable Implant Overdenture Treatment Options

Only two treatment options are available for maxillary IODs, whereas five treatment options are available for the mandibular IOD. The difference is due primarily to the biomechanical disadvantages of the maxilla compared with the mandible. As such, the two treatment options are limited to an RP-5 with four to six implants with soft tissue support, or an RP-4 restoration with six to eight implants (which is completely supported, retained, and stabilized by implants). The crown height space is critical for maxillary overdentures, and more often a lack of space may compromise tooth position compared with the mandibular situation. The maxillary anterior crown height space requirement is greater than the posterior dimension. A minimum of 14 mm of anterior crown height space and 12-14 mm of posterior space is required for IOD (i.e., bar-retained) because of the greater anterior teeth coronal dimensions and specific locations (Fig. 25.13).

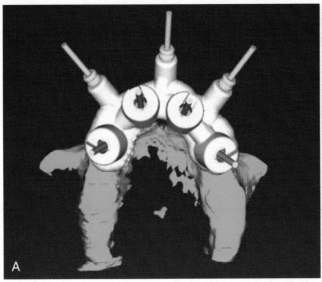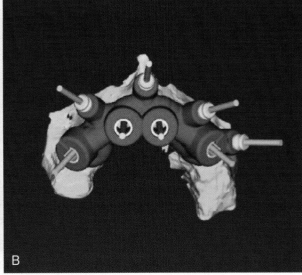

• **Fig. 25.12** All-on-Four Protocol. (A and B) Two implants placed axially in the anterior and two implants placed posterior, which are angulated less than 45 degrees to avoid the maxillary sinus.

TABLE 25.2

Comparison of Maxillary Prostheses

Factor	Fixed Prosthesis (FP-1,2, or 3)	Removable Prosthesis (RP-4)	Removable Prosthesis (RP-5)
Psycho-logical	+++	++	+
Material	Zirconia, Porcelain Fused Metal Acrylic Hybrid	Titanium or Gold Bar Acrylic Prosthesis	Titanium / Gold Bar or Independent Attachments Acrylic Prosthesis
Lip Support	+	+++	+++
Esthetics	Zirconia or Porcelain	Acrylic	Acrylic
	++	++	++
Phonetics	+++	++	+
Function	+++	++	+
Long Term Success	+++	++	+
Biting Force	+++	++	+
Hygiene	+	++	++

+++, Best; ++, Better; +, Good.

Option 1: Removable Maxillary RP-4 Implant Overdenture

The first option for a maxillary IOD is an RP-4 prosthesis with six to eight implants, which is rigid during function (i.e., primary support is by implants, no soft tissue support) (Box 25.5). This option is the preferred IOD design because it maintains greater bone volume and provides improved retention and confidence to the patient compared with a denture or RP-5 prosthesis. Because the palate is removed from this prosthesis (i.e., horseshoe-shaped),

soft tissue support is lost, thereby requiring increased number of implants. The cost of treatment is similar to a fixed prosthesis because of the increased number of implants required.

Unfortunately, many clinicians believe that the RP-4 overdenture requires fewer implants and less attention to the biomechanics of occlusal load, just because the prosthesis is removable. In the author's opinion, this is a primary reason for such a high implant failure rate in maxillary IODs. Combined factors such as reduced cost, patient fear of bone grafting, and lack of advanced training of the doctor are often the determining factors motivating the choice for a maxillary IOD.

Treatment planning for RP-4 maxillary overdentures is similar to a fixed prosthesis, because the IOD is fixed during function. Two of the key implant positions for the RP-4 maxillary IOD are in the bilateral canines and distal half of the first molar positions. These implant positions usually require sinus augmentation in the molar position. Additional posterior implants are located bilaterally in the premolar position, preferably the second premolar site. In addition, at least one anterior implant between the canines often is required. Six implants is the minimum number for an RP-4 treatment option. When force factors are greater, the next most important sites are the second molar positions (bilaterally) to increase the A-P spread and improve the biomechanics of the system. The occlusal scheme for the RP-4 prosthesis is similar to a fixed prosthesis: mutually protected occlusion (unless opposing a mandibular complete denture) (Fig. 25.14).

Option 2: Removable Maxillary RP-5 Implant Overdenture

The second treatment option for the maxillary arch is the RP-5 prosthesis (Box 25.6). A maxillary conventional complete denture usually has good retention, support, and stability. Although an RP-5 maxillary IOD is superior to a complete denture, many patients do not see much of a difference. The major advantages of an RP-5 maxillary IOD are the maintenance of the anterior bone and it being a less expensive treatment option in comparison with an RP-4 or fixed prosthesis. The treatment is far less expensive because bilateral sinus grafts are not required and molar implants are not indicated. Therefore this treatment plan is often used as a transition to an RP-4 or FP-3 prosthesis when financial considerations of the patient require a staged treatment over several years.

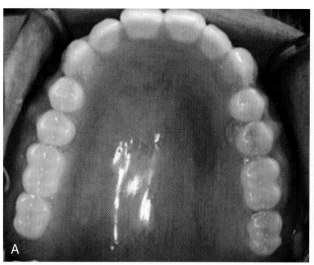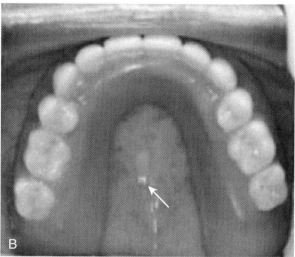

• **Fig. 25.13** Maxillary Overdentures. (A) RP-5: full palatal coverage for which the soft tissue provides primary support and the implants are for secondary support. (B) RP-4: horseshoe-shaped prosthesis that receives its primary support from the implants and no support from the soft tissue. Note the lack of palatal support (primary stress bearing area).

• BOX 25.5 Removable Maxillary Prosthesis Treatment Plan 1 (RP-4)

Indications:
- Patients who cannot tolerate full palatal coverage
- Gag reflex
- Patients who require prosthesis with no movement

Prosthesis design: bar-supported horseshoe shape prosthesis

Advantages
- Less palatal coverage (horseshoe shape)
- Increased speech, taste
- No soft tissue support, completely implant supported
- Hygiene easier than fixed

Disadvantages
- Palate removed: lack of acrylic bulk > fracture
- Cost: more implants
- Posterior bone needed: sinus grafts

Positions (Based on Dental Arch Form)
- **Square:** 6 implants: bilateral canine, bicuspids, and first molar
- **Ovoid:** 7 implants: bilateral canines, bicuspids, and first molars
- **Tapering:** 8 implants: bilateral canines, bicuspids, first molars, and incisor

---

The first treatment option for a completely edentulous maxilla uses four to six implants supporting an RP-5 prosthesis, of which at least three are positioned in the premaxilla. Based on the poor success rates reported in the literature, specific biomechanical requirements, and poor bone quality, the fewest number of implants for an RP-5 maxillary overdenture should be four, with a wide A-P spread. The key implants are positioned in the bilateral canine regions and at least one central or lateral incisor position. In some cases, implant placement in the central incisor region may reduce the amount of available space for the prosthesis. Additional secondary implants may be placed in the first or second premolar region. In such cases, because of the reduced A-P spread and the lateral incisor in the anterior-most implant site, the second premolar position also should be used on the contralateral side (along

with the canine) to improve the A-P spread. Six implants are often indicated for an RP-5 prosthesis when force factors are greater.

The maxillary RP-5 IOD is designed exactly as a complete denture with fully extended palate and flanges. When Locators or O-rings attachments are used to retain the prosthesis, they may be positioned more distal than a Hader clip, often immediately distal to the canine position. The prosthesis should be allowed to move slightly in the incisal region during function so that the restoration may rotate toward the posterior soft tissue around a fulcrum located in the canine or premolar position. The benefits of an RP-5 maxillary overdenture primary support from the soft tissue and secondary support from the implants. In addition, the benefit of premaxillary bone maintenance is seen because prosthesis of the implant stimulation (Figs. 25.15 and 25.16).

Summary

Maxillary IODs may be as predictable as mandibular overdentures when biomechanical considerations specific to the maxilla are incorporated in the treatment plan. In general this requires implants in greater numbers and a greater awareness of prosthetic principles.

Only two maxillary IOD treatment options are available. The fewest number of implants for this restoration is four to six implants to support an RP-5 prosthesis. A rigid IOD (RP-4) most often requires the placement of seven or more implants. In other words, maxillary IODs are completely different from their mandibular counterpart. In the completely edentulous maxilla, an IOD is often the treatment of choice. Unlike in the mandible, the maxillary lip often requires additional support as a consequence of bone loss. An ideal high lip line exposes the interdental papillae between the anterior teeth. Using overdentures to replace the hard and soft tissue is easier than attempting to do this with bone and soft tissue or zirconia prostheses.

A completely implant supported IOD (RP-4) requires the same number and position of implants as a fixed restoration. Thus sinus grafts and anterior implants usually are indicated, regardless of whether the prosthesis is fixed or removable. A common complication arises when four to six implants are placed, and an RP-4 palateless IOD is fabricated. Without the primary stress bearing area palatal support, the implants are often subjected to increased force factors, thus increasing complications and morbidity.

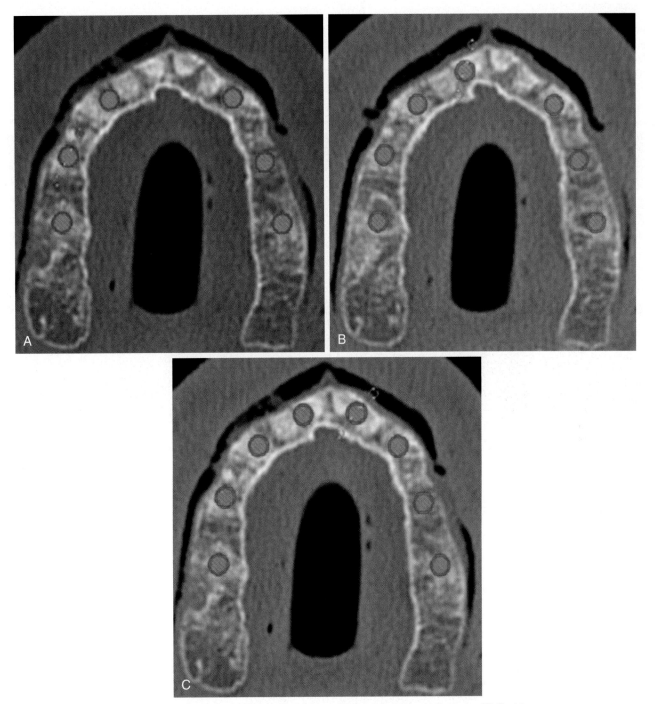

• **Fig. 25.14** RP-4 Overdenture Treatment Options. (A) Square arch—six implants. (B) Ovoid—seven implants. (C) Tapered—eight implants. An RP-4 is treatment planned similar to a maxillary fixed prosthesis.

• BOX 25.6 Removable Maxillary Prosthesis Treatment Plan 1 (RP-5)

Indications:
- Shorter treatment time required
- Contraindication to bone grafting

Prosthesis design: attachments only—complete palatal coverage (primary support from the soft tissue)

Advantages
- Increased retention and stability in comparison to a denture
- Maintain premaxilla bone
- Reduced fee (~RP-4)

Disadvantages
- Requires full palate (~soft tissue primary support)
- Must have adequate bone in anterior and bicuspid area
- Need adequate crown height space

Positions (Based on Dental Arch Form)
- **Square:** 4 implants: bilateral canine, bicuspids and/or incisor
- **Ovoid:** 5 implants: bilateral canine, bilateral bicuspid, and incisor
- **Tapering:** 6 implants: bilateral canines, incisors, and bicuspids

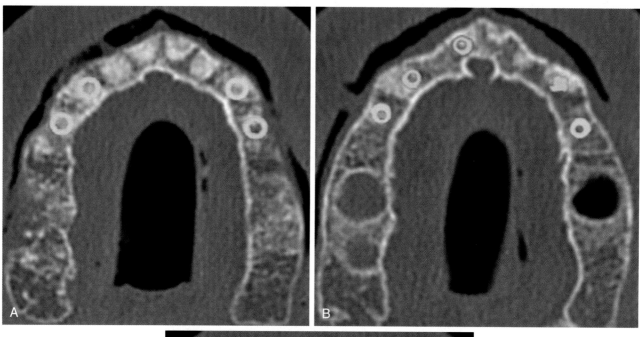

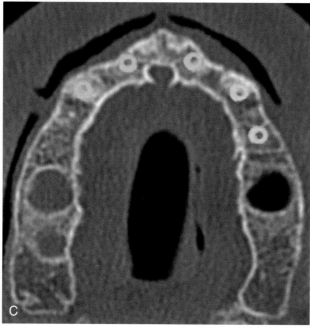

• **Fig. 25.15** RP-5 Treatment Options. (A) Four implants in canine and first premolar positions. (B) Five implants in canine, first premolars, and in the central/lateral incisor position. (C) Five implants in canines, one in premolar, and central/lateral incisors positions. Caution should be exercised to not remove palatal coverage from an RP-5 prosthesis.

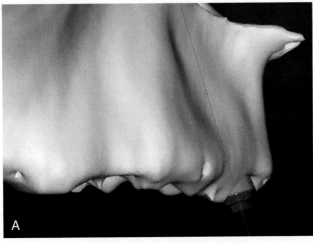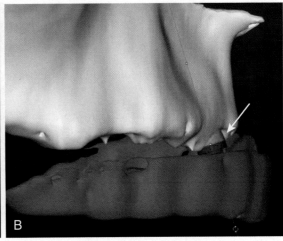

• **Fig. 25.16** Central Incisor Implant Placement. (A) In tapered arch forms, placement of an implant in the central incisor region may impinge on the prosthesis. (B) Implant positioning that results in inadequate space for a prosthesis. Therefore, implants may be required to be positioned in the central-lateral or lateral position to allow for increased prosthetic room.

References

1. Tjan AH, Miller GD, The JG. Some aesthetic factors in a smile. *J Prosthet Dent.* 1984;51:24–28.
2. Misch CE. *Premaxilla Implant Considerations: Surgery and Fixed Prosthodontics. Contemporary Implant Dentistry.* St. Louis, MO: Mosby Year Book; 1993:427–431.
3. Block Michael S. Maxillary fixed prosthesis design based on the preoperative physical examination. *J Oral Maxillofac. Surg.* 2015;73(5):851–860.
4. Lee CK, Agar JR. Surgical and prosthetic planning for a two-implant-retained mandibular overdenture: a clinical report. *J Prosthet Dent.* 2006;95:102–105.
5. Trakas Theodoros, et al. Attachment systems for implant retained overdentures: a literature review. *Implant Dentistry.* 2006;15(1):24–34.
6. Jivraj S, Chee W, Corrado P. Treatment planning of the edentulous maxilla. *Br Dent J.* 2006;201:5.
7. Naert I, DeClercq M, Theuniers G, et al. Overdentures supported by osseointegrated fixtures for the edentulous mandible. A 2.5 year report. *Int J Oral Maxillofac Impl.* 1988;3:191–196.
8. Jemt T. Fixed implant–supported prostheses in the edentulous maxilla. A five-year follow-up report." *Clin Oral Implants Res.* 1994;5(3):142–147.
9. Hutton JE, Heath MR, Chai JY, et al. Factors related to success and failure rates at 3-year follow-up in a multicenter study of overdentures supported by Brånemark implants. *Int J Oral Maxillofac Implants.* 1995;10:33–42.
10. Enquist B, Bergendal T, Kallus T. A retrospective multicenter evaluation of osseointegrated implants supporting overdentures. *Int J Oral Maxillofac Implants.* 1988;3:129–134.
11. Johns RB, Jemt T, Heath MR, et al. A multicenter study of overdentures supported by Brånemark implants. *Int J Oral Maxillofac Implants.* 1992;7:513–522.
12. Bergendal T, Enquist B. Implant-suppported overdentures: a longitudinal prospective study. *Int J Oral Maxillofac Implants.* 1998;13:253–262.
13. Hooghe M, Naert I. Implant supported overdentures—The Leuven experience. *J Dent.* 1997;25(1):25–32.
14. Smedberg JI, Nilner K, Frykholm A. A six-year follow-up study of maxillary overdentures on osseointegrated implants. *Eur J Prosthodont Restor Dent.* 1999;7:51–56.
15. Kiener P, Oetterli M, Mericske E, Mericske-Stern R. Effectiveness of maxillary overdentures supported by implants: maintenance and prosthetic complications. *I J Prosthodont.* 2001;14:133–140.

16. Mericske-Stern R, Oetterli M, Kiener P, Mericske E. A follow-up study of maxillary implants supporting an overdenture: clinical and radiographic results. *Int J Oral Maxillofac Implants.* 2002;17:678–686.
17. Narhi TO, Hevinga M, Voorsmit RA, Kalk W. Maxillary overdentures retained by splinted and unsplinted implants: a retrospective study. *Int J Oral Maxillofac Implants.* 2001;16:259–266.
18. Widbom C, Soderfeldt B, Kronstrom M. A retrospective evaluation of treatments with implant-supported maxillary overdentures. *Clin Implant Dent Relat Res.* 2005;7:166–172.
19. Shannon IL, Terry JM, Nakamoto RY. Palatal coverage and parotid flow rate. *J Prosthet Dent.* 1970;24:601–607.
20. Strain JC. The influence of completed dentures upon taste perception. *J Prosthet Dent.* 1952;2:60–67.
21. Giddon DB, Dreisbach ME, Pfaffman C, Manley RS. Relative abilities of natural and artificial dentition patients for judging the sweetness of solid foods. *J Prosthet Dent.* 1954;4:263–268.
22. Watson RM, Jemt T, Chai J, et al. Prosthodontic treatment, patient response and the need for maintenance of complete implant-supported overdentures: an appraisal of 5 years of prospective study. *Int J Prosthodont.* 1997;10:345–354.
23. Ekfeldt A, Johansson LA, Isaksson S. Implant-supported overdenture therapy: a retrospective study. *Int J Prostho- dont.* 1997;10:366–374.
24. Bryant SR, MacDonald-Jankowski D, Kwonsik K. Does the type of implant prosthesis affect outcomes for the completely edentulous arch? *Int J Oral Maxillofac Implants.* 2007;22:117–139.
25. Ivanoff CH, Grondahl K, Bergstrom C, et al. Influence of bicortical or monocortical anchorage on maxillary implant stability: a 15-year retrospective study of Brånemark system implants. *Int J Oral Maxillofac Implants.* 2000;15:103–110.
26. Jemt T, Bergendal B, Arvidson K, et al. Implant-supported welded titanium frameworks in the edentulous maxilla: a 5-year prospective multicenter study. *Int J Prosthodont.* 2002;15:544–548.
27. Engfors I, Ortorp A, Jemt T. Fixed implant-supported prostheses in elderly patients: a 5-year retrospective study of 133 edentulous patients older than 79 years. *Clin Implant Dent Relat Res.* 2004;6:190–198.
28. Maló Paulo, Rangert Bo, Dvärsäter Lisbeth. Immediate function of Brånemark implants in the esthetic zone: a retrospective clinical study with 6 months to 4 years of follow-up. *Clin Implant Dent Relat Res.* 2000;2(3):138–146.
29. Fortin Y, Sullivan RM, Rangert BR. The Marius implant bridge: surgical and prosthetic rehabilitation for the completely edentulous upper jaw with moderate to severe resorption: a 5-year retrospective clinical study. *Clin Implant Dent Relat Res.* 2002;4:69–77.

30. Rocci A, Martignoni M, Gottlow J. Immediate loading in the maxilla using flapless surgery, implants placed in predetermined positions, and prefabricated provisional restorations. A restrospective 3-year clinical study. *Clin Implant Dent Relat Res.* 2003;5:S29–S36.

31. Olsson M, Urde G, Andersen E, Sennerby L. Early loading of maxillary fixed cross-arch dental prostheses supported by six or eight oxidized titanium implants: results after 1 year of loading, case series. *Clin Implant Dent Relat Res.* 2003;5:S81–S87.

32. Fischer K, Stenberg T. Three-year data from a randomized, controlled study of early loading of single-stage dental implants supporting maxillary full-arch prostheses. *Int J Oral Maxillofac Implants.* 2006;21:245–252.

33. Zampelis A, Rangert B, Heijl L. Tilting of splinted implants for improved prosthodontic support: a two-dimensional finite element analysis. *J Prosthet Dent.* 2007;97:S35–S43.

34. Goodacre CJ, Bernal G, Rungcharassaeng K, et al. Clinical complications with implants and implant prostheses. *J Prosthet Dent.* 2003;90:121–132.

35. Palmqvist S, Sondell K, Swartz B. Implant-supported maxillary overdentures: outcome in planned and emergency cases. *Int J Oral Maxillofac Implants.* 1994;9:184–190.

36. Jemt T, Lekholm U. Implant treatment in edentulous maxillae: a 5-year follow-up report on patients with different degrees of jaw resorption. *Int J Oral Maxillofac Implants.* 1995;10:303–311.

37. Jemt T, Chai J, Harnett J, et al. A 5-year prospective multi-center follow-up report on overdentures supported on osseointegrated implants. *Int J Oral Maxillofac Implants.* 1996;11:291–298.

38. Chan MF, Narhito, de Bart C, et al. Treatment of the atrophic edentulous maxilla in the implant supported overdentures: a review of the literature. *Int J Prosthodont.* 1998;11:7–15.

39. Cox JF, Zarb GA. The longitudinal clinical efficacy of osseointegrated dental implants: a 3-year report. *Int J Oral Maxillofac Implants.* 1987;2:91–100.

40. Misch CE. *Dental Implant Prosthetics-E-Book.* St. Louis, MO. Elsevier. 2004.

PART VI

Implant Surgery

26
Basic Surgical Techniques and Armamentarium

CHRISTOPHER R. RESNIK AND RANDOLPH R. RESNIK

Basic dental surgical methods were practiced in the early Roman times when diseased gingival tissues were excised with instruments and no local anesthetic. Today, many of the principles of modern-day surgical procedures are based on the teachings of William Stewart Halsted, MD, the "Father of Modern-Day Surgery." Halsted, an American surgeon and cofounder of Johns Hopkins Hospital, developed surgical principles in the late 19th century that are still universally used today. He emphasized a strict aseptic technique and tissue-handling principles to obtain predictable soft tissue surgical success rates. He determined that the gentle handling of lacerated tissues would aid healing by causing less damage to the blood and nerve supply in the operative field. With his work, the "Tenets of Halsted" resulted that have helped to guide the principles of surgery in all medical disciplines[1] (Box 26.1).

Dental implant surgery encompasses a broad range of procedures involving the hard and soft tissues of the oral cavity. The procedures vary from simple exodontia to technically challenging full-mouth, bone augmentation and implant procedures. The implant clinician must have a strong foundation for basic surgical principles so that potential complications are avoided. For most implant procedures, specific instruments and armamentarium, as well as protocols, have been developed to facilitate the procedures. With these basic principles in mind, surgical protocols and biologic principles have been developed in the field of oral implantology. Over the years the surgical management of the dental implant patient has led to a more evidence-based practice and the introduction of improved techniques and instrumentation. Therefore this chapter will emphasize basic surgical principles that should ideally be used during implant-related procedures. In addition, a comprehensive review of the surgical armamentarium will be discussed.

Flap Design

Surgical flaps are made to gain access to a surgical area or to relocate tissue from one area to another. Over the years the mucogingival flap design used in oral implantology has changed dramatically. The use of technology has allowed for more accurate and ideal placement of implants and bone grafts, along with better techniques for handling tissue and preserving blood supply. In the early years of oral implantology, most surgeries were completed with an aggressive full reflection of the surgical area including full releasing incisions that traumatized the tissue and compromised the blood supply. Following the original Brånemark protocol, implants were buried below the tissue and left to integrate for 4 to 6 months before a second surgery to uncover and place a healing abutment (stage 2 technique). In the 1990s a more conservative, one-stage surgery technique became popular that involved placement of a healing abutment at the time of implant placement. This procedure showed remarkable results, with decreased morbidity. Then in the 2000s immediate implant placement became popular, and advancements in guided surgery allowed the advent of "flapless" surgery, which resulted in much less trauma. With advanced technology, clinicians are now able to 3D print surgical guides in their office that are based on cone beam computed tomographic imaging for ideal implant placement and accurate anatomy, which has led to more accuracy with flapless techniques. However, flapless surgery is not indicated in all cases and certainly may lead to higher morbidity. Therefore it is imperative that the implant surgeon understand the basic principles of flap design.

The type of flap used in surgery varies dramatically, with much of the design criteria based on the purpose and anatomic area of the surgical site. Flap designs may be classified by the type of tissue (full versus partial thickness) and the number and type of incisions used to create them (envelope, papilla sparing, triangular, trapezoidal, vestibular, etc.).

When developing the ideal flap design, a few basic principles pertain to all flaps used in implant dentistry.

Maintain Blood Supply

The primary goal of any flap design is to retain and maximize the native blood supply to continuously nourish the

• BOX 26.1   Tenets of Halsted

1. The gentle handling of tissues
2. An aseptic technique
3. Sharp anatomic dissection of tissues
4. Careful hemostasis, using fine, nonirritating suture material in minimal amounts
5. The obliteration of dead space in the wound
6. The avoidance of tension
7. The importance of trauma to the surgical site postoperatively

602

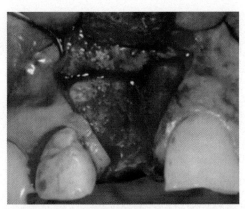

● **Fig. 26.1** Ideal flap design with broad base incision that preserves the blood supply. Note how the width of the incision base is much greater than the ridge.

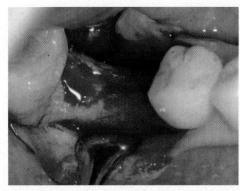

● **Fig. 26.2** Flap design provides sufficient access to visualize the entire surgical field. Too small of a flap will lead to stretching of the tissue and an increase in inflammation.

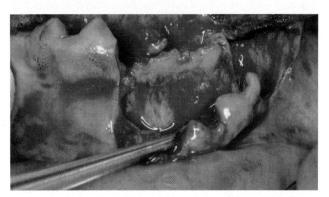

● **Fig. 26.3** Full-thickness reflection with 2–4 Molt instrument.

surrounding tissue and bone.[2] If the blood supply is disrupted to the wound margin, in theory the health of the tissue may be compromised, which may lead to poor wound healing. It has been shown that three essential factors are required to maintain and regenerate soft tissue quality with implant-related procedures: (1) preservation of the blood supply to the adjacent papilla, (2) preservation of the bone on the adjacent teeth, and (3) minimal scar tissue formation during surgery.[3] When soft tissue becomes rigid and nonflexible as a result of traumatic surgical manipulation or previous surgical interventions, it may not allow for ideal adaptation or flexibility around the dental implant or prosthesis.[4]

Most importantly in the esthetic zone, it is imperative to maintain the papilla. The vascularity of the papilla tissue is supplied by various vascular anastomoses that cross the alveolar ridge. If repeated incisions and trauma to the vascular supply occur, scar tissue formation will result as fibroblasts become prematurely activated to form excess fibrotic tissue. This type of tissue is usually difficult to manipulate and may lead to recession and esthetic complications. An exaggerated level of erythema, edema, and discomfort may be indicative of compromised blood supply.[5]

The base of the flap is important in maintaining the blood supply. Ideally the flap should always be broader than the free margin (i.e., ridge area) to preserve the blood supply. All areas of the flap must have a source of uninterrupted vasculature to prevent ischemic necrosis of the flap.[6] Ideally flaps should have sides that converge, moving from the base to the apex (ridge). The length of the flap should generally not exceed twice the width of the base. The base of the flap should not have significant pressure or be excessively stretched or twisted, which may compromise the blood supply (Fig. 26.1).

Flap Design to Provide Access

The flap design must provide sufficient access to provide necessary visualization of the entire surgical area. Adequate access must also exist for the insertion of instruments required to perform the surgery and to reflect the tissue to maintain access. The flap must be held out of the operative field by a retractor that ideally would rest on intact bone without tension. Excess tension most likely will result in tissue trauma and an increase in swelling.[7] If increased edema is present, the patient may experience greater discomfort, and there is a greater possibility of incision line opening or compromised wound healing (Fig. 26.2).

Full-Thickness Reflection

The flap should be a full-thickness mucoperiosteal flap that will include the surface mucosa, submucosa, and periosteum. Because implant surgery usually requires access to the underlying alveolar bone, all tissue must be sufficiently reflected. In addition, full-thickness flaps are ideal because the periosteum is the primary tissue responsible for the bone healing process, and replacement of the periosteum in its original position hastens that healing process. In addition, torn, split, and macerated tissue heals much slower than a cleanly reflected full-thickness flap, thereby delaying the healing process.[8]

A sharp scalpel should be used to score the bone to obtain a full-thickness reflection, thus ensuring complete penetration through the tissue layers. When reflecting the tissue, the underlying bone should be "scraped," thus minimizing the possibility of a partial-thickness flap. Care must be taken when reflecting the tissue to separate the tissue away from the bone. When using a periosteal elevator (e.g., 2–4 Molt), the tip edge should always rest on the bone to prevent tearing through of the tissue flap (Fig. 26.3).

Minimize Trauma to Tissue

Meticulous handling is required to minimize trauma to the soft tissue. Proper use of appropriate tissue forceps, avoidance of excessive suctioning by the assistant, and "tieback" sutures all contribute to improved flap management. Nonlocking tissue pickups (e.g., Adson forceps) are commonly used to hold soft tissues in place when retracting tissue or during the suturing process. Various designs of tissue forceps exist, most commonly having smooth tips, cross-hatched tips, or serrated teeth (often called *mouse's teeth*). Serrated teeth forceps used on tissues will result in more tissue damage because they may tear the tissue, whereas smooth surface forceps tend to be much gentler to the tissue.

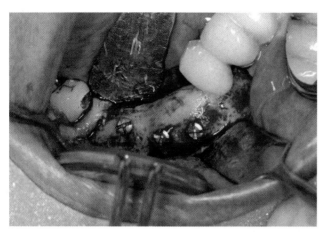

• **Fig. 26.4** Tissue retractors should ideally be positioned on bone to provide ideal access to the surgical field and minimize trauma to the tissue and vital structures.

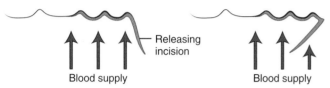

• **Fig. 26.5** Vertical release incisions are required to provide access to the surgical field and prevent excess pressure on tissue flaps. The correct release incision is on the left which maintains the blood supply. The incorrect flap design is illustrated on the right as the blood supply is cut off because of the location of the release incision.

Tissue retractors should be selected and placed in a position to prevent undue pressure on the flap. Maintaining the retractors on bone and not on the tissue will minimize trauma to the tissue. Excessive pressure and tension on the tissue flap will impair blood circulation, alter the physiologic healing of the surgical wound, and predispose the wound to bacterial colonization, which may lead to incision line opening (Fig. 26.4).[9]

Vertical Release Incisions

Vertical release incisions may be used to maintain the blood supply and decrease the tension to the flap. Usually the primary blood supply is to the facial flap, which is from the unkeratinized mobile mucosa. Vertical release incisions are often made to the height of the mucogingival junction, and flared 45 degrees to allow for spreading of the tissue and maintenance of the blood supply.[10] Vertical release incisions should not be made over bony prominences (e.g., canine eminence) because this will increase tension on the incision line and may increase the possibility of incision line opening. In addition, it is often difficult to suture over these areas because the tissue tends to be very thin (Fig. 26.5).

Maintain Flap Margins Over Bone

The soft tissue flap design should also have the margins of the wound over host bone whenever possible. This is especially important when approximating tissue over bone grafts or barrier membranes. The host bone provides growth factors to the margins and allows the periosteum to regenerate faster to the site.[11] The margins distal to the elevated flap should exhibit minimal reflection. The palatal flap and the facial tissues distal to the reflected flap usually are not elevated from the palatal bone (i.e., unless augmentation is required) because the blood supply to the incision line

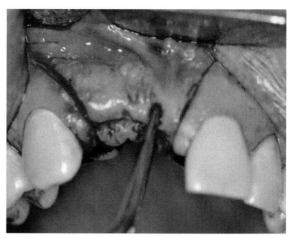

• **Fig. 26.6** Flap with excess tension increases possibility of incision line opening.

will be compromised. In some cases the soft tissue reflection distal to the surgery site may be split thickness to maintain periosteum on the bone around the incision line. This will improve the early vascularization to the incision line and adhesion of the margins to reduce retraction during initial healing.

Prevent Desiccation of Tissue

The tissues should be maintained in a moist environment without prolonged periods of desiccation.[12] If excessive drying of the tissues occurs, there is less likelihood that complete wound closure will occur. If the tissue margins become desiccated, periodic irrigations with sterile saline (0.9% sodium chloride) or saline-moistened gauze may be used.

Flap Mobility

The passivity of the flap is paramount for the successful wound healing of the soft tissues. When sutures are positioned too tight to overcome the residual tension of the flap, they may alter the blood supply, thereby reducing the vessel patency and impairing vascularization.[13] Excessive flap tension is the most frequent causative factor leading to incision line opening.[14] This is best prevented by appropriate incision and flap design, the use of periosteal releasing incisions (PRIs), and blunt dissection ("tissue stretching").

Past techniques to expand tissue primarily used a more apical tissue reflection and horizontal scoring of the periosteum parallel to the primary incision. Historically the vestibular approach by Brånemark allowed for optimal visualization of anatomic landmarks, suturing remote from the surgical area, complete tissue coverage, as well as predictable primary closure and healing.[15] The postoperative disadvantages of this approach include distortion of the vestibule and other anatomic landmarks, edema, difficult suture removal, and cumulative patient discomfort.[16]

Langer and Langer[17] documented the use of overlapping partial-thickness flaps. This approach results in extension of the coronal aspect of the buccal or palatal flap, allowing primary intention closure around the site in an overlapping manner. This is usually effective for primary closure when less than 5-mm advancement of the flap is necessary (Fig. 26.6).

A submucosal space technique developed by Misch[18] in the early 1980s is an effective method to expand tissue over larger grafts (greater than 15 Å ~10 mm in height and width) (Box 26.2).

The utility of periosteal incision for gaining flap release was studied by Park.[19] He found flaps could be advanced up to 171.3% (more than 1½ longer than its original length) by two vertical incisions and a PRI under a minimal tension of 5 g, whereas one or two vertical incisions without PRI could advance the flap only 113.4% and 124.2%, respectively. These results suggested that PRI can be predictably used to attain tension-free primary closure under a minimal pulling tension of flaps (Fig. 26.7). A sharp scalpel blade at a 45 degree angle or Metzenbamm scissors are used to score the periosteum to create greater flap extension. This will allow tension-free primary closure.

• BOX 26.2 Submucosal Space Technique

Procedure

1. A full-thickness facial flap first is elevated off the facial bone approximately 5 mm above the height of the vestibule.
2. One incision with a scalpel, 1 to 2 mm deep, is made through the periosteum, parallel to the crestal incision and 3 to 5 mm above the vestibular height of the mucoperiosteum. This shallow incision is made the full length of the facial flap and may even extend above and beyond the vertical release incisions. Care is taken to make this incision above the mucogingival junction; otherwise the flap may be perforated and delay soft tissue healing.
3. Soft tissue scissors (e.g., Metzenbaum) are used in a blunt dissection technique to create a tunnel apical to the vestibule and above the unreflected periosteum. The scissors are closed and pushed through the initial scalpel incision approximately 10 mm deep, then opened slowly.
4. This submucosal space is parallel to the surface mucosa (not deep toward the overlying bone) and above the unreflected periosteum. The thickness of the facial flap should be 3 to 5 mm because the scissors are parallel to the surface. This tunnel is expanded with the tissue scissors several millimeters above and distal to the vertical relief incisions.
5. The submucosal space is developed and the flap is advanced the distance of the "tunnel" and draped over the graft to approximate the tissue for primary closure without tension. Ideally the facial flap should be able to advance over the graft and past the lingual flap margin by more than 5 mm. The facial flap may then be returned to the lingual flap margin and sutured. This soft tissue procedure is performed before preparing the host region for any type of bone grafting or augmentation around an implant.

Types of Flaps

Flapless

Flapless implant surgery has become popular because of the associated decreased pain and morbidity. In the flapless technique a tissue punch is used to remove the gingival tissue over the osteotomy site. Mainly this technique has been advocated because of the preservation of the blood flow to the papilla and decreased postoperative pain. Oliver[20] has shown that flapless surgery is advantageous for preserving the crestal bone and is reduced when the gingival tissue is thick (>3 mm).[21] However, when performing flapless surgery, adequate bone quantity must be present, along with sufficient keratinized tissue. The associated disadvantage of this technique is the inability to visualize the underlying bone. Cone beam computed tomographic imaging and guided surgery have made flapless surgery more predictable; however, inherent errors still exist. In most flapless surgery cases a tissue punch is used to expose the bone. The gingival tissue will be removed in the area of the osteotomy. Care should be exercised in using a tissue punch when an inadequate amount of keratinized tissue is present. Flapless surgery has been shown to result in overheating the bone because it is often difficult to irrigate the osteotomy adequately when a flap is not raised (Fig. 26.8 and Box 26.3).[22]

Papilla Sparing

The interproximal soft tissue in sites next to adjacent natural teeth may be classified into three categories: (1) papillae have an acceptable height in the edentulous site, (2) papillae have less than acceptable height, or (3) one papilla is acceptable and the other papilla is depressed and requires elevation.[23] When the interproximal papilla has an acceptable height, "papilla-saving" incisions are made adjacent to each neighboring tooth. The vertical incisions are made on the facial aspect of the edentulous site and begin 1 mm below the mucogingival junction, within the keratinized tissue. Extending the vertical incisions beyond the mucogingival junction increases the risk for scar formation at the incision site. The full-thickness incision then approaches the crest of the edentulous site, leaving 1.0 to 1.5 mm of the interproximal papilla adjacent to each tooth. This maintains the blood supply to the papillae and will help to preserve the papillae after healing. The goal is for the facial flap to be advanced over the implant or in approximation to a permucosal extension at the conclusion of the procedure, with no voids at the

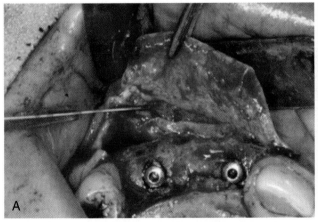
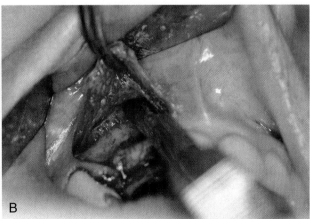

• **Fig. 26.7** Tissue tension reduction: (A, B) Severing periosteal fibers with a 15 blade parallel; to the flap.

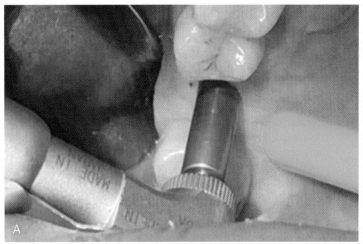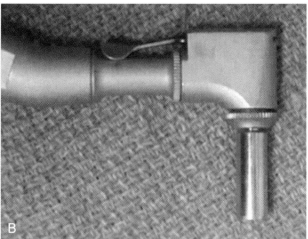

• **Fig. 26.8** Flapless Incision. (A) Tissue punch bur which corresponds to diameter of the intended implant size, (B) Slow-speed latch type handpiece used to remove tissue.

• **BOX 26.3** Flapless Surgery

Advantages
- Less invasive
- Maintains tissue vasculature
- No vertical incisions
- Less patient discomfort

Disadvantages
- Limited visibility
- Overheating bone
- Limited access to evaluate bone
- Malpositioning is more common (unless guided)

---

incision line and primary closure (Fig. 26.9). Bilateral buccal vertical releasing incisions should extend obliquely at an angle and connect to the horizontal incision. This flap is indicated in the esthetic zone, areas where you need to increase the amount of keratinized gingiva on the buccal, or in patients with a thin gingival biotype (Box 26.4).

Envelope

An envelope flap is designed with a midcrestal incision over the implant site, followed by sulcular incisions on the buccal and palatal that extend at least one tooth to the mesial and distal. A full-thickness flap is reflected using blunt dissection. One of the benefits of this flap is that scarring from vertical incisions will be avoided. On reflection, if more access is required for osseous defects or implant placement complications, a vertical releasing incision may be added to create a triangular or trapezoidal flap. The envelope flap is contraindicated in cases where extensive bone grafting is required because of the limited access and the increased risk for tension on closure (Fig. 26.10 and Box 26.5).

Triangular and Trapezoidal

The triangular and trapezoidal incisions are more aggressive incisions that are initiated over the implant site and sulcular incisions that continue horizontally to at least one adjacent tooth. Both the triangular and trapezoidal incisions involve

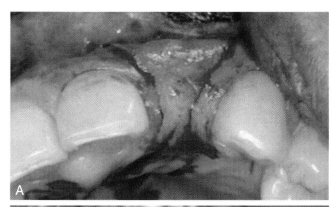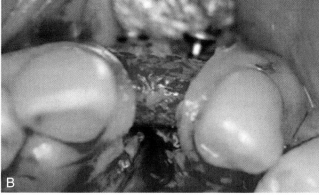

• **Fig. 26.9** Papilla-Sparing Incision. (A) Incision maintaining 1 mm of papilla tissue. (B) Reflected flap maintaining papilla tissue intact.

• **BOX 26.4** Papilla-Sparing Surgery

Advantages
- No disruption of the papillae
- Less morbidity
- Minimal disruption of vasculature

Disadvantages
- No access to additional sites
- Need additional skill set
- Minimal reflected space for implant placement
- Difficulty in bone grafting
- Possible scarring in nonkeratinized tissue

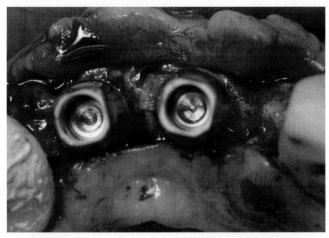

• **Fig. 26.10** Envelope Flap. Minimal flap that maintains blood supply.

• BOX 26.5   Envelope Flap Surgery

Advantages
- No vertical incisions
- Easy to suture
- Easy to modify

Disadvantages
- Limited access
- Moderate disruption of vasculature
- Increased risk for tension upon closure
- Guided bone regeneration not possible

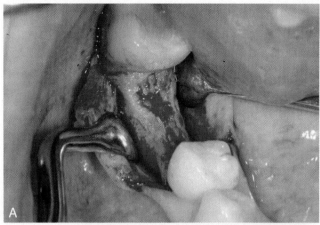

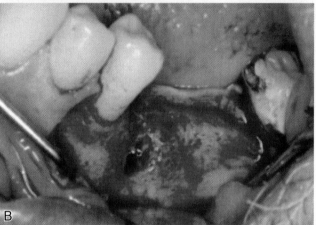

• **Fig. 26.11** Examples are larger, more aggressive flap designs: (A) triangular and (B) trapezoidal.

• BOX 26.6   Triangular/Trapezoidal Flap Surgery

Advantages
- Better visibility
- Increased possibility of tension-free closure
- Access to additional sites

Disadvantages
- Increased bone loss and recession
- Increased disruption of blood supply
- Reflection/Suturing of adjacent papilla
- Increased patient morbidity

---

a sulcular incision and vertical releasing incisions (i.e., triangular: one vertical release; trapezoidal: two vertical release incisions). A vertical releasing incision is then extended apically above the mucogingival junction. By placing the vertical releasing incision as distal as possible, scarring may be spared that may occur during healing.[24] PRIs are placed to aid in flap advancement to gain tension-free primary closure. The main advantage of these flaps is direct visibility of the bone, which allows access to bone recontouring, as well as bone grafting. These flaps are contraindicated in patients with a thin gingival biotype because of the tension placed on the flap[25] (Fig. 26.11 and Box 26.6).

Vestibular

The vestibular flap incision is a minimally invasive technique that allows preservation of the interproximal tissue and allows access for buccal ridge recontouring and soft tissue grafting.[26] This technique involves one or more full-thickness vertical incisions in the vestibule away from the gingival margin and sulcus. After tissue elevation a subperiosteal pouch is created to allow space for a bone graft. The main limitation of this flap is the lack of visualization and access to the alveolar ridge (Box 26.7).

Proper Incision Technique

The design of the surgical incision is based on many factors such as anatomic location, tissue quality, type of procedure, and desired

---

• BOX 26.7   Vestibular Flap Surgery

Advantages
- Less invasive
- No disruption of papillae
- May use with bone-grafting procedures

Disadvantages
- Limited access
- Low visibility
- Not indicated for implant placement

healing outcome.[27] Flap designs may be further classified as to the type of tissue (full versus partial thickness), the number of incisions used to create them (envelope, papilla sparing, triangular, trapezoidal), or secondary incisions that dictate the flap's direction (rotating versus coronally versus apically advancing).[25]

Over the years the mucogingival flap design used in oral implantology has changed dramatically. Technology has allowed for the more accurate and ideal placement of implants and bone grafts. Better techniques and methods with tissue handling and preserving the blood supply have become reality. In the early years of oral implantology, most surgeries were completed with an aggressive full reflection of the surgical area with multiple release incisions. Most implants were placed with a submerged (stage 2) technique. In the 1990s a more conservative one-stage surgery technique became popular that involved placement of a healing abutment at the time of implant placement. This procedure showed remarkable results with a decreased morbidity. In the early 2000s advancements in guided surgery allowed the advent of "flapless" surgery, which resulted in much less trauma and patient complications.

With most dental implant procedures, surgical incisions are required. With a properly placed incision, the implant clinician may obtain adequate access to the surgical site for implant placement, identify necessary landmarks, and prevent unnecessary complications. The design of the surgical incision is based on numerous factors such as anatomic location, tissue quality, amount of keratinized tissue, procedure, amount of access required, and the desired healing outcome. There exist numerous principles that must be adhered to for the majority of incisions.

Proper Incision Positioning

The primary incision should ideally be located in keratinized tissue whenever possible. This will allow for an increased wound surface area and a resultant increase in vascularity to the incision line.[28] Not only does this reduce significant initial intraoral bleeding, it also will result in severing less blood vessels. A reduction in postoperative edema will result, which decreases tension to the incision line and possible incision line opening. If there exists 3 mm or more of attached gingiva on the crest of the edentulous ridge, the incision should ideally bisect the soft tissue. This places half of the attached gingiva width on each side of the incision (i.e., 1.5 mm), thereby strengthening the incision line. If there is less than 3 mm of attached keratinized tissue on the ridge crest, the incision should be made more lingually so that at least 1.5 mm of attached tissue is placed to the facial aspect of the implant. This concept is especially important in the posterior mandible because attached tissue is required to prevent tension and pulling from the buccinator muscle (Fig. 26.12).

Incisions made through attached gingiva and over healthy bone are more desirable than those through unattached gingiva and over unhealthy or missing bone contours. When osseous defects are present, properly placed incisions allow the wound margins to be sutured over intact, healthy bone that are a minimum of a few millimeters away from the bone defect. This will result in supporting the healing wound. In esthetic zones a papilla-sparing flap may be used to preserve the papilla and minimize possible tissue recession (Fig. 26.13).

In summary, the incision location may vary depending on multiple factors. The goal of any incision is to allow for adequate exposure of the operative field and to minimize possible damage or tearing of the tissue margins. This will lead to a better chance of obtaining primary closure, which results in better healing and less chance of postoperative complications.[29]

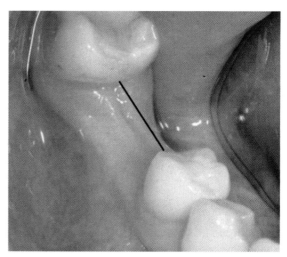

• **Fig. 26.12** Incision design based on amount of attached tissue. If less than 3 mm of attached tissue is present, then the incision is positioned more lingually.

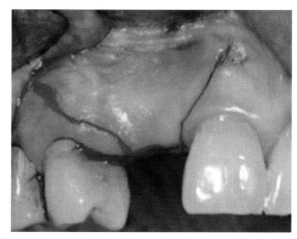

• **Fig. 26.13** Incision made more lingual to increase attached tissue to the buccal. Note the broad based papilla sparing incision.

Use of a Sharp Scalpel Blade

A sharp scalpel blade allows incisions to be made cleanly without unnecessary damage from repeated strokes, especially if not in the same plane. Many factors dictate how fast the scalpel blade will dull, such as contacting teeth, titanium (e.g., implants, abutments, healing cover screws), and dense bone, which tend to lead to accelerated dulling. The resistance and thickness of the tissues may dull the blade at different rates; therefore the surgeon should change the scalpel blade whenever a difference is noted in blade sharpness. Sharp dissections tend to minimize trauma to the incision line, which will result in less tissue trauma and postoperative swelling (Fig. 26.14).

Scalpel Technique

Clean, precise incisions allow for optimal wound closure. An ideal incision includes a single stroke through the tissue in one direction with firm, even pressure on the scalpel. Tentative strokes, especially in different planes, will increase the amount of damaged tissue and increase the amount of bleeding and inflammation. Long, continuous strokes are preferable to shorter,

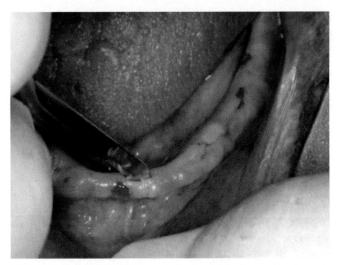

• **Fig. 26.14** Incision should be made to "score" the bone; this allows for full-thickness reflection of the tissue.

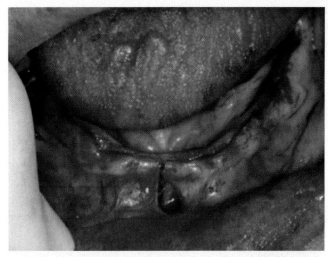

• **Fig. 26.16** Incisions should be made to avoid any vital structures, for example, the mental foramen and lingual nerve in the mandible.

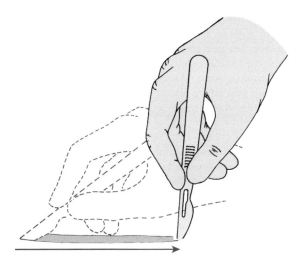

• **Fig. 26.15** Proper method of making incision using no. 15 scalpel blade. Note the scalpel motion is made by moving the hand at the wrist and not by moving the entire forearm. (*From Hupp JR, Ellis E, Tucker MR. Contemporary Oral and Maxillofacial Surgery. 7th ed. Philadelphia: Elsevier; 2020.*)

inconsistent, interrupted strokes. Ideally the incision should always be over bone.

In most cases the blade should be held perpendicular to the epithelial surface. This will result in an angle that produces square wound margins, which are easier to reapproximate during suturing and less likely for surgical wound necrosis and incision line opening to occur[30] (Fig. 26.15).

Avoid Vital Structures

The incision and flap should be designed to avoid possible injuries to vital structures. The two most important structures in the mandible include the mental nerve and lingual nerve. When making incisions in the mandibular premolar area, care should be exercised with the anatomy of the mental nerve. Usually three to four branches of the mental nerve will ascend from the mental foramen and are superficially located in the soft tissue. In mandibular edentulous cases the scalpel blade should always remain on the bone. This will prevent "slipping" off the ridge and damaging

deeper vital structures. In mandibular severe atrophy cases the mandibular canal may be dehisced, which can lead to direct transection of the nerve fibers. In instances where the nerve lies on top of the ridge, the incision is carried lingual to the ridge to avoid severing the nerve. In the posterior mandible the lingual nerve may be closely adhered to the lingual aspect of the mandible. Therefore in the retromolar pad area, incisions should always be positioned lateral to the pad.

In the maxilla, rarely will an incision damage a vital structure. On the buccal, there exist no vessels that would be problematic, except for the infraorbital nerve, which exits the infraorbital foramen. However, direct trauma is usually rare in this area. On the palatal aspect the nasopalatine vessels exit the incisive foramen and supply the anterior palatal gingiva. If this area is incised, minimal bleeding will result, and the neural tissue regenerates rather quickly.[31] Posterior palatal release incisions should be avoided because the greater palatine nerve and artery may be traumatized, which may lead to increased bleeding episodes (Fig. 26.16).

Proper Scalpel Grip

Pencil Grip

The scalpel is grasped close to the blade between the tips of the thumb and the index finger, with the remaining handle resting on the web of the thumb, much like grasping a pencil. With this grip the motion is predominately from the thumb and index finger, allowing for precise cutting of tissue. A finger rest may be used to increase the accuracy of the fine cutting. This grip may also be "backhanded" by reversing the direction of the blade without changing the upper arm position. The pencil grip is best used for short, fine movements for precise incisions, because the muscles of the hand are used significantly more than the muscles of the forearm. The blade edge is usually held at 30 to 40 degrees to the tissue. One of the limitations of this technique is the greater angle, which results in less cutting-edge contact, and limits the depth of the incision (Fig. 26.17).

Fingertip Grip

With this technique the scalpel is held between the thumb and the middle finger, while the index finger is placed on the body of the scalpel blade to apply downward pressure, much like grasping a butter knife. This grip technique uses more arm motion and is primarily used for making long skin incisions. The main advantage is the increased blade-to-tissue contact, which provides good depth and direction control. The greater the length of tissue contact with the scalpel, the more

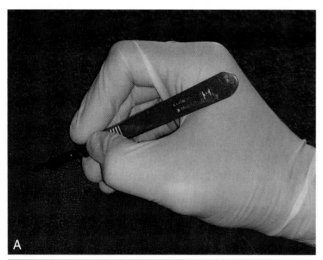

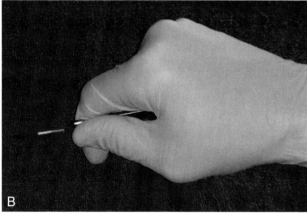

• **Fig. 26.17** Scalpel Grip. (A) Pencil grip: ideal scalpel grip because maximum control is obtained. (B) Palm grip: nonideal scalpel grip with minimal control which is rarely used in implant dentistry.

the walls of the incision resist minute or sudden changes in direction, allowing for smoother, straighter incisions. The main disadvantage of the fingertip grip is that it does not allow for precise blade cuts.

Palm Grip

The palm grip is used when strong pressure in indicated to incise the tissue. The scalpel is held in the palm of the dominant hand with the index finger on top of the handle. The cutting pressure is derived from the palm and fingers as well as the entire arm. However, this grip is rarely used in implant dentistry (Fig. 26.17).

Surgical Armamentarium

A full array of instruments may be used in oral implantology, and usually the clinician will over time develop personal preferences with respect to various procedures. The following is a summary of some of the most popular instruments used today.

Instrument to Incise Tissue

Scalpel/Surgical Blades

The scalpel is the ideal instrument for making incisions and separating tissue. Scalpels are basically manufactured in two forms: disposable and metal reusable handle. The most used scalpel in oral implantology is the #3 scalpel, which commonly has a metric ruler on one side, which allows for intraoperative measurements. As stated earlier, the scalpel must be held in a way that permits full control of the instrument and at the same time freedom of movement. The handle of the scalpel is grasped between the thumb and the third and fourth fingers, and the index finger is placed over the back of the blade to provide firm control.

The most common scalpel blade used in oral implantology is the #15 blade or #15c blade. The #15 blade has a short, rounded cutting edge, combined with an angled point. In addition, the #12 or #12b blade is commonly used, mainly around teeth or in difficult access areas. These blades are small, pointed, and crescent shaped, which are end cutting on the inside edge of the curve. Blades can be either carbon steel or stainless steel. Carbon-steel surgical blades are sharper than stainless-steel blades but may dull quicker (Fig. 26.18).

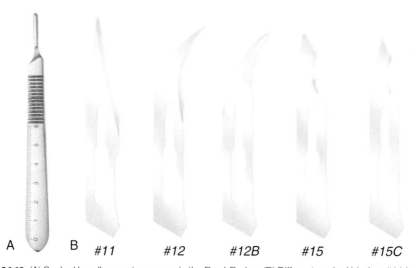

A   B   #11   #12   #12B   #15   #15C

• **Fig. 26.18** (A) Scalpel handle: most common is the Bard-Barker. (B) Different scalpel blades: #11 is used for incision of abscesses or infections; #12 and #12b are used around teeth to connect incisions in difficult access areas; #15 is the most common blade used in oral implantology; and #15c has a smaller neck that allows for easier access around teeth.

Instruments to Reflect Tissue

Once the incision is made, the mucosa and periosteum must be reflected to expose the bone. The Molt periosteal elevator (#9) is one of the more common instruments to complete this task. The periosteal elevator usually has a sharp, pointed end and a broad, flat end. Normally the pointed end is used to initiate the reflection, followed by the broad end, which allows for a larger volume of tissue to be reflected. In the authors opinion an easier and more efficient instrument to use to reflect tissue is the 2/4 Molt. This double-ended instrument has two small, rounded, sharp areas, 2/4 (4 mm/6 mm), and is positioned in a dished-out fashion to allow for tissue to be reflected easier (Fig. 26.19).

In general, tissue can be reflected three different ways: (1) prying motion—pointed end used in a prying motion to elevate the soft tissue; (2) push stroke—used after full thickness incision to slide underneath the flap; and (3) pull or scrape stroke—used to remove tissue tags from the bone in a scraping motion (Fig. 26.20).

Instruments to Grasp Tissue

Tissue forceps are used to stabilize soft tissue flaps for suturing and reflection of flaps. The most common tissue forceps used in implant dentistry include the Adson and Allison forceps.

Adson forceps (pickups): to grasp and stabilize soft tissue flaps during suturing or implant and bone graft procedures. These delicate forceps have small teeth or serrations to gently hold tissue for stability. Care should be exercised to not crush the tissue because the tissue can be irreversibly damaged (Fig. 26.21).

Allison forceps: these forceps have larger and more aggressive teeth used to hold heavy or high-tension tissue. In implant dentistry these types of forceps are rarely used.

Instruments to Remove Bone/Tissue

Rongeur forceps

A rongeur is a heavy-duty surgical instrument with a sharp-edged, scoop-shaped tip, used for gouging or snipping away the bone. The word *rongeur* is a French word meaning "gnawer." In oral implantology the rongeur is used to cut or contour tissue, or to remove pieces of bone. Rongeur forceps have a spring between the handles, which increases the magnitude of the removal force. A common type used is termed *double-action* rongeur, which significantly generates more force than a single-action rongeur. Because the blades are concave toward the inside, harvested bone is easily retained to be used in grafting areas.

1. *Side Cutting* to cut and contour bone, remove sharp edges; will retain bone for grafting purposes
2. *End Cutting* to cut and contour bone; one beak may engage bone to shave bone from the ridge (Fig. 26.22)

Surgical burs

Surgical burs can also be used to remove bone. It is important to always use irrigation when using the surgical burs. The tissue must be adequately reflected to prevent trauma to the tissue with the burs. Cross-cut fissure burs may be used to make pilot holes in the host bone that will allow the bone to be removed with a chisel. Additional burs used to remove bone (i.e., alveoplasty) include special ridge reduction burs, straight handpiece (HP) acrylic barrel shaped burs, or HP round burs (Fig. 26.23).

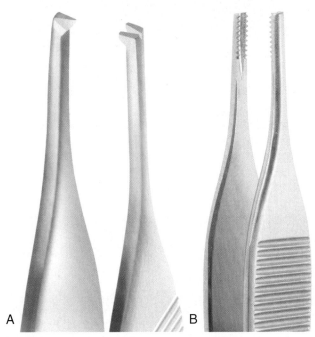

• **Fig. 26.21** Adson Forceps. (A) Teeth: may perforate and tear thin tissue; however, it allows for better grasping of the tissue. (B) Serrated: less chance of perforating tissue.

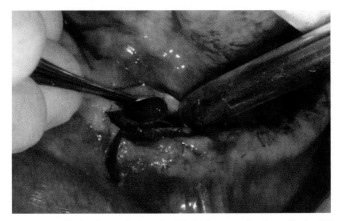

• **Fig. 26.19** Reflection technique for full-thickness reflection with the 2/4 molt instrument.

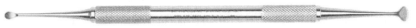

• **Fig. 26.20** Recommended periosteal reflection instrument: 2 to 4 Molt.

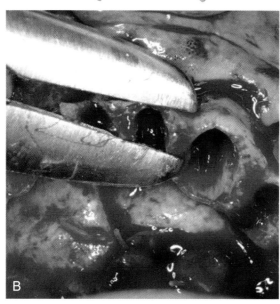

Fig. 26.22 Rongeur. (A) Double-action rongeur allows for greater force for bone removal. (B) Bone removal using a "rocking" motion.

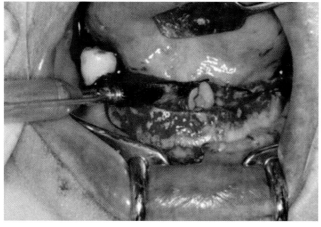

Fig. 26.23 Bone removal using carbide HP bur in a straight 1:1 handpiece.

Bone file

A bone file is a double ended serrated instrument used to remove sharp, spiny ridges within the bone (Fig. 26.24).

Instruments to Remove Tissue From Extraction Sockets or Bony Defects

The *surgical curette* is an instrument used to ensure removal of debris and diseased tissue. These instruments are usually spoon shaped and have sharp edges that allow scraping of the bony walls. Not only will the scraping remove soft tissue, the curettes will also initiate the regional acceleratory phenomenon (RAP). The most commonly used and recommended surgical curette has serrated edges (e.g., Lucas 86 Currette) (Figs. 26.25 and 26.26).

Bone-Grafting Instruments

Bone scrapers

Bone scrapers are mainly used by clinicians to harvest autogenous bone from the oral cavity and allow the collected bone particles to be delivered to the surgical site. These instruments consist of a harvesting blade and collection chamber, with a narrow-tipped syringe for access-restricted areas (Fig. 26.27).

Grafting spoon and condenser

These instruments hold bone to be placed at a specific area with a spoon-type of instrument. Usually a condenser is present on the other side of the instrument, which allows for the condensing of the bone graft material into the defect (Fig. 26.28).

Surgical Scissors

There exists a full array of scissors used in oral implantology: straight, curved, serrated, and nonserrated. Surgical scissors are used to cut tissue, spread tissue, and cut sutures. Usually the thumb and ring finger are placed in the scissor rings, with the index finger to steady the scissor. Curved scissors are usually preferred by most surgeons because they provide a better field of view and access to restricted areas.

Dean: the most commonly used scissors in oral implantology, which have slightly curved handles and offset serrated blades that allow for easy access to cut sutures and to remove diseased tissue. Dean scissors feature angled blades that are approximately 3 cm in length from midscrew. They have one serrated blade, with a slightly curved handle.

Iris: very small, extremely sharp scissors with a fine tip. Some iris scissors have curved blades for certain types of precision tasks, whereas others may have straight blades.

Kelly: commonly used to trim tissue or cut sutures because they have one serrated cutting side to the scissors.

Metzenbaum: surgical scissors that are designed for delicate tissue and blunt dissection. The scissors are available in variable lengths and have a relatively long shank-to-blade ratio. They are constructed of stainless steel and may have tungsten carbide cutting surface inserts. Blades can be curved or straight (Fig. 26.29).

Hemostats

The hemostat is an instrument that has serrated tips that allow for the "clamping" of tissue or small materials. Directly above the

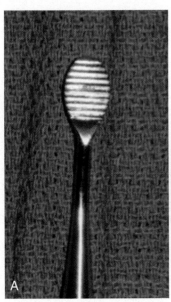
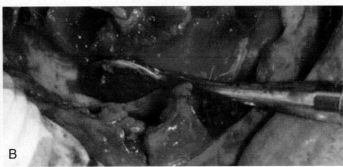

• **Fig. 26.24** Bone file (A) used to smooth out sharp ridges, (B) which may lead to postoperative tissue irritation especially after osteoplasty procedures have been performed.

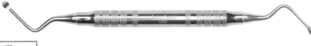

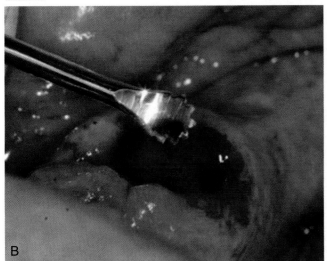

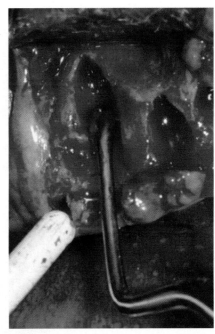

• **Fig. 26.25** (A) Lucas 86 Surgical Curette (Salvin), which is a serrated spoon excavator. (B) Removing tissue within an extraction site and initiating the regional acceleratory phenomenon.

• **Fig. 26.26** Technique for curetting the extraction socket before grafting or addition of bone graft material.

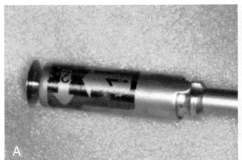
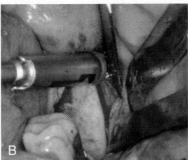
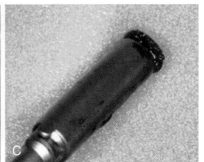

• **Fig. 26.27** (A) Bone Scraper, (B) Bone scraper being used to harvest bone from tuberosity area, (C) Harvested bone in bone scraper.

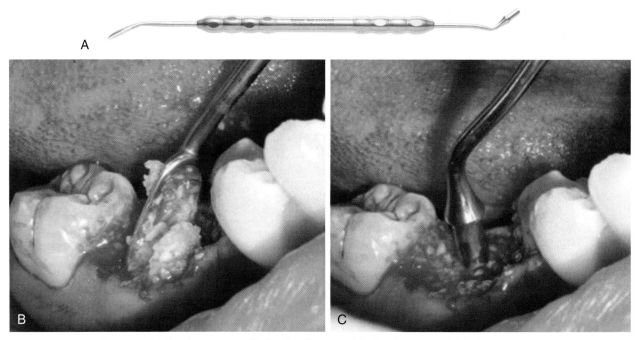

• **Fig. 26.28** Grafting Instruments. (A) Grafting Spoon and Packer Instrument, (B) Spoon to transport graft material to surgical site, (C) Packer to augment the surgical site.

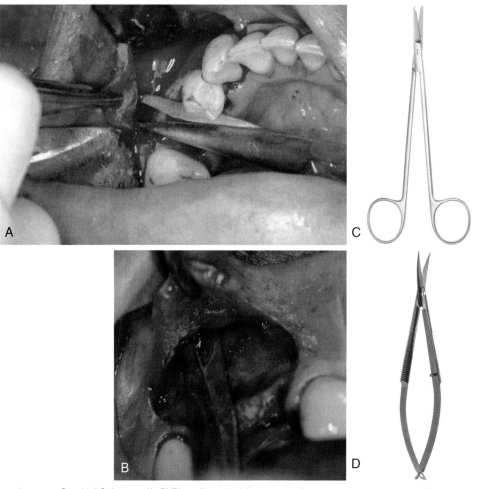

• **Fig. 26.29** Surgical Scissors. (A, B) Blunt dissection tissue spreading for tension free closure. (C) Suture scissors. (D) Castroviejo scissors.

finger rings is a ratchet to control the degree of force or restriction. In oral implantology, hemostats are used to constrict blood vessels (i.e., bleeding), retrieve loose objects in the oral cavity, and securely hold small items (Fig. 26.30).

Instruments to Retract Tissue

Retractors are used to hold back the cheek, tongue, or flap, which permit visibility to the surgical site. Examples include:

Mirror—conventional mouth mirror to retract tongue

Weider tongue retractor—broad, heart-shaped retractor with grooves and perforations that hold tongue and cheek away from surgical site

Seldin retractor—double ended with round blunted ends, used to retract a tissue flap from bone after an incision

Minnesota retractor—to retract tongue or cheek away from surgical site and has the advantage of reflecting both at the same time

Misch "Spoon" cheek and tongue retractor—to hold tongue or cheek away from surgical site, ergonomically designed to reduce hand fatigue

Sinus graft cheek retractor—broad-based flap retractor that reduces force to the infraorbital foramen area, thus reducing the possibility of a neuropraxia (Fig. 26.31)

Instruments to Hold Mouth Open

Bite block—sterilizable rubber block in multiple sizes to keep mouth open during procedures

Molt mouth prop—ratchet-designed instrument with rubber tips that allows variation on opening

Orringer retractor—spring-loaded mouth prop that self-maintaining spring-loaded mouth prop which maintains upper and lower soft tissue retraction (Fig. 26.32)

Suctions/Aspirators—suctioning is crucial to keeping the surgical field clear from debris to allow the surgeon to have clear visibility

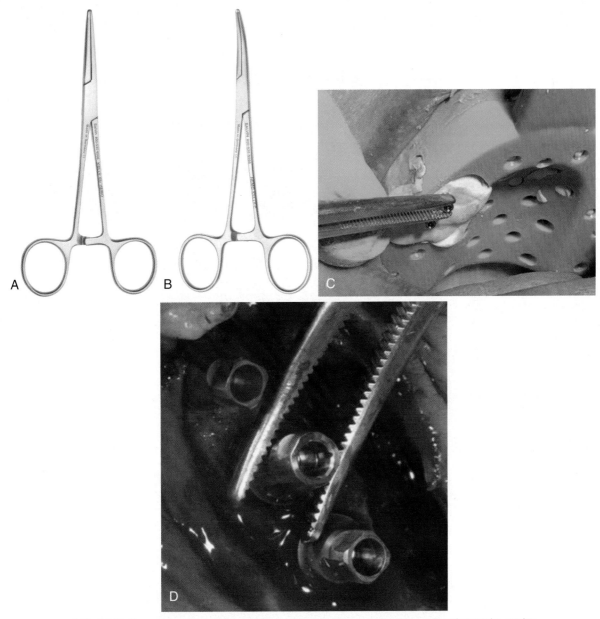

• **Fig. 26.30** Hemostats. (A) Straight. (B) Curved. (C) Hemostats used to remove direct impression coping screws. (D) Curved hemostats used to hold abutment to prevent countertorque.

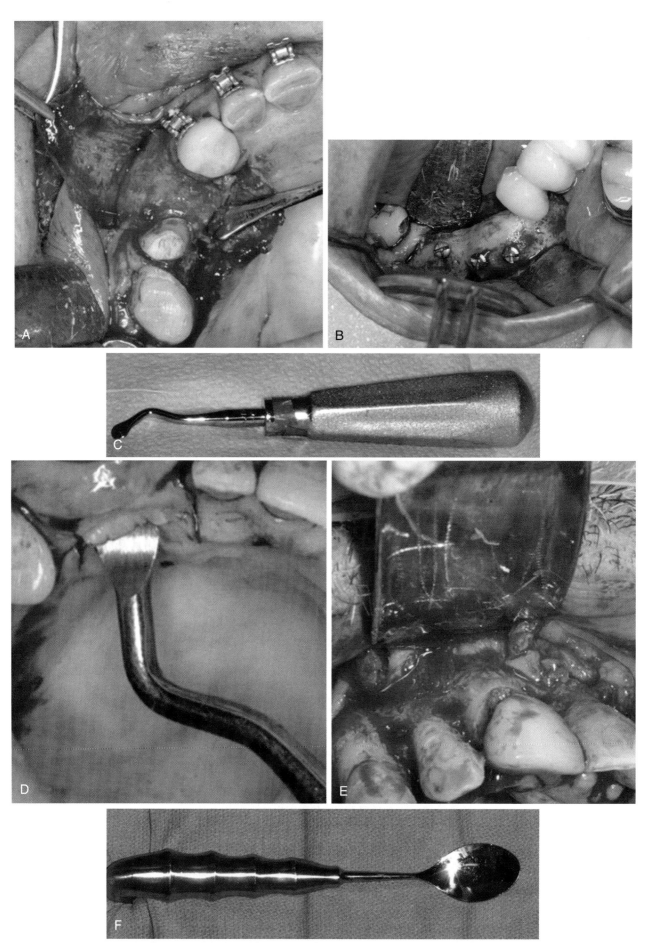

• **Fig. 26.31** Tissue Retraction. (A) Tissue pickups and molt retracting the tissue, (B) Seldin retractors, or holding tissue (C) Misch Ridge Elevator. (D) Clinical image of Misch Ridge Elevator reflecting tissue. (E) Minnesota. Retractor (F) Misch Spoon.

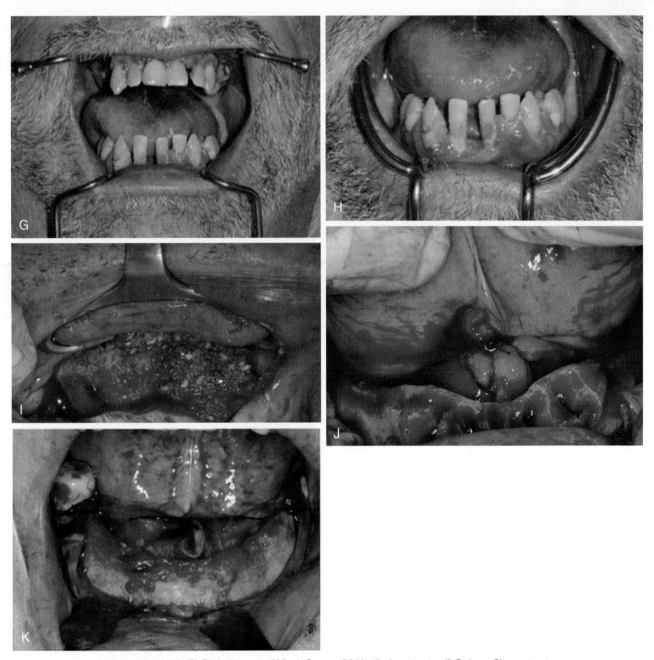

• **Fig. 26.31, cont'd** (G) Clinical image of Misch Spoon. (H) Vestibular retractor. (I) Orringer Sinus retractor. (J and K) Sutures used to tie back lingual tissue.

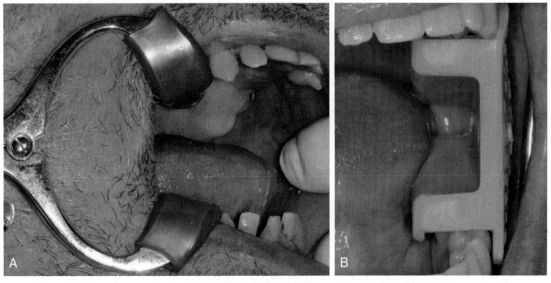

• **Fig. 26.32** Instruments to Hold Mouth Open. (A) Molt mouth prop. (B) Rubber mouth prop.

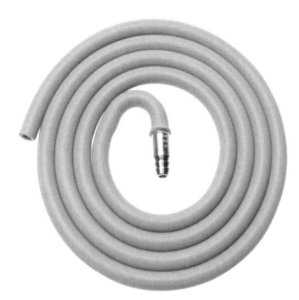

• **Fig. 26.33** Flexible Suction Tubing.

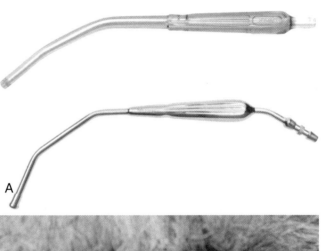

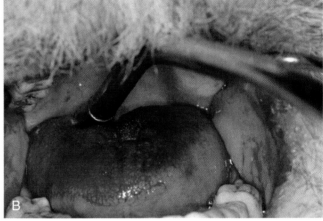

General surgical suction—used to clear the airway or surgical site; may be made of metal, which is autoclavable, or plastic, which is disposable

Fraser suction—suction that contains a hole in the handle that can be covered; vacuum relief hole controls suction by covering or uncovering the hole with fingertip; when uncovered, very little suction will result, which is important when working with bone or membranes (Fig. 26.33)

Yankauer tonsil aspirator—angled, long suction that has a perforated ball-type end for suctioning the posterior throat; a Yankauer is used to suction oropharyngeal secretions very effectively to prevent aspiration (Fig. 26.34)

• **Fig. 26.34** Yankauer Suction. (A) Extended suction for in posterior oropharynx. (B) Yankauer suction is used to suction debris from the posterior palate area.

Instruments to Hold Drapes

Towel clamp—a nonperforating clamp used to secure instruments and surgical materials, such as suction tubing to the surgical drapes (Fig. 26.35)

Handpieces/Motors

1. *Surgical motor console:* Composed of a console, foot pedal, and motor cord, which allows for the use of a contraangle or straight handpiece.
   • *1:1 handpieces:* usually straight handpieces that run at higher revolutions per minute (i.e., 40,000–50,000 revolutions/min); used for bone-grafting procedures
   • *16:1 or 20:1 handpieces:* contraangle reduction implant handpieces to drill osteotomies and/or place implants (Fig. 26.36)
2. *Piezosurgery units:* Piezoelectric bone surgery is an innovative technology that selectively cuts mineralized tissue without damaging soft tissue. This technology uses a high-frequency vibration (i.e., 25–35 kHz) that is transmitted to specialized surgical tips. The major advantages of this technology are the high precision accuracy, minimal thermal damage, increased healing, and less soft tissue trauma. There exist many uses of Piezosurgery in oral implantology, which

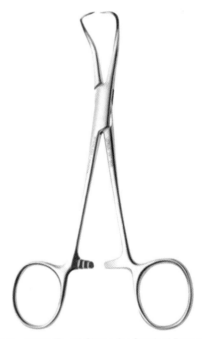

• **Fig. 26.35** Towel Clamp for Surgical Drapes.

differ in various and versatile tips that are interchangeably used on the handpiece. This type of surgical unit may be used for atraumatic extractions, removal of implants, bone-grafting procedures, and sinus augmentation procedures (Fig. 26.37).

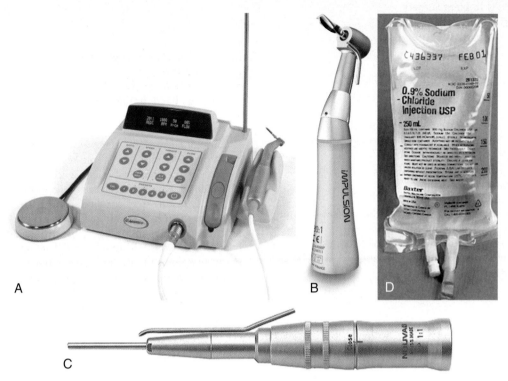

• **Fig. 26.36** (A) Aseptico surgical motor (Aseptico, Woodinville, Wash.). (B) 20:1 reduction handpiece for drilling osteotomy and placing implants (Aseptico). (C) 1:1 handpiece that is used for bone removal or harvesting autogenous bone grafts (Nouvag, Goldach, Switzerland). (D) Irrigation solution should be 0.9% sodium chloride or sterile saline. (Baxter, Deerfield, Ill.).

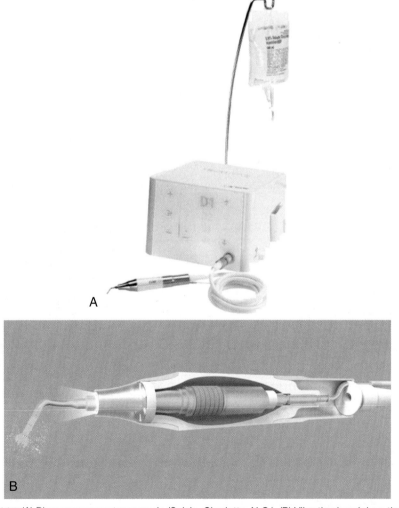

• **Fig. 26.37** (A) Piezosurgery motor console (Salvin, Charlotte, N.C.). (B) Vibrating handpiece that uses ultrasound frequency technology, resulting in precision and safe cutting of hard tissue.

Osteotomes

An osteotome is a surgical instrument which is used to cut, expand, or divide bone. There exists multiple types which are procedure specific.

Pointed: designed for progressive circumferential (circular) expansion (i.e., bone spreading) of the alveolar ridges which are compromised in width (i.e., Division B).

Progressive osteotomes: to incrementally widen or expand bone before implant placement

1. *Concave:* Concave osteotomes are used to infracture the floor of the maxillary sinus through the implant osteotomy. The concave tip retains bone graft material.

2. *Convex:* Convex osteotomes are used to raise the floor of the maxillary sinus after fracturing (SA-2 technique) (Fig. 26.38).

Sinus Curettes

Membrane curettes: Used to aid in the elevation of the sinus membrane, these curettes feature a rounder smooth tip for lifting the sinus with minimal puncture risk (Fig. 26.39).

Aseptic Technique

Ideally any surgical procedure where there may be an increased bacterial insult should use a sterile technique. There is much misunderstanding, though, when it comes to the terms *clean*, *aseptic*, and *sterile*.

- *Clean technique:* The clean technique includes routine hand washing, hand drying, and use of nonsterile gloves.
- *Aseptic technique:* The aseptic technique is used for short invasive procedures. It includes antiseptic hand wash, sterile gloves, antiseptic rinse, and use of a clean, dedicated area.
- *Sterile technique:* The sterile technique includes measures to prevent the spread of bacteria from the environment to the patient by eliminating all microorganisms in that environment. This is mainly used for any procedure in which the bacterial count needs to be lowered and an increase in infection rate will lead to significant morbidity. This includes surgical hand scrub, hands dried with sterile towels, complete sterile field, sterile gown, mask, and gloves (Table 26.1; Boxes 26.8 and 26.9).

Achieving surgical asepsis requires multiple steps, including surgical gloving and gowning, along with maintaining a sterile field. Each member of the team involved in a sterile procedure is responsible for maintaining the aseptic environment.

Sterile Field

Sterile drapes are most often used within the sterile field to cover any surgical area used during the surgery (Fig. 26.40). Drapes come in various sizes and are most easily purchased in a kit. The inner surface of the sterile field, except for a 1-inch border, is considered the sterile field that may be used to add sterile items. This 1-inch

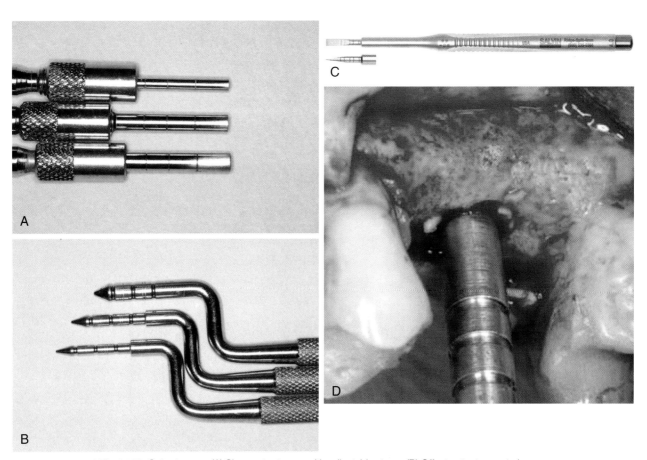

• **Fig. 26.38** Osteotomes. (A) Sinus osteotomes with adjustable stops. (B) Offset osteotomes to increase osteotomy diameter. (C) Straight osteotome for bone spreading. (D) Clinical image of crestal bone graft using an osteotome.

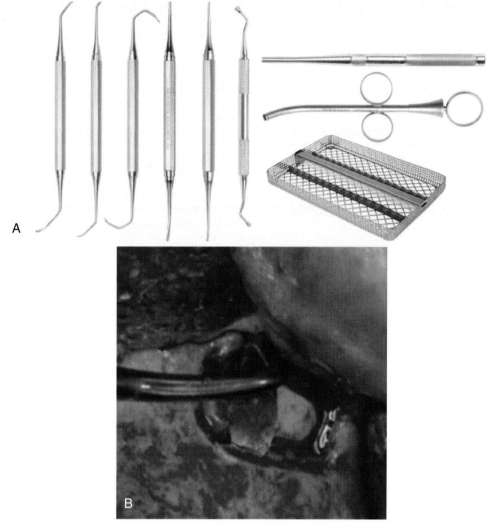

• **Fig. 26.39** (A) Basic sinus surgery kit. (B) Sinus curette reflecting sinus membrane.

TABLE 26.1	Clean Versus Aseptic Versus Sterile		
	Clean	**Aseptic**	**Sterile**
Procedure space	Dental operatory	Surgical suite	Surgical suite
Gloves	Nonsterile	Sterile	Sterile surgical
Hand hygiene before the procedures	Routine	Aseptic (e.g., alcohol)	Surgical scrub iodophors, chlorhexidine
Skin antisepsis	No	Alcohol	Chlorhexidine
Sterile field	No	No	Yes
Sterile gown, mask, head covering	No	No	Yes

From Suzuki JB, Resnik RR. Wound dehiscence: incision line opening. In: Resnik RR, Misch CE, eds. *Misch's Avoiding Complications in Oral Implantology*. St. Louis, MO: Mosby; 2018.

• **BOX 26.8** General Principles for a Sterile Technique

- Only sterile materials and instruments are placed within the sterile field.
- Check for chemical indicators to verify sterility of items placed onto the sterile field, along with package integrity and package expiration (if appropriate).
- Above and below the sterile field table is considered "nonsterile."
- Materials that display a manufacturer's expiration date should be considered unsafe for use after that date. (Rationale: Expiration dates do not guarantee either sterility or lack of sterility.)
- If any sterile item (material, instrument, gown, glove) has been compromised, the package contents, gown, or the sterile field is considered contaminated. This may happen when:
  - nonsterile items contact sterile items; or
  - liquids or moisture soak through a drape, gown, or package (strikethrough).
- Single-use materials should only be used on an individual patient for a single procedure and then discarded.
- Reusable medical devices shall be reprocessed and sterilized according to the manufacturer's directions.
- Any item that falls below table level is considered unsterile.

• BOX 26.9 Sterile Scrub Technique

Step 1: Prescrub Wash

A short prescrub wash is completed, including the hands up to the elbow. This is to remove superficial microorganisms and gross debris.

- Before the scrub, make sure surgical attire is worn and remove all jewelry. Glasses (loops, lights, etc.) should be placed in the ideal position.
- Perform a rinse from the fingertips to the elbows so the water flows from the cleanest area (fingertips) to the less clean area (elbows). Use a sink that is wide and deep so that both arms are contained within the borders so that water is not splashed out of the sink.
- Open the scrub brush and perform a preliminary scrub from fingers to the elbows. The next part of the prescrub is to clean the subungual area of each cuticle. With the disposable nail cleaning device, remove any debris from under each cuticle. The brush side of the scrub brush may be used over each cuticle.

Step 2: Primary Scrub

Depending on the hospital or surgical center, scrubbing methods and protocol will vary. The counted stroke method seems to be the most efficient to guarantee sterility. With the sponge side of the scrub brush, complete five strokes for each side of each finger (four sides), five strokes for each side of the hand, and five strokes for each forearm side. Rinse hands and arms under running water in only one direction, from fingertips to elbows. Care must be exercised to ensure fingers, hands, and arms do not touch any nonsterile surface (e.g., faucet). The hands should remain above the waist and below the axilla. If the water is controlled by hand-control levers, a nonsterile surgical assistant should turn the water off. Usually the prescrub and primary scrub will take approximately 3 minutes.

Step 3: Gowning

The hands should be dried with a sterile towel. Care should be exercised to prevent the sterile gown or gloves from water contamination. When moving from the scrub sink to the sterile area, keep hands in front of the body, above the waist, and below the axilla. The neckline, shoulders, underarms, and sleeve cuffs are considered nonsterile.

The sterile gown should be immediately donned after complete drying of the hands and forearms, before gloving. Even though the complete gown is sterile when placed on the sterile table, once the gown is donned, only the front from the waist to the axilla is sterile. The gown should be lifted upward and away from the table, and allowed to open by locating the neckline and armholes. Hold the inside front of the gown at the level of the armholes to allow the gown to unfold. Do not touch the outside of the gown with bare hands. Extend both arms into the armholes, and the gown and sleeves will unfold. The gown is pulled onto the body with the cuffs of the sleeves extended over the hands. Do not push the hands completely through the cuffs.

Surgical gowns establish a barrier that minimizes the possibility of contamination from nonsterile to sterile areas, which is commonly referred to as a "strikethrough" barrier. They are made of a material that is resistant to blood and fluid penetration.

Step 4: Sterile Gloving

Sterile gloves are packaged in a sterile package. The closed gloving technique is most widely used. It ensures the hands touch only the inside of the gown and gloves. With the dominant hand, pick up the nondominant glove by the inner wrap straight up, placing it on the nondominant hand. Guide and wiggle the fingers into the glove. Using the gloved hand, pick up the remaining glove and guide it on the nondominant hand, making sure the gown cuff is covered. The nondominant glove will then pull the dominant glove cuff over the gown.

Step 5: Tying of the Gown

After the gown and gloves are in place, the front tie of the gown must be secured. The surgeon holds the left string with the left hand and holds the right large string and tag with the right hand. The tag is separated from the small string and handed to an assistant. The surgeon rotates 360 degrees and the assistant tears off the tag, leaving the right and left for the surgeon to tie.

---

border may also be used to position the drape within the surgical field. When placing sterile items onto the surgical field, items may be "dropped" from approximately 6 inches above the sterile field.

Surgical Scrub

The surgical scrub is the process that removes as many microorganisms as possible from the nail beds, hands, and forearms by mechanical washing and chemical antisepsis for a surgical procedure. This will result in a decrease in microbial count, and it inhibits the regrowth of bacteria. There are two different types of scrubbing techniques: a sterile sponge/brush with antimicrobial agent or a brushless technique with alcohol/chlorhexidine gluconate (Figs. 26.41 and 26.42). All rings, watches, bracelets, and jewelry should be removed before starting the hand scrub. Surgical hats, protective eyewear, headlights, and a surgical mask must be donned before surgical hand asepsis. Drying of the hands and arms is a priority because moist surfaces allow bacteria to multiply. Gowning, gloving, and tying the front tie of the gown occur after the hand scrub (Figs. 26.43 and 26.44).

Utilization of Ideal Suturing

Materials and Techniques

The objective of the proper suturing of the surgical wound is to position and secure the margins of the incisions to promote ideal and optimal healing. The goal of the suture material and technique is to hold the margins of the wound in close apposition until the wound has healed enough to withstand normal functional tension and stress on the incision line.[32] If surgical wounds are not properly approximated, separation of the margins will occur, which leads to increased postsurgical morbidity. The clinician must select a suture with qualities that include high tensile strength,[33] tissue biocompatibility that prevents tissue irritation, ease of knot tying, and the ability to prevent minimal knot slippage (Table 26.2).

Suture Type

Absorbable

Absorbable sutures are popular and advantageous in implant dentistry because of the elimination of a suture removal appointment. There are two types of resorbable sutures: natural and synthetic.

Natural Natural sutures are mainly broken down by body enzymes. The most common natural sutures are plain and chromic gut (Fig. 26.45).

Plain gut. Plain gut is a monofilament derived from highly purified collagen from sheep intestinal submucosa. It is highly antigenic, losing 50% of tensile strength after 24 hours. Gut has unpredictable absorption because of the enzymes and macrophages that break it down. This type of suture has been shown to have a high incidence of tissue reactions, which impede healing.

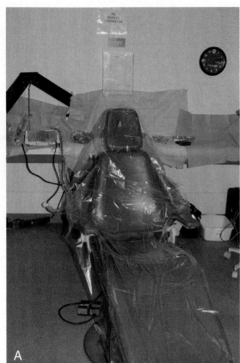

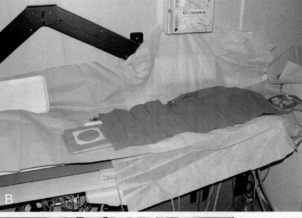

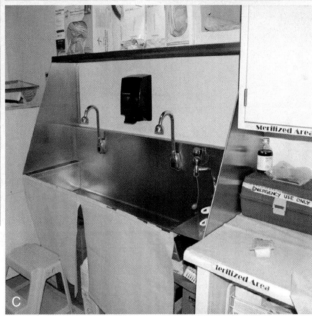

• **Fig. 26.40** Sterile Operatory Setup. (A) A sterile surgical field includes sterile table drapes to cover any areas that are going to contain surgical materials. Ideally the chair is covered; however, it is considered nonsterile. (B) All sterile supplies are placed within the confines of the sterile drapes. (C) A sink area should be present to allow for a sterile scrub area and gowning.

Chromic gut. Chromic gut is also derived from purified collagen from sheep intestinal submucosa that is treated with chromic salts, which decrease absorption. This material is highly antigenic and loses 50% of tensile strength after 5 days. As a monofilament, it causes significant tissue reactivity. Chromic gut causes inflammation, loses tension, and resorbs too quickly to maintain soft tissue approximation over an augmented site. It is not recommended when the tissues are advanced for a bone augmentation. Hypersensitivity reactions have been shown to occur because of the chromate particles present in the suture.[34]

Synthetic Synthetic sutures are broken down by hydrolysis because of their hydrophobic nature. The most common synthetic, absorbable suture in implant dentistry is polyglycolic acid (PGA) (Fig. 26.46).

PGA (Vicryl). Because PGA sutures are absorbed by hydrolysis breakdown, they are not affected by a low pH. Because they are manufactured by synthetic polymers, their resorption is slower and they will maintain the incision line with a tensile strength much longer than most suture materials. This suture material

will maintain sufficient tension over the first 2 weeks (75%), 50% after 3 weeks, and 25% after 2 weeks. PGA sutures have varying resorption rates, which consist of regular breakdown (≈21–28 days) and fast absorbing (≈7–14 days). The suture material is inert and has a relatively low tissue reaction.

Nonabsorbable

Nonabsorbable sutures are composed of human-made materials, which are not metabolized by the body. The most commonly used nonresorbable suture in dentistry is a natural fiber, silk, which undergoes a special manufacturing process to make it adequate for its use in surgery. Other nonabsorbable sutures are made of artificial fibers (e.g., polypropylene, polyester, nylon), which may contain coatings to enhance their performance characteristics (Fig. 26.47).

Silk: Over time, silk has been the most universally used suture material in dentistry because of its low cost and ease of handling. However, silk has many disadvantages with respect to implant dentistry. First, it is nonresorbable and must be removed. Because silk is a multifilament, is has been shown to "wick," which results

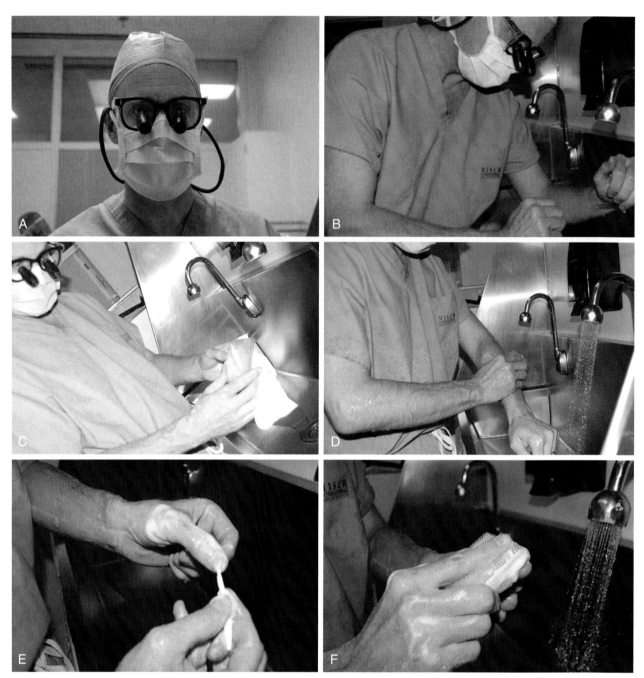

● **Fig. 26.41** Prescrub Technique. (A) Make sure hat, mask, glasses, and light source are worn and in place before the initiation of the scrub technique. (B) With lukewarm water, prerinse from fingertips to elbow. (C) Open surgical scrub brush with fingertip cleaner. (D) Complete a preliminary scrub from hands to the elbow with the soap brush. (E) Use fingertip cleaner to clean under fingernails, and (F) use the "brush" side of the scrub brush to complete fingernail cleansing.

in accumulating bacteria and fluid to the surgical wound.[35] And lastly, silk has been shown to release less tension during early retraction of the flap from healing, along with eliciting greater inflammation reactions, which may contribute to incision line opening more often than synthetic materials.[36,37]

Polypropylene (i.e., PROLENE): This suture, which is a monofilament, will not lose tensile strength over time. It is inert, has very little tissue reaction, possesses a low coefficient of friction, passes through tissue very easily, and has good knot security. The main disadvantage of this suture material tissue is irritation from the cut ends of the suture material.

Polytetrafluoroethylene: The polytetrafluoroethylene (PTFE) suture material is a monofilament, which has a relatively high tensile strength and is nonwicking (low bacteria accumulation). In addition, PTFE sutures have good handling qualities, are easy to tie with excellent knot security, are soft and comfortable for patients, and are biologically inert.

The main disadvantage of PTFE is that it is very expensive. PTFE sutures are slippery and have poor frictional resistance to knot loosening. At least seven equally tensioned, flat square throws are required to produce a secure knot when using PTFE material.

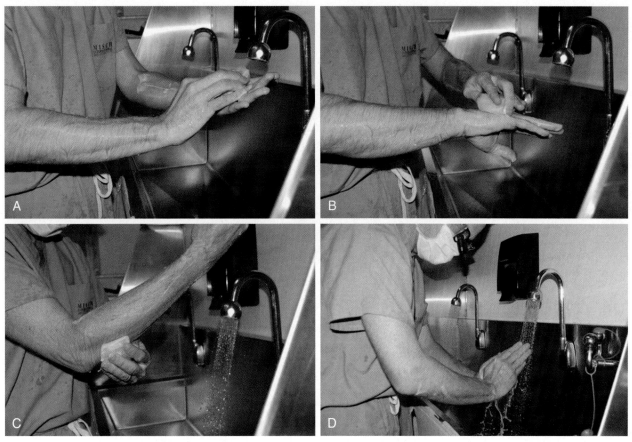

• **Fig. 26.42** Scrub Technique. (A) Scrub each side of the finger approximately five times. (B) Scrub each side of hand. (C) Scrub up to the wrist, then up to the elbow. (D) Rinse from the fingertips to the elbows. The theory is to remove all debris/bacteria away from the fingertips to the wrist. The entire scrub process should take approximately 3 minutes.

Suture Qualities

The selection of the suture material should be made with regard to the location and type of surgical procedure provided. However, an ideal suture material should exhibit high tensile strength, low tissue reactivity, and be absorbable.

High Tensile Strength

High tensile strength is the measured force, in pounds, that the suture will withstand before breaking. A suture material with low tensile strength will lead to suture breakdown, which will most likely compromise the healing of the incision line. The tensile strength of the tissue to be sutured will ideally determine the tensile strength of the suture selected. The tensile strength of the suture should be at least as strong as the tensile strength of the tissue being sutured.

Low Tissue Reactivity

Tissue reaction from the suture material has been shown to be exhibited through an inflammatory response, which will usually develop during the first 2 to 7 days after suturing the tissue. The suture material selected should have an inherent low tissue reactivity.[38] Low tissue reactivity means that the suture material should exhibit a minimal inflammatory response, which will not delay wound healing or increase infection rate. Tissue reaction is reflected through

an inflammatory response, which develops during the first 2 to 7 days after suturing the tissue. Several studies published over the past forty years have reported that synthetic materials exhibit superior behavior to oral tissues in terms of tissue inflammatory reactions compared with nonsynthetic suture material.

Absorbable

Absorbable suture material allows for the convenience of no suture removal. These types of sutures undergo degradation and absorption in the tissues; thus the sutures do not have to be removed. There are two mechanisms of degradation of absorbable sutures: enzymatic breakdown or degradation by hydrolysis (PGA). Sutures derived from a biologic origin (i.e., plain and chromic gut) are digested by intraoral enzymes. Usually these types of sutures lose their tensile strength quickly (within days of surgery) and are not ideal for dental implant procedures. Secondly, these sutures may break down even faster when the intraoral pH is low. A decreased pH may result from infection, medications, metabolic disorders, or dry mouth. Trauma from suture removal may sometimes lead to incision line opening.

Treatment Implications

For dental implant procedures involving dental implant placement and bone grafting, the ideal suture material should exhibit a

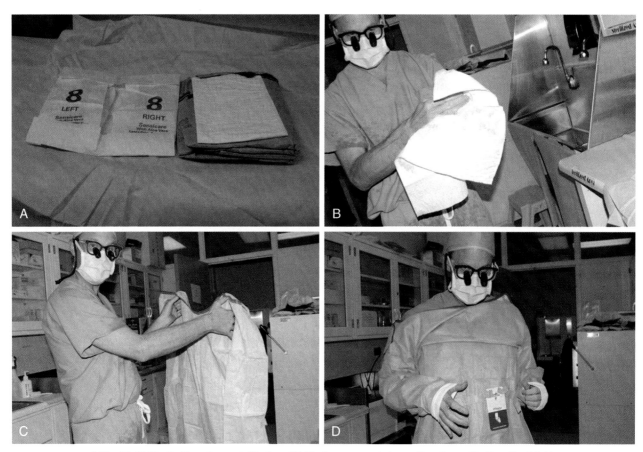

• **Fig. 26.43** Sterile Gowning and Gloving. (A) Sterile gown and gloves (Sensicare, Medline, Northfield, Ill.). (B) Dry hands thoroughly, because moist hands will impair glove positioning; always maintain hands between waist and chin for sterility. (C) Pick up the gown from the sterile field from the inside surface of the gown; step back from the sterile field, allowing the gown to unfold from the body; and place arms into the sleeves of the gown. (D) When gown is in the ideal position, hands are at the seam of the inside cuff. Keep hands between waist and neck level to maintain sterility.

high tensile strength, low tissue reactivity, and be absorble or easily removed. The most common today include the use of PGA ("Vicryl"). A nonresorbable alternative would be a PTFE suture (e.g., Cytoplast), which exhibits a high tensile strength and is nonwicking.

Suture Size

Surgical threads are classified by diameter, ranging from 1 to 10, with the highest number being the smallest thread size. In implant dentistry the most common diameter is 3-0 for incision lines and 4-0 or 5-0 around tissue release margins or areas that exhibit thinner tissue. In some situations a 2-0 suture will be used, usually as a tie-back for the lingual tissue when performing mandibular surgery. Ideally the smallest-diameter suture material that will adequately hold the tissue in approximation should be used. As diameters of suture decrease, so do their respective tensile strengths (Fig. 26.48).

Suture Needle

The surgical needle is composed of three parts: (1) point, (2) needle body, and (3) swaged end. The needle type is classified by the curvature, radius, and shape. The most commonly used suture needles in implant dentistry are the 3/8 and 1/2 circle needles.[37] The 3/8 needle allows for the passage of the needle from buccal to lingual in one pass. The 1/2 is usually used in more restrictive

areas such as maxillary molars and in periosteal and mucogingival surgery.[39] The clinician should always be aware that there exist two types of needle designs: reverse cutting and conventional. In implant dentistry the reverse cutting should always be used because this will minimize severing of the tissues. The reverse cutting needle has a smooth inner curvature, with its third cutting edge located on its convex (outer) edge (Fig. 26.49).

Suturing Technique

Interrupted

Simple loop. The simple loop is the most common suture used in implant dentistry. It is used to approximate mobile surgical flaps in edentulous areas. Each suture is tied and cut after insertion through the tissue. The disadvantage of this suture is it is more time consuming than a continuous suture. However, it does have the advantage that, if one of the sutures would loosen or break, the remaining sutures would most likely hold the wound together to minimize wound dehiscence (Fig. 26.50).

Figure-eight. The figure-eight suture is placed as a simple loop on the buccal; however, on the lingual the needle passes through the outer aspect of the flap. The main disadvantage of the figure-eight is the suture material is interposed between the flaps after full closure. The figure-eight suture is most commonly used with extraction sites and around papilla (Fig. 26.51).

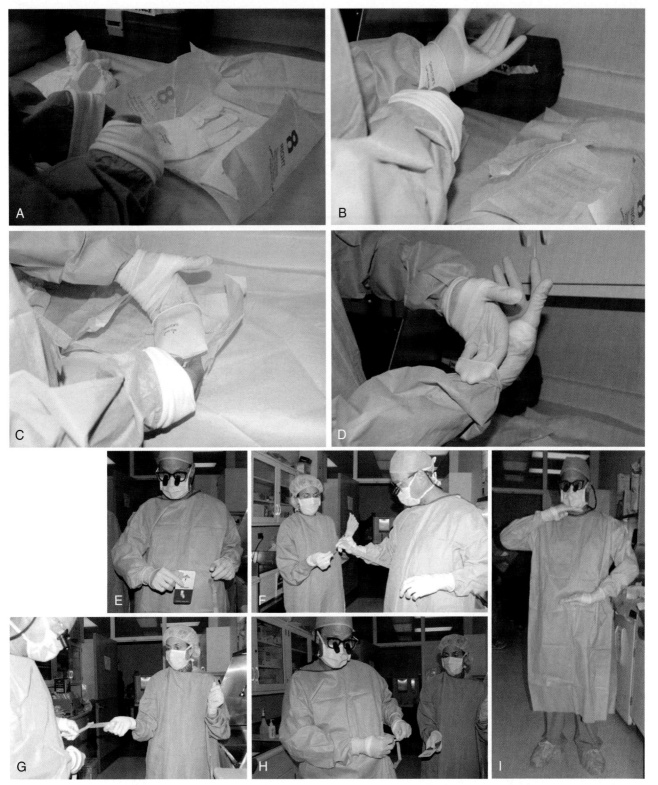

• **Fig. 26.44** Gloving and Gown Tying. (A) Pick up the first glove by the cuff, touching only the inside portion of the cuff. (B) While holding the cuff in one hand, slip your other hand into the glove. (C) Pick up the second glove by sliding the fingers of the gloved hand under the cuff of the second glove. (D) Put the second glove on the ungloved hand by using the cuff. (E) The surgeon holds left string (short) with left hand, holds tag and right string (long) with right hand, then pulls off tag with right hand. (F) The surgeon hands the tag to the assistant. (G) The surgeon spins around 360 degrees, and the assistant hands the long string to the surgeon, who ties the front of the gown. (H) The surgeon ties the front ties, and the assistant or circulator ties the Velcro back. (I) The surgeon is gowned and the hands sure below the sterile area. The sterile area is below the axilla and above the waist.

TABLE 26.2 Suture Materials Used in Oral Implantology

Suture	Types	Color of Material	Raw Material	Tensile Strength Retention In Vivo	Absorption Rate	Tissue Reaction	Contraindications	Warnings
Surgical gut	Plain	Yellowish-tan, Blue dyed	Collagen derived from healthy mammals (i.e., cow, sheep)	Lost within 3–5 days; individual patient characteristics can affect rate of tensile strength loss	Digested by proteolytic body enzymes within 7–10 days	Moderate	Should not be used in tissues that heal slowly and require support or under high-tension areas	Absorbs relatively quickly
Surgical gut	Chromic	Brown, Blue dyed	Collagen derived from healthy mammals (i.e., cow, sheep); treated to resist digestion by body tissues	Lost within 7–10 days; individual patient characteristics can affect rate of tensile strength loss	Digested by body enzymes within 7–10 days	Moderate, but less than plain surgical gut	Being absorbable, should not be used where prolonged approximation of tissues under stress is required	Protein-based absorbable sutures have a tendency to fray when tied
Coated VICRYL (polyglactin 910)	Braided	Violet undyed (natural)	Copolymer of lactide and glycolide coated with polyglactin 370 and calcium stearate	Approximately 60% remains at 2 weeks; approximately 30% remains at 3 weeks (dependent on the type)	Minimal until about 40th day; essentially complete between 60 and 90 days; absorbed by slow hydrolysis	Mild	Even though a high tensile strength, may not be sufficient for high-stress areas	None known
PDS (polydioxanone)	Monofilament	Violet, Clear	Polyester polyethylene terephthalate coated with polybutilate	Approximately 70% remains at 2 weeks; approximately 50% remains at 4 weeks; approximately 25% remains at 6 weeks	Minimal until about 90th day; essentially complete within 210 days; absorbed by slow hydrolysis	Slight	Being absorbable, should not be used where prolonged approximation of tissues under stress is required	None known
Surgical silk	Braided	Black, White	Natural protein fiber of raw silk spun by silkworm (i.e., fibroin)	Loses all or most in about 1 year	Usually cannot be found after 2 years; encapsulation by fibrous connective tissue may result	Acute inflammatory reaction	Should not be used in any area where suture removal would be difficult	Slowly absorbs, tissue reaction
e-PTFE (expanded polytetrafluoroethylene)	Monofilament	White	Cytoplast	Nonresorbable	Nonresorbable	Biologically inert, Comfortable to patients	None	None
Surgical steel	Monofilament, Multifilament	Silver metallic	An alloy of iron-nickel-chromium	Indefinite	Nonabsorbable: remains encapsulated in body tissues	Low	Should not be used when a prosthesis of another alloy is implanted	May corrode and break at points of bending, twisting, and knotting

TABLE 26.2 Suture Materials Used in Oral Implantology—cont'd

Suture	Types	Color of Material	Raw Material	Tensile Strength Retention In Vivo	Absorption Rate	Tissue Reaction	Contraindications	Warnings
ETHILON nylon	Monofilament	Black Green Clear	Polyamide polymer	Loses 15%–20% per year	Degrades at a rate of about 15%–20% per year	Extremely low	None	None
NUROLON nylon	Braided	Black White	Polyamide polymer	Loses 15%–20% per year	Degrades at a rate of about 15%–20% per year	Extremely low	None	None
MERSILENE polyester fiber	Braided	Green White	Polyester polyethylene terephthalate	Indefinite	Nonabsorbable: remains encapsulated in body tissues	Minimal	None	None
ETHIBOND polyester fiber	Braided	Green White	Polyester polyethylene terephthalate coated with polybutilate	Indefinite	Nonabsorbable: remains encapsulated in body tissues	Minimal	None	Has not been evaluated in ophthalmic surgery
PROLENE polypropylene	Monofilament	Clear blue	Polymer of propylene	Indefinite	Nonabsorbable: remains encapsulated in body tissues	Minimal transient acute inflammatory reaction	None	None

Adapted from Suzuki JB, Resnik RR. Wound dehiscence: incision line opening. In: Resnik RR, Misch CE, eds: *Misch's Avoiding Complications in Oral Implantology.* St. Louis, MO: Mosby; 2018.

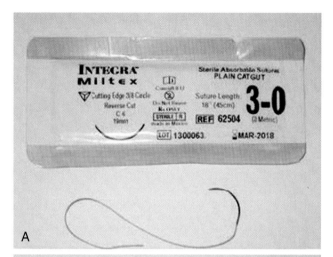

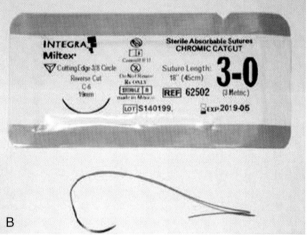

• **Fig. 26.45** Resorbable fast-resorbing sutures (Integra LifeSciences, Plainsboro, N.J.) with low tensile strength. (A) Plain gut. (B) Chromic gut.

Second-Stage Surgery: Permucosal Abutment Suturing. A modification of the interrupted suture may be completed on second-stage surgery with a permucosal abutment that has a suture groove. A suture groove 3 to 5 mm above the platform connection may be incorporated in the healing abutment (e.g., External implant system, previously known as the Maestro dental system [BioHorizons IPH, Inc.]) (Fig. 26.52). When the tissue requires apical repositioning or when it is 3 to 4 mm thick and may grow over the healing abutment, the suture groove may be used. A suture is placed next to the healing abutment. Tissue forceps lift the suture from the incision line, and the suture is then rotated to form a loop. The loop is placed over the enlarged healing abutment and into the suture groove or under the healing cap. The suture may then be tied, securing the tissue at the height of the suture groove. A similar technique is used on the other side of the healing abutment. These two sutures (one on each side) hold the tissue at the level of the suture groove and prevent it from lifting up and over the healing cap during soft tissue healing.

Continuous

Soft tissue spans necessitating four or more interrupted sutures are best approximated with continuous nonlocking sutures. This suture design places less tension on the suture line and soft tissue, and allows faster vascularization of the reflected soft tissue flaps. However, whether locking or nonlocking, this suture knot has a tendency to loosen with uneven distribution of tension, which results in a compromise to the integrity of the suture knot (Fig. 26.53).

Horizontal/Vertical Mattress

Mattress sutures are a variation of the interrupted suture and are used most commonly where there exists muscle pull or

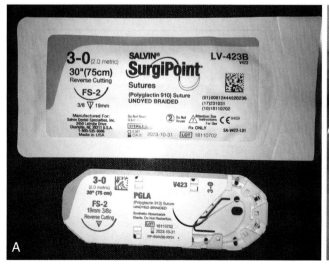

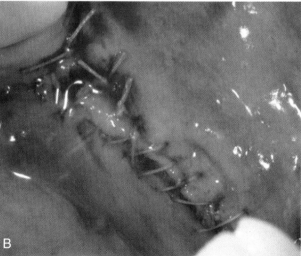

• **Fig. 26.46** Resorbable Fast-Resorbing Sutures With High Tensile Strength. (A) Synthetic absorbable suture: polyglycolic acid (PGA) sutures, which are supplied in various resorption rates (Salvin, Charlotte, N.C.). (B) Clinical image of PGA suture, which has the advantage of being resorbable with excellent tensile strength.

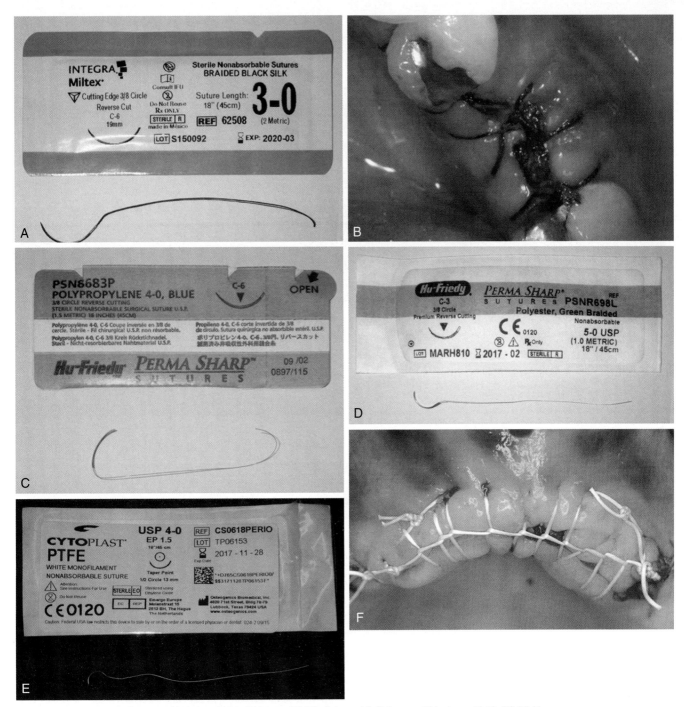

• **Fig. 26.47** Nonabsorbable Sutures. (A) Silk (Integra LifeSciences, Plainsboro, N.J.). (B) Wicking present on silk sutures. (C) Polypropylene (Hu-Friedy, Chicago, Ill.). (D) Polyester (Hu-Friedy, Chicago, Ill.). (E) Polytetrafluoroethylene (PTFE) (Osteogenics Biomedical, Lubbock, Tex.). (F) Clinical image of PTFE suture that exhibits exceptional tensile strength.

high tension. This type of suturing technique will evert the surgical wound edges, which keeps the epithelium away from underlying structures and maintains the tissue flaps to the underlying structures (i.e., dental implant, graft material, membrane).[40]

There are two types of mattress suture, horizontal and vertical. Both of these suture types allow for greater tension to be applied on the soft tissue closure without risk for tearing the soft tissue flap. It should be emphasized they are not used to obtain primary closure when tension on the soft tissue flaps is present at surgery. The tissues should rest passively together before suturing. However, during functional/parafunctional movement of the tissues, the tension on the incision line may be reduced with a horizontal mattress suture. They are often used in the mandible when the floor of the mouth is in proximity to the lingual flap and the tissue is thin. They may also be used on a facial flap with a strong muscle pull on the soft tissue. In addition, horizontal mattress sutures evert the soft tissue margin and ensure primary closure without epithelium entrapment. A combination of a few horizontal mattress sutures with a continuous suture may be indicated to close large soft tissue spans (Figs. 26.54 and 26.55; Box 26.10).

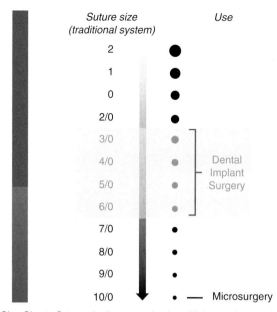

• **Fig. 26.48** Suture Size Chart. Suture size increases in size with increasing number. The most common suture size in oral implantology is 3-0 and 4-0. For finer tissue procedures, 5-0 and 6-0 are most commonly used.

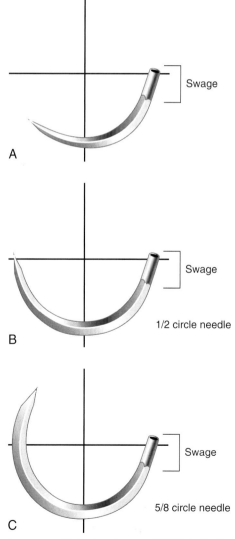

• **Fig. 26.49** Common needle sizes used in implant dentistry: (A) 3/8 circle; (B) 1/2 circle; and (C) 5/8 circle. (*From Suzuki JB, Resnik RR. Wound dehiscence: incision line opening. In: Resnik RR, Misch CE, eds. Misch's Avoiding Complications in Oral Implantology. St. Louis, MO: Mosby; 2018.*)

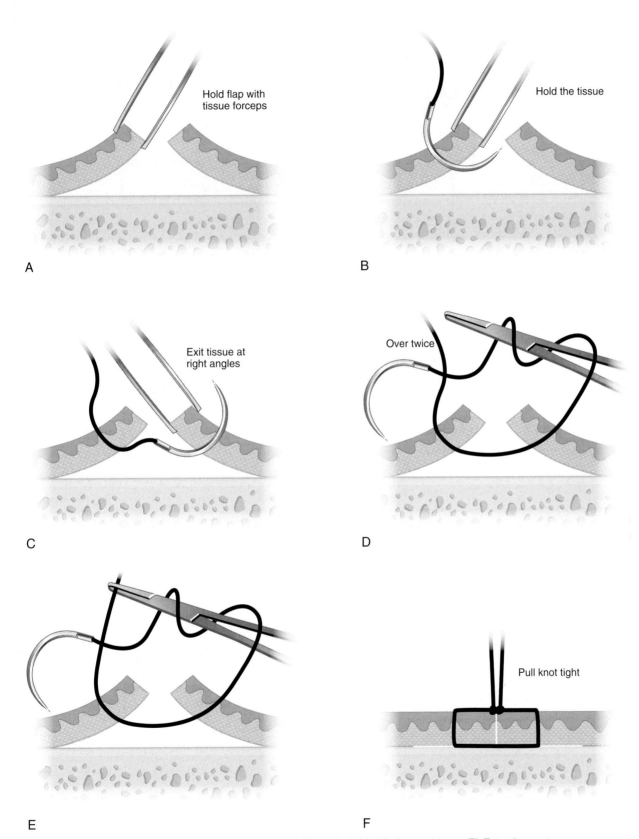

Hold flap with
tissue forceps

A

Hold the tissue

B

Exit tissue at
right angles

C

Over twice

D

Pull knot tight

E

F

• **Fig. 26.50** Simple Interrupted Suture. (A) Tissue is held with tissue pickups. (B) Enter tissue at a 90-degree angle. (C) Exit tissue at a 90-degree angle. (D) Two throws over needle holders. (E) Needle holders engage the opposite end of the suture. (F) The first knot is pulled tight to lay flat.

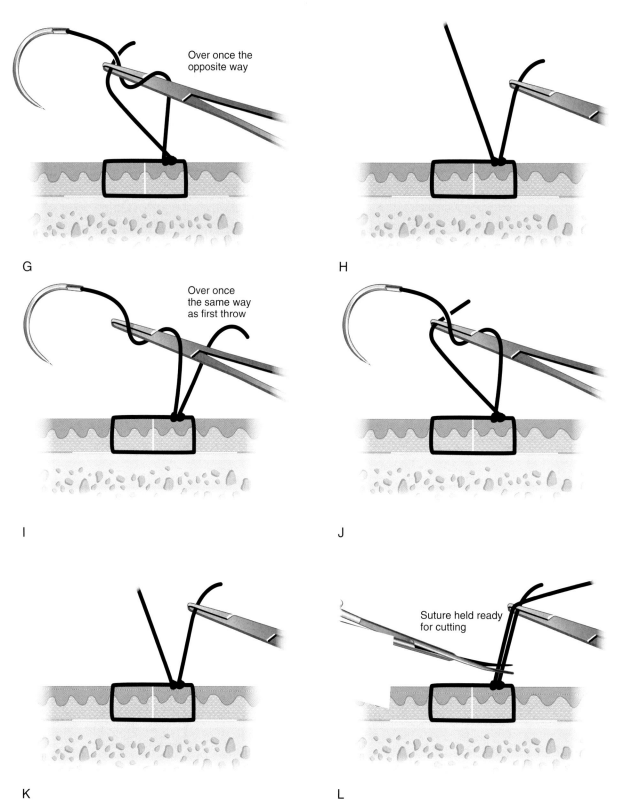

G

Over once the opposite way

H

I

Over once the same way as first throw

J

K

L

Suture held ready for cutting

Fig. 26.50, cont'd (G) One throw the opposite way from the first throw. (H) Second knot is secured. (I) One throw the same way as the first throw. (J) Needle holders engage opposite end of suture. (K) Third knot secured. (L) Suture ends are cut approximately 3 mm in length. (*From Suzuki JB, Resnik RR. Wound dehiscence: incision line opening. In: Resnik RR, Misch CE, eds.* Misch's Avoiding Complications in Oral Implantology. *St Louis, MO: Mosby; 2018.*)

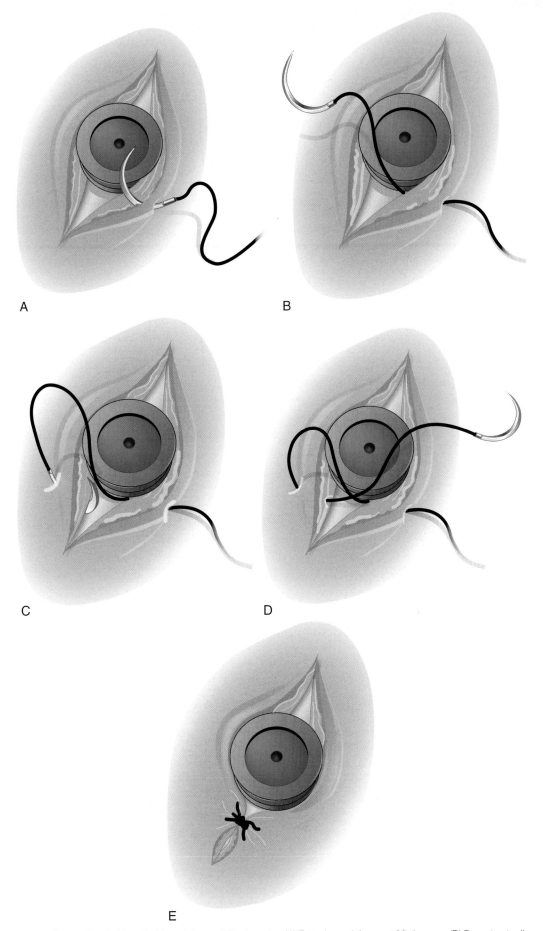

A

B

C

D

E

• **Fig. 26.51** Figure-Eight Suture That Is Usually Placed Around Abutments. (A) Enter buccal tissue at 90 degrees. (B) Do not enter lingual flap. (C) Enter from lingual at 90 degrees. (D) Do not enter buccal flap. (E) Tie suture ends. (*From Suzuki JB, Resnik RR. Wound dehiscence: incision line opening. In: Resnik RR, Misch CE, eds.* Misch's Avoiding Complications in Oral Implantology. *St. Louis, MO: Mosby; 2018.*)

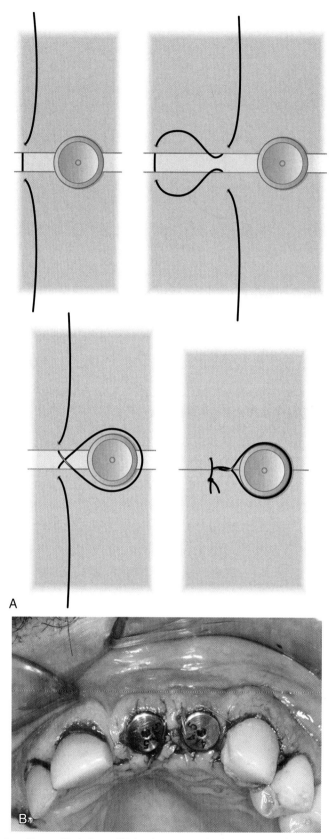

A

B

• **Fig. 26.52** Suture Groove Technique. (A) A suture groove in the permucosal extension may be positioned 3 to 5 mm above the bone. (B) The suture groove helps to apically reposition the tissue, so it will remain less than 3 to 5 mm thick, therefore to reduce the sulcus depth.

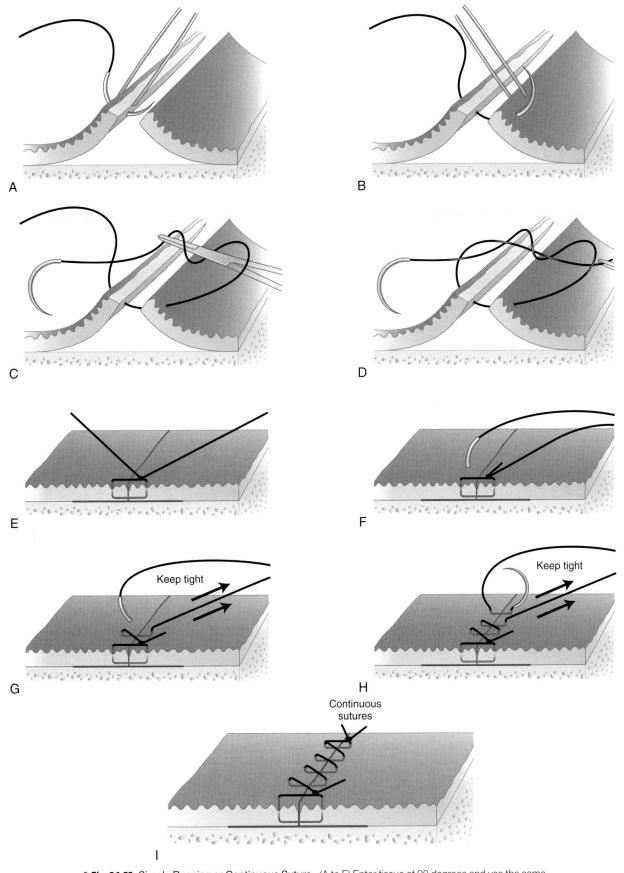

• **Fig. 26.53** Simple Running or Continuous Suture. (A to E) Enter tissue at 90 degrees and use the same protocol as a simple interrupted suture. (F) Instead of both strands (ends) being cut, cut only the short strand, leaving a 2- to 3-mm tail. The second stitch should be made approximately 3 mm from the first suture. (G and H) Multiple stitches are made encompassing the entire incision line. (I) The last stitch is not pulled completely through the tissue. Instead the loop is held with the needle holder and used as the short strand to tie off the distal end of the suture closure.

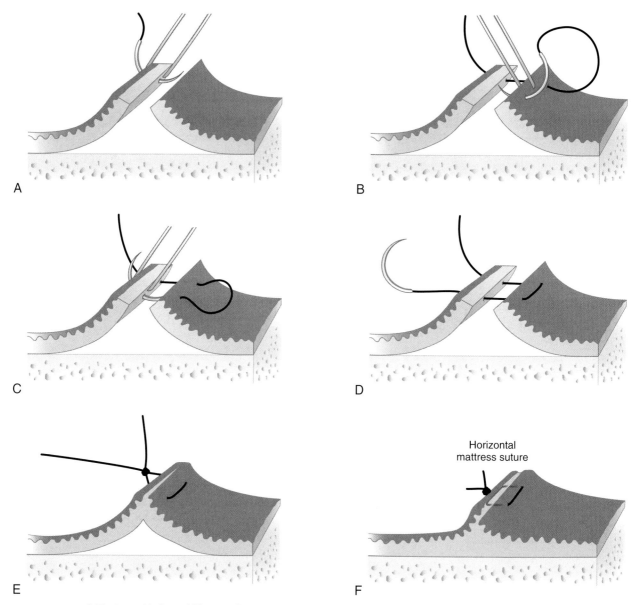

A

B

C

D

E

F

• **Fig. 26.54** Horizontal Mattress Suture. (A) The needle enters the tissue at 90 degrees and exits on the lingual side of the incision. (B to E) The needle is then placed backward in the needle holder and is inserted approximately 4 mm farther down from the first stitch. The needle passes from the far side to the near side (buccal). (F) The suture is then tied gently on the side of the wound where the suturing originated.

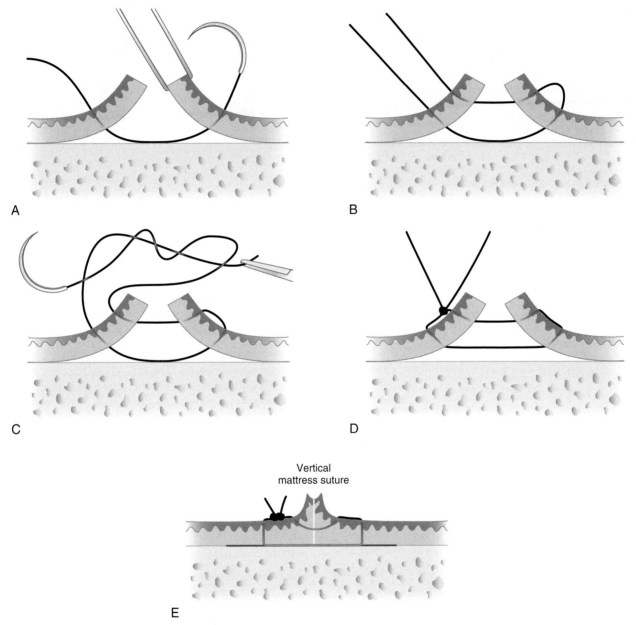

A

B

C

D

Vertical
mattress suture

E

• **Fig. 26.55** Vertical Mattress Suture (Far-Far-Near-Near). (A) The needle should enter the tissue at 90 degrees approximately 5 to 6 mm from the margin of the incision and exits on the opposite side (same distance on the lingual aspect of the tissue as the facial). (B and C) The needle is placed backward in the needle holder and enters the lingual tissue toward the buccal (approximately the distance from the incision line). (D and E) The stitch is then tied off on the facial aspect.

• BOX 26.10 Basic Suturing Principles

1. Suture from mobile to immobile tissues: This allows for better control and manipulation of the tissue.
2. Do not hold needle at swage: This may result in bending of the needle.
3. Enter tissue at 90 degrees: This allows for easier passage of the needle through the tissue and prevents tearing.
4. Keep fingers in needle holder (index finger for security): Usually the thumb and index fingers are used to hold the needle holder. The fingers should always remain in the needle holders because this will expedite the suturing process, along with allowing for better control.
5. Enter 2 to 3 mm and exit from tissue margin: Less than 2 mm will lead to tearing of the tissue margin.
6. Suture 3 to 5 mm apart: Too many sutures will impair blood supply to the incision line and increase possibility of incision line opening (ILO).
7. First throw must lie flat: After the first loop is tied, it is mandatory the loop lie flat. If folded, the loop will lose tension and knot security will be lost. Final tension of the first tie should be as horizontal as possible.
8. Avoid excessive tension: Tying knots too tight leads to tissue ischemia and ILO. Knot tension should not cause tissue blanching. In tying the knot, a "sawing" motion should be avoided because this may result in weakening the integrity of the suture.
9. Evert tissue, not invert: This makes it less likely that ILO will occur.
10. Cut sutures approximately 2 to 3 mm at completion of knot: Less than 2 mm leads to loss of knot tension, and more than 3 mm leads to patient irritation. When the ends are too long, patients will tend to irritate the area with their tongue.
11. Complete knot: The final knot should be tight and firm so that slippage will not occur. Ideally the smallest knot possible should be used to prevent tissue and foreign body reactions.

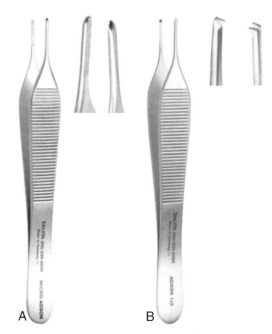

• **Fig. 26.56** Tissue Pickups. (A) Serrated. (B) 1 Å~ 2 tips. (*Courtesy Salvin Dental Specialties, Inc., Charlotte, N.C.*)

Suturing Instruments

It is imperative that the implant clinician has a complete understanding of the instrumentation used in the suturing technique.

Tissue Pickups

The goal of the tissue pickup is to hold tissue (i.e., flap) while suturing. Care should be exercised not to crush or sever the tissue. There are various types of tissue pickups, with the serrated being the most popular. The 1 x 2 teeth pick-ups will usually result in tearing of the tissue, especially when the tissue is thin (Fig. 26.56).

Needle Holders

Most needle holders are made from stainless steel, titanium, and tungsten carbide tipped. The tungsten carbide tipped needle holders tend to deform the suture needle the least amount. Correct use of needle holders includes:

- Always use the appropriate-size needle holder for the size of the needle. The larger the needle size, the wider and heavier

the needle holders should be. In contrast, with thinner tissue with a smaller size needle and suture material, smaller, more delicate needle holders are recommended (e.g., Castroviejo).

- Avoid placement of the needle holders near the swage or eye of the needle. Needles should be grasped approximately one-fourth to half their length from the swaged area.
- Check the alignment of the needle holder tips, making sure there is no opening between the tips. The needle should not be able to rock, twist, or turn within the needle holder tips.
- Always close the needle holder on the first or second ratchet. If the needle is grasped too tightly, the needle may break or weaken. Hemostats should never be used as a replacement for needle holders because they will damage the suture needle and material (Fig. 26.57).

Suture Scissors

Many different types of scissors may be used in the suturing process. There are straight, curved, and special suture scissors that are used for cutting sutures, especially for removing sutures postoperatively (Fig. 26.58). When using suture scissors to cut the ends of the tied knot, make sure both tips of the scissors are visible to avoid inadvertently cutting tissue beyond the suture.

Suturing Knots

Surgical suture knot tying is the most important aspect of suturing and often the most common problematic area. Surgical knots in the oral cavity must be particularly secure to overcome the potential of loosening with saliva and normal function.[41] There are three components of a sutured knot: (1) loop, which is created by the knot; (2) knot, which is composed of multiple throws, each of which represents a weave of two strands; and (3) ears, which are composed of the cut ends of the suture.[41] For knots to be effective, they must contain all three parts and possess attributes of both knot security and loop security. Knot security is defined as the efficacy of the knot at resisting slippage when load is applied. This depends on three factors: friction, internal interference, and slack between suture throws.

Loop security is the ability to maintain a tight suture loop as a knot is tied.[42] Any tied knot may have good knot security but poor loop security (a loose suture loop). Loose suture loops may be ineffective in approximating tissue edges to be secured. Ideally the knot should have minimal volume and be tied so that it fails only by breakage, rather than by slippage. A three-throw surgeon's knot square (2/1/1) should be used.[43] Security of the knot will depend on the material used, the depth and location of the wound, and the amount of stress that will be placed on the wound postoperatively. Operator experience is an important factor because considerable variation may result between knots tied by different surgeons and even between knots tied by the same individual on different occasions (Fig. 26.59).[44]

Treatment Implications

The type of surgical knot is directly related to the suture material being used. When using silk, expanded PTFE, chromic, or plain gut, a slip (granny) knot should be used. With synthetic resorbable and nonabsorbable synthetic suture materials, a modified surgeon's knot is recommended.[45]

For most dental implant procedures the surgical knot of choice is the modified surgeon's knot. The basic surgeon's knot is composed of two overhand knots. The first overhand knot is a double (i.e., composed of two loops or throws) and the second overhand knot is a single (loop) wound in the opposite direction. Additional knot security can be achieved with the common modification to the surgeon's knot, consisting of the addition of a third knot (composed of two loops) in the same direction as the first loop.[46]

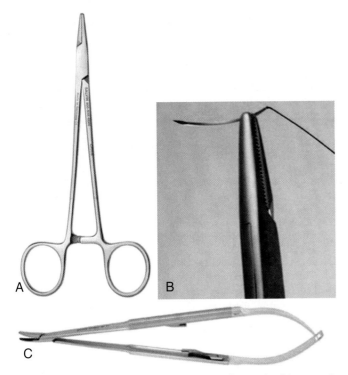

• **Fig. 26.57** Needle Holders for Suturing. (A) Convention Mayo needle holder. (B) Ideal needle holder placement. *(A and B: Courtesy Hu-Friedy Mfg. Co., LLC, Chicago, Ill.)* (C) Castroviejo needle holder.

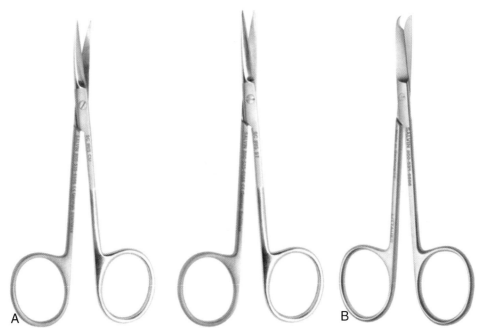

• **Fig. 26.58** (A) Various types of straight versus curved scissors. (B) Postoperative scissors. *(B: Courtesy Salvin Dental Specialties, Inc., Charlotte, N.C.)*

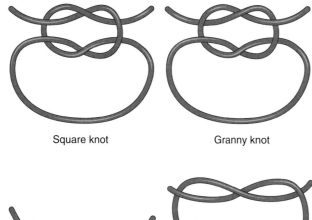

Square knot   Granny knot

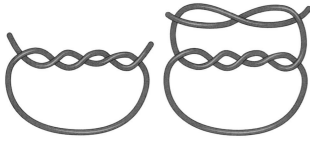

Surgeon's knot

• **Fig. 26.59** Various Suture Knot Types. Most knots in implant dentistry use a modification of the surgeon's knot. (*From Suzuki JB, Resnik RR. Wound dehiscence: incision line opening. In: Resnik RR, Misch CE, eds.* Misch's Avoiding Complications in Oral Implantology. *St. Louis, MO: Mosby; 2018.*)

References

1. Cameron J. Williams Stewart Halsted: Our Surgical Heritage. *Ann Surg.* 1997;225(5). 265–258.
2. Mormann W, Ciancio SG. Blood supply of human gingiva following periodontal surgery. A fluoresceinangiographic study. *J Periodontol.* 1977;48:681–692.
3. Froum SJ, Wang WC, Hafez T, et al. Incision design and soft tissue management to maintain or establish an interproximal papilla around integrated implants: a case series. *Int J Periodontics Restorative Dent.* 2018;38(1):61–69.
4. Tsutsui J, Wang J, Suzuki M, et al. Incision Design and Soft Tissue Management to Establish an Interproximal Papilla Around Integrated Implants: A Case Series. *Int J Periodontics Restorative Dent.* 2018;38(1):61–69.
5. Hunt BW, Sandifer JB, Assad DA, Gher ME. Effect of flap design on healing and osseointegration of dental implants. *Int J Periodontics Restorative Dent.* 1996;16(6).
6. Hupp J. Principles of more complex exodontia. In: *Contemporary Oral and Maxillofacial Surgery.* Elsevier; 2014.
7. Hunt WB, Sandifer JB, Assad DA, Gher ME. Effect of flap design on healing and osseointegration of dental implants. *Int J Periodontics Restorative Dent.* 1996;16:583–593.
8. Pfeifer J. The reaction of alveolar bone to flap procdeures in man. *Periodontics.* 1965;3:135–141.
9. Burkhardt R, Lang NP. Role of flap tension in primary wound closure of mucoperiosteal flaps: a prospective cohort study. *Clin Oral Implants Res.* 2010;21(1):50–54.
10. Koymen R, Karacayli U, Gocmen-Mas N, et al. Flap and incision design in implant dentistry: clinical and anatomical study. *Surg Radiol Anat.* 2009;31(4):301–306.
11. Hermann JS, Buser D. Guided bone regeneration for dental implants. *Curr Opin Periodontol.* 1996;3:168–177.
12. Velvert P, Peters IC, Peters AO. Soft tissue management: flap design, incision, tissue elevation, and tissue retraction. *Endodontic Topics.* 2005;11:78–97.
13. de Sanctis M, Clementini M. Flap approaches in plastic periodontal and implant surgery: critical elements in design and execution. *J Clin Periodontol.* 2014.
14. Greenstein G, Greenstein B, Cavallaro J, Elian N, Tarnow D. Flap advancement: practical techniques to attain tension-free primary closure. *J Periodontol.* 2009;80(1):4–15.
15. Zarb GA, Albrektsson T, Branemark PI. *T Issue-Integrated Prostheses: Osseointegration in Clinical Dentistry Illinois.* Quintessnce; 1985.
16. Buser D, Dahlin C, Schenk R. *Guided Bone Regeneration.* Chicago: Quintessence; 1994.
17. Langer B, Langer L. Overlapped flap: a surgical modification for implant fixture installation. *Int J Periodontics Restorative Dent.* 1990;10:208–215.
18. Misch CE. Bone augmentation for implant placement: keys to bone grafting. In: Misch CE, ed. *Contemporary Implant Dentistry.* 2nd ed. St Louis: Mosby; 1999. 421–267.
19. Park JC, Kim CS, Choi SH, et al. Flap extension attained by vertical and periosteal-releasing incisions: a prospective cohort study. *Clin Oral Implants Res.* 2012;23:993–998.
20. Oliver R. Flapless dental implant surgery may improve hard and soft tissue outcomes. *J Evid Based Dent Pract.* 2012;12(3):87–88.
21. Sclar AG. Guidelines for flapless surgery. *J Oral Maxillofac Surg.* 2007;65:20–32.
22. Misir AF, Sumer M, Yenisey M, Ergioglu E. Effect of surgical drill guide on heat generated from implant drilling. *J Oral Maxillofac Surg.* 2009;67:2663–2668.
23. Greenstein G, Tarnow D. Using papillae-sparing incisions in the esthetic zone to restore form and function. *Compendium.* 2014.
24. Park JC, Kim CS, Choi SH, et al. Flap extension attained by vertical and periosteal-releasing incisions: a prospective cohort study. *Clin Oral Implants Res.* 2012;23:993–998.
25. Hutchens LH, Beauchamp SD, Mcleod SH, et al. Considerations for Incision and Flap Design With Implant Therapy in the Esthetic Zone. *Implant Dentistry.* 2018;27(3):381–387.
26. Zadeh HH. Minimally invasive treatmetn of maxillary anterior gingival recession defects by vestibular incision subperiosteal tunnel access and platelet derived growth factor BB. *Int J Periodontics Restorative Dent.* 2011;31:653–660.
27. Kleinheinz J, Buchter A, Kruse-Losler B, Weingart D, Joos U. Incision design in implant dentistry based on vascularization of the mucosa. *Clin Oral Impl Res.* 2005;16:518–523.
28. Flanagan D. An incision design to promote a gingival base for the creation of interdental implant papillae. *J Oral Implantol.* 2002;28:25–28.
29. Al-Juboori MJ, bin Abdulrahaman S, Dawood HF. Principles of flap design in dental implantology. *Dent Implantol Update.* 2012;23:41–44.
30. Peterson LJ, Ellis E, Hupp JR, et al. *Oral and Maxillofacial Surfery.* St Louis: Mosby; 1998.
31. Cavallaro J, Tsuji S, Chiu TS, Greenstein G. Management of the nasopalatine canal and foramen associated with dental implant therapy. *Compend Contin Educ Dent.* 2016;38(6):367–372.
32. Wound Closure Manual, Somerville, NJ: Ethicon Inc;1985:1–101.
33. Silverstein LH. *Principles of Dental Suturing: The Complete Guide to Surgical Closure.* Mahwah, NJ: Montage Medgia; 1999.
34. Engler RJ, Weber CB, Turnicky R. Hypersensitivity to chromated catgut sutures: a case report and review of the literature. *Ann Allergy.* 1986;56:317–320.
35. Manor A, Kaffe I. Unusual foreign body reaction to a braided silk suture: A case report. *J Periodontol* 1981;53:86–88.
36. Leknes KN, Selvig KA, Boe OE, et al. Tissue reactions to sutures in the presence and absence of antiinfective therapy. *J Clin Periodontol.* 2005;32:130–138.
37. Cohen ES. *Atlas of Cosmetic and Reconstructive Periodontal Surgery.* New York: PMPH-USA; 2007.
38. Lilly GE, Armstrong JH, Salem JE, et al. Reaction of oral tissues to suture materials, Part II. *Oral Surg Oral Med Oral Pathol.* 1968;26(4):592–599.

39. Silverstein LH. Suture selection for optimal flap closure and tissue healing. Perio-implant showcase. *Pract Periodontics Aesthet Dent.* 2005;16:2–3.
40. Silverstein LH, Kurtzman GM. A review of dental suturing for optimal soft-tissue management. *Compend Contin Educ Dent.* 2005;26:163–166.
41. Edlich RF, Rodeheaver GT, Morgan RF, et al. Principles of emergency wound management. *Ann Emerg Med.* 1988;17:1284–1302.
42. Burkhart SS, Wirth MA, Simonich M, et al. Knot security in simple sliding knots and its relationship to rotator cuff repair: how secure must the knot be? *Arthroscopy.* 2000;16:202–207.
43. Drake DB, Rodeheaver PF, Edlich RF, et al. Experimental studies in swine for measurement of suture extrusion. *J Long Term Eff Med Implants.* 2004;14(3):251–259.
44. Herrmann J. Tensile strength and knot security of surgical suture materials. *Am Surg.* 1971;37:209.
45. Silverstein LH. *Principles of Dental Suturing: The Complete Guide to Surgical Closure.* New York: Montage Media; 1999.
46. Alzacko SM, Majid OW. "Security loop" tie: a new technique to overcome loosening of surgical knots. *Oral Surg Oral Med Oral Pathol Oral Radiol Endod.* 2007;104:e1–e4.

27

Implant Placement Surgical Protocol

RANDOLPH R. RESNIK

Pre-Implant Placement Protocols

The technique for dental implant surgery has evolved over the years from the original protocol pioneered in the 1970s by Per-Ingvar Brånemark, a Swedish physician and researcher. With Brånemark's delayed approach, implant placement was completed, then after a healing period, the implants were exposed and prosthetically rehabilitated. Today, with the integration of computer and digitized technology, dental implant clinicians now have a full array of choices with the placement of dental implants.

Flap Design

Prior to the placement of implants, the underlying bone and osteotomy site must be exposed for implant osteotomy preparation and insertion (Chapter 26).

Full-thickness flap: The most common technique includes a mucoperiosteal flap, which may involve the buccal, lingual, and crestal areas.

Flapless: This technique does not reflect the crestal soft tissue. Instead, a core of keratinized tissue (the size of the implant crest module diameter) is removed over the crestal bone. The implant osteotomy is then performed in the center of the core of the exposed bone. This protocol requires no sutures around the healing abutment after implant placement. The advantages of this technique include less discomfort, tenderness, and swelling, which are usually minimal.

The primary disadvantage of the flapless approach is the inability to assess the bone volume before or during the implant osteotomy or insertion. Therefore this technique should only be used when the bone width is abundant (>7 mm). In addition, bone grafting needs and procedures cannot be precisely evaluated. The soft tissue around the implant site should be ideal in the amount of attached keratinized mucosa because the soft tissue pouch is over the bone site, not in a region related to the soft tissue. Often, the keratinized tissue is reduced on the buccal half of the ridge and the tissue punch may inadvertently remove all the keratinized tissue on the facial aspect of the implant. Because the crest of the ridge is below the soft tissue, it is difficult to see lines on the drill to access the depth of drilling. Therefore stops on the drill are particularly beneficial. The clinician may have difficulty in assessing the location of the implant crest module in relation to the crest of bone because it is also below the soft tissue. And lastly, the interdental papillae may not be elevated with this technique. Therefore the soft tissue drape should be ideal in volume of keratinized tissue, both faciolingually and mesiodistally.

Surgical Approaches

Freehand surgery: This may include the flap or flapless technique, with the clinician placing the implant with the diagnostic information available (i.e., position of adjacent teeth, radiographs). Freehand surgery may include the use of nonlimiting surgical templates, which allow the surgeon the dimensional variability in implant location because the template will indicate the position of the final prosthesis; however, it will not specifically guide the placement of the implant (see Chapter 15 for surgical approaches).

Guided: This type of surgery, which may be performed flap or flapless, guides the osteotomy from a digitally designed and printed surgical template. This type of surgery allows the highest level of precision and control because the implant position is dictated via a comprehensive three-dimensional evaluation of the anatomy. Guided surgery may be differentiated by the type of support of the template:

Bone supported: The template rests on the alveolar bone and this technique requires the reflection of a full thickness flap.

Tissue (mucosa) supported: The template is supported by the soft tissue. This type of template is most commonly used with a flapless technique.

Tooth-supported: This is the most accurate technique and includes placement of the template directly on the natural teeth for support.

Guided surgery may also be classified according to the amount of drill guidance:

Pilot template: Allows guidance for the position and angulation for only the first drill in the surgical protocol. After the first drill, the osteotomy is completed freehand.

Universal template: This type of template is compatible with all implant systems and allows for depth, position, and angulation. However, the final osteotomy drill, along with implant placement, is completed freehand.

Fully guided template: Template that allows for depth, position, angulation, and implant placement via the guide.

Navigational directed surgery: Computerized navigation surgery has evolved from neurosurgical procedures into the field of dental implantology. This technique allows the clinician to precisely transfer a detailed presurgical implant plan to the patient. The clinician uses computerized navigation to adjust the position and angulation of the surgical drill according to the presurgical digital implant plan. The real-time imaging of the surgical drill allows for continuous updates on the positioning of the drill to avoid critical anatomic structures.

Dental Implant Osteotomy Preparation

Decreasing Heat During Osteotomy Preparation

The heat generated during an implant osteotomy is related to the presence and temperature of irrigation,[1-3] amount of bone being prepared,[4,5] drill sharpness and design,[5,6] time of preparation,[7] depth of the osteotomy,[8,9] pressure on the drill,[5] drill speed,[10] and variation in cortical thickness (bone density).[11]

Bone cell survival is very susceptible to heat. Eriksson has demonstrated that, in animal studies, bone temperature as low as 3°C above normal (40°C) can result in bone cell necrosis.[12] Therefore a conscious effort is made to control temperature elevation every time a rotary instrument is placed in contact with bone. Many dental implant preparation variables need to be addressed in understanding the reduction of heat during the osteotomy process.

Irrigation versus No Irrigation

Although some authors have advocated implant osteotomy preparation without irrigation, the literature does not support it.[13] Yacker and colleagues showed that, without irrigation, drill temperatures greater than 100°C are reached within seconds of the osteotomy, and consistent temperatures greater than 47°C are measured several millimeters away from the implant osteotomy.[14] Benington and colleagues have reported that the osteotomy temperature may rise up to 130.1°C without irrigation after monitoring changes in bone temperature during the sequence of drilling for implant site preparation.[15]

To minimize heat generation, at least 50 mL/min of cooled irrigation of sterile saline (0.9% NaCl) should be used as a profuse irrigant and is a critical factor in the osteotomy process. The more dense the bone, the greater the need for copious irrigation. Distilled water should not be used because rapid cell death may occur in this medium.[4,9] The irrigant also may act as a lubricant and removes bone particles from the implant osteotomy site. The temperatures of the irrigant can also affect the bone temperature. Barrak and colleagues reported that cooling the irrigation fluid to 10°C, no mean temperature change >1°C will occur. Therefore placing the irrigation fluid into a refrigerator before implant surgery will help to prevent heat generation during implant placement[16,17] (Fig. 27.1).

Graduated versus One-Step Drilling

The amount of heat produced in the bone is directly related to the amount of bone removed by each drill.[18] For example, a 2-mm pilot drill generates greater heat than a 1.5-mm pilot drill.[4] As a result, most manufacturers suggest that the first drill (pilot) should be approximately 1.5 mm in diameter. In a similar fashion, the amount of heat generated by successive drills is also directly related to the increase in drill diameter.[19] For example, a 3-mm drill after a 2-mm drill removes 0.5 mm on each side of the drill. A 2.5-mm drill after a 2-mm drill only cuts 0.25 mm of bone on each side of

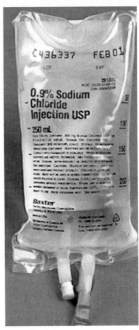

● **Fig. 27.1** Irrigation should use 0.9% NaCl (sterile saline), which may be cooled to reduce heat generation. The irrigation bags may be stored in a refrigerator.

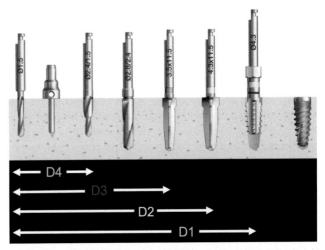

● **Fig. 27.2** Number of steps in the preparation of the osteotomy is related to the bone density. Usually D1 will require all drills including the bone tap, the D2 protocol uses all drills except the bone tap, D3 requires the standard protocol stopping at the second to last drill, and D4 uses only the first or second drills.

the osteotomy. The smaller incremental drill size allows the clinician to prepare the site faster, with less pressure and less heat generation.[6] In addition, when larger increases in drill diameter are used to prepare bone, the clinician may inadvertently change the angulation of the drill because the larger drill is removing a greater bone volume and the tactile sense is decreased. As a result, an elliptical osteotomy may be prepared that does not correspond accurately to the round implant diameter. The gradual increase in osteotomy size also reduces the drill shatter at the crestal opening, which can inadvertently fragment the bony crest in which complete bony contact is especially desired. The gradual increase in drill diameter also maintains the sharpness of each drill for a longer period, which also reduces the heat generation (Fig. 27.2).

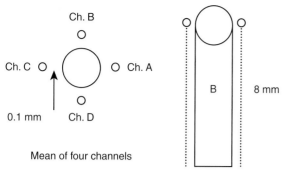

• **Fig. 27.3** Thermocouples were positioned within 1 mm of the drill site and inserted into bone for a depth of 8 mm. The wires were connected to a computer to measure the temperature, time of preparation, and time the bone temperature was elevated.

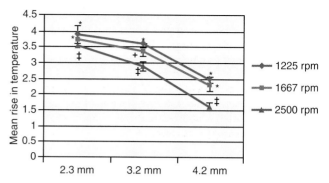

• **Fig. 27.4** Internally cooled drill of the Paragon implant system recorded 41°C with the first drill at 1225 rpm; 2500 rpm reduced the bone temperature preparation for all drill diameters.

Drilling Speed

The subject of drilling speed has become very controversial in implant dentistry today. Eriksson and colleagues originally recommended drilling speeds of 1500 to 2000 rotations per minute (rpm) with irrigation.[20] Most recently in implant dentistry, the rotational speed of the drill has been suggested to be less than 2000 rpm, and several manufacturers have recommended speeds as low as 50 rpm. Kim and colleagues suggested drilling osteotomies at 50 rpm without irrigation and stated that the bone temperature may not significantly increase.[13]

However, Yeniyol and colleagues showed that excessively low drilling speeds (less than 250 rpm) increased the degree of fragmentation of the osteotomy edge. It has been shown that low speed drills will "wobble," which leads to overpreparation of the osteotomy site.[21]

A controversial subject in implant dentistry is whether higher drilling speed is correlated with higher bone temperature during preparation. Although some reports have shown this, the majority of well-documented studies disprove this. For example, if high-speed preparation was detrimental, then slow-speed handpieces would be used to prepare natural teeth. A high-speed handpiece (~300,000 rpm) can remove bone over an impacted tooth or during an apicoectomy and still allow bone regeneration. Rafel prepared bone at 350,000 rpm in a human mandible and found a temperature of only 23.5°C at a distance of 3 mm from the drill periphery.[22] High-speed drills at 300,000 rpm have been used to prepare blade implant osteotomies for years, yet studies proved bone grew over the blade shoulder and was in direct contact with the implant.[23]

A study by Sharawy and colleagues compared four drill designs (two internal irrigated and two external irrigated) at speeds of 1225, 1667, and 2500 rpm.[4] Thermocouples connected to a computer to record temperature and time were placed within 1 mm of the osteotomy site in D2-type bone (Fig. 27.3). All drill designs in the study recorded lower bone temperatures with the greatest rotations per minute and, conversely, found the highest bone temperatures with the lowest rotations per minute (Figs. 27.4 and 27.5). As important, the slowest rotations per minute resulted in bone temperatures at or greater than 40°C, which may be a threshold of bone cell death. The highest rotations per minute (2500) increased the bone temperature by 2° to 3.5°C, whereas the 1225 rpm recorded a bone temperature greater than 41°C. Therefore the higher speed of 2500 rpm may prepare bone at a lower temperature than 1500 rpm, especially when in dense bone. The rotational speed of the drill is one of the more critical criteria to reduce bone temperatures.

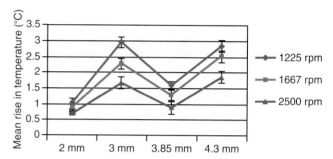

• **Fig. 27.5** Externally cooled drills of the Brånemark implant system recorded reduced temperatures at 2500 rpm, compared with slower speeds.

Sharawy and colleagues demonstrated that, regardless of the drill design or method of irrigation, 2500 rpm prepared bone at a lower temperature than slower speeds.[4] The clinician should allow the cutting surface of the drill to contact D1 and D2 bone fewer than 5 of every 10 seconds. Ideally, a pumping up-and-down motion (i.e., bone dancing) is used to prepare the osteotomy and provide constant irrigation to the drill cutting surface. It also maintains a constant drill speed and reduces the friction time against the bone, all of which reduce heat.

Drilling Time

Eriksson reported bone cell death when a temperature of 40°C was applied for 7 minutes, or when a temperature of 47°C was applied for 1 minute.[12] In other words, time and temperature are interrelated critical factors in implant site preparation. As the temperature increases, the time the bone temperature is elevated must be reduced. In the study by Sharawy and colleagues, the time the bone temperature remained elevated was recorded for each rotation per minute evaluated.[4] When the drill prepared an 8-mm depth osteotomy, the temperature remained elevated for 45 to 58 seconds (Fig. 27.6). The slower the rotations per minute (1225), the longer the bone temperature remained above the baseline. Because two to three drills are used to prepare an implant site, at 1225 rpm the first drill may increase the temperature to 41°C, the second drill to 45°C, and the third drill to 49°C, when the time between each sequence is not extended more than 1 minute. In the study by Sharawy and colleagues, the first drill diameter recorded the longest preparation time and the highest temperature, and the longest recovery time. Therefore to reduce the preparation time within the bone to a minimum in D1 bone, the clinician should not apply constant pressure to the drill, but "bone dance" with

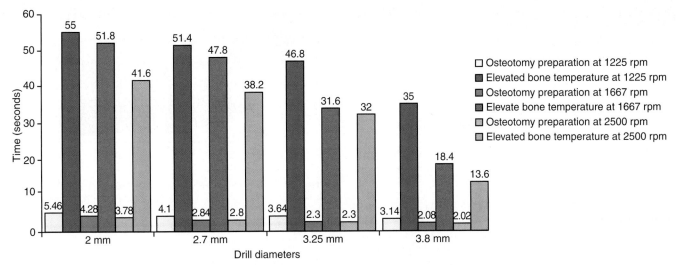

• **Fig. 27.6** Internally cooled drills of the Nobel Biocare, Steri-Oss implant system demonstrate the temperature in the bone remains elevated for an extended period (up to 58 seconds) after site preparations in D2 bone. The lower the rotations per minute are the longer the temperature remains elevated.

intermittent pressure for 1 second in the D1 bone and 1 to 2 seconds out of the bone while the cooled irrigation is allowed to perfuse the site.

In summary, in D1 and D2 bone, a higher speed (1500–2000 rpm) should be used in the preparation of bone. In poorer quality bone (e.g., D3 and D4) drilling speed is not as crucial, therefore a lower speed maybe use (~1000 rpm).

Drilling Pressure

The pressure exerted when preparing the osteotomy should not result in heat generation. Hobkirk and Rusiniak found that the average force placed on a handpiece during preparation of an osteotomy is 1.2 kg.[11] Matthews and Hirsch concluded that the force applied to the handpiece was more influential than the drill speed in temperature elevation.[24] When the pressure on the handpiece was increased appropriately, drill speeds from 345 to 2900 rpm did not affect the temperature. Matthews and Hirsch found that increasing both speed and pressure allowed the drill to cut more efficiently and generated less heat. The effect of drill speed and pressure related to bone temperature was also reported by Brisman.[10] In cortical bone, speeds of 1800 rpm with a load of 1.2 kg produced the same heat as when speed increased to 2400 rpm with a pressure of 2.4 kg. The greater speed and greater pressure was more efficient than low speeds. Increasing pressure alone increased heat; increasing speed alone also increased heat. Different amounts of pressure are therefore used in response to the density of the bone. Sufficient pressure should be used on the drill to proceed at least 2 mm every 5 seconds. If this is not achieved, then new (sharper) or smaller diameter drills are indicated for each site preparation. The pressure on the drills should not reduce the rotations per minute, which makes the drill less efficient and increases heat. Handpieces of sufficient torque should be used to prevent this complication.

Intermittent versus Continuous Drilling

When preparing an osteotomy site, continuous drilling (i.e., no pumping motion) results in numerous possible negative consequences. When constant pressure is applied, irrigation cannot enter the osteotomy site; therefore this may result in heat-related damage. In addition, by not removing the drill from the osteotomy site during preparation, bone debris is maintained within the flutes of the surgical burs, resulting in potential heat generation. This also leads to less efficient drilling.

When intermittent drilling or bone dancing (i.e., continuously bringing the surgical bur in and out of the osteotomy site), less heat generation is seen. By bringing the bur in and out of the osteotomy site, irrigation may enter the site along with allowing any debris to be removed, thus making the cutting process more efficient. The only disadvantage of the bone dancing technique is the possibility of changing angulation or inadvertent widening of the osteotomy site.[25] Care should be exercised in withdrawing and inserting the implant drill at the same trajectory or angulation.

Insertion Torque

The insertion torque (IT) is the force used to insert a dental implant into a prepared osteotomy. The amount of torque is expressed in units of newton centimeters (N/cm), which ultimately determines the loading protocol. IT is the primary most important factor in determining primary stability, with higher torque values leading to higher primary stability.[26]

Lower values of IT have been shown to be associated with implant failures.[27]

Many studies have indicated IT near the range of 35-45 N/cm to be ideal for implant integration.[28,29] To standardize the amount of torque, calibrated torque wrenches, physiodispenser instruments with integrated electronic torque control settings, and preset torque settings on the implant electric motor systems should be used (Box 27.1).

Bone Density Factors Related to Implant Preparation

As discussed in Chapter 18, the density of the available bone has a significant effect on the predictability and success of dental implants. In the past, clinical reports that did not alter the surgical and prosthetic protocol had variable survival rates. In this chapter, a generic surgical protocol will be discussed, which is directly

- **Irrigation:** copious amounts of 0.9% NaCl
- **Irrigation solution temperature:** refrigerate before use
- **Drilling technique:** graduated protocol (more drills)
- Intermittent (bone dancing)
- **Drilling speed:** D1, D2 bone is 1500–2000 rpm; D3, D4 bone is ~1000 rpm
- **Drilling time:** greater drilling time, greater heat generation
- **Drilling pressure:** minimize pressure, never allow rotations per minute to decrease from excess pressure
- **Insertion torque:** 35-45 N/cm

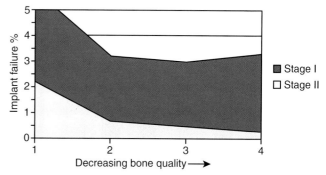

• **Fig. 27.7** A study by the Dental Implant Research Group represented 33 different hospitals that place dental implants. The highest surgical failure rate was quality 1 bone, followed by quality 4 bone. The fewest surgical failures were observed in quality 3 bone.

related to bone density that has been shown to increase success of dental implants.

The density of available bone in an edentulous site has a primary influence on treatment planning, implant design, surgical approach, healing time, and initial progressive bone loading during prosthetic reconstruction. The quality of the recipient bone directly influences the amount of trauma generated during osteotomy preparation. This in turn provokes a cascade of reactions at the bone–implant interface that directly affect the quality of the load-bearing surface.

Once the implant is initially integrated with the bone, the bone-loading process from occlusal forces becomes a critical factor in long-term implant survival. The bone density under load is directly related to the bone strength and is therefore a critical parameter for long-term survival.[30,31] The occlusal stresses applied through the implant to the bone must remain within the physiologic to mild overload zone; otherwise, pathologic overload with associated bone loss and microfracture leading to implant failure may occur. The treatment planning and scientific rationale of strength, modulus of elasticity, bone-implant contact (BIC) percentage, and stress transfer difference related to bone density has been addressed in Chapter 18. This chapter addresses the modifications of the surgical and healing aspects related to each bone density in the oral environment.

Literature Review

Lekholm and Zarb listed four bone qualities found in the anterior regions of the jawbone: quality 1, comprises homogeneous compact bone; quality 2, a thick layer of compact bone surrounding a core of dense trabecular bone; quality 3, a thin layer of cortical bone surrounding dense trabecular bone of favorable strength; and quality 4, a thin layer of cortical bone surrounding a core of low-density trabecular bone.[32] Irrespective of the different bone qualities, all bone was treated with the same implant design and standard surgical and prosthetic protocols.

After the proposed protocols of Brånemark and colleagues, it was found that implant survival in initial surgical success was related to the quality of bone.[33] A higher surgical failure was observed in softer bone types, especially in the maxilla. For example, Engquist reported the surgical loss of 38 of 191 implants in the maxilla in D4 bone (20% loss) compared with 8 of 148 mandibular implants (5% loss) before stage II surgery.[34] Jaffin and Berman reported an overall 8.3% surgical and initial healing loss in 444 maxillary implants with softer bone.[35] Friberg and colleagues reported a 4.8% implant failure at stage II uncovery for 732 maxillary posterior implants, which was greater than mandibular failure.[36] Quirynen et al. also reported a 4.1% implant loss at stage II uncovery out of 269 implants in the maxilla.[37] Fugazzotto and

colleagues reported 22 failures out of 34 implants placed in quality 4 bone.[38] Hutton and colleagues identified poor bone quantity and quality 4 as the highest risk of implant failure in a study of 510 implants, with an overall failure rate in the maxilla nine times greater than in the mandible.[39] Sullivan and colleagues indicated a 6.4% stage II failure rate in the maxilla (12/188) and a 3.2% failure in the mandible (7/216).[40] Snauwaert and colleagues reported more frequent early failures in poor density maxillae.[41] Herrmann and colleagues correlated failure factors such as poor bone quality and volume.[42] A number of reports in the literature demonstrated that the greatest risk of surgical failure was observed in the softest bone type (D4), especially when found in the maxilla.

On the other extreme, a large clinical study from 33 US Department of Veterans Affairs (VA) hospitals by the Dental Implant Clinical Research Group (DICRG) states quality 1 bone had the highest surgical failure rate (4.3%), followed by quality 4 (3.9%), quality 2 (2.9%), and quality 3 with the fewest failures at 2.6% (Fig. 27.7). The overall implant surgical failure was 3%; the maxilla had better success at stage II surgery (98.1%) than the mandible (96.4%).[43] It must be emphasized that these reports only present implant failures up to stage II uncovery. The DICRG also noted that the failure rate was twice as great for surgeons who had placed fewer than 50 implants, compared with more experienced surgeons. The literature contains many published reports that indicated an implant surgical failure range from 3.2% to 5% in the mandible and 1.9% to 20% in the maxilla, with most reports indicating the greatest failure rates in maxillary implants with soft bone. It is clear from these reports that a wide range of results may be achieved; therefore consideration should be given to methods that improve surgical survival.

Misch developed a different surgical protocol for different bone qualities in 1988. The Misch classification of bone density includes four classifications, D1, D2, D3, and D4, which are based on the amount of cortical and cancellous bone. D1 bone is primarily composed of dense cortical bone and found mainly in the anterior mandible, with basal bone. D2 bone has dense-to-porous cortical bone on the crest and, within the bone, has coarse trabecular bone. D3 bone types have a thinner porous cortical crest and fine trabecular bone in the region next to the implant. D4 bone has almost no crestal cortical bone. The fine trabecular bone composes almost all of the total volume of bone next to the implant.

After these specific methods, prospective and retrospective multicenter clinical studies in a wide range of office settings found surgical survival to be greater 99%, regardless of the density type of bone, the arch (mandible versus maxilla), and gender and age of

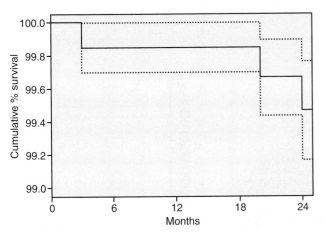

• **Fig. 27.8** Multicenter study reported a surgical success of 99.6%, regardless of bone quality. (Data from Misch CE, Hoar JB, Beck G, et al. A bone quality based implant system: a preliminary report of stage I and stage II. *Implant Dent.* 1998;7:35–42.)

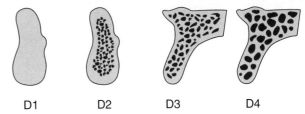

• **Fig. 27.9** Misch Classification for Bone Density. *D1,* dense cortical bone; *D2,* dense-to-porous cortical bone with coarse trabecular bone; *D3,* thinner porous cortical crest and fine trabecular bone; and *D4,* minimal crestal cortical bone with fine trabecular bone.

• BOX **27.2**   **Determination of Bone Density**

1. CBCT Radiographic (Hounsfield units)
2. Location
3. Past history of surgery in area
4. Tactile sensation

• BOX **27.3**   **Hounsfield Unit Numbers Related to Bone Density**

D1: >1250
D2: 850 – 1250
D3: 350 – 850
D4: 0 – 350

---

the patient.[44,45] Therefore a different surgical protocol for different bone densities appears warranted. The implant design, surgical protocol, healing, treatment plans, and progressive loading time spans are unique for each bone density type. More recently the use of improved rotary instruments, implant designs, and surgical approaches for different bone qualities has been recognized as a valid recommendation. A multicenter prospective clinical study by Misch and colleagues of 364 consecutive implants in 104 consecutive patients found a surgical survival rate (up to abutment connection) at stage II of 100% for D1, 98.4% for D2, 99.8% for D3, and 100% for D4 implants[46] (Fig. 27.8). Altering the surgical approach for each bone density can yield an overall implant surgical survival of 99.8% and a 2-year survival of 99.4%. In this chapter the surgical considerations and optimal healing time are discussed relative to each bone category, based on the literature, prospective clinical studies, and long-term experience.

Bone Density Classifications

Misch defined four bone density groups in all regions of the jaws that vary in both macroscopic cortical and trabecular bone types.[47] The regions of the jaws are divided into (1) the anterior maxilla (second premolar to second premolar), (2) posterior maxilla (molar region), (3) anterior mandible (first premolar to first premolar), and (4) posterior mandible (second premolar and molars). The regions of the jaws often have similar bone densities (Fig. 27.9).

In general, the anterior mandible is usually D2 bone, the posterior mandible is D3 bone, the anterior maxilla is D3 bone, and the posterior maxilla is often D4 bone. This generalization is used for the initial treatment plan. However, resorbed anterior mandibles may be D1 bone in approximately 25% of male patients and the posterior maxilla may have D3 bone after 6 months in the majority of sinus graft patients. The regional locations of the different densities of cortical bone are more consistent than the highly variable trabecular bone. Bone density may be most precisely determined before surgery by a computed tomography (CT) scan of the edentulous site (accompanied by Hounsfield values of the bone). Reformatted software allows "electronic surgery" of the CBCT images and relates the Hounsfield values at the implant–bone interface. Conventional dental radiographs, such as periapical, panoramic,

or lateral cephalometric images, are usually not diagnostic (Boxes 27.2 and 27.3) in the assessment of bone density.

A common point at which to evaluate bone quality is during surgery. The presence and thickness of a crestal cortical plate and the density of trabecular bone are easily determined during implant osteotomy preparation. The density of bone is determined by the initial bone drill, and evaluation continues until the final osteotomy preparation.

It should be emphasized that the bone density (D1–D4) classification of Misch is slightly different from Lekholm and Zarb's bone quality types (Q1–Q4). According to Misch and colleagues, D3 bone has fine trabeculae that is 47% to 68% weaker than D2 trabeculae, and 20% stronger than D4 trabeculae, whereas Lekholm and Zarb stated that Q3 bone has favorable-strength trabeculae similar to Q2.[34,36] In other words, the actual strength of the trabecular bone is different for each bone density, regardless of the presence or absence of cortical bone adjacent to the implant. In addition, the Lekholm and Zarb bone quality only evaluated bone in the anterior maxilla and mandible. The Misch bone density scale also evaluated the posterior molar regions of the jaws. As a result, a primary difference between D3 and D4 bone is also the presence of cortical bone in D3, which increases its overall strength and modulus of elasticity.[32] The quality 4 bone of Lekholm and Zarb is similar to Misch's D3, whereas D4 bone is even weaker because little to no cortical bone is present to improve the strength or the elastic modulus of the fine trabecular bone.

Osseodensification

A new method of implant preparation, termed osseodensification (OD), has recently been introduced to implant dentistry.

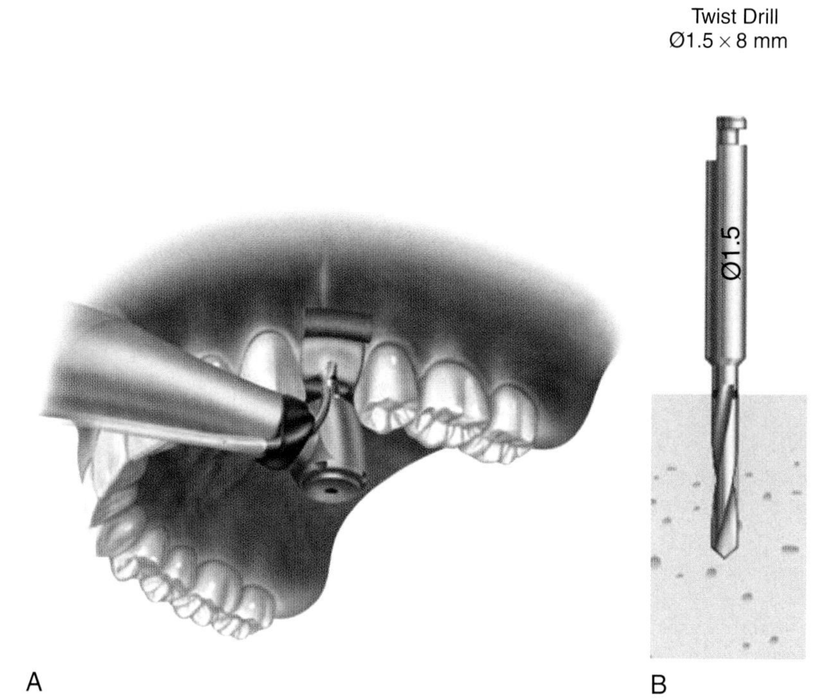

Twist Drill
Ø1.5 × 8 mm

A   B

• **Fig. 27.10** Pilot drill. (A and B) With most surgical systems, the first drill includes a pilot drill with an approximate diameter of 1.5 mm. This initial drill is usually not prepared to final depth to allow for direction modification if needed.

Huwais and colleagues, in 2013, introduced a surgical protocol that includes the use of special densifying burs, which results with low plastic deformation of the bone. The specially designed burs (Densah burs) result in bone densification as the osteotomy is prepared, thereby increasing bone at the implant interface.[48]

The Densah burs utilize the concept of osteotomes, along with drilling speed to laterally compact bone during preparation. Bone is preserved and condensed through compaction autografting, increasing the bone density and improving the mechanical stability of the implant.[49] Conventional surgical drills excavate bone during implant osteotomies, which requires approximately 12 weeks of bone remodeling to repair. Because the OD protocol preserves bone while increasing density, the healing time may be shorter.[46]

Other methods of OD by use of undersizing the drills has been established. Degidi and colleagues showed a significant increase in primary stability by decreasing the preparation size by 10%.[50] Alghamdi and colleagues used an adapted bone site preparation technique by undersizing the osteotomy sites in poor bone density and showed favorable implant survival rates.[51] Therefore in the Misch implant placement protocol, the implant placement surgical protocol is specific for each bone density and varies with the amount of overpreparation and underpreparation of the osteotomy sites.

Generic Drilling Sequence

Before discussing the surgical implant protocol specific to bone density, the clinician must understand the generic protocol for dental implant osteotomy preparation and placement.

Step 1: Pilot Drill

With most surgical systems, a 1.5-mm or 2.0-mm surgical pilot drill is used to initiate the osteotomy. Pilot drills are end-cutting starter drills used to most commonly initiate an osteotomy in the center of the ridge in a mesiodistal and buccolingual dimension. The osteotomy should be completed with a reduction handpiece (e.g., 16:1 or 20:1 high-torque handpiece) and an electric motor at a preferred speed of 2000 rpm (i.e., for D1 and D2 bone) and >1000 rpm (i.e., for D3 and D4) under copious amounts of chilled saline irrigant. The osteotomy is made no greater than 7 to 9 mm deep in the bone (Fig. 27.10). The rationale for preparation of only 7 to 9 mm is if the angulation is determined to be nonideal, then it is easier to modify.

Step 2: Position Verification

Once the initial osteotomy is prepared, it is assessed for ideal position (see Chapter 28). If incorrect, the osteotomy location may be "stretched" to the proper location by a side-cutting Lindemann bur. This bur makes the hole oblong toward the corrected center position. After the new position is obtained, it should be deepened 1 to 2 mm beyond the depth of the initial osteotomy. This will prevent the second surgical bur from entering the first nonideal implant osteotomy.

Usually a direction indicator (depth gauge), which corresponds to the initial bur diameter, is then inserted into the osteotomy and the angulation and position assessed (Fig. 27.11). If direction indicators are not available, then older surgical burs may be used after slight modification (i.e., shortened 2–4 mm to allow for radiographic ease). A periapical radiograph should be obtained to determine proximity to any vital structures. The clinician should be well aware of the "Y" factor of their surgical drill system. The Y factor corresponds to the additional length of the bur that is inherent with surgical drills (i.e., a 10-mm depth drill may drill to a length that exceeds 11.0 mm).

Ideal final implant positioning should be a minimum of 1.5 mm from an adjacent tooth, 3.0 mm from another implant, and 2.0 mm from a vital structure such as the inferior alveolar canal or mental foramen.

Step 3: Second Twist Drill

The second drill used is approximately 2.5 mm in diameter, and is an end-cutting twist drill required for the initial osteotomy to the required depth. The osteotomy location and angulation are reassessed at this point. A slight correction of

position or angulation with a Lindemann drill may be completed; however, it should ideally be accomplished after the first drill (Fig. 27.12).

Step 4: Final Shaping Drills

Depending on the surgical system used, most shaping drills are used to sequentially widen the osteotomy to the matching diameter of the implant being placed. Depending on the diameter, multiple twist drills maybe used. The desired depth, along with the ideal location and angulation of the osteotomy, should be verified. Most implant drill kits will clearly identify the drill sequence and final osteotomy diameter related to each diameter implant (Fig. 27.13). Usually, the final drill will be within 1.0 mm of the final diameter of the implant diameter (i.e., a 4.0-mm implant will have a final drill size of approximately 3.2 mm).

Step 5: Crest Module and Bone Tap Drills

Most implant crest modules (implant neck) are larger in diameter than the implant body. The larger diameter often requires a side-cutting crest module drill in D1 (and some D2) crestal bone situations to prepare the crestal aspect of the implant osteotomy. This drill is not recommended when the bone density is poor (D3 and D4) (Fig. 27.14). This drill is used to open up the crestal area of the ridge to accommodate the wider crest module. When used, copious amounts of saline should be used.

In addition, usually in D1 bone, some implant systems will require the use of a bone tap or threadformer to prepare the threads in the bone before implant insertion. Most often for single-tooth implants, the threadformers or taps should use a high-torque, slow-speed handpiece and be rotated at less than 30 rpm into the bone. Irrigation also helps to lubricate and clean the bone tap and osteotomy site of debris during this process.

Parallel Pin
Ø4.3 mm

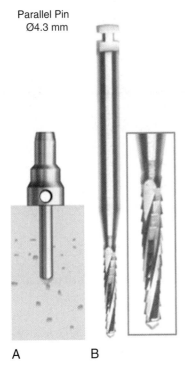

A   B

• **Fig. 27.11** (A) Parallel pin placed into pilot drill osteotomy to verify positioning clinically and radiographically.. (B) If modification of osteotomy is indicated, use of a Lindemann bur should be used to reposition osteotomy.

Twist Drill
Ø2.4/1.5 × 8 mm

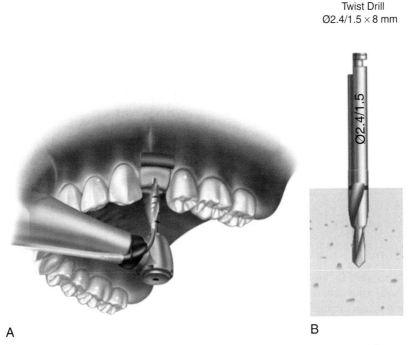

A   B

• **Fig. 27.12** (A and B) Second twist drill is used to widen the osteotomy to allow for larger diameter drills.

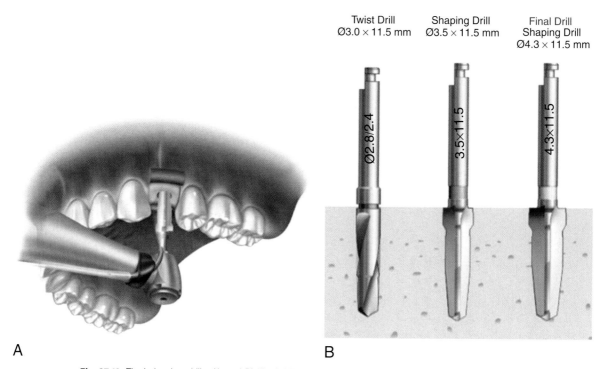

Twist Drill
Ø3.0 × 11.5 mm

Shaping Drill
Ø3.5 × 11.5 mm

Final Drill
Shaping Drill
Ø4.3 × 11.5 mm

A

B

• **Fig. 27.13** Final shaping drills. (A and B) Final drills used to widen the osteotomy to accommodate the diameter of the intended implant.

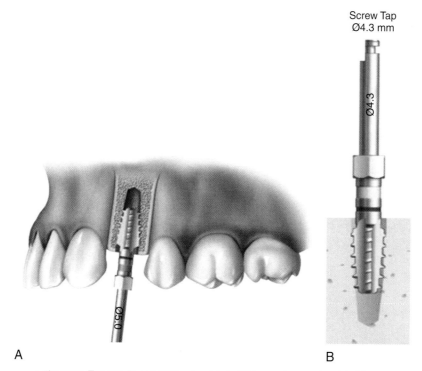

Screw Tap
Ø4.3 mm

A

B

• **Fig. 27.14** Tap drill. (A and B) Used mainly in D1 bone at approximately 30 rpm.

Step 6: Implant Insertion

The implant site may then be prepared for implant insertion. The osteotomy is lavaged with sterile saline and aspirated to remove bone debris and stagnant blood. This reduces the risk of these materials being forced into the bone marrow spaces or neurovascular channels during implant insertion, causing hydrostatic pressure. This pressure may increase the devital zone of bone around the implant or even cause short-term neurosensory impairments when the implant site is in the vicinity of the mandibular canal.

The implant may be inserted with a hand ratchet or handpiece. The advantage of inserting an implant with a handpiece is that the placement will be more ideal and deviation is less likely, especially in poorer quality of bone (e.g., D3 and D4 bone). However, in better quality of bone, especially D1, difficulty in insertion may

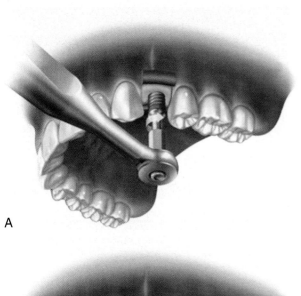

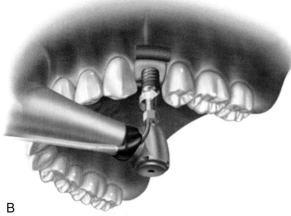

• **Fig. 27.15** Implant insertion. (A) Placement of implant with a hand ratchet, which is usually used only in D1 and D2 bone. (B) Placement of implant with handpiece, which is usually indicated in D2, D3, and D4 bone.

sometimes occur. When placing an implant with a hand ratchet, good apical pressure should be used to decrease the possibility of deviating the path of the implant. If the implant is tightened into the osteotomy and significant stress occurs at the crestal area, pressure necrosis may occur and an increase in the devital zone of bone around the implant during healing will occur. If this should occur, the implant may be unthreaded 1 to 2 mm and then reinserted back into the osteotomy. When the implant is placed into the final position, a post-insertion periapical radiograph is taken to verify ideal positioning (Fig. 27.15).

Dental Implant Surgical Protocol 1 (D1 Bone)

Dense Cortical (D1) Bone

The dense D1 bone (i.e., similar to the hardness of oak or maple wood) is composed of almost all dense cortical bone. The maxilla almost never presents with D1 bone. In division A bone, approximately 4% of the anterior mandibles and 2% of the posterior mandibles have this dense bone category. In division C–h bone of an anterior mandible, these numbers increase and may reach 25% in males, whereas weaker bone density D3 and D4 bone are less commonly encountered.

The Hounsfield unit numbers are usually greater than 1250 HU.

Advantages of D1 Bone

The homogeneous, dense D1 bone type presents several advantages for implant dentistry. Composed histologically of dense lamellar bone with complete haversian systems, it is highly mineralized and able to withstand higher occlusal loads. The cortical lamellar bone may heal with little interim woven bone formation, ensuring excellent bone strength while healing next to the implant.[52,53]

D1 bone is more often found in anterior mandibles with moderate to severe resorption and greater crown/implant ratios. Implants placed into this bone density improve the dissipation of stresses in the crestal cortical region despite higher moments of force from the greater crown height to sustain long-term functional stress.

The percentage of light microscopic contact of bone at the implant interface is greatest in D1 bone type and greater than 80% (Fig. 27.16). In addition, this bone density exhibits greater strength than any other bone type. The strongest bone also benefits from the greatest BIC. Because of the density of this bone, less stress is transmitted to the apical third of the implants than in other bone types. As a result, shorter implants can better withstand greater loads than in any other bone densities. In fact, the placement of longer implants may decrease surgical survival rates because overheating during osteotomy preparation is a primary concern in this bone type. Greater heat is often generated at the apical portion of the osteotomy, especially when preparing dense cortical bone.[54]

Disadvantages of D1 Bone

Increased Crown-Implant Ratio. Dense cortical bone also presents several disadvantages. Because these cases are usually seen with mandibles with limited height (i.e., usually less than 12 mm), the crown height space is often greater than 15 mm. As a result, additional force-multiplying factors (i.e., such as cantilevers or lateral forces) are further magnified on the implant-prosthetic system. It is imperative that stress-reducing factors may be incorporated in the prosthesis design to reduce these effects, not only on the bone, but also on the prosthetic components (Fig. 27.17).

Poorer Blood Supply. D1 bone has fewer blood vessels than the other three types; therefore it is more dependent on the periosteum for its nutrition. The cortical bone receives the outer one-third of all its arterial and venous supply from the periosteum.[55] This bone density is almost all cortical, and the capacity of regeneration is impaired because of the poor blood circulation. Therefore delicate and minimal periosteal reflection is indicated. When D1 density is present, the bone width is usually abundant and the mandible widens apically. Fortunately, there are few occurrences when facial or lingual undercuts are observed with D1 bone densities, and flap reflection can be safely kept to a minimum. The precise closure of the periosteum and the overlaying tissue has been shown to help recover the blood supply and is encouraged.[56] Because of the compromised blood supply, this type of bone will actually take longer time to heal compared with D2 bone.

Overheating the Bone. The primary surgical problem of D1 bone is the dense cortical bone is more difficult to prepare for endosteal implants than any other bone density. The most common cause of implant failure in this bone quality is surgical trauma resulting from overheating the bone during the implant osteotomy procedures because surgical drills progress with more difficulty.

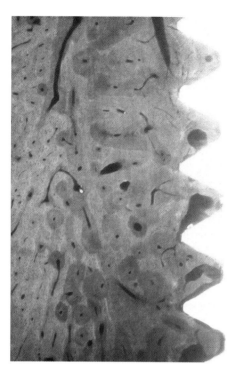

• **Fig. 27.16** D1 bone has the highest bone-implant contact (BIC), which is usually greater than 80% after initial bone healing. Thus the strongest bone is also the bone with the greatest BIC. Both these conditions make D1 bone the most suitable for occlusal loading.

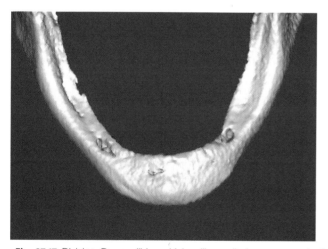

• **Fig. 27.17** Division D mandible, which will usually be composed of D1 bone. Because of the extensive atrophy, the crown-implant ratio is increased.

The zone of devitalized bone that forms around the implant is larger in this bone density and must be remodeled and replaced by vital bone for the interface to be load bearing (Fig. 27.18). As a result, implant surgical failure may be greater in D1 bone than any other bone density. Therefore it is imperative the clinician strive to minimize the thermal trauma.

Pressure Necrosis. Because of the thick, dense cortical bone, placement of an implant may lead to an increase in internal stresses at the crestal area. Therefore after implant placement to the height of the bone level, the implant may be unthreaded 1 to 2 mm, the bone allowed to relieve the stresses, and then it is reinserted to the final placement level. By allowing the bone to expand from creep,

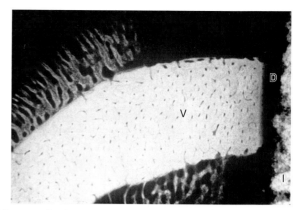

• **Fig. 27.18** Devital zone (D) of bone next to the implant (I) is primarily created by heat generated during surgery, which radiates from the site, especially in cortical bone. Other contributing factors include lack of blood supply, pressure necrosis from implant placement, microfracture from bone tapping, and implant insertion. V, Vital bone.

it is less likely that pressure necrosis, which leads to bone loss or die-back, will occur (Box 27.4).

Implant Osteotomy Drilling Sequence

In D1 bone, all the drills of the surgical system should be utilized. Because of the density of this bone type, more graduated drills will result in less heat generation. A secondary cause of lack of osseous integration may be related to mechanical trauma of the bone. There are several methods to reduce mechanical trauma in D1 bone, and one of these is related to final drill size selection. In D1 bone, the final bone preparation may be sized slightly larger in both width and height, especially for a threaded implant, than the manufacturer-recommended surgical protocol. This reduces the risk of microfracture trauma between the implant threads during insertion, which may lead to fibrous tissue formation at the bone–implant interface. In addition, a final drill dimension only used in D1 bone remains sharper for this critical step.

If a surgical drill of slightly greater diameter is not available with the implant system, the clinician can use the final drill size available and pass it within the osteotomy several times. By entering the osteotomy site multiple times, the osteotomy diameter will become slightly oversized. In fact, all drills for the D1 drilling sequence may use this method, therefore, less bone is removed with future drills, resulting in less heat generation.

A bone tap should be used in D1 bone before insertion of a threaded implant. There are several reasons for the use of a bone tap. Because the final drill osteotomy is almost 1 mm smaller than the outer diameter of the implant, the bone tap creates the space for the thread of the implant. This drill has open flutes, which permit the shaving of the bone to accumulate and be removed before placing the implant. A self-tapping implant insertion compresses the bone in the region of the threads. This is an advantage in softer bone types, but not in cortical bone. The tap reduces the mechanical trauma to the bone while the implant is inserted. The bone is also able to slightly recover from the trauma of the tap once it is removed and permits a more passive implant placement. Watzek and colleagues found a higher woven bone interface (i.e., a sign of bone trauma) when a self-threading implant design was used, compared with a pretapped implant site.[57] Satomi and colleagues found a higher BIC after initial healing with pretapped implant osteotomies compared with a self-tapping site, which is also indicative of less bone trauma. The use of a self-tapping implant insertion technique in dense bone

Bone Necrosis
Prevention:
- Final implant placement at or above bone level
- Unthread ½ turn to relieve internal stresses

Decreased Blood Supply
Prevention
- Primarily from periosteum
- Increased healing time
- Minimal reflection

Should Use Bone Tap
Prevention:
- Decreases pressure necrosis
- Allows passive implant fit
- Prevents internal implant–body/implant–bone interface microfracture
- Removes drill remnants

Overheating during Osteotomy
Prevention:
- New drill designs, flutes, geometry
- Abundant external irrigation
- Intermittent pressure on drill (bone dancing)
- Pause every 3–5 seconds; keep irrigating
- Incremental drill sequence *(more drills; pass same drill more than once to widen osteotomy in preparation of next drill)*

---

qualities has demonstrated a significantly higher degree of hard tissue trauma; therefore it is not recommended in D1 bone.[58]

The bone tap should be used with a hand ratchet and irrigation. The slow-speed, high-torque handpiece is very efficient and has several advantages in D2 bone. However, D1 bone is so strong that the handpiece gears may strip, and the handpiece is more likely to require repeated repair.

The hand position of the surgeon is important in maintaining constant force and direction on the hand ratchet during the bone-tapping process. When using a ratchet, the horizontal rotation on the tap causes it to tip back and forth around the vertical axis. Therefore, when using a ratchet the ratchet is held while the thumb of the other hand is placed directly over the bone tap, the index finger of the same hand retracts the lip for improved access and vision. The ratchet rotates the tap with one hand while the thumb and middle finger of the other hand apply constant pressure and direction to the tap so it does not tip back and forth or strip the osteotomy site (which may happen if the tap does not continue to advance within the osteotomy each turn of the tap).

A bone tap in D1 bone prevents the antirotational component of the implant body from being damaged during implant insertion in this dense bone type. A minor advantage to tapping may be the fact that drill remnants are more likely to be left in the implant osteotomy during preparation in dense bone or with a new drill and cutting edge. The bone tap may remove these remnants and decrease the risk of long-term corrosion from dissimilar metals contacting within the bone, although no reports in the literature have indicated this to be a problem.

Once the tapping process is complete, the osteotomy is irrigated and suctioned. The implant should be inserted with a hand ratchet, minimizing damage to the handpiece and allowing the clinician to gauge the IT of the implant. The implant should not be tightened with a high-torque pressure (>75 N/cm) to the full depth of the osteotomy; this causes it to "bottom out" and may set up microfractures along the implant interface. Instead, once the threaded implant is introduced into the osteotomy and in final position, it is often unthreaded 1 to 2 mm to ensure that there is no residual pressure along the bone interface. Then, after 20 to 30 seconds, the implant may be reinserted to its final position. This step is primarily used in D1 bone because excessive initial strain may form at the interface of the cortical bone with even one extra rotation of the implant.[59] The rotational stress is usually highest at the crestal region, which may even cause mechanical bone microfracture and marginal bone loss.

Use of Copious Amounts of Irrigation. As the depth of the osteotomy increases, the risk of the inadequate irrigation increases.[60] Therefore the bone dancing method of preparation is paramount, especially when reaching the apical area of the osteotomy. Copious amounts of either external irrigating drilling techniques should be used; however, many other factors should be understood. Irrigation, drill design, rotations per minute, and drill sizing are paramount to reduce heat. In addition, the chilling of the saline bags (i.e., placed in refrigerator before use) allow for the decrease in heat generation (Fig. 27.19).

Bone Debris Removal. During osteotomy preparation of D1 bone, fragments of bone often adhere to the flutes of the surgical burs. This bone is a great source for grafting around compromised sites after implant placement. Also, bone chips in the osteotomy may cause an increase in frictional heat and should be removed by irrigation in D1 bone to maintain optimal cutting action (Fig. 27.20). The bone debris should be frequently wiped off the cutting flutes of the drill with a surgical sponge. These bone shavings prevent coolant from reaching the bone and result in the drill being less efficient. The color of these bone shavings is important to evaluate. Any beige coloration to the bone debris indicates excessive heat is being generated and the bone debris is nonvital (Fig. 27.21). A brownish color indicates the bone cell death extends several millimeters away from the implant osteotomy. The color of the bone debris should be reddish or white, which indicates vital bone (Fig. 27.22).

Use of New Drills. The use of new drills with a sharp cutting flute is most critical for D1 bone surgery. Bone drills become dull after repeated use, especially if autoclaved frequently. Chacon and colleagues evaluated three different drill systems after repeated drilling and sterilization. The bone temperature 0.5 mm from the osteotomy preparation increased every 25 uses of the system, even though light microscopic evaluation showed little wear.[6] When the drills become dull, the clinician may not appreciate it in softer bone, but when D1 bone is prepared, the drill sharpness can become critical.

Larger Crest Module. Most implant designs have a larger crest module compared with the body of the implant. This design feature ensures a bone "seal" around the top portion of the implant after it is threaded into position. For example, a crest module is usually 4.1 mm for a 3.75-mm-diameter implant. Because the final osteotomy drill of many systems is in the 3.2-mm-diameter range, the 0.9-mm difference is substantial, especially in crestal cortical bone. As a result, a crestal bone drill is used in D1 bone, which prepares the larger diameter at the top of the osteotomy (Fig. 27.23). In a study by Novaes and colleagues, the difference in crestal bone loss after an initial healing period of 3 months was 1.5 mm between using a crestal drill compared with no crestal drill.[61] The additional bone trauma from compressing a larger crest module into the osteotomy is significant and may increase surgical

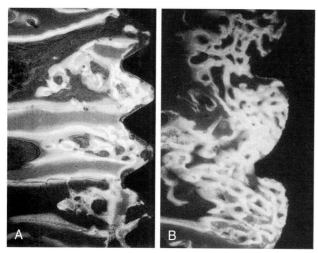

● **Fig. 27.19** (A) Pretapped bone site has less woven (newly generated) bone and illustrated less trauma on implant insertion. (B) A self-tapping implant insertion causes greater bone trauma and exhibits massive woven regenerative bone formation as a consequence. (From Watzek G, Danhel-Mayhauser M, Matejka M, et al. Experimental comparison of Brånemark and TPS dental implants in sheep [abstract]. In: *UCLA Symposium: Implants in the Partially Edentulous Patient*; 1990.)

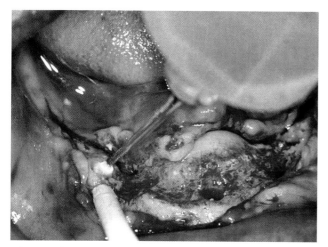

● **Fig. 27.20** Bone chip debris should be frequently removed by irrigation in D1 bone to improve efficiency of the drill and before implant insertion after bone tapping.

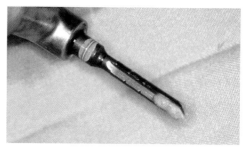

● **Fig. 27.21** Bone debris in the drill should be evaluated. A brown or beige color indicates the temperature is too high and the bone is devitalized.

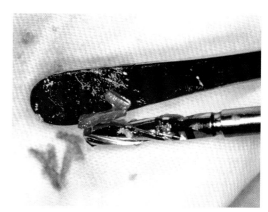

● **Fig. 27.22** Bone debris in the drill should be white or reddish, which indicates vital bone and ideal preparation conditions.

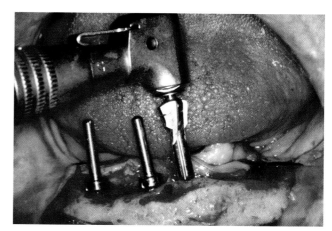

● **Fig. 27.23** Crestal bone tap should be used in D1 bone to prepare marginal bone to receive the crest module of the implant body, which is larger in diameter than the implant body.

bone loss around the implant (i.e., pressure necrosis). Therefore a crestal bone drill should be used in D1 bone as the last drilling step in the preparation of the osteotomy.

Final Implant Positioning. The ideal implant length for D1 bone is 10 mm for a 4-mm-diameter implant. There is little, if any, benefit to increased implant length beyond 10 mm in D1 bone for a threaded implant body because most all the stresses after healing are limited to the crestal half of the implant, with occlusal loading (Fig. 27.24). The longer implant makes bone preparation more difficult and generates more heat in this bone type. The final placement of the implant in relation to the crest of the ridge is related to its design and the bone density. A one-stage surgical approach is often used in D1 bone. A healing abutment may be added to permit the implant to heal above the soft tissue, thus eliminating a second-stage surgery.

The D1 dense compact bone is often of decreased height. Therefore the actual support system of the implant may be increased in division C–h limited-height bone type by not countersinking the smooth portion of the implant crest module below the crest of the ridge. The smooth portion of the implant body may be placed above the ridge if no load is applied to the implant during initial healing, and the risk of micromovement during this period is minimal.

Bone Healing

Many of the cutting cones that develop from monocytes in the circulating blood and are responsible for bone remodeling at the implant interface. These blood cells originate from the blood vessels found in well-vascularized trabecular bone, which has a greater capacity for regeneration than compact bone. Therefore in some aspects cortical bone requires greater healing time compared with trabecular bone.

On the other hand, because of the load-bearing capability of D1 bone and the excellent Bone-Implant Contact (BIC), prosthetic loading of D1 bone may start before the completion of the initial healing phase. Conditions that contribute to a lack of movement during healing are primordial to achieve a direct bone–implant interface. D1 bone is strong and often able to resist micromovement, regardless of whether an implant is loaded. As a result, immediate implant loading is often possible when multiple implants are splinted together, without compromise to the overall survival rate of the implant. However, most often, a blend of treatment conditions result in a minimum 3-month unloaded healing period in this bone type.

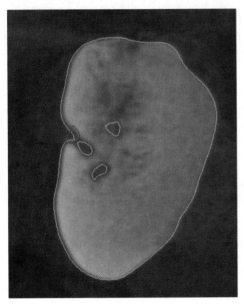

Fig. 27.24 D1 Bone: Mandibular cross-sectional image depicting mainly dense D1 bone.

Once the bone–implant interface is established, it exhibits the strongest load-bearing properties of any bone type. As a result, progressive bone loading is not necessary to develop a stable condition. The restoring clinician may proceed without delay as desired to the final prosthesis (Box 27.5; Fig. 27.25).

Dental Implant Surgical Protocol 2 (D2 Bone)

Dense-to-Thick Porous Cortical and Coarse Trabecular Bone (D2)

The second density of bone found in the edentulous jaws (D2) is a combination of dense-to-porous cortical bone on the crest and coarse trabecular bone within the cortical plates (Fig. 27.26). The Hounsfield values on reformatted CBCT images are 750 to 1250 units for this bone quality. The tactile feeling when preparing this bone density is similar to preparations in spruce or white pine wood (i.e. soft wood). The D2 bone trabeculae are 40% to 60% stronger than D3 trabeculae. This bone type occurs most frequently in the anterior mandible, followed by the posterior mandible. On occasion it is observed in the anterior maxilla, especially for a single missing tooth, although the dense-to-porous cortical bone is then found primarily on the lingual surface of the implant site.[62]

• BOX 27.5 Implant Placement Surgical Protocols

D1 Bone Surgical Protocol
- Drilling speed: ~2000 to 2500 rpm
- Bone tap: 25 rpm
- Irrigation: copious amounts of saline
- Bone dance: very critical to reduce heat
- Drill osteotomy multiple times with each drill to *oversize osteotomy*
- Ideally use new drills
- Always insert implant with hand wrench, not a handpiece

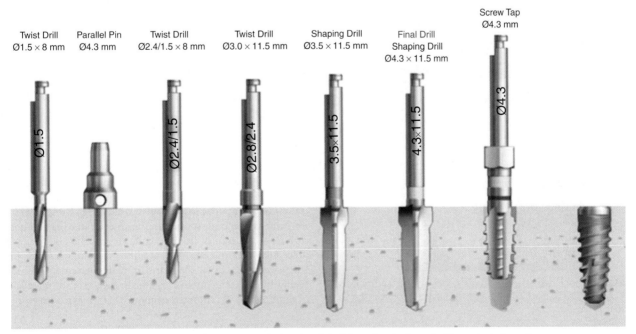

| Twist Drill Ø1.5 × 8 mm | Parallel Pin Ø4.3 mm | Twist Drill Ø2.4/1.5 × 8 mm | Twist Drill Ø3.0 × 11.5 mm | Shaping Drill Ø3.5 × 11.5 mm | Final Drill Shaping Drill Ø4.3 × 11.5 mm | Screw Tap Ø4.3 mm |

Fig. 27.25 D1 implant placement surgical protocol. In this protocol, all surgical burs, including a bone tap are used.

Advantages of D2 Bone

D2 bone provides excellent implant interface healing, and osteo-integration is very predictable; therefore it is the ideal type of bone. There exist no disadvantages in D2 bone.

Most implant systems refer to this density of bone for their generalized surgical protocol. The dense-to-porous cortical bone on the crest or lateral portions of the implant site provide a secure initial rigid interface. The implant may even be placed slightly above the crest of the ridge, with decreased compromise or risk of movement at the interface during healing compared with softer bone types. The intrabony blood supply allows bleeding during the osteotomy, which helps control overheating during preparation and is most beneficial for bone–implant interface healing.[63]

Implant Osteotomy Surgical Sequence

The drill sequence for D2 bone is similar to D1 bone, with a few exceptions. Therefore all drills in the surgical sequence are used except the bone tap. The use of a bone tap for D2 bone is dependent on the final osteotomy size, the implant body size, the depth of the thread, and the shape of the thread. A bone tap most often will lead to a decreased primary stability in D2 bone. A crestal bone drill should be used for most implant designs in D2 bone.[64] The osteotomy preparation should proceed at a higher speed (e.g., ~2000 rpm). Sharawy and colleagues showed that D2 bone with an osteotomy depth of 8 mm could be prepared in 4 to 8 seconds, dependent on drill design and rpm.[39] Therefore the osteotomy depth should not proceed slowly, creating additional heat. Enough pressure should be placed on the handpiece to proceed approximately at least 5 mm every 5 seconds.

The implant may be threaded into position with a low-speed (less than 30 rpm), high-torque (75 N/cm) handpiece, rather than using a hand ratchet. The handpiece allows a more precise implant rotation, and a constant pressure ensures the implant will progress into the site without risk of stripping the bone within the threads. During this process, the irrigation may be stopped so the patient does not attempt to close the mouth and swallow, which may contaminate the implant and cause it to be pushed off the axis of the implant osteotomy. However, if minimal bleeding is present, then a small amount of irrigation may be used.

A threaded implant placed in the anterior mandible engages the cortical bone at the edentulous crest, and often the lingual lateral side. In division C–h bone, the implant may also engage the apical cortical region; however, in the mandible, care should be exercised to not perforate the inferior border. This provides immediate stability and proven long-term survival.

When the anterior maxilla presents this bone density, it is treated similarly to the D2 mandible. A threaded implant should engage the palatal cortical plate rather than the labial cortical bone, which is thinner and porous. However, care should be exercised because the implant may be pushed more labial, even stripping the facial plate. The anterior maxilla usually has less available bone height than does the anterior mandible. As a result, the apex of the implant may engage the thin cortical plate of the floor of the nose when a solid, traditional screw-type system is used. Because the greatest stresses after healing are primarily transmitted around the crest, the primary advantage of the apical end of the implant engaging cortical bone is initial stability during healing.

Healing

The excellent blood supply and rigid initial fixation of D2 bone permits adequate bone healing within 4 months. The lamellar bone–implant interface is more than 60% established at the 4-month healing interval. BIC is approximately 70% at this point in time, especially when cortical bone engages the lateral and lingual portions of the implant (Fig. 27.27). Abutment placement and prosthodontic therapy may then commence. It should be noted that the time frame for initial bone healing is based on the density of the bone and not on the location in the jaws. Therefore a 4-month rigid healing phase is adequate for porous cortical and coarse trabecular (D2) bone, even when found in the maxilla. Progressive bone loading is usually not required for D2 bone, although an increase in BIC takes place during the initial loading period (Box 27.6; Fig. 27.28).

Dental Implant Surgical Protocol 3 (D3 Bone)

Thin Porous Cortical and Fine Trabecular Bone (D3)

The third density of bone (D3) is composed of thinner porous cortical bone on the crest and fine trabecular bone within the ridge (Fig. 27.29). The CBCT-reformatted images may have a range of 375 to 750 HU. This bone quality provides the clinician with a tactile sense similar to drilling in compressed balsa wood. The trabeculae are approximately 50% weaker than those in D2 bone. D3 bone is found most often in the anterior maxilla and posterior regions of the mouth in either arch. It may also be found in the division B edentulous ridge, modified by osteoplasty to provide adequate width for a root-form implant placement. Sinus augmentation grafts are often D3 bone in the posterior maxilla after a healing period of 6 months or more.[65] D3 bone is least prevalent

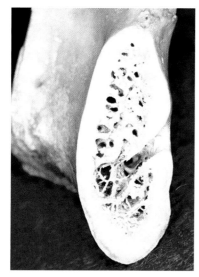

• **Fig. 27.26** D2 bone has a dense to porous cortical crest, and inner trabecular bone is coarse. It is found most often in the anterior mandible.

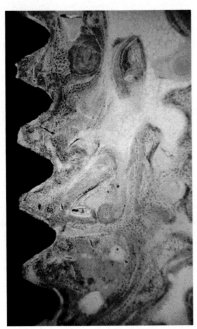

• **Fig. 27.27** Bone-implant contact is approximately 70% in D2 bone after initial healing and is excellent for load-bearing capability.

- Drilling speed: ~2000 to 2500 rpm
- Bone tap: usually not needed
- Irrigation: copious amounts of saline
- Bone dance: very critical to reduce heat
- Implant placement: with insertion wrench or handpiece

in division C–h or division D anterior mandibles. Larger diameter implants (5 mm or 6 mm) are more essential in D3 bone in the molar regions than in the previous categories. A roughened implant body (i.e., such as acid-etched media or resorbable blast media) presents advantages in this bone density, regardless of design, to compensate for the limited initial bone contact and decreased bone strength inherent in the trabecular architecture.

The porous cortical layer is thinner on the crest and labial aspect of the maxilla, and the fine trabecular pattern is more discrete in wide edentulous sites. The D3 anterior maxilla is usually of less width than its mandibular D3 counterpart. The D3 bone is not only 50% weaker than D2 bone, but the BIC is also less favorable in D3 bone. These additive factors can increase the risk of implant failure. Therefore small-diameter implants are not suggested in most situations. Instead, bone spreading in this bone density is mechanically easier to perform (i.e. less cortical thickness) and allows the placement of greater diameter implants. The increased-diameter implants lead to improved prognosis, especially when lateral forces or greater force magnitudes are expected. In addition, bone spreading compacts the trabecular bone and increases its density after initial healing (e.g., OD).

Advantages of D3 Bone

The main advantage of D3 porous compact and fine trabecular bone is that the implant osteotomy preparation time and difficulty is minimal for each drill size and is usually less than 10 seconds. The crest module drill and bone tap may be eliminated in the surgical protocol. Blood supply is excellent for initial healing, and intraosseous bleeding helps cool the osteotomy during preparation. As a result, this bone density is usually associated with a high surgical survival rate.

Disadvantages of D3 Bone

D3 bone also presents several disadvantages. It is more delicate to surgically manage than the previous two bone density types as its preparation takes minimal effort.

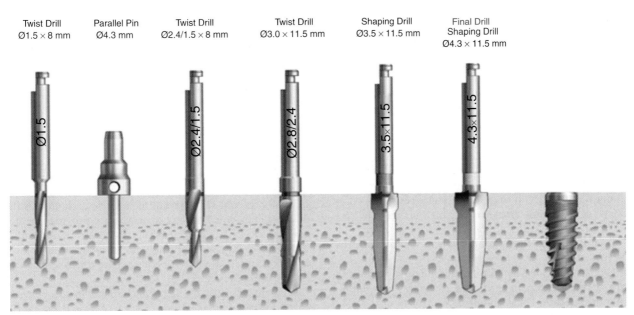

Twist Drill Ø1.5 × 8 mm | Parallel Pin Ø4.3 mm | Twist Drill Ø2.4/1.5 × 8 mm | Twist Drill Ø3.0 × 11.5 mm | Shaping Drill Ø3.5 × 11.5 mm | Final Drill Shaping Drill Ø4.3 × 11.5 mm

Ø1.5 | Ø2.4/1.5 | Ø2.8/2.4 | 3.5×11.5 | 4.3×11.5

• **Fig. 27.28** D2 surgical protocol. Note the use of all surgical burs except the bone tap.

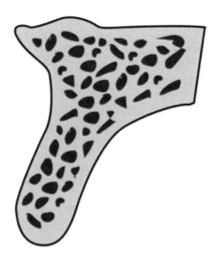

D3

• **Fig. 27.29** D3 bone exhibits minimal cortical bone and thin trabecular bone.

The motor speed in drilling the osteotomy is not as important as in D1 or D2 bone. Therefore bone preparation in D3 bone can range from 1000 to 2000 rpm and must be made with constant care of direction to avoid enlargement or elliptical preparation of the site.

A common mistake that causes an elliptical site (i.e., over-sized osteotomy) to form is the pronation of the wrist, which redirects the handpiece direction. In dense bone, the side of the drill encroaches on the dense cortical crest, which opposes the movement and stops the rotation before the crestal osteotomy is enlarged. In D3 bone the arc pathway is not stopped and the osteotomy at the level of the crestal bone is of greater diameter than the drill. If the implant design does not increase at the crestal region, then the surgical defect created around the crestal area of the implant may heal with fibrous tissue rather than bone and cause an initial bony pocket.

Therefore the osteotomy should be drilled with the arm in a "drill press" type of motion (i.e., in one plane). To improve rigid fixation of traditional root-form designs during healing, the opposing thin cortical bone of the nasal or antral floor is often engaged in the maxilla or the apicolingual plate in the mandible, when immediate loading (IL) is considered. If the original implant height determined before surgery does not engage the opposing cortical bone, then the osteotomy is increased in depth until it is engaged. Slightly longer implants may be placed in this approach to further increase surface area of support. However, it should be remembered that this technique improves stability during healing but does not decrease the crestal loads to bone after healing. Instead, implant crest module design and the crestal one-third of the implant body design are necessary to decrease stress when the implant prosthesis is loaded.

The clinician must be careful to avoid undesired lateral perforations of the cortical bone during osteotomy procedures, especially on the thin, labial porous cortical plate of the maxilla. A common mistake is the stripping of the thin facial plates

during the osteotomy. The initial and intermediate drills proceed through the fine trabecular bone without incident. However, the lingual aspect of the end-cutting drill contacts the thick palatal cortical bone within the osteotomy, which resists preparation, and pushes the drill facially, which may strip the facial plate. A very firm hand, which prevents lateral displacement of the drill and handpiece during the implant osteotomy and does not permit the drill to move facially, is mandatory to prevent this unwanted complication.

Implant Osteotomy Surgical Sequence

In D3 bone, the final drill (i.e., in some systems the final two drills) is not used because the placement of the implant allows for the lateral displacement of the bone, increasing bone density. A crestal bone drill should not be used in D3 bone. The thin, porous cortical bone on the crest provides improved initial stability of the implant when it is compressed against the crest module of the implant. Unlike D1 and D2 bone, the final drill diameter (3.0–3.4 mm for a standard-diameter implant) is of benefit for the 4.1-mm to 4.2-mm crest module dimension to compress the weaker bone. The compressed soft bone not only provides greater stability, but it heals with a higher BIC, which is a benefit during the initial bone-loading process.

A bone tap is never indicated in D3 bone because the fine trabeculae are 50% weaker than D2 trabeculae, and when the implant is threaded into position, it compresses the bone. This provides improved initial stability and increases the BIC during initial healing. Bone compaction is a benefit when the bone density is poor. Because crest module drills and a bone tap are usually not used in D3 bone, the number of steps and time of preparation are reduced. With any drill in D3 bone, it should only be passed once in the osteotomy to avoid oversizing the preparation. On the other hand, a complication often occurs when inserting the threaded implant into the prepared bone site of the anterior maxilla. The threaded implant does not completely thread into the more dense palatal plate of bone in this region, and the implant may be pushed facially, often stripping the facial bone because the implant is threaded into position. This often occurs when a ratchet is used instead of a handpiece when placing the implant. A hand ratchet often will distort and widen the top of the osteotomy and impair proper bone contact with the crest module of the implant. In addition, the hand ratchet will often push the implant toward the facial bone, into the softer bone. This causes the implant to be positioned more facially than originally prepared and may even strip the thin cortical plate on the facial aspect of the osteotomy.

In abundant bone volume, the implant may self-tap the soft, thin, trabecular bone to enhance initial stability. An implant with a wider crest module can compress the crestal bone when inserted without using a countersink drill. The implant should not be removed and reinserted because initial rigid fixation may be compromised. If the only cortical bone is on the crest of the ridge, as in a posterior mandible, the implants are not countersunk below the crest in this density of bone. The thin, porous cortical plate provides greater initial stability than the fine trabecular bone underneath. This is especially important in the posterior mandible of a clenching parafunctional patient because bone torsion occurs during heavy biting pressures.

Therefore for placement of an implant in D3 bone, a low-speed (30 rpm), high-torque handpiece should be used rather than a hand wrench for self-tapping implant insertion. This

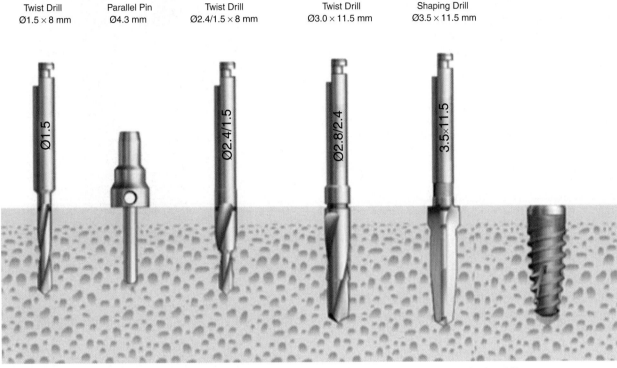

Twist Drill
Ø1.5 × 8 mm

Parallel Pin
Ø4.3 mm

Twist Drill
Ø2.4/1.5 × 8 mm

Twist Drill
Ø3.0 × 11.5 mm

Shaping Drill
Ø3.5 × 11.5 mm

• **Fig. 27.30** D3 surgical protocol. Note the use of all surgical burs except the last shaping drill.

decreases the risk of oversizing the osteotomy with an elliptical implant insertion, which usually results from hand wrench placement in softer bone. A firm hand during handpiece insertion also can prevent the implant from being pushed facially and away from the thicker lingual cortical plate. Tightening a threaded implant to increase fixation once completely inserted is not recommended because stripping of the threads and decreased fixation may occur.

A roughened surface condition or coating on a threaded implant body is advantageous in this soft bone condition to enhance initial stability and the amount of initial trabecular bone at the bone–implant interface. The amount of bone initially at the bone–implant interface is reduced compared with bone types D1 and D2. If the lingual and apical cortical bone are not engaged at the time of implant placement, then less than 50% of the implant surface may actually contact bone. An additional implant may be used to improve load distribution and prosthodontic support during the early loading period. Often a two-stage technique is recommended to minimize premature loading of the implant (Fig. 27.30; Box 27.7).

Healing

The time frame for atraumatic healing is usually 5 months or more. The actual implant interface develops more rapidly than D2 bone; however, the extended time permits the regional acceleratory phenomenon (RAP) from implant surgery to stimulate the formation of more trabecular bone patterns. In addition, the more advanced bone mineralization within the extra months also increases its strength before loading. An extended gradual loading period (e.g., progressive bone loading) is also recommended to further improve this bone density during the initial bone loading (Box 27.8).

> ### • BOX 27.7 Disadvantages of D3 Bone
>
> **Bone-Implant Contact**
> - Approximately 50%
> - Longer healing period
> - Additional implants recommended
>
> **Implant Placement**
> - One chance, widen osteotomy
> - Thin crestal cortical bone which decreases primary stability
> - Greater risk of overload during healing

> ### • BOX 27.8 D3 Bone Surgical Protocol
>
> - Underprep: no last bur (osseodensification)
> - Drilling speed: ~1000 to 2500 rpm (speed not as important in poorer quality bone)
> - Final drill and bone tap: not used
> - Irrigation: copious amounts of saline
> - Bone dance: not as critical in comparison to better quality bone
> - Implant placement: handpiece

Dental Implant Surgical Protocol 4 (D4 Bone)

Fine Trabecular Bone (D4)

Fine trabecular (D4) bone has very little density and little or no cortical crestal bone. It is the opposite spectrum of dense cortical (D1) bone. The most common locations for this type of bone are the posterior molar region of a maxilla in the long-term edentulous patient, or in an augmented ridge in height and width with particulate bone or substitutes, or in a sinus graft. It is rarely observed in the mandible but on occasion does exist. These edentulous ridges are often very wide but have reduced vertical height. This bone type is also present after osteoplasty in wide D3 ridges because the crestal cortical bone is removed during this procedure.

The tactile sense during osteotomy preparation of this bone is similar to stiff, dense Styrofoam. The bone trabeculae may be up to 10 times weaker than the cortical bone of D1. The BIC after initial loading is often less than 25% (Fig. 27.31). A CBCT scan with reformatted images of D4 bone has a Hounsfield number of 0 - 350 HU. units.

Division B implants are not suggested in this bone type. Bone spreading is easiest in this bone density, and larger diameter implants are suggested whenever possible. A roughened implant surface coating is almost mandatory to improve the amount of BIC in this bone quality after initial healing.

Disadvantages of D4 Bone

Fine trabecular bone presents the most arduous endeavor to obtain rigid fixation. Bone trabeculae are sparse and, as a result, initial fixation of any implant design presents a surgical challenge (Fig. 27.32).

Additional implants are placed to improve implant-bone loading distribution and prosthodontic rehabilitation, especially during the first critical year of function. For fixed restorations, no cantilever on the prosthesis is used with this bone density. An additional implant may be placed at the time of surgery in the second molar region to further improve support. The implant of choice in the wide posterior maxilla with D4 bone is a greater diameter and roughened surface. or HA-coated threaded implant. When properly inserted, the-threaded implant can be more stable and provides greater surface area. The larger diameter implant offers greater surface area for support, further compresses the fine trabecular bone for greater initial rigidity, has a greater chance to engage the lateral regions of cortical bone for support, and improves stress transfer during loading (Box 27.9).

Implant Osteotomy Drilling Sequence

The initial drill and possibly the second drill are used to determine site depth and angulation is the only one that should be used in this bone type, after which osteotomes may be used with a surgical mallet or handpiece to compress the bone site, rather than remove bone, as the osteotomy increases in size (Figs. 27.33 and 27.34).

The compaction technique of the site is prepared with great care. The bone site may be easily distorted, resulting in reduced initial stability of the implant. The final osteotomy diameter is similar to the D3 preparation. The residual ridge is easily expanded in this bone type. The osteotomy may both compress the bone trabeculae and expand the osteotomy site.

The implant should self-tap the bone or shape the implant receptor site while being seated with a slow-speed, high-torque handpiece. A hand wrench is contraindicated because it may deviate the positioning of the implant. The pressure on the implant during insertion corresponds to the speed of rotation, and the implant proceeds to self-tap the soft bone. It is difficult to thread an implant in soft bone in difficult access regions. If there is any cortical bone in the opposing landmark, it is engaged to enhance stability and simultaneously ensure the maximum length of

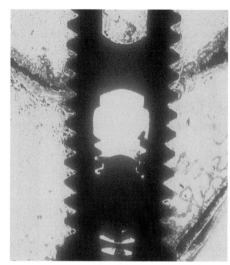

• **Fig. 27.31** Posterior maxillary region may be D4 bone, with bone-implant contact after initial loading no greater than 25%.

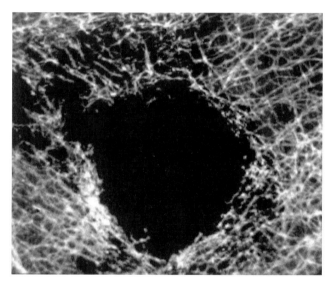

• **Fig. 27.32** Conventional drilling procedure uses an extraction technique that removes bone from the site. Note fragmentation of the osteotomy margin.

• BOX **27.9** **Disadvantages of D4 Bone**

Bone Anatomy

Location:
- Minimal cortical crest, decreased primary stability cortical crest
- Decreased bone height (i.e. maxillary posterior)
- Requires more implants

Osteotomy
- Must undersize osteotomy for osseodensification
- Surgical Access (i.e. posterior maxilla)

---

implant. An implant with a greater crestal diameter presents the added benefit to further compress the crestal bone for stability.

Once inserted, the implant should not be removed and reinserted; instead, one-time placement is mandatory. The implant is countersunk in this bone if any risk of loading is expected during healing (e.g.,

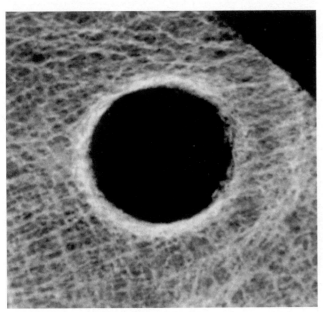

• **Fig. 27.33** Bone compaction technique to prepare the implant site, which results in osseodensification.

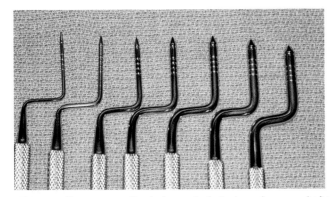

• **Fig. 27.34** Bone compaction instruments (osteotomes) are used after the initial pilot drill to prepare the osteotomy.

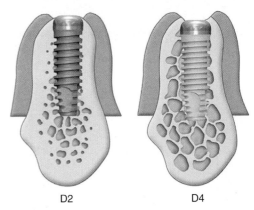

D2   D4

• **Fig. 27.35** In D4 bone, the implant is often countersunk below the crest of the ridge, wherever a soft tissue–borne restoration is worn during the initial healing phase. In D2 bone, the implant is usually placed at the crest of the bone.

• BOX 27.10 D4 Bone Surgical Protocol

- Underprep (osseodensification)
- Drilling speed: ~1000 to 2500 rpm (speed not as important in poorer quality bone)
- Irrigation: copious amounts of saline
- Bone dance: not recommended as will enlarge osteotomy
- Implant placement: handpiece (do not deviate from original osteotomy)

---

under a soft tissue–borne prosthesis). Countersinking the implant below the crest reduces the risk of micromovement during healing in this very soft bone No countersink drill is used before countersinking. A two-stage technique is recommended because this will minimize premature loading of the implant (Fig. 27.35; Box 27.10).

Healing

The healing and progressive bone-loading sequence for D4 bone require more time than the other three types of bone. Time is needed to allow bone to remodel at the surface and to intensify its trabecular pattern. The additional time also allows a more advanced bone mineralization and increased strength. Six or more months of undisturbed healing is suggested. The compression technique for surgery, the extended healing time, and progressive bone-loading protocol allow the remodeling of this bone into a more organized and load-bearing quality similar to D3 bone before the final prosthetic loading of the implants (Fig. 27.36).

Primary Stability

Accurate assessment of primary stability is crucial in the implant placement protocol. Methods of measuring implant stability

include percussion testing, IT, reverse torque testing, resonance frequency analysis (RFA), and surgical experience.

Periotest

In the early days of implantology, instrumented percussion testing used the Periotest system. Periotest evaluations have been used to gauge primary stability. The system is composed of a metallic tapping rod in a handpiece, which is electromagnetically driven and electronically controlled. Signals produced by tapping are converted to unique values called Periotest values. These results are expressed in arbitrary units with acceptable Periotest values in the ranges of –4 to –2 and –4 to +2. However, today this device has been supplanted by RFA because of the lack of reproducibility of results derived from Periotest measurements (Fig. 27.37).

Resonance Frequency Analysis

In implantology today, the more common method of determining primary stability is resonance frequency analysis (RFA). RFA is a testing method that provides objective and reliable measurements of lateral micromobility at various stages of the implant treatment process. The method analyzes the first resonance frequency of a small transducer attached to an implant or abutment. It can be used to monitor the changes in stiffness and stability at the implant–tissue interface and to discriminate between successful implants and clinical failures. The Implant Stability Quotient (ISQ) is the scale of measurement for use with the RFA method.

This more objective assessment of stability may help improve a clinician's learning curve and is useful for future comparison. Multiple studies[66,67] have determined that an acceptable stability range lies between 55 and 85 ISQ, with an average ISQ level of 70.[68]

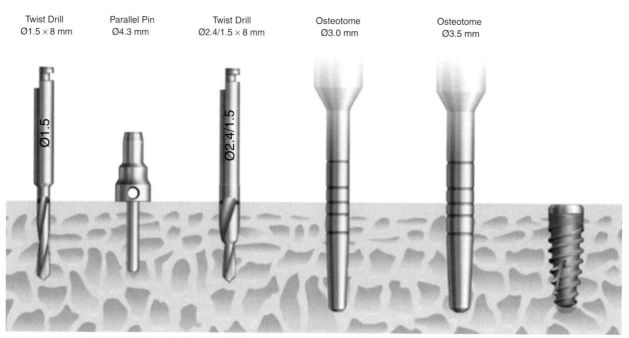

Twist Drill	Parallel Pin	Twist Drill	Osteotome	Osteotome
Ø1.5 × 8 mm	Ø4.3 mm	Ø2.4/1.5 × 8 mm	Ø3.0 mm	Ø3.5 mm

• **Fig. 27.36** D4 surgical protocol. Only one to two burs are used, then osteotomes osseodensify the osteotomy, which results in an increased bone density.

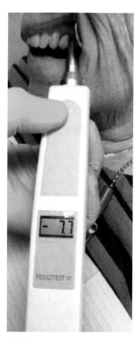

• **Fig. 27.37** Periotest, which uses a tapping rod to evaluate implant stability.

Various studies have shown that the RFA protocol can provide the clinician with important information about the current status of the bone-implant interface via ISQ values. In combination with clinical and radiographic findings, the use of RFA can be used as a valuable diagnostic adjunct with regards to the bone density, healing protocols, and loading protocols for dental implants, as well as recognizing the potential failure of implants.

Sennerby reported on a classification of ISQ values in relation to the health of dental implants. The ISQ values were placed into three zones based on RFA measurements at the time of implant placement. Recommendations include the "safe zone" which includes ISQ values of 70 or above. These high ISQ values are usually suitable for immediate load protocols. The second classification includes "questionable" implants, which represent values from 55 – 70 ISQ. Values in this range require continuous monitoring to determine if ISQ numbers increase after longer healing. It is recommended that implants with ISQ's in this range should undergo progressive bone loading techniques. The last zone includes implants with an ISQ value of less than 55. These implants are compromised and may be associated with an increased failure rate. Therefore, increased healing times are recommended along with progressive bone loading protocols. If subsequent readings still remain low after healing and progressive bone loading protocols, further healing may be warranted.[69]

Numerous studies have shown the successful use of RFA in the evaluation of implant health. Sjöström et al.[70] evaluated the primary stability of maxillary implants of successful vs. failed implants. The average ISQ for the successful implants were 62 ISQ and the failed implants were 54 ISQ. Turkyilmaz and McGlumphy in a retrospective study of 300 implants over three years showed failed implants with an average ISQ of 46 and successful implants an average of 67 ISQ. In the evaluation of Hounsfield units and insertion torque, similar significant differences were found.[71] (Fig. 27.38; Box 27.11).

In general, the RFA technique via ISQ values provide valuable information on the current status of the implant–bone interface. The ISQ values correlate to the micromobility of the implant, which is directly related to the biomechanical properties of the surrounding bone tissue and the quality of the bone-implant interface. Through various studies, it has been shown that lower ISQ values are directly associated with eventual implant failure. Therefore, the RFA technique is a valuable modality in evaluating dental implant health during any phase of the implant process.[72]

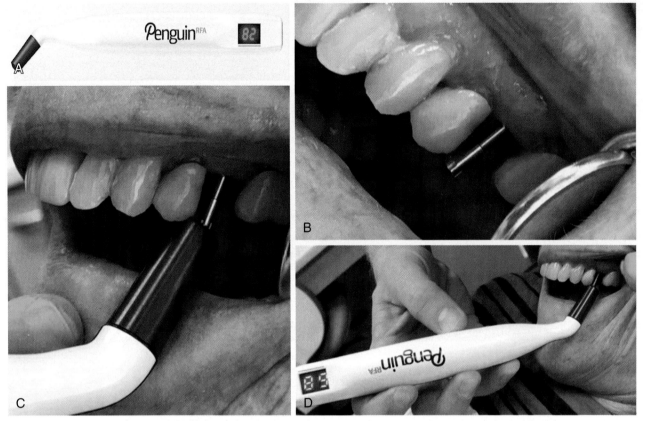

• **Fig. 27.38** Penguin RFA. (A) Penguin RFA measures implant stability and osseointegration. (B) Reusable MulTipeg is inserted into the implant body. (C) Penguin is placed in approximation to the reusable MulTipeg. (D) Final reading of the RFA, ideally the Implant Stability Quotient reading will be greater than 55.

• BOX 27.11 Resonance Frequency Analysis

- Autoclavable
- Calibrated transducers used are SmartPegs
- Magnetic peg is fixed to the implant fixture or abutment
- Peg is excited through magnetic pulses and starts to vibrate, inducing an electric volt that is picked up by the magnetic RFA
- Establishment of a new unit to describe the frequencies = ISQ
- Readings are taken in two directions (MD) and BL and the average is recorded as the ISQ

BL, buccal-lingual; *ISQ,* Implant Stability Quotient; *MD,* mesial-distal; *RFA,* radiofrequency analysis.

One-Stage versus Two-Stage

The clinician is often confronted with the choice of completing the dental implant procedure with a one-stage or a two-stage protocol. Numerous studies have shown no difference in success rates between the two techniques.[73,74]

Two-Stage Surgery

The two-stage surgery technique involves the placement of the implant and a low-profile cover screw, which is inserted into the implant body. When the cover screw is in final position, it may be slightly tightened, loosened, and tightened again. No tissue, blood coagulants, or bone particles should prevent the complete seating of the cover screw. In addition, the cover screw should not be tightened with significant force because this may result in the implant rotating, which increases the possibility of nonintegration.

The two-stage surgical approach offers several advantages. By submerging the implant below the tissue, no pressure is placed on the surgery site, allowing the implant to heal undisturbed. In addition, there exists less chance of infection, and overloading the implant prematurely is less likely. However, with a two-stage approach, a second-stage surgery is required, which usually will lead to longer healing times. Studies have shown that less keratinized tissue is present compared with a one-stage protocol.

The indications for a two-stage surgery include anytime primary stability is in question, such as compromised bone density. If excessive parafunctional habits are present, then submerging the implant is an ideal treatment to minimize the possibility of biomechanical overloading. Last, if bone grafting procedures are used in conjunction with the implant placement, then undisturbed healing via a two-stage technique is ideal (Fig. 27.39; Box 27.12).

One-Stage Surgery

A one-stage surgical protocol involves the placement of a healing abutment that extends slightly above the crest of the tissue. The soft tissue is then sutured around the healing abutment to form a soft tissue drape during the healing period. There are numerous advantages to the one-stage surgery technique.

One advantage is that the soft tissue matures while the bone interface is healing. This permits the restoration to be fabricated with complete assessment of the soft tissue profile. In the two-step

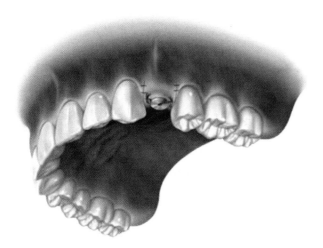

• **Fig. 27.39** After implant placement, a cover screw is inserted into the implant. A second-stage surgery is indicated to expose the implant for prosthetic rehabilitation.

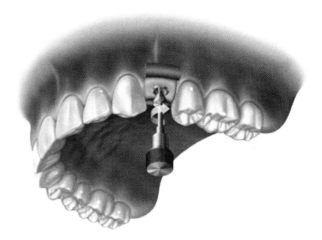

• **Fig. 27.40** After implant placement, a healing abutment is inserted into the implant to allow for ideal soft tissue healing.

• **BOX 27.12** **Two-Stage Surgical Protocol**

Advantages:
• Submerged implant
• No pressure on surgery site
• Less chance of infection

Disadvantages:
• Second-stage surgery needed
• Longer healing times
• Less keratinized tissue versus one-stage

Indications:
• ? Primary stability
• Bone grafting/membranes
• Parafunction/force issues

• **BOX 27.13** **One-Stage Surgical Protocol**

Advantages:
• No second surgery
• Shortens treatment time
• Better tissue health

Disadvantages:
• Healing abutments can be loose
• Force-related issues
• Less space for interim prosthesis

Indications:
• Favorable primary stability
• No bone grafting/membranes
• No parafunction/force Issues

---

procedure, the soft tissue is less mature when the prosthesis is fabricated because a stage II surgery is required to uncover the implant and place a healing abutment.

Because a healing abutment has been placed on the implant, a second surgical procedure and suture removal appointment are not necessary. This saves the patient discomfort and results in two less appointments (stage II uncovery and suture removal).

The abutment to implant connection may be placed above the crest of bone in the one-stage surgery. This higher location of the implant–abutment connection may reduce some of the early crestal bone loss in a developing implant interface. In addition, Weber observed an improved hemidesmosome soft tissue–implant connection when the components above the bone were not removed and reinserted, such as when the healing gap connection is below the bone.[75] Depending on the crest module design, the one-stage surgical approach may have less early crestal bone loss.

The one-stage technique also has numerous disadvantages. The higher profile permucosal extension (PME) is more at risk of loading during healing, especially when an overlying soft tissue–borne transitional restoration is worn. Therefore a disadvantage may be a higher healing failure rate. However, clinical studies of one-stage surgery indicate similar implant survival rates in good bone volumes and quality.

Because the healing abutment is placed with finger pressure, patients may tend to place unnecessary force on the abutment via their tongue. This may result in the loosening of the abutment and possible aspiration. If the healing abutment becomes partially loose, then soft tissue will often grow in between the abutment and implant, preventing complete seating of the prostheses. When a bone graft is placed at the time of implant insertion, primary closure of the soft tissues improves the environment to grow bone. Therefore the one-stage approach is indicated less often under these conditions.

A one-stage surgical protocol is indicated when implant placement involves excellent primary stability. The patient should not exhibit any parafunctional or force-related habits and there should be no bone grafting procedures completed in conjunction with the implant placement (Fig. 27.40; Box 27.13; Table 27.1).

Summary

Bone remodels in relation to the forces exerted on it. Depending on the location of the edentulous ridge and the amount of time the area has been edentulous, the density of bone is variable. Clinically, the surgeon can correlate the hardness of the trabecular bone and the presence of a cortical plate with four different densities of bone. The typical locations of these different densities, the alteration in surgical technique with each type, and the advantages and

TABLE 27.1	**Surgical Preparation and Implant Insertion Protocol**						
Bone Density	Location	Similar Density	Drilling Protocol	Drilling Speed	Insertion Level	Insertion Technique	Ideal Healing
D1	Anterior mandible	Maple/oak wood	All drills + bone tap	2000 rpm (bone dancing)	At or slightly above crest	Hand ratchet	3–4 months
D2	Anterior mandible Posterior mandible, Anterior maxilla	White pine wood	All drills (possible bone tap)	2000 rpm (bone dancing)	Level with crest	Hand ratchet or handpiece	4 months
D3	Anterior maxilla Posterior mandible	Balsa wood	All drills except last shaping drill	~1000 rpm	At or slightly below crest	Handpiece (30 rpm)	4–5 months
D4	Posterior maxilla	Styrofoam	Only one to two beginning burs, then osteotomes	~1000 rpm	Slightly below crest	Handpiece (30 rpm)	5–6 months

disadvantages of each have been related to each density classification. The dense cortical bone of D1 is the strongest bone, approximately 10 times greater than D4 bone, and is the most difficult to prepare. The thick, porous cortical and coarse trabecular D2 bone is twice as strong as D3 bone and is ideal for implant support. The thin, porous cortical and fine trabecular D3 bone is similar to preparations in compressed balsa wood. The fine trabecular bone of D4 is similar to osteotomies in dense Styrofoam. The initial drills may be used to distinguish among the four bone density types.

A surgical preparation and implant insertion protocol has been discussed which relates specifically to the bone density. D1 bone heals with a lamellar bone interface and has the greatest percentage of bone at the implant body contact regions. D2 bone heals with woven and lamellar bone, is adequately mineralized at 4 months, and often has approximately 70% bone in initial contact after healing with the implant body. D3 bone has about 50% bone at the initial implant interface after healing and benefits from a roughened surface on the screw-shaped implant body to increase initial fixation and bone contact. An additional 1 month (total of 5 months) is used for initial bone healing, compared with D2 bone, to permit a greater percentage of bone trabeculae to mineralize and form around the implant. D4 bone density has the least amount of trabeculae at implant placement. Additional time for bone healing and incremental bone loading will improve the density and result in implant survival similar to that of other bone densities.

References

1. Eriksson AR, Albrektsson T, Albrektsson B. Heat caused by drilling in cortical bone. Temperature measured in vivo in patients and animals. *Acta Orthop Scand*. 1984;55:629–631.
2. Schroeder A. Preparation of the implant bed. In: Schroeder A, Sutter F, eds. *Oral Implantology*. New York: Thieme; 1996.
3. Ercoli C, Funkenbusch PD, Lee HJ, et al. The influence of drill wear on cutting efficiency and heat production during osteotomy preparation for dental implants: a study of drill durability. *Int J Oral Maxillofac Implants*. 2004;19:335–349.
4. Sharawy M, Misch CE, Weller N, et al. Heat generation during implant drilling: the significance of motor speed. *Oral Maxillofac Surg*. 2002;60:1160–1169.
5. Matthews J, Hirsch C. Temperatures measured in human cortical bone when drilling. *J Bone Joint Surg*. 1972;45A:297–308.

6. Chacon GE, Bower DL, Larsen PE, et al. Heat production by 3 implant drill systems after repeated drilling and sterilization. *J Oral Maxillofac Surg*. 2006;64:265–269.
7. Adell R, Lekholm U, Brånemark PI. Surgical procedures. In: Brånemark PI, Zarb GA, Albrektsson T, eds. *Tissue-integrated Prostheses Osseointegration in Clinical Dentistry*. Chicago: Quintessence; 1985.
8. Wiggins KL, Malkin S. Drilling of bone. *J Biomech*. 1976;9:553–559.
9. Rafel SS. Temperature changes during high-speed drilling on bone. *J Oral Surg Anesth Hosp Dent Serv*. 1962;20:475–477.
10. Brisman DL. The effect of speed, pressure, and time on bone temperature during the drilling of implant sites. *Int J Oral Maxillofac Implants*. 1996;11:35–37.
11. Hobkirk J, Rusiniak K. Investigation of variable factors in drilling bone. *J Oral Surg*. 1977;35:968–973.
12. Eriksson RA, Albrektsson T. Temperature threshold levels for heat-induced bone tissue injury: a vital-microscopic study in the rabbit. *J Prosthet Dent*. 1983;50:101–107.
13. Kim SJ, Yoo J, Kim YS, Shin SW. Temperature change in pig rib bone during implant site preparation by low-speed drilling. *J Appl Oral Science*. 2010;18(5):522–527.
14. Yacker M, Klein M. The effect of irrigation on osteotomy depth and bur diameter. *Int J Oral Maxillofac Implants*. 1996;11:635–638.
15. Benington IC, Biagioni PA, Briggs J, Sheridan S, Lamey PJ. Thermal changes observed at implant sites during internal and external irrigation. *Clin Oral Implants Res*. 2002;13(3):293–297.
16. Barrak I, et al. Effect of the combination of low-speed drilling and cooled irrigation fluid on intraosseous heat generation during guided surgical implant site preparation: an in vitro study. *Implant Dentistry*. 2017;26(4):541–546.
17. Boa K, et al. Intraosseous generation of heat during guided surgical drilling: an ex vivo study of the effect of the temperature of the irrigating fluid. *Br J Oral Maxillofac Surg*. 2016;54(8):904–908.
18. Davidson SR, James DF. Drilling in bone: modeling heat generation and temperature distribution. *J Biomech Eng*. 2003;125:305–314.
19. Yacker M, Klein M. The effect of irrigation on osteotomy depth and bur diameter. *Int J Oral Maxillofac Implants*. 1996;11:635–638.
20. Eriksson RA, Adell R. Temperatures during drilling for the placement of implants using the osseointegration technique. *J Oral Maxillofac Surg*. 1986;44:4–7.
21. Yeniyol S, Jimbo R, Marin C, et al. The effect of drilling speed on early bone healing to oral impl Oral. *Surg Oral Med Oral Pathol Oral Radiol*. 2013;116:550–555.

22. Rafel SS. Temperature changes during high-speed drilling on bone. *J Oral Surg Anesth Hosp Dent Serv.* 1962;20:475–477.

23. Babbush CA. The endosteal blade vent implant—the histology of animal studies and scanning electron microscope observations. In: Babbush CA, ed. *Surgical Atlas of Dental Implant Techniques.* Philadelphia: WB Saunders; 1980.

24. Matthews J, Hirsch C. Temperatures measured in human cortical bone when drilling. *J Bone Joint Surg.* 1972;45A:297–308.

25. Watcher R, Stoll P. Increase of temperature during osteotomy. In vitro and in vivo investigations. *Int J Oral Maxillofac Surg.* 1991;20:245–249.

26. Meredith N. A review of implant design, geometry and placement. *Appl Osseointegr Res.* 2008;6:6e12.

27. Ottoni JM, Oliveira ZF, Mansini R, Cabral AM. Correlation between placement torque and survival of single-tooth implants. *Int J Oral Maxillofac Implants.* 2005;20(5):769–776.

28. da Cunha HA, Francischone CE, Filho HN, de Oleviera RC. A comparison between cutting torque and resonance frequency in the assessment of primary stability and final torque capacity of standard and TiUnite single-tooth implants under immediate loading. *Int J Oral Maxillofac Implants.* 2004;19(4):578–585.

29. Horwitz J, Zuabi O, Peled M, Machtei EE. Immediate and delayed restoration of dental implants in periodontally susceptible patients: 1 year results. *Int J Oral Maxillofac Implants.* 2007;22(3):423–429.

30. Qu Z. *Mechanical Properties of Trabecular Bone in Human Mandible [doctoral Thesis].* Birmingham, Ala: University of Alabama at Birmingham.; 1994.

31. Misch CE, Qu Z, Bidez MW. Mechanical properties of trabecular bone in the human mandible: implications for dental implant treatment planning and surgical placement. *J Oral Maxillofac Surg.* 1999;57:700–706.

32. Lekholm U, Zarb GA. Patient selection and preparation. In: Brånemark PI, Zarb GA, Albrektsson T, eds. *Tissue-integrated Prostheses.* Chicago: Quintessence; 1985.

33. Adell R, Lekholm U, Rockler B. A 15-year study of osseointegrated implants in the treatment of the edentulous jaw. *Int J Oral Surg.* 1981;10:387–416.

34. Engquist B, Bergendal T, Kallus T, et al. A retrospective multicenter evaluation of osseointegrated implants supporting overdentures. *Int J Oral Maxillofac Implants.* 1988;3:129–134.

35. Jaffin RA, Berman CL. The excessive loss of Brånemark fixtures in type IV bone: a 5-year analysis. *J Periodontol.* 1991;62:2–4.

36. Friberg B, Jemt T, Lekholm U. Early failures in 4,641 consecutively placed Brånemark dental implants: a study from stage I surgery to the connection of completed prostheses. *Int J Oral Maxillofac Implants.* 1991;6:142–146.

37. Quirynen M, Naert I, van Steenberghe D, et al. A study of 589 consecutive implants supporting complete fixed prostheses: dental and periodontal aspects. *J Prosthet Dent.* 1992;68:655–663.

38. Fugazzotto PA, Wheeler SL, Lindsay JA. Success and failure rates of cylinder implants in type IV bone. *J Periodontol.* 1993;64:1085–1087.

39. Hutton JE, Heath MR, Chai JY, et al. Factors related to success and failure rates at 3 year follow up in a multicenter study of overdentures supported by Branemark implants. *Int J Oral Maxillofac Implants.* 1995;10:33–42.

40. Sullivan DY, Sherwood RL, Collins TA, et al. The reverse-torque test: a clinical report. *Int J Oral Maxillofac Implants.* 1996;11:179–185.

41. Snauwaert K, Duyck D, van Steenberghe D, et al. Time dependent failure rate and marginal bone loss of implant supported prostheses: a 15-year follow-up. *Study Clin Oral Invest.* 2000;4:13–20.

42. Herrmann I, Lekholm U, Holm S, et al. Evaluation of patient and implant characteristics as potential prognostic factors for oral implant failures. *Int J Oral Maxillofac Implants.* 2005;20:220–230.

43. Truhlar RS, Morris HF, Ochi S, et al. Second stage failures related to bone quality in patients receiving endosseous dental implants: DICRG Interim Report No. 7. Dental Implant Clinical Research Group. *Implant Dent.* 1994;3:252–255.

44. Misch CE, Hoar JB, Beck G, et al. A bone quality based implant system: a preliminary report of stage I and stage II. *Implant Dent.* 1998;7:35–42.

45. Misch CE, Poitras Y, Dietsh-Misch F. Endosteal implants in the edentulous posterior maxilla—rationale and clinical results. *Oral Health.* 2000:7–16.

46. Frost HM. A brief review for orthopedic surgeons: Fatigue damage (microdamage) in bone (its determinants and clinical implications). *J Orthop Sci.* 1998;3:272–281.

47. Misch CE. Density of bone: effect on treatment plans, surgical approach, healing, and progressive bone loading. *Int J Oral Implantol.* 1990;6:23–31.

48. Huwais S. *Inventor; Fluted osteotome and surgical method for use.* US Patent Application US2013/0004918. 2013.

49. Huwais S, Meyer E. Osseodensification: a novel approach in implant osteotomy preparation to increase primary stability, bone mineral density and bone to implant contact. *Int J Oral Maxillofac Implants.* 2016;32:27–36.

50. Degidi M, Giuseppe Daprile, Piattelli A. Influence of underpreparation on primary stability of implants inserted in poor quality bone sites: an in vitro study. *J Oral Maxillofac Surg.* 2015;73(6):1084–1088.

51. Alghamdi H, Anand PS, Anil S. Undersized implant site preparation to enhance primary implant stability in poor bone density: a prospective clinical study. *J Oral Maxillofac Surg.* 2011;69(12):e506–e512.

52. Roberts EW, Turley PK, Brezniak N, et al. Bone physiology and metabolism. *J Calif Dent Assoc.* 1987;15:54–61.

53. Roberts WE. Fundamental principles of bone physiology, metabolism and loading. In: Naert I, van Steenberghe D, Worthington P, eds. *Osseointegration in Oral Rehabilitation.* Carol Stream: Ill: Quintessence; 1993.

54. Haider R, Watzek G, Plenk Jr H. Influences of drill cooling and bone structure on primary implant fixation. *Int J Oral Maxillofac Implants.* 1993;8:83–91.

55. Chanavaz M. Anatomy and histophysiology of the periosteum: classification of the periosteal blood supply to the adjacent bone with 855r and gamma spectrometry. *J Oral Implantol.* 1995;21:214–219.

56. Crock JG, Morrisson WA. A vascularized periosteal flap: anatomical study. *Br J Plast Surg.* 1992;45:474–478.

57. Watzek G, Danhel-Mayhauser M, Matejka M, et al. *Experimental Comparison of Brånemark and TPS Dental Implants in Sheep [Abstract]Presented at Ucla Symposium: Implants in the Partially Edentulous. Patient* Palm Springs, CA; 1990.

58. Satomi K, Akagawa Y, Nikai H, et al. Bone implant interface structures after nontapping and tapping insertion of screw type titanium alloy endosseous implants. *J Prosthet Dent.* 1988;59:339–342.

59. Beer A, Gahleitner A, Holm A, et al. Adapted preparation technique for screw-type implants: explorative in vitro pilot study in a porcine bone model. *Clin Oral Implants Res.* 2007;18:103–107.

60. Watzek G, Haider R, Gitsch M, et al. *Influence of Drill Cooling and Bone Structure on Primary Implant Fixation.* Boston: American Academy of Osseo-integration; 1991. [abstract].

61. Novaes Jr AB, de Oliveira RR, Taba Jr M, et al. Crestal bone loss minimized when following the crestal preparation protocol: a histomorphometric study in dogs. *J Oral Implantol.* 2005;31:276–282.

62. Orenstein IH, Synan WJ, Truhlar RS, et al. Bone quality in patients receiving endosseous dental implants: DICRG Interim Report No. 1. *Implant Dent.* 1994;3:90–94.

63. Rhinelander FW. The normal circulation of bone and its response to surgical intervention. *J Biomed Mater Res.* 1974;8:87–90.

64. Degidi M, Daprile G, Piattelli A. Determination of primary stability: a comparison of the surgeon's perception and objective measurements. *Int J Oral Maxillofac Implants.* 2010;25(3):558–561.

65. Misch CE. Maxillary sinus augmentation for edentulous arches for implant dentistry: organized alternative treatment plans. *Int J Oral Implantol.* 1987;4:7–12.

66. Bischof M, et al. Implant stability measurement of delayed and immediately loaded implants during healing. *Clin Oral Implants Res.* 2004;15(5):529–539.

67. Sennerby L, Meredith N. Resonance frequency analysis: measuring implant stability and osseointegration. *Compend Contin Educ Dent.* 1998;19(5):493–498, 500, 502; quiz 504.

68. Konstantinović VS, Ivanjac F, Lazić V, et al. Assessment of implant stability by resonant frequency analysis. *Military Med Pharm J Serbia.* 2015;72(2):169.

69. Lars S. Resonance frequency analysis for implant stability measurements. A review. *Integration Diagn Update.* 2015;1:11.

70. Sjöström M, Lundgren S, Nilson H, Sennerby L. Monitoring of implant stability in grafted bone using resonance frequency analysis. A clinical study from implant placement to 6 months of loading. *Int J Oral Maxillofac Surg.* 2005;34:45–51.

71. Turkyilmaz I, McGlumphy EA. Influence of bone density on implant stability parameters and implant success: a retrospective clinical study. *BMC Oral Health.* 2008;8:32.

72. Östman PO, Hellman M, Wendelhag I, Sennerby L. Resonance frequency analysis measurements of implants at placement surgery. *Int J Prosthodont.* 2006;19(1).

73. Cardelli P, et al. Clinical assessment of submerged vs non-submerged implants placed in pristine bone. *Oral Implantol.* 2013;6(4):89.

74. Byrne G. Outcomes of one-stage versus two-stage implant placement. *J Am Dent Assoc.* 2010;141(10):1257–1258.

75. Weber HP, Fiorellini JP. The biology and morphology of the implant-tissue interface. *Alpha Omegan.* 1992;85:61–64.

28

Ideal Implant Positioning

RANDOLPH R. RESNIK AND CARL E. MISCH[†]

To obtain ideal esthetics and function of an implant-supported prosthesis, the three-dimensional positioning of the dental implant within the bone is critical. The malposition of the dental implant can lead to significant implant complications and increased morbidity. Nonideal implant positioning may result in undesirable outcomes that may ultimately affect the success and longevity of prosthetic rehabilitation.[1] To achieve an ideal result for the patient, a clinician must be conscious of the implant placement with respect to the ideal and correct orientation of the final prosthesis design. Optimal dental implant positioning is dictated by the three-dimensional placement of implants with respect to the biomechanical and prosthetic principles related to the final implant prosthesis.

Recently advances in implant dentistry technology have created a greater appreciation for the esthetic results of the implant restoration. Implant dentistry has experienced a profound shift from a functional thought process with a surgical approach to esthetics, to a more prosthetically and biologically driven protocol.[2] The dental implant should be positioned in ideal relationship to the position of the existing teeth, vital structures, and other implants, as well as the buccolingual, mesiodistal, and apicocoronal dimensions. When implants are positioned with no emphasis to the three-dimensional location, any of the following detrimental effects may occur (Fig. 28.1) Box 28.1:

> • **BOX 28.1** **Non-Ideal Implant Positioning Complications**
>
> * Increased implant morbidity
> * Increased prosthetic complications (e.g., esthetics, prosthesis)
> * Increased prosthetic costs (e.g., implant parts, laboratory costs)
> * Increased peri-implant complications
> * Decreased longevity of prosthesis
> * Less patient acceptance

The ideal three-dimensional positioning of a dental implant needs to be addressed before the surgical procedure. Lack of proper planning may lead to malpositioning which may be evaluated in the three spatial planes. The placement of a dental implant in available bone is comparable to an object in space that is defined by "x," "y," and "z" coordinates. In implant dentistry, the x-axis is defined by the mesiodistal plane, the y-axis is the buccolingual dimension, and the z-axis is known as the apicocoronal (length of implant body in relation to the osseous crest).[3] Unfortunately,

many dental implants are placed within the existing available bone without respect to the three dimensions. In this chapter, the proper positioning of implants will be discussed according to the final prosthetic needs and demands of the patient and the treatment protocols for implants that are placed in nonideal positions.

"X"-Axis (Mesial-Distal) Positioning

Insufficient Implant–Tooth Distance (Apical)

Ideal Positioning

Ideally, it is best to allow at least a minimum of 1.5 mm from the adjacent tooth root or tooth structure.[4] Maintaining this amount of space from a tooth root decreases the possibility of causing damage to the tooth and postoperative complications (Fig. 28.2).

Pretreatment Evaluation

Preoperatively, the most accurate technique to determine available space for an implant adjacent to a tooth is with a cone beam computerized tomography (CBCT) axial image. The ideal x-axis angulation and position needs to be determined via interactive CBCT treatment planning and transferred to the surgical procedure. This is most easily accomplished with a CBCT-generated surgical template. If the implant placement is being completed freehand, then an intraoral radiograph (e.g., periapical) should be used after the first pilot drill to determine ideal positioning with respect to the adjacent teeth. After initial evaluation, the osteotomy positioning may be changed or modified via a Lindemann drill (i.e., side-cutting bur) (Fig. 28.3).

Implants that are positioned too close to an adjacent tooth root are usually the result of poor treatment planning (inadequate space), poor surgical technique (improper angulation), or placement of an implant body that is too wide. This may also occur when root dilacerations of an adjacent tooth exist or if a tooth has been orthodontically repositioned to where the tooth root has encroached on the intraroot space.

The maxillary lateral incisor position may pose a significant challenge in some cases, especially if the area is replacing a congenitally missing lateral incisor. Often, after orthodontic treatment, there exists an ideal mesiodistal distance of the clinical crowns; however, compromised intraroot distance may result because of tilting the teeth orthodontically into position (i.e., clinical crown of the central incisor moves mesially and apical root moving distally). Lack of space may contraindicate implant placement or require orthodontic treatment for repositioning of the roots (Fig. 28.4).

Another common area for root approximation complications is the maxillary first premolar edentulous site. Careful consideration for the angulation of a natural canine must be evaluated. The 11-degree

[†]Deceased

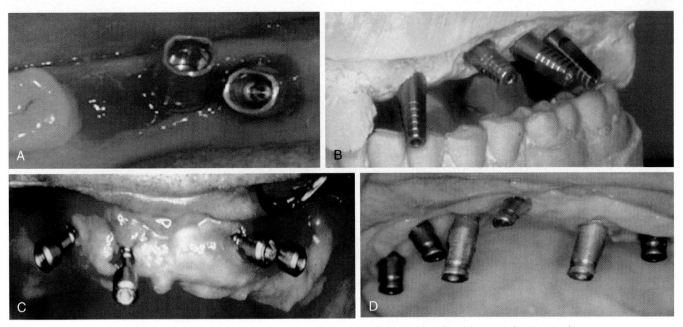

• **Fig. 28.1** Malpositioned implants. (A) Mandibular posterior implants placed too close together, too much distance from anterior adjacent tooth, and poor angulation. (B) Maxillary left implant with poor positioning and angulation. (C and D) Maxillary implant placement with no regards to positioning and final prosthesis.

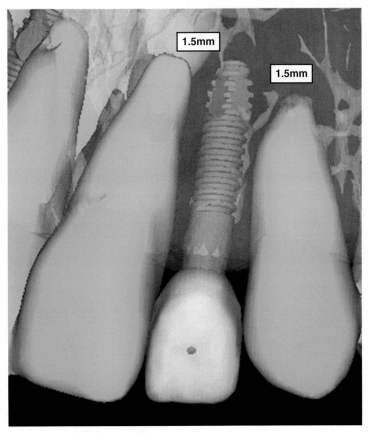

1.5mm

1.5mm

• **Fig. 28.2** Ideal implant placement with regards to the apical area of the adjacent teeth (>1.5 mm). If the implant encroaches upon the root, complications may result.

average distal inclination and distal curvature of the canine root frequently place the apex of the root into the first premolar implant area. The implant should be angled to follow the root of the canine and prevent contact or perforation of the natural root. A shorter implant often is indicated, especially when a second premolar is also present. In some cases, an implant may be contraindicated (Fig. 28.5).

Complications

Implants positioned too close to a tooth risk damage to the periodontal ligament (PDL) and surrounding structures. This may cause displacement of bone into the PDL space and result in altered blood supply to the adjacent tooth, loss of tooth vitality, apical periodontitis, and internal or external resorption (Fig. 28.6).[5]

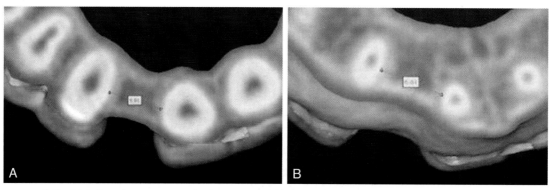

• **Fig. 28.3** Cone beam computerized tomography (CBCT) evaluation. (A) Axial three-dimensional CBCT view measuring midroot distance. (B) Axial view measuring at the most apical extent of the tooth roots.

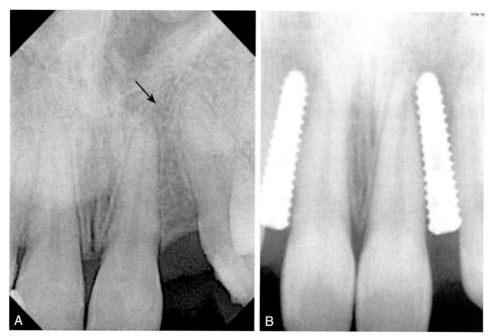

• **Fig. 28.4** (A) Postorthodontic treatment exhibiting tilting of the maxillary central crown mesially, which results in the root apex tilting distally, resulting in less available space for a lateral incisor implant. (B) Poor treatment plan of two congenitally missing lateral incisors with insufficient space resulting in impingement on the adjacent tooth roots.

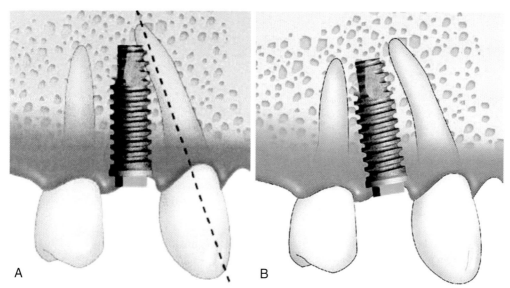

• **Fig. 28.5** Maxillary first bicuspid area. (A) Often the maxillary first bicuspid is placed and may encroach on the natural curvature of the maxillary cuspid. (B) Ideally the implant should be placed parallel to the cuspid root or a shorter implant to minimize the possibility of root encroachment.

Because of the close proximity of implants to an adjacent tooth, the implant may fail because of infection or bone resorption. If less than 1.5 mm of space exists between the implant and the root apex, then the PDL may be damaged, which can result in irreversible trauma and internal or external resorption of the natural tooth. Therefore placing an implant too close to the root surface may ultimately lead to implant or tooth loss, which can occur in the short term or the long term.

In the field of orthodontics today, temporary anchorage devices (TADs) have become popular for cases requiring anchorage. TAD implants are smaller diameter implants (<1.8 mm) that are inserted perpendicular to the long axis of the tooth in the interradicular spaces of the maxilla and mandible. TADs are used for tooth movement (e.g., labial segment retraction or mesial movement of teeth) or for intraoral anchorage, in which tooth movement in all three planes may be accomplished. Interradicular orthodontic implant complications may include loss of tooth vitality, tooth loss, osteosclerosis, and dentoalveolar ankylosis.[6,7] These implants should be cautiously placed because they often are positioned in areas of minimal intraroot distance and above the mucogingival line in attached tissue, which often leads to detrimental effects on adjacent tooth structure[8] (Fig. 28.7).

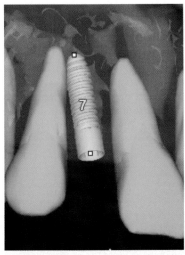

• **Fig. 28.6** Nonideal positioning with respect to the root apex. Implant has an ideal crestal positioning; however, apical positioning results in the implant being too close to the root apex.

Treatment

Initial placement. If there is insufficient space between an implant and the root apex after initial placement, then the implant should be removed and repositioned, especially if the adjacent tooth becomes symptomatic. If available space is compromised, then the roots should be repositioned via orthodontics or the treatment plan changed to a different type of prosthesis.

Past placement. If an implant has been restored and root approximation (<1.5 mm) exists, then the tooth/implant should be monitored on a more stringent clinical and radiographic recall basis along with informing the patient of possible morbidity. The patient should be made aware of the proximity and possible complications that may result. If symptomatic or radiographic pathology is present, then the implant should be removed and repositioned along with vitality testing of the tooth (Fig. 28.8; Box 28.2).

Insufficient Implant–Tooth Distance (Coronal)

Ideal Positioning

For tissue health and ideal emergence profile, a minimum of 2.0 mm should be present from the implant neck to the adjacent tooth[9] (Fig. 28.9). When the implant is closer than mm to the adjacent tooth, any bone loss related to the microgap, the biologic width, or stress concentration may cause the implant and adjacent tooth to lose bone. More space is required at the coronal area (1.5 mm vs. 2.0 mm) to accommodate a papilla.

Within an edentulous space, the implant should be placed in the middle of the space, with an equal amount of interproximal bone toward each adjacent tooth. Ideally, there should exist 2.0 mm or more from the adjacent cement-enamel junction (CEJ) of each tooth. When evaluating defect width around an implant with bone loss, it is usually less than 1.5 mm wide. Hence, if bone loss around the implant occurs, then the bone loss will remain a vertical defect and is less likely to cause bone loss on the adjacent natural tooth. If bone is maintained and no bone loss occurs around the adjacent tooth, then the interdental papilla height will be maintained.

Pretreatment Evaluation

The coronal implant–tooth distance may be determined by evaluating CBCT images (i.e., axial images) or the use of study casts in conjunction with diagnostic wax-ups. On preoperative evaluation, if inadequate space exists for implant placement, then the following treatment may be completed to increase mesiodistal distance:

1. Enameloplasty (modification of the interproximal contact areas) may be completed on the proximal contours of the

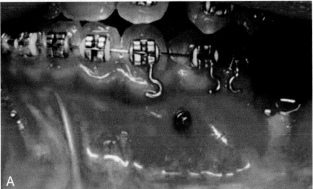
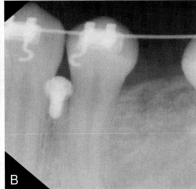

• **Fig. 28.7** Orthodontic implants (temporary anchorage devise [TADs]) that are used for anchorage usually will be very close to adjacent roots. (A) Clinical image depicting a TAD that is placed in between two tooth roots and perpendicular to the bone. (B) Intraoral radiograph showing minimal space for implant placement between tooth roots.

adjacent teeth to increase mesiodistal dimensions. However, care should be exercised in the amount of enamel removed because aggressive modification may lead to hypersensitivity and possible endodontic intervention (Fig. 28.10A, 28.10D).

2. Orthodontic intervention may be used to upright a tilted adjacent tooth to increase the intratooth space. For larger spaces (multiple spaces), one implant may be placed, and an orthodontic spring incorporated in the transitional crown. The spring pushes the distal tooth more distal and, after orthodontic movement, the second implant may be inserted with less risk and improved hygiene between each implant. Another option is to reduce the space orthodontically and place only one implant and crown (see Fig. 28.10B).

3. For larger spaces (multiple implants) the implants may be offset, with one implant placed buccal and the other implant on a diagonal toward the lingual.[9] The diagonal dimension increases the mesiodistal space by 0.5 to 1 mm. In the mandible, the most anterior implant is placed to the lingual aspect of the midcrest and the more distal implant is placed to the facial aspect to facilitate access of a floss threader from the vestibule into the intraimplant space. The occlusal contacts also are slightly modified on the buccal aspect of the mesial implant to occlude over the central fossa. In the maxilla, the anterior implant is placed facially and the distal implant palatally to improve esthetics. The distal occlusal contact is placed over the lingual cusp, and the mesial occlusal contact is located in the central fossa position. The cervical esthetics of the maxillary molar are compromised on the distal half of the tooth to achieve greater intratooth distance and easier access for home care. This maxillary implant placement requires the intraimplant furcation to be approached from the palate, rather than the buccal approach, as for the mandible Fig. 28.10D.

Prevention

A common technique to avoid placing implants too close to a tooth is the use of a surgical template. A pilot, universal or fully guided surgical template may be used that will prevent the implant from being placed too close to the tooth. In addition, if a template is not used, there exist multiple positioning devices that allow for ideal osteotomy positioning (i.e., 1.5–2.0 mm from the adjacent tooth). A surgical spacer may be used, which enables the initial osteotomy site to be placed at the correct position, allowing for adequate space between the tooth and final implant position (Fig. 28.11A–B). Surgical guidance systems (Salvin, Charlotte, North Carolina) also may be used to ensure ideal implant placement (buccolingual and mesiodistal spacing) and may be used with any surgical drill system (see Fig. 28.11C–D). However, the most accurate positioning adjunct is the use of CBCT-generated surgical templates (tooth supported) (see Fig. 28.11E).

Complications

Lack of space between the implant platform and the coronal aspect of the adjacent tooth occurs most likely from poor initial osteotomy positioning, poor treatment planning, or the use of

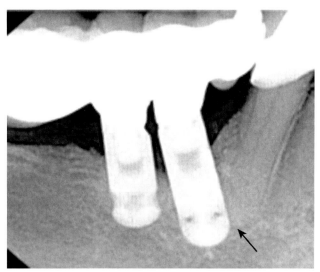

• **Fig. 28.8** Tooth root proximity existing on a final prosthesis. Patients should be informed and a more frequent evaluation should be completed along with regular pulp vitality testing.

• **BOX 28.2** **Lack of Space Between Tooth/Implant (Apical)**

Complication:
• Tooth hypersensitivity
• Loss of tooth vitality
• Periapical pathology
• Tooth loss
• Implant loss

Prevention:
• Ideal positioning (>1.5 mm)
• Accurate radiographic evaluation (cone beam computerized tomography)
• Diagnostic wax-up/interactive treatment planning

Treatment:
• Preprosthetic
  • Remove implant
  • Check tooth vitality
• Postprosthetic
  • Strict recall evaluation
  • Monitor tooth vitality

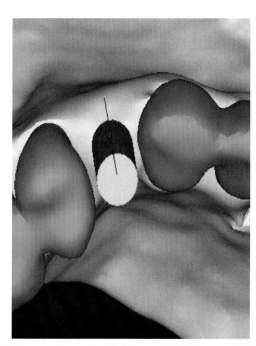

• **Fig. 28.9** In some cases, insufficient mesial-distal space will be present which decreases clinical crown space. Ideally, 2.0 mm should be present between implant and adjacent tooth (crestally).

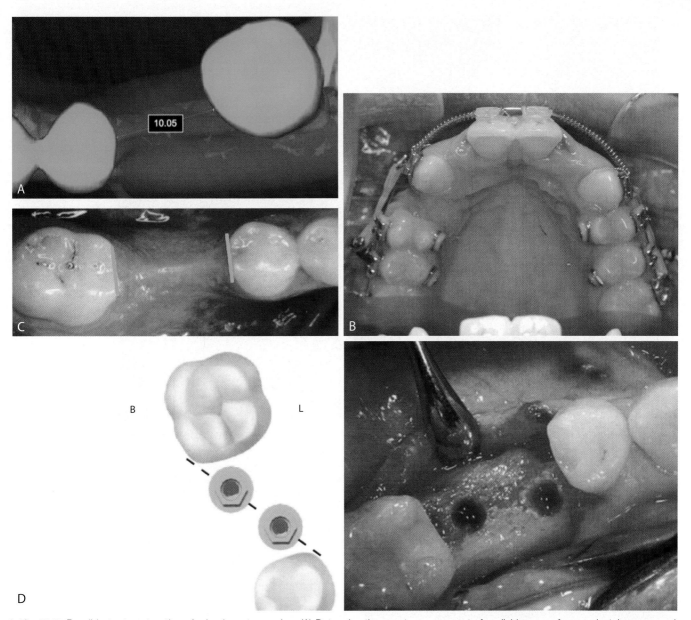

• **Fig. 28.10** Possible treatment options for inadequate spacing. (A) Determine the exact measurement of available space for an edentulous space via cone beam computerized tomographic images. (B) Orthodontic repositioning allowing additional spacing. (C) Enameloplasty of adjacent tooth allows for additional space for prosthesis emergence. (D) In some cases two smaller diameter implants may be placed to replace one molar, however care should be exercised not to position implants too close to each other or too close to adjacent tooth.

an implant body that is too large. This will lead to a situation in which the implant encroaches on the adjacent tooth. Implant clinicians must be aware that most implant crestal platforms are larger than the implant body, which will result in decreased space between the adjacent tooth (e.g., a 3.8-mm implant may have a 4.1-mm platform) (Fig. 28.12; Table 28.1).

Prosthetically, when there exists a lack of space between the adjacent clinical crown and implant, it may be difficult, if not impossible, to form an ideal emergence profile in the new final prosthesis. Lack of proper emergence profile leads to esthetic, hygienic, and soft tissue complications, which increases implant morbidity (Fig. 28.13A–C). Hygiene difficulties will become more frequent because of the unnatural contours of the prosthesis and the lack of space for cleansability. This usually will result in

plaque buildup and related peri-implant complications. Normal hygiene techniques will be modified to access the areas for proper cleansability.

Also, because of the lack of space between the implant and coronal portion of the tooth, bone loss will likely occur. Interproximal bone loss may result from lack of sufficient blood supply. Esposito and colleagues have shown a correlation between increased bone loss and decreased distance of the implant from the adjacent tooth.[10] They reported bone loss increased with decreasing distance, especially in the maxillary incisor region. Because of interproximal bone loss caused by the proximity of the implant to the coronal portion of the tooth, a lack of or reduction in the size of papilla will be present. This will result in peri-implant conditions and resultant esthetic issues (see Fig. 28.13D).

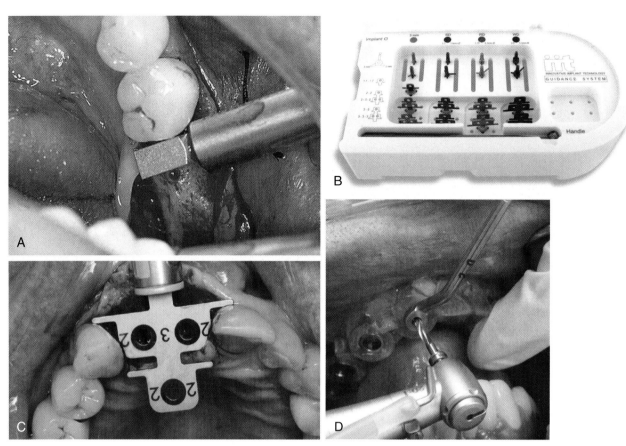

• **Fig. 28.11** Ideal implant placement. (A) Positioning device placed on the distal contact of the adjacent tooth allows for the ideal osteotomy site in the edentulous space. (B and C) Surgical guidance systems may be used for various situations and spacing between teeth. (Courtesy Salvin Dental Specialties, Inc., Charlotte, NC.) (D) Tooth-supported surgical template allowing for accurate implant positioning.)

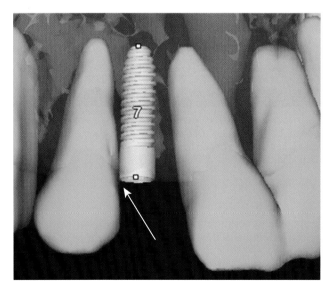

• **Fig. 28.12** Implant placement too close to the clinical crown of the adjacent tooth (<2.0 mm).

TABLE 28.1	Average Mesiodistal Width of Permanent Teeth	
Tooth	**Mandibular (mm)**	**Maxilla (mm)**
Central incisor	5.3	8.6
Lateral incisor	5.7	6.6
Cuspid	6.8	7.6
First bicuspid	7.0	7.1
Second bicuspid	7.1	6.6
First molar	11.4	10.4
Second molar	10.8	9.8

From Hebel MKS, Gajjar R. Anatomic basis for implant selection and positioning. In: Babbush C, ed. *Dental implants: The art and science.* 2nd ed. Philadelphia, PA: Saunders; 2001.

Treatment

Initial placement. On surgical implant placement, if the position of the implant is less than 2.0 mm from the adjacent clinical crown, removal and reposition of the implant should be completed. If the implant is positioned 1.5–2.0 mm from the adjacent tooth,

a possible option would include modifying (enameloplasty) the adjacent tooth, as long as irreversible damage to the tooth is not done and an ideal emergence profile can be established.

Past placement. If the implant has been restored and approximation (<1.5 mm) exists, then the tooth/implant should be strictly monitored. If the natural tooth becomes symptomatic, then the implant should be removed and repositioned, along with long-term vitality testing of the tooth (Box 28.3).

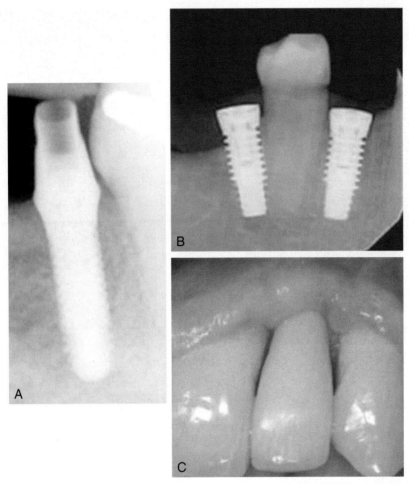

• **Fig. 28.13** Complications resulting from impingement on adjacent teeth. (A and B) Poor implant positioning resulting in inability to create an emergence profile for crowns. (C) Implant body that is too wide results in bone loss followed by tissue loss.

• **BOX 28.3** Lack of Space Between Tooth/Implant (Coronal)

Complication:
- Interproximal bone loss
- Compromised emergence profile
- Complicates prosthetic procedures
- Reduced papilla height
- Hygiene difficulties

Prevention:
- Ideal positioning (~ 2.0 mm)
- Accurate radiographic evaluation (cone beam computerized tomography)
- Diagnostic wax-up/interactive treatment planning
- Use of a surgical template

Treatment:
- Preprosthetic
  - Enameloplasty, crown natural tooth
  - Possible removal of implant and reposition

Excessive Implant–Tooth Distance (Coronal)

Ideal Positioning

If excessive space (>4.0 mm) exists between the implant body and adjacent tooth, a biomechanical disadvantage will result because of the cantilever effect (i.e., contact area of the adjacent tooth). Ideally, the implant should be loaded along the long axis of the implant body. Because of the excessive space between the implant and tooth, overcontouring of the final prosthesis is required to achieve a contact area with the adjacent tooth (Fig. 28.14).

Pretreatment Evaluation

To prevent the placement of an implant too far from an adjacent tooth, a CBCT-generated template may be used to accurately place the implant. Because teeth are present, a tooth-supported guide would be the most accurate template compared with bone-borne or tissue-borne guides. In addition, special positioning devices allow for ideal osteotomy placement and adherence to the ideal placement of 1.5 to 2.0 mm from the adjacent tooth. These predetermined distance spacers will minimize the possibility of placing the implant too close or too far from the adjacent tooth (Fig. 28.15).

Complications

The excessive space present between the implant and adjacent tooth will result in biomechanical issues and possible esthetic complications. Loading of the cantilever area will produce - a resultant shear force. Because bone is weakest with shear forces, bone loss will most likely occur around the crestal area of the implant. Cantilevers present on implant prostheses are more problematic than on natural teeth for several reasons. Forces are magnified to the

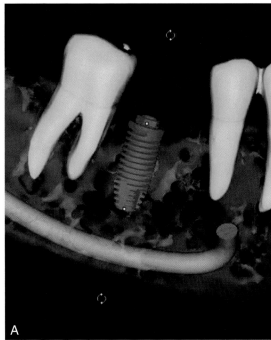

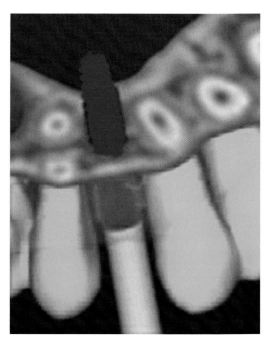

• **Fig. 28.15** Implant should be placed in the midpoint of the mesiodistal distance via three-dimensional cone beam computerized tomographic interactive treatment planning.

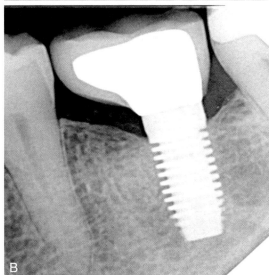

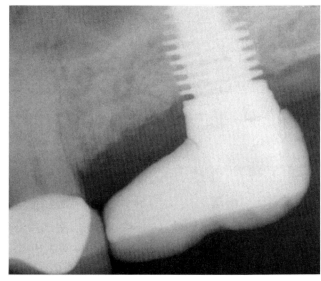

• **Fig. 28.14** Implant placed too far from the adjacent tooth. (A) The implant should be placed at the midpoint of the mesiodistal distance. (B) Nonideal placement may result in cantilever effect biomechanical disadvantages.

• **Fig. 28.16** Clinical image depicting poor implant positioning leading to a significant cantilever effect. Forces placed on the mesial cantilever will result in shear forces to the implant crestal area.

entire implant system, which may result in implant screw loosening, cement retention failure, or even possibly the mobility and failure of the implant itself. Second, because the implant is void of a PDL, there is no stress release system in place to protect the implant. Studies have shown a 1-mm increase in the horizontal offset of an implant restoration may produce a 15% increase in torque during function, and a 1-mm increase in the vertical offset introduces a 5% increase.[11] The overcontoured crown leads to resultant shear forces, which may lead to component failure (i.e., screw loosening, screw fracture, implant fracture).

Because of the need to obtain interproximal contact, the final prosthesis will be atypical, which may lead to increased difficulty in prosthetic impression, laboratory, and insertion procedures (Figs. 28.16 and 28.17). Food impaction is a common complaint from patients with an increased implant–tooth distance because periodontal maintenance is difficult as a result of related soft tissue complications. The chronic soft tissue problems may lead to

peri-implant disease (i.e., peri-mucositis, peri-implantitis) which results in an increased implant morbidity.

Treatment

Initial placement. If nonideal placement is determined during surgery, the implant should be repositioned in the ideal position (i.e., 1.5–2.0 mm from the adjacent tooth). To prevent malposition the following osteotomy formula may be used: ½ diameter of the implant + 2.0 mm from tooth = osteotomy site initiation.

In other words, a 4.0-mm implant pilot osteotomy would be 2.0 mm + 2.0 mm = 4.0 mm from the adjacent tooth. If the initial osteotomy is not ideal, then a Lindemann drill (side cutting) is used to reposition the osteotomy into the correct position.

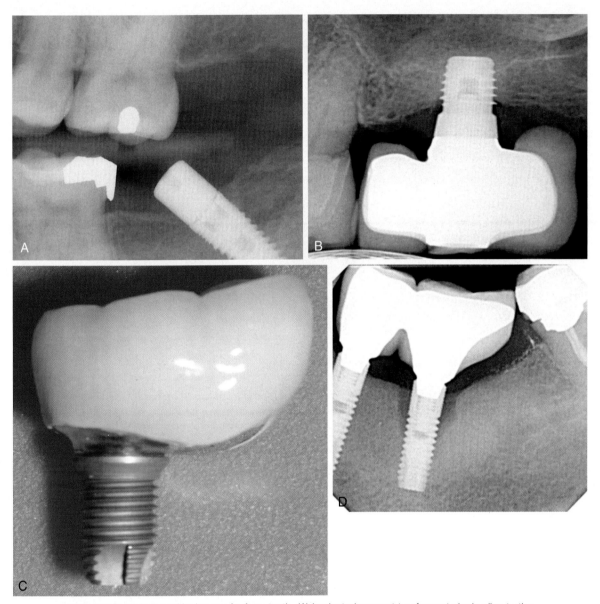

• **Fig. 28.17** Implant positioning too far from tooth. (A) Implant placement too far posterior leading to the implant being non-restorable, (B) Poor implant positioning resulting in prosthesis that has resultant anterior and posterior cantilevers. (C and D) Atypical prosthesis because of nonideal implant placement and need to obtain contact area, which results in biomechanical complications and food impaction.

Past placement. If the implant has already been placed and is ready to be restored, then the amount of occlusal force should be assessed to determine the ideal treatment:

Minimal occlusal forces: If favorable force factors exist (e.g., opposing removable prosthesis, lack of parafunction) then a cantilever (overcontoured crown) may be fabricated with (Fig. 28.18A) the following:
- Narrow occlusal table
- Minimal cusp height: It has been reported that every 10-degree increase in cusp inclination leads to a 30% increase in the torque applied to the restoration during function[10]
- No lateral contacts
- Strong, long contact area

High occlusal forces: If unfavorable forces (e.g., opposing fixed or implant prosthesis, parafunction) are present, then a cantilever is contraindicated and the mesiodistal distance is reduced by either:

- Overcontouring adjacent crown (e.g., crown, composite) (see Fig. 28.18B)
- Remove implant and reposition (Box 28.4).

Lack of Implant–Implant Distance

Ideal Positioning

The distance between two implants has been determined to be a significant factor with respect to crestal bone loss, the presence of interimplant papilla, and generalized tissue health. Ideally, there should exist 3 mm or more space between any two adjacent implants. This will allow adequate room for interdental papilla and tissue health, cleansability, transfer copings during prosthetic impressions, and minimizing horizontal bone loss. When implants are placed too close together, it is usually the result of poor treatment planning or surgical technique (Fig. 28.19).

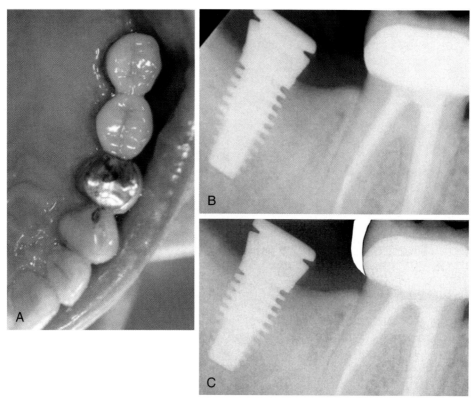

• **Fig. 28.18** Treatment of excessive distance. (A) Prosthesis with narrow occlusal table, minimal cusp height, and no lateral contacts maintains implant-protected occlusion. (B and C) To decrease implant–tooth distance, the natural tooth may be elongated or overcontoured by the use of a crown or bonding.

• **BOX 28.4** **Excessive Space Between Tooth/Implant**

Complication
- Overcontoured crowns
- Atypical prosthetics
- Cantilever effect (biomechanics)
- Food impaction
- Periodontal complications

Prevention
- Ideal positioning (1.5–2.0 mm from tooth)
- Accurate radiographic evaluation (cone beam computerized tomography)
- Diagnostic wax-up/interactive treatment planning
- Parallel long axis of adjacent tooth
- Use of a surgical template

Treatment
Minimal occlusal forces:
1. Narrow occlusal table
2. Minimal cusp height
3. No lateral contacts
   - Cantilever (overcontoured crown)
   High occlusal forces:
1. Overcontour adjacent tooth
   - Reduce mesiodistal distance
2. Remove implant and reposition

Pretreatment Evaluation

The preliminary evaluation to determine distance for multiple implants is the evaluation and measurement of space in the axial dimension. This may be accomplished by use of a CBCT image (axial) depicting the adjacent tooth roots for measurement (Fig. 28.20).

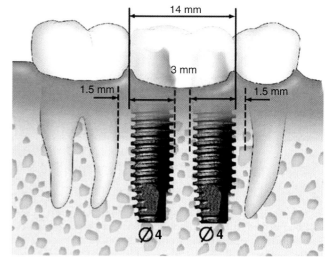

• **Fig. 28.19** Ideal interimplant distance: 3.0 mm between implants and 1.5 mm 1.0-2.0 mm from adjacent teeth.

Osteotomy Measurement. A formula exists for ideal placement of initial osteotomies in anticipation of the final implants. For example, when placing 5.0- and 4.0-mm implants, add ½ diameter of implant + 3.0 mm between implants and 2.5 mm + 2.0 mm + 3.0 mm = 7.5 mm between osteotomy sites. In this example, the initial osteotomy sites may be placed at approximately 7.5 mm between the two pilot holes. In addition, special spacing guides may be used for ideal positioning. Ideally, the implant diameter width should correspond to the width of the natural tooth at the level 2 mm below the CEJ.

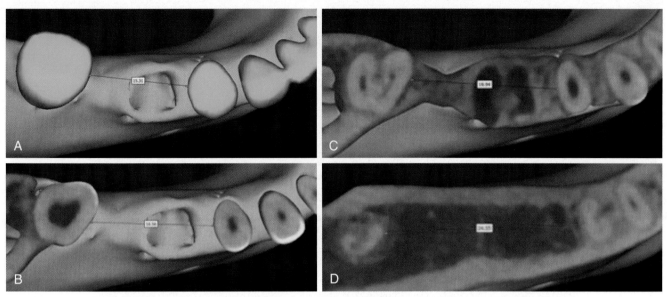

• **Fig. 28.20** Evaluation of intertooth distance. (A) Clinical crown measurement. (B) Cement-enamel junction measurement. (C) Midroot distance. (D) Apical distance.

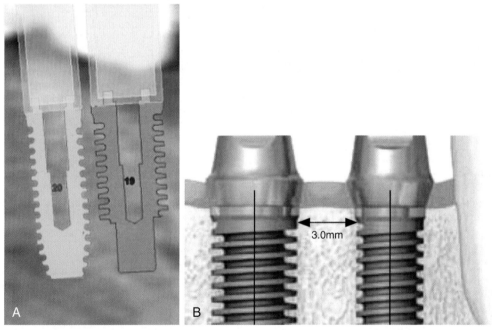

• **Fig. 28.21** (A) Implants placed too close together. (B) Ideally, the space should be 3.0 mm.

Complications

When lack of interproximal bone (i.e., <3.0 mm) is present, a decreased blood supply will result, eventually leading to bone loss. Tarnow and colleagues have shown that implants placed less than 3.0 mm apart may have adequate stability and function; however, this placement will likely result in crestal bone loss. In this study, implants with a greater than 3-mm distance between implants resulted in a 0.45-mm bone loss, whereas implants positioned less than 3 mm had over twice the amount of bone loss, or approximately 1.04 mm[12] (Fig. 28.21).

In addition, when lack of space exists between the implants, the resultant bone loss will be responsible for the loss of the papilla. As the bone resorbs, the distance between the contact point of the crowns and the bone level increases. As this distance increases (i.e., >5 mm), the papilla will become smaller in size and contour.

Lack of space may also lead to difficulty in hygiene access, which will result in poor tissue health. The resultant tissue condition will most likely lead to peri-mucositis or peri-implantitis. Prosthetically, lack of space may result in difficulty in obtaining a final impression (i.e., placement of impression transfer copings) and seating the final prosthesis. With some implant systems, the transfer copings may be adjusted to allow for impression of the implant bodies. Additionally, an unconventional implant prosthesis (irregularly contoured) will most likely need to be fabricated (Fig. 28.22).

Treatment

Initial placement. If implants are not ideally positioned, then the osteotomy should be repositioned to ideal positions (3 mm between implants). The implant positions may be altered with the side-cutting Lindemann drill (Fig. 28.23).

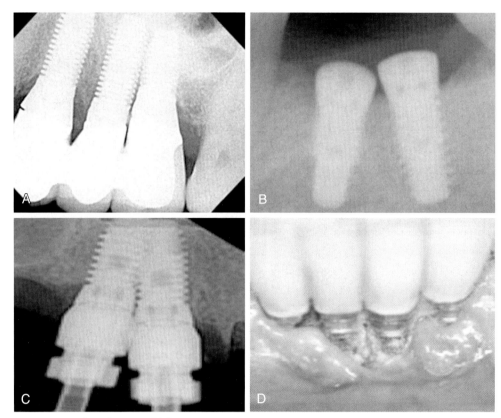

• **Fig. 28.22** Complications. (A) Close proximity of posterior implants resulting in bone loss. (B and C) When implants are too close together, the prosthetic procedures may be difficult or impossible to complete. (D) Implant proximity resulting in hygiene difficulty and resultant peri-implant disease.

Past placement. If implants have been restored, then removal of implants and repositioning should be completed if the patient cannot adequately clean the prosthesis. In some situations, the abutment/implant body may be minimally modified to gain extra space, usually with a flame-shaped diamond bur. This is best completed with external hex implants because modification of internal hex implants may alter structural integrity of the implant, leading to possible fracture (Box 28.5).

Buccolingual Positioning("Y-Axis")

The faciopalatal (buccolingual) positioning of the dental implant is crucial to the esthetic and biomechanical effectiveness of the final prosthesis. Frequently, implant positioning is dictated by the resulting available bone, leading to angulation complications. Bone remodeling after tooth extractions is common, with resorption occurring from the buccal plate initially, decreasing the width of bone and shifting the ridge position more lingual. When evaluating the faciopalatal positioning, two dimensions need to be investigated:
1. Faciopalatal ridge position
2. Faciopalatal angulation position

Ideal Positioning (Faciopalatal Ridge Dimensions)

The faciopalatal position of the implant with adequate bone width is mid to slightly palatal of the edentulous ridge. This approach permits the use of the largest diameter implant to be placed in the space with respect to the natural tooth dimensions. Ideally, after implant placement, the crestal bone should be at least 2.0 mm wide on the facial aspect of the implant and 1.0 mm or more on the palatal aspect (Fig. 28.24).[13]

Pretreatment Evaluation

With this positioning protocol, if implant bone loss occurs, then the facial plate will remain intact and not cause recession on the facial aspect of the implant crown. Therefore for a 4-mm-diameter implant, a minimum of 7-mm faciopalatal width of bone is required (i.e., 4.0-mm-diameter implant + 2.0 mm buccal bone + 1.0 mm lingual bone). Bone spreading in conjunction with implant placement or bone grafting on the facial aspect of the edentulous site may be indicated when the ridge is compromised in width.

When evaluating the CBCT images, the available bone width may be determined via the cross-sectional images. With the use of interactive treatment planning, implant positions can be evaluated to ensure a minimum of 2.0 mm present on the buccal and 1.0 mm on the lingual aspects of the ridges (Fig. 28.25). The faciopalatal width is not as critical on the palatal aspect (i.e., with respect to the buccal bone) of the implant because it usually contains dense cortical bone, which is more resistant to bone loss and is usually not in the esthetic zone.

When present, the buccal cortical bone minimizes future hard and soft tissue recession. In this scenario, if bone loss occurs on the implant, the facial plate will remain intact, and minimal recession on the facial aspect of the implant will result. Spray and colleagues have shown that if the facial bone is more than 1.8 mm in

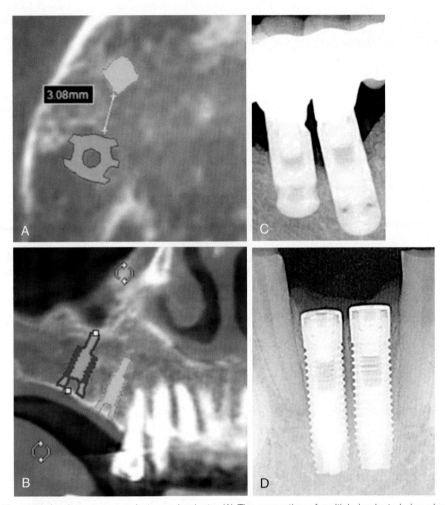

• **Fig. 28.23** Inadequate space between implants. (A) The prevention of multiple implants being placed too close together includes the use of interactive treatment planning (multiple cone beam computerized tomography views) to ensure ideal spacing. (B) Inadequate space between implants; ideally one of the implants should be removed and replaced in a more ideal position. (C) When implants are already restored, a strict recall should be followed to monitor bone loss and related periodontal complications. (D) Two implants placed in anterior mandible with insufficient space between implants (> 3.0mm) and lack of space between adjacent teeth (1.5–2.0 mm).

thickness (after implant placement), recession infrequently results. However, if the facial plate is less than 1.8 mm, vertical resorption occurs quickly, mainly because of the lack of blood supply.[14] Therefore improper buccolingual positioning has a direct effect on the long-term health of the implant and prosthesis.

A common mistake, especially with clinicians early on their learning curve, is to use solely two-dimensional radiographs or clinical evaluation of the soft tissue thickness. Often this is misleading and may pose a significant change to the implant placement or final prosthesis. Thus viewing the third dimension of bone (i.e., CBCT survey) will allow for the accurate assessment of available bone width and ideal position of the implant (Fig. 28.26).

Ideal Positioning (Faciopalatal Angulation)

The faciopalatal angulation is a crucial factor in the long-term success of the dental implant and prosthesis. One area that faciopalatal positioning is most critical is the maxillary anterior region. Because of the inherent angulation issues (i.e., trajectory of the natural teeth with respect to the available bone), coupled with being in the esthetic zone, there is very little room for error when placing implants in this area. In the literature, three different protocols for the buccolingual (faciopalatal) angulations of the implant body have been discussed: (1) similar to the facial position of the adjacent natural teeth, (2) under the incisal edge of the final restoration, and (3) within the cingulum position of the implant crown (Fig. 28.27).

Facial Implant Body Angulation (Anterior). In theory, a maxillary anterior implant body angulation should be positioned at the facial emergence of the final crown, and this position should be in the same position as a natural tooth.

However, the facial crown contour of a natural tooth has two planes, and its incisal edge is palatal to the facial emergence of the natural tooth by 12 to15 degrees (Fig. 28.28). This is why maxillary anterior crown preparations are in two or three planes (Fig. 28.29). In addition, because the implant is narrower in diameter than the faciopalatal root dimension, when the implant body is oriented as a natural tooth and has a facial emergence, a straight abutment is not wide enough to permit the two-plane or three-plane reduction to bring the incisal edge of the preparation more palatal. As a result, the incisal edge of the preparation remains too facial and will require significant modification or an angled abutment.

Therefore the implant body should be more palatal than a natural root, so 2.0 mm of bone exists on the facial aspect. Many

Complication:
- Increased bone loss
- Loss of interdental papilla
- Hygiene issues
- Prosthesis complications (Poor emergence profile/impression)

Prevention:
- Ideal positioning (3.0 mm between implants)
- Accurate radiographic evaluation (cone beam computerized tomography)
- Diagnostic wax-up/interactive treatment planning
- Use of a surgical template

Treatment:
- Custom abutments
- Strict recall
- Remove implants and reposition
- Minimal occlusal forces

implant clinicians, especially early on their learning curve, will attempt to align the implant body with the facial aspect of adjacent teeth and the implant may inadvertently be inserted too facial. When this occurs, no predictable method exists to restore proper esthetics. At best, the final crown will appear too long. This problem is compounded when the implant is also inserted too shallow and insufficient room is present to obtain a proper emergence profile. To correct a maligned implant with soft tissue grafts or bone augmentation is rarely successful after the implant is already inserted in a final position (Fig. 28.30).

In the maxillary anterior area, natural teeth are loaded at an angle because of their natural angulation compared with the mandibular anterior teeth. This is one reason why maxillary anterior teeth are wider in diameter than mandibular anterior teeth (i.e., which are loaded in their long axis). The facial angulation position of the implant body often corresponds to an implant body angulation, often with up to 15 degrees off-axial loads. This angled load increases the force to the abutment screw–implant–bone complex by 25.9% compared with a long-axis load.[15] These offset loads increase the risks of abutment screw loosening, crestal bone loss, and cervical soft tissue marginal

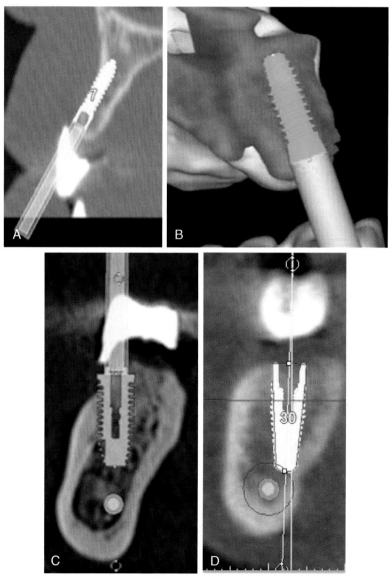

• **Fig. 28.24** Buccal-Lingual Positioning: (A) Non-ideal maxillary positioning, (B) Ideal maxillary positioning, (C) Non-ideal positioning in mandible too facial, (D) Ideal positioning in central fossa of restoration.

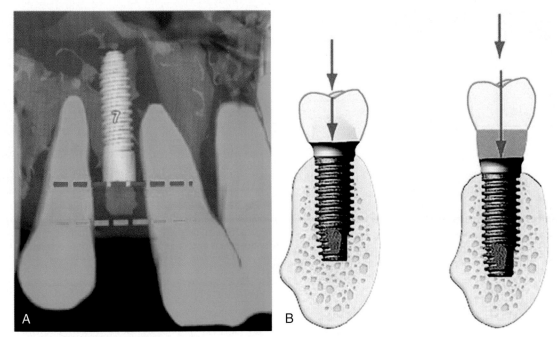

• **Fig. 28.25** Implant placement too deep. (A) Implant placed greater than 4.0 mm from free gingival margin, which increases potential complications. (B) The crown height is not a multiplier of force when the load is in the long axis of the implant. However, any angled force or cantilever increases the force and the crown height magnifies the effect.

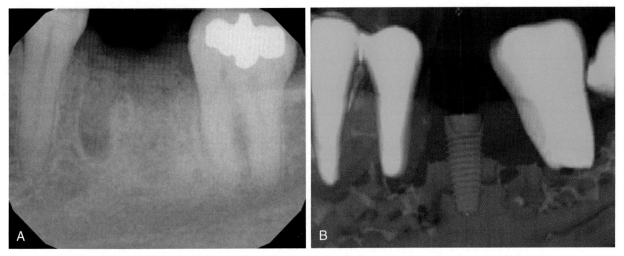

• **Fig. 28.26** (A) Two-dimensional radiograph not depicting the true bone dimensions because of inherent inaccuracies. (B) Cone beam computerized tomography cross-sectional image allowing for the accurate representation of bony dimensions.

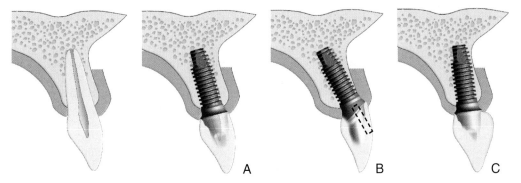

• **Fig. 28.27** Three implant angulation positions are suggested in the literature for a maxillary anterior single-tooth implant. (A) Under the incisal edge. (B) Similar to the facial position of the adjacent teeth (B). (C) Under the cingulum position of the implant crown. (From Misch CE. Single-tooth implant restoration: maxillary anterior and posterior regions. *Dental Implant Prosthetics*. St Louis, MO: Elsevier Mosby; 2015.)

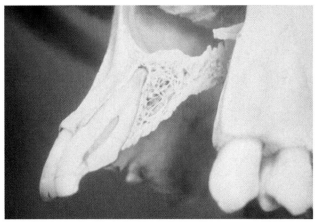

• **Fig. 28.28** Maxillary anterior teeth have an incisal edge 12 to 15 degrees more palatal than the facial emergence position of the crown. (From Misch CE. Single-tooth implant restoration: maxillary anterior and posterior regions. *Dental Implant Prosthetics*. St Louis, MO: Elsevier Mosby; 2015.)

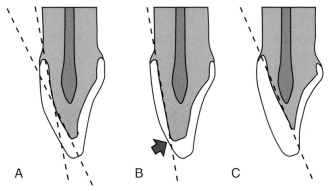

• **Fig. 28.29** (A) Maxillary anterior crown preparations are made in two or more planes. (B, C) When the plane of the emergence profile is only used, the incisal edge of the preparation is too facial. (From Misch CE. Single-tooth implant restoration: maxillary anterior and posterior regions. *Dental Implant Prosthetics*. St Louis, MO: Elsevier Mosby; 2015.)

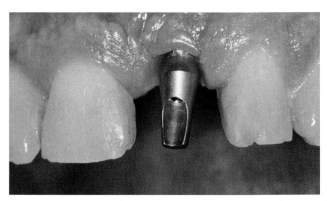

• **Fig. 28.30** Implant positioned too facial and too shallow. The angled abutment must be prepared to make room for restorative materials and to allow a more apical position of the crown margin. (From Misch CE. Single-tooth implant restoration: maxillary anterior and posterior regions. *Dental Implant Prosthetics*. St Louis, MO: Elsevier Mosby; 2015.)

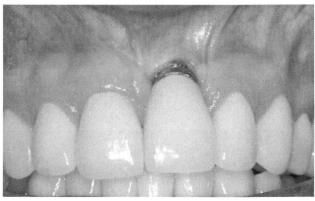

• **Fig. 28.31** Implant placed too facial and the thin tissue receded after crestal bone loss. (From Misch CE. Single-tooth implant restoration: maxillary anterior and posterior regions. *Dental Implant Prosthetics*. St Louis, MO: Elsevier Mosby; 2015.)

shrinkage.[16] As a result, implants angled facially may compromise the esthetics and increase the risk of complications (Fig. 28.31).

Cingulum Implant Body Angulation. A second angulation suggested in the literature is more palatal, with an emergence under the cingulum of the crown. This may also be the result of an implant insertion in a width-deficient ridge (division B) because the bone is lost primarily from the facial aspect and the ridge shifts toward the lingual. This position is also often the goal when a screw-retained crown is used in the final restoration. The prosthesis fixation screw (i.e., to retain a maxillary anterior crown) cannot be located in the incisal or facial region of the crown because this will compromise the esthetics.

This position also is suggested to increase the bone thickness on the facial aspect of the implant body. However, the cingulum implant position may cause a considerable hygiene compromise.[17] The implant body in the anterior maxilla is round and usually 3.5 to 5.5 mm in diameter. The labial cervical contour of the implant crown must be similar to the adjacent teeth for the ultimate esthetic effect. Because the long axis of the implant for a screw-retained crown must emerge from the cingulum position, this requires a facial projection of the crown or "buccal correction" facing away from the implant body. The facial ridge lap must extend 2 to 4 mm and is often similar in contour to the modified ridge lap pontic of a three-unit fixed prosthesis.

The modified ridge lap crown has become a common solution to correct the esthetics of the restoration when the implant is placed in narrow bone or follows a palatal angulation position.[18,19] However, plaque control on the facial aspect of the implant is almost impossible. Unlike a pontic for a fixed partial denture (FPD), the ridge lap crown has a gingival sulcus that requires sulcular hygiene. Even if the toothbrush (or probe) could reach under the facial ridge lap to the gingival sulcus, no hygiene or measuring device could be manipulated to a right angle to proceed into the facial gingival sulcus. As a result, although an acceptable esthetic restoration may be developed, especially with the additional cervical porcelain, the hygiene requirements render this approach less acceptable (Fig. 28.32).

Some authors argue that an improved contour may be developed subgingivally rather than supragingivally with a palatal implant position. To create this contour, the implant body must be positioned more apical than desired. This position may prevent food from accumulating on the cervical "table" of the crown. However, the "subgingival ridge lap" does not permit access to the facial sulcus of the implant body for the elimination of plaque and to evaluate the bleeding index or facial bone loss (Fig. 28.33). Therefore the maintenance requirement for the implant facial sulcular region suggests this modality is not a primary option.

Greater interarch clearance is often needed with an implant palatal position because the permucosal post exits the tissue in a more palatal position. Inadequate interarch space may especially

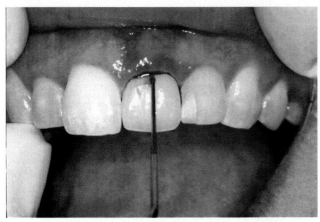

Fig. 28.32 Implant crown with a "modified ridge lap." The tissue periodically becomes inflamed because hygiene aids (or a dental probe) cannot enter the sulcus of the implant; instead, it can only slide along the facial ridge lap to the free gingival margin. (From Misch CE. Single-tooth implant restoration: maxillary anterior and posterior regions. *Dental Implant Prosthetics*. St Louis, MO: Elsevier Mosby; 2015.)

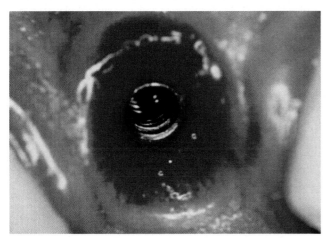

Fig. 28.33 Implant with a "subgingival ridge lap crown" and an inflamed gingival sulcus. (From Misch CE. Single-tooth implant restoration: maxillary anterior and posterior regions. *Dental Implant Prosthetics*. St Louis, MO: Elsevier Mosby; 2015.)

hinder the restoration of Angle's class II, division 2 patients with the implant in this position.

Ideal Implant Angulation. The third implant angulation in the literature describes the most desirable implant angulation. The clinician determines the line for the best angulation by the point of the incisal edge position of the implant crown and the midfaciopalatal (i.e., or slightly palatal) position on the crest of the bone. The center of the implant is located directly under the incisal edge of the crown so that a straight abutment for cement can be used. Because the crown profile is in two planes, with the incisal edge more palatal than the cervical portion, the incisal edge position is ideal for implant placement and accommodates some of the facial bone loss that often occurs before implant placement.

The facial emergence of the crown mimics the adjacent teeth, proceeding from the implant body under the tissue (Fig. 28.34). The angle of force to the implant is less from the long axis, which decreases the crestal stresses to the bone and abutment screws. When in doubt, the implant surgeon should err toward the palatal aspect of the incisal edge position, not to the facial aspect,

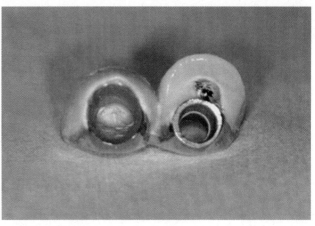

Fig. 28.34 *Left:* Implant crown is positioned under the incisal edge and has a facial emergence profile similar to the adjacent teeth. *Right:* The implant was positioned under the cingulum and requires a screw-retained crown with a facial ridge lap to have a similar facial crown emergence as the adjacent teeth. (From Misch CE. Single-tooth implant restoration: maxillary anterior and posterior regions. *Dental Implant Prosthetics*. St Louis, MO: Elsevier Mosby; 2015.)

because it is easier to correct a slight palatal position in the final crown contour, compared with the implant body angled too facial.

The implant body angulation slightly lingual to the incisal edge may also be used for cement or screw-retained restorations. In screw-retained restorations, an angled abutment for screw retention is inserted, and the coping screw for the crown may be located within the cingulum. This method does not require a facial ridge lap of the final crown, which decreases the risk of compromised hygiene. However, it should be noted that prosthetic screw loosening is one of the more common complications of maxillary anterior screw-retained crowns.[20] When this occurs, there is an increased risk of marginal bone loss as a result of the crown movement and microgap created by the loose screw. When ideal bone volume is present, a surgical template that indicates the incisal edge and facial contour of the final prosthesis may be used.

Faciopalatal Positioning

A. Angulation with Respect to Prosthesis Type

1. FP-1 & FP-2 Prosthesis

Cement-retained (anterior). The ideal angulation for an FP-1 or FP-2 in the anterior is slightly lingual to the incisal edge. This is advantageous for two reasons. First, a straight abutment may be used, which is esthetically more pleasing and prosthetically less complex. When an FP-1/FP-2 prosthesis is indicated, precise buccolingual angulation implant placement is necessary to obtain an ideal esthetic result. In the anterior region, the ideal implant position allows the placement of a straight abutment slightly lingual to the incisal edge of the final crown for a cemented prosthesis. The resulting forces are concentrated along the long axis of the implant, minimizing damaging shear forces. In addition, if access is ever required to treat screw loosening, the existing crown may be retained, preventing a new crown from having to be fabricated.

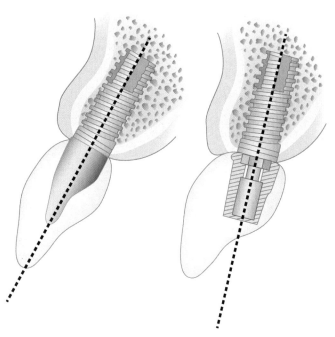

A Cemented   B Screw retained

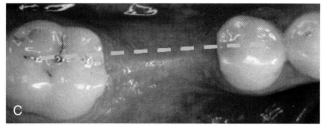

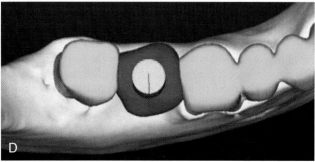

• **Fig. 28.35** (A, B) Ideal implant placement for a cement and screw-retained prosthesis in the anterior, (C, D) Ideal posterior implant placement in line with the adjacent teeth central fossa's.

Screw-retained (anterior). For screw-retained prostheses in the anterior, the implant should emerge within the cingulum area of the anterior tooth so the access hole does not affect the esthetics of the restoration. If the implant is placed too facially, then the access hole will impinge on the esthetics of the restoration (i.e., screw hole through the facial of the restoration). If the implant is placed too far lingually, overcontouring of the final crown may result in biomechanical issues and possible occlusal interferences (Fig. 28.35A–C).

Posterior region (cement retained or screw retained). In the posterior region, the long axis of the implant should emerge within the approximate center (central fossa) of the prosthesis for a screw-retained or cement-retained FP-1 or FP-2. This allows occlusal

forces to be directed ideally along the long axis of the implant (see Fig. 28.35D–E).

Complications

Facial. If the implant is placed too facial for an FP-1 or FP-2 prosthesis, then esthetic issues will result from overcontouring of the prosthesis. Bone dehiscence usually will be accompanied by tissue recession, and this complication is more pronounced in thin biotype patients. Facial positioning is often a complication when implants are placed in immediate extraction sites. To correct the facial position of the implant, an angled abutment must be used. However, because of the access hole, the facial of the abutment is more bulky. This results in overcontouring of the facial aspect of the prosthesis, which will lead to tissue recession and bone loss (Fig. 28.36).

Lingual. Implants placed too far to the lingual can result in facial overcontouring of the final prosthesis (ridge lap) for esthetic reasons. The prosthetic impression and placement of the prosthesis is also complicated, which results in difficulty with the seating of the abutments. Because of the overcontouring of the lingual contours, patients often complain of lack of space for the tongue, which may impede speech. In the anterior region, a lingual-placed implant may make the implant nonrestorable if the patient has a deep bite occlusion and insufficient interocclusal space (Fig. 28.37).

FP-3 Prosthesis

Screw retained. After evaluation of the articulated setup, arch form, available bone, and force factors, the FP-3 prostheses should be determined to be either screw retained or cement retained. For screw-retained prostheses, ideal positioning should be slightly lingual to the denture/porcelain/zirconia teeth to minimize tooth fractures and delamination in the anterior. In the posterior, the implant positioning should be within the central fossa of the Prostheses teeth.

Cement retained. For cement-retained restorations, implant positioning should be located slightly lingual to the incisal edge in the anterior region and in the central fossa area in the posterior. If force factors are a concern, then ideal implant placement is crucial to minimize biomechanical overload. However, if force factors are low, then nonideal placement is less of a problem with cement-retained prostheses because abutment angulation may be modified (Fig. 28.38).

Complications

Facial. Implants positioned too facially will impinge on the esthetics, complicate screw insertion, and result in increased prosthesis component fractures. Because the access holes will extrude through the facial contours of the teeth, the access will need to be covered with composite. This predisposes the prosthesis to loss or discoloring of the composite plugs. Also, facially inclined implants may lead to soft tissue irritation because of lack of attached tissue.

Lingual. Implants placed too far lingually will result in an overcontoured prosthesis, resulting in possible speech problems in the maxilla and crowding of the tongue in the mandible. Because the bulk of the material is needed for strength of the prosthesis, often this overcontouring results in an atypical prosthesis. In addition, lingually placed implants usually will result in lack of attached tissue, which may lead to chronic soft tissue problems (Figs. 28.39 and 28.40).

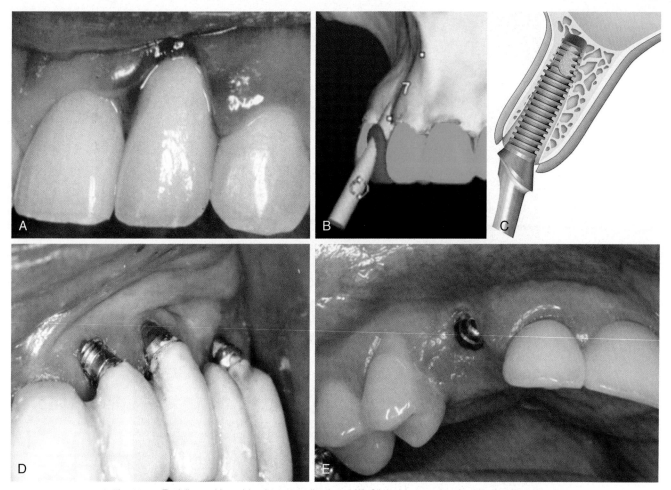

• **Fig. 28.36** Facially positioned implant complications. (A) Clinical image showing the facial positioning which results in peri-mucositis, (B) Pre-treatment evaluation should be completed to avoid malposition. (C) Facially positioned anterior implant often will require an angled or custom abutment. (D) Facially inclined implants resulting in esthetic and bone loss issues. (E) Facial positioning leading to the implant being non-restorable.

RP-4 and RP-5. The faciopalatal angulation for implants placed for removable overdentures should be positioned to emerge within the body of the denture base. This is crucial so the components (e.g., attachments, bar) that are attached to the implant do not impinge on the ideal setting of the denture teeth. Denture acrylic requires a minimum of 2.0 mm of bulk for strength and resistance form to prevent fractures and delamination.

Malpositioning

Lingual. Implants that are positioned too far lingually for an overdenture will result in overcontouring the lingual surface of the denture. This may interfere with phonetics, and often patients will complain of lack of space for the tongue. If the lingual aspect of the denture is thinned too much during adjustment, this will result in an area of possible fracture or loss of attachment.

Facial. Implants placed too far facially will interfere with ideal denture tooth placement, leading to possible denture tooth "pop offs." Often the esthetics are compromised because of the required malpositioning of the denture teeth. In addition, facially positioned implants often result in lack of adequate attached tissue and potential periodontal concerns because gingival irritation and recession are more likely to result. This may

lead to chronic pain, and remediation is usually unsuccessful (Fig. 28.41; Boxes 28.6 and 28.7).

Apicocoronal (Z-Axis)

The depth of implant placement in the bone is a significant factor in relation to the longevity of the implants. Whether the implant is placed too deep or not apical enough, prosthetic and periodontal complications may increase implant morbidity.

Ideal Positioning

In most regions of the mouth, it has been suggested that the implant platform be placed approximately 2 to 4 mm apical to the adjacent cemento-enamel junction (CEJ) or free gingival margin (FGM). Most recently, the free gingival margin is used as the anatomic landmark as this will allow for more accurate representation when soft and hard tissue recession is present.[21] (Fig. 28.42).

The best platform level for a two-stage implant is similar to the most desirable bone level before the loss of a natural tooth, which is 2 mm below the adjacent tooth CEJ.[22] This positions the platform of the implant approximately 3 mm below the facial FGM

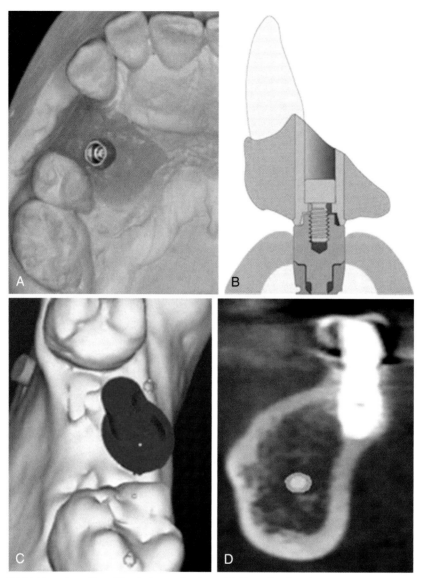

• **Fig. 28.37** Lingual positioned implant complications. (A) Lingually placed abutment requiring overcontouring and possible tongue impingement complications. (B) Usually lingually placed implants can be restored with a screw-retained prosthesis. (C) Posterior implant placed too far to the lingual requiring angled abutment. (D) Lingually placed posterior implant perforating the lingual plate.

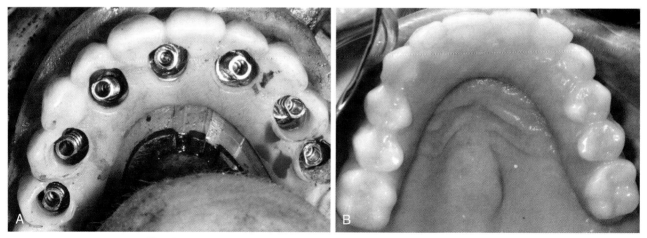

• **Fig. 28.38** FP-3 Ideal Implant Positioning (A) Immediate placement/load positioning, (B) Final monolithic zirconia prosthesis.

of the implant crown. This position will allow for 3 mm of soft tissue for the emergence of the implant crown on the midfacial region and more as the soft tissue measurements proceed toward the interproximal regions. This depth also increases the thickness of the soft tissues over the facial aspect of the titanium implant

body, which masks the darker color. It is easier to use the FGMs of the adjacent teeth to help determine the depth than it is to attempt to use the CEJ as a landmark (Fig. 28.43).

In conclusion, the ideal anterior and posterior implant body position is 2 to 4 mm below the facial FGM of the adjacent teeth. The depth of an implant platform greater than 4 mm below the adjacent CEJ is too deep. An implant platform position less than 2 mm below the FGM of the crown is too shallow. Therefore the ideal depth position of the implant platform is more than 2 mm and less than 4 mm below the FGM.

Excessive Depth

Some authors have suggested that the implant be deepened (countersunk) below the crestal bone more than 4 mm below the facial CEJ of the adjacent teeth to develop a crown emergence profile similar to a natural tooth (Fig. 28.44).[22,23] This provides a subgingival emergence transition of about 5 mm on the facial aspect to achieve the width of the natural tooth (4 mm below the CEJ, and the ideal FGM on the facial is 1 mm above the CEJ). This concept was originally developed for a 4-mm-diameter implant, and the diameter of a central incisor root is 4 mm at a position 4 mm below the CEJ[24] (Fig. 28.45). Very esthetic restorations may be fabricated with this implant depth position because the bulk of subgingival porcelain provides good color and contour for the crown. However, several concerns arise regarding the long-term sulcular health around the implant when it is seated greater than 4 mm below the CEJ.

Various studies have shown during the first year of function, a mean bone loss range of 0.5 to 3.0 mm, depending partly on implant design. The bone maybe lost at least 0.5 mm below the connection of the abutment to the implant body and extends to any smooth or machined surface beyond the crest module.[25] For example, Malevez and colleagues noted more pronounced bone loss for conical implants that had long, smooth, tapered crest modules.[26] This may lead to facial sulcular probing depths of 7 to 8 mm or greater. Grunder evaluated single-tooth

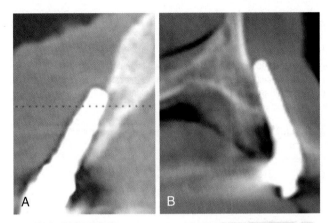
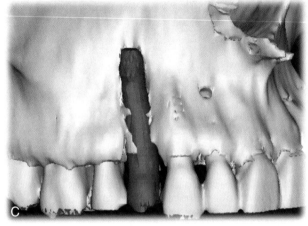
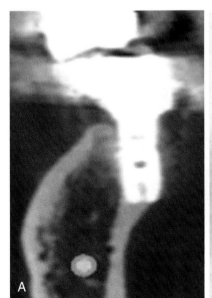

• **Fig. 28.39** (A and B) Facially positioned implants. (C) 3D CBCT image showing lack of bone from facially inclined implant.

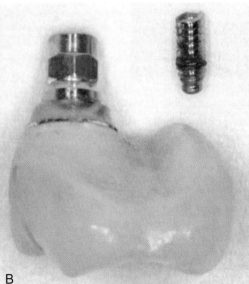
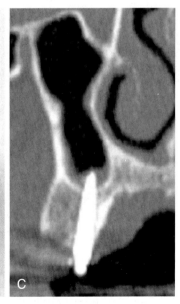

• **Fig. 28.40** (A) Lingually placed implant impinging on the tongue space. Note the overcontoured buccal cantilever for occlusal purposes, (B) Lingual placed implant requiring large ridge lap pontic and fractured screw. (C) Maxillary lingually angled implant.

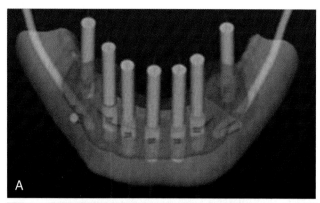

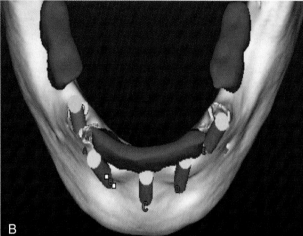

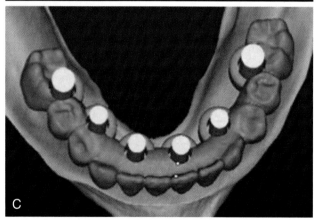

• **Fig. 28.41** (A) Pretreatment planning for ideal implant placement. (B) Facially angled implant impinging on the esthetics and prosthesis. (C) Ideal implant placement.

• **BOX 28.6** Excessive Angulation (Facially)

Complication:
- Bone loss (dehiscence)
- Esthetics (overcontour)
- Thin tissue (recession)
- Prosthetic complications
- Implant failure

Prevention:
- Understand ideal angulation with respect to final prosthesis type
- Accurate radiographic evaluation (cone beam computerized tomography)
- Diagnostic wax-up/interactive treatment planning
- Use of a surgical template

Treatment:
- Custom abutments
- Possible removal of implant

• **BOX 28.7** Excessive Angulation (Lingual)

Complication:
Maxilla:
- Ridge-lap
- Crown bulky

Mandible:
- Lack of tongue space
- Speech issue
- Overcontour

Prevention:
- Understand ideal angulation with respect to final prosthesis type
- Accurate radiographic evaluation (cone beam computerized tomography)
- Diagnostic wax-up/interactive treatment planning
- Use of a surgical template

Treatment:
- Modified ridge lap screw retained
- Decrease occlusal force factors
- Remove/reposition implant

implants in function for 1 year and noted the bone levels were 2 mm apical to the implant–abutment connection, and sulcular probing depths were 9.0 to 10.5 mm, using a Brånemark implant design.[27] As a result, daily care devices cannot maintain the sulcus health, and anaerobic bacteria are more likely to develop. The interproximal regions of the implant crown, which correspond to the incidence or absence of interdental papillae, usually exhibit even greater probing depths. As a result, gingival shrinkage of the tissue is more likely to occur when the implant is placed more than 4 mm below the facial position of the adjacent CEJ.

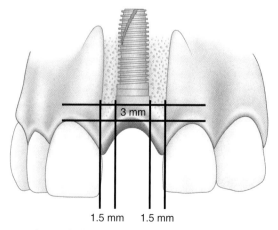

• **Fig. 28.42** Image depicting ideal implant positioning (1.5 mm from adjacent teeth and 3 mm below the free gingival margin).

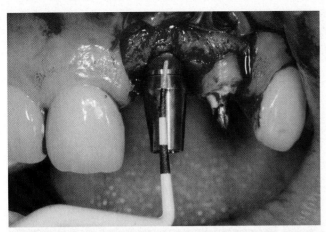

• **Fig. 28.43** Ideal implant depth is 3 mm below the free gingival margin of the future implant crown. This implant is too shallow for an ideal placement. (From Misch CE. Single-tooth implant restoration: maxillary anterior and posterior regions. *Dental Implant Prosthetics.* St Louis, MO: Elsevier Mosby; 2015.)

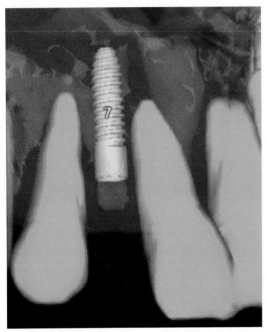

• **Fig. 28.44** Implant position too deep in apicocoronal position.

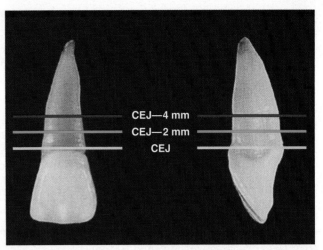

• **Fig. 28.45** Central incisor root is 4 mm in diameter when it is measured 4 mm below the cement-enamel junction. (From Misch CE. Single-tooth implant restoration: maxillary anterior and posterior regions. *Dental Implant Prosthetics.* St Louis, MO: Elsevier Mosby; 2015.)

The attachment mechanism of the soft tissue above the bone is less tenacious compared with a tooth, and the defense mechanism of the peri-implant tissues may be weaker than that of teeth.[28] To err on the side of safety for the best sulcular health conditions, it is recommended that the clinician should limit sulcular depths adjacent to implants to less than 5 mm.[29] This may be even more relevant for single-tooth implants because of the devastating consequences of gingival shrinkage for long-term esthetics. In addition, the interproximal regions of the single-tooth implant crown is shared with the adjacent teeth, and anaerobic bacteria that form in the region next to the implant may affect the adjacent natural tooth as a result of a horizontal defect (especially when the implant is closer than 1.5 mm to the tooth).

When the implant is countersunk below the crestal cortical bone (as with this depth technique), the trabecular bone around the crest module is weaker against occlusal loads. In addition, when the implant is placed below the crestal bone, the resultant initial crown height is increased, as are moment forces. An increased risk of additional bone loss also is present from the increased moment loads applied to weaker trabecular bone, which may also result in soft tissue shrinkage over the long term. The end result is longer clinical crowns, which also decrease gradually in width (as the narrowing dimensions approach the implant body). The interproximal region may result in black triangular spacings in lieu of interdental papillae.

The increased crown height also increases forces to the abutment screw and increases the risk of screw loosening.

FP-1, FP-2, and FP-3

Placement Too Deep. When implant placement results in positioning deeper than 4 mm below CEJ or FGM, many complications may result:

1. Unfavorable crown height space (CHS; crown-implant ratio).
2. Periodontal complications because of the inability to perform proper hygiene and associated bone loss on adjacent teeth.
3. Higher moment forces, which cause biomechanical overload with resultant crestal bone loss.
4. Prosthetics are more complicated, with difficulty in impression taking, placing abutments, and seating the prosthesis.
5. With deeply placed implants, often the facial plate will resorb, especially if facial inclination is present.
6. Long-term sulcular health is decreased because there is minimal to no cortical bone present. The trabecular bone around the crest module is weaker against occlusal loads.
7. Resultant initial crown height and moment forces are increased. A further increased risk of soft tissue shrinkage occurs long term, with additional bone loss at the crest module. The result is longer clinical crowns, which also decrease gradually in width (as the narrowing dimensions approach the implant body), with resultant black triangular spacings in lieu of interdental papillae and compromised long-term esthetics (Figs. 28.46 and 28.47).

Treatment

Treatment planning phase. During the treatment planning phase, if it is determined there exist no alternatives to placing the implants at a compromised depth (i.e., bone grafting contraindicated), the following can be completed to decrease the possible of complications:

1. Increase the number of implants.
2. Increase the diameters of implants.

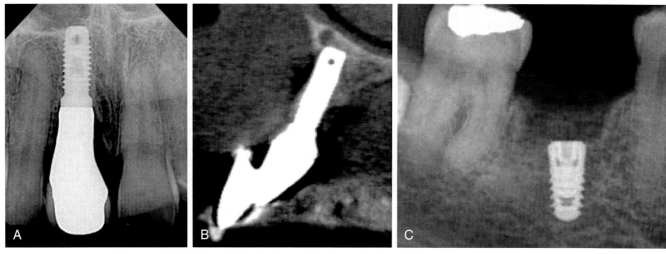

● **Fig. 28.46** (A) Apically positioned implant resulting in atypical prosthesis and predisposing the implant to bone loss and peri-implant disease. (B) Resultant prosthesis from apically positioned implant. (C) Mandibular implant apically positioned too close to mandibular canal.

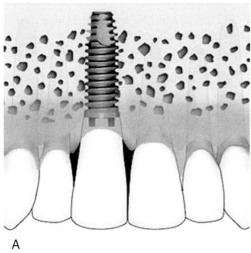

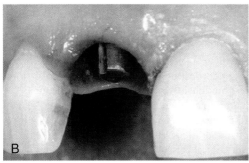

● **Fig. 28.47** (A) Black triangle formation as a result of apical positioned implant. (B) Implant placement too deep resulting in significantly larger clinical crown.

3. Design implants to maximize the surface area.
4. Fabricate removable restorations (less retentive) and incorporate soft tissue support.
5. Remove the removable restoration during sleeping hours to reduce the noxious effects of nocturnal parafunction.
6. Splint implants together, regardless of whether they support a fixed or removable prosthesis (Fig. 28.48).

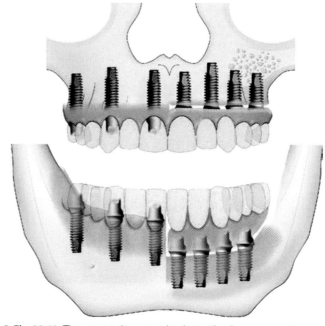

● **Fig. 28.48** The greater the crown-implant ratio, the greater is the need for more implants and splinting the implants.

At the time of surgery. If an implant is inserted and the position is known to be excessively deep, ideally the implant should be removed, site bone grafted, and then the implant replaced at an ideal position after sufficient healing. If rigid fixation cannot be accomplished, then the implant should be removed and grafting allowed to heal, with future implant placement.

Integrated implant. If it is determined after integration that the implant position is compromised, then the risk versus benefit of removing the implant needs to be determined. If the morbidity of removing the implant is too significant, then the implant may be restored with the following guidelines:

1. Shorten cantilever length.
2. Minimize buccal and lingual offset loads.

3. Ideal emergence profile.
4. Occlusal contact load should be reduced on any offset load from the implant support system.
5. Occlusal contact load should be reduced on any offset load from the implant support system.

Occlusal contacts in centric relation (CR) occlusion may be eliminated on the offset load area. A parafunction load may be reduced because the most cantilevered portion of the prosthesis is loaded only during functional activity while eating food.[30]

NOTE: Questionable treatments, including segmental osteotomies, are not recommended because of the invasiveness, length of treatment time, and questionable prognosis (Box 28.8).

Inadequate Depth

When the implant body is positioned less than 2 mm below the facial FGM of the crown, the cervical esthetics of the restoration are at an increased risk because limited space is present subgingivally to develop the facial emergence profile of the crown. The porcelain or zirconia of the crown may not be subgingival enough to mask the titanium color of the abutment or implant below the crown margin (Fig. 28.49A). If bone loss occurs, then the titanium implant abutment or body may

• BOX 28.8 Implant Placement Too Deep (Apicocoronally)

Complication:
- Unfavorable crown height space
- (Crown:implant ratio)
- Higher moment forces: bone loss
- Periodontal complications
- Prosthetics more difficult

Prevention:
- Ideal:
  - 3 mm below free gingival margin (2–4 mm)
- Options:
  - Graft
  - Change to fixed partial denture

Treatment:
1. Remove implant
2. Ideal emergence profile
3. Monitor
4. ? Treatment

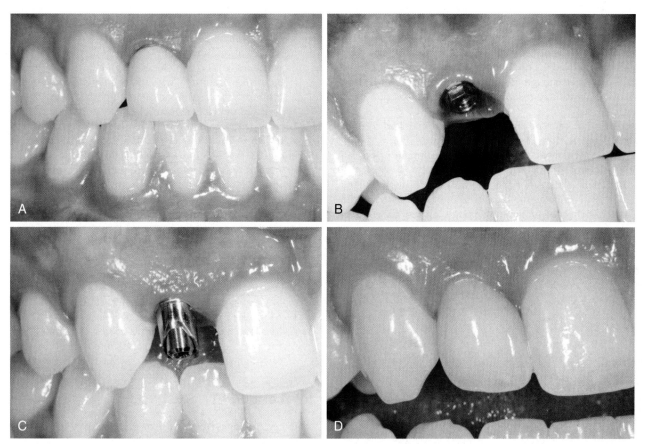

• **Fig. 28.49** (A) An implant replacing a maxillary lateral incisor that is inserted too shallow. The implant crown is not placed subgingival enough to develop an emergence profile or to mask the color of the abutment. (B) The implant is positioned too shallow. (C) An abutment is inserted, and a subgingival margin is created on the implant body. (D) The final implant crown is inserted below the tissue 1.5 mm and on the implant body. (From Misch CE. Single-tooth implant restoration: maxillary anterior and posterior regions. *Dental Implant Prosthetics*. St Louis, MO: Elsevier Mosby; 2015.)

also cast a dark shadow on the gingival tissues. If apical shrinkage of tissue occurs, then the dark titanium abutment and implant body may become directly visible. Periodontal surgical procedures to position soft tissue over the exposed titanium are unpredictable.

On occasion, the crestal bone height is coronal to the ideal bone height (3 mm below the facial FGM). The two most common conditions that result in this finding are (1) when the adjacent teeth are closer than 6 mm (in agenesis of a lateral incisor) and (2) when a block bone graft regenerated excess width and height of bone. Ideally, the midcrestal bone is 3 mm below the interproximal bone and follows the interproximal scallop of the CEJ of the missing tooth. When the teeth are closer than 6 mm (i.e., a lateral incisor in the maxilla), the interproximal bone height of each adjacent tooth to the missing space is able to stimulate and maintain bone at the interproximal bone level. The same conditions may occur when bone augmentation gains height to the interproximal height of bone.

When a single-tooth implant replaces a missing tooth with these conditions, an osteoplasty should be performed so that the midcrestal region is 3 mm apical to the FGM of the adjacent tooth; otherwise, the implant position will be too shallow and result in a short crown height at the gingival margins.

To solve the problem of an implant body placed too shallow, the restoring dentist may need to prepare the implant crest module and place the margin of the crown directly on the implant body (even if esthetic crown lengthening of the surrounding bone and soft tissue is necessary) (see Fig. 28.49B–D). Also feather edge margin should be used to minimizes this weakening of the abutment or implant body.

The following may occur when implant positioning is not deep enough (<3 mm from CEJ, <2 mm from FGM):

1. Inadequate emergence profile (transition from the narrower diameter of the implant compared with the wider dimension of the crown).
2. Decreased retention of the implant, which may lead to uncementable restorations or component fracture.
3. Poor resultant esthetics because implant abutment or implant body will show through, resulting in cervical darkness, and if this occurs in the anterior region, it may be unpleasant for the patient. Normally, the facial margin of the crown will not be able to be placed subgingival enough to mask the titanium color of the abutment below the margin.

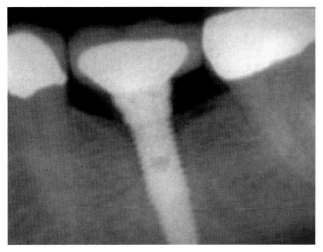

• **Fig. 28.50** Poor emergence profile as a result of inadequate implant depth.

4. Inadequate running room because the location of the crest module will leave inadequate room for adequate hygiene. An abrupt change from the prosthetic platform to the diameter of the restoration will result. Normally, this will most likely result in hygiene difficulty (Fig. 28.50).

Treatment

Treatment planning phase. If it is determined during the treatment planning phase that implant positioning would result in an implant being in a nonideal location with respect to the FGM, modifications to the treatment plan or final prosthesis may be indicated. Skeletal discrepancies (deep bite), reduced occlusal vertical dimension (OVD) from attrition or abrasion, minimal bone atrophy after tooth loss, and supraeruption of unopposed teeth may all result in less than ideal space for prosthetic replacement of the dentition. Traditional prosthetic and restorative procedures are indicated to restore the proper OVD and plane of occlusion and increase the CHS:

1. Modification or adjustment of opposing occlusion should always be explained to the patient at the initiation of treatment to prevent miscommunication issues. This is extremely important, especially if alteration of the opposing tooth would result in the need for endodontic therapy.
2. Ideally, 8.0 mm of space is required for a cementable prosthesis. The 8-mm requirement for CHS consists of 2 mm of occlusal material space, 4 mm minimum abutment height for retention, and 2 mm above the bone for the biologic width dimension (which does not include the sulcus because a crown margin may be 1 mm subgingival for retention or esthetics). If this cannot be accomplished, a screw-retained prosthesis or change to an FPD treatment plan is indicated.

At time of surgery. If the implant is inserted and the position is known to be excessively shallow, removal of the implant is indicated, the osteotomy should be deepened if available bone is present, and the implant is reinserted at a more favorable depth. The location of vital structures should always be determined before deepening of the osteotomy.

Integrated implant. After implant integration, if the implant is determined to be of inadequate depth, the implant should be ideally removed. However, if the morbidity of removing the implant is too significant, then the following may be evaluated as possible treatment options:

- A screw-retained prosthesis
- Shorten cantilever length/Narrow occlusal table
- Minimize buccal and lingual offset loads
- Ideal emergence profile (Fig. 28.51)
- Increase mechanical and chemical retention of the abutment by roughening the abutment surface or retentive grooves.

RP-4 and RP-5

When evaluating a treatment plan for a removable implant prosthesis, numerous factors need to be addressed. First, it must be determined that adequate interocclusal space is present, especially is a connecting bar is to be utilized. For a bar and overdenture with attachments, 15 mm of space is required from the crest of the ridge to the incisal edge is suggested. If interocclusal space is insufficient, then an osteoplasty at the time of surgery should be completed to increase space for the final prosthesis. Interactive

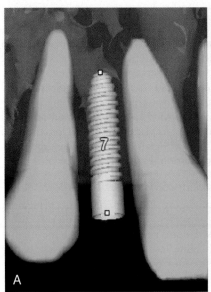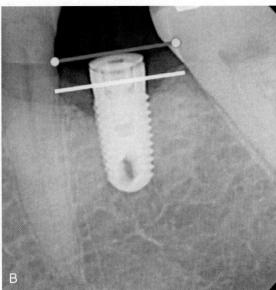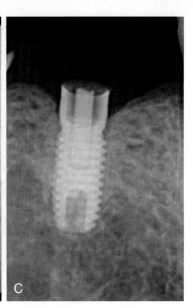

● **Fig. 28.51** Implant positioning that is too shallow. (A) Cone beam computerized tomography image depicting an implant placement that is too shallow. (B) Periapical radiograph showing insufficient depth *(red)* and ideal placement *(yellow)*. (C) Inadequate depth, which led to fracture of implant abutment screw.

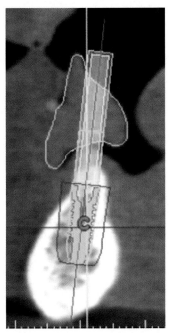

● **Fig. 28.52** Interocclusal space (Crown-Height Space) evaluated via CBCT 3D imaging.

treatment planning may be used to fabricate a reduction guide, which will allow the implant clinician to remove the ideal amount of bone. A minimum of 2.0 mm of acrylic is required to adequately retain denture teeth and maintain structural integrity of the prosthesis.

Complications: More than 15 mm

For an RP-5 prosthesis, greater interocclusal space is usually not problematic because of the soft tissue support. However, with an RP-4 (implant-supported) prosthesis, greater interocclusal space may pose a problem, with increased "rocking" of the prosthesis because of the lack of soft tissue support (i.e., RP-4 is completely implant supported). With removable prostheses, two prosthetic levels of height should be taken into consideration. The first is the height of the attachment system to the crest of the bone. The greater the height distance, the greater the forces applied to the bar, screws, and implant structures. The second CHS to consider is the distance from the attachment to the occlusal plane. This distance represents the increase in prosthetic forces applied to the attachment. For example, in a CHS of 15 mm, a locator attachment may be 7 mm from the crest of bone, resulting in a lever action of 7 mm applied to the implants. The distance from the rotation point of the locator attachment to the occlusal plane may be an additional 8 mm. Under these conditions, a greater lever action is applied to the prosthesis than to the implant interface. This results in increased instability of the restoration under lateral forces (Fig. 28.52).[30]

Treatment

If more than 15 mm of space is present, an RP-5 prosthesis should have ideal interocclusal space for the final prosthesis. Peripheral extension and the primary stress-bearing area support (maxilla–horizontal palate, residual ridge; mandible–buccal shelf) should be used to decrease excessive loading force. The occlusion should include bilateral balanced contacts with no occlusal prematurities. If excessive force exists (i.e., excessive CHS and/or parafunction), then an RP-4 (totally implant supported) may be changed to an RP-5 (soft tissue supported) to decrease the force.

Complications: Less than 15 mm

When sufficient CHS is lacking and the prosthesis is more prone to component fatigue and fracture, an overdenture is more difficult to fabricate than a porcelain-to-metal fixed prosthesis or zirconia monolithic prosthesis. The 15-mm minimum CHS provides an adequate bulk of acrylic to resist fracture; space to set denture teeth without modification; and room for attachments, bars, soft tissue, and

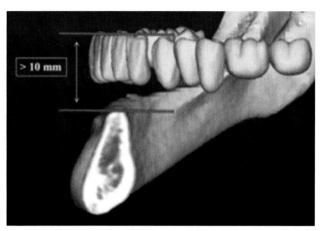

• **Fig. 28.53** Minimum interocclusal space for an FP-3 prosthesis.

hygiene. In the mandible (Fig. 28.53) the soft tissue is often 1 to 3 mm in thickness above the bone, so the occlusal plane to soft tissue should be at least 9 to 11 mm in height. An osteoplasty to increase CHS before implant placement or a fixed restoration is often indicated when abundant bone height and width are present (Fig. 28.54).

Treatment

If less than 15 mm of CHS is present, then an RP-4 and RP-5 may present issues. Without sufficient space for tissue health, attachment space, bulk of acrylic, and nonmodified denture teeth, the overdenture may undergo fatigue and possible fractures. An RP-4 may be changed to an RP-5 to obtain soft tissue support to minimize forces to the attachments. Additionally, the overdenture prosthesis should be changed to a metal base, metal reinforced, or fiber mesh to increase the strength of the prosthesis, to prevent prosthesis fracture (Box 28.9).

Implant Position with Respect to Vital Structures

Inferior Alveolar Nerve Canal or Mental Foramen

Accurate positioning of implants in approximation to the inferior alveolar canal and mental foramen is crucial in preventing neurosensory impairment. The correct location of the nerve and canal should be ascertained via three- dimensional imaging, especially when the implant may be within 2 mm of the nerve. After identification of the vital structures, the implant should be placed greater than 2 mm from the inferior alveolar canal or mental foramen. Implant placement less than 2 mm increases the risk of compression or traumatic injuries to the nerve trunk, which may result in neurosensory deficits (Fig. 28.55)

Inferior Border of Mandible

Placement of dental implants in the anterior mandible can lead to significant and even life-threatening complications. Care should be noted to evaluate the angulation and trajectory of the anterior mandible with three-dimensional imaging to minimize the possibility of perforating the lingual cortex. Two-dimensional radiographs (i.e., panoramic) may lead to false representation of the amount of bone available. If the inferior border of the mandible is perforated, then bleeding may become evident from the sublingual and submental blood vessels. Because this area is difficult to access, dangerous sublingual bleeding complications may arise (Fig. 28.56).

Nasal Cavity

The anterior maxilla is often a very challenging area to place implants. Because of the compromised bone in width and height, along with angulation issues, implants are often malpositioned. Placement of implants in the anterior maxilla may be very challenging, especially when a minimal height of bone is present. Ideally, implants should be positioned just short of the nasal floor, without engaging the thin inferior floor of the nasal cavity. There do exist more advanced surgical techniques in which the implants may extend into the nasal cavity 1 to 2 mm via a subnasal graft; however, these procedures should be completed with caution (Fig. 28.57).[31]

Distance from the Maxillary Sinus (Inferior Border)

One of the more challenging areas for implant placement involves the posterior maxilla. The implant dentist often encounters compromised bone height and poor bone quality in this area because of bone loss and pneumatization of the maxillary sinus. There are four treatment options (Misch classification) for implants placed in this area, with respect to the quantity of bone from the crest of the ridge to the inferior border of the sinus (Fig. 28.58):[32]

1. SA-1: Implant placement that does not penetrate the maxillary sinus proper
2. SA-2: Implant placement with penetration into the sinus approximately 1 to 2 mm without bone grafting.
3. SA-3: Implant placement along with bone grafting, either with the crestal or lateral approach
4. SA-4: Sinus augmentation from a lateral approach with delayed implant placement

Prevention of Implant Malposition

Ideal Treatment Planning

The surest way to minimize errors in positioning during implant surgery is to develop a comprehensive strategy during the preoperative assessment phase of treatment. CBCT analysis offers the clinician an excellent evaluation of the patient's anatomy to properly plan implant position, diameter, and length, which helps to prevent positional, spacing, and depth issues.

Ideal Available Bone

The amount of available bone width (faciopalatal) should be at least 3.0 mm greater than the implant diameter at implant insertion (i.e. 2.0 mm of buccal bone and 1.0 mm of lingual bone). For example, a 4.0-mm implant requires at least 7.0 mm of bone width (minimum). Augmentation has become very predictable and accepted in the profession, therefore the clinician should never compromise when adequate bone is not available. Various bone grafting techniques and materials are available that the clinician should implement in treating these compromised cases.

Understanding the Prosthesis Type and Associated Ideal Positioning

When treatment planning, the final prosthesis should always be evaluated first, before implant placement. The implant clinician must have a strong understanding of the various prosthesis types (e.g., FP-1, FP-2, FP-3, RP-4, RP-5) along with the positional and prosthesis demands and needs. The prosthesis type

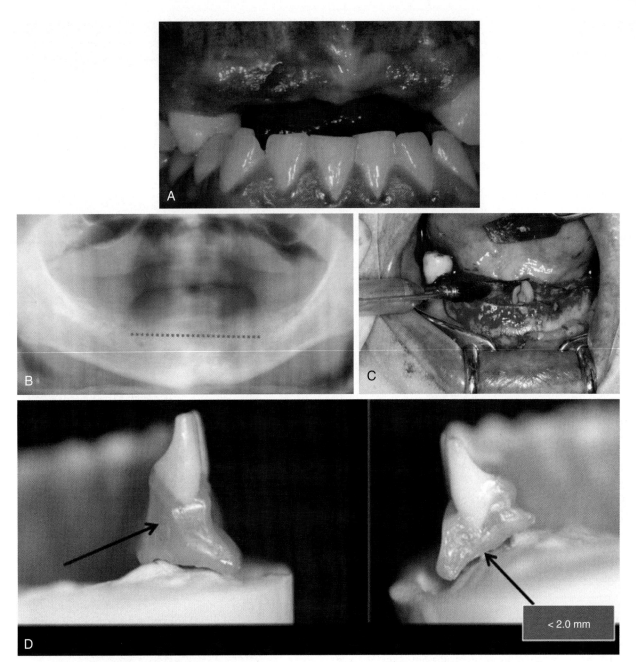

• **Fig. 28.54** Lack of interocclusal space for removable prosthesis. (A) Evaluation in the treatment planning phase with patient occluding in centric occlusion. (B) The amount of osteoplasty should be determined preoperatively *(red line)*. (C) Osteoplasty via course acrylic bur. (D) Lack of acrylic bulk leads to poor retention of denture teeth and possible fracture of denture base (<2 mm); at least 2 mm of acrylic is required for adequate strength.

(fixed [FP-1, FP-2, FP-3] or removable [RP-4, RP-5]) dictates the ideal placement of implants. It is imperative the patient be fully informed of the various prosthesis types along with the advantages and disadvantages.

Soft Tissue Evaluation

The biotype (thin versus thick) tissue should always be evaluated before implant placement. Thin biotypes are at higher risk of gingival recession and esthetic issues, especially in the anterior part of the mouth. Thin biotype patients are more susceptible to malpositioning issues, and greater emphasis should be noted on

ideal conditions. If needed, soft tissue augmentation should be completed before implant placement.

Condition of the Adjacent Teeth

Before implant placement in edentulous sites, the adjacent natural teeth should be evaluated for restorability and existing pathology that may be present. A 5- to 10-year prognostic window should be established for each natural tooth before the completion of an implant treatment plan. If a tooth does not possess a favorable 5- to 10-year prognosis, extraction should be discussed or alternative treatment options.

• BOX 28.9 **Implant Placement Insufficient Depth (Apicocoronally)**

Complication:
- Decrease retention
- Poor emergence profile
- Component fracture

Prevention:
- Ideal:
  - 3 mm below free gingival margin (2–4 mm)
- Options:
  - Change to fixed partial denture

Treatment:
- Screw retained
- Remove implant, replace with deeper implant

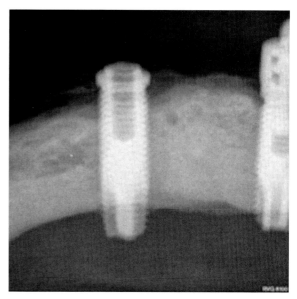

• **Fig. 28.56** Poor positioning leading to perforation of the inferior border of mandible.

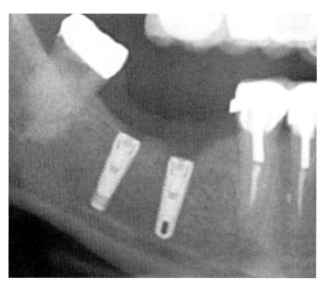

• **Fig. 28.55** Poor positioning leading to inferior alveolar canal impingement.

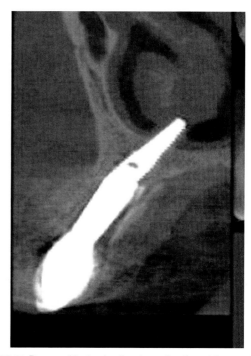

• **Fig. 28.57** Poor positioning leading to perforation of the nasal cavity.

Presence of Pathology

The intended implant site should be carefully evaluated for the presence of pathology at the site or latent adjacent pathology associated with natural teeth, which may lead to increased implant morbidity. It is common to have residual bacteria present, especially if a recently infected natural tooth extraction was performed. Additionally, the adjacent teeth should be evaluated for periapical pathology, because this may lead to a retrograde peri-implantitis.

Good Surgical Technique

To minimize the possibility of improper positioning, the implant clinician should evaluate the osteotomy location after the use of the first pilot drill. Usually, the pilot drill is used to a depth of 6 to 8 mm. A direction indicator is placed and should be evaluated both radiographically and with a surgical template for proper positioning. The position can also be evaluated by having the patient close lightly to determine the interocclusal positioning with the direction indicator. Any modifications of the angulation should be completed with a Lindemann drill.

Poorly Dense Bone

In poorly dense bone (~D4), overpreparation of the osteotomy site may lead to redirection of the implant on placement. Additionally, implants should be inserted with a handpiece rather than a hand ratchet. When implants are placed in poorly dense bone with a ratchet, the implant may be easily redirectioned by placing it in a more elliptical direction.

Understand the True Location of Vital Structures

Knowing the exact location of the vital structures is paramount in avoiding complications. Impinging on vital structures such as the mandibular canal, maxillary sinus, or nasal cavity may

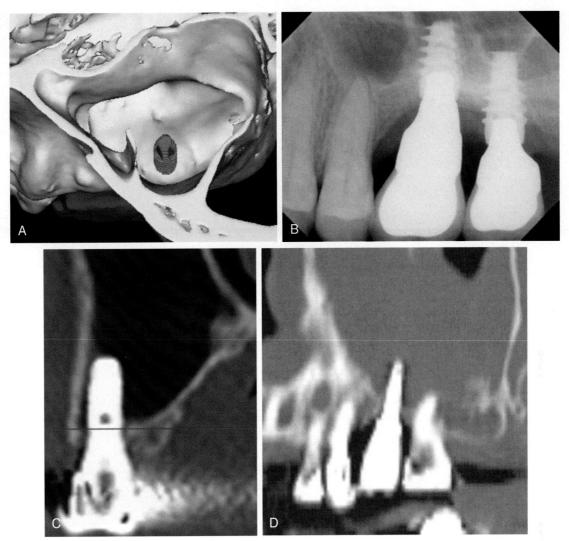

• **Fig. 28.58** Implant placement in posterior maxilla without bone grafting. (A and B) Implant penetration into the sinus cavity. (C) Implant placed into the sinus depicting no bone in the sinus, leading to inadequate support for the prosthesis. (D) Implant placed into sinus causing rhinosinusitis.

increase morbidity and place the patient at risk for irreversible complications.

Use of Surgical Templates

A surgical template is defined by the prosthodontics glossary as a guide used to assist in ideal surgical placement and angulation of dental implants.[21] The objective of using a surgical template is to provide accurate placement of the implant according to a surgical treatment. There are many different types of surgical templates used today. Stumpel classified surgical templates according to the amount of surgical restriction that is used in the template. The design categories are (1) nonlimiting, (2) partial limiting, and (3) complete limiting.[33]

Non-Limiting Design

The nonlimiting template allows the implant surgeon dimensional variability in the implant location because the template indicates the ideal space (location) for the final restoration, not the actual mesiodistal angulation. The nonlimiting template is advantageous because of the ease in fabrication and the low cost involved.

These templates allow the implant surgeon only an initial location of the proposed prosthesis, not the exact angulation (buccolingual) and position (mesiodistal). A great deal of flexibility and latitude regarding the final position of the implant is inherent with this type of template (Fig. 28.59).

Partial Limiting Design

The partial limiting design incorporates a guided sleeve or a slot that allows for angulation of one drill size (usually the pilot drill). After the first drill is used, the rest of the osteotomy sites are completed freehand. Various techniques can be used in fabricating a partial limiting template, including manual laboratory-fabricated templates or templates fabricated from a radiographic template, which is then converted to a surgical guide template.

Complication. Although the partial limiting design is more accurate than the nonlimiting design, these templates still do not allow for final, positioning of the implant. Clinical studies have shown these types of templates to have a high degree of error in the buccolingual orientation (Fig. 28.60).[34]

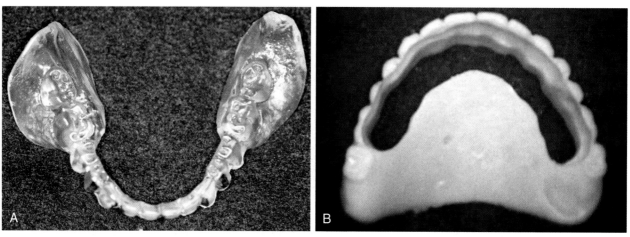

• **Fig. 28.59** Nonlimiting surgical templates: (A) Mandibular prosthesis with lingual contour removed. (B) Maxillary prosthesis with lingual contour removed and retention of the palate for support.

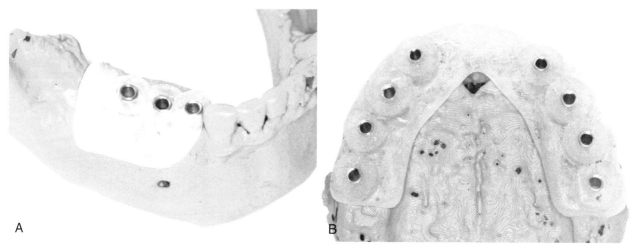

• **Fig. 28.60** Complete limiting surgical templates. (A and B) Complete fabricated limiting templates, which allows for accurate placement in the mesiodistal and buccolingual dimensions.

Complete Limiting Design

With the complete limiting template design, the position, angulation, and depth of the osteotomy are dictated by the guided tubes or sleeves, restricting any variation by the implant surgeon. This type of guide prevents any osteotomy error in the buccolingual and mesiodistal planes. Additionally, drill stops can be incorporated to prevent overpreparation in depth of the site. Basically, with the complete limiting design, the final position of the implant is known before the actual surgery. This technique is extremely popular because the prosthetic final abutment or provisional restoration can be prefabricated for immediate provisionalization after implant placement.

Complication. The use of complete limiting surgical templates that are fabricated from interactive treatment planning with cone beam technology has been shown to be highly accurate. However, caution must be used when employing surgical templates that are fabricated conventionally (not from CBCT) on dental study casts, which are rigid, nonfunctional surfaces without information of the soft tissue thickness and bone morphology. These types of surgical templates, usually made from study casts, allow for placement of implants according to an estimate of location of teeth, soft and hard tissue, and vital structures without three-dimensional guidance (Figs. 28.61, 28.62, and 28.63).[35]

Use of CBCT Surgical Guides

To overcome the limitations and complications inherent with conventional surgical templates, the use of CBCT-generated templates has evolved in implant dentistry today. A computer-generated surgical guide (partial limiting or complete limiting) provides a link between the CBCT treatment plan and the actual surgery by transferring the interactive plan accurately to the surgical site.

With the use of CBCT-generated software programs, this anatomic relationship can be predictably determined before surgery. After the scan is completed the data must be converted into a format that can be used by the scanning software. Every treatment-planning software program has its own specific protocol, but all software is compatible with Digital Imaging and Communication in Medicine (DICOM) files that are generated and downloaded from the scanner. Although many third party companies complete the interactive treatment planning process, it is highly recommended the implant dentist be involved in the process. After the files have been converted into the software program, evaluation of potential implant sites in the desired prosthetic locations can be completed. Virtual implants may be placed via comprehensive implant libraries, which include the implant brand, type, diameter, and length. The available bone

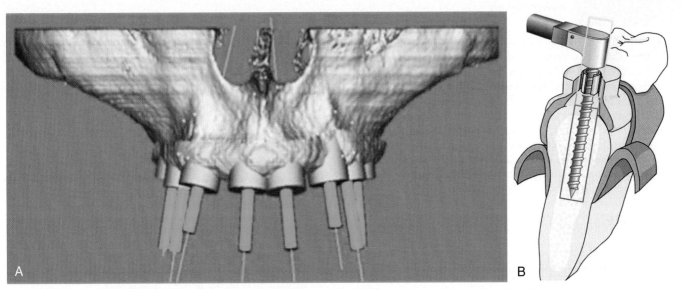

• **Fig. 28.61** Bone-supported surgical template. (A and B) Template requires the exposure of the bone and the complete seating of the surgical template.

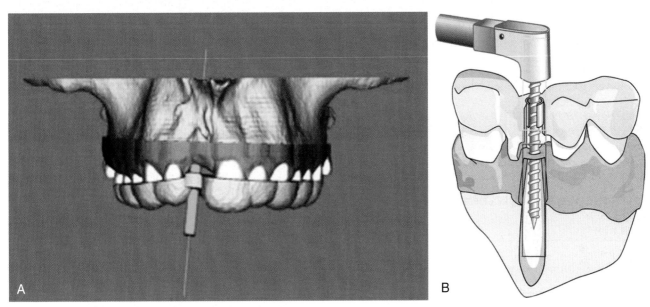

• **Fig. 28.62** Tooth-supported surgical template. (A and B) Template requires adequate remaining teeth for complete seating and stabilization over the teeth.

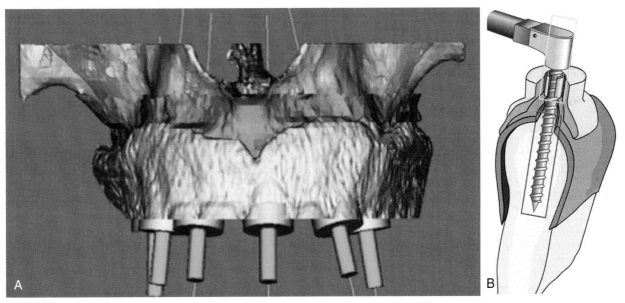

• **Fig. 28.63** Soft tissue–supported surgical template. (A and B) Template requires adequate soft tissue to allow for complete seating and stabilization.

dimensions may be ascertained, along with the density and angulation with respect to the planned prosthesis. After completion of the final implant positions, the treatment plan is saved, and the surgical template is designed.[29] it is well documented in the literature that surgical templates are significantly more accurate than freehand insertion.[36] With all types of guides the implant clinician must show good judgment regarding the accuracy of the template and must be able to determine any discrepancies (especially in bone volume) between the intended osteotomy site and the actual current bony architecture of the patient.

Summary

One of the most critical skills in the practice of implant dentistry is the ability to place an implant in the ideal and correct position. The complexity of this skill set is underrated; the clinician needs to understand the three planes of placement, along with maintaining a safe distance from vital structures. Malpositioning may result in a successful integration of the implant, but it may place the intended restoration at significant risk for complication and/or failure. Technological advances such as guided surgery and surgical templates have proven to be helpful to implant clinicians, especially those early on their surgical learning curve or in cases in which space tolerances are low. However, even these techniques have margins of error and

tolerances that need to be fully understood. With a combination of proper treatment planning and ideal positioning guidelines, the implant clinician can ensure a predictable surgical and prosthetic outcome (Box 28.10).

References

1. Katona TR, Goodacre CJ, Brown DT, et al. Force-moment systems on single maxillary anterior implants: effects of incisal guidance, fixture orientation, and loss of bone support. *Int J Oral Maxillofac Implants*. 1993;8:512–522.
2. Priest GF. The esthetic challenge of adjacent implants. *J Oral Maxillofac Surg*. 2007;65(suppl 1):2–12.
3. Stumpel L. Model-based guided implant placement; planned precision. *Inside Dent*. 2008;4(9):72–77.
4. Buser D, Martin W, Belser UC. Optimizing esthetics for implant restorations in the anterior maxilla: anatomic and surgical considerations. *Int J Oral Maxillofac Implants*. 2004;19(suppl):43–61.
5. Margelos JT, Verdelis KG. Irreversible pulpal damage of teeth adjacent to recently placed osseointegrated implants. *J Endod*. 1995;21:479–482.
6. Asscherickx K, Vannet BV, Wehrbein H, et al. Root repair after injury from miniscrew. *Clin Oral Implants Res*. 2005;16:575–578.
7. Kravitz ND, Kusnoto B. Risks and complications of orthodontic miniscrews. *Am J Orthod Dentofacial Orthop*. 2007;131:S43–S51.
8. Brisceno CE, Rossouw PE, Carrillo R. Healing of the roots and surrounding structures after intentional damage with miniscrew implants. *Am J Orthod Dentofacial Orthop*. 2009;135:292–301.
9. Buser D, Martin W, Belser UC. Optimizing esthetics for implant restorations in the anterior maxilla: anatomic and surgical considerations. *Int J Oral Maxillofac Implants*. 2004;19(suppl):43–61.
10. Esposito M, Ekestubbe A, Grondahl K. Radiologic evaluation of marginal bone loss at tooth surfaces facing single Branemark implants. *Clin Oral Implants Res*. 1993;4:151–157.
11. Rieger MR, Mayberry M, Brose MO. Finite element analysis of six endosseous implants. *J Prosthet Dent*. 1990;63:671–676.
12. Tarnow DP, Cho SC, Wallace SS. The effect of inter-implant distance on the height of inter-implant bone. *J Periodontol*. 2000;71:546–549.
13. Su CY, Fu JH, Wang HL. The role of implant position on long–term success. *Clin Adv Periodontics*. 2014;4(3):187–193.
14. Spray JR, Black CG, Morris HF. The influence of bone thickness on facial marginal bone response: stage 1 placement through stage 2 uncovering. *Ann Periodontol*. 2000;5:119–128.
15. Misch CE, Bidez MW. Occlusion and crestal bone resorption:etiology and treatment planning strategies for implants. In: McNeil C, ed. *Science and Practice of Occlusion*. Chicago: Quintessence; 1997.
16. Ha CY, Lim YJ, Kim MJ, et al. The influence of abutment angulation on screw loosening of implants in anterior maxilla. *J Oral Maxillofac Implants*. 2011;26:45–55.
17. Misch CE. The maxillary anterior single tooth implant aesthetic–health compromise. *Int J Dent Symp*. 1995;3:4–9.
18. Perel S, Sullivan Y, eds. *Esthetics and Osseointegration*. Chicago: Quintessence; 1994.
19. Saadouin AP, Sullivan DY, Korrschek M, et al. Single tooth implant management for success. *Pract Periodontics Aesthet Dent*. 1994;6:73–82.
20. Goodacre CJ, Kan JK, Rungcharassaeng K. Clinical complications of osseointegrated implants. *J Prosthet Dent*. 1999;81:537–552.
21. Nisapakultorn K, Suphanantachat S, Silkosessak O, Rattanamongkolgul S. Factors affecting soft tissue level around anterior maxillary single-tooth implants: soft tissue level at single-tooth implants. *Clin Oral Implants Res*. 2010;21(6):662–670. https://doi.org/10.1111/j.1600-0501.2009.01887.x.
22. Misch CE. The maxillary anterior single tooth implant aesthetic–health compromise. *Int J Dent Symp*. 1995;3:4–9.
23. Saadouin AP, Sullivan DY, Korrschek M, et al. Single tooth implant management for success. *Pract Periodontics Aesthet Dent*. 1994;6:73–82.

• BOX 28.10 Ideal Implant Positioning Summary

Implant Distances:
- Implant-Tooth: 1.5 mm (apical), 2.0 mm (coronal)
- Implant–implant: 3.0 mm

Bone Thickness: (after implant placement)
- Buccal = 2.0 mm
- Lingual = 1.0 mm

Ideal Positioning:
- Apicocoronal: 2.0–3.0 mm apical to free gingival margin

Prosthesis Type: (Cement vs. Screw Retained)
- Anterior
  - Cement: Slightly lingual to incisal edge
  - Screw: Cingulum Area
- Posterior
  - Cement/Screw: Central Fossa

Interocclusal Space: (minimum)
- Cement-Retained Prosthesis
  - 7–8.0mm (Zirconia), 8–10.0 mm (Porcelain Fused Metal)
- Screw-Retained Prosthesis
  - 5.0–6.0 mm (Zirconia/PFM)
- Overdenture
  - Bar-Retained: 14–16 mm (depending on attachment)
  - Independent Attachment: 9 mm (e.g. Locator)

Vital Structure Distance:
- Nasal Cavity: may engage cortical bone without perforation
- Maxillary Sinus: (into sinus proper)
  - SA-1: Implant placement below sinus floor
  - SA-2: 1.0 – 2.0 mm membrane elevation
  - SA-3: Transcrestal (3.0-4.0 mm), Lateral Wall (> 4.0 mm)
  - SA-4: Lateral Wall: minimum of 5 mm host bone
- Mandibular Anterior: No cortical bone perforation
- Mandibular Posterior: 2.0 mm from mandibular canal/mental foramen

24. Perel S, Sullivan Y, eds. *Esthetics and Osseointegration*. Chicago: Quintessence; 1994.

25. Hansson S. The implant neck smooth or provided with retention elements. *Clin Oral Implants Res*. 1999;10:394–405.

26. Malevez C, Hermans M, Daelemans P. Marginal bone levels at Brånemark system implants used for single tooth restoration: the influence of implant design and anatomical region. *Clin Oral Implants Res*. 1996;7:162–169.

27. Grunder U. Stability of the mucosal topography around single tooth implants and adjacent teeth: 1 year results. *Int J Periodontics Restorative Dent*. 2000;20:11–17.

28. Berglundh T, Lindhe J, Ericsson I, et al. The soft tissue barrier at implants and teeth. *Clin Oral Implants Res*. 1991;2 :81–90.

29. Yukna RA. Periodontal considerations for dental implants. In: Block MS, Kent JN, eds. *Endosseous Implants for Maxillofacial Reconstruction*. Philadelphia: WB Saunders; 1995.

30. Misch CE, Goodacre CJ, Finley JM, et al. Consensus conference panel report: crown-height space guidelines for implant dentistry—part 2. *Implant Dent*. 2006;15:113–121.

31. Naitoh M, Ariji E, Okumura S, et al. Can implants be correctly angulated based on surgical templates used for osseointegrated dental implants? *Clin Oral Implants Res*. 2000;11:409–414.

32. Ha CY, Lim YJ, Kim MJ, et al. The influence of abutment angulation on screw loosening of implants in anterior maxilla. *Int J Oral Maxillofac Implants*. 2011;26:45–55.

33. Stumpel 3rd LJ. Cast-based guided implant placement: a novel technique. *J Prosthet Dent*. 2008;100:61–69.

34. Almog DM, Torrado E, Meitner SW. Fabrication of imaging and surgical guides for dental implants. *J Prosthet Dent*. 2001;85:504–508.

35. Ramasamy M, Giri RR, et al. Implant surgical guides: from the past to the present. *J Pharm BioAllied Sci*. 2013;5(suppl 1):S98–S102.

36. Nickenig HJ, Wichmann M, Hamel J, et al. Evaluation of the difference in accuracy between implant placement by virtual planning data and surgical guide templates versus the conventional free-hand method—a combined in vivo—in vitro technique using cone-beam CT (Part II). *J Cranio-Maxillo-Fac Surg*. 2010;38(7):488–493.

29

Maxillary Anterior Implant Placement

RANDOLPH R. RESNIK AND CARL E. MISCH*

Maxillary Anterior Implant Placement

Contrary to missing a posterior tooth, most patients have an emotional response regarding a maxillary anterior missing tooth. Because the premaxillary teeth are directly within the smile line, no question exists regarding the need to replace the tooth, and financial considerations are usually less important. When posterior teeth are extracted, little resistance to the preparation of adjacent teeth may be given to the dentist. However, when anterior, normal-looking teeth must be prepared to serve as fixed partial denture (FPD) abutments, the patient is more anxious and often looks for an alternative. In the patient's perspective, anterior FPD prostheses are never as esthetic as natural teeth. This in part is because they are able to distinguish between the esthetics of a natural tooth versus a porcelain/zirconia restoration.

Therefore the profession and patients are gravitating to implant replacement instead of conventional prosthetics. Single-tooth implants are now one of the most common implant procedures performed in the United States. In the nonesthetic posterior region, the single-tooth implant is one of the simplest procedures in implant surgery and prosthetics. However, it should be noted, the maxillary anterior single-tooth replacement is often the most difficult procedure in all of implant dentistry.

The highly esthetic zone of the premaxilla often requires both hard (bone and teeth) and soft tissue restoration. The soft tissue drape is usually the most difficult aspect of treatment to develop and maintain. As a consequence, maxillary anterior single-tooth replacement is often a significant challenge, regardless of the experience and skill of the clinician.

Maxillary Anterior Implant Studies

In general, the single-tooth implant has the highest success rate compared with any other treatment option to replace missing teeth with an implant restoration (e.g., short-span FPD, full-arch FPD, single-tooth implant).[1-4] Misch and colleagues reported on 276 anterior maxillary single implants used to restore missing teeth from agenesis. In 255 adolescent patients, the implants were monitored for a range of 2 to 16 years, with a 98.6% implant and crown survival rate.[5] In the same year, Wennstrom and colleagues

reported on a 5-year prospective study with 45 single-tooth implants, with a 97.7% implant survival rate with minimal bone loss.[6] In 2006, Zarone and colleagues reported on lateral maxillary agenesis replacement with 34 implants, with a 97% survival rate at 39 months.[7] A review of the literature by Goodacre and colleagues found that single-tooth implant studies had the highest survival rate of any prosthesis type and averaged 97%.[8] Therefore the maxillary anterior implant has been well researched and most studies show a very high success rate.

More recently, a trend toward single-stage and immediate-placement implants has emerged, appearing especially attractive in the maxillary anterior region. This is preferable because the soft tissue drape is easier to retain, and with this type of treatment shorter treatment time is advantageous. Kemppainen and colleagues in a prospective study of 102 single-tooth implants in the anterior maxilla, reported a 99% success rate using one- and two-stage implant protocols.[9] Other studies have recommended one-stage and immediate load with overwhelming success.[10,11]

Maxillary Anterior Teeth Evaluation

The maxillary anterior implant is successful only if the final restoration it supports is fully supported functionally and esthetically with the adjacent dentition. The exponential growth of the field of implant dentistry has been paralleled by exciting new advancements in esthetic dentistry and plastic regenerative surgery. This growth has made the profession realize that the restoration of the peri-implant soft and hard tissue to an optimal architecture is the key to a successful implant restoration. It is no longer acceptable practice to only achieve osseointegration with an implant. The implant restoration complex in the esthetic zone should ideally be achieved in a context that respects all biological tissues (Fig. 29.1).

When the goal for a maxillary incisor single-tooth replacement is to obtain an ideal result, the clinician should first evaluate not only the edentulous site but also the remaining anterior teeth. Because only one tooth is missing, the adjacent teeth most often dictate its length, contour, shape, and position. If this is not satisfactory, then a potential modification may need to be integrated into the overall treatment plan.

Parameters for a healthy esthetic anterior restoration have been established. The following guidelines have been proposed by esthetic and cosmetic dentistry colleagues. These parameters

*Deceased.

706

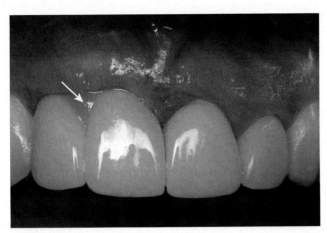

• **Fig. 29.1** Maxillary anterior implants that may be functional; however, in some situations (i.e., high smile line) they may not be esthetically pleasing to patients because of the addition of pink porcelain between the lateral and central incisor.

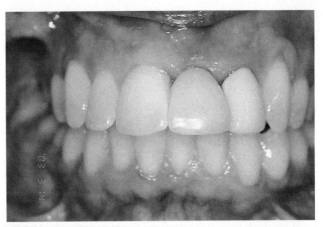

• **Fig. 29.2** Patient's left maxillary central incisor was replaced with an implant and crown. The tooth is wider than the right central incisor. Orthodontics could have reduced the horizontal overjet of the lateral and central incisors and resulted in more symmetric teeth. A second option is a veneer on the right central incisor to correct the rotation and make the natural tooth more symmetric to the implant crown.

play a determinant role in the final result and should not be overlooked. The patient must be educated about their present condition before the onset of treatment, and the starting point should be documented. The patient, once fully informed of the existing discrepancies and their potential negative effect on the envisioned result, may decide to address and correct the existing problems of the adjacent teeth or simply elect to accept the compromise. Correction may be as simple as bleaching the remaining teeth or as complex as full esthetic rehabilitation with crown lengthening, soft tissue plastic surgery, veneers or crowns, and orthodontic therapy (or a combination of these procedures).

Maxillary Tooth Size

The two maxillary central incisors should appear symmetric and of similar size, most importantly when the patient has a high smile line. This is most critical to evaluate when the missing tooth is one central incisor (Fig. 29.2). Outline asymmetry is visually acceptable the more distal from the midline the eye travels. When one maxillary tooth is missing, the remaining space may be compromised from drifting of the adjacent teeth. Orthodontic intervention may be indicated when the missing tooth is a central incisor with a mesiodistal space less or more than the size of the corresponding central incisor. The other option is to modify the existing central incisor with a veneer or composite to make it similar in size and shape to the missing tooth restoration. This has the advantage of lowering the mesial interproximal contact and making the two centrals more square shaped, which decreases the height requirement of the papilla. The shades of the two centrals is easier to match when made at the same time in the laboratory. To understand ideal tooth size, the clinician should have a clear understanding of the normal and average tooth dimensions.

Central Incisor. The average clinical crown length of the maxillary central incisor is 10.2 mm for a male patient and 9.4 mm for a female patient.[12] In some cases, surgical crown lengthening and longer anterior teeth may be indicated to reduce gingival exposure during a high-smile lip position. Because the clinical crown height of an implant-supported central incisor is often longer than the adjacent tooth, an esthetic crown lengthening on the natural tooth may be used to align the gingival margins. When an implant crown is longer than the corresponding natural tooth, a crown-lengthening procedure may be more predictable on the natural tooth than attempting to augment the implant crown with soft tissue.

However, the clinical crowns of natural teeth are rarely more than 12 mm high. The width of the average maxillary central is 8.6 mm for a male patient and 8.1 mm for a female patient. Although male teeth are usually slightly longer and wider, the length to width ratio is similar to female teeth, (0.85 for male patients and 0.86 for female patients). A ratio range of 0.70 to 0.86 has been reported to be acceptable for the central incisors when they are similar. When the anterior teeth are made longer and both centrals have the same width, an acceptable result may be obtained.

Lateral Incisor. The average clinical crown length of the maxillary lateral incisor is 8.7 mm for a male patient and 7.8 mm for a female patient. Therefore the average lateral incisor is almost 1.5 mm shorter than the central incisor (at both the gingival region and the incisal edge). Gingival margins of the maxillary lateral incisors may be similar to centrals and canines, but they should not be higher than the neighboring teeth. Therefore an implant crown on the lateral incisor should not be longer than the central or canine. The average width of a lateral incisor is 6.6 mm for a male patient and 6.1 mm for a female patient, but this is more variable than for any other anterior tooth. The length to width ratio is slightly greater for a female patient (0.79, compared with the male patient ratio of 0.76). A lateral incisor space may be slightly narrower than the other natural tooth; however, when replacing the lateral incisor, it may be preferable to perform a slight mesial stripping of the adjacent canine to duplicate and make symmetric the lateral incisors.

Canine. The average male canine clinical crown length is 10.1 mm and width is 7.6 mm, with a ratio of 0.77. The canine is usually the same height as the central but 1 mm narrower. Usually the lateral incisor is 1 mm narrower than the cuspid. The female canine height averages 8.9 mm (0.5 mm shorter than the central) and 7.2 mm in width (1 mm narrower), with a ratio of 0.81. As a general rule, regardless of sex, the central incisor is 2 mm wider than the lateral incisor and 1 mm wider than the canine. However, on the horizontal plane, the canine is 1 to 2 mm shorter than the central incisor and corresponds to the curvature of the lower lip during smiling.

Tooth Shape

Three basic shapes of maxillary anterior teeth exist: (1) square, (2) ovoid, and (3) triangular. The tooth shape will directly influence the interproximal contact area and the gingival embrasure. The

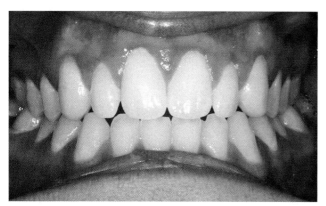

• **Fig. 29.3** Triangular tooth shape has the steepest gingival scallop, and the interproximal bone is farthest from the tip of the papilla. After an extraction, shrinkage of the tissue makes the soft tissue drape in this tooth shape the most difficult to restore.

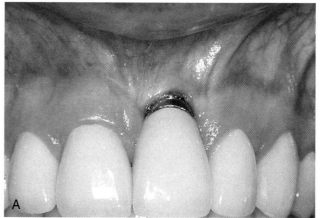

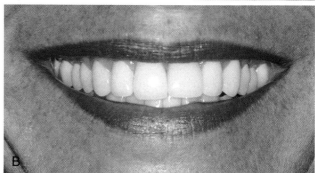

• **Fig. 29.4** (A) The maxillary left central incisor was restored with an implant restoration. The patient desired a soft tissue graft to cover the implant crest module. (B) The high lip position during smiling did not display the cervical region of the patient's central incisors. Although this is not an ideal result, additional surgeries would not improve the crown's appearance within the esthetic zone, and the soft tissue pocket created may increase the risk of peri-implantitis.

square tooth shape is the most favorable to obtain an ideal soft tissue drape and papillae around the crown because the interproximal contact is further apical and more tooth structure will fill the interproximal region. In contrast, a triangular tooth shape has a more incisal interproximal contact, a steeper gingival scallop, and is farther from the interproximal bone (Fig. 29.3). As a result, a space often exists between the interproximal contact and the interdental papilla of the remaining teeth. This is especially noteworthy to observe at the initial examination. When the soft tissue fills the interproximal space of the remaining anterior teeth that have a triangular shape, the tissues may be very liable and easily disappear during the healing phases after implant surgery. Care should be taken if the adjacent soft tissue requires reflection for a bone graft before the implant insertion. The ideal restoration of the soft tissue with a triangular-shaped tooth is less predictable.

The cervical embrasure of the adjacent teeth to the edentulous site should be particularly evaluated. A triangular tooth is narrow at the cervical embrasure, and the base of the interproximal tissue is wide. In addition, the adjacent tooth contact is often higher off the tissue, with an increased risk of a black triangular space. When such a condition is present on the adjacent teeth of the missing tooth, it is likely that the interdental papillae region will also be compromised on the implant crown. The tooth shape also affects the topography of the underlying hard tissues. The roots of triangular tooth shapes are positioned farther apart; therefore they have thicker facial and interproximal bone. This may decrease the amount of crestal bone loss after an extraction. In addition, the prognosis for an immediate implant insertion is more favorable in these situations because the bone defect is smaller in diameter and the interproximal bone more likely to provide the recommended 1.5 mm or more of interproximal bone from the adjacent tooth. The square-shaped tooth is more likely to have less interproximal bone between the roots. Therefore it presents a greater risk of crestal or interproximal bone loss with an immediate implant insertion, making it less favorable for immediate implant insertion after extraction.

Soft Tissue Drape

The height of the maxillary lip when smiling (high lip line) is one of the most important criterion to evaluate when observing the cervical region of the maxillary anterior teeth. Its position is usually related to age, with older men showing the least amount of teeth and soft tissue and younger female patients displaying the most. Some patients (15% of male patients and 6% of female

patients) show only the incisal half of the anterior teeth when they smile.[13] Those patients should be identified and it should be explained in detail that an ideal soft tissue result in the gingival region is not mandatory. Clinical results in emergence contours, interdental papilla presence, and even shade and contour of the crown are much less demanding. Therefore the additional surgical intervention and cost may not be necessary when these patients are willing to accept a slight compromise in ideal esthetics (Fig. 29.4).

Ideally the height of the maxillary lip should rest at the junction of the free gingival margin on the facial aspect of the maxillary centrals and canine teeth.[14,15] Thus the interdental papillae are visible, but little gingival display is seen over the clinical crowns. Almost 70% of patients have this ideal smile position. A "gummy" smile is defined as showing more than 2 mm of soft tissue above the clinical maxillary crowns and is more acceptable in the female patient. It may occur in more than 14% of the female population and 7% of the male population. The higher the high lip line, the more ideal the esthetic requirements are for the remaining teeth and the single-tooth replacement. Therefore the existing maxillary anterior teeth condition is closely scrutinized when a high lip line exists and ideal results are desired.

The soft tissue drape of the remaining teeth should be evaluated, especially if exposed during the high lip position of smiling. Under ideal conditions, soft tissue completely fills the interproximal space, with no dark triangles from the absence of light within the oral cavity. The interproximal contact between the maxillary central incisors should begin in the incisal third of the teeth and

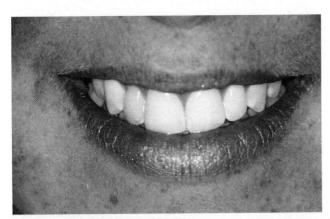

● **Fig. 29.5** Interdental papillae are often highest between the central incisor, with progressively less height as they proceed distal. The high lip line during smiling shows the interdistal papillae in more than 85% of the patients. (NOTE: The maxillary right lateral incisor is an implant restoration.)

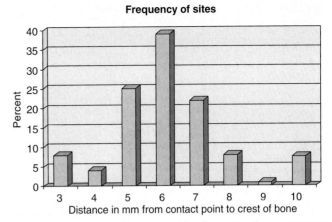

● **Fig. 29.6** Distance from the interproximal contact to the crest of bone with natural teeth most often measures 5 mm, 6 mm, or 7 mm.[58] (Tarnow, D. P., Magner, A. W., & Fletcher, P. (1992). The effect of the distance from the contact point to the crest of bone on the presence or absence of the interproximal dental papilla. *Journal of periodontology*, 63(12), 995-996.)

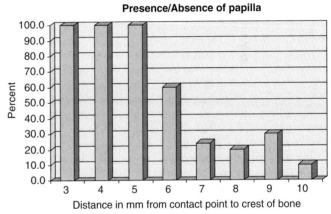

● **Fig. 29.7** When the interproximal contact-to-bone distance is 5 mm or less, the interdental papilla completely fills (100%) the space between the teeth. When the contact–bone distance is 6 mm (the most common measurement), almost 40% of the time a black triangular space occurs between the teeth from the absence of papilla filling the space. A 7-mm or greater contact–bone distance nearly always has an incomplete fill of the interproximal space with the soft tissue. (From Tarnow DP, Magner AW, Fletcher P. The effect of the distance from the contact point to the crest of bone on the presence or absence of the interproximal dental papilla. *J Periodontol.* 1992;63(12):995-996.)

continue to the height of the central interdental papilla. In a healthy patient, very little to no space is seen between the papillae and interproximal contact. According to Kois, the distance from the facial free gingival margin to the height of the central midinterproximal papilla is usually 4 to 5 mm; therefore the interdental papilla height is approximately 40% to 50% of the exposed tooth length.[16] Interproximal contacts at the incisal position start progressively more gingivally from central to canine. The greatest papilla height is often between the centrals, slightly lower between the centrals and laterals, and even lower between laterals and canines (Fig. 29.5).

However, the papilla height is often similar between the centrals and from the centrals to the laterals. Under ideal conditions the osseous scallop of bone in the maxillary anterior region begins 2 mm below the cement-enamel junction (CEJ) midfacial to a point 3 mm more incisal in the interproximal region. The soft tissue follows this osseous scallop. A soft tissue biological dimension of approximately 3 mm in height above the bone is present at the midfacial position (1 mm above the CEJ) and 3 to 5 mm above the interproximal bone. Therefore if the interproximal contact is within 3 to 5 mm of the interproximal bone, then the interdental papilla will most often completely fill the space. Tarnow and colleagues[17] and Norland and Tarnow[18] measured the distance from the bottom of the interproximal contact to the vertical height of interproximal bone on natural teeth and observed how frequently the interproximal space would be completely filled by soft tissue. The distances ranged from 3 to 10 mm, with 88% of the contacts to the bone at 5 mm, 6 mm, or 7 mm; the most common measurement was 6 mm (40%), followed by 5 mm (25%), and then 7 mm (22%) (Fig. 29.6).

When the contact point to bone was 3 to 5 mm, the papilla almost always filled the space. When the contact was 6 mm, an absence of papilla was noted almost 45% of the time; at a 7-mm distance the papilla did not fill the space 75% of the time (Fig. 29.7). In other words, a difference of 1 to 2 mm from the interproximal contact to the interseptal bone is very significant in relation to the interproximal soft tissue. Therefore it is critical to evaluate this dimension before implant surgery. If the height of the interproximal bone is lost or the interproximal contact is more incisal, then the soft tissue will less likely fill the interproximal space. In addition, contact distances to bone of 7 mm sometimes present a papilla initially, but after surgical reflection the chance this papilla will return to the original position may be less than 25%.

The higher the gingival scallop, or difference between the height of the papilla and the free gingival margin, the higher the risk for gingival loss after extraction. Likewise, once the tooth is extracted and an edentulous site is healed, the less likely the surgical and restorative procedures will be able to restore an ideal soft tissue contour. In contrast, a flatter gingival scallop and an interproximal tissue close to the osseous crest are conducive to minimal tissue shrinkage and a more ideal outcome. The height of the facial gingival contour is in the middle of the tooth for the maxillary lateral incisors and the four mandibular anterior teeth; however, it is slightly to the distal on the central incisors and canines. The height of the free gingival margins of the two centrals are similar to both canines. The cervical height of the lateral incisors may be level or below the centrals and canines but symmetric to each other. It may be easier to lengthen the cervical contour of the contralateral incisor when replacing a missing lateral incisor with an implant

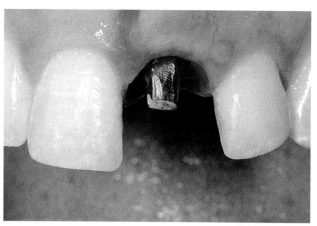

• **Fig. 29.8** Single missing central incisor is often the most challenging surgical and prosthetic implant to complete. The soft and hard tissues need to be ideal to obtain an acceptable esthetic result.

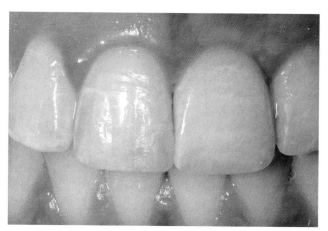

• **Fig. 29.9** Maxillary left central incisor implant crown in position. The soft tissue drape is established through both surgical and prosthetic methods.

instead of attempting to lower the gingival contour on the implant crown when gingiva and bone shrinkage has occurred. The least desirable gingival contour is seen when one anterior tooth is higher than the rest. Unfortunately this is a common occurrence with an implant crown when the bone and/or soft tissue is not augmented in conjunction with implant insertion or uncovery.

The color and texture of the tissue is also evaluated in the edentulous tooth site. The attached keratinized gingival tone and coral-pink color should be similar around the implant abutment compared with the healthy adjacent teeth. The biotype of the gingiva is usually classified as either thick or thin. Thicker tissue is more resistant to the shrinkage or recession and more often leads to the formation of a periodontal pocket after bone loss. Thin gingival tissues around the teeth are more prone to shrinkage after tooth extraction and are more difficult to elevate or augment after tooth loss. Gingival recession is the most common esthetic complication of thin biotypes after anterior single-tooth extraction and is also a concern after implant surgery, uncovery, or both. According to Kois,[19] predictability of the maxillary anterior single-tooth implant is ultimately determined by the patient's own presenting anatomy. Favorable conditions include (1) when the tooth position is more coronal relative to the full gingival margin, (2) square tooth shapes, (3) flat scallop periodontium forms, (4) thick periodontium biotypes, and (5) high (<3 mm) facial osseous crest positions of the teeth and midcrestal. Unfavorable patient anatomy includes (1) aligned or apical preexisting tooth (relative to the free gingival margin), (2) triangular tooth shapes, (3) high scallop periodontium form, (4) thin periodontium types, and (5) low (>4 mm) facial osseous crest positions in relation to adjacent teeth and the midcrestal area.

Anatomic Challenges

Natural Tooth Size Versus Implant Diameter

The esthetics of a maxillary anterior single crown on a natural tooth is often one of the most difficult procedures in restorative dentistry. When an implant is being restored, the challenges are even greater (Figs. 29.8 and 29.9). When comparing the size and shape of an implant versus natural tooth, the implant is often 5 mm or less in diameter and round in cross section. A natural maxillary anterior crown cervix region is approximately 4.5 to 7 mm in mesiodistal cross section and is never completely round. In fact, the natural central incisor and canine teeth are often larger

in their faciopalatal dimension at the CEJ than in the mesiodistal dimension. Because the bone is lost first in the faciopalatal width, the greater width of implants in this dimension would require even greater augmentation than presently advocated. As a result, the cervical esthetics of a single-implant crown must accommodate a round-diameter implant and balance hygiene and esthetic parameters. Additional prosthetic steps and components with varied emergence profiles or customized tooth-colored abutments are often required to render the illusion of a crown on a natural abutment.

Compromised Bone Height

The available bone should be closely evaluated because it will greatly influence the soft tissue drape, implant size, implant position (angulation and depth), and ultimately the final esthetic outcome. Hard tissue topography is a prerequisite to an optimal, esthetic implant restoration. Therefore a comprehensive cone beam computerized tomography (CBCT) evaluation of the available bone volume present is mandatory to determine the ideal implant position. The osseous midcrestal position of the edentulous site should be approximately 2 to 3 mm below the facial CEJ or free gingival margin of the adjacent teeth. The interproximal bone should be scalloped 3 mm more incisal than the midcrestal position.

The position of the interproximal crest of bone is an important anatomic consideration, especially for the development of the interproximal soft tissue height. Becker and colleagues classified the range of interproximal bone height above the midfacial scallop from less than 2.1 mm (flat) to scalloped (2.8 mm) to pronounced scalloped (<4.1 mm).[20] The flat anatomy should correspond to a square-shaped tooth, the scalloped to an ovoid-shaped tooth, and the pronounced scalloped to a triangular-shaped tooth (Fig. 29.10). However, these relationships do not always exist. When a flat interdental-to-crest dimension is found on triangular teeth, the interproximal space will usually not be filled with soft tissue because the dimension of the interproximal contact to the bone will be greater than 5 mm (Fig. 29.11).[21]

Often the osseous crest may be more apical than ideal in both the implant site and the adjacent tooth roots. Under these conditions, ideal crown contour, soft tissue emergence, and interproximal tissue conditions are less likely (Figs. 29.12 and 29.13). Instead of the expected FP-1 prosthesis, most likely an FP-2 prosthesis will be the end result. Bone and soft tissue changes after maxillary anterior tooth loss are rather rapid and of considerable consequence. As a result, many maxillary anterior edentulous sites require at least some bone and/or soft tissue modification before, in conjunction with, and/or at implant uncovery.

Compromised Mesiodistal Space

An adequate mesiodistal space is necessary for an esthetic outcome of an implant restoration and the interproximal soft tissue health of the adjacent teeth. A traditional two-piece implant should be a minimum of 1.5 mm from an adjacent tooth. When the implant is closer to an adjacent tooth, any bone loss related to the microgap, the biological width, and/or stress may result in loss of bone around the implant or adjacent tooth. This may compromise interproximal esthetics and/or sulcular health of the implant and natural tooth (Fig. 29.14).[22] In addition, when an implant is less than 1.5 mm from a natural tooth, inadequate room is available for an ideal emergence profile of the implant restoration.

Compromised Faciopalatal Width

In most cases in which a maxillary anterior single tooth is lost, the facial plate of bone will be compromised. Studies have shown a 25% decrease in faciopalatal width occurs within the first year of tooth loss and rapidly evolves into a 30% to 40% decrease within 3 years. As a result, even an intact alveolus 6 to 8 mm wide is often inadequate in width after 1 year for a division A root-form

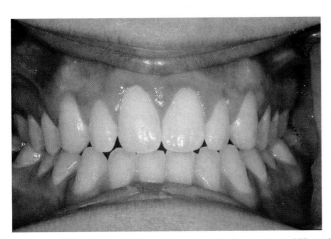

● **Fig. 29.10** Triangular tooth form corresponds to the greatest width and height of interdental papillae and the most incisal interproximal contact position on the crown.

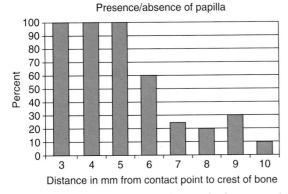

● **Fig. 29.11** When natural teeth have an interproximal crown contact to interseptal bone distance of 5 mm or less, the interdental papilla almost always fills the interproximal space. When the distance is 6 mm, the interproximal space is not filled with soft tissue almost 40% of the time; at 7 mm the interproximal space is filled with an interproximal papilla 25% of the time.

implant in a central incisor position, and after 3 years it almost never presents adequate available bone for an ideal sized implant. The bone width loss is primarily from the facial region, because the labial plate is very thin compared with the palatal plate, and facial undercuts are often found over the roots of the teeth (Fig. 29.15).[23] Studies have shown the median buccal alveolar thickness in the maxillary anterior region to be; 1 mm apical to alveolar bone margin = 0.83 mm, midroot = 0.70 mm, and 1 mm from the tooth apex = 0.88. A bone graft is often necessary to restore the

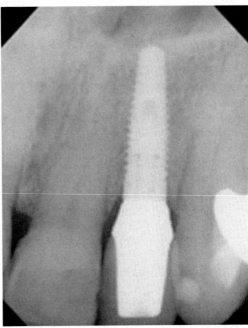

● **Fig. 29.12** Implant position slightly apical to the ideal 3 mm below the free gingival margin resulting in an FP-2 prosthesis (elongated clinical crown compared with adjacent teeth).

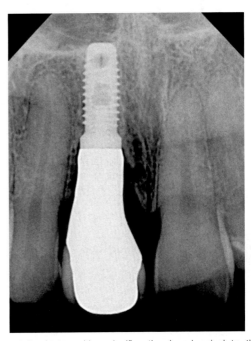

● **Fig. 29.13** Implant position significantly placed apical to the adjacent teeth, which will result in remodeling of the crestal bone. Note the increased crown height space leading to an FP-3 prosthesis (prosthesis replacing clinical crown and soft tissue with pink porcelain or zirconia).

proper anatomy of the ridge and to avoid a compromised implant position more palatal and apical.

The amount of available bone width (faciopalatal) should be at least 3.0 mm greater than the implant diameter at implant insertion. Therefore a 3.5-mm implant requires at least 6.5 mm of bone width. Bone augmentation in width is very predictable. In many instances it is performed before implant placement; however, in some cases, it may be performed at the time of implant insertion, especially when minimal dehiscence of the implant is visible. It should be emphasized that the implant diameter measurement is at the crest module of the implant. Most 3.75-mm-diameter implant bodies are 4.1 mm at the crest module. In these situations, the mesiodistal limitation is 7.1 mm and the faciolingual width limitation is 7.1 mm.

Selection of the Implant Size

The first factor that influences the size of an implant is the mesiodistal dimension of the missing tooth. The average mesiodistal dimension of a central incisor is 8.6 mm (male) and 8.1 mm (female), a lateral incisor is 6.6 mm (male) and 6.1 mm (female), and a canine is 7.6 mm (male) and 7.2 mm (female). In general, the implant body should not be as wide as the natural tooth or clinical crown because the emergence contour and interdental papillae region cannot be properly established.

The mesiodistal dimensions of the maxillary central incisor at the cervix (preferably 1 mm below the free gingival margin) averages 6.4 mm, the lateral incisor dimension is 4.7 mm, and canine natural teeth at the cervix are 5.6 mm (Table 29.1).[24] However, these dimensions are also too large for an implant. The bone level on natural teeth is approximately 2 mm below the CEJ;

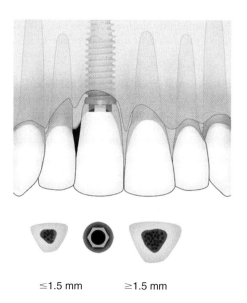

≤1.5 mm ≥1.5 mm

• **Fig. 29.14** If bone loss occurs on an implant placed closer than 1.5 mm to a tooth (on the distal), then bone and soft tissue drape will also be lost on the tooth. As a result, the distance from the interproximal crown contact to the interproximal bone increases, and the risk of soft tissue shrinkage and loss of interdental papilla increases. When the implant is greater than 1.5 mm from the tooth (on the mesial); bone loss on the implants does not cause bone loss on the tooth root. The interproximal crown contact to interproximal bone relationship remains ideal, and the interdental papilla is maintained.

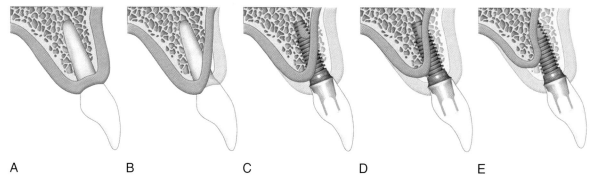

A   B   C   D   E

• **Fig. 29.15** Bone Resorption in the Maxillary Anterior (A) Before the loss of a maxillary anterior tooth, the bone around the roots most often is present. (B) Extraction often causes a loss of the thin labial plate of bone over the root. After extraction, the residual ridge most often is decreased in width (division B). (C) After 6 months to 1 year, the residual ridge continues to resorb and becomes division B–w. (D) Eventually, the residual ridge forms a C–w bone volume that is slightly deficient in height and less than 2.5 mm in width. (E) This bone volume often extends almost to the floor of the nose.

TABLE 29.1	**Maxillary Teeth Dimensions**				
Type of Tooth	Mesiodistal Crown (mm)	Mesiodistal Cervix (mm)	Faciolingual Crown (mm)	Faciolingual Cervix (mm)	2 mm Below Cement-Enamel Junction
Central incisor	8.6	6.4	7.1	6.4	5.5
Lateral incisor	6.6	4.7	6.2	5.8	4.3
Canine	7.6	5.6	8.1	7.6	4.6

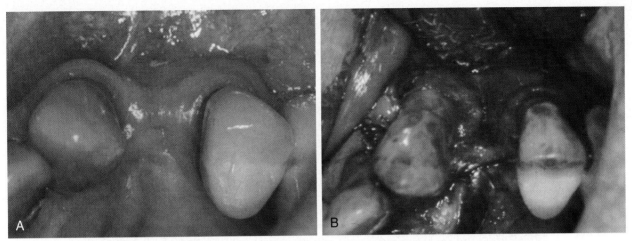

• **Fig. 29.16** Compromised bone width. (A) Preoperative view is very deceiving and can give a false positive on the amount of bone present. (B) Reflection of the ridge tissue reveals a significant defect present.

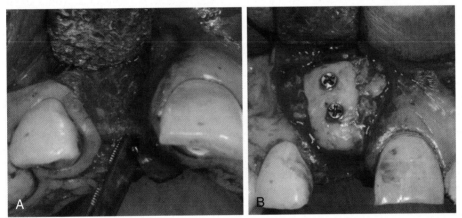

• **Fig. 29.17** (A) Large ridge defect. (B) To gain adequate width of bone, a symphysis bone graft is completed.

the natural tooth dimensions at this bone level are reduced to 5.5 mm for central incisors, 4.3 mm for lateral incisors, and 4.6 mm for canines. Therefore, in theory, the latter dimensions most closely resemble the consummate implant diameter to mimic the emergence profile of a natural tooth. However, this dimension is usually too large to adequately restore the soft tissue drape of the missing anterior tooth.

The second factor that determines the mesiodistal implant diameter is the necessary distance from an adjacent tooth root.[25] Initial vertical bone loss around an implant during the first year of loading is variable and ranges from 0.5 to more than 3.0 mm. The height of the interseptal (interimplant) bone in part determines the incidence of presence or absence of the interdental papillae between the teeth. When the distance from the interseptal bone to interproximal contact is 5 mm or less, the papilla fills the space. When the distance is 6 mm, a partial absence of papilla is seen 45% of the time, and at 7 mm the risk of a compromise in the interproximal space is 75%.[26] Therefore the intraseptal bone height is relative to the maintenance of the interdental papilla and should be preserved. As a consequence, the implant should be at least 1.5 mm from the adjacent teeth whenever possible, and the interseptal bone on the adjacent teeth should be within 5 mm of the desired interproximal crown contact position.

In summary, two mesiodistal parameters determine the preferable implant size. The suggested width of the single-tooth implant should correspond to the width of the missing natural tooth, 2 mm below the CEJ. The distance between the roots of the adjacent teeth should also be measured. The implant diameter + 3 mm (1.5 mm on each side) should be equal to or less than the distance between the adjacent roots, at the crest of the ridge (which is 2 mm below the interproximal CEJ).

The next dimension that determines the width of an anterior implant is the faciopalatal dimension of bone. The width of bone should allow at least 1.5 mm on the facial aspect of the implant so that if a vertical defect forms around the crest module, then that defect would not become horizontal and change the cervical contour of the facial gingival (Fig. 29.16). Because of its initial reduced volume, facial bone tends to be labile, and its resorption is responsible for most of the compromised long-term esthetic results in the anterior maxilla. The faciopalatal width dimension is not as critical on the palatal aspect of the implant because it is dense cortical bone, more resistant to bone loss, and not within the esthetic zone. Facial bone grafting at the time of implant insertion is frequently indicated because the bone volume in width is often compromised (Figs. 29.17 and 29.18).

The width of the implant should mimic the emergence of a natural tooth and help preserve the bone and health of the adjacent teeth. The natural intraroot distance of the two central incisors distance is approximately 2 mm. However, the natural roots of the central to lateral and lateral to canine are usually less than 1.5 mm

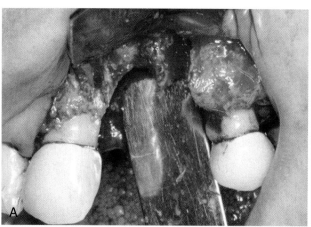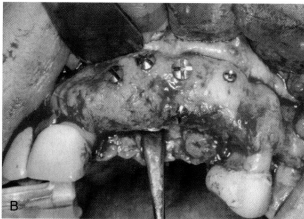

• **Fig. 29.18** (A) Compromised ridge with significant deficiency in width. (B) Guided bone regeneration required to obtain sufficient width and height for implant placement.

• **BOX 29.1** **Ideal Average Implant Diameter**

Central incisor: 4.0–5.2 mm
Lateral incisor: 3.0–3.5 mm
Canine: 3.7–4.2 mm

---

apart and often only 0.5 mm of space exists between them. As a consequence, the typical size of the single-tooth implant is usually smaller in diameter than the natural tooth root.

The typical diameters of the implant used to replace the average-size tooth often results in a 4.0- to 5.2-mm implant for a central incisor, a 3.0- to 3.5-mm implant for a lateral incisor, and a 3.7- to 4.2-mm implant for a canine. The difference in the emergence profile of a 4-mm-diameter implant and a 5-mm-diameter implant is negligible and often not clinically relevant for an anterior tooth because a 0.5-mm difference occurs on each side of the implant. Therefore, when in doubt, the clinician should use a smaller diameter implant. As such, a 4-mm-diameter implant may often be used in the central-implant position for a single-tooth replacement. Likewise, a 3.0- to 3.5-mm implant is often used for a lateral incisor single-tooth restoration (Box 29.1).

Implant Position

The maxillary anterior single-tooth implant should be positioned precisely in three planes. From a mesiodistal aspect, the implant most often is placed in the middle of the space, with an equal amount of interproximal bone toward each adjacent tooth. On occasion, the central incisor implant is positioned slightly to the distal of the intratooth space (Fig. 29.19) when the incisive foramen is enlarged and encroaches on the ideal placement. When a central incisor implant is planned and the foramen between the existing central incisor root and implant site is larger than usual, the remaining bone may be inadequate for placement.

The nasopalatine foramen may also expand off to one side of the midline within the bony canal. When the central incisor implant is placed, the implant may encroach on the canal and result in a soft tissue interface on the mesiopalatal surface of the implant. As a precaution, the clinician should reflect the palatal tissue when placing a maxillary central incisor implant and, if necessary, place the implant in a more distal position (Fig. 29.20). This usually requires a smaller diameter implant than usual to remain 1.5 mm or more from the lateral incisor. On occasion, the contents of the foramen maybe be removed and a bone graft inserted to decrease the size of the incisive canal.

The midfaciopalatal position of the implant is in the middle to slightly palatal 0.5 mm of the edentulous ridge of adequate contour. This approach permits the use of the greatest diameter implant. The crestal bone should be at least 1.5-2.0 mm wider on the facial aspect of the implant and 1.0 mm on the palatal aspect. Therefore for a 4-mm-diameter implant, a minimum 6.5-mm faciopalatal width of bone is required for the central or canine position, and 6.0 mm of bone width is required for a lateral incisor with a 3.5-mm implant. Bone spreading in conjunction with implant placement or bone grafting on the facial aspect of the edentulous site may be indicated when the ridge is less wide than is desirable. The thickness of bone on the facial aspect of a natural root is usually 0.5-0.7 mm thick in the anterior region. As a result, if the implant is placed in the center of the ridge, the implant will be 1 mm or more palatal than the facial emergence of the adjacent crowns at the free gingival margin.

The implant center is positioned in the faciopalatal center of the edentulous ridge and the midmesiodistal position. The implant body angulation from this point is considered next. In the literature, three faciopalatal angulations of the implant body are suggested: (1) a facial angulation so that emergence of the final crown will be similar to adjacent teeth, (2) under the incisal edge of the final restoration, and (3) within the cingulum position of the implant crown (Fig. 29.21).

Facial Implant Body Angulation

Researchers often theorize that a maxillary anterior implant body angulation should be positioned at the facial emergence of the final crown. The facial implant position is predicated on the concept that the facial emergence of the implant crown at the cervical should be in the same position as a natural tooth. At first, this makes some sense. However, the crown of a natural tooth has two planes, and its incisal edge is palatal to the facial emergence of the natural tooth by 12 to 15 degrees (Fig. 29.22). This is why anterior crown preparations are in two or three planes. The implant body is more palatal than a natural root, so 1.5 mm of bone exists facially. In addition, because the implant is narrower in diameter than the faciopalatal root dimension, when the implant body is oriented as a natural tooth and has a facial emergence, a straight abutment is not wide enough to permit the two or three plane reduction to bring the incisal edge of the preparation more palatal. As a result, the incisal edge of the preparation remains too facial. Therefore when the implant is angled to the facial emergence of a tooth, an angled abutment of 15 degrees must be used to bring the incisal edge more palatal. Most two-piece angled abutments have a design flaw that compromises facial cervical esthetics. The metal flange facial to the abutment

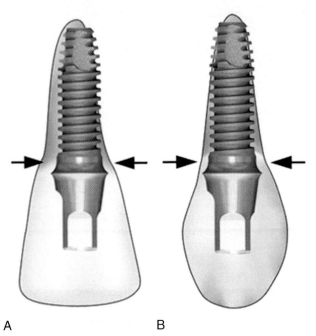

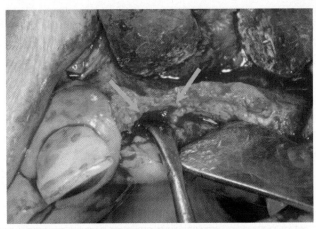

• **Fig. 29.20** Complete reflection of lingual tissue to determine the position and size of the nasopalatine foramen and canal. The enlarged nasopalatine canal and foramen has led to compromised bone for implant placement.

• **Fig. 29.19** (A) The ideal mesiodistal implant position for a central incisor is 0.5 to 1.0 mm more distal than the midtooth position. This decreases the risk of encroachment on the incisive canal. (B) The best mesiodistal position for a cuspid is centered in the cuspid position.

screw is thinner than a straight abutment and may result in fracture (especially because angled loads are placed on the facial-positioned implant). The manufacturers thicken the profile of the abutment on the facial aspect to reduce the risk of fracture. However, this design flaw brings the cervical facial margin more facial and wider than the implant body, which is already as facial as the adjacent tooth. As a result, the implant crown margin is facially overcontoured. The restoring doctor then has to prepare the facial aspect of the abutment metal flange for esthetics, which weakens it and makes it prone to fracture. When the implant clinician attempts to align the implant body with the facial aspect of adjacent teeth, the implant may inadvertently be inserted too facial. No single method exists to restore proper esthetics when the implant abutment is located above the free gingival margin of the adjacent teeth. At best, the final crown appears too long and too facial. Soft tissue grafts and/or bone augmentation do not improve the condition once the implant is already incorrectly inserted (Fig. 29.23).

The natural maxillary anterior teeth are loaded at a 12- to 15-degree angle because of their natural angulation compared with the mandibular anterior teeth. This is one reason the maxillary anterior teeth are wider in diameter than mandibular anterior teeth (which are most commonly loaded in their long axis). The facial angulation of the implant body often corresponds to an implant body angulation, which leads to 15-degree off-axial loads and increases the force to the abutment screw-implant-bone complex by 25.9% compared with a long axis load. These offset loads increase the risks of abutment screw loosening, crestal bone loss, and cervical soft tissue marginal shrinkage. In summary, implants angled too facially compromise the esthetics and increase the risk of complications (Fig. 29.24).

Cingulum Implant Body Angulation

A second angulation suggested in the literature is more palatal, with an emergence under the cingulum of the crown. This also

may be the result of an implant insertion in a width-deficient ridge (division B) because the bone is lost primarily on the facial. This position is often the goal when a screw-retained crown is used for the prosthesis. The prosthesis fixation screw (to retain a maxillary anterior crown) cannot be located in the incisal or facial region of the crown as this will impinge on the esthetics.

The cingulum implant position may result in a considerable compromise. The implant body is round and usually 4.0 to 5.5 mm in diameter. The labial cervical contour of the implant crown must be similar to the adjacent teeth for the ultimate esthetic effect. Because the long axis of the implant for a screw-retained crown must emerge in the cingulum position, this most often requires a facial projection of the crown or "buccal correction" facing away from the implant body. The facial ridge lap must extend 2 to 4 mm and is often similar in contour to the modified ridge lap pontic of a three-unit fixed prosthesis (Fig. 29.25).

The modified ridge lap crown has become a common solution to correct the esthetics of the restoration when the implant is placed in narrow bone or follows a palatal angulation position. However, plaque control on the facial of the implant is almost impossible. Even if the toothbrush could reach the gingival sulcus, no hygiene device could be manipulated to a right angle to proceed into the facial gingival sulcus. As a result, although an acceptable esthetic restoration may be developed, especially with the additional cervical porcelain, the hygiene requirements and present implant dentistry standards render this approach nonideal (Fig. 29.26).

Some authors argue that an improved contour may be developed subgingivally with a palatal implant position. To create this contour, the implant body must be positioned more apical than desired. This position may prevent food from accumulating on the cervical "table" of the crown. However, the subgingival ridge lap does not permit access to the facial sulcus of the implant body for the elimination of plaque and to evaluate the bleeding index or facial bone loss. Therefore the maintenance requirements for the implant facial sulcular region do not permit the clinician to consider this modality as a valid primary option.

Greater interarch clearance is often required with an implant palatal position because the permucosal post exits the tissue in a more palatal position. Inadequate interarch space may especially hinder the restoration of Angle's class II, division 2 patients, with the implant in this position. The bony ridge should be augmented if too narrow for the ideal implant diameter and position, or an alternate treatment option should be selected.

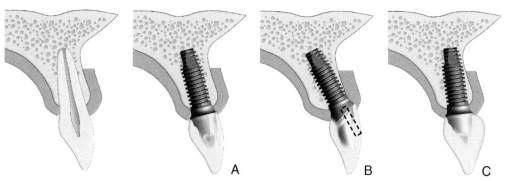

• **Fig. 29.21** Three implant positions are found in the literature related to the final crown position. (A) A position below the incisal edge is best used for a cemented crown in the esthetic zone. (B) An implant is in the position of the natural root of the tooth. Although this makes sense, it places the implant too facial, and an angled abutment is usually necessary. (C) An implant in the cingulum position that is used when a screw-retained crown is the treatment of choice. This position requires a facial ridge lap of porcelain when used for FP-1 prostheses in the esthetic zone.

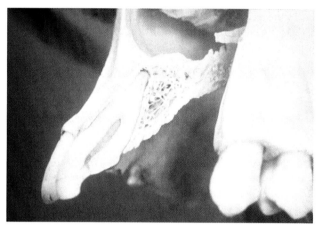

• **Fig. 29.22** Natural tooth has very thin facial cortical bone over the root, and the incisal edge of the crown is 12 to 15 degrees palatal to the facial emergence profile. This is not an ideal position for an implant. The bone to the palatal region is better suited for an implant and allows the implant to be positioned under the incisal edge.

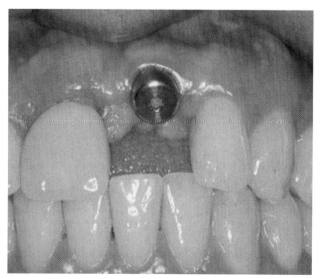

• **Fig. 29.23** Implant placement too facially positioned. Soft tissue grafts will not correct the malpositioning and usually the most ideal treatment is implant removal and re-positioned in a more ideal position.

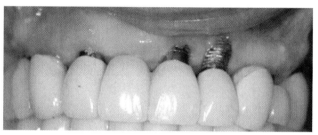

• **Fig. 29.24** Facially positioned implant leading to compromised esthetics.

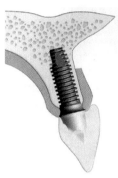

• **Fig. 29.25** Implant placed in the cingulum position will usually require a ridge lap on the implant crown to restore the facial contour of the tooth.

Ideal Implant Angulation

The third implant angulation in the literature describes the most desirable implant angulation. A straight line is determined by connecting two points. The clinician determines the line for the best angulation by the point slightly lingual to the incisal edge position of the implant crown and the midfaciopalatal position on the crest of the bone. The center of the implant is located slightly lingual to the incisal edge of the crown so that a straight abutment for cement retention emerges directly below the incisal edge (Fig. 29.27). Because the crown profile is in two planes, with the incisal edge more palatal than the cervical portion, the incisal edge position is perfect for implant placement and accommodates some of the facial bone loss that often occurs prior to implant placement. The facial emergence of the crown mimics the adjacent teeth, proceeding from the implant body under the tissue. The angle of force to the implant is also improved, which decreases the crestal stresses to the bone and abutment screws. When in doubt, the

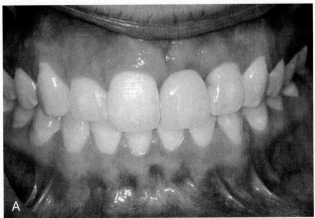

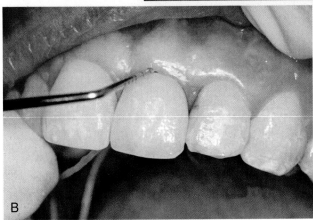

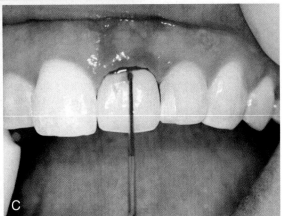

• **Fig. 29.26** (A) The maxillary left central incisor *(right side)* with a ridge lap crown presents acceptable esthetics. (B) However, probing on the facial aspect measures the distance to the implant but cannot evaluate facial bone loss because it cannot be directed apically to the pocket depth. (C) Periodically, the left central incisor implant becomes inflamed, and the bleeding index increases as a result of the inability to clean the implant sulcus on the facial.

clinician should err toward the palatal aspect of the incisal edge position, not to the facial aspect, because it is easier to correct a slight palatal position in the final crown contour compared with the implant body angled too facial.

The implant abutment selected for a maxillary anterior single-tooth implant is most commonly used for a cemented restoration; however, screw-retained prostheses are becoming more popular. A greater range of corrective options exists with a cement-retained crown for implants, especially if it is not ideally positioned. The location of the cervical margin of a cemented crown can be anywhere on the abutment post or even on the body of the implant provided it is 1 mm or more above the bone.

The implant body angulation under the incisal edge may also be used for screw-retained restorations. In these cases an angled abutment for screw retention is placed, and the coping screw for the crown may be located within the cingulum. This method does not require a facial ridge lap of the final crown, which decreases the risk of compromised hygiene. When ideal bone volume is present, a surgical template that ideally correlates the incisal edge and facial contour of the final prosthesis may be used.

Soft Tissue Incision: Surgical Protocol

Obtaining and maintaining the ideal tissue drape is often the most difficult aspect of maxillary anterior single-tooth replacement within the esthetic zone. Several different approaches

have been advocated to enhance the soft tissue appearance. The approaches may be surgical (addition or subtraction) or prosthetic and include (1) a soft tissue graft before bone augmentation, (2) a soft tissue augmentation in conjunction with a bone graft before implant insertion, (3) soft tissue augmentation in conjunction with implant insertion, (4) soft tissue manipulation at the implant uncovery procedure, (5) a prosthetic modification of interproximal contact position, (6) creeping attachment around the implant crown, or (7) a prosthetic replacement of the soft tissue with pink-colored porcelain (Box 29.2).

Surgical additive techniques such as pouch procedures, interpositional grafts, sliding flaps, and connective tissue grafts (autogenous or acellular dermal matrix) have all been proposed. A soft tissue graft may be performed as a separate procedure before any other surgery when the patient has a high lip dynamic and the soft tissue color and/or volume is grossly deficient. Most often, a connective tissue graft to improve the soft tissue drape is indicated.

A bone graft and soft tissue augmentation is indicated when the bone on the adjacent teeth is within normal limits (2 mm below the CEJ) but deficient in width and midcrestal volume. When the interproximal bone is not within normal limits, orthodontic extrusion maybe an option, followed by a crown and possibly endodontic therapy. The goal of a soft tissue augmentation for either of the two previous procedures is to obtain soft tissue on the crest of the ridge at the height of the interproximal papilla height.

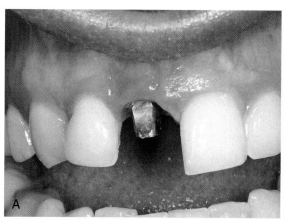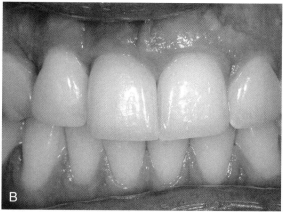

• **Fig. 29.27** (A) The perfect position for an anterior single-tooth implant is under the incisal edge to the approximate midcrest position. A central incisor should have the position slightly distal and slightly toward the palate. (B) The implant crown has a 1.0- to 1.5-mm subgingival margin and begins a facial, mesial, and distal contour at this point to exit the tissue similarly to the contour of the adjacent tooth.

• BOX 29.2   Soft Tissue Contouring and Emergence Profile

Preprosthetic Surgery
- Soft tissue graft before bone augmentation
- Soft tissue graft in conjunction with bone graft before implant surgery

Surgery Stage I
- Soft tissue augmentation
- Nonresorbable hydroxyapatite graft
- Lingually oriented incision to position more tissue to the facial
- Papilla saving incisions

Surgery Stage II
- Connective tissue graft (subepithelial)
- Soft tissue plastic surgery
- Gingivoplasty (coarse diamond)
- Prosthetics
- Wide healing abutment
- Temporary contouring through provisional restoration
- Anatomic abutment, tooth-colored abutment
- Pink porcelain/zirconia on abutment
- Lingually oriented incision to position more tissue to the facial

---

When elevating the interproximal tissue in the anterior maxilla, "papilla-saving" incisions are made adjacent to each neighboring tooth (Fig. 29.28). The vertical incisions are made on the facial aspect of the edentulous site and begin 1 mm below the macrogingival junction, within the keratinized tissue. Extending the vertical incisions beyond the macrogingival junction increases the risk of scar formation at the incision site. The full-thickness incision then approaches the crest of the edentulous site, leaving 1.0 to 1.5 mm of the interproximal papilla adjacent to each tooth. The vertical incisions are not wider at the base than the crestal width of tissue. This permits the facial flap to be advanced over the implant or short and adjacent to a healing abutment at the conclusion of the procedure, with no voids at the incision line and primary closure.

When the papillae are depressed in the edentulous site, vertical-release incisions are made along the root angle of each adjacent tooth, beginning 1 mm below the macrogingival junction and

in the sulcus of each adjacent tooth. Therefore the interproximal papilla region becomes part of the facial soft tissue flap.

The crestal incision is made on the palatal incline of the edentulous site to provide greater thickness of keratinized tissue on the facial aspect of the flap. This also allows more interproximal tissue to be elevated to enhance the papilla height.

The soft tissue is reflected, and the crestal bone width of the ridge is evaluated. When a central incisor site is reflected, the palatal flap is reflected to the incisive foramen for identification and evaluation. On occasion, its position may require the soft tissue to be enucleated and a graft positioned in its site. An initial pilot drill is positioned in the midmesiodistal and faciopalatal aspect of the ridge and proceeds approximately 7 to 9 mm within the bone under copious cooled sterile saline. A direction indicator is positioned into the site for evaluation to determine the implant position with respect to the facial, palatal, mesial, and distal implant position. A periapical radiograph is taken, and the initial osteotomy in relation to the adjacent roots and opposing landmark (i.e., floor of nose) is assessed. If adjustments are required, then a side-cutting drill (i.e., Lindemann drill) may be used.

The second drill is used to increase the depth and width of the osteotomy at approximately 2000 rotations per minute (rpm) (in D1 and D2 bone) under copious amounts of cooled sterile saline. The osteotomy drilling should be completed with a "bone-dancing" preparation to avoid overheating the bone. If the bone density is D3 or D4, lower rotations per minute may be used (~1000 rpm). If a surgical guide is not used, then the angulation of the drill should be within the long axis of the intended implant position to coincide with the lingual aspect of the incisal edge. If the osteotomy is not ideally positioned, then the side-cutting drill (Lindeman) is introduced into the osteotomy, and the palatal bone is removed by "shaving" up and down in the palatal aspect of the preparation.

The final size osteotomy drill is used to complete the osteotomy according to the bone density surgical protocol. In general, a crestal bone drill and bone tap should not be used in the maxillary anterior region because the maxillary bone usually has little to no cortical bone present on the bony crest. Using a crestal bone bur will often lead to a decreased primary stability of the implant and reduced facial bone thickness.

The threaded implant is inserted with a handpiece at 30 rpm because this is the most accurate insertion technique. Placing an

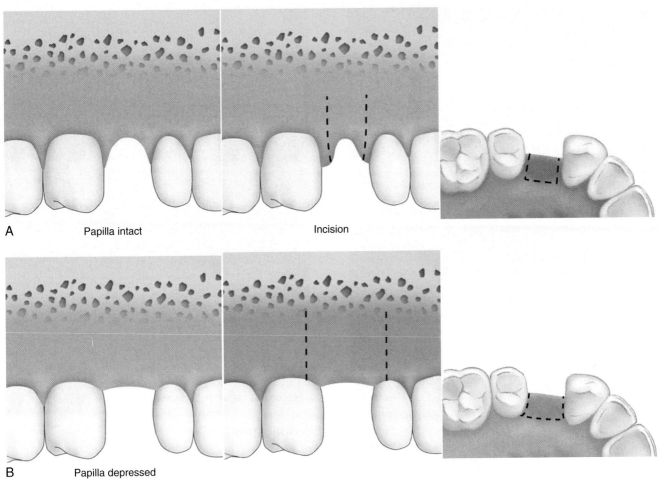

A   Papilla intact   Incision

B   Papilla depressed

• **Fig. 29.28** (A) When the interdental papillae are in an acceptable position, papilla-saving incisions are made to minimize soft tissue reflection. The incisions are vertical to allow primary closure. When the papillae are depressed, the vertical release incisions include the papilla in the edentulous site. (B) In situations with a more depressed soft tissue, facial soft tissue and papillae over each adjacent tooth are also reflected. The crestal incision is positioned towards the palatal incline on the ridge.

implant with an insertion wrench may lead to possible misdirection of the implant, most commonly being pushed to the facial. When a handpiece is used, counterforces on the handpiece handle and the fingers of the other hand on the handpiece head may permit the implant to be inserted without compromise to angulation or position.

The implant is rotated in final position, with a flattening of the antirotational component to the facial (i.e., depending on the implant type and design). The implant mount may be removed, and the clinician decides whether a low-profile cover screw (two stage) or healing abutment (one stage) is used within the implant. When the hard and soft tissue contours are ideal and a papilla-saving incision was made, a healing abutment may be used. When a bone graft is placed and/or the crestal tissue elevated to increase the height of the papilla, a low-profile cover screw is more often used to allow for undisturbed healing. Once the cover screw is inserted, the clinician decides whether a bone graft on the facial bone is indicated. When the facial bone over the implant is less than 1.5 mm thick, bone from the osteotomy is ideally used over the facial aspect along with a collagen membrane. If tissue thickness is required, an acellular dermal matrix may be used instead of the collagen membrane (Fig. 29.29) to increase the bulk of tissue, therefore allowing for a more esthetic result.

Soft Tissue Closure

The soft tissue is approximated and sutured with a resorbable suture material (most commonly 4-0 or 5-0) around the healing abutment or over the cover screw, depending on whether the tissue is at the ideal position or is being augmented. The increased tissue thickness from augmentation facilitates the sculpting of interdental papillae at stage II surgery, improves ridge contour, and prevents the grayish hue of the titanium implant body from showing through the labial mucosa in the event of crestal bone loss in the future.

Transitional Prosthesis

A soft tissue–borne transitional prosthesis is not recommended because this may increase crestal bone loss during the healing period. In addition, it may depress the interdental papillae of the adjacent teeth. For a single tooth edentulus area, a resin-bonded fixed restoration may be fabricated to provide esthetics and improve speech and function, especially when crestal bone regeneration is performed. When a resin-bonded restoration is used, the adjacent teeth are not prepared and the prosthesis is bonded to the tooth regions below the centric occlusal contacts of the teeth.

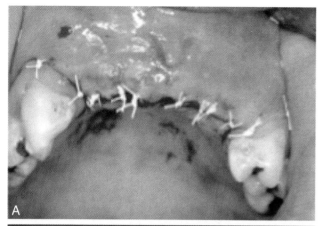

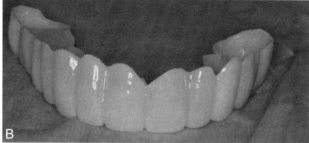

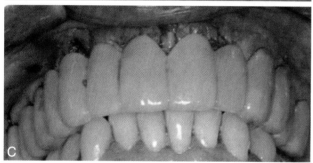

● **Fig. 29.29** Removable Interim Prosthesis: (A) Maxillary anterior surgery site, (B) Smile Transitions interim prosthesis which is durable and highly esthetic that prevents pressure on the surgical site, (C) Removable prosthesis in place.

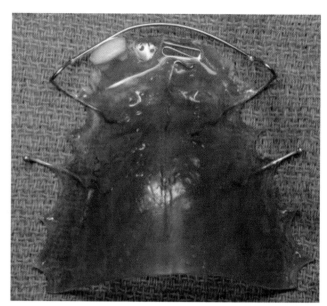

● **Fig. 29.30** Hawley appliance with the addition of a denture tooth, may be used as an interim prosthesis

For multiple missing maxillary anterior teeth, a removable partial or full arch prosthesis (Smile Transitions™ - Glidewell Laboratories) maybe utilized during the healing period. The prosthesis is retained by the remaining natural teeth, thereby preventing pressure or impingement on the soft tissues overlying the surgery site. (Fig. 29.29).

Other options include an Essix appliance, which is an acrylic shell, similar to a bleaching tray, that has a denture tooth attached to replace the missing tooth. This prosthesis is the easiest for tooth replacement after surgical procedures. Another option may include a cast-clasp removable partial denture (RPD) with indirect rest seats to prevent rotation movements on the surgical site (Fig. 29.30).

In some cases, an immediate placement/loaded prosthesis may be used; however, this needs to be completed under ideal conditions (e.g., favorable primary stability and insertion torque, bone density, lack of parafunction). The benefits of immediate implant insertion after tooth extraction are related to an improved preservation of the soft tissue drape and the bone architecture compared with their collapse after tooth extraction. As a result, bone augmentation and soft tissue grafts may be avoided. The procedure has been described as a preservation technique aiming at maintaining the harmonious gingival architecture. The procedure also reduces the number of surgical procedures, which may decrease the cost to the patient.

Complications

The primary esthetic complications of maxillary anterior single-tooth implants include interdental papillae deficiency and gingival shrinkage after crown delivery.

Interdental Papilla Deficiency

The interproximal CEJ of a natural tooth exhibits a reverse scallop toward the incisal edge. The same pattern is followed by the alveolar interproximal bone, which is more coronal in the interproximal regions than in the facial or lingual plates. As a consequence, the probing depth in the papilla region of a natural tooth is quite similar to the facial or palatal probing depths. Interproximal bone around an implant does not follow such a contour. As a result, the interdental papillae, which look natural and rise to fill the interproximal regions between healthy adjacent teeth, exhibit greater probing depths than the other surfaces of the implant crown. In fact, because the interproximal bone height also may be lost next to the adjacent teeth, the dental and implant papilla also correspond to a greater proximal probing depth next to the natural tooth. A greater sulcus depth increases the risk of shrinkage after gingivoplasty, or later, even with good daily hygiene care. As a result, even years later the tissue may shrink and result in a poor interproximal esthetic situation (Fig. 29.31).

As previously addressed, four surgical time sequences exist to address the interproximal tissue height: (1) before a bone graft with a connective tissue graft; (2) in conjunction with a bone graft, often using an acellular tissue graft (i.e., OrACELL; Salvin, Charlotte, North Carolina); (3) at implant insertion, with an elevation of the tissue over a healing abutment and (4) at implant uncovery (i.e., split-finger technique). There are several other methods to improve the soft tissue drape. These approaches used to modify the soft tissue are prosthetic-related methods.

The most common prosthodontic solution to alleviate soft tissue limitations is helpful when soft tissue surgery has not recreated

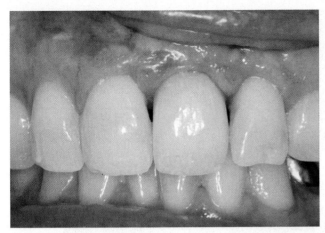

• **Fig. 29.31** Most common esthetic complication in the premaxilla is the inadequate soft tissue drape around an implant crown. The patient's left central incisor exhibits black interproximal spaces.

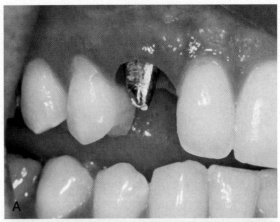

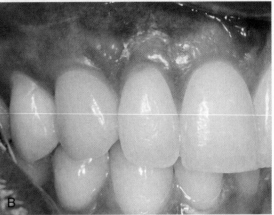

• **Fig. 29.32** (A) A prosthetic solution for inadequate papilla height is to lower the interproximal contact of the crown by reshaping the adjacent teeth. (B) The canine implant crown fills the space and eliminates the interdental spaces caused by the lack of papilla height.

an ideal interproximal papilla height. The interproximal region may be treated similarly to the pontic interproximal region of a three-unit FPD (Fig. 29.32). Rarely are interdental papillae present next to the pontics of a fixed prosthesis. Instead, rather than raising the tissue to the interproximal contact of the crown, the interproximal contact is extended toward the tissue, and the cervical region of the pontic is slightly overcontoured. A similar approach may be applied to the single-tooth implant. The interproximal contacts of the adjacent teeth are recontoured, especially on the palatal line angle, to become oblong and extend toward the tissue. The contact areas of the single-tooth crown are extended, especially on the palatal line angle, toward the gingiva. The cervical region of the single-tooth implant is slightly overcontoured in width, similarly to the pontic of a fixed prosthesis. This concept does slightly compromise the interproximal esthetics. The papilla is not as high next to the implant crowns as it is between the natural teeth, and the cervical width of the crown is 0.5 mm wider.

However, the sulcus depth is reduced on the tooth and implant crown, and the daily hygiene conditions are improved. In addition, long-term shrinkage of the tissue is less likely to occur. This option should be the method of choice whenever possible and especially when the high lip position during smiling does not display the gingival regions around the teeth.

Nasopalatine (Incisive) Foramen and Canal

Anatomy

The nasopalatine (incisive) canal connects the oral cavity (nasopalatine foramen) with the floor of the nasal cavity. The soft tissue overlying the foramen is often associated with two lateral canals, which often fuse before exiting the foramen.[27] The maxillary division of the trigeminal nerve gives off the nasopalatine nerve branch, which enters the posterior nasal cavity via the sphenopalatine foramen, transverses the roof of the nose and proceeds along the nasal septum in between the periosteum and mucosa before exiting the nasopalatine foramen.[28] Mraiwa and colleagues reported that the nasopalatine foramen is located approximately 7.4 mm from the labial surface of an unresorbed maxillary anterior ridge and that the distance will vary after the amount of osseous resorption after extractions. The mean diameter of the nasopalatine foramen was shown to be approximately

4.6 mm (range, 1.5–9.2 mm).[29] The length of the nasopalatine canal has been reported to be approximately 9 mm, with a range of 3 to 14 mm.[30] The average height has been documented to be approximately 10.08 to 10.86 mm.[31,32] However, as the premaxilla resorbs, the nasopalatine canal decreases in size.[33] When the maxillary premaxilla alveolus resorbs in height, the incisive canal reduces in length; therefore division A, B, and C–w bone has greater canal length than division C–h and D bone. The angle of the nasopalatine canal has been shown to vary from 46 to 99 degrees with respect to the horizontal plane with a mean angulation of 66 degrees.[34] A vertical projection above the incisive canal along the nasal floor is called the premaxillary wing. The nasal process of the maxillary premaxilla rises 2 to 3 mm above the nasal floor (Fig. 29.33).

Surgical Approaches to the Nasopalatine Canal

In most cases, an implant may be positioned to replace a central incisor without encroaching on the nasopalatine canal. However, if extensive resorption or a large canal is present, then the nasopalatine canal may have a direct effect on the implant positioning. Therefore ideally the implant should never contact any soft tissue contents of the canal. To avoid this from occurring, there exist several approaches when the nasopalatine directly affects the implant positioning. Kraut et al reported that approximately 4% of nasopalatine canals directly affect the ideal positioning of implants in the premaxilla.

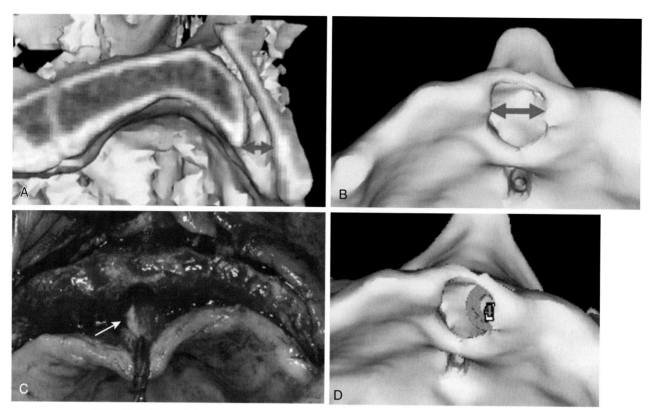

• **Fig. 29.33** Nasopalatine canal and foramen. (A) Large nasopalatine canal. (B) Large nasopalatine foramen. (C) Clinical image of nasopalatine foramen exposure, which compromises implant placement in the central incisor region. (D) Attempting to place implant in cases with large nasopalatine canal leads to penetration into the canal and a soft tissue interface.

Bone Grafting the Nasopalatine Canal with Delayed Implant Placement

One option when the size and position of the nasopalatine canal impinges on the implant placement is to enucleate and bone graft the canal. The nasopalatine canal is exposed by full-thickness reflection and the soft tissues within the canal are entirely curetted. Serrated spoon excavators (e.g. Lucas 86) may be used along with a round carbide bur to completely remove any soft tissue remnants from the canal. Rosenquist and colleagues first reported on removing the contents of the nasopalatine canal and autogenous bone grafting the area. Implant placement was delayed for approximately 5 months with a 100% success.[35] Since then, numerous additional studies have shown positive outcomes with this procedure including guided bone regeneration techniques along with grafting the nasopalatine canal (Fig. 29.34).[36,37]

Removal of the Canal Contents + Implant Placement

A second option includes the enucleation of the nasopalatine canal followed by immediate implant placement. The incisive foramen is first reflected and identified, and a periodontal probe evaluates the angle and depth of the bony canal to ensure a minimum length of 9 mm. The soft tissues in the incisive canal are curetted from the canal site, which is approximately 4 mm in diameter at its apex. A round carbide bur (e.g. # 6 or # 8 round bur) in a straight handpiece may be used to remove the soft tissue remnants. In addition, the trauma from the round bur initiates the regional acceleratory phenomenon (RAP), which allows for more predictable healing (Fig. 29.35).

Once the soft tissue is removed, drills progressively increase the diameter to the final implant osteotomy diameter 2 mm below the final height of the canal. A blunt osteotome and gentle, sudden impact force with a mallet then prepares the apical 2 mm of the implant site. A large-diameter threaded implant (>5 mm) is generally used and should be greater than the diameter of the foramen (Fig. 29.36). When the foramen diameter is greater than that of the implant available, the canal is augmented with an autologous or allograft bone graft, and the implant insertion is delayed for several months. This technique is often clinically challenging.

Positioning the Implant Away From the Nasopalatine Canal

In the literature, some authors have suggested placing the implant in a nonideal position to avoid the nasopalatine canal. If the intended prosthesis is an RPD, the implant may be positioned to avoid penetration into the canal. The most common position would be in the embrasure area of the central and lateral position. This would result in maintaining the anteroposterior spread, along with not penetrating into the canal. However, care should be exercised not to angulate the implant too far to the facial as this may impinge on the esthetics of the prosthesis.

Kraut and colleagues evaluated CBCT scans and found that 4% of the time the nasopalatine canal would interfere with the normal preparation of an osteotomy for an implant.[38]

Mardinger and colleagues reported that after extraction the average length of the canal shortened from 10.7 to 9 mm and the nasopalatine foramen encompassed 36.5% of the ridge width (range, 13%–58%) as it enlarges in all directions. In severely resorbed ridges, the nasopalatine foramen enlarged by 32%

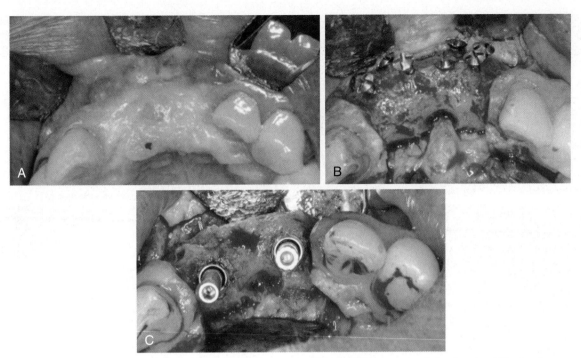

• **Fig. 29.34** Bone graft with delayed implant placement. (A and B) Ridge augmentation to gain width of bone so implant placement does not impinge on the nasopalatine foramen. (C) Ideal implant placement.

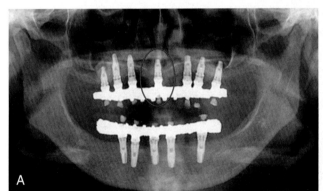

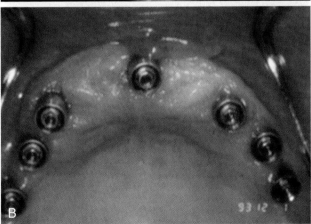

• **Fig. 29.35** (A) Implant placement into the nasopalatine canal for a removable implant-supported overdenture. By placing an implant in the nasopalatine canal, the anteroposterior spread is increased. (B) Clinical image depicting implant in the nasopalatine canal.

(1.8 mm) and reached approximately 5.5 mm in diameter, which could occupy up to 58% of the ridge.[39]

Another technique for a fixed prosthesis is to angulate the implant intentionally, often placing the implant at an increased apical position. The theory includes allowing more space (i.e., running room) for the prosthesis that creates a more favorable emergence profile. However, this technique does increase the crown height space, which is a force magnifier. In addition, adjacent teeth may be compromised periodontally.

Complications of Nasopalatine Implants

Migrated Implant

Some rather significant complications may be associated with incisive canal implants. The first surgical complication of an incisive foramen implant is related to the implant that is too small for the foramen and not properly fixated (i.e., inadequate primary stability). The implant may be inadvertently pushed through the incisive canal and into the nares proper. Because patients are in a supine position during the surgery, the implant may fall back into the soft plate, then into the trachea or esophagus. If the implant disappears from the oral site, the patient's head should be turned to the side immediately, then down and forward. A nasal speculum and tissue forceps may then be used to recover the implant or immediate medical referral.

Excessive Bleeding

A second surgical complication may include excessive bleeding from the incisive foramen. Although this complication is very rare, it is possible. When reflection of the palatal tissue off the incisive canal is associated with arterial bleeding, a blunt bone tap (mirror handle) may be placed over the canal and a mallet used to hit the instrument firmly, crushing the bone over the artery. After several minutes the procedure may continue, and the implant insertion

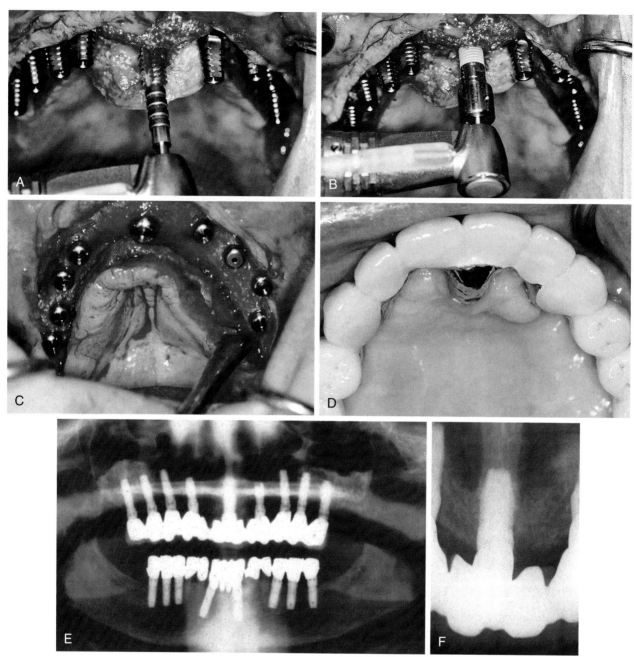

• **Fig. 29.36** (A) The incisive foramen was excavated and prepared for an implant. The site may be bone tapped before implant insertion. (B) A 5-mm-diameter implant is inserted into the incisive foramen after implant preparation. (C) A stage II reentry reveals bone around the incisive foramen implant. (D) On occasion, a fixed prosthesis may be fabricated with the anterior implants in the canine and incisive foramen position. (E) A panoramic radiograph of the incisive foramen implant, bilateral sinus grafts, and nine implants (including the canine positions). (F) A periapical radiograph of an incisive foramen implant after 5 years of function.

will obdurate the site and arrest the bleeding. Additional techniques include the use of injecting epinephrine 1:50,000 directly into the foramen. An electrocautery unit may also be used with a ball type of attachment.[40]

Neurosensory Impairment

A third complication of an nasopalatine foramen implant is associated with enucleation of the soft tissue from the foramen, which may result in neurologic impairment of the soft tissues in the anterior palate. These complications may be anesthesia or paresthesia to the soft tissue or a dysesthesia, resulting in a burning sensation,

which have been reported in numerous reports.[41,42] In most cases, collateral innervation from the greater palatine nerve to the anterior palate is present which eliminates any possible neurosensory disturbances.

Tissue Regeneration

The fourth complication is a long-term complication which may include the regeneration of the soft tissue in the incisive canal, resulting in bone loss and failure of the implant (Fig. 29.37). When the implant is removed and the soft tissue biopsied, nerve fibers can be seen reinvading the site. This most likely occurs because the implant

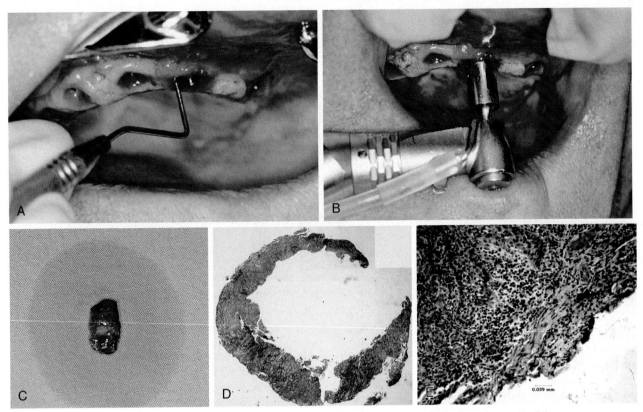

• **Fig. 29.37** (A) A long-term complication of an incisive foramen implant may be bone loss around the implant that extends the full length of the implant. (B) When more than 50% of the implant has been lost, it should most often be extracted. A trephine bur may remove the integrated portion of the implant. (C) The implant removed is surrounded by soft tissue. (D) Histologic examination of the soft tissue around the implant reveals that the contents of the incisive canal are reforming around the implant. (E) Histologic examination demonstrates nerve fibers in the soft tissue around the implant.

was too small for the size of the foramen, and the soft tissue can reform around the implant. Treatment of this complication includes removing the implant and, if necessary for the treatment plan, regrafting and/or reimplantation at a later date.

Implants in Approximation to the Nasal Cavity

Anatomic Considerations

The anterior nasal spine has an anterior component that averages 4.1 mm (0–9 mm) in adults.[27] Posterior and lateral to it, two flat processes, the alae of the premaxilla, project superiorly and laterally. The piriform aperture is bounded below and laterally by the maxilla. The breadth of the piriform aperture in adults ranges from 20 to 28 mm and averages 23.6 mm.[43,44] The lower border of the inferior piriform rim may be sharp or rounded. This border often rises from the premaxillary bone and ends anteromedially in the anterior nasal spine. The anatomy of the nasal floor is variable in relation to the inferior turbinate and is typically situated 5 to 9 mm below the level of this structure (Fig. 29.38).[45]

When maxillary anterior teeth are present or have maintained the residual bone, the inferior piriform rim is usually level or a few millimeters above the floor of the nose in the central and lateral region.[46] The inferior piriform rim above the nasal floor forms a prenasal fossa, which is found in 12% of patients.[47] In these cases a shallow depression extends toward the alveolar arch behind a sharp border of the inferior piriform rim. As a result, when the

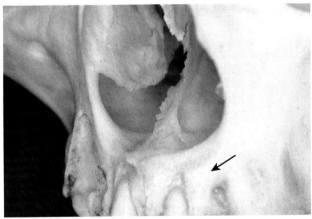

• **Fig. 29.38** Natural canine root is distal to the lateral piriform rim of the nose. However, a nasal recess extends distal, behind the piriform rim and over the canine site of a resorbed maxilla, which is more palatal than the tooth root position. The inferior concha of the nose is 4 to 6 mm superior to this recess region.

inferior piriform rim is used as a guideline for the height of the opposing cortical plate from the crest of the ridge in the maxilla during surgery to determine implant length, the lowest portion of the nasal floor and nasal mucosa may be inadvertently perforated during the implant osteotomy and placement. Ideally, implant placement should be short of the nasal floor.

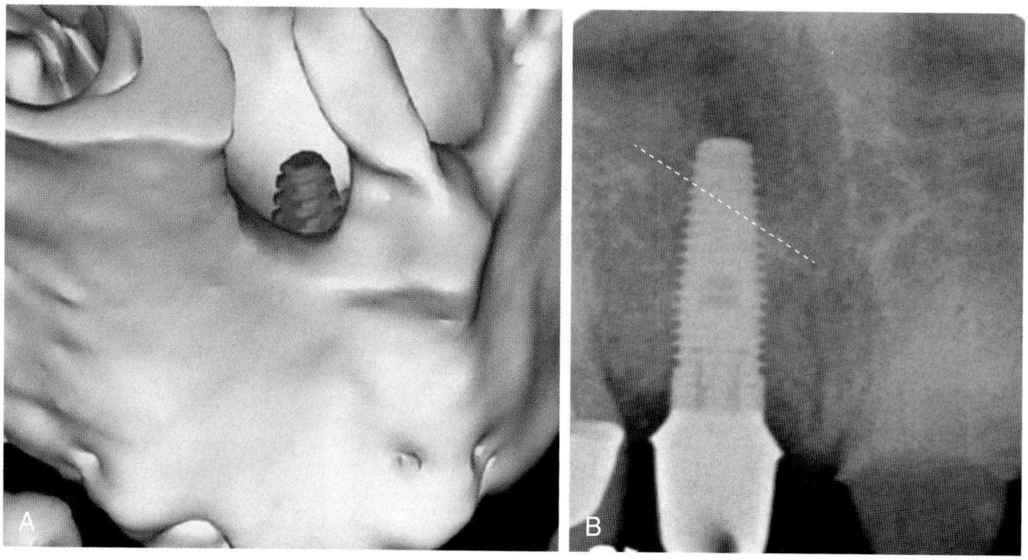

• **Fig. 29.39** (A and B) Implant placement into the nasal cavity proper is not recommended because irritation and nasal congestion problems may result.

The canine tooth position is immediately distal to the lateral piriform rim. The canine eminence in this area is lost after several years of edentulism, and the crest of the residual C–h bone volume ridge is palatal to the original tooth position. The nasal cavity is usually above, medial, and palatal to the canine position in the dentate patient. However, a nasal recess is present behind the lateral piriform rim. This nasal recess corresponds to the apical region of the canine position in the C–h maxilla, which has resorbed palatally and is now under the nasal cavity. Implants placed in the canine position of a C–h bone volume may extend more superiorly than the natural canine root.

The arterial blood supply to the nose is derived from both the external and internal carotid arteries. The terminal branch of the maxillary artery (a branch of the external carotid) supplies the sphenopalatine artery, which supplies the lateral and medial wall of the nasal chamber. The anterior and posterior ethmoid arteries (branches of the ophthalmic artery) supply the nasal vestibule and the anterior portion of the septum. In addition, a few vessels from the greater palatine artery pass through the incisive canal of the palate to reach the anterior part of the nose. At the junction between the squamous epithelium of the nasal vestibule and the respiratory epithelium of the nasal cavity lies a strip about 1.5 mm wide covering a region of wide and long capillary loops, known as Kiesselbach's plexus.[48] It extends to the lower and central part of the cartilaginous septum and is a common region for nose bleeds (Fig. 29.39).

Ideally, dental implants should be positioned short of the nasal cavity. Wolff and colleagues reported a case report describing an implant placed into the nasal cavity resulting in severe congestion postop. Therefore dental implants protruding into the nasal cavity may cause alterations in airflow. If this should occur, the implant should be removed or the apical portion of the protruding implant may be removed via a transnasal approach (Fig. 29.40).[49]

Maxillary Anterior Anodontia

The most common maxillary anterior tooth replaced by an implant is a central incisor lost from trauma (e.g., endodontic failure, fracture, root resorption) and/or a lateral incisor absent as a result of agenesis. The absence of one or more teeth is known as anodontia and may be complete (very rare) or partial (also called hypodontia). It is many times more common than supernumerary teeth. The primary cause of partial anodontia is familial heredity, and incidence ranges from 1.5% to as high as 10% in the US population.[50] The genetic predisposition has been associated with PAX9 promoter polymorphisms.[51] In addition, a number of syndromes exist in the literature that include multiple missing teeth, of which ectodermal dysplasia is the most common.

A high correlation is found between primary tooth absence and a permanent missing tooth; however, a missing tooth occurs more frequently in the permanent dentition. Caprioglio and colleagues[52] evaluated the records of almost 10,000 patients between the ages of 5 to 15 years of age. Of all the missing single teeth, the mandibular second premolar was most often missing (38.6%), followed by the maxillary lateral incisor (29.3%), the maxillary second premolar (16.5%), and the mandibular central incisor (4.0%). The remaining teeth were absent at a rate of only 0.5% to 1.8%, with the maxillary first molar being the least affected. The missing mandibular second premolar primarily occurred in male patients, whereas the maxillary lateral incisor primarily occurred in female patients. The most common multiple teeth lost (other than third molars) are the maxillary lateral incisors, followed by the mandibular second premolars and maxillary second premolars. Congenitally missing teeth are therefore a common scenario seen in dental practices today. Fortunately, less than 1% of those missing teeth are missing more than two teeth, and less than 0.5% of this group are missing more than five permanent teeth.

When acceptable conditions can be created, an anterior single-tooth implant is the treatment of choice for a congenitally missing anterior tooth. However, the treatment of congenitally missing teeth are very challenging with significant esthetic and functional demands.

The replacement of congenitally missing teeth usually occurs during the adolescence period. Because of this patient population, many issues complicate the treatment including (1) interdisciplinary approach, (2) postorthodontic retention, (3) implant placement timing, (4) ideal placement is required, and (5) associated esthetic and soft tissue problems exist.

This condition is especially beneficial for a lateral incisor because the ideal cervical region of the tooth is similar to the implant diameter. However, the roots of the adjacent natural teeth often impinge

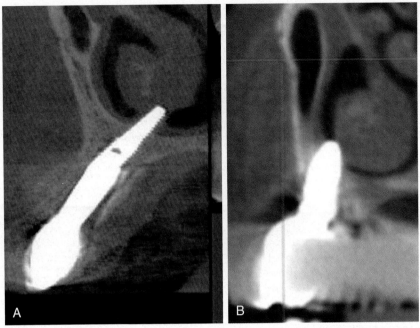

• **Fig. 29.40** (A and B) Implant placement into the nasal cavity may result in compromised crown height space and irritation from violating the inferior meatus and turbinate. Note the implants are actually in contact with the turbinate.

on the edentulous space, resultying in insufficient mesial-distal space for a dental implant. As a consequence, orthodontic therapy before implant placement should often be considered. An additional advantage of orthodontics before or in conjunction with implant treatment for the congenital missing tooth is that the missing lateral incisor may be restored provisionally by a denture tooth attached to the orthodontic wire to provide an esthetic replacement without trauma to the augmented ridge or implant during healing.

The missing maxillary lateral incisor is most often replaced with a dental implant because the other orthodontic or prosthetic options are usually poor alternatives. The clinician should first determine whether space-opening (maintenance) procedures or space closure (orthodontics) is the treatment of choice for the missing tooth. The treatment options are usually different for a mandibular second premolar compared with a maxillary lateral incisor.

Graber[53] noted a strong correlation between a missing single tooth and altered tooth size, shape, or both. A common condition is a missing lateral incisor, in which the contralateral lateral incisor is smaller than usual or a peg lateral. As such, the mesiodistal space is often limited to less than 6.5 mm. In these instances, a nonfunctional, small-diameter implant of 3.0 mm may be considered. When the intratooth space is less than 5 mm, other treatment options should be considered including a cantilevered FPD from the canine abutment.

Congenitally Missing Lateral Incisor Treatment Protocol

In most cases of congenitally missing lateral incisors, orthodontic intervention is required. There usually are three phases of treatment for the replacement of congenitally missing lateral incisors, (1) orthodontic treatment, (2) postorthodontic treatment, and (3) final implant treatment.

Orthodontic

There are two different orthodontic treatments for the restoration of a congenitally missing lateral incisor: cuspid substitution (space closing)[54] and conventional treatment (space opening).[55]

With cuspid substitution, the permanent cuspid is orthodontically repositioned into the lateral incisor space and the first premolar into the canine space. The advantage of this treatment is that it uses conventional orthodontic treatment, which usually entails comprehensive orthodontic care. The disadvantage of this treatment is that most patients end up with a class 1 occlusion, therefore a malocclusion results. Usually, the patient will not have a cuspid disocclusion, but a group function will result. In addition, esthetically, the cuspid differs greatly in shape, size, and color compared to a lateral incisor. Usually the cuspid shade is one to two shades darker than the lateral, and if recontouring of the cuspid is completed, usually the show-through of the dentin will make the tooth even darker. The canine is normally 1 mm wider than the lateral incisor; reducing the interproximal areas of the tooth will result in further darkening.[56] Last, the permanent cuspid is more convex than a lateral; therefore reshaping often will result in hypersensitivity and esthetic issues. The first premolar is normally shorter and narrower than the contralateral cuspid (Fig. 29.41).

Conventional orthodontic treatment includes opening the space to allow for a future restoration, which usually includes an endosseous implant. The goal of conventional orthodontic treatment is to achieve ideal coronal and apical space for an implant, along with a favorable occlusal scheme for the final prosthesis (Fig. 29.42).

The amount of space required is a minimum of 6 mm, which results from the "golden ratio."[57] The golden ratio describes the relationship between the central and lateral incisor, which states that the lateral incisor is ⅔ the size (mesiodistal width) of the central incisor. The average central incisor is 9 mm wide; therefore the lateral width would be 6 mm. Chu described another method of determining the width of the lateral incisor. With this method, the central incisor is determined to be "x." The lateral incisor then is calculated as "x – 2 mm" and the cuspid is "x – 1 mm."[58] Last, the author uses a method that measures the contralateral side and duplicates that space in the final restoration. In some cases, cosmetic bonding may need to be completed to make the spaces ideal.

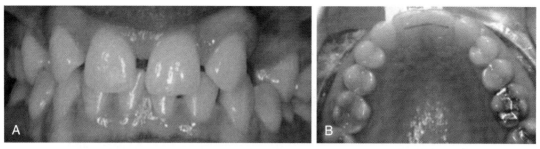

• **Fig. 29.41** Canine substitution. (A) Preoperative image depicting congenitally missing lateral incisors. (B) Final postoperative image showing canine repositioned into the lateral position and first premolar repositioned into the cuspid position.

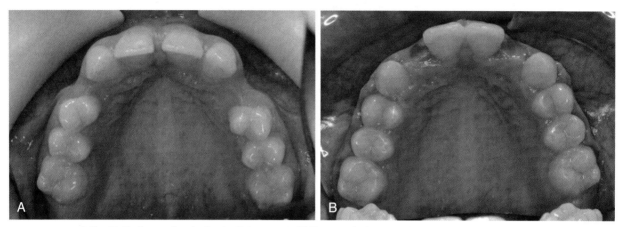

• **Fig. 29.42** Conventional orthodontic treatment, (A) Preoperatively, congenitally missing laterals. (B) Postoperatively, canines repositioned into their ideal position allowing for future implant placement.

Spacing Requirements

Before placing an implant into a congenitally missing space, a CBCT should be obtained to determine the exact space between the adjacent teeth, both coronally and apically. In many cases, clinicians will determine whether there is adequate coronal space; however, the apical space is compromised. This often occurs when space is obtained by use of a palatal expander, and then the central incisors are "tipped," instead of "bodily" moved back into position. By closing the space between the central incisors, the root apexes will be approximate, leaving inadequate space for a dental implant. In most cases, the interroot distance should be a minimum of 6 mm (Fig. 29.43).[59,60] The minimum space required should be verified via a CBCT examination by measuring the coronal, midroot, and apical areas.

Postorthodontic Retention

In most cases of postorthodontic treatment, the patient is usually too young for implant treatment. Therefore it is imperative that patients are maintained during this period to prevent relapse. Postorthodontic retention usually is via a removable or rigid prosthesis. Common removable prostheses include a Hawley appliance or an Essix appliance.[61] Unfortunately, apical relapse or reapproximation has been shown to occur in approximately 11% of postorthodontic cases because of retainer noncompliance, compensatory eruption, and increased vertical growth.[62] Ideally, to prevent root approximation, a rigid, nonremovable prosthesis should be used. Rigid retention usually involves the insertion of a resin-bonded bridge, which is advantageous because it is a nonremovable prosthesis; however, a high debonding rate is seen.[63]

Final Prosthesis

For a congenitally missing lateral incisor, an implant retained prosthesis is advantageous over all other options (e.g., resin-bonded prosthesis, FPD, cantilevered fixed prosthesis, RPD). The clinician must evaluate and take into consideration the following factors when treatment planning for an implant prosthesis: timing, available bone present, coronal and apical space, positioning, esthetics, and gingival contours.

Timing. A common complication occurs when clinicians use chronologic age as the determining factor for the timing of implant placement. Ideally, implant placement should be completed when the patient has facial growth cessation. In the literature, growth cessation has been documented to be determined with the use of dental development,[64] voice changes,[65] hand–wrist radiographs,[66] cervical vertebrae maturation,[67] and serial lateral cephalometric radiographs.[68] Unfortunately, most of the accurate options to determine growth cessation are via radiation exposure. Therefore to reduce the radiation exposure to adolescent implant patients, the author recommends measuring growth cessation by monitoring stature growth, usually with the assistance of the patient's pediatrician. Studies have shown that less than a 0.5-cm growth in a 6-month period is an ideal time to initiate dental implant treatment.[69]

If implants are placed before growth cessation, the downward growth of the maxilla results in the implants being in infraocclusion compared with the natural teeth. When facial growth occurs, changes will result in tooth position. Because of the osseointegration (i.e., ankylosis) of the dental implant, the dental implant cannot change position, which may result in esthetic complications.[70] Westwood and colleagues reported implants placed at age 12 will

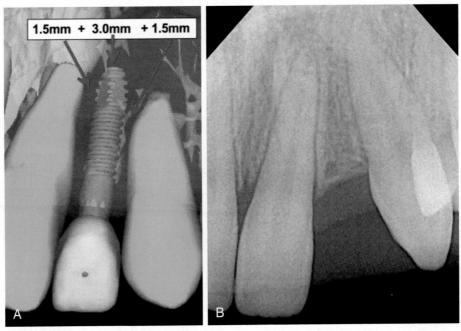

• **Fig. 29.43** (A) Ideal implant placement for lateral incisor, 1.5 mm from teeth and a 3.0-mm implant diameter. (B) Nonideal space caused by orthodontic tipping of the central incisors.

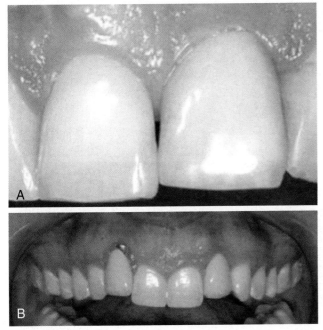

• **Fig. 29.44** (A) Implant placement too early. Because of continued growth of the maxilla, the implant *(left central incisor)* is positioned in infraocclusion. (B) Bilateral lateral incisors in infraocclusion. Note the tissue recession and implant exposure of the maxillary right lateral incisor.

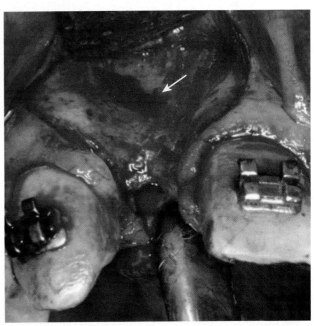

• **Fig. 29.45** Maxillary right lateral incisor showing compromised bone. Note the large concavity adjacent to the midroot of the adjacent teeth.

be in infraocclusion 5 to 7 mm 4 years later.[71] Ranly showed that at age16 teeth are located approximately 10 mm coronally from their position at age 7.[72] In general, implant submergence is not easily correctable. It may be possible to place a new prosthesis on the implant to correct the occlusal discrepancy, increased crown-implant ratio, and the poor esthetics. However, significant biomechanical issues along with potential peri-implant disease may result. If eruption of the adjacent teeth occurs, remediation of the implant usually involves explantation of the implant, bone augmentation, and placement of a new implant (Fig. 29.44).

Available Bone Present. Because the congenitally missing tooth does not have a permanent tooth bud, the available bone in the area most often is compromised in quality and quantity. In most cases, a division B or a division C–w is present. To obtain adequate bone for implant placement, bone augmentation is usually recommended. Bone augmentation maybe completed before growth cessation; however, it should be timed correctly with implant placement at the time of no future growth. In some cases, the permanent cuspid may be allowed to erupt mesially through the alveolus into the lateral incisor position. Because of its significant buccolingual dimensions, the edentulous ridge is maintained. When the permanent canine is moved orthodontically into the ideal canine position, an increased buccolingual width will be retained (Figs. 29.45 and 29.46).[73]

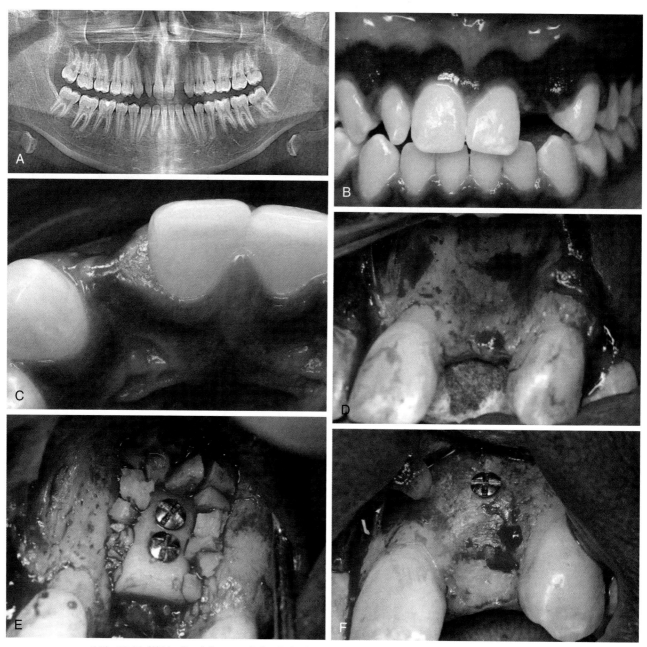

• **Fig. 29.46** (A) Maxillary left congenitally missing lateral incisor. (B and C) Clinical images of compromised available bone and soft tissue. (D) Tissue reflection showing large osseous defect, (E) autogenous bone graft, (F) postgraft healing,

Continued

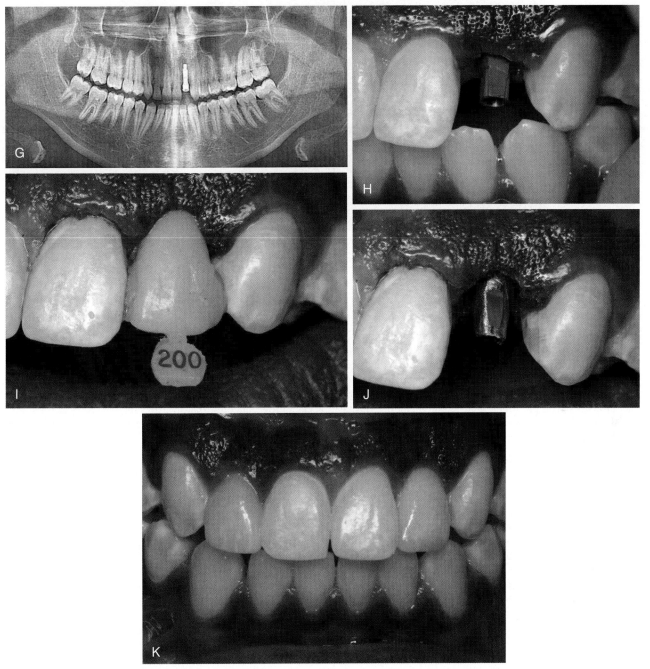

• **Fig. 29.46, cont'd** (G) implant placement, (H) second-stage surgery with implant post placement to develop the soft tissue drape, (I) interim prosthesis fabricated to develop soft tissue, (J) papilla developed, and (K) final implant prosthesis.

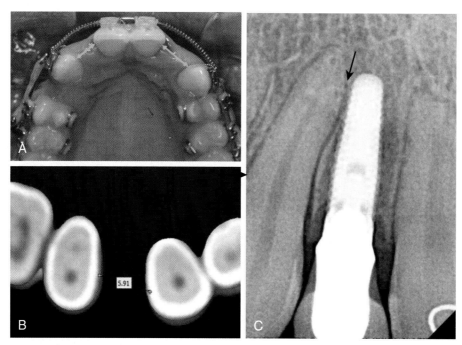

• **Fig. 29.47** Coronal space. (A) Nonsymmetric coronal space that is being remedied via conventional orthodontic treatment. (B) Cone beam computerized tomographic three-dimensional image measuring ideal space for implant. (C) Nonideal space for implants. The placement of implants places the adjacent teeth at significant risk.

Coronal and Apical Space. A CBCT examination should be completed to verify that a minimum of 6 mm of space is present coronally and apically. A minimum of 1.5 mm of space needs to be present between the final implant position and an adjacent tooth root. If implant placement is too close to an adjacent tooth root, a number of complications may result, including devitalization of teeth, development of pathology around the teeth or implant, sensitivity of teeth, and loss of teeth or implant. If the coronal space is compromised, apical migration of the papilla will occur, leading to open gingival embrasures and compromised gingival scallop (Figs. 29.47 and 29.48).[74]

Implant Positioning. Often, implants placed in the premaxilla are positioned too facially. This occurs because of a thin buccal plate and the existing bone trajectory. If an implant is facially positioned, then esthetic issues may result including tissue showthrough of the implant or abutment and gingival recession (Fig. 29.49). In addition, bone loss may occur from unfavorable force factors. For a cement-retained prosthesis, the implant should be placed slightly lingual to the incisal edge of the tooth. For a screw-retained prosthesis, the implant should be positioned in the cingulum area. In the apicocoronal position, the implant body should ideally be positioned 2 to 3 mm below the free gingival margins of the central incisor and cuspid (Fig. 29.50).[75]

Soft Tissue Complications. Usually when a tooth is missing congenitally, the associated papilla will not be present. To increase the thickness of the tissue, acellular dermis (OrACELL) may be used at the time of bone augmentation or implant placement.

After implant placement, tissue grafting is more difficult and less predictable. Another option to increase tissue thickness is the use of the split-finger technique, which is completed at the second-stage surgery appointment and uses a healing abutment to increase the size of the papilla.[76] Last, the tissue can be guided via a provisional restoration. After implant healing is complete, a provisional restoration may be placed on the implant to prosthetically guide the soft tissue into an ideal position. The subgingival contours of a provisional prosthesis have been shown to influence the final position of the prosthesis (Fig. 29.51).[77]

Summary

The replacement of missing teeth in the premaxilla is very challenging because of the highly specific soft and hard tissue criteria, in addition to all other esthetic, phonetic, functional, and occlusal requirements. Maxillary anterior tooth loss usually compromises ideal bone volume and position for proper implant placement. Implant diameter, compared with that of natural teeth, results in challenging cervical esthetics. Unique surgical and prosthetic concepts are implemented for proper results. In spite of all the technical difficulties that the surgical and restoring clinician may face, the anterior single-tooth implant is the ideal modality of choice to replace a missing anterior maxillary tooth. However, the clinician must have a strong foundation for the inherent complications that are involved with replacing maxillary anterior teeth.

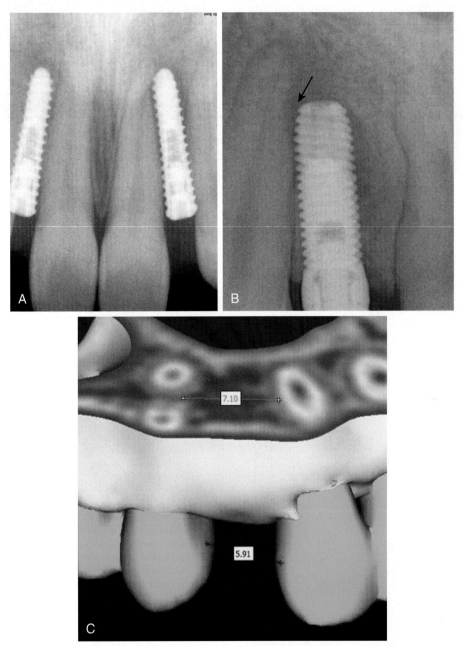

• **Fig. 29.48** (A) Lack of Available bone for implants encroaching upon periodontal ligament space of adjacent teeth, (B) Poor positioning leading to pathology involving the implant and natural tooth, (C) A CBCT examination should always be utilized to determine the available bone for implant placement.

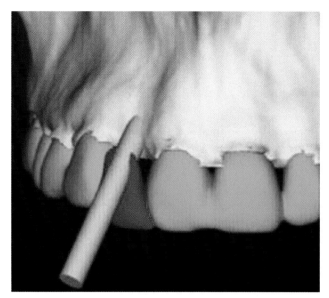

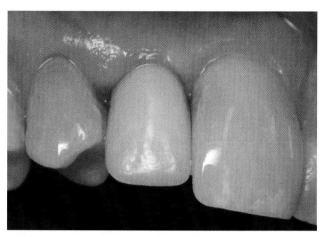

• **Fig. 29.51** Maxillary right lateral incisor with compromised papilla showing the start of black triangles.

• **Fig. 29.49** Implant placement too facial leading to inability to fabricate a screw-retained prosthesis or requiring a custom angled abutment.

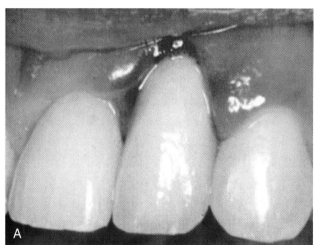

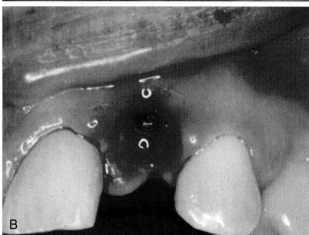

• **Fig. 29.50** (A) Implant placement too far apical leading to increased crown height space and peri-implant disease, (B) Image depicting the bleeding, diseased tissue resulting from inability to maintain proper hygiene.

References

1. Priest GF. Failure rates of restorations for single tooth replacements. *Int J Prosthodont (IJP)*. 1996;9:38–45.
2. Watson MT. Implant dentistry, a 10 year retrospective report. *Dent Prod Rep*. 1996:25–32.
3. Scurria MS, Bader JD, Shugars DA. Meta-analysis of fixed partial denture survival: prostheses and abutments. *J Prosthet Dent*. 1998;79:459–464.
4. Goodacre CJ, Bernal G, Rungcharassaeng K, et al. Clinical complications with implants and implant prostheses. *J Prosthet Dent*. 2003;90:121–132.
5. Misch CE, D'Alessio R, Misch-Dietsh F. Maxillary partial anodontia and implant dentistry—maxillary anterior partial anodontia in 255 adolescent patients: a 15-year retrospective study of 276 implant site replacement. *Oral Health*. 2005;95:45–57.
6. Wennstrom JL, Ekestubbe A, Grondahl K, et al. Implant supported single-tooth restorations: a 5-year prospective study. *J Clin Periodontol*. 2005;32:567–574.
7. Zarone F, Sorrentino R, Vaccaro F, et al. Prosthetic treatment of maxillary lateral incisor agenesis with osseointegrated implants: a 24-39 month prospective clinical study. *Clin Oral Implants Res*. 2006;17:94–101.
8. Goodacre CJ, Bernal G, Rungcharassaeng K, et al. Clinical complications in fixed prosthodontics. *J Prosthet Dent*. 2003;90:31–41.
9. Kemppainen P, Eskola S, Ylipaavalniemi P. A comparative prospective clinical study of two single tooth implants: a preliminary report of 102 implants. *J Prosthet Dent*. 1997;77:382–387.
10. Kan JY, Rungcharassaeng K. Immediate implant placement and provisionalization of maxillary anterior single implants: a surgical and prosthodontic rationale. *Pract Periodont Aesthet Dent*. 2000;12:817–824.
11. Groisman M, Frossard WM, Ferreira H, et al. Single tooth implants in the maxillary incisor region with immediate provisionalization: 2-year prospective study. *Pract Proced Aesth Dent*. 2003;15:115–122.
12. Sterett JD, Olivier T, Robindon F, et al. Width and length ratios of normal clinical crowns of maxillary anterior dentition in man. *J Clin Periodontol*. 1999;26:153–157.
13. Tjan AH, Miller GD. The JG: some esthetic factors in a smile. *J Prosthet Dent*. 1984;51:24–28.
14. Kokich V. Esthetics and anterior tooth position: an orthodontic perspective. Part I. Crown length. *J Esthet Dent*. 1993;5:19–23.
15. Kokich Jr VO, Kiyak AH, Shapiro PA. Comparing the perception of dentists and lay people to altered dental esthetics. *J Esthet Dent*. 1999;11(6):311–324.
16. Kois MCJ. Altering gingival levels: the restorative connector. I. Biologic variables. *J Esthet Dent*. 1994;6:3–9.

17. Tarnow DP, Magner AW, Fletcher P. The effect of the distance from the contact point to the crest of bone on the presence or absence of the interproximal papilla. *J Periodontol.* 1992;63:995–996.

18. Nordland WP, Tarnow DP. A classification system for loss of papillary height. *J Periodontol.* 1998;69:1124–1126.

19. Kois JC. Predictable single tooth peri-implant esthetics—five diagnostic keys. *Compend Contin Educ Dent.* 2001;22:199–218.

20. Becker W, Ochsenbein C, Tibbetts L, et al. Alveolar bone anatomic profi les as measured from dry skulls: clinical ramifi cations. *J Clin Periodontol.* 1997;24:727–731.

21. Tarnow DP, Magner AW, Fletcher P. The effect of the distance from the contact point to the crest of bone on the presence or absence of the interproximal papilla. *J Periodontol.* 1992;63:995–996.

22. Tarnow DP, Eskow RM. Preservation of implant esthetics, soft tissue and restorative considerations. *J Esthet Dent.* 1996;8:12–19.

23. Vera C, De Kok IJ, Reinhold D, Yap AK, et al. Evaluation of buccal alveolar bone dimension of maxillary anterior and premolar teeth: a cone beam computed tomography investigation. *Int J Oral Maxillofac Implants.* 2012;27(6).

24. Wheeler RC. *A Textbook of Dental Anatomy and Physiology.* 4th ed. Philadelphia: Lea & Febiger; 1965.

25. Tarnow DP, Cho SC, Wallace SS. The effect of interimplant distance on the height of inter-implant bone crest. *J Periodontol.* 2000;71:546–549.

26. Tarnow DP, Magner AW, Fletcher P. The effect of the distance from the contact point to the crest of bone on the presence or absence of the interproximal papilla. *J Periodontol.* 1992;63:995–996.

27. Allard RH, van der Kwast WA, van der Waal I. Nasopalatine duct cyst. Review of the literature and report of 22 cases. *Int J Oral Surg.* 1981;10(6):447–461.

28. Liang X, Jacobs R, Martens W, et al. Macro- and micro-anatomical, histological and computed tomography scan characterization of the nasopalatine canal. *J Clin Periodontol.* 2009;36(7):598–603.

29. Mraiwa N, Jacobs R, Van Cleynenbreugel J, et al. The nasopalatine canal revisited using 2D and 3D CT imaging. *Dentomaxillofac Radiol.* 2004;33(6):396–402.

30. Thakur, Arpita Rai, Krishna Burde, Kruthika Guttal, and Venkatesh G. Naikmasur. Anatomy and morphology of the nasopalatine canal using cone-beam computed tomography. *Imaging science in dentistry.* 2013;43(4):273–281.

31. Tozum TF, Guncu GN, Yildirim YD, et al. Evaluation of maxillary incisive canal characteristics related to dental implant treatment with computerized tomography: a clinical multicenter study. *J Periodontol.* 2012;83(3):337–343.

32. Thakur AR, Burde K, Guttal K, et al. Anatomy and morphology of the nasopalatine canal using cone-beam computed tomography. *Imaging Sci Dent.* 2013;43(4):273–281.

33. Cavallaro J, et al. Management of the nasopalatine canal and foramen associated with dental implant therapy. *Compend Contin Educ Dent. (Jamesburg, NJ: 1995).* 2016;38(6):367–372.

34. Thakur AR, Burde K, Guttal K, et al. Anatomy and morphology of the nasopalatine canal using cone-beam computed tomography. *Imaging Sci Dent.* 2013;43(4):273–281.

35. Rosenquist JB, Nystrom E. Occlusion of the incisal canal with bone chips. A procedure to facilitate insertion of implants in the anterior maxilla. *Int J Oral Maxillofac Surg.* 1992;21(4):210–211.

36. Scher ELC. Use of the incisive canal as a recipient site for root form implants: preliminary clinical reports. *Implant Dent.* 1994;3(1):38–41.

37. Verardi S, Pastagia J. Obliteration of the nasopalatine canal in conjunction with horizontal ridge augmentation. *Compend Contin Educ Dent.* 2012;33(2):116–120. 122.

38. Kraut RA, Boyden DK. Location of incisive canal in relation to central incisor implants. *Implant Dent.* 1998;7(3):221–225.

39. Mardinger O, Namani-Sadan N, Chaushu G, et al. Morphologic changes of the nasopalatine canal related to dental implantation: a radiologic study in different degrees of absorbed maxillae. *J Periodontol.* 2008;79(9):1659–1662.

40. Cavallaro J, et al. Management of the nasopalatine canal and foramen associated with dental implant therapy. *Compend Contin Educ Dent. (Jamesburg, NJ: 1995).* 2016;38(6):367–372.

41. Peñarrocha D, Candel E, Guirado JL, et al. Implants placed in the nasopalatine canal to rehabilitate severely atrophic maxillae: a retrospective study with long follow-up. *J Oral Implantol.* 2014;40(6):699–706.

42. Raghoebar GM, den Hartog L, Vissink A. Augmentation in proximity to the incisive foramen to allow placement of endosseous implants: a case series. *J Oral Maxillofac Surg.* 2010;68(9):2267–2271.

43. Lang J, Baumeister R. Uber das postnatale Wachtumder Nasenhohle. *Gegenbaurs Morphol Jahrb.* 1982;128:354–393.

44. Lang J. *Clinical Anatomy of the Nose, Nasal Cavity and Paranasal Sinuses.* New York: Thieme; 1989.

45. Bell WH, Proffit WR, White RP. *Surgical Corrections of Dental Facial Deformities.* Philadelphia: WB Saunders; 1980:1.

46. Blitzer A, Lawson W, Friedman W, eds. *Surgery of the Paranasal Sinuses.* Philadelphia: WB Saunders; 1985.

47. Hovorka O. *Die Aussere Nase.* Vienna: Hohler; 1893.

48. Kiesselbach W. Uber nasenbluten. *Wien Med.* 1885;2:501.

49. Wolff J,KHK, et al. Altered nasal airflow: an unusual complication following implant surgery in the anterior maxilla. *Int J Imp Dent.* 2016;2(1):6.

50. Stamatiou J, Symons AL. Agenesis of the permanent lateral incisor: distribution, number and sites. *J Clin Pediatr Dent.* 1991;15:244–246.

51. Shimizu T, Maeda T. "Prevalence and genetic basis of tooth agenesis. *Jpn Dent Sci Rev.* 45 (1):52-58.

52. Caprioglio D, Vernole B, Aru G, et al. *Leagenesie Dentali.* Milan, Italy: Masson; 1988:1–14.

53. Graber LW. Congenital absence of teeth: a review with emphasis on inheritance patterns. *J Am Dent Assoc.* 1978;96(2):266–275.

54. Millar BJ, Taylor NG. Lateral thinking: the management of missing upper lateral incisors. *Br Dent J.* 1995;179(3):99–106.

55. Pinho T. Agenesis of upper lateral incisors- case study: orthodontic and restaurative procedures. *Gnathos.* 2003;2(2):35–42.

56. Chu SJ. Range and mean distribution frequency of individual tooth width of maxillary anterior dentition. *Pract Proced Aesthet Dent.* 2007;19:209–215.

57. Lombardi RE. The principles of visual perception and their application to dental esthetics. *J Prosthet Dent.* 1973;29:358.

58. Chu SJ. Range and mean distribution frequency of individual tooth width of the maxillary anterior dentition. *Pract Periodontics Aesthet Dent.* 2007;19(4):209.

59. Thilander B, Odman J, Gröndahl K, Friberg B. Osseointegrated implants in adolescents. An alternative in replacing missing teeth? *Eur J Orthod.* 1994;16:84–95.

60. Esposito M, Ekkestube A, Gröndahl K. Radiological evaluation of marginal bone loss at tooth surfaces facing single-tooth implants. *Clin Oral Implants Res.* 1993;4:151.

61. Park JH, Okadakage S, et al. Orthodontic treatment of a congenitally missing maxillary lateral incisor. *J Esthet Restor Dent.* 2010;22(5):297–312.

62. Olsen TM, Kokich VG Sr. Postorthodontic root approximation after opening space for maxillary lateral incisorImplants. *Am J Orthod Dentofacial Orthop.* 2010;137:158.e1–158.e8.

63. Zarone F, Sorrentino R, et al. Prosthetic treatment of maxillary lateral incisor agenesis with osseointegrated implants: a 24-39-month prospective clinical study. *Clin Oral Implants Res.* 2006;17(1):94–101.

64. Lewis AB, Garn SM. The relationship between tooth formation and other maturation factors. *Angle Orthod.* 1960;30:70–77.

65. Hägg U, Taranger J. Menarche and voice changes as indicators of the pubertal growth spurt. *Acta Odontol Scand.* 1980;38:179–186.

66. Hägg U, Taranger J. Skeletal stages of the hand and wrist as indicators of the pubertal growth spurt. *Acta Odontol Scand.* 1980;38:187.

67. O'Reilly M, Yanniello GJ. Mandibular growth changes and maturation of cervical vertebrae—a longitudinal cephalometric study. *Angle Orthod.* 1988;58:179–184.

68. Nanda RS. The rates of growth of several facial components measured from serial cephalometric roentgenograms. *Am J Orthod*. 41:658–673

69. Heij, GOp D, Opdebeeck H, et al. Facial development, continuous tooth eruption, and mesial drift as compromising factors for implant placement. *Int J Oral Maxillofac Implants*. 2006;21(6).

70. Bernard JP, Schatz JP, Christou P, Belser U, Kiliaridis S. Long-term vertical changes of the anterior maxillary teeth adjacent to single implants in young and mature adults. A retrospective study. *J Clin Periodontol*. 2004;31:1024–1028.

71. Westwood R, Mikel, James M, Duncan. Implants in adolescents: a literature review and case reports. *Int J Oral Maxillofac Implants*. 1996;11(6).

72. Ranly DM. Early orofacial development. *J Clin Pediatr Dent*. 1998;22(4):267–275.

73. Kokich VG. Managing orthodontic- restorative treatment for the adolescent patient. In: McNamara JA, Brudon WL, eds. *Orthodontics and Dentofacial Ortho- Pedics*. Ann Arbor, MI: Needham Press; 2001:423–452.

74. Esposito M, Ekestubbe A, Gr€ondahl K. Radiological evaluation of marginal bone loss at tooth surfaces facing single Br#anemark implants. *Clin Oral Implants Res*. 1993;4:151–157.

75. Kokich VG. Maxillary lateral incisor implants: planning with the aid of orthodontics. *Int J Oral Maxillofac Surg*. 2004;62:48–56.

76. Misch CE, Al-Shammari KF, Wang H-L. Creation of interimplant papillae through a split-finger technique. *Implant Dent*. 2004;13(1): 20–27.

77. Yamamoto M, Miyoshi Y, Kataoka S. Special discussion—fundamentals of esthetics: contouring techniques for metal ceramic restorations. *Quintessence Dent Technol*. 1990/1991;14:10–81.

30

Mandibular Anatomic Implications for Dental Implant Surgery

RANDOLPH R. RESNIK

In dental implantology today it is imperative the clinician have a strong understanding of the surgical anatomy and variations with respect to implant placement in the mandible. Before the commencement of dental implant surgery, a careful and detailed evaluation should be completed of the mandibular vital structures. This may be accomplished by including a clinical evaluation, a visual examination, along with palpation of the anatomic areas. The clinician should have a clear and concise three-dimensional (3D) vision of the anatomic structures in relation to the intended implant surgical procedure.

A thorough radiographic examination needs to be completed to provide information concerning the location and topography of the 3D anatomy. In this chapter a comprehensive evaluation of the important mandibular anatomic areas will be discussed, together with their clinical relevance in dental implant surgery (Fig. 30.1).

Mandibular Anterior

Hourglass Anterior Mandibles

The mandibular anterior region has historically been considered one of the safest and most predictable regions for implant placement. The predictability stems from the favorable quality of bone (i.e., thick cortical and dense trabecular bone) most commonly present in this area. The morphology of the mandibular anterior has been classified as the following shapes: hourglass, ovoid, pear, sickle, and triangular. The pear shape, which is usually abundant with bone, has been shown to be the most common among edentulous and dentate patients.[1]

However, this anatomic area may be compromised by a narrow alveolar width or severe osseous constriction. These types of bony variations have been termed an *hourglass effect*, which is usually indicative of a developmental abnormality. Hourglass mandibles, which have been shown to have an incidence rate of approximately 4%, should always be concerning to the clinician because of possible perforations during implant placement surgery.[2] The position of the alveolar constriction may vary significantly because they have been shown to be high, low, or variable within the alveolus. A thorough 3D cone beam computed tomographic (CBCT) examination should be completed to prevent complications in this area, and guided surgery is recommended to minimize the possibility of perforations[3] (Fig. 30.2).

Butura et al.[4] classified mandibular anterior constrictions as: (1) facial constriction, (2) lingual constriction, and (3) hourglass constriction. They discussed various treatment options to include alveoplasty to a level beyond the constriction, staged bone graft reconstruction, posterior and anterior angled implants to avoid the site, and extra-long implants to bypass the constriction and engage the inferior border of the mandible.[4]

Clinical Relevance

Due to the variable expression of hourglass mandibles, treatment strategies are based on the location and extent of the undercut. In some cases implant placement in this area will be contraindicated. In less severe constrictions an osteoplasty may be performed, together with implant placement. However, the crown height space may be increased significantly, leading to possible biomechanical issues. In addition, other constrictions may require grafting procedures to increase bone volume for implant placement (Fig. 30.3).

If the positioning of a dental implant leads to perforation of the bony mandibular plates, possible life-threatening hemorrhage episodes may occur. These events have been reported when a drill perforates the lingual plate of the sublingual region of the mandible and traumatizes a sublingual or submental artery, especially in the canine region.[5,6] If perforation of the lingual cortical plate is associated with arterial bleeding, it is critical to identify its origin and treat aggressively. The origin of bleeding in the floor of the anterior region of the mouth may be from the lingual artery, facial artery, or one of its branches. Perforation of either the submental artery (originates from the facial artery) or the sublingual artery (originates from the lingual artery) may lead to bony perforation and bleeding, causing an expanding ecchymosis (sublingual hematoma) and compromising the airway. If this should occur, the patient should be repositioned in an upright position, and bimanual pressure should be applied to the area of bleeding. If the airway is compromised, immediate emergency assistance should be summoned (Fig. 30.4).

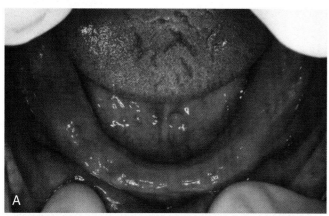

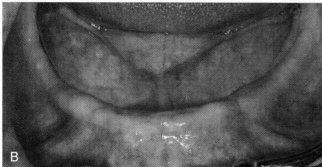

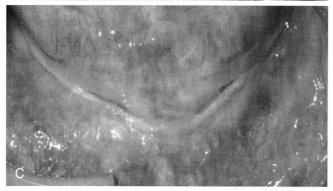

• **Fig. 30.1 Variable Mandibular Anatomy.** The mandibular arch varies dramatically with respect to the amount of hard and soft tissue resorption. (A) Mandibular arch with a significant amount of bone and keratinized tissue. (B) As bone resorption occurs, the loss of the attached tissue results. (C) Advanced resorption of the hard and soft tissues resulting in a severely atrophic mandible with minimal attached tissue.

Median Vascular Canal

In the mandibular midline, radiographic examination often reveals the presence of a radiolucent canal, which is termed a *median vascular canal*. This canal houses the bilateral sublingual arteries that enter the lingual foramen, which is located on the lingual aspect of the mandible. The lingual foramen is seen as a radiopacity below the genial tubercles, which is visible on approximately 52% of CBCT scans.[7] This arterial anastomosis may transverse anteriorly, inferiorly, or superiorly within the anterior mandible, in some instances exiting the facial aspect of the symphysis area. Various studies have shown median vascular canals to be present in 100% of cases, detected on CBCT examinations. Two-dimensional (2D) panoramic radiographs observe their presence only 4.2% of the

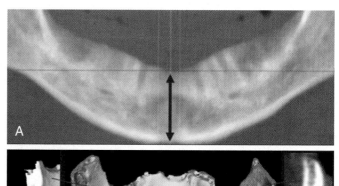

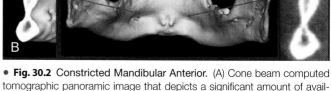

• **Fig. 30.2 Constricted Mandibular Anterior.** (A) Cone beam computed tomographic panoramic image that depicts a significant amount of available bone; however, it does not indicate a constriction is present. (B) Cross-sectional images showing the hourglass appearance of the anterior mandible, which contraindicates implant placement.

time.[8] This is most likely due to the superimposition of the cervical vertebrae and to the orientation of the panoramic beam in relation to the position of the canals. Gahleitner et al.[9] reported one to five canals per patient with an average diameter of 0.7 mm, with a range of 0.4 to 1.5 mm (Fig. 30.5).

The presence and size of the sublingual anastomosis and the median vascular canal are easily seen on a cross-sectional or axial image of a CBCT scan. In approximately 31% of lingual vascular canals the diameter exceeds at least 1 mm.[10] The sublingual artery is a branch of the lingual artery that originates from the external carotid artery. The lingual artery courses medially to the greater horn of the hyoid bone and crosses inferiorly and facially around the hypoglossal nerve. It then transverses deep to the digastric and stylohyoid muscles, and courses between the hyoglossus and genioglossus muscles. There exist four main branches of the lingual artery: the suprahyoid, dorsal lingual, deep lingual, and sublingual (Fig. 30.6).

Clinical Relevance

When planning implants in the anterior mandible, if a large anastomosis is present, the position may be modified to prevent encroachment on the structure. If this area is violated, excessive bleeding may result. The intraosseous bleeding is usually well controlled by placing an implant, direction indicator, or surgical bur in the osteotomy site. There will be no neurosensory issue with encroaching on this area because there are no sensory fibers within the canal (Fig. 30.7).

Severely Angled Anterior Mandible

There exists one uncommon subcategory of Division C, namely C–a (i.e. Division C bone with excessive angulation). In this category, available bone is adequate in height, but angulation is greater than 30 degrees regardless of implant placement. When present, this condition is most often found in the anterior mandible. For ideal implant placement, usually bone augmentation is required. However, a diagnostic wax-up should be completed first because Division C–a mandibles are usually associated with skeletal Class III patients (Fig. 30.8).

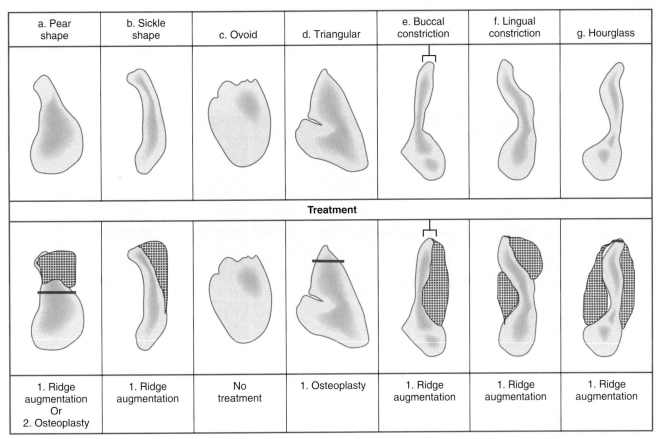

a. Pear shape	b. Sickle shape	c. Ovoid	d. Triangular	e. Buccal constriction	f. Lingual constriction	g. Hourglass

Treatment

1. Ridge augmentation Or 2. Osteoplasty	1. Ridge augmentation	No treatment	1. Osteoplasty	1. Ridge augmentation	1. Ridge augmentation	1. Ridge augmentation

• **Fig. 30.3** Anterior Mandible Cross-Sectional Morphology and Treatment. (A) Pear shape. (B) Sickle shape. (C) Ovoid. (D) Triangular. (E) Buccal constriction. (F) Lingual constriction. (G) Hourglass.

Clinical Relevance

Root form implants placed in Division C–a will lead to poorly positioned implants that will most likely be nonrestorable for a fixed prosthesis. This will most likely result in an overcontoured prosthesis, speech difficulty, compromised tongue space, and inability to obtain an ideal occlusion. Therefore in most cases, a staged bone graft and implant treatment plan should be formulated.

Lack of Keratinized Tissue

As the mandibular osseous process progresses, the presence of keratinized tissue becomes more compromised. In general, implants are healthiest when there exists sufficient keratinized tissue. Some reports indicate the lack of keratinized tissue may contribute to implant failure.[11] Mobile, nonkeratinized mucosa has been shown to exhibit greater probing depths, which has been confirmed histologically. The absence of keratinized mucosa also increases the susceptibility of peri-implant regions to plaque-induced destruction.[12] Additional studies have shown that mobile mucosa may disrupt the implant-epithelial attachment zone and contribute to an increased risk for inflammation from plaque.[13] For larger edentulous ridges the zone of attached tissue on the facial flap (mandible) provides greater resistance for the sutures against tension of the mentalis muscle in the anterior region and the buccinator muscle in the molar and premolar regions, which often cause

incision line opening. As a result, an incision made facial to the attached tissue may cause partial ischemia to some of the crestal tissue. In addition, the incision in unkeratinized facial tissue may sever larger blood vessels, which increases bleeding and decreases vision during surgery, while also potentially complicating final suturing (Fig. 30.9).

Clinical Relevance

For implant sites, an evaluation of the quality and quantity of keratinized tissue should be completed. If insufficient attached tissue is present, tissue augmentation procedures should be completed before implant placement. For larger edentulous sites, especially in the mandible, the incision may be modified to maintain the attached tissue in some cases. If the crest of the ridge is above the floor of the mouth, and there exists greater than 3 mm of attached, keratinized gingiva on the crest of the ridge, a full-thickness incision is made, bisecting the attached tissue. If less than 3 mm of attached gingiva exists on the ridge, the full-thickness incision is made more to the lingual so that at least 1.5 mm of the attached tissue is to the facial aspect of the incision line. Another treatment option includes the use of an acellular dermis (e.g., OraCell; Salvin Dental Corp.). Acellular dermis may be placed at the time of implant placement, thereby increasing the thickness and quality of the tissue while the integration of the implants is taking place (Fig. 30.10).

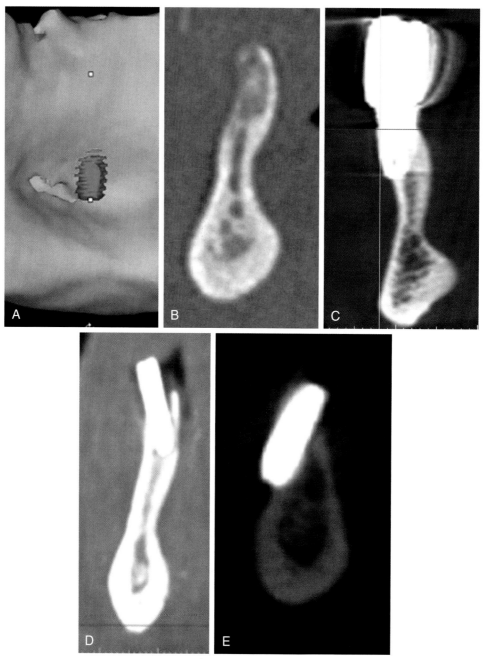

• **Fig. 30.4** Mandibular Anterior Perforation. (A) Implant treatment plan showing perforation of the inferior border of the mandible. (B) Lingual constriction that may lead to bleeding complications, along with chronic tissue irritation. (C to E) Implant placement in a constricted ridge leading to nonideal implant placement.

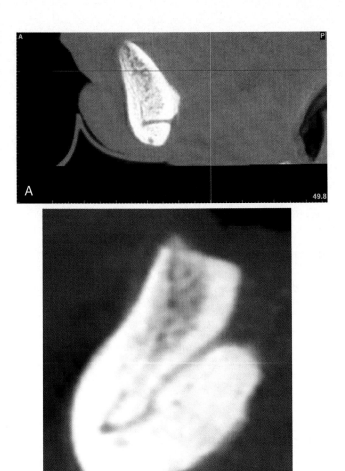

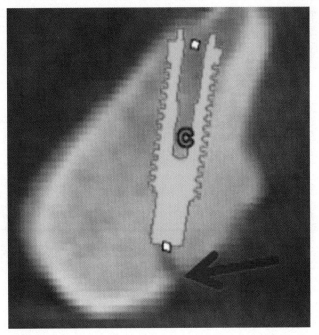

• **Fig. 30.7** Implant placement into the canal may result in bleeding episodes.

• **Fig. 30.5** Median Vascular Canal. (A) Canal extending close to buccal plate and then superiorly to almost the crestal area. (B) Canal extending inferiorly and then superiorly.

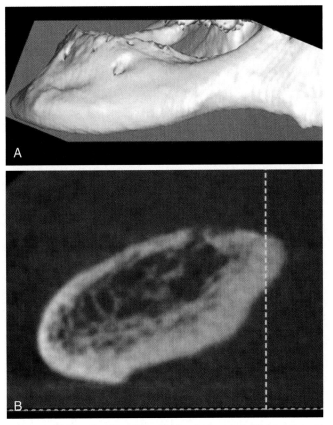

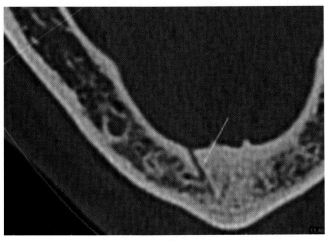

• **Fig. 30.6** Rare off-midline vascular canal.

• **Fig. 30.8** Division C–a Mandible. (A) Mandibular anterior Division C–a with extreme angulation. (B) Cross-sectional image of a Division C–a mandible.

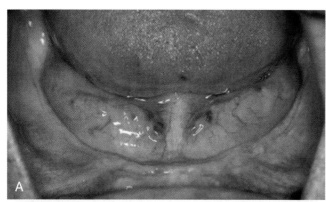

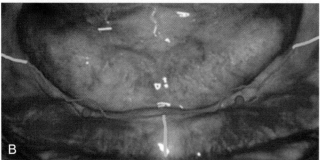

• **Fig. 30.9** (A) Maxillary anterior ridge with compromised attached tissue. (B) When less than 3 mm of attached gingiva is present, the incision for a full-arch mandible should include making the incision more lingual and extending to the lingual aspect of the mandible when there is nerve dehiscence.

Inadequate Width of Bone

A common consequence of tooth loss and bone remodeling in the mandibular anterior region is the resultant narrowing and knife-edge configuration of the mandibular bony ridges (i.e., Division B available bone). Pietrokovski et al.[14] evaluated edentulous ridges in human jaws and found that 43% of mandibular anterior ridges were knife-edge and 38% in the premolar region. Nishimura et al.[15] reported a higher incidence of mandibular knife-edge ridges in females compared with males, mainly because of increased osteopenia changes with unfavorable bone mineral density values.

Clinical Relevance

Therefore before implant placement, it is often necessary to reduce the bone width (i.e., osteoplasty), which results in an increased horizontal width of available bone. An osteoplasty may be carried out with various methods, including osteoplasty burs, barrel burs (i.e., acrylic burs), rongeurs, bone chisels, and Piezosurgery units. By increasing the width of bone, dental implants may be placed with sufficient bone on the buccal (~2.0 mm) and on the lingual (~1.0 mm).

Although an osteoplasty increases available bone for implant placement, many detrimental effects may result. Reduction of a knifelike ridge will decrease the amount of cortical bone present. The cortical bone is a crucial component for primary stability of the implant and is responsible for a greater stress distribution. In addition, as the bony height is reduced, the crown height space increases. The increased crown/implant ratio results in greater strain at the peri-implant interface, which predisposes the implant to biomechanical complications.

The amount of osteoplasty required should be determined before surgery via the use of CBCT treatment planning. In general, if a fixed prosthesis (e.g., FP-1, FP-2, FP-3) is indicated, a minimal osteoplasty is recommended. By minimizing the reduction of bone height, the possibility of a crown/implant ratio problem resulting is decreased. In some cases bone augmentation may be required to maintain the height of bone and increase the bone width, rather than reducing the ridge by means of an osteoplasty. If a removable prosthesis (e.g. RP-4, RP-5) is indicated, a more aggressive osteoplasty is recommended, because this will allow for increased space for the removable prosthesis (i.e., thickness of acrylic, attachment space). In general, the greater the interocclusal space, the less likely a prosthesis or attachment fracture can occur (Box 30.1 and Fig. 30.11).

Mandibular Posterior

Although the posterior mandible is considered a predictable anatomic area for implant placement, there are many drawbacks that include compromised available bone in height and width, significant undercuts, difficult access, and numerous vital structures that may be damaged (e.g., inferior alveolar nerve [IAN], mental nerve, submandibular gland). Iatrogenic violation of these vital structures may result in neurosensory disturbance, pain, infection, excessive bleeding, and compromised implant positioning (Fig. 30.12).

Lack of Bone Height

The posterior mandible resorbs from buccal to lingual, transforming from a Division A to a Division B rather rapidly. Because of the trajectory of the posterior mandible, implant placement in an ideal position for prosthetic rehabilitation may be difficult. When limited alveolar ridge height exists, four options are usually available: (1) no treatment, (2) vertical ridge augmentation with delayed implant placement, (3) vertical bone augmentation with simultaneous implant placement, and (4) the use of short implants.[16-19]

Vertical Bone Augmentation (With Simultaneous or Delayed Implant Placement)

With severely resorbed alveolar ridges in the posterior mandible, the available bone height for standard implant placement is often limited by the proximity of the mandibular canal. Vertical bone augmentation is an option for increasing the ridge dimensions, thereby allowing for placement of standard-length implants. By increasing the bone height, esthetics and biomechanical complications are less likely to complicate the longevity of the implant prosthesis.

However, increasing bone height in the posterior mandible is one of the most challenging procedures in implant dentistry. To increase the available bone, various techniques, including autogenous block grafts, guided bone regeneration, and distraction osteogenesis, have been discussed in the literature. However, an increased rate of surgical complications and enhanced patient morbidity have been associated with these types of procedures.

Shorter Implants

Recently the use of short implants (~8 mm) in the atrophic posterior mandible has been introduced to circumvent the need for vertical bone augmentation. Because the loss of vertical bone height is often associated with inadequate available bone for implant

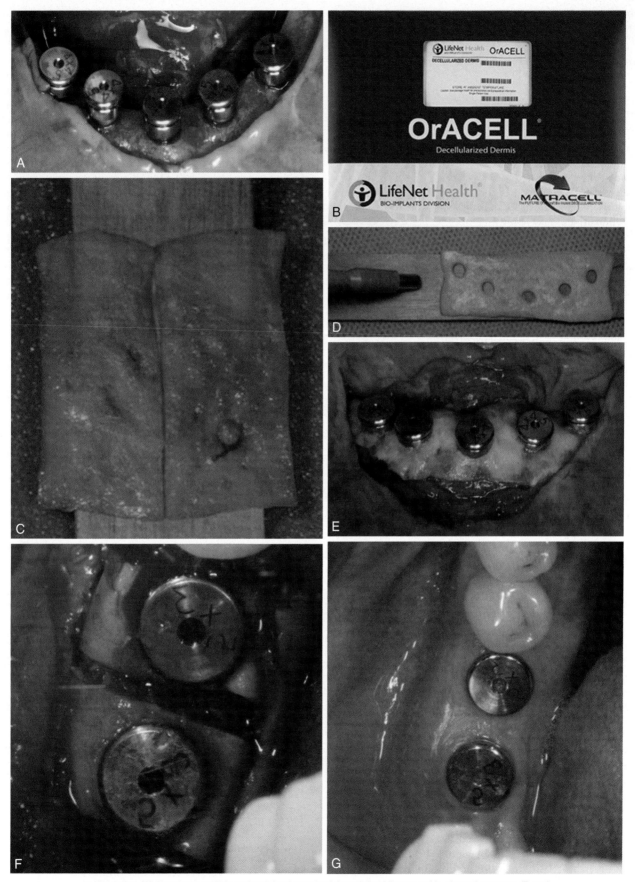

• **Fig. 30.10** (A) Anterior mandible with minimal attached, keratinized tissue and implant placement. (B and C) OrACELL acellular dermis. (D) Four-millimeter holes are made with a biopsy punch to fit over the neck of the implants. (E) Acellular dermis placed with healing abutments. This technique has the advantage of increasing tissue quantity in conjunction with implant healing. (F and G) Before and after case of implant placement and acellular dermis.

1. **Fixed implant prosthesis (FP-1, FP-2, FP-3)**
   a. Porcelain fused to metal: 10 mm
   b. Zirconia: 8 mm
2. **Removable implant prosthesis (RP-4, RP-5)**
   a. Attachments (no bar): 9 mm (e.g., Locator)
   b. Bar + attachment: 15 mm

placement, the safety zone (2-mm distance between the implant and nerve canal) is sometimes compromised with conventional length implants. If this occurs, an increased possibility of a neurosensory impairment may result.

Therefore the use of shorter length implants offers the clinician many advantages in comparison with vertical bone augmentation: it is a less invasive surgery, less surgical experience is required, it is less expensive, and it has a faster treatment time. However, shorter implants do have drawbacks: they may result in an increased crown height space, less surface area in comparison with standard length implants, and a possible higher rate of biological and technical complications from occlusal overload.

In summary, studies on the use of short implants (~8 mm) are promising.[20,21] Many factors should be evaluated when deciding whether short implants should be used instead of vertical bone augmentation. Force factors (e.g., opposing occlusion, parafunction) must be favorable, and an implant-protected occlusion should adhered to. In addition, with short implants, the widest diameter implant possible should be selected, along with an increased number of implants. The final prosthesis involving multiple implants should always be splinted for greater force distribution (Fig. 30.13).

Mandibular Deformation (Flexure of the Mandible)

Full-arch implant-supported prostheses with a rigid substructure have become controversial in implant dentistry because of the associated increased strain at the bone-implant interface. Because of the rigid bone-implant interface that is associated with dental implants, jaw deformation may transmit excessive stress, which can result in complications. In the literature, pain has been associated with full-arch rigidly splinted prostheses.[22,23] Gates and Nicholls[24] reported on deformation of impression material when full-arch impressions are taken with the mouth wide open. The inaccuracies may result in ill-fitting or nonpassive superstructures in different jaw positions. In addition, mandibular deformation has been associated with loosening of full-arch implant-supported prostheses and possible fractures of prostheses during mastication.[25,26]

Etiology

Flexure. The body of the mandible flexes distal to the foramen on opening and has torsion during heavy biting, with potential clinical significance for full-arch implant prostheses. Many reports have addressed the dimensional changes of the mandible during jaw activity as a result of masticatory muscle action. Five different movements have been postulated. Medial convergence is the one most commonly addressed.[27] The mandible between the mental foramina is stable relative to flexure and torsion. However, distal to the foramina, the mandible exhibits considerable movement toward the midline on opening.[28] This movement is caused primarily by the attachment of the internal pterygoid muscles on the

medial ramus of the mandible. The distortion of the mandible occurs early in the opening cycle, and the maximum changes may occur with as little as 28% opening (or about 12 mm). This flexure has also been observed during protrusive jaw movements.[29] The greater the active opening and protrusive movements, the greater the amplitude of mandibular flexion. The amount of movement varies among individuals and depends on the density and volume of bone and the location of the site in question. In general the more distal the sites, the more medial is flexure. The amplitude of the mandibular body flexure toward the midline has been measured to be as much as 800 μm in the first molar-to-first molar region to as much as 1500 μm in the ramus-to-ramus sites.

Torsion. Torsion of the mandibular body distal to the foramina has also been documented in both animal and human studies. Hylander[30] evaluated larger members of the rhesus monkey family (macaque) and found the mandible twisted on the working side and bent in the parasagittal plane on the balancing side during the power stroke of mastication and unilateral molar biting. Parasagittal bending of the human jaw during unilateral biting was confirmed by Abdel-Latif et al.,[31] who showed patients with implant prostheses measured up to 19 degrees of dorsoventral shear.

The torsion during parafunction is caused primarily by forceful contraction of the masseter muscle attachments. Parafunctional bruxism and clenching may cause torsion-related problems in the implant support system and prosthesis when the mandibular teeth are splinted from the molar-to-molar regions.

Implants placed in front of the foramina and splinted together or implants in one posterior quadrant joined to anterior implants have not shown these complications related to the flexure or torsion of the mandible. Complete implant-supported fixed restorations can halt the posterior bone loss associated with edentulism, improve psychological health, and produce fewer prosthetic complications than removable restorations. All edentulous mandibular patients should be given the option of having a fixed prosthesis. However, the increase in forces of mastication, increase in force with patients of greater force factors (e.g., parafunction, crown height space, opposing arch type), or reduced bone density in the implant sites warrant an increase in implant number or implant position in anterior and posterior implant sites (Fig. 30.14).

Prevention

The concept of flexure and torsion does not affect the maxilla, where all implants are often splinted together, regardless of their positions in the arch. Prevention of mandibular flexure should include the following treatment plans:

Bilateral posterior implants: If implants are positioned bilaterally in the premolar/molar regions of the mandible, the final prosthesis should be fabricated with two sections. This will minimize the possibility of flexure/torsion issues. Usually, the prosthesis is. splint in the premolar area.

Anterior implants with unilateral implants posterior: With implant support on only one posterior side, full-arch splinted prostheses will not be subject to the flexure/torsion problems.

Anterior implants with no posterior implants: With no posterior implant support, full-arch splinted prostheses may be fabricated without concern regarding flexure/torsion problems.

Treatment

If a full-arch splinted prosthesis is fabricated and the patient exhibits complications (e.g. pain, difficulty opening, posterior

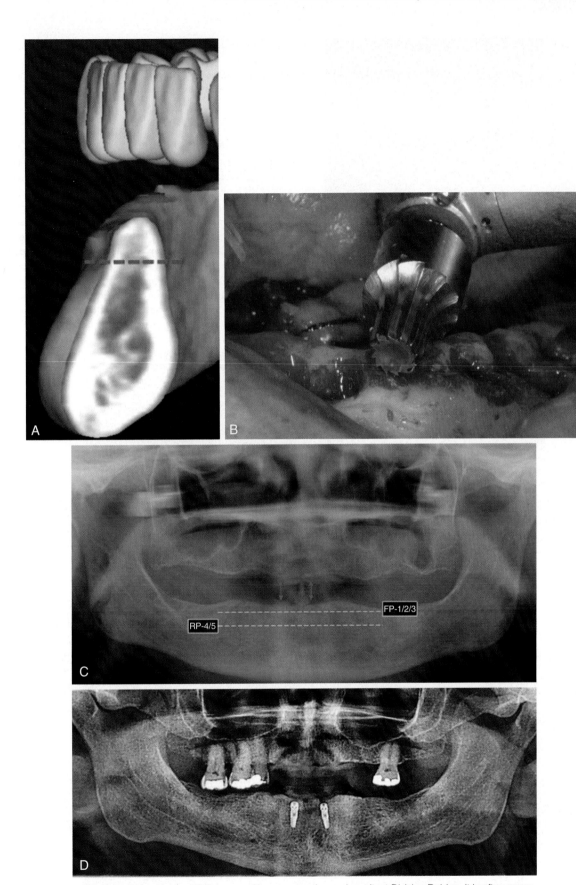

• **Fig. 30.11** Osteoplasty. (A) Because of bone resorption and resultant Division B ridge, it is often necessary to reduce the height of bone via osteoplasty. (B) Osteoplasty of the mandibular anterior ridge to gain width of bone and increase interocclusal space. (C) In general, for a fixed prosthesis (e.g., FP-1, FP-2, FP-3), minimal osteoplasty should be completed to minimize crown height space issues. For a removable prosthesis (e.g., RP-4, RP-5), a more aggressive osteoplasty should be performed to increase space for prosthetic rehabilitation. (D) Implant placement for a removable implant overdenture with insufficient interocclusal space leading to the nonrestorability of the implants.

bone loss) related to the flexure/torsion of the mandible, the prosthesis should ideally be re-fabricated to allow for stress relieve for flexure and torsion forces. This is most likely completed by making the prosthesis in more than one piece.

Bony Anatomic Areas

Posterior Lingual Undercut

In the posterior mandible, it is imperative the implant clinician have detailed knowledge of the three-dimensional anatomy of the area. A lingual undercut is often present, which may lead to complications with life-threatening consequences.

Parnia et al.[32] classified posterior lingual concavities into three types: type 1 (20%): flat depressions less than 2 mm in depth, type 2 (52%) occur with 2 to 3 mm in depth, type 3 (28%) showed significant concavities of more than 3 mm. Nickenig et al.[33] classified posterior mandible morphology to be U-shaped (undercut), P-shaped (parallel), and C-shaped (convex). Lingual undercuts had a prevalence rate of 68% in the molar region, with the prevalence rate far greater in the second

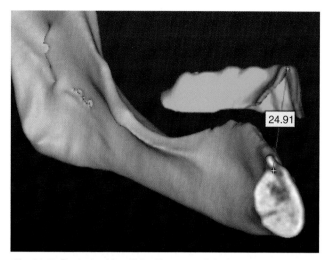

• **Fig. 30.12** Posterior Mandible. Because of the bone morphology and resorptive patterns of the posterior mandible, this anatomic area is often difficult to treat.

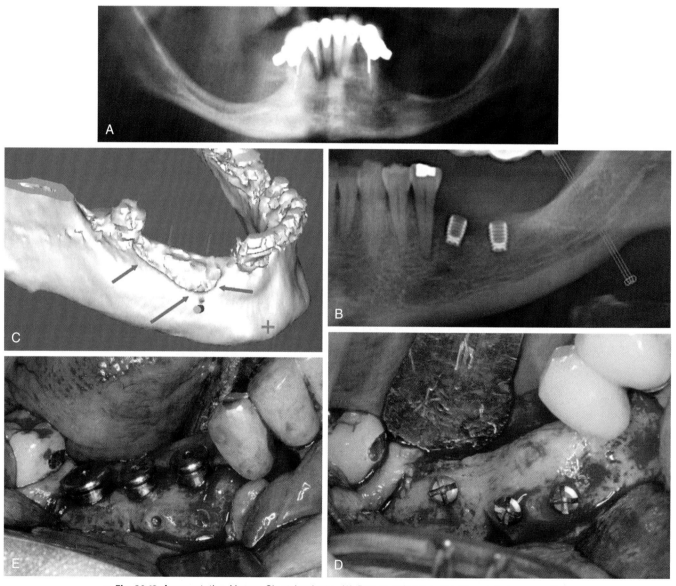

• **Fig. 30.13** Augmentation Versus Short Implants. (A) Due to extensive atrophy, posterior resorption results in a Division D ridge that contraindicates bone augmentation. (B) Short implant placement that prevents nerve impairment, but predisposes patient to biomechanical issues. (C to E) Vertical augmentation graft: large defect augmented with autogenous bone, with delayed implant placement.

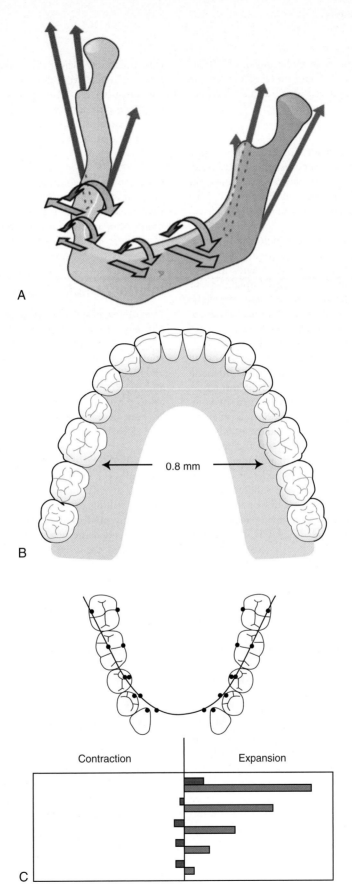

• **Fig. 30.14** (A) The mandible flexes toward the midline on opening or during protrusive movements as a result of the internal pterygoid muscle attachments on the ramus. The mandible also torques, with the inferior border rotating out and up, and the crestal region rotating lingually. The movement is caused by the masseter muscles during forceful biting or parafunction. (B) The amount of flexure depends on the amount of the bone volume and the sites in question. The medial movement from the first molar to the first molar region may be 800 μm. (C) Unilateral molar biting causes the mandible to undergo torsion with the bottom of the mandible expanding outward and the crest of the mandible rotating medially. (*Adapted from Hylander WL. Mandibular function in Galago crassicaudatus and Macaca fascicularis: an in vivo approach to stress analysis of the mandible. J Morphol. 1979;159:253-296.*)

molar region (90%) than in the first molar region (56%).[33] Other studies have shown that lingual undercuts occur in approximately 66% of the population, with a mean undercut of 2.4 mm (Fig. 30.15).[34]

Clinical Relevance

If perforation of the lingual plate is made with either the surgical drill or implant placement, life-threatening situations may result from sublingual bleeding. Within the lingual undercut area, the sublingual and submental arteries are present. Trauma to either of these arteries can result in a sublingual hematoma and airway compromise.

If the perforation were to occur above the mylohyoid muscle, damage to the lingual nerve may result in a neurosensory impairment. If an implant is inserted in this area that extends into the undercut, constant irritation from the extruded implant in the soft tissue may cause the patient chronic pain. In some cases violation may predispose the patient to infection. A clinical examination should always be carried out to determine whether an osseous undercut exists. This may be confirmed with a CBCT examination because cross-sectional images are an effective way of observing lingual undercuts. Violation of this area may cause infection or constant irritation from the extruded implant in the soft tissue.

In addition to the blood vessels in the sublingual area, two salivary glands are also present. The submandibular fossa is a depression on the medial surface of the posterior mandible, which is inferior to the mylohyoid ridge. Within this fossa the submandibular gland is present. Anterior to the submandibular gland is the sublingual fossa, which is present on both sides of the mental spine. The sublingual gland is found in the sublingual fossa. The submandibular and sublingual fossae should be palpated and evaluated before implant osteotomies. In this area, perforation of the lingual plate may damage either of the glands, resulting in possible infection.

Accurate measurements must be determined to prevent overpreparation of the osteotomy site in the posterior mandible. This is most easily completed with a CBCT examination. A clinical examination and palpation of the bone ridge at the proposed implant sites should also be completed. Osteotomy angulation should be carefully evaluated because improper drilling angulation may also lead to perforations. Perforations may lead to infection that can spread to the parapharyngeal and retropharyngeal space. Infections in these spaces progress to severe complications, such as mediastinitis, mycotic aneurysm, internal jugular vein thrombosis, or upper airway obstruction.[35] These complications may occur immediately or can be delayed and should be treated aggressively.

Shorter implants with a tapered design have been shown to be beneficial in avoiding lingual bone perforations.[36] Ideally, implants should always be positioned along the long axis of the occlusal forces, therefore implants should not be placed at an excessive angulation (>30 degrees) to avoid undercuts. de Souza et al.[37] has shown that the submandibular fossa has a direct influence on implant placement (i.e., implant size, position, and angulation) 20% of the time (Fig. 30.16).

Vascular Considerations

Incisive Canal Vessels

The incisive artery is the second terminal branch of the inferior alveolar artery, which is a branch of the maxillary artery. The incisal branch continues anteriorly after supplying the mandibular

first molar area, where it innervates the incisor teeth and anastomoses with the contralateral incisal artery. In rare cases the incisive canal is large, lending to greater bleeding during osteotomy preparation or bone-grafting procedures. The exact location of the incisive canal is easily determined via a CBCT evaluation in the panoramic or sagittal views.

Clinical Relevance

Clinicians often confuse the incisive canal with an anterior loop of the mental nerve. The nerve, artery, and vein within this canal may cause bleeding episodes if traumatized. Usually the placement of the implant, a direction indicator, or surgical bur can be placed into osteotomy to apply pressure to allow for the clotting process.

Inferior Alveolar Artery

The inferior alveolar artery is a branch of the maxillary artery, one of the two terminal branches of the external carotid. Before entering the mandibular foramen, it gives off the mylohyoid artery. In approximately the first molar region, it divides into the mental and incisal branches. The mental branch exits the mental foramen and supplies the chin and lower lip, where it eventually will anastomose with the submental and inferior labial arteries. The exact location of the inferior alveolar artery is easily determined via a CBCT evaluation in the panoramic or sagittal views.

Clinical Relevance

Normally the inferior alveolar artery is located superiorly to the Inferior alveolar nerve (IAN) IAN within the bony mandibular canal. Drilling or placing an implant into the inferior alveolar canal may predispose to significant bleeding. Some authors have recommended the placement of an implant or direction indicator short of the canal to control the bleeding; however, this may lead to possible neurosensory disturbances from hematoma or local irritation to the IAN canal. A 2.0-mm safety zone should be established to prevent complications in this area. If bleeding does occur, follow-up postoperative care is essential because hematoma formation within the canal may lead to a neurosensory impairment. This condition should be monitored because it may progress to respiratory depression via a dissecting hematoma in the floor of the mouth.

Buccal Artery

A common donor site for autogenous grafting is the lateral ramus area in the posterior mandible. When making the incision lateral to the retromolar pad, a common blood vessel to sever is the buccal artery. The buccal artery is a branch of the maxillary artery and will most likely cause a significant bleeding episode. This artery runs obliquely between the internal pterygoid and the insertion of the temporalis on the outer surface of the buccinator.

Clinical Relevance

In most cases, damage to the buccal artery is very difficult to avoid. Incision and reflection will usually encompass the area of buccal artery location. When performing surgery in this area, a hemostat should always be available for immediate access to clamp the vessel. A curved hemostat should be used to clamp the vessel, thus decreasing the bleeding. It should be left in place for 3 to 5 minutes. If bleeding persists, a ligature may be placed with Vicryl suture material (i.e., resorbable) (Fig. 30.18).

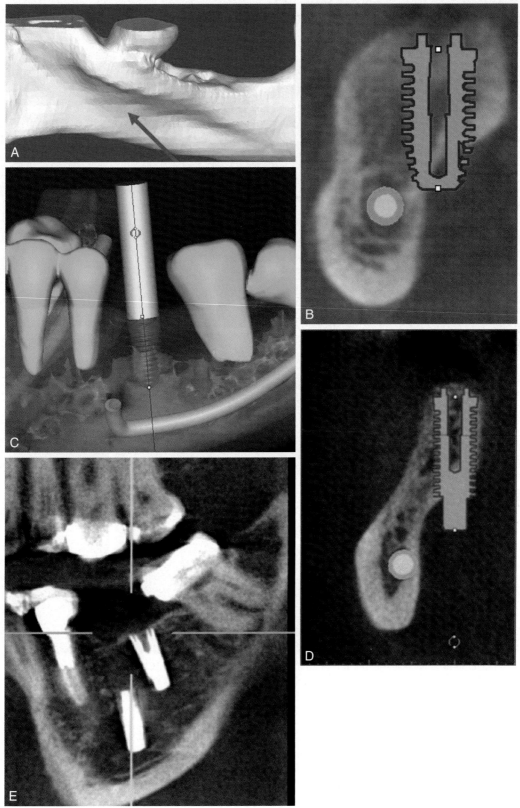

• **Fig. 30.15** Posterior Lingual Undercut. (A) Large sublingual posterior undercut. (B) Of concern is the possibility of lingual perforation. (C and D) Implant dimension measurements should never be made from cone beam computed tomographic panoramic views because third dimension of bone needs to be determined. (E) Implant placement without regard to sublingual undercut results in migration of the dental implant into sublingual space.

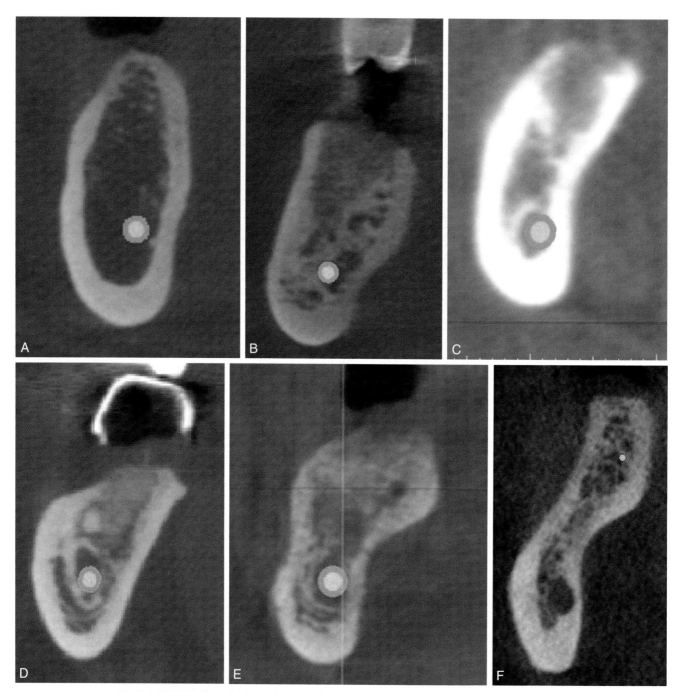

• **Fig. 30.16** Variable Posterior Bony Anatomy.   (A) Straight, no angulation. (B) Slight angulation with minimal lingual undercut. (C) Larger lingual undercut resulting from more extensive atrophy. (D) More significant angulation resulting from buccal bone resorption. (E and F) Extensive lingual undercuts.

Facial Artery

The facial artery is a branch of the external carotid artery, lying superior to the lingual artery and medial to the ramus of the mandible. It courses below the digastric and stylohyoid muscles, and passes through a groove in the submandibular gland before it becomes superficial around the inferior border of the mandible. There are two main branches of the facial artery: the facial and cervical. The facial branch encompasses five branches, which supply the eye, nose, and lips. There are four branches of the cervical region, supplying the pharynx, soft palate, auditory tube, and submandibular gland.

Clinical Relevance

Excessive retraction in this area may lead to trauma to the facial artery. If bleeding from the facial artery exists, pressure should immediately be applied to the angle of the mandible over the vessel. Usually immediate medical assistance will need to be summoned.

Neural Considerations

Lingual Nerve

The lingual nerve is a branch of the trigeminal nerve that provides sensory innervation to the mandibular lingual tissue and the

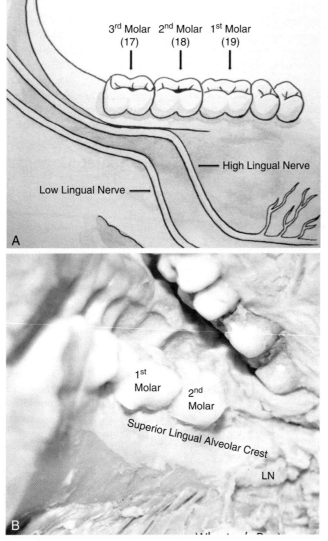

3rd Molar (17)   **2nd Molar (18)**   **1st Molar (19)**

High Lingual Nerve

Low Lingual Nerve

A

1st Molar

2nd Molar

Superior Lingual Alveolar Crest

LN

B

• **Fig. 30.17** Lingual Nerve Anatomy and Variant Positions. (A,B) Note the proximity to the crest of the ridge in the "high" variant position. A lingually placed incision or excessive retraction may cause damage to the lingual nerve. (*From Benninger B, Kloenne J, Horn JL. Clinical anatomy of the lingual nerve and identification with ultrasonography. Br J Oral Maxillofac Surg. 2013;51:541-544.*)

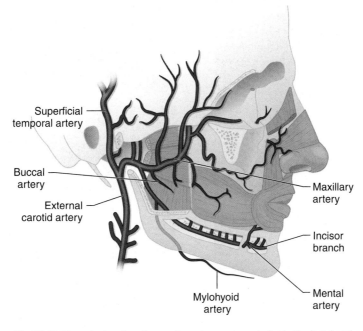

Superficial temporal artery

Buccal artery

External carotid artery

Maxillary artery

Incisor branch

Mylohyoid artery

Mental artery

• **Fig. 30.18** Buccal artery location and most common arteries in the head and neck.

anterior two-thirds of the tongue. The lingual nerve is a concern for implant clinicians because it may be damaged during reflection of the lingual flap. The lingual nerve is most commonly found 3 mm apical to the alveolar crest and 2 mm horizontal from the lingual cortical plate. However, 22% of the time, it may contact the lingual cortical plate.[38] Variations of this nerve have reported it to be located lingual to the third molar area, at or above the crest of the bone.[39]

Clinical Relevance

When elevating tissue in the posterior mandible, always maintain the retractor on the bone and minimize stretching of the tissue on the lingual aspect of the mandible. The lingual nerve is very susceptible to neuropraxia types of nerve impairments. In addition, no lingual vertical release incisions should be used because of the variant lingual nerve anatomy. In addition, in the posterior ramus area, incisions shoudl always be lateral lateral to the retromolar pad because the lingual nerve transverses this area in 10% of cases (Fig. 30.17).

Inferior Alveolar Nerve

Prevention of iatrogenic injuries to the third division of the trigeminal nerve is paramount in implant dentistry today. A resultant neurosensory impairment in the head and neck region may affect the patient's quality of life and may present potentially significant medicolegal problems for the clinician. To prevent damage to these vital nerve structures, it is imperative for the implant dentist to have a comprehensive radiographic survey of the region, thorough knowledge of the normal versus variant anatomy, and awareness of intraoperative surgical techniques to minimize the possibility of nerve impairment (Fig. 30.19).

Radiographic Considerations

Two-Dimensional Radiography

Today the use of 2D radiography is becoming less common for dental implant treatment planning. Two-dimensional radiographs, mainly panoramic, have many inherent disadvantages in evaluating potential implant sites. All panoramic (2D) radiographs exhibit some degree of distortion, nonuniform magnification, and image superimposition, which can potentially lead to incorrect measurement and assessment of neural structures. Studies have shown periapical and panoramic radiography to be unreliable in assessing the true location of the inferior alveolar canal and the mental foramen.[40] Extreme caution should be exercised when using 2D radiography as the only modality for implant site evaluation (Fig. 30.20). Two-dimensional radiographs may be used for initial assessment of potential implants sites.

Even with the generalized acceptance of CBCT radiography in the diagnosis and treatment planning of dental implants, numerous manufacturers still make available to implant dentists magnification guides and digital software programs for intraoral

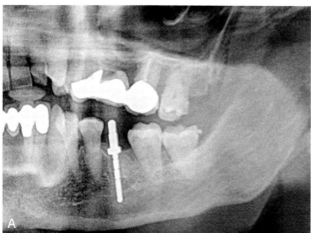
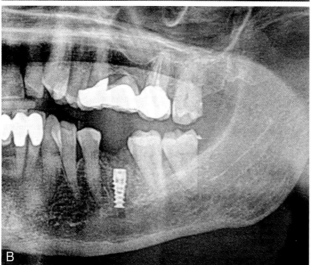

• **Fig. 30.19** Posterior Mandible Complication. (A) Implant osteotomy violating the inferior alveolar canal from poor preoperative planning. (B) Implant placement resulting in a neurosensory deficit.

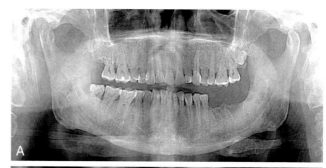
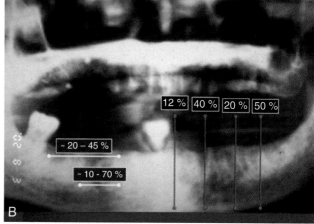

• **Fig. 30.20** Two-Dimensional Radiographs. (A) Panoramic radiographs are inherently inaccurate and do not show the accurate position of the inferior alveolar canal or mental foramen. (B) Panoramic radiographs have a variable magnification factor in the vertical and horizontal planes.

radiographs to assist in the placement of implants over vital structures. The clinician should be aware that panoramic radiographs have variable magnification (i.e., not 25% as related by many implant and panoramic companies), and even calibrated intraoral software programs cannot accurately assess true distances because of their 2D origin. Both periapical and panoramic radiography are associated with magnification that is inconsistent and difficult to determine. Schropp et al.[41] have shown that in more than 70% of cases in which implant size was initially determined via panoramic radiographs, the implant size had to be altered after CBCT evaluation. Magnification guides should never be used as the sole criteria for implant site evaluation because they may lead to overestimation of available bone dimensions.

Three-Dimensional Radiography

In most cases a 3D radiographic modality is recommended for evaluation of the mandibular arch and related nerve anatomy. Studies have shown approximately 50% of nerve injuries resulted from inadequate radiographic assessment.[42,43] Therefore to determine the ideal location and measurement parameters associated with the dental implant placement, the clinician must be able to accurately measure the distance between the alveolar crest and the superior border of the mandibular canal, as well as the width of bone in the proposed implant site. Medical slice computed tomography (MSCT) and CBCT images have been shown to be the most accurate radiographic modalities in the assessment of available bone and identification of the IAN.[44] A thorough knowledge of the relative 3D position of the IAN is crucial in preventing mandibular nerve impairment before implant placement (Fig. 30.21).

Because MSCT and CBCT have been shown to be 1:1 (no magnification), the implant dentist has the ability to place implants, measure available bone, evaluate bone density, determine the prosthetic treatment plan, and order surgical templates directly from their computerized treatment plan. Interactive treatment planning software programs available today contain libraries of most implants systems, which allow the clinician to accurately access the size, type, and ideal placement of the implant in relation to anatomic structures. This virtual treatment plan may then be transferred to the patient's surgery by means of a surgical template or computer-assisted navigation system.

For clinicians early on their learning curve, the fabrication of a bone model can be an invaluable preoperative diagnostic tool. Bone models are made directly from the CBCT dicom (.dcm) data, which are easily fabricated with in-office 3D printers. The

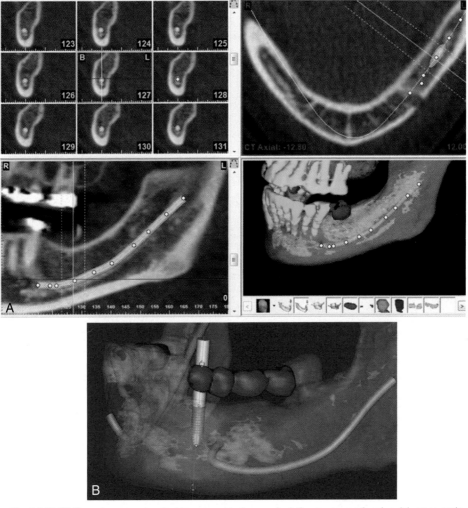

• **Fig. 30.21** (A) Cone beam computed tomographic image depicting cross-sectional, axial, panoramic, and three-dimensional images. (B) Virtual treatment plan showing the mandibular nerve in relation to placement of an implant.

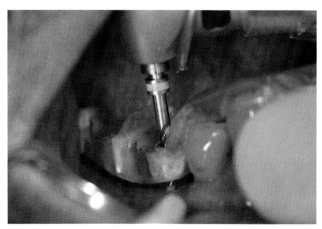

• **Fig. 30.22** Guided-Implant Surgery. With the use of surgical templates, implants may be positioned more accurately, thereby avoiding possible nerve complications.

clinician is able to evaluate the exact osseous morphology (width of bone, undercuts, bony landmarks) and location of vital structures (color coded within the model) before the actual surgery. Implant osteotomies may be performed in a laboratory setting to allow the implant dentist to complete the procedure before surgery.

Neurosensory impairment issues are most frequently an inadvertent sequela of improper diagnosis, treatment planning, or surgical technique. Many of these complications can be overcome by using 3D surgical guides for the ideal positioning and placement of implants. Basically the surgical guide is the conduit for transferring the interactive treatment plan from the computer to the patient's actual surgical procedure. This allows the implant dentist to be able to place the implants in the exact location as per the treatment plan. Surgical guides are categorized based on method of retainment: tooth, bone, or mucosa supported. In addition, guides are distinguished by the surgical technique involved: fully guided—all osteotomies and implant placement is completed through the guide; universal guide—all osteotomies except for the final drill and implant placement are completed through the guide; and pilot—only the first or initial drill is used through the guide. Guided surgery with surgical templates has been reported to improve the accuracy of implant placement in clinical situations in comparison with conventional surgical methods (Fig. 30.22).[45] Nickenig et al.[46] showed that implants placed with surgical templates were within 0.9 mm of the planned positions, whereas free-hand placement resulted in deviations of approximately 2 to 3 mm.

Anatomic Considerations

To avoid damage to the IAN, the clinician must have a thorough understanding of the normal versus variant anatomy of the posterior mandible.

Inferior Alveolar Canal

Inferior-Superior Plane

There is a common belief that the vertical position of the IAN is relatively constant within the mandible. Normally the IAN runs a concave path from posterior to anterior, with anterior terminal segments exiting the mental foramen (mental nerve) and a branch that ascends to the midline of the mandible (incisive nerve). However, numerous anatomic studies have confirmed the

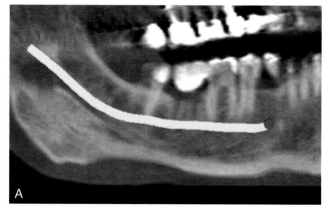

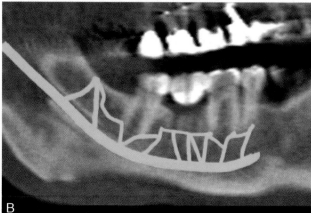

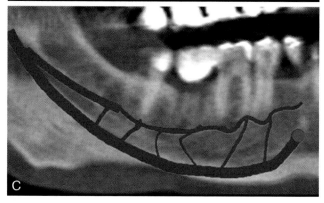

• **Fig. 30.23** Inferior Alveolar Nerve (Inferior-Superior Plane). (A) Type 1 (high): positioned close to tooth apex. (B) Type 2 (intermediate): most common position within the middle of the mandible. (C) Type 3 (low): positioned in the inferior border of the mandible.

inferior-superior (vertical) positions of the IAN are not consistent.[47,48] An early classification of the vertical positions of the course of the alveolar nerve was reported by Carter and Keen.[49] They described three distinct types: (1) in close approximation to the apices of the teeth, (2) a large nerve approximately in the middle of the mandible with individual nerves supplying the mandibular teeth, and (3) a nerve trunk close to the inferior cortical plate with large plexuses to the mandibular teeth. In type 1 nerves, impairment is common because of the close proximity to the nerve bundle. Three percent of patients can have the IAN directly contacting one or both of the roots of the mandibular first molar.[50] It is highly recommended that a comprehensive radiographic survey be completed to evaluate the IAN in a vertical plane, especially with type 1 and 2 nerves (Fig. 30.23). Juodzbalys et al.[51] categorized the inferior-superior positioning as either: (1)

high, within 2 mm of teeth apices; (2) intermediate; or (3) low. Heasman[52] reported that 68% of patients exhibit an intermediate zone path of the IAN canal, with an average distance of 3.5 to 5.4 mm from the first and second molar roots.

Buccal-Lingual Plane

Studies have shown the buccal-lingual location of the IAN as it progresses anteriorly is not constant. The nerve paths have been described in a buccal-lingual direction with a high degree of variability and are dependent on the amount of bone resorption, as well as age and race variables.[53]

Kim et al.[54] evaluated and classified the buccolingual IAN location into three types: type 1, IAN canal is in close proximity to the lingual plate (~70%); type 2, IAN canal follows the middle of the ramus from the second molars to first molars (~15%); and type 3, IAN canal follows the middle or lingual thirds of the mandible from the ramus to the body (~15%).

In addition, older and Caucasian patient groups have shown less distance between the buccal aspect of the nerve and the inferior border of the mandible. Other studies have shown the most common area for the IAN to be in the middle of the buccal and lingual cortical plates is the first molar region.[55] Thus, in the buccal-lingual plane, the IAN is highly variable, therefore 3D cross-sectional images should be used to determine the true position of the nerve (Fig. 30.24).

Mental Foramen

Determining the exact location of the mental foramen is crucial when placing implants in the posterior mandible. Although the foramen has been thought to be symmetric to the contralateral side in most patients, the location has been shown to be highly variable.[56] The mental nerve passes through the mental foramen with three to four nerve branches that exit with an average diameter of 1 mm.[57] This nerve will innervate the skin of the mental area, and the other two proceed to innervate the skin of the lower lip, mucous membranes, and the gingiva as far posteriorly as the second premolar. Any trauma to this nerve may result in neurosensory impairment in this area.

The size, shape, location, and opening angulation of the mental foramen are variable. Usually the mental nerve exits the mental foramen from the mental canal. The mental canal is most commonly angled in a superior direction from the mandibular canal (i.e., average is approximately 50 degrees, with a range from 11 to 70 degrees).[58] The size of the mental foramen in the literature has been reported to range from 2.5 to 5.5 mm. The most common shape is ovoid (~65%) and round (~23%).[59]

The positioning of the mental foramen is also extremely variable in the vertical and horizontal planes. Clinically there are many different techniques in identifying the foramen, with a wide variation of predictability.

Visualization of the Mental Nerve

Two-dimensional Radiographs. Studies have shown that in more than 50% of periapical and panoramic radiographs the mental foramen is not in the location depicted on the 2D image.[60] Conventional 2D radiography should never be used as the sole diagnostic modality in evaluating the foramen position (Fig. 30.25).

Three-dimensional Radiography. The literature has shown that 3D imaging is the most accurate diagnostic tool to ascertain the exact location of the mental foramen. CBCT panoramic and cross-sectional images, together with 3D images, are the easiest

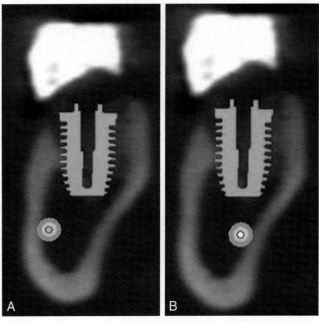

• **Fig. 30.24** Buccal-Lingual Inferior Alveolar Nerve Canal Position. The position in the buccal-lingual position is variable: (A) buccal positioned; (B) lingual positioned.

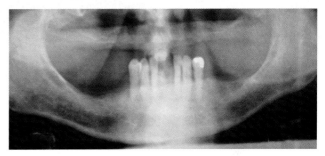

• **Fig. 30.25** Two-dimensional radiograph that has been shown to depict the true location of the mental foramen only 50% of the time.

and most accurate techniques in determining the exact foramen location (Fig. 30.26).[61]

Palpation. In rare cases the clinician may be able to palpate the location of the mental foramen. Most notably, when bone resorption has caused the nerve to be exposed on the residual ridge, the concavity formed by the exposure of the nerve can be determined. In these cases the location of the mental foramen may be marked with a surgical pen. When the nerve is located on the buccal surface of the mandible, the palpation method of identification has very low utility.

Anatomic Eandmarks. In the literature, many authors have postulated that landmarks such as teeth and mandibular bony areas may help identify the location of the mental foramen. With respect to teeth, the location cannot conclusively be associated with a particular tooth (e.g., first premolar, second premolar, between apices of the premolars) because studies have shown the location to be dependent on gender, age, and race.[62] In addition, patients exhibit different types of facial and skeletal growth, along with orthodontic factors that make dentition landmarks completely inaccurate. Numerous studies have shown a high correlation between mental foramen location and race. However, most of these studies associate the location of the mental foramen with a specific tooth[63-66] (Fig. 30.27).

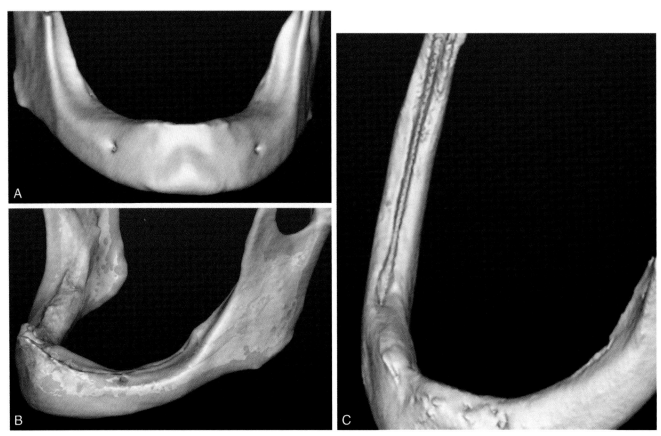

• **Fig. 30.26** (A and B) Cone beam computed tomographic three-dimensional image showing true position and size of mental foramen. (C) Complete dehiscence of mandibular canal.

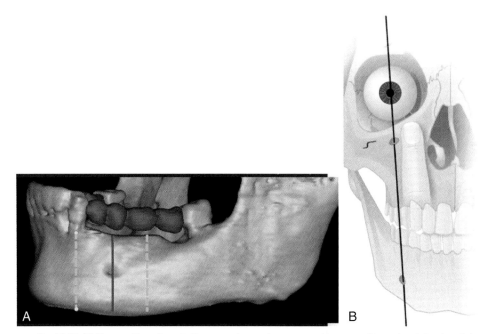

• **Fig. 30.27** (A) The position of mental foramen does not correspond to a specific anatomic landmark (e.g., first premolar, second premolar). The mental foramen may be positioned as far anterior as the cuspid and as far posterior as the first molar. (B) In the literature a vertical line drawn from the pupil of the eye and infra-orbital foramen will be in close approximation to the mental foramen. However, this technique has inherent inaccuracies because many patients have different skeletal relationships.

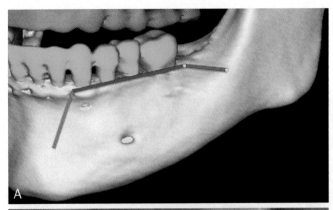

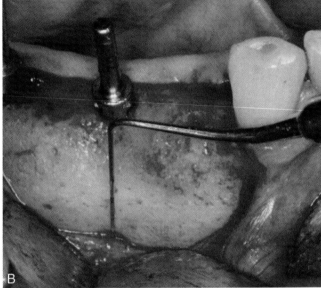

● **Fig. 30.28** (A) Incision outline to expose foramen consists of a crestal incision to the mesial of the canine and distal of the molar, with an anterior and a posterior vertical release incision. (B) After foramen exposure the height of available bone may be determined.

Direct Evaluation. The most precise technique available today to determine the exact location of the mental foramen is by direct evaluation. Exposing the mental foramen may be intimidating to some clinicians, especially early on their learning curve. This can be accomplished with very low morbidity; however, the technique's success depends on the clinician's training and experience.

Technique to Expose Mental Foramen

1. Crestal incision is made from the canine position (mesial) to the first molar position, with vertical 45-degree release incisions anterior and posterior (Fig. 30.28).
2. Full-thickness reflection is completed below the mucogingival junction: A moist 4 × 4 gauze is placed over the index finger, and the flap is elevated apically until the superior aspect of the foramen is located (Fig. 30.29).
3. The gauze may be used anterior and posterior to the foramen to confirm the foramen location.
4. Once the foramen is located, a periodontal probe may be used to measure the ridge height. The implant length is usually 2 mm less than the measured distance.

Three-dimensional Ultrasound. The most promising imaging technique for the future is ultrasound. Ultrasound has the advantage of no ionizing radiation and the ability to reconstruct 3D images of bone surfaces to within an accuracy level of 24 μm. At this time, ultrasound units are not available specifically for dental use.[67]

Mental Nerve Variants

Accessory and Double Foramen. Studies have shown that in approximately 6.62% to 12.5% of patients, an accessory foramen is present.[68,69] In the majority of cases, small accessory foramina usually contain a small branch of the mental nerve or a nutrient branch that supplies the teeth. These are usually not problematic because of cross-innervation or actually contain nutrient branches and no sensory fibers to the soft tissue. Accessory foramens are usually radiographically differentiated from a double foramen in the accessory foramen, which will be seen on a CBCT as a very small foramen, usually anterior to the larger main mental foramen.

However, in a small percentage of cases, a larger branch of the mental nerve (equal or larger-size foramen) may exit the second mental foramen, which is termed a *double foramen.* Special care should be extended in this situation because it may contain components of one of the three branches of the mental nerve. Accessory foramina are believed to be the result of early branching of the IAN, before exiting the mental foramen during the 12th week of gestation.[70] Double foramens are easily seen in 3D images, or the coronal CBCT images are depicted as two larger size foramens, often being of the same size (Fig. 30.30).

Anterior Loops of the Mental Nerve. As the mental nerve proceeds anteriorly in the mandible, it sometimes runs inferior and anterior to the mental foramen. This anterior and caudal component of the mental nerve will curve cranially back to the mental foramen and is termed the *anterior loop.*[71] Recently, CBCT and dissection studies have shown a rather high (70%) prevalence rate of anterior loops, with a mean of 1.16 mm distance anteriorly. The anterior loop may be depicted most predictably on axial CBCT images, with 2D radiographs being totally unreliable.

Determining the presence of an anterior loop is critical when placing implants anterior to the mental foramen. Inability to ascertain the presence of an anterior loop may result in damage to the mental nerve (Fig. 30.31). The anterior loop measurement should be added to the safe zone to avoid damaging the mental nerve. For example, if a 1.0-mm anterior loop is present, then the safety zone should be calculated to be 3.0 mm (1.0 mm anterior loop + 2.0 mm safety zone).

Incisive Nerve Branch. The incisive nerve branch, a continuation and terminal branch of the IAN, supplies the mandibular canine and incisor teeth, and is seen as a radiolucent canal in the anterior mandible. The canal is most commonly present in the middle third of the mandible and narrows toward the midline, reaching the midline only 18% of the time.[72] The incisive nerve is often mistaken for an anterior loop in the mandible. Because there is no soft tissue sensory component to this nerve, implants may be placed in proximity to it without nerve impairment. Studies have shown incisive canals have a mean diameter of 1.8 mm and location 9.7 mm from the lower cortical border.[73] The incisive nerve has been recognized as an important anatomic structure that must be taken into consideration when performing surgery in this area. Excessive bleeding has been reported as a significant intraoperative complication in this area when it is perforated during osteotomy preparation (Fig. 30.32). However, this is usually remedied by placing the implant, direction indicator, or surgical bur into the osteotomy site.

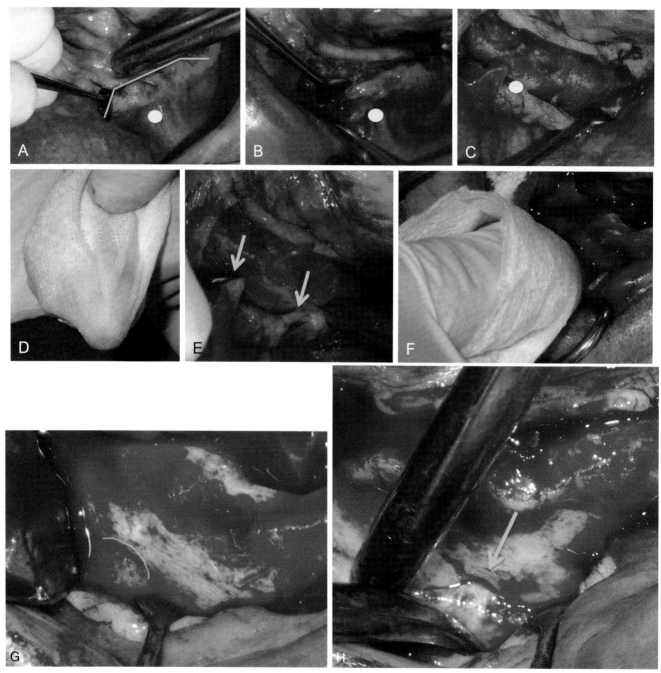

● **Fig. 30.29** Exposure of the Mental Foramen. (A) General incision outline with mental foramen high-lighted in yellow. (B) Anterior full-thickness reflection. (C) Posterior full-thickness reflection. (D) Moist 4 × 4 gauze placed over index finger. (E) Tissue anterior and posterior (green arrows) is reflected apically with gauze. (F) Tissue reflected apically with gauze. (G) Superior margin of foramen identified. (H) Verification of exposed foramen.

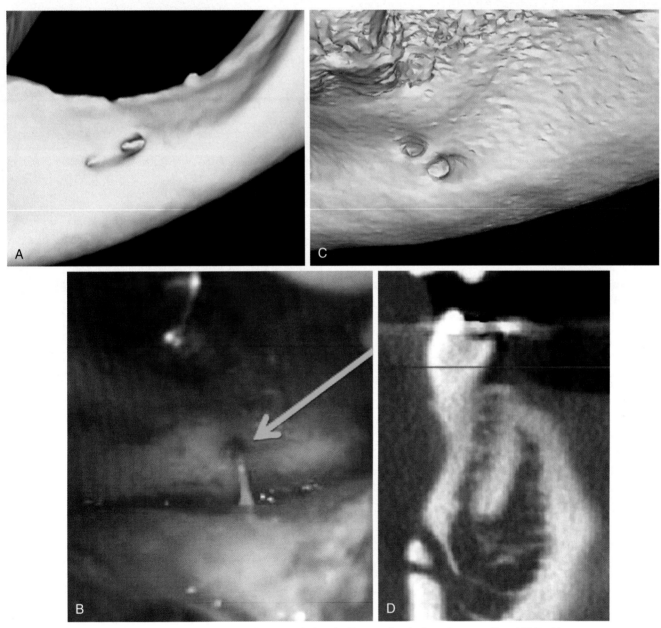

• **Fig. 30.30** (A and B) Accessory foramen, depicted with a small and a large foramen. (C and D) Double foramen, depicted with two large foramina.

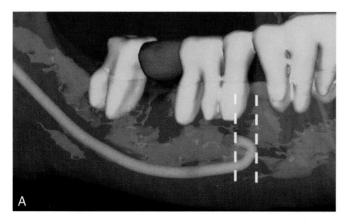

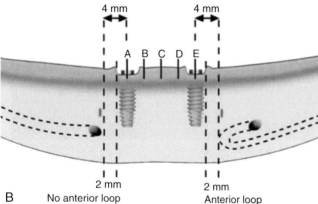

- **Fig. 30.31** Anterior Loop. (A) Anterior loop of mental nerve that is consistent with the mental nerve anterior to the mental foramen. (B) The anterior loop measurement should be added to the 2-mm safety zone to ensure adequate space between the implant and the foramen.

Surgical Principles to Decrease Neurosensory Complications

Safety Zone

A 2-mm safety zone with osteotomy preparation and final implant placement is paramount in preventing neurosensory impairments.[74] Therefore the final implant position should always maintain a minimum distance of 2 mm from the IAN canal. Compression-related injuries (neuropraxia) can occur by encroaching on the IAN without actual contact. Nerve impairments have been reported when implants are placed less than 2 mm from the canal without actual invasion of the canal.

Bleeding and resultant hematomas have been shown to cause nerve damage because of final positioning of the implant too close to the neurovascular canal.[75] In addition, the IAN superior cortical bone can be compressed, causing pressure necrosis with resultant nerve impairment.[76] Interactive treatment planning software programs allow the implant clinician to accurately assess the ideal placement with respect to this vital structure (Fig. 30.33).

Always Take Into Account the Y Dimension of the Implant Burs

Care should always be exercised in knowing the exact drilling depth when performing osteotomies over vital structures, especially in the posterior mandible. The implant clinician should double-check the marking depth on the burs before initiating the osteotomy. The principle of "measure twice, drill once" should be followed to prevent iatrogenic overpreparation of the implant site.

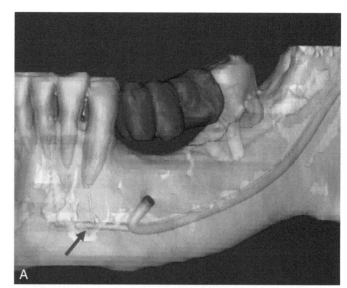

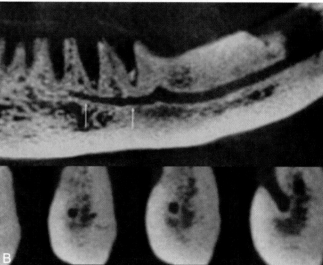

- **Fig. 30.32** Incisive Nerve. (A) Three-dimensional image depicting the incisive nerve, which is the second terminal branch of the inferior alveolar nerve. (B) Cone beam computed tomographic panoramic and cross-sectional images showing the incisive nerve canal (green arrows).

In addition, the Y dimension of the implant system being used must be known. With many implant surgical systems, the depth of the millimeter lines inscribed on surgical drills do not always coincide with the actual depth of the drill. Most drills contain a V-shaped apical portion designed for cutting efficiency (Y dimension). Usually the wider the drill, the greater the Y dimension. The implant clinician should always evaluate the manufacturer's drill length with respect to the length of the implant before performing the osteotomy. If this concept is not adhered to, overpreparation of the site may occur, resulting in nerve damage (Fig. 30.34).

Use Drill Stop Burs to Prevent Overpreparation

An additional technique to prevent overpreparation of the osteotomy site is the use of stop drills. These drills have a predetermined depth marking that prevents overpreparation. Stop drills are beneficial in the mandibular posterior area, especially when visibility and access are compromised. Generic drill stop kits are also available that may be used with most implant surgical systems (Salvin Dental Corp.). These autoclavable, reusable kits

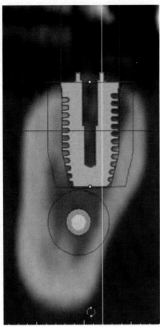

• **Fig. 30.33** Safety Zone. A 2-mm safety zone should always be present between the implant and the inferior alveolar canal.

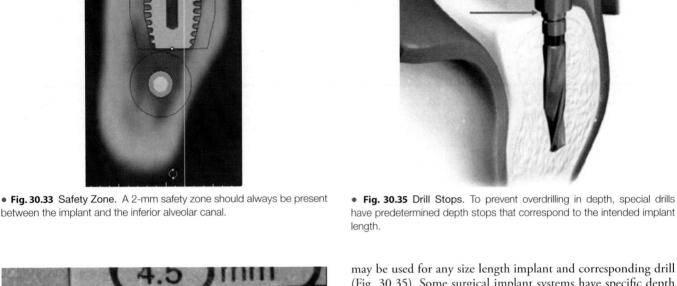

• **Fig. 30.35** Drill Stops. To prevent overdrilling in depth, special drills have predetermined depth stops that correspond to the intended implant length.

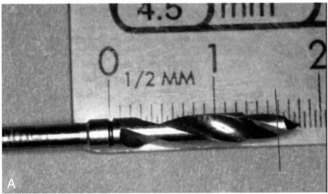

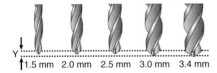

Drill diameter	Y dimension
1.5 mm	0.43 mm
2.0 mm	0.58 mm
2.5 mm	0.74 mm
3.0 mm	0.86 mm
3.2 mm	0.94 mm
3.4 mm	0.99 mm
3.7 mm	1.07 mm
4.0 mm	1.17 mm
4.2 mm	1.22 mm
4.4 mm	1.27 mm
4.7 mm	1.35 mm

B

• **Fig. 30.34** "Y" Dimension. (A) All surgical drills have an inherent Y dimension, which results in a greater drill length to each drill. (B) Y dimension increases as the surgical drills increase in size.

may be used for any size length implant and corresponding drill (Fig. 30.35). Some surgical implant systems have specific depth burs that coincide with the actual implant depth (e.g., Hahn Implants; Glidewell Corp.).

Understand Bony Crest Anatomy

Due to resultant bone resorption after extraction, the alveolar ridge becomes compromised in width (Division B bone) at the expense of the buccal plate. When measuring available bone height, special consideration should be given to the final location of the superior aspect of the implant platform, not the existing crest of the ridge. It will often appear there is adequate vertical height for implant placement; however, when the osteotomy is initiated, the thin crest will be lost (i.e., because the diameter of the drill exceeds the width of the bone) and the implant will be placed inferior to where it was originally intended. This can lead to unexpected depth drilling and an implant that is placed too close to the vital structure. The clinician should either augment the ridge to maintain vertical height or reduce the height calculation by the amount of osteotomy-induced osteoplasty (Fig. 30.36).

Maintain Total Control of the Handpiece

When performing osteotomies in the posterior mandible, special care should be noted to maintain complete control of the surgical handpiece. Large marrow spaces (i.e., where there is a lack of or thin trabecular bone) are often present, which may allow the osteotomy site to become deeper than intended. This will result in the implant being placed more apically, leading to neurosensory impairment. A CBCT comprehensive evaluation allows the implant dentist to view the bone quality before surgery. Most software programs associated with CBCT units allow the clinician to ascertain the density in the intended site. The implant clinician may also determine the bone density by tactile sensation when drilling. In addition, when drilling the osteotomy near the mental foramen, care should be exercised not to bend the wrist. This can

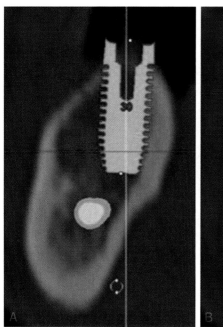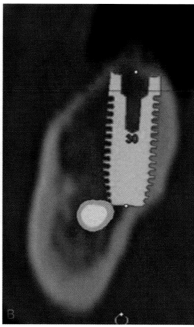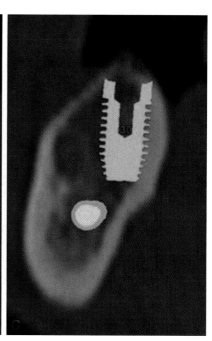

• **Fig. 30.36** Division B Ridge. (A) Incorrect measurement from superior crest to inferior alveolar nerve (IAN) canal. (B) Because the thin crest was not taken into consideration, implant placement will lead to encroachment of the IAN canal. (C) Ideal selection of implant length and positioning.

potentially redirect the drill or implant placement in an unwanted direction (e.g., near the mental foramen, into a tooth root). Surgical templates and guides are beneficial in preventing this malpositioning complication.

Do Not Place Bone Graft Material in Close Approximation to Nerve

After tooth extractions, especially in the mandibular premolar areas, care should be exercised in placing bone graft material (autologous, allogenic, xenogenic) in direct contact with an exposed IAN. Whether socket grafting or in conjunction with implant placement, case studies have shown resultant neurosensory impairment from bone graft material causing compression, crushing, or chemical burn injuries.[77] When grafting sockets with an exposed IAN canal, excessive pressure should be avoided. In addition, a small piece of fast resorbing collagen (e.g., OraTape, OraPlug) may be placed before the addition of grafting material. This will decrease the chance of particulate graft being in direct approximation to the nerve canal (Fig. 30.37).

Use Copious Amounts of Irrigation

Overheating the bone during osteotomy preparation may produce thermal stimuli that may lead to peri-implant necrosis and secondary postoperative nerve damage. Neural tissue is extremely sensitive and may be damaged by heat stimuli. The thickness of the necrotic area is proportional to the amount of heat generated during preparation.[78] The implant dentist must be cautious not to overheat the bone. This can be minimized by "bone dancing," which involves drilling in short intervals and allowing irrigation to enter the osteotomy, preventing heat generation. In addition, new (sharp) and intermediate-size drill burs may be used to reduce heat generation. This is more crucial with harder bone density (e.g., D1 or D2) or bone with compromised vascularity.

Avoid Incision-Related Injuries

Avoid incision-related injuries when making incisions in close approximation to the mental foramen and associated nerve structures in the posterior mandible. In cases of severe bone atrophy the presence of nerve dehiscence may inadvertently result in a transected nerve during the initial incision (i.e., making the incision on the crest of the ridge). Anatomic landmarks, 3D models, accurate measurements from CBCT scan, and palpation of the nerves are ways to avoid this complication. In addition, incisions in the posterior of the oral cavity should never be made over the retromolar pad. This can result in possible injury to the lingual nerve, which in 10% of cases transects this area[79] (Fig. 30.38).

Avoid Flap/Retraction–Related Injuries

Neurosensory impairments may also occur from overzealous use or incorrect placement of retractors. Broad-base (not sharp) retractors should be used to retract tissue that is not directly over the mental foramen because excessive stretching of the nerve trunk may cause irreversible damage. It is imperative that the mental foramen and associated branches of the mental nerve be identified in this area when placing retractors. Retractors should always be placed and held on the bone to prevent slippage or excessive soft tissue pressure, which can lead to a neuropraxia type of nerve damage (Fig. 30.39). Excessive stretching of the tissue may also lead to neurosensory impairments. It has been shown the perineurium protects the fascicles; however, if greater than 30% elongation of the nerve occurs, structural damage will occur to the nerve fibers.[80]

Use Special Care When Releasing Periosteum Over Mental Foramen

It is a common procedure during closure after implant placement or bone grafting to stretch the periosteal tissue to allow primary and "tension-free" closure.

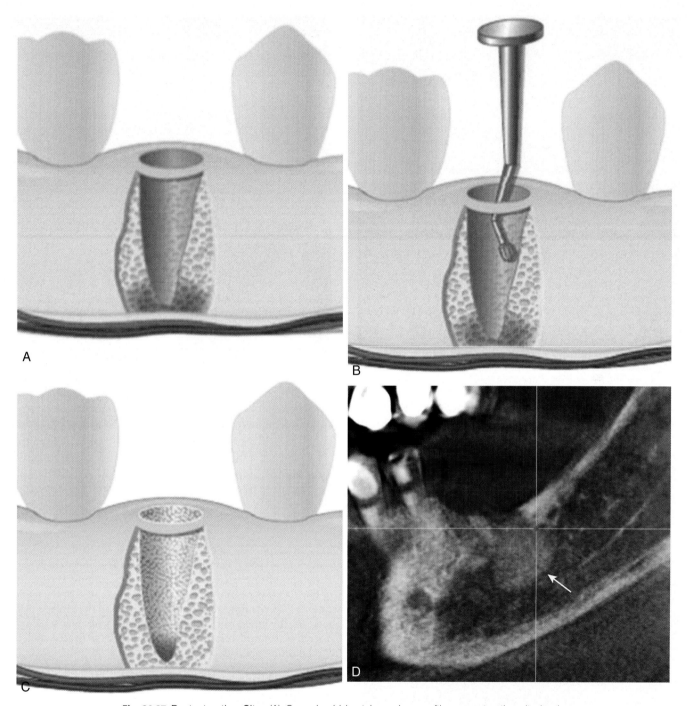

• **Fig. 30.37** Postextraction Site. (A) Care should be taken when grafting an extraction site in close approximation to the inferior alveolar nerve. (B) A curette should be used with caution because direct damage to the nerve may occur. (C) Grafting in close approximation to the canal may lead to nerve trauma. (D) Bone graft material placed into an extraction socket resulting in a nerve impairment.

Various techniques are used to "release" the tissue to improve vascularization of the incision line and adhesion of the margins to prevent incision line opening. The submucosal technique developed by Misch in 1988 is an effective method to expand the tissue. This procedure involves the use of a #15 scalpel blade and soft tissue scissors (i.e., Metzenbaum) to create a blunt dissection. Knowledge of the location of the three mental nerve branches is necessary because inadvertent incisions over the mental nerve branches may result in neurotmesis (transection) types of nerve injuries (Fig. 30.40).

Careful Suturing

When the mental nerve is exposed, care should be exercised to prevent nerve tissue from being entrapped within the sutures. The mental nerve emerges from the mental foramen and divides into three branches below the depressor anguli oris muscle. Caution must be exercised to prevent any of the mental nerve branches from becoming entrapped within the suture material, potentially causing a neuropraxia (compression) type of nerve injury. In addition, nerve fibers may be damaged from the passage of the extremely sharp suture needle through the tissue.

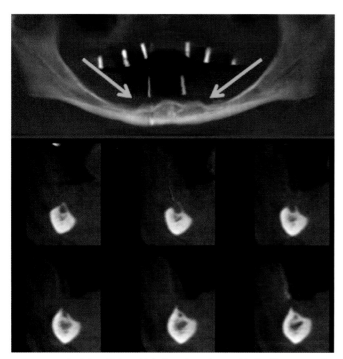

• **Fig. 30.38 Incision-Related Injuries.** In patients with significant mandibular atrophy and dehiscence of the nerve canal, possible incision-related injuries may result. The incision should be modified to avoid exposed nerves by extending to the lingual when approaching the exposed nerves.

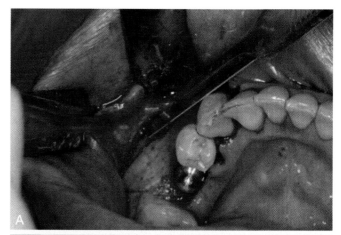

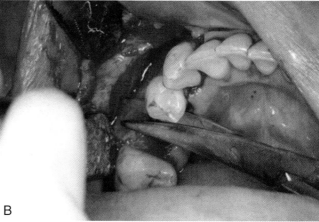

• **Fig. 30.40** (A and B) Periosteal release incision (A) and blunt dissection (B) should never be completed in close approximation to the mandibular nerve.

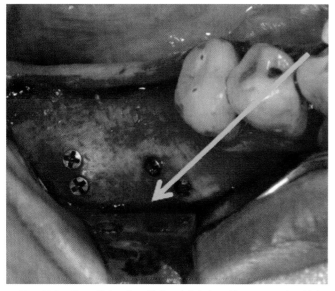

• **Fig. 30.39 Flap Retraction–Related Injuries.** Retractors should be carefully positioned to avoid stretching or damaging the inferior alveolar nerve.

Verify Correct Positioning of CBCT SurgiGuides

Studies have shown that the most precise and accurate surgical templates are tooth supported. When using bone- or tissue-supported surgical guides, care must be exercised to correctly position the guide because an error in placement may result in direct damage to the IAN. Tooth-supported guides should always be the first choice if possible because they are clinically proven to give rise to the fewest positioning errors. The least accurate is the

mucosa supported, which are usually used for flapless surgery.[66] Studies have shown that flapless surgical guides consistently show deviations of implant positions from ideal locations. Perforations of the buccal plate can be found in more than 50% of the flapless cases.[81] A very minor discrepancy (anteroposterior) in the placement of the guide can lead to impingement on vital structures. Therefore surgical templates should always be fixated and the ideal position verified.

Surgical Procedures That Increase Neurosensory Complications

Immediate Implants in the Mandibular Premolar Area

Immediate implants have gained overwhelming popularity in implant dentistry today. Extreme caution must be exercised when extracting and immediately placing implants in the mandibular premolar area. As noted earlier, many variables dictate the position of the mental foramen, with the foramen being highly variable. Studies have shown that 25% to 38% of the time the mental foramen is superior to the premolars apex.[82] Because most immediate implant osteotomy sites involve drilling the osteotomy site deeper for stability (~2–4.0 mm), the odds of nerve trauma are greatly increased. Because of this the implant clinician must be very selective in cases involving extraction and immediate implant placement in this anatomic area (Fig. 30.41).

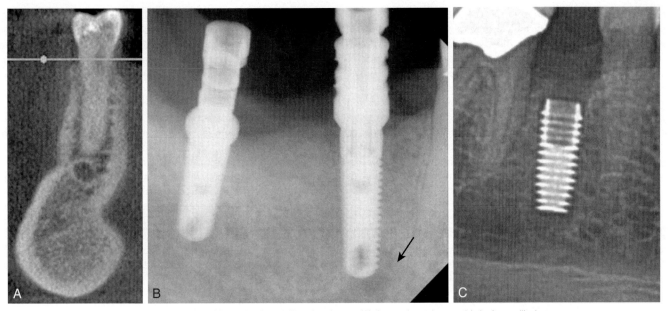

• **Fig. 30.41** Mandibular Premolar Immediate Implants. (A) Approximately one-third of mandibular premolars root apexes are inferior to the mental foramen. (B and C) Implant placement into the mental foramina leading to neurosensory impairment.

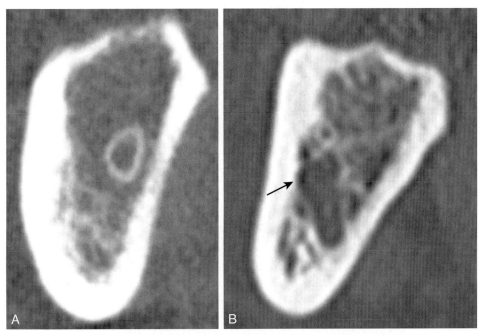

• **Fig. 30.42** Superior Cortical Plate of Inferior Alveolar Nerve (IAN) Canal. (A) Mandibular canal with thick cortical plate, which is uncommon. (B) Thin to no cortical bone is present over the IAN canal.

Drill Until the Superior Cortical Plate Is "Felt"

It has been advocated in the literature that the osteotomy depth may be determined by "feeling" the superior cortical plate of the inferior alveolar canal. A 2-mm safety zone should always be adhered to because research has shown that in approximately 28% of posterior mandibles there is no superior cortical plate over the inferior alveolar canal.[83] In addition, studies have shown it to be impossible to use tactile sense to ascertain the presence of superior cortical bone surrounding the mandibular canal. Clinical reports have revealed hemorrhage into the canal, or bone fragments may

cause compression or ischemia of the nerve from engaging the superior cortical plate. Dependence on the ability to "feel" the superior cortical plate through tactile sense increases the likelihood of nerve complications (Fig. 30.42).

Infiltration Technique

An alternative technique in placing implants in the posterior mandible is not using mandibular nerve block anesthesia. Instead, infiltration is accomplished in the soft tissue surrounding the osteotomy site, and the patient is asked to alert the implant clinician on the proximity of the drill to the nerve bundle.[84] This alternative technique results in a very high degree of subjectivity concerning patients' responses, because of varying degrees of pain thresholds. In addition, disadvantages of this surgical method include inconsistent mandibular nerve anatomy, with varying locations of dental-alveolar nerve branches. With the success of CBCT radiography in implant dentistry today in determining the exact location of the IAN, this technique should be avoided because of the high degree of false-negative and false-positive results from patients. Etoz et al.[85] showed this supraperiosteal infiltration technique to be safe in 91% of cases. However, according to this study, approximately 1 patient in 10 ended up with a neurosensory deficit.

Placing Implants Lingual to the Inferior Alveolar Nerve Canal or Foramen

Many authors have advocated placing implants lingual to the neurovascular bundle (Kumar; Stellar). As stated previously, the buccal-lingual nerve position within the mandible is extremely variable, along with the incidence and trajectory of lingual osseous concavities.

Attempting to place implants buccal or lingual to the inferior alveolar canal or mental foramen is associated with a high degree of morbidity, even with the use of CBCT-guided surgery. In addition, perforation of the cortical plate can occur, which may lead to sublingual bleeding or formation of a sublingual hematoma (Fig. 30.43).

Place Implants at the Depth of the Adjacent Root Apexes

Many implant clinicians use the location and length of the adjacent teeth as a guide in determining the size (length) of the implant to be placed. Usually a Panorex or periapical radiograph is used in determination of this length. When this technique is used in anatomic type 2 or 3 (i.e., more apically positioned in the vertical dimension) nerve courses, the incidence of nerve impairment is low. However, in mandibles that exhibit a type 1 nerve course (close to root apex), close approximation of the implant to the canal is likely, leading to a higher probability of neurosensory impairment. Ideally the implant clinician should ascertain the available bone above the mandibular canal via 3D radiographic analysis (Fig. 30.44).

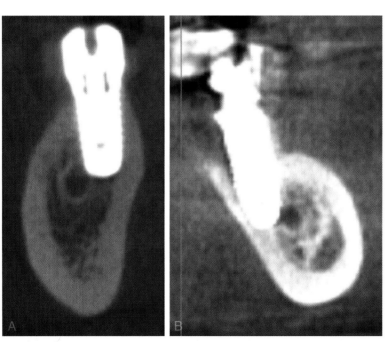

• **Fig. 30.43** Lingual Placed Implant. (A and B) Implants should never be placed lingual to the inferior alveolar nerve canal because nerve injury or perforation of the lingual plate may occur.

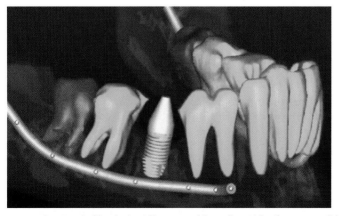

• **Fig. 30.44** In type 1 nerves, placement of implants at the apex of the adjacent tooth may result in direct nerve trauma.

"As Long as There Is Not Excessive Bleeding, the Mandibular Canal Has Not Been Violated"

Another unconventional technique in avoiding nerve impairment is the evaluation of the amount of bleeding from the osteotomy site. Many practitioners correlate the amount of hemorrhage with the proximity of the neurovascular bundle (IAN, artery, vein, and lymphatic vessels). Anatomic studies have shown that the inferior alveolar artery may lie parallel to the nerve and lingual as it traverses anteriorly. Its position varies with respect to the IAN within the mandibular canal. Other studies show the inferior alveolar artery appears to be solitary and lies superior and lingual to the IAN, slightly above the horizontal position.[86] In addition, there exist multiple inferior alveolar veins positioned superior to the nerve, which may cause venous oozing if directly traumatized. A false-positive result may occur if this area is damaged because large marrow spaces, which can cause excessive bleeding, are common in the posterior mandible (D3 bone). The degree of bleeding should not be used as an indication of nerve proximity or violation of the mandibular canal.

Replacing Second Molars

There are many prosthetic and surgical disadvantages when evaluating edentulous, second mandibular molar sites for implant placement. Disadvantages include high incidence of sublingual bony undercuts, which can result in perforation of the lingual plate or angulation issues, decreased interocclusal space (especially with supraeruption of the adjacent tooth), difficult access for surgery and prosthetic component insertion, and the fact that there is 10% greater occlusal force on the second molar versus the first molar. Function is not a primary reason for replacement because 90% of masticatory efficiency is generated anterior to the mesial half of the mandibular first molar, and cheek biting is more common in this area because of the proximity of the buccinators muscle. One of the most important disadvantages is the close approximation of the mandibular canal in the second molar area, which leads to difficulty in placement of implants in this area. When implants are placed, usually the available bone present is compromised in height. As a result the second molar is often not replaced when the only posterior teeth missing are the second and third molars. The primary disadvantage of not replacing the second molar is extrusion of the opposing maxillary second molar. If extrusion is a significant concern, a full-coverage crown on the mandibular first molar may include occlusal contact with the mesial marginal ridge of the maxillary second molar (Fig. 30.45).

Nerve Repositioning

Treatment of patients who exhibit compromised alveolar crest height in the posterior mandibular area can be very challenging. Techniques include the use of shorter implants, which become biomechanically compromised, or the use of bone grafting to increase available bone for future implant placement. An alternative technique is to reposition the IAN laterally, either by nerve lateralization or nerve transposition. In nerve lateralization the IAN is exposed and retracted laterally while the dental implants are placed. The transposition technique, first published in 1987 by Jensen and Nock,[87] includes the mental foramen in the osteotomy, resulting in the IAN being positioned more posterior. The inherent risk with these complex procedures is neurosensory impairment (anesthesia, paresthesia, or dysesthesia) to the mental nerve branch. Although this is a valid treatment option in significantly atrophied cases, this technique should be reserved for practitioners with advanced training and experience with these procedures (Fig. 30.46).

Conclusion

Prior to implant or bone grafting procedures in the mandible, a careful and detailed clinical and radiographic evaluation is paramount to identify vital structures in the mandible. The use of cone beam computed tomography is essential to determine the location of normal and variant anatomic structures such as bone undercuts, poor bone density, extreme bony angulation, blood vessels, and the mandibular canal and mental foramen. The complications that may result can range from very minor issues to life

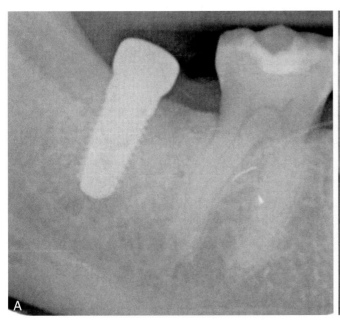
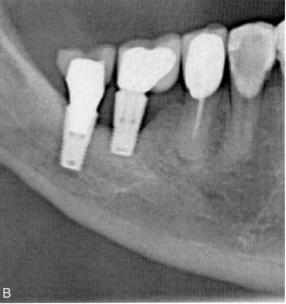

• **Fig. 30.45** Second Molar Implants. (A and B) Implants in the second molar region have a high incidence of nerve trauma because of the location of the mandibular nerve in relation to the second molar implant site.

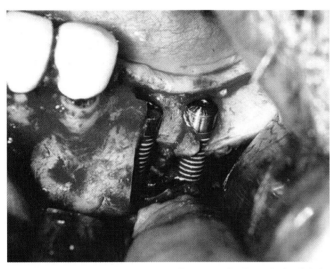

• **Fig. 30.46 Nerve Repositioning.** The repositioning of the inferior alveolar nerve should be completed only by experienced clinicians with advanced training in the technique.

threatening circumstances. Therefore, the clinician must understand the possible sequalae and management if violation of one of these mandibular vital structures is compromised.

References

1. Wright DMD, Roberta A. *An Analysis of Anterior Mandibular Anatomy Using Cone Beam Computed Tomography: A Study of Dentate and Edentulous Mandibles*; 2016.
2. Butura CC, Galindo DF, Cottam J, Adams M, Jensen O. Hourglass mandibular anatomic variant incidence and treatment considerations for all-on-four implant therapy: report of 10 cases. *J Oral Maxillofacial Surg*. 2011;69(8):2135–2143.
3. Greenstein G, Cavallaro J, Tarnow D. Practical application of anatomy for the dental implant surgeon. *J Periodontol*. 2008;79(10):1833–1846.
4. Butura CC, Galindo DF, Cottam J, Adams M, Jensen O. Hourglass mandibular anatomic variant incidence and treatment considerations for all-on-four implant therapy: report of 10 cases. *J Oral Maxillofacial Surg*. 2011;69(8):2135–2143.
5. Kalpidis CD, Anthony B. Konstantinidis. Critical hemorrhage in the floor of the mouth during implant placement in the first mandibular premolar position: a case report. *Implant Dentistry*. 2005;14(2):117–124.
6. Rosano G, Taschieri S, Gaudy Jean François, Testori T, Del Fabbro M. Anatomic assessment of the anterior mandible and relative hemorrhage risk in implant dentistry: a cadaveric study. *Clinical Oral Implants Res*. 2009;20(8):791–795.
7. Sheikhi M, Mosavat F, Ahmadi A. Assessing the anatomical variations of lingual foramen and its bony canals with CBCT taken from 102 patients in Isfahan. *Dental Res J*. 2012;9(suppl 1):S45.
8. Babiuc IULIANA, Tarlungeanu I, Mihaela P. Cone beam computed tomography observations of the lingual foramina and their bony canals in the median region of the mandible. *Rom J Morphol Embryol*. 2011;52(3):827–879.
9. Gahleitner A, Hofschneider U, et al. Lingual vascular canals of the mandible: evaluation with dental CT. *Radiology*. 2001;220(1):186–189.
10. Babiuc IULIANA, Tarlungeanu I, Mihaela P. Cone beam computed tomography observations of the lingual foramina and their bony canals in the median region of the mandible. *Rom J Morphol Embryol*. 2011;52(3):827–879.
11. Kirsch A, Ackermann KL. The IMZ osteointegrated implant system. *Dent Clin North Am*. 1989;33:733–791.
12. Warrer K, Buser D, Lang NP, et al. Plaque-induced periimplantitis in the presence or absence of keratinized mucosa: an experimental study in monkeys. *Clin Oral Implants Res*. 1995;6:131–138.
13. Listgarten M, Lang NP, Schroeder HE, et al. Periodontal tissues and their counterparts around endosseous implants. *Clin Oral Implants Res*. 1991;2:81–90.
14. Pietrokovski J, Ruth S, Arensburg B, Kaffe I. Morphologic characteristics of bony edentulous jaws. *J Prosthodontics*. 2007;16(2):141–147.
15. Nishimura I, Hosokawa R, Atwood DA. The knive-edge tendency in mandibular residual ridges in women. *J Prosthetic Dentistry*. 1992;67(6):820–826.
16. Felice P, Checchi V, Pistilli R, Scarano A, Pellegrino G, Esposito M. Bone augmentation versus 5-mm dental implants in posterior atrophic jaws. Four-month post-loading results from a randomized controlled clinical trial. *Eur J Oral Implantol*. 2009;2:267–281.
17. Simion M, Jovanovic SA, Tinti C, Benfenati SP. Long-term evaluation of osseointegrated implants inserted at the time or after vertical ridge augmentation. A retrospective study on 123 implants with 1–5 year follow-up. *Clin Oral Implants Res*. 2001;12:35–45.
18. Simion M, Dahlin C, Rocchietta I, Stavropoulos A, Sanchez R, Karring T. Vertical ridge augmentation with guided bone regeneration in association with dental implants: an experimental study in dogs. *Clin Oral Implants Res*. 2007;18:86–94.
19. Rocchietta I, Fontana F, Simion M. Clinical outcomes of vertical bone augmentation to enable dental implant placement: a systematic review. *J Clin Periodontol*. 2008;35(suppl):203–215.
20. Amine M, Guelzim Y, Benfaida S, Bennani A, Andoh A. Short implants (5–8 mm) vs. long implants in augmented bone and their impact on peri-implant bone in maxilla and/or mandible: systematic review. *J Stomatol, Oral Maxillofacial Surg*. 2018.
21. Thoma DS, Cha JK, Jung UW. Treatment concepts for the posterior maxilla and mandible: short implants versus long implants in augmented bone. *J Periodontal Implant Sci*. 2017;47(1):2–12.
22. Gates GN, Nicholls JI. Evaluation of mandibular arch width change. *J Prosthet Dent*. 1981;46:385.
23. Grant AA. Some aspects of mandibular movement: acceleration and horizontal distortion. *Ann Acad Med Singap*. 1986;15:305.
24. Gates GN, Nicholls JI. Evaluation of mandibular arch width change. *J Prosthet Dent*. 1981;46:385.
25. Meijer HJA, Starmans FJM, Steen WHA, et al. A comparison of three finite element models of an edentulous mandible provided with implants. *J Oral Rehab*. 1993;20:147.
26. Gregory M, Murphy WM, Scott J, et al. A clinical study of the Branmark dental implant system. *Br Dent J*. 1995;168:18.
27. Hylander WL. The human mandible: lever or link? *Am J Phys Anthropol*. 1975;43:227–242.
28. Osborne J, Tomlin HR. Medial convergence of the mandible. *Br Dent J*. 1964;117:112–114.
29. De Marco TJ, Paine S. Mandibular dimensional change. *J Prosthet Dent*. 1974;31:482–485.
30. Hylander WL. Mandibular function in Galago crassicaudatus and macaca fascicularis: an in vivo approach to stress analysis of the mandible. *J Morphol*. 1979;159:253–296.
31. Abdel-Latif HH, Hobkirk JA, Kelleway JP. Functional mandibular deformation in edentulous subjects treated with dental implants. *Int J Prosthodont (IJP)*. 2000;13:513–519.
32. Parnia F, Fard EM, Mahboub F, Hafezeqoran A, Gavgani FE. Tomographic volume evaluation of submandibular fossa in patients requiring dental implants. *Oral Surg Oral Med Oral Pathol Oral Radiol Endod*. 2010;109:e32–e36.
33. Nickenig HJ, Wichmann M, Eitner S, Zöller JE. Matthias Kreppel. "Lingual concavities in the mandible: a morphological study using cross-sectional analysis determined by CBCT. *J Cranio-Maxillofacial Surg*. 2015;43(2):254–259.

34. Chan HL., Brooks SL, et al. "Cross–sectional analysis of the mandibular lingual concavity using cone beam computed tomography. *Clinical Oral Implants Res.* 2011;22(2):201–206.

35. Chan HL, Brooks SL, Fu JH, Yeh CY, Rudek I, Wang HL. Cross-sectional analysis of the mandibular lingual concavity using cone beam computed tomography. *Clin Oral Implants Res.* 2011;22:201–206.

36. Leong DJ, Chan HL, Yeh CY, Takarakis N, Fu JH, Wang HL. Risk of lingual plate perforation during implant placement in the posterior mandible: a human cadaver study. *Implant Dent.* 2011;20:360–363.

37. de Souza, Azevedo L, et al. Assessment of mandibular posterior regional landmarks using cone-beam computed tomography in dental implant surgery. *Ann Anat.* 2016;205:53–59.

38. Behnia H, Kheradvar A, Shahrokhi M. An anatomic study of the lingual nerve in the third molar region. *J Oral Maxillofacial Surg.* 2000;58(6):649–651.

39. Pogrel MA, Goldman KE. Lingual flap retraction for third molar removal. *J Oral Maxillofacial Surg.* 2004;62(9):1125–1130.

40. Yosue T, Brooks SL. The appearance of mental foramina on panoramic and periapical radiographs. II. Experimental evaluation. *Oral Surg Oral Med Oral Pathol.* 1989;68:488–492.

41. Schropp L, Wenzel A, Kostopoulos L. Impact of conventional tomography on prediction of the appropriate implant size. *Oral Surg Oral Med Oral Pathol Oral Radiol Endod.* 2001;92:458–463.

42. Yilmaz Z, et al. A survey of the opinion and experience of UK dentists: Part 1: the incidence and cause of iatrogenic trigeminal nerve injuries related to dental implant surgery. *Implant Dent.* 2016;25(5):638–645.

43. Pinchi V, et al. Analysis of professional malpractice claims in implant dentistry in Italy from insurance company technical reports, 2006 to 2010. *Int J Oral Maxillofac Implants.* 2014;29:1177–1184.

44. Ylikontiola L. Comparison of three radiographic methods used to locate the mandibular canal in the buccolingual direction before bilateral sagittal split osteotomy. *Oral Surg Oral Med Oral Pathol Oral Radiol Endod.* 2002;93:736–742.

45. Fortin T, Bosson JL, Coudert JL, Isidori M. Reliability of preoperative planning of an image-guided system for oral implant placement based on 3-dimensional images: an in vivo study. *Int J Oral Maxillofac Implants.* 2003;18:886–893.

46. Nickenig HJ, et al. Evaluation of the difference in accuracy between implant placement by virtual planning data and surgical guide templates versus the conventional free-hand method—a combined in vivo–in vitro technique using cone-beam CT (Part II). *J Cranio-Maxillofacial Surg.* 2010;38(7):488–493.

47. Anderson LC, Kosinski TF. A review of the intraosseous course of the nerves of the mandible. *J Oral Implantol.* 1991;17:394–403.

48. Narayana K, Vasudha S. Intraosseous course of the inferior alveolar (dental) nerve and its relative position in the mandible. *Indian J Dent Res.* 2004;15:99–102.

49. Carter RB, Keen EN. The intramandibular course of the inferior dental nerve. *J Anat.* 1971;108(Pt 3):433–440.

50. Simonton JD. Age- and gender-related differences in the position of the inferior alveolar nerve by using cone beam computed tomography. *J Endod.* 2009;35:944–949.

51. Juodzbalys G, Wang HL, Sabalys G. Anatomy of mandibular vital structures. Part I: mandibular canal and inferior alveolar neurovascular bundle in relation with dental implantology. *J Oral Maxillofacial Research.* 2010;1(1).

52. Heasman PA. Variation in the position of the inferior dental canal and its significance to restorative dentistry. *J Dentistry.* 1988;16(1):36–39.

53. Kim ST, Hu KS, Song WC, et al. Location of the mandibular canal and the topography of its neurovascular structures. *J Craniofac Surg.* 2009;20:936–939.

54. Kim ST, Hu KS, et al. Location of the mandibular canal and the topography of its neurovascular structures. *J Craniofacial Surgery.* 2009;20(3):936–939.

55. Miller CS, Nummikoski PV, Barnett DA, Langlais RP. Cross-sectional tomography. A diagnostic technique for determining the buccolingual relationship of impacted mandibular third molars and the inferior alveolar neurovascular bundle. *Oral Surg Oral Med Oral Pathol.* 1990;70:791–797.

56. Narayana K, Vasudha S. Intraosseous course of the inferior alveolar (dental) nerve and its relative position in the mandible. *Indian J Dent Res.* 2004;15:99–102.

57. Mraiwa N, Jacobs R, Daniel van Steenberghe, Quirynen M. Clinical assessment and surgical implications of anatomic challenges in the anterior mandible. *Clini Implant Dentistry Related Res.* 2003;5(4):219–225.

58. Solar P, Ulm C, Frey G, Matejka M. A classification of the intraosseous paths of the mental nerve. *Int J Oral Maxillofacial Implants.* 1994;9(3).

59. Gershenson A, Nathan H, Luchansky E. Mental foramen and mental nerve: changes with age. *Acta Anat.* 1986;126(1):21–28.

60. Yosue T, Brooks SL. The appearance of mental foramina on panoramic and periapical radiographs. II. Experimental evaluation. *Oral Surg Oral Med Oral Pathol.* 1989;68:488–492.

61. Beshtawi KR. *The Accuracy of the Mental Foramen Position on Panoramic Radiographs and CBCT*; 2017.

62. Juodzbalys G, Wang HL, Sabalys G. Anatomy of mandibular vital structures. Part II: mandibular incisive canal, mental foramen and associated neurovascular bundles in relation with dental implantology. *J Oral Maxillofac Res.* 2010;1:e3.

63. Fishel D, Buchner A, Hershkowith A, Kaffe I. Roentgenologic study of the mental foramen. *Oral Surg Oral Med Oral Pathol.* 1976;41(5):682–686.

64. Wang TM, Shih C, Liu JC, Kuo KJ. A clinical and anatomical study of the location of the mental foramen in adult Chinese mandibles. *Acta Anat.* 1986;126(1):29–33.

65. Shankland 2nd WE. The position of the mental foramen in Asian Indians. *J Oral Implantol.* 1994;20(2):118–123.

66. al Jasser NM, Nwoku AL. Radiographic study of the mental foramen in a selected Saudi population. *Dentomaxillofac Radiol.* 1998;27(6):341–343.

67. Tsui BCH. Ultrasound imaging to localize foramina for superficial trigeminal nerve block. *Can J Anaesth.* 2009;56(9):704–706.

68. Shankland WE 2nd. The position of the mental foramen in Asian Indians. *J Oral Implantol.* 1994;20:118–123.

69. Haghanifar S, Rokouei M. Radiographic evaluation of the mental foramen in a selected Iranian population. *Indian J Dental Res.* 2009;20:150–152.

70. Apostolakis D, Brown JE. The anterior loop of the inferior alveolar nerve: prevalence, measurement of its length and a recommendation for interforaminal implant installation based on cone beam CT imaging. *Clin Oral Implants Res.* 2012;23:1022–1030.

71. Apostolakis D, Brown JE. The anterior loop of the inferior alveolar nerve: prevalence, measurement of its length and a recommendation for interforaminal implant installation based on cone beam CT imaging. *Clin Oral Implants Res.* 2012;23:1022–1030.

72. Mraiwa N, Jacobs R, Moerman P, Lambrichts I, Daniel van Steenberghe, Quirynen M. Presence and course of the incisive canal in the human mandibular interforaminal region: two-dimensional imaging versus anatomical observations. *Surg Radiol Anat.* 2003;25(5–6):416–423.

73. Mraiwa N, Jacobs R, Moerman P, et al. Presence and course of the incisive canal in the human mandibular interforaminal region: two-dimensional imaging versus anatomical observations. *Surg Radiol Anat.* 2003;25:416–423.

74. Misch CE, ed. *Contemporary Implant Dentistry*. St Louis: Mosby; 2008.

75. Lamas Pelayo J, Peñarrocha Diago M, Martí Bowen E, Peñarrocha Diago M. Intraoperative complications during oral implantology. *Med Oral Patol Oral Cir Buca.* 2008;13:E239–E243.

76. Khawaja N, Renton T. Case studies on implant removal influencing the resolution of inferior alveolar nerve injury. *Br Dent J.* 2009;206: 365–370.

77. Bagheri SC, Meyer RA. Management of mandibular nerve injuries from dental implants. *Atlas Oral Maxillofac Surg Clin North Am.* 2011;19:47–61.

78. Tehemar SH. Factors affecting heat generation during implant site preparation: a review of biologic observations and future considerations. *Int J Oral Maxillofac Implants.* 1999;14:127–136.

79. Mendes, Marcelo Breno Meneses, Carla Maria de Carvalho Leite Leal, Maria Cândida de Almeida Lopes Nunes. Anatomical relationship of lingual nerve to the region of mandibular third molar. *J Oral Maxillofacial Res.* 2013;4(4).

80. Hubbard JH. The quality of nerve regeneration. Factors independent of the most skillful repair. *Surg Clin North Am.* 1972;52(5): 1099–1105.

81. Van de Velde T, Glor F, De Bruyn H. A model study on flapless implant placement by clinicians with a different experience level in implant surgery. *Clin Oral Implants Res.* 2008;19:66–72.

82. Juodzbalys G, Wang HL, Sabalys G. Anatomy of mandibular vital structures. Part II: mandibular incisive canal, mental foramen and associated neurovascular bundles in relation with dental implantology. *J Oral Maxillofac Res.* 2010;1:e3.

83. Khawaja N, Renton T. Case studies on implant removal influencing the resolution of inferior alveolar nerve injury. *Br Dent J.* 2009;206:365–370.

84. Heller AA, Shankland II WE. Alternative to the inferior alveolar nerve block anesthesia when placing mandibular dental implants posterior to the mental foramen. *J Oral Implantol.* 2001;27: 127–133.

85. Etoz OA, Er N, Demirbas AE. Is supraperiosteal infiltration anesthesia safe enough to prevent inferior alveolar nerve during posterior mandibular implant surgery? *Med Oral Patol Oral Cir Bucal.* 2011;16(3):e386–e390.

86. de Oliveira-Santos C, Rubira-Bullen IR, Monteiro SA, et al. Neurovascular anatomical variations in the anterior palate observed on CBCT images. *Clin Oral Implants Res.* 2013;24:1044–1048.

87. Jensen O, Nock D. Inferior alveolar nerve repositioning in conjunction with placement of osseointegrated implants: a case report. *Oral Surg Oral Med Oral Pathol.* 1987;63:263–268.

31
Dental Implant Complications

RANDOLPH R. RESNIK

In implant dentistry today, most procedures are completed free of complications. However, complications do occur and may have devastating, long-lasting effects for the patient and the clinician. Ideally the clinician should have a strong understanding of surgical and prosthetic implant principles, which minimizes the possibility of complications. However, even if the clinician follows the most strict and predictable protocols, unexpected situations may occur. Therefore this chapter provides a comprehensive summary of the etiology, prevention, and management of possible complications resulting from the treatment planning, intra-operative, post-operative, and maintenance situations.

Intraoperative Complications

Malpositioned Initial Osteotomy Site

In performing the initial osteotomy for a dental implant, in some cases the initial implant position may not be placed in the ideal location. The osteotomy may need to be repositioned to allow for ideal placement. The use of a Lindemann bur (i.e., side-cutting fissure bur) is ideal for the repositioning of an osteotomy because of its side-cutting capabilities. Lindemann burs allow for easy and efficient positional change with minimal trauma to the bone.

Once the initial osteotomy is prepared, it is assessed for proper position with a direction indicator. If nonideal placement occurs, the osteotomy site may need to be "stretched" or repositioned to a more ideal location.

Prevention

Surgical templates or implant-positioning devices for ideal implant positioning should be used to prevent the improper placement of the initial osteotomy. A pilot surgical guide (i.e., guide that allows only for the drilling of the first pilot drill) can be used for the clinician to obtain the accurate mesial-distal and buccal-lingual position of the osteotomy site. This is especially useful for decreasing the possibility of malpositioning for clinicians who are early on their learning cure.

Treatment

The use of conventional drills (non-side-cutting) is difficult to horizontally reposition an osteotomy site because of the end-cutting capabilities of the burs. The use of a side-cutting Lindemann bur will allow for repositioning to a new, corrected site. It is imperative the new osteotomy position should be deepened so that subsequent end-cutting drills will not reposition back into the original osteotomy site.

However, when using the Lindemann bur, always use copious amounts of saline because this bur will generate a significant amount of trauma and heat to the bone[1] (Fig. 31.1).

Facial Dehiscence After Implant Placement

After implant placement, it is not uncommon to have facial plate dehiscence on the buccal aspect of the implant, usually in the crestal area. Because bone resorbs from the facial to lingual, in some cases after implant placement, less than 2.0 mm of facial bone is present. A minimum of 2.0 mm of bone is recommended to maintain ideal hard and soft tissue surrounding the implant. If the implant is allowed to heal with a known facial dehiscence, the implant will be more susceptible to peri-implant disease and increased implant morbidity.

Ridges that are compromised (i.e., Division B, C, or D) should be modified to obtain a Division A bone (e.g., >7 mm width and >10 mm of bone height) before osteotomy initiation. This may be accomplished by either osteoplasty or lateral bone augmentation. After implant placement, a minimum of 2.0 mm of facial bone should be present over the implant or the compromised facial area should be grafted.

Treatment

After implant placement, if there exists less than 2.0 mm of bone on the facial aspect of the ridge, the site may be grafted with autogenous bone (ideally). The autogenous bone is most easily obtained from bone fragments gathered from the flutes of the surgical drills during the osteotomy preparation. The consistency of this bone allows for ease of packing, and the graft will have less chance of migrating. Ideally, the autogenous bone should be red or white colored as this signifies live, viable bone. If the bone fragments are black or brown, the bone should be discarded as it is most likely necrotic. Allograft bone is not the most ideal bone to graft in this area as it tends to migrate easily after placement and is an added expense (Fig. 31.2).

Loss of Facial Plate When Placing an Implant

When placing implants in bone that is compromised in width (i.e., Division B bone), it is not uncommon to fracture or lose the facial plate of the supporting bone. This leads to a compromise in the healing of the implant and the longevity of the implant and final prosthesis.

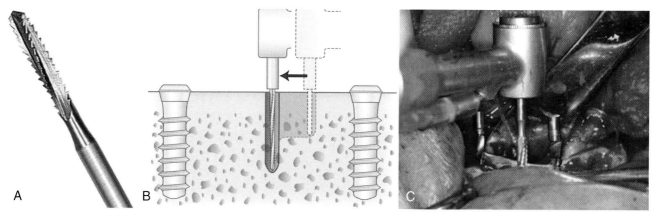

• **Fig. 31.1** Repositioning Osteotomy Site. (A) Side-cutting Lindeman bur. (B) Use of a Lindeman bur to reposition the osteotomy should always deepen the new osteotomy site because this will prevent subsequent burs from falling into the original site. (C) Clinical image of repositioning osteotomy more distal.

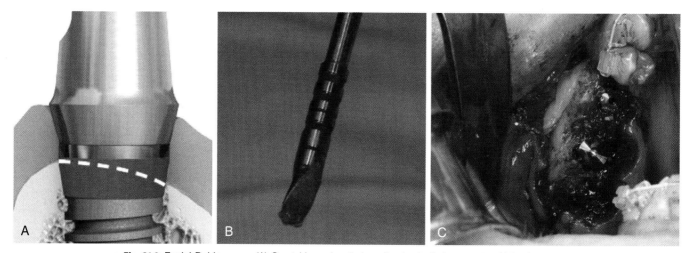

• **Fig. 31.2** Facial Dehiscence. (A) Crestal bone is missing after implant placement, which often occurs because of buccal and lingual crestal height discrepancies. (B) Autogenous bone fragments within the bur flutes. (C) Grafting after implant placement.

Prevention

Ideally the width of bone needs to exceed 7.0 mm for placement of a 4.0-mm diameter implant. When compromised width of bone exists, the trauma of the osteotomy or the placement of the implant may fracture or "pop off" the buccal plate. This is most likely the result of the buccal plate being thinner than the lingual plate, which results in the facial plate being more fragile and susceptible to fracture (Fig. 31.3).

The available bone before implant placement should be evaluated via a cone beam computed tomography (CBCT) examination. If nonideal width of bone is present, site development, including grafting, is indicated to obtain a Division A bone. The osteotomy preparation should be in one plane, and care should be exercised not to deviate from the original angulation. If Division B bone is present, ridge augmentation is recommended to achieve a Division A ridge before implant placement.

Treatment

After implant placement, if a fracture or loss of the buccal plate exists, treatment will depend on the extent of the deficit.

Loss of Entire Buccal Plate. If the entire buccal plate is lost or if mobility of the implant exists, the ideal treatment should include removing the implant, followed by grafting the site. After sufficient healing occurs, implant placement may be completed.

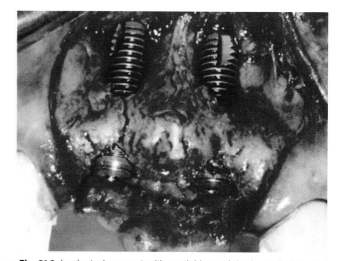

• **Fig. 31.3** Implant placement with partial loss of the buccal plate. Note the fractures present in the host bone.

Partial Buccal Plate Still Intact. If no mobility of the implant is present and the facial plate is partially intact, the facial area can be grafted, ideally with autogenous bone from the osteotomy site (e.g., bone from the surgical drill).

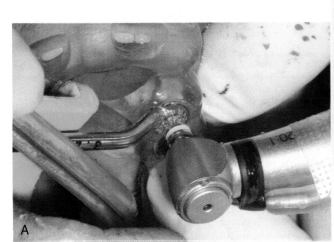
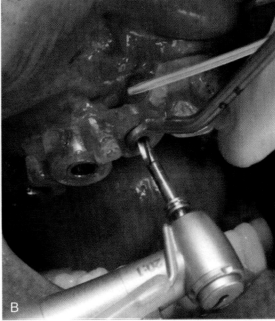

● **Fig. 31.4** Overheating of the osteotomy site often occurs when using a surgical template. (A) With most surgical templates, minimal irrigation enters the osteotomy site. (B) Ideally supplemental irrigation can be used to decrease heat generation. Note the modification of the template which allows for external irrigation.

Overheating the Bone

One of the most common complications that has been associated with early implant failure and bone loss is overheating of the bone during the osteotomy preparation. This is usually the result of osteotomy preparation in dense bone with a nonideal surgical osteotomy protocol. The Misch osteotomy preparation protocol has been developed to minimize heat generation in D1 and D2 bone density types. Bone tissue has been shown to be very susceptible to thermal related injuries, with studies showing the temperature threshold to be 47 °C for tissue survival when drilling is maintained for more than 60 seconds. If heat generation is higher than this limit, then osseointegration is in question because of the resulting necrosis of the surrounding bone cells.[2] In addition, resultant hyperemia, fibrosis, osteocytic degeneration and increased osteoclast activity may occur which may lead to a necrotic zone around the implant.[3]

Prevention

Intermediate Burs. In addition to the surgical protocol, multiple intermediate drills may be used in the drilling protocol (See Chapter 27). A decrease in the heat and trauma generated is seen when gradual increases in drill diameter are used. This technique reduces the amount of pressure and heat transmitted to the bone, especially in the presence of dense and thick cortical bone.

Copious Amounts of Saline. Together with external irrigation from the surgical drills, increased irrigation may be obtained by using internal irrigation (through the surgical bur) or with supplemental irrigation via a syringe. In addition, the use of chilled saline allows for a significant reduction of heat generation.

Bone Dance. The bone-dancing technique was introduced by Misch in 1988 to reduce the amount of heat generation. When preparing the osteotomy, small increments of bone are removed by using an up-and-down motion of the drill. This will allow increased irrigation into the osteotomy, along with removing bone fragments, which decreases frictional heat.

Use of Sharp, New Drills. Drills that are dull will increase heat generation, causing the possibility of overheating the bone. Surgical drills should be replaced approximately every 20 to 30 autoclave cycles; however, this is highly dependent on past use.

Drill Speed. Sharawy et al.[4] have shown the drill speed in hard, dense bone (e.g. D1 and D2 bone types) should be approximately 2000 to 2500 rpm. Osteotomy preparation at higher speeds with sharp drills elicits less risk for osseous damage and a decreased amount of devitalized zone adjacent to the implant. Yeniyol et al.[5] have shown that drilling at very slow speeds results in a higher degree of bone fragmentation. However, in poorer bone density, lower speed (e.g., ~1000 rpm) may be used with little concern for overheating the bone.

Surgical Templates. Surgical templates often result in overheating of the bone because of the inability of saline to enter the osteotomy because of the minimal space between the guide tubes in the template and the drill size. Ideally the template should be modified to open up the facial aspect of the template so supplemental irrigation may be used (Fig. 31.4).

Treatment

If known excess heat generation occurs during implant placement, ideally the implant should be removed, regional acceleratory phenomenon (RAP) initiated, and the site grafted for future implant placement. If bone width is available after sufficient RAP is completed, a wider implant may be placed.

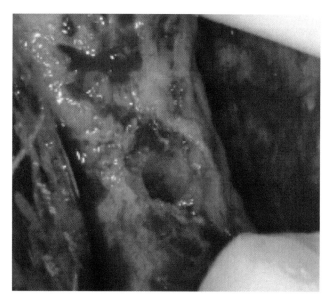

• **Fig. 31.5** Overheating the bone from improper surgical drilling protocol; note the lack of bleeding from the osteotomy site.

Implant Pressure Necrosis

When placing implants in bone with thick cortical components (i.e., D1 and D2 bone), possible early implant failure may occur from pressure necrosis. Numerous studies have shown that the overcompression of the crestal bone is a contributing factor in peri-implant disease and implant failure.[6] It is suggested that excessive tightening of the implant creates compression forces within the crestal bone around the implant. This may impair the microcirculation and lead to bone resorption.

Pressure necrosis from implant placement may increase the devital zone of bone around the implant, or even cause short-term neurosensory impairment when the implant site is in the vicinity of the mandibular canal. This most often occurs where there exists a cortical component of bone in the crestal region (~D1–D2 bone). If a crestal bone drill is not used or surgical steps to alleviate the internal stresses are not completed, excess stress will be generated on insertion of the implant, which will lead to "die-back" or a devitalized zone (Fig. 31.5).

Prevention

Torque. The implant should not be "tightened" into the osteotomy with excessive torque pressure. A torque value of 35 N-cm is considered safe with most threaded implant designs. If excessive pressure is present, the implant should be unscrewed 3 to 4 mm and then reinserted.

Crestal Bone Bur. Because most implants have a wider crest module (wider diameter of the neck of the implant in comparison with the implant body), greater stress can be concentrated upon placement in D1 and D2 types of bone. To decrease crestal pressure, a crestal bone bur can be used to minimize the stress at the ridge crest.

Use of Insertion Wrench. To decrease the crestal stress, the implant may be inserted with a hand ratchet to depth, then unthreaded 3 to 4 mm, and then reinserted to ideal depth. By unscrewing the implant 3 to 4 mm, the bone is given time to "creep," which on reinsertion, will have less force at the crestal region.

Treatment

Ideally the thickness of crestal bone and bone quality type should be ascertained before implant osteotomy preparation. This may be determined via a CBCT radiographic examination.

If a large cortical component of bone is present and the implant placed is known to contain excess pressure, the implant should be removed and the crestal bone modified. The implant then should be reinserted at a lower insertion torque.

Injury to Adjacent Teeth

Damaging adjacent natural teeth during dental implant placement may lead to adverse effects on adjacent tooth structures and can result in dental implant failure or adjacent tooth loss. The injury to the root structure of adjacent teeth may be direct (i.e., damage to tooth by the drill or implant) or indirect (i.e., thermal damage from the osteotomy process). The direct trauma may result in bone loss, natural tooth or implant loss, infection, internal or external resorption, loss of tooth vitality, or prosthetic failure.

Trauma to adjacent teeth may occur upon the placement of dental implants because of poor surgical technique including improper angulation, implant sites with insufficient available space or bone quantity, or placement of implants with an incorrect diameter. Dilacerated roots and excessive tilting of natural teeth in the mesiodistal direction may impinge on the intended implant space and prevent ideal placement. In addition, available space discrepancies often exist between the coronal space and the apical space. Studies of orthodontic mini-implants placed in contact with teeth (<1.0 mm) have been shown to cause root resorption. However, if the implant is removed in a timely fashion, cementum repair may occur.[7]

Prevention

The location of adjacent teeth to the implant site should be evaluated before implant placement. This is most accurately determined by evaluating CBCT images, usually in the axial plane. Accurate spacing is easily determined by measuring the intertooth distance. The angulation should always be evaluated after the initial osteotomy with a direction indicator (i.e., radiograph with known diameter and length guide pin in osteotomy) to assess proper positioning and angulation. CBCT surgical templates may be used to avoid damaging adjacent root surfaces. Ideally a minimum of 1.5 mm of space between the implant and root surface is recommended.

Treatment

Perioperative. If after placement of the dental implant, it appears the implant is too close (<1.5 mm) from the periodontal ligament or tooth structure, ideally it should be removed and repositioned. If the implant is removed and another is inserted, care should be exercised to verify adequate primary stability. If primary stability is not obtained, then an implant with a larger diameter or length may be inserted. If that is not feasible, then the osteotomy site should be grafted and implant placement delayed.

Postoperative/Post-healing. If the implant has been previously placed and is asymptomatic and not encroaching on the periodontal ligament/tooth structure, strict monitoring should be completed on a regular basis, with vitality testing of the adjacent teeth. If the adjacent tooth is sensitive to thermal stimulation or percussion, the implant should be removed immediately (Fig. 31.6).

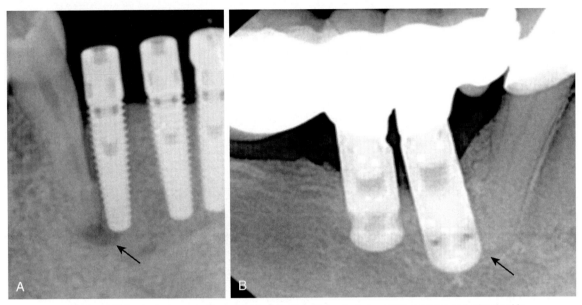

• **Fig. 31.6** (A) Implant placement too close to a tooth root; implant should be removed and reinserted in a more ideal position. (B) Implant that was placed many years ago should be closely monitored clinically and radiographically.

Swallowing/Aspiration of Implant Components

Because of the nature of dental implant procedures, the aspiration or ingestion of dental components or materials may occur. Accidental inhalation of dental instruments (drills, burs, direction indicators, root tips, crowns, etc.) can result in many complications, including life-threatening situations. Because of the small size of abutments, screws, drivers, and other implant components, a significant risk for the implant clinician exists. This may occur during any dental implant procedure, including the surgical and prosthetic phases.

There is usually two possibilities: the patient may swallow the foreign object into the stomach or aspirate the foreign object into the lungs.

Swallow: If the object is swallowed, usually the patient will be asymptomatic. However, depending on the shape and size of the object, it may need to be removed because of the complication of blockage within the gastrointestinal system.

Aspiration: The object may be aspirated into the lungs, in which case the patient will usually be symptomatic. The patient will exhibit signs of coughing, wheezing, hoarseness, choking, stridor, or cyanosis. The patient will often complain of pain and discomfort.

Prevention

Various techniques are available for the implant clinician to prevent aspiration or swallowing of a foreign object. There is no one technique that will guarantee this complication will be avoided; however, extreme caution should always be exercised.

Techniques to prevent swallowing or aspiration include:
- Floss ligatures to all implant components.
- Use of special prosthetic instruments (e.g., EasyReach Wrench; Salvin Dental).
- Use throat packs (4 × 4 gauze) or pharyngeal screens.
- Utilize high-vacuum suction.
- Use curved hemostats for retrieval of objects.

Treatment

When swallowing or aspiration of implant components occurs, the clinician must act proactively to avoid complications and medicolegal issues. First, if an instrument is lost in the mouth, the patient should be instructed not to sit straight up because this will ensure the swallowing or aspiration of the instrument. The patient should turn to the side and attempt to "cough" the instrument up. If the instrument is lost, symptoms usually will determine whether aspiration into the lungs or swallowing into the stomach has occurred. If the instrument has been swallowed into the stomach, usually the patient will exhibit no symptoms. If the patient has aspirated the instrument, this will most likely be accompanied with coughing, wheezing, pain, and cyanosis. This may be life-threatening and should be treated accordingly as a medical emergency. In all swallowing/aspiration situations the patient should be referred immediately to his or her physician or emergency room for a chest x-ray. If the instrument has been aspirated, it will usually be located in the right bronchus because the right main bronchus has a more acute angle than the left. Rigid bronchoscopy is usually used for the removal of the instrument under general anesthesia (Fig. 31.7).

Air Emphysema

Because of the attachment apparatus difference between implants and teeth, air extruded into the sulcular area around implants may lead to air emphysema. Subcutaneous emphysema is a condition in which air is introduced into the subcutaneous or fascial spaces. The two most common ways for this to occur is the use of an air-driven handpiece or an air-water syringe in which air is forced into the sulcular area. Symptoms will include swelling that increases over time, with a "crackling" feeling with pain. Crepitus to palpation will confirm the diagnosis of air emphysema. The patient will usually be apprehensive, with a feeling of difficulty in breathing.

Subcutaneous air emphysema can lead to many devastating complications during and after dental implant surgery. Early recognition and management of this condition is crucial to preventing

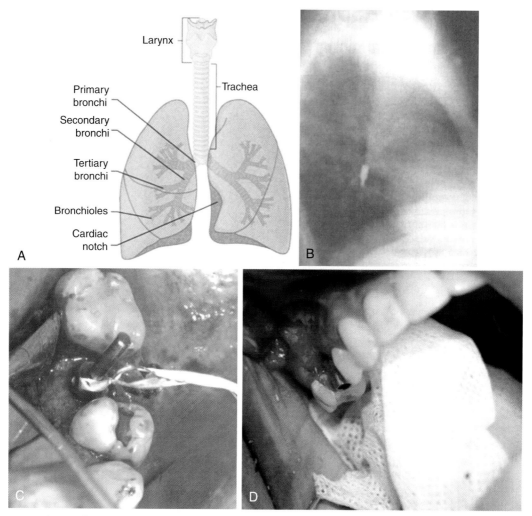

• **Fig. 31.7** Aspiration of Foreign Bodies. (A) Pulmonary system anatomy. (B) Implant driver lodged in the right bronchus. (C) Floss should be tied to all implant components to minimize aspiration. (D) Use a 4 × 4 throat pack; never use a 2 × 2 pack because the patient can easily swallow it.

progression of the problem. As the air accumulates subcutaneously, dissection occurs along the connective tissue that joins the adjacent muscle planes. Via the fascial spaces, air from the oral cavity may extend into the mediastinum space, where it can communicate with parapharyngeal and retropharyngeal spaces, which leads to airway compromise. From the retropharyngeal space, air may lead into the pleural space and pericardium, which could result in heart and lung failure.

Prevention

When placing implants, modifying abutments in the oral cavity, or removing bone around an implant body, an electric handpiece should always be used (i.e., never use an air-driven handpiece). In addition, air-water syringes should never be used to place air into the sulcular area parallel to the long axis of the implant.

Treatment

Usually symptoms arise immediately; however, cases have been described in the literature that have occurred minutes to hours after a procedure. Patients with significant emphysema should be monitored closely before discharge, for respiratory or cardiac distress. Treatment should include supportive therapy with heat and analgesics. Antibiotic therapy should always be administered because infection may result from bacteria being induced into the

fascial spaces, with resultant cellulitis or necrotizing fascitis. Resolution usually occurs in 4 to 7 days, with minimal morbidity. In isolated cases, exploratory surgery, emergency tracheotomy, and the placement of chest tubes have been reported (Fig. 31.8).[8]

Electric Handpiece Burns

Electric handpieces, the most common type of handpiece used in implant dentistry today, have a tendency to overheat, which may result in significant soft tissue complications. In 2007 and 2010, the U.S. Food and Drug Administration (FDA) released warnings to health professionals concerning possible serious burns related to electric dental handpieces. The FDA has requested manufacturers to decrease these issues by design modification, overheating alarms, warning labels, and clinician training to avoid overheating.

Because electric handpieces have insulated housings, the clinician may not be aware of the extent of the heat generated in the handpiece. Compounding the problem is that the patient may be anesthetized and unaware of the thermal injury. Injuries have been reported ranging from first- to third-degree burns and may require reconstructive surgery. Unlike conventional air-driven handpieces that decrease efficiency when overworked, electric handpieces will maintain higher efficiency, thus generating a greater amount of heat.

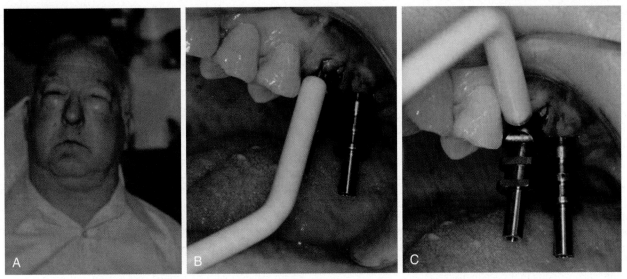

• **Fig. 31.8** (A) Facial air emphysema. (B) Air-water syringes should never be directed along the long axis of the implant. (C) Proper air-water syringe positioning, perpendicular to the long-axis of the dental implant.

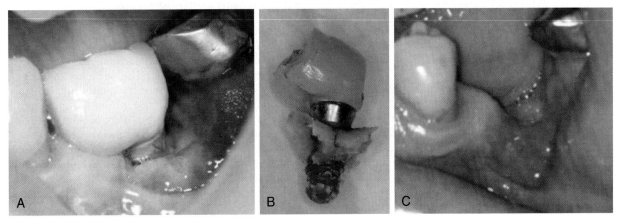

• **Fig. 31.9** (A) Implant site that was treated with an electrosurgery unit. (B) Implant loss and bone necrosis. (C) Resultant large bony defect.

Prevention

Awareness is most crucial for avoiding this complication. The clinician should be conscious of the possibility of the handpiece overheating, take frequent breaks during treatment, and check continuously for the implant motor becoming hot during treatment. Electric handpieces should have routine maintenance according to the manufacturer's recommendations. Usually the straight 1:1 handpieces have a greater incidence than the 16:1 or 20:1 reduction handpieces.

Treatment

If a burn occurs, treatment will vary depending on the severity. Treatments range from over-the-counter ointment to a physician referral. For severe burns, systemic antibiotics are warranted. If the burn does not penetrate the vermillion border, healing will usually result without a defect.

Monopolar Electrosurgery Units

Monopolar electrosurgical units are a common soft tissue modality used in dentistry today. However, in implant dentistry, when these units are used around dental implants, significant complications may arise. Monopolar electrocautery should never be used in the proximity of a dental implant or implant prosthesis.

Electrosurgery is defined as the controlled passage of high-frequency waveforms, or currents, for the purpose of altering the surrounding soft tissue. The action of monopolar electrocautery is cutting the tissue by means of an advancing spark with a grounded patient. This results in sparking, current spread, and thermal damage in the tissues because of the generation of heat.

Prevention

In implant dentistry, monopolar electrosurgery units are contraindicated. The monopolar electrodes should not contact an implant or electrical shock osteoradionecrosis and possible implant loss may result. However, bipolar electrosurgical units have been shown to be effective around dental implants. Bipolar electrocautery uses molecular resonance with a sine-wave current that prevents sparking and thermal damage. These types of units may be used continuously around implants because they produce progressive coagulation rather than a single high-output discharge, thus creating no spark.[9]

Treatment

Treatment is usually palliative in nature because electrosurgery damage is usually irreversible in nature (Fig. 31.9).

Salivary Gland Injury

The sublingual gland may be injured when an implant is poorly positioned in the posterior mandible, which may cause the formation of a ranula. Ranulas are defined as an accumulation of extravasated salivary secretions that form pseudocysts in the submandibular area. When the ranulas form above the mylohyoid muscle, they appear as a translucent, bluish swelling in the sublingual space. Most ranulas are visible on a clinical examination and are considered "plunging" when they extend inferiorly from the sublingual space into the neck area. Ranulas are usually not fixed, and they are rarely painful unless they become secondarily infected. In some cases they develop into larger lesions and may compromise the airway.

The proximity of the sublingual gland to the lingual cortical plate of the mandible makes it susceptible to injury. Trauma usually occurs from improper angulation during dental implant surgery, which perforates the lingual cortex and causes damage to the sublingual gland. In addition, the gland may be injured during aggressive reflection and retraction when working in the sublingual area.

Prevention

To prevent damage to the salivary glands, ideal preoperative treatment planning, good surgical technique, proper implant angulation, and careful retraction will avoid these complications.

In addition, the anatomy of the sublingual area must be understood. The sublingual gland is positioned adjacent to the lingual cortex and seated below the mylohyoid muscle.

The submandibular duct is positioned inferior and medial to the sublingual gland. The lingual nerve will cross the submandibular duct from medial to lateral and then cross back at the first premolar area, where it branches into the tongue musculature.

Treatment

Treatment should include referral to an oral and maxillofacial surgeon, which usually involves the complete removal of the sublingual gland. In some cases, where the ranulas are very small and asymptomatic, no surgery may be indicated or marsupialization to reestablish connection with the oral cavity (Fig. 31.10).[10]

Bleeding-Related Complications

Prevention/Treatment of Bleeding

The ideal management of intraoperative hemorrhage is prevention. Although the clinician should be capable of handling potential bleeding complications, the best course of action is avoidance, which is aided by taking the appropriate preventive measures. A preoperative assessment of the patient is mandatory, including a thorough preoperative patient history, and medical consultation when indicated. The clinician also should be familiar with managing patients receiving anticoagulants and those who have bleeding issues, should use meticulous intraoperative surgical technique, and should provide appropriate postoperative instructions, care, and follow-up. Patients need to be instructed on the importance of compliance with prescribed medication and proper postoperative instructions and care.

Incision/Reflection of Tissue

The dental implant clinician must carefully plan the location of incisions with respect to surgical anatomy to maintain hemostasis and minimize bleeding. Ideally incisions should always be made over host bone when possible. This will allow for pressure to be applied over bone in the event of uncontrolled bleeding. The flap design should incorporate release incisions so that excessive pressure and stretching is reduced to decrease possible tearing of the tissue and resultant blood vessel trauma.

Reflection and elevation of the mucosa and periosteum should be carefully completed with full-thickness and atraumatic reflection. Split-thickness flaps should be avoided to minimize potential bleeding sites. Anatomic areas containing vital structures, which may be highly vascular, should be carefully evaluated and avoided if possible (Fig. 31.11).

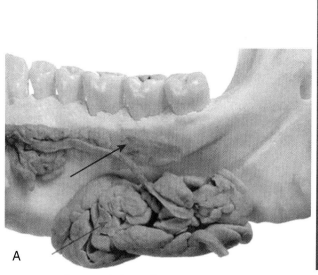
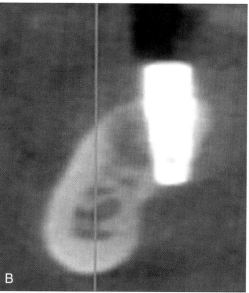

• **Fig. 31.10** Salivary Gland Damage. (A) Anatomic depiction of the sublingual gland (red) and submandibular gland (green). (B) Implant perforation of the lingual plate may result in gland damage.

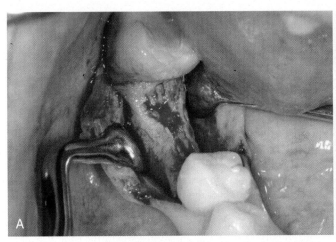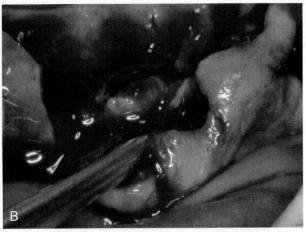

• **Fig. 31.11** (A) Ideal incision location and full-thickness reflection will reduce bleeding with atraumatic reflection of the tissue. (B) Split-thickness flap, which results in increased bleeding and tissue trauma.

Anatomy/Anatomic Variants

Strategic planning of potential implant sites is extremely important, with a thorough understanding of anatomic structures and variants with the use of CBCT. The lack of distortion of the CBCT images allows the clinician to better plan surgical sites, while maintaining relatively safe zones from anatomic structures.

Mandibular Anterior: Intraosseous Vessels

Median Vascular Canal. On occasion, in the mandibular midline, copious bleeding may be present (e.g., C position, even though no bone perforation has occurred). Bilateral sublingual arteries enter through the lingual foramen within the lingual plate below the genial tubercles in the mandible. As this anastomosis transverses within the anterior mandible, the canal is termed the *median vascular canal.* Bleeding in this area may be significant; however, it is not associated with any type of neurosensory impairment. The presence and size of the sublingual anastomosis and the median vascular canal is most commonly seen on a cross-sectional or axial image of a CBCT scan. If a large anastomosis is present, the position of the planned osteotomy may need to be modified.

Management. If significant bleeding occurs after implant osteotomy in the midline, a direction indicator or surgical bur can be placed in the osteotomy site to apply pressure. If the osteotomy is completed, an implant may also be introduced into the site, which will compress the walls of bone, thus slowing the bleeding process (Fig. 31.12). In most cases intraosseous bleeding is more easily controlled in comparison with soft tissue hemorrhage.

Inferior Alveolar Artery. The inferior alveolar artery is a branch of the maxillary artery, one of the two terminal branches of the external carotid. Before entering the mandibular foramen, it gives off the mylohyoid artery. In approximately the first molar region, it divides into the mental and incisal branches. The mental branch exits the mental foramen and supplies the chin and lower lip, where it eventually will anastomose with the submental and inferior labial arteries. The exact location of the inferior alveolar artery is easily determined via a CBCT evaluation in the panoramic or sagittal views.

Management. Normally the inferior alveolar artery is located superiorly to the inferior alveolar nerve within the bony mandibular canal. Drilling or placing an implant into the inferior alveolar canal may predispose to significant bleeding. Hemorrhage

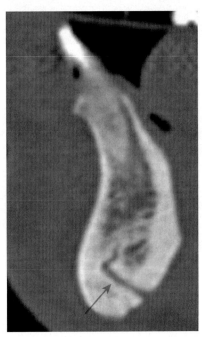

• **Fig. 31.12** Median Vascular Canal. In the mandibular midline, the radiolucent canal that houses the right and left sublingual anastomosis.

may be controlled by placement of an implant or direction indicator short of the canal. A 2.0-mm safety zone between the implant and canal should be adhered to. If bleeding does occur, follow-up postoperative care is essential because hematoma formation within the canal may lead to a neurosensory impairment. This condition should be monitored because it may progress to respiratory depression via a dissecting hematoma in the floor of the mouth (Fig. 31.13).

Incisive Artery. The incisive artery is the second terminal branch of the inferior alveolar artery, which is a branch of the maxillary artery. The incisal branch continues anteriorly after supplying the mandibular first molar area, where it innervates the incisor teeth and anastomoses with the contralateral incisal artery. In rare cases the incisive canal is large, lending to greater bleeding during osteotomy preparation or bone-grafting procedures.[11] The exact location of the incisive canal is easily determined via a CBCT evaluation in the panoramic or sagittal views.

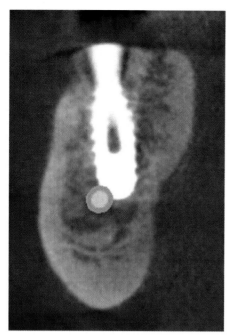

• **Fig. 31.13** Implant placement into the mandibular canal, which may result in excessive bleeding from the inferior alveolar artery.

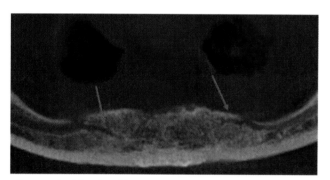

• **Fig. 31.14** Incisive Canal Vessels. The incisive canal is the radiolucent canal extending anterior from the mental foramen and mandibular canal. Implants placed into this area may cause increased bleeding.

Management. Bleeding complications can occur when implants are placed into the mandibular incisive canal, which contains the incisive artery. If bleeding does occur during placement of the implant, a direction indicator, surgical bur, or implant can be placed into the osteotomy to apply pressure (Fig. 31.14).

Mandibular Anterior: Extraosseous Vessels

The anterior mandible is usually known as a safe area for implant placement, but in certain situations it may present with a significant undercut on the lingual aspect between the foramina. Life-threatening hemorrhage has been reported when a drill perforates the lingual plate of the sublingual region of the mandible and traumatizes a sublingual or submental artery, especially in the canine region.[12,13]

If perforation of the lingual cortical plate is associated with arterial bleeding, it is critical to identify its origin and treat aggressively. The origin of bleeding in the floor of the anterior region of the mouth may be from the lingual artery, facial artery, or one of its branches. The submental artery originates from the facial artery and courses along the inferior border of the mandible. The sublingual artery, a branch of the lingual artery, runs along the inferior border of the mandible and terminates in the midline. Perforation in this area may lead to bleeding, causing an expanding ecchymosis (sublingual hematoma) and compromising the airway.

Sublingual Artery (Lingual Artery). The lingual artery is a branch of the external carotid artery between the superior thyroid and facial arteries. The lingual artery courses medially to the greater horn of the hyoid bone and crosses inferiorly and facially around the hypoglossal nerve. It then transverses deep to the digastric and stylohyoid muscles, and courses between the hyoglossus and genioglossus muscles. There exist four main branches of the lingual artery: the suprahyoid, dorsal lingual, deep lingual, and sublingual.

Of clinical significance to oral implantology is the sublingual artery, which supplies the sublingual salivary gland, mylohyoid and surrounding muscles, and the mucous membranes and gingiva of the mandible. A distal branch runs medially in the anterior lingual mandibular gingiva and anastomoses with the contralateral artery. An additional branch connects with the submental artery under the mylohyoid muscle.[14] The lingual artery will anastomose throughout the tongue area, with more anastomoses occurring anteriorly.[15]

Submental Artery (Facial Artery). The most important branch of the facial artery associated with oral implantology is the submental branch, which is the largest of the branches of the facial artery. The submental branch exits the submandibular gland and proceeds anteriorly on the surface of the mylohyoid muscle, just inferior to the body of the mandible. The submental branch terminates as an anastomosis with the sublingual branch of the lingual artery and the mylohyoid branch of the inferior alveolar artery.[14]

Studies have shown that the floor of the mouth and lingual gingiva are supplied approximately 53% by the submental artery and the remaining by the sublingual artery.[16] Perforation of the lingual cortical plate may result in trauma to the submental artery. Treatment should include immediate repositioning of the patient in an upright position followed by the application of bimanual pressure. This should be immediately applied, followed by airway management and emergency protocol.

Bleeding from the submental artery may be decreased by applying finger pressure over the lower border of the mandible. Doppler ultrasonography studies have shown this to reduce the arterial blood by 25% to 50% at the oral commissure level and 33% to 50% at the inferior border of the nares.[17]

Prevention. Clinical and radiographic evaluation should be completed to ascertain the amount of available bone and osseous angulation in the anterior mandible. The length of implants should be carefully evaluated because bicortical stabilization (which may lead to perforation of the lingual plate) is no longer advocated for implant success. This is most important in the mandibular canine position as the arteries are close to the lingual cortical plate. In addition, care should be exercised in elevation of the lingual flap and manipulation of the lingual tissue.

Clinical Significance. Bleeding into the sublingual and submaxillary spaces will cause elevation of the tongue and floor of the mouth. Bleeding in these spaces will proceed to airway obstruction because the anterior extension of the hematoma is limited by the superficial layers of the cervical fascia.[18] The signs and symptoms of sublingual swelling include immediate or delayed (up to 4–8 hours after surgery) elevation of the floor of the mouth, protrusion of the tongue, profuse intraoral bleeding, difficulty in swallowing, and respiratory depression. The submandibular swelling may dislocate the trachea to the contralateral side and compromise the airway.[19] In addition, pulsatile hematomas (pseudoaneurysms) of the lingual artery may result from the injury (Fig. 31.15).[20]

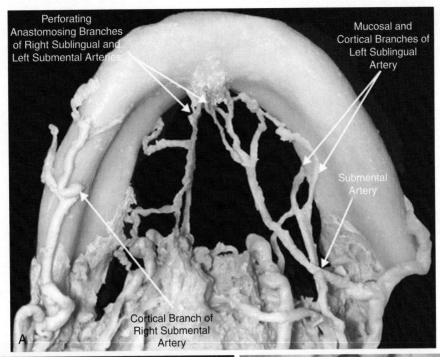

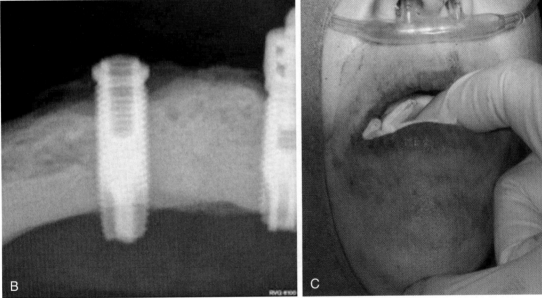

• **Fig. 31.15** (A) Sublingual and submental artery anatomy in the floor of the mouth. (B) Perforating lingual plate, which may cause sublingual bleeding. (C) To slow the bleeding, bimanual pressure with a 4 × 4 gauze on the lingual surface of the mandible and extraoral pressure on the inferior mandible. (*From Loukas M, Kinsella CR Jr, Kapos T, et al: Anatomical variation in arterial supply of the mandible with special regard to implant placement. Int J Oral Maxillofac Surg 37(4):367–371, 2008.*)

Management. Immediate bimanual pressure should be applied to the bleeding area if the location can be determined. A 4 × 4 gauze may be used to apply the bimanual compression downward from the floor of the mouth (lingual surface of the mandible) and in an upward direction from the submental skin area. The patient should be repositioned from a supine to an upright position. Young forceps may be used to pull the tongue outward, which will slow the bleeding. Airway obstruction should be of vital concern because this may lead to a life-threatening situation. If any clinical signs of airway obstruction exist (e.g., dyspnea, dysphagia, wheezing, stridor, cyanosis), emergency intervention should be summoned immediately. Ligation of the bleeding vessel is the ideal treatment to control the hemorrhage. This may be difficult in an office setting because of the location and surgical access of the bleeding vessel. To obtain definitive control of sublingual artery bleeding, surgical intervention with selective ligation of the branches, along with arterial embolization via interventional angiography, is indicated (Fig. 31.16).[21]

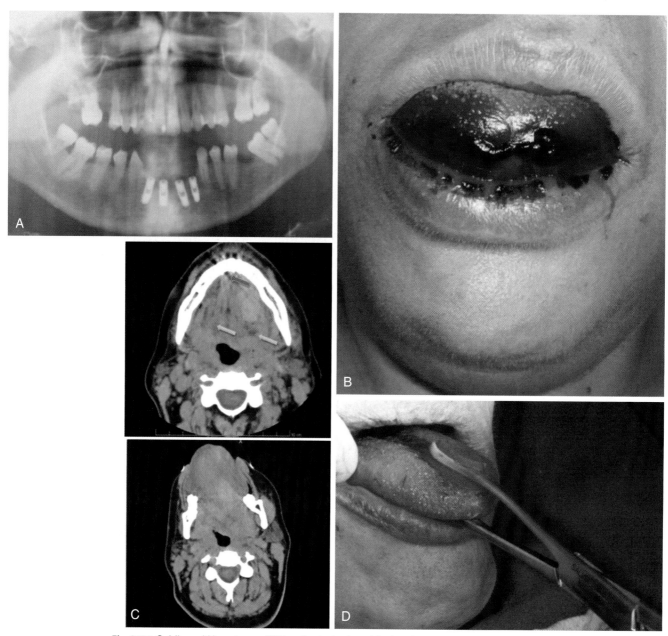

• **Fig. 31.16** Sublingual Hematoma. (A) Four implants placed flapless in the anterior mandible. (B) Resultant sublingual hematoma with airway compromise. (C) Axial computed tomography images showing extent of hematoma (blue arrows) with airway compromise. Note perforation of lingual cortical plate (red arrow). (D) Young forceps may be used to pull tongue out to decrease the bleeding and helps maintain airway until medical assistance arrives. (*From Limongelli L, Tempesta A, Crincoli V, et al: Massive lingual and sublingual haematoma following postextractive flapless implant placement in the anterior mandible. Case Rep Dent. 2015;2015:839098.*)

Mandibular Posterior: Extraosseous Vessels

Posterior Lingual Undercut. In the mandibular posterior area a lingual undercut may be problematic and difficult to manage. In this area, perforation of the lingual plate can occur easily, thereby causing bleeding episodes, with an origin that may be difficult to locate. Life-threatening situations may result from sublingual bleeding. Violation of this area may cause infection or constant irritation from the extruded implant in the soft tissue. If the perforation were to occur above the mylohyoid muscle, damage to the lingual nerve could result in a neurosensory impairment.

Prevention. A clinical examination should always be carried out to determine whether an osseous undercut exists. This may be confirmed with a CBCT examination because cross-sectional images are an effective way of observing lingual undercuts. In addition, angulation and positioning must be continuously verified to prevent inadvertent perforation. Studies have shown that lingual undercuts occur in approximately 66% of the population, with a mean undercut of 2.4 mm.[22] Accurate measurements must be made to prevent overpreparation of the osteotomy site in the posterior mandible.

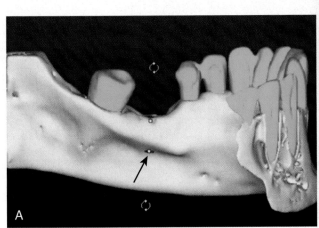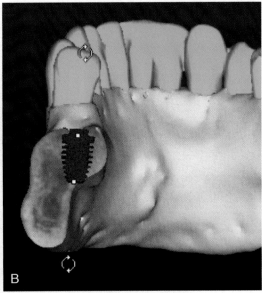

● **Fig. 31.17** Mandibular Posterior Undercut. (A) Three-dimensional image depicting the posterior undercut. (B) When an undercut is present, limited available height is present for implant placement. This will often lead to a crown/implant ratio issue.

Accurate visualization of this area is most easily completed with a CBCT examination. Osteotomy angulation should always be carefully evaluated because improper drilling angulation may lead to perforations. In addition, hourglass mandibles, which have been shown to have an incidence rate of approximately 4%, should always be concerning because perforation will occur.[23]

In addition, clinical palpation of the ridge during osteotomy preparation will minimize perforations and decrease complications. During osteotomy preparation, handpiece control must be maintained to minimize inadvertent lingual plate perforation.

Management. If sublingual posterior bleeding (submental or sublingual arteries) occurs, the patient should be repositioned in an upright position and bimanual pressure should be applied to the area of bleeding. If the airway is compromised, immediate emergency assistance should be summoned (Fig. 31.17).

Buccal Artery. A popular donor site for autogenous grafting is the lateral ramus area in the posterior mandible. When making the incision lateral to the retromolar pad, a common blood vessel to damage is the buccal artery. The buccal artery is a branch of the maxillary artery and will most likely cause a significant bleeding episode. This artery runs obliquely between the internal pterygoid and the insertion of the temporalis on the outer surface of the buccinator.

Prevention. In most cases damage to the buccal artery is impossible to avoid. Incision and reflection will usually encompass the area of buccal artery location. When performing surgery in this area, a curved hemostat should always be available for immediate access to clamp the vessel.

Management. A curved Kelly hemostat should be used to control the bleeding. It should be left in place for 3 to 5 minutes until clotting is complete. If bleeding persists, a ligature may be placed with Vicryl suture material (Fig. 31.18).

Maxilla: Lateral Wall/Nasal Bleeding

Significant bleeding from the lateral approach sinus elevation surgery is rare; however, when it occurs, it has the potential to

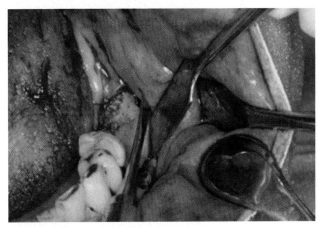

● **Fig. 31.18** Buccal Artery. The buccal artery is often traumatized when making incisions in the retromolar area.

be troublesome. Three main arterial vessels should be of concern with the lateral approach sinus augmentation. Because of the intraosseous and extraosseous anastomoses that are formed by the infraorbital and posterior superior alveolar arteries, intraoperative bleeding complications of the lateral wall may occur. In some cases this bleeding may be significant.

Extraosseous Anastomosis. The soft tissue vertical release incisions of the facial flap in a resorbed maxilla may sever the extraosseous anastomoses during lateral wall osteotomy preparation for sinus graft surgery. The extraosseous anastomosis on average is located 23 mm from the crest of the dentate ridge; however, in the resorbed maxilla, it may be within 10 mm of the crest. When this artery is severed, significant bleeding has been observed. These vessels originate from the maxillary artery and have no bony landmark to compress the vessel. Vertical release incisions in the soft tissue should be kept to a minimum height, with delicate reflection of the periosteum. Hemostats are usually difficult to place on the facial flap to arrest the bleeding. Significant pressure at the

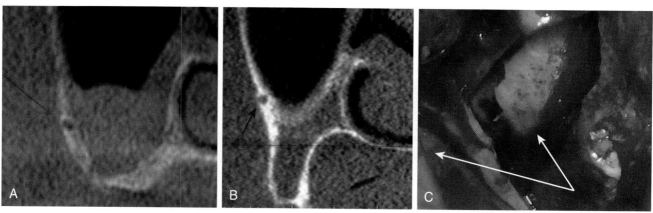

• **Fig. 31.19** Intraosseous Anastomosis. (A) Cross-sectional image showing radiolucent notch on the lateral wall of the sinus. (B) Intraosseous notch (red arrow). (C) Intraosseous anastomosis pulsating bleed (white arrows).

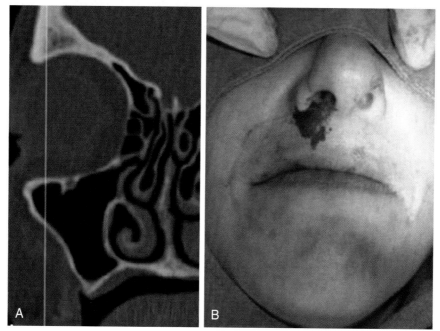

• **Fig. 31.20** (A) Posterior lateral nasal artery (red line) in close approximation to the lateral wall of the nasal cavity (medial wall of maxillary sinus). (B) Nasal bleed during sinus augmentation procedure.

posterior border of the maxilla and elevation of the head to reduce the blood pressure to the vessels usually slows the bleeding. The elevation of the head may reduce nasal mucosal blood flow by 38%.[24]

Intraosseous Anastomosis. The vertical component of the lateral access wall for the sinus graft often severs the intraosseous anastomoses of the posterior alveolar artery and infraorbital artery, which is on average approximately 15 to 20 mm from the crest of a dentate ridge. Methods to limit this bleeding, which is far less of a risk, include cauterization with the use of a handpiece and diamond bur without water, electrocautery, or pressure on a surgical sponge while the head is elevated. In some cases a second window is made distal to the bleeding area source for access to ligate (Fig. 31.19).

Posterior Lateral Nasal Artery. The third artery that implant surgeons should be cautious of is the posterior lateral nasal artery (Fig. 31.20). This artery is a branch of the

sphenopalatine artery, which is located within the medial wall of the antrum. As it courses anteriorly, it anastomoses with terminal branches of the facial artery and ethmoidal arteries. A significant bleeding complication may arise if this vessel is severed during elevation of the membrane off the thin medial wall.

If the excessive bleeding occurs while the medial wall is elevated, the sinus may be packed with hemostatic agents, followed by packing with large 4 × 4-inch surgical sponges and elevation of the head. Once the bleeding is arrested, the sponges are removed, the layered graft materials may be inserted, and the procedure completed.

Epistaxis (active bleeding from the nose) after sinus graft surgery is rather common. This may occur with or without a known membrane perforation. Usually epistaxis is limited to the first 24 hours after surgery, and the patient should always be warned of this potential complication.

If bleeding should occur through the nose, there exist numerous techniques to obtain hemostasis. Placing a cotton roll, coated with petroleum jelly with dental floss tied to one end, within the nares may obtund nose bleeding after the surgery. After 5 minutes the dental floss is gently pulled and the cotton roll removed. The head is also elevated, and ice is applied to the bridge of the nose. If bleeding cannot be controlled, reentry into the graft site and endoscopic ligation by an ENT (ear, nose, and throat) surgeon may be required.

If the orbital wall of the sinus is perforated or if an opening into the nares is already present from a previous event (i.e., previous sinus surgery), the sinus curette may enter the nares and initiate bleeding. The arteries involved in this site are composed of branches of the sphenopalatine and descending palliative arteries, which are branches of the internal maxillary artery. The posterior half of the inferior turbinate has a venous network, the Woodruff plexus, which is highly vascular. A cotton roll with silver nitrate or lidocaine with 1:50,000 epinephrine is also effective in obtaining hemostasis.

Postoperative Bleeding Control

Patient Education

It is imperative that patients understand that minor oozing may persist for up to 24 hours after dental implant surgery. If the patient is taking anticoagulants, this may persist for up to 48 hours. The patient should be instructed on the use of pressure dressings, and special care should be taken to minimize any trauma to the surgical site (e.g., eating, pulling on lip to see surgical site). The patient should avoid rinsing the mouth vigorously. All postoperative instructions should be reviewed with the patient and given in writing before surgery.

Patients should be instructed to limit their activities for a minimum of 24 hours, depending on the extent of the surgery. The head should be elevated as much as possible during the daytime hours, and the use of two pillows (i.e., elevate head) during sleeping will reduce secondary bleeding episodes.

Postoperative hemorrhage in anticoagulated patients may lead to significant issues. Studies have shown bleeding episodes in anticoagulant patients will most likely occur within 6 days of the surgery.[25] In patients who have exhibited significant bleeding during surgery, hemorrhagic shock, although rare, should be evaluated. If the patient displays any signs or symptoms of shock (e.g., tachycardia, hypotension, lethargy, disorientation, cold/clammy skin), immediate medical assistance should be summoned. Treatment would include intravenous fluid replacement to replenish the intravascular volume and restore tissue perfusion. Finally, caution should be exercised on the postoperative use of medications that may increase bleeding. A comprehensive review of the patient's medications should be completed to determine whether any drug interactions may exist that would increase bleeding. Agents that interfere with platelet function should be avoided for routine analgesia (e.g., nonsteroidal antiinflammatory drugs [NSAIDs], aspirin) unless the benefit outweighs the increased risk for bleeding. The routine perioperative use of aspirin should usually be avoided because of an increased risk for bleeding and lack of benefit. However, if these medications are administered for a separate indication under the recommendation of a physician (e.g., recent stroke, acute coronary syndromes, implanted coronary stent), they should be continued.

Techniques to Decrease and Control Bleeding

The need to control gross bleeding is paramount for successful surgery because insidious and continuous loss of blood from arteries, veins, or capillaries can become significant if bleeding is not controlled. Dental implant clinicians have numerous options for maintaining hemostasis, which include mechanical, thermal, pharmacologic, and topical agents.

Mechanical Methods

The most common primary mechanical method to control bleeding is to apply direct pressure or compression on the bleeding site, along with repositioning the patient. Secondary mechanical methods include suturing, clamping the blood vessel with hemostats, and ligating the bleeding vessel with suture material.

Positional Changes. When significant bleeding occurs, maintaining the patient in a supine position is not recommended because of increased bleeding (head below the heart). Hydrostatic pressure occurs within the vascular system because of the weight of the blood vessels and is dependent on gravity. The pressure is decreased in any vessel above the heart and increased in blood vessels below the heart. Studies have shown that in an upright position, the average pressure at the level of the heart is 100 mm Hg. Vessels in the head and neck averaged 49 and 186 mm Hg, respectively, at the foot level.[26] Repositioning the patient to an upright position (head above the heart) will not stop the bleeding; however, it will significantly decrease the hemorrhage (studies have shown a decrease up to 38%).[27]

Direct Pressure. If significant intraoperative bleeding occurs, the ideal treatment should involve immediate application of pressure to the surgical site. Pressure or compression directly on the blood vessel will allow for platelet aggregation and initiation of the coagulation cascade. Pressure may be applied manually or by the patient biting forcefully on a gauze dressing. Pressure should be maintained for at least 3 to 5 minutes to allow the formation of a blood clot. Caution should be exercised not to remove the gauze too early because this may dislodge the clot.

Ideally 3 × 3 or 4 × 4 gauze should be used because 2 × 2 gauze may be accidentally aspirated. In primary bleeding, pressure is the simplest and fastest method to control bleeding before the use of hemostatic measures.

Suturing. Suturing plays a significant role not only in obtaining primary closure for ideal healing but also for maintaining hemostasis (direct versus indirect). Direct placement of a suture (ligation) is used when there is access to a deep bleeding vessel. The suture is placed by entering the tissue at least 4 mm from the bleeding vessel, 3 mm below the vessel, and 4 mm exiting the tissue. This will ligate or occlude the vessel as long as it is placed proximal to the bleeding area. A figure-eight suture technique is ideally used. Indirect suture placement is used to retract the tissue and minimize bleeding via pressure from the accumulated tissue. This is most often used as tie-backs when reflecting an edentulous mandible (cuspid to molar bilaterally). And lastly, good suturing technique is paramount for preventing reactionary bleeding after surgery. Ideally interrupted or mattress sutures should be placed in conjunction with continuous sutures to maintain closure. A suture material that exhibits high tensile strength is recommended, such as polyglycolic acid (e.g., Vicryl). The interim prosthesis should be modified to have no direct pressure on the wound site, as this may dislodge the sutures (Fig. 31.21).

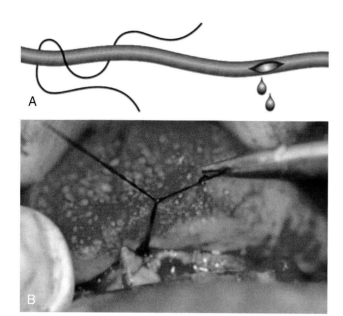

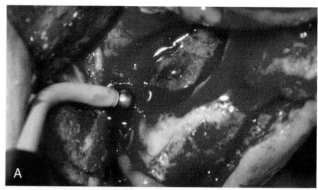

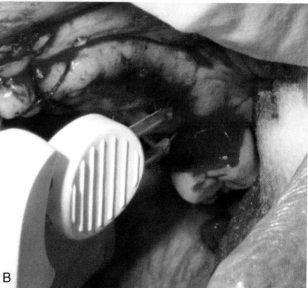

• **Fig. 31.21** Suturing. (A) Direct ligation with figure-eight suturing technique. (B) Indirect tie-back of the mandibular lingual tissue from cuspid-molar contralaterally, which decreases bleeding, allows for ease of retraction, and prevents tissue trauma.

Clamped Vessel With Hemostat Forceps. When local measures are not successful in controlling bleeding, a hemostat may be used to clamp the blood vessel. Usually a curved Kelly hemostat may be used to clamp the vessel to control the bleeding via two mechanisms:

1. The first mechanism is occluding the vessel and damaging the blood vessel's wall to stimulate clotting. This clamping pressure should be maintained for approximately 2 to 3 minutes, which will usually allow for hemostasis. However, this method may be unreliable because the clot may become dislodged and postoperative bleeding may occur after removal of the hemostat.
2. A more successful technique in controlling bleeding is to use fine-pointed hemostats (Kelly hemostats) and ligate the bleeding vessel with suture material. The vessel should be clamped to obtain immediate hemostasis, with the tip of the hemostat extending beyond the vessel. A clamped vessel may be ligated with suture material such as an absorbable suture with high tensile strength (e.g., Vicryl). A tie should be placed around the hemostat, extending to the vessel. The hemostats are then removed, and two additional throws are made with the suture. Usually bleeding from vessels of 2 mm or greater diameter should be ligated. Direct ligation of the bleeding blood vessel is usually the most effective technique in stopping arterial blood flow. However, exposure and identification of the bleeding vessel may sometimes be extremely difficult. In addition, the bleeding may occur from multiple capillaries, which may result in difficult hemostasis.

Electrocautery. Electrocauterization, developed in the 1930s, has been one of the most common hemostatic techniques because of its low cost, accessibility, ease of use, and effectiveness. Electrocautery is the process of destroying tissue using heat conduction, with a probe that is heated by an electric current. Different procedures may be completed with the use of high radiofrequency alternating current for cutting, coagulating, and vaporizing tissues.

• **Fig. 31.22** Electrocautery. (A) Monopolar electrocautery, which uses current to establish hemostasis. A ball electrode is the most common to be used; however, access is sometimes difficult. (B) A battery-operated disposable cautery unit that does not use current, however generates heat to ligate the blood vessel.

Electrocautery is most effective on small vessels and may be used in two modes: monopolar and bipolar (Fig. 31.22).

Monopolar electrosurgery delivers current using different types of waveforms (i.e., modes). The coagulation mode uses an interrupted waveform, which generates heat, thereby coagulating a cell, a phenomenon also termed *fulguration*. The cutting mode is low energy, which produces a cutting effect to vaporize tissue with minimal hemostasis. The blend mode simultaneously cuts tissue and coagulates bleeding. This technique is often difficult to use in implant surgery because access and a relatively dry field is needed to cauterize the vessel. A dry field is needed for the effective electrical current to pass through the tissues. A high-speed plastic, not metal, suction tip should be used to maintain a dry field.

Buzzing the Hemostat (Electrocautery + Hemostat Ligation). Usually on larger vessels the combination of a clamped vessel (with curved hemostat) and electrocautery will allow for the cauterizing of the blood vessel, thus stopping blood flow in the vessel. The protocol is as follows:

1. Use the lowest possible setting to achieve the desired effect.
2. Use the CUT mode, not the COAG mode. COAG has a higher peak-to-peak voltage and is more prone to alternate (small) current pathways.

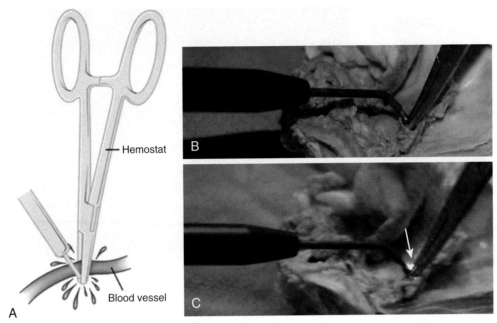

• **Fig. 31.23** (A–C) "Buzzing the hemostat" usually used for larger-vessel ligation (arterial). The vessel is clamped with the hemostat, and the electrocautery unit is placed on CUT mode and lightly touches the hemostat. A spark will usually result (arrow). Before its use, supplemental oxygen (nasal cannula) should be discontinued to prevent a patient airway fire.

3. After clamping the vessel, touch the active electrode to the hemostat closer to the patient (below the hand holding the hemostat) and then activate the electrode. This minimizes sparking and the subsequent demodulation of current, while encouraging a path of least resistance.

NOTE: Care should be exercised because the implant clinician may receive burns or be shocked even when wearing protective gloves. When the surgeon clamps a bleeding vessel and the electrode is touched to the hemostat, the tissue between the clamped hemostat is coagulated. The "buzzing" may cause high-voltage breakdown of the surgeon's glove, leading to a burn. To minimize this possibility, the surgeon's glove should be changed, if wet, because hydrated gloves show a lower resistance. In addition, the electrode should be placed in contact with the hemostat before activation of the electrosurgical current, to minimize the production of a spark (Fig. 31.23).

Lasers. Lasers, which are gaining popularity as a tool in dental surgery, may also be used to achieve hemostasis. Laser is an acronym for "light amplification by stimulated emission of radiation," which produces laser light energy. Laser energy delivered to an area of bleeding may be reflected, scattered, transmitted, or absorbed. The extent of the tissue reaction depends on the laser wavelength, power settings, spot size, and length of contact time with the bleeding area. Lasers have been shown to be a safe or useful modality in treating dental surgery patients with bleeding disorders.[28]

Pharmacologic Techniques

Although pharmacologic techniques may be used in implant dentistry to control bleeding, the success of maintaining hemostasis is questionable, with varying results.

Epinephrine. Epinephrine may be used to enhance hemostasis in combination with local anesthesia (e.g., 2% Lidocaine 100,000, 1/50,000 epinephrine). When locally placed, epinephrine will reduce bleeding, slow the absorption of the local anesthetic, and prolong the anesthetic and analgesic effect. The hemostatic properties are related to platelet aggregation, which leads to a decrease in the adrenoreceptors within the vessel walls, thus producing vasoconstriction. However, rebound hyperemia may result postoperatively, which will increase bleeding. Various studies have shown that topical application of a 1/100,000 concentration of epinephrine creates vasoconstriction and controls hemostasis with sinus graft procedures, with no appreciable changes in systemic hemodynamics.[29]

Tranexamic Acid Solution. Tranexamic acid 4.8% is an antifibrinolytic oral rinse that facilitates clot formation by inhibiting the activation of plasminogen to plasmin. Plasmin prevents the clotting process from initiating fibrinolysis. Tranexamic acid solution may be used as a mouthwash postoperatively and has been shown to enhance clotting in patients with coagulopathies or anticoagulant therapy. Sindet-Pedersen and Ramstrom[30] showed a significant reduction in postoperative bleeding with a 10-mL rinse, four times a day for 7 days postoperatively. Choi et al.[31] reported a significant decrease in bleeding during maxillary surgery after a bolus of tranexamic acid was given preoperatively (Fig. 31.24).

Topical Hemostatic Agents. Absorbable topical hemostatic agents are used when conventional methods of hemostasis are ineffective. These agents may be placed directly into the bleeding site to decrease bleeding during the procedure or during the postoperative interval. They work either mechanically or by augmenting the coagulation cascade. The topical hemostatic agents have the added benefit of minimizing the possibility of systemic blood clots, which are drawbacks of systemic hemostatic agents. There are two types: active and passive (Table 31.1).

Active Hemostatic Agents

Thrombin. Active topical hemostatic agents have biologic activity that induces clotting at the end of the coagulation cascade. Most active agents used in dental implant surgery contain the coagulant thrombin. Thrombin is a naturally derived

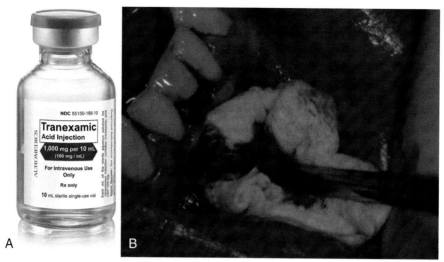

• **Fig. 31.24** Tranexamic Acid Injection. (A) Injection solution (Auromedics, East Windsor, N.J.). (B) Injectable tranexamic acid placed under bleeding flap.

TABLE 31.1   Active and Passive Hemostatic Agents

COMMON HEMOSTATIC AGENTS			
Type	**Product**	**Advantages**	**Disadvantages**
Collagen	OraTape, OraPlug (Salvin), CollaTape, CollaPlug (Zimmer)	Inexpensive; resorbs in 10–14 days; highly absorbent to many times its own weight	None
Microcellular collagen	Avitene (Davol), Helitene (Integra), Instat (Ethicon)	Good application for large surfaces; superior hemostasis to gelatin and cellulose	Difficult to handle; expensive
Gelatin	GelFoam (Baxter), Surgiform (Ethicon)	Swelling after application results in tamponade effect; neutral pH	May cause tissue/neural damage due to compression from swelling; possible dislodgement from bleeding site
Cellulose	Surgicel (Ethicon), Blood Stop (Salvin), Oxycel (Becton Dickinson), ActCel (Coreva Health Sciences)	Easy to handle; low pH provides antimicrobial coverage; expands three to four times its original size and converts to a gel	Possible foreign body reaction; low pH may lead to possible postoperative irritation; needs to be removed
Thrombin	Thrombin-JMI Bovine (Pfizer), Evithrom-human (Ethicon), Recothrom-recombinant (ZymoGenetics)	Can be added to collagen products, good for small-vessel bleeding	Bovine has been shown to be immunogenic; leads to severe coagulopathy
Thrombin + gelatin	FloSeal (Baxter)	Very good for arterial bleeding areas because it acts as an adhesive	Can result in significant swelling from the compression; can cause neural disturbance
Fibrin sealant	Tisseel (Baxter) Evicel (Ethicon)	Good for larger bleeding areas because it acts as an adhesive	Expensive; preparation time
Kaolinite	QuikClot (Z-Medica)	Kaolin is a natural occurring mineral	Limited use in dental surgery; needs to be poured into wound; exothermic reaction causes heat
Synthetic bone hemostatic agents	Bone wax Ostene (Ceremed)	Ostene is soluble; it dissolves in 48 hours and is not metabolized, with a low bacterial adhesion and infection rate	Bone wax is insoluble; must be removed or will cause inflammation and a foreign body giant cell reaction; should not be used in implant dentistry

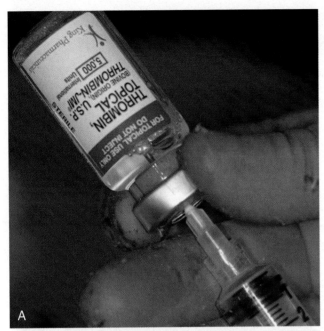
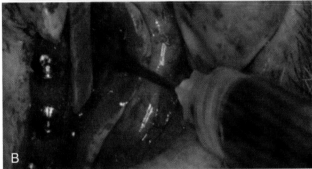

• **Fig. 31.25** (A) Topical thrombin (King Pharmaceuticals, Bristol, Tenn.). (B) Injected under a flap.

enzyme that is formed from prothrombin and acts as the basis for a fibrin clot by converting fibrinogen to fibrin. It is mainly used as a topical hemostatic agent in 5000- to 10,000-unit solutions, which accelerates capillary bleeding. It may be used as a powder or combined with a gelatin sponge during surgical procedures.

Thrombin bypasses the initial enzymatic process, thereby exerting its effect by impairing aspects of the coagulation cascade. For thrombin to maintain hemostasis, circulating fibrinogen is needed because it is necessary for the formulation of a clot. Therefore when a patient exhibits the absence of fibrinogen, thrombin will not be effective. Fibrinogen is less susceptible to coagulopathies caused by clotting factor deficiencies and platelet dysfunction.[32] However, thrombin does work in the presence of antiplatelet and anticoagulation medications, which are quite prevalent in the population (Fig. 31.25).

Types of Thrombin. Thrombin is available in many forms as a hemostatic agent and has been purified from numerous sources and classified according to the plasma used to create it. Bovine thrombin (e.g., Thrombin-JMI) is available as a powder that may be used dry, reconstituted with sterile saline, or added to gelatin sponges or collagen. Antibody formation has been associated with bovine thrombin, and this may lead to coagulopathies.[33]

Human plasma thrombin (e.g., Evithrom) is available as a frozen liquid that can be reconstituted via an absorbable gelatin sponge. Human plasma thrombin has been associated with the potential risk for viral or disease transmission.[34]

Recombinant thrombin (e.g., Recothrom) is a genetically engineered thrombin available in a powder form. It may be applied via a spray kit or with an absorbable gelatin sponge. The use of recombinant thrombin eliminates the risk for antibody formation and disease and virus transmission.[35]

Advantages. Thrombin use is advantageous in patients receiving antiplatelet or anticoagulation medications. Thrombin does not need to be removed from the bleeding site because degeneration and reabsorption of the fibrin clot is achieved during the normal healing process. Usually thrombin-containing active agents have a rapid onset of action, providing hemostasis within 10 minutes in most patients.[36]

Disadvantages. Thrombin is ineffective in patients who suffer from afibrinogenemia because fibrinogen will not be present in the patient's blood. Care should be exercised not to use thrombin directly on larger vessels because systemic absorption may lead to intravascular thrombosis.

Passive Hemostatic Agents. Passive hemostatic agents provide hemostasis by accelerating the coagulation process. These agents form a physical, lattice-like matrix, which activates the extrinsic clotting pathway and provides a platform for platelets to aggregate and form a clot. Passive hemostatic agents are effective only on patients who have an ideal coagulation process. If the patient suffers from any type of coagulopathy, other hemostatic techniques should be used.

Passive hemostatic agents are available in many different forms (e.g., bovine collagen, cellulose, gelatins) and application methods (e.g., absorbable sponge, foam, pads that may absorb several times their own weight). Expansion may lead to complications, specifically pressing on neural tissue (e.g., inferior alveolar nerve). Therefore after hemostasis is obtained, passive hemostats should be removed to minimize postoperative complications. Passive hemostatic agents are readily available and inexpensive.

Collagen. Collagen-based hemostatic agents work by contact activation and promotion of platelet aggregation, which occurs as a result of contact between blood and collagen. Collagen is available in many carrier forms such as a powder, paste, or sponge. Studies have shown that between 2% and 4% of the total population is allergic to bovine collagen.[37]

Bovine Collagen (OraPlug, OraTape; Salvin Dental Specialties, Inc.). Products such as OraPlug and OraTape are soft, white, pliable, nonfriable, coherent, spongelike structures that are fabricated from bovine collagen (usually from deep flexor tendons). They are nontoxic, nonpyrogenic, and highly absorbent. Indications include the control of oozing or bleeding from clean oral wounds. They help control bleeding, by stabilizing blood clots, and protect the wound bed to facilitate the healing process. When applied, the products should be held in place for approximately 2 to 5 minutes to achieve ideal hemostasis and then may be removed, replaced, or left in place. Most collagen materials are completely resorbed within 14 to 56 days (Fig. 31.26).[38]

Cellulose. The most common cellulose-based hemostatic agent is regenerated oxidized cellulose that initiates clotting via contact activation. Oxidized cellulose has been shown to be poorly absorbed and may cause healing complications postoperatively.

Regenerated Cotton Cellulose (BloodSTOP; LifeScience PLUS, Inc.). BloodSTOP is a biocompatible, nonirritating, water-soluble, regenerated cotton cellulose hemostatic agent that resembles traditional gauze. When applied to a bleeding surgical site, BloodSTOP quickly absorbs blood and transforms into a gel to seal the

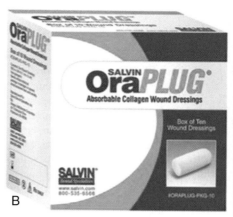
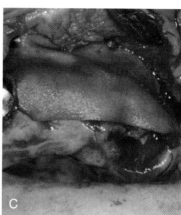

• **Fig. 31.26** Collagen Hemostatic Agents. (A) OraTape. (B) OraPlug. (C) Collagen hemostatic agent placed to control bleeding. (*A and B: Courtesy Salvin Dental Specialties, Charlotte, N.C.*)

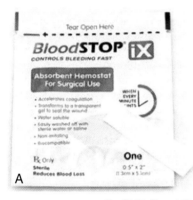
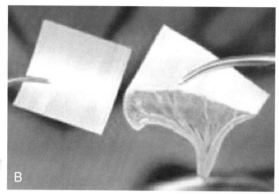
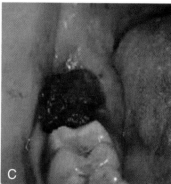

• **Fig. 31.27** (A and B) BloodSTOP hemostatic agent (LifeScience PLUS, Inc., Mountain View, Calif.). (C) BloodSTOP placed in extraction site.

wound with a protective transparent layer, actively aids in blood coagulation, and creates a positive environment for wound healing. Because BloodSTOP is 100% natural cellulose and is water soluble, it is easily removed without disruption of the wound surfaces after hemostasis. It is manufactured in a single-use, sterile package with a 0.5 × ~2-inch size (Fig. 31.27).

Mechanical
Beeswax. Bone wax, a soft, malleable, nonbrittle wax, was invented in 1886 by Sir Victor Horsley. The material is a combination of beeswax, salicylic acid, and almond oil.[39] It is most commonly used when the bleeding is visualized as having an origin from within the bone. This type of bleeding most commonly occurs during osteotomy preparation and extractions. Bone wax exhibits no hemostatic quality; it obliterates the vascular spaces in cancellous bone. However, caution should be exercised with the use of bone wax because it is water insoluble and will not be absorbed. It may predispose the area to infection or inhibit bone healing. Studies have shown that bone wax, when removed from an osseous defect after 10 minutes, completely inhibited further bone regeneration.[40] Bone wax also increases inflammation, which may cause a foreign body giant cell reaction and infection at the site (Fig. 31.28).[41]

Synthetic Bone Hemostat Material (Ostene; Ceremed Inc.). Ostene is a synthetic bone hemostat material approved in 2004 by the FDA for use in cranial and spinal procedures. This material is a mixture of water-soluble alkylene oxide copolymers that elicits minimal postoperative inflammation. It has many advantages over

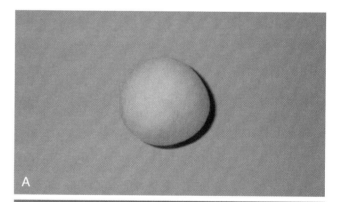
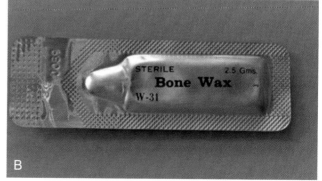

• **Fig. 31.28** (A and B) Bone wax. (*B: Courtesy Surgical Specialties, Wyomissing, Pa.*)

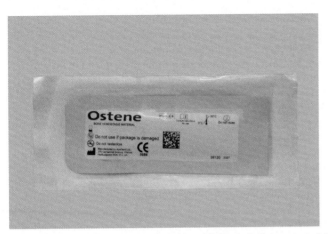

• **Fig. 31.29** Ostene (Bone Hemostasis Material) (Baxter). Ostene material is a sterile water-soluble surgical implant material. It can be used for the control of bleeding from bone surfaces by acting as a mechanical barrier.

bone wax because it is water soluble and dissolves in 48 hours. It has been associated with a decreased infection rate and positive bone cultures.[42] Ostene is supplied in sterile peel pouches and is applied in a manner similar to bone wax, without the associated disadvantages (Fig. 31.29).

Postoperative Complications

Edema (Postoperative) Surgical Swelling

Postoperative edema is a direct result of tissue injury and is defined as an accumulation of fluid in the interstitial tissue. Two variables determine the extent of edema: (1) the amount of tissue injury is proportional to the amount of edema; and (2) the looser the connective tissue at the surgery site, the more edema is most likely to be present. Because postoperative swelling can adversely affect the incision line (i.e., result in incision line opening [ILO]), measures should be taken to minimize this condition. Usually edema will peak at approximately 48 to 72 hours; therefore patients should always be informed. Increased swelling after the fourth day may be an indication of infection, rather than postsurgical edema.

Etiology

The mediators of the inflammatory process include cyclooxygenase and prostaglandins, which play a significant role in the development of postoperative inflammation and pain. When tissue manipulation or damage occurs, phospholipids are converted into arachidonic acid by way of phospholipase A_2 (PLA_2). Arachidonic acid, which is an amino acid, is released into the tissue, which produces prostaglandins via enzymatic breakdown via cyclooxygenases. The end result is the formation of leukotrienes, prostacyclins, prostaglandins, and thromboxane A_2, which are the mediators for inflammation and pain.

Prevention

Good surgical technique must be used with minimal tissue trauma to decrease postoperative swelling. Additional factors include patient systemic disorders, excessive retraction, and long surgical duration, which will all contribute to increased inflammation after surgery. Postoperative prophylactic medications such as ibuprofen (NSAIDs) and glucocorticosteroids (steroids) are used as prophylactic medications, which counteract the negative effects of the edema cascade.

Nonsteroidal Anti-inflammatory Drugs. NSAIDs have an analgesic effect, as well as an anti-inflammatory effect. This drug class reduces inflammation by inhibiting the synthesis of prostaglandins from arachidonic acid. Therefore the use of the popular analgesic drug ibuprofen has a secondary beneficial anti-inflammatory effect. NSAIDs do not have a ceiling effect for inflammation (i.e., ceiling effect for analgesia is 400 mg); however, higher doses to achieve anti-inflammatory qualities are accompanied by serious side effects.

Recommendation: Ibuprofen 400 mg for type 1 to 4 procedures (see Chapter 14).

Glucocorticosteroids. The adrenal cortex, which uses cholesterol as a substrate, synthesizes and secretes two types of steroid hormones—the androgens and corticosteroids. The corticosteroids are classified additionally by their major actions: (1) glucocorticoids, which have effects on carbohydrate metabolism and have potent anti-inflammatory actions; and (2) mineralocorticoids, which have sodium-retaining qualities. The use of synthetic glucocorticosteroids has become popular in the postoperative management of inflammation after oral surgical procedures. These synthetic glucocorticoids have greater anti-inflammatory potency in comparison with natural steroids, with very little sodium and water retention. Most steroids have similar chemical structures; however, they differ in their milligram potency.[43] The anti-inflammatory effects are achieved by altering the connective tissue response to injury, causing a decrease in hyperemia, which results in less exudation and cellular migration, along with infiltration at the site of injury.[44]

Glucocorticoids bind to glucocorticoid receptors within cells and form a glucocorticoid receptor (GR) complex. This complex alters the synthesis of messenger RNA from the DNA molecule, affecting the production of different proteins. By suppressing the production of proteins that are involved in inflammation, glucocorticoids also activate lipocortins, which have been shown to inhibit the action of Phospholipase A2 (PLA_2).

PLA_2 is a key enzyme involved in the release of arachidonic acid from cell membranes.

Arachidonic acid is an omega-6 fatty acid that is incorporated into cell membranes. When a cell is damaged, arachidonic acid is released from cell membranes and is converted into inflammatory and pain prostaglandins by cyclooxygenase-2 enzymes. The release of arachidonic acid requires the activation of enzyme PLA_2. However, lipocortins, which cause the inhibition of PLA_2, prevent the release of arachidonic acid, thereby reducing the amounts of inflammatory prostaglandins.

A wide range of glucocorticoid preparations are available for local, oral, and parenteral administration. In relation to the naturally occurring cortisol (hydrocortisone), synthetic glucocorticoids are longer acting and more potent. The main differences are based on the classification as short acting (<12 hours), intermediate acting (12–36 hours), and long acting (>36 hours). A summary of the most common glucocorticosteroids is shown in Table 31.2.

The ideal synthetic glucocorticoid for dental implant surgery should maintain high anti-inflammatory potency with minimal mineralocorticoid effects. The glucocorticoid that best suits the requirements is the long-acting glucocorticoid dexamethasone (Decadron). It is imperative this drug be administered before surgery so that adequate blood levels are obtained. Also, it should be given in the morning in conjunction with the natural release of cortisol (~8:00 a.m.). This timing will interfere the least with the adrenocortical system. Because inflammation usually peaks between 48 and 72 hours, the postoperative regimen of dexamethasone should not exceed 3 days after surgery. This high-dose, short-term gluco-corticoid therapy has been shown not to significantly affect the hypothalamic-pituitary-adrenal axis, which controls many of the body's processes, including reactions to stress.[45]

A significant additional benefit of the administration of dexamethasone is the potent antiemetic effects for the prophylactic treatment of postoperative nausea and vomiting. This is now an accepted medication for hospital-based outpatient surgery, usually given in doses of 8 to 10 mg intravenously.[46]

Contraindications to the use of corticosteroids include active infections (viral, bacterial, fungal), tuberculosis, ocular herpes simplex, primary glaucoma, acute psychosis, and diabetes mellitus. Special attention must be given to patients with diabetes because glucocorticoids have an anti-insulin action that results in increased serum glucose and glycosuria.[47] Usually corticosteroids are contraindicated with patients with insulin-dependent diabetes. For patients with oral and diet-controlled diabetes, a medical consult should be completed before any treatment.

Recommendation: Decadron 4 mg for type 1 to 4 procedures (see Chapter 14).

Cryotherapy. Cryotherapy (application of ice) is one of the simplest and most economical modalities in the management of postoperative soft tissue inflammation. The use of ice to reduce pain and swelling dates back to the ancient Egyptians, more than 4000 years ago.[48]

The use of cryotherapy is highly advised in any dental implant procedure in which excessive inflammation is expected. The mechanism of action involves a reduction in fluid accumulation within the body tissues, slowing of metabolism, control of hemorrhage, and a decrease in the excitability of peripheral nerve fibers leading to an increase in pain threshold.[49]

Caution must be taken to limit the application of ice to no longer than 2 days because prolonged use may cause rebound swelling and cell destruction. Improper and prolonged use of ice may result in cell death caused by prolonged vasoconstriction, ischemia, and capillary thrombosis.[50]

After 2 to 3 days, moist heat may be applied to the region to increase blood and lymph flow to help clear the area of the inflammatory consequences. This also helps reduce any ecchymosis that may have occurred from the tissue reflection. Although usually safe, the application of ice is cautioned in patients suffering from cold hypersensitivities and intolerances and peripheral vascular diseases. In addition, ice application may be problematic in patients who are elderly or very young because they may have impaired thermal regulation and limited ability to communicate.

Care should be exercised in using facial bandages because prolonged ice administration may result in soft tissue injury.

Recommendation: Cold dressings (ice packs) should be applied extraorally (not directly on skin: place a layer of dry cloth between ice and skin) over the surgical site for 20 minutes on/20 minutes off for the first 24 to 36 hours (Fig. 31.30).

Decrease Activities. Patients should be instructed to decrease activities after surgery because this will minimize swelling postoperatively. The more active the patient and the more strenuous activity the patient engages in, the greater the extraoral swelling.

TABLE 31.2	Synthetic Glucocorticoids		
Glucocorticoids	Anti-inflammatory Potency	Equivalent Dose (mg)	Duration (hr)
Short acting			
Hydrocortisone	1.0	20	<12
Cortisone	0.8	25	<12
Intermediate acting			
Prednisone	4.0	5	24–36
Prednisolone	4.0	5	24–36
Long acting			
Dexamethasone	25	0.75	48

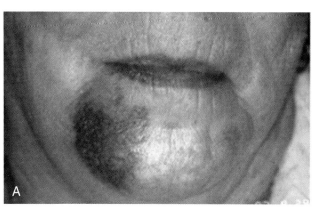
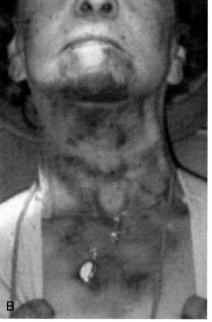

• **Fig. 31.30** (A and B) Common postoperative complications of (A) edema and (B) ecchymosis.

Recommendation: Activities should be limited for the first 3 days. Elevation of the head (sitting upright) and sleeping on multiple pillows will minimize the postoperative swelling.

Treatment

Swelling is self-limiting and once it occurs, it is usually difficult to treat (time dependent). The earlier mentioned medications/therapy (Decadron, NSAIDs, cryotherapy) will help to reduce postoperative inflammation, especially after longer, more invasive surgeries.

Ecchymosis (Bruising)

Ecchymosis is subcutaneous extravasation of blood within the tissues, which results in discoloration of the skin from the seepage of blood in the tissues. The location of the ecchymosis may be distant to the surgical site because of gravity (i.e., always inform patients preoperatively). Ecchymosis that presents in the inferior mandibular area or neck may be from bleeding under the flap and traveling via fascial spaces because of gravity.

Etiology

The cause of ecchymosis (bruising) is not confined to an existing hematologic disease or to medication-induced bleeding. Moderate bruising should be expected after dental implant surgery, especially after longer, more invasive surgeries. Female and elderly patients are more susceptible to bruising.

The ecchymosis cascade includes:
1. Blood vessels rupture.
2. Red blood cells die and release hemoglobin.
3. Macrophages (white blood cells) degrade hemoglobin via phagocytosis.
4. Hemo > bilirubin = bluish-red color.
5. Bilirubin > hemosiderin = golden-brown color.

Ecchymosis may appear as bright red, black, blue, purple, or a combination of the above colors. It usually consists of nonelevated, rounded, and irregular areas that increase in intensity over 3 to 4 days postsurgery and will diminish and become yellow as they disappear. It may take 2 to 3 weeks for complete resolution.

Prevention

Unfortunately, even with gentle handling of tissues and good surgical technique, ecchymosis may be unavoidable. To minimize ecchymosis, avoid postoperative aspirin, herbal remedies, and food supplements that may increase bleeding. Always inform the patient preoperatively (preferably in written postoperative instructions) that bruising may occur. Elderly patients are more susceptible to ecchymosis because of decreased tissue tone and weaker intracellular attachment.

Treatment

Ecchymosis is self-limiting and usually resolves without treatment. However, the patient may treat the ecchymosis in the following ways:

Rest/avoid strenuous activity: promotes tissue healing and decreases inflammation

Elevation: helps decrease inflammation, facilitates proper venous return, and improves circulation to the site

Analgesics: helps reduce pain associated with the onset of ecchymosis

Sun exposure: inform patient to avoid sun exposure to the area of bruising because excessive sunlight may cause permanent discoloration

Dental Implant Periapical Lesions (Retrograde Peri-implantitis)

After implant placement and recall examinations, case reports have shown the genesis of periapical lesions (radiolucency), which may suggest a possible precursor to failure of the endosseous implant.[51] These periapical lesions have been termed *apical peri-implantitis* and *retrograde peri-implantitis.*[52] The lesions have been defined as symptomatic or asymptomatic periapical radiolucency developing after implant placement with a normal coronal bone-to-implant interface.

Etiology

Asymptomatic. A clinically asymptomatic periapical radiolucency is considered to be inactive when radiographically there exists evidence of bone destruction with no clinical symptoms.

This may result from placing an implant into a site in which the osteotomy was prepared deeper than the implant length, resulting in an apical space. Also, when implants are placed adjacent to a tooth with an apical scar, this may result in a radiolucency. Inactive lesions may be caused by thermal bone necrosis, which is a direct result of overheating the bone. The thermal injury may result in a fibrous tissue interface, which may compromise the prognosis of the implant.

Symptomatic. A clinically symptomatic lesion is most commonly caused by bacterial contamination during implant placement. This may occur when an implant is placed into a preexisting area with bacteria (existing infection, cyst, granuloma, or abscess). When lesions are initiated at the apex, they may spread coronally or facially. Clinical symptoms with active lesions include intense pain, inflammation, percussion, mobility, or possible fistulas tract formation (Fig. 31.31).[53]

Prevention

Prevention of periapical lesions includes the following:
1. Clear evaluation of adjacent tooth structure to rule out preexisting infection or pathology
2. Pulp testing of adjacent teeth
3. Caution when placing immediate implants into sites with possible pathology
4. Extensive debridement of pathologic tissue and decortication of immediate extraction sites

Treatment

Because of the multifactorial etiology of periapical lesions around dental implants, there is no accepted general consensus on the treatment. Nonsurgical antibiotic treatment of periapical lesions has been shown to be unsuccessful.[54] The following have been shown to be effective treatments of periapical lesions:

Exposure: Tissue reflection is completed to expose the apical implant area (buccal or lingual access).

Debridement: The granulation tissue is completely removed to expose the bony walls of the apical area.

Removal of implant apex (elective): The apical portion of the implant may be removed to gain better access to the bony walls. This should be completed only if there is no biomechanical compromise for the implant.

Surface decontamination: The implant surface may be detoxified with various chemicals such as tetracycline (250 mg) grafting,[55] citric acid (40%),[56] chlorhexidine, and hydrogen peroxide.[57,58]

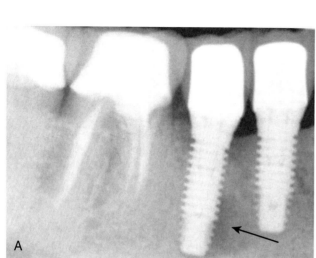
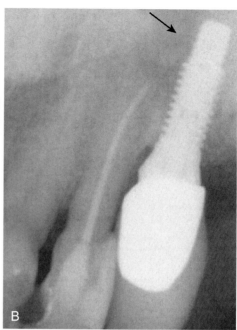

● **Fig. 31.31** Retrograde Periapical Lesion. (A) Radiolucency on mesial of implant of mandibular implant. (B) Radiolucency on mesial of maxillary implant.

Allograft: The defect area is grafted with allograft material, along with a resorbable membrane. A local antibiotic (e.g., Ancef, Cleocin) should be added to the graft for additional antimicrobial coverage.

Systemic antibiotics: Systemic prophylactic antibiotics (e.g., amoxicillin) should be used, together with 0.012% chlorhexidine oral rinse.

Titanium Allergy/Hypersensitivity

Hypersensitivity to titanium (Ti) is an ever-increasing reportable complication in medicine today that has been associated with a wide range of situations. In orthopedic medicine there are many case reports of titanium alloy hypersensitivity. Witt and Swann[59] reported 13 cases of failed total hip prostheses and concluded the tissue reaction in response to metal-wear debris may have been the causative factor of the failed implants. This process has been termed *repassivation* and may produce an oxide that surrounds and turns the peri-implant tissues black. Yamauchi et al.[60] reported a titanium-implanted pacemaker caused an allergic reaction. The patient experienced development of a distinct erythema over the implantation site, which resulted in a generalized eczema. Titanium sensitivity was confirmed by intracutaneous and lymphocyte stimulation testing.

In the dental literature, allergic reactions to pure titanium are rare. However, many authors have suggested there is a higher incidence of titanium alloy allergy with respect to dental implants; it is most likely underreported because of a poor understanding of failure or allergy.[61] Preez et al.[62] have reported a case of implant failure caused by a suspected titanium hypersensitivity reaction around a dental implant. Histologic results showed a chronic inflammatory reaction with concomitant fibrosis. Egusa et al. reported a titanium implant overdenture case that resulted in generalized eczema that fully resolved after implant removal.[46] Sicilia et al.,[63] in a clinical study of 1500 consecutive implant patients, reported approximately nine implants with a positive reaction to titanium allergy.

Etiology

Sensitivity to titanium has been shown to be a result of the presence of macrophages and T lymphocytes with the presence of B lymphocytes, which results in a type IV hypersensitivity reaction.[64] All metals, when in a biologic environment, undergo corrosion, which may lead to the formation of metallic ions and trigger the immune system complex with endogenous proteins.[65] Titanium alloy dental implants have been shown to contain many "impurities" that may trigger type IV hypersensitivity reactions. Harloff et al.[66] used spectral analysis to investigate various titanium alloy implants. The results showed that all of the titanium alloy samples contained small amounts of other elements such as beryllium (Be), cobalt (Co), chromium (Cr), copper (Cu), iron (Fe), nickel (Ni), and palladium. These impurity elements have been shown to be the cause of the hypersensitivity reactions.

Prevention

A thorough medical history involving any history of titanium hypersensitivity is strongly recommended.

Treatment

When titanium hypersensitivity is suspected the implants should be removed and the patient should be referred to his or her physician for appropriate testing. Case reports have shown that after complete removal of the implants, complete resolution results.[67] Metal sensitivity is usually diagnosed using a "patch test," which involves placement of titanium (allergen) to the skin for approximately 3 to 4 days. A positive test would include the appearance of an erythematous reaction. However, there is a possibility of false-negative results because the sealing qualities of the skin against direct contact may make the test unreliable (Fig. 31.32).

Incision Line Opening

ILO is one of the most common complications resulting from dental implant and bone graft surgery, occurring when a wound dehisces along a suture line (Fig. 31.33). The prevalence

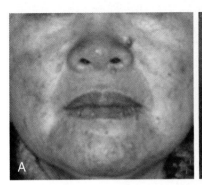
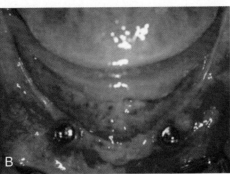
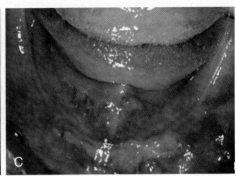

• **Fig. 31.32** Titanium Dental Implant Allergy. (A) Facial eczema after implant placement. (B) Intraoral view of type IV hypersensitivity reaction. (C) Complete resolution after implant removal. (*From Egusa H, Ko N, Shimazu T, et al. Suspected association of an allergic reaction with titanium dental implants: a clinical report.* J Prosthet Dent. *2008;100:344-347.*)

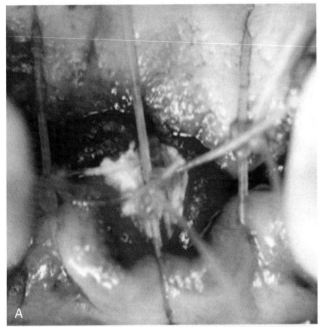
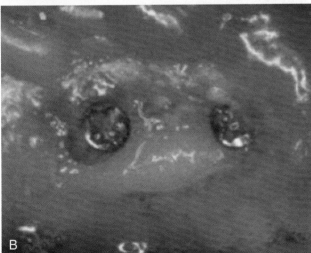

• **Fig. 31.33** Incision Line Opening (ILO). (A) Breakdown of the suture line leading to ILO. (B) Bone graft with ILO.

• BOX 31.1   Clinical Dental Implant Wound Opening Categories

Class 0: The mucosa covering the implant is intact.
Class 1: A breach in the mucosa covering the implant is observed. Oral implant communication may be detected with a periodontal probe, but the implant surface cannot be observed without mechanically interfering with the mucosa.
Class 2: The mucosa above the cover screw is fenestrated; the cover screw is visible. The borders of the perforation do not reach or overlap the borders of the cover screw.
Class 3: The cover screw is visible. In some areas of the cover screw the borders of the perforation aperture overlap the borders of the cover screw.
Class 4: The cover screw is completely exposed.

---

rate of ILO has been shown in studies to range from 4.6% to 40% around submerged implants.[68,69] Mendoza et al.[70] reported 37% of postimplant surgery patients exhibited no ILO, whereas 43% had partial ILO and 20% had complete ILO. However, when evaluating soft tissue dehiscence around membranes (barriers), studies have shown a 30% incidence rate when part of guided bone regeneration procedures.[71] Therefore ILO is a common postoperative complication after dental implant and bone-grafting surgery. In this chapter the causative factors, prevention, and management of ILO will be discussed, together with a treatment protocol that is procedure and time specific.

Classification of Incision Line Opening Complications

When placing root form implants with a two-stage approach, spontaneous early exposure of submerged implants has the potential for complications that may affect healing and osseointegration of the implants. A classification and nomenclature system for these exposures is useful for communication and recordkeeping. Clinical wound opening has been categorized by Tal[69] (Box 31.1 and Fig. 31.34).

Considering that spontaneous early exposures are complications that can potentially lead to mucositis or peri-implantitis, Barboza and Caula[72] proposed classification for spontaneous early

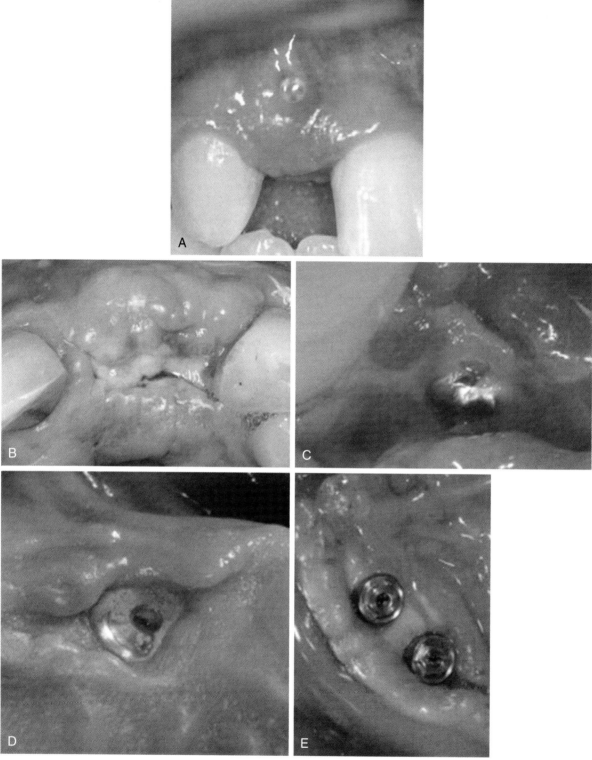

• **Fig. 31.34** Incision Line Opening Classification. (A) Class 0 wound healing. (B) Class 1 wound healing. (C) Class 2 wound healing. (D) Class 3 wound healing. (E) Class 4 wound healing.

exposure of submerged implants based on diagnostic methods and treatment modalities to prevent or intercept such complications. They suggested that implants with spontaneous exposure should immediately be surgically exposed as early as possible to prevent mucositis. A healing abutment should be placed after the cover screw is removed.[72]

Morbidity Consequences of Incision Line Opening With Implants and Bone Grafting

The resultant consequences of ILO can vary depending on the type of implant or bone-grafting procedure. For implant placement with good initial fixation, primary closure is favored for one-stage surgery, with placement of a permucosal abutment. For bone augmentation procedures, primary closure is of paramount importance for clinicians when performing guided bone regeneration techniques and autogenous onlay grafting procedures. When ILO occurs during autogenous block grafting, there tends to be a greater potential for delayed healing, loss of graft into the oral cavity, and increased risk for infection.

Exposure of nonresorbable membranes adds additional risk for infection and unsatisfactory results. If guided bone regeneration is performed in conjunction with implant placement, ILO may also lead to loss of the implant. ILO most likely will result in a bacterial smear layer on the implant body, which may inhibit bone formation. Bone resorption resulting from infection may require implant removal. The same degree of ILO, without simultaneous implant placement, could possibly be managed and compensated for by bone expansion, use of slightly narrower implants, increased number of implants, and/or additional augmentation.

In addition, ILO can negatively affect esthetic clinical outcomes. The placement of implants simultaneous with regenerative procedures adds the risk for a functional and esthetically compromised result. For multistage bone augmentation procedures, primary soft tissue healing allows for the most predictable outcomes. Incision technique, flap design, soft tissue handling, and avoidance of transitional prosthesis pressure are key factors in avoiding ILO.

Wound dehiscence may be associated with increased discomfort and the need for closer monitoring. More postoperative appointments are required. These are financially nonproductive and negatively impact practice profitability. Some patients may seek care or a second opinion because of loss of confidence in the primary clinician. When ILO occurs, the clinician should be proactive in follow-up care and educating the patient on the complication consequences.

Prevention of Incision Line Opening

Good Surgical Technique

The implant clinician should adhere to the following surgical principles to minimize and promote optimum wound healing and decrease the possibility of ILO.

Incision in Keratinized Tissue. The primary incision should ideally be located in keratinized tissue whenever possible. This permits increased wound surface area and a resultant increase in vascularity to the incision. Not only does this reduce the initial intraoral bleeding, it also severs smaller blood vessels and reduces postoperative edema, which may add tension to the incision line. If there is 3 mm or more of attached gingiva on the crest of the edentulous ridge, the incision bisects this tissue. This places half of the attached gingiva width on each side of the incision. If there is less than 3 mm of attached keratinized tissue on the crest, the incision is made more lingually so that at least 1.5 mm of the attached tissue is placed to the facial aspect of the implant. This concept is very important in the posterior mandible because attached tissue is needed to prevent tension and pulling from the buccinator muscle (Fig. 31.35).[73]

Broad-Based Incision Design. The apex or tip of the flap should never be wider than the base (e.g., diverge from incision base to the apex). This will maintain adequate vasculature that will prevent ischemic necrosis to the flap, decreasing the possibility of ILO. The length of the flap should generally not exceed twice the width of the base. In addition, the base of the flap should not have significant pressure or be excessively stretched or twisted, which may compromise the blood supply (Fig. 31.36).[74]

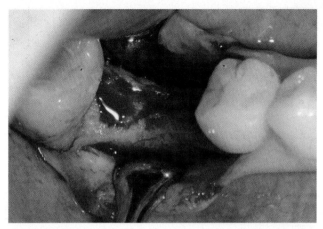

● **Fig. 31.35** Incision should always maintain attached tissue on the facial.

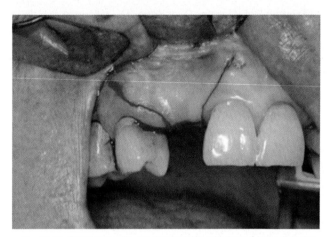

● **Fig. 31.36** Anterior papilla-sparing incision with broad-based design.

Allow for Adequate Access. The flap should be large enough to provide adequate visualization of the surgical site and allow for the insertion of instruments to perform the surgical procedure. If the flap is too small, a retractor will not be able to maintain the flap without excessive pressure. Excessive retraction pressure will lead to increased inflammation, which may compromise the healing of the incision line.

Vertical Release Incision to Maintain Blood Supply and Decrease Tension on Flap. The blood supply to the reflected flap should be maintained whenever possible. The primary blood supply to the facial flap, which is most often the flap reflected for an implant or bone graft, is from the unkeratinized mobile mucosa. This is especially true where muscles of facial expression or functional muscles attach to the periosteum. Therefore vertical release incisions are made to the height of the mucogingival junction, and the facial flap may be reflected approximately 5 mm above the height of the mucogingival junction. Both of these incision approaches maintain more blood supply to the facial flap. In addition, incisions and reflection in the mobile alveolar mucosa increase flap retraction during initial healing, which may contribute to ILO and may increase risk for scar formation and delayed healing of the incision line as a consequence of reduced blood supply.

Vertical release incisions should not be made over bony prominences (e.g., canine eminence) because this will increase tension on the incision line and may increase the possibility of ILO (Fig. 31.37).

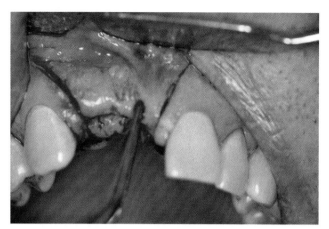

• **Fig. 31.37** Vertical release incisions to allow for tension-free closure.

Maintain Flap Margins Over Bone. The soft tissue flap design should also have the margins of the wound over host bone whenever possible. This is especially important when approximating tissue over bone grafts or barrier membranes. The host bone provides growth factors to the margins and allows the periosteum to regenerate faster to the site. The margins distal to the elevated flap should have minimal reflection. The palatal flap and the facial tissues distal to the reflected flap should not be elevated from the palatal bone (unless augmentation is required) because the blood supply to the incision line will be delayed. In addition, the unreflected flap does not retract during initial healing, which could place additional tension on the incision line. The soft tissue reflection distal to the graft site may be split thickness to maintain periosteum on the bone around the incision line. This improves the early vascularization to the incision line and adhesion of the margins to reduce retraction during initial healing.

Clean, Concise Incision. A clean incision is made through the tissue in one direction with even pressure of the scalpel. A sharp blade of proper size (i.e., #15 blade) should be used to be make clean, concise incisions without traumatizing the tissue from repeated passes or strokes. Tentative strokes, especially in different planes, will increase the amount of damaged tissue and increase the amount of bleeding. Long, continuous strokes are preferable to shorter, inconsistent, and interrupted strokes.[75]

Sharp dissection will minimize trauma to the incision line, which will result in easier closure. Care should be noted of vital underlying nerves, blood vessels, and associated muscles. Scalpel blades dull rather easily, especially when used on bone and tissue with greater resistance. The clinician should change blades when dulling is suspected to decrease tissue trauma. The incision should be made with the blade held perpendicular to the epithelial surface. This will result in an angle that produces square wound margins that are easier to reorient during suturing and less likely for surgical wound necrosis to occur.

Full-Thickness Reflection and Ideal Flap Elevation. Ideally the flap should be full thickness and include the surface mucosa, submucosa, and periosteum. The periosteum is necessary for healing; the replacement of the periosteum in its original position will increase healing.

Tissue elevation should be completed with extreme care. Meticulous handling is required to minimize trauma to the soft tissue. Proper use of appropriate tissue forceps, avoidance of excessive suctioning by the assistant, and "tie-back" sutures all contribute to improved flap management. Nonlocking tissue pick-ups, also called "thumb forceps," are commonly held between the thumb

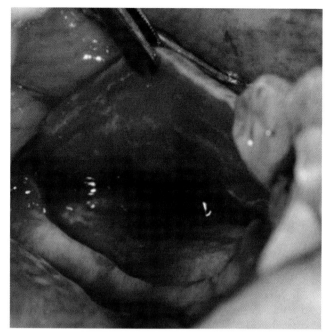

• **Fig. 31.38** Full-thickness flap and reflection.

and two or three fingers of one hand. Spring tension at one end holds the grasping ends apart until pressure is applied. These forceps are used to hold tissues in place when applying sutures and to gently retract tissues during exploratory surgery. Tissue forceps can have smooth tips, cross-hatched tips, or serrated tips (often called "mouse's teeth"). Serrated forceps used on tissues will cause less tissue damage than smooth surface forceps because the surgeon can grasp with less overall pressure.

Smooth or cross-hatched forceps are used to move dressings, remove sutures, and perform similar tasks.

During flap elevation, elevators should rest on bone and not on soft tissue. Care should be exercised not to continuously suction the tissue because this may irritate and traumatize the tissue margins. Use of variable-suction tips with fingertip control can help minimize tissue damage. After flap replacement, it is advantageous to apply pressure to the tissue for several minutes to minimize blood clot thickness and to ensure bleeding has stopped.

Minimizing surgical operating time will directly benefit soft tissues and will reduce the risk for infection.[76] The tissue retractors should be selected and placed in a position to prevent undue pressure on tissues. Maintaining the retractors on bone and not on the tissue will minimize trauma to the tissue. Excessive pressure and tension on the tissue flap will impair blood circulation, alter the physiologic healing of the surgical wound, and predispose the wound to bacterial colonization (Fig. 31.38).

Papilla-Saving Incisions. The interproximal soft tissue in sites next to adjacent natural teeth may be classified into three categories: (1) papillae have an acceptable height in the edentulous site, (2) papillae have less than acceptable height, or (3) one papilla is acceptable and the other papilla is depressed and requires elevation.

When the interproximal papilla has an acceptable height, "papilla-saving" incisions are made adjacent to each neighboring tooth. The vertical incisions are made on the facial aspect of the edentulous site and begin 1 mm below the mucogingival junction, within the keratinized tissue. Extending the vertical incisions beyond the mucogingival junction increases the risk for scar formation at the incision site. The full-thickness incision then approaches the crest of the edentulous site, leaving 1.0 to 1.5 mm of the interproximal papilla adjacent to each tooth. The vertical incisions are not wider at the base than the crestal width of tissue. This permits the facial flap to be advanced over the implant or short and adjacent to a permucosal extension at the conclusion of the procedure, with no voids at the incision line and primary closure.

Hemostasis. Hemostasis is important for many reasons, such as providing a clean surgical field for accurate dissection and flap elevation, along with decreasing trauma. Bleeding can occur from arteries, veins, or capillaries and may result in diffuse, continuous oozing. Ideally complete hemostasis should be achieved before the closure of the wound. If not, the continuous bleeding or hematoma will prevent the apposition of the surgical wound. There are many mechanical, thermal, and chemical methods that may be used to achieve adequate hemostasis. Care should be noted that the use of active or passive hemostatic agents, along with electrocauterization of the wound margins, may decrease the normal physiologic healing of the wound margins and predispose the site to infection and possible wound dehiscence. If hemostatic agents are used (e.g., cellulose), they should be removed after hemostasis is accomplished because this may interfere with surgical wound healing.

Prevent Desiccation of the Tissue. The tissues should be maintained in a moist environment without prolonged periods of desiccation. If drying of the tissues occurs, there is less likelihood that complete wound closure will occur. If the tissue margins become desiccated, periodic irrigations with sterile saline (0.9% sodium chloride) or a saline-moistened gauze may be used.

Relieving Tissue (Tension Free). Excessive flap tension is the most frequent causative factor of ILO. This is best prevented by appropriate incision and flap design, the use of periosteal releasing incisions (PRIs), and blunt dissection ("tissue stretching"). Past techniques to expand tissue primarily used a more apical tissue reflection and horizontal scoring of the periosteum parallel to the primary incision. Historically the vestibular approach by Brånemark allowed for optimal visualization of anatomic landmarks, suturing remote from the surgical area, complete tissue coverage, as well as predictable primary closure and healing.[77] The postoperative disadvantages of this approach include distortion of the vestibule and other anatomic landmarks, edema, difficult suture removal, and cumulative patient discomfort.[78] Langer and Langer[79] documented the use of overlapping partial-thickness flaps. This approach results in extension of the coronal aspect of the buccal or palatal flap, allowing primary intention closure around the site in an overlapping manner. This is usually effective for primary closure when less than 5-mm advancement of the flap is necessary.

A submucosal space technique developed by Misch[80] in the early 1980s is an effective method to expand tissue over larger grafts (greater than 15 × 10 mm in height and width) (Box 31.2).

The utility of periosteal incision for gaining flap release was studied by Park et al.[81] They found that flaps could be advanced up to 171.3% (>1.5 times longer than its original length) by two vertical incisions and a PRI under a minimal tension of 5 g, whereas one or two vertical incisions without PRI could advance the flap only 113.4% and 124.2%, respectively. These results suggested that PRI can be predictably used to attain tension-free primary closure under a minimal pulling tension of flaps (Fig. 31.39).

• BOX 31.2 Submucosal Space Technique[153]

1. The full-thickness facial flap first is elevated off the facial bone approximately 5 mm above the height of the vestibule.
2. One incision with a scalpel, 1 to 2 mm deep, is made through the periosteum, parallel to the crestal incision and 3 to 5 mm above the vestibular height of the mucoperiosteum. This shallow incision is made the full length of the facial flap and may even extend above and beyond the vertical release incisions. Care is taken to make this incision above the mucogingival junction; otherwise the flap may be perforated and delay soft tissue healing.
3. Soft tissue scissors (e.g., Metzenbaum) are used in a blunt dissection technique to create a tunnel apical to the vestibule and above the unreflected periosteum. The scissors are closed and pushed through the initial scalpel incision approximately 10 mm deep, then opened slowly.
4. This submucosal space is parallel to the surface mucosa (not deep toward the overlying bone) and above the unreflected periosteum. The thickness of the facial flap should be 3 to 5 mm because the scissors are parallel to the surface. This tunnel is expanded with the tissue scissors several millimeters above and distal to the vertical relief incisions.
5. The submucosal space is developed and the flap is advanced the distance of the "tunnel" and draped over the graft to approximate the tissue for primary closure without tension. Ideally the facial flap should be able to advance over the graft and past the lingual flap margin by more than 5 mm. The facial flap may then be returned to the lingual flap margin and sutured. This soft tissue procedure is performed before preparing the host region for any type of bone grafting or augmentation around an implant.

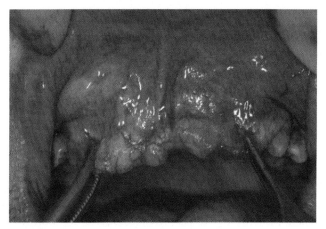

• Fig. 31.39 Tension-Free Closure. Facial flap can be pulled over the lingual flap by a minimum of 5 mm.

Decreasing "Dead Spaces"

Gentle pressure is applied to the reflected soft tissue flaps for 3 to 5 minutes. This pressure may reduce postoperative bleeding under the flap, which may cause "dead spaces" and delayed healing. Any stagnant blood under the flap is "milked" from under the soft tissue by gentle pressure. This also allows the fibrin formation from the platelets to help "glue" the flap to the graft site.

Decrease Inflammation

Systemic corticosteroids or NSAIDs may be administered before and after surgery to decrease soft tissue edema because edema has been shown to contribute to ILO.

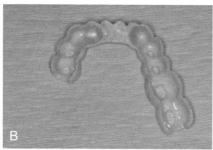
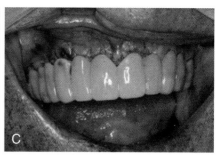

• **Fig. 31.40** Ideal Provisional Prosthesis. (A) Postsuturing image. (B) Snap-On Smile prosthesis. (C) Insertion of prosthesis.

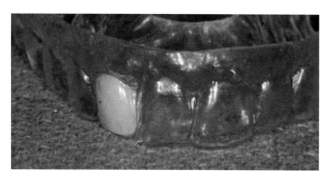

• **Fig. 31.41** Essix Appliance.

Transitional and Interim Prosthesis Design

Occlusal forces applied to a removable prosthesis over a healing implant or graft site may also cause ILO of soft tissues and delay wound healing. Without appropriate adjustment, these forces can easily result in ILO by compressing the surgical area during function before suture removal. The potential for crestal bone loss is increased during any graft healing or around implants during stage I healing, which may lead to implant failure from early loading. Although use of such prostheses should be discouraged, other strategies to minimize or eliminate this possibility would include extensive relief of the intaglio surface, flange elimination, and use of tissue conditioners.

Much more preferable provisional tooth replacement(s) would be either tooth or implant (transitional) supported (Fig. 31.40).

Other examples of fixed transitional prostheses would include the bonding of natural tooth crowns or denture teeth to the teeth bounding the edentulous space and modification of existing fixed partial denture, that is, pontic shortening. Removable transitional prostheses, such as an Essix retainer or Snap-On Smile prosthesis, are frequently used because of their rigid support and resultant lack of pressure on the incision line. A resin-bonded fixed restoration can also be fabricated to provide improved function, especially when crestal bone regeneration is performed.

The prosthesis may depress the interdental papillae of adjacent teeth. As a result a resin-bonded fixed prosthesis is fabricated for the extended healing, and a removable device may be used short term for cosmetic emergencies (if the prosthesis debonds) (Fig. 31.41).

When a resin-bonded restoration is used, the adjacent teeth are not prepared and the device is bonded to teeth below the centric occlusal contacts. The interdental papillae are often depressed after initial socket healing. This type of transitional restoration for the single-tooth implant has the multiple benefits of being off the soft tissue drape, the developing bone augmented site, and the healing implant-bone interface.

Several options to the resin-bonded device permit these goals. An Essix appliance is an acrylic shell, similar to a bleaching tray, that has a denture tooth attached to replace the missing tooth. This prosthesis is the simplest treatment for tooth replacement postsurgery.

When an adjacent tooth requires a crown be added to the orthodontic wire, a cast-clasp RPD with indirect rest seats, which prevents rotational movements on the surgical site, is an excellent option.

Atraumatic Suture Removal

Removing sutures too early or traumatically may result in ILO and cause delayed healing, leading to morbidity of the implant or bone graft.

Normally nonresorbable sutures or extended absorbable sutures are removed within 10 to 14 days after surgery. Suture removal should include the following steps:

1. Patient rinses lightly with 0.12% chlorhexidine gluconate.
2. With tissue pick-ups, hold up the knot end of the suture and cut the suture closest to the tissue. Care should be exercised not to traumatize or irritate the surgical wound.
3. Gently pull the suture out with the knot outside of the tissue. Do not pull the knot through the tissue to remove.
4. Have the patient rinse with 0.12% chlorhexidine. Evaluate and make sure the interim prosthesis does not impinge on the surgical wound. The adjacent tooth may be prepared and a cantilevered transitional fixed partial denture with a pontic over the surgical site may be used. When the patient requires orthodontics, a denture tooth and an attached bracket may be added to the orthodontic wire.

Management of Incision Line Opening

In the dental implant literature there are two treatment recommendations discussed with respect to ILO. The first is to allow the surgical wound to heal via secondary intention with the use of antimicrobials and hygiene measures. The second treatment modality is to resuture the opened surgical wound, which is not recommended by the author (Table 31.3).

To allow the site to heal by secondary intention, there needs to be significant discipline and patient cooperation for a successful outcome. This treatment technique is dictated by many variables, such as the health of the existing tissue, tissue thickness, location, age of the patient, and size of the dehiscence.

For an incision line opening to heal correctly, strict post-op instructions and procedures must be adhered to by the clinician and the patient. First, the clinician should make sure that no external influence may directly traumatize or delay the healing. If an interim prosthesis is being used, care should be exercised to minimize any direct contact with the incision line. The intaglio surface of the prosthesis over the incision line should be modified

TABLE 31.3 Treatment of Incision Line Opening

Surgical Procedure	TREATMENT	
	Early (<1 Week)	Late (~>3 Weeks)
Implant:		
One stage	Secondary intention protocol (resuture ONLY if favorable conditions)	Secondary intention protocol
Two stage	Secondary intention protocol	• Remove overlying tissue with tissue punch bur or scalpel • Place permucosal extension (≈1 mm above tissue; higher extension may lead to excessive force on the implant) (Fig. 31.42)
Bone Graft:		
Particulate graft	Secondary intention protocol	Secondary intention protocol
Block graft	Secondary intention protocol	• Check for mobility of graft • Reduce sharp bony edges • Freshen wound edges with diamond bur
Membrane:		
Collagen (regular)	Secondary intention protocol	Secondary intention protocol
Collagen (extended)	Secondary intention protocol	Secondary intention protocol • Trim excess membrane above tissue level with scissors
Acellular dermal matrix (AlloDerm)	Secondary intention protocol	Secondary intention protocol • Trim excess membrane above tissue level with scissors
Nonresorbable (cytoplast, titanium)	Secondary intention protocol	• Remove membrane if chronic tissue irritation or infection • Ideally attempt to maintain for at least 6 weeks

accordingly to be concave, not convex. The stress bearing areas (i.e. Maxilla – horizontal palate and residual ridge, Mandible- buccal shelf) should be maintained to absorb the occlusal forces. In addition, the ILO should be locally cleaned with 0.12% chlorhexidine. The patient should be placed on a strict recall, ideally seen every week for the first month.

The patient should be instructed to rinse non-vigorously with 0.12% chlorhexidine twice a day. Strict avoidance of smoking and alcohol use as this will delay healing. If an interim prosthesis is being used, no denture adhesive should be positioned over the ILO area. And lastly, the patient should be instructed to not evaluate the site, especially by pulling the lip up to inspect the area. This will stretch the incision line and most likely will result in further dehiscence (Box 31.3).

Resuturing Protocol

Resuturing is most often not recommended because it is an unpredictable technique and in some cases increases the amount of dehiscence. When attempting to resuture a fresh wound, usually the epithelium is thin and friable, which often leads to tearing of the incision line. This may result in a larger dehiscence or infection. If completed, the margins of the tissue should be "freshened" with a scalpel or a diamond bur. Greenstein et al.[82] have recommended that, when the dehiscence is small and occurs within 24 to 48 hours, the clinician may immediately resuture the dehiscence. Once the wound is large (2–3 cm) or the time elapsed is more than 2 to 3 days, it becomes more difficult for the margins of the wound to be excised and resutured. It is the author's recommendation to be cautious with resuturing incision lines that may end up resulting in increased morbidity of the surgical wound (Fig. 31.42).

• BOX 31.3 Secondary Intention Protocol

Clinician
1. Relieve prosthesis to have no buccal flange and no contact on the surgical wound area.
2. Maintain stress-bearing areas on the prosthesis with the use of a tissue conditioner; however, material should be removed from the dehisced area.
3. Locally clean the dehiscence area with 0.12% chlorhexidine.
4. Employ closer observation of the patient to include recall appointments a minimum of once a week for the first month.

Patient Instructions
1. Nonvigorous rinse with 0.12% chlorhexidine twice daily and plaque control.
2. Minimize the use of interim prosthesis.
3. No direct mastication on the area of dehiscence.
4. Avoid smoking and the use of alcohol.
5. Avoid peroxide and alcohol-based mouth rinses.
6. Avoid acidic foods.
7. Avoid inspection of dehiscent site (pulling on lip to see area).
8. Do not use any denture adhesive with the interim prosthesis.

Biomechanical Complications

Screw Loosening

Abutment screw loosening has been shown to be associated with an approximately 6% of implant prostheses fabricated.[83] Screw loosening is the most common implant prosthetic complication, accounting for approximately 33% of all post-implant prosthodontic complications.[84] More recent studies indicate this

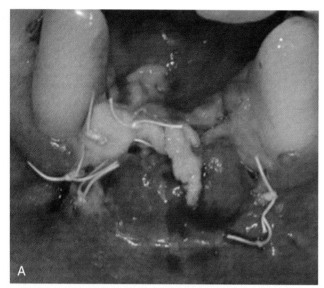

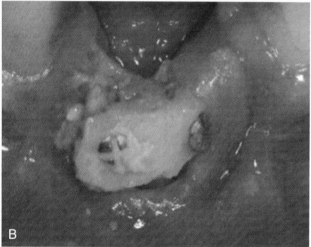

• **Fig. 31.42** Resuturing Complication. (A) Two weeks postoperatively showing suture breakdown. (B) After resuturing, complete bone graft is exposed. This is why resuturing is not recommended.

complication occurs in approximately 8% of single crowns, 5% of multiple-unit fixed prostheses, and 3% of implant overdentures. De Boever et al.[85] have shown that 12% of prostheses exhibit loosening within 3 years, whereas Chaar et al.[86] have shown an incidence rate of 4.3% within 5 years and approximately 10% long term (5–10 years). Screw loosening may cause considerable complications. A loose screw may contribute to crestal bone loss because bacteria are able to colonize and harbor in the open interface. When an abutment screw becomes loose on a cemented crown, the crown may need to be cut off the abutment to gain access to the abutment screw, which results in patient disappointment and unproductive clinician time. If a loose abutment screw is not treated appropriately, fracture of the prosthesis, implant components, or the implant body may occur.

Etiology

External Force Factors. External forces that act on a screw joint greatly increase the risk for screw loosening. These forces may be called *joint-separating forces* when related to screw loosening; however, they are the same forces that are risk factors for implant failure, crestal bone loss, and component fracture. When the external joint-separating forces are greater than the force holding the screws together (called *clamping forces*), the screw will become loose. The external forces from parafunction, crown height, masticatory dynamics, position in the dental arch, and opposing dentition are factors that can dramatically increase the stress to the implant and the screw joint. In addition, conditions that magnify or increase these factors are cantilevers, angled loads, and poor occlusal designs. External forces applied to the joint system are important to account for when the aim is to decrease the incidence of screw loosening. The endurance limit of a material is the amount of force required to fracture the object when enough cycles are applied. The greater the force, the fewer cycles required before fracture occurs. It is the combination and relationship of both the amount of force and the number of cycles that is the cause of the screw loosening complication.

Cantilevers/Increased Crown Height Space. One of the most common causative factors resulting in screw loosening is excessive continuous occlusal forces. The most common example occurs in prostheses with improper occlusal contacts. The greater the stress applied to the prostheses, the greater the risk for abutment screw loosening. A nonideal prosthetic design may potentiate the force applied. Cantilevers increase the risk for screw loosening because they increase the magnitude of forces to the implant system: there is a direct relationship between the length of the cantilever and force applied to the prosthesis.[87] Any of these external forces applied to a cantilever will further magnify the joint-separating forces. For example, cantilevers on prostheses lead to uneven occlusal loads. Uneven occlusal loads cause repeated cycles of compression and then tension and shear of implant components. Screws are especially vulnerable to tensile and shear forces. Both of these are dramatically increased with cantilever forces or angled loads. Because the screw is an inclined plane, the continued vibration causes it to unthread.

The greater the range of external forces, the fewer the number of cycles necessary before screw loosening. When an increased crown height space exists (poor crown/implant ratio), there is a resultant greater force applied to the screw. This usually results in a greater risk for screw loosening (or fracture). Boggan et al.[88] demonstrated that the force that is applied to the screw is directly related to the crown height. The crown height acts as a vertical cantilever, which magnifies the force on the abutment screw.

Parafunction. Of all the external forces that cause screw loosening, the primary factor is parafunction related. A horizontal bruxing patient loads the implant crown with an angled force repeatedly. This increases the magnitude of force, cycles to fatigue failure, and the angle of the force that places shear on the interface. Abutment screw loosening can be expected in a patient with a severe bruxing habit. A parafunction patient increases the amount of force to the system while also increasing the number of cycles to the system.

Hence fractures of porcelain and cement seals and also screw loosening or fracture are inevitable. When the adjacent natural teeth are mobile to lateral or angled forces, the rigid implant and implant crown may be overloaded. A heavy bite force occlusal adjustment, which allows the adjacent teeth to move before implant crown contact, is recommended to reduce the risk for overload. Continuous occlusal loads can have a cumulative effect on the preload, and the screw material may undergo deformation.[89] When the force exceeds the yield strength, plastic deformation occurs, and the screw begins to deform. This material deformation causes the screw to loosen and leads to potential failure of the prosthesis.

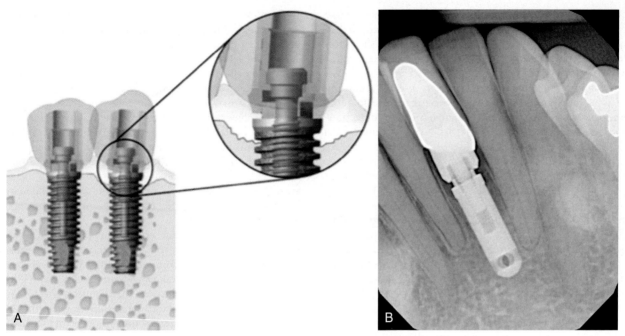

• **Fig. 31.43** (A) Nonpassive or improperly seated screw-retained restorations may be distorted when seated into position when the prosthetic screw is threaded. The distortion of the superstructure causes stresses that are concentrated at the crestal bone level and may result in bone loss. (B) Radiographic image depicting incomplete seating of abutment, which predisposes prosthesis to screw loosening.

Screw loosening is also affected by the amount of the force and the number of cycles, and is similar to fatigue. External methods to limit screw loosening include factors that reduce the biomechanical stress. These include key implant positions (i.e., to distribute forces evenly), sufficient number of implants (i.e., adequate surface area), passive prosthetic frameworks, and adequate occlusal schemes.[90]

Splinted Versus Nonsplinted Crowns. Screw loosening of abutment or prosthetic screws occurs more often on individual implant crowns than on crowns that are splinted together. For example, in a report for single molar replacement, the abutment screw-loosening rate was 40% during a 3-year period. When two splinted implants were used to replace the molar space, the screw loosening was reduced to 8%.[91] The stress distribution of splinted prosthetic units results in less force applied to the screw system. Studies have shown that splinted implant-retained overdentures have far less screw loosening in comparison with fixed prostheses.[92]

Crown/Abutment Not Fully Seated. If the abutment is not fully seated because of improper abutment placement, tissue impingement, or bone impingement, a poor distribution of force in the screw system will result, which leads to increased screw loosening. When the abutment is not fully seated and completely tightened, the prosthetic screw will be distorted, which leads to inadequate preload and subsequent screw loosening or fracture (Fig. 31.43).

Insufficient/Excessive Torqueing. When improper preload via the torqueing process is applied to the abutment screw, screw loosening will often occur. This may be caused by either excessive or insufficient tightening of the abutment screw. An implant screw is similar to a bolt joint in engineering. There is a preload (tightening force) placed on the screw, which develops a force within the screw. As the screw is tightened, it elongates, producing tension, which results in the implant screw acting like a spring. The preload stretch of the screw is maintained by frictional force, and the tension between the screw and the implant/abutment is termed a clamping force.

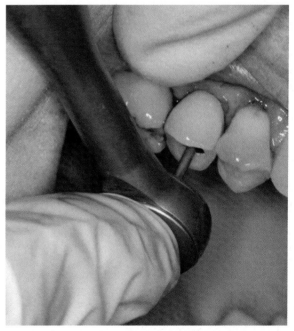

• **Fig. 31.44** Nonideal torque applied to the screw leads to a greater incidence of screw loosening. If the screw is not torqued sufficiently or overtorque occurs, insufficient preload will result, which will most likely result in screw loosening. The proper torque wrench and technique should be used according to the manufacturer's specifications because implant systems have various recommended torque values.

When insufficient preload is applied to the screw, there is insufficient clamping force, which ultimately leads to screw loosening, especially under occlusal loading. When excessive force is applied, the clamping force is easily released, and screw loosening will occur (Fig. 31.44).

Screw Diameter. The diameter of the abutment screw may have a significant effect on the amount of preload applied to the system before deformation occurs. The greater the screw diameter, the higher the preload that may be applied, which results in a greater clamping force on the screw joint. However, the coping and prosthetic screws vary greatly according to the type, size, and material. The strength of the material increases by a power of 4 when the diameter of the screw doubles (a screw with twice the diameter is 16 times stronger). As a result, abutment screws loosen less often because they can take a higher preload compared with coping and prosthetic screws. Some companies offer similar diameters for abutment and prosthetic screws. As a result a similar clamping force may be used for either component.

Screw Material. The composition of the screw is another factor that modifies its performance. The composition of the metal may influence the amount of strain in the screw from preload and the point of fracture, directly affecting the amount of preload that can be safely applied. Screw material and yield strength vary greatly when all other factors are similar (e.g., 12.4 N for a gold screw to 83.8 N for a titanium alloy screw fixation).[93]

The deformation or permanent distortion of the screw is the endpoint of the elastic modulus. Titanium alloy has four times the bending fracture resistance of grade 1 titanium. Abutment screws made of grade 1 titanium deform and fracture more easily than the alloy. Titanium alloy is 2.4 times stronger than grade 4 titanium. As such, a higher torque magnitude can be used on the titanium alloy abutment screw and female component (found within the implant body), less on grade 4 titanium, less on grade 1 titanium, and the least on gold screws.

The elongation of metal is related to the modulus of elasticity, which depends on the type of material, width, design, and the amount of stress applied. The material of which the screw is made (e.g., titanium alloy, titanium, or gold) has a specific modulus of elasticity. A prosthetic gold screw exhibits greater elongation than a screw made of titanium alloy but has a lower yield strength.

Although the strengths of titanium grades are dramatically different, the modulus of elasticity is similar for grade 1 to 4 titanium. Hence the strain of the abutment screw is similar with each grade of titanium, but the safety load relative to fracture is different. Titanium alloy (grade 5) has a slightly higher modulus of elasticity. Although not clinically relevant to metal-bone osseointegration, the titanium alloy screw should have a slightly higher preload value. This is not a consequence relative to permanent deformation or fracture because it is more than twice as strong as the other grades of titanium.

The metal for the screwdriver used in the torque wrench is also important to consider. Stripping of the screw head prevents the clinician from tightening or removing the screw. Some manufacturers fabricate the torque wrench driver out of titanium alloy, and the screw is made of gold or titanium. The concept is that the torque wrench will not deform the hexagon and will not strip, so the device lasts longer. However, this is not ideal. It is easier to replace the torque wrench driver than the abutment or prosthetic screw.

From a clinical standpoint the receptor site for the torque wrench is also a feature of the screw head to consider. The screw head has a rotation feature, most commonly a hexagonal design. The more sides to the rotation feature, the more often the head will strip. A slot or triangular feature will strip less than a hexagon.

Component Fit. In the science of machining metal components there is a range of dimensions that manufacturers use. For instance, an implant 4 mm in diameter may actually range from 3.99 to 4.01 mm. Likewise the abutment and prosthetic coping connection also has a range. As a result, if a smaller implant body hex dimension is mated with a larger abutment connection, the components may not ideally fit together. Most implant manufacturers allow for a misfit range that results in the abutment or coping being able to rotate 10 degrees on the implant body. Components between the abutment and implant body may have a misfit of 10 degrees in a rotational dimension, and horizontal discrepancies have been reported up to 99 μm.[94,95] These ranges are different with respect to each implant system. The more accurate the component fit, the less force is applied to the abutment or prosthetic screw.

The incidence of screw loosening is also a function of the accuracy of fit of the flat-to-flat connection of the implant and abutment or prosthetic component. Implant abutment connections or prosthetic connections with an unstable mating interface place undue stress on the screw that connects the components. Mechanical testing has demonstrated a direct correlation between the tolerance of the flat-to-flat dimension of the external hexagon and the stability of the abutment or prosthetic screw. Binon[96] showed that a mean flat-to-flat range of less than 0.005 mm exists on the hexagon, and a flat-to-flat range of less than 0.05 mm for the entire sample would result in a more stable screw joint. Studies have shown plastic castable patterns, which can be highly inaccurate, to have a vertical misfit as high as 66 μm.[97] The same manufacturing conditions apply to impression transfer copings and analogs. Many manufacturers have a wider machining range (+ or – variance) for the prosthetic components to reduce the cost of manufacturing. When transfer copings and analogs are used in impressions and then to fabricate the prosthesis in the laboratory and the implants are splinted together, the prosthesis may not passively seat.

Many manufacturers recommend the use of plastic (nonmetal) burnout posts. Plastic burnout prosthetic copings cost less, but they exhibit much greater laboratory variance and poor fit because of irregularities and settling of the superstructure. Besides cost, another advantage of a plastic burnout pattern for a coping is that one type of metal is used for the coping and superstructure, lessening the risk for metal corrosion or separation between the coping and superstructure.

A machined coping may be used to fit the implant abutment more accurately to reduce settling. Some manufacturers suggest a titanium coping to reduce the risk for misfit. However, oxides form on the titanium-machined coping surface and impair metal adherence when the prosthesis or abutment metal work is cast to the coping. Mechanical retentive features on the coping improve this metal-to-metal attachment. Laboratory studies demonstrate that an alloy-cylinder compatibility exists when noble-metal alloys are used rather than titanium for a superior metal-to-metal connection. A machine coping connection is still present, so it is superior to the plastic components used to cast one metal.[98] The risk of oxides forming between the coping and metal of the prosthesis is also reduced.

Implant Design. The type and design of the dental implant has a significant impact on screw loosening. As a general rule, most implant bodies have an antirotational feature for the abutment connection. The most common designs are an external hexagon, an internal hexagon, a Morse taper, and a Morse taper with threads.

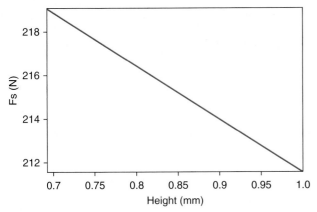

• **Fig. 31.45** The higher (or deeper) the antirotational hexagon component (x component on the graph), the less the force applied to the abutment screw (Fs) on the y axis. A 0.7-mm hexagon height is standard in the industry and was used first by Nobel Biocare. A 1-mm hexagon height has less risk for screw loosening because the force on the screw is decreased.

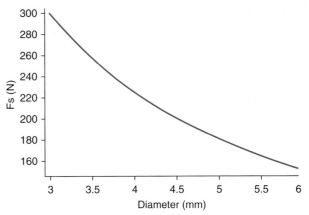

• **Fig. 31.46** To reduce forces on the abutment screw, the platform diameter of the implant is more important than the hexagon height. The larger the diameter (x-axis), the less the force applied to the screw (y axis).

Factors that affect the abutment screw connection and screw loosening include the height (or depth) of the hexagon and the platform diameter. Boggan et al.[88] studied the influence of design factors on the mechanical strength and quality of fit of the implant abutment interface. Whereas failure mode for static test samples was bending or deformation of the abutment screw, fracture of the abutment screw was the common failure mode for the fatigue test samples. The static failure load was greater for the external hex implants of 1 mm in height, compared with implants with an internal hexagon of 1.7 mm. The larger-diameter implant had the greatest static load before failure.[88] As the hexagon height (or depth) increases, the load on the abutment screw decreases. Likewise, as the diameter of the implant platform increases, the force on the abutment screw decreases. Reduction of the lateral load (P) on the abutment screw is crucial to prevent the load on the screw to be beyond the yield strength of the material.

The height (or depth) of the antirotational hexagon is directly related to the force applied to the abutment screw with any lateral load. Because the crown is connected to the abutment and the abutment rests on the implant platform, a lateral force on the crown creates a tipping force on the abutment. This tipping force is resisted by the hexagon height or depth, the platform, and the abutment screw. When the arc of rotation is above the hexagon height, all of the force is applied to the abutment screw. For the hexagon height to be above the arc of tipping forces, the hexagon height must be at least 1 mm for a 4-mm-diameter implant. Yet many implant manufacturers feature a hexagon height of only 0.7 mm, so almost all of the force is directed to the abutment screw, increasing the occurrence of screw loosening and fracture (Fig. 31.45).

The difference between external (EC) versus internal connections (IC) has been well documented. Studies have shown that the incidence rate associated with EC implants was 18.3% at a mean of 5.3 years (217 of 1183 restorations; maximum, 59.9%).[99,100] The complication rate with internal connection (IC) implants was 2.7% at a mean of 4.5 years (142 of 5235 restorations; maximum, 31.6%).[101,102] Other studies have shown the external hex to have a significantly higher incidence of screw loosening than the internal hex (MA-EC, 15.1%; Zr-EC, 6.8%; MA-IC, 1.5%; Zr-IC, 0.9%).[103]

The platform dimension on which the abutment is seated is also an important factor in screw loosening. Larger-diameter implants, with associated larger platform dimensions, reduce the forces applied to an abutment screw and change the arc of displacement of the abutment on the crest module. For example, in a report by Cho et al.,[104] abutment screw loosening over a 3-year period was almost 15% for a 4-mm implant diameter but less than 6% for the 5-mm implant diameter (Fig. 31.46).

Screw Versus Cement Retained. When evaluating the prosthesis type (cement versus screw), studies have shown screw retained (8.5%) had a much higher incidence of screw loosening in comparison with cement retained (3.1%). These complications have a greater incidence with screw-retained restorations compared with cement-retained restorations because cement-retained restorations are more passive and have less strain on the implant system.[105] Although a cement-retained restoration is more common, screw-retained restorations are indicated when low-profile retention is necessary on a short abutment or when the implant bodies are more than 30 degrees from each other and splinting is required to restore the patient.

In addition, a screw-retained prosthesis has the advantage of less chance of tissue irritation because of the high incidence of retained cement with a cement-retained prosthesis. Screw loosening and partially unretained restorations are common complications of nonpassive castings. The more passive the fit on the implant abutment for screw retention and the more controlled the occlusal forces, the more secure is the prosthesis. The repeated compressive and tensile forces from nonpassive castings under occlusal loads cause vibration and loosening of the screw components. Accuracy in design and fabrication of the metal superstructure are determining factors for the reduction of forces at the implant abutment and implant-bone interface. Passive screw-retained restorations are more difficult to fabricate than passive cement-retained restorations. When the screw is threaded into position, the superstructure may distort, the implant may move within the bone, or the abutment screw may distort. The distortion of the superstructure and implant system may reach a level such that a 500-μm original gap may not be detectable.[106] As a result the casting may appear to fit the implant abutment for screw retention. However, the superstructure, bone, and components do not bend beyond their elastic limit, and compression, tensile, and shear forces are placed on the bone-implant interface.[107] The bone must remodel to eliminate these forces. If the forces are beyond physiologic or ultimate strength limits, resorption of the bone-implant interface occurs. As a result, greater crestal bone loss has been associated with nonpassive castings. Creep (a constant force applied over time on a material) or fatigue also can contribute to fracture of the components over time because of a constant load or cyclic load frequency.

Anatomic Location. The location of the prosthesis in the oral cavity is also a significant factor in the incidence of screw loosening. Sadid-Zadeh et al.[108] showed a significant incidence difference with respect to anatomic locations, anterior (12.8%; 51 of 398 restorations) and posterior positioning (4.8%; 144 of 2972 restorations). However, when evaluating internal connection implants, they had an associated higher incidence of screw loosening in the posterior region (4.3%) than the anterior region (0.7%).

Prevention

Decreased Force. Because of the directional relationship between force and screw loosening, the evaluation, diagnosis, and modification of treatment plans related to stress conditions are of considerable importance. After the clinician has identified the source of excessive force on the implant system, the treatment plan is altered in an attempt to minimize the negative impact on the longevity of the implant, bone, and final restoration.

Prosthetic Design. The prosthetic design may be altered to minimize the possibility of screw loosening. Ideal implant placement in the key implant positions should be adhered to.

Cantilevers should be eliminated or reduced, especially when high occlusal forces are present. In addition, implant protection principles should be adhered to, including reduction of cuspal inclines of the prosthesis (decreased cusp height), decreased occlusal table, and no lateral contacts, especially in the posterior.

Ideal Preload. The ideal torque force on an abutment screw varies by manufacturer and may range from 10 to 35 N-cm. This preload is determined by many variables, including the screw material, screw head design, abutment material, abutment surface, and possible lubricant. To reduce the incidence of screw loosening, the abutment screw should be torqued by the following protocol:
1. Light finger-tighten with driver (~10 N-cm).
2. Maximum finger-tighten with driver (~20 N-cm).
3. Implant screw should be torqued to the manufacturer's specifications (~30-35 N/cm).
4. After 5 to 10 minutes, the screw should be retorqued to the same manufacturer's specifications.

NOTE: For cases of expected increased force, the implant screw may be retorqued a third time after 30 to 60 days.

Screw-Tightening Sequence. When screw-tightening a multiunit fixed implant prostheses, a proper sequence and technique is crucial to obtain the correct torque. The torque should be applied incrementally among all screws so that not one screw is tightened fully. This is based on the fact that a multi-unit prosthesis is unlikely to be "completely" passive. A nonideal tightening sequence will lead to either an insufficient or excessive amount of torque placed onto a specific screw thread. Undertorque will lead to insufficient clamping force and lack of ideal stretching of the screw. This will most often lead to screw loosening. Overtorque will lead to permanent deformation of the screw, which may lead to screw fracture.

Settling Effect. Settling is a term used to describe the effect of various implant parts wearing and fitting closer together. Minor irregularities on or within a casting that incorporates the top of an abutment or screw can cause slight elevation of the casting or the screw head. Over time, micromovement wears down the

irregularities, and the parts fit closer together. However, this settling relaxes the preload force on the prosthetic screw and is more likely to cause screw loosening. This embedment relaxation or loss of preload has been shown to be approximately 2% to 10% of the initial preload within the first few seconds or minutes after tightening. This is the reasoning for the earlier protocol to include a second retorque after 5 to 10 minutes to regain the lost preload due to settling.[109]

Torque Under Moist Conditions. Studies have shown when placing and torqueing abutment screws, more accurate torque values result under wet conditions versus dry.[110] Saline may be used to lubricate the screw before placement of preload to maximize the accuracy of the preload.

Wider Implant Bodies. The use of wider implant bodies results in decreased force on the screw. Graves et al.[111] have shown increasing implant size from 3.75 to 5.0 mm results in 20% greater strength, whereas increasing implant size from 3.75 to 6.0 mm increases the strength by 33%.

Treatment

When confronted with a mobile prosthesis, it is important to determine whether the mobility is a result of screw loosening or the actual implant being mobile (implant failure). Box 31.2 illustrates a technique to determine the cause of the prosthesis movement (Fig. 31.47).

Implant Movement. Mobility of the implant body indicates failure of the implant and necessitates immediate removal. A radiograph may reveal a circumferential radiolucency. The site should then be re-evaluated after adequate healing for the need of bone grafting, implant placement, or change in prosthetic treatment planning.

Abutment Screw Movement

Option 1. Removing a cemented crown from a mobile abutment is very challenging with conventional crown removal techniques (e.g., crown bumper). The impact force that is applied to the mobile crown is dissipated because of the loose screw. This may result in damage to the internal threads of the implant body. In addition, when an implant crown margin is subgingival, it is often difficult to obtain access for the crown remover. In poorer bone densities, overzealous use of a crown remover may result in loss of the bone-implant interface.

Option 2. The safest and most predictable treatment option to treat abutment movement is accomplished with making an occlusal access and transforming the cement-retained crown into a screw-retained crown (Fig. 31.48).

Following are the steps for completing this procedure:
1. Evaluate and determine the location and angulation of the implant abutment screw (buccal-lingually and mesial-distally). An intraoral radiograph is often helpful.
2. With a round diamond bur (≈#8 round), access is made through the occlusal surface to remove the abutment screw (i.e., central fossa: posterior teeth and lingual aspect of crown in anterior teeth).
3. After the screw is located, the screw is engaged with the appropriate hex driver, reverse-torqued, and the screw is removed.
4. Discard old screw and place new screw.
5. Torque to the manufacturer's specifications with ideal protocol.
6. Cover access hole with filler (polytetrafluoroethylene) and opaque composite.

In situations where the access hole is through the facial aspect of the prosthesis (i.e., anterior crowns), the crown will need to be removed and a new crown fabricated. Care should be exercised

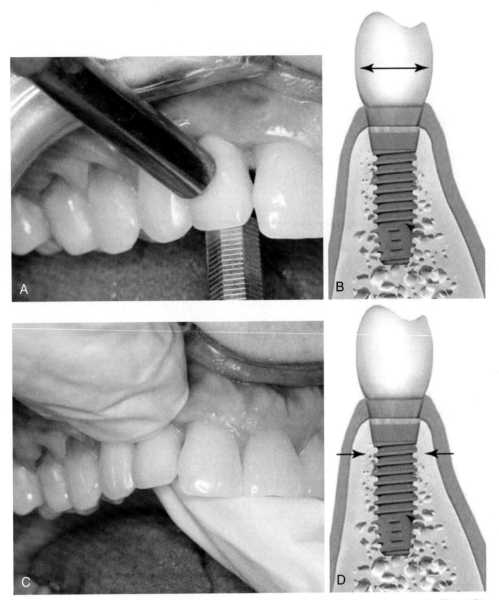

• **Fig. 31.47** (A and B) Checking buccal-lingual mobility of the prosthesis with a mirror handle. (C and D) Palpation of buccal and lingual cortical plates to evaluate the presence of pain.

when cutting the crown off because in most cases it is difficult to determine the cement location (Fig. 31.49).

This may result in sectioning the crown too deep, causing damage to the abutment, abutment screw, or implant body. A safer method includes the earlier technique (access with screw removal) with fabrication of a new prosthesis. If the abutment remains fixated to the prosthesis, the prosthesis can be easily removed by gently heating the prosthesis with a Bunsen burner.

Screw Fracture

Etiology

The causative factor most likely to induce screw fractures is biomechanical stress to the implant system. The biomechanical stress leads to partially unretained restorations or fatigue, which is directly related to an increased amount of force. Prosthesis screw fracture has been shown to occur with a mean incidence rate of 4% with a range of 0% to 19%. Abutment screw fracture is directly related to the screw diameter, with larger-diameter screws fracturing less often, and a mean incidence rate of 2% and a range of 0.2% to 8% (Fig. 31.50).[112]

Prevention

Immediate Treatment of Loose Screw. If an abutment screw is determined to be mobile, immediate treatment is recommended. The longer the period that force is applied to a mobile prosthesis, the greater the chance the abutment screw will be deformed and possibly fracture. The loose screw follows a fatigue curve that is related to the number of cycles and the intensity of the repeated forces.

Treatment

Explorer Removal. The easiest method to remove a screw is to rotate the screw counterclockwise with a sharp explorer tip.

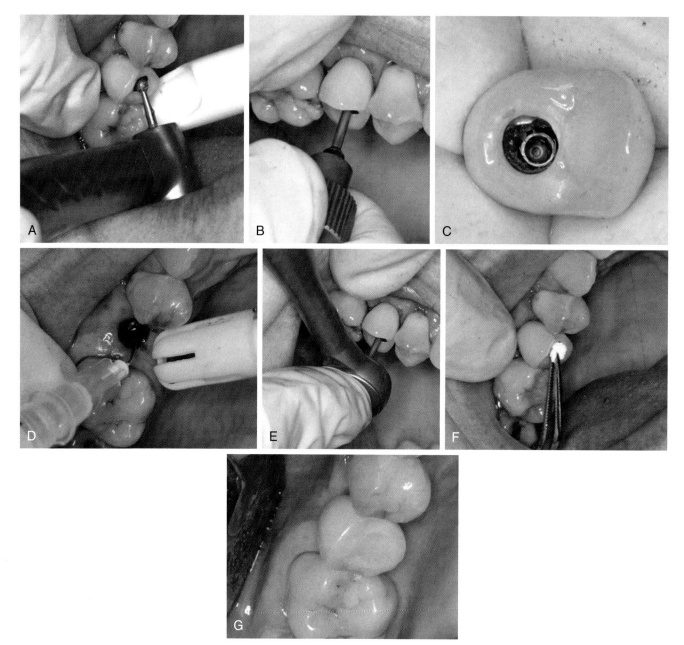

• **Fig. 31.48** Loose Screw Removal Technique. (A) Occlusal access is made with a #8 round diamond bur. (B) Screw is easily removed with implant driver. (C) Access needs to be large enough to allow for screw removal. (D) Chlorhexidine irrigation of the internal threads. (E) A new screw is torqued into position according to the manufacturer's recommendations. (F) Sterile polytetrafluoroethylene is placed in the access hole after final torque. (G) Opaque composite placed into access.

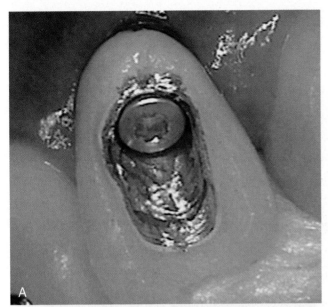

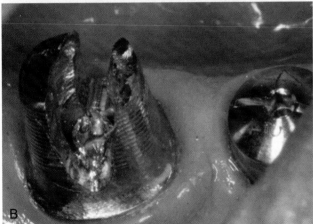

• **Fig. 31.49** (A) Most commonly in the maxillary anterior the access may need to be made through the facial surface. (B) Care should be exercised in cutting cement-retained crowns off because the abutment screw may be irreversibly damaged.

Because a loose screw has no preload, the fractured component remains passive in the implant body. If the screw has been deformed or debris has been introduced between the screw and the implant body, this technique may not be successful (Fig. 31.51).

Ultrasonic/Cavitron Device. If debris is present between the threads, an ultrasonic or Cavitron device may be used. The vibration (≈20,000–30,000 rpm) will usually dislodge the debris, and the screw can then be removed via the explorer method.

Round Bur (205LN). A very small round bur or 205LN can be used in a slow-speed handpiece or AS123 screwdriver. The tip of the bur is placed at the seam of the fractured screw and abutment (implant). As the bur spins clockwise, the friction placed on the screw makes it turn counterclockwise, and the screw unthreads.

Inverted Cone Bur (~33½ Bur). With an inverted cone bur in a high-speed handpiece (ideally electric handpiece in reverse), gently touch the top of the screw. This will usually result in the screw being extruded from the implant body. Care should be exercised to not touch the implant body with the bur because this will result in damage to the implant body threads. With this technique, always use a throat pack to prevent loss (Fig. 31.52).

Slot the Top of the Screw. A slot 1 mm deep is made through the center of the screw with a high-speed handpiece and a very narrow fissure bur (or 33½ bur). A small screwdriver is then used to unthread the screw. Be careful using this technique because the bur may inadvertently perforate the side of the implant body. There is no predictable method to repair the implant body if this occurs. The patient should be informed that implant failure may result as a consequence of this technique (Fig. 31.53).

Manufactured Retrieval Instruments. Multiple retrieval kits are on the market that are used to remove fractured screws. These are usually specific for the type of implant body type (internal, external, trilobe, etc.) (Fig. 31.54).

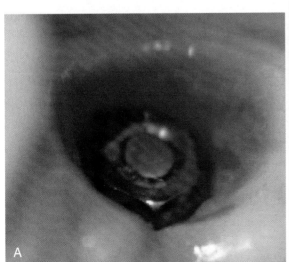

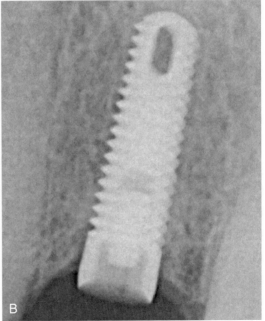

• **Fig. 31.50** (A and B) Fractured screws that usually occur from occlusal overload.

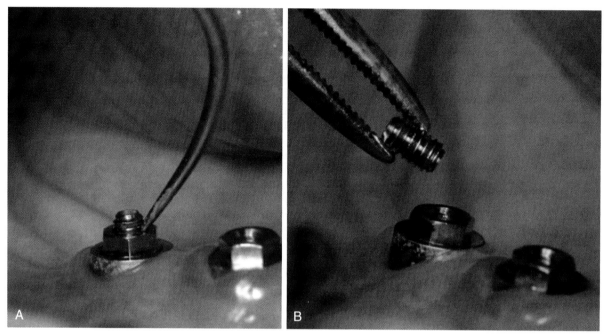

• **Fig. 31.51** Explorer Technique to Remove Broken Screw. (A and B) The screw may be easily removed if preload is lost by using the explorer in a counterclockwise direction.

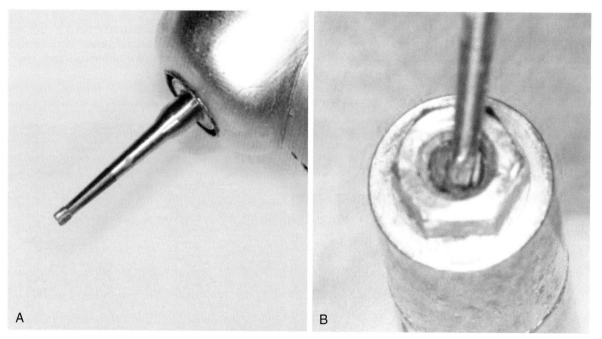

• **Fig. 31.52** (A) Inverted cone (33½ bur) with handpiece. (B) The fractured screw is lightly tapped in the center of the screw, which will usually dislodge the screw. A throat pack should be used, and care should be exercised to not touch the internal walls of the implant.

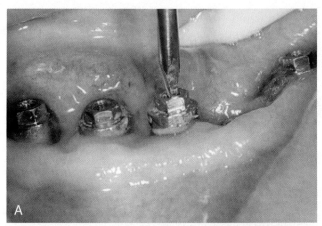

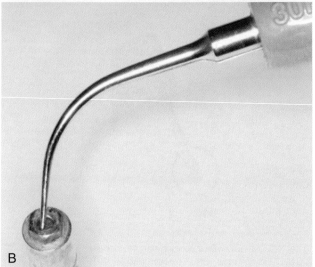

• **Fig. 31.53** (A) Slot the top of the screw. A slot is made in the screw with a high-speed handpiece and narrow fissure bar. A screwdriver is then used to unthread the screw. (B) Use of an ultrasonic scaler to loosen debris between the screw and the internal threads of the implant.

Neurosensory Impairment

The iatrogenic injury of any of the branches of the trigeminal nerve is a major concern in implant dentistry. As the number of implants being placed each year keeps increasing, along with a greater number of clinicians performing the procedures, the incidence of nerve impairments will most likely continue to increase. The reported incidence of such nerve injuries after dental implant procedures is highly variable (0%–44%) in the literature.[113] Studies have shown that approximately 73% of doctors who perform implant surgery have experienced postoperative nerve complications.[114] Libersa et al.[115] evaluated transient versus permanent nerve injuries after implant placement and reported a permanent injury 75% of the time (Fig. 31.55).

When a nerve injury occurs, it is paramount the dental implant clinician be able to recognize the type and extent of injury, and provide the most appropriate postoperative care. Traumatic and iatrogenic nerve complications may involve total or partial nerve resection, crushing, thermal, stretching, or entrapment injuries. The resulting sensory deficits may range from a nonpainful, minor loss of sensation (hypoesthesia), to a more permanent and severe debilitating pain dysfunction (dysesthesia). The sensory complications from a nerve injury will usually result in an overall decreased

quality of life for the patient and potential long-standing psychological problems.[116] Not only do these complications affect the patient, the clinician is often confronted with patient dissatisfaction, embarrassment, and possible medicolegal implications.

In the field of oral implantology today the clinician must have a thorough understanding of the cause, prevention, and treatment of neurosensory impairments. A postoperative classification and guidelines for the diagnosis and management of neurosensory deficits have been developed by the author, which is dependent on the history, type, and nature of the injury.

Specific Anatomic Areas Susceptible to Nerve Injury

Inferior Alveolar Nerve

Nerve impairment to the inferior alveolar nerve (mental nerve) is a common clinical complication with major medicolegal implications. Because of its anatomic location, the mental nerve is the most common nerve to be damaged via implants or bone graft procedures. Trauma usually occurs from placement of implants directly into the foramen or into the inferior alveolar canal in the posterior mandible. Sensory nerve injury may result in altered sensation, complete numbness, and/or pain, which may interfere with speech, eating, drinking, shaving, or makeup application and lead to social embarrassment.

The mandibular division of the trigeminal nerve (cranial nerve V) exits the skull base via foramen ovale and then divides into an anterior and posterior division. The anterior division of the mandibular nerve has mainly motor branches that innervate the temporalis, lateral pterygoid, and masseter muscles. The posterior division of the mandibular nerve is mainly sensory, which provides branches including the lingual nerve, inferior alveolar nerve, and auriculotemporal nerve. The inferior alveolar nerve divides into two terminal branches, the mental and incisive nerves.[117] The mental nerve courses anteriorly until it exits through the mental foramen, which is sensory to the soft tissues of the chin, lip, and anterior gingiva. The incisive nerve continues anterior and innervates the mandibular anterior teeth.

Most nerve injuries that occur in relation to dental implant surgery involve the inferior alveolar nerve. Accurately determining the exact location of the inferior alveolar nerve as it courses through the body of the mandible is imperative to avoid neurosensory disturbances secondary to implant placement. Histologically this inferior alveolar nerve consists of connective tissue and neural components in which the smallest functional unit is the individual nerve fiber. The inferior alveolar nerve fibers may be either myelinated or unmyelinated. The myelinated nerve fibers are the most abundant; they consist of a single axon encased individually by a single Schwann cell. The individual nerve fibers and Schwann cells are surrounded by the endoneurium, which acts as a protective cushion made up of a basal lamina, collagen fibers, and endoneurial capillaries.

Lingual Nerve

Within the infratemporal fossa the lingual nerve divides from the posterior division of the mandibular nerve (V3) as a terminal branch. As the lingual nerve proceeds anteriorly, it lies against the medial pterygoid muscle and medial to the mandibular ramus. It then passes inferiorly to the superior constrictor attachment and courses anteroinferiorly to the lateral surface of the tongue. As it runs forward deep to the submandibular gland, it terminates as the sublingual nerve.

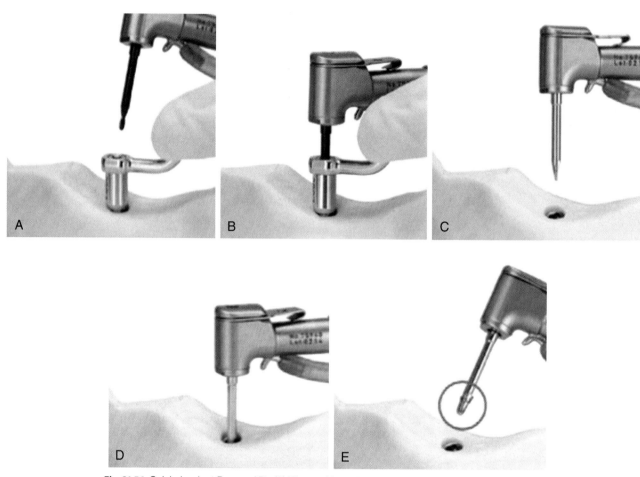

• **Fig. 31.54** Salvin Implant Rescue Kit. (A) Place guide on implant and hold with stabilizing handle. Insert drill into implant handpiece. Set motor to REVERSE at 1000 to 1250 rpm and 50 to 70 N-cm torque. (B) Drill in REVERSE using "up and down" motion to prepare 1- to 2-mm deep dimple into top of broken screw. (C) Insert tap into implant handpiece; set motor to REVERSE at 70 to 80 rpm and 50 to 70 N-cm torque. (D) Insert tap into the 1- to 2-mm dimple in the top of the broken screw. Use the tap in REVERSE to remove broken screw. (E) Screw removed. (*Courtesy Salvin Dental Specialties, Inc., Charlotte, N.C.*)

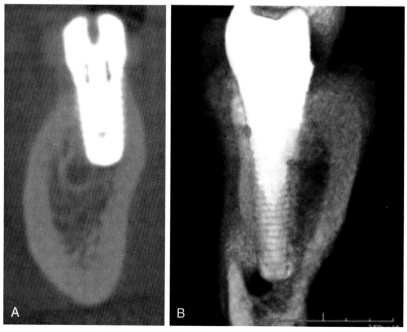

• **Fig. 31.55** (A and B) Implant-induced nerve impairment.

The lingual nerve is sensory to the anterior two-thirds of the tongue, floor of the mouth, and lingual gingiva. It also contains visceral afferent and efferent fibers from cranial nerve VII (facial nerve) and from the chorda tympani, which relays taste information. With the prevalence of second molar implants, care should be taken to note the possible position of the lingual nerve on the medial ridge of the retromolar triangle, where it courses anteriorly along the superior lingual alveolar crest, which is slightly lingual to the teeth.[118]

Due to the lingual nerve's variable anatomic location, it may be iatrogenically traumatized during various implant surgical procedures. Usually the lingual nerve is not damaged from the actual osteotomy preparation of implants unless the lingual plate is perforated. This sensory nerve is most likely traumatized during soft tissue reflection during implant placement in the second molar area or incision/reflection over the retromolar pad for bone graft procedures.

In addition, the lingual nerve can suffer damage from lingual flap retraction and inferior alveolar nerve blocks. Studies have shown that lingual nerve impairment after nerve blocks occurs twice as often as inferior alveolar nerve damage.[119] This is most likely due to the fact the lingual nerve is most commonly unifascular at the site of the injection. Sensory damage to the lingual nerve may cause a wide spectrum of complications ranging from complete anesthesia to paraesthesia, dysesthesia, drooling, tongue biting, change in taste perception, and change in speech pattern.

Nasopalatine Nerve

The incisive canals fuse and form a common Y-shaped canal that exits lingual to the central incisor teeth (incisive foramen or incisive fossa). The nasopalatine nerve passes through these canals and provides sensation to the anterior palate. These nerves (also termed *incisive nerves*) terminate at the nasal floor and enter the oral cavity via the incisive canal, which is underneath the incisive papilla. To prevent trauma to these nerves, ideal presurgical planning of implant placement in the maxillary incisor region should be carefully evaluated.

In the literature, many authors have advocated removing the contents of the nasopalatine canal and grafting with a high success rate.[120] Although this nerve is often affected by the placement of implants or bone grafting in the incisor region, sensory disturbances are rare. Nerve damage reported in the literature caused by complete removal[121] or flap surgery[122] is of short duration. This is most likely due to cross-innervation of the greater palatine nerve on the anterior palatal area.

Anterior Superior Alveolar Nerve

The anterior superior alveolar nerve branches from the infraorbital canal on the lateral face. This small canal may be seen lingual to the cuspid and is denoted as the canalis sinuosus. The canal runs forward and downward to the inferior wall of the orbit and after reaching the edge of the anterior nasal aperture in the inferior turbinate, it follows the lower margin of the nasal aperture and opens to the side of the nasal septum. Studies have shown that in approximately 15% of the population, this canal is approximately 1 to 2 mm in diameter. The canals present as a direct extension of the canalis sinuosus and may be clinically relevant when greater than 2.0 mm (Fig. 31.56).[123]

The canine pillar region is a key implant position for dental implants. Care should be exercised to evaluate for the presence of neurovascular bundles. Insertion of implants in approximation to the canal may be problematic because this may lead to a soft tissue interface and failure of the implant and temporary or permanent sensory dysfunction and possible bleeding issues. However, significant sensory impairments are rare because of cross-innervation. Many clinicians are unaware of the canalis sinuosus and may misdiagnose this radiolucency as apical pathology of the maxillary cuspid.

Infraorbital Nerve

The infraorbital nerve emerges from the infraorbital foramen and gives off four branches: the inferior palpebral, external nasal, internal nasal, and the superior labial branches, which are sensory to the lower eyelid, cheek, and upper lip. The inferior palpebral branches supply the skin and conjunctiva of the lower eyelid. The nasal branches

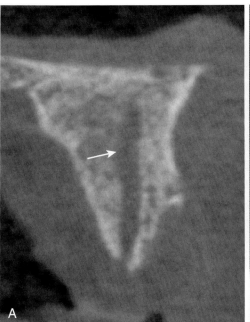
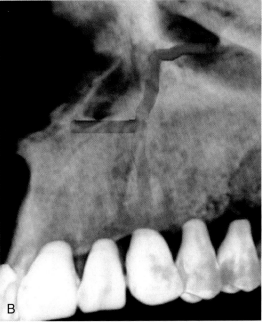

• **Fig. 31.56** Canalis sinuosus. (A) Anatomic variant that may lead to the placement of implants into the canal, leading to a soft tissue interface. Cross-sectional cone beam computed tomographic image showing location in center of the residual ridge. (B) Three-dimensional view of the canalis sinuosus.

supply the lateral nose soft tissue and the movable part of the nasal septum, and the superior labial branches supply the skin of the cheek and upper lip. Normally the average distance of the inferior border of the orbital rim to the infraorbital foramen is 4.6 to 10.4 mm.

Impairment of the infraorbital nerve may be very traumatic to patients. Damage to branches of the infraorbital nerve usually will result from retraction-related trauma (neuropraxia). Procedures involving the maxillary cuspid-bicuspid area are most susceptible to injuries. Anatomic variants of the infraorbital foramen have been shown to be up to 14 mm from the orbital rim. This is most likely seen in elderly female patients with extensive alveolar atrophy.

Etiology of Nerve Injuries

Most implant-related nerve impairments are the direct result of poor treatment planning and inadequate radiographic evaluation. Trauma to associated nerves in the oral cavity occurs when the implant clinician is not aware of the amount of bone or does not know the location of nerve canals or foramina. The preoperative evaluation and assessment are crucial to determine the amount of available bone in approximation to nerve anatomy. A CBCT examination is most commonly used for the three-dimensional planning in these areas.

Neurosensory impairment injuries may result from a wide array of intraoperative and postoperative complications. For example, nerves may be mechanically injured by indirect or direct trauma via retraction, laceration, pressure, stretching, and transection. Thermal trauma may cause inflammation and secondary ischemia injuries with associated degeneration. And lastly, peripheral nerves have been shown to be susceptible to chemical injuries, where the nerve is directly traumatized by chemical solutions.

Administration of Local Anesthesia

Adequate local anesthesia is paramount for successful dental implant surgery and stress reduction protocol. However, although rare, the use of nerve blocks may result in trauma to various branches of the trigeminal nerve. The exact cause of local anesthesia nerve damage is unclear, and various theories such as injection needle trauma, hematoma formation, and local anesthetic toxicity have been discussed.

Although the true incidence is difficult to quantify because of reporting difficulties, studies have shown permanent injury occurs in approximately 1 in 25,000 inferior nerve blocks. Most patients do recover fully without deficits, with full recovery in 85% of patients with complete remission in 8 to 10 weeks.[124]

Damage From Injection Needle. Complications resulting from needle trauma are likely the most common theory on why nerve injury results after administering nerve blocks. First, it is not uncommon for the tip of the needle to become barbed (damaged) when contacting bone. Stacy et al.[125] showed that 78% of needles became barbed after initial injection, increasing the possibility of damaging the nerve. Two-thirds of the needles developed outward-facing barbs, which have been shown to rupture the perineurium, damage the endoneurium, and cause transection of nerve fibers. The lingual nerve has been associated with the highest percentage of nerve impairment cases as a result of an anesthetic injection (~70%).[126] Because of the lingual nerve's anatomic location, it is predisposed to nerve injuries because it is commonly contacted when using the pterygomandibular raphe as an injection landmark because of the nerve being positioned shallow in the tissue (~3–5 mm from the mucosa).[127]

Hematoma. The anesthetic needle may also cause damage to the epineurial blood vessels, which may result in hemorrhage-related compression on the nerve fibers. The accumulation of blood may lead to fibrosis and scar formation, which may cause pressure-related trauma.[128] The extent of impairment to the nerve is directly related to the amount of pressure exerted by the hematoma and recovery time of the axonal and connective tissue damage.

Anesthetic Toxicity. If the anesthetic is injected within the fascicular space, chemical irritation and damage may occur. Studies have shown articaine to comprise 54% of mandibular nerve block injuries,[129] and it is 21 times more likely to cause injury in comparison with other nerve injuries.[130] Theories concerning articaine toxicity include the high concentration of articaine solution and the increased resultant inflammatory reaction.[131] Lidocaine has been shown to be the least toxic anesthetic, followed by articaine, mepivacaine, and bupivacaine.[132] Chemical trauma from local anesthetics has been shown to cause demyelination and axonal degeneration of nerve fibers.[134]

Soft Tissue Reflection

Injury to nerves and nerve fibers may occur during the reflection, retraction, or suturing of the soft tissue. This is most noted when the mental nerve is dehisced or exposed on the mandibular ridge. Special caution should be exercised when making incisions over these areas because complete transection injuries may occur from incisions through the nerve or foramen. Stretching injuries (neuropraxia) may occur from excessive retraction, so care should be noted as to the proximity of neural vital structures within the retracted tissue. A common stretching injury occurs with the infraorbital nerve, especially when implants or bone grafting are being performed in the canine and bicuspid region. Complete transection of the nerve may result from attempting to reduce the tissue tension over the surgery flap without regard to the anatomic location of the nerve (Fig. 31.57).

Implant and Implant Drill Trauma

The surgical drilling for implant placement may result in a direct or indirect neurosensory impairment.

Trauma. Direct trauma from surgical drilling may occur from overpreparation of the osteotomy site or lack of knowledge of the true bur length. The implant clinician must know and understand the true length of the surgical burs used in the osteotomy site preparation. For many surgical drill systems, the marked millimeter gauge lines inscribed on the shank of the drills most often do not include the cutting edge of the drill and do not correspond to the actual depth of the drill. Most surgical implant drills have a sharp, V-shaped apical portion to improve their cutting efficiency and allow adequate depth of drilling. The V-shaped apical portion of the drill (termed the *Y dimension* in engineering) is often not included in the depth measurements of the commercial drills and may measure as much as 1.5 mm longer than the intended depth. Therefore the clinician may inadvertently drill deeper than anticipated because of the drill design.

In addition, overpreparation may occur, especially in less dense bone. The implant clinician should use the initial implant osteotomy twist drill as a gauge for bone density type and for an evaluation of the position of the surgical drill relative to the mandibular canal or vital structure. In implant dentistry today the popularity of immediate placement implants has been associated with an increase in drilling-related trauma. To gain primary stability, most immediate implant osteotomy sites require drill preparation and implant placement apical to the extraction site. When placing implants in the mandibular premolar area, violation of the canal

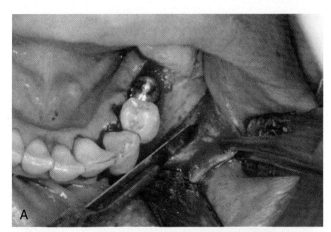

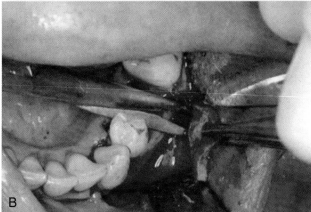

• **Fig. 31.57** Periosteal release of the tissue to obtain tension-free closure, which may cause nerve injury. (A) The use of a #15 blade to release the periosteal fibers. (B) Blunt dissection to release tissue with Metzenbaum scissors.

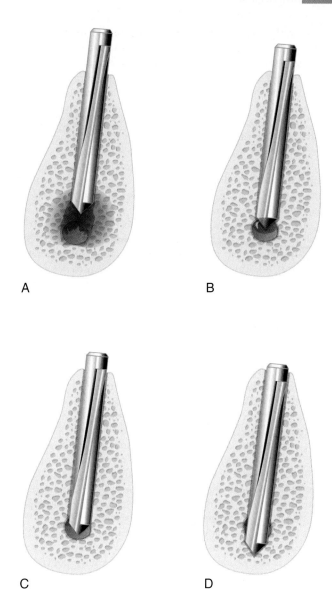

• **Fig. 31.58** Drill Impingement Trauma. (A) Encroachment: even though the surgical drill is short of canal, thermal damage and bone necrosis (brown/green) result in nerve damage. (B) Partial penetration (hematoma): the surgical drill partially penetrates the superior aspect of the canal, resulting in bleeding and hematoma formation. (C) Partial penetration (laceration): the surgical drill penetrates deeper into the canal, which results in laceration of nerve fibers. (D) Transection: the surgical drill may penetrate the entire canal, leading to complete transection of the nerve fibers.

may occur, causing nerve damage. Therefore in this anatomic area, immediate implant placement is not recommended unless adequate bone is available below the root apex. The following subsections describe the various types of surgical drill trauma that may lead to a neurosensory impairment.

Thermal Trauma. The surgical drill may cause a nerve impairment from thermal damage even though the surgical drill does not violate the mandibular canal. Most commonly this is the result of insufficient irrigation, which leads to overheating the bone. The associated thermal trauma may lead to nerve impairment via bone necrosis from overheating the bone during preparation. Nerve tissue has been shown to be more sensitive to thermal trauma than bone (osseous) tissue. In the literature, excessive temperatures have been reported to produce necrosis, fibrosis, degeneration, and increased osteoclastic involvement.[30] To minimize this complication, the bone density should be evaluated preoperatively via CBCT examination, tactile evaluation, and location. In harder bone densities (e.g., D1 and D2), special care should be exercised in reducing the possibility of overheating the bone (see Chapter 27).

Partial Penetration. The surgical drill may also cause direct trauma to the neurovascular bundle by penetrating the mandibular canal or mental foramen. The neurosensory impairment will be directly related to the specific nerve fascicles that are damaged. Normally the vein and artery, which are positioned more superiorly than the nerve, will be damaged when penetration of the canal results. This indirect trauma leads to nerve damage from the excessive bleeding (hematoma), as well as thermal and chemical injuries from the penetration into the canal.

Transection. The most severe type of nerve injury, with the lowest probability of regeneration, is when the implant drill transects the canal. In a true transection the nerve is completely severed. When this occurs, repair and regeneration of the traumatized nerve are highly variable. Complete transection of the nerve occurs when surgical error involves the preparation of an osteotomy too deep because of inaccurate measurements or slippage of the handpiece. This type of injury results in the most severe of response, a total nerve impairment (anesthesia) and neuroma formation. Usually this type of nerve injury results in a complete anesthesia and retrograde degeneration, resulting in possible future dysesthesia.[135] The extent of neurosensory impairment is directly related to the extent of fascicle injury and is dependent on the time the implant is left to irritate the nerve fibers (Fig. 31.58).

Implant Encroachment on the Mandibular Canal. Injuries to vital nerve structures caused by implant positioning are most common in the posterior mandible. These injuries may be caused by direct trauma (mechanical) and indirect trauma or infection (pressure). Placement of an implant into or near the mandibular canal is associated with many types of neurosensory impairments (Fig. 31.59). When an implant is too close to the mandibular canal, a compression or secondary ischemia injury may occur. To prevent these complications, the implant clinician should always adhere to a 2.0-mm safety zone of the implant in proximity to the canal or mental foramen. Studies have shown that implant pressure on the canal occurs with increasing stress as the bone density decreases.[136] Khaja and Renton showed that placing an implant too close to the canal may induce hemorrhage or deposition of debris into the canal, causing ischemia of the nerve. Even removing the implant or repositioning may not alleviate and decrease pressure-related symptoms. Additional studies have shown the presence of postoperative severe pain after implant placement in close approximation to the canal, resulting in chronic stimulation and debilitating chronic neuropathy.[137]

Partial Penetration Into the Mandibular Canal. Placement of the implant body into the mandibular canal is associated with a high degree of morbidity. Even though the sensory nerve fascicles are usually inferior to blood vessels within the canal, a partial penetration may result in an injury that is usually related to the fibers that are damaged. This is why in some clinical situations the implant is directly within the canal; however, no neurosensory symptoms exist.

In addition, implant placement into the canal may cause hematoma formation (severing of the inferior alveolar artery or vein), leading to a pressure-induced nerve impairment.

Infection. Placement of implants in approximation to the canal may cause neurosensory impairments via peri-implant infections. Infectious processes after implant placement may result from heat generation, contamination, or prior existence of bone pathology. This may lead to spread of infection that may extend into the neural anatomy. Case reports have shown nerve impairment issues resulting from an implant infected by chronic peri-implantitis.[33]

Mandibular Socket Grafting. After mandibular tooth extractions, grafting into the socket may effectively expose the inferior alveolar nerve to socket medicaments. This may lead to chemical neuritis, and if the irritation persists, an irreversible neuropathy may occur (Fig. 31.60). In addition, care should be exercised when removing pathology and granulation tissue from extraction sockets in close proximity to the nerve canal (type 1 nerve).[138] Overzealous curetting of the socket apex may lead to direct traumatic injury of the canal.

Delayed Nerve Damage (Canal Narrowing). Nerve damage may result even when ideal implant placement is performed (>2.0 mm from the nerve canal). Shamloo et al.[139] reported an implant placement case in which the implant body resulted in compression and bone to be forced into the superior aspect of the mandibular canal (canal narrowing). This led to delayed healing and remodeling within the canal and resulted in excessive narrowing of the canal, with compression of the nerve fibers. The narrowed aspect of the canal was shown be approximately 0.2 mm, with an average diameter in the nonaffected sites being approximately 3.2 mm.[139] The nerve impairment (paresthesia and anesthesia) occurred 2 years after implant placement surgery.

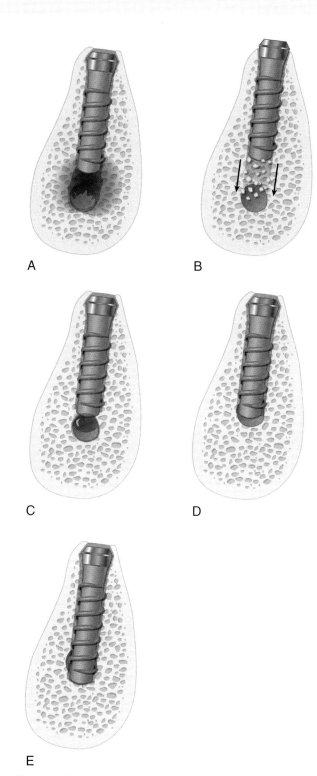

A B

C D

E

• **Fig. 31.59** Implant Impingement Trauma. (A) Encroachment: even though the implant body is short of the canal, thermal damage may occur from overheating the bone. (B) Bone fragments (trabeculae) may be pushed apically, resulting in a pressure necrosis nerve injury. (C) Partial penetration (hematoma): the implant body may partially penetrate the superior aspect of the canal, resulting in bleeding and hematoma formation. (D) Partial penetration (laceration): the implant body may penetrate deeper into the canal, which results in laceration of nerve fibers. (E) Transection: the implant body may penetrate the entire canal, leading to complete transection of the nerve fibers.

Nerve Healing Physiology

After nerve injury, there exist two phases of healing: degeneration and regeneration.

Degeneration

There are two types of nerve degeneration: segmental degeneration and Wallerian degeneration. Segmental demyelination occurs when the myelin sheath is damaged and causes a slowing of the conduction velocity, which may prevent the transmission of nerve impulses. The resulting effects will clinically be paresthesia, dysesthesia, or hyperesthesia. The second type of degeneration is termed *Wallerian degeneration*, in which the axons and myelin sheath distal (away from the central nervous system) to the injury undergo complete disintegration. The axons proximal to the site of injury (toward the central nervous system) undergo less degeneration, but many nodes of Ranvier (periodic gaps in the myelin sheaths of axons that facilitate the rapid conduction of nerve impulses) are affected. Wallerian degeneration usually occurs after complete transection of the nerve and results in a dysesthesia type of symptoms.

Regeneration

Usually regeneration occurs immediately after nerve injury. The proximal nerve area sprouts out new fibers that grow at a rate of 1.0 to 1.5 mm/day. This will continue until the site innervated by the nerve is reached or blocked by fibrous connective tissue, bone, or an object (e.g., dental implant). During the regeneration process, new myelin sheaths form as axons increase in size. In some situations the continuity of the Schwann cells is disrupted, and connective tissue may enter the area. The growth may find an alternative path, or it may form a traumatic neuroma, which is usually characterized by significant pain. Studies have shown that the administration of steroids may minimize the formation of neuromas, especially the administration of high doses within the first week of nerve injury (Fig. 31.61).[140]

Neurosensory Deficit Classification

There are two widely accepted classifications of nerve injuries. In 1943 Seddon[141] postulated a three-stage classification, which was later reclassified by Sunderland in 1951 into five different subclassifications. These nerve injury classifications are described by the resultant morphophysiologic type of injury, which is based on the time course and amount of sensory recovery (Fig. 31.62).

Neuropraxia, or first-degree injury, is characterized by a conduction block with no degeneration of the axon or visible damage of the epineurium. Usually this type of injury is consistent with stretching or manipulation (reflection of tissue) of the nerve fibers, which results in injury to the endoneurial capillaries. The degree of trauma to the endoneurial capillaries will determine the magnitude of intrafascicular edema, which results in various degrees of conduction block. Usually resolution of sensation and function will occur within hours to weeks.

Axonotmesis (second-, third-, or fourth-degree injury) consists of degeneration or regeneration axonal injuries. The injury classification depends on the severity of axonal damage. This type of injury involves the endoneurium, with minimum disruption to the perineurium and epineurium. The most common types of injury are traction, stretching, and compression, which can lead to severe ischemia, intrafascicular edema, or demyelination of the nerve fibers. Initially complete anesthesia is most common,

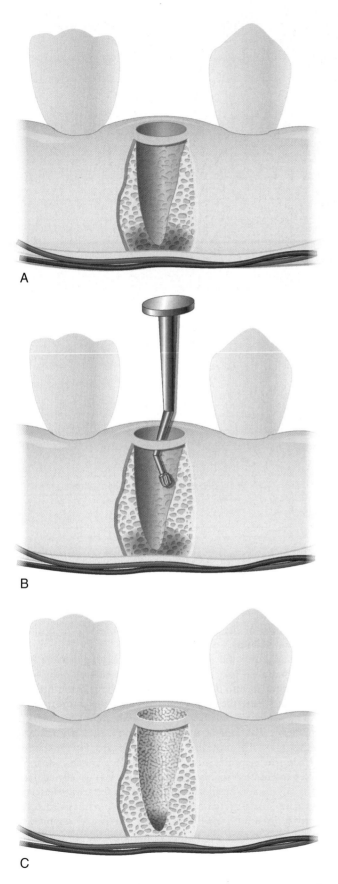

• **Fig. 31.60** Post-extraction Site. (A) Care should be taken when grafting an extraction site in close approximation to the inferior alveolar nerve. (B) A curette should be used with caution because direct damage to the nerve may occur. (C) Grafting in close approximation to the canal may lead to nerve trauma.

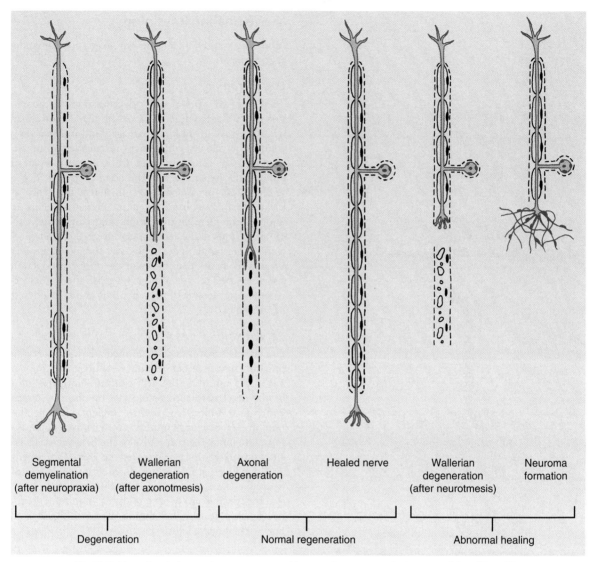

• **Fig. 31.61** Normal and abnormal nerve responses (degeneration, regeneration) to nerve injury. (*From Hupp JR, Tucker MR, Ellis E. Contemporary Oral and Maxillofacial Surgery. 6th ed. St. Louis, MO: Mosby; 2014.*)

which is followed by paresthesia as recovery begins. Improvement of the related sensory deficits occurs within approximately 2 to 4 months, with complete recovery usually within 12 months. In some cases painful dysesthesias are possible, with resulting neuroma formation.

Neurotmesis (fifth-degree injury) is the most severe type of injury, resulting from severe traction, compression, or complete transection injuries. Initially patients exhibit anesthesia, followed by paresthesia with possible dysesthesia. A very low probability of neurosensory recovery exists, with immediate referral for a neurosurgical evaluation recommended.[142] The axon and encapsulating connective tissue will lose their continuity. There is usually complete loss of motor, sensory, and autonomic function. Neuroma formation is common if transection has occurred.

The literature involving peripheral nerve injuries is vast, with a significant variation in the nomenclature used to describe the associated clinical signs and symptoms. Neurosensory impairments are classified from complete numbness to severe pain of the facial soft tissues to the intraoral anatomy. Because of these deficits, severe complications result for the patient and the clinician. A thorough

understanding of the associated classifications and definitions is necessary (Tables 31.4 and 31.5).

To standardize the nomenclature concerning nerve injuries, the International Association for the Study of Pain reduced sensory impairment into three categories: anesthesia, paresthesia, and dysesthesia.[42] Anesthesia is characterized by the complete lack of "feeling," which is usually consistent with complete transection of the nerve. This type of altered sensation is most severe because anesthesias are the most difficult and unpredictable to treat, with a high incidence of neuroma formation. Paresthesia is defined as an altered sensation that is not unpleasant. It is usually characterized as a "pins and needles" feeling. Within the paraesthesia category, many subcategories exist, including hypoesthesia (decreased sensitivity to stimulation), hypoalgesia (decreased response to a stimulus that is normally painful), and synesthesia (sensation in an area when another is stimulated). Dysesthesias are classified as an altered sensation that is unpleasant. Usually pain is associated with this type of impairment, which may be spontaneous or mechanically evoked. Subcategories include hyperalgesia (painful response to nonpainful stimuli), hyperpathia (delayed or prolonged painful response), anesthetic dolorosa (pain in an area that

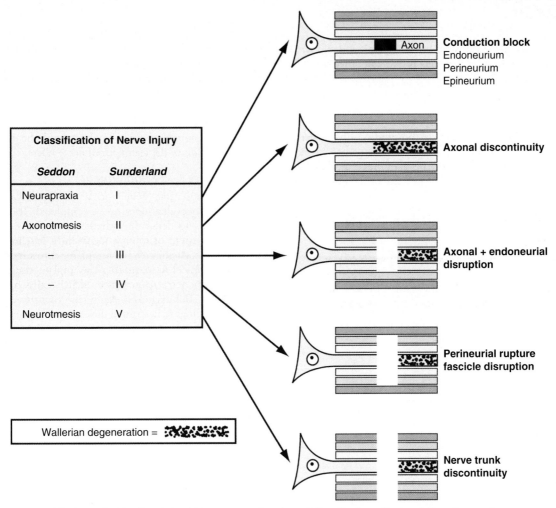

Classification of Nerve Injury

Seddon	Sunderland
Neurapraxia	I
Axonotmesis	II
–	III
–	IV
Neurotmesis	V

Conduction block
Endoneurium
Perineurium
Epineurium

Axon

Axonal discontinuity

Axonal + endoneurial disruption

Perineurial rupture fascicle disruption

Wallerian degeneration =

Nerve trunk discontinuity

• **Fig. 31.62** Seddon/Sunderland Neurosensory Impairment Classification with description of nerve damage. (*From Ellenbogen RG, Sekhar LN, eds.* Principles of Neurological Surgery. *3rd ed. Philadelphia: Saunders; 2012.*)

TABLE 31.4 **Neurosensory Impairment Classification and Injury Response**

Sunderland	Seddon	Description	Causes	Responses	Recovery Rate
I	Neurapraxia	Temporary interruption of nerve transmission (conduction block)	• Nerve compression • Edema • Hematoma • Minor stretching • Thermal	• Neuritis • Paresthesia	Complete (fast—days to weeks)
II	Axonotmesis	Endoneurium, perineurium, and epineurium remain intact; some axonal degeneration may occur	• Nerve compression • Traction • Hematoma • Partial crush • Edema • Stretching	• Paresthesia • Episodic • Dysesthesia	Complete (slow—weeks)
III		Disruption of axon and connective tissue (endoneurium), causing disorganized regeneration; Wallerian degeneration occurs	• Crush • Puncture • Severe hematoma • Stretching	• Paresthesia • Dysesthesia	Variable (slow—weeks to months)
IV		Damage involves entire fascicle; axonal, endoneurium, and perineurium changes occur; the epineurium is intact; scar tissue formation	• Full crush • Extreme stretching • High thermal • Direct chemical trauma	• Hypoesthesia • Dysesthesia • Neuroma formation	Unlikely
V	Neurotmesis	Complete transaction or tear of the nerve with amputation neuroma forming at injury site	• Complete • Transection (overpreparation with implant drill)	• Anesthesia • Intractable pain • Neuroma	None

is anesthetized), causalgia (persistent burning pain), and allodynia (pain in response to a stimulus that usually does not provoke pain).

Treatment

Nerve Impairment at Time of Surgery

During surgery, if known traction or compression of the nerve trunk has occurred, the topical application of dexamethasone may be used to minimize deficits. Upon removal of the surgical deill or implant from the mandibular canal, 1 to 2 mL of the intravenous

TABLE 31.5	Description of Neurosensory Impairment Deficits[154]
Paresthesia	Abnormal sensation that is not unpleasant
Anesthesia	Total loss of feeling or sensation
Dysesthesia	Abnormal sensation that is unpleasant
Allodynia	Pain due to a stimulus that does not normally provoke pain
Hyperpathia	Abnormally painful reaction to a stimulus
Causalgia	Persistent burning pain
Anesthesia dolorosa	Pain in an area that is Anesthetized
Hyperesthesia	Increased sensitivity to stimulation
Hyperalgesia	Increased response to a stimulus that is normally painful
Hypoesthesia	Decreased sensitivity to stimulation
Hypoalgesia	Decreased response to a stimulus that is normally painful
Synesthesia	Sensation felt in an area when another area is stimulated

form of dexamethasone (4 mg/mL) is topically applied into the osteotomy site (Fig. 31.63). This direct steroid application will reduce neural inflammation and may enhance recovery from neurosensory deficits. Studies have shown no morbidity associated with the topical application of glucocorticoids at the injury site, and postsurgical recovery has also been shown to improve significantly.[143] No bone grafting or implant should be placed that may lead to irritation of the traumatized nerve fibers.

Postoperative Nerve Impairment

When a neurosensory deficit occurs postoperatively, a comprehensive sensory evaluation must be completed. This initial examination is used to determine whether a sensory deficit exists, to quantify the extent of injury, document a baseline for recovery, and determine whether referral for microneurosurgery is indicated.

Step 1: Clinical Assessment. The implant clinician must first determine whether a neurosensory deficit exists by mapping the area of deficit. This diagnostic examination consists of objective and subjective findings to determine the extent of impairment, to use as a baseline for future evaluation, and to determine when referral for surgical intervention is required. The subjective clinical sensory tests involve nociceptive and mechanoceptive examinations. Nociceptive tests trigger a variety of autonomic responses that result in the subjective experience of pain. Mechanoceptive tests use mechanical stimuli to trigger sensory neurons that elicit various responses such as touch, position, and motion (Table 31.6 and Fig. 31.64).

Clinical Examination Complications. There exist many inherent problems with relying on the credibility of the patient's subjective responses. Because there may exist a high degree of false-positive and false-negative results, clinicians should use clear and concise instructions when administering these tests. For instance, when administering the "directional movement" test, the clinician should complete this test on the contralateral side first so the patient understands the technique and response. The results of the subjective clinical examination will depend on good communication between the implant clinician and the patient, with the outcome of the results related to the patient's perceived interpretation and how to relate their

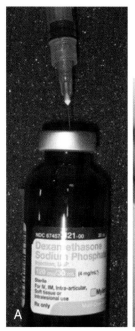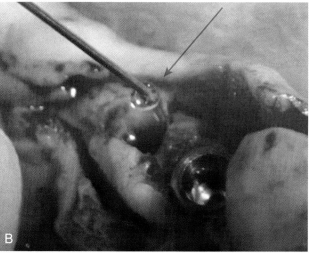

• **Fig. 31.63** (A) Dexamethasone 4 mg/mL (Mylan, Canonsburg, Pa.). (B) One to two milliliters of dexamethasone placed into the osteotomy site.

TABLE 31.6	Diagnostic Testing for Neurosensory Impairment	

Diagnostic Test	Description
Nociceptive	
Pin pressure (A-delta, C-fiber)	Determination of feeling from pin pressure using a blunted explorer. A normal response (distinct sharp pain) is a positive sign of feeling (in relation to an unaffected area) with no pain. If no feeling is present in comparison with an unaffected side, the area is termed *hypoalgesia*. If an exaggerated response is noted in relation to an unaffected side, the area is termed *hyperalgesia*.
Thermal discrimination (warm: A-delta, cold: C-fibers)	Ice chips or ethyl chloride spray and a heated mirror handle (warmed to 43°C) are used to determine the patient's ability to feel cold and hot.
Mechanoceptive	
Static light touch	Cotton tip applicator with the patient's eyes closed to test tactile stimulation by gently touching the skin and determining the threshold of the patient (A-beta afferent axons). Directional movement: Soft brush is used to determine the patient's ability to detect both sensation (A-beta and A-alpha axons) and direction of movement. The soft brush is swiped from left to right, as well as in the reverse direction.
Two-point discrimination	With the patient's eyes closed, the patient's ability to discriminate varying (myelinated A-alpha fibers) distances between two points is determined using a caliper. The normal values vary significantly, with the average being approximately 5 mm.[73]

perceptions. In addition, the tests should be administered with the patient's eyes closed, so as to minimize the possibility of incorrect responses.

Step 2: Radiographic Evaluation/Removal or Repositioning of the Implant. A thorough and comprehensive radiographic examination should be completed, including (ideally) a CBCT radiograph. If the implant (or bone screw) is in close approximation of the nerve bundle, removal or repositioning should be completed. Care should be exercised in "backing" the implant out (repositioning farther from the nerve) because trauma to the nerve may still be present from hematoma formation or pressure from cancellous bone crushed into the neural space. In addition, backing the implant out may lead to the implant being positioned undesirably because of lack of interocclusal space for the restoration (i.e., too coronally positioned). In these cases the implant should be removed and the osteotomy site irrigated with 4% dexamethasone (1–2 mL). No graft materials should be added to the osteotomy site because they may interfere with the reinnervation and repair of the nerve trunk.[144]

Step 3: Pharmacologic Intervention. Immediately after the nerve is traumatized, the inflammatory process begins with the activation of cytokines and inflammatory mediators. These inflammatory mediators will contribute to the development of nerve trauma by activating the neurons and their nociceptors.[145]

With any type of nerve impairment, corticosteroids or nonsteroidal anti-inflammatory agents should be used immediately. Studies have shown that the use of systemic adrenocorticosteroids (e.g., dexamethasone) minimizes neuropathic symptoms after nerve trauma if administered in high doses within 1 week of injury.[146] It has been advocated that a tapering dose of a corticosteroid for 5 to 7 days after trigeminal nerve injury is beneficial.[147] Dexamethasone (~8 mg) is specifically recommended because of its greater anti-inflammatory effects, in comparison with other corticosteroids such as methylprednisolone or prednisone. Additional pharmacologic agents include antidepressants, neurologic drugs, antisympathetic agents, and topical agents.

In addition, cryotherapy (ice packs) should be applied to the paraneural tissues for the first 24 hours and then episodically for the first week. Cryotherapy has been shown to be beneficial in minimizing secondary nerve injury from edema-induced compression, decreasing the metabolic degeneration rate of trigeminal ganglion cells, and slowing potential neuroma formation.[148] Additional physiologic agents include transcutaneous electric nerve stimulation, acupuncture, and low-level laser therapy.

Step 4: Possible Referral. In certain situations patients may need to be referred in a timely manner to a practitioner experienced in nerve injury assessment and repair. The decision and timing to refer should be based on the patient's symptoms and the type of injury, together with the experience of the implant dentist in treating nerve injuries. Usually sufficient time is given for neurosensory recovery. In cases of dysesthesia, anesthesia, or known nerve transection, prompt surgical intervention may allow for the best chance of neurosensory recovery. Early, aggressive treatment has been shown to minimize possible transition to chronic refractory neuropathies (Table 31.7).[149]

Step 5: Follow-Up Care. Follow-up care should always be a component of the treatment of a patient with nerve impairment. The interval between appointments is determined by the extent and type of nerve injury. Usually after the 1-week postoperative appointment, patients are seen every 2 weeks with mapping and documentation of the deficits noted.

Surgical Intervention. Surgical repair is indicated in some cases of neurosensory impairment. In general, early treatment is crucial to success and decreased morbidity. Microneurosurgical procedures include direct nerve repair via primary anastomoses of the two severed nerve ends for transection injuries. For nerve splits, reestablishment and proper alignment of nerve stumps will allow for the best chance to correct regeneration of the damaged nerves.

Fractured Implant

Although rare with today's dental implants, fractured implant bodies may cause significant problems for both clinicians and patients. Dental implant fractures may be one of the major causes of late implant failures and may include possible medicolegal issues. Studies by Goodacre et al.[150] relate the risk for implant body fracture in the early to intermediate period for implants 3.75 mm in diameter to be approximately 1%, the abutment screw fracture risk at 2%, and the prosthetic screw risk at 4% (Fig. 31.65).

Etiology

The incidence of implant body fracture dramatically increases when force conditions are greater. Cantilevers, angled loads, and parafunction increase the risk for fracture. The risk for fracture also increases over time. Typical mechanical failures are due to either

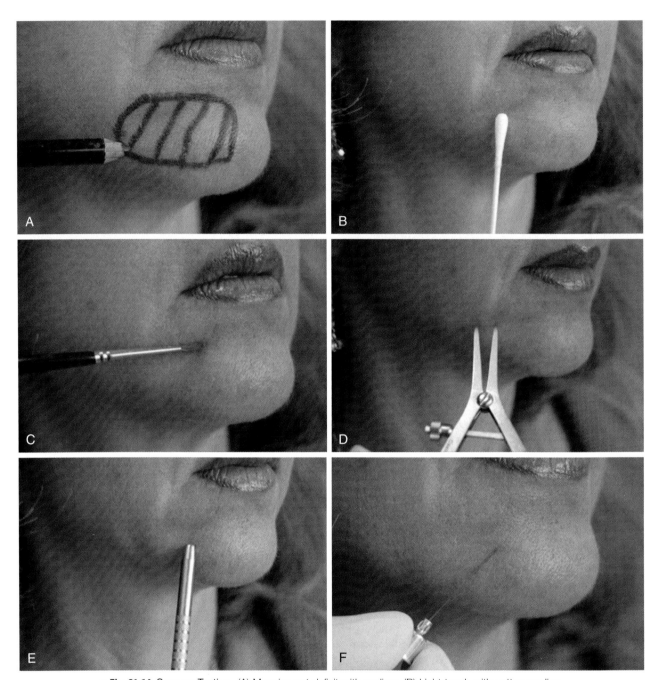

• **Fig. 31.64** Sensory Testing. (A) Mapping out deficit with eyeliner. (B) Light touch with cotton applicator. (C) Directional test with brush. (D) Two-point discrimination using calipers. (E) Thermal test with mirror handle. (F) Pinpoint tests with explorer or dull needle.

static loads or fatigue loads. Static load (i.e., one load cycle) failures cause the stress in the material to exceed its ultimate strength after one load application. Fatigue load failures occur if the material is subjected to lower loads but repeated cycles of that load. The endurance limit or fatigue strength is the level of highest stress a material may be repetitively cycled through without failure. The endurance limit of a material is often less than half of its ultimate tensile strength. Therefore fatigue and ultimate strength values are related, but fatigue is a more critical factor, especially for patients with parafunction because they impose higher stress magnitude and greater cycles of load. Different materials have varying degrees of resistance to repeated loading and subsequent fatigue-related failures. The

fatigue strength of titanium alloy (Ti-6Al-4V) is four times greater (and safer) than grade 1 titanium and almost two times greater than grade 4 titanium. Long-term fracture of implant bodies and components may be dramatically reduced with the use of titanium alloy rather than any grade of commercially pure titanium.

Prevention

A titanium alloy implant should ideally be used to reduce the possibility of implant body fracture. Parafunctional habits should be addressed with occlusal guards, narrow occlusal tables, no lateral contacts, and an ideal occlusal scheme.

TABLE 31.7 Neurosensory Impairment Treatment Protocol

NEUROSENSORY DEFICIT TREATMENT ALGORITHMS				
Postsurgery	Documentation	Pharmacological Intervention	Treatment	Referral
~48 hours	Three-dimensional radiographic examination (cone beam computed tomography); neurosensory examination	Corticosteroids: (dexamethasone 4 mg) 2 tabs a.m. for 3 days 1 tab a.m. for 3 days	Implant evaluation: • Removal and reposition if impingement within the mandibular canal • No bone grafting • Cryotherapy (1 week)	None, unless unfamiliar with neurosensory testing
1 week	Neurosensory examination (testing should be continued every 2 weeks thereafter)	High-dose NSAIDs (600–800 mg ibuprofen TID)	Palliative	Refer to oral surgeon or neurosurgeon if: • Known nerve transection • Dysesthesia • Complete anesthesia
8 weeks	Neurosensory examination	NSAIDs PRN	Palliative	IF NO SIGN OF IMPROVEMENT, refer to OMFS or microsurgeon

NSAID, Nonsteroidal antiinflammatory drug; *OMFS,* Oral and Maxillofacial Surgery Foundation; *PRN,* as needed; *TID,* twice daily.

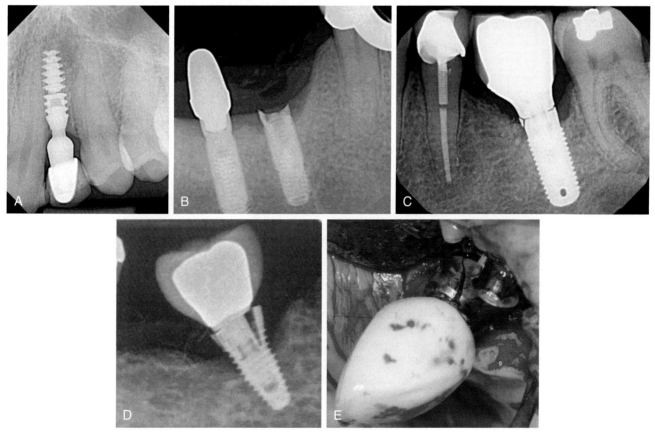

• **Fig. 31.65** Fractured Implants. (A) Midimplant fracture. (B and C) Implant neck fracture. (D) Crestal implant fracture. (E) Clinical image of implant neck fracture.

Treatment

The ideal treatment for a fractured implant includes the removal and possible replacement of the implant. Alternative treatments include modification of the prosthesis to not include the implant and possible modification of the fractured implant (cementable abutment).

Explantation of Dental Implants

In some situations a failing implant or the position of the implant necessitates removal with reinsertion in an ideal position. The following are possible reasons why dental implants may need to be removed:

- Mobility of the implant
- Extensive bone loss
- Chronic pain
- Advanced peri-implantitis
- Fractured implant
- Malpositioned implant

Potential Complications

Taking an aggressive approach to removing an implant may lead to further bone loss and jeopardize the future site for reimplantation. Because an implant does not contain a periodontal ligament, placing too much force and pressure on it may lead to buccal or lingual plate failure. Loss of bony plates or excessive bone loss may result in the need for extensive bone augmentation in the future.

Treatment

The removal of dental implants is dictated by the location, amount of bone present, type of implant, and presence of mobility.

Mobile Implant

The loss of the bone-implant integration necessitates immediate removal because infection and further loss of bone may result. In certain cases the implant may migrate within tissue spaces or may be swallowed or aspirated.

Countertorque Ratchet. This technique involves placing an abutment or an engaging extraction tool into the implant and reverse torqueing the implant counterclockwise. This technique is usually atraumatic, however caution should be exercised to not use excess force as this may lead to bony plate fracture.

Convention Extraction Techniques. This method uses conventional forceps and elevators, and should be used only with minimal luxation to prevent possible fracture of the buccal or lingual plate. After removal, all soft tissue should be removed from the implant site before grafting or reimplantation. A throat pack should always be used to minimize the possibility of aspiration of the implant upon removal.

Nonmobile Implant

A partial or fully integrated implant is usually more problematic and can be in some cases very difficult to remove. Conventional extraction techniques should never be used because they may lead to significant bone loss or fracture. If a final crown and abutment is present, they should be removed to allow for easier access.

Countertorque Ratchet. This technique involves placing an abutment or an engaging extraction tool into the implant and reverse torqueing the implant counterclockwise. This should be used only in poorly dense bone (~maxilla). Care should be exercised in higher-density bone because damage or fracture of the implant body or adjacent bone may occur with this type of removal technique. The existing bone density is the most critical factor which affects the ease of implant removal via the countertorque technique.

Implant Type. In general, an internal hex implant is easier to remove via the countertorque method. External hex implants, because they engage coronal to the implant body, are more difficult to remove because of lack of leverage. Trilobe internal connections, especially those with smaller diameters, have been shown to fracture when greater than 45 N-cm of torque is applied.[151] Care should be exercised to prevent fracturing the implant on removal.

Implant Thread Shape. There are generally four types of implant thread designs: buttress, square, V-shaped, and reverse buttress. The square thread shape has the highest bone-implant contact and will be the most difficult to remove via the countertorque method.

Implant Body Design. A tapered implant design will be easier to remove than a square implant design. The thread depth and surface area decrease in the apical area, which minimizes the torque force necessary for removal. In addition, less chance of fracturing the bony plates exists.

Antirotational Design. Some implant designs contain a vent or opening, usually at the apical end, that will allow for bone growth integration. This will complicate the removal of a partially or fully integrated implant. A trephine or surgical bur technique may be indicated in the removal of these types of implants.

Reverse Screw Techniques. A reverse screw removal drill is usually inidcated when the internal aspect of the implants (threads) are damaged or when the countertorque method is unsuccessful.

Caution should be exercised with smaller-diameter internal implants (~3.0 mm) because fracture of the implant body may occur (Fig. 31.66).

High-Speed Burs. The use of a high-speed bur is a fast, efficient technique to remove an integrated implant. Ideally a tapered surgical bur (extra long: 700 XXL) is used to minimize bone removal. The bur is used 360 degrees around the implant to a depth of half to three-fourths the length of the implant to be removed. Copious amounts of saline should be used to minimize thermal damage and the possibility of osteomyelitis. This helps to maintain bone and minimize damage to vital structures. After removal, the implant site should be irrigated to remove any particles (Fig. 31.67).

Piezo Surgical Units. A piezo surgical unit uses piezoelectric vibrations to cut bone tissue. By adjusting the ultrasonic frequency of the unit, it is possible to remove hard tissue while leaving soft tissue untouched by the process. Studies have shown that piezo units cause less soft tissue damage compared with other extraction techniques.[151]

Trephine Burs. Trephine burs are barrel-shaped burs that are available in various diameters. The bur selected should be slightly larger than the implant crest module because too large of a trephine bur will result in excessive bone removal. Too small of a trephine may result in implant body particles being removed and becoming embedded in the implant site. Copious amounts of saline should

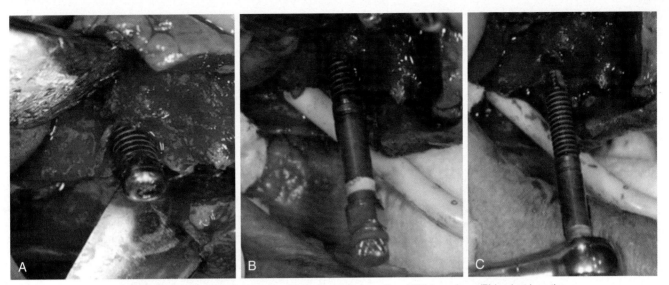

● **Fig. 31.66** Reverse Screw Technique. (A) Implant with more than 50% bone loss. (B) Implant insertion tool inserted into implant. (C) Reverse torque with hand ratchet.

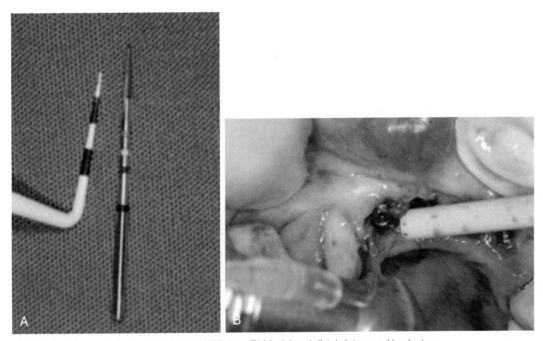

● **Fig. 31.67** (A) 700XXL bur. (B) Mesial and distal slot around implant.

be used to minimize thermal damage and the possibility of osteomyelitis. If the apex of the implant is in approximation to a vital structure, the trephine bur should not be used at the apex to avoid vital structure damage.

After the implant is removed, the implant site should be irrigated to remove any retained titanium particles (Fig. 31.68).

Combination of Techniques. In some cases it is prudent to remove bone half to three-fourths the length of the implant (using a trephine, piezo, or high-speed bur), together with the use of conventional extraction techniques or the countertorque method.

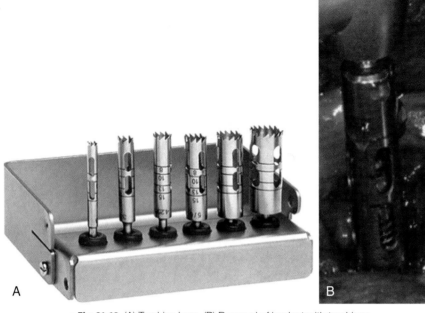

• **Fig. 31.68** (A) Trephine burs. (B) Removal of implant with trephines.

References

1. Simonetti M, Facco G, Barberis F, et al. Bone characteristics following osteotomy surgery: an in vitro SEM study comparing traditional Lindemann drill with sonic and

2. Eriksson R, Albrektsson T. Temperature threshold levels for heat induced bone tissue injury: a vital-microscopic study in the rabbit. *J Prosthet Den.* 1983;50:101–107. doi: 10.1016/0022-3913(83)90174-9.

3. Weinlaender, M. "Bone growth around dental implants." Dental Clinics of North America 35, no. 3 (1991): 585-601.

4. Sharawy M, Misch CE, Weller N, et al. Heat generation during implant drilling: the significance of motor speed. *J Oral Maxillofac Surg.* 2002;60:1160–1169.

5. Yeniyol S, Jimbo R, Marin C, et al. The effect of drilling speed on early bone healing to oral implants. *Oral Surg Oral Med Oral Pathol Oral Radiol.* 2013;116:550–555.

6. Bashutski JD, D'Silva NJ, Wang HL. Implant compression necrosis: current understanding and case report. *J Periodontol.* 2009;80:700–704.

7. Kim H, Kim TW. Histologic evaluation of root-surface healing after root contact or approximation during placement of mini-implants. *Am J Orthod Dentofacial Orthop.* 2011;139:752–760.

8. McKenzie WS, Rosenberg M. Iatrogenic subcutaneous emphysema of dental and surgical origin: a literature review. *J Oral Maxillofac Surg.* 2009;67:1265–1268.

9. Shuman IE. Bipolar versus monopolar electrosurgery: clinical applications. *DEnt Today.* 2001;20:74.

10. Newlands C, Kerawala C. *O Ral and Maxillofacial Surgery.* Oxford: Oxford University Press; 2010.

11. Loukas M, Kinsella CR, Kapos T, et al. Anatomical variation in arterial supply of the mandible with special regard to implant placement. *Int J Oral Maxillofac Surg.* 2008;37:367–371.

12. Laboda G. Life-threatening hemorrhage after placement of an endosseous implant. Report of a case. *J Am Dent Assoc.* 1990;121:559–600.

13. Kalpidis CE, Konstantinidis AB. Critical hemorrhage in the floor of the mouth during implant placement in the first mandibular premolar position: a case report. *IMplant Dent.* 2005;14:117–124.

14. Flanagan D. Important arterial supply of the mandible, control of an arterial hemorrhage, and report of a hemorrhagic incident. *J Oral Implantol.* 2003;29:165–173.

15. Vujaskovic G. Anastomosis between the left and the right lingual artery in Serb-Croatian (Roman). *S tomatol Glas Srb.* 1990;37:267–274.

16. Bavitz JB, Harn SD, Homze EJ. Arterial supply to the floor of the mouth and lingual gingiva. *Oral Surg Oral Med Oral Pathol.* 1994;77:232–235.

17. Zhao Z, Li S, Xu J, et al. Color Doppler flow imaging of the facial artery and vein. *Plast Reconstr Surg.* 2000;106:1249–1253.

18. Rosenbaum L, Thurma P, Krantz SB. Upper airway obstruction as a complication of oral anticoagulation therapy. *Arch Intern Med.* 1979;139:1151–1153.

19. Saino M, Akasaka M, Najajima M, et al. A case of a ruptured lingual artery aneurysm treated with endovascular surgery. *Noshinkeigeka.* 1997;25:835–839 [in Japanese].

20. Mitchell RB, Pereira KD, Lazar RH, et al. Pseudoaneurysm of the right lingual artery: an unusual cause of severe hemorrhage during tonsillectomy. *Ear Nose Throat J.* 1997;76:575–576.

21. Lee CYS, Yanagihara LC, Suzuki JB. Brisk, pulsatile bleeding from the anterior mandibular incisive canal during implant surgery: a case report and use of an active hemostatic matrix to terminate acute bleeding. *Implant Dent.* 2012;21:368–373.

22. Chan HL, Brooks SL, Fu JH. Cross-sectional analysis of the mandibular lingual concavity using cone beam computed tomography. *Clin Oral Implants Res.* 2011;22:201–206.

23. Butura CC, et al. Hourglass mandibular anatomic variant incidence and treatment considerations for all-on-four implant therapy: report of 10 cases. *J Oral Maxillofac Surg.* 2011;69:2135–2143.

24. Gurr P, Callahan V, Baldwin D. Laser-Doppler blood flowmetry measurement of nasal mucosa blood flow after injection of the greater palatine canal. *J Laryngol Otol.* 1996;110:124–128.

25. Morimoto Y, Niwa H, Minematsu K, et al. Risk factors affecting postoperative hemorrhage after tooth extraction in patients receiving oral antithrombotic therapy. *J Oral Maxillofac Surg.* 2011;69:1550–1556.

26. Martin-Du Pan RC, Benoit R, Girardier L. The role of body position and gravity in the symptoms and treatment of various medical diseases. *Swiss Med Wkly.* 2004;134:543–551.

27. Gurr P, Callahan V, Baldwin D. Laser-Doppler blood flowmetry measurement of nasal mucosa blood flow after injection of the greater palatine canal. *J Laryngol Otol.* 1996;110:124–128.

28. Horch HH, Deppe H. Laser in der Zahnärztlichen Chirurgie und Mund-, Kiefer-und Gesichtschirurgie. Angew. Lasermedizin. Lehr-und Handbuch für Praxis und Klinik. *Losebl.-Ausg Landsberg Ecomed.* 2004;3:1.

29. Degerliyurt K, Denizci S. Does the topical use of epinephrine for sinus floor augmentation affect systemic hemodynamics? *Implant Dent.* 2013;22(3):289–294.

30. Sindet-Pedersen S, Ramstrom G. Hemostatic effect of tranexamic acid mouthwash in anticoagulant-treated patients undergoing oral surgery. *New Engl J Med.* 1989;320:840–843.

31. Choi WS, Irwin MG, Samman N. The effect of tranexamic acid on blood loss during orthognathic surgery: a randomized controlled trial. *J Oral Maxillofac Surg.* 2009;67:125–133.

32. Oz MC, Rondinone JF, Shargill NS. FloSeal Matrix: new generation topical hemostatic sealant. *J Card Surg.* 2003;18:486–493.

33. Pfizer Injectables product fact sheet. Thrombin-JMI syringe spray kit thrombin, topical (bovine origin), USP Not for Injection. Available at: http://www.pfizerinjectables.com/factsheets/Thrombin-JMI_all%20SKUs.pdf.

34. Evithrom. Available at: *http://www.ethicon.com/healthcare-professionals/products/biosurgery/evithrom-thrombin-topical-human.*

35. Recothrom. Available at: http://www.recothrom.com.

36. Bochicchio G, Dunne J, Bochicchio K, Scalea T. The combination of platelet-enriched autologous plasma with bovine collagen and thrombin decreases the need for multiple blood transfusions in trauma patients with retroperitoneal bleeding. *J Trauma.* 2004;56:76–79.

37. Lynn AK, Yannas IV, Bonfield W. Antigenicity and immunogenicity of collagen. *J Biomed Mater Res B Appl Biomater.* 2004;71:343–354.

38. Ogle OE. Perioperative hemorrhage. In: Dym H, Ogle OE, eds. *Atlas of Minor Oral Surgery.* Philadelphia: Saunders; 2010.

39. Tan TC, Black PM. Sir victor horsley (1857–1916): pioneer of neurological surgery. *Neurosurgery.* 2002;50:607–611, discussion 611–612.

40. Ibarrola JL, Bjorenson JE, Austin BP, et al. Osseous reactions to three hemostatic agents. *J Endod.* 1985;11:75–83.

41. Allison RT. Foreign body reactions and an associated histological artifact due to bone wax. *BR J Biomed Sci.* 1994;51:14–17.

42. Wellisz T, Yuehuei H, Wen X, et al. Infection rates and healing using bone wax and a soluble polymer material. *Clin Orthop Relat Res.* 2008;466:481–486.

43. American Dental Association. *Accepted Dental Therapeutics.* 40th ed. Chicago: ADA; 1984.

44. Esen E, Tasar F. Determination of the anti-inflammatory effects of methylprednisolone on the sequelae of third molar surgery. *J Oral Maxillofac Surg.* 1999;57:1201–1206.

45. Neuper EA, Lee JW, Philput CB, et al. Evaluation of dexamethasone for reduction of postsurgical sequelae of third molar removal. *J Oral Maxillofac Surg.* 1992;50:1177–1182.

46. Wang JJ, Ho ST, Lee SC, et al. The prophylactic effect of dexamethasone on postoperative nausea and vomiting in women undergoing thyroidectomy: a comparison of droperidol with saline. *Anesth Analg.* 1999;89:200–203.

47. Misch CE, Moore P. Steroids and the reduction of pain, edema and dysfunction in implant dentistry. *Int J Oral Implantol.* 1989;6:27–31.

48. Bull MJV. Cutaneous cryosurgery: principles and clinical practice. *Brit J Gen Pract.* 1995;45:399–566.

49. Forouzanfar T, Sabelis A, Ausems S, et al. Effect of ice compression on pain after mandibular third molar surgery: a single-blind, randomized controlled trial. *Int J Oral Maxillofac Surg.* 2008;37:824–830.

50. Cameron MH. *Physical Agents in Rehabilitation—From Research to Practice.* Philadelphia: Saunders; 1999.

51. Ayango L, Sheridan PJ. Development and treatment of retrograde peri-implantitis involving a site with a history of failed endodontic and apicoectomy procedures: a series of reports. *Int J Oral Maxillofac Implants.* 2001;3:412–417.

52. Quirynen M, Gijbels F, Jacobs R. An infected jawbone site compromising successful osseointegration. *Periodontol 2000.* 2003;33:129–144.

53. Temmerman A, Lefever D, Teughels W, et al. Etiology and treatment of periapical lesions around dental implants. *Periodontol 2000.* 2014;66(1):247–254.

54. Dahlin C, Nikfarid H, Alsen B, et al. Apical peri-implantitis: possible predisposing factors, case reports, and surgical treatment suggestions. *Clin Implant Dent Relat Res.* 2009;3:222–227.

55. Ashley ET, Covington LL, Bishop BG, et al. Ailing and failing endosseous dental implants: a literature review. *J Contemp Dent Pract.* 2003;4(2):35–50.

56. Suarez F, Monje A, Galindo-Moreno P, et al. Implant surface detoxification: a comprehensive review. *Implant Dent.* 2013;22(5):465–473.

57. Meffert RM. How to treat ailing and failing implants. *Implant Dent.* 1992;1(1):25–26.

58. Artzi Z, Tal H, Chweidan H. Bone regeneration for reintegration in peri-implant destruction. *Compend Contin Educ Dent.* 1998;19(1):17–20.

59. Witt JD, Swann M. Metal wear and tissue response in failed titanium alloy total hip replacements. *J Bone Joint Surg Br.* 1991;73:559–563.

60. Yamauchi R, Morita A, Tsuji T. Pacemaker dermatitis from titanium. *Contact Dermatitis.* 2000;42:52–53.

61. Siddiqi A, Payne AG, De Silva RK, et al. Titanium allergy: could it affect dental implant integration? *Clin Oral Implants Res.* 2011;22:673–680.

62. du Preez LA, Bütow KW, Swart TJ. Implant failure due to titanium hypersensitivity/allergy? Report of a case. *SADJ.* 2007;62:24–25.

63. Sicilia A, Cuesta S, Coma G, et al. Titanium allergy in dental implant patients: a clinical study on 1500 consecutive patients. *Clin Oral Implants Res.* 2008;19:823–835.

64. Holgers KM, Roupe G, Tjellström A, Bjursten LM. Clinical, immunological and bacteriological evaluation of adverse reactions to skin-penetrating titanium implants in the head and neck region. *Contact Dermatitis.* 1992;27:1–7.

65. Hallab N, Merritt K, Jacobs JJ. Metal sensitivity in patients with orthopaedic implants. *J Bone Joint Surg Am.* 2001;83A:428–436.

66. Harloff T, Hönle W, Holzwarth U, et al. Titanium allergy or not? "Impurity" of titanium implant materials. *Health.* 2010;2:306–310.

67. Egusa H, Ko N, Shimazu T, Yatani H. Suspected association of an allergic reaction with titanium dental implants: a clinical report. *J Prosthet Dent.* 2008;100:344–347.

68. Adell R, Lekholm U, Rockler B, et al. Marginal tissue reactions at osseointegrated titanium fixtures (I). A 3-year longitudinal prospective study. *Int J Oral Maxillofac Surg.* 1986;15:39–52.

69. Tal H. Spontaneous early exposure of submerged implants: I. Classification and clinical observations. *J Periodontol.* 1999;70:213–219.

70. Mendoza G, Reyes JD, Guerrero ME, et al. Influence of keratinized tissue on spontaneous exposure of submerged implants: classification and clinical observations. *J Osseointegr.* 2014;6:47–50.

71. Lekovic V, Kenney EB, Weinlaender M, et al. A bone regenerative approach to alveolar ridge maintenance following tooth extraction. Report of 10 cases. *J Periodontol.* 1997;68:563–570.

72. Barboza EP, Caula AL. Diagnoses, clinical classification, and proposed treatment of spontaneous early exposure of submerged implants. *Implant Dent.* 2002;11:331–337.

73. Gapski R, Wang HL, Misch CE. Management of incision design in symphysis graft procedures: a review of the literature. *J Oral Implantol.* 2001;26:134–142.

74. Hupp JR, Tucker MR, Ellis E. *Contemporary Oral and Maxillofacial Surgery.* Philadelphia: Elsevier Health Sciences; 2013.

75. Peterson LJ, Ellis E, Hupp JR, et al. *Oral and Maxillofacial Surgery.* St. Louis: Mosby; 1998.

76. Leong G, Wilson J, Charlett A. Duration of operation as a risk factor for surgical site infection: comparison of English and US data. *J Hosp Infect*. 2006;63:255–262.

77. Zarb GA, Albrektsson T, Branemark PI. *T Issue-Integrated Prostheses: Osseointegration in Clinical Dentistry*. Illinois: Quintessence; 1985.

78. Buser D, Dahlin C, Schenk R. *G Uided Bone Regeneration*. Chicago: Quintessence; 1994.

79. Langer B, Langer L. Overlapped fl ap: a surgical modification for implant fixture installation. *Int J Periodontics Restorative Dent*. 1990;10:208–215.

80. Misch CE. Bone augmentation for implant placement: keys to bone grafting. In: Misch CE, ed. *Contemporary Implant Dentistry*. 2nd ed. St Louis: Mosby; 1999:421–447.

81. Park JC, Kim CS, Choi SH, et al. Flap extension attained by vertical and periosteal-releasing incisions: a prospective cohort study. *Clin Oral Implants Res*. 2012;23:993–998.

82. Greenstein G, Cavallaro J, Romanos G, et al. Clinical recommendations for avoiding and managing surgical complications associated with implant dentistry: a review. *J Periodontol*. 2008;79:1317–1329.

83. Goodacre CJ, Bernal G, Rungcharassaeng K. Clinical complications with implants and implant prostheses. *J Prosthet Dent*. 2003;90:121–132.

84. Kourtis SG, Sotiriadou S, Voliotis S, Challas A. Private practice results of dental implants. Part I: survival and evaluation of risk factors—Part II: surgical and prosthetic complications. *Implant Dent*. 2004;13(4):373–385.

85. De Boever AL, Keersmaekers K, Vanmaele G, et al. Prosthetic complications in fixed endosseous implant-borne reconstructions after an observations period of at least 40 months. *J Oral Rehabil*. 2006;33(11):833–839.

86. Chaar MS, Att W, Strub JR. Prosthetic outcome of cementretained implant-supported fixed dental restorations: a systematic review. *J Oral Rehabil*. 2011;38:697–711.

87. Kallus T, Bessing C. Loose gold screws frequently occur in full-arch fixed prostheses supported by osseointegrated implants after 5 years. *Int J Oral Maxillofac Implants*. 1991;9:169–178.

88. Boggan S, Strong JT, Misch CE, et al. Influence of hex geometry and prosthetic table width on static and fatigue strength of dental implants. *J Prosthet Dent*. 1999;82:436–440.

89. Wie H. Registration of localization occlusion and occluding material for failing screw joints in the Brånemark implant system. *Clin Oral Implants Res*. 1995;6:47–53.

90. Hurson S. Practical clinical guidelines to prevent screw loosening. *Int J Dent Symp*. 1995;3(1):23–25.

91. Balshi TJ, Hernandez RE, Pryszlak MC, et al. A comparative study of one implant versus two replacing a single molar. *Int J Oral Maxillofac Implants*. 1996;11:372–378.

92. Hemming KW, Schmitt A, Zarb GA. Complications and maintenance requirements for fixed prostheses and overdentures in the edentulous mandible: a 5-year report. *Int J Oral Maxillofac Implants*. 1994;9:191–196.

93. McGlumphy EA, Elfers CL, Mendel DA. A comparison of torsional ductile fracture in implant coronal screws (abstract), Academy of Osseointegration Proceedings. *Int J Oral Maxillofac Implants*. 1992;7:124.

94. Binon PP, McHugh MJ. The effect of eliminating implant abutment rotational misfit on screw-joint stability. *Int J Prosthodont*. 1996;9:511–519.

95. Binon PP. The evolution and evaluation of two interference fit implant interfaces. *Postgrad Dent*. 1996;3:3–13.

96. Binon PP. The effect of implant/abutment hexagonal misfit on screw joint stability. *Int J Prosthodont*. 1996;9:149–160.

97. Binon PP. Evaluation of three slip fit hexagonal implants. *Implant Dent*. 1996;5:235–248.

98. Carr AB, Brantley WA. Characterization of noble metal implant cylinders: as received cylinders and cast interfaces with noble metal alloys. *J Prosthet Dent*. 1996;75:77–85.

99. Bonde MJ, Stokholm R, Isidor F, et al. Outcome of implantsupported single-tooth replacements performed by dental students. A 10-year clinical and radiographic retrospective study. *Eur J Oral Implantol*. 2010;3:37–46.

100. Jemt T. Single implants in the anterior maxilla after 15 years of follow-up: comparison with central implants in the edentulous maxilla. *Int J Prosthodont*. 2008;21:400–408.

101. Mangano C, Mangano F, Piattelli A, et al. Prospective clinical evaluation of 307 single-tooth Morse taper-connection implants: a multicenter study. *I nt J Oral Maxillofac Implants*. 2010;25:394–400.

102. Duncan JP, Nazarova E, Vogiatzi T, et al. Prosthodontic complications in a prospective clinical trial of single-stage implants at 36 months. *Int J Oral Maxillofac Implants*. 2003;18:561–565.

103. Sadid-Zadeh R, Ahmad K, Hyeongil K. Prosthetic failure in implant dentistry. *Dent Clin North Am*. 2015;59(1):195–214.

104. Cho SC, Small PN, Elian N, Tarnow D. Screw loosening for standard and wide diameter implants in partially edentulous cases: 3- to 7-year longitudinal data. *Implant Dent*. 2004;13(3):245–250.

105. Clelland NL, Van Putten MC. Comparison of strains produced in a bone stimulant between conventional cast and resin-luted implant frameworks. *Int J Oral Maxillofac Implants*. 1997;12:793–799.

106. Clelland NL, Papazoglou E, Carr AB, et al. Comparison of strains transferred to a bone stimulant among implant overdenture bars with various levels of misfi t. *J Prosthodont*. 1995;4:243–250.

107. Jemt T. In vivo measurement of precision fit involving implant supported prostheses in the edentulous jaw. *Int J Oral Maxillofac Implants*. 1996;11:151–158.

108. Sadid-Zadeh R, Ahmad K, Hyeongil K. Prosthetic failure in implant dentistry. *Dent Clin North Am*. 2015;59(1):195–214.

109. Yao K-T, Kao H-C, Cheng C-K, et al. The effect of clockwise and counterclockwise twisting moments on abutment screw loosening. *Clin Oral Implants Res*. 2011;23:1–6.

110. Nigro F, Sendyk CL, Francischone Jr CE, Francischone CE. Removal torque of zirconia abutment screws under dry and wet conditions. *Braz Dent J*. 2010;21(3):225–228.

111. Graves SL, Jansen CE, Saddiqui AA, et al. Wide diameter implants: indications, considerations and preliminary results over a two-year period. *Aust Prosthodont J*. 1994;8:31–37.

112. Goodacre CJ, Bernal G, Rungcharassaeng K. Clinical complications with implants and implant prostheses. *J Prosthet Dent*. 2003;90:121–132.

113. Alhassani AA, AlGhamdi AS. Inferior alveolar nerve injury in implant dentistry: diagnosis, causes, prevention, and management. *J Oral Implantol*. 2010;36:401–407.

114. Misch CE, Resnik R. Mandibular nerve neurosensory impairment after dental implant surgery: management and protocol. *Implant Dent*. 2010;19:378–386.

115. Libersa P, Savignat M, Tonnel A. Neurosensory disturbances of the inferior alveolar nerve: a retrospective study of complaints in a 10-year period. *J Oral Maxillofac Surg*. 2007;65:1486–1489.

116. Abarca M, van Steenberghe D, Malevez C, et al. Neurosensory disturbances after immediate loading of implants in the anterior mandible: an initial questionnaire approach followed by a psychophysical assessment. *Clin Oral Investig*. 2006;10:269–277.

117. Wadu SG, Penhall B, Townsend GC. Morphological variability of the human inferior alveolar nerve. *CLin Anat*. 1997;10:82–87.

118. Benninger B, Kloenne J, Horn JL. Clinical anatomy of the lingual nerve and identifi cation with ultrasonography. *Br J Oral Maxillofac Surg*. 2013;51:541–544.

119. Pogrel MA, Thamby S. Permanent nerve involvement resulting from inferior alveolar nerve block. *J Am Dent Assoc*. 2000;131:901–907.

120. Artzi Z, Nemcovsky CE, Bitlitum I, Segal P. Displacement of the incisive foramen in conjunction with implant placement in the anterior maxilla without jeopardizing vitality of nasopalatine nerve and vessels: a novel surgical approach. *Clin Oral Implants Res*. 2000;11:505–510.

121. Filippi A, Pohl Y, Tekin U. Sensory disorders after separation of the nasopalatine nerve during removal of palatal displaced canines: prospective investigations. *Br J Oral Maxillofac Surg*. 1999;37:134–136.

122. Magennis P. Sensory morbidity after palatal flap surgery–fact or fiction? *J Ir Dent Assoc.* 1990;36:60–61.

123. de Oliveira-Santos C, Rubira-Bullen IR, Monteiro SA, et al. Neurovascular anatomical variations in the anterior palate observed on CBCT images. *Clin Oral Implants Res.* 2013;24:1044–1048.

124. Bagheri SC, Bell B, Khan HA. Nerve damage in dentistry. In: Pogrel MA, ed. *Current Therapy in Oral and Maxillofacial Surgery.* Philadelphia: Elsevier Health Sciences; 2011:421–468.

125. Stacy GC, Hajjar G. Barbed needle and inexplicable paresthesias and trismus after dental regional anesthesia. *Oral Surg Oral Med Oral Pathol.* 1994;77:585–588.

126. Malamed SF. *H Andbook of Local Anesthesia.* 4th ed. St Louis: Mosby; 1997.

127. Smith MH, Lung KE. Nerve injuries after dental injection: a review of the literature. *J Can Dent Assoc.* 2006;72:559.

128. Harn SD, Durham TM. Incidence of lingual nerve trauma and postinjection complications in conventional mandibular block anesthesia. *J Am Dent Assoc.* 1990;121:519–523.

129. Hillerup S, Jensen R. Nerve injury caused by mandibular block analgesia. *Int J Oral Maxillofac Surg.* 2006;35:437–443.

130. Haas DA, Lennon D. A 21 year retrospective study of reports of paresthesia following local anesthetic administration. *J Can Dent Assoc.* 1995;61:319–320. 323–326, 329–330.

131. Kanaa MD, Whitworth JM, Corbett IP, Meechan JG. Articaine buccal infiltration enhances the effectiveness of lidocaine inferior alveolar nerve block. *Int Endod J.* 2009;42:238–246.

132. Ribeiro Jr PD, Sanches MG, Okamoto T. Comparative analysis of tissue reactions to anesthetic solutions: histological analysis in subcutaneous tissue of rats. *Anesth Prog.* 2003;50:169–180.

133 Khawaja, N., and T. Renton. "Case studies on implant removal influencing the resolution of inferior alveolar nerve injury." British dental journal 206, no. 7 (2009):365.

134. Juodzbalys G, Wang HL, Sabalys G. Injury of the inferior alveolar nerve during implant placement: a literature review. *J Oral Maxillofac Res.* 2011;2:e1.

135. Kim, Hyun Jeong. Peripheral Nerve Injuries Related to Local Anesthesia in the Dental Clinic. *J Korean Dent Soc Anesthesiol.* 2014;14(2):89–94.

136. Sammartino G, Marenzi G, Citarella R, et al. Analysis of the occlusal stress transmitted to the inferior alveolar nerve by an osseointegrated threaded fixture. *J Periodontol.* 2008;79:1735–1744.

137. Al-Ouf K, Salti L. Postinsertion pain in region of mandibular dental implants: a case report. *IMplant Dent.* 2011;20:27–31.

138. Renton T. Oral surgery: part 4. Minimising and managing nerve injuries and other complications. *Br Dent J.* 2013;215:393–399.

139. Shamloo N, Safi Y, Fathpour K, et al. Lower lip numbness due to the mandibular canal narrowing after dental reimplantation: a case report. *Dent Res J (Isfahan).* 2015;12:386.

140. Misch CE, Resnik R. Mandibular nerve neurosensory impairment after dental implant surgery: management and protocol. *Implant Dent.* 2010;19:378–386.

141. Seddon JJ. Three types of nerve injury. B rain 66:237, 1943 .40. Sunderland S. A classification of peripheral nerve injuries produced by a loss of function. *Brain.* 1951;74:491.

142. Sunderland S. The anatomy and physiology of nerve injury. *Muscle Nerve.* 1990;13(9):771–784.

143. de Oliveira-Santos C, Rubira-Bullen IR, Monteiro SA, et al. Neurovascular anatomical variations in the anterior palate observed on CBCT images. *Clin Oral Implants Res.* 2013;24:1044–1048.

144. Misch CE, ed. *Contemporary Implant Dentistry.* St Louis: Mosby; 2008.

145. Costigan M, Scholz J, Woolf CJ. Neuropathic pain: a maladaptive response of the nervous system to damage. *Annu Rev Neurosci.* 2009;32:1–32.

146. Vecht CJ, Haaxma-Reiche H, Van Putten WL. Conventional versus high-dose dexamethasone in metastatic spinal cord compression. *Neurology.* 1989;39(suppl 1):220.

147. Seo K, Tanaka Y, Terumitsu M, et al. Efficacy of steroid treatment for sensory impairment after orthognathic surgery. *J Oral Maxillofac Surg.* 2004;62:1193.

148. Olson J. A review of cryotherapy. *Phys Ther.* 1972;52:840.

149. Pogrel MA, Thamby S. Permanent nerve involvement resulting from inferior alveolar nerve block. *J Am Dent Assoc.* 2000;131:901–907.

150. Goodacre CJ, Bernal G, Runcharassaeng K, et al. Clinical complications with implants and implant prostheses. *J Prosthet Dent.* 2003;90:121.

151. Froum S, Yamanaka T, Cho SC, et al. Techniques to remove a failed integrated implant. *Compend Contin Educ Dent.* 2011;32:22–26.

152. Preti G, Martinasso G, Peirone B, et al. Cytokines and growth factors involved in the osseointegration of oral titanium implants positioned using piezoelectric bone surgery versus a drill technique: a pilot study in minipigs. *J Periodontol.* 2007;78:716–722.

153. Misch CE. Bone augmentation for implant placement: keys to bone grafting. In: Misch CE, ed. *Contemporary Implant Dentistry.* 2nd ed. St Louis: Mosby; 1999:421–447.

154. Misch Carl E, Resnik R. *Misch's Avoiding Complications in Oral Implantology.* Elsevier Health Sciences; 2017.

32
Immediate Implant Placement Surgical Protocol

RANDOLPH R. RESNIK

The traditional dental implant placement protocol is a proven and reliable treatment modality to restore edentulous spaces. However, a healing period is usually required after extraction and/or graft, which delays the implant placement and ultimately the placement of the final prosthesis. This extended treatment time leaves the patient without teeth and usually an interim prosthesis. Since the 1980s these conventional treatment protocols have been challenged to be replaced with other options that are geared toward shorter treatment times. Classifications have been reported to clarify the placement of dental implants according to various time intervals after tooth extraction.

The placement of dental implants at the time of tooth extraction (immediate implants) has been shown to be a viable treatment protocol in implant dentistry today.[1-4] The objectives of immediate implant placement are the same as for conventional staged treatment: implant primary stability, sufficient rigid fixation after healing, ideal positioning for implant restoration, and an ideal esthetic result. Immediate implant placement has become extremely popular because these objectives can be obtained with fewer procedures, less treatment time, and less cost to the patient. However, immediate placement implants are more demanding and require a special skill set from the implant clinician. The surgical procedure and prosthetic rehabilitation are more complex, with multiple factors that may lead to an increased morbidity or complications. Therefore this chapter will address the immediate placement protocol with a comprehensive evaluation of treatment planning and specific factors related to site-specific recommendations and the prevention of complications (Fig. 32.1) Box 32.1.

• BOX 32.1 Implant Placement Definitions[1]

- Immediate = at time of extraction
- Early = 4–6 weeks after extraction
- Delayed = 3–4 months after extraction
- Late = >4 months after tooth extraction

Advantages of Immediate Implant Placement

Decreased Treatment Time and Cost

The immediate placement procedure reduces the number of surgical appointments because no postoperative healing period is required. Because of the decreased number of surgical appointments, patient discomfort and morbidity are decreased. In addition, less chair time is required, which reduces the overall cost of the procedure.

Decreased Need for Bone Augmentation

Because the implant is placed at the same time as extraction, the bone remodeling process does not take place in which bone resorbs from the facial to the lingual, often resulting in compromised bone dimensions. If no immediate implant or grafting is completed at the time of extraction, resorption has been shown to result in approximately 1 to 2 mm of vertical bone height and 4 to 5 of horizontal bone width within 1 to 3 years.[5] Additional studies have shown that at 6 months after extraction, bone healing averages approximately 1.24 mm vertical bone loss (range 0.9–3.6 mm) and 3.79 mm horizontal bone decrease (range 2.46–4.56 mm) (Fig. 32.2).[6]

Preservation of the Soft Tissue Drape

An additional benefit of immediate implant insertion after tooth extraction is related to the preservation of the soft tissue drape. Most often after tooth extraction, the soft tissue drape is lost and becomes compromised. The immediate implant placement technique has been described as a "preservation technique," because the gingival architecture is preserved. If the soft tissue drape is not maintained, "black triangles" will result in the interproximal areas, which compromises long-term esthetics and/or contributes to peri-implant disease (Fig. 32.3).

Improved Implant Positioning

Because the implant is placed into the existing extraction site, the ideal implant positioning is much easier for the clinician. In a staged implant protocol, often the available bone is not in the

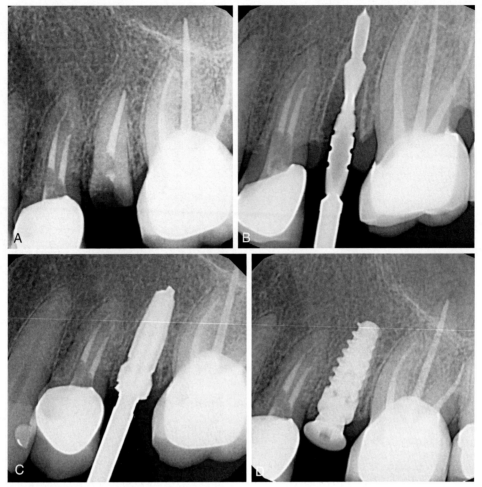

• **Fig. 32.1 Immediate Placement Implant.** (A) Nonrestorable maxillary second bicuspid fracture. (B and C) Verification of initial pilot and final drill engaging bone apical to root apex. (D) Final immediate implant placement.

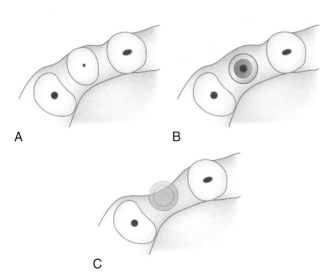

• **Fig. 32.2** (A) Existing tooth root supporting the buccal plate. (B) Immediate implant supports the buccal plate. (C) Diagram depicting resorption of buccal bone requiring bone graft before implant placement.

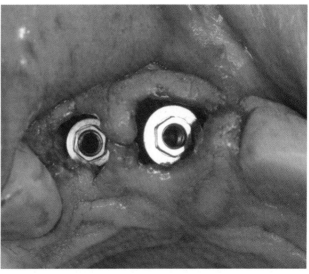

• **Fig. 32.3** Immediate implant placement with minimal soft tissue reflection allows for the preservation of the soft tissue drape and results in minimal recession.

- Decreased treatment time and cost
- Decreased need for bone augmentation
- Preservation of the soft tissue drape
- Improved implant positioning
- High patient satisfaction

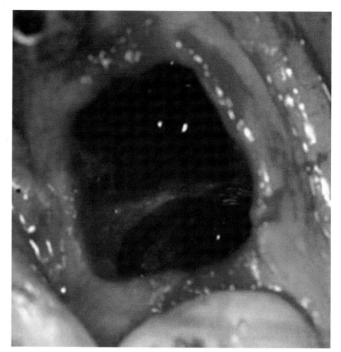

• **Fig. 32.4** Poor Site Morphology: Mandibular extraction resulting in minimal bone for immediate implant placement.

ideal position (i.e., the ridge is positioned more lingually), which leads to nonideal implant placement, with resultant implant prosthesis complications (Box 32.2).

Disadvantages of Immediate Placement

Site Morphology

After tooth extraction the dimensions of the remaining socket (i.e., mesial-distal and buccal-lingual dimensions) are usually much different from the implant diameter. Therefore a discrepancy is present between the implant diameter and the morphology of the socket, which results in bony defects. For example, the maxillary molar has an 8.0-mm mesial-distal average cervix diameter and a 10.0-mm buccal-lingual diameter. After extraction, usually a 5.0- or 6.0-mm diameter is inserted that leaves a 2.0- to 3.0-mm (mesial-distal) and a 4.0- to 5.0-mm buccal-lingual discrepancy (Fig. 32.4).

Surgical Technique Is More Complicated

Placement of an implant into an extraction site is usually much more surgically demanding. The techniques are site specific and usually do not follow standard manufacturers' surgical placement protocols. Most notably, it is often difficult to achieve primary stability because of poor bone density or compromised bone quantity (Fig. 32.5).

Anatomic Limitations

It is often necessary to deepen the osteotomy 2 to 4 mm apical to the existing extraction socket (apical wall) to obtain primary stability. This may result in impingement on vital structures, resulting in neurosensory impairments, perforation into the maxillary sinus or nasal cavity, or perforation of the cortical plates. In the maxillary anterior the nasal cavity may be penetrated, and in the posterior the maxillary sinus may be violated, which can predispose the patient to rhinosinusitis. In the mandibular posterior, extending the osteotomy deeper may lead to violation of the mandibular canal and resultant nerve damage (i.e., especially common in type 1 nerve positions) or lingual plate perforation (Fig. 32.6).

Lack of Primary Closure

It is usually difficult or even impossible to obtain primary closure after tooth extraction and immediate implant placement. Unless a large incision is made and the tissue stretched, it is often challenging to approximate the tissues. Therefore usually a membrane will be required to be placed over the extraction site. Making larger broad-based incisions with vertical releases incisions results in compromised blood supply and is usually not

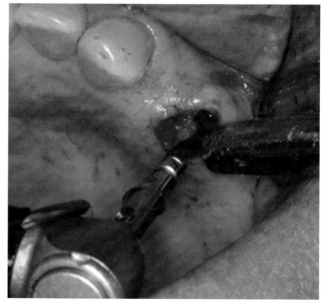

• **Fig. 32.5** Surgical placement into an extraction site requires an increased skill set.

warranted. In some cases, when compromised keratinized tissues exist, free tissue, subepithelial, or connective tissue grafts may be indicated after stage I healing to restore the facial attached keratinized tissue.

Presence of Acute/Chronic Pathology

Although studies have shown immediate implants may be successfully placed after extraction of teeth into infected sites, there is obviously an increased risk. Because residual bacteria may be present after an extraction, healing may be affected and morbidity higher. If exudate is present, the pH is lowered, which

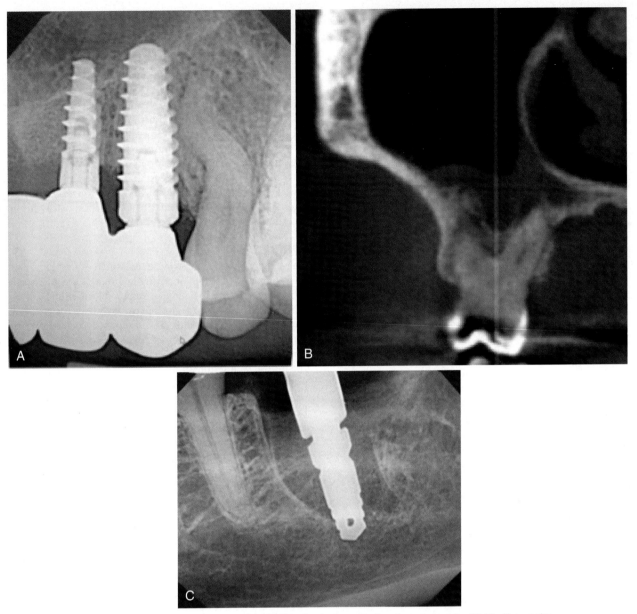

• **Fig. 32.6 Anatomic Limitations.** (A) Maxillary implant penetrating the nasal cavity. (B) Maxillary molar showing no host bone present for immediate implant placement because of the maxillary sinus location. (C) Implant placement positioned more apical to root socket, which impinges on the mandibular canal.

may cause solution-mediated resorption of the grafted bone and contamination of the implant body because of a bacterial smear layer. Therefore implant placement into an infected site is a controversial topic in implant dentistry, and the implant clinician must be conscious of the possible associated complications (Fig. 32.7).

Consequences of Implant Failure

If implant failure results from an immediate implant, significant complications may occur. Usually the need for bone augmentation will result, which delays treatment and increases costs. Studies have shown that a replacement implant (second time) has a success rate of approximately 71%, and a third replacement has a success rate of approximately 60% (Fig. 32.8 and Box 32.3).[7,8] Therefore, implant failure may lead to many financial and patient related issues.

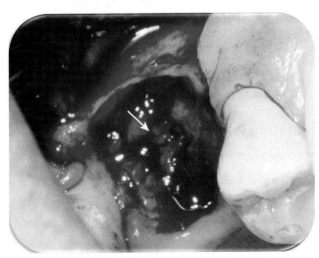

• **Fig. 32.7** Postextraction site exhibiting acute pathology.

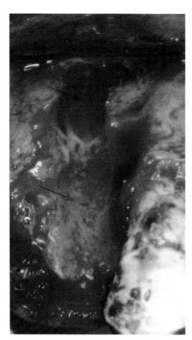

• **Fig. 32.8** Immediate Implant Failure: Large defect resulting from the loss of an immediate implant resulting no buccal plate remaining and missing mesial bone.

Immediate Implant Studies

Immediate placement implants were first reported by Lazzara in 1989.[1] In his studies, he documented the placement of implants at the time of extraction with the use of barrier membranes. Becker et al.[9,10] in 1999 reported a 93.3% survival rate for implants placed at the time of extraction and grafted with barrier membranes after 1 and 5 years after loading. Since then, a full array of studies has confirmed the success and predictability of placing implants at the time of extraction.[11,12] Peñarrocha-Diago et al.[13] evaluated immediate versus nonimmediate placement of implants for full-arch fixed restorations. They determined that the immediate group had a higher success rate (97.7%) versus the nonimmediate group (96.3%).

Treatment Planning Considerations

Available Bone

The concept of available bone is generally accepted as a primary determinant of implant placement viability. Available bone describes the amount of bone in an extraction site considered for implantation. It is measured in width, height, length, angulation, and crown height space (Fig. 32.9). As a general guideline, 1.5 to 2 mm of surgical error is maintained between the implant and any adjacent landmark or vital structure. This is especially critical when the opposing landmark is the mandibular inferior alveolar nerve.

When evaluating available bone in an immediate extraction site, the implant clinician must consider the dimension of the extraction socket and the defect between the labial plate of bone and the proposed position of the implant. The resultant defect may be deceiving. For example, most anterior teeth have a faciopalatal dimension that is far greater than its mesiodistal dimension. When an anterior tooth requires extraction, during the extraction process the thin facial cortex often becomes compromised or lost. As a result the buccal cortex is almost always several millimeters apical to the palatal cortical plate, and frequently bone grafting and/or membrane placement in conjunction with the implant insertion are indicated.

Bone Height

The height of available bone is measured from the crest of the edentulous ridge to the opposing landmark. The anterior regions are limited by the maxillary nares or the inferior border of the mandible. The anterior regions of the jaws have the greatest height because the maxillary sinus and inferior alveolar nerve limit this dimension in the posterior regions. The maxillary canine eminence region often offers the greatest height of available bone in the maxillary anterior.[1] In the posterior jaw region there is usually greater bone height in the maxillary first premolar than in the second premolar, which has greater height than the molar sites because of the concave morphology of the maxillary sinus floor. Likewise, the mandibular first premolar region is usually anterior to the mental foramen and provides the most vertical column of bone in the posterior mandible. However, on occasion, this premolar site may present a reduced height compared with the anterior region because of the presence of an anterior loop of the mandibular canal. The nerve courses anteriorly below the foramen and proceeds superiorly, then distally, before its exit through the mental foramen. Posterior nerve anatomy has particular significance with regard to immediate implant placement. Primary stability for immediately placed implants is frequently achieved using bone apical to the extraction site. In the posterior mandible the course of the inferior alveolar nerve can vary from type 1 to type 3, with associated available apical bone ranging from nonexistent to sufficient and surgical risk varying accordingly. In addition, variants of the mental foramen exist that can increase the possibility of injury to the inferior alveolar nerve during immediate implant placement in the region (Fig. 32.10). The available bone height in an edentulous site is the most important dimension for implant consideration because it affects both implant length and crown height. Crown height affects force factors and esthetics. In addition, vertical bone augmentation, if needed, is less predictable than width augmentation.

Bone Width

The width of available bone is measured between the facial and lingual plates at the crest of the potential implant site. It is the next most significant criterion affecting long-term survival of endosteal implants. The crestal aspect of the residual ridge is often cortical in nature and exhibits greater density than the underlying trabecular bone regions, especially in the mandible.

Accordingly, the lack of crestal bone at an extraction site makes the achievement of primary stability more challenging for immediate implant placement. Facial dehiscence defects commonly found after tooth extraction and immediate implant placement

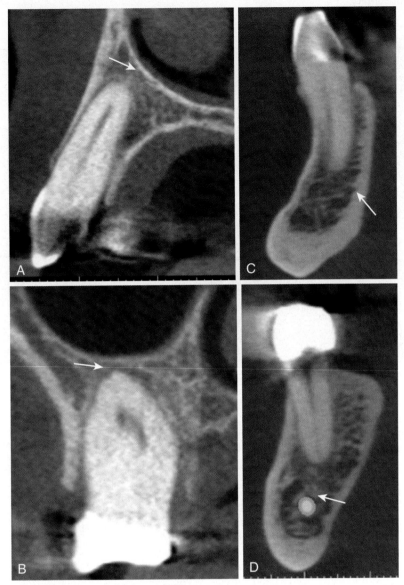

• **Fig. 32.9** Anatomic limitations for immediate implant treatment planning: (A) Floor of the nasal cavity. (B) Inferior border of the maxillary sinus. (C) Lingual cortical plate of the inferior mandible. (D) Inferior alveolar canal.

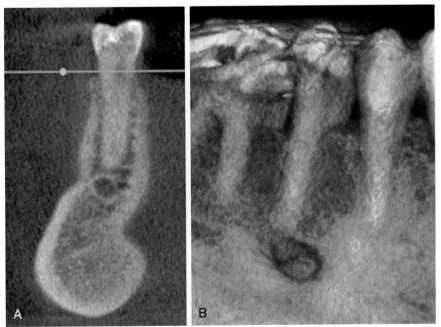

• **Fig. 32.10** Proximity of the Mental Foramen to the Premolar Apices. (A) In 25% to 38% of cases the mental foramen is superior to the premolar apex. (B) Three-dimensional image depicting a premolar root in the mental foramen.

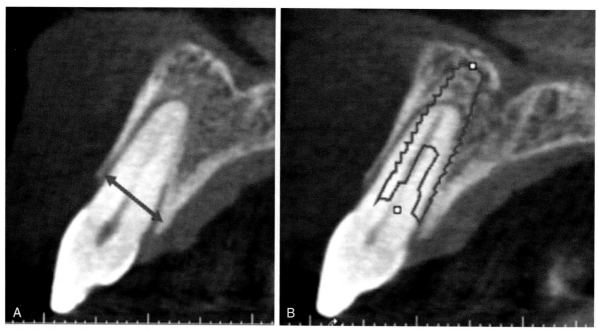

• **Fig. 32.11** Evaluation of Width: (A) Bone width may be measured on CBCT cross-section, (B) Evaluation by interactive treatment planning with implant placement.

have been shown to have more compromised healing compared with infrabony defects (Fig. 32.11).[9]

Bone Length

Bone length is defined as the mesiodistal length of bone in a postextraction area. It is most often limited by adjacent teeth or implants. As a general rule the implant should be at least 1.5 mm from an adjacent tooth and 3 mm from an adjacent implant. These measurements not only allow surgical error but also compensates for the width of an implant or tooth crestal defect, which is usually less than 1.4 mm and may vary with implant diameter and thread design. As a result, if bone loss occurs around the crest module of an implant or around a tooth with periodontal disease, the associated vertical bone defect will not typically expand into horizontal defect and thereby cause bone loss on the adjacent structure (Fig. 32.12).

Bone Angulation

Bone angulation is an additional determinant for available bone (Fig. 32.13). The initial alveolar bone angulation represents the natural tooth root trajectory in relation to the occlusal plane. Ideally it is perpendicular to the plane of occlusion, which is aligned with the forces of occlusion and is parallel to the long axis of the prosthodontic restoration. The incisal and occlusal surfaces of the teeth follow the curve of Wilson and curve of Spee. As such, the roots of the maxillary teeth are angled toward a common point approximately 4 inches away. The mandibular roots flare, so the anatomic crowns are more lingually inclined in the posterior regions and labially inclined in the anterior area compared with the underlying roots. The mandibular first premolar cusp tip is usually vertical to its root apex. The maxillary anterior teeth are the only segment in either arch that does not receive a long axis load to the tooth roots, but instead are usually loaded at a 12-degree angle. As such, their root diameter is greater than the mandibular anterior teeth. In all other regions the teeth are loaded perpendicular to the curves of Wilson or Spee. The anterior sextants may have labial undercuts that often mandate greater

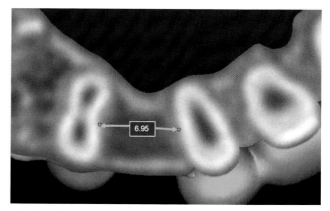

• **Fig. 32.12** Cone beam computed tomographic three-dimensional axial image measuring the length between two root tips.

angulation of the implants or concurrent grafting of the site after insertion. The narrower width ridge often requires a root form implant design that is likewise narrower. Compared with larger diameters, smaller-diameter designs cause greater crestal stress and may not offer the same range of custom abutments. In addition, the narrower width of bone does not permit as much latitude in placement regarding angulation within the bone. This limits the acceptable angulation of bone in the narrow ridge to 20 degrees from the axis of the adjacent clinical crowns or a line perpendicular to the occlusal plane.[14] The angulation of available bone in the maxillary first premolar region may place the adjacent cuspid at risk during implant placement.

Esthetic Risk

Especially in the anterior region, extracting a tooth with the immediate implant placement may result in nonideal esthetic issues. Therefore the patient should be evaluated preoperatively for the following esthetic parameters: lip line in relation to the

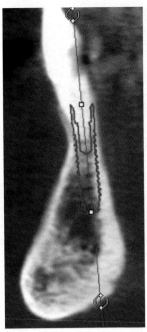

• **Fig. 32.13** Cone beam computed tomographic image determining ideal angulation.

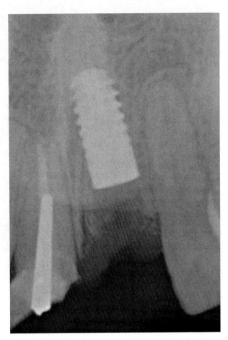

• **Fig. 32.15** Immediate placement resulting in poor esthetics and periodontal complications because of positioning too deep and poor angulation.

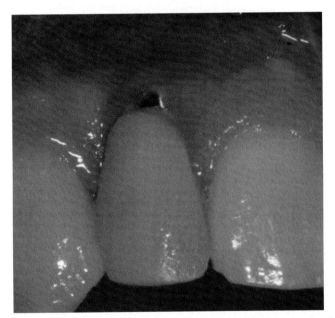

• **Fig. 32.14** Maxillary lateral incisor resulting in poor esthetics because of a facially placed immediate implant placement.

teeth and gingival margins, presence and position of interproximal papilla, shape and shade of adjacent teeth, presence of restorations on adjacent teeth, and a hard and soft tissue thickness analysis. In some cases, even with an ideal esthetic result, possible limitations may deem the placement of implants nonideal (Fig. 32.14).

Type of Prosthesis

The clinician must always be proactive in the evaluation and anticipation of the final prosthesis and its associated dimensions of crown height space, whether for a single-tooth crown or full-arch prosthesis. In clinical situations where tooth extraction will

result in an edentulous arch, an alveoloplasty may need to be completed to satisfy the need for additional space. In completely edentulous patients, alveoplasty may result in the complete obliteration of the residual socket. This is imperative because sufficient crown height space is needed for an overdenture and attachment, whereas minimal reduction is required when a type 3 fixed prosthesis (FP-3) is treatment planned. When considering immediate implant placement for partially edentulous patients, the anatomic dimensions of the edentulous space must be evaluated. In some cases the opposing arch may need to be modified, or possible orthodontic treatment to realign or reposition the dentition (Fig. 32.15).

Bone Density

Bone quality or density refers to the internal structure of bone and reflects a number of its biomechanical properties, such as strength and modulus of elasticity. The density of available bone in a potential implant site is a determining factor in treatment planning, implant design, surgical approach, healing time, and initial progressive bone loading during prosthetic reconstruction. The quality of bone is often dependent on the arch position. The densest bone is usually observed in the anterior mandible, with less dense bone in the anterior maxilla and posterior mandible, and the least dense bone typically found in the posterior maxilla. In addition to arch location, several authors have reported different failure rates related to the quality of the bone. Johns et al.[15] reported a higher failure rate in the maxilla (poorer bone quality) in comparison with the mandible (more favorable bone density). Smedberg et al.[16] reported a 36% failure rate in the poorest bone density. The reduced implant survival most often is more related to bone density than arch location. In a 15-year follow-up study, Herrmann et al.[17] found implant failures were strongly correlated to patient factors, including bone quality, especially when coupled with poor bone volume. Bone quality is directly related to the ability to achieve an acceptable level of primary fixation for

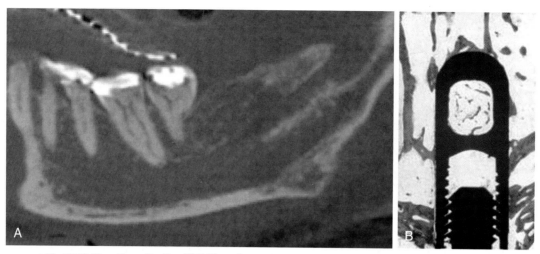

● **Fig. 32.16** Poor Bone Quality. (A) D4 bone has an increased failure rate with immediate placement. (B) D4 bone has less than 30% bone-implant contact.

immediate implant placement, as well as long-term success for all placement protocols (Fig. 32.16).

Existing Crown Form

When evaluating teeth for immediate placement, tapered crown forms usually are associated with a higher risk for soft tissue compromise after extraction. The tapered crown also has more interproximal bone between the teeth and more facial bone over the tapered root. As such, under perfect conditions, the tapered tooth form may be more advantageous for extraction and immediate implant insertion. A square tooth form has less gingival shrinkage after extraction and exhibits less scalloping of the interproximal and facial bone with adjacent tooth roots. There is also less bone between the roots and larger spaces between the extraction site and the implant. As a result an immediate implant insertion after extraction offers less benefit for the soft tissue and greater risk for the implant-bone interface.[18]

Anatomic Location

For immediate implant placement an awareness of the bone characteristics of the proposed anatomic location will help dictate the appropriate treatment plan modifications for short- and long-term success. Regional variations in both available bone and bone density have already been described. The initial treatment plan before surgery suggests the anterior maxilla be treated as D3 bone, the posterior maxilla as D4 bone, the anterior mandible as D2 bone, and the posterior mandible as D3 bone. Bone remodeling, including loss of bone density, is primarily related to the length of time the region has been edentulous and therefore not loaded, the initial density of the bone, and mandibular flexure and torsion.

Immediate implant placement can take advantage of the fact that implant placement can be performed before the bone density in the jaws begins its usual decline after tooth loss.

Tissue Thickness

The patient's biotype is crucial in evaluating the susceptibility to increased tissue recession. Patients with a thin biotype are more predisposed to gingival recession and bone loss. Usually patients

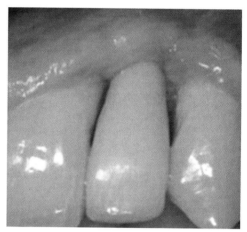

● **Fig. 32.17** Thin biotype leads to postoperative tissue recession and black triangles.

with a thin biotype will require bone and possible tissue grafting to minimize recession.

Kan et al.[19] reported marginal tissue levels around immediate implants may continue up to 8.2 years (mean 4 years) after placement. In addition, thin biotypes were found to recede three times more than thick biotypes. For patients exhibiting a thin biotype, the use of orthodontic forced eruption procedures before tooth removal and implantation. This will result in bone and soft tissues to move coronally, thereby increasing mucosal tissue adjacent to the implant (Fig. 32.17).

Buccal Bone Thickness

In general the buccal bone is thinner than the lingual bone, and the buccal bone is usually compromised after extraction. For example, Januario et al.[20] evaluated facial bone thickness in the anterior maxillae at various measurements from the bone crest. They determined the bone thickness in the tooth sites to be approximately ≤1 mm thick (≤0.6 mm on average). In addition, they found the marginal portion of the wall was <0.5 mm wide.[20] After extraction, bone resorbs naturally from buccal to the lingual. There exist three main sources of blood supply to the bone surrounding the teeth: the periodontal ligament blood vessels, the periosteal blood vessels, and the alveolar bone blood vessels. After an extraction, 20% of the blood supply from periodontal ligament blood vessels is lost and over the buccal plate of bone loses 50% of its blood supply.[21] In addition, if a buccal flap is elevated on the buccal side, the periosteal blood supply will be discontinued for approximately 4 to 6 days, until the formation of a new anastomoses. The cortical bone buccal plate contains no endosteal blood vessels; therefore, complete resorption of the buccal plate may occur after extraction if implant placement or grafting is not completed. Socket grafting is frequently used in the treatment postextraction to prevent collapse and to minimize resorption of the thin buccal plate (Fig. 32.18).

Implant Position

The immediate implant positioning is dictated by the anatomic position. For implants placed in the maxillary anterior, immediate implants should not be placed close to the buccal plate; instead they should be positioned more in the lingual aspect of the extraction socket. Evans and Chen[22] evaluated the esthetic outcomes of immediate anterior implants and found implants placed more buccally had three times more soft tissue recession than lingually placed implants (1.8 versus 0.6 mm). Spray et al.[23] reported that when 2 mm of facial bone thickness was present, vertical bone loss height was minimal. When <2 mm of bone thickness was present, tissue recession and failure resulted. In the mandibular anterior, implants should be positioned more toward the lingual, but not as much lingual version as the maxillary anterior. In the maxillary and mandibular posterior region the implants should be positioned in the center of the extraction socket, with a buccal lingual trajectory similar to the central fossas of the adjacent teeth.

Requirements for Immediate Implant Placement

1. A CBCT evaluation confirms sufficient bone quantity (buccal plate bone, bone apical to root apex, palatal bone); in addition, sufficient proximal bone to avoid encroachment on adjacent roots
2. An esthetic risk evaluation should be completed before immediate implant placement. The following factors should be taken into consideration (i.e., smile line, soft tissue drape, adjacent teeth shade stable and free of large restorations)
3. Ability to position implant in an ideal location for prosthetic rehabilitation, which is dependent on the anatomic location and the available bone.
4. Ideal primary implant stability is achieved (35–45 N/cm), which is dictated by bone density, surgical technique (i.e., drilling and osseodensification protocols), and implant design
5. If any of the above requirements are not satisfactory, the clinician should determine if other treatment options exist.

Immediate Implant Placement Technique

Step 1: Clinical and Radiographic Examination

A thorough clinical and radiographic examination should be completed as the first step of the immediate placement technique. Preferably a comprehensive CBCT scan is taken of the associated areas in question. The type of extraction defect (e.g., walls of bone present) may be anticipated with a careful preoperative clinical examination that includes periodontal probing, evaluation

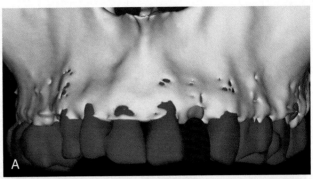
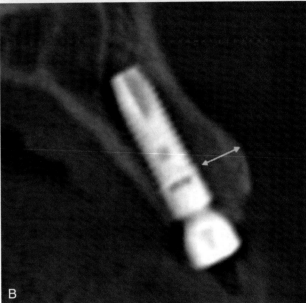

• **Fig. 32.18** Buccal Bone Thickness. (A) Thin buccal bone leading to poor immediate implant candidate. (B) Postoperative radiograph depicting thick buccal bone, which results in higher success and better soft tissue healing.

of mobility, infection, and fractures, along with two- and three-dimensional radiographs. These collective clinical data are useful in evaluating for possible factors that would lead to immediate placement contraindications (Fig. 32.19).

Step 2: Atraumatic Tooth Extraction

Once the extraction of a natural tooth is indicated, methods to maintain or preserve the surrounding hard and soft tissues should be of utmost importance. Avoiding soft tissue injury reduces the dimensional loss of the underlying bone as the periosteum supplies more than 80% of the blood supply to surrounding cortical bone.[24] The atraumatic extraction of a natural tooth should ideally begin with a sulcular incision, preferably with a thin scalpel blade or periotome 360 degrees around the tooth. This will ensure all connective tissue attachment fibers above the bone level are severed. Failure to cut these fibers before extraction will result in increased tissue trauma and possible fracture of the buccal plate of bone. For an atraumatic extraction, the less soft tissue reflection the better as to minimize disruption of the blood supply.

The next step in an atraumatic extraction process is to evaluate the crown and root anatomy for ease of removal, especially with multirooted teeth. Proximal reduction of the tooth will increase the space so bone expansion can be completed and also will prevent damage from the adjacent teeth. If the roots of the tooth to

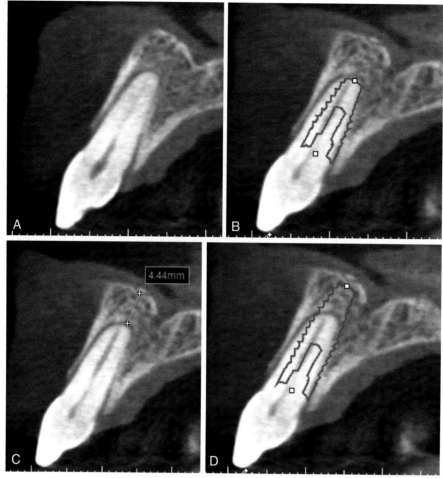

● **Fig. 32.19** Cone Beam Computed Tomography (CBCT) Interactive Treatment Planning for Immediate Implant. (A) CBCT cross section of maxillary central incisor. (B) Interactive treatment plan depicting implant length coinciding with root length. Placement of implant this length would lead to decreased prognosis. (C) Measurement of apical bone is available. (D) Ideal-length immediate implant.

be extracted are divergent, they should be sectioned and removed as individual units, because this will decrease the risk of fracturing a root or the surrounding bone. Elevation from the mesiolingual, direct lingual, or distolingual is most beneficial in avoiding the alteration of the buccal hard and soft tissue including the papillae.

Periotomes and dental elevators, which both use the mechanical advantage of a wedge, can then be used to initiate the luxation of teeth for their removal. A traditional dental forceps is used to grasp the tooth for any needed additional luxation before tooth removal. Ideally forceps should not be used until mobility of the tooth is present. Alternatively, a biomechanically based forceps (physics forceps) can be used. Its increased mechanical advantage may allow for tooth removal without application of rotational forces, minimizing potential fracture of the facial plate of bone (Fig. 32.20).[25]

Step 3: Curetting the Extraction Socket

The debridement of the extraction socket is imperative in the immediate implant process. Any remnants of periodontal ligament, bacteria, residual infection, dental material (i.e., gutta percha), and tooth fragments may affect the osseointegration process. Therefore the extraction socket should be thoroughly debrided and irrigated with saline to ensure the socket is free of contaminants.

A serrated spoon curette (Salvin Dental) should be used to scrape the walls of the socket (degranulation) and also initiate the regional acceleratory phenomenon (RAP), which enhances the healing process. This will initiate multiple areas of bleeding, which will promote a greater initiation of angiogenesis to the area (Fig. 32.21).

Step 4: Evaluating the Extraction Socket for Remaining Walls

The easiest and simplest technique for evaluating the remaining walls of bone after an extraction is with a blunted probe. The index finger may be placed over the buccal plate of bone, and the probe is introduced into the socket and run up and down within the socket. If the probe is felt (i.e., most commonly on a missing buccal plate), then no bone is present and the socket is missing a wall of bone (Fig. 32.22).

Classification of Bony Defects

Thick Five-Bony-Wall Defects. The most ideal condition for a successful immediate implant is the presence of five thick, bony walls around the extraction site. Most of the keys for predictable bone formation are present under these conditions, and the socket usually will form bone in the extraction socket without loss of width or height (Fig. 32.23).

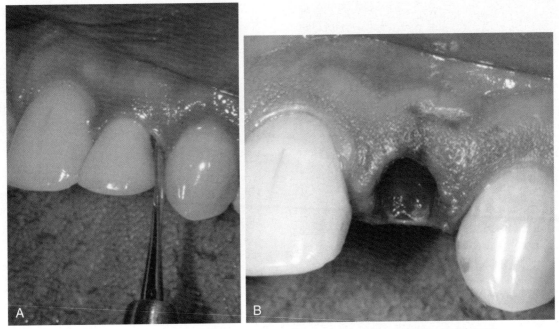

• **Fig. 32.20** (A and B) Periotome atraumatic extraction; note minimal tissue reflection and damage.

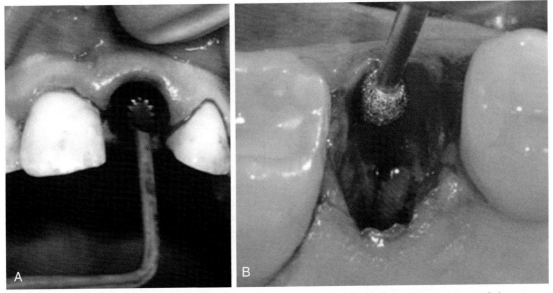

• **Fig. 32.21** (A) Curetting the extraction socket with serrated spoon. (B) #10 round bur to remove soft tissue within the extraction socket and to initiate the regional acceleratory phenomenon technique.

Four-Wall Bony Socket. When a labial plate around a socket is missing, the absence of the wall prevents space maintenance, reduces host bone vascularization, and is replaced with soft tissue. In most cases bone augmentation procedures must be used to obtain an ideal volume and contour of bone. Sockets with a missing wall are significantly compromised and heal by repair rather than regeneration.

The first determination after the tooth extraction is complete is the assessment of the thickness of labial and palatal plates of bone and their relative height to the ideal volume desired. When one of the plates of bone is thinner than 1.5 mm or when height is desired, a socket graft is indicated, even in the presence of five bony walls (Fig. 32.24).

There exist three treatment options after tooth removal and bony wall evaluation:
1. *No treatment:* The most likely reason the option of no treatment would be chosen is if there is active infection present in the extraction site that cannot be completely eradicated.
2. *Bone grafting:* If the remaining walls of bone are not advantageous, then grafting the socket is completed. Usually one- to three-wall, and in many cases four wall defects should be grafted instead of attempting immediate placement.
3. *Immediate implant placement:* If favorable conditions exist, the implant is placed immediately after the extraction of the tooth.

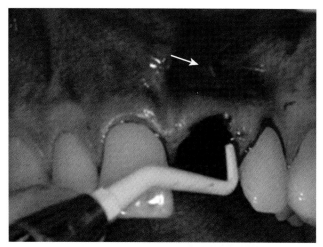

• **Fig. 32.22** Evaluating the number of walls remaining with a colored periodontal probe. Note the lack of buccal plate.

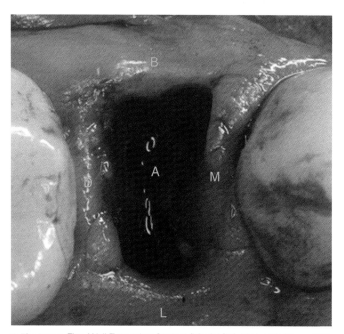

• **Fig. 32.23** Five-Wall Extraction Socket (Mesial [*M*], Distal [*D*], Buccal [*B*], Lingual [*L*], and Apical [*A*] Present).

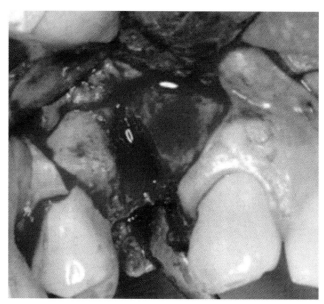

• **Fig. 32.24** Four-Wall Extraction Socket (Mesial, Distal, Lingual, and Apical Present). The buccal plate is missing which is the most common wall to be lost after extraction.

Step 5: Immediate Implant Placement Technique

Flap Design

Three types of flap designs are used for immediate implants: open (buccal and lingual tissue reflected), minimal flap (no buccal or lingual reflection, but minimal flap to expose crestal area), or flapless (tissue punch). Caneva et al.[26] evaluated flap versus flapless implant placement into extraction sockets and determined there is no difference in bone loss between the two techniques (Fig. 32.25).

Implant Osteotomy

The immediate implant placement surgical technique is initiated with either a surgical template or freehand technique.

a. *Surgical template:* If a surgical template is used, it should be placed over the adjacent teeth (i.e., ideally tooth supported) and standard drilling procedures completed according to the manufacturer's instructions (i.e., pilot, universal, fully guided surgical templates.) (Fig. 32.26).

b. *Freehand:* The initial osteotomy is directly related to the anatomic area and remaining socket anatomy. For example, in the maxillary anterior region it is crucial to avoid placing the implant directly in the center of the extraction socket. Placement of the implant in this position may perforate the buccal plate and increase morbidity. In addition, the implant is often too facial, which compromises esthetics. It is imperative the implant's final trajectory is within the incisal edge.

In the posterior regions, implants usually may be placed within the extraction site, along a trajectory in line with the central fossa of the adjacent teeth (Fig. 32.27 and Table 32.1).

Heat generation. Site preparation should always be performed with copious amounts of irrigation with cold saline (i.e., refrigerated) to reduce heat generation. It is often difficult to avoid heat generation when using a guided template or a flapless procedure. Therefore, a "bone dancing" technique should always be followed to allow saline to enter the osteotomy site.

Prevention of perforation. During the osteotomy process for an immediate implant placement, the clinician should use their index finger over the buccal plate for tactile sense to confirm no buccal vibration or fenestration.[27]

Ideal Positioning

Ideal depth. In general it has been accepted in the literature that 2 to 4 mm of bone is ideally required apical to the inferior part of the socket to obtain primary stability for an immediate implant.[28] Madani et al.[29] reported in a retrospective study that implant placement 1.08 mm subcrestally is the ideal depth of the neck of the implant. Subcrestal placement of the implant greater than 2 mm led to and increased bone loss. The vertical position of the implant shoulder should be 1 mm apical to the buccal crest to allow for adequate space for an emergence profile of the final restoration. Ideally a tapered design implant is used to avoid buccal fenestration, which is highly likely with a straight-walled design (Fig. 32.28).[30,31]

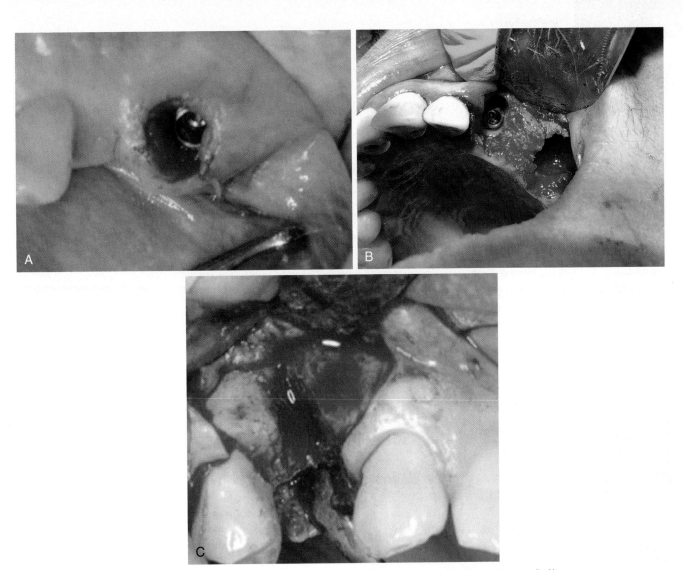

• **Fig. 32.25** Flap Design. (A) Flapless. (B) Minimal flap. (C) Open flap is usually utilized when a wall of bone is missing and bone grafting is indicated.

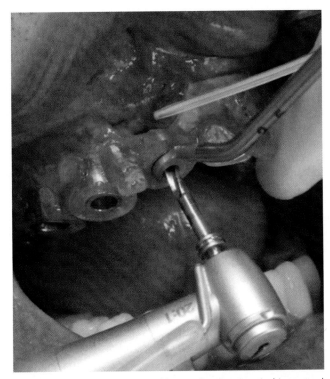

• **Fig. 32.26** Surgical placement with cone beam computed tomography tooth-supported template into the immediate extraction site.

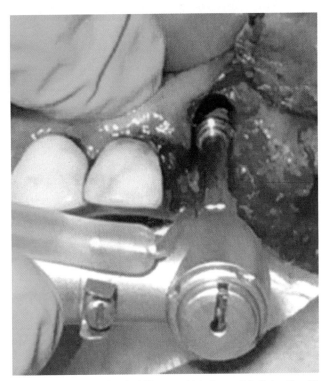

• **Fig. 32.27** Freehand Surgical Placement Into Immediate Extraction Site.

TABLE 32.1 Surgical Protocol for Various Anatomic Areas

Anatomic Area	Initial Osteotomy Location	Apical Implant positioning	Horizontal Implant Positioning	Miscellaneous
Maxillary anterior	Engage lingual plate	Engage 2–4 mm of bone past apex	Engage mesial, distal, and palatal	No engagement of buccal wall
Maxillary premolar	First: palatal socket Second: lingual of socket	Engage 2–4 mm of bone past apex	Engage mesial, distal, and palatal	No engagement of buccal wall
Maxillary molars	Lateral to septal bone in "sawing" motion	Rarely can engage apically without sinus penetration	Difficult to obtain because of socket morphology	Use extreme caution because rarely sufficient bone is present
Mandibular anterior	Center to lingual of socket	Engage 2–4 mm of bone past apex	Engage mesial, distal, and palatal	Angulation and thin buccal bone are of concern
Mandibular premolar	Center to lingual of socket	Difficult to engage more apical because of mental foramen	Engage mesial, distal, and palatal	Use extreme caution as close proximity to mental foramen
Mandibular molars	Lateral to septal bone in "sawing" motion	Difficult to engage more apical because of mandibular foramen	Difficult to obtain because of socket morphology	Use extreme caution as close proximity to mandibular canal

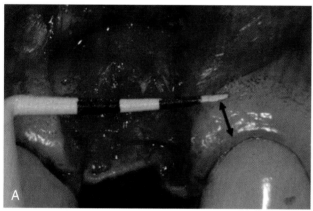

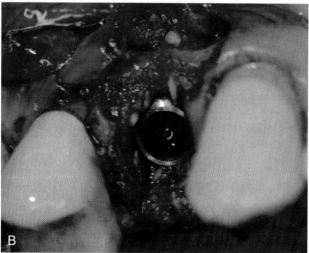

• **Fig. 32.28** (A, B) Ideal depth to coincide with 2 to 3 mm below the free gingival margin.

Jumping distance (maxillary anterior). The horizontal bone defect ("Jumping Distance," "Gap") is defined as the distance between the implant and the surrounding wall of the defect. Multiple animal and human studies have shown that the gap will fill with bone, regardless of whether graft materials and barriers are used.[32-35] Botticelli et al.[33-35] reported that in defects of 2 mm or larger, no grafting was needed to grow bone. Tarnow et al.[36] concluded that as long as the buccal plate is intact after the extraction, no bone graft, membrane, or primary closure is needed, irregardless of how large the defect is. In most cases, care should be exercised not to completely fill the extraction socket with the implant. Many studies have shown conflicting results with the aftermath of filling the void between the implant and buccal socket wall.[26,37] In the author's opinion, the gap should always be grafting with a bone substitute that will maintain the space long enough for bone to regenerate, which ultimately will maintain the hard and soft tissue. Therefore a slower resorbing material (i.e., mineralized freeze-dried bone or xenograft), not a faster resorbing material (i.e., demineralized freeze-dried bone and autograft), should be used to augment the gap.

Too large an implant diameter for the tooth in question should not be used because they will reduce the gap space, thereby risking future soft and hard tissue recession (i.e. immediate implant placement in maxillary central incisor should not exceed 5 mm in diameter) (Fig. 32.29).[38] In addition, if the diameter of the implant is too large, a compromised emergence profile will result with the final prosthesis.

Lindeman drill. In most extraction sites the standard round or starter drill will have a tendency to "chatter," which makes initial placement of the osteotomy difficult. The author advocates the use of a Lindeman drill (side cutting surgical bur) to initiate osteotomies in extractions side. This type of bur when used in a "sawing" motion allows for an initial groove to be made that provides for proper and more precise positioning (Fig. 32.30).

Maxillary anterior position. Multiple studies have shown that postoperative gingival recession in the anterior region is associated with buccal implant positioning, which usually occurs when the implant is placed in the center of the extraction socket.[22] In the most esthetic area of the oral cavity (maxillary anterior), it is imperative that the positioning of the implant be lingually oriented. This will allow the buccal gap to be >2 mm, which has been shown to be vital in preventing hard and soft tissue recession.[39,40] A lingually placed implant will also minimize the possibility of apical perforation, which is common when implants are placed in the socket and a parallel walled implant is used.[41] In addition, oversize implants should not be placed in the maxillary anterior because the buccal gap will be obliterated and the implant will encroach on the proximal area.[42] If the proximal area is compromised, a poor emergence profile will result, which may lead to peri-implant disease (Fig. 32.31).

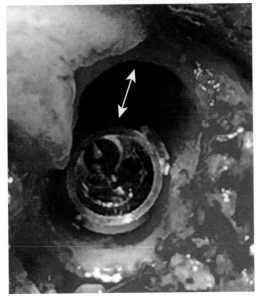

• **Fig. 32.29** Jumping Gap Present on Facial of Implant.

Minimum torque. To achieve primary stability, a minimum torque value has been shown to be one of the most important factors in the success of immediate implants. The minimum torque has been shown to be approximately 35-45 N/cm in the literature.[43,44]

Final Emergence Position Based on Prosthesis. For a cement-retained prosthesis, the implant should exit slightly lingual to the incisal edge in the anterior and in the central fossa in the posterior. For a screw-retained prosthesis, the implant should exit in the cingulum area in the anterior and in the central fossa of the posterior. For a removable prosthesis, the implants should exit slightly lingual to the anterior teeth and within the central fossa of the posterior teeth.

Implant Design

Tapered versus parallel. Many studies have evaluated the implant design (tapered versus parallel) in the immediate implant protocol. McAllister et al.[45] showed a high success with tapered implants with a high initial implant stability. Tapered implants have been reported to be superior with immediate implants because the implants are narrow apically, which result in less chance of perforation. Because they are wider coronally, their jumping distance is less, therefore requiring less augmentation. However, Lang et al.[46] found that parallel and tapered implants have very positive short-term success rates with improved wound healing and primary stability.

Implant surface. Many researchers have evaluated rough versus machined surfaces for immediate implants. Wagenberg and Froum[47]

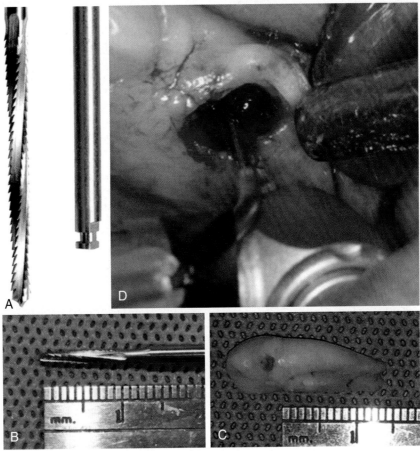

• **Fig. 32.30** (A) Lindeman side-cutting drill (Salvin). (B) As a guide for depth preparation, measure the flutes of the drill (i.e. use this measurement as a depth guide for osteotomy preparation, (C) Extracted tooth may be measured to determine socket depth, (D) Lindeman bur initiating the osteotomy.

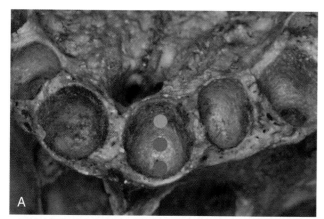

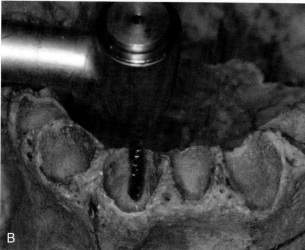

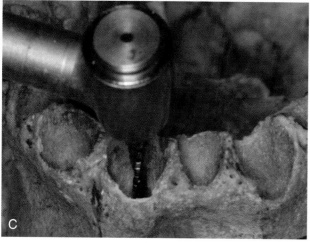

• **Fig. 32.31** Maxillary Anterior Placement. (A) Osteotomy should be initiated within the lingual wall. (B) A groove is placed in the lingual wall. (C) From the lingual groove position, the handpiece is rotated facially to allow for ideal implant angulation.

completed a clinical study with 1925 implants and reported higher success rates with roughened surfaces. Results concluded machined-surface implants were twice as likely to fail as roughened surface implants (4.6% versus 2.3%). In addition, studies have verified that roughened surfaces with a microthreaded neck result in less crestal bone loss than implants with non-microthreaded necks.[48]

Implant neck/collar design. When evaluating the implant collar or neck of the implant to be placed in an immediate extracting

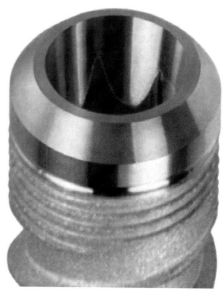

• **Fig. 32.32** Tapered and platform switch implant has been shown to be the ideal implant for immediate implants.

site, studies have shown a tapered platform-switched internal connection to be superior for healing and implant survival.[49-52] Linkevicius et al.[53] determined that the use of a platform switching implant in a one-stage implant placement approach does not prevent crestal bone loss when the tissue is thin (≤2 mm). However, when the tissue is thick (>2 mm), use of a platform-switch implant shows minimal bone recession at the 1-year time frame.[53] Puisys and Linkevicius,[54] in a two-stage protocol, showed similar results with the thin versus thick tissue. Thin tissues (≤2 mm) lost minimal amount of crestal bone, whereas thick tissues (>2 mm) or thin tissues augmented with acellular dermal matrix (LifeNet; Salvin) had similar crestal bone maintenance with minimal bone loss at 1 year postoperatively (Fig. 32.32).[54]

Implant length. Schnitman et al.[55] reported that implant lengths greater than 10 mm provide significantly higher success rates for immediate implants. However, the implant length is directly related to the bone density. In favorable bone densities (e.g., D1, D2), implant length is not as important. When poor bone density is present (e.g., D3, D4), longer implants are required because of the greater need for primary stability and rigid fixation (Fig. 32.33 and Box 32.3).

Implant Stability

The initial stability of the immediate implant is one of the most critical factors in the success of the implant. When micromovement occurs, the implant-bone interface is reduced, thereby resulting in loss of primary stability. Micromovement greater than 100 μm may cause fibrous encapsulation of the implant.[56] There exist two types of implant stability, primary and secondary.

Primary. Primary stability is defined as the stability of the dental implant immediately after placement; it is derived from mechanical friction of the implant threads and the surrounding bone. Several methods have been advocated in the literature to determine primary stability.

a. *Percussion* is the first test method in the literature to be used to assess primary stability and estimate the amount of bone-implant contact. This technique is based on vibrational-acoustic science, where a "high pitched" sound signifies integration and a "low-pitched" sound may be indicative of lack of integration.

Unfortunately, this test is highly dependent on the clinician's experience level and subjective beliefs. Therefore although still used, it is not the most ideal testing method (Fig. 32.34).[57,58]

b. *Periotest* (Seimens, Bensheim, Germany) is a testing method that has been proposed to be a more objective method for assessment of implant stability. Although much better than the percussion test, the Periotest has been shown to have inaccuracies in the lack of resolution, poor sensitivity, and subject to operator variability (Fig. 32.35).[59]

c. A more recent method is the use of *insertion torque* that can be measured with low-speed insertion tools (i.e., surgical handpiece) or manual wrench ratchet. It has been shown that for a successful immediate loading protocol, the insertion torque should be between 35 and 45 N/cm.[60,61]

d. *Resonance frequency analysis* (RFA) is a diagnostic tool that allows for detecting implant stability as a function of the stiffness of the bone-implant interface. This test can be used in a continuous and objective manner during the healing phases of the implant. RFA was initially presented by Meredith et al.[62] in 1996. RFA has been shown to have quantitative and reproducible measurements on the presence of integration, immediate load feasibility, and follow-up evaluation at the prediction of an implant failure.[63]

RFA is a technique that is based on continual excitation of the implant interface through the use of dynamic vibration analysis (piezo effect). A specialized transducer, which contains two

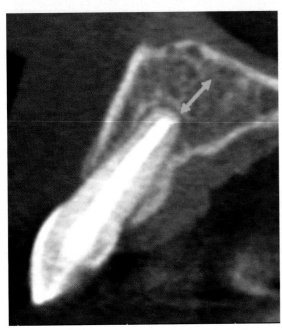

• **Fig. 32.33** Implant Length. Ideally an immediate implant needs to extend 2 to 4 mm beyond the apex of the tooth root, especially when poor bone density is present.

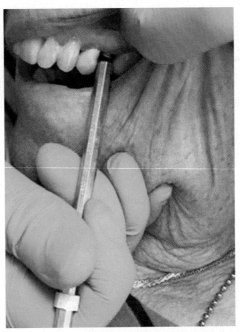

• **Fig. 32.34** Percussion test may be used to evaluate the initial primary stability; however, this test is very subjective.

• BOX 32.3   Root Lengths[20]

Maxillary
Central incisor: 13.0 mm
Lateral incisor: 13.0 mm
Canine: 17.0 mm
First premolar: 14.0 mm
Second premolar: 14.0 mm
First molar: 12.0 mm (B), 13.0 mm (L)
Second molar: 11.0 mm (B), 12.0 mm (L)

Mandible
Central incisor: 12.5 mm
Lateral incisor: 14.0 mm
Canine: 16.0 mm
First premolar: 14.0 mm
Second premolar: 14.5 mm
First molar: 14.0 mm
Second molar: 13.0 mm

B, Buccal; L, lingual.

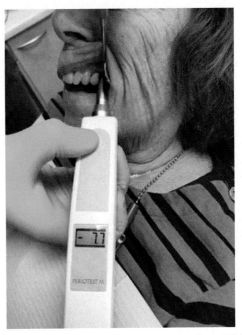

• **Fig. 32.35** Periotest was a more objective test to evaluate initial stability; however, it gives inconsistent results.

piezoceramic elements, is either attached directly to the implant or abutment. The first piezo element generates an excitation signal that is a sinusoidal wave (5–15 kHz), leading to vibration of a whole transducer-implant-tissue complex. The oscillation response is measured by the second piezo element.[64]

The RFA technique measures implant stability as a function of stiffness of the bone-implant complex. The health of the implant is measured on an implant stability quotient (ISQ) that is calculated on a scale from 1 to 100. The full integration of an implant is usually measured in the range from 45 to 85 ISQ. Measurements of less than 45 are indicative of implant failure, whereas an ISQ value of 60 to 70 indicates success.[65]

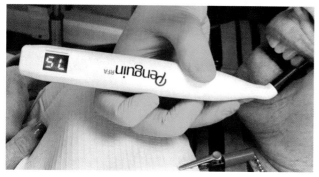

• **Fig. 32.36** Resonance Frequency Analysis (RFA). The Penguin RFA (Glidewell) is a noninvasive resonance frequency analysis test that results in reliable, accurate numerical results concerning the stability of immediate placed implants.

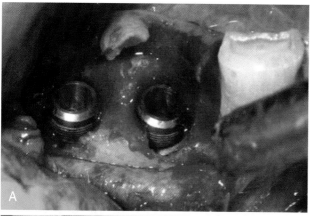

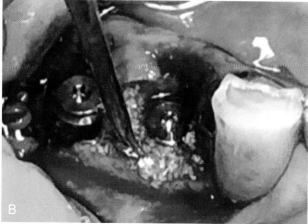

• **Fig. 32.37** (A) Grafting of the jumping gap and other bony defects. (B) Membrane placement to prevent migration of bone graft material.

Secondary. During the healing process, the primary stability process is replaced by the biological process of bone healing. The main factors that influence secondary stability are the initial primary stability, bone remodeling process, bone-implant contact, and implant surface characteristics.

The use of RFA after the initial healing has shown great success. Han et al.[66] reported a decrease in ISQ values within the first 3 weeks after implant placement; then a return to the original ISQ values is observed approximately 8 weeks after surgery.

When comparing implants placed into immediate extraction sites vs. healed sites, Han et al.[67] showed implants immediately loaded performed the same, whether in postextraction or healed sited. In addition, they showed that tapered implants with strong self- cutting threads provides an excellent initial stability, with high insertion torque and ISQ values (Fig. 32.36).

Grafting/Membrane

After implant stability is confirmed, the present osseous defects are evaluated and grafted accordingly. Ideally the bone-grafting material should include a slower resorbing material that will maintain the space to allow for bone regeneration (e.g., demineralized/mineralized allograft, allograft + autograft, or xenograft). The membrane selection is dictated by the defect present. If the buccal wall is missing or very thin, then a longer-acting collagen membrane is recommended. It is more predictable if the membrane is placed on the buccal along with grafting before implant placement. If all five walls are present, then a collagen plug (or collagen tape) is placed over the socket (Fig. 32.37).

Closure

In most immediate placement sites it is difficult to obtain primary closure unless the flap is advanced. However, advancement of the flap will result in less keratinized tissue to the facial of the prosthesis. When inadequate keratinized tissue results, tissue grafts are usually indicated (Fig. 32.38).

Immediate Load or Staged Treatment

After implant placement a healing abutment (1-stage) or a cover screw (2-stage) may be placed. In immediate load cases a provisional restoration may be inserted, allowing the pontic (ovate design) to heal the soft tissue. De Rouck et al.[68] demonstrated that using single immediate implants with immediate provisionalization aids in

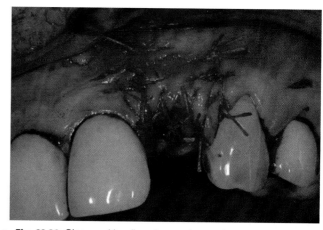

• **Fig. 32.38** Closure. Usually primary closure is not completed, and extending the flap to obtain primary closure is not generally recommended.

optimizing the esthetic results. They concluded that the provisional will mold the soft tissue and will limit the amount of soft tissue loss. Tarnow et al.[69] reported that immediate implant placement with a bone graft and a well-contoured provisional crown resulted in the least amount of facial-palatal contour change (<1 mm).

Immediate Implants Into Infected Sites

Placing implants into infected sites has been controversial. Villa and Rangert[70] reported on a series of cases where implants were placed immediately after extraction and had exhibited periodontal or endodontic infections. After 2 years the cumulative survival rate was 100%. The theory includes that after extraction, infections and microorganisms present can be eliminated with proper socket degranulation. Novaes et al.[71] evaluated immediate implant placement of implants placed in chronically infected sites. They determined that as long as antibiotics are used, meticulous debridement is completed, and alveolar bone preparation before implant placement is properly performed, immediate implants in infected sites are not contraindicated. Crespi et al.[72] evaluated immediate implant associated with a chronic periapical lesion; they did not demonstrate an increased rate of complications, and showed favorable soft and hard tissue postoperatively (Fig. 32.39).

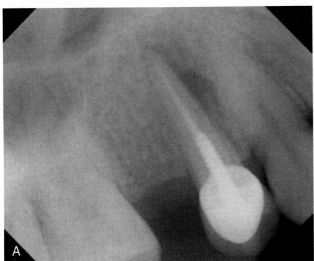

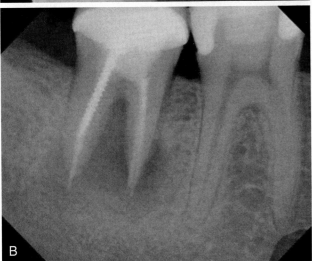

• **Fig. 32.39** (A and B) Extreme caution should be exercised when placing immediate implants into sites with active infection.

Complications

Not Recognizing 4-Wall Socket

One of the most common complications for immediate implant placement is for the clinician to not diagnosis the loss of the buccal socket wall. A five wall socket is ideal and is treated with the conventional surgical technique (Fig. 32.40). In contrast, a four-wall socket requires a longer acting collagen membrane that is positioned over the buccal aspect of the extraction site. (Fig. 32.41).

Not Understanding Specific Anatomical Factors

Each tooth in the maxillary and mandibular arch is associated with factors which may make conditions ideal for an immediate implant placement or contraindicate placement. The author has formulated a protocol for each tooth based on specific anatomic and treatment planning criteria. Each speciifc tooth has ideal conditions (green), cautious conditions (yellow), or contraindication (red). (Fig. 32.42 and Fig. 32.43).

Inability to Obtain Primary Stability

Primary implant stability may be difficult to achieve in extraction sites where the trabecular bone density is less than ideal. Unlike a healed ridge of desirable bone volume, primary stability in fresh extraction sites is more difficult to achieve in general because of the lesser quantity of native bone present, as well as the fact that the anatomic challenge of the coronal aspect of the extraction site is often wider than the implant being placed. Potential variations in bone density may necessitate multiple modifications to osteotomy preparation and implant placement protocols compared with procedures performed in homogeneous bone density. As a result, after attempted implantation, the clinician may be faced with an implant with a questionable level of primary stability (Fig. 32.44).

Prevention

Complete Osteotomy Preparation in Appropriate Location and Surgical Sequence. Depending on the size of the extracted tooth and the implant to be placed, the implant in most cases extend past the original dimensions of the root apex and provide mechanical retention of the implant. In the anterior maxillary region, immediate implant placement often requires the osteotomy and implant insertion engage the lingual wall of the alveolus for rigid fixation. For maxillary posterior teeth the initial bur should be positioned off-center toward the lingual side of the interradicular septum. For mandibular posterior teeth the initial bur should be positioned on the mesial aspect of the interradicular septum. A Lindemann bur is useful for initiating and modifying osteotomies. The objective of this multiplane preparation process is to create an osteotomy in a prosthetically correct position without compromising the buccal wall of bone.

Underprepare Osteotomy Width and Overprepare Osteotomy Length. Misch[14] initially outlined a protocol that adapts the treatment plan, implant selection, surgical approach, healing regimen, and initial prosthetic loading to all bone densities and all arch positions, which resulted in similar implant success for all bone densities. The density of the residual native bone can influence the ability to achieve adequate primary fixation. With anterior single-rooted teeth, using bone beyond the apex and the lateral engagement of some or all of the tooth socket walls is instrumental in obtaining sufficient primary stability. With posterior implants, vital structures such as the inferior alveolar nerve and the maxillary sinus limit stability derived from bone beyond the tooth apices. Furthermore, the limited native bone present undergoes remodeling after the surgical trauma of osteotomy preparation and implant insertion. This trauma leads to a weakening of the bone-implant interface and may have an adverse effect on the initial implant stability (Fig. 32.45).

Often inadequate primary stability may manifest itself only after 4 to 6 weeks; the bone interface is stronger on the day of implant placement compared with 3 months later. The surgical process of the implant osteotomy preparation and implant insertion cause a RAP of bone repair around the implant interface. As a result of the surgical placement, organized, mineralized lamellar bone in the preparation site becomes unorganized, less mineralized, woven bone of repair next to the implant. The implant-bone interface is weakest and most at risk for overload at 3 to 6 weeks after surgical insertion because the surgical trauma causes bone remodeling at the interface that is least mineralized and unorganized during this time frame. A clinical report by Buchs et al.[73] found immediately loaded implant failure occurred primarily between 3 and 5 weeks after implant insertion from mobility without infection. At 4 months the bone is still only 60% mineralized, organized lamellar bone. With time, bone formation and mineralization will lead to increased interlocking with the implant surface and a stronger implant-bone interface. However, this has proved to be sufficient in most bone types and clinical situations

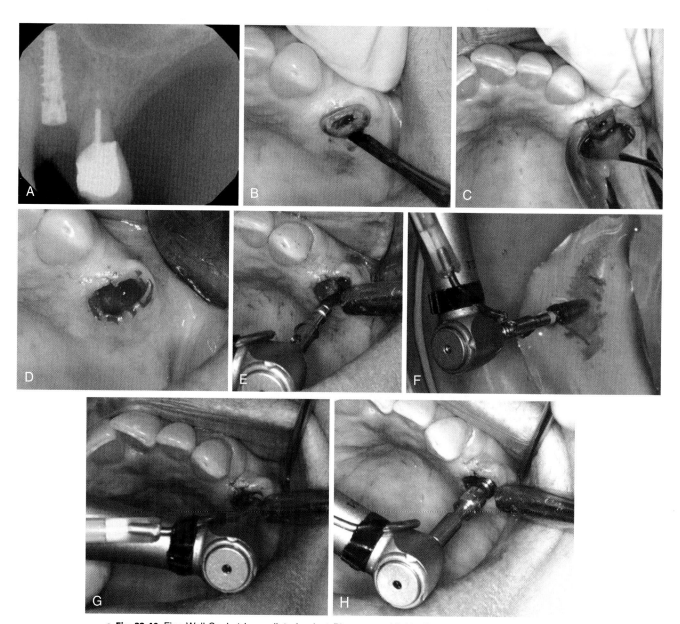

• **Fig. 32.40** Five Wall Socket Immediate Implant Placement. (A) Maxillary second premolar depicting sufficient apical bone for immediate implant placement. (B) Atraumatic extraction with a periotome. (C) Mobile root removed with forceps. (D) Five-wall socket remaining after extraction. (E) Osteotomy initiated with Lindeman drill slightly lingual. (F) Bone chips from bur flutes is saved for grafting the buccal gap after implant placement. (G) Osteotomy diameter is increased. (H) Implant insertion with handpiece. (I) Final implant positioning.

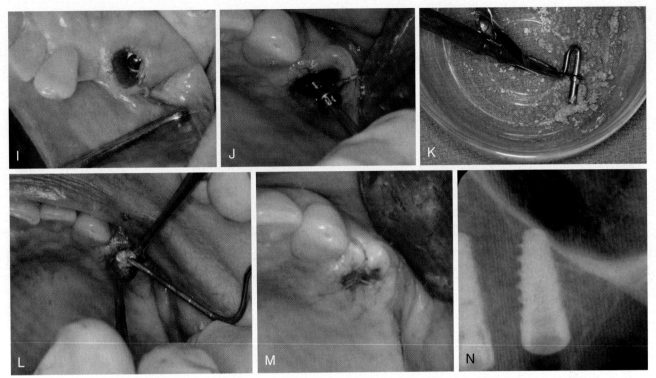

• **Fig. 32.40, cont'd** (J) Cover screw or healing abutment should be placed before bone graft placement. (K) Bone graft is used to fill the jumping gap and any bony defects; amalgam plugger allows for easy placement into small voids. (L) Grafting material packed into voids and membrane placement. (M) Final closure. (N) Final radiograph.

for two-stage healing and delayed implant loading. The relative lack of native bone (compared with a healed site) suggests the osteotomy should frequently be undersized in width, the degree of which is dependent on bone density. In addition, for less dense bone, immediate implant fixation can be facilitated if the clinician can use osteotomes or osseodensification techniques for radial compaction. Dependent on tooth socket size and anatomy, sufficient implant stability can sometimes be achieved by lateral wall engagement only. However, extending the osteotomy 2 to 4 mm past the socket apex (without encroaching on vital structures) is more commonly completed for primary stability.[74]

Implant Design and Initial Stability. The clinical perception of primary implant stability is frequently based on the cutting resistance of the implant during its insertion. The feeling of "good" stability may be accentuated if there is the sense of an abrupt stop at the seating of the implant. Although root form tapered implants often have a geometry that will provide a firm stop, the resultant stability may be a false perception.[75] In addition, in a tapered, threaded implant, threads at the apical half are often not as deep because the outer diameter of the implant body continues to decrease. This limits the initial fixation of the implant and further reduces the functional surface area. For immediate implant placement, the tapered/conical body design may be of benefit during initial insertion because it is positioned within the osteotomy halfway before engaging bone. The choice of implant body with regard to primary stabilization is equivocal and may be more influenced by osteotomy preparation than implant body design. A study by Sakoh et al.[76] concluded that the combination of both conical implant design and the procedure of under dimensioned drilling appeared to be associated with increased primary stability (Fig. 32.46).

Treatment Options

Redirection dependent on bone density. If the implant has poor primary stability, the implant can sometimes be redirected into denser bone; the redirection may be needed in more than one plane and kept within the ideal three-dimensional boundaries for prosthetic reconstruction. Often a subtle tap of the (threaded) implant in an axial direction will gain the needed initial primary stability without putting the implant at risk from excessive apical positioning relative to the osseous crest and any adjacent teeth. A mallet and straight or offset osteotome can be used over top of the implant body.

Use of larger diameter implant. The dimensions, longer and/ or wider, of the "rescue" implant may allow for satisfactory better primary fixation; however, it must still be in an acceptable position in relation to the crestal bone, adjacent teeth, and planned final prosthesis.[77] This may be placed in a redirected manner described earlier. An increased implant surface area can engage more cortical bone. It has also been shown in an experimental study in rabbit tibia that wider implant diameters resulted in increased removal torque values.[78] Matsushita et al.[79] used a two-dimensional finite element method to analyze the effect of different implant diameters on stress distribution within the alveolar bone using HA-coated implants. They found that stress in cortical bone decreased with increased implant diameter. Ivanoff et al.,[80] however, reported a lower survival rate and a tendency for higher bone loss for 5.0-mm-diameter implants, compared with 3.75-mm- or 4.0-mm-diameter implants. Resultant decreased facial bone dimensions associated with wider implant dimensions increase the probability of soft tissue recession. However, caution should be exercised in placing too wide of an implant because it

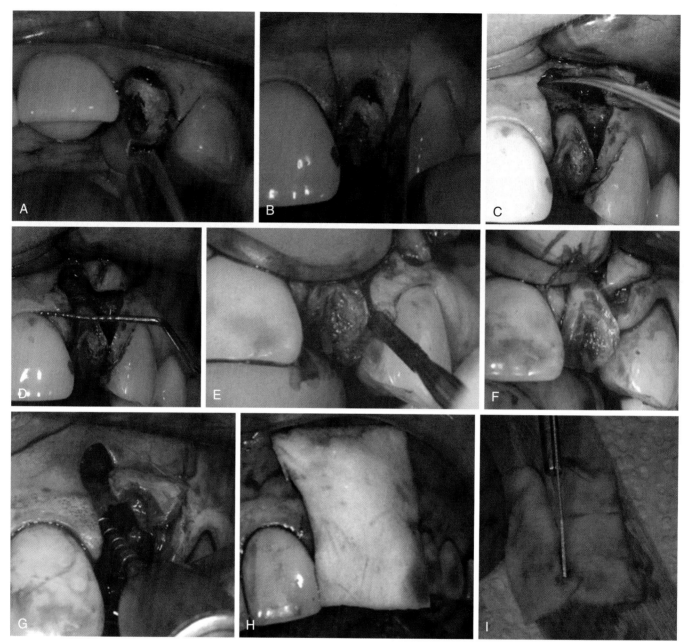

• **Fig. 32.41** Four-Walled Socket Immediate Implant Placement. (A) Maxillary left lateral incisor cone beam computed tomography showing no buccal bone present. (B) Sulcular and broad-based release incisions. (C) Reflection. (D) Lack of buccal bone remaining and evaluation of the 2- to 4-mm measurement from the free gingival margin. (E) Atraumatic extraction. (F) Root removal. (G) Osteotomy with Lindeman drill in lingual wall. (H) Extended collagen membrane measurement. (I) Collagen cut with scalpel to fill socket.

may encroach on the buccal plate or result in a nonideal prosthetic outcome.

Leave implant in place. An implant with loss of rotational stability (spinner) and minimal, if any, surrounding ridge deficiencies may be left in place. If replacement is not possible (e.g., in cases of inadequate bone dimensions or where a larger implant is unavailable), the implant clinician must then decide whether to leave the implant in place or remove it and reevaluate the site for further implant therapy after healing is complete. Ivanoff et al.[81] reported osseointegrated implants that have been mobilized because of a traumatic disruption of the bone-implant interface may reintegrate if allowed to heal for an additional period. Orenstein et al.[82]

reported a 79.8% survival rate after 3 years of implants that were mobile at placement. A significant factor for most of these implants was the presence of a HA coating. Almost half of the noncoated, initially mobile implants failed by 3 years postplacement. Even if initially mobile implants are found to integrate, precautions are advised to avoid implant overload. Clinicians may want to use strategies such as long-term temporization to promote bone maturation and evaluate the viability of initially mobile implants in function before inserting the definitive prosthesis.

Abort the procedure. The clinician may consider aborting the procedure and proceeding with bone grafting and delayed implant placement (Fig. 32.47).

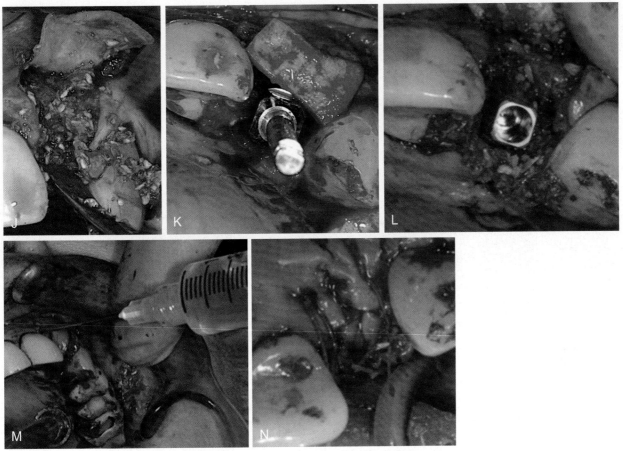

• **Fig. 32.41, cont'd** (J) Positioning of collagen along buccal wall. (K) Implant placement. (L) Abutment placement to check angulation. (M) platelet rich fibrin (PRF) placed underneath the flap. (N) Final closure.

Postoperative Complications

Transitional Prosthesis Impingement

The transitional prosthesis over an immediate implant should not rest or apply pressure to the soft tissue over the site. Implants and particulate grafts are more prone to movement during healing, which prevents blood vessels from entering and forming bone in the site. If possible, a fixed provisional or a pressure-free prosthesis is ideal for successful healing (Fig. 32.48).

Neurosensory Impairment

The close proximity of inferior alveolar nerve to the apices of the mandibular posterior teeth poses the possibility of neurosensory impairment when preparing osteotomies and during implant insertion. In most cases, the immediate implant gains its primary stability from the bone beyond the root apices. This risk is greater in the posterior mandible extraction site than in a healed site with its increased volume of bone and associated likelihood of the more abundant bone achieving primary stability without nerve encroachment. Preventive strategies include preoperative three-dimensional imaging, guided surgery, and having a heightened awareness of local anatomy (Fig. 32.49). Neurosensory impairment is most common in Type 1 nerve positions (i.e. anterior posterior position close to root apexes.

For this discussion, care must be taken to distinguish between a compromise(s) that could be present after a delayed/two-stage procedure (e.g., increased final crown height) versus a compromise that could be solely attributed to implant placement at the time of extraction. Examples of the latter are characterized by excessive positions in one or more of the potential three reference planes. Nonideal positioning can also result after multistage procedures; however, the need for native bone for primary stability in immediate placement cases increases the likelihood of positioning error. Management of cases with resultant excessive mesial-distal space/length can be frequently treated by placement of additional (usually narrower-diameter) implants. Use of surgical templates or guided surgery are recommended for clinicians desiring physical reference points during surgery (Fig. 32.50).

Conclusion

Placement of immediate implants into an extraction site has been shown through the literature to be very successful. Technological advances have led to an array of options for the patient and clinician as an alternative to the traditional two-stage technique. Immediate placement implants pose many challenges to clinicians, especially when treating patients with preexisting hard and soft tissue deficiencies. In this chapter, the advantages and disadvantages of immediate implants were explained in detail along with numerous treatment planning factors that should be ideally evaluated prior to treatment. With appropriate patient selection and treatment planning, complications may be minimized, and success rates increased with immediate placement implants. In addition, each specific tooth position is discussed in detail with a treatment planning protocol which allows the clinician to understand when ideal conditions exist, cautious variables are present, and when immediate placement is contraindicated.

	Maxillary Central			Maxillary Lateral			Maxillary Cuspid		
	IDEAL	CAUTION	HIGH RISK	IDEAL	CAUTION	HIGH RISK	IDEAL	CAUTION	HIGH RISK
Available Bone Height	> 4mm below nasal floor	2-3 mm below nasal floor	< 2mm below nasal floor	>4mm below nasal floor	2 -3 mm below nasal floor	< 2mm below nasal floor	> 4mm below nasal floor	2-3 mm below nasal floor	< 2mm below nasal floor
Available Bone Width	> 7mm	6mm	< 6mm	> 6mm	5 mm	< 5mm	> 7mm	6 mm	< 6 mm
Smile Line Position	Low	Medium	High	Low	Medium	High	Low	Medium	High
Esthetic Demands	None	Minimal	High	None	Minimal	High	None	Minimal	High
Gingival Index	Favorable		Unfavorable	Favorable		Unfavorable	Favorable		Unfavorable
Vertical Bone Loss	None Present	Minimal	Significant	None Present	Minimal	Significant	None Present	Minimal	Significant
Facial Bone Concavity	None	Minimal	Significant	None	Minimal	Significant	None	Minimal	Significant
Mesial Distal Space	8.0 mm	7.0 - 8.0 mm	< 7mm	> 6.0 mm	5.0 – 6.0 mm	< 5.0 mm	8.0 mm	7.0 –8.0 mm	< 7.0 mm
Nasopalatine Canal Position	Small	Medium	Large	N/A	N/A	N/A	N/A	N/A	N/A
Occlusal Relationship	Not Present	Moderate Deepbite	Significant Deepbite	Not present	Moderate Deepbite	Significant Deepbite	Not Present	Moderate Deepbite	Significant Deepbite
Bone Density	D2	D3	D4	D2	D3	D4	D2	D3	D4
Ideal Implant Size	4.0 - 4.5 mm	4.0 – 4.5 mm	4.0– 4.5 mm	4.0 - 4.5 mm	4.0 – 4.5 mm	4.0– 4.5 mm	4.0 - 4.5 mm	4.0– 4.5 mm	4.0– 4.5 mm

A

	Maxillary 1st Premolar			Maxillary 2nd Premolar			Maxillary 1st / 2nd Molar		
	IDEAL	CAUTION	HIGH RISK	IDEAL	CAUTION	HIGH RISK	IDEAL	CAUTION	HIGH RISK
Available Bone Height	>4mm above root apex	2-3 mm above root apex	< 2mm above root apex	>4mm above root apex	2-3 mm above root apex	< 2mm above root apex	< 4 mm above root apex	2-3 mm above root apex	< 2mm above root apex
Available Bone Width	> 7 mm	6mm	< 6mm	> 7 mm	6 mm	< 6 mm	> 8 mm	7 mm	< 7 mm
Smile Line	Low	Medium	High	Low	Medium	High	Low	Medium	High
Esthetic Demands	None	Minimal	High	None	Minimal	High	None	Minimal	High
Gingival Index	Favorable		Unfavorable	Favorable		Unfavorable	Favorable		Unfavorable
Vertical Bone Loss	None	Minimal	Significant	None	Minimal	Significant	None Present	Minimal	Significant
Maxillary Sinus Position	Posterior to 1st Premolar Apex	Apex within 1-2 mm of sinus	< 1mm apex to sinus	> 4 mm beyond apex	2 – 3 mm beyond apex	< 1 mm apex to sinus	> 4 mm beyond apex	2 – 3 mm beyond apex	< 1 mm apex to sinus
Mesial Distal Space	7.0 mm	6.0 mm	< 6.0 mm	7.0 mm	6.0 mm	< 6.0 mm	11.0 mm	9 - 11.0 mm	< 9.0 mm
Bone Density	D2	D3	D4	D2	D3	D4	D2	D3	D4
Ideal Implant Size	4.0 - 5.0 mm	4.0 - 5.0 mm	4.0 - 5.0 mm	4.0 - 5.0 mm	4.0 - 5.0 mm	4.0 - 5.0 mm	5.0 – 6.0 mm	5.0 – 6.0 mm	5.0 – 6.0 mm

B

• **Fig. 32.42** Maxillary Immediate Implant Treatment Factors: (A) Maxillary Anterior, (B) Maxillary Posterior.

A

	Mandibular Central			Mandibular Lateral			Mandibular Cuspid		
	IDEAL	CAUTION	HIGH RISK	IDEAL	CAUTION	HIGH RISK	IDEAL	CAUTION	HIGH RISK
Available Bone Height	> 4mm beyond root apex	2-3 mm beyond root apex	<2mm beyond root apex	> 4mm beyond root apex	2-3 mm beyond root apex	<2mm beyond root apex	> 4mm beyond root apex	2-3mm beyond root apex	<2mm beyond root apex
Available Bone Width	> 6 mm	5 mm	< 5 mm	> 6mm	5 mm	< 5mm	> 7 mm	6 mm	< 6 mm
Esthetic Demands	None	Minimal	High	None	Minimal	High	None	Minimal	High
Gingival Index	Favorable		Unfavorable	Favorable		Unfavorable	Favorable		Unfavorable
Vertical Bone Loss	None	Minimal	Significant	None	Minimal	Significant	None	Minimal	Significant
Facial Bone Concavity	None	Minimal	Significant	None	Minimal	Significant	None	Minimal	Significant
Mesial Distal Space	5.0 – 6.0 mm	4.5 – 5.0 mm	< 4.5 mm	5.0 – 6.0 mm	4.5 – 5.0 mm	< 4.5 mm	7.0 mm	6.0 – 7.0	< 6.0 mm
Bone Density	D2	D3	D4	D2	D3	D4	D2	D3	D4
Ideal Implant Size	3.0 – 3.5 mm	3.0 – 3.5 mm	3.0 – 3.5 mm	3.0 – 3.5 mm	3.0 – 3.5 mm	3.0 – 3.5 mm	4.0 – 4.5 mm	4.0 – 4.5 mm	4.0 – 4.5 mm

B

	Mandibular 1st Premolar			Mandibular 2nd Premolar			Mandibular 1st/2nd Molars		
	IDEAL	CAUTION	HIGH RISK	IDEAL	CAUTION	HIGH RISK	IDEAL	CAUTION	HIGH RISK
Available Bone Height	> 4mm beyond root apex	2-3 mm beyond root apex	<2mm beyond root apex	> 4mm beyond root apex	2-3 mm beyond root apex	<2mm beyond root apex	> 4mm beyond root apex	2-3mm beyond root apex	<2mm beyond root apex
Available Bone Width	> 7 mm	6 mm	< 6 mm	> 7 mm	6 mm	< 6 mm	> 8 mm	7 mm	< 7 mm
Foramen/Canal Location	> 4mm below apex	2- 4mm below apex	< 2mm below apex	> 4mm below apex	2- 4mm below apex	< 2mm below apex	> 4mm below apex	2- 4mm below apex	< 2mm below apex
Gingival Index	Favorable		Unfavorable	Favorable		Unfavorable	Favorable		Unfavorable
Vertical Bone Loss	None	Minimal	Significant	None	Minimal	Significant	None	Minimal	Significant
Mesial Distal Space	7.0 mm	6.0-7.0 mm	< 6.0 mm	7.0 mm	6.0-7.0 mm	< 6.0 mm	11.0 mm	9 - 11.0 mm	< 9.0 mm
Bone Density	D2	D3	D4	D2	D3	D4	D2	D3	D4
Ideal Implant Size	4.0 – 5.0 mm	4.0 – 5.0 mm	4.0 – 5.0 mm	4.0 – 5.0 mm	4.0 – 5.0 mm	4.0 – 5.0 mm	5.0 – 6.0 mm	5.0 – 6.0 mm	5.0 –6.0 mm

• **Fig. 32.43** Maxillary Immediate Implant Treatment Factors: (A) Mandibular Anterior, (B) Mandibular Posterior.

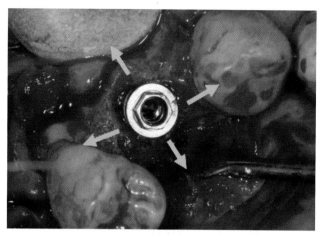

• **Fig. 32.44** Immediate Implant Complication. Lack of primary stability that increases complication and failure rate.

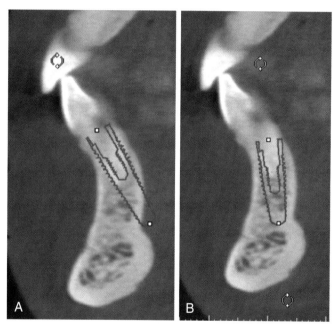

• **Fig. 32.45** (A) The trajectory should not be dictated on the natural tooth because this may be misleading. (B) Ideal trajectory based on host bone.

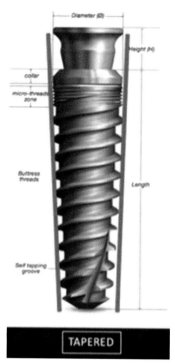

TAPERED

• **Fig. 32.46** Tapered implants have been shown to have better immediate implant fixation.

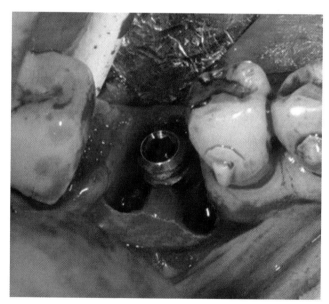

• **Fig. 32.47** Implant with inadequate primary stability and minimal adjacent host bone. If adequate primary stability cannot be obtained, the implant should be removed and the site grafted.

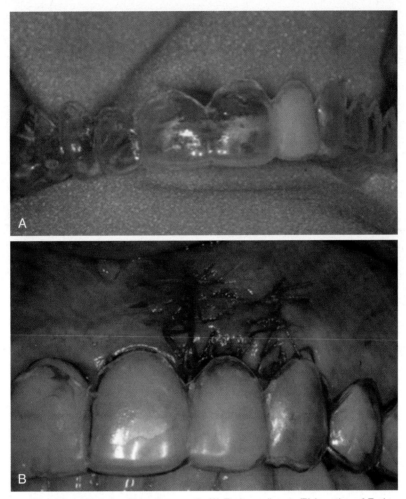

• **Fig. 32.48** Transitional Prosthesis Impingement. (A) Essix appliance. (B) Insertion of Essix appliance depicting no pressure on surgical site.

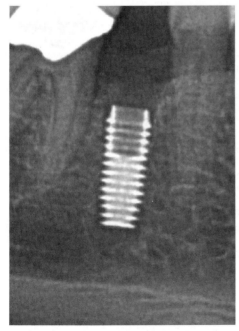

• **Fig. 32.49** Neurosensory Impairment resulting from immediate implant placement too deep which penetrated the mandibular canal.

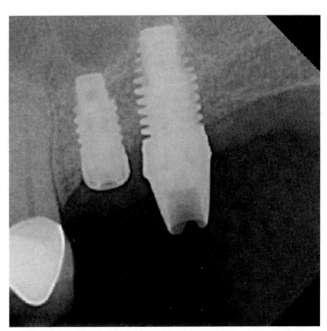

• **Fig. 32.50** Management of malpositioning error by addition of narrow implant. (*From Jividen GJ, Misch CE. Complications associated with immediate implant placement. In: Resnik RR, Misch CE, eds.* Misch's Avoiding Complications in Oral Implantology. *St. Louis, MO: Elsevier; 2018.*)

References

1. Lazzara RJ. Immediate implant placement into extraction sites: surgical and restorative advantages. *Int J Periodontics Restorative Dent.* 1989;9(5):332–343.
2. Gelb DA. Immediate implant surgery: three-year retrospective evaluation of 50 consecutive cases. *Int J Oral Maxillofac Implants.* 1993;8(4):388–399.
3. Hammerle CH, Chen ST, Wilson Jr TG. Consensus statements and recommended clinical procedures regarding the placement of implants in extraction sockets. *Int J Oral Maxillofac Implants.* 2004;19(suppl):26–28.
4. Lang NP, Pun L, Lau KY, et al. A systematic review on survival and success rates of implants placed immediately into fresh extraction sockets after at least 1 year. *Clin Oral Implants Res.* 2012;23(suppl 5):39–66.
5. Schropp L, Wenzel A, Kostopoulos L, et al. Bone healing and soft tissue contour changes following single-tooth extraction: a clinical and radiographic 12-month prospective study. *Int J Periodontics Restorative Dent.* 2003;23(4):313–323.
6. Tan WL, Wong TL, Wong MC, et al. A systematic review of post-extractional alveolar hard and soft tissue dimensional changes in humans. *Clin Oral Implants Res.* 2012;23(suppl 5):1–21.
7. Grossmann Y, Levin L. Success and survival of single dental implants placed in sites of previously failed implants. *J Periodontol.* 2007;78(9):1670–1674.
8. Machtei EE, Horwitz J, Mahler D, et al. Third attempt to place implants in sites where previous surgeries have failed. *J Clin Periodontol.* 2011;38(2):195–198.
9. Becker W, Dahlin C, Becker BE, et al. The use of e-PTFE barrier membranes for bone promotion around titanium implants placed into extraction sockets: a prospective multicenter study. *Int J Oral Maxillofac Implants.* 1994;9:31–40.
10. Becker W, Dahlin C, Lekholm U, et al. Five-year evaluation of implants placed at extraction and with dehiscences and fenestration defects augmented with ePTFE membranes: results from a prospective multicenter study. *Clin Implant Dent Relat Res.* 1999;1:27–32.
11. Rosenquist B, Ahmed M. The immediate replacement of teeth by dental implants using homologous bone membranes to seal the sockets: clinical and radiographic findings. *Clin Oral Implants Res.* 2000;11:572–582.
12. Schwartz-Arad D, Chaushu G. Immediate implant placement: a procedure without incisions. *J Periodontol.* 1998;69:743–750.
13. Peñarrocha-Diago MA, Maestre-Ferrín L, Demarchi CL, et al. Immediate versus nonimmediate placement of implants for full-arch fixed restorations: a preliminary study. *J Oral Maxillofac Surg.* 2011;69(1):154–159.
14. Misch CE. *Contemporary Implant Dentistry.* 3rd ed. St Louis: Mosby; 2008.
15. Johns RB, et al. A multicenter study of overdentures supported by Branemark implants. *Int J Oral Maxillofac Implants.* 1992;7(4):513–522.
16. Smedberg JI, et al. A clinical and radiological two-year follow-up study of maxillary overdentures on osseointegrated implants. *Clin Oral Implants Res.* 1993;4(1):39–46.
17. Herrmann I, et al. Evaluation of patient and implant characteristics as potential prognostic factors for oral implant failures. *Int J Oral Maxillofac Implants.* 2005;20(2):220–230.
18. McAllister BS, Cherry JE, Kolinski ML, et al. Two-year evaluation of a variable-thread tapered implant in extraction sites with immediate temporization: a multicenter clinical trial. *Int J Oral Maxillofac Implants.* 2012;27(3):611.
19. Kan JY, Rungcharassaeng K, Lozada JL, Zimmerman G. Facial gingival tissue stability following immediate placement and provisionalization of maxillary anterior single implants: a 2- to 8-year follow-up. *Int J Oral Maxillofac Implants.* 2011;26(1):179–187.
20. Januario AL, Duarte WR, Barriviera M, et al. Dimension of the facial bone wall in the anterior maxilla: a cone-beam computed tomography study. *Clin Oral Implants Res.* 2011;22(10):1168–1171.
21. Araujo MG, Lindhe J. Dimensional ridge alterations following tooth extraction. An experimental study in the dog. *J Clin Periodontol.* 2005;32(2):212–218.
22. Evans CD, Chen ST. Esthetic outcomes of immediate implant placements. *Clin Oral Implants Res.* 2008;19:73–80.
23. Spray JR, Black CG, Morris HF, Ochi S. The influence of bone thickness on facial marginal bone response: stage 1 placement through stage 2 uncovering. *Ann Periodontol.* 2000;5(1):119–128.
24. Roberts WE, et al. Implants: bone physiology and metabolism. *CDA J (Calif Dent Assoc).* 1987;15(10):54–61.
25. Misch CE, Perez HM. Atraumatic extractions: a biomechanical rationale. *Dent Today.* 2008;27(8):100–101. 98.
26. Caneva M, Salata LA, de Souza SS, et al. Hard tissue formation adjacent to implants of various size and configuration immediately placed into extraction sockets: an experimental study in dogs. *Clin Oral Implants Res.* 2010;21(9):885–890.
27. Levine RA. Surgical and prosthetic treatment of a failed maxillary central incisor. *Inside Dent.* 2016;12(6):64–70.
28. Schwartz D, Chaushu. The ways and wherefores of immediate placement of implants into fresh extraction sites: a literature review. *J Periodontol.* 1997;68:915–923.
29. Madani E, Smeets R, Freiwald E, et al. Impact of different placement depths on the crestal bone level of immediate versus delayed placed platform-switched implants. *J Cranio-Maxillofacial Surg.* 2018;46(7):1139–1146.
30. Advanced surface and material enable Straumann's bone level implants to overcome placement challenges. *Compend Contin Educ Dent.* 2015;36(8):628.
31. Kan JY, Roe P, Rungcharassaeng K. Effects of implant morphology on rotational stability during immediate implant placement in the esthetic zone. *Int J Oral Maxillofac Implants.* 2015;30(3):667–670.
32. Scipioni A, et al. Healing at implants with and without primary bone contact. An experimental study in dogs. *Clin Oral Implants Res.* 1997;8:39–47.
33. Botticelli D, Berglundh T, Buser D, et al. The jumping distance revisited: an experimental study in the dog. *Clin Oral Implants Res.* 2003;14:35–42.
34. Botticelli D, Berglundh T, Lindhe J, et al. Appositional bone formation in marginal defects at implants. *Clin Oral Implants Res.* 2003;14:1–9.
35. Botticelli D, Berglundh T, Lindhe J. Hard-tissue alterations following immediate implant placement in extraction sites. *J Clin Periodontal.* 2004;31:820–828.
36. Tarnow DP, Chu SJ. Human histologic verification of osseointegration of an immediate implant placed into a fresh extraction socket with excessive gap distance without primary flap closure, graft, or membrane: a case report. *Int J Periodontics Restorative Dent.* 2011;31(5).
37. Sanz M, et al. A prospective, randomized-controlled clinical trial to evaluate bone preservation using implants with different geometry placed into extraction sockets in the maxilla. *Clin Oral Implants Res.* 2010;21(1):13–21.
38. Chen ST, Darby IB, Reynolds EC. A prospective clinical study of non-submerged immediate implants: clinical outcomes and esthetic results. *Clin Oral Implants Res.* 2007;18(5):552–562.
39. Caneva M, Salata LA, de Souza SS, et al. Influence of implant positioning in extraction sockets on osseointegration: histomorphometric analyses in dogs. *Clin Oral Implants Res.* 2010;21(1):43–49.
40. Lee EA, Gonzalez-Martin O, Fiorellini J. Lingualized flapless implant placement into fresh extraction sockets preserves buccal alveolar bone: a cone beam computed tomography study. *Int J Periodontics Restorative Dent.* 2014;34(1):61–68.
41. Buser D, Martin W, Bleser UC. Optimizing esthetics for implant restorations in the anterior maxilla: anatomic and surgical considerations. *Int J Oral Maxillofac Implants.* 2004;19(suppl):43–61.
42. Chen S, Buser D. Advantages and disadvantages of treatment options for implant placement in post-extraction sockets. In: Buser D, Wismeijer D, Belser U, eds. ITI Treatment Guide. Vol. 3. *Implant Placement in Post-Extraction Sites: Treatment Options.* Berlin:Quintessenz Verlag;2008:29–42.

43. Wöhrle PS. Single-tooth replacement in the aesthetic zone with immediate provisionalization: fourteen consecutive case reports. *Pract Periodontics Aesthet Dent.* 1998;10(9):1107–1114.

44. Kan JY, Rungcharassaeng K. Immediate placement and provisionalization of maxillary anterior single implants: a surgical and prosthodontic rationale. *Pract Periodontics Aesthet Dent.* 2000;12(9):817–824.

45. McAllister BS, Cherry JE, Kolinski ML, et al. Two-year evaluation of a variable-thread tapered implant in extraction sites with immediate temporization: a multicenter clinical trial. *Int J Oral Maxillofac Implants.* 2012;27(3):611.

46. Lang NP, Tonetti MS, Suvan JE, et al. Immediate implant placement with transmucosal healing in areas of aesthetic priority: a multicentre randomized–controlled clinical trial I. Surgical outcomes. *Clin Oral Implants Res.* 2007;18(2):88–196.

47. Wagenberg B, Froum SJ. A retrospective study of 1925 Consecutively placed immediate implants from 1988 to 2004. *Int J Oral Maxillofac Implants.* 2006;21(1):71.

48. Levine RA, Ganeles J, Gonzaga L, et al. 10 keys for successful esthetic-zone single immediate implants. *Compend Contin Educ Dent.* 2017;38(4):248–260.

49. Atieh MA, Ibrahim HM, Atieh AH. Platform switching for marginal bone preservation around dental implants: a systematic review and meta-analysis. *J Periodontol.* 2010;81:1350–1366.

50. Aguilar-Salvatierra A, Calvo-Guirado JL, Gonzalez-Jaranay M, et al. Peri-implant evaluation of immediately loaded implants placed in esthetic zone in patients with diabetes mellitus type 2: a two-year study. *Clin Oral Implants Res.* 2016;27(2):156–161.

51. Cooper LF, Reside GL, Raes F, et al. Immediate provisionalization of dental implants placed in healed alveolar ridges and extraction sockets: a 5-year prospective evaluation. *Int J Oral Maxillofac Implants.* 2014;29(3):709–717.

52. Buser D, Chappuis V, Belser UC, Chen S. Implant placement postextraction in esthetic single tooth sites: when immediate, when early, when late? *Periodontol 2000.* 2017;73(1):84–102.

53. Linkevicius T, Puisys A, Steigmann M, et al. Influence of vertical soft tissue thickness on crestal bone changes around implants with platform switching: a comparative clinical study. *Clin Implant Dent Relat Res.* 2015;17(6):1228–1236.

54. Puisys A, Linkevicius T. The influence of mucosal tissue thickening on crestal bone stability around bone–level implants. A prospective controlled clinical trial. *Clin Oral Implants Res.* 2015;26(2):123–129.

55. Schnitman PA, et al. Ten-year results for Branemark implants immediately loaded with fixed prostheses at implant placement. *Int J Oral Maxillofac Implants.* 1997;12:495–503.

56. Brunski JB. Biomechanical factors affecting the bone-dental implant interface: review paper. *Clin Mater.* 1992;10:153–201.

57. Mall N, Dhanasekar B, Aparna IN. Validation of implant stability: a measure of implant permanence. *Indian J Dent Res.* 2011;22:462–467.

58. Meredith N. Assessment of implant stability as a prognostic determinant. *Int J Prosthodont (IJP).* 1998;11:491–501.

59. Atsumi M, Park SH, Wang HL. Methods used to assess implant stability: current status. *Int J Oral Maxillofac Implants.* 2007;22:743–754.

60. Ostman PO, Hellman M, Sennerby L. Immediate occlusal loading of implants in the partially edentate mandible: a prospective 1-year radiographic and 4-year clinical study. *Int J Oral Maxillofac Implants.* 2008;23:315–322.

61. Lekholm U. Immediate/early loading of oral implants in compromised patients. *Periodontol 2000.* 2003;33:194–203.

62. Meredith N, Alleyne D, Cawley P. Quantitative determination of the stability of the implant-tissue interface using resonance frequency analysis. *Clin Oral Implants Res.* 1996;7:261–267.

63. Huang HM, Chiu CL, Yeh CY, et al. Early detection of implant healing process using resonance frequency analysis. *Clin Oral Implants Res.* 2003;14:437–443.

64. Zix J, Hug S, Kessler-Liechti G, et al. Measurement of dental implant stability by resonance frequency analysis and damping capacity assessment: comparison of both techniques in a clinical trial. *Int J Oral Maxillofac Implants.* 2008;23(3):525–530.

65. Sennerby L, Roos J. Surgical determinants of clinical success of osseointegrated oral implants: a review of the literature. *Int J Prosthodont (IJP).* 1998;11:408–420.

66. Han J, Lulic M, Lang NP. Factors influencing resonance frequency analysis assessed by Osstell mentor during implant tissue integration: II. Implant surface modifications and implant diameter. *Clin Oral Implants Res.* 2010;21:605–611.

67. Han CH, Mangano F, Mortellaro C, Park KB. Immediate loading of tapered implants placed in postextraction sockets and healed sites. *J Craniofac Surg.* 2016;27(5):1220–1227.

68. De Rouck T, Collys K, Wyn I, Cosyn J. Instant provisionalization of immediate single-tooth implants is essential to optimize esthetic treatment outcome. *Clin Oral Implants Res.* 2009;20(6):566–570.

69. Tarnow DP, Chu SJ, Salama MA, et al. Flapless postextraction socket implant placement in the esthetic zone: Part 1. The effect of bone grafting and/or provisional restoration on facial-palatal ridge dimensional change—a retrospective cohort study. *Int J Periodontics Restorative Dent.* 2014;34(3):323–331.

70. Villa R, Rangert B. Early loading of inerforaminal implants immediately installed after extraction of teeth presenting endodontic and periodontal lesions. *Clin Imp Dent and Related Res.* 2005;7:S28–S35.

71. Novaes Jr AB, Vidigal Jr GM, Novaes AB, et al. Immediate implants placed into infected sites: a histomorphometric study in dogs. *Int J Oral Maxillofac Implants.* 1998;13(3).

72. Crespi R, Cappare P, Gherlone E, Romanos GE. Immediate versus delayed loading of dental implants placed in fresh extraction sockets in the maxillary esthetic zone: a clinical comparative study. *Int J Oral Maxillofac Implants.* 2008;23:753–758.

73. Buchs AU, Levine L, Moy P. Preliminary report of immediately loaded Altiva Natural Tooth Replacement dental implants. *Clin Implant Dent Relat Res.* 2001;3(2):97–106.

74. Greenstein G, Cavallaro J. Immediate dental implant placement: technique, part I. *Dent Today.* 2014;33(1):100–104, 98; quiz 105.

75. Sennerby L, Meredith N. Implant stability measurements using resonance frequency analysis: biological and biomechanical aspects and clinical implications. *Periodontol 2000.* 2008;47:51–66.

76. Sakoh J, et al. Primary stability of a conical implant and a hybrid, cylindric screw-type implant in vitro. *Int J Oral Maxillofac Implants.* 2006;21(4):560–566.

77. Langer B, et al. The wide fixture: a solution for special bone situations and a rescue for the compromised implant: Part 1. *Int J Oral Maxillofac Implants.* 1993;8(4):400–408.

78. Ivanoff CJ, Sennerby L, Johansson C, et al. Influence of implant diameters on the integration of screw implants: an experimental study in rabbits. *Int J Oral Maxillofac Surg.* 1997;26(2):141–148.

79. Matsushita Y, Kitoh M, Mizuta K, et al. Two-dimensional FEM analysis of hydroxyapatite implants: diameter effects on stress distribution. *J Oral Implantol.* 1990;16(1):6–11.

80. Ivanoff CJ, Grondahl K, Sennerby L, et al. Influence of variations in implant diameters: a 3- to 5-year retrospective clinical report. *Int J Oral Maxillofac Implants.* 1999;14(2):173–180.

81. Ivanoff CJ, Sennerby L, Lekholm U. Reintegration of mobilized titanium implants: an experimental study in rabbit tibia. *Int J Oral Maxillofac Surg.* 1997;26(4):310–315.

82. Orenstein IH, Tarnow DP, Morris HF, et al. Three-year post-placement survival of implants mobile at placement. *Ann Periodontol.* 2000;5(1):32–41.

83. Nelson SJ. Wheeler's Dental Anatomy. *Physiology and Occlusion.* 10th ed. Elsevier; 2015.

33

Immediate Load/Restoration in Implant Dentistry

RANDOLPH R. RESNIK AND CARL E. MISCH

For years the two-stage surgical protocol established by Brånemark et al.[1] to accomplish osseointegration was considered a prerequisite for achieving osseointegration and long-term success. This traditional surgical protocol consisted of placing dental implants slightly below the crestal bone, obtaining and maintaining a soft tissue covering over the implant, and allowing for a nonloaded implant environment for 3 to 6 months. The success of the two-stage technique was highly documented; however, many in the field still strived for shorter treatment times and fewer surgical interventions. With advances in implant technology, the traditional protocol in implant dentistry has been reevaluated, which has led to a growing interest in the immediate-loading protocol. An abundance of clinical studies have shown positive outcomes and success with loading implants immediately or within a short period after implant placement.[2,3]

The immediate-loaded implant concept has become popular in the dental profession because it allows patients to have the ability to combine the surgical and prosthetic procedures into a single appointment. As a result of the immediate-loading technology, advances have led to an array of new implant designs and treatment protocols. In this chapter the concept of immediate-loading protocol will be discussed in detail, together with various immediate-loading protocols for single-tooth replacement, multiteeth replacement, and full-arch rehabilitation.

Immediate-Loading Terminology

The concept of immediate-loading implants involves a nonsubmerged first-stage surgery, with the immediate loading of the implants with an interim or final prosthesis. The terminology and nomenclature for these techniques are poorly understood, with little consistency. Therefore in an attempt to standardize the language in which immediate loading is discussed, Misch et al.[4] suggested a terminology for immediate restoration and/or occlusal loading (Box 33.1).

Advantages of Immediate Load Protocol

Less Discomfort for Patients

When the immediate loaded principle is used, patient discomfort and morbidity are reduced. No second-stage surgery (i.e., uncover) is required, therefore fewer appointments will be necessary for the patient. In many delayed loading situations, it is necessary for the patient to wear a removable prosthesis throughout the healing period. Not only does this lead to increased discomfort and inconvenience for the patient, but also the possibility of overloading the tissue and/or implant is greater. With the immediate load technique, a removable prosthesis is not worn, therefore decreasing the morbidity to the patient.

Faster Treatment

The immediate-loading protocol reduces the need for second-stage surgery and subsequent healing of the tissue. Therefore a more simplified surgical workflow is indicated that leads to shorter treatment time. In addition, in most cases, surgical intervention and complex bone augmentation procedures are not required to restore resorbed ridges that result from the postextraction bone remodeling process. This results in far fewer appointments and shorter treatment time.

More Ideal Soft Tissue Drape

In some clinical situations, placing a prosthesis at the time of surgery will allow for better soft tissue healing. The surrounding tissue is given the opportunity to mature and heal to the existing prosthesis. This is most important in esthetic areas, where soft tissue shrinkage after second-stage surgery may compromise the soft tissue margins and papilla contours.

Immediate Satisfaction and Patient Acceptance

Placing a prosthesis immediately after implant placement has been associated with increased psychological acceptance and patient satisfaction. In cases of full arch extractions, inserting a prosthesis immediately not only improves esthetics, but also will maintain masticatory function and muscle mass. Blomberg and Lindquist[5] evaluated patients undergoing extractions and immediate placement of an implant-supported bridge and their overall satisfaction to the procedure. Overwhelmingly, patients stated a significant improvement in their quality of life and increased self-confidence.[5]

Immediate occlusal loading: Insertion of an implant-supported interim prosthesis (e.g., polymethylmethacrylate [PMMA] temporary) or final restoration in occlusal contact within *2 weeks* of the implant insertion.

Early occlusal loading: Refers to an implant-supported prosthesis in occlusion between *2 weeks and 3 months* after implant placement (i.e., occlusal loading implants after a short healing period, ~5 weeks).

Delayed or staged occlusal loading: An implant prosthesis with an occlusal load after *more than 3 months* after implant insertion. The delayed occlusal loading approach may use either a two-stage surgical procedure that covers the implants with soft tissue or a one-stage approach that exposes the implant with a healing abutment.

Nonfunctional immediate prosthesis: This describes an implant prosthesis with no direct occlusal load *within 2 weeks* of implant insertion and is primarily considered in partially edentulous patients (i.e., congenitally missing maxillary lateral incisor).

Nonfunctional early prosthesis: Describes a prosthesis delivered between 2 weeks and 3 months after the implant insertion.[114]

Occlusal loading: The prosthesis is in contact with the opposing dentition in centric occlusion.

Nonocclusal loading: The prosthesis is not in contact in centric occlusion with the opposing dentition in the natural jaw position.

Provisional prosthesis: A fixed or removable dental prosthesis designed to enhance esthetics, stabilization, and/or function for a limited period, after which it is to be replaced by a definitive dental prosthesis. This type of prosthesis assists in the determination of the therapeutic effectiveness of a specific treatment plan or the form and function.[115]

Greater Bone-Implant Contact

Numerous studies are available that report positive success rates with immediate-loaded implants that are exposed to the oral cavity during the healing phase.[6,7] Histologic studies have shown an improved bone-implant contact (BIC) with immediate-loaded implants compared with conventional protocol implants.[8,9] Piattelli et al.[10] evaluated the histology of nonsubmerged, unloaded, and early-loaded titanium implants in monkeys. They determined that early-loaded implants exhibited lamellar cortical bone that was thicker in comparison with unloaded implants.[10] Testori et al.[11] reported a BIC of 64.2% for a single immediate-loaded implant and a BIC of 38.9% for a single submerged implant.

Disadvantages of Immediate Load Implants

Increased Skill Level Required

Especially when extracting teeth and placing implants at the same time, an increased skill level is required. These types of cases require significant preplanning, most commonly with advanced cone beam computed tomography (CBCT) interactive treatment planning. In addition, CBCT bone reduction and placement guides may be indicated, which increases the complexity of the surgery and prosthetic protocols.

Initial Surgical/Prosthetic Appointment Longer

In some cases the surgical placement of implants and the prosthetic procedures may require a longer appointment duration than normal. This may lead to increases exceeding the patient's tolerance for appointment length. With some patients, this may predispose them to an increased possibility of medical complications.

Possible Increased Implant Morbidity

An often talked about disadvantage for the immediate load concept is the risk for implant bone loss or implant failure. In general this is not supported by clinical studies and research. Chen et. al. in a systemic review and meta-analysis compared immediate loaded implants vs. conventional loading and found no difference in marginal bone loss between the two techniques. However, if failure does occur, this will often lead to the patient's loss of confidence in the doctor, increased costs and treatment time, together with a longer treatment period.

Prerequisites for Immediate-Loading Protocol

For the immediate-loading protocol to be successful, various treatment planning and patient factors need to be taken into consideration implemented in the patients treatment.

Adequate Bone Density

Ideally the bone density should be favorable for an immediate-loaded prosthesis (~D1, D2, D3). However, in some cases of poor bone quality, even with modified surgical protocols, achieving an insertion torque greater than 35 N-cm is unachievable. In these clinical situations the immediate-loading protocol is not recommended, and a healing period of 4 to 6 months is suggested before loading the dental implants. In addition, the prosthetic rehabilitation should include a progressive bone-loading protocol, which increases bone density around the implants.[12]

Sufficient Bone Dimensions

For immediate load cases, it is imperative that sufficient height and width of bone are available for the placement of implants. Lazzara et al.[13] stated that 12 mm of available bone height is recommended (i.e., for a 10-mm implant) and 6 mm of available bone width is required for adequate support. In clinical cases of compromised bone quantity, immediate-loaded implants may be at higher risk for bone loss or failure, therefore more implants or implants with a greater surface area are recommended.

Ideal Insertion Torque

In the literature it is generally accepted that the immediate-loading concept is based on obtaining an insertion torque of greater than 35 N-cm to provide sufficient implant stability when the prosthesis is placed under loading situations.[14-16] However, studies have shown successful implant integration at insertion torques of 30 N-cm or less.[17] Maló et al.[18] stated that implants inserted with <30 N-cm of torque in an All-on-4 protocol have similar short-term success outcomes and marginal bone loss compared with implants inserted with ≥30 N-cm of torque.

In most clinical situations with favorable bone quality (i.e., D1, D2, D3), insertion torque of greater than 35 N-cm is usually attainable. In clinical situations of less dense bone (i.e., D3, D4), this is often difficult, if not impossible, to obtain without surgical placement protocol revision. Therefore modified surgical drilling protocols should be used in less dense bone, which may include underpreparation of the osteotomy sites, use of osteotomes, or osseodensification protocols.

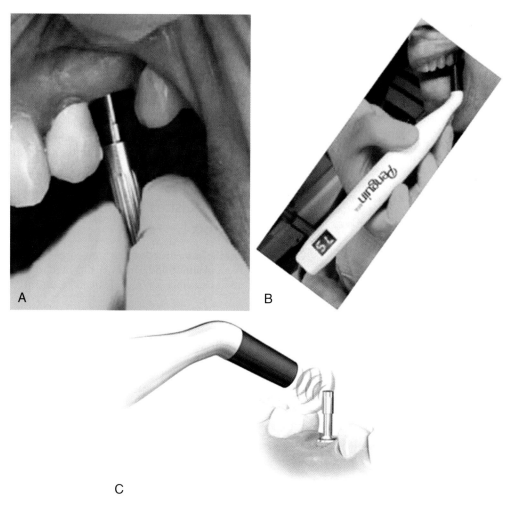

A

B

C

• **Fig. 33.1** Resonance Frequency Analysis with Penguin RFA. (A) MultiPeg placed into Implant Body, (B) Penguin RFA reading, (C) The Penguin RFA measures the resonance frequency of the reusable Multipeg. The frequency is displayed as an ISQ-value (Implant Stability Quotient).

Ideal Resonance Frequency Analysis Readings

The primary stability of an inserted dental implant can be measured via resonance frequency analysis (RFA). The RFA values will give a numerical assessment on the lateral movement (i.e., micromotion) of the implant during the healing phase. The micromotion differs for each implant system, mainly dictated on the implant design. For example, for implants with roughened surfaces, tolerance is in the range of 50 to 150 μm,[19,20] and with machined surfaces is approximately 100 μm of micromovement.[21] Studies have confirmed an implant stability quotient (ISQ) of 70 or greater is needed for an immediate-loaded prosthesis, 65 to 70 for early loading, and 60 to 65 for traditional healing (Fig. 33.1).[22,23]

Ability to Achieve an Adequate Anteroposterior Spread

The anteroposterior (A-P) spread (i.e., distance between the middle of the most anterior implant and the distal of the posterior implants) is important in increasing the mechanical advantage and force distribution of the prosthesis. In general the A-P spread is related to the ability to cantilever the prosthesis. The larger the A-P spread distance, the greater the force distribution for forces

applied to the immediate-loaded prosthesis. However, force factors play a significant role in determining if a prosthesis may be cantilevered.[24]

Rational for Implant Immediate-Loading Protocol

Effect of Surgical Trauma on Healing

The immediate implant-loading concept challenges the conventional healing period of 3 to 6 months of no loading before the restoration of the implant. Often the risks of this procedure are perceived to be during the first week after the implant insertion surgery. In reality the bone interface is stronger on the day of implant placement compared with 3 months later[23] (Fig. 33.2).

The surgical process of the implant osteotomy preparation and implant insertion result in a regional acceleratory phenomenon of bone repair around the implant interface.[24] As a result of the surgical placement, organized, mineralized lamellar bone next to the implant site becomes unorganized, less mineralized, and mainly made up of woven bone.[25] The implant-bone interface is weakest and most at risk for overload at 3 to 6 weeks after surgical insertion because the surgical trauma causes bone remodeling at the interface that is least mineralized and unorganized during this

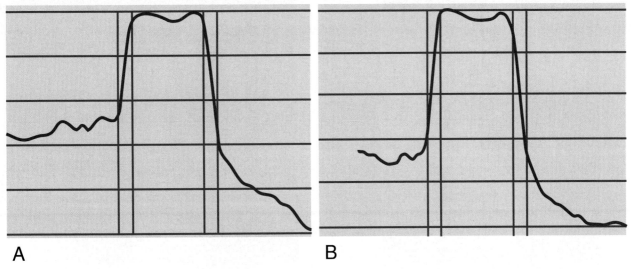

Fig. 33.2 (A) A densitometry profile of an implant 10 days after insertion. The two parallel lines at the interface represent the bone-implant contact. (B) After 3 months the densitometry profile was repeated. The implant interface is weaker at this time than the initial radiograph showed. (*Data are from Strid KG: Radiographic results. In Brånemark PI, Zarb GA, Albrektsson T, eds.* Tissue Integrated Prostheses. *Chicago: Quintessence; 1985.*)

time frame. A clinical report by Buchs et al.[27,28] found immediate-loaded implant failure occurred primarily between 3 and 5 weeks after implant insertion from mobility without infection. At 4 months the bone is still only 60% mineralized, organized lamellar bone.[28] However, this has proved to be sufficient in most bone types and clinical situations for two-stage healing and delayed implant loading.

One method to decrease the risk for immediate occlusal overload is to decrease the surgical trauma and amount of initial bone remodeling at implant placement. Roberts et al.[29,30] reported a devital zone of bone for 1 mm or more around the implant as a result of the surgical trauma (Fig. 33.3). Causes of trauma include thermal injury and microfracture of bone during implant placement. Excessive surgical trauma and thermal injury may lead to osteonecrosis and result in fibrous encapsulation around the implant.[31] Eriksson and Albrektsson[32,33] have reported bone cell death at temperatures as low as 40°C, which relate to surgical factors of the amount of bone prepared, drill sharpness, depth of the osteotomy, and variation in cortical thickness.

Studies have shown a self-tapping implant causes greater bone remodeling (woven bone) around the implant during initial healing compared with a bone tap and implant placement technique.[34] The implant should be nonmobile on insertion; however, pressure necrosis from increased torque may increase the risk for microdamage at the interface and result in bone loss. Pressure necrosis may occur from placing excessive torque on the implant, which results in an increased amount of strain at the interface. When this occurs, an increase in the amount of bone remodeling will take place, which decreases the strength of the bone-implant interface. Therefore it is prudent to minimize factors related to thermal injury and surgical trauma when considering the immediate-loading protocol.

Bone-Loading Trauma

Cortical and trabecular bone have been shown to be modified by modeling or remodeling.[25] Remodeling, or bone turnover, permits

the repair of bone after trauma or allows the bone to respond to its local mechanical environment. The bone most often is lamellar in nature; however, it may become woven bone during the repair or remodeling process. Lamellar bone and woven bone are the primary bone tissue types found around a dental implant. Lamellar bone is organized, highly mineralized, is the strongest bone type, has the highest modulus of elasticity, and is called load-bearing bone. By comparison, woven bone is unorganized, less mineralized, weaker, and more flexible (lower modulus of elasticity). Woven bone may form at a rate of 60 µm/day, whereas lamellar bone forms at a rate of 1 to 5 µm/day.[28] The classic two-stage surgical approach to implant dentistry permitted the surgical repair of the implant to be separated from the early loading response by 3 to 6 months. Therefore the majority of the woven bone that formed to repair the initial surgical trauma was replaced with lamellar bone. Lamellar bone is stronger and able to respond to the mechanical environment of occlusal loading. The rationale for immediate loading is not only to reduce the risk for fibrous tissue formation (i.e., which results in clinical failure), but also to minimize woven bone formation and promote lamellar bone maturation to sustain occlusal load.

The woven bone of surgical trauma has been called *repair bone*, and the woven bone formed from the mechanical response may be called *reactive woven bone*.[35] Remodeling also is called *bone turnover*, and not only repairs damaged bone but also allows the implant interface to adapt to its biomechanical situation (Fig. 33.4). The interface-remodeling rate is the period of time for bone at the implant interface to be replaced with new bone. Once the bone is loaded by the implant prosthesis, the interface begins to remodel again. However, this time the trigger for this process is strain, rather than the trauma of implant placement. Strain is defined as the change in length of a material divided by the original length, and it is measured as the percentage of change. When the surgical trauma is too great or the mechanical stress is too severe, fibrous tissue may form rather than bone. Fibrous tissue at an implant interface will usually result in clinical mobility rather than rigid fixation.

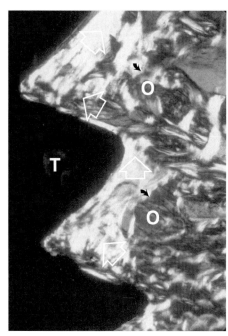

• **Fig. 33.3** Bone remodeling around an implant after surgery replaces a 1-mm or more devital zone of bone. Arrows indicate the devital zone of bone replacement. *O,* Original bone; *T,* implant.

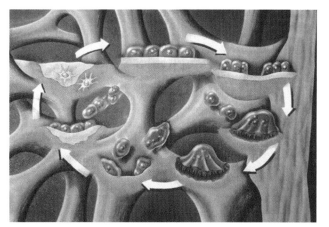

• **Fig. 33.4** Bone remodeling replaces the existing bone with new bone and is controlled primarily by the amount of microstrain within the bone. The rate of the bone remodeling also is related directly to the amount of microstrain.

Histologic Evaluation of Immediate-Loaded Implants

Short-Term Evaluation

General agreement is that excess stresses to an implant interface may cause overload and implant failure. However, immediate loading of an implant does not necessarily result in excessive stresses. The initial histologic response of bone at the implant interface has been evaluated on immediate-loaded implants. A direct BIC with favorable bone quality around the implants has been reported. Romanos et al.[25] demonstrated no statistical difference between immediate- and delayed-loaded implants. Sharawy[27] evaluated the immediate- versus delayed-healing interface of 20 dental implants

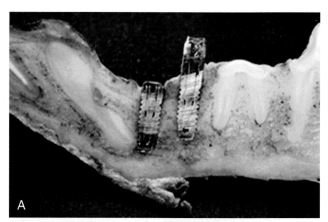

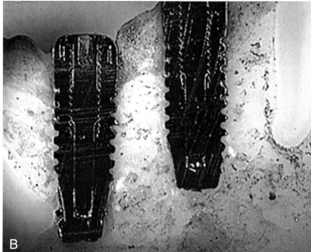

• **Fig. 33.5** (A,B) Paired implants inserted into a canine model, with one implant not loaded and the other immediately placed into function for 4 weeks.

in five adult beagle dogs (Fig. 33.5). All implants were inserted into premolar grafted bone defect sites. The implants were paired, so half of the implants were submerged, and the adjacent implants received an abutment and were subjected to immediate function for 4 weeks. The implants then were evaluated with histometric analyses of plastic embedded calcified sections. No statistically significant difference ($P > 0.05$) was found in the BIC ratios between the submerged and loaded implants (Fig. 33.6). Similarly, the volume fractions of the interface bone were not significantly different. The bone next to the implants appeared mature and showed evidence of remodeling.[27]

Suzuki et al.[28] performed a clinical and histologic evaluation of immediate-loaded posterior implants in nonhuman primates. After loading 10 implants for 90 days, they were compared with 5 control implants with no loading. The BIC percentage ranged from 50.3% to 64.1%, with an average of 56.3% for the controls. The immediate-loaded group had one implant failure, seven implants with an average of 67.6% BIC, and two implants with 43.2% and 45.6% BIC, respectively. Therefore the study demonstrated immediate-loaded implants may have a higher BIC than nonloaded implants, most likely a response to the strain conditions in the bone. However, three implants had less BIC or failure compared with controls. Although benefits exist related to immediate loading, it appears some risks are involved in the procedure.[28]

Testori et al.[30] reported on the histologic interface of two implants in humans that were immediately loaded after 4 months.

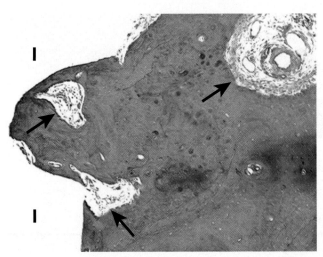

• **Fig. 33.6** No statistical difference in bone-implant contact percent and the volume fractions of the interface were found between the implants immediately loaded and those with no load for 1 month.

The bone contact ranged from 78% to 85%, with no epithelial migration. Therefore immediately loading an implant interface apparently does not necessarily place the interface at increased risk for fibrous tissue formation.[30]

Long-Term Evaluation

Piatelli et al.[31] evaluated bone reactions and the bone and titanium interface in early loaded implants in monkeys, compared with unloaded implants in the same arch several months after immediate loading. No statistically significant differences were detected in the BIC after 8 months.[31] However, loaded implants had less marrow spaces and more compact bone. A later study by the same group demonstrated greater bone contact in immediately loaded implants at 9 months.[33] No fibrous tissue was found at the interface. After 15 months, unloaded and immediately loaded implants were compared, and loaded implants exhibited greater (almost twice) direct bone contact at the interface. In particular, early loaded screws demonstrated thicker lamellar and cortical bone than unloaded implants. This finding suggests that early occlusal loading may enhance bone remodeling and further increase bone density.[36]

Randow et al.[39] evaluated the bone interface in a human patient after 18 months in an immediate-loading situation. They noted a direct bone-implant interface. Ledermann[37,38] confirmed these results in a 95-year-old patient who had an immediate-loaded, bar-connected overdenture in function for 12 years. Thus a long-lasting direct BIC relationship appears to be possible.[39]

Immediate Occlusal Loading: Factors That Decrease Risks

Bone Microstrain

When bone is loaded, its shape may change. This change may be measured as strain. Microstrain conditions 100 times less than the ultimate strength of bone may trigger a cellular response. Frost[40] has developed a microstrain language for bone based on its biological response at different microstrain levels (Fig. 33.7). Bone fractures at 10,000 to 20,000 microstrain (me) units (1%–2% strain). However, at levels of 20% to 40% of this value, bone

already starts to disappear or form fibrous tissue and is called the *pathologic overload zone.* The ideal microstrain for bone is called the physiologic or adapted zone. The remodeling rate of the bone in the jaws of a dentate canine or human that is in the physiologic zone is about 40% each year.[42] At these levels of strain, the bone is allowed to remodel and remain an organized, mineralized lamellar bone. This is called the *ideal load-bearing zone* for an implant interface. The mild overload zone corresponds to an intermediate level of microstrain between the ideal load-bearing zone and pathologic overload. In this strain region, bone begins a healing process to repair microfractures, which are often caused by fatigue. Histologically the bone in this range is called *reactive woven bone.* Rather than the surgical trauma causing this accelerated bone repair, the microstrain causes the trauma from overload. In either condition the bone is less mineralized, less organized, weaker, and has a lower modulus of elasticity.

One goal for an immediate-loaded implant-prosthesis system is to decrease the risk for occlusal overload and its resultant increase in the remodeling rate of bone. Under these conditions the surgical regional acceleratory phenomenon may replace the bone interface without the additional risk for biomechanical overload. When strain is placed on the horizontal axis and stress is positioned on the vertical axis, the relationship between these two mechanical indexes results in the flexibility or modulus of elasticity of a material. Therefore the modulus conveys the amount of deformation in a material (strain) for a given load (stress) level. The lower the stress applied to the bone (force divided by the functional surface area that receives the load), the lower the microstrain in the bone (Fig. 33.8). Therefore one method to decrease microstrain and the remodeling rate in bone is to provide conditions that increase functional surface area to the implant-bone interface.[43] The surface area of load may be increased in a number of ways: implant number, implant size, implant design, and implant body surface conditions. The force to the prosthesis also is related to the strain and may be altered in magnitude, duration, direction, or type. Methods that affect the amount of force include patient conditions, implant position, and direction of occlusal load.

Increased Surface Area

Implant Number

The clinician may increase the functional surface area of occlusal load at an implant interface by increasing implant number. Therefore rather than three to five implants to support a fixed prosthesis, use of additional implants when immediate loading is planned is more prudent. Immediate-loading reports in the literature with the lowest percentage survival correspond to fewer implants loaded.[34,44]

In numerous studies, 10 to 13 implants were inserted and splinted together per arch, and implant survival rate may be greater than 97%.[35,40-42] The increased number of implants also increases the retention of the restoration and reduces the number of pontics. The increased retention minimizes the occurrence of partially unretained restorations during healing, which can overload the implants still supporting the restoration. The decrease in pontics may decrease the risk for fracture of the transitional prosthesis, which also may be a source of overload to the remaining implants supporting the prosthesis. In general the maxilla typically requires more implants in comparison with the mandible. This approach helps compensate for the less dense bone and increased directions of force often found in the maxillary arch.

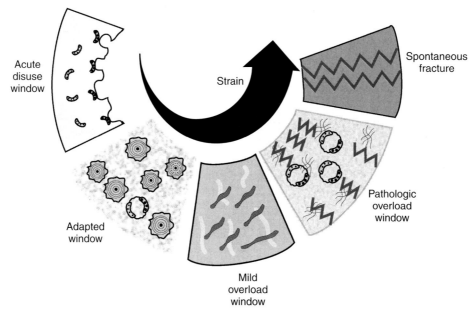

• **Fig. 33.7** Frost has reported on four distinct microstrain patterns within the bone. The acute disuse window results in atrophy, the adapted window is the physiologic response of organized bone, the mild overload zone corresponds to fatigue fractures with reactive woven bone formation, and the pathologic overload zone causes bone resorption. (*Data are from Frost HM. Mechanical adaption of Frost's mechanostat theory. In: Martin DB, Burr DB, eds.* Structure, Function and Adaption of Compact Bone. *New York: Raven Press; 1989.*)

Implant Size

The surface area may also be increased by the size of the implant. Each 3-mm increase in length can improve surface area support by more than 20%.[48] The benefit of increased length is not found at the crestal-bone interface but rather in initial stability of the bone-implant interface. Most of the stresses to an implant-bone interface are concentrated at the crestal bone, so the increased implant length does little to decrease the stress that occurs at the transosteal region around the implant.[49] Therefore length is not an effective method to decrease stress because it does not address the problem in the functional surface area region of the bone-implant interface. However, because the implant is loaded before the establishment of a histologic interface, implant length is more relevant for immediate-load applications, especially in softer bone types. The additional implant length also may permit the implant to engage the opposing cortical plate, which further increases the initial stability of the implant.

The functional surface area of each implant support system is related primarily to the width and the design of the implant. Wider root form implants provide a greater area of bone contact than narrow implants (of similar design). The crest of the ridge is where the occlusal stresses are greatest. As a result, width is more important than length of implant (once a minimum length has been obtained for initial fixation). Bone augmentation in width may be indicated to increase implant diameter when forces are greater, as in cases of moderate-to-severe parafunction. The major increase in tooth size occurs in the molar regions for natural teeth, where root surface area doubles compared with the rest of the dentition (Fig. 33.9). Therefore implant diameter often is increased in the molar region. When a larger-diameter implant is not possible without additional augmentation surgery, more implants may be inserted (i.e., two for each molar), which also is a method to double the overall surface area in the posterior region.

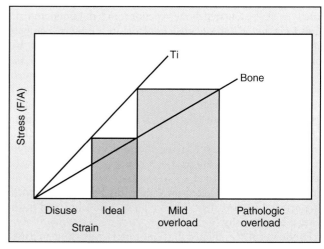

• **Fig. 33.8** When stress is applied to a material, a change in shape occurs (strain). The modulus of elasticity of a material represents the interaction of stress and strain. Titanium (Ti) has a higher modulus of elasticity than bone. When stress is applied to both of these materials, the microstrain difference between the two in the Frost microstrain zone at the interface at 50 units or less is disuse atrophy. When the microstrain difference is 50 to 2500 units, the ideal loading zone is present; between 2500 and 4000 units, the zone is in mild overload; and at more than 4000 units, the zone is in pathologic overload.

Implant Body Design

The implant body design should be more specific for immediate loading because the bone has not had time to mature and grow into recesses or undercuts in the design or attach to a surface condition before the application of occlusal load. For a threaded implant, bone is present in the depth of the threads from the day of insertion. Therefore the functional surface area is greater during the immediate-load format. The number of

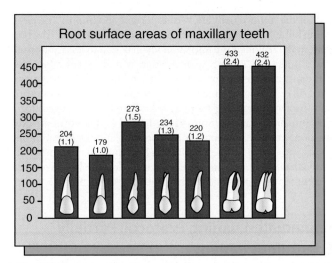

Root surface areas of maxillary teeth

• **Fig. 33.9** The natural dentition root surface area is two times greater in the molar region compared with any other tooth position. Treatment plans for immediate loading should consider implant size or number to increase surface area in this region, especially in the maxilla.

the threads also affects the amount of area available to resist the forces during immediate loading. The greater the number of threads, the greater the functional surface area at the time of immediate load.

Another variable in implant design is the thread depth, which varies in implant design. The greater the thread depth, the greater the functional surface area for immediate-load application. In general the thread depth of most threaded implants is approximately 0.2 mm, whereas the thread depth of other implant designs may reach 0.42 mm.[49] Therefore one threaded implant may have more than two times the overall functional surface area compared with other implants of similar length and width.

The functional surface area of an implant body may affect the remodeling rate of bone during loading. A macrosphere implant with reduced surface area may have twice the remodeling rate of a typical threaded implant design. A square-threaded implant design, with deeper threads in greater number, is reported to have a 10-fold reduction in remodeling rate under similar loading conditions and approximates 50% per year. The higher the remodeling rate, the weaker is the bone interface. The teeth have a bone remodeling rate of 40% per year, which maintains lamellar bone at the interface.[50]

The thread geometry also may affect the strength of early osseointegration and the bone-implant interface. Steigenga[51] placed 72 implants into 12 rabbits and reverse-torque tested the unloaded implants after 12 weeks. One-third of the implants had a V-thread, one-third had a reverse buttress shape, and one-third had a square thread. The number and depth of threads were the same, as were the width and length of each implant. The V-thread and reverse buttress thread geometry yielded similar values for reverse-torque and BIC values. The square thread demonstrated statistically significantly higher values for both of these evaluations.

Implant thread design may affect the bone turnover rate (remodeling rate) during occlusal load conditions. For a V-shaped thread design, a 10-fold greater shear force is applied to bone compared with a square thread shape.[49] Bone is strongest to compression and weakest to shear loading.[52] Compressive forces decrease the microstrain to bone compared with shear forces. Therefore the thread shape and implant design may decrease the early risks of immediate loading while the bone is repairing the surgical trauma.

A few clinical trials have compared immediate loading with different implant thread designs and tapered-implant bodies in the completely edentulous patient. The short-term clinical reports indicate a high success rate, regardless of implant design. As a result, overall shape and thread geometry apparently may not be the most important aspects for immediate occlusal load survival. Implant number, implant position, and patient factors most likely are more relevant components of success. Future studies in this area certainly are needed.

Decreased Force Conditions

The clinician may evaluate forces by magnitude, duration, direction and type. Ideally these conditions should be reduced to minimize the magnification of noxious effects of these forces.

Patient Factors. The greater the occlusal force applied to the prosthesis, the greater is the stress at the implant-bone interface and the greater the strain to the bone. Therefore force conditions that increase occlusal load increase the risks of immediate loading. Parafunction such as bruxism and clenching represents significant force factors because magnitude of the force is increased, the duration of the force is increased, and the direction of the force is more horizontal than axial to the implants with a greater shear component.[38] Balshi and Wolfinger[41] reported that 75% of all failure in immediate occlusal loading occurred in patients with bruxism. In their report, 130 implants were placed in 10 patients, with 40 implants immediately loaded and 90 implants following the traditional two-stage approach. The authors reported an 80% survival rate for immediately loaded implants compared with 96% for the traditional protocol. Grunder[42] appraised immediate loading in eight edentulous patients, four of whom exhibited bruxism. Overall success rates were 87% in the maxilla and 97% in the mandible, with five of the seven implant failures in the bruxism group. Parafunctional loads also increase the risk for abutment screw loosening, unretained prostheses, or fracture of the transitional restoration used for immediate loading. If any of these complications occur, then the remaining implants that are loaded are more likely to fail.

Occlusal Load Direction. The occlusal load direction may affect the remodeling rate. An axial load to an implant body maintains more lamellar bone and has a lower remodeling rate compared with an implant with an offset load. In an animal study, Barbier and Schepers[43] observed osteoclasts and inflammatory cells at the interface of offset-loaded implants and noted lamellar bone and a lower remodeling rate around axially loaded implants in the same animal. Therefore the clinician should eliminate posterior cantilevers in the immediate-load transitional restoration because they magnify the detrimental effects of force direction.

Implant Position. Dental implants have been used widely to retain and support cross-arch fixed partial dentures (FPDs). Implant position is often as important as implant number. For example, elimination of cantilevers on two implants supporting three teeth is recommended, rather than positioning the implants next to each other with a cantilever.[53] The cross-arch splint forming an arch is an effective design to reduce stress to the entire implant support system. Therefore the splinted-arch position concept is advantageous for the immediate-load transitional prosthesis in completely edentulous patients.

Implant position is one of the more important factors in immediate loading for completely edentulous patients. The mandible may be divided into three sections around the arch: the canine-to-canine area and the bilateral posterior sections. Several clinical reports discuss immediate load in a mandible with only three

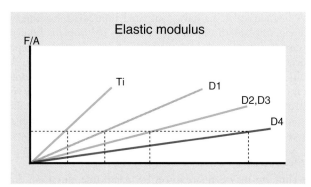

• **Fig. 33.10** The modulus of elasticity is related to the bone density. Therefore the microstrain mismatch between titanium (Ti) and Division 4 (D4) bone is greater than that between titanium and D1 bone, even when the stress amount is the same. Force/Area (F/A)

implants, as long as the implants are positioned in the midline and each posterior region.[54,55]

The maxilla requires more implant support than the mandible because the bone is less dense and the direction of force is outside of the arch in all eccentric movements. The maxilla is usually divided into five sections, depending on the intensity of the force conditions and the shape of the arch. The minimum five sections include the incisor region, the bilateral canine areas, and the bilateral posterior regions. At least one implant should be inserted into each maxillary section and splinted together during the immediate-loading process.

Concerns have been raised regarding cross-arch splinting in the mandible because of mandibular flexure and torsion distal to the mental foramens. Clinical reports indicate the acrylic used in the transitional prosthesis is flexible enough to alleviate these concerns. However, the final restoration should be fabricated in at least two independent sections when implants are placed in both posterior molar positions.[56]

Mechanical Properties of Bone

The modulus of elasticity is related to bone quality (Fig. 33.10). The less dense the bone, the lower is the modulus. The amount of BIC is also less for less dense bone. The strength of the bone also is related directly to the density of the bone. The softer the bone, the weaker are the bone trabeculae.[56,57] In addition, the remodeling rate of cortical bone is slower than that of trabecular bone. As such, the cortical bone is more likely to remain lamellar in structure during the immediate-loading process, compared with trabecular bone.

The bone in the anterior regions of the jaw may have cortical bone at the crestal and apical region of the root form implant, whenever the implant is long enough to engage both cortices. The anterior root form implants should attempt to engage the opposing cortical plate when immediate load is contemplated. The improved biomechanical condition of the cortical bone and the additional implant surface area are advantageous. The maxillary cortical bone is thin compared with the mandibular counterpart at the crestal region and the opposing landmark. In the posterior regions the maxillary sinus and mandibular canal usually negate the apical engagement of the opposing cortex of bone, which is also thin in the maxilla.

Cortical bone is also present on the lateral aspects of the residual ridge. Root form implants do not typically engage these plates unless the edentulous ridge is narrow. Bone grafting must depend on several factors to be predictable. Adequate blood supply and a

lack of micromovement are two important conditions. The developing bone is woven bone and more at risk for overload. The bone graft in the region of the implant body may lead to less fixation and lower initial BIC. Bone augmentation is more predictable when soft tissue completely covers the graft (and membranes when present). All of these conditions make bone grafting, implant insertion, and immediate loading more at risk. Therefore the suggestion is that implants that are immediately loaded be placed in an existing bone volume adequate for early loading and the overall proper prosthetic design. Bone grafting, before implant placement and immediate loading, is suggested when inadequate bone volume is present for proper reconstructive procedures (Fig. 33.11).

Immediate-Loading Protocol: Partially Edentulous Patients

Single Implants

Immediate dental implants for single implants is well documented in the literature, with numerous clinical trials showing satisfactory survival and success rates. However, a major difference with the longevity of single immediate implants is the loading protocol. In a meta-analysis study there was a five times higher failure rate with immediate-load single implants in comparison with delayed healing. No evaluated studies showed superior soft tissue and esthetic advantages in comparison with delayed surgical protocols. In 1998 Misch[58,59] published the first article during the "reinvention" of immediate "load" for partially edentulous patients. Because most patients have adequate remaining teeth in contact to function, his protocol included a provisional prosthesis primarily for esthetics, and the implant prosthesis is completely void of any occlusal contacts. This concept was termed N-FIT, or nonfunctional immediate teeth (Boxes 33.2 to 33.4).

Literature Review for Single Implants

Early Loading With Single Implants

Andersen et al.[60] evaluated early loading of eight implants in the maxilla. After implant placement, impressions were completed and interim acrylic resin restorations were fabricated approximately 1 week after surgery. At 6 months the interim crowns were removed and a final single tooth prosthesis was inserted. After 5 years a 100% success rate was reported, along with a 0.53-mm bone gain between the implant placement and final evaluation. Cooper et al.[61] reported on the 3-year implant success rate of immediate placed maxillary anterior implants after surgery. Peri-implant bone levels, along with papilla growth, were evaluated. The authors concluded that the gingival zenith increased from year 1 to 3, and marginal bone loss was minimal at an average of 0.42 mm.

Immediate Loading With Single Implants

Gomes et al.[62] published an initial report of immediate loading on a single implant. This report included the fabrication of a screw-retained provisional crown on an immediate-placed implant. Ericsson et al.[63] reported on a prospective study with single tooth implants with an immediate loading protocol compared with a two-stage implant procedure. In the immediate-loaded group, an interim single crown prosthesis was inserted within 24 hours of placement. Within 6 months the implants were restored with a final prosthesis. Two implants (14%) in the

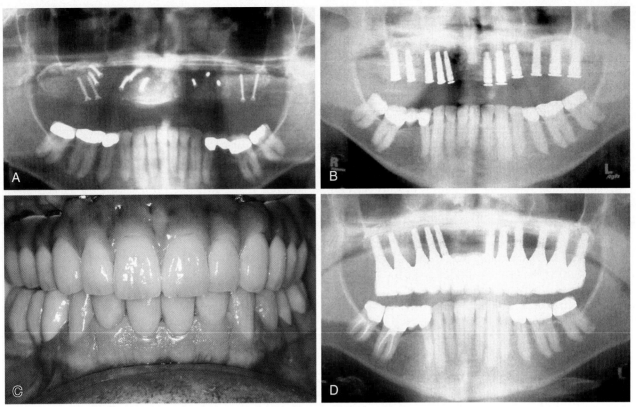

• **Fig. 33.11** (A) An iliac crest bone graft to the maxilla restores the bone volume of this type 2 DIVISION C-height (C–h), D maxilla. (B) Eleven implants were inserted, and an impression was made for the delivery of the temporary restoration at the suture removal appointment. (C) The final restoration is fabricated after at least 6 months. This intraoral photograph illustrates the definitive maxillary porcelain-metal restoration. (D) A panoramic radiograph of the final maxillary restoration and the corrected mandibular occlusal plane.

• BOX 33.2 **Nonfunctional Immediate Teeth**

Indications
- Edentulous area with favorable available bone and bone density
- Partially edentulous patients with centric occlusal contacts and excursions on natural teeth (or healed implants)
  - No parafunctional habits
  - Ideal implant position and implant dimensions (i.e., diameter and length)

Contraindications
- Patients with parafunctional oral habits (i.e., anterior and lateral tongue thrust, or biting on a pipe while smoking)
- Occlusal contacts that would result in functional contacts on implant prosthesis

---

• BOX 33.3 **Advantages of Nonfunctional Immediate Teeth**

- Patient has a fixed esthetic tooth replacement after stage I surgery.
- No stage II surgery is necessary (eliminates discomfort for the patient and decreases overhead for the doctor).
- The soft tissue emergence may be developed with the transitional prosthesis and the tissue allowed to mature during the bone-healing process.
- The soft tissue hemidesmosome attachment on the implant body below the microgap connection may heal with an improved interface.
- The patient is able to evaluate the esthetics of the provisional prosthesis during the healing phase.

• BOX 33.4 **Disadvantages of Nonfunctional Immediate Teeth**

- If force is applied to the provisional prosthesis, micromovement of the implant may cause crestal bone loss or implant failure.
- Parafunction from tongue or foreign habits (i.e., pen biting) may cause trauma and crestal bone loss or implant failure.
- Impression material or acrylic may become trapped under tissue or between the implant and crestal bone.
- Bone that is too soft, small implant diameters, or implant designs with less surface area may cause too great crestal stress contours and cause bone loss or implant failures.
- The duration of the surgery and/or postoperative appointment is longer.

---

immediate-loaded group failed, and no implant loss was seen in the two-stage protocol. Average bone loss was approximately 0.1 mm for both implant groups. Hui[65] evaluated 24 patients who received implant restorations on single teeth after tooth extraction in the esthetic zone. After a 1.5-year follow-up, all implants remained integrated.[63]

Degidi et al.[65] evaluated single implants that were nonfunctionally immediately loaded. All implants were placed with a minimum insertion torque of 25 N-cm, and after 5 years of follow-up a 95.5% survival rate was reported. When comparing healed versus immediate extraction sites, 100% and 92.5% success rates, respectively, were reported. A 100% success rate was reported in favorable bone quality (type 1), whereas a 95.5% rate was found in poor bone quality (type 4).[65]

Chaushu et al.[66] compared the success of immediate-loaded implants in fresh extraction sites compared with sites that were healed. Provisional restorations were placed immediately the day of surgery. The authors concluded that immediate loading in an extraction site did increase the failure rate (i.e., approximately 20%) in comparison with immediate-loaded healed sites. Mankoo[67] described the immediate implant placement and provisionalization in the anterior region of the oral cavity. He reported this technique was advantageous, not only because of the lack of a stage 2 surgery required, but also the esthetic benefits provided from a provisional restoration.

In addition, a removable prosthesis is not required, which is usually difficult for the patient to adapt to and has associated esthetic issues.

A meta-analysis identifying more than 5000 studies was completed by Pigozzo et al.[68] and concluded no significant differences between immediate- and early-loading protocols with single-implant crowns. The success and survival rate together with marginal bone loss was evaluated up to 3 years.

Surgical/Prosthetic Protocol for Single Implants

After placement of a single tooth implant the clinician has three options at his or her disposal:

1. *Two-stage technique:* involves delayed healing and a second surgery to expose the implant before prosthetic rehabilitation
2. *One-stage technique:* a healing abutment is placed after implant placement, healing is completed, and prosthetic rehabilitation is delayed
3. *Immediate restoration with a provisional prosthesis:* may be loaded or nonfunctional; rarely will a single-tooth immediate implant be placed directly into function because of increased biomechanical forces that may result in poor healing or failure of the implant

Single-Tooth Nonfunctional Immediate-Restoration Procedure

The N-FIT concept presents a similar approach to the immediate-loading technique, except the implant-supported transitional prosthesis is placed out of all direct opposing occlusal contacts during the bone healing period. As a result the implant clinician may fabricate an esthetic tooth replacement immediately for the patient, but with no occlusal contact. By placing an immediate prosthesis, the soft tissue contours, as well as the esthetics, may be developed via the provisional prosthesis and bone-healing process (Fig. 33.12).

After implant placement, there exist multiple treatment options for the clinician to provisionalize the implant restoration.

1. Implant crown fabricated by the dental laboratory where the clinician relines the provisional prosthesis to a stock type abutment placement; this may be a cement or screw-retained prosthesis.
2. Prefabricated crown that is relined by the clinician; usually a stock or prefabricate abutment is inserted and prepared, after which the provisional restoration is fabricated to the esthetics and functional demands of the area
3. Composite that is bonded to a stock or prefabricated abutment and the adjacent teeth

4. The clinician takes an impression of the implant after insertion, together with jaw records and opposing impressions; a healing abutment is placed; at the suture removal, which is usually 2 weeks after placement, the healing abutment is removed and replaced with a laboratory-modified abutment and provisional prosthesis; this is an example of early loading

No matter what technique is used to fabricate a provisional prosthesis, it is imperative that the occlusion is strictly monitored. After placement of the interim crown the prosthesis should be evaluated in all centric and eccentric excursions to verify no contact. Of special concern is in the maxillary anterior region, because horizontal movement of the anterior teeth is far greater than the posterior teeth. Therefore the excursive movements should be evaluated with all degrees of force (i.e., clenching and bruxing movements) (Fig. 33.13 and Box 33.5).

Partially Edentulous (Greater Than One Edentulous Space)

With partially edentulous spaces, immediate-loaded implants is a controversial topic. Most studies consist of patient treatment in load-based areas such as the posterior part of the oral cavity. Few studies have been completed in the esthetic zone. Until more detailed studies are available, clinicians should be conscious of placing immediate implants, especially in the esthetic in partially edentulous patients.

Literature Review of Partially Edentulous Arches

Early Loading in the Partially Edentulous Arch

Testori et al.[69] reported on a 3-year 97.7% success rate in a longitudinal, prospective, multicenter study of early implant loading. All implants were placed in the posterior region of the oral cavity and were loaded within 8 weeks. Cochran et al.,[70] in a longitudinal, prospective, multicenter study, reported a 99.1% success rate after 1 year. Implants were placed in the posterior regions of the jaws, with various healing times based on the density of bone. Luongo et al.[71] evaluated the immediate and early loading (11 days) of implants in the posterior maxilla and mandible. A 98.8% success rate was reported, and the results were similar to those with delayed-loaded implants. Vanden Bogaerde et al.,[72] in a multicenter study, placed interim prostheses between 9 and 16 days after implant placement in the maxilla. An implant survival rate of 99.1% after 18 months was reported, with bone loss less than 0.8 mm.

Immediate Loading in the Partially Edentulous Arch

Drago and Lazzara[73] related a study involving restored fixed provisional implant crowns without occlusion immediately after implant placement. The implants were immediately restored with prefabricated stock abutments and cement retained. No occlusal contacts or interferences were present. Final prostheses were inserted 8 to 12 weeks after implant placement. After 18 months the implant survival rate was 97.4%, and an average bone loss of 0.76 mm was reported.[73] Interestingly, Machtei et al.[74] evaluated implants placed in the mandible in patients with chronic periodontitis. They concluded that immediate-loading protocols are a predictable treatment; however, caution should be exercised in the molar regions. Schincaglia et al.[75] reported a split-mouth study with bilateral, partially edentulous posterior mandibles. The overall success rate was 95%; an insertion torque of 20 N-cm or greater and an ISQ value more than 60 N-cm was recommended (Fig. 33.14).

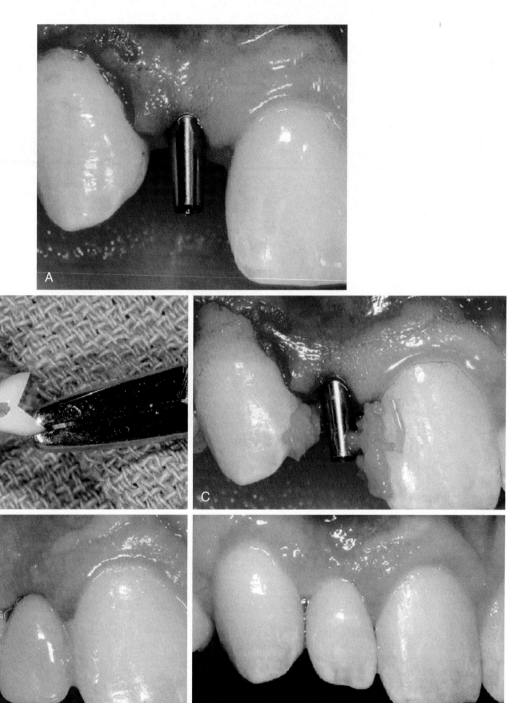

• **Fig. 33.12** Nonfunctional Immediate Prosthesis. (A) Maxillary right lateral incisor implant placement. (B) A acrylic temporary prosthesis is fabricated chairside and relined to fit the inserted abutment. (C) The adjacent teeth are acid-etched. (D) The provisional prosthesis is bonded to the adjacent teeth, and the occlusion is confirmed to include no contacts. (E) After 4 months of healing the provisional prosthesis is removed and the final prosthesis completed.

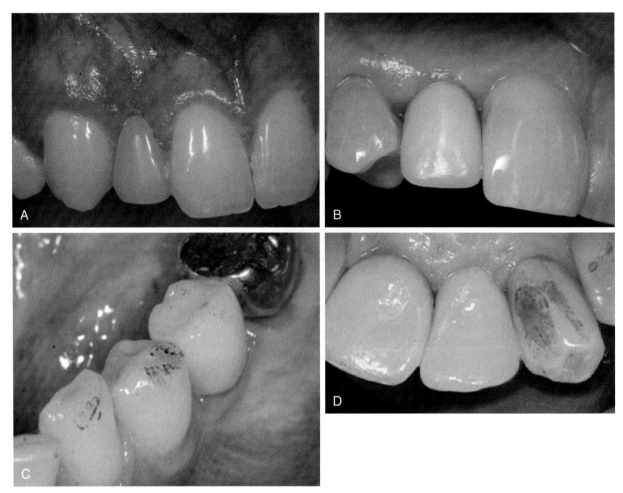

• **Fig. 33.13** Single-Tooth Provisional Prostheses. (A) Prosthesis may be bonded to adjacent teeth, however only when no horizontal mobility of the adjacent abutment teeth is present. (B) Provisional with no contact with adjacent teeth because of heavy excursive contacts on the canine. (C) Provisional placed on an immediate mandibular premolar; note the slight contact in light occlusion, all contacts should be removed to remain nonfunctional, (D) Lateral incisor immediate load showing no occlusal contacts and ideal contacts on cuspid.

• BOX 33.5 **Protocol for Stage I Nonfunctional Early Loading Immediate Teeth**

Appointment #1: Surgery

1. Make impression of opposing arch and obtain tooth shade and centric bite registration.
2. Perform stage I implant surgery (use wider implants when possible).
3. Make an impression with additional silicone material or polyether. Verify that no impression material is entrapped underneath the flap.
4. Place a healing abutment approximately 2 mm above the tissue.
5. Suture (tissue thickness should be less than 4 mm).

Laboratory Procedure

1. Impressions are mounted on an articulator with correct jaw records.
2. An abutment is selected and prepared for either a cement or screw-retained prosthesis.
3. Provisional prosthesis is fabricated with narrow occlusal table, minimal cusp height, and no occlusal or excursive contacts.

Appointment #2: Suture Removal/Prosthesis Insertion

1. Sutures are removed atraumatically.
2. The healing abutment is removed and the internal opening of the implant is irrigated with chlorhexidine.
3. The laboratory-fabricated abutment is inserted (if cement retained).
4. Use countertorque (hemostat) and tighten to abutment screw 20 to 30 N-cm (which is less than final preload).
5. Insert provisional prosthesis and evaluate contour and occlusion (no occlusal contacts).
6. Instruct patient to eat soft foods (e.g., pasta, fish, cooked meat). No raw vegetables or hard bread are allowed until final prosthesis delivery. No oral habits, such as gum chewing, are permitted. When possible the patient should avoid chewing food in implant regions.

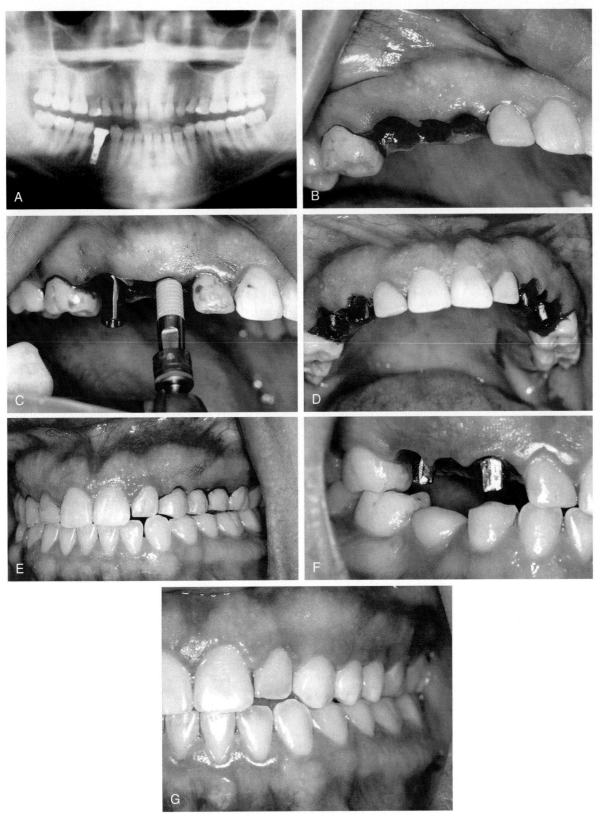

• **Fig. 33.14** (A) A panoramic radiograph of a patient with partial anodontia missing the bilateral permanent canines, first premolar, and second premolars. (B) The deciduous teeth have been extracted. (C) Two implants are used to support the prosthesis on each side. The mesiodistal space is inadequate for three implants. (D) The four implants are prepared for a cemented transitional prosthesis. (E) The transitional N-FIT restorations are primarily for esthetics and are completely out of occlusion in centric relation and all excursions. (F) The final restoration is made after 4 to 6 months. At this point the soft and hard tissues are mature. (G) The final restoration of the three-unit fixed partial denture supported by two immediate-loaded implants.

Completely Edentulous Arches

The immediate placement and loading of implants in the edentulous arches has become popular in implant dentistry today. In comparison with conventional implant procedures, the success of immediate placement and loading in the maxilla and mandible is dependent on patient selection, the preoperative treatment planning, and the skill set of the clinician in completing the surgical and prosthetic phases of treatment. These types of procedures tend to be more complex and can be associated with a higher degree of complications. The concept of immediate placement/load first originated with the mandibular arch and has been well studied. However, even though studies are limited in the maxilla, the maxillary arch is becoming more popular in implant dentistry today.

Literature Review of Edentulous Arches

Early Loading in the Mandibular Edentulous Arch

Numerous studies have shown favorable results with the early loading of the mandibular edentulous arch. Engquist et al.[76,77] reported on more than 100 edentulous mandible patients. Each patient was treated with four Nobel Biocare implants in the anterior mandible for a fixed implant prosthesis. They evaluated four groups: one-stage surgery, two-stage surgery, one-piece abutments, and early loading. The permanent prosthesis was loaded between 10 days and 3 weeks. With the early loading group, approximately 7% of the implants failed; however, this group exhibited less marginal bone loss than the control group.[76,77] Friberg et al.[78] evaluated more than 750 implants in the edentulous mandible, with the fixed prosthesis being placed approximately 13 days after implant placement. A 97.5% success rate was reported, with mean marginal bone resorption of approximately 0.4 mm.

Immediate Loading in the Mandibular Edentulous Arch

In 1990 Schnitman et al.[79] reported for the first time the immediate loading of dental implants in the anterior mandible. Five to six implants were placed in the interforaminal region, with additional implants placed posterior. Three of the implants were used for an interim prosthesis, which was converted from the patient's denture. The authors concluded the immediate loading of implants was a viable treatment option for patients because the long-term success was not impacted by the early loading of the implants. In a follow-up study, Schnitman et al.[80] treated 10 patients with an immediate-loaded fixed prosthesis. About 15.3% of the immediate implants failed, and all conventional loaded implants were successful. Schnitman et al.[80] concluded that immediate-loaded implants in the short term are successful; however, in the long term, they may have a questionable prognosis. Tarnow et al.[81] evaluated patients treated with a minimum of 10 implants, with 5 of the implants submerged, with no loading. A fixed interim prosthesis was inserted and later replaced with a fixed provisional prosthesis. Although three of the implants failed (two immediate loaded and one submerged), Tarnow et al. concluded that immediate implants splinted together are a viable treatment option.

More recently, studies have shown four to six implants placed in the mandible have favorable success rates. Chow et al.[82] placed four implants in patients with a screw-retained interim prosthesis. After 1 year the implants had a 100% success rate. In a prospective four-center study, Testori et al.[83] evaluated 62 patients in which an interim prosthesis was inserted within 4 hours of implant surgery. A success rate of 99.4% was reported, with crestal bone loss similar to the traditional delayed technique. Aalam et al.[84] evaluated 16 patients who received mandibular implants for screw-retained hybrid prostheses. After 3 years the implant success rate was 96.6%, and the prosthetic success rate was 100% (Fig. 33.15).

Early Loading in the Maxillary Edentulous Arch

Fischer and Stenberg[85] reported on early implant loading of 24 maxillary edentulous patients. After 3 years the implant success rate was 100%, and a 3-year study showed less radiographic bone loss in the early loaded than the control group.

Olsson et al.[86] studied for 1 year 10 patients who had received a fixed full-arch provisional prosthesis 1 to 9 days after implant placement. A permanent prosthesis was placed 2 to 7 months after implant placement. About 6.6% of the implants failed, all from infection, and an associated 1.3-mm marginal bone loss was reported.

Immediate Loading in the Maxillary Edentulous Arch

Bergkvist et al.[87] reported on a provisional prosthesis placed on immediate-loaded maxillary implants. After a mean healing period of 15 weeks, a final screw-retained prosthesis was fabricated. Approximately 2% of the implants failed during the healing period, and the mean marginal bone loss was 1.6 mm after 8 months.[87] Ibanez et al.[88] evaluated 26 patients who had fully edentulous maxillae, with implants that were loaded within 2 days of placement with either a provisional or final prosthesis. The success rate was 100% after a healing period of 1 to 6 years. The radiographic bone level change was a loss of 0.56 mm at 12 months and 0.94 mm at 72 months. Degidi et al.[89] reported on a 5-year follow-up of implants immediately loaded with an interim prosthesis followed by a final prosthesis. A 98% success rate was shown, with most failures occurring in the first 6 months of healing. In addition, they concluded that wider implants were associated with an increased failure rate. Balshi et al.,[90] in evaluation of 55 patients who received immediate implants, along with immediate-loaded implants, found a 99.0% survival rate of the implants and a 100% survival rate of the prosthesis. The interim prostheses consisted of an all-acrylic screw-retained prosthesis that was replaced approximately 4 to 6 months later (Fig. 33.16).

Provisional Implants

The use of provisional implants, which are defined as implants placed to retain an interim prosthesis, are not necessarily indicated for a permanent prosthesis. Originally these implants were thought not to achieve osseointegration. However, Balkin et al.[91] evaluated miniimplants for light microscopy evaluation after 4 to 5 months of immediate function. They reported that osseointegration did occur with mature and healthy bone. Iezzi et al.[92] reported on three provisional implants that were placed to retain a provisional prosthesis for 4 months. They concluded the existence of bone trabeculae around the implants, as well as the occurrence of the bone remodeling process. Heberer et al.[93] followed 254 provisional implants that were placed in 64 patients and remained functional up to 462 days. The total success rate reported was 82%, and patient factors such as gender, opposing occlusion, and implant position did not appear to be significant. Simon and Caputo[94] completed removal torque tests on provisional implants in 31 patients. They concluded that osseointegration may pose

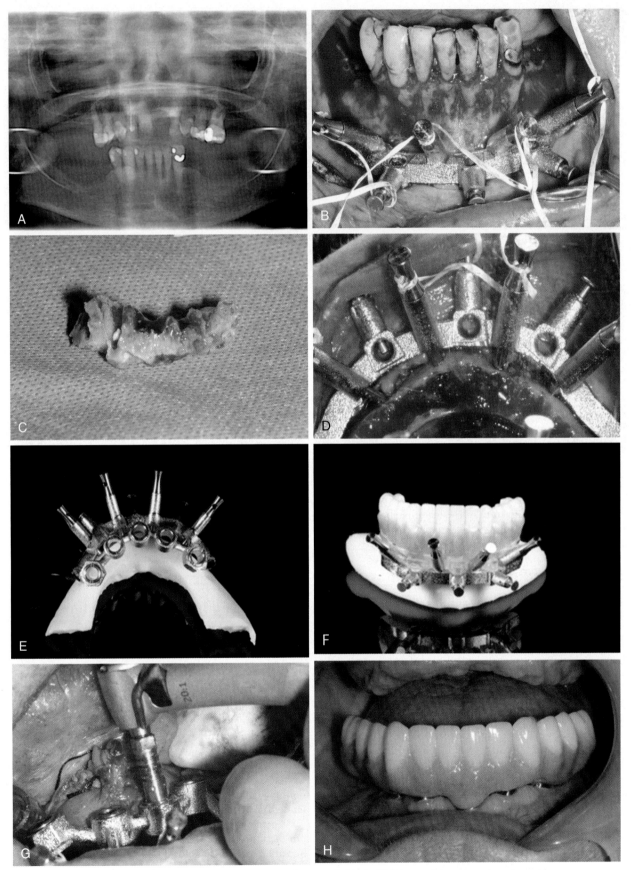

• **Fig. 33.15** Mandibular Immediate Loading (Chrome Guides). (A) Preoperative panoramic radiograph. (B) Reduction guide fixated into position. (C) Bone removed from anterior mandible to gain sufficient height for implant placement. (D) Post-osteotomy. (E) Implant guide on bone model. (F) Polymethylmethacrylate provisional prosthesis. (G) Fully guided implant placement. (H) Final hybrid prosthesis.

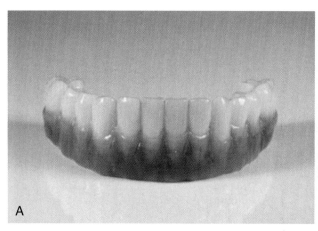 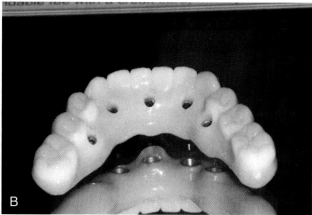

• **Fig. 33.16** Zirconia Final Prosthesis. (A and B) The monolithic zirconia prosthesis has the advantages of greater flexural strength and higher fracture resistance.

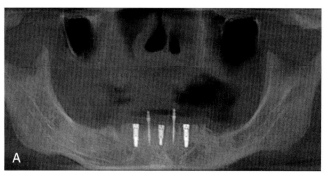 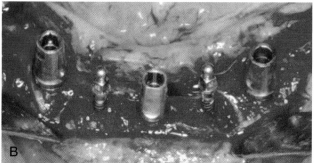

• **Fig. 33.17** Provisional Implants. (A and B) Implants placed into "B," "C," and "D" implants with two miniimplants between the implants to retain an interim prosthesis (O-Ring Attachments).

an increased possibility of fracture in the mandible because they reported that implants left in after 10 months showed a higher possibility of fracture on removal (Fig. 33.17).

All-on-4 Surgical/Prosthetic Protocol

Malo et al.[95,96] originally introduced the concept of the All-on-4 protocol, which involves the immediate loading of a fixed prosthesis on four implants placed in the maxilla or mandible. Although numerous options are available, in general two parallel implants are placed anteriorly and two angled implants are placed posteriorly. The posterior implants are accurately positioned to avoid key vital structures (e.g., maxillary sinus, inferior alveolar canal), increase A-P spread, and minimize cantilever length. Because of these positioning protocols, a significant treatment time savings is seen as sinus augmentation and bone-grafting procedures in the mandible are avoided. Usually in the maxilla, two posterior implants are positioned at up to 45 degrees of angulation to avoid the maxillary sinus. In the mandible the position of the implants is dictated by the mental foramen position (i.e., possible anterior loop); however, they are usually angulated anteriorly 30 to 45 degrees. Multiunit abutments are placed into the implants with varying degrees of angulation, usually consisting of 0, 17, or 30 degrees.[95,96]

Requirements of the All-on-4 Technique

1. Minimum of 35 N-cm insertion torque: If this cannot be achieved, then a conventional healing phase is recommended.
2. No significant parafunction habits

3. Available bone dimensions:
   Maxilla: >5 mm of width and >10 mm of height
   Mandible: >5 mm of width and >8 mm of height
4. Favorable bone density of D1, D2, or D3

Advanced Fully Guided Immediate Placement/Loading Protocols (Box 33.6, Box 33.7, Fig. 33.18)

There exist various surgical/prosthetic protocols (e.g., 3D Diagnostix, nSequence) that allow a fully guided surgical and prosthetic protocol, which combines three-dimensional CBCT-guided surgery with a definitive fixed immediate prosthesis. These protocols allow the clinician to maximize the precision of CBCT technology, together with having the capability of delivering a provisional fixed prosthesis with precision and accuracy. These techniques, compared with a freehand two-dimensional approach, have increased precision, predictability, and time-saving consistency. The fully guided, immediate placement/loading protocols allow for three-dimensional (3D) precision digital implant planning with virtual surgical and prosthetic protocols, 3D modification of bony anatomy to optimize implant placement and positioning, implant placement with a fully guided technique, and same-day delivery of a screw-retained immediate fixed prosthesis. In addition, this protocol allows for definitive control for surgical treatment planning, especially in immediate extraction cases where the bony anatomy requires alteration[97] Fig. 33.19 (Box 33.8; Figs. 33.20 through 33.22).

• BOX 33.6 Generic All-on-4 Protocol

1. Preoperative Records

Initially, maxillary and mandibular impressions are obtained conventionally or digitally (i.e., intraoral scanner), along with an accurate bite registration. A tooth shade is selected. Intraoral and extraoral photographs may be taken to assist in the diagnosis and treatment planning. Maxillary and mandibular cone beam computed tomography (CBCT) scans are obtained, with the patient wearing the bite registration in maximum intercuspation. The impressions, along with the CBCT scans are uploaded to a third-party manufacturer for processing.

2. Three-Dimensional Data Conversion

The digital three-dimensional (3D) data are merged with the 3D bony anatomy, which results in the formation of a 3D-specific dataset of tooth position, bony anatomy, occlusal considerations, prosthesis fabrication, and ideal biomechanical implant positioning. This is usually accomplished with a specialized software and third-party manufacturer (e.g., 3D Diagnostix).

3. Prosthetic and Surgical Treatment Plan

With an interdisciplinary team approach, the 3D data is used in formulating a prosthetic and surgical treatment plan. The prosthesis type should always be identified first and then the surgical plan formulated to fulfill the requirements of the prosthesis. The treatment planning factors should include: (1) type of prosthesis; (2) available bone; (3) bone density; (4) parafunctional forces; (5) anteroposterior spread; (6) occlusion; (7) implant dimensions and positions; (8) osteoplasty, if indicated; (9) path of prosthesis insertion; and (10) multiunit abutments and access holes.

4. Fabrication of Surgical Guides and Provisional Prosthesis

After treatment planning is complete, the finalized data set is sent for milling and rapid prototyping by the third-party manufacturer. A bone reduction guide (if indicated), implant surgical guide, and abutment guide are usually fabricated via stereolithography. The provisional prosthesis is most commonly milled in a monolithic polymethylmethacrylate (PMMA) block material. The manufacturer will provide a detailed surgery report on the guide sequence, along with implant size and position protocols.

5. Surgery

After anesthesia a bone reduction guide or bone foundation is positioned, usually with the aid of a registration and existing teeth. In some cases this guide will be fixated to the bone. The teeth are then extracted. After extraction a surgical implant guide will be positioned, which will assist in implant placement. This may include a universal or a fully guided template. After implant placement, multiunit abutments, which have been predetermined from the CBCT plan, are placed into the implant bodies.

6. Provisional Prosthesis Insertion

Temporary, stock abutments are placed into each multiunit abutment. The PMMA provisional prosthesis is then inserted and evaluated for fit. The PMMA prosthesis is then luted to the temporary abutment via light-cured acrylic. The PMMA can then be removed and polished for final insertion. Soft tissue closure is accomplished with a resorbable suture material with high tensile strength (e.g., Vicryl).

7. Final Prosthesis Fabrication

After sufficient healing a final prosthesis (i.e., monolithic zirconia) is fabricated. The function, phonetics, and design of the PMMA provisional can be used as a guide for any future modifications of the permanent prosthesis.

• BOX 33.7 All-on-4 Surgical/Prosthetic Approaches

The All-on-4 treatment may be performed with two approaches:
1. **Conventional surgery:** full-thickness flap and freehand implant placement
   a. After flap elevation a midline osteotomy is completed in which the All-on-4 guide is placed.
   b. *Posterior surgical osteotomy:* The posterior sites are prepared at approximately 45 degrees, using the guide as an angulation tool. Implants are inserted at a final torque of 35 to 45 N-cm. Thirty-degree multiunit abutments are placed into both posterior sites. The abutments are tightened to the manufacturer's recommendations.
   c. *Anterior surgical osteotomy:* Prepare and place two anterior implants in the approximate "B" and "D" positions. Implants are inserted at a final torque of 35 to 45 N-cm. Multiunit abutments are placed into both anterior sites. The abutments are tightened to the manufacturer's recommendations.
2. **Guided: tissue- or bone-supported guide**
   a. Implant placement: Four implants are placed according to the type of guide (tissue supported—flapless) or bone supported (flap is raised to expose residual ridge). The four implants are placed according to the interactive CBCT treatment plan. NOTE: the angulation of the posterior implants is dictated by anatomic landmarks evaluated on the 3D CBCT.

Prosthetic Procedure
1. Temporary multiunit abutment copings are placed on each implant and hand tightened.
2. The fabricated prosthesis is tried in to verify proper seating and occlusion. Light-cured composite/acrylic is used fixate the interim prosthesis to the temporary abutments. The prosthesis is removed, and any voids present between the abutments and prosthesis are filled with composite/acrylic.
3. The prosthesis is polished and reinserted for final insertion. The abutment screws are placed with a final torque as per the manufacturer's recommendations. Polytetrafluoroethylene (PTFE) tape is placed in the access holes and light-cured composite/acrylic is used to cover the holes (Fig. 33.18).

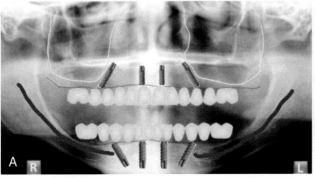
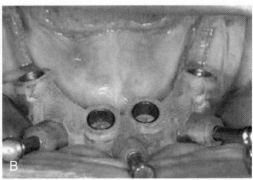

• **Fig. 33.18** (A and B) All-on-4 protocol, which includes two anterior implants and two posterior angled implants.

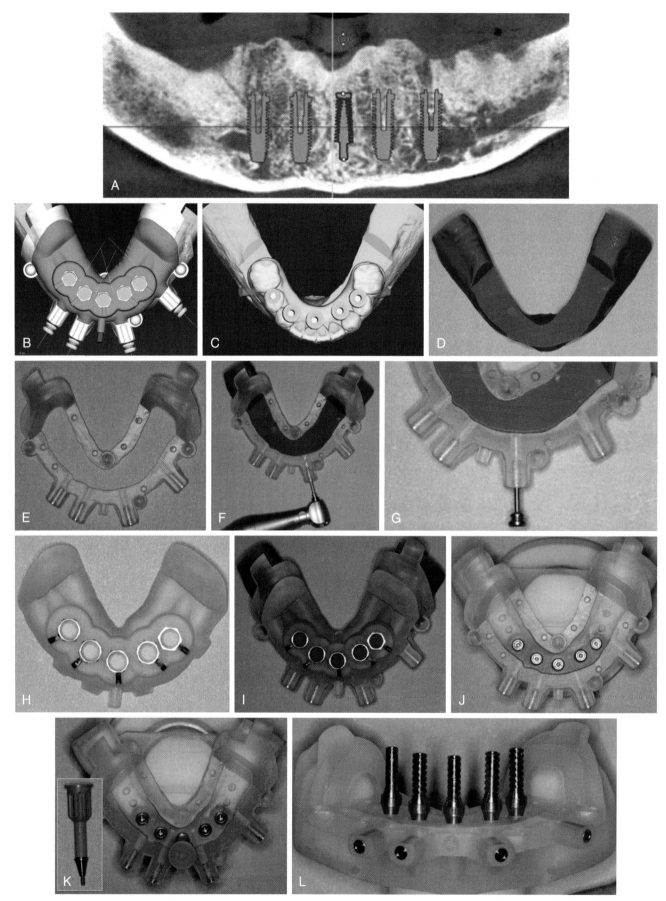

Continued

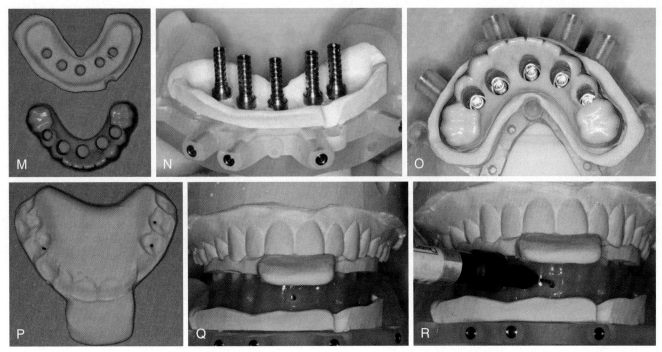

• **Fig. 33.19** Stackable Guide (3ddx): (A) Interactive treatment plan including five mandibular implants, (B) Computerized Surgical Guide Design, (C) Computerized PMMA Prosthesis Design, (D) CADS/CAM model depicting osteoplasty requirement, (E) Foundation Guide which is also is used as the osteoplasty or bone reduction guide, (F) Fixation Pin Drill, (G) Fixation Pin Insertion, (H) Stackable Surgical Guide, (I) Stackable Surgical Guide placed on foundation guide, (J) Implant Placement, (K) Multi-Unit Abutment Placement into implants, (L) Temporary Abutment Placement into multi-unit abutments, (M) Gasket and PMMA Interim Prosthesis, (N) Gasket Placement over Abutments, (O) Interim Prosthesis Placement, (P) Bite Registration, (Q) Patient Bites into Occlusion with Bite Registration, (R) Flowable composite / acrylic inserted through holes to fixate PMMA prosthesis to Temporary Abutments.

• BOX 33.8 Immediate Placement/Immediate-Loading Protocol

A. Bone-Supported Surgical Guide

Clinician (Preoperative Appointment #1)
1. Conventional impressions + bite registration or digital impressions
2. Obtain cone beam computed tomographic (CBCT) scan
   - Make sure bite registration is in place and patient closes into centric occlusion.
3. Tooth shade is selected

Preplanning
1. The case is reviewed via three-dimensional interactive CBCT software and preplanned according to ideal implant position, biomechanical force factors, and prosthesis type (Fig. 33.19A, B, C,D).
2. The treatment planned case, along with impressions (or digital impressions), is sent to a laboratory or manufacturer for fabrication of the following:
   - The working study casts are fabricated and mounted on an articulator, using the surgical template as a reference.
   - The surgical template is fabricated from the CBCT plan via CAD/CAM or a 3D printer.
   - Multiunit abutments and prefabricated temporary abutments are attached to the implant analogs on the working cast.
   - A polymethylmethacrylate (PMMA) is fabricated and hollowed out, which correspond to the abutment positions.

The laboratory furnishes the implant clinician with:
   a. *Bone foundation guide*—Fixated guide that is bone supported and is used as the primary guide that holds all additional stackable guides that are used. In addition, if ridge reduction is indicated, this guide may be used as a stackable bone reduction guide (Fig. 33.19E).

   b. *Stackable surgical guide*—This stackable (i.e., attaches into the bone foundation guide) template is fabricated from the CBCT treatment and corresponds to the position of the implants. Usually this is a fully guided template, which allows for all osteotomy preparation and implant placement through the guide (Fig. 33.19H, I, J).
   c. *Multiunit abutments*—Prefabricated abutments are specific to the implant system being used, which allows for the ideal angulation correction between the implants. Usually multiunits can be standard (no angulation) or angled with various angles (Fig. 33.19K, 33.20A).
   d. *Temporary abutments*—These are nonengaging screw-retained abutments placed into the multiunit abutments that are used to allow for fixation of the prosthesis to the multiunit abutments (Fig. 33.19L, 33.20B).
   e. *Stackable abutment guide*—A stackable abutment guide fits into the foundation guide and allows for the final positioning of the abutments, which are inserted into the implants and used to fixate the prosthesis.
   f. *Silicone gasket*—This is a flexible gasket that is placed over the temporary abutments to prevent flow of acrylic/composite into the tissue space when fixating the provisional prosthesis into the abutments (Fig. 33.19M, N).
   g. *Bite registration*—Used to verify proper positioning and seating of the provisional prosthesis (Fig. 33.19P, Q).
   h. *Provisional prosthesis*—This prosthesis (usually a PMMA prosthesis) is inserted at the time of implant placement. It is used during the healing period to verify esthetic, vertical dimension, occlusion, and patient acceptance (Fig. 33.19O, R).

• BOX 33.8 Immediate Placement/Immediate-Loading Protocol—cont'd

i. *Fixation Pins*—usually 3 -4 fixation pins are used to fixate the foundation guide to the bone. The pins prevent any movement of the guide during the osteotomy process. (Fig. 33.19F, G).

Clinician (Surgery: Appointment #2)

1. Remaining teeth are extracted if indicated, along with debridement of the extraction sockets (Fig. 33.21A–C).
2. The tissue is reflected to expose the residual ridge. The flap design is dictated on the size of the guide.

NOTE: The guide should be evaluated so that it is fully seated, with no rocking or movement. Caution should be exercised to verify no tissue impingement underneath the guide. The *bone foundation guide* is fixated with fixation pins to prevent movement of the guide during osteotomy preparation. Usually three to four fixation pins are used, which are based on the implant positions (Fig. 33.21D).

3. If bone reduction is indicated, the bone is reduced to the level of the guide with bone reduction burs. Therefore the bone foundation guide acts as a bone reduction guide.
4. The *stackable surgical guide* is placed over the bone foundation guide. The osteotomies are prepared according to the fully guided surgical protocol that is specific to the implant system being used. All implants are placed into the final position and the stackable surgical guide is removed (Fig. 33.21E–G).
5. The *stackable multi-unit guide* is then positioned onto the bone foundation guide. This guide allows for the ideal positioning and placement of the multiunit abutments. Note that multiunit abutments may be straight or angled depending on the implant system being used. The multiunit abutments are torqued according to the manufacturer's instructions and the stackable guide is removed.

NOTE: A periapical radiograph may be taken to verify complete seating of the abutments.

6. The *temporary screw-retained abutments* are placed into the multiunit abutments. The abutment screws should not be finally torqued into place and only tightened with finger pressure (Fig. 33.21H).
7. The *soft silicone jig* is positioned over the temporary abutments. Complete seating of the jig should be verified because this may prevent complete seating of the interim prosthesis (Fig. 33.21I).
8. The *interim prosthesis* (e.g., PMMA, acrylic) is positioned over the temporary abutments and gasket. Complete seating of the prosthesis is verified, along with ideal occlusion. The *bite registration index* is inserted to confirm ideal vertical dimension and centric occlusion. Adjustments are made accordingly to the PMMA prosthesis or occlusal anatomy (Fig. 33.21J).
   • Alternative technique: A duplicate prosthesis may be used to obtain a bite registration or esthetic modification to be used in the final prosthesis.

9. Fixating Interim Prosthesis to Temporary Abutments: The interim prosthesis is then luted to the temporary abutments via light-cure composite (i.e., also may use self- or dual-cure acrylic) through injection vents present in the interim prosthesis. Patient closes in centric occlusion; light-cured composite is flowed through predrilled holes. The flowable acrylic is cured via a curing light. The silicone jig will prevent composite/acrylic from flowing into the abutment/sulcus area (Fig. 33.21K and 33.21L).
10. The screws holding the interim prosthesis to the abutments are loosened and removed. The prosthesis is inspected for voids between the temporary abutments and the interim prosthesis. Composite/acrylic is added accordingly. The prosthesis is then polished and reseated, with screws torqued to the manufacturer's recommendations. Access holes are filled with sterilized polytetrafluoroethylene tape (plumber's tape) and light-cured composite.
    • NOTE: Alternative treatment: Before the final seating of the interim prosthesis, a clear duplicate prosthesis can be used to obtain jaw records and final impression for the final prosthesis fabrication.

Clinician (Prosthetic: Appointment #3)

• After sufficient healing, the clinician confirms the correct vertical dimension, occlusion, shade, and contours of the prosthesis. The interim prosthesis is removed and a final impression completed. A verification jig maybe used for the obtaining an accurate impression. Sectioned acrylic blocks which contain titanium cylinder are secured onto each implant. Each cylinder is luted together and the final impression is taken. If no changes are indicated, the laboratory is instructed to complete the final prosthesis, which most commonly is a monolithic zirconia full-arch prosthesis.

Clinician (Prosthetic: Appointment #4)

• The clinician inserts the final prosthesis after removal of the interim prosthesis.
• The interim prosthesis is saved as a backup prosthesis or may be used as a possible future provisional if the need should arise (Fig. 33.21M).

B. Tissue-Supported Surgical Guide

Same procedure as described in part A with the following exceptions:
1. Dual Scan CBCT is utilized for the fabrication of the tissue supported guide.
2. A tissue foundation guide is used instead of the bone foundation guide (Fig. 33.2L).
3. The tissue is not reflected and the procedure is completed flapless.
4. No bone reduction guide is used.

Complications of Fixed Provisional Prostheses

If basic prosthodontic principles are not adhered to when placing a provisional prosthesis, complications may become more prevalent. Ideally the prosthesis should not interfere with soft tissue healing, cantilevers should be limited and avoided if possible, occlusal tables narrowed buccal-lingually, and even and ideal occlusal contacts. Suarez-Feito et al.[98] evaluated the complications in 242 consecutively treated patients, with more than 1000 implants supporting a provisional prosthesis. During the first 60 to 90 days, 8.3% of patients had at least one fracture, with 7.4% occurring within the first 4 weeks. In total, 8.3% of the patients had at least one fracture and 7.4% of the restorations fractured, of which more than half occurred during the first 4 weeks. When the opposing occlusion was an implant-supported prosthesis, the fracture risk

was 4.7 times higher. The maxillary arch had a 3.5 times greater fracture risk.[98] Nikellis et al.[99] reported similar results, which included a 16.6% fracture rate with provisional prostheses when the opposing dentition was an implant-supported prosthesis. To combat the higher complication rate in the maxilla, Collaert and De Bruyn[100] suggested a metal framework to reinforce the provisional reconstruction, as their study showed seven out of nine provisional prostheses resulted with early fractures. After changing their protocol to include a cast metal bar, no additional fractures were seen.[100] In addition, speech-related issues have been shown to be problematic. In the maxilla, usually because of implant position and increased structural reinforcement, compromised space for the tongue has been shown. Therefore because of the bulkiness, patients often reported this problem. Molly et al.[101] reported that

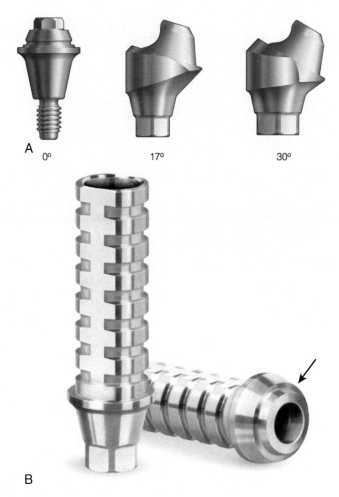

A   0°   17°   30°

B

• **Fig. 33.20** (A) Multiunit abutments with varying angulations that depend on implant trajectory. Most commonly, the multi-unit abutments are available in 0°, 17°, and 30° (B) Temporary abutments that insert into the multiunit abutments that secure the prosthesis to the implants. Usually, non-engaging abutments (arrow) are used for full arch cases.

10% of maxillary immediate-loaded implant prostheses resulted in patients exhibiting nonadaptable speech deterioration. Van Lierde et al.[102] showed similar results with immediate-loaded All-on-4 prostheses, where 53% of patients had related speech issues. The most common reason was the palatal positioning of implants with angulated abutments (Fig. 33.23).

Immediate Load Implant Overdentures

The immediate-load concept for mandibular overdentures has been discussed in the literature for more than 50 years. The subperiosteal implant and the mandibular staple implant were loaded immediately after insertion and fulfilled the immediate-load definition. Babbush et al.[103] reported on immediate-loaded overdentures in the early 1980s, with threaded root form implants. More recently, Chiapasco et al.[104] documented implant success rates of 88% to 97% over 5 to 13 years. In theory the risk of joining implants together with a bar for an implant overdenture is less than for a fixed prosthesis, because the patient may remove the restoration at night to eliminate the risk for nocturnal parafunction. In addition, the overdenture may have some inherent movement and load to the soft tissue, which adds a stress relief system for the rigid implants.

The treatment plan for implant number and position for implant overdentures that are completely implant supported (i.e., RP-4 prosthesis) should be similar to a fixed restoration. If the prosthesis has no movement while in place, then it cannot gain support from the soft tissue. Although the prosthesis may be removed, it is completely implant supported during function or parafunction.

In contrast, a RP-5 prosthesis primarily loads the soft tissue with secondary support from the implants. Implant overdentures with hard and soft tissue support may be at increased risk for immediate loading because the biomechanical torque to the implants may be increased compared with completely implant-supported restorations. One should exercise care relative to the amount and direction of prosthesis movement during the initial loading period.

The use of a single immediate implant has been documented by numerous authors in the literature. Cordioli et al.[105] and Krennmair and Ulm[106] both concluded that one implant placed in the mandibular midline was a credible treatment, in particular for elderly patients with dentures who are experiencing masticatory complications. In addition, positive outcomes such as satisfaction and improved health-related quality of life, along with good functional outcomes, were reported to be greater.

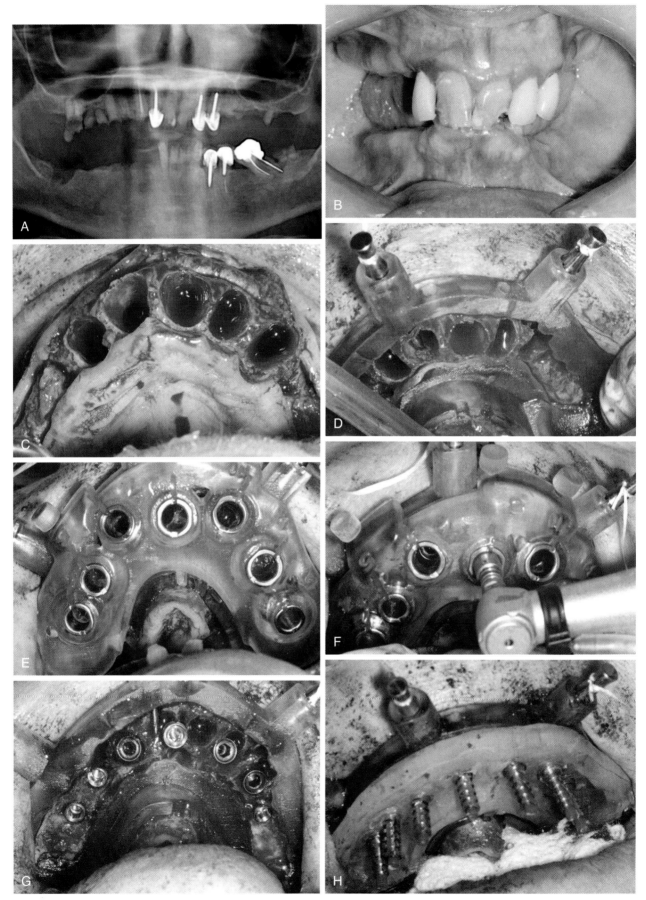

Continued

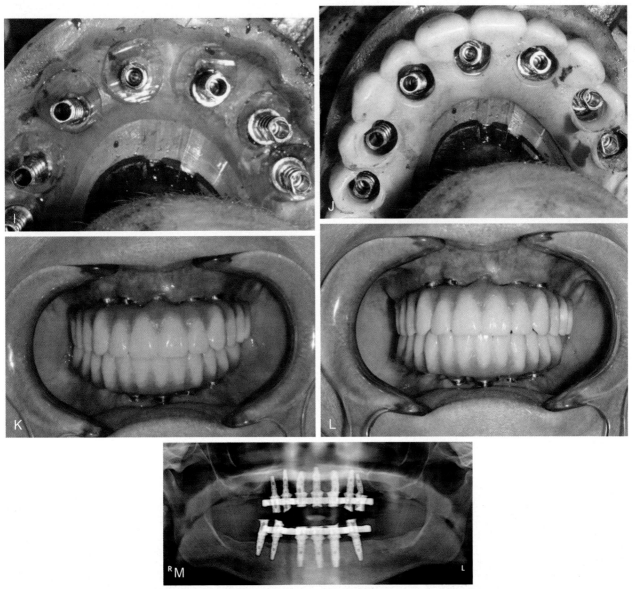

• **Fig. 33.21** (A) Preoperative panoramic displaying nonrestorable maxillary and mandibular teeth. (B) Intraoral view of nonrestorable teeth. (C) Extraction of maxillary teeth. (D) Bone foundation guide fixated on the residual ridge. This guide is also used as a bone reduction guide. (E) Stackable surgical guide: guide that inserts into the bone foundation guide, which is used to prepare osteotomies and placement of implants. (F) Implant placement via fully guided template. (G) Implant placement in maxilla. (H) Temporary screw-retained abutments inserted into the multiunit abutments. (I) Soft silicone jig is placed over the abutments to prevent composite/acrylic from flowing into the tissue spaces. (J) Polymethylmethacrylate (PMMA) provisional prosthesis: try-in of the PMMA prosthesis to verify complete seating. (K) Final insert of maxillary and mandibular PMMA interim prostheses. (L) Final insert of maxillary and mandibular zirconia prostheses. (M) Final postoperative prosthesis panoramic radiograph.

Liddelow and Henry[107] reported on a 36-month prospective study evaluating a single-implant overdenture that is restored immediately into function. They concluded that a single implant with an oxidized surface may provide beneficial outcomes with minimal financial outlay for the patient (Fig. 33.24).

Ormianer et al.[108] reported on a modified loading protocol with two implants that were immediately loaded in the mandible. A success rate of 96.4% was achieved with a modified fixation technique. Impregum (3M ESPE) was used to provide retention for the prosthesis during the early phases of treatment, as the impression material was changed every 2 weeks for the first 3 months (Fig. 33.25).

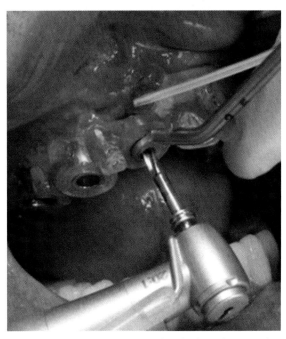

• **Fig. 33.22** A Tissue-supported immediate implant placement is a flapless procedure which has a high incidence of complications and does not allow for ideal bone grafting of defects around placed implants.

Immediate Load Overdenture Treatment Protocol

Immediate Load Implant Overdentures

a. *Immediate loading:* After implant placement, abutments are placed into the implant bodies. The patient's current prosthesis is modified to seat completely, without interferences from the denture. The appropriate female attachment is directly secured to the denture base with light-cured attachment acrylic/composite. After adequate healing, conventional prosthetic protocols may be used to fabricate a new prosthesis with either single or splinted implant attachments.

b. *Early loading:* At the time of implant placement a final impression is made of the existing implants. At the postoperative appointment, jaw records are completed, with the correct vertical dimension and bite registration. Conventional prosthetic protocol is then adhered to complete the final prosthesis with either single or splinted attachments.

Immediate Loading: Postoperative Instructions

Diet

If the immediately loaded prosthesis becomes partially uncemented or fractures, the remaining implants attached to the restoration are at increased risk for overload failure. Therefore the diet of the patient should be limited to only soft foods during the immediate-loading process. Pasta and fish are acceptable, whereas hard crusts of bread, meat, and raw vegetables or fruits are contraindicated.

Final Prosthesis

After sufficient healing is completed (~ 4 - 8 months), The interim prosthesis is removed and a final impression is obtained to fabricate the final prosthesis.

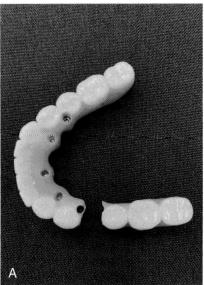
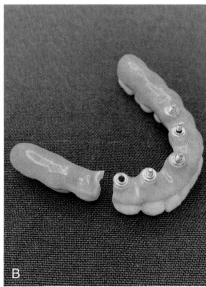
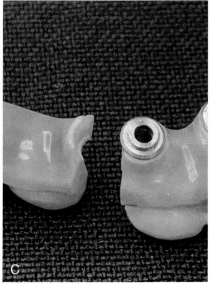

• **Fig. 33.23** Fractured Polymethylmethacrylate (PMMA) Prosthesis. (A to C) The most common complication for a PMMA interim prosthesis is a fractured substructure. The enclosed images depict a fracture, mainly because of the large cantilever that is present.

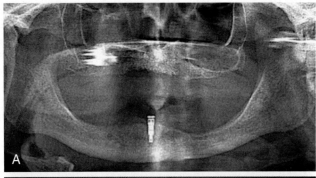

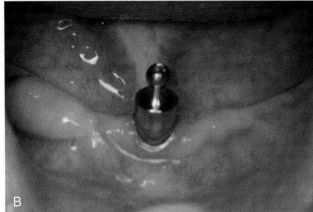

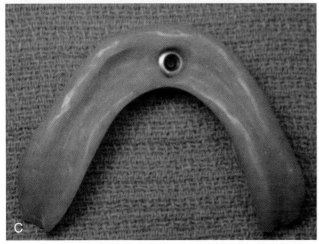

• **Fig. 33.24** Immediate Single-Implant Overdenture. (A) One implant placed in the midline that results in varying results of patient satisfaction. (B) O-ring attachment placed. (C) Prosthesis with O-ring attachment.

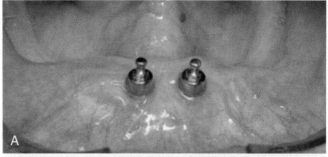

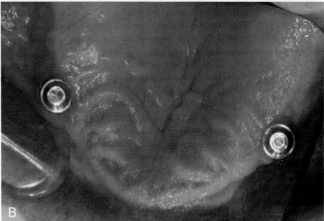

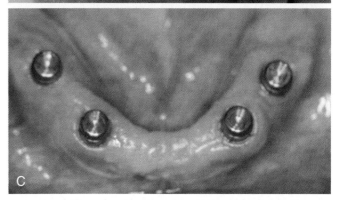

• **Fig. 33.25** Immediate-Loading Overdenture. (A) Mandibular Two-Implant O-Ring Attachment Overdenture, (B) Maxillary Two Implant Overdenture which is usually inadeqaute support for a Maxillary Overdenture, (C) Four Implant Overdenture will allows for greater support.

Immediate Loading: Postoperative Complications

Full-Arch Immediate Prosthesis (Multiunit Abutments)

Göthberg et al.[109] compared two types of multiunit abutments (one oxidized and the other machined) versus implant prostheses without abutments supporting fixed prosthesis (i.e., FP-3) with either an immediate- or delayed-loading protocol. There was no significant difference in marginal bone loss between the distinct loading protocols. However, implants with machined multiunit abutments presented significantly less marginal bone loss after 3 years in comparison with oxidized abutments or no abutments.

Full-Arch Immediate Prosthesis (Connection/ Disconnection of Healing Abutments)

Numerous researchers have evaluated the effect of placing the definitive (final) abutment at the time of the implant placement versus at a later stage on the soft and hard tissues. Molina et al.[113] evaluated the connection and disconnection of healing abutments versus the final abutment being placed at the time of insertion with early-loaded implants. They determined that the continued connection/disconnection of the abutment led to bone loss during the healing phase. This study supported other immediate-placed implant studies with similar outcomes.[110-112] Therefore throughout the full-arch immediate prosthesis protocol, the fewer the number of times healing abutments are connected/disconnected, the less bone loss will result. The connection of the abutment at the time of implant placement seems to reduce bone level changes during the 6- month healing period, compared with the use of standard healing abutments (which are continuously removed during the prosthetic process).

Summary

The delivery of care for patients missing one or all of their teeth often requires implants to restore function, esthetics, bone and soft tissue contours, speech, and intraoral health. The delayed occlusal-loading protocol, either the one- or two-stage approach, has been evaluated for more than 30 years by a number of clinical settings and situations. However, in some patient conditions the delayed healing process can cause psychological, social, speech, and/or function problems. A full range of treatment options relative to the initial hard and soft tissue healing is available. Immediate restoration of a patient after implant surgery is one of these alternatives.

A benefit/risk ratio may be assessed for each patient condition to ascertain whether immediate occlusal loading is a worthwhile alternative. The greater the benefit and/or the lower the risk, the more likely that immediate loading is considered. A complete edentulous mandible restored with an overdenture supported by four or more implants is a very low-risk condition. If the patient cannot tolerate a mandibular denture and does not wear the device, then an immediate-load protocol would be a high benefit. The highest risk for immediate loading would be a posterior single-tooth implant. Implant number cannot be increased, and implant length cannot engage cortical bone. When the single-tooth replacement is out of the esthetic zone, very low benefit is obtained with the immediate-restoration approach.

Additional clinical studies to evaluate the associated risks, especially in the maxillary arch, are expected over the next several years. Until the profession has longer-term evidence and more multicenter studies, immediate occlusal loading will be a secondary treatment option, restricted on a case-by-case basis.

A biomechanical rational for immediate loading may decrease the risk for occlusal overload during initial healing. The stresses applied to the implant support system result in strain to the bone interface. The greater the stress, the higher is the strain. Increasing implant area and/or reducing the forces applied to the prosthesis may reduce stress. The implant size, design, and surface condition all affect the area over which the occlusal forces are dissipated. The forces may be reduced by patient factors, implant position, reducing force magnifiers such as crown height or cantilever length, reducing the occlusal contacts, decreasing angled forces to the prostheses, and altering the diet. The mechanical properties of bone also affect the risk for overload, because the bone density is directly related to the strength of bone, its elastic modulus, and the amount of BIC. All of these factors are important in the traditional two-stage approach. They are especially noteworthy for immediate loading, because the surgical trauma of placing the implant also modifies the mechanical properties of bone during initial healing.

The majority of clinical reports reveal similar survival rates between immediate-loaded and two-stage unloaded healing approaches in the completely edentulous patient. Nonetheless, these findings do not imply that a submerged surgical approach is no longer necessary or prudent in many cases. Future studies may find indications based on surgical, host, implant, and occlusal conditions more beneficial for one versus the other. For example, the strength of bone and the modulus of elasticity are related directly to bone density. The softest bone type may be 10 times weaker than for the densest types. The microstrain mismatch of titanium and the softest bone is much greater than the densest bone. As a result, higher implant failure and greater crestal bone loss seem likely but as yet are not reported in the literature. The biomechanical treatment approach to increase surface area and decrease forces applied to the immediate restorations is most likely the major reason for the high implant survival.

References

1. Brånemark PI, Hansson BO, Adell R, et al. Osseointegrated implants in the treatment of edentulous jaw: experience from a 10 year period. *Scand J Plast Reconstr Surg.* 1977;2(10):1–132.
2. Adell R, Lekholm U, Rockler B, et al. A 15-year study of osseointegrated implants in the treatment of the edentulous jaw. *Int J Oral Surg.* 1981;10:387–416.
3. Van Steenberghe D, Lekholm N, Bolender C, et al. The applicability of osseointegrated oral implants in the rehabilitation of partial edentulism: a prospective multi-center study of 558 fixtures. *Int J Oral Maxillofac Implants.* 1990;5:272–281.
4. Misch CE, Wang HL, Misch CM, et al. Rationale for the application of immediate load in implant dentistry. I. *Implant Dent.* 2004;13:207–215.
5. Blomberg S, Lindquist LW. Psychological reactions to edentulousness and treatment with jawbone-anchored bridges. *Acta Psychiatr Scand.* 1983;68:251–262.
6. Becker W, Becker BE, Israelson H, et al. One-step surgical placement of Braºnemark implants: a prospective multicenter clinical study. *Int J Oral Maxillofac Implants.* 1997;12:454–462.
7. Schroeder A, van der Zypen E, Stich H, Sutter F. The reactions of bone, connective tissue, and epithelium to endosteal implants with titanium-sprayed surfaces. *J Maxillofac Surg.* 1981;9:15–25.
8. Piattelli A, Ruggeri A, Franchi M, Romasco N, Trisi P. An histologic and histomorphometric study of bone reactions to unloaded and loaded non-submerged single implants in monkeys: a pilot study. *J Oral Implantol.* 1993;19:314–320.
9. Piattelli A, Corigliano M, Scarano A, Quaranta M. Bone reactions to early occlusal loading of two-stage titanium plasma-sprayed implants: a pilot study in monkeys. *Int J Periodontics Restorative Dent.* 1997;17:162–169.
10. Piattelli A, Corigliano M, Scarano A, Costigliola G, Paolantonio M. Immediate loading of titanium plasmasprayed implants: an histologic analysis in monkeys. *J Periodontol.* 1998;69:321–327.
11. Testori T, Szmukler-Moncler S, Francetti L, Del Fabbro M, Trisi P, Weinstein RL. Healing of Osseotite implants under submerged and immediate loading conditions in a single patient: a case report and interface analysis after 2 months. *Int J Periodontics Restorative Dent.* 2002;22:345–353.
12. Chrcanovic BR, Albrektsson T, Wennerberg A. Reasons for failures of oral implants. *J Oral Rehabil.* 2014;41:443–476.
13. Lazzara RJ, Testori T, Meltzer A, Craig M, Porter S, Goené RJ. "Immediate Occlusal Loading (IOL) of dental implants: predictable results through DIEM guidelines." *Pract Proced Aesthet Dent: PPAD.* 2004;16(4):3–15.
14. Malo P, de Araújo Nobre M, Lopes A, Francischone C, Rigolizzo M. "All-on-4" immediate-function concept for completely edentulous maxillae: a clinical report on the medium (3 years) and long-term (5 years) outcomes. *Clin Implant Dent Relat Res.* 2012;14(suppl 1):e139–e150. https://doi. org/10.1111/j.1708-8208.2011.00395.x.
15. Malo P, de Araújo Nobre M, Lopes A, Moss SM, Molina GJ. A longitudinal study of the survival of All-on-4 implants in the mandible with up to 10 years of follow-up. *J Am Dent Assoc.* 2011;142:310–320.
16. Schimmel M, Srinivasan M, Herrmann FR, Müller F. Loading protocols for implant-supported overdentures in the edentulous jaw: a systematic review and meta-analysis. *Int J Oral Maxillofac Implants.* 2014;29:S271–S286.

17. Douglas de Oliveira DW, Lages FS, Lanza LA, Gomes AM, Queiroz TP, Costa Fde O. Dental implants with immediate loading using insertion torque of 30 Ncm: a systematic review. *Implant Dent.* 2016;25:675–683.

18. Maló P, Lopes A, de Araújo Nobre M, Ferro A. Immediate function dental implants inserted with less than 30 N·cm of torque in full-arch maxillary rehabilitations using the All-on-4 concept: retrospective study. *Int J Oral Maxillofac surgery.* 2018;47(8):1079–1085.

19. Szmuckler-Moncler S, Piatelli A, Favero GA, Dubruille JH. Considerations preliminary to the application of early and immediate loading protocols in dental implantology. *Clin Oral Impl Res.* 2000;11(1):12–25.

20. Soballe K. Hydroxyapatite ceramic coating for bone implant fixation. Mechanical and histological studies in dogs. *Act Orthop Scan Suppl.* 1993;255:1–58.

21. Vaillancourt H, Pilliar RM, McCammond D. Finite element analysis of crestal bone loss around porous-coated dental implants. *J Appl Biomater.* 1995;6(4):267–282.

22. Sennerby L, Meredith N. Analisi della freuqenza di resonanza (RFA). Conoscenze attuali e implicazioni cliniche. In: Chiapasco M, Gatti C, eds. *Osteointegrazione E Carico Immediato. Fondamenti Biologici e Applicazioni Cliniche.* Milan: Masson; 2002:19–31.

23. Balshi SF, Allen FD, Wolfinger GJ, Balshi TJ. A resonance frequency analysis assessment of maxillary and mandibular immediately loaded implants. *Int J Oral Maxillofac Implants.* 2005;20(4).

24. Lazzara RJ, Testori T, Meltzer A, Craig M, Porter S, Goené RJ. "Immediate Occlusal Loading (IOL) of dental implants: predictable results through DIEM guidelines." *Pract Proced Aesthet Dent PPAD.* 2004;16(4):3–15.

25. Romanos G, Tok CG, Sias CH, et al. Peri-implant bone reactions to immediately loaded implants: an experimental study in monkeys. *J Periodontol.* 2001;72:506–511.

26. Buchs AU, Levine L, Moy P. Preliminary report of immediately loaded Altiva Natural Tooth Replacement dental implants. *Clin Implant Dent Relat Res.* 2001;3(2):97–106.

27. Sharawy M. *Immediate vs Delayed Loading in a Canine Model: A Histometric and Volume Fraction Analysis, Unpublished Data*; 2000.

28. Suzuki JB, Misch CE, Sharawy M, et al. Clinical and histological evaluation of immediate loaded posterior implants in non-human primates. *Implant Dent.* 2007;16:176–186.

29. Roberts WE. Bone tissue interface. *J Dent Educ.* 1988;52(12):804–809.

30. Testori T, Szmukler-Moncler S, Francetti L, et al. The immediate loading of Osseotite implants: a case report and histologic analysis after 4 months of occlusal loading. *Int J Perio Restorative Dent.* 2001;21:451–459.

31. Piatelli A, Corigliano M, Scarano A, et al. Bone reactions to early occlusal loading of two-stage titanium plasma-sprayed implants: a pilot study in monkeys. *Int J Periodontics Restorative Dent.* 1997;17:162–169.

32. Eriksson AR, Albrektsson T, Albrektsson B. Heat caused by drilling cortical bone: temperature measured in vivo in patients and animals. *Acta Orthop Scand.* 1984;55(6):629–631.

33. Piatelli A, Corigliano M, Scarano A, et al. Immediate loading of titanium plasma-sprayed implants: an histologic analysis in monkeys. *J Periodontol.* 1998;69:321–327.

34. Romanos G, Tok CG, Sias CH, et al. Peri-implant bone reactions to immediately loaded implants: an experimental study in monkeys. *J Periodontol.* 2001;72:506–511.

35. Horiuchi K, Uchida H, Yamamoto K, et al. Immediate loading of Brånemark system implants following placement in edentulous patients: a clinical report. *Int J Oral Maxillofac Implants.* 2000;15:824–830.

36. Piatelli A, Ruggeri A, Franchi M, et al. An histologic and histomorphic-metric study of bone reactions to unloaded and loaded non-submerged single implants in monkeys: a pilot study. *J Oral Implantol.* 1993;19:314–320.

37. Ledermann PD, Hassell TM, Hefti AF. Osseointegrated dental implants as alternative therapy to bridge construction or orthodontics in young patients: seven years of clinical experience. *Pediatr Dent.* 1993;15(5):327–333.

38. Misch CE. Patient force factors. In: Misch CE, ed. *Contemporary Implant Dentistry.* St Louis: Mosby; 1993.

39. Randow R, Ericsson I, Nilner K, et al. Immediate functional loading of Brånemark dental implants: an 18-month clinical follow-up study. *Clin Oral Implants Res.* 1999;10:8–15.

40. Frost HM. Wolff's Law and bone's structural adaptations to mechanical usage: an overview for clinicians. *Angle Orthod.* 1994;64(3):175–188.

41. Balshi TJ, Wolfinger GJ. Immediate loading of Brånemark implants in edentulous mandible: a preliminary report. *Implant Dent.* 1997;6:83–88.

42. Grunder U. Immediate functional loading of immediate implants in edentulous arches: two-year results. *Int J Periodontics Restorative Dent.* 2002;21:545–551.

43. Barbier L, Schepers E. Adaptive bone remodeling around oral implants under axial and non axial loading conditions in the dog mandible. *Int J Oral Maxillofac Implants.* 1997;12:215–223.

44. Parfitt AM. The physiological and clinical significance of bone histomorphometric data. In: Reck RR, ed. *Bone Histomorphometry, Techniques and Interpretation.* Boca Raton, Fla: CRC Press; 1983.

45. Ganeles J, Rosenberg MM, Holt RL, et al. Immediate loading of implants with fixed restorations in the completely edentulous mandible: report of 27 patients from a private practice. *Int J Oral Maxillofac Implants.* 2001;16:418–426.

46. Jaffin RA, Kumar A, Berman CL. Immediate loading of implants in partially and fully edentulous jaws: a series of 27 case reports. *J Periodontol.* 2000;71:833–838.

47. Misch CE, Degidi M. Immediate loading implants with fixed prostheses in the completely edentulous patient. *Clin Implant Dent Relat Res.* 2003;5:100–203.

48. Misch CE. Divisions of available bone. In: Misch CE, ed. *Contemporary Implant Dentistry.* St Louis: Mosby; 1993.

49. Strong JT, Misch CE, Bidez MW, et al. Functional surface area: thread form parameter optimization for implant body design. *Compend Contin Educ Dent.* 1998;19:4–9.

50. Misch CE, Bidez MW, Sharawy M. A bioengineered implant for an ideal bone cellular response to loading forces: a literature review and case report. *J Periodontol.* 2001;72:1276–1286.

51. Steigenga J. *Thread Geometry and its Effect on Initial Osteointegration Using Reverse Torque Testing and Histometric Analysis* [master's thesis]. Ann Arbor, Mich: University of Michigan; 2003.

52. Reilly DT, Burstein AH. The elastic and ultimate properties of compact bone tissue. *J Biomech.* 1975;80:393–405.

53. Brunski JB. Biomechanical factors affecting the bone-dental implant interface: review paper. *Clin Mater.* 1992;10:153–201.

54. Schnitman DA, Wohrle PS, Rubenstein JE, et al. Brånemark implants immediately loaded with fixed prostheses at implant placement: ten year results. *Int J Oral Maxillofacial Implants.* 1997;12:495–503.

55. Brånemark PI, Engstrand P, Ohrnell LO, et al. Brånemark Novum: a new treatment concept for rehabilitation of the edentulous mandible—preliminary results from a prospective clinical follow-up study. *Clin Implant Dent Relat Res.* 1999;1:2–16.

56. Misch CE. Mandibular full-arch implant fixed prosthetic options. In: Misch CE, ed. *Dental Implant Prosthetics.* St Louis: Mosby; 2005.

57. Misch CE. Density of bone: effect on treatment plans, surgical approach, healing and progressive bone loading. *Int J Oral Implantol.* 1990;6:23–31.

58. Misch CE. Non-functional immediate teeth in partially edentulous patients: a pilot study of 10 consecutive cases using the Maestro dental implant system. *Compend Contin Educ Dent.* 1998;19:25–36.

59. Misch CE. Non-functional immediate teeth. *Dent Today.* 1998;17:88–91.

60. Andersen E, Haanaes HR, Knutsen BM. Immediate loading of single-tooth ITI implants in the anterior maxilla: a prospective 5-year pilot study. *Clin Oral Implants Res.* 2002;13:281–287.

61. Cooper LF, Ellner S, Moriarty J, et al. Three year evaluation of single-tooth implants restored 3 weeks after 1-stage surgery. *Int J Oral Maxillofac Implants.* 2007;22(5):791–800.

62. Gomes A, Lozada JL, Caplanis N, Kleinman A. Immediate loading of a single hydroxyapatite-coated threaded root form implant: a clinical report. *J Oral Implantol.* 1998;24(3):159–166.

63. Ericsson I, Nilson H, Lindh T, Nilner K, Randow K. Immediate functional loading of Bra°nemark single tooth implants. An 18 months_ clinical pilot follow-up study. *Clin Oral Implants Res.* 2000;11:26–33.

64. Hui E, Chow J, Li D, Liu J, Wat P, Law H. Immediate provisional for single-tooth implant replacement with Brånemark system: preliminary report. *Clin Implant Dent Relat Res.* 2001;3(2):79–86.

65. Degidi M, Piattelli A, Gehrik P, Felice P, Carinci F. Five-year outcome of 111 immediate non-functional single restorations. *J Oral Implantol.* 2006;32:277–285.

66. Chaushu G, Chaushu S, Tzohar A, Dayan D. Immediate loading of single-tooth implants: immediate versus nonimmediate implantation. A clinical report. *Int J Oral Maxillofac Implants.* 2001;16(2):267–272.

67. Mankoo T. Contemporary implant concepts in aesthetic dentistry—Part 2: immediate single-tooth implants. *Pract Proced Aesthet Dent.* 2004;16(1):61–68. quiz 70.

68. Pigozzo MN, Rebelo da Costa T, Newton S, Cruz Laganá D. "Immediate versus early loading of single dental implants: a systematic review and meta-analysis". *J Prosthet Dent.* 2018.

69. Testori T, Del Fabbro M, Feldman S, et al. A multicenter prospective evaluation of 2-months loaded Osseotite implants placed in the posterior jaws:3-year follow-up results. *Clin Oral Implants Res.* 2002;13:154–161.

70. Cochran DL, Morton D, Weber HP. Consensus statements and recommended clinical procedures regarding loading protocols for endosseous dental implants. *Int J Oral Maxillofac Implants.* 2004;19:109–113.

71. Luongo G, Di Raimondo R, Filippini P, Gualini F, Paoleschi C. Early loading of sandblasted, acid-etched implants in the posterior maxilla and mandible: a 1-year follow-up report from a multicenter 3-year prospective study. *Int J Oral Maxillofac Implants.* 2005;20:84–91.

72. Vanden Bogaerde L, Pedretti G, Dellacasa P, Mozzati M, Rangert B, Wendelhag I. Early function of splinted implants in maxillas and posterior mandibles, using Bra°nemark System Tiunite implants: an 18-month prospective clinical multicenter study. *Clin Implant Dent Relat Res.* 2004;6:121–129.

73. Drago CJ, Lazzara RJ. Immediate provisional restoration of Osseotite implants: a clinical report of 18-month results. *Int J Oral Maxillofac Implants.* 2004;19:534–541.

74. Machtei EE, Frankenthal S, Blumenfeld I, Gutmacher Z, Horwitz J. Dental implants for immediate fixed restorations of partially edentulous patients: a 1-year prospective pilot clinical trial in periodontally susceptible patients. *J Periodontol.* 2007;78:1188–1194.

75. Schincaglia GP, Marzola R, Scapoli C, Scotti R. Immediate loading of dental implants supporting fixed partial dentures in the posterior mandible: a randomized controlled split-mouth study—turned versus titanium oxide implant surface. *Int J Oral Maxillofac Implants.* 2007;22:35–46.

76. Engquist B, Astrand P, Anze´n B, et al. Simplified methods of implant treatment in the edentulous lower jaw. A controlled prospective study. Part II: early loading. *Clin Implant Dent Relat Res.* 2004;6:90–100.

77. Engquist B, A°strand P, Anze´n B, et al. Simplified methods of implant treatment in the edentulous lower jaw: a 3-year follow-up report of a controlled prospective study of one-stage versus two-stage surgery and early loading. *Clin Implant Dent Relat Res.* 2005;7:95–104.

78. Friberg B, Henningsson C, Jemt T. Rehabilitation of edentulous mandibles by means of turned Bra°nemark System implants after one-stage surgery: a 1-year retrospective study of 152 patients. *Clin Implant Dent Relat Res.* 2005;7:1–9.

79. Schnitman PA, Wohrle PS, Rubenstein JE. Immediate fixed interim prostheses supported by two-stage threaded implants: methodology and results. *J Oral Implantol.* 1990;16:96–105.

80. Schnitman PA, Wohrle PS, Rubenstein JE, DaSilva JD, Wang NH. Ten-year results for Bra°nemark implants immediately loaded with fixed prostheses at implant placement. *Int J Oral Maxillofac Implants.* 1997;12:495–503.

81. Tarnow DP, Emtiaz S, Classi A. Immediate loading of threaded implants at stage 1 surgery in edentulous arches: ten consecutive case reports with 1- to 5-year data. *Int J Oral Maxillofac Implants.* 1997;12:319–324.

82. Chow J, Hui E, Liu J. Immediate loading of Bra°nemark system fixtures in the mandible with a fixed provisional prosthesis. *Appl Osseointegration Res.* 2001;1:30–35.

83. Testori T, Szmukler-Moncler S, Francetti L, et al. Immediate loading of Osseotite implants: a case report and histologic analysis after 4 months of occlusal loading. *Int J Periodontics Restorative Dent.* 2001;21:451–459.

84. Aalam AA, Nowzari H, Krivitsky A. Functional restoration of implants on the day of surgical placement in the fully edentulous mandible: a case series. *Clin Implant Dent Relat Res.* 2005;7:10–16.

85. Fischer K, Stenberg T. Three-year data from a randomized, controlled study of early loading of single-stage dental implants supporting maxillary full-arch prostheses. *Int J Oral Maxillofac Implants.* 2006;21:245–252.

86. Olsson M, Urde G, Andersen JB, Sennerby L. Early loading of maxillary fixed cross-arch dental prostheses supported by six or eight oxidized titanium implants: results after 1 year of loading, case series. *Clin Implant Dent Relat Res.* 2003;5(1):81–87.

87. Bergkvist G, Sahlholm S, Karlsson U, Nilner K, Lindh C. Immediately loaded implants supporting fixed prostheses in the edentulous maxilla: a preliminary clinical and radiologic report. *Int J Oral Maxillofac Implants.* 2005;20:399–405.

88. Ibanez JC, Tahhan MJ, Zamar JA, et al. Immediate occlusal loading of double acid-etched surface titanium implants in 41 consecutive full-arch cases in the mandible and maxilla: 6- to 74-month results. *J Periodontol.* 2005;76:1972–1981.

89. Degidi M, Piattelli A. Immediate functional and nonfunctional loading of dental implants: a 2- to 60-month follow-up study of 646 titanium implants. *J Periodontol.* 2003;74:225–241.

90. Balshi SF, Wolfinger GJ, Balshi TJ. A prospective study of immediate functional loading, following the Teeth in a Day protocol: a case series of 55 consecutive edentulous maxillas. *Clin Implant Dent Relat Res.* 2005;7:24–31.

91. Balkin BE, Steflik DE, Naval F. Mini-dental implant insertion with the auto-advance technique for ongoing applica- tions. *J Oral Implantol.* 2001;27:32–37.

92. Iezzi G, Pecora G, Scarano A, Perrotti V, Piattelli A. Histologic evaluation of 3 retrieved immediately loaded implants after a 4-month period. *Implant Dent.* 2006;15:305–312.

93. Heberer S, Hildebrand D, Nelson K. Survival rate and potential influential factors for two transitional implant systems in edentulous patients: a prospective clinical study. *J Oral Rehabil.* 2011;38:447–453.

94. Simon H, Caputo AA. Removal torque of immediately loaded transitional endosseous implants in human subjects. *Int J Oral Maxillofac Implants.* 2002;17:839–845.

95. Malo P, Rangert B, Nobre M. "All-on-Four" immediate-function concept with Brånemark system implants for completely edentulous mandibles: a retrospective clinical study. *Clin Implant Dent Relat Res.* 2003;5(1):2–9.

96. Malo P, Rangert B, Nobre M. All-on-4 immediate-function concept with Brånemark system implants for completely edentulous maxillae: a 1-year retrospective clinical study. *Clin Implant Dent Relat Res.* 2005;7(1):S88–S94.

97. Pikos MA, Magyar CW, Llop DR. "Guided full-arch immediate-function treatment modality for the edentulous and terminal dentition patient." *Compend Contin Educ Dent (Jamesburg, NJ: 1995).* 2015;36(2):116–119.

98. Suarez-Feito JM, Sicilia A, Angulo J, Banerji S, Cuesta I, Millar B. Clinical performance of provisional screw-retained metal-free acrylic restorations in an immediate loading implant protocol: a 242 consecutive patients' report. *Clin Oral Implants Res.* 2010;21:1360–1369.

99. Nikellis I, Levi A, Nicolopoulos C. Immediate loading of 190 endosseous dental implants: a prospective observational study of 40 patient treatments with up to 2-year data. *Int J Oral Maxillofac Implants.* 2004;19:116–123.

100. Collaert B, De Bruyn H. Immediate functional loading of TiOblast dental implants in full-arch edentulous maxillae: a 3-year prospective study. *Clin Oral Implants Res.* 2008;19:1254–1260.

101. Molly L, Nackaerts O, Vandewiele K, Manders E, van Steenberghe D, Jacobs R. Speech adaptation after treatment of full edentulism through immediate-loaded implant protocols. *Clin Oral Implants Res.* 2008;19:86–90.

102. Van Lierde K, Browaeys H, Corthals P, Mussche P, Van Kerkhoven E, De Bruyn H. Comparison of speech intelligibility, articulation and oromyofunctional behaviour in subjects with single-tooth implants, fixed implant prosthetics or conventional removable prostheses. *J Oral RehaBil.* 2012;39:285–293.

103. Babbush CA, Kent JN, Misiek DJ. Titanium plasma spray (TPS) screw implants for the reconstruction of the edentulous mandible. *J Oral Maxillofac Surg.* 1986;44:274–282.

104. Chiapasco M, Gatti C, Rossi F, et al. Implant-retained mandibular overdentures with immediate loading: a retrospective multicenter study on 226 consecutive cases. *Clin Oral Implants Res.* 1997;8:48–54.

105. Cordioli G, Majzoub Z, Castagna S. "Mandibular overdentures anchored to single implants: a five-year prospective study." *J Prosthet Dent.* 1997;78(2):159–165.

106. Krennmair G, Ulm C. "The symphyseal single-tooth implant for anchorage of a mandibular complete denture in geriatric patients: a clinical report." *Int J Oral Maxillofac Implants.* 2001;16(1).

107. Liddelow G, Henry P. "The immediately loaded single implant—retained mandibular overdenture: a 36-month prospective study." *Int J Prosthodont.* 2010;23(1).

108. Ormianer Z, Garg AK, Ady P. "Immediate loading of implant overdentures using modified loading protocol." *Implant Dentistry.* 2006;15(1):35–40.

109. Göthberg C, André U, Gröndahl K, Thomsen P, Slotte C. Bone response and soft tissue changes around implants with/without abutments supporting fixed partial dentures: results from a 3-year prospective, randomized, controlled study. *Clin Implant Dent Relat Res.* 2016;18:309–322.

110. Canullo L, Bignozzi I, Cocchetto R, Cristalli MP, Iannello G. Immediate positioning of a definitive abutment versus repeated abutment replacements in post-extractive implants: 3-year follow-up of a randomised multicentre clinical trial. *Eur J Oral Implantol.* 2010;3:285–296.

111. Degidi M, Nardi D, Daprile G, Piattelli A. Nonremoval of immediate abutments in cases involving subcrestally placed postextractive tapered single implants: a randomized controlled clinical study. *Clin Implant Dent Relat Res.* 2014;16:794–805.

112. Grandi T, Guazzi P, Samarani R, Maghaireh H, Grandi G. One abutment/one-time versus a provisional abutment in immediately loaded post-extractive single implants: a 1-year follow-up of a multicentre randomised controlled trial. *Eur J Oral Implantol.* 2014;7:141–149.

113. Molina A, Sanz-Sánchez I, Martín C, Blanco J, Sanz M. The effect of one-time abutment placement on interproximal bone levels and peri-implant soft tissues: a prospective randomized clinical trial. *Clin Oral Implants Res.* 2016;00:1–10.

114. ÖStman PO. "Immediate/early loading of dental implants. Clinical documentation and presentation of a treatment concept." *Periodontol 2000.* 2008;47(1):90–112.

115. Ferro Keith J, Morgano SM, Driscoll CF, et al. "The glossary of prosthodontic terms." *J Prosthet Dent.* 2017.

PART VII

Soft and Hard Tissue Rehabilitation

34

Atraumatic Tooth Extraction and Socket Grafting

RANDOLPH R. RESNIK AND JON B. SUZUKI

It is imperative that the implant clinician has a strong understanding of the extraction socket healing process and options for the socket graft site preservation technique. In most cases the extraction process will initiate a sequence of bony resorptive morphologic changes that negatively alters the alveolar ridge. This chapter will discuss the process of atraumatic extraction and a decision process on when no graft is indicated and when to graft (i.e., protocol on various bone substitutes, membranes, and healing periods).

Extraction Socket Healing

In understanding the healing process of the extraction site, the terminology is often misrepresented (Box 34.1). The process of bone repair occurs when there is injury or conditions of the bone that cause incomplete bone volume to form in the residual ridge. The most common conditions that cause bone repair are the absence of a labial plate before or as a consequence of tooth extraction. Other factors include a bony wall that is less than 1.5 mm thick (usually the facial), exudate, gross apical pathology, or excessive heat from a dental drill during root extraction.

The tooth socket with five bony walls (i.e., mesial, distal, buccal, lingual, and apical) will heal by bone regeneration (Fig. 34.1). The process of bone regeneration heals by secondary intention, and bone healing in many aspects is similar to secondary intention soft tissue healing. The healing sequence in both hard and soft tissue includes inflammation, epithelialization, fibroplasia, and remodeling. However, socket healing presents unique microvascular features and a sequential pattern of bone formation before remodeling.

Numerous authors in the literature have proposed the healing sequence and various stages of bone regeneration after a tooth is extracted with a healthy surrounding alveolus.

Stage 1: Granulation Stage: After a tooth is extracted, an initial clot forms within the socket which consists of a "coagulum" of red and white blood cells. At approximately the third day, the coagulum is slowly replaced by highly vascular granulation tissue. The blood clot begins to shrink, and capillaries form sinusoids and granulation tissue, starting from the socket apex and spreading laterally and crestally along the socket walls. Granulation tissue replaces the clot over a 4-to 5-day period.[1,2]

Stage 2: Initial Angiogenic Stage: The initial angiogenic stage starts approximately a week after extraction. This stage develops from the broken ends of blood vessels in the residual periodontal ligament covering the cribriform plate. Blood plasma leaks from the broken vessels, and immature fibroblasts aggregate at the plasma-rich regions. Fibroplasia begins early in the sequence during the first week as a result of the ingrowth of capillaries and fibroblasts. White blood cells kill bacteria and begin to dissolve foreign bodies and bone fragments. With few exceptions the angiogenesis begins at the bottom of the socket because this area is not severely injured during the extraction and has the greatest source of blood vessels.[3]

Stage 3: Early Bone Formation Stage: This stage starts approximately three to four weeks after extraction. The granulation tissue gradually is replaced by connective tissue (collagen fibers, spindle shaped fibroblasts). The capillary activity begins the early phases of trabeculae development. This capillary activity is initiated at the socket apex, and trabeculae of woven bone growth will occur following the formation of blood vessels. During this stage, the cortical bone of the crestal area of the socket will start to resorb, along with the interseptal regions and the thinner facial plate.[4]

Stage 4: Bone Growth Stage: The bone growth stage starts at approximately four to six weeks after the extraction. This period demonstrates the greatest sinusoid formation activity. The forming trabeculae of woven bone first start from the bottom of the socket after the meshwork of newly formed anastomosing sinusoidal capillaries. Bone formation is more rapid at this point, creating a three-dimensional lattice pattern of woven bone. New bone trabeculae form on the walls and approximately two-thirds of the socket is filled at four – five weeks. At this stage, the center of the socket is primarily composed of woven bone. The more-organized lamellar bone starts to form from the lining of the socket, moving toward the center. At approximately 6 weeks, bone trabeculae almost completely fill the socket.[5]

Stage 5: Bone Reorganization Stage: The bone reorganization stage starts at about 6 weeks after extraction. Usually complete epithelial closure of the socket is completed by this time. The primary bone trabeculae remodel to form thicker secondary cancellous bone. This process always begins at the apex of the extraction socket. At approximately 60 days, woven bone has completely bridged the defect and at 90 days, woven bone is resorbed by osteoclasts which is replaced by lamellar bone. The bridged woven bone is usually completely remodeled to lamellar bone by 16

- **Bone remodeling**—the replacement of old bone tissue by new bone tissue; natural phenomena to maintain healthy bone mass
- **Bone modeling**—adapts bone size and shape to stress or loading
- **Bone repair**—a physiologic process in which the body facilitates the repair of a bone fracture
- **Bone regeneration**—requires the use of surgical protocols that enable bone growth within deficient sites, using the principles of osteogenesis, osteoinduction, and osteoconduction
- **Socket restoration versus preservation**—difficult to differentiate; both terms are used
  - Bone is restored in the socket (generally for the placement of an implant)
  - Bone preservation indicates long-term stability of the alveolar ridge

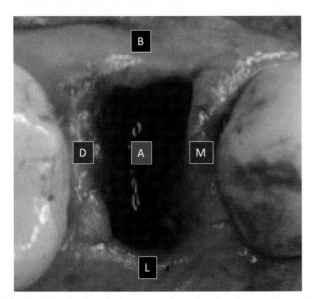

• **Fig. 34.1** The treatment plan and protocol for a post-extraction socket is dictated by five bony walls: mesial (*M*), distal (*D*), buccal (*B*), lingual (*L*), and apical (*A*).

weeks and most osteogenic activity is complete at this time. A new periosteum is established by 180 days.[6,7,8]

The timing for these stages varies among individuals and clinical situations. The number of bony walls around the socket and size of the alveolus greatly influence the regeneration process. In general, larger molar extraction sites (i.e. molar) take longer to completely form bone compared with smaller-diameter anterior sites. Although the period of regeneration for an extraction socket is variable, the clinical sign that the socket regeneration is complete is when the radiographic lamina dura (which represents the cribriform plate) is no longer present. This healing period usually takes between 3 to 6 months, dependent on tooth size, root number, and extent of trauma during the extraction (Fig. 34.2).

Importance of the Buccal Plate

One of the most important factors in the regeneration and repair of bone is the buccal plate. The buccal plate of bone is more susceptible to bone loss. Studies have shown the buccal plate may lose up to 56% horizontal bone loss and 30% vertical bone loss within the first year after extraction.[9,10] In addition, when the buccal plate is thicker, the ridge tends to resorb less. The buccal plate is also more susceptible to trauma. When iatrogenic buccal plate damage occurs, the socket no longer heals by regeneration, however will heal by repair. This is usually a slower healing process and more unpredictable (Fig. 34.3).

Atraumatic Tooth Extraction

Theory of Atraumatic Tooth Extraction

There exists a full array of reasons teeth are deemed unrestorable; periodontal, endodontic, prosthetic, or orthodontic failures. Once the extraction of a natural tooth is indicated, methods to maintain or obtain the surrounding hard and soft tissues are indicated. It is the primary goal of the implant clinician to extract the nonrestorable tooth while minimizing associated trauma and maintaining the hard and soft tissue.

The atraumatic tooth extraction technique and socket grafting has become a popular procedure in implant dentistry. The process of atraumatic tooth extraction and preservation of soft and hard tissues begins with the surrounding soft tissue. The cells of the inner layer of the periosteum are responsible for bone remodeling. When the bone volume is ideal, the periosteum should be minimally reflected in preservation of the blood supply. However, the periosteum can also be a limiting factor in the volume of bone formation. When the periosteum is separated from the bone graft by a barrier membrane, more volume of bone is regenerated. The periosteum helps bone remodeling or bone repair, but may also limit bone modeling and regeneration.

Atraumatic Tooth Extraction Technique

Many techniques and protocols exist for removing teeth; however, some basic principles should be applied to all extractions.

Severing the Connective Tissue Fibers

The soft tissue drape surrounding the teeth is affected by the reflection of the periosteum and often shrinks to adapt to the residual ridge form. In fact, the soft tissue is more labile to the trauma and reflection of the tissues than the hard tissues. Therefore the sulcular and surrounding soft tissue should ideally remain undisturbed during tooth extraction to prevent further dimensional loss. The extraction of a natural tooth begins with an incision within the sulcus, preferably with a thin scalpel blade or a blunt periotome. The incision should encompass the entire tooth (i.e., 360 degrees around the tooth) to sever the connective tissue attachment fibers above the bone (Fig. 34.4). There exist 13 different connective tissue fiber groups around a tooth, of which 6 directly insert into the cementum of the tooth above the bone. If these fibers are not severed before the extraction, trauma to the soft tissue is imminent. The soft tissue may tear, causing a delay in the healing process and increases bleeding (Fig. 34.5).

Minimizing Soft Tissue Reflection

The soft tissue should ideally be minimally reflected, because soft tissue retraction and shrinkage during initial healing are more evident, especially in the interdental papilla region. Usually a flap is raised when the buccal plate is not intact or surgical extraction of the tooth is indicated. If a tissue flap needs to be raised, an envelope flap (no vertical extension) is used. The vertical

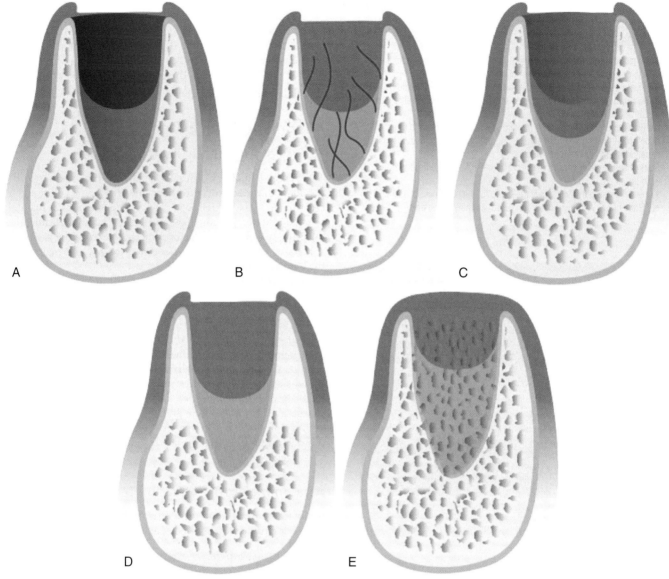

• **Fig. 34.2** The Five Stages of Extraction Site Healing: (A) Granulation Stage: Initial blood clot forms and is gradually replaced with granulation tissue, (B) Initial Angiogenic Stage: Blood vessel formation integrates into the graft which starts at approximately one week, (C) Early Bone Formation Stage: At approximately 3-4 weeks, the granulation tissue is replaced by connective tissue. Woven bone starts to form at apex, (D) Bone Growth Stage: Greater woven bone growth continues as the center of the socket is primarily woven bone. Lamellar bone starts to form around the apex and lining of the socket, (E) Bone Reorganization Stage: Complete epithelial closure is usually complete by week 6. Woven bone is gradually replaced by lamellar and is complete by 16 weeks.

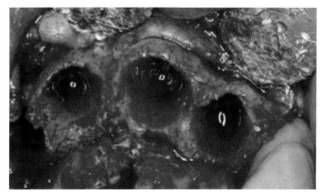

• **Fig. 34.3** The buccal plate is susceptible to fracture during extraction because the buccal plate is usually thinner than the lingual plate.

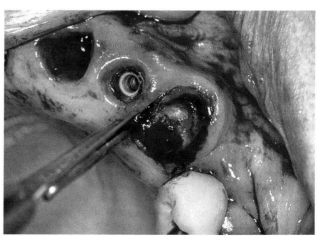

• **Fig. 34.4** The extraction of the tooth begins with a scalpel to incise the sulcular connective tissue fibers above the bone, which are attached to the cementum of the tooth.

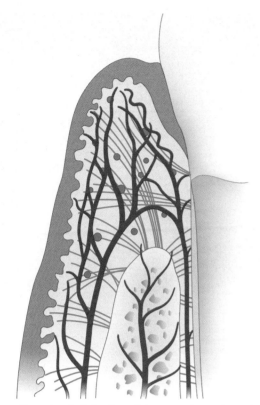

• **Fig. 34.5** Illustration depicting the soft tissue attachment to a natural tooth. Thirteen different fibers insert into the tooth root and if not severed during the atraumatic extraction technique, hard and soft tissue damage will result.

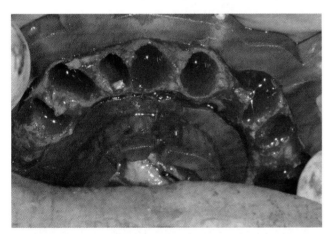

• **Fig. 34.6** When a bone supported and reduction guide is indicated, a more extensive reflection is required for access and seating of the template.

incisions may compromise the blood supply and may delay the healing of the area. Whenever the periosteum is reflected, the cells are injured and need to regenerate before the remodeling process begins. The cortical bone receives more than 80% of its arterial blood supply and facilitates 100% of its venous blood return through the periosteum.[11] In some situations reflection of the tissue is necessary such as the use of bone-supported surgical templates (Fig. 34.6).

Evaluating the Anatomy of the Tooth to Be Extracted

The next step in the atraumatic extraction process is to evaluate the crown and root anatomy. This is especially important for divergent, multirooted teeth. If the roots of the tooth to be extracted are divergent, they should be sectioned and removed as individual units, rather than risking fracture of the roots or surrounding bone (Fig. 34.7). When the roots are fractured, there is an increased risk for bone fracture/removal to retrieve them. If bone removal around the tooth is necessary (because the tooth is fractured or decayed to the bony crest), it ideally should be at the expense of the lingual alveolus, not the more labial bone. The buccal plate of bone is almost always thinner than the lingual plate. Another option to reduce trauma when taking out teeth is modification of the contact (proximal) areas. When adjacent teeth are present the pathway of removal is often obstructed by the position of the adjacent tooth. If the tooth to be extracted is not reduced (i.e., mesial and distally), instruments or pressure may chip the enamel (or restoration) of the adjacent tooth and may cause the extraction of the tooth to take an altered pathway of removal, which is more likely to fracture the roots, bone, or both (Fig. 34.8).

Atraumatic Removal of the Tooth

Basic Principles. Biomechanic concepts have been used to extract teeth for thousands of years and date back to the days of Aristotle (384–322 BCE),[12] who described the mechanics of the extraction forceps, including the advantages of "two levers acting in contrary sense having a single fulcrum." This was 100 years before Archimedes reported on the principles of the lever. Pierre Fauchard[13] (1678–1761) is credited with being the pioneer of scientific dentistry and gave specific instructions for extracting teeth using a dental elevator, a "pelican," or pincers (forceps). He describes loosening the tooth with an elevator, then using the claw of the "pelican" (invented by Chauliac[14] in the fourteenth century). The pelican handle was positioned both on the tooth and on the gum below the tooth while it was rocked back and forth (which he called "shaking") before the extraction. Taft described a similar technique using the dental key, which had

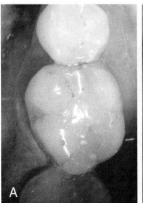 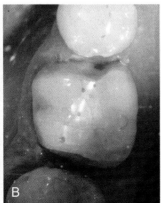 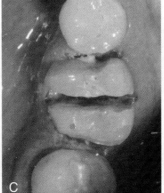 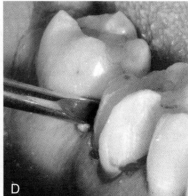

• **Fig. 34.7** Atraumatic Extraction: (A) Mandibular first molar to be extracted, (B) Proximal contacts removed to allow for easier extraction, (C) Sectional of roots to minimize trauma, (D) Use of periotome to remove roots.

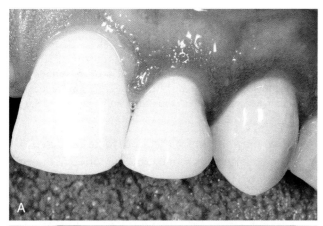

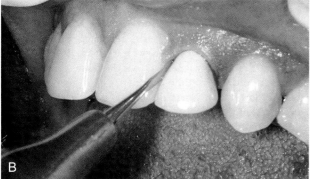

• **Fig. 34.8** (A) The maxillary lateral incisor requires extraction. The pathway of removal may restrict the extraction or chip an adjacent tooth. (B) The distal portion of the lateral incisor was reduced to allow the tooth to move distal, which allows pressure to the periodontal ligament and bone. In addition, there is less risk for adjacent tooth damage.

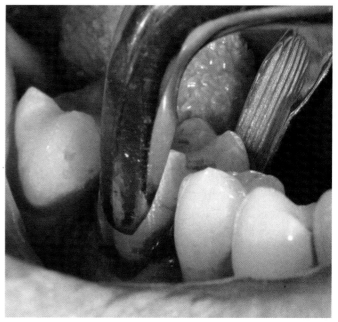

• **Fig. 34.9** Improper Extraction Technique: may often lead to retained fractured root tips or loss of buccal plate.

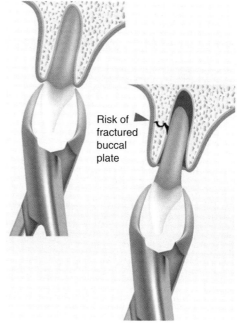

Risk of fractured buccal plate

• **Fig. 34.10** Conventional extraction forceps often will result in the fracture the buccal plate leading to a compromised future implant site.

left and right claws that provided twisting and rocking in both directions.[15] This allowed the tooth to be loosened sufficiently to be pulled from the socket with "pincers" (forceps). Modern extraction forceps date from Tomes in 1840, with the development of the anatomic forceps, complete with a handle and beak to fit the neck of the tooth.

Biomechanics of Tooth Removal. The principle of the dental elevator is also not a modern development. Abulkasim (AD 1050–1122) was the first to apply a single lever (elevator) under the tooth to force it from its "bed." It was improved by Ambroise Paré in the sixteenth century to lift out the tooth before using the pelican. Although these biomechanical methods to remove teeth are effective, a review of the biomechanical principles is in order to decrease the trauma during the tooth extraction process.

The term "simple machine" is often used to describe basic devices that increase the amount of force applied (e.g., the lever, inclined plane, wheel, screw, pulley). They each transmit or modify force or torque. The most common devices used in the extraction of teeth include levers and inclined planes.

The wedge is technically a moving double inclined plane, which overcomes a large resistance by applying a relatively smaller force than the load necessary to move an object. The mechanical advantage of a wedge depends on the ratio of its length to its thickness. A short wedge with a wide angle moves an object faster; however, it requires more force than a long wedge with a smaller angle. Dental elevators use the mechanical advantage of a wedge to initiate the luxation of teeth for their removal (Figs. 34.9 and 34.10).

Periotomes. Periotomes are usually longer and thinner wedges compared with dental elevators and often are used to begin the atraumatic extraction process. Periotomes may be used in a similar manner for extraction of intact teeth or removal of retained root fragments.

Technique.

1. The long axis of the periotome blade should be inserted into the interproximal region along the root long axis (to protect the facial plate of bone), with the tip of the periotome blade located within the crest of the alveolar bone. The instrument is then pushed or tapped with a mallet into the periodontal ligament space along the mesial and distal root, severing the periodontal

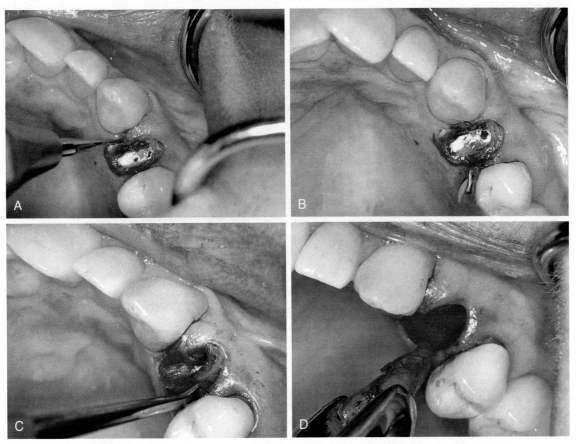

• **Fig. 34.11** (A) A periotome is inserted along the tooth root on the mesial and pushed (or tapped with a mallet) to wedge the tooth against the opposing cribriform plate. A similar process is performed on the distal interpositional region of the tooth root. (B) Once the periotome acts as a wedge and is in place for 10 to 30 seconds, it is tapped (with a mallet) farther down along the mesial and distal interproximal root surface. (C) The periotome is converted into a lever by rotating the handle several degrees, which magnifies the force against the root. The tooth becomes slightly mobile at this stage. (D) A traditional dental forceps may remove the tooth after initial mobility is created by the periotome.

ligament immediately below the alveolar crest and wedging the tooth against the opposing cribriform plate (Fig. 34.11A). The periotome should never be used on the facial plate because this may damage the host bone.

2. A period of 10 to 30 seconds is allowed to elapse while the instrument is in place. This allows biomechanical creep to occur to the ligament and reduces its strength, and because the tooth is pushed against the opposing alveolus, it also will begin to expand the bone. This process is much more effective when there is no adjacent tooth contact. Reducing the mesial and distal proximal contacts of the tooth to be extracted not only decreases the risk for damage to the adjacent tooth crown, but also aids in the extraction hopeless tooth.

3. The periotome is then pushed farther down into the periodontal ligament space toward the root apex, often using a mallet and light tapping force. This process continues along the crestal third of the tooth. At the completion of this step the tooth is often slightly mobile (Fig. 34.11B).

4. Once the periotome is used as a moving wedge, it may then be converted to a lever (Fig. 34.11C). The blade of the periotome is often 3 to 4 mm wide. When the handle is rotated, one side of the periotome is applied to the tooth root, the other side to the cribriform plate, and the width of the "wedge" is now the length of a lever, which magnifies the rotation force (moment). The rotation of the periotome handle increases both tooth

mobility and the force against the opposite cortical plate to further expand it within physiologic limits.

5. A single-rooted tooth is most often tapered. As the periotome is tapped further apically toward the cribriform plate, it is slightly rotated. Because the socket is tapered, the lateral force on one side of the tooth is converted to a coronal direction force on the other side and the root is pushed out of the socket. As a result the periotome may now be pushed farther apical, toward the root apex. When time elapses between each force application, the tooth may even slide up and completely out of the socket. Additional time and elevation may be required if significant tooth mobility is not achieved.

Use of Conventional Forceps. Traditional dental forceps should not be applied to the tooth until significant tooth mobility is achieved. Once the wedge and lever action of the dental elevator is applied to a tooth, most often dental forceps are used to ultimately grasp and deliberately rock the tooth back and forth, and to rotate it as much as conditions will allow. The combination of these tooth movements expands the bony socket and separates the periodontal ligaments. As a consequence the tooth may be removed (Fig. 34.11D). Conventional dental forceps are actually two first-class levers connected with a hinge. The forces applied to the forceps handles are the long side of the lever and the beaks on the tooth are the short side of the lever, with the hinge acting as a fulcrum. The force on the handles is magnified to allow the

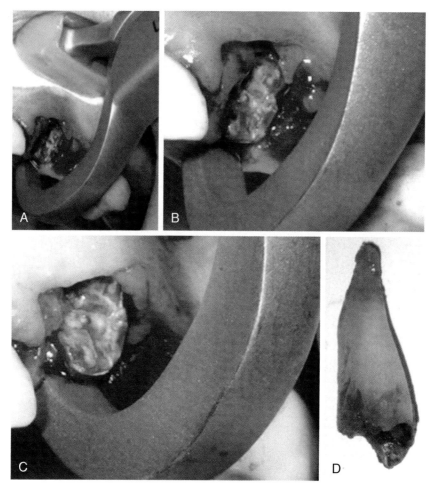

• **Fig. 34.12** The Physics (Atraumatic) Forceps. (A) A "bumper" (one beak) is placed on the facial of the tooth to be extracted at or below the mucogingival junction. The second beak is placed on the lingual, engaging the tooth root. The handles of the forceps act as a lever to rotate (avulse) the tooth from the socket. The bumper is placed below the tooth, usually at or above the mucogingival junction. The beak is placed low on the tooth root in the gingival sulcus. (B) Once the forcep is in position on the tooth root, the Physics Forceps is used as one unit (no squeezing of the handles). A few degrees of rotation to the facial places moment force on the tooth, which is held for 30 to 60 seconds. (C) Once the tooth releases from the socket, it is removed with a pincer-like device (e.g., pick-ups, extraction forceps, hemostat). (D) After removal of the tooth root, inspection of the root is completed to verify complete removal.

beaks of the forceps to grasp the tooth with great force. None of the force on the forceps handles is used to extract the tooth. Rather, the increased force on the forceps beaks often crushes or fractures the tooth. The forceps hold the tooth, and the surgeon's hand, wrist, and arm are used to move and extract the tooth. This action would be similar to forcibly pulling a bottle cap off a bottle or pulling a nail from a piece of wood using only a pair of pliers.

Alternative Extraction Forceps. The principles of biomechanics are the basis for the development of a different type of dental forceps called *Physics Forceps* (Golden-Misch Instruments, Detroit, Mich.). A *moment of force* in physics represents the magnitude of force applied to a rotational system at a distance from the axis of rotation. The principle of moment M is derived from Archimedes' discovery of the operating principle of the lever and is defined as

$$M = rF$$

where F is the applied force and r is the distance from the force applied to the object. The concept of a moment arm is key to the operation of the lever, which is capable of generating mechanical advantage. This means that the force applied to an object is affected by the length of the lever arms. The lever arm is the distance from the force input to the fulcrum or from the fulcrum to the force output.

The Physics Forceps is a dental extractor that uses first-class lever mechanics. One beak of the forcep is connected to a "bumper," which acts as a fulcrum during the extraction. The bumper is placed most often on the facial aspect of the dental alveolus, at or above the mucogingival junction. The second beak of the forcep is positioned as low as practical on the tooth root, most often on the palatal (lingual) into the gingival sulcus.

Once the forcep is in position around the tooth root, no squeezing pressure is applied to the tooth. Instead, the handles, once in position, are rotated as one unit facially for a few degrees and stopped for approximately 30-60 seconds (Fig. 34.12). The torque force generated on the tooth, periodontal ligament, and bone is related to the length of the handle to the bumper (8 cm), divided by the distance from the bumper to the forceps beak (1 cm). As a result a force on the handle connected to the bumper will increase the force on the tooth periodontal ligament and bone by eight times. No force is required to be placed on the forceps beak,

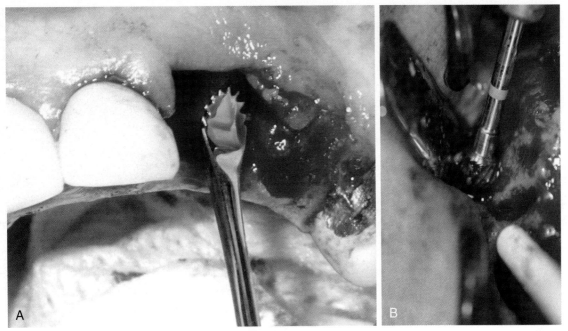

• **Fig. 34.13** Postextraction Debridement. (A) Serrated curette removing debris and soft tissue from within the socket. (B) Round carbide bure debriding the socket.

which is on the tooth. Therefore the tooth does not split, crush, or fracture. The 30-60 seconds of constant force cause biomechanical creep into the bone and periodontal ligament. Once creep has expanded and weakened the periodontal ligament and bone, the forceps handle may be slowly rotated another few degrees. This usually releases and elevates the tooth a few millimeters from the socket within an additional 10 seconds. At this point the tooth is loose and ready to be removed from the socket using any pincer-like device (e.g., pick-ups, an extraction forceps, a hemostat).

The extraction of a tooth using the Physics Forceps is similar to the removal of a nail from wood with use of a carpenter's hammer (instead of pliers). The handle of the hammer is a lever, and the beaks of the hammer fit under the head of a nail (they do not squeeze the head). The hammer head acts as a fulcrum. A rotational force applied to the hammer handle magnifies the force by the length of the handle, and the nail is elevated from the wood. Unlike a nail in wood, which is parallel and has friction for its full length, a tooth is tapered. Therefore after it is elevated a few millimeters, the periodontal ligament fibers are broken, and the tooth may be easily removed, without additional rotational force. This is important to note, because further rotational force on the forceps may fracture the facial plate of bone.

Creep is a phenomenon whereby a material continues to change shape over time under a constant load. In a tooth extraction, creep may occur to bone and the periodontal ligament. Reilly established the creep curve of bone, whereby under a constant load of 60 MPa, the bone over time responds in three different stages.[12] The majority of bone changes occur within the first minute, whereby the initial strain of bone (the change of length divided by the original length) is modified. The greater the force, the greater the deformation of the bone. This process allows the tooth socket to expand and the tooth to exit the socket. A secondary creep curve allows the bone to further deform when the force is applied for 1 to 5 minutes. The longer the time, the greater the deformation. However, the secondary deformation is only a 10% to 20% difference compared with the initial strain over the first

minute. Eventually the bone will fracture if the load is applied over a longer time frame, representing creep rupture.

The creep curve of the periodontal complex is similar to the creep curve of the bone, whereby the constant load on a tooth over time increases the strain and decreases the strength of the periodontal complex. Therefore the clinician should not underestimate the values of time and constant force to the tooth ligament and bone in the extraction process.

Socket Debridement After Extraction

Once the tooth is extracted, the tooth socket should be thoroughly debrided to remove all remnants of the periodontal ligament and any other soft tissue debris (e.g., granulation tissue). In addition, all fibrous tissue from periodontal disease or endodontic origin should be completely removed, because these tissues impair bone formation and delay bone healing for extended periods. Bleeding must ideally be present to allow for bone growth factors to enter the site. If bleeding is inadequate, the cribriform plate should be perforated with either a periodontal curette or a small carbide bur (i.e., #2 round bur) to promote bleeding and potentiate the healing process. Care should be exercised to not fenestrate the buccal or lingual walls and Fig. 34.15 or penetrate any vital structures (e.g., teeth, nerves, sinus, nasal cavity). A serrated curette (i.e., Lucas 86; Salvin Dental) can be used to remove the soft tissue and, secondarily, initiates bleeding. If lateral ridge augmentation is required, then bone decortication holes should be made over the recipient site to initiate angiogenesis and the regional acceleratory phenomenon (RAP) (Figs. 34.13 and 34.14).

Socket Grafting of the Extraction Site

Socket-Grafting Technique. Multiple bone graft procedures and studies have been evaluated for socket augmentation at the time of extraction. In most cases clinicians use one technique for socket grafting, without regard to the number of walls of bone remaining. Therefore rather than using the same technique regardless of clinical conditions, when bone repair rather than

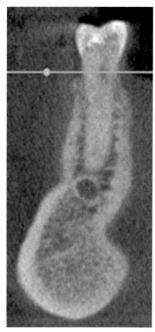

• **Fig. 34.14** Care should be exercised when debriding sockets in the mental foramen area because this may cause neurosensory impairment.

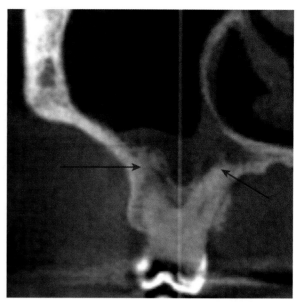

• **Fig. 34.15** The proximity of the maxillary posterior teeth to the maxillary sinus may lead to perforation of the sinus and possible infectious episodes.

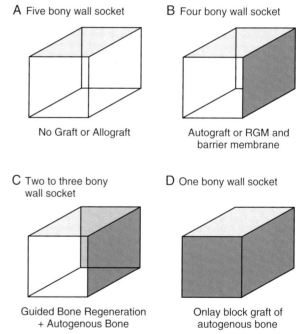

• **Fig. 34.16** The graft materials and techniques for socket grafting are related to the remaining number of bony walls. (A) A thick, five-wall bony socket may remain ungrafted or use of an allograft. A thin wall bony socket used an allograft and collagen membrane. (B) Four-wall socket requires an allograft and a longer-acting membrane. (C, D) A Three-Two- or One wall socket will most likely require autogenous bone, usually in the form of an onlay block.

regeneration is likely, the clinician should provide as many keys to bone grafting as possible to increase the socket.

What Type of Bone?. Misch and Dietsh[16] have suggested different graft materials and techniques based on the number of bony walls that remained after the tooth is removed. A thick five bony wall defect will grow bone with almost any resorbable graft material, for example, an alloplast, allograft, or autograft. When a wall of bone is less than 1.5 mm or a labial plate is missing (four bony wall defect), an autograft or freeze-dried bone (FDB) with barrier membrane (BM) and guided bone regeneration increased the predictability of restoring the original bony contour. Becker et al.[17] evaluated demineralized freeze-dried bone (DFDB) alone in extraction sockets, and no evidence of bone formation was observed. It appears DFDB alone may be a poor choice for socket grafting. LeKovic et al.[18] compared extractions alone with BM with extractions. At 6 months, crestal bone loss (0.38 versus 1.50 mm) and horizontal ridge resorption (−1.31 versus −4.56 mm) were found.[18] A two or three bony wall defect usually will require the placement of a regenerative material, and autogenous bone or possibly a block graft of cortical autogenous bone fixated into the host bone position is suggested for one bony wall defect therefore, debridement should be completd with great care (Figs 34.16).

In the literature there exists no consensus with respect to the type of bone and the ideal membrane. Most studies completed on the type of bone include either allografts or xenografts. Allografts include demineralized (DFDBA) or mineralized freeze-dried bone allograft (FDBA). Because of the remaining calcium and phosphate salts, FDBA tends to resorb much slower and therefore maintains space much better than DFDBA. Xenografts resorb very slow, as some studies have shown them to last more than 44 months.[19]

What Type of Membrane?. The indication for the ideal membrane is dictated on the presence of a buccal wall. If all walls of the extraction socket are intact, then a fast-acting collagen is used (e.g., CollaTape, CollaPlug). If the buccal plate is missing, the membrane must be placed olver the buccal wall and should consist of a longer-acting material (e.g., longer-acting collagen or

polytetrafluoroethylene [PTFE]). The advantage of the absorbable membrane (i.e., collagen) is that no reentry is required. The use of a dense PTFE attracts bone cells more readily; however, it is nonresorbable and needs to be removed.

Thick Five Bony Wall Socket (>1.5 mm). The bone regeneration process will restore complete morphology and bone volume to the residual ridge. This most often occurs when there are five thick bony walls around the extraction site (i.e., all remaining walls intact). Most of the keys for predictable bone formation are present under these conditions, and the socket often forms bone in

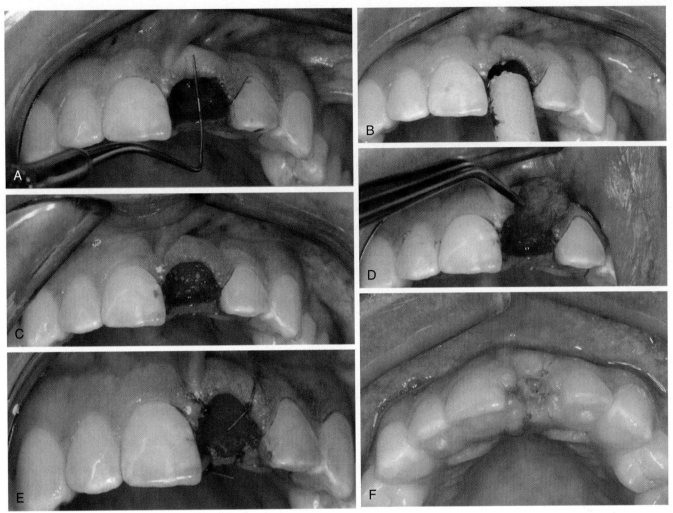

• **Fig. 34.17** Five-Walled Socket (< 1.5 mm). (A) Atraumatic Extraction. (B) Grafting with allograft. (C) Condensation of the graft. (D) Collagen membrane. (E) Final closure. (F) Six-week healing.

the extraction socket without loss of width or height. The atraumatic extraction of a tooth without pathology provides many of the keys necessary for predictable bone regeneration. The extraction process sets up the regional acceleratory phenomenon (RAP) for healing (which increases the rate of repair and adds bone morphogenetic protein to the site); the five bony walls protect the graft from mobility; the torn blood vessels in the periodontal complex leak growth factors into the region (platelet-derived growth factor, transforming growth factor); the space is maintained by the five walls of the bone; the bony walls provide blood vessels from bone into the site; and the defect size is small (i.e., one tooth). As a result the only key initially missing is soft tissue closure. The soft tissue around the extraction site begins to grow over the clot, and granulation tissue of the socket and within 2 to 3 weeks covers the extraction site (Fig. 34.17). There exist three treatment options for a few thick five bony wall socket;

Treatment Options (Five-Walled) ->1.5 mm)
1. Immediate Placement Implant.
2. No Treatment (Delayed implant Placement). In most thick bony wall sockets, bone will regenerate without bone graft material added; however, if the buccal plate is less than 1.5 mm, a socket graft is indicated to minimize collapse of the socket and to ensure adequate bone for future implant placement.
3. *Socket Grafting:* When the extraction socket is grafted, the selection of bone graft material is very important. The graft material

selected should coincide with the normal regeneration process. Therefore a material that resorbs too fast (e.g., autogenous bone, demineralized bone) or a material that resorbs too slow (e.g., cortical mineralized graft, xenograft) is not ideal for use in a five-walled defect. A much better choice would include a mineralized freeze-dried graft (cortico-cancellous 50-50) or a 70% mineralized/30% demineralized graft material that will maintain the space.

Five-Walled Bone-Grafting Technique. After complete socket debridement the socket is filled with the bone graft material in small increments. The bone graft material is compressed into the socket to avoid air spaces (i.e., should have "pushback"). Once the socket is completely filled, a collagen plug is hydrated in saline and then cut in half and compressed. The collagen is then inserted over the bone graft. Another option is cutting a piece of collagen tape (i.e., small oval piece) and positioning it over the grafted socket. The collagen is placed over the coronal aspect of the socket and the reflected tucked under the minimal flap on the buccal and lingual. The tissue is then closed with a crisscross suture. Ideally the suture technique should include the use of a high-tensile suture material (Fig. 34.18 and Box 34.2) similar to vicryl or PTFE.

Thin Five Bony Wall Socket (< 1.5 mm). For thin five bony wall sockets, the lack of socket grafting will result in unpredictable healing results. Therefore, it is recommended that these types of sockets be treated with a conventional socket grafting technique (# 3 Treatment Option for Thick Five Bony Wall Socket).

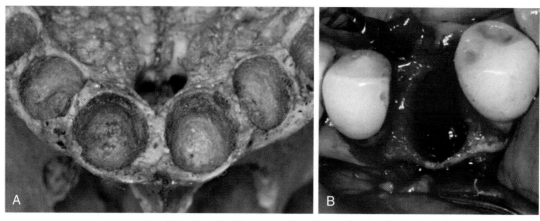

• **Fig. 34.18** Five Wall Socket: (A, B) All five walls remaining.

• **BOX 34.2**   **Five-Walled Socket (> 1.5 mm)**

Three Treatment Options:
1. Immediate Implant Placement
2. No Socket Graft (delayed implant placement)
3. Socket Graft

Reflection: conservative
Allograft: cortico-cancellous mineralized allograft or 70% mineralized/30%demineralized allograft
Membrane: regular collagen (~collagen plug)
Closure: primary closure is unachievable
Suture: crisscross suture (polytetrafluoroethylene or Vicryl)
Immediate implant: fair to good candidate
Prosthesis: Usually an FP-1 fixed prosthesis

*Thin Five-Walled Socket is treated with option # 3.

Four-Wall Bony Socket. Most often in a four-walled defect, the buccal wall is missing. When a labial plate around a socket is missing, the absence of the wall prevents space maintenance, reduces host bone vascularization, and replaces it with soft tissue vascularization. The facial bone level will never regenerate above the height of bone on the facial cortical plate of the tooth. Bone augmentation procedures must be used to obtain an ideal volume and contour of bone. Sockets with a missing lateral wall are significantly compromised and heal by repair rather than regeneration.

When conditions of repair instead of regeneration are present, socket grafting for ridge augmentation at the time of extraction is indicated.[20] Tooth extraction without grafting in four-walled defects will result in residual bone loss from resorption. For example, the maxillary anterior region may be reduced 23% in the first 6 months after an extraction and another 11% over the following 5 years.[21] Within 2 years an average of 40% to 60% of the original height and width of bone may be lost with multiple extractions.[22]

The first determination after the tooth extraction is complete is the assessment of the thickness of labial and palatal plates of bone and their relative height to the ideal volume desires. A curette or explorer may be used with the index finger over the buccal plate. If the buccal plate is missing, it will be easy to detect by tactile sensation. When the buccal plate is missing or when it is less than 1.5 mm thick, a socket graft is indicated. The two techniques of choice include a bone graft or a modified socket seal surgery (Figs. 34.19 and 34.26).

Four-Walled Bone-Grafting Technique. After complete debridement, a collagen membrane is contoured into a modified "V-Shape Cone," where the narrow part is placed on the inner surface of the buccal wall. Placing the membrane on the external aspect of the remaining buccal wall may compromise the blood supply and healing. The wider part of the membrane is trimmed to cover the socket opening and extend slightly to the lingual to "tuck" under the lingual marginal tissue. After the membrane is in place, the socket is filled with the bone graft material in small increments. The material is compressed into the socket to avoid air spaces (i.e., should have "pushback"). The suture technique should include the use of a high-tensile suture material. A crisscross suture is recommended, which encompasses the membrane and graft material. This will prevent the loss of the membrane and will contain the graft material. In some cases the membrane may be sutured to the tissue (Fig. 34.20 and Box 34.3).

NOTE: The membrane should cover only the missing buccal wall; the other walls should not have membrane coverage as this will decrease the healing of the area. The goal of the membrane is to prevent the soft tissue from repopulating the defect. If a membrane is not used, there is a greater chance of the graft particles migrating, resulting in unpredictable results.

One, two, and three bony wall sockets. When multiple walls of bone are missing, the greater the need for autogenous bone. A particulate graft is unpredictable in these situations. Therefore a donor site is most often used to obtain the autogenous bone: mandible (i.e., ramus, symphysis) or maxilla (i.e., tuberosity). In some cases (i.e. three bony wall sockets) a membrane tent screw may be used for space maintenance (Fig. 34.21) via guided bone regeneration protocols (GBR).

Obtaining Autogenous Grafting: Secondary Sites

Mandibular Ramus Donor Site: "Scraping Technique"

When autogenous bone is indicated, there exists many possible locations to harvest. One option which is easy, simple, and minimal morbidity is to obtain autogenous bone is to expose the mandibular ramus and remove bone from the external oblique ridge with double-action rongeurs. The "scrapings" may be placed in a surgical bowl with sterile saline. A second option to obtain smaller autogenous chips is to remove a block graft from the lateral ramus. Ramus block grafts may be taken; however, the blocks need to be reduced into smaller pieces, which is rather time consuming. In addition, a ramus block graft (i.e., veneer graft of the lateral ramus) has a greater morbidity rate and far greater postoperative complications (Fig. 34.22).

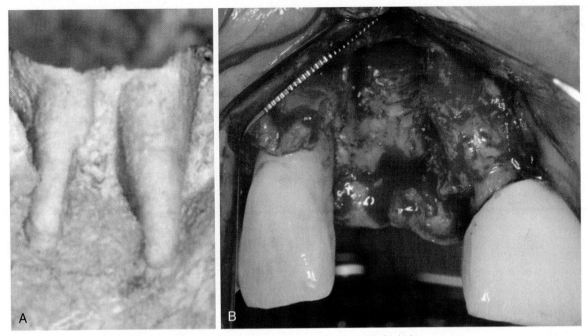

• **Fig. 34.19** Four Wall Socket: (A, B) Buccal wall missing.

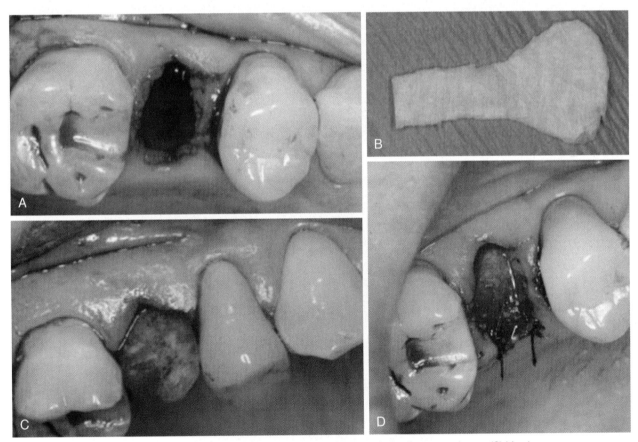

• **Fig. 34.20** Four-Walled Socket. (A) Postextraction. (B) Extended collagen membrane. (C) Membrane in place. (D) Postsuturing.

Mandibular Ramus Donor Site: "Trephine Bur Bone Harvest"

A more aggressive technique to obtain autogenous bone cores from the ramus with trephine burs. Trephine burs are end-cutting burs that are available in various diameters with the 6- to 8-mm trephine being the most popular to harvest bone from the ramus. For this technique, the ramus has become a more popular site in comparison with the symphysis area because of less morbidity. Once the ramus site (i.e., external oblique) is reflected, the trephine bur is used to harvest the autograft. Half of the trephine bur

• BOX 34.3 **Four-Walled Bony Socket**

Reflection: conservative
Allograft: cortico-cancellous mineralized allograft or 70% mineralized/30% demineralized allograft
Membrane: extended collagen or cytoplast (PTFE), (acellular dermis—thin biotype)
Closure: primary closure is usually unachievable
Suture: crisscross Suture (PTFE or Vicryl)
Immediate implant: poor to fair candidate
Prosthesis: Most likely a FP-2 or FP-3 prosthesis

*Autogenous bone can be used with allograft bone to accelerate healing and increase predictability.

is placed over the external oblique bony ridge, whereas the other half is lateral to the bone and above the reflected masseter muscle, which is elevated off the anterior lateral aspect of the ramus. Strict reflection of the soft tissues is warranted. The trephine bur is used with latch type angled surgical drill at 2000-2500 rpm with copious saline irrigation, 5 to 8 mm deep, making sure it is above and lateral to the position of the inferior alveolar nerve, artery, and vein. The inferior alveolar canal position may be identified via a cone beam computed tomography (CBCT) examination survey.

After the first trephine osteotomy is completed, the second site is completed above the half circle created by the first osteotomy and overlays the circle in the top third, or 3 mm from the top. This is repeated in the bottom third of the initial half circle, 3 mm above the bottom. Three interlacing semicircles are created along

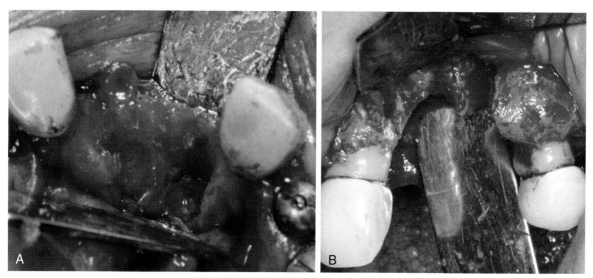

• **Fig. 34.21** (A) 3 - Wall socket - missing lingual and mesial walls, (B) 1 - Wall socket - missing all walls except the apical wall.

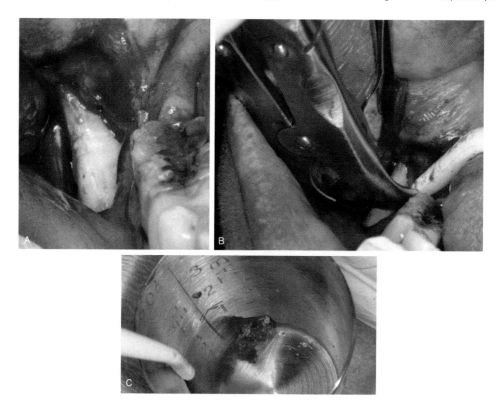

• **Fig. 34.22** Mandibular Ramus Scraping Technique. (A) Ramus exposed. (B) Double-action rongeur. (C) Autograft stored in sterile saline.

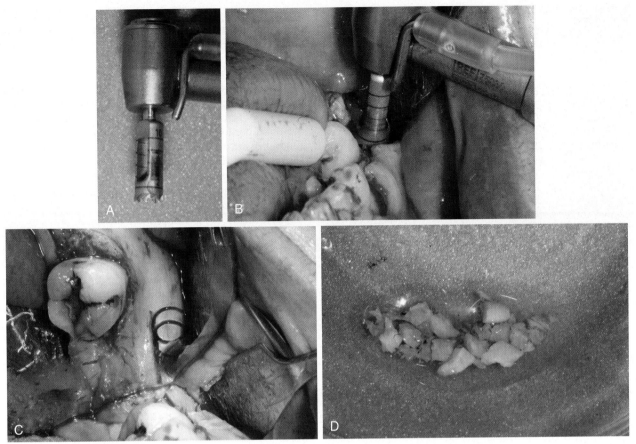

• **Fig. 34.23** Ramus Trephine Harvest - (A) 6 mm Trephine bur in latch handpiece, (B, C) Osteotomy performed over external oblique ridge, (D) Autogenous bone fragments.

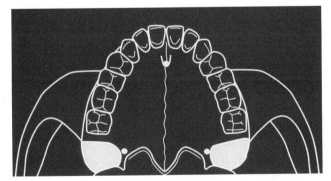

• **Fig. 34.24** The maxillary tuberosity region is a common bone donor site for bone grafting when trabecular bone is the desired product. Trabecular bone has growth factors for blood vessels and for regeneration of a bone defect.

the external oblique of the ascending ramus. A large No. 8 round carbide in a straight handpiece then may score the lateral aspect of the ramus, corresponding to the depth of the trephine bur semicircle cuts. A chisel or surgical curette then may greenstick fracture the donor bone pieces from the ramus. These harvested pieces are usually an ideal size to use in the graft site, because they are approximately 5 × 3 × 5 mm large. A collagen sponge (e.g., OraTape, OraPlug) may be placed in the donor site and the tissues approximated for primary closure. One disadvantage of the trephine ramus technique is the loss of bone from the multiple osteotomies of the burs (Fig. 34.23).

Maxillary Tuberosity Donor Site

The tuberosity offers a variable amount of trabecular bone, which is dependent on the amount of maxillary bone atrophy and maxillary sinus pneumatization. This area is convenient and often the first choice of autogenous donor sites for maxillary sinus grafting[23,24]; it also may be considered for smaller areas of ridge augmentation[25,26] (Fig. 34.24). The cancellous nature of the bone allows it to be molded into an alveolar defect, such as an extraction socket.[17] The trabecular graft will more often require the use of a barrier membrane to minimize resorption and stabilize the graft.[27] The tuberosity autograft has growth factors for osteoinduction and to accelerate blood vessel growth in the host site.

The thicker soft tissue in the tuberosity region can mislead the assessment of this donor site. The tuberosity should be evaluated with a CBCT survey to determine the maxillary sinus location and the amount of host bone present. The anatomic limitations of this area include the maxillary sinus, pterygoid plates, adjacent teeth when present, and the greater palatine canal.

The tuberosity technique includes making a vertical incision a posteriorly at the lateral aspect of the maxilla and is extended anteriorly across the tuberosity into the molar region. After reflection of a mucoperiosteal flap, bone may be harvested from the tuberosity with a rongeur or chisel. Removing the graft with a chisel will allow the harvesting of a larger piece of bone. However, the sinus may inadvertently be entered during removal of the graft, with resultant oroantral communication. If this is observed at suture removal, the patient is instructed to avoid creating high nasal

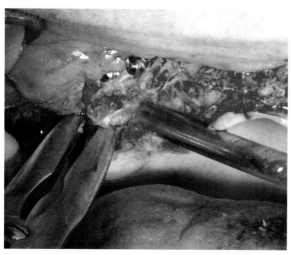

• **Fig. 34.25** Tuberosity Harvest with Double Action Rongeurs.

pressures and should be placed on antibiotics to prevent infection and ensure normal drainage. Most often, the oroantral opening will close on its own (Fig. 34.25). If the oral-antral opening does not close, surgical closure is usually indicated.

Socket Seal Surgery

A composite graft socket seal surgery was developed by Misch et al.[28,29] composed of connective tissue, periosteum, and trabecular bone used to seal a fresh extraction socket. A connective tissue graft has the advantage over a keratinized graft by blending into the surrounding attached gingival regions, offering similar color and texture of the epithelium. This is most advantageous in the maxillary anterior region and other esthetic areas. The composite graft also contains autogenous bone. The major advantage of autologous bone is a more rapid and predictable bone formation via osteogenesis. The main disadvantage is the tuberosity bone resorbs rather fast, therefore unpredictable bone growth in quantity may result.

First, a CBCT evaluation should be completed to determine if adequate bone is present in the tuberosity location. A 6- to 10-mm trephine bur corresponding to the extraction site diameter is used in a slow-speed, high-torque handpiece (e.g., 16:1 or 20:1) to harvest a gingival graft with underlying bone. The most common site for the intraoral composite graft harvest is the maxillary tuberosity region (see Fig. 34.10). The trephine bur will drill through the unreflected, keratinized, attached gingiva and into the bone of the tuberosity region at the prescribed depth related to the thickness of the tissue and the amount of donor bone available. Care should be exerted not to enter the antrum. A trephine bur may be used as a lever to greenstick fracture the bone core from its base, once it is in position within the bone. A Molt elevator may also be used for this purpose. The bone core (usually 5–10 mm in height) and the attached soft tissue (about 3 mm in height) is trimmed of its epithelium with tissue scissors, leaving 3 to 6 mm of connective tissue attached to the bone core. If the bone core does not fill the extraction socket completely, a mineralized bone graft material (e.g., cortico-cancellous FDBA) may be used in the apical portion of the socket, provided the labial plate is still intact. Because the new bone forms from the apical portion of the socket, this is the least important region to augment.

If no bone plate remains in the apical half of the socket, additional autogenous bone should be harvested from an additional

intraoral site to overfill the apical half of the socket. The bone of the composite graft (connective tissue attached to periosteum and bone) is compressed and fitted into the remaining portion of the socket.

The tissue of the composite graft will seal the socket and remain above the surrounding gingiva. A mallet and blunt instrument should be used to lightly tap it into place and compress the bony core to conform to the crestal contour of the socket. The connective tissue portion of the graft is then sutured to the surrounding gingival tissue with facial and palatal interrupted 4–0 PTFE or Vicryl sutures (Fig. 34.26). A removable transitional prosthesis should not be permitted to load the tissue during the first 6-8 weeks after extraction; otherwise the composite graft may become mobile and sequestrate.

The benefits of the composite graft socket seal surgery technique permit the surrounding keratinized gingival tissues to migrate and form a similar color and texture of keratinized tissue over the socket. The blood supply to the composite graft is established from the surrounding soft tissue. In addition, because autogenous bone is used as the graft in the coronal half of the socket, where the facial bone is most often very thin or absent, more predictable results will occur than if an allograft were used. The transfer of the bone graft with an intact periosteal layer expedites revascularization and may decrease the healing time.[30,31] As a result, reentry may be in 4 to 5 months, and placement of an ideal implant diameter is often made possible.

Use of Bone Growth Factors in Extraction Site

Blood Concentrates

An option for faster healing and possibly better bone regeneration is the use of blood concentrates alone or in combination with bone graft material. Many authors have discussed the use of blood concentrates in the post-extraction site. Choukroun et al. described the use of his second generation platelet concentrate platelet rich fribrin (PRF) with socket grafting.[32] PRF is a natural fibrin biomaterial that allows for greater microvascularization and cell migration into the wound. Growth factors have been shown to be released up to 28 days after placement in extraction sites.[33] Histologically, the fibrin clot stimulates the extraction socket environment for more ideal bone regeneration and remodeling.[34,35] Rao et al. reported better bone regeneration and increased bone density in extraction sites with PRF alone compared to a control group.[36] However, the authors advocate if PRF is to be used, it is combined with bone graft material, which has been shown in the literature to facilitate more ideal and faster bone regeneration.[37]

Bone Morphogenic Protein

The use of bone morphogenic protein (BMP) has been investigated with the treatment of post-extraction sockets. BMP's are members of a family of proteins that are highly osseoinductive and stimulate mesenchymal cells to enhance bone growth. Fiorellini et al.[38] conducted controlled studies with the use of rhBMP-2 (bone morphogenic protein) with acellular collagen sponge in extraction sites. They concluded the use of BMP induced significant bone formation for the future placement of dental implants. Histologically, the bone was similar to native bone and was load bearing. Rh-BMP is commercially availability as an osteoinductive alloplastic bone graft material (Infuse Bone Graft, Medtronic Spinal and Biologics, Memphis, TN, USA).

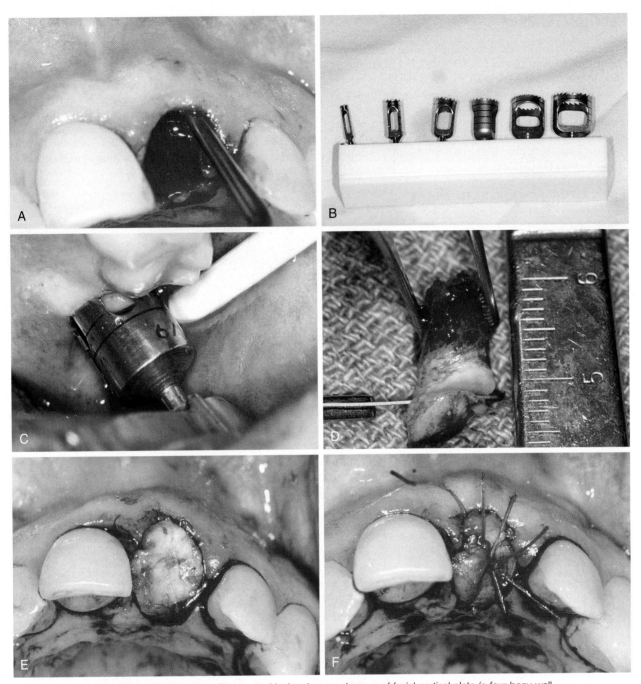

• **Fig. 34.26** (A) The left maxillary central incisor has an absence of facial cortical plate (a four bony wall defect). (B) A trephine bur diameter is selected that corresponds to the size of the extraction site (Biohorizons, Birmingham, Ala.). (C) The trephine bur performs an osteotomy directly through the keratinized attached gingiva and into the tuberosity, and proceeds to the floor of the antrum. (D) The keratinized tissue, mucosa, periosteum, and bone of the composite graft are removed from the trephine bur. The tissue thickness is reduced to 2 to 3 mm above the bone. The surface of the tissue is connective tissue. (E) The composite graft is inserted into the extraction socket, and a blunt instrument (e.g., mirror handle) and mallet taps the composite graft into the socket so that the connective tissue is level with the surrounding tissues. (F) Sutures are positioned to maintain the composite graft in place.

Provisional Restorations

In most cases of socket-grafting site preservation, the patient will require a provisional restoration to maintain esthetics and function, and to protect the surgery site. For an interim removable prosthesis the implant clinician should ensure the prosthesis is tooth supported (i.e., has vertical stops on the adjacent teeth to prevent the partial denture tooth from exerting pressure directly on the tissues around the extractions site), and the surface area over the surgical site should be hygienic in contour. If a fixed prosthesis is used (e.g., resin bonded bridge), the undersurface should not impinge on the tissue (Fig. 34.27).

Socket Graft Healing

There exist many variables when determining when a socket graft site is healed for implant placement. Care should be exercised to place the implant only after adequate hard and soft tissue healing is obtained. Healing of the hard and soft tissues is determined by the size of the defect, type of graft material, type of bone graft, use of a membrane, and blood supply to the area. Usually a healing time ranging from 4 - 8 months is required. Radiographically, usually when the cribriform plate is not seen on the x-ray, adequate healing is achieved (Fig. 34.28).

Socket Grafting Contraindications

Infected Site

A relative contraindication to the socket-grafting protocol is the presence of an acute infection. A tooth demonstrating active infection (i.e., exudate or fistula) should be extracted without placement of bone graft material. The patient's acute infection should be managed by drainage of the infection, lavage of the infected area, and the use of systemic antibiotics. The bone grafting may be delayed for a minimum of 8 weeks postextraction to decrease the possibility of a graft infection. In addition, this delay will ensure better tissue quality (i.e., primary closure of the grafted site with keratinized tissue), elevated osteoblast activity, and a newly formed woven bone within the socket. The disadvantage of this surgical approach is the need for an additional surgery and a extended total treatment time (Fig. 34.29).

Proximity to Vital Structure (Mental Foramen, Mandibular Canal)

In the mandibular premolar area, 25% to 38% of the time the mental foramen is superior to the apex of either of the premolars. The location of the mental foramen is highly variable; however, it is most commonly located in the first or second premolar area. If a premolar is extracted, CBCT measurements need to confirm adequate bone below the apex. The clinician must be careful in debriding this area because nerve impairment may occur.

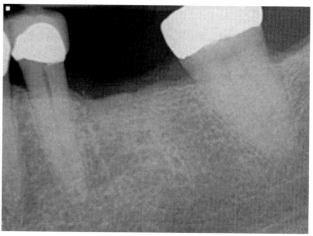

• **Fig. 34.28** Healed graft site exhibiting lack of cribriform plate present.

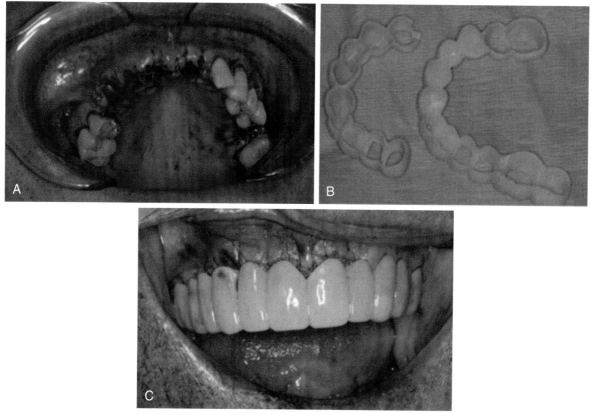

• **Fig. 34.27** Provisional Restoration. (A) Postextraction. (B) Overlay temporary bridge (i.e., Snap-On Smile). (C) Interim prosthesis inserted placing no pressure on extraction site.

In the mandibular molar area, especially in type 1 nerve locations (i.e., mandibular canal close to mandibular teeth apexes), after extraction it is important not to curette or place graft material in close proximity to the nerve canal (Fig. 34.30). In many cases, no superior cortical bone is present over the mandibular canal.

Maxillary Sinus

In the maxillary first molar area, approximately 42% of the maxillary roots are located in the sinus proper.[39] When the tooth is extracted the sinus membrane may be perforated, and an exposure may occur. If grafting is completed, bone graft material may be introduced into the sinus proper, leading to the possibility of acute rhinosinusitis or oral-antral fistula formation (Fig. 34.31).

Socket Graft Complications

Inadequate Fill

Care should be exercised in filling the entire socket from the apex to the ridge with no voids. This is most often to occur in multirooted teeth, especially when root diameter is small. Small increments of graft material should be introduced into the socket at a time to avoid inadequate fills. Complications occur when too large of a syringe or too much volume of material is introduced into the socket and it becomes difficult to condense properly. Amalgam carriers with small amalgam pluggers can be used to graft smaller sized sockets (Fig. 34.32).

Too Dense of Socket Fill

Avoid excessive pressure when condensing the graft material into the socket. Too dense of a particulate graft fill may compromise the vascularity within the socket and final healing (Fig. 34.33). Usually when "push-back" of the material occurs, the socket is grafted sufficiently.

Overfilling the Extraction Socket

Excess graft material in height placed in the socket may compromise the soft tissue healing over the extraction socket. The graft material should be placed into the socket to the level of the surrounding socket walls. When excess bone is placed into an extraction site, it will usually be slowly lost postoperatively (Fig. 34.34). In addition, soft tissue healing over the extraction site will be delayed.

Leaving Soft Tissue or Root Fragment

After extraction the tooth and root structure should always be evaluated to verify no tissue or root tip is inadvertently left in the socket. Grafting over soft tissue or a root tip will increase the possibility of infection, decrease the amount of bone formation, and delay the healing process (Fig. 34.35).

Use of Incorrect Bone Graft Material

Certain bone substitutes are not ideal for socket grafting. Some of these materials include nonresorbable hydroxyapatite, calcified copolymer alloplast (Bioplant HTR; Bioplant

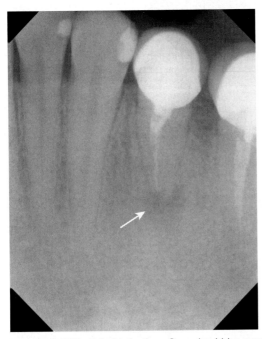

• **Fig. 34.29** Tooth With Apical Infection. Care should be exercised in grafting into an infected socket.

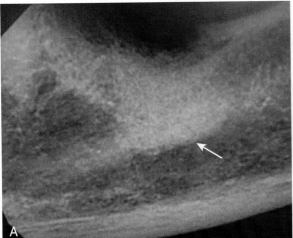
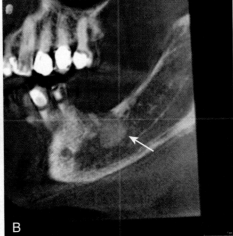

• **Fig. 34.30** Neurosensory Impairment (A and B) Socket graft material in close approximation to the mandibular canal. Care should be exercised in type 1 nerve paths.

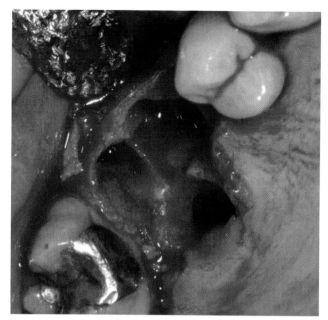

• **Fig. 34.31** Maxillary Sinus Approximation. Approximately 42% of molar roots are into the sinus floor, leading to possible perforation and extrusion of graft material into the sinus. Note the lingual root perforation into the maxillary sinus.

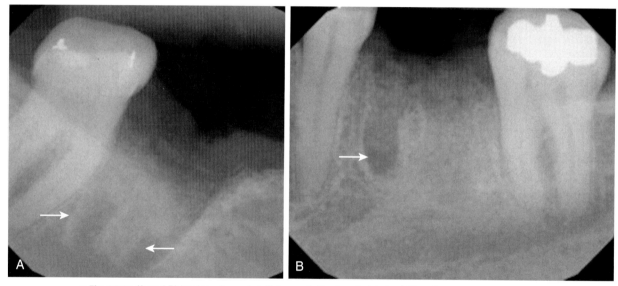

• **Fig. 34.32** (A and B) Inadequate socket fill (arrows). Graft material should be placed into the extraction sockets in small increments so that voids and inadequate fill do not occur.

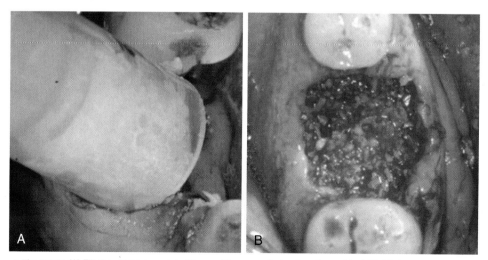

• **Fig. 34.33** (A) Fill should be completed in small increments to allow for an ideal fill. (B) Adequate density is achieved when "pushback" occurs when packing the graft material.

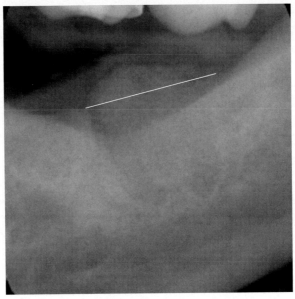

• **Fig. 34.34** Overfilling the Extraction Socket. Bone should not be grafted above the cortical plate levels. This will result in poor wound healing migration of the graft material and incision line opening.

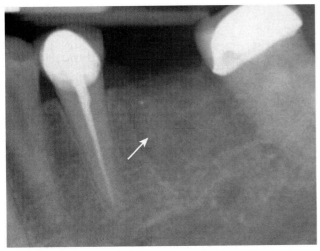

• **Fig. 34.35** Retained Root Tip. After the extraction, radiographic evidence should verify no retained roots in the socket.

Inc.), and "bioactive" glasses. Most of the alloplasts either do not resorb or resorb slowly with a fibrous encapsulation, thereby making them nonideal for subsequent implant placement (Box 34.4). Ideally, the bone graft material should resorb at the same rate that bone formation occurs (i.e. mineralized cortico-cancellous allograft or 70% mineralized/30% demineralized allograft).

Conclusion

The extraction of a natural tooth is one of the most widely performed procedures completed in dentistry today. After tooth extraction, it is well documented in the literature significant morphologic and dimensional changes occur to the extraction socket. When hard and soft tissue is lost, an increased difficulty in implant placement results, which compromises the final prosthetic outcome. Therefore, it is imperative that extraction sites are treatment predictably to maintain the hard and soft tissue volume. Many clinicians treat all sockets the same, with a set treatment

---

• **BOX 34.4** **Summary of Post-Extraction Options**

1. Immediate implant placement (Usually for 5-walled sockets)
2. No Socket Graft - Delayed Implant Placement
   a. Five-walled socket (> 1.5 mm of buccal plate)
   b. Infected site
3. Socket graft—five-walled socket (< 1.5 mm of buccal plate)
   • Allograft + CollaTape/CollaPlug
4. Socket graft—four-walled socket
   • Allograft + extended collagen/dense polytetrafluoroethylene membrane
5. Socket graft—one-, two-, three-walled socket
   • Autograft + allograft

---

protocol to provide for placement of a future implant. However, the morphology, most specifically the number of remaining bony walls, play a significant role in the amount of resorption after extraction. Therefore, an extraction socket treatment protocol has been established which is dictated on the number of remaining walls. Each classification involves a different treatment protocol with the goal of maintaining the available bone and regenerating bone within the socket area so that ideal implant placement may be completed at a later date. In addition, the clinician must have a strong understanding of the indications and contraindications of socket grafting along with the ideal treatment of associated complications.

References

1. Irinakis, T., & Tabesh, M. (2007). Preserving the socket dimensions with bone grafting in single sites: an esthetic surgical approach when planning delayed implant placement. *J Oral Implantol.* 33(3), 156-163.
2. Ohta Y. Comparative changes in microvasculature and bone during healing of implant and extraction sites. *J Oral Implant.* 1993;3:184–198.
3. Lin WL, McCulloch CA, Cho MI. Differentiation of periodontal ligament fibroblasts into osteoblasts during socket healing after tooth extraction in the rat. *Anat Rec.* 1994;240:492–506.

4. Araujo MG, Berglundh T, Lindhe J. On the dynamics of periodontal tissue formation in degree III furcation defects. An experimental study in dogs. *J Clin Periodontol*. 1997;24:738–746.
5. Cardaropoli G, Araujo M, Lindhe J. Dynamics of bone tissue formation in tooth extraction sites. An experimental study in dogs. *J Clin Periodontol*. 2003;30:809–818.
6. Evian CI, Rosenberg ES, Coslet JG, Corn H. The osteogenic activity of bone removed from healing extraction sockets in humans. *J Periodontol*. 1982;53:81–85.
7. Schropp L, Wenzel A, Kostopoulos L, Karring T. Bone healing and soft tissue contour changes following single-tooth extraction: a clinical and radiographic 12-month prospective study. *Int J Periodontics Restorative Dent*. 2003;23:313–323.
8. Cardaropoli G, Araújo M, Lindhe J. Dynamics of bone tissue formation in tooth extraction sites: an experimental study in dogs. *J Clin Periodontol*. 2003;30(9):809–818.
9. Ohta Y. Comparative changes in microvasculature and bone during healing of implant and extraction sites. *J Oral Implant*. 1993;3:184–198.
10. Araujo MG, Lindhe J. Dimensional ridge alterations following tooth extraction. An experimental study in the dog. *J Clin Periodontol*. 2005;32(2):212–218.
11. Botticelli D, Berglundh T, Lindhe J. Hard-tissue alterations following immediate implant placement in extraction sites. *J Clin Periodontol*. 2004;31(10):820–828.
12. Roberts WE, Turley PK, Brezniak N, et al. Bone physiology and metabolism. *Calif Dent Assoc J*. 1987;15:54–61.
13. Reilly, DT, Burstein AH. The elastic and ultimate properties of compact bone tissue. *J Biomech*. 1975;8(6):393–405.
14. Fauchard P. *Le Chirurgien Dentiste, Oú Traité Des Dents*. Paris: PJ Mariette; 1728.
15. Chauliac G. *De La Grande Chirurgie*. Rouen, France: David du Petit val; 1649.
16. Glenner RA, Davis AB, Burns SB. *The American Dentist*. Missoula. Mont: Pictorial Histories; 1990.
17. Misch CE, Dietsh F. Bone grafting materials. *Implant Dent*. 1993;2:158–167.
18. Becker W, Becker BE, Caffesse R. A comparison of demineralized freeze-dried bone and autologous bone to induce bone formation in human extraction sockets. *J Periodontol*. 1994;65:1128–1133.
19. LeKovic V, Keeney EB, Weinlaender M, et al. A bone regeneration approach to alveolar ridge maintenance following tooth extraction: report of 10 cases. *J Periodontol*. 1997;68:563–570.
20. Skoglund A, Hising P, Young C. A clinical and histologic examination in humans of the osseous response to implanted natural bone mineral. *Int J Oral Maxillofac Implants*. 1997;12(2):194–199.
21. Misch CE, Dietsh F. Bone grafting materials. *Implant Dent*. 1993;2:158–167.
22. Artzi Z, Tal H, Dayan D. Porous bovine bone mineral in healing of human extraction sockets, part I: histo-morphometric evaluations at 9 months. *J Periodont*. 2000;71:1015–1023.
23. McCall RA, Rosenfeld AL. Influence of residual ridge resorption patterns on implant fixture placement and tooth position. *Int J Periodontics Restorative Dent*. 1991;11:8023.
24. Tatum H. Maxillary and sinus implant reconstruction. *Dent Clin North Am*. 1986;30:207–229.
25. Misch CE. Divisions of available bone. In: Misch CE, ed. *Contemporary Implant Dentistry*. 2nd ed. St Louis: Mosby; 1993.
26. Misch CM. Comparison of intraoral donor sites for onlay grafting prior to implant placement. *Int J Oral Maxillofac Implants*. 1997;12:767–776.
27. ten Bruggenkate CM, Kraaijenhagen HA, van der Kwast WAM, et al. Autogenous maxillary bone grafts in conjunction with placement of I.T.I. endosseous implants: a preliminary report. *Int J Oral Maxillofac Surg*. 1992;21:81–84.
28. Buser D, Dula K, Belser UC, et al. Localized ridge augmentation using guided bone regeneration. II. Surgical procedure in the mandible. *Int J Periodontics Restorative Dent*. 1995;15:11–29.
29. Misch CE, Dietsh F, Misch CM. A modified socket seal surgery: a composite graft approach. *J Oral Implantol*. 1999;25:244–250.
30. Tischler M, Misch CE. Extraction site bone grafting in general dentistry: review of application and principles. *Dent Today*. 2004;23:108–113.
31. Knize D. The influence of periosteum and calcitonin on on-lay bone graft survival. *Plast Reconstr Surg*. 1974;53:190–199.
32. Zucman P, Mauer P, Berbesson C. The effects of autographs of bone and periosteum in recent diaphyseal fractures. *J Bone Joint Surg*. 1968;50B:409.
33. Choukroun J, Diss A, Simonpieri A, et al. Plateletrich fibrin (PRF): a second-generation platelet concentrate. Part IV: clinical effects on tissue healing. *Oral Surg Oral Med Oral Pathol Oral Radiol Endod*. 2006;101:E56–E60.
34. He L, Lin Y, Hu X, Zhang Y, Wu H, et al. A comparative study of platelet-rich fibrin (PRF) and platelet-rich plasma (PRP) on the effect of proliferation and differentiation of rat osteoblasts in vitro. *Oral Surg Oral Med Oral Pathol Oral Radiol Endod*. 2009;108:707–713.
35. Dohan DM, Choukroun J, Diss A, et al. Platelet-rich fibrin (PRF): a second-generation platelet concentrate. Part II: platelet-related biologic features. *Oral Surg Oral Med Oral Pathol Oral Radiol Endod*. 2006;101:E45–E50.
36. Dohan DM, Choukroun J, Diss A, et al. Platelet-rich fibrin (PRF): a second-generation platelet concentrate. Part III: leucocyte activation: a new feature for platelet concentrates?.
37. Girish Rao S, Bhat P, Nagesh KS, et al. Bone regeneration in extraction sockets with autologous platelet rich fibrin gel. *J Maxillofac Oral Surg*. 2013;12(1):11–16.
38. Marx R, Carlson ER, Eichstaedt RM, et al. Platelet rich plasma growth factors enhancement for bonegrafts. *Oral Surg Oral Med Oral Pathol Oral Radiol Endod*. 1998;85:638–646. doi: 10.10.
39. Fiorellini JP, Howell TH, Cochran D, et al. Randomized study evaluating recombinant human bone morphogenetic protein-2 for extraction socket augmentation. *J Periodontol*. 2005;76(4):605–13.
40. Kang SH, Kim BS, Kim Y. Proximity of posterior teeth to the maxillary sinus and buccal bone thickness: a biometric assessment using cone-beam computed tomography. *J Endod*. 2015;41(11):1839–1846.

35

Bone Substitutes and Membranes

RALPH POWERS

Since acknowledging titanium as an inert substance capable of binding to bone in humans, implant dentistry has flourished.[1,2] Dr. Per-Ingvar Brånemark is known as the "father of the modern dental implant" for taking a serendipitous finding in orthopedic research and applying it to dentistry.[3] It took decades for him to convince the medical and dental communities that titanium could be integrated into living tissues, a process he called *osseointegration*. Now dental implants are considered a standard of care and enjoy a very high success rate. Having a reliable implant system is only part of the equation. It is well understood that both bone volume and bone quality are essential for implant placement and survival.[4]

Most dental implants require some type of bone augmentation. For many years autograft (considered the gold standard) was the only material available as a bone void filler, and it still has a place in many applications.[5] However, dramatic discoveries in biomaterials and improvements in processing, preservation, and packaging have made bone graft substitutes (BGS) available that are safe, effective, accessible in sufficient quantities, and suitable for almost all clinical situations. In fact, the global BGS and dental membrane market is expected to grow at a compound annual growth rate of 9.9% per year through 2025.[6] Much of this increase is driven by the large expected increase in dental implant and prosthetics work. The key factors driving the growth of this market include the growing geriatric population and corresponding dental disorders, rising incidence of tooth decay and edentulism, and the ability for more dental practitioners to place implants and provide more complete treatment solutions.

It is up to the clinician to create an osseo-adaptive situation when grafting, that is, having a host site prepared and a patient sufficient in health to allow for natural and predictable healing after any type of augmentation procedure. The wise clinician will be familiar with many types of BGS, as well as membranes, and their properties. The clinician should develop a decision tree for every clinical scenario based on a combination of empirical and scientific support. It is hoped the following information will provide a basis for understanding the many bone graft and membrane materials currently available.

Terminology for Bone Repair and Regeneration

Bone remodeling is the ongoing process by which bone is resorbed and replaced in a dynamic steady-state process that maintains the health of bone. The process affects the entire skeleton all of the time. Although bone may appear superficially as a static tissue, it is actually very dynamic, undergoing constant remodeling throughout the life of the vertebrate organism. Bone remodeling is triggered by a need for calcium in the extracellular fluid, but it also occurs in response to mechanical stresses (microfracture) on the bone tissue.

For the remodeling to occur, appropriate cell signaling occurs to trigger osteoclasts to resorb the surface of the bone, followed by deposition of bone by osteoblasts. Together the cells in any given particular region of the bone surface that are responsible for bone remodeling are known as the basic multicellular unit (BMU). The action of osteoclasts and osteoblasts is synchronized: cells that resorb and deposit bone, respectively.

To understand bone remodeling, you need to know about three cell types found in bone:

- Osteoclasts are bone-resorbing cells (*-clast* means "to break"; osteoclasts break down bone). They are large, multinucleate cells that form through the fusion of precursor cells. Unlike osteoblasts, which are related to fibroblasts and other connective tissue cells, osteoclasts are descended from stem cells in the bone marrow that also give rise to monocytes (macrophages). One essential feature is the ingrowth of vascular tissue (neovascularization); this is an essential feature of remodeling in that the new vessels will carry cells and nutrients.
- Osteoblasts are bone-forming cells. They are connective tissue cells found at the surface of bone. They can be stimulated to proliferate and differentiate as osteocytes. They are recruited to the area and form the lining of the newly created tunnel.
- Osteocytes are mature bone cells. Osteocytes manufacture type I collagen and other substances that make up the bone extracellular matrix. Osteocytes will be found enclosed in bone[7] (Fig. 35.1).

Fig. 35.2 includes multiple cells and shows the phases of bone remodeling. The group of cells creating the tunnel through the bone is the BMU (forming the "cutting cone"). Osteoclasts are followed by preosteoblasts that adhere to the new wall of the area resorbed. As they mature to osteoblasts, they begin to secrete osteoid (immature bone matrix) in which they eventually are trapped and where they live out the remainder of their existence as osteocytes. This marks the start of reversal of the resorptive phase. The final product is the formation of Haversian canals (Fig. 35.3), or "osteons," familiar to all as a normal observation in bone histology.

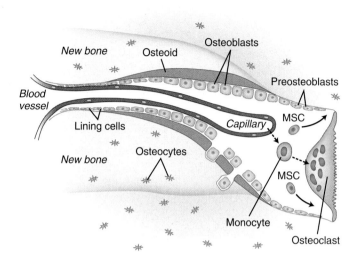

Fig. 35.1 The Basics of Bone Remodeling. Involved are osteoclasts (removing old or impaired bone), preosteoblast and osteoblasts (forming new immature bone), and osteocytes trapped within the new bone matrix. None of this can occur without new vasculature to bring in essential cells and fluids. Mesenchymal stme cells (MSC) are the precursors to the bone forming "blast" cells.

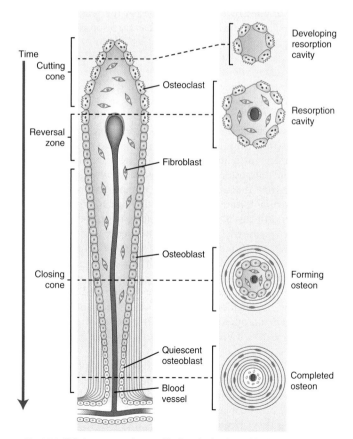

Fig. 35.2 This is a more advanced look at the basic multicellular unit forming the "cutting cone." (*Adapted from: Roberts WE Garetto LP, Arbuckle GR et al: What are the risk factors of osteoporosis? Assessing bone health, J Am Dent Assoc 122:59-61, 1991. Source: https://basicmedicalkey.com/functional-anatomy-of-the-musculoskeletal-system/*)

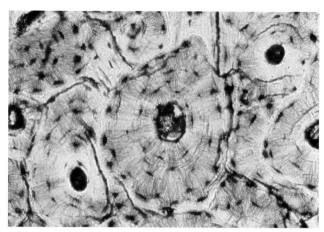

Fig. 35.3 Osteons, or Haversian canals. Evidence that bone remodeling occurred in the area.

In infants, bone "turnover" is rapid and may result in a 100% new skeleton within 1 year; in adults, it is approximately 10%.[8] Statistics of adult bone remodeling are as follows:

- Life span of BMU is ~6 to 9 months.
- Speed of BMU is ~ 25 μm/day.
- Bone volume replaced by a single BMU is ~0.025 mm^3.
- Life span of osteoclasts is ~2 weeks.
- Life span of osteoblasts is ~3 weeks.
- Interval between successive remodeling events at the same location is ~2 to 5 years.
- Rate of turnover of whole skeleton is ~10% per year.

The 10% per year approximation for the entire skeleton is based on an average 4% turnover per year in cortical bone, which represents roughly 75% of the entire skeleton, and an average 28% per year in trabecular (cancellous) bone, which represents roughly 25% of the skeleton. As you can see, remodeling occurs slowly and continuously.

Bone modeling adapts structure to loading and removes damage as to maintain bone strength. It involves independent sites of resorption and formation that change the size and shape of bones. The stimulus is additional localized stress (as in orthodontic tooth movement and weight training). This is described by Wolff's law, which proposes that bone in a healthy person or animal will adapt to the loads under which it is placed.[9] Modeling occurs at the cellular level in a fashion similar to that described for remodeling.

Bone repair is a proliferative physiologic process in which the body facilitates the repair of a bone fracture. Repair occurs in response to trauma (fracture or overuse) and is the result of a complicated cascade of events.

Bone regeneration is the regrowth of lost tissue. This requires the use of surgical protocols that enable regeneration of the deficient sites, using the principles of osteogenesis, osteoinduction, and osteoconduction (see more detailed definitions later in this chapter).

- *Guided bone regeneration* (GBR) refers to alveolar ridge augmentation or bone redevelopment (for implant placement or to preserve the site for fixed or removable bridgework); this often requires the presence of a membrane to protect the grafted area and restrict the entrance of unwanted cells. When a graft is placed into a site (in, for example, a fresh extraction socket), a competition occurs between soft tissue and bone-forming cells to fill the surgical site. Soft tissue cells (epithelial cells and fibroblasts) migrate at a very fast rate compared with bone-formers. A properly chosen and placed membrane will reduce the competition. Below the membrane, regeneration occurs. It involves the proliferation of new blood vessels (angiogenesis) and the migration of bone-forming cells (osteogenesis). An initial blood clot will form, which is replaced by fibrous bone. This material (called *woven bone*) is characterized by a haphazard organization of collagen and is mechanically weak. Later this will be transformed into a better organized, load-bearing "lamellar bone" (via normal bone remodeling).[10]

- *Guided tissue regeneration* (GTR) involves the same techniques used in GBR, but for redeveloping (regenerating) lost periodontal tissues (cementum, periodontal ligament, alveolar bone) to retain the natural dentition. Early research in this area was instrumental in the development of the modern membrane.[11]

The concept of GBR was described first in 1959 when cell-occlusive membranes were employed for spinal fusions.[12] The terms *guided bone regeneration* (GBR) and *guided tissue regeneration* (GTR) often are used synonymously and rather inappropriately. GTR deals with the regeneration of the supporting periodontal apparatus, including cementum, periodontal ligament, and alveolar bone, whereas GBR refers to the promotion of bone formation alone. GBR and GTR are based on the same principles that use barrier membranes for space maintenance over a defect, promoting the ingrowth of osteogenic cells and preventing migration of undesired cells from the overlying soft tissues into the wound. Protection of a blood clot in the defect and exclusion of gingival connective tissue and provision of a secluded space into which osteogenic cell from the bone can migrate are essential for a successful outcome. The sequence of bone healing is affected not only by invasion of nonosteogenic tissue but more so by the defect size and morphology.

Bone preservation indicates long-term stability of the alveolar ridge. This is a general term for all of the previous terms in this section.

Mechanisms of Bone Repair and Regeneration

From the time of Hippocrates it has been known that bone has considerable potential for regeneration and repair. Nicholas Senn,[13] a surgeon at Rush Medical College in Chicago, described the utility of antiseptic decalcified bone implants in the treatment of osteomyelitis and certain bone deformities. Pierre Lacroix[14] proposed that there might be a hypothetical substance, osteogenin, that might initiate bone growth.

Marshall R. Urist provided the biological basis of bone morphogenesis. Urist[15] made the key discovery that demineralized, lyophilized segments of bone induced new bone formation when implanted in muscle pouches in rabbits. This discovery was published in 1965 in *Science*.[15] The term *bone morphogenetic protein* (BMP) first appeared in the scientific literature via the *Journal of Dental Research* in 1971.[16] Bone morphogenetic (or morphogeneic) proteins are now referred to as BMPs for convenience.

Bone induction is a sequential multistep cascade. The key steps in this cascade are *chemotaxis, mitosis,* and *differentiation*. Chemotaxis is movement of a motile cell in a direction corresponding to a gradient of increasing or decreasing concentration of a particular substance (such as a BMP). Mitosis is a type of cell division that results in two daughter cells each having the same number and kind of chromosomes as the parent nucleus. This is typical of ordinary tissue growth. Differentiation is the process by which a

cell becomes specialized to perform a specific function, as in the case of a bone cell, a blood cell, or a neuron. There are more than 250 general types of cells in the human body. For bone induction, BMPs (uncovered by normal bone remodeling or exposed in the matrix of a properly demineralized graft) signal for chemotaxis of bone-forming cells to the bone void. The cells divide to increase their number and mature to a more specialized form to produce new immature bone material (osteoid). Over time this area is remodeled to provide a better structure.

Early studies by Hari Reddi unraveled the sequence of events involved in bone matrix–induced bone morphogenesis. On the basis of this work, it seemed likely that "morphogens" were present in the bone matrix. A systematic study, using a battery of bioassays for bone formation, was undertaken to isolate and purify putative bone morphogenetic proteins.[17] It is well recognized that BMPs can be found in properly prepared demineralized bone products in the correct proportion to induce the sequential steps needed for bone regeneration. To date, 20 BMPs have been identified.[18] Now laboratory-produced recombinant human BMPs (rhBMPs) are used in orthopedic applications (rhBMP-2 and rhBMP-7), such as spinal fusions and nonunions. rhBMP-2 is U.S. Food and Drug Administration (FDA) approved for some dental use.

In general, osteoinduction is the process by which osteogenesis is induced. It is a phenomenon regularly seen in any type of bone healing process. Osteoinduction implies the recruitment of immature cells and the stimulation of these cells to develop into preosteoblasts. In a bone healing situation such as a fracture the majority of bone healing is dependent on osteoinduction. Osteoconduction means that bone grows on a surface.

Currently *osteogenesis* can occur only with autografts. Examples are the use of the rib, grafts from the chin, ascending ramus, ilium, tibia, or outer table of the cranium, or from bone collected during extraction or other dental procedure. Osteogenesis occurs when vital osteoblasts originating from the bone graft material contribute to new bone growth along with bone growth generated via osteoinduction and osteoconduction.[19]

Osteoinduction has a rich research history and has been well studied. Osteoinductive materials will recruit the proper bone cells to a site, and these cells will form bone. Osteoinduction can produce bone where bone is not normally found (ectopic or heterotropic sites). In fact, the early tests for a material's osteoinductive "potential" were placement of that material into the muscle pouch of an animal. An example of a test animal is the "nude" mouse. A nude mouse is a laboratory mouse from a strain with a genetic mutation that causes a deteriorated or absent thymus, resulting in an inhibited immune system because of a greatly reduced number of T cells. The phenotype (main outward appearance) of the mouse is a lack of body hair, which gives it the "nude" nickname. The nude mouse is valuable to research because it can receive many different types of tissue grafts, as it mounts no rejection response. Therefore if new bone forms in the muscle pouch of a nude mouse, it provides evidence of the potential for osteoinductivity. Now *in vitro* tests have been developed to assess potential osteoinductivity, although the *in vivo* animal assay is considered the gold standard.[20]

Osteoconduction is the formation of bone on a surface. All inert materials possess this characteristic. In bone regeneration, healthy bone must be present adjacent to the site where the graft is placed. Because bone will move from the healthy host site through the grafting material placed in the bone void, this is commonly referred to as "creeping substitution." Fig. 35.4 illustrates this phenomenon with a cancellous-based product.

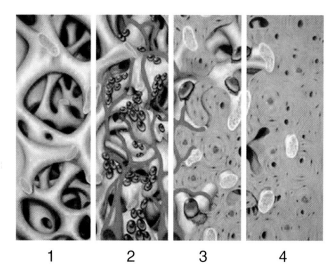

• **Fig. 35.4** "Creeping substitution." This occurs with all materials to some extent because all BGSs are osteoconductive. It requires the presence of healthy host bone in close proximity to the graft. Neovascularization occurs in cells that will remove/repopulate the space. (*Source: https:// pocketdentistry.com/basics-of-bone-grafting-and-graft-materials/*)

It occurs similarly with a cortical material, but at a slower rate. The rate of creeping substitution is based on the available space for vascular ingrowth. Available space is based on particle spacing (if a "powder" type material is used), as well as macroporosity and microporosity of the material.[21]

- Macroporosity (pore size greater than 100 μm) is usually required to facilitate the osteogenesis and angiogenesis. Interconnected macropores are necessary to promote body fluid circulation and cell migration to the core of the implant. An example of macroporosity is the normal marrow space formed by trabeculation in the cancellous portion of bone, or the interparticle spacing that is created when particulate grafts are placed.
- Microporosity (pore size less than 10 μm) has importance, as does the unique surface properties of microporous scaffolds. These have considerable influence on fluid distribution and protein adsorption. Moreover, capillary force generated by the microporosity can improve the attachment of bone-related cells on the scaffolds surface and even make the cells achieve penetration into the micropores smaller than them (Fig. 35.5).

Osteopromotion involves the enhancement of osteoinduction without the material possessing osteoinductive properties. As an example, enamel matrix derivative (xenograft based) has been

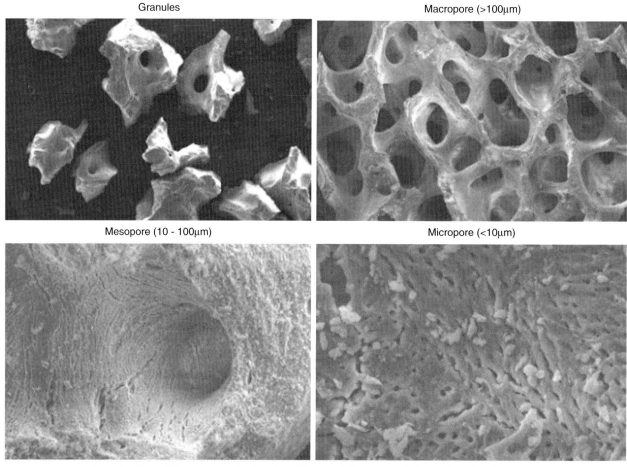

• **Fig. 35.5** Different Types of Porosity. (*Courtesy SigmaGraft Biomaterials, Fullerton, Calif.: http://sigmagraft. com/inteross/*)

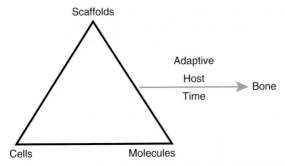

• **Fig. 35.6** The Bone Healing Triad. (*Adapted from Murphy CM, O'Brien FJ, Little DG, Schindeler A. Cell-scaffold interactions in the bone tissue engineering triad. Eur Cell Mater. 2013;26:120-132.*)

shown to enhance the osteoinductive effect of demineralized freeze-dried bone allograft (DFDBA) but will not stimulate new bone growth alone.[22] Platelet-rich plasma and other substances derived from the patient's own blood are also examples.

Ideal Bone Graft Substitute

Reconstruction of bone defects or preparation of a site for implant placement remains a challenge. On the one hand, autografts harbor most features of "ideal" BGS; on the other hand, they have a lot of insurmountable disadvantages (higher level of surgical skill needed, insufficient quantity, second-site morbidity, increased operative time, etc.). An ideal bone graft substitute should:

• be biomechanically stable;
• degrade within an appropriate time frame;
• exhibit osteoconductive, osteogenic, and osteoinductive properties; and
• provide a favorable environment for invading blood vessels and bone-forming cells.

Even though osteoconductivity of biomaterials for bone tissue engineering (BTE) strategies can be directed by their composition, surface character, and internal structure, osteoinductive and osteogenic features (discussed later) can be enhanced by the addition of osteopromotive materials.[23]

Having the ideal substitute would address only a part of what is needed for successful bone regeneration. As illustrated in Fig. 35.6, the bone healing triad is based on the complex process involved in tissue repair, wherein the matrix/scaffold (osteoconductive materials), signaling proteins (osteoinductive, located within the matrix), and tissue-forming cells (osteogenic, osteoclasts and osteoblasts) work in concert to form new tissue (bone) in the healthy (osseo-adaptive) host over time.

Ideal Membrane Material

GBR is a common technique in implant dentistry for the treatment of bone defects. As discussed earlier, a critical component of the GBR procedure is the use of a barrier membrane. These materials are used to prevent the invasion of cells that are not needed or would interfere with bone formation. The primary goal is selective cell repopulation.[24] An ideal barrier membrane should:

• Be biologically compatible. There should be no inflammation or interaction between the barrier material and the host.
• Provide space maintenance. When desired, the membrane should have the ability to prevent defect collapse.

• Stabilize the blood clot that forms as part of natural healing. This will allow the regeneration process to progress and reduce unwanted tissue integration into the defect.
• Provide cell occlusion. This is the primary function of the membrane, but many membranes allow the passage of fluid that may assist in healing.
• Have some degree of mechanical strength (based on end-user needs). Strength is needed, and in some cases shape memory is desired.
• Resorb predictably, per the end-user requirements. Fortunately, many configurations with varying rates of resorption exist.
• Be easy to modify and manipulate.

As you will see, there are many types of membranes to choose from, most of which possess those properties. It is up to the clinician to choose the barrier membrane that best provides for the desired clinical outcome.

Classification of Bone Graft Substitutes and Membranes

Transplant refers to the transfer of an organ from one body to another, or from a certain section of the patient's own body to another area. This procedure is usually performed to replace a damaged or missing organ. Tissues can be transferred from one individual to another, and because they are generally placed to encourage the body to heal itself, thus being incorporated into the host, they are considered transplants.

Implants are medical devices intended to replace a missing body part, support a damaged part, or enhance the body in some way. Titanium dental implants are a good example. Some researchers consider allografts and xenografts (biological material) to be implants because they are nonliving. It is acceptable to call them either transplants or implants.

Autograft (or autotransplantation) is the transplantation of functioning organs, tissues, or even particular proteins from one part of the body to another in the same person. Examples in implant dentistry are grafts from the ascending ramus, chin, or iliac crest.

Allograft (or homograft) is the transplantation of cells, tissues, or organs to a recipient from a genetically nonidentical donor of the same species. It can also be called an *allogeneic transplant*. Related to this are isografts—a graft of tissue between two individuals who are genetically identical (i.e., monozygotic twins). Demineralized freeze-dried bone and acellular dermis are examples used in implant dentistry.

Xenograft (or heterograft) is a tissue graft or organ transplant from a donor of a different species from the recipient. Bovine or porcine sourced materials (cancellous bone or collagen membranes) are good examples. An interesting example of xenografts is coral-derived materials. These are considered xenografts (as opposed to alloplasts) because of their organic nature.

Alloplast is an inorganic material used as a bone substitute or an implant. Hydroxyapatite (HA) and tricalcium phosphate (TCP) materials are examples.

Oversight

A *510(k)* is a premarket submission made to the FDA to demonstrate that a medical device is as safe and effective, that is, substantially equivalent, as a legally marketed device. Once the device is determined to be substantially equivalent, it can then be marketed in the United States. Two years after the Medical Device Amendments of 1976 were enacted, the FDA issued its final draft of the medical device Good Manufacturing Practice (GMP) regulation, a series of requirements that prescribed the facilities, methods, and controls to be used in the manufacture, packaging, and storage of medical devices. All 510(k) products must be manufactured under GMP, and proof that they are is part of the process for obtaining approval. Xenograft and alloplast materials fall under the 501(k) requirements. Products going through the 510(k) pathway can have intended applications or claims.

An *investigational device exemption* (IDE) allows the investigational device to be used in a clinical study to collect safety and effectiveness data. Clinical studies are most often conducted to support a premarket approval. Only a small percentage of 510(k)s require clinical data to support the application. Investigational use also includes clinical evaluation of certain modifications or new intended uses of legally marketed devices. All clinical evaluations of investigational devices, unless exempt, must have an approved IDE before the study is initiated. It is rare that a product intended to be used as a BGS or membrane in dentistry requires an IDE and premarket approval. If the device does need clinical evaluation and has not been cleared for marketing, these are required:

- an investigational plan approved by an institutional review board
- informed consent from all patients
- labeling stating that the device is for investigational use only
- monitoring of the study
- required records and reports

Good Clinical Practice refers to the regulations and requirements that must be complied with while conducting a clinical study. These regulations apply to the manufacturers, sponsors, clinical investigators, institutional review boards, and the medical device.

Products containing or consisting of human cells or tissues that are intended for implantation, transplantation, infusion, or transfer into a human recipient, and are considered minimally manipulated, are called *human cellular and tissue-based products* (HCT/Ps). HCT/Ps must also be intended for homologous use and cannot be combined with another article (except for water, crystalloids, or a sterilizing, preserving, or storage agent). The product must have no systemic effect and cannot be dependent on the metabolic activity of living cells for the primary function.

Allograft products are considered medical devices when the FDA determines that they have been more than minimally processed. To be considered beyond minimally processed, an original characteristic of a structural tissue must be altered, and that characteristic has to be relevant in that it has a potential effect on the utility of the tissue for reconstruction, repair, or replacement.

Manufacturers of HCT/Ps (i.e., tissue processors) are required by the FDA to comply with Current Good Tissue Practice. This includes proper handling, processing, labeling, and recordkeeping procedures. Under these regulations, tissue banks must screen and test all donors for risk factors and clinical evidence of relevant communicable disease agents.

With the rapid growth of all areas of tissue banking, there has been an increasing need for accountability and for measures that ensure that safe, quality tissues are available for clinical use. Quality improvement can be affected through voluntary standards, and most tissue banks have incorporated the achievement of high standards into their goals. The American Association of Tissue Banks (AATB) has established comprehensive standards for donor screening, recovery and processing of musculoskeletal, cardiac,

vascular, and skin tissues, and reproductive cells.[25] In addition, the standards contain institutional requirements; descriptions of required functional components of a tissue bank; requirements for construction and management of records and development of procedures; requirements for informed consent, tissue labeling, storage, and release; expectations for handling adverse outcomes, investigations, and tissue recalls; requirements for establishment of a quality program; specifications for equipment and facilities; and guidelines for tissue-dispensing services and tissue distribution intermediaries. AATB's *Standards for Tissue Banking* are consulted not only by tissue bankers but also by end-user healthcare facilities, other standard-setting organizations, and regulators worldwide. In 2018, more than 100 tissue banks in North America held AATB accreditation. Best practice for checking a tissue bank's accreditation status is to perform an accredited bank search on the AATB website.[26]

The Joint Commission has standards for storage and issuance of tissue for hospitals and ambulatory surgery centers. These standards apply to bone, tendon, fascia, and cartilage, as well as cellular tissues of both human and animal (xenograft) origin. The standards address key functions, including the need to develop procedures for tissue acquisition and storage, recordkeeping and tracking, and follow-up of adverse events and suspected allograft-caused infections, which must be reported to the tissue bank from which the tissue was obtained. Similar to federal regulations and AATB *Standards*, the minimal record retention period is specified to be 10 years from the date of transplantation, distribution, other disposition, or expiration, whichever is latest.

FDA authority to create and "enforce regulations necessary to prevent the introduction, transmission, or spread of communicable diseases between the States or from foreign countries into the States" under Section 361(a) of the U.S. Public Health Service Act (42 USC 264) applies to human tissue intended for transplantation. Formal enforcement policy and regulations did not exist until December 14, 1993 (codified in 21 CFR Parts 16 and 1270), when the "Interim Rule: Human Tissue Intended for Transplantation," which required donor screening, infectious disease testing, and recordkeeping "to prevent transmission of infectious diseases through human tissue used in transplantation," was adopted in response to reports of HIV transmission by human tissue and of potentially unsafe bone imported into the United States.[27]

These regulations were supplanted by a series of federal regulations, published in stages, first announced in the Proposed Approach to the Regulation of Cellular and Tissue-Based Products in March 1997. A final rule, "Human Cells, Tissues, and Cellular and Tissue-Based Products: Establishment Registration and Listing," published in January 2001, required organizations that are engaged in tissue recovery, donor qualification, tissue processing, and/or tissue-related laboratory testing to register as a tissue establishment with the FDA. The rule (21 CFR Part 1271) became effective for all tissue banks on March 29, 2004.

A final rule, "Eligibility Determination for Donors of Human Cells, Tissues, and Cellular and Tissue-Based Products," published May 25, 2004, set forth donor eligibility requirements, including health history screening and laboratory testing. Another final rule, "Current Good Tissue Practice for Human Cell, Tissue and Cellular and Tissue-Based Product Establishments; Inspection and Enforcement," published on November 24, 2004, established elements of good tissue practice, analogous to GMP for blood banks. Both rules became effective May 25, 2005.

Sterility

Sterility will be discussed from the viewpoint of allografts because they are the most difficult to sterilize because of their fragile biologic nature and variety.[28]

Tissue sterilization is defined as the killing or elimination of all microorganisms from allograft tissue, whereas disinfection refers to the removal of microbial contamination. The Association for the Advancement of Medical Instrumentation, a standard-setting organization for the medical instrumentation and technology industry, defines sterility assurance level (SAL) as the probability that an individual device, dose, or unit is nonsterile (i.e., one or more viable microorganisms being present) after it has been exposed to a validated sterilization process. Although absolute sterility in theory would represent an absence of any pathogen, SAL is generally applied only to the level of possible contamination with bacteria or parasites. In contrast with log reduction of viruses determined in assessments of virus reduction methods, SAL is an absolute determined by the ability of the method to eradicate or reduce microorganisms, the susceptibility of organisms that may be present to the sterilization method applied, and the maximal bioburden that could occur in the initial material. For example, a SAL of 10^{-6} means that there is less than a 1 in 1,000,000 chance of a viable microorganism remaining after the sterilization procedure. The FDA requires that medical devices be sterilized using a method validated to achieve a SAL of 10^{-6}. A medical device derived from or that includes a biological product component must also meet a SAL of 10^{-6} if it is to be labeled sterile. A SAL of 10^{-3}, or a 1 in 1000 chance of a viable microorganism being present, is a more achievable goal selected by some processors for aseptically processed tissues if the processor has been unable to validate their process to the more stringent SAL of 10^{-6} level, or if the tissues are unable to withstand the harsh treatment needed to achieve a more restrictive SAL without an impairment of tissue function. Such tissues may not then be labeled as sterile.

The complex physical structures and density of musculoskeletal tissues pose challenges for adequate penetration of antimicrobial agents to eradicate microorganisms. Allografts will not tolerate methods usually applied to metal and plastic medical devices because such treatment would impair the mechanical and biologic properties necessary for clinical utility. As an alternative, sterilization of tissues has been accomplished by several methods, including heat, chemicals, ethylene oxide gas, supercritical CO_2, and gamma or electron beam irradiation. However, not all sterilants have adequate tissue penetration. This is particularly the case for gases and liquids. The initial bioburden, which may be high in some tissues, must be considered. Some tissues are treated with antibiotics in vitro before storage, but this treatment decontaminates only the surface and may be effective against bacteria only.

A variety of methods, including chemical treatments and irradiation, has been used to reduce or eliminate pathogens in tissue intended for transplantation. The introduction of bone sterilization by ethylene oxide gas simplified bone processing and facilitated the widespread use of sterilized air-dried and lyophilized bone products. The effects of ethylene oxide treatment on the biomechanical and osteoinductive capacity of bone allografts have been questioned, although animal studies have yielded inconsistent results. These concerns, combined with those regarding the carcinogenic potential of ethylene oxide and its breakdown products, have largely led to abandonment of this method in the United States and the United Kingdom.

First introduced in the 1960s, gamma irradiation of bone is still used widely, usually employing a cobalt-60 source. The gamma rays penetrate bone effectively and work by generating free radicals, which may have adverse effects on collagen and limit utility in soft tissues unless performed in a controlled dose fashion at ultra-low temperature. The minimal bactericidal level of gamma irradiation is 10 to 20 kGy (1 kGy = 100,000 rad). Uncontrolled human studies have shown irradiated, calcified, and demineralized bone grafts to be clinically effective. Numerous studies have shown that mineralized bone allografts irradiated at 25 to 30 kGy are also clinically effective, with high success rates reported. In controlled studies the clinical effectiveness of bone allografts subjected to 25 kGy irradiation was comparable with that of nonirradiated bone grafts, although doses exceeding 25 kGy for cortical bone and 60 kGy for cancellous bone have been found to induce cross-linking of collagen and to impair mechanical function in a dose-dependent fashion. There is *in vitro* evidence that high irradiation reduces osteoclast activity and increases osteoblast apoptosis (programmed cell death), and that residual bacterial products induce inflammatory bone resorption after macrophage inactivation. However, the clinical significance of these findings has not been established. Newer processes employing radioprotectants have preserved bone allograft integrity when doses $\geq$25 kGy are applied, and controlled-dose methods permit successful irradiation at lower doses (see Proprietary Sterilization Methods to follow). Irradiated demineralized bone has potential osteoinductive activity and has been effective in nonstructural clinical applications.

Concerns about pathogen transmission and the limitations of irradiation, especially for soft tissues, have prompted improvements in sterilization methods and in the validation of these methods. A number of proprietary chemical-based processing methods have been developed with aims of effectively penetrating tissues and reducing, killing, or inactivating microorganisms and viruses without unacceptable adverse effects on the tissue's biomechanical properties. In addition, for use in transplantation, the agents must either be able to be effectively removed or be nontoxic. All methods in current use are applied only to tissue from donors who have met stringent criteria for medical history and behavioral risk assessment as well as negative results on infectious disease marker testing.

Proprietary Sterilization Methods

The Tutoplast process (Tutogen Medical, Gainesville, Fla.) was the first process to sterilize and preserve tissue without affecting biological or mechanical properties. The process has been in use since the early 1970s for a variety of hard and soft tissues, including bone, fascia lata, pericardium, skin, amniotic membrane, and sclera. Initially lipids are removed in an ultrasonic acetone bath that also inactivates enveloped viruses and reduces prion activity. Bacteria are destroyed using alternating hyperosmotic saline and purified water baths that also wash out cellular debris. Soluble proteins, nonenveloped viruses, and bacterial spores are destroyed in multiple hydrogen peroxide baths, and a 1N sodium hydroxide treatment further reduces prion infectivity by 6 logs. A final acetone wash removes any residual prions and inactivates any remaining enveloped viruses. Vacuum extraction dehydrates the tissue before the grafts are shaped and then double-barrier packaged. Terminal sterilization using low-dose gamma irradiation yields a SAL of 10^{-6}.

The Allowash XG process (LifeNet Health [LNH], Virginia Beach, Va.) employs six steps: (1) bioburden control, (2) bioburden assessment, (3) minimization of contamination during processing, (4) rigorous cleaning, (5) disinfection steps, and (6) a final step of low-temperature, controlled-dose gamma irradiation. The process has been validated to achieve a SAL of 10^{-6}. Holtzclaw et al.[29] in 2008 compared the Allowash XG and Tutoplast methods, and found that each achieved medical-grade sterility with no effect on biological or biomechanical properties.

The BioCleanse process (Regeneration Technologies, Alachua, Fla.) uses low-temperature addition of chemical sterilants, such as hydrogen peroxide and isopropyl alcohol, which permeate the tissue's inner matrix, followed by pressure variations intended to drive the sterilants into and out of the tissue. Regeneration Technologies reports a SAL of 10^{-6} for soft tissues without adverse effects on the initial allograft mechanical properties.

The Clearant process (Clearant, Los Angeles, Calif.) is designed to avoid the negative effects of gamma irradiation through addition of free radical scavengers, using pretreatment dimethyl sulfoxide and propylene glycol as radioprotectants. Although the process subjects tissue to 50 kGy radiation and achieves a SAL of 10^{-6} for bacteria, fungi, yeast, and spores, the tissue's biomechanical properties are retained.

The Musculoskeletal Transplant Foundation (Edison, N.J.) uses a series of chemicals, including nonionic detergents, hydrogen peroxide, and alcohol, to treat cortical and cancellous bone grafts. For soft tissues an antibiotic mixture containing gentamicin, amphotericin B, and Primaxin is added and then washed out to a nondetectable concentration. The Musculoskeletal Transplant Foundation claims a SAL of 10^{-3} for its products. Incoming tissues whose bioburden exceeds prescribed parameters are pretreated with low-dose gamma irradiation.

NovaSterilis (Lansing, N.Y.) has developed a sterilization technique that uses supercritical carbon dioxide at low temperatures and relatively low pressures, resulting in transient acidification, which is lethal to bacteria and viruses, with good penetration reported. However, this technique only recently became available for clinically available allografts, and data on clinical efficacy and retention of allograft mechanical properties are limited.

End-User Responsibilities

Informed Consent. The clinician is, as defined by the AATB and other organizations, the end-user. As such, the clinician's responsibility is the safest and most efficacious treatment for his or her patient. This begins with a complete understanding of the characteristics and limitations of any material used in treatment. Second, the patient expectations and concerns must be assessed. This is part of the process of informed consent. It is important that proper informed consent is obtained.

The Doctrine of Informed Consent[30] is based on significant history:
- *Schloendorff* v. *Society of New York Hospital* in 1914: An operation was performed against the patient's wishes.
- *Salgo* v. *Leland Stanford Jr. University Board of Trustees* in 1957: The patient had not been informed of the risks involved with the surgery performed.
- *Natanson* v. *Kline* in 1960: This verdict established a standard that the risks as understood by a reasonable practitioner must be disclosed.
- *Canterbury* v. *Spence* in 1972: This verdict required practitioners to disclose the risks that a reasonable patient would want to know.
- AMA Position Paper on "informed consent" in 1981: This document established the "best standards" concerning informed consent in medicine.

Consent is to reflect all applicable local, state, and federal laws and regulations, as well as internal policies and evolving best practices. The informed consent discussion has several components[31]:
- the nature of the proposed treatment, including necessity, prognosis, time element, and cost;
- viable alternatives to the proposed treatment, including what a specialist might offer or the choice of no treatment; and
- what are the foreseeable risks, including things likely to occur and risks of no treatment?

When obtaining informed consent, the dental professional should:
- Use language that is easily understandable.
- Provide opportunities for patient questions, such as "What more would you like to know?" or "What are your concerns?"
- Assess patient understanding by stating, "If I have not explained the proposed dentistry clearly or if you have difficulty understanding, please tell me so we can discuss anything you do not understand."

When gaining consent for the use of allografts, please use language that does not degrade the spirit of the gift of donation (i.e., use "deceased donor" instead of "cadaver" and "recovered" instead of "harvested"). Remember that all tissue is recovered "aseptically" (not "sterile" and not necessarily in an operating room). For all types of materials (allograft, xenograft, alloplast), processors and manufacturers often provide patient education materials for use by the end-user. These do not replace the informed consent discussion but exist to augment the effort. In addition, most companies that provide materials have a toll-free number or website for answering patient inquiries. Patients' ability to recollect and comprehend treatment information plays a fundamental role in their decision making.[32] Although patients in general report that they understand information given to them, they may have limited comprehension. Additional media may improve conventional informed consent processes in dentistry in a meaningful way.

Proper Handling of Materials. The end-user is responsible for reviewing the "product insert" (also known by other names, e.g., "instructions for use," "package insert"). This document provides valuable information on storage, indications, contraindications, tracking, among others. Some materials have been treated with chemicals or antibiotics, and this must be listed to avoid allergic reactions in their patients.

Materials should be inspected on receipt. Are the materials the ones ordered? Is the packaging intact? Were the materials protected from extremes in temperature during shipment? What is the expiration date? If the material appears to be compromised in any way, or is not what was expected, the distributor should be notified.

Materials should be stored as indicated until time of use. It is imperative that certain material not be frozen or kept in areas with extreme heat (both conditions can destroy the characteristics of some materials). In addition, materials should be "logged" or tracked internally at time of receipt, when used on a patient, or when discarded or returned. All materials bear a unique identifier, and it is the responsibility of the end-user to have a system for identifying when and where each material is used. In the case of allografts, federal law states that each allograft unit have a distinct identifier, and that a system exists to track the graft from processor to consignee (and back). This makes it the responsibility of the end-user to track from his or her office inventory to the patient, meaning that the unique identifier can be associated with the patient's unique identifier (chart number, etc.).[33]

Tracking of xenograft and alloplast, although not always required, is a good practice. Take the example of a patient who experiences a localized reaction at a site where augmentation occurred; allograft bone was mixed with alloplast, and the site was covered with a xenograft membrane. Identification numbers for each material would be needed to determine, with the help of the individual processors, the root cause of the localized reaction. In this case, having the information at hand as part of the patient surgical notes would be a great advantage.

In the unlikely chance that a recall occurs, it is much easier to determine patients receiving affected units if that information is in a central database or log. Therefore in addition to information in the patient's operative note, it is wise to have a central log where grafts received into inventory are logged (date and time), as well as their final disposition (used on a patient [and ID of that patient], returned to distributor, discarded, etc., noting date and time).

Expiration Dates. Materials are not to be used past their expiration date. Disposition should be recorded in the office log, and the material should be discarded in a proper manner.

Material Safety Data Sheets. Material Safety Data Sheets (MSDS) are not required for BGSs and membranes. The Occupational Safety & Health Administration requires chemical manufacturers and importers to develop an MSDS for each hazardous chemical produced or imported, and these must be provided to a distributor or end-user before or at the time of shipment. "Hazardous" chemicals are defined as any chemical that is a physical or health hazard. A "physical hazard" is a chemical where scientific evidence shows that it is combustible, a compressed gas, explosive, flammable, an oxidizer, or unstable (reactive). A "health hazard" is a chemical for which statistical evidence exists that shows acute or chronic health effects in exposed individuals. BGSs and membranes do not pose a physical or health hazard.

As always, refer to the Instructions for Use document accompanying any BGS or membrane. This will contain specific information on indications for use, contraindications, precautions, and preparation instructions.

"Single-Patient Use". All BGSs and membranes, if packaged individually, are designated for single patient use. This means that the material cannot be used for treatment of more than one patient. The AATB demands that "Single-Patient Use" appears on the label of every allograft produced by AATB-accredited tissue processors. Processors are working with the AATB to ensure that each graft is used for treatment of only one patient, and that each graft can be tracked (personal communication, Jon Boyd, Director of Certification and Online Learning, AATB, McLean, Va.). Although the terminology may differ (e.g., "single use"), similar intent exists for xenografts and alloplasts (and this information may appear on a package insert). Consider the following:

- To reuse a single-use device or material without considering the consequences could expose patients and staff to risks that outweigh the perceived benefits.
- A device or material designated as "single use" must not be reused. It should be used only on an individual patient during a single procedure and then discarded. It is not intended to be reprocessed and used again, even on the same patient.
- The reuse of single-use devices can affect their safety, performance, and effectiveness, exposing patients and staff to unnecessary risk.
- The reuse of single-use devices has legal implications: Anyone who reprocesses or reuses a device intended by the manufacturer for use on a single occasion bears full responsibility for its safety and effectiveness.

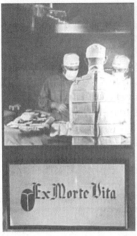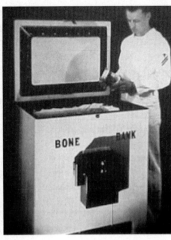

● **Fig. 35.7** Photographs from the first tissue bank, U.S. Navy at Bethesda Naval Hospital in Bethesda, Maryland. The picture on the left shows technicians at work processing deceased donor material. Out of respect for the donor, processing was done in silence with technicians communicating nonverbally. The sign on the door translates to "from death, life." The right photograph shows a technician removing frozen grafts from a –80°C chest freezer. (*From Strong DM. The US Navy Tissue Bank: 50 years on the cutting edge.* Cell Tissue Bank. *2000;1:9-16.*)

End-User Queries. When in doubt, the end-user should contact his or her product distributor for additional information. It is the responsibility of the distributor to find answers, or to refer the end-user to a subject matter expert, which may include direct discussion with the manufacturer. In most cases the well-trained distributor representative or customer service representative can answer questions related to manufacture, clinical use, and safety.

Allograft Source, Processing, and Distribution

Allograft tissue banking has a rich history. The first tissue bank was established by the U.S. Navy in 1949 by Dr. George Hyatt.[34] Hyatt was an orthopedic surgeon at the Naval Medical Center in Bethesda, Maryland. The navy program was the first of its kind in the world and established many of the standards that are followed today (Fig. 35.7). During the 1950s, the identification of appropriate donor criteria for tissue donation, the development of procurement and processing methods, the establishment of a graft registry and documentation, and the clinical evaluation of a variety of tissues were pioneered at this facility. Cryopreservation, freeze-drying, irradiation sterilization of tissue, and immunologic principles of tissue transplantation were developed during the 50 years of research and development by navy scientists. Organ preservation, cadaveric bone marrow recovery, and immunosuppressive protocols were also developed at the Navy Tissue Bank. The navy was also instrumental in the establishment of the National Marrow Donor Program and the AATB in the United States. Although the Navy Tissue Bank has ceased activity after 50 years of excellence, it should be recognized as the first standard setter for the world community of tissue banks. The first civilian tissue banks were formed by ex-navy surgeons who trained at Bethesda.

At this time, all tissue banking in the United States is dependent on organ procurement organizations (OPOs). The OPOs are the mechanism through which families can elect to donate not only their loved one's lifesaving organs but also eyes, skin, heart valves, veins, arteries, bone, tendon, ligaments, and other "tissue" that can be used to improve health.

OPOs represent a unique component of health care.[35] By federal law, they are the only organizations that can perform the lifesaving mission of recovering organs from deceased donors for transplantation. When the National Organ Transplant Act was signed into law in 1984, it created the national Organ Procurement and Transplantation Network (OPTN) for matching donor organs to waiting recipients. The OPTN both standardized the process through which organs are donated and shared across the country, and created the system of federally designated OPOs throughout the United States and its territories. The OPTN includes all OPOs and transplant centers, and is managed under contract by the United Network for Organ Sharing located in Richmond, Virginia. There are currently 58 OPOs in the United States, and all are nonprofit entities.

Because the focus of the OPO is organ donation, tissue recovery and processing are managed by separate entities (tissue, eye, skin, heart valves) as designated by each OPO (through a contract). It is the responsibility of the OPO to make sure *every* family has the opportunity to fulfill their loved one's donation wishes.

Tissue processors may use either the OPO or regional recovery programs for the recovery of tissue. All donor suitability assessment, recovery, transport, storage, processing, postproduction testing, and distribution are the responsibility of the tissue processor.

Donor suitability is standardized throughout the United States and consists of three parts: initial medical interview with next of kin, physical assessment by the recovery team, and laboratory testing for communicable disease. The medical history and history of present illness are critical, and findings result in a high number of decisions not to proceed with tissue donation. When a potential donor is approved for recovery, they are assigned a unique identifier; this number will be associated with all tissue grafts subsequently produced. Tissue recovery *must* take place quickly: within 15 hours from time of asystole, or up to 24 hours from asystole if the deceased donor was refrigerated within 12 hours of death. Therefore laboratory testing is performed after recovery has occurred. The laboratory assessments not only test for donor suitability (communicable disease and systemic infection), but a representative culture from each piece of tissue is tested for microbiologic contamination via aerobic and anaerobic means at both room and body temperatures. Any biologic contaminant found is known as bioburden.

Recovery occurs, when possible, in an operating room at the hospital of the deceased donor. Many recovery programs and OPOs have dedicated recovery facilities, and the donor can be transported there for recovery. Some medical examiner offices have dedicated facilities in cooperation with the local recovery program or OPO. Recovery is done under aseptic conditions just like any surgical procedure. The donor is prepped, draped, and recovery occurs in a particular sequence via zones. Each zone uses new equipment. Tissue removed is swabbed for culturing, wrapped in special materials (impervious to fluids), tagged with the assigned unique identifier, and placed on ice for transport to the tissue processor.

After arriving at the processor, tissue is placed in quarantine (−80°C) until all serologic and microbiologic tests are complete. In addition, some donors have autopsies, the results of which must be obtained before processing. A final chart review and additional information must be assessed and approved before processing into usable grafts. The tissue bank medical director has full responsibility for release of tissue for processing.

Processing occurs in clean rooms or laminar flow hoods under strict aseptic conditions. One set of technicians processes one donor at a time—no donor pooling or cross-contamination is allowed. Different tissues undergo processing in different ways. Regardless of the tissue processor, the end product is the same: preparation and preservation of tissue without changing the biochemical or biological characteristics.

Grafts (now in quarantine) undergo postproduction review and testing (e.g., residual moisture if freeze-dried, residual calcium if demineralized) before final "in-package" sterilization (see earlier Sterility section). Poststerility review occurs (review of dosimetry and last look at all processing records) before approval by the quality team for release into the "bank" for distribution. Finished grafts are based on surgeon demand. Because the demand in many cases outweighs the supply, every effort is taken to maximize the donor gift. The time from receipt of donor tissue to grafts ready to distribute, at most tissue processors, takes approximately 90 days.

Regarding the "average donor" and the types of grafts produced for dental use, my research shows that two tissue banks provide the majority (>50%) of "full-line" allograft offering to the dental implant community. These two are Community Tissue Services (CTS) based in Dayton, Ohio, and LNH in Virginia Beach, Virginia. In addition, both offer branded and private label allograft options to the two largest dental implant suppliers in the world (Nobel Biocare and Straumann, respectively). Both use similar processing technology, and both have a long history of cooperation in tissue banking (CTS was founded in 1986, and LNH was founded in 1982). These two nonprofit organizations are innovative and active as leaders in AATB. I queried both processors regarding donors and grafts produced for the dental segment in 2017 (personal communication, Paul Lehner, Dental Product Manager, CTS, and David Adamson, General Manager Dental and Craniomaxillofacial, LNH).

Regarding donors, it is interesting that if you look at all donors received, the range is 12 to 80 years old (these are "musculoskeletal" donations that can be turned into grafts for a variety of surgical specialties, including dental). An average age cannot be calculated because the distribution is bimodal, that is, with two different "peaks." One peak occurs from about age 18 to 24 years, and the other appears from age 45 to 65 years. About 86.5% of the donors were younger than 70 years, and nearly three of every four donors are male. What is most interesting is that the donor age and gender statistics have not changed since the late 2000s (compared with my data from 2007), except that the number of donors has greatly increased. The increase is due to active donation awareness programs[36] and an increase in the number of individuals signing up on the national donor registry—that number is currently 130 million.[37] There were approximately 30,000 tissue donors in the United States in 2017.

Finally, all dental allograft processors in the United States are AATB accredited. Accreditation is a rigorous program that requires adherence to AATB standards, membership in the national organization, and periodic inspections. The AATB restricts distribution of allografts to hospitals, certain healthcare facilities, dentists, and podiatrists. Distribution intermediaries can receive and store allografts for redistribution, but they must follow AATB guidelines, be registered with the FDA, and are subject to state registration(s) and inspection(s).

Xenograft Source, Production, and Distribution

Clinicians and researchers have experimented with ways to correct skeletal defects in the modern era. Nothing exemplifies this search better than the early experiences with xenografts. Orell[38] in 1937 reported his clinical experiences with the surgical grafting of os purum, os novum, and boiled bone. Os purum was ox bone prepared by a complicated physicochemical procedure that freed the bone of lipids, connective tissue, and some protein but still left some of the collagen matrix. It was used to fill various skeletal defects, and the author claimed that it was resorbed and replaced by host bone in 2 to 3 years.[38] In 1956, Forsberg[39] used finely ground, sterile os purum as an implant material for periodontal osseous defects. He reported 11 cases and claimed excellent results in 1, satisfactory results in 7, and poor results in the remaining 3 cases after a postoperative period of up to 12 months.[39]

University studies on laboratory-produced anorganic xenograft bone began in earnest in the 1950s. Anorganic means that the organic portion (~40% by weight) is totally removed, leaving pure HA. Scopp et al.[40,41] in the 1960s reported experimental and clinical work with the first commercially available xenogeneic implant material called Boplant (Squibb Pharmaceuticals; this product is no longer available). It was derived from calf bone, and processing consisted of detergent extraction, followed by chloroform and methanol extraction to reduce the lipid content, washing with sterile deionized water, sterilization by immersions in a liquid sterilizing agent, and finally lyophilization and vacuum packaging.[40,41] This work was the precursor to the modern xenograft. Notably, xenografts can be demineralized, freeze-dried, and/or deproteinized, but most distribution is of a calcified matrix form. To date, sources for xenograft material used in dentistry include bovine, porcine, equine, and species of coral. In general, bovine and porcine use cancellous bone. Both materials mimic human bone in density, porosity, and calcium content.[42-44]

The best example of xenograft processing and use can be seen with anorganic bovine materials such as Bio-Oss (Geistlich Pharma North America, Inc.).[45] The Geistlich Pharma website includes a searchable database for Geistlich Pharma materials and associated clinical studies. Of all of the available BGS materials, Bio-Oss has the greatest number of published studies. Since its beginnings in 1851 the company has dealt with the processing and refining of bone and collagen materials, and up to now they have the most researched biomaterials.

Geistlich Pharma manufactures its biomaterials in its own production department at the company's headquarters in Switzerland. The entire production process is subject to the strictest safety standards and quality checks: from the selection of the raw material suppliers to the delivery of the end products. Safety during the manufacture of the products is guaranteed thanks to extensive hygiene measures in a sophisticated zone system with different safety levels and permanent controls.

Geistlich Bio-Oss is made from the mineral part of bovine bone (and is also known as deproteinized bovine bone material). The strictly controlled manufacturing process ensures high quality and safety standards by:

- a defined origin of the raw material;
- a restricted country of origin, for example, Australia, which is historically and currently free of bovine spongiform encephalopathy (a prion disease, or "mad cow");
- using selected and certified slaughterhouses;
- performing of pre and post mortem health inspection for each individual animal;
- restricting source to extremity bone (according to World Health Organization Guidelines on tissue infectivity classified as tissues with no detected infectivity or infectious prions), as opposed to axial skeleton bones that may be associated with the spinal column;

- effective inactivation methods with 15-hour treatment at high temperature and cleaning with strong alkaline solutions;
- medical-grade sterilization and double sterile packaging; and
- official controls by international authorities.

Many of the controls placed on xenograft production are similar to what is seen with allograft. GMP must be followed and international manufacturers are subject to International Organization for Standardization rules.[46] International materials coming to the United States must obtain FDA clearance, most often via 510(k) approvals. Distribution of most xenograft materials in dentistry is accomplished through dental supply companies.

Alloplast Production and Distribution

The category of alloplastic implants includes any nonosseous material placed into a bony defect for the purpose of stimulating repair or regeneration. It includes a very wide range of materials, both biologically and nonbiologically derived, and is limited only by the imagination of the investigator and the tolerance of living host tissue. Albee[47] in 1920 reviewed the literature to date and reported that osmic acid, fibrin, blood, gelatin with lime salts, zinc chloride, thyroidin, glacial acetic acid, tincture of iodine, adrenaline, extract of hypophysis, copper sulfate, oil of turpentine, ammonia, lactic acid, silver nitrate solution, alcohol, carbolic acid, oak bark extract, vaccines, and sera had been used to stimulate bone growth without any appreciable success.

Historically the oldest known alloplast used in medicine is calcium sulfate. Calcium sulfate, also known as "gypsum" or "plaster of paris," was first implanted in humans by Dreesman in 1892 as a void filler of tuberculous osteomyelitis.[48]

A great many materials are used today as the basis of alloplasts. These include (but are not limited to): HA (and its many derivatives), tricalcium phosphates, biphasic configurations, calcium sulfates, bioactive glass (BG), polymer-based materials, and composite materials.[49] In recent years more attention has been placed on macroporosity and microporosity (and interconnectivity of pores), interparticle spacing, mechanical qualities, and rate of resorption.

Alloplast production follows the guidelines of the pharmaceutical industry. Materials are "manufactured" under GMP, subject to FDA and International Organization for Standardization regulations, and their use is restricted to medical facilities and licensed health professionals. Distribution to dental practitioners in the United States is predominantly through medical and dental supply companies.

Graft Descriptions[50-60]

Allograft

Mineralized Cortical Particulate. Also known as freeze-dried bone allograft (FDBA) (Fig. 35.8), mineralized cortical particulate grafts still contain all of the natural bone components (inorganic and organic including BMPs hidden within the bone matrix). Even though it is called *mineralized*, there is no mineral added; it is simply "not" demineralized. FDBA is sourced from extremity bone (femur, tibia, fibula, humerus, radius, ulna, etc.). It can be processed, ground, and sieved to any desired particle range. A common range is 250 to 1000 μm. Particles smaller than 50 μm are quickly removed from the site by macrophages. Some processors offer particles up to 3 mm for filling of larger defects. Because FDBA still contains its calcified portion, it has mechanical strength. For that reason it is a popular graft material in implant dentistry. FDBA is osteoconductive.

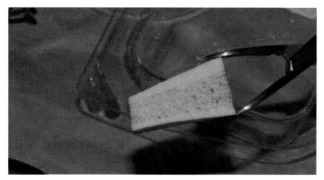

• **Fig. 35.8** This is a common allograft from the ilium. It is shown as a reminder that there are only two types of bone—cortical and cancellous—from which bone grafts are fashioned. Cortical has little macroporosity, whereas cancellous has much. The cancellous portion is made of interconnecting pores and is created from trabeculae oriented as per Wolff's law (form and function). New vessel formation can occur much quicker in cancellous bone. *(From Sfasciotti GL, Trapani CT, Powers RM. Mandibular ridge augmentation using a mineralized ilium block: A case letter. J Oral Implantol 42(2):215-219, 2016.)*

Mineralized Cancellous Particulate. Also known as FDBA, mineralized cancellous particulate is made solely from the cancellous portion of bone. Graft source is the metaphyseal region of long bones. It shares many of the characteristics of mineralized cortical particulate but has greater macroporosity because of the marrow space. In addition, the trabecular surface of cancellous is covered with endosteum that, like periosteum, probably plays a role in bone regeneration. Because of the porous nature of cancellous bone, new vessel growth (in theory) is more rapid through the graft; therefore regeneration will be quicker. Another benefit is that cancellous particles tend to lock together better than equivalently sized cortical particles, and this will reduce micromotion in a graft site. Mineralized cancellous grafts are osteoconductive.

Mineralized Cortical/Cancellous Mix. The mineralized cortical/cancellous mix is a combination of the two previous graft types. It can be manufactured in two ways: first is mixing together each component 50:50 (v/v), which requires cortical and cancellous material from a single donor, which requires additional quality-control measures; and the second way is to grind and sieve bone from the metaphysis of a long bone, which is known as a "natural" mix (called *corticocancellous*) and results in a graft with varying and undetermined proportions of cancellous component. Cortical/cancellous mix is gaining in popularity because these grafts provide good mechanical support and provide for faster incorporation.

According to information provided by tissue processors CTS and LNH (personal communication, Paul Lehner and David Adamson), in 2017 the previous three graft types (combined) accounted for >80% of the total allograft units distributed. In contrast, in the early 1990s >80% of the grafts distributed were demineralized cortical particulate (unpublished data). This shift is directly related to the increase in graft use to support implant placement.

Demineralized Cortical Particulate. Demineralized cortical particulate is also known as DFDBA or demineralized bone matrix (DBM). This historically was the first graft produced in great numbers by tissue processors for the periodontal market. Demineralized grafts have osteoinductive potential because processing removes the mineralized portion of the graft, thus exposing the noncollagenous proteins (e.g., BMPs) associated with the collagen matrix. These proteins recruit bone-forming cells to the site, thus inducing new bone growth. To be called *demineralized*, the AATB

specifies that residual calcium in the final graft cannot exceed 8% by weight. Normal cortical bone, for example, has ~30% residual calcium. If a graft is over- or under-demineralized, it will not possess its full osteoinductive potential. DFDBA is often just called *demineralized*. The other term, *DBM*, is reserved for DFDBA that is put with a carrier or is packaged in a convenience device such as a syringe. When reading market reports, DFDBA is considered nonproprietary, made by many processors; DBM is proprietary and made by few processors, usually under patent protection. Because DFDBA (and DBM) have their mineral component removed, they have little mechanical strength and often will not maintain space. Both forms, if prepared correctly, are compressible, have osteoinductive potential, and are osteoconductive.

Mineralized Cortical/Demineralized Cortical Combination. One of the newest grafts, mineralized cortical/demineralized cortical combination (70:30 v/v) takes advantage of the best characteristics of its components. Unlike DFDBA, this version will maintain space and incorporates quickly compared with mineralized graft forms. It is both osteoconductive and osteoinductive.

Laminar Bone. Laminar bone is a graft form that was popular in the 1990s that has undergone a resurgence. It is made by preparing cortical sheets (from the diaphysis portion of long bones) and demineralizing. This flexible graft not only induces new bone to grow but acts as its own membrane.

Irradiated Cancellous (Vertebral Body). Vertebral bodies possess marrow and cancellous with extremely dense trabeculation (per Wolff's law). Cortical particulate, cancellous particulate, and block grafts can be produced from vertebral materials. These materials receive a 25 to 38 kGy gamma irradiation.

Mineralized Cortical and Cancellous Blocks and Cubes. Blocks and cubes in almost any dimension can be made from solid sections of cortical and cancellous bone. These would be used in larger cases where missing walls must be replaced, among other cases. These materials arrive freeze-dried, and clinicians must take care when rehydrating and during fixation. In the freeze-dried state, these grafts are brittle. When properly rehydrated, these have the same biomechanics as natural bone. Most often, fixation is by a lag screw method.

Gel, Pastes, and Putties. Gel, pastes, and putties are all made with DBM as the main component with an inert carrier substance. The first such graft came out in the early 1990s and used glycerol as a means of dispensing the DBM particles. This was formulated for convenience: the DBM needed no rehydration, there were no loose particles to deal with, and the graft was ready to go off the shelf. Many gels, pastes, and putties currently exist in the market. There is overlap in the naming of these materials. In general, gel means very thin (low viscosity), with the possibility of being delivered via a syringe or other device. Paste is thicker and may lend itself to delivery in an open-bore device. Putty is moldable and can be hand-delivered to a site. Many describe it like the modeling compound Play-Doh (Hasbro Corp., Cincinnati, Ohio) used by children and artists. Putty has additional utility in that it can often be combined with other graft materials (e.g., autograft) or osteopromotive materials. Gels, pastes, and putties also may come in various formulation. Some have only DBM and a carrier, whereas others have DBM, a mineralized component, and a carrier. These materials would maintain space much better than a pure demineralized material.

Rib, Mandible, Bone Pins, and Sheets. A variety of additional skeletal grafts can be found at different tissue processors. Ribs are processed by most tissue banks. Mandibles are restricted to a few banks—these being difficult to recover and process. Bone pins (solid cortical) have become more popular in recent years and are used much like tenting screws. Cortical sheets are available, but not by all tissue processors. Most tissue banks, if contacted, will work to assist a clinician in finding who has the graft available.

Cell-Based Materials. Osteocel (Nuvasive, Inc., distributed by ACE Surgical, Brockton, Mass.) is an excellent example of a cell-based material. From a single donor, DFDBA, mineralized cancellous, and cells from the bone marrow are processed and recombined into this specialized graft. The resulting material is osteoinductive, osteoconductive, and osteogenic. Other processors are researching similar solutions, and this is a fast-growing area of tissue regeneration.

Placental Tissues. The placenta is the source of valuable membranes and cells. Human amniotic membrane is the most commonly used and is derived from the fetal membranes. It consists of the inner amniotic membrane made of single layer of amnion cells fixed to collagen-rich mesenchyme. Human amniotic membrane has low immunogenicity, antiinflammatory properties, and can be isolated without the sacrifice of human embryos. Amniotic membrane has various clinical applications in the field of dermatology, ophthalmology, ENT (ear, nose, and throat) surgery, orthopedics, and dental surgery.

Fascia Lata. Fascia lata is the deep fascia of the thigh. It invests the whole of the thigh but varies in thickness in different parts (the section used for dentistry is around 1 mm thick). Since the 1920s, fascia lata from deceased donors has been used in reconstructive surgery. In 1993, Callan[55] described cases where freeze-dried fascia lata was used as a membrane. Although still available from many tissue banks for orthopedic applications, it has largely been replaced by acellular dermis in dental applications.

Pericardium. Pericardium is the membrane enclosing the heart, consisting of an outer fibrous layer and an inner double layer of serous membrane. The material resembles fascia lata and can be used in a similar fashion. Pericardium is recovered from only heart valve donors; therefore it is in short supply and not processed by most tissue banks. Xenograft pericardium can be substituted (see later discussion).

Acellular Dermis. Acellular dermal matrix has been used as a soft tissue replacement since its introduction in 1994. Its first dental use was correcting areas with insufficient attached gingiva, but in 1999, Crook[56] reported using it as a barrier membrane. Even though the material is in high demand, few tissue banks produce acellular dermis because most methods of production are proprietary. Acellular dermal matrices are soft tissue matrix grafts created by a process that results in decellularization but leaves the extracellular matrix intact. It starts with a full-thickness skin graft from a deceased donor. The full-thickness graft is exposed to chemicals that remove the epidermis. A secondary step exposes the remaining dermis to chemicals (detergents and endonucleases) that removed the cells and DNA. This is the "decellularization" step that renders the graft acellular. As a result, an immunologic response in the host is unlikely. Extracellular matrix is preserved, as well as biomechanical properties. These materials have found great use in burns treatment, plastic and reconstructive surgery, podiatry, orthopedics, and dentistry.

Xenograft

Particulate Form. Processing and production considerations for xenograft is similar to what has been described for allograft. However, cancellous (also known as spongiosa or trabecular bone) seems to be the preferred form. Xenograft is most often

deproteinized (removing all immunogenic factors) by a variety of methods. What is left is a calcified matrix resembling natural inorganic component (HA) in all ways. Macroporosity and microporosity are preserved. As discussed previously, both bovine and porcine bone resemble human bone from a biochemical and biomechanical perspective. Xenograft particulate is available in a variety of particle ranges. Because xenograft is pure mineral, it does resorb slowly and is an excellent material for long-term space preservation.

Block Form. Solid and porous blocks of xenograft HA can be formed based on desired characteristics. These will function to preserve space for much longer than with an allograft. Macroporosity and microporosity can be controlled, as well as surface characteristics. As a pure HA product the grafts tend to be more brittle than natural bone, so care should be taken when modifying shape or using fixation screws.

Pericardium. As mentioned previously, allograft pericardium is in short supply. As a result, bovine and porcine pericardium substitutes have been developed and introduced into the dental market. Bovine has a greater collagen content than the porcine version. They generally consist of three layers with collagen and elastic fibers in an amorphous matrix. Their surface is porous, which allows for cellular attachment and proliferation, yet has an increased density for soft tissue exclusion. Pericardium membranes have shown a prolonged resorption in comparison with collagen membranes.

Collagen-Based Products. Resorbable collagen membranes (Fig. 35.9) are manufactured from xenogeneic tendon and skin to manage oral wounds such as extraction sockets, for sinus-lift procedures and repairs, and for periodontal or endodontic surgeries. They act as scaffolds for bone deposition in GBR, promote platelet aggregation, stabilize clots, and attract fibroblasts, facilitating wound healing. They are designed to resorb within 2 weeks to 6 months and are biocompatible, easy to manipulate, and only weakly immunogenic. For ease of use, collagen-based products are available in a wide variety of forms such as membranes, plugs, or tape. Extended collagen membranes resorb in 4 to 6 months and are used for larger bony defects that require longer healing periods. These membranes are modified by increasing the cross-link density.

Coralline Grafts. *Madrepore* ("stone coral") and *millepora* ("fire coral") are harvested and treated to become "coral-derived granules" and other types of coralline xenografts. Coral-based materials are mainly calcium carbonate (and an important proportion of fluorides, useful in the context of grafting to promote bone development), whereas natural human bone is made of HA, along with calcium phosphate and carbonate. The coral material is transformed industrially into HA through a hydrothermal process, yielding a nonresorbable xenograft. If the process is omitted, the coralline material remains in its calcium carbonate state for better resorption of the graft by the natural bone.

Alloplast

Hydroxyapatite. HA is a commonly used calcium phosphate biomaterial for bone regeneration applications due to having a composition and structure similar to natural bone mineral. HA-based grafts form a chemical bond directly to bone once implanted. Synthetic HA is available and used in various forms: (1) porous nonresorbable, (2) solid nonresorbable, and (3) resorbable (nonceramic, porous). HA functions as an osteoconductive graft material. These grafts show slow and limited

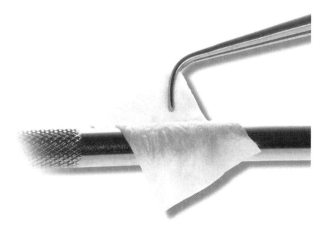

• **Fig. 35.9** Collagen Membrane. Collagen materials come in a variety of shapes and vary in their resorption time. (*Courtesy Humanus Dental AB, Malmö, Sweden: https://www.humanusdental.com/conform-resorbable-collagen-membrane-1520-mm*)

resorptive potential and generally are dependent on passive dissolution in tissue fluid and cell-mediated processes such as phagocytosis of particles for resorption. The degradation rate of HA depends on the method of ceramic formation, the calcium/phosphate ratio, crystallographic structure, and porosity. The ability of HA to resorb is also heavily dependent on the processing temperature. HA grafts synthesized at high temperatures are very dense with very limited biodegradability. These dense grafts are usually used as inert biocompatible fillers. At lower temperatures the particulate HA is porous and undergoes slow resorption.

Tricalcium Phosphates. Over the last few years, TCP has been used and extensively investigated as a bone substitute. TCP has two crystallographic forms: α-TCP and β-TCP. β-TCP exhibits good biocompatibility and osteoconductivity, and is used commonly as a partially resorbable filler allowing replacement with newly formed bone. Resorption of TCP grafts is thought to be dependent on dissolution by biological fluids and by presence of osteoclast-mediated resorption. In terms of bone regenerative potential, β-TCP grafts have been shown to be similar to autogenous bone, FDBA, DFDBA, and collagen sponge.

Biphasic Configurations. Biphasic configurations refer to grafts made from biphasic calcium phosphate, material composed of HA and β-TCP. The combinations are interesting in that the ratio of HA to β-TCP can be modified to provide for desired (slow versus fast) resorption. Also, by modifying the carrier and the characteristics of the granules, macroporosity and microporosity can be affected. These materials have a long history of use in orthopedics.

Calcium Sulfate. Calcium sulfate compounds have a compressive strength greater than that of cancellous bone. Calcium sulfate is usually applied as a barrier material to improve the clinical outcomes of periodontal regeneration therapy. When used as a barrier, calcium sulfate materials work as an adjunct with other graft materials.

Bioactive Glass. BG is a wide-open and fast-growing field in tissue engineering. BG has been widely studied since the 1970s. Since 45S5 BGs were discovered by Hench in 1969, they have been used for interface bonding of implant, and tissue repair and regeneration of bone. Glasses are noncrystalline amorphous solids that are commonly composed of silica-based materials with other minor additives. Compared with soda-lime glass (commonly used, as in windows or bottles), Bioglass 45S5 (trademarked by the University of Florida) contains less silica and higher amounts of calcium and phosphorus. The 45S5 name signifies glass with 45 weight % of SiO_2 and a 5:1 molar ratio of calcium to phosphorus. This high ratio of calcium to phosphorus promotes formation of apatite crystals. Lower Ca:P ratios do not bond to bone. Bioglass 45S5's specific composition is optimal in biomedical applications because of its similar composition to that of HA, the mineral component of bone.

The necessity of finding a material that forms a living bond with tissues led Hench to develop bioglass repair tissues during the Vietnam War. Bioglass offers advantages such as control of rate of degradation, excellent osteoconductivity, bioactivity, and capacity to deliver cells, but they present limitations in certain mechanical properties, such as low strength, toughness, and reliability. It can chemically bond with host tissue by forming a bonelike apatite layer between materials and bone tissue. Ionic dissolution products of BG can promote proliferation and differentiation of osteoblasts by activating a series of genes that regulate cellular behaviors. The first generation of BG was prepared by the melting-quenching method. Although traditional melting-derived BGs have excellent bioactivity, it was fired at a very high temperature (>1300°C), so it had a dense structure and small specific surface area, which limits its application. Compared with the melting-quenching method, the sol-gel method is a chemistry-based synthesis route, of which a solution containing the compositional precursors undergoes polymer-type reactions at room temperature to form a gel. The second generation of sol-gel BGs possesses uniform composition, composed of numerous nanoparticles with microporous and mesoporous structure, and thus it has high specific surface area. These advantages grant sol-gel BGs excellent bioactivity. However, up to now, there is no commercial product made of pure sol-gel BG in clinical application.

Synthetic Polymers. Synthetic polymers are discussed later in the Membranes section.

Titanium Mesh. Guided bone regenerative membranes can help in treating moderate-to-severe osseous defects, but the inherent physical property of the membrane to collapse toward the defect because of the pressure of the overlying soft tissues (thus reducing the space required for regeneration) makes the overall amount of regenerated bone questionable. The use of titanium mesh, which can maintain the space, can be a predictable and reliable treatment modality for regenerating and reconstructing a severely deficient alveolar ridge. The main advantages of the titanium mesh are that it maintains and preserves the space to be regenerated without collapsing, and it is flexible and can be bent. It can be shaped and adapted so it can assist bone regeneration in non-space-maintaining defects. Due to the presence of holes within the mesh (Fig. 35.10), it does not interfere with the blood supply directly from the periosteum to the underlying tissues and bone-grafting material. It is also completely biocompatible to oral tissues. Titanium mesh performs dual duty as a bone replacement and a barrier product.

Membranes

GTR and GBR membranes can be found in every graft source category previously listed. Each can be viewed as being either "resorbable" or "nonresorbable" based on whether the membrane can be left in the surgical site. There are advantages and disadvantages to each, and it is up to the clinician to understand where each type will have applicability.

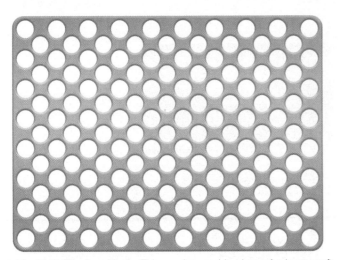

● **Fig. 35.10** Titanium Mesh. This can be used in place of a bone graft substitute when severe defects are encountered. The material acts as its own membrane. (*Courtesy Salvin Dental*)

Resorbable Membranes. There are three types of biologically resorbable (degradable) membranes: (1) polyglycolide synthetic copolymers, (2) collagen, and (3) calcium sulfate.

The most commonly used biodegradable synthetic polymers for three-dimensional scaffolds in tissue engineering are saturated poly(α-hydroxy esters), including poly(lactic acid) (PLA) and poly(glycolic acid) (PGA), as well as poly(lactic-coglycolide) copolymers. The chemical properties of these polymers allow hydrolytic degradation through deesterification. Once degraded, the monomeric components of each polymer are removed by natural pathways. PGA is converted to metabolites or eliminated by other mechanisms, and PLA can be cleared through the tricarboxylic acid cycle. Due to these properties, PLA and PGA have been used in biomedical products and devices, such as degradable sutures, which have been approved by the FDA. Their properties can be highly modified through each product's final material design, surface topography, and porosity. In addition, dissolution rates can be controlled with resorption occurring in weeks to months.

Collagen membranes, as well as all resorbable membranes, do not normally require a second surgery for retrieval. Patients appreciate the elimination of a second surgery, in addition to less morbidity. Collagen is the principal component of connective tissue and provides structural support for tissues throughout the body. Collagen is a hemostatic agent. It possesses the ability to stimulate platelet attachment and to enhance fibrin linkage, which may assist initial clot formation and stabilization, leading to enhanced regeneration. In addition, collagen is chemotactic for fibroblasts. Collagen membranes are easy to manipulate and adapt nicely to the alveolar topography. Although collagen is a weak immunogen, it is very well tolerated by patients.

Calcium sulfate with its long use in medicine provides an inexpensive solution in a variety of clinical situations. As previously discussed, when used as a resorbable barrier, calcium sulfate materials work as an adjunct with other graft materials.

Nonresorbable Membranes. Materials such as cellulose acetate laboratory filters (Millipore; Merck KGaA, Darmstadt, Germany, operating as MilliporeSigma in the United States), silicone sheets, and expanded polytetrafluoroethylene (e-PTFE) laboratory filters were the first nonresorbable biomaterials used for investigating barrier membranes for regenerative therapy. Although these materials demonstrated some therapeutic potential, limitations such as inability to integrate with surrounding tissue, brittleness, and the need to remove them after a certain period were observed. The function of nondegradable (nonresorbable) membranes is temporary, as they maintain their structural integrity on placement and are later retrieved via surgery. Although this gives the clinician greater control over the length of time the membrane will remain in place, the retrieval procedure increases the risk for surgical site morbidity and leaves the regenerated tissues susceptible to damage and postsurgery bacterial contamination. However, in situations such as alveolar ridge augmentation before placement of dental implants, it may be desirable for the membrane to retain its functional characteristics long enough for adequate healing to occur, and then be removed. Hence in specific situations a nonresorbable membrane provides more predictable performance.

e-PTFE was originally developed in 1969, and it became the standard for bone regeneration in the early 1990s. The e-PTFE membrane was sintered (sintering is the process of compacting and forming a solid mass of material by heat or pressure without melting it to the point of liquefaction), and it had pores between 5 and 20 μm in the structure of the material. The most popular commercial type of e-PTFE was Gore-Tex (W.L. Gore & Associates, Newark, Del.). The e-PTFE membrane acts as a mechanical hindrance. Fibroblasts and other connective tissue cells are prevented from entering the bone defect so that the presumably slower migrating cells with osteogenic potential are allowed to repopulate the defect.

In time, clinicians discovered that e-PFTE exposed to the oral cavity resulted in migration of microorganisms through the highly porous membrane. With an average pore size of 5 to 20 μm and the diameter of pathogenic bacteria generally less than 10 μm, migration of microorganisms through the highly porous e-PTFE membrane at exposure was a common complication. A high-density polytetrafluoroethylene (d-PTFE) membrane with a nominal pore size of less than 0.3 μm was developed (Cytoplast; Osteogenics Biomedical, Lubbock, Tex.) to address this problem. The increased efficacy of d-PTFE membranes in GTR has been proved with animal and human studies. Even when the membrane is exposed to the oral cavity, bacteria is excluded by the membrane, whereas oxygen diffusion and transfusion of small molecules across the membrane is still possible. Thus the d-PTFE membranes can result in good bone regeneration even after exposure. Because the larger pore size of e-PTFE membranes allows tight soft tissue attachment, it usually requires sharp dissection at membrane removal. On the contrary, removal of d-PTFE is simplified because of lack of tissue ingrowth into the surface structure. In 1995, Bartee[58] reported that the use of d-PTFE is particularly useful when primary closure is impossible without tension, such as alveolar ridge preservation, large bone defects, and the placement of implants immediately after extraction. In those cases d-PTFE membranes can be left exposed, and thus preserve soft tissue and the position of the mucogingival junction.

Comparing Bone Graft Substitutes and Membrane Characteristics

When comparing bone graft substitutes and membrane characteristics, the choices are many. Fortunately there are suppliers who have developed regenerative portfolios that offer a "full range" of choices, allowing the clinician latitude in providing their patient with the best treatment. Fig. 35.11 illustrates a small sample of available material diversity from one such supplier.

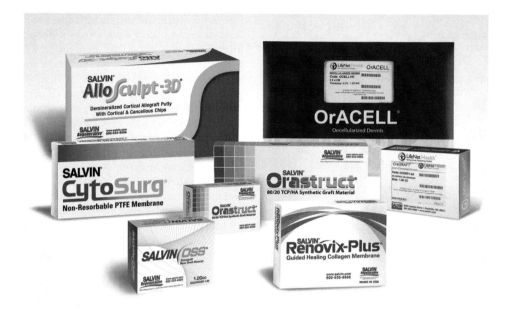

● **Fig. 35.11** Today's clinician has many products to choose from. (*Courtesy Salvin Dental*)

The clinician is faced with a wide variety of materials in the market. Many appear to be similar, whereas many others appear to be markedly superior or inferior. As pointed out in this chapter, there are but a few product categories. The products in all categories are made under the strictest of regulations. Industry strives to provide safe and effective grafts for all surgical specialties.

Information on any graft type is easy to find thanks to the World Wide Web. The end-user has a responsibility to keep up to date on materials and techniques. Companies supplying the specialty of implant dentistry have expanded their regenerative portfolios and gained the technical knowledge to support the doctor in making grafting choices. This ensures the best treatment option for every patient.

The following tables are provided as a quick summary of materials covered in this chapter. Table 35.1 examines the materials regulated as HCT/Ps (donated human tissue). Table 35.2 lists the materials that are on the market via the 510(k) route (xenografts and alloplasts).

Looking to the Future

In the area of hard tissue replacement, significant advancements are being made related to milled "custom" graft materials. Most of the strides are a result of improvements in scanning, tomography, and manufacturing technologies. Also, advances in cell culture and the ability to create three-dimensional print scaffolds from biologic materials provide unlimited opportunities for both hard and soft tissues. Soft tissue augmentation shows promise in several areas, mainly from improved understanding in the area of wound healing and improved manufacturing. Cell-based grafts will play a big part in regeneration.

Milling of "custom" blocks is currently available.[61] Patient selection is a great part of the success and at the time of this writing, only dental surgeons who have received special training on the technique can use the service. Fabrication requires cone beam computed tomography and a tissue processor with the ability to mill bone using computer-aided design and computer-aided manufacturing (Fig. 35.12). The technology originated in Europe, is now available in the United States, and resultant grafts:
- are sourced from processed human allograft;

- are composed of natural mineralized collagen (normal trabecular bone);
- have 65% to 80% macroporosity, pore size 100 to 1800 μm (mean 600 to 900 μm);
- can be produced to a maximum size: 23 × 13 × 13 mm;
- show fast graft incorporation and complete remodeling potential;
- possess no antigenicity;
- result in no donor site morbidity;
- heal/integrate in 5 to 6 months;
- can be stored at ambient temperature for long periods; and
- are safe and sterile.

Cell culture technology is one of the fastest-growing areas of regenerative innovation.[62] It is part of BTE, the specific field of tissue engineering that mainly focuses on enhancing bone regeneration and repair by creating substitutes to traditional bone-grafting materials. BTE started about three decades ago and has witnessed tremendous growth ever since. Bone serves as a paradigm for general principles in tissue engineering because of its high regenerative potential compared with other tissues in the body. Classic BTE paradigm includes the following three key components: biomaterials to provide a scaffold for new tissue growth, cells, and signaling molecules. It is quite possible that components can be made from different classes of materials (e.g., a xenograft combined with an alloplast), thus taking advantage of the best properties of each.

Scaffolds can be either acellular or cellular on implantation within this model. In the former, the architecture and geometry promote the recruitment of local stem cell and or/osteoprogenitor cells, which could be possible with attachment motifs and chemical "smart" cues placed within the scaffold architecture. On the other hand, the latter strategy involves implantation of a scaffold combined with stem cell and or/osteoprogenitor cells, which can be incorporated by two methods: (1) cell seeding into a "prefabricated" scaffold, a commonly applied tissue engineering strategy; and (2) cell encapsulation during scaffold fabrication made of hydrogel polymer matrix, based on the immobilization of cells within a semipermeable membrane. This technique protects cells from the immune system and permits uniform cell distribution within the construct.[63]

TABLE 35.1   Allograft-Derived Materials

HCT/P Products	Function	Space Maintaining	Mode	Time to Remodel
Mineralized cortical	BGS particulate	Yes	Osteoconductive	6 months
Mineralized cancellous	BGS particulate	Yes	Osteoconductive	<6 months
Mineralized cortical/cancellous mix	BGS particulate	Yes	Osteoconductive	<6 months
Demineralized cortical	BGS particulate	No	Osteoconductive/osteoinductive	4–5 months
Mineralized cortical/demineralized cortical mix	BGS particulate	Yes	Osteoconductive/osteoinductive	4–5 months
Laminar bone	BGS structural	N/A	Osteoconductive/osteoinductive	4–5 months
DBM gel, putty, paste	BGS particulate	Varies	Osteoconductive/osteoinductive	Varies
Mineralized block, cube, rib, mandible, pins	BGS structural	Yes	Osteoconductive	Slow
Cell-based material	BGS particulate	Yes	Osteoconductive/osteoinductive/osteogenic?	Varies
Placental tissue	Membrane	N/A	Resorbable	Fast
Fascia lata	Membrane	N/A	Resorbable	4–6 months
Pericardium	Membrane	N/A	Resorbable	4–6 months
Acellular dermis	Membrane	N/A	Resorbable	4–6 months

BGS, Bone graft substitutes; *DBM*, demineralized bone matrix; *N/A*, not applicable.

TABLE 35.2   Xenograft- and Alloplast-Derived Materials [510(k) Regulated]

510(k) Products	Function	Space Maintaining	Mode	Time to Remodel
Xenograft mineralized cancellous	BGS particulate	Yes	Osteoconductive	Slow
Xenograft mineralized cancellous block	BGS structural	Yes	Osteoconductive	Slow
Xenograft pericardium	Membrane	N/A	Resorbable	4–6 months
Xenograft collagen forms	Membrane	N/A	Resorbable	Varies, weeks to months
Coralline based	BGS particulate	Yes	Osteoconductive	Slow to medium
Hydroxyapatite	BGS particulate and structural	Yes	Osteoconductive	Varies (generally slow)
Tricalcium phosphates	BGS particulate	Yes	Osteoconductive	Varies (generally fast)
Biphasic (hydroxyapatite + tricalcium phosphate)	BGS particulate	Yes	Osteoconductive	Varies (can be controlled by ratio of mix
Calcium sulfate	BGS (additive) and membrane	Yes	Osteoconductive (resorbable when used as membrane)	Fast
Bioactive glass	BGS (mainly as particulate)	Yes	Osteoconductive	Varies (generally slow)
Synthetic polymers	Membrane	N/A	Resorbable and nonresorbable forms	Varies based on composition
Titanium mesh	BGS (in severe cases) and membrane	Maintains space	Nonresorbable	Never resorbs

BGS, Bone graft substitutes; *N/A*, not applicable.

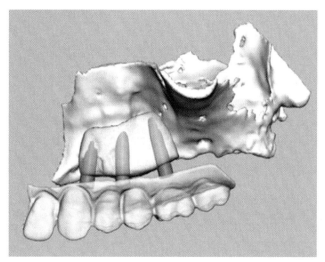

• **Fig. 35.12** A custom solution created from cone beam computed tomography and computer-aided design/computer-aided manufacturing milling (botiss.com).

Regarding BTE created scaffolds, the following characteristics are desired:
• hydrophilicity, roughness, and surface topography
• porosity, pore size, and interconnectivity
• mechanical strength close to native tissues and a predictable degradation rate (5 to 6 months is desired for dental use)
• biocompatible and bioactive
• ability to bind and release drugs or chemicals that can affect the healing microenvironment

Much work remains in this area, but the technologies show great promise.

Soft tissue grafts and membranes will benefit from a better understanding of clinical need. Manufacturers now know that collagen-based membranes can be modified by cross-linking to affect the rate of resorption. In addition, collagen-based materials can be preformed in molds to increase utility in cases with extreme anatomic variations. Thickness can be modified to produce "dead soft" materials that lack any memory and adhere perfectly to local anatomy. Naturally, research is going on with all material types for membranes that can be left "predictably" exposed to the oral cavity in cases where primary closure cannot be achieved. Much work with d-PTFE has already occurred in this area.[64]

Rowe et al.[65] in 2016 discussed work with electrospinning. This is a process by which microfibers/nanofibers can be formed from a viscous polymer solution exposed to an electric field. Although widely used in tissue engineering applications, biocompatible PLA and poly(ε-caprolactone) electrospun meshes have displayed properties that might enable its application as a GTR/GBR membrane. In initial tests it performed better than a current commercially available product.

Controllable osteoinduction maintained in the original defect area is the key to precise bone repair. In 2018, Ma et al.[66] reported on research involving the development of a dual-sided ("Janus") membrane that acts as a membrane on one side and is osteoinductive on the other.

Allografts (acellular dermis, fascia lata, and pericardium) are constantly being modified. The main focus for the future will be processing innovations resulting in consistency of thickness, sterility of the product (to a SAL 10^{-6}—not all products are at this desired level), and an increase in the length of time materials can be stored at ambient temperature. Acellular dermis will be highly studied because of its unique makeup and utility in many surgical disciplines. A unique reticular dermis is already available that retains architectural elements (open structure), mechanical properties (elasticity, organized collagen, and elastin), and key matrix proteins to support physiologic cellular responses during regenerative remodeling.[67] Of course a great deal of attention is being given to placental-based materials (chorion and amnion), with many products being marketed at the time of this writing.

Cell-based products for use in dentistry are currently available.[68] These feature (generally) three components: demineralized cortical bone, mineralized cancellous bone, and marrow cells; therefore these products mimic the biologic profile of autograft (osteoinductive, osteoconductive, and osteogenic). Currently these products require special shipping and storage at ultracold temperatures (not usually available in the typical dental office). Future efforts with these grafts will be to create shipping solutions that can act as short-term storage for those offices without ultralow-temperature freezers or the ability to store at lower temperatures for short periods. In addition, ways to increase the number and viability of bone-forming cells are being studied. Cell-based grafts are the most difficult of all BGS materials to produce because each component must come from a single donor, and processing must occur quickly to protect the viability of the osteogenic component.

Summary

Bone graft substitutes and membranes make up a significant portion of the dental implant market. Most patients who need implant therapy will need either an autograft or a substitute. The industries and regulatory bodies responsible for the manufacture of these materials, and instruments and technologies that augment their use, have reached a high level of maturity. Patient safety and graft performance are the focus of industry while always striving for improvement. Patients are active participants in their own treatment, and the most appropriate grafting decisions can be made collaboratively through the informed consent process.

The use of autografts, allografts, xenografts, or alloplasts, alone or in combination, should be based on the individual's systemic healing capacity, the osteogenic potential of the recipient site, time available for graft maturation, and the patient's expectations. Clinicians have a responsibility to their patients to understand the many products available for use in GBR. It must also be understood that no one ideal BGS or membrane exists.

Although product comparisons may seem difficult, the process is made easier by realizing the best patient outcome. Each graft class has characteristics unique to that group, and it is up to the end-user to evaluate each characteristic against patient needs. Also, the end-user has a responsibility to handle and use each material as intended to protect his or her patients and staff.

What has been presented in this chapter covers the basics of BGS and membranes. The next 10 to 15 years will see dramatic changes in biomaterials and techniques, and will provide the clinicians even more options for successful implant treatment.

Acknowledgments

The author thanks Paul Lehner, David Adamson, Karen Colella, William Simmons, Greg Slayton, and Jonathan Boyd for their technical assistance and their dedication to the dental specialty. He also expresses his appreciation to the employees of CTS, LNH, Salvin Dental Specialties, and the AATB. They have been friends and mentors for many years.

References

1. Leventhal GS. Titanium, a metal for surgery. *J Bone Joint Surg Am.* 1951;33-A(2):473–474.

2. Brånemark PI, Hansson BO, Adell R, et al. Osseointegrated implants in the treatment of the edentulous jaw. Experience from a 10-year period. *Scand J Plast Reconstr Surg Suppl.* 1977;16:1–132.

3. Dr. Brånemark, father of modern dental implant, dies at 85. https://www.ada.org/sitecore/content/home-ada/publications/ada-news/2015-archive/january/dr-branemark-father-of-modern-dental-implant-dies-at-85#.WuCOuw1S4-8.email. Accessed May 30, 2018.

4. Chrcanovic BR, Albrektsson T, Wennerberg A. Bone quality and quantity and dental implant failure: a systematic review and meta-analysis. *Int J Prosthodont.* 2017;30(3):219–237. https://doi.org/10.11607/ijp.5142.

5. Misch CM. Autogenous bone: is it still the gold standard? *Implant Dent.* 2010;19(5):361. https://doi.org/10.1097/ID.0b013e3181f8115b.

6. Global Dental Membrane and Bone Graft Substitute Market Dynamics 2018: Industry Analysis, Competitors Size & Share, Trends, Demand, Global Research to 2025 – Healthcare News. https://journalhealthcare.com/156676/global-dental-membrane-and-bone-graft-substitute-market-dynamics-2018-industry-analysis-competitors-size-share-trends-demand-global-research-to-2025/. Accessed May 30, 2018.

7. Bone Remodeling. https://courses.washington.edu/conj/bess/bone/bone2.html. Accessed May 30, 2018.

8. Parfitt AM, Drezner MK, Glorieux FH, et al. Bone histomorphometry: standardization of nomenclature, symbols, and units. Report of the ASBMR Histomorphometry Nomenclature Committee. *J Bone Miner Res.* 1987;2(6):595–610. https://doi.org/10.1002/jbmr.5650020617.

9. Wolff J. Concerning the interrelationship between form and function of the individual parts of the organism. By Julius Wolff, 1900. *Clin Orthop.* 1988;(228):2–11.

10. Khojasteh A, Kheiri L, Motamedian SR, Khoshkam V. Guided bone regeneration for the reconstruction of alveolar bone defects. *Ann Maxillofac Surg.* 2017;7(2):263–277. https://doi.org/10.4103/ams.ams_76_17.

11. Nyman S, Gottlow J, Karring T, Lindhe J. The regenerative potential of the periodontal ligament. An experimental study in the monkey. *J Clin Periodontol.* 1982;9(3):257–265.

12. Hurley LA, Stinchfield FE, Bassett AL, Lyon WH. The role of soft tissues in osteogenesis. An experimental study of canine spine fusions. *J Bone Joint Surg Am.* 1959;41-A:1243–1254.

13. Senn on the healing of aseptic bone cavities by implantation of antiseptic decalcified bone. *Ann Surg.* 1889;10(5):352–368.

14. Lacroix P. Recent investigations on the growth of bone. *Nature.* 1945;156:576–577.

15. Urist M. Bone: formation by autoinduction. *Science.* 1965;150:893–899.

16. Urist MR, Strates BS. Bone morphogenetic protein. *J Dent Res.* 1971;50(6):1392–1406. https://doi.org/10.1177/00220345710500060601.

17. Reddi H. Bone morphogenetic proteins. *Adv Dent Res.* 1995;9(suppl 3):13. https://doi.org/10.1177/08959374950090030401.

18. Sheikh Z, Javaid MA, Hamdan N, et al. Bone regeneration using bone morphogenetic proteins and various biomaterial carriers. *Mater Basel Switz.* 2015;8(4):1778–1816. https://doi.org/10.3390/ma8041778.

19. Wozney JM. The bone morphogenetic protein family and osteogenesis. *Mol Reprod Dev.* 1992;32(2):160–167. https://doi.org/10.1002/mrd.1080320212.

20. Edwards JT, Diegmann MH, Scarborough NL. Osteoinduction of human demineralized bone: characterization in a rat model. *Clin Orthop.* 1998;357:219–228.

21. Zhang K, Fan Y, Dunne N, Li X. Effect of microporosity on scaffolds for bone tissue engineering. *Regen Biomater.* 2018;5(2):115–124. https://doi.org/10.1093/rb/rby001.

22. Boyan BD, Weesner TC, Lohmann CH, et al. Porcine fetal enamel matrix derivative enhances bone formation induced by demineralized freeze dried bone allograft in vivo. *J Periodontol.* 2000;71(8):1278–1286. https://doi.org/10.1902/jop.2000.71.8.1278.

23. Janicki P, Schmidmaier G. What should be the characteristics of the ideal bone graft substitute? Combining scaffolds with growth factors and/or stem cells. *Injury.* 2011;42(suppl 2):S77–81. https://doi.org/10.1016/j.injury.2011.06.014.

24. Rakhmatia YD, Ayukawa Y, Furuhashi A, Koyano K. Current barrier membranes: titanium mesh and other membranes for guided bone regeneration in dental applications. *J Prosthodont Res.* 2013;57(1):3–14. https://doi.org/10.1016/j.jpor.2012.12.001.

25. American Association of Tissue Banks. *Standards for Tissue Banking.* 14th ed. McLean, VA: AATB; 2016.

26. Accredited Bank Search. https://www.aatb.org/?q=content/accredited-bank-search.

27. CFR—Code of Federal Regulations Title 21. https://www.accessdata.fda.gov/scripts/cdrh/cfdocs/cfcfr/CFRSearch.cfm?CFRPart=1271. Accessed May 30, 2018.

28. Powers R, Linden J. Tissue Banking. In: *Rossi's Principles of Transfusion Medicine.* 5th ed. West Sussex, UK: Wiley-Blackwell; 2016.

29. Holtzclaw D, Toscano N, Eisenlohr L, Callan D. The safety of bone allografts used in dentistry: a review. *J Am Dent Assoc 1939.* 2008;139(9):1192–1199.

30. Green D, McKenzie R. Nuances of informed consent: the paradigm of regional anesthesia. *Hosp Spec Surg.* 2007;3(1):115–118. https://doi.org/10.1007/s11420-006-9035-y.

31. Watterson D. Informed consent and informed refusal in dentistry. https://www.rdhmag.com/articles/print/volume-32/issue-9/features/informed-consent-and-informed-refusal.html.

32. Moreira NCF, Pachêco-Pereira C, Keenan L, et al. Informed consent comprehension and recollection in adult dental patients: a systematic review. *J Am Dent Assoc 1939.* 2016;147(8):605–619.e7. https://doi.org/10.1016/j.adaj.2016.03.004.

33. Strong DM, Shinozaki N. Coding and traceability for cells, tissues and organs for transplantation. *Cell Tissue Bank.* 2010;11(4):305–323. https://doi.org/10.1007/s10561-010-9179-3.

34. Strong DM. The US Navy Tissue Bank: 50 years on the cutting edge. *Cell Tissue Bank.* 2000;1(1):9–16. https://doi.org/10.1023/A:1010151928461.

35. About OPOs. AOPO. http://www.aopo.org/about-opos/. Accessed May 29, 2018.

36. Donate Life America: Organ, Eye, and Tissue Donation Registration. Donate Life America. https://www.donatelife.net/. Accessed May 29, 2018.

37. Organ Donation, Organ Donor Registry | organdonor.gov. https://organdonor.gov/index.html. Accessed May 29, 2018.

38. Orell S. Surgical bone grafting with "os purum," "os novum," and "boiled bone. *J Bone Joint Surg.* 1937;19:873.

39. Forsberg H. Transplantatin of os purum and bone chips in the surgical treatment of periodontal disease (preliminary report). *Acta Odont Scandinav.* 1956;13:235.

40. Scopp IW, Kassouny DY, Morgan FH. Bovine bone (Boplant). *J Periodontol.* 1966;37(5):400–407.

41. Scopp I, Morgan J, Dooner J, et al. Bovine Bone (Boplant) implants for infrabony oral lesions. *Periodontics.* 1966;4:169–176.

42. Pietrzak WS, Ali SN, Chitturi D, et al. BMP depletion occurs during prolonged acid demineralization of bone: characterization and implications for graft preparation. *Cell Tissue Bank.* 2011;12(2):81–88. https://doi.org/10.1007/s10561-009-9168-6.

43. Pietrzak WS, Woodell-May J. The composition of human cortical allograft bone derived from FDA/AATB-screened donors. *J Craniofac Surg.* 2005;16(4):579–585.

44. Aerssens J, Boonen S, Lowet G, Dequeker J. Interspecies differences in bone composition, density, and quality: potential implications for in vivo bone research. *Endocrinology.* 1998;139(2):663–670. https://doi.org/10.1210/endo.139.2.5751.

45. America GPN. Geistlich Biomaterials - USA Pharma. https://www.geistlich-na.com/en-us/.

46. ISO - International Organization for Standardization. https://www.iso.org/home.html. Accessed May 30, 2018.

47. Albee FH. Studies in bone growth: triple calcium phosphate as a stimulus to osteogenesis. *Ann Surg*. 1920;71(1):32–39.

48. Peltier LF, Bickel EY, Lillo R, Thein MS. The use of plaster of paris to fill defects in bone. *Ann Surg*. 1957;146(1):61–69.

49. Campana V, Milano G, Pagano E, et al. Bone substitutes in orthopaedic surgery: from basic science to clinical practice. *J Mater Sci Mater Med*. 2014;25(10):2445–2461. https://doi.org/10.1007/s10856-014-5240-2.

50. Samsell B, Moore M, Bertasi G, et al. Are bone allografts safe and effective for today's dental practitioners? *Dentistry*. 2014;4(9):1–6. https://doi.org/10.4172/2161-1122.1000260.

51. Liu J, Kerns DG. Mechanisms of guided bone regeneration: a review. *Open Dent J*. 2014;8:56–65. https://doi.org/10.2174/1874210601408010056.

52. Sheikh Z, Hamdan N, Ikeda Y, et al. Natural graft tissues and synthetic biomaterials for periodontal and alveolar bone reconstructive applications: a review. *Biomater Res*. 2017;21:9. https://doi.org/10.1186/s40824-017-0095-5.

53. Tomlin EM, Nelson SJ, Rossmann JA. Ridge preservation for implant therapy: a review of the literature. *Open Dent J*. 2014;8:66–76. https://doi.org/10.2174/1874210601408010066.

54. Mohan R, Bajaj A, Gundappa M. Human amnion membrane: potential applications in oral and periodontal field. *J Int Soc Prev Community Dent*. 2017;7(1):15–21. https://doi.org/10.4103/jispcd.JISPCD_359_16.

55. Callan DP. Guided tissue regeneration without a stage 2 surgical procedure. *Int J Periodontics Restorative Dent*. 1993;13(2):172–179.

56. Crook K. GBR and sinus augmentation using autogenous and DFDB Allograft and Alloderm as the barrier. *N M Dent J*. 1999;50(2):24–26.

57. Almazrooa SA, Noonan V, Woo S-B. Resorbable collagen membranes: histopathologic features. *Oral Surg Oral Med Oral Pathol Oral Radiol*. 2014;118(2):236–240. https://doi.org/10.1016/j.oooo.2014.04.006.

58. Bartee BK. The use of high-density polytetrafluoroethylene membrane to treat osseous defects: clinical reports. *Implant Dent*. 1995;4(1):21–26.

59. Gentile P, Chiono V, Carmagnola I, Hatton PV. An overview of poly(lactic-co-glycolic) acid (PLGA)-based biomaterials for bone tissue engineering. *Int J Mol Sci*. 2014;15(3):3640–3659. https://doi.org/10.3390/ijms15033640.

60. Chen J, Zeng L, Chen X, et al. Preparation and characterization of bioactive glass tablets and evaluation of bioactivity and cytotoxicity in vitro. *Bioact Mater*. 2018;3(3):315–321. https://doi.org/10.1016/j.bioactmat.2017.11.004.

61. Otto S, Kleye C, Burian E, et al. Custom-milled individual allogeneic bone grafts for alveolar cleft osteoplasty-A technical note. *J Craniomaxillofac Surg*. 2017;45(12):1955–1961. https://doi.org/10.1016/j.jcms.2017.09.011.

62. Oryan A, Alidadi S, Moshiri A, et al. Bone regenerative medicine: classic options, novel strategies, and future directions. *J Orthop Surg*. 2014;9(1):18. https://doi.org/10.1186/1749-799X-9-18.

63. Asa'ad F, Pagni G, Pilipchuk SP, et al. 3D-printed scaffolds and biomaterials: review of alveolar bone augmentation and periodontal regeneration applications. *Int J Dent*. 2016:1239842. https://doi.org/10.1155/2016/1239842.

64. Barboza EP, Stutz B, Ferreira VF, Carvalho W. Guided bone regeneration using nonexpanded polytetrafluoroethylene membranes in preparation for dental implant placements—a report of 420 cases. *Implant Dent*. 2010;19(1):2–7. https://doi.org/10.1097/ID.0b013e3181cda72c.

65. Rowe MJ, Kamocki K, Pankajakshan D, et al. Dimensionally stable and bioactive membrane for guided bone regeneration: an in vitro study. *J Biomed Mater Res B Appl Biomater*. 2016;104(3):594–605. https://doi.org/10.1002/jbm.b.33430.

66. Ma B, Han J, Zhang S, et al. Hydroxyapatite nanobelt/polylactic acid Janus membrane with osteoinduction/barrier dual functions for precise bone defect repair. *Acta Biomater*. 2018;71:108–117. https://doi.org/10.1016/j.actbio.2018.02.033.

67. Dasgupta A, Orgill D, Galiano RD, et al. A novel reticular dermal graft leverages architectural and biological properties to support wound repair. *Plast Reconstr Surg Glob Open*. 2016;4(10). https://doi.org/10.1097/GOX.0000000000001065.

68. Maksoud M. Stem cell bone allografts in maxillary sinus and ridge augmentation, report of a case. *J Dent Oral Biol*. 2016;1(1):1–4.

36

Particulate Membrane grafting/ Guided Bone Regeneration

C. STEPHEN CALDWELL

The field of restorative dentistry has been through a paradigm shift in recent years that has completely changed treatment planning and the prospects for reconstruction of severely compromised dental cases. The use of dental implants in most treatment plans today offers the possibility of restorative success using fixed prostheses in many situations that would have previously been impossible. Meeting the demands and expectations of our enthusiastic patient population requires the multidisciplined implant team to perform at new and challenging levels of sophistication. As we attempt to restore these progressively more difficult cases, the severely compromised bony ridge defects that we encounter will continue to challenge team members to develop new and predictable grafting techniques (Fig. 36.1).

The goal of any dental implant procedure is to restore the patient to optimal form, function, and esthetics. Through the combined efforts of a great number of clinicians and researchers, guidelines have been established in regard to proper implant numbers and positioning based on possible prosthetic designs. The patient's existing bone volume often makes the proper placement and positioning of implants difficult, if not impossible. Ideal treatment planning in implant dentistry often requires the correction of significant alveolar ridge defects in regions where dental implants are indicated to support critical prostheses. Alveolar ridge defects are caused by a variety of factors including developmental anomalies, trauma, and most commonly, tooth extraction. After tooth loss a predictable resorptive process of the alveolar bone occurs in both a horizontal and a vertical dimension[1] (Fig. 36.2).

The loss of alveolar bone can pose a challenge both from the perspective of supporting a conventional removable prosthesis or placement of dental implants in an ideal position for functional and esthetic results. Before development of effective bone-grafting techniques, implants were placed in regions where there was available bony support, often leaving the restorative dentist with the task of restoring an implant in a less than ideal position within the arch. The success of implant dentistry today has been largely related to the advent of bone augmentation techniques that allow regeneration of an ideal ridge form and placement of implants in their ideal functional and esthetic positions[2–6] (Fig. 36.3).

The augmentation of bone volumes through grafting is an effective, but technique-sensitive process. It requires meticulous surgical skill, practice, and knowledge to become proficient in creating predictable bone growth before implant placement. Complications are plentiful in this discipline, leading to treatment delays, patient and provider frustration, as well as possible neurosensory, vascular, and infectious issues. The dental implant surgeon must have a firm understanding of the limitations encountered in various bone-grafting techniques to develop appropriate treatment plans. Clinicians must be able to not only prevent complications during the procedure, but also properly address complications related to these issues should they arise (Box 36.1).

Indications for Bone Grafting

The presence of an adequate volume of available bone is one of the most important prerequisites for predictable implant placement and osseointegration. Although loss in bone volume may result from trauma, bone deficiency is most frequently due to the normal physiologic process that occurs after tooth loss or extraction. Studies have shown that resultant bone resorption after tooth removal can be approximately 1.5 to 2 mm vertically and 3.8 mm in the horizontal plane within 6 months.[7,8]

Currently, bone regeneration procedures are widely accepted as a viable option for the treatment of edentulous deficiencies to be restored with an implant-supported prosthesis. Implant clinicians have a wide range of bone-grafting materials and procedures at their disposal. For years the gold standard in bone regeneration has been the use of autogenous (autograft) bone because of its inherent osteoconductive, osteoinductive, and osteogenic properties (Box 36.2). Because autogenous bone is composed of the patient's own tissue, there is a reduction in the likelihood of immunoreactions and possible infectious transmission. However, autogenous bone grafting has disadvantages, including the need for a secondary surgical site, a potential increase in pain and discomfort, bone-harvesting quantity restrictions, increased costs, and longer surgical procedures. Studies have shown that only 61% of patients accept grafting with autogenous bone.[9] Methods

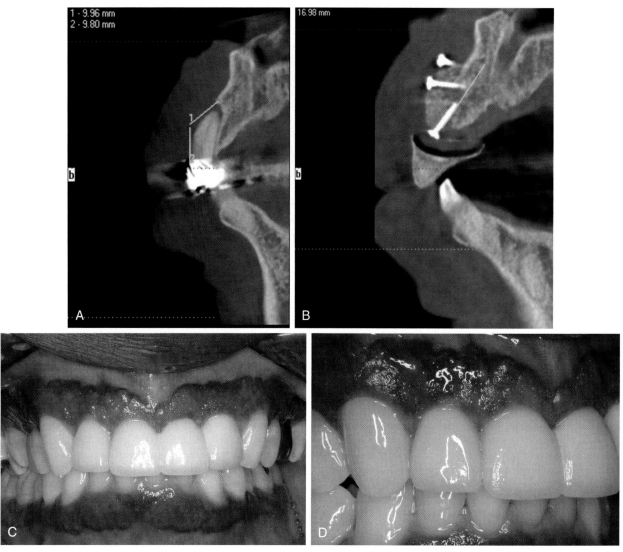

• **Fig. 36.1** Careful planning and surgical execution can provide patients with the opportunity to replace their missing teeth with restorations that are not only functional, but also esthetically pleasing. (A Preoperative CBCT Cross-section of severely compromised central incisor B) Cross-section of the same site after completing a large ridge augmentation. (C and D) Final restorations in the anterior graft site.

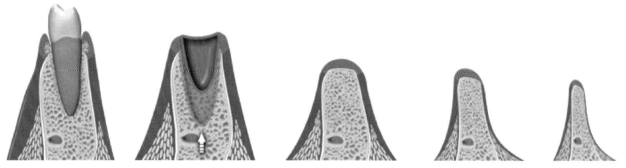

• **Fig. 36.2** The progressive resorption of the bony ridge after an extraction leads to a situation that compromises all aspects of the restorative process. As resorption advances, less bone is available for implant placement, thus compromising the final result.

that minimize the inconvenience related to autogenous bone harvests allow the surgical team the opportunity to use the boost of autogenous grafts without putting their patients through excessive discomfort. As tempting as it may be, the lack of incorporation of at least some autogenous bone in a large ridge augmentation (> 3 mm) can ultimately change the density of the final graft, its resistance to unpredictable remodeling, the overall ability to regenerate vertical volume, and to some degree the width of a

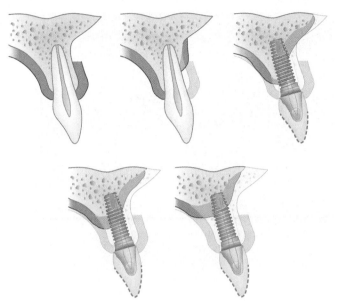

● **Fig. 36.3** Loss of Soft and Hard Tissue. After tooth loss, bone loss occurs with respect to the prosthesis position. As the bone resorbs, the vertical and horizontal soft tissue support around teeth and implants disappears. This results in the exposure of the failing implant body, together with a future nonesthetic implant prosthesis.

● **BOX 36.1   Hard Tissue Considerations With Implant Treatment Planning**

- Alveolar ridge width
- Alveolar ridge height
- Alveolar ridge angulation
- Available restorative space
- Maxillary/Mandibular alveolar ridge relationship
- Proximity to vital structures
- Bony undercuts/defects
- Maxillary Sinus pneumatization
- Available autogenous donor sites

● **BOX 36.2   Biologic Bone Healing Classification**

1. **Osteogenic Grafts**
- Osteogenic bone grafts originate from autogenous origin and are comprised of live, viable cells capable of differentiation and formation of bone.

2. **Osteoinductive Grafts**
- Osteoinductive grafting materials provide a biological stimulus (proteins and growth factors) that *induce* the progression of mesenchymal stem cells and other osteoprogenitor cells toward osteoblast lineage.

3. **Osteoconductive Grafts**
- Osteoconduction is the process that allows the bone graft to be conducive to forming bone, thereby acting as scaffolding for bone growth.

---

large horizontal graft site. Therefore ideally 50% autogenous bone should be used in vertical regeneration cases and in large-volume horizontal grafts.

Success in any implant prosthesis requires the implants to be placed in positions that provide ideal esthetics, function, comfort,

and support. To be successful in the development of a favorable prosthesis, the number and positions of implants in an edentulous space must be determined with a careful analysis of the relationship between the restorative prosthesis and the forces that will be exerted on the final prosthesis. This is then combined with the functional and esthetic aspects of the case, ultimately dictating the relationship between the implants, bone, and opposing forces. All of these factors must be considered in planning support for a prosthesis that functions well while maintaining the bone volume around its implant abutments. Clinicians too often try to bypass the grafting process, either to save time or because they are not experienced in advanced grafting techniques. Insufficient bone in recipient sites leads to placement of implants with inadequate diameters, shorter lengths, insufficient numbers, or less than ideal angulations. Compromises such as these can eventually lead to significant damage around an implant and the prosthesis it supports. Due to the fact that resorption and remodeling occur in every edentulous site, the need for adjunctive bone grafting must be considered and is often vital for a successful outcome.

Failure to recognize the need for bone grafting leads to numerous treatment issues, ranging from esthetic complications to implant and prosthetic failure. Placing implants of suboptimal sizes or in less than ideal numbers to bypass the grafting process is a compromise that often leads to force-related failures of implant components, failure of the prosthesis itself, or accompanied bone loss. Ultimately, prosthetic and implant morbidities may result. A multidisciplinary approach should be taken to assess the optimal prosthetic solution for the patient, based on the patient's wishes, available bone, and other factors. After a prosthetic plan has been established, the clinician should begin planning the implant positions required to execute the prosthetic option. Once the sites for the specific implants have been determined, the associated regions are evaluated for bony foundational support in that specific site. If inadequate bone is available to successfully place an implant in a key location for the prosthesis, grafting should then be included in the treatment plan to build the appropriate bone volumes (Fig. 36.4).

Cellular Bone Regeneration Process

The cellular development of bone in a deficient site involves a delicate process that occurs over an extended period. This series of steps can be easily disrupted by cellular ingrowth, micromovement, infection, or bacterial contamination. Therefore the process of guided bone regeneration (GBR) is always carried out in a protected space where the natural step-by-step process of bone development can occur. The first phase of this regeneration process involves the recruitment of osteoblast precursors and growth factors to the recipient area. This is accomplished primarily through the existing bony recipient bed, its vasculature, and the graft material (i.e., autograft, allograft, xenograft). The second phase of the process is the resorption/deposition process. Host osteoprogenitor cells will infiltrate the graft within 7 days, and resorption and deposition will occur via creeping substitution and osteoconduction. The osteoblast precursors differentiate into mature osteoblasts under the influence of osteoinductors and synthesize new bone during the first weeks. Growth factors involved in the bone formation process act on fibroblast and osteoblast proliferation, extracellular matrix deposition, mesenchymal cell differentiation, and vascular proliferation (Fig. 36.5 and Box 36.3).

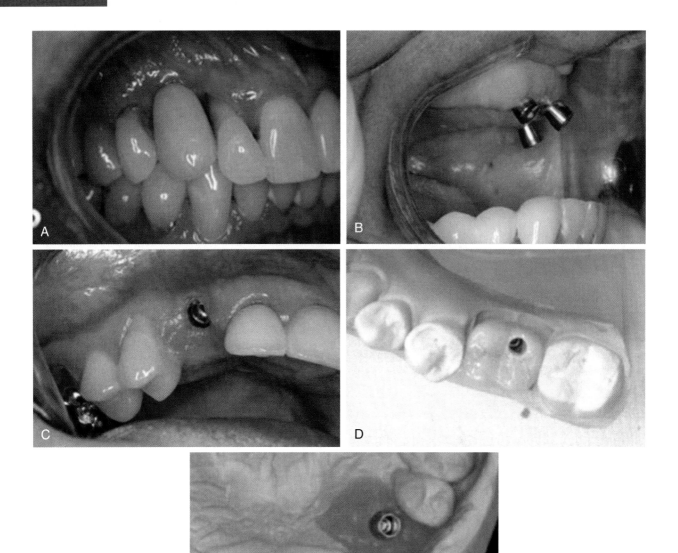

• **Fig. 36.4** Malpositioned Implants. (A) Implants placed in compromised bone sites result in a compromised final prosthesis. (B and C) Implants positioned too far facially will increase prosthesis morbidity and compromise esthetics. (D and E) Implants positioned too far lingual will result in an overcontoured prosthesis, but also will place the implants at a biomechanical disadvantage.

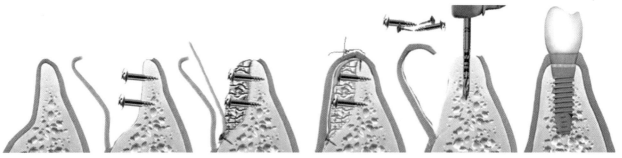

• **Fig. 36.5** Guided bone regeneration combines the science of bone regeneration with the management of space maintenance for development of planned bony configurations. With the use of bone screws and a barrier membrane, bone regeneration may take place.

Treatment Planning in the Compromised Edentulous Ridge

Treatment planning for implant-supported restorations in edentulous spaces requires a clear understanding of the resorptive patterns of bone loss. As a ridge resorbs, available bone for support of dental implants disappears, preventing placement of implants in key locations for restorative success. After tooth loss the initial pattern of bone resorption starts with loss of the lateral (buccal) aspect of the ridge, eventually leading to a decrease in

---

• BOX 36.3 Bone Healing and Grafting Definitions

Bone Remodeling—the natural phenomena in which old bone is continually replaced with new bone. This balanced process is critical for maintenance of healthy bone mass.

Bone Modeling—these changes in size and shape of bone in a region are adaptations in response to stress or loading forces directed to the bone.

Bone Repair—the physiologic process in which the body facilitates the repair of a bone fracture.

Bone Regeneration—the development of new bone growth in deficient sites using surgical protocols that apply the principles of osteogenesis, osteoinduction, and osteoconduction for directed bone growth.

Guided Bone Regeneration (GBR): technique to reconstruct alveolar bone deficiencies via the use of a barrier membrane to exclude epithelial cells and allow slower-growing cells to form bone.

Guided Tissue Regeneration (GTR): technique to regenerate lost periodontal structures via the use of a barrier membrane to exclude epithelial or connective tissue ingrowth.

---

vertical ridge height. As this resorptive process occurs, the position of implant-supported restorations can change substantially secondary to the new interarch relationship between the maxilla and the mandible. For instance, the loss of maxillary posterior teeth with the accompanied loss of the buccal bony ridge width will often lead to development of a posterior crossbite. This is compounded as the mandible deteriorates into a division C or D ridge, resorbing until the remaining mandibular basal bone is actually positioned laterally, away from the remaining maxillary bone. Treatment planning must combine final restorative loading of implants in a manner that will not place unreasonable forces on the implant-bone interface leading to excessive bone remodeling and implant failure. The current ability of the implant team to regenerate bone in critical sites has increased the predictability of final prostheses and in doing so has reduced the number of implant failures (Fig. 36.6).

Edentulous Site Assessment

The treatment planning process begins with a reasonable assessment of the extent of the bony deficiency and the capacity of a regenerative procedure to create adequate support for implants in their ideal positions for comfort, esthetics, function, and support. As the extent of bone regeneration is evaluated, care must be taken in the beginning stages to identify the expected positions of each restoration or prosthesis using accurate restorative wax-ups. Evaluation of the relationship between the required restorative positions and the bony deficiency will then provide insight into the volume and shape of the bone that will need to be regenerated. At this

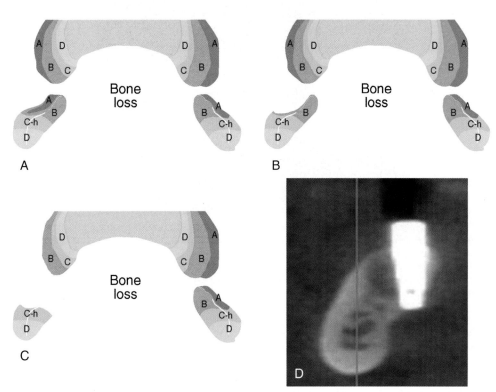

• **Fig. 36.6** Resorptive Pattern in Posterior Mandible. (A) The normal bony contours in a coronal view of the maxillary and mandibular arches. (B) The initial resorption of bone in the mandibular arch from Division A to Division B. (C) As bone resorbs further (Division B to Division C), the resultant mandibular position is more lingually (medially) inclined in comparison with the maxillary arch. Further loss in the lower arch leaves the remaining bone in a more lateral position than the maxillary arch. (D) Often when bone resorbs, the position of the implant is compromised, as can be seen by the cross-sectional image depicting a perforation.

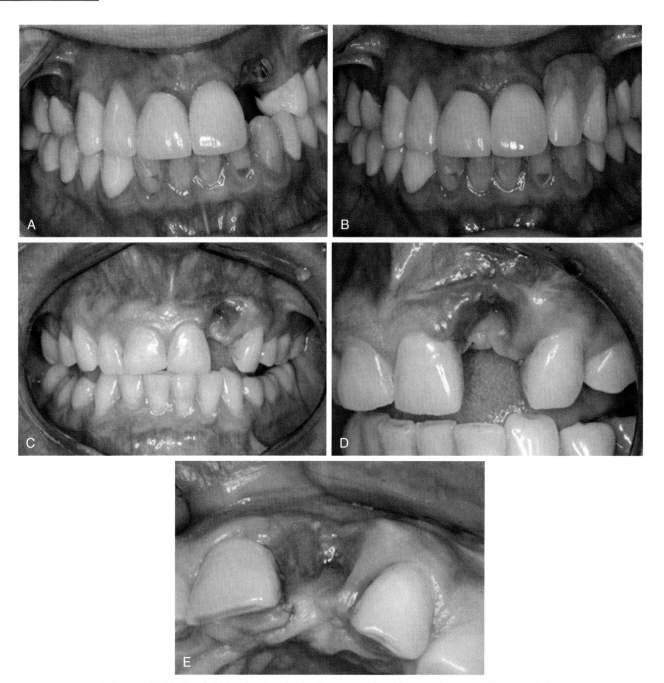

• **Fig. 36.7** (A) Maxillary left lateral and canine implants were placed in a poorly executed bone graft site, leading to a devastating esthetic situation. (B) Because of the malpositioned implants, a removable partial denture was placed to hide the implant position. (C) Maxillary left lateral incisor replacement resulted in a defect after two unsuccessful attempts to graft a missing facial cortical plate. (D) The loss of the cortical bone raised the defect to the level of the apices of the adjacent teeth. (E) The only remaining bone is found along the palatal cortical plate.

stage the most predictable surgical approach and bone graft material (e.g., autograft, allograft, xenograft) is selected to ensure adequate bone support can be developed for ideal implant placement.

In site assessment treatment planning, complications often result when the clinician fails to understand the relationship between the limitations of various regenerative grafting techniques and the predictable development of the required bone contours and bone volume needed for overall restorative success. It is not possible to treat every bony defect with simple or limited techniques that a clinician learns early in his or her learning curve. This discipline requires a variety of approaches to meet the reality of advanced bone resorption, and as the surgeon gains experience, correct application of techniques will lead to predictable outcomes. When the incorrect technique is used, inadequate bone volume will be regenerated, leading to either compromised restorative results or a potential failure of the prosthesis. These problems not only compromise the local grafting site, but they can also destroy bone around surrounding teeth, creating a worse situation than was originally encountered (Fig. 36.7).

In an ideal setting, prevention of ridge resorption starts with aware-ness of ridge preservation and limiting bone loss before major ridge defects occur. This starts with atraumatic extraction techniques, aggres-sive socket grafting, and communication among the members of the implant team in respect to the need for timely preservation of the ridge. The longer the patient remains without an implant in an extrac-tion site, the greater the chance that adjunctive grafting procedures will be necessary. Use of effective grafting materials is critical for successful results. For patients with long-term edentulism, the surgeon needs to be fully aware of the patterns of bone resorption to understand the current underlying bony architecture and to correctly choose a grafting protocol that will build the correct volume for the intended prosthesis. This working knowledge of ridge resorption and expertise in the use of effective diagnostic imaging to accurately assess bone volumes gives the clinician the opportunity to correctly organize a reasonable and predictable implant treatment plan (Fig. 36.8).

The use of cone beam computed tomographic (CBCT) imaging, together with proper diagnostic digital or cast models, allows the cli-nician to create a clear prosthetic plan. The restorative wax-up can easily be interlaced into computed tomographic (CT) imaging soft-ware for assessment of the bone volumes needed for proper implant support in key positions. This whole process has been advanced with digital scans and virtual crowns/implants. The digital plans, once inte-grated into CBCT images, allow the team to visualize the relation-ships between bone volume and restorative components. Once the dimensions and volume of the graft have been determined, proper application of bone-grafting techniques and materials is necessary to ensure that the intended volume can be achieved. At this point the patient should be educated on the details of the regenerative pro-cedures and a timeline of treatment. Advanced grafting procedures delay completion of the final prosthesis, and patients should be aware of the extent of the inconveniences that will need to be tolerated dur-ing this surgical sequence (Fig. 36.9, Fig. 36.10).

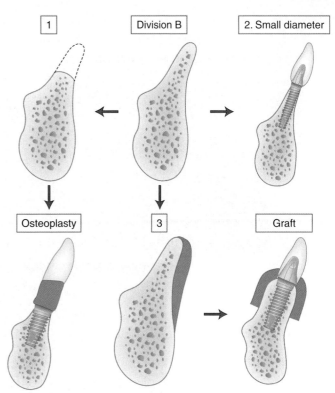

Fig. 36.8 Treatment Planning Decision Tree. In a Division B ridge, various treatment options are possible, including osteoplasty, Division B implants, or bone grafting. However, each treatment plan has advan-tages and disadvantages that should be taken into consideration with respect to the final prosthesis (e.g., type 1 fixed prosthesis [FP-1], FP-2, or FP-3).

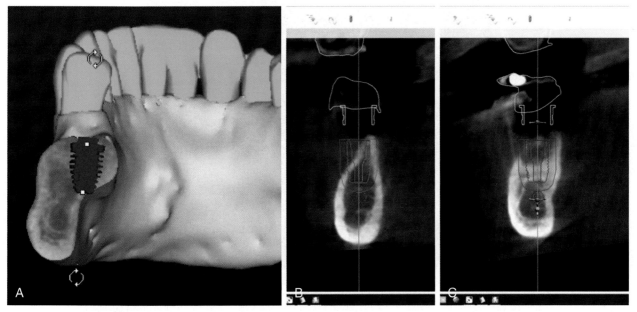

Fig. 36.9 (A) Use of three-dimensional imaging allows the implant team the opportunity to visualize the relationship between the osteotomy and the surrounding bone and teeth. (B) Examination of cone beam computed tomography cross sections allows assessment of proposed implant sites and their relationship to available bone. In this case there is not enough bone to support an implant without additional grafting in the site. (C) The absence of adequate buccal bony support indicates the need to regenerate at least 5mm of bone. Bone around this coronal 5mm of the implant is critical for functional support during loading.

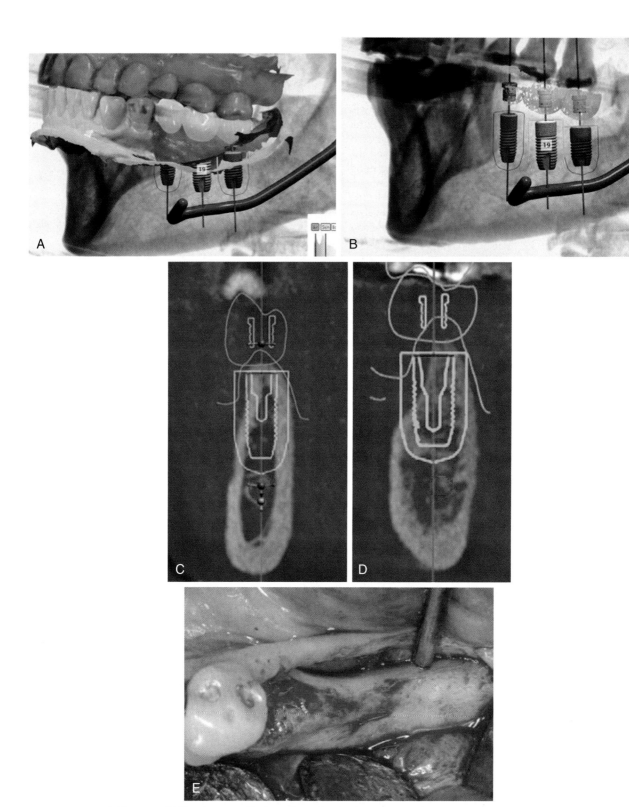

• **Fig. 36.10** (A) Planning a case in three-dimensional software starts with incorporation of the restorative wax-up into the cone beam computed tomographic image. (B) Implants are then introduced in positions that will support the crowns in their required restorative positions. (C and D) As the cross sections are evaluated in this particular case, it is apparent that there is not enough ridge width for placement of implants in the existing bone. This preliminary view indicates that augmentation of the ridge will be necessary for proper implant alignment and support. (E) Evaluation of the actual bony ridge at the time of surgery confirms the previous digital assessment of the bony deficiency.

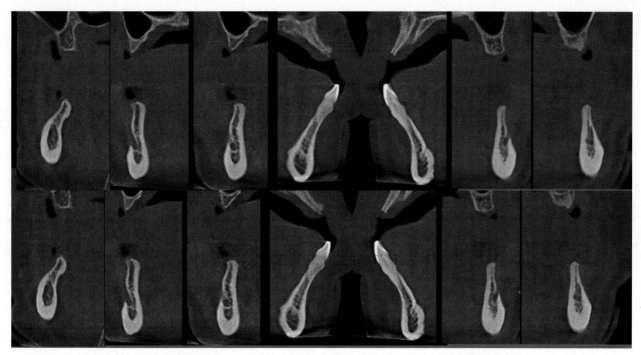

• **Fig. 36.11** This series of cross sections was prepared from a mandible showing a patient who has a very thin overall ridge width throughout the anterior and posterior regions. As this case is considered for augmentation, concern should be directed to the potential for graft failure because of the overall discrepancy between the thin basal bone width and the required width for implant positioning.

Bony Defect Morphology Considerations and Classification

One of the most difficult components of bone augmentation treatment planning is learning how to predict the amount of bone that will actually be required to develop the proper foundational support that the restorative treatment plan requires. Evaluation of the clinical situation, review of two-dimensional radiographs, assessment of models with restorative wax-ups, and information from CBCT all play a role in determining where bone will be required and how much bone will be needed to successfully graft the site. The concept of determining graft volume is even more important when autogenous bone is incorporated into the regenerative process. The location of an autogenous bone harvest often determines how much volume of bone can be retrieved. The chin and ramus are the primary sites for significant donor volumes used in block grafting, but these sites can provide only a limited volume of bone. If these local donor sites are inadequate, bone can be taken at the apex of many osteotomy sites. In addition, the use of a Piezosurgery unit and bone scrapers may be utilized to harvest cortical shavings. (Fig. 36.11)

In cases where a previous procedure fails to properly develop adequate bone volumes for ideal implant positioning, reflection of tissue over the grafted site will reveal inadequate bony support for the intended implant size and position. At this time, critical decisions must be made to prevent the chance of compromising the overall case success because of this shortfall. The easiest solution is to stop and regraft the site, but this causes inconvenience for the patient, embarrassment for the surgeon, and an overall increase in the treatment time and expense. The alternative is to either ignore the deficiency, placing the implant in a deficient site or attempting supplemental grafting around the exposed implant surfaces. Implant placement in compromised sites without grafting ultimately limits the implant size or forces improper positioning of the implant in the alternative position. This option then leads to a compromised result and incurs unnecessary risk for future failure. For more experienced surgeons, simultaneous implant placement with additional grafting can be attempted, but this is limited to cases where the surrounding basal bone allows proper implant positioning application of grafting principles. (Fig. 36.12), (Fig. 36.13).

Bony Defect Classification

Determining if an edentulous site will require augmentation should start with an initial assessment of the bony defect. Careful review of the topography of the recipient site includes review of the bone levels on adjacent teeth, bony protuberances, the depth of the actual defect itself, variations in the vertical height of the remaining walls of the ridge, and the condition of the surrounding soft tissue. A successful graft depends on the passage of various cellular components from the surrounding recipient site's bony walls and vascular components into the developing graft site. The larger the distance from these bony surfaces to the peripheral graft components, the greater is the challenge for the various cells to migrate to the outer limits of the particulate graft. The surrounding prominent bony contours also provide additional support and protection for the graft particles, limiting micromovement that usually results in compromised bone growth. These fixed bony surfaces can also help with containment of graft particles and eventual support of membranes. Depending on the morphology and topography of the defect, the clinician may determine the difficulty and potential success of augmentation procedures. The following classification system is based on the bony contours of the deficient area.

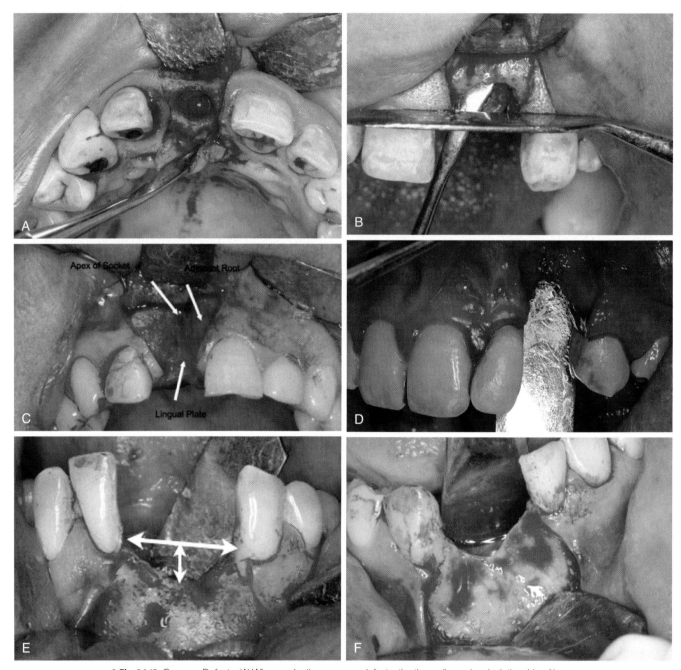

• **Fig. 36.12** Osseous Defects. (A) When evaluating osseous defects, the three-dimensional relationship of bone loss versus adjacent tooth positioning is crucial. (B) Severe vertical resorption requires regeneration to avoid complications with support, esthetics, and poor healing. (C) The position of the adjacent teeth and roots should be evaluated to determine the prognosis of an implant-related restoration. (D) Defects that destroy both the facial and palatal cortical plates limit the choice of regenerative procedures that can be used. (E and F) When there is a sharp declining ridge adjacent to a natural tooth, placement of an implant 1.5 mm away creates a failing situation beginning at time of the initial implant placement. As time passes, both the tooth and the implant will be compromised. Positioning the implant away from the natural tooth can limit this proximity problem; however, the implant body position will be too apical, which affects the esthetics and biomechanics.

Bone Defect Classification
1. Depression
2. Concavity
3. Trough
4. Elevation/Prominence
5. Vertical (Height)
6. Buccal & Lingual Cortical Destruction
7. Complex/Multi-Dimensional
   (Fig. 36.14), (Fig. 36.15).

Depression

A simple depression in a potential implant site is a bony defect measuring less than 3.0 mm. If these types of defects are left untreated, they can contribute to either a ridge dehiscence or a fenestration when an implant is placed in the region. These depressed areas are usually grafted at the time of implant placement and they do not require the use of extensive space maintenance techniques. When a depression is noted, it can

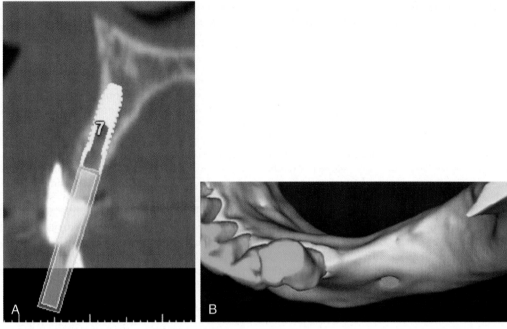

• **Fig. 36.13** Cone Beam Computed Tomography (CBCT) Evaluation of Osseous Defects. (A) The use of interactive treatment planning should be completed to determine any possible bony deficiencies. (B) Three-dimensional CBCT can be used to obtain a better ideal of the bone morphology.

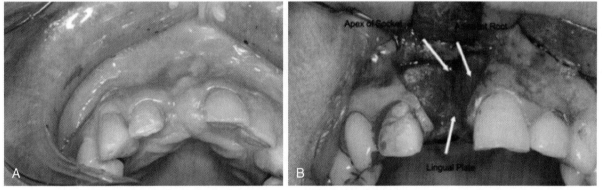

• **Fig. 36.14** (A) Evaluation of the clinical appearance of an edentulous space can easily mislead clinicians with respect to the underlying bony contours. (B) Flap reflection reveals a severely resorbed facial aspect of the edentulous ridge.

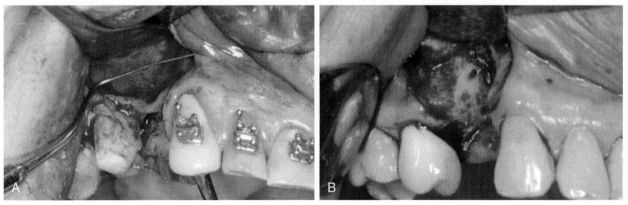

• **Fig. 36.15** (A) Facial and palatal ridge resorption with coronal and apical defects. This will require facial and palatal regeneration. (B) Severe facial resorption with some remaining palatal bony cortical plate.

be covered with a layer of allograft material and covered with a collagen membrane. Long-term isolation of the particles is not as critical in these situations as compared to larger defects where fibrous in-growth can be catastrophic. Depression type bony defects are the most predictable types of grafts and advanced surgical expertise is not as critical as in other defect types.

Concavity

The concave shaped ridge defect has a significant horizontal depression or bony defect in the middle of the ridge that exceeds 3.0 mm in overall depth. These defects have reasonable remnants of bone surrounding the site that can be used for graft support, containment of particles, and delivery of an adequate supply of cells for angiogenesis. Regeneration in these sites is relatively predictable and most of the implant support will still be provided by the surrounding autogenous bone. A concave defect will require adequate space maintenance for the development of significant horizontal bony growth requiring the use of a static support system (e.g. bone screws, a titanium supported membrane) that is maintained for at least 5 months. (Fig. 36.16A, Fig. 36.16B).

Trough

Severe ridge defects may on occasion destroy the ridge to the depth of the lingual/palatal cortical plate. These are most commonly seen in single tooth defects, especially after a traumatic extraction. The resulting defect provides clearly defined lateral walls of bone formed by the roots of the adjacent teeth and most of these sites also have an apical wall of bone that approximates the prior apex of the tooth. Although these are deep and involved defects, they provide protection for the graft components through their actual configuration. Fixation of tenting screws in the middle of these defects assures maintenance of the needed space for regeneration. The presence of four actual bony walls provides a ready source of cellular components and the resulting regenerative potential is excellent. Therefore, grafting in these defects can be completed more predictably than a wide and exposed concave defect that requires complex vertical support for development of graft depth,

protection from removeable prostheses, and general exposure to micromovement (Fig. 36.17).

Elevation/Prominence

When ridge defects extend across the span of several teeth, the topography of the lateral and vertical surfaces of potential graft sites can vary significantly. A horizontal concavity or isolated depression in a recipient site can be complicated by adjacent elevated prominences of cortical bone. The maxillary cuspid region would be a typical site where the original tooth extended beyond the surrounding basal bone. The loss of the cortical plate on an adjacent premolar would be a distinct contrast to the prominent cortical support over a cuspid. Other examples would be changes in the overall facial contours created by malpositioned teeth. Situations like this also can develop as various teeth are lost over an extended period of time and the resulting loss of ridge support emphasizes the facial contours of the remaining compromised teeth. Grafting around these prominent regions does not require much support in the elevated area, but good space maintenance is needed directly adjacent to the elevated portion of the recipient site (Fig. 36.18).

Vertical (Height)

Accurate assessment of the vertical ridge height in a potential augmentation site is critical from a treatment planning standpoint. As the vertical defect height is increased, the crown-implant ratio becomes problematic with respect to esthetics and biomechanical factors. Regeneration of vertical height is a complex grafting procedure and that is usually reserved for clinicians with advanced experience and skills in complex soft tissue manipulation. A true vertical defect is in essence a through and through defect with the loss of both cortical plates. These defects will require that the concept of space maintenance be moved into a 3rd dimensional skill. A thin sharp-edged ridge top is usually present, with two dense cortical surfaces approximating each another with little to no medullary component between them. The resulting surface area requiring regeneration involves the palatal/lingual aspect, the vertical height defect region, and the highly resorbed facial/buccal portion of the ridge. The limiting factor with these types of defects is the level of the bone on the interproximal aspect of the adjacent

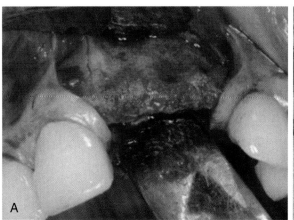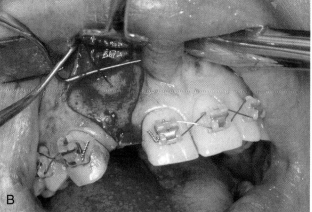

• **Fig. 36.16** (A). Concave Ridge Defect: This ridge has multiple contours to the generalized horizontal defect. There is an angular coronal defect at the top of the ridge, as well as a serious apical defect that leaves a large region that will need to be regenerated. (B). This Concave defect requires significant support for the membrane to regenerate adequate bone in the deeper portions.

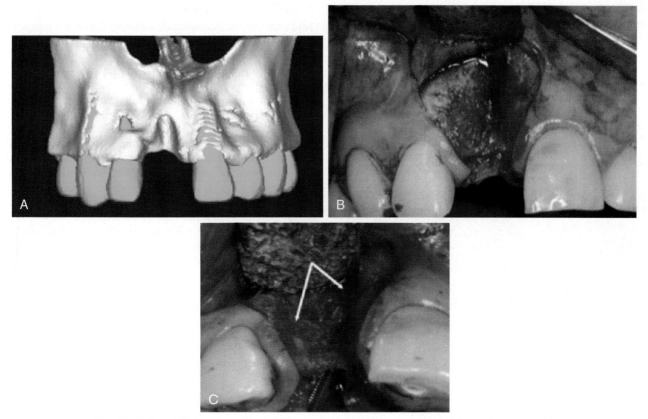

• **Fig. 36.17** Trough Defect Type: (A) 3D CBCT image demonstrating the loss of interproximal bone. This will greatly limit development of adequate height of the interproximal papilla in the final restoration. (B and C) Three-dimensional and clinical images of severe horizontal defect with loss of bone on adjacent teeth. There is still fairly good vertical height of the palatal cortical plate.

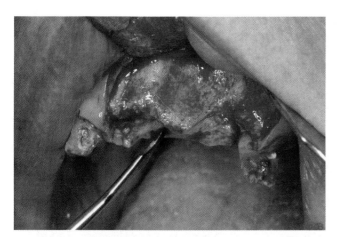

• **Fig. 36.18** This ridge defect has a complex nature to its topography. The prominent portions of the facial aspect of the ridge will help with support and regenerative components to the more compromised adjacent areas. Careful evaluation of the remaining surfaces demonstrate examples of other defect types.

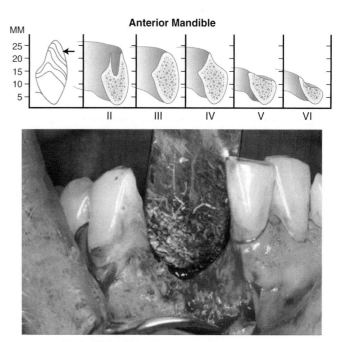

• **Fig. 36.19** Vertical Ridge Defect Type: Lower anterior complex ridge defect with serious vertical component that destroyed both the facial and lingual cortical plates. The precipitous vertical drop in bone height from the interproximal tooth bone to the base of the defect requires correction of the vertical defect for reasonable implant placement and esthetics. Placement of an implant in the middle of the depressed region would still involve a horizontal deficiency. Preservation of the bone levels on the adjacent teeth is a priority.

teeth. Clinicians must understand that it is not possible to raise a ridge higher than the adjacent bony level. In complex cases, this limitation can often require removal of an adjacent tooth to provide a higher adjacent interproximal height for potential vertical development. This is most often seen in anterior areas of the maxilla and mandible where the aesthetic demands of a case require as much vertical regeneration as possible (Fig. 36.19).

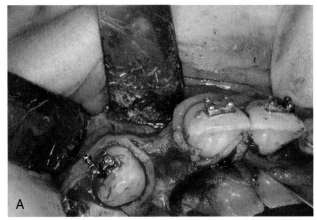

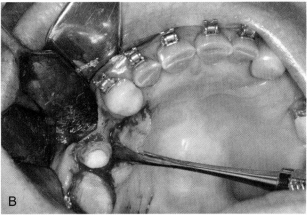

• **Fig. 36.20** Hour-glass Ridge Defect: The images in examples (A) and (B) demonstrate the destruction of the facial and palatal cortical plates. Regeneration in these sites will require growth in both dimensions. Failure to regenerate the palatal portion of the site will lead to facial positioning of the implant and most likely, a facial bony deficiency.

Buccal/Lingual (Palatal)

Ridge assessment must include a three-dimensional review of the bony resorption on the lingual/palatal aspects as well as on the facial and vertical regions. Severe ridge defects can often include a significant lingual/palatal component that moves the regenerative procedure into a complex surgical category. The most common site for a true "Hour Glass" ridge defect is in the anterior portion of the maxilla or mandible. Unfortunately, these sites are technically challenging with respect to tissue release, space maintenance, and graft containment. In general, the palatal tissue is very thick and dense, limiting any significant stretching or expansion of tissue over a graft and membrane. For example, the lingual tissue in the mandible is paper-thin and procedures to release and extend lingual tissue over a graft has a potential for button-holing a flap or for potential complications in the region of vessels, salivary components, and muscle attachments. Fixation of tenting screws in palatal defects requires extensive reflection of the palatal tissue and accurate anchorage of the membrane beyond the borders of the bony defect. Membrane fixation on the lingual aspect of the mandible is a delicate process and awareness of the vital structures if critical. Regeneration in these sites is limited to clinicians with extensive surgical and bone grafting experience (Fig. 36.20 A, B).

Complex/Multi-Dimensional

Complex ridge defects are made up of a combination of the configurations described above. These sites will more than likely have deep horizontal destruction that is combined with at least one vertical component. These type of defects vary from a severe single tooth site to a complete section of a quadrant. It is the recognition of the complexity of these situations that is critical for success. The sheer volume of bone that needs to be regenerated can only be determined with advanced integration of 3D Imaging and CBCT surveys. The restorative requirements then dictate the actual locations for implant support and subsequently the areas where specific volumes of bone will be need to be regenerated. At that point, the specific technique can be chosen by its potential for development of large volumes of bone. These cases require harvesting significant volumes of autogenous bone and use of isolating membranes capable of separating the developing graft sites from soft tissue infiltration. Complex cases should be avoided until a clinician has extensive experience in development of bone in each of the basic situations described above (Fig. 36.21).

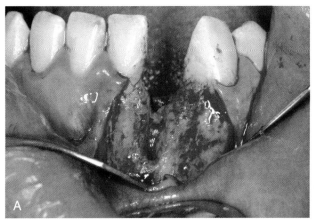
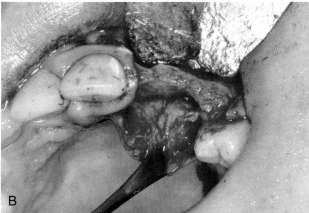

• **Fig. 36.21** Complex Ridge Defect: The images in (A) and (B) demonstrate the severity of bone loss that can occur over time and in highly destructive situations. These defects require advanced training and experience for predictable grafting success.

Soft Tissue Considerations

Patient-to-patient comparisons of the soft tissue drape surrounding the natural teeth often demonstrate significant differences in color, surface consistency, tissue thickness, and overall esthetics. This is emphasized when a very thin and friable tissue drape surrounds an anterior tooth. Differentiation of patients into either a "thick biotype" or a "thin biotype" is a critical tool that should be used during routine restorative care and anterior implant–related treatment planning. Cook et al.[10] demonstrated the simplest way to determine a patient's tissue biotype is through the evaluation of the visibility of a periodontal probe in the sulcus of an anterior tooth. A patient with a thick biotype will not show any translucence of the probe through the sulcular tissue. In contrast, a thin biotype will allow visualization of the coloration of a probe through the sulcular tissue.[10]

A patient with a thick biotype has tissue with a robust pink stippled appearance. This dense tissue drape forms a thick layer of tissue that is very forgiving when dental restorations are placed around natural teeth and when dental implants are involved. The thin biotype patient, however, presents a much more difficult challenge. These patients often have a thinner labial plate thickness, a narrower keratinized tissue width, and a greater distance from the cement-enamel junction to the initial alveolar crest. This delicate layer of tissue is so thin that the periodontal probe can be visualized when it is lightly placed in the sulcus. Patients with a thin biotype are also more prone to tissue recession, complicating the predictability of restorative esthetics around anterior teeth. As teeth migrate out of position or rotate in the arch, the prominence of the roots can increase, complicating the soft tissue situation even more. Thin layers of tissue around the maxillary anterior teeth require meticulous planning to hide underlying crown margins (Box 36.4 and Fig. 36.22).

Patient biotype and bony architecture must be considered early in all implant treatment planning to avoid a variety of issues that become very complex compared with similar situations around natural teeth. This early planning allows the surgical team the opportunity to incorporate tissue grafting into each surgical stage, allowing deficiencies to be avoided or to at least be minimized. These problems can be significantly complicated when major bone grafting has been completed in the region, resulting in elevation of the mucogingival junction and repositioning of the mucosa into the zone surrounding implant restorative margins. The tissue thickness in postoperative graft sites is often very thin, and development of an adequate emergence profile for crowns requires development of at least 3 mm of keratinized tissue thickness over the top of the implant body prior to restoring the implant. Restorative dentists often find it difficult to mask the dark tones in the coronal portions of natural teeth with endodontic-related color changes. This problem is compounded in a patient with a thin biotype as the color passes through the thin facial bone and thin tissue consistency. This problem with translucence is a reoccurring issue with implant restorations. Problems related to the translucence of the dark hue of the implant body and the abutment through thin tissue can significantly complicate the esthetics surrounding the final restoration.[11] A patient with a thick biotype and thick facial cortical

> **• BOX 36.4 Soft Tissue Evaluate and Assessment Considerations**
>
> - Gingival biotype
> - Width of keratinized tissue
> - Soft tissue thickness
> - Vestibular depth
> - Smile Line
> - Frenum attachments

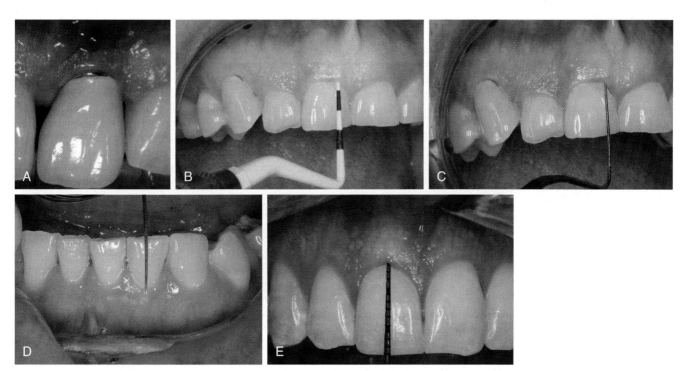

• **Fig. 36.22** (A) Thin biotype exhibiting metal show-through. Tissue biotype can be defined by the translucence of a probe through the sulcus. (B) Thick biotype yellow probe (i.e., no-show through). (C) Thick biotype with dark probe (i.e., no show-through). (D) Intermediate biotype with visible probe through sulcular tissue (i.e., show-through). (E) Thin biotype with probe (i.e., show-through).

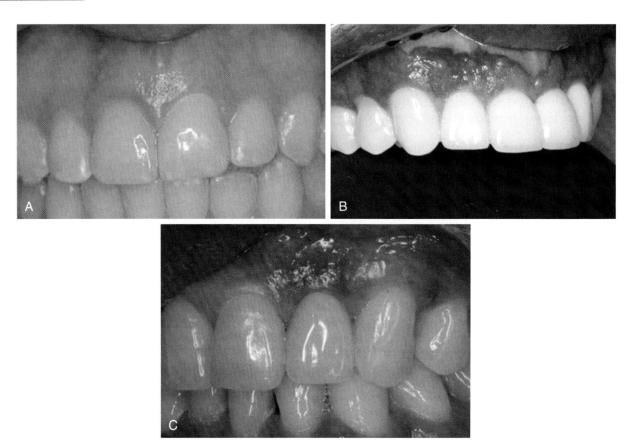

• **Fig. 36.23** Tissue Biotypes. (A and B) Thick biotype. (C) Thin biotype.

bone makes an ideal implant patient when restorations are placed and minor deficiencies can be hidden behind the thickened tissue mass. A patient with a thin biotype does not usually have a robust facial bone thickness, and any remodeling changes in facial bone density or thickness can greatly alter the restorative esthetics (Fig. 36.23).

Additional problems related to tissue thickness develop in implant cases as time passes and bony changes occur around the implant body. Esthetics around an implant restoration often change because there is an active bone remodeling process around implants that often results in a loss of facial cortical thickness. This can be a serious problem if an implant is placed in a site with very thin facial bone or in a site where the quality of bone lateral to the implant resorbs as the prosthesis is loaded and the functional forces are centered on the coronal 5 mm of the implant body. If recession or slight bone loss occurs, the facial aspect of the implant can be exposed, creating a dark hue that shows through the overlying tissue and contributes to a poor esthetic situation.

As anterior immediate implants are considered, recommendations for the actual location of the implant in the socket have changed significantly as resorptive patterns in immediate implants have been studied over time. An immediate implant currently should be placed significantly palatal to the facial cortical plate to allow for bone remodeling. This paradigm shift has occurred over time as the recommendations for implant diameters in anterior spaces have steadily decreased to accommodate for these changes in facial bone thickness and complications related to color translucence through the soft tissue. Current recommendations specify that the facial aspect of the implant body should be placed at least 3 mm palatal to the inner edge of the facial cortical plate. Additional authors currently recommend grafting on the facial aspect of anterior immediate implant sites with

bovine particulate grafts and connective tissue graft to minimize long-term changes.

When a clinician is preoperatively aware of a problem related to tissue biotype, it is possible to plan ahead procedurally to maintain or possibly change the biotype, leading to optimal esthetic outcomes. Patients with a very thin biotype can be evaluated for intraoperative supplementation using connective tissue grafts and facial bone grafts to create a more forgiving tissue drape over the implant site. Because thicker cortical bone volumes promote thicker biotypes, the bony architecture and soft tissue drape may be modified in an esthetic zone before implant placement and restoration. Advance planning also provides the implant team an opportunity to inform the patient about these issues and to point out potential esthetic complications before commencing treatment. Any compromise in a patient's expectations must be addressed, especially if the patient is not interested in grafting to modify the tissue type.

Implant restorative care in thin biotypes often requires tissue augmentation as the case ages to create a thick, dense layer of fibrous tissue over the implant body and any deficiencies involving the adjacent natural teeth. Connective grafting procedures are readily available to increase the thickness of the tissue drape in situations such as this. Subepithelial connective grafting procedures may use palatal connective tissue, dense connective tissue from the maxillary tuberosity, or acellular dermal matrix (i.e., OrACELL [Salvin Dental Specialties], AlloDerm [BioHorizons IPH, Inc.], PerioDerm) as the source of donor tissue. A thick layer of connective tissue is inserted into the deficient regions with tunneling procedures, allowing the repositioned tissue flap to provide the blood supply to the developing graft site. The use of the subepithelial approach allows the implant clinician to produce a final tissue tone and color that matches the adjacent natural tissue (Fig. 36.24A, B and C).

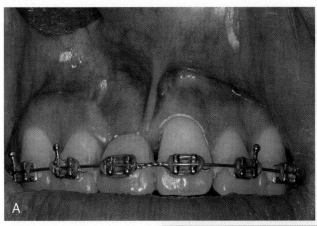
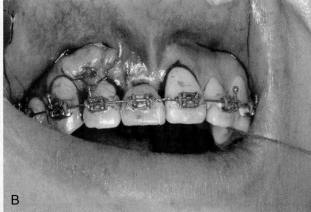
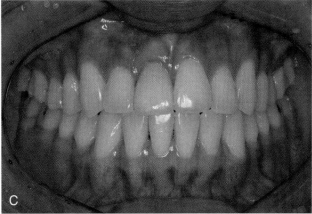

• **Fig. 36.24** Soft Tissue Augmentation over the facial aspect of an implant site with "grey tone" to the overlying soft tissue. (A). Grey coloration over the facial of the implant site. (B) A connective tissue graft is drawn into a tunnel prepared over the facial of the implant site. (C). The final restoration in place following the successful grafting procedure.

Large edentulous regions in the posterior portions of both arches often have little, if any, remaining keratinized tissue. These deficient regions can be augmented "before" the bone grafting procedure using "free tissue grafting techniques." In these cases, the epithelial layer of the palate is used as the source of the donor tissue. This usually creates large zones of thicker keratinized tissue with a distinct pinkish white color, duplicating the color of the tissue where the graft was harvested. This dense tissue is not always acceptable from an esthetic standpoint when it is placed in the anterior maxilla. Some of this color issue can be reduced by taking the graft from the posterior portion of the vault of the palate, away from the rugae found in the anterior palate. Use of thinner palatal grafts can also limit some of these annoying color issues. It is still important to keep in mind that the actual "thickness of the tissue" is important in the development of an emergence profile for the final restorations. At least 3 mm of tissue thickness is needed for not only this emergence pattern but is also important from the standpoint of implant health as the implant is restored and maintained.

The importance of the depth of soft tissue above the platform height has been described by Linkevicius et al.[12] in respect to maintenance of crestal bone height. Implants with less than 3 mm of tissue height over an implant were shown to be susceptible to crestal bone loss. The authors compared both regular root form implant and platform switch designs, and all implants were shown to be susceptible to this specific soft tissue related bone loss.[12]

Most anterior treatment plans involving major bone-grafting today incorporate the addition of layers of connective tissue,

allograft, or bovine graft particles with membrane coverage to limit excessive bone remodeling in these critical regions. These concepts are critical in "immediate implant" cases, where many cases require both soft tissue and hard tissue supplementation.

Augmentation and implant treatment planning should include a careful assessment of any frenum attachments that could interfere with the grafting process. Grafting in regions where there is still a highly placed frenum can be compromised during the healing phase when remnants of the frenum place tension on the closed incision line, contributing to incision line opening. The maxillary frenum should routinely be removed if it appears to be problematic for future tissue health. The lower frenum and lateral frenum attachments can create a similar tension effect, but the routine periosteal release incision in these graft sites usually eliminates this particular problem in most cases (Fig. 36.25).

Guided Bone Regeneration Protocol

Regeneration of bone in a specified area requires that a protected zone be created where the development process can be completed without interference. Block grafting and other approaches have previously been described for development of significant amounts of bone regeneration in appropriate sites. This chapter describes various protocols that use the principle of "space maintenance and tissue exclusion" for defined bone development. One of the most important components of the GBR process is space maintenance via the use of barrier membranes. Dahlin et al.[13] and many other authors have described the

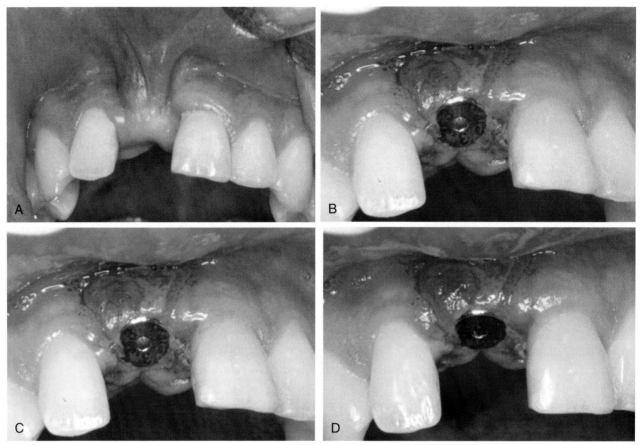

• **Fig. 36.25** (A) High frenum attachment. (B to D) Removal of frenum and placement of healing abutment.

• **BOX 36.5** "PASS" Principles for Predictable Bone Regeneration[69]

Primary closure
Angiogenesis for necessary blood supply and undifferentiated mesenchymal cells
Space maintenance/creation to facilitate adequate space for bone ingrowth
Stability of wound to induce blood clot formation

• **BOX 36.6** Growth Rates of Soft Tissue Versus Hard Tissue

Woven bone = 60–100 µm/day
Lamellar bone = 1 µm/day
Fibrous tissue = 1000 µm/day (1 mm/day)

---

development of new bone growth using membranes that contained grafts materials, allowing only neighboring bone or bone marrow cells to migrate into the bony defect, without ingrowth of competing soft tissue cells from the overlying mucosa.

In general, membranes are used in GBR procedures to act as biological and mechanical barriers, preventing the invasion of non–bone-forming cells (e.g., epithelial cells), whereas slower-migrating bone-forming cells are drawn into the defect sites.[14] As bone defects heal over time, there is a competition between soft tissue ingrowth and slower action bone-forming cells that are trying to migrate into the area. Soft tissue cells tend to migrate at a much faster rate than bone-forming cells and if left unchecked, they will infiltrate the developing site. Therefore the primary goal of barrier membranes is to allow for selective cell repopulation and to guide the proliferation of various tissues during the healing process.[15] Below the protective membrane, the regeneration process proceeds with angiogenesis and migration of osteogenic cells into the site. This initial blood clot is replaced by woven bone after vascular ingrowth, and later is transformed into load-bearing lamellar bone. This ultimately assists in the support of hard and soft tissue regeneration.[16] If a barrier membrane is not used, the bony defect will fill in with soft tissue, resulting in compromised bone growth (Boxes 36.5 and 36.6).

In the following guided bone regeneration protocol, there exists nine distinct steps for successful and predictable outcomes;
1. Incision and Flap Design
2. Flap Reflection
3. Removal of Residual Soft Tissue
4. Recipient Bed Preparation
5. Tissue Release
6. Membrane Placement
7. Space Maintenance
8. Bone Graft Placement
9. Closure

Step 1: Incision and Flap Design

Incision design is one of the keys to a predictable regenerative result. Ideal incision designs provide complete access to the surgical site without compromising the integrity of the surrounding tissue. As the incision is planned the anatomy of the adjacent papilla must be considered to prevent any damage that will compromise the esthetics and function of the tissue postoperatively. The patient's biotype and the amount of keratinized tissue is always reviewed, and any deficiencies in attached tissue must be accounted for in the incision design. The incision must be planned in a way that keeps incision lines away from critical regions where graft particles or blocks could become exposed. Observation of sound surgical principles in preparation of incisions is critical for maintenance of the blood supply to all of the involved tissues. Wide-based incisions are always important to prevent interruptions in the vascular supply to the flap.

Failure to properly plan the incision design of a flap during grafting can pose numerous issues, mainly related to incision line opening postoperatively. Incision line opening exposes the regeneration site to an influx of oral pathogens, soft tissue ingrowth, and loss of the graft materials that were intended to be isolated during the maturation process (Fig. 36.26A, B and C and Box 36.7).

The coronal incision is usually placed on the crest of the ridge, favoring a location closer to the palatal aspect if possible. It is important that the scalpel make a continuous full-thickness cut through the tissue and the periosteum, ending on the actual bone. Incisions that are irregular and leave regions of attached tissue and periosteum will lead to maceration of the flap as it is reflected. This shredding of tissue also compromises the periosteal layer that is the primary source for blood to the underlying bone. A survey of the available keratinized tissue must be completed before making an incision. In regions of bountiful attached tissue, the surgeon can use his discretion in the location of the incision through the keratinized regions. In regions where the keratinized tissue is limited, the incision should at least "split" the distance between the two edges of the keratinized tissue. It is always best to try to keep incision lines away from areas that are key to regenerative volume and protection (Fig. 36.27A,B, C, D).

When possible, the papillae should be preserved while incisions are prepared. If there is a good papilla adjacent to a graft site, the incision should be designed to avoid involvement of the papilla or it should be moved to the adjacent interproximal space. If the papilla is absent or is flat, the incision can be directed to the root approximating the graft or it can be moved to the adjacent space. It should be kept in mind that regeneration of a compromised interproximal papilla is still one of the most difficult endeavors in soft tissue surgery today. An incision in the middle of an anterior space of a "thin biotype" patient can either permanently scar the region or can completely destroy the papilla form and esthetics in the final restoration.

The positioning of vertical releasing incisions is one of the most important parts of the incision. A broad-based releasing incision should be prepared to maintain the blood supply to the flap and to allow elevation, retraction, repositioning, and suturing without tension. It should be kept in mind that most graft sites have a compromised soft tissue component that becomes a greater issue as the complexity of the underlying architecture increases. Most of these sites have a minimal keratinized band of tissue at the crest of the ridge, tapering quickly to the mobile mucosa of the vestibule. Full-thickness vertical release incisions should generally be planned to extend to the apical portion of mucogingival junction. In larger bone graft sites the vertical release will often extend deeper into the vestibule to help with complete release of the flap

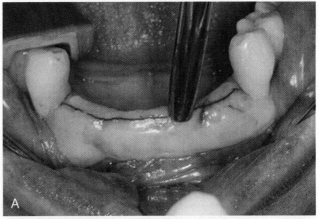
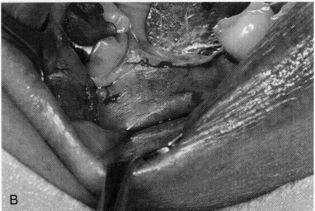
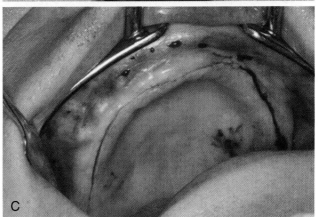

● **Fig. 36.26** Incision Design. (A) Ideal crestal incision when adequate attached tissue is present. (B) Crestal or more lingually placed incision that preserves the limited amount of keratinized tissue. (C) Crestal full-arch incision designed to preserve the limited facial zone of keratinized tissue.

● BOX 36.7 **Principle Concepts to Be Practiced in Grafting Incisions**

- Consideration of tissue biotype as incision is planned
- Maintain ideal papilla forms and levels
- Preservation and utilization of keratinized tissue in region
- Maintain the integrity of the full-thickness flap during reflection
- Design of lateral releasing incisions in locations that minimize exposure of graft particles
- Maintaining wide-based incisions to provide adequate blood supply to flap

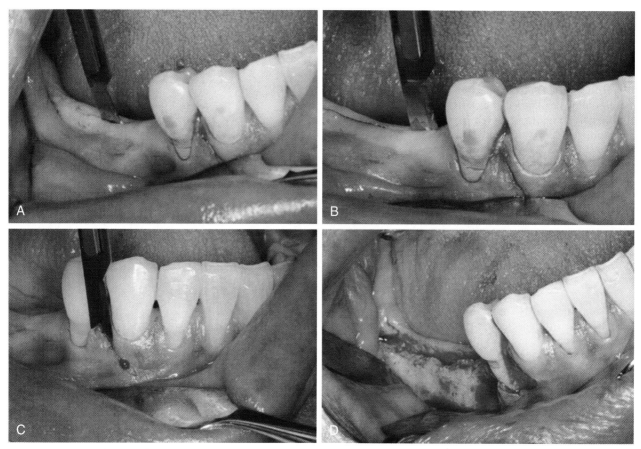

• **Fig. 36.27** Design for Papilla Preservation. (A and B) Ridge incision, making sure to "score" the bone to obtain full-thickness flap; (C and D) incision continued to include a vertical release.

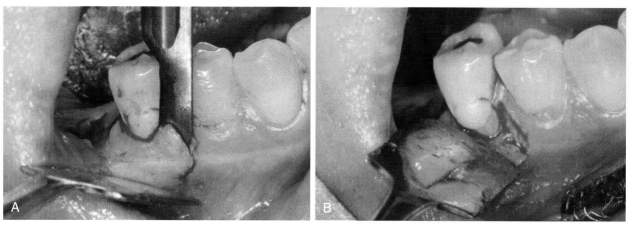

• **Fig. 36.28** Papilla-Sparing Incision. (A) Initial incision. (B) Full-thickness reflection.

during a tension-free closure. The location of vertical releases should be moved away from the most critical zones of the graft, limiting encroachment of the incision closure on the bulk of the graft particles and membrane margin. This is very important in cases where the barrier membrane is nonresorbable and exposure of a margin of the membrane can contribute to graft failure. In those cases, it is best to completely move the release to a completely different interproximal space. Properly placed incisions will position the margins of the flap over host bone instead of the graft particles and the membrane (Figs. 36.28 A and B). Vertical incisions have been related to scar formation in the surgical sites

after healing. Most scars are related to irregular incisions and poor adaptation of the wound edges at the time of suturing.

The goal of any implant treatment plan would be placement of restorations in the middle of a zone of attached keratinized tissue that is at least 3 mm thick from the level of the platform of the implant to the margin of the tissue surrounding the implant. Few resorbed ridges have an abundance of keratinized, and in most situations the surgeon will need to incorporate development of a thick tissue zone that will provide an emergence profile for the restoration and protection of the implant-bone interface. As the incision is prepared, the keratinized tissue dictates the path of the

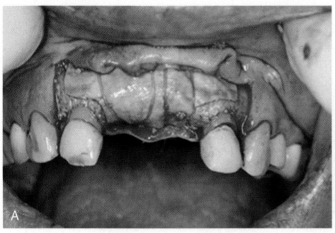
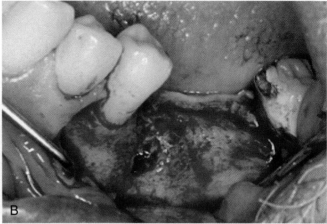

• **Fig. 36.29** Alternative Release Incisions. (A) The vertical releasing incision is often moved laterally to the adjacent papilla space to obtain adequate access. This will minimize incision line opening when larger graft volumes are obtained. (B) Extending the incision to an adjacent tooth also minimizes the possibility of the incision over top of the graft site.

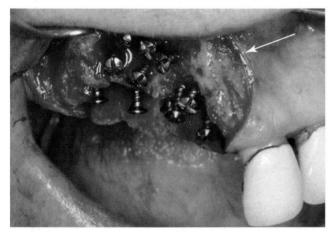

• **Fig. 36.30** Poorly Placed Release Incision. The incision should be positioned away from the graft site and also be more lateral to obtain a more broad-based flap design.

incision line and often determines how easily the wound will be to close and to withstand the strain on the incision line during healing. If adequate attached tissue is not present, soft tissue grafting should be completed either before the augmentation procedure, as a portion of the grafting protocol, or after the implants are placed. Tissue development options include autogenous free tissue grafts, autologous connective tissue grafts, acellular dermal matrix (Allo-Derm, OrACELL), or combinations of Mucograft and soft tissue grafts. In addition, when inadequate keratinized tissue is present, the incision should be placed toward the lingual portion of the remaining keratinized tissue, preserving as much attached tissue on the facial as possible. This allows for greater resistance to muscle pull and will decrease incision line opening (Fig. 36.29 A and B) (Fig. 36. 30).

Step 2: Flap Reflection and Site Preparation

Full-Thickness Reflection

Elevation of the tissue to expose the recipient site requires reflection of a full-thickness mucoperiosteal flap. This should be completed in an uninterrupted release of the flap that includes the surface mucosa, submucosa, and periosteum. This initial release is accomplished with an angled curette or a scalpel that is used to score the bone, ensuring complete penetration through the tissue layers and the periosteum. As the tissue is reflected, the underlying bone should be "scraped" with the curette or periosteal elevator in a side-to-side motion. It is important to confirm at this stage that the complete flap has been freed from the bone and that it is freely drawing away from the bony surface. Partial-thickness reflection leads to tissue trauma or shredding of the flap itself. Tissue that has been compromised in this manner results in slower healing and a higher morbidity. When using a periosteal elevator (i.e., 2–4 Molt) for this flap release, the edge should always rest on the bone to prevent tearing through of the tissue flap.

The tissue thickness on the lingual aspect of the mandible is very thin and friable. This tissue can be easily torn during reflection of the flap and manipulation of the tissue during the grafting procedures. Resulting "buttonhole" openings compromise the blood supply to the surrounding tissue that is needed for coverage over the graft site, leading to compromised results postoperatively. Tearing or buttonholing the lingual flap may also expose the graft site and increase the possibility of margin necrosis coronal to the tear. This exposure may lead to a total graft failure (Fig. 36.31 A and B).

If the lingual flap is torn during the procedure, it can sometimes be repaired using 5–0 chromic suture, approximating the edges of the tear and preventing tension on the weak site. It is recommended to use a collagen membrane below these fenestrations to assist with healing and to isolate the graft materials. Maintenance of the blood supply to the tissue flap is important, requiring that all tension on the flap be minimized.

A flap covering a graft that does not have complete release of pressure on the two margins of the flap will often pull open during the healing process (incision line opening). Tension on the flap compromises the blood supply to the tissue along the suture line that is under pressure. This pressure leads to necrosis and eventual separation of the two edges of the flap closure. Once this has occurred the flap cannot be sutured back into place, and the graft site is open for contamination and tissue ingrowth. The success of bone grafting is largely dependent on the maintenance of space for bone development and isolation of the graft particles during the slow process of osteogenesis. Soft tissue ingrowth, bacterial contamination, and migration of graft particles predictably compromise regenerative results.

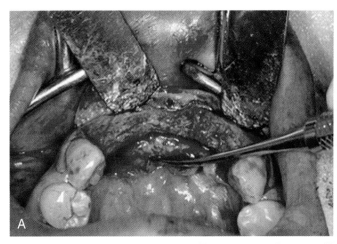
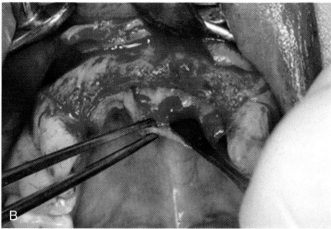

• **Fig. 36.31** Lingual Flap Design and Exposure. (A) The lingual should be reflected to expose the entire lingual surface; however, care must be exercised not to tear the flap. Perforating or a buttonhole in the flap will compromise the graft site. (B) If this occurs, it is very difficult to mend the tear, potentially compromising the closure of the graft site or predisposing the region to incision line opening over the healing graft. Incision line opening leads to an increased morbidity of the graft site.

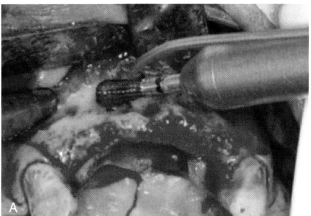
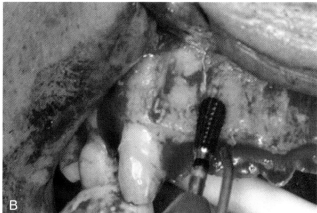

• **Fig. 36.32** (A and B) Removal of fibrous/soft tissue with course barrel bur.

The typical graft site requires that the overlying flap be released enough for extension of the flap at least 5 mm beyond the edge of the adjacent margin for a tension-free flap closure. The only way to achieve this free flap release is complete release of the periosteal layer, allowing the elastic fibers of the underlying flap to stretch as the flap is drawn over the graft site.

Step 3: Removal of Residual Soft Tissue and Pathology

Before bone grafting, all evidence of soft tissue remnants should be eradicated. Soft tissue fibers left on the recipient site can limit proper attachment of the newly regenerated bone to the underlying basal layer. These fibrous tissue remnants are the same tissue that the barrier membrane is attempting to exclude from the site. Early fibrous tissue growth in the wound simply bypasses that critical barrier and starts fresh tissue development right in the center of the graft site (Fig. 36.32 A and B).

Step 4: Recipient Bed Preparation

Preparation of the recipient site for an augmentation is very important in the development of a healthy ridge. The recipient site is usually covered with a dense layer of cortical bone that does not easily provide a blood supply to a developing graft. The process of decortication of the recipient base is used to open multiple pathways through this thick layer of bone. These pilot holes create an open pathway to the underlying trabecular bone where blood flow into the graft site will increase revascularization (angiogenesis) and introduce bone growth factors into the graft site.[17] The decortication is usually accomplished with the use of cross-cut fissure burs or small, round burs that are used to perforate the cortical plate. Copious amounts of chilled saline should be used to prevent thermal trauma (Fig. 36.33 A and B).

The decortication process initiates the regional acceleratory phenomenon, which describes the cellular stimulating technique used to accelerate the healing rate of a graft site. In this process, bone decortication is used as a "noxious stimulus," and it has been shown that the healing rate of a graft site can be increased 2 to 10 times the normal healing rate by initiating the regional acceleratory phenomenon (RAP).[18] This acceleration is accomplished by the introduction of platelets to the area that ultimately release growth factors including platelet-derived growth factor (PDGF) and transforming growth factor (TGF). Ultimately the decortication process will lead to better integration of the graft to the host bone.

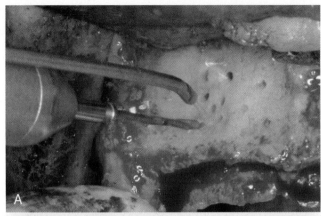

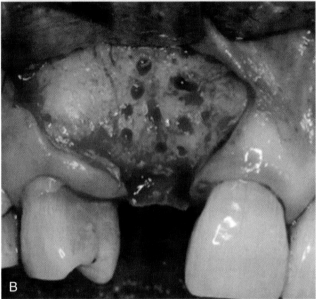

• **Fig. 36.33** Host Site Decortication. (A) The host site is prepared with a tapered cross-cut fissure bur (e.g., 169 L) to initiate angiogenesis. (B) The decortication must be deep enough to initiate bleeding, thus allowing blood vessels into the area (i.e., angiogenesis).

Step 5: Tissue Release

Successful augmentation procedures require maintenance of an intact tissue closure along the incision line during the healing process. One of the most common surgical complications that clinicians will experience early in their learning curve is incision line opening. The failure of maintaining this tissue union is directly related to an inadequate release of tension on the tissue flap as it is stretched over the widened graft space. Clinicians will find that it is highly unlikely to pull a tissue flap over any sizable graft site without first altering the integrity of the flap itself.

The most important concept in augmentation procedures is total membrane coverage of grafting materials from the time of membrane placement to completion of the graft maturation process. Success is directly related to the overall management of the soft tissue flap during flap closure. A successful case starts with the incision and continues with proper flap reflection of an intact periosteal layer, proper membrane positioning, and completion with a tension-free flap closure.

Tissue Release Technique

Examination of the exposed inner surface of a reflected flap will reveal a smooth, shiny layer of the periosteum. The periosteum is composed of a thin, firm layer of dense tissue that has no elastic fibers. This binding layer limits any significant elongation of the flap as it is stretched over a graft site. A shallow incision through the dense tissue "releases" the tight band of pressure on the underlying tissue flap. The tissue directly below the periosteum is primarily composed of elastic-type fibers, and once the periosteum has been released, the entire flap can be stretched. This simple releasing incision ultimately allows tension-free closure over the graft site (Fig. 36.34 A B and C) site (Fig. 36.35 A and B).

Step 6: Membrane Selection and Placement

Barrier membranes are generally used in guided bone regeneration procedures to act as biological and mechanical barriers against the invasion of fibrous tissue into the developing graft site. The membrane also will allow for the migration of the slower-migrating bone-forming cells into the defect sites During the bone regeneration process, there is a competition between soft-tissue and bone-forming cells to invade the surgical site. In general, soft-tissue cells migrate at a much faster rate than bone-forming cells. Therefore, the primary goal of barrier membranes is to allow for selective cell repopulation and to guide the proliferation of various cells during the healing process. Below the protection of the membrane, the regeneration process is allowed to continue unchecked with early angiogenesis and migration of osteogenic cells. The initial blood clot is replaced by woven bone after vascular ingrowth, which later is transformed into load-bearing lamellar bone. This will ultimately support the hard- and soft-tissue regeneration. If a barrier membrane is not utilized, lack of isolated space maintenance will result in soft-tissue integration and compromised bone growth.

Types of Membranes

Membranes are typically classified as resorbable or nonresorbable. Nonresorbable membranes have included titanium foils, expanded polytetrafluoroethylene (e-PTFE), and dense polytetrafluoroethylene (d-PTFE) with or without titanium reinforcement. Resorbable membranes are typically made of polyesters (e.g., polyglycolic acid, polylactic acid) or tissue-derived collagens (e.g., AlloDerm GBR, Pericardium, Ossix Plus). Non-resorbable membranes are bio-inert materials and require a second surgical procedure for removal after bone regeneration is complete. Resorbable membranes are naturally biodegradable and have varying resorption rates. However, all membranes, non-resorbable or resorbable, differ in their biomaterial and physical characteristics. These varied characteristics can often be associated with advantages and disadvantages in various clinical situations (Box 36.8).

Non-Resorbable Membranes. Non-resorbable membranes exhibit excellent biocompatibility, superior mechanical strength, increased rigidity, and generally achieve more favorable space maintenance than unsupported resorbable membranes. However, wound dehiscence is more common with non-resorbable membranes, and these membranes have the disadvantage of the need for a second surgery. This second procedure can result in an increased morbidity, higher costs, and over-all patient discomfort. The most common types of non-resorbable membranes include polytetrafluoroethylene (PTFE) and titanium mesh.

a. **Expanded PTFE membranes** — The expanded PTFE membrane (e-PTFE) was the first type of membrane used in implant dentistry and was the gold standard for bone regeneration in the 1990s. The e-PTFE membrane was advantageous as it prevented fibroblasts and connective-tissue cells from invading the

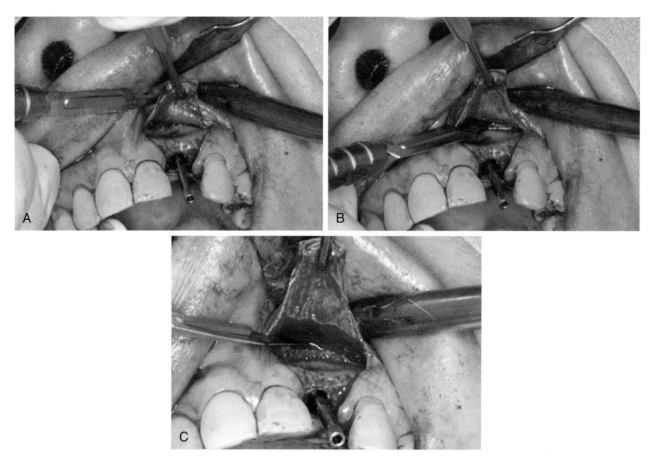

• **Fig. 36.34** Tissue Release Procedure. (A) Adequate flap release around bone graft sites is the most critical step for tension-free flap closure and predictable graft success. (B) A single shallow incision through the periosteum is prepared inside the flap while maintaining tension from elevating the flap. (C) The clear separation of the periosteal edges as the flap is extended and the elastic fibers allow the flap to stretch (i.e., tension-free).

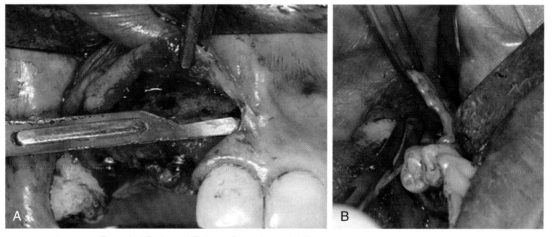

• **Fig. 36.35** Extended Periosteal Release Procedures. (A) The incision may be extended on the mesial and distal aspect of the graft site to allow increased mobility of the flap when it is extended. (B) After blunt dissection of the periosteal release with scissors (i.e., scissors should be parallel to the flap), the flap can be freely extended over the graft site. This release must be completed until the flap can be repositioned at least 5 mm beyond the lingual aspect of the graft site.

bone defect, yet they allowed the osteogenic cells to repopulate the graft area. The most common e-PTFE membrane in implant dentistry was GORE-TEX® (W.L. Gore & Associates, Inc.; Flagstaff, Ariz.).

The two sides of e-PTFE membranes were composed of different layers. One side was approximately 1 mm thick with 90 percent porosity, which impeded the growth of epithelium; The other side was approximately 0.15 mm thick with 30 percent

• BOX 36.8 Ideal Barrier Membrane Characteristics

1. *Tissue compatibility* — Ideally, the membrane should be biocompatible, resulting in no inflammation or interaction between the membrane and the host tissue that could lead to wound dehiscence or a local infection.
2. *Space maintenance* — The membrane should have a generally firm consistency to help maintain the regenerative space and to prevent loss of the defined ridge shape required by the restorative plan.
3. *Stabilization of the blood clot* — The membrane should provide stabilization of the blood clot, allowing the regeneration process to progress and reducing connective tissue integration into the defect.
4. *Cell Occlusiveness* — The porosity of the membrane should prevent fibrous tissue from invading the graft site. A larger pore size may inhibit bone formation by allowing the in-growth of faster-growing soft tissue cells. When the pore size is too small, limited cell migration inhibits collagen deposition and ultimately contributes to poor graft development.
5. *Mechanical Strength* — The membrane should have high durability and mechanical strength to protect the blood clot and resist passage of unwanted cells and bacteria. This same material strength is important when the membrane is tacked to the apical portion of the recipient site. A fragile membrane can easily tear around the fixation tack, releasing the anchorage of the membrane.
6. *Predictable resorption rate* — The resorption time of the membrane should coincide with the regeneration rate of bone tissue. The continued presence of the membrane is dependent on the location of the graft, the available vascularity in the region, and the quantity of graft material.
7. *Easy to modify and manipulate* — The membrane should be capable of size and shape alteration while maintaining adequate stiffness to prevent collapse into the graft site.

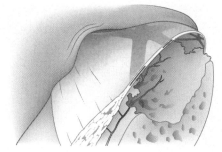

• **Fig. 36.36** D-PTFE membrane with titanium reinforcement depicting space maintenance principle, which allows for angiogenesis and the bone regeneration to progress. (Image adapted from Osteogenic Biomedical).

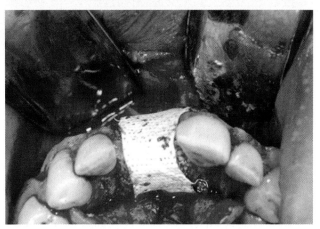

• **Fig. 36.37** Polytetrafluoroethylene (d-PTFE) Membrane. Clinical view of d-PTFE membrane.

porosity, which provided space for new bone growth and limited fibrous tissue ingrowth.[19]

The e-PTFE membranes had a high incidence of exposure, thereby resulting in an increased infection rate because of the ingrowth of bacteria into the highly porous structure. Additionally, the porous structure, with an approximate pore size of 5–20 micrometers, allowed for soft-tissue ingrowth, leading to increased difficulty in removal.

b. **High-density PTFE membranes** — Because of the associated complications of e-PTFE membranes, a higher density material — less than 0.3 microns — was developed in the early 1990s under the name Cytoplast™ (Osteogenics Biomedical; Lubbock, Texas). This high-density PTFE (also termed dense PTFE or d-PTFE) has been shown to have a lower risk of bacterial colonization in comparison to e-PTFE membranes, therefore resulting in fewer infections. The high density and small pore size of the membrane prevents passage of bacteria through the membrane, while allowing oxygen diffusion and passage of small molecules. Because of the lack of tissue ingrowth into the 0.3 micron pores, d-PTFE membranes are much easier to remove. Clinical use of d-PTFE has demonstrated that localized membrane exposure does not always dictate failure of the developing graft. If the d-PTFE membrane can be maintained for at least 6 weeks, removal at that time or later will often be followed with development of a reasonable bony ridge. (Fig. 36.36).

c. **Titanium-reinforced PTFE membranes** — The addition of a Titanium strut to a PTFE membrane allows the membrane to be shaped into a form that will develop bone in the contour and volume required by the restorative plan. These types of membranes are especially useful in the treatment of large osseous defects where varied thicknesses of bone are dictated by

an irregular recipient topography. Studies of GBR procedures using titanium-reinforced nonresorbable membranes have shown great success with horizontal and vertical alveolar ridge augmentation because of their ability to maintain space, minimize graft mobility, and exclude soft tissue ingrowth.[20–24] (Fig. 36.37) (Fig. 36.38).

d. **Titanium Mesh** Titanium mesh is a non-resorbable barrier that has been shown to be effective in maintaining space without collapsing. Titanium foils are flexible and can be bent and manipulated to mold around a bony defect. Titanium mesh has demonstrated predictable biocompatibility and features holes within the mesh that allow for maintenance of the blood supply from the periosteum. The primary disadvantage of titanium mesh is related to an increased incidence of wound dehiscence's and overall difficulty in maintaining soft-tissue coverage during the lengthy healing process. Exposure of the mesh may lead to an increased rate of infection and patient discomfort, leading to early removal of the mesh.

Resorbable Membranes. Resorbable membranes exhibit the advantage of no second-stage surgery for removal, thus decreasing discomfort and morbidity to the patient. However, the drawbacks of collagen include an unpredictable resorption time, which may adversely affect the amount of bone formation. Resorbable membranes derived from xenogeneic collagen for use in GBR procedures are the most popular membranes utilized in implant dentistry today. The various types of resorbable membranes include collagen, pericardium, and acellular dermal matrix.

Resorbable collagen membranes consist of either type I or type III collagen from bovine or porcine origin. Collagen membranes are easy

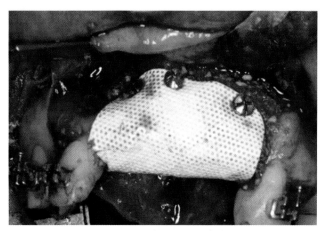

• **Fig. 36.38** Polytetrafluoroethylene (PTFE) Membrane: Clinical image depicting dense PTFE membrane prior to modification of the 2mm free zone adjacent to each tooth (Photo courtesy of Dr. John Hamrick).

to manipulate and have favorable effects on coagulation and wound healing, variable cross-linking, low antigenicity and high tensile strength.[25] Additionally, they inhibit epithelial cells, promote the attachment of connective-tissue cells, and increase platelet aggregation, which leads to wound stabilization and increased healing.

Collagen constitutes over 50 percent of the proteins in the human body. As the collagen membrane is degraded through enzymatic reactions, the process resembles normal tissue turnover.[26–33] Today, most collagen membranes are derived from allogenic or xenogeneic sources, which have become popular in implant dentistry. They act as scaffolding for osteoconduction, increase platelet aggregation and stability of clots, and allow for the attraction of fibroblasts for healing. Collagen membranes are manufactured with a variable resorption rate, which occurs through inflammatory cell biodegradation. The resorption rate is altered via the manufacturing process by the amount of cross-linking.

Collagen barriers are available in various forms:

a. **Collagen tape / plugs** are mainly used to control bleeding and maintain the blood clot within extraction sites. Collagen tape/plugs are usually a soft, pliable, sponge-like material that rapidly absorbs blood, thereby creating an artificial clot. The collagen allows aggregation of platelets, which results in the degranulation and release of bone-growth factors. Collagen tape/plugs have a resorption time of approximately 10–14 days are not indicated for guided bone regeneration procedures.

b. **Regular collagen membranes** resorb in three to four months and are mainly used in guided bone regeneration for small- to medium size bony defects. Ideally, primary closure is recommended to decrease graft morbidity.

d. **Extended collagen membranes** resorb in four to six months and are used for larger bony defects that require longer healing periods. These membranes are modified by increasing the cross-link density. Cross-linked collagen membranes are most commonly used in guided bone regeneration procedures for larger bony defects requiring longer healing time and graft containment.

e. **Pericardium Membranes** are most commonly of either bovine or porcine origin, with bovine having a greater collagen content. They generally consist of three layers with collagen and elastic fibers in an amorphous matrix. Their surface is porous, which allows for

cellular attachment and proliferation, yet has an increased density for soft-tissue exclusion. (Fig. 36.39 A, B, and C).

f. **Acellular Dermal Matrix (ADM)** is a biocompatible human (allograft) connective-tissue matrix derived through a process of removing all cells within the dermis. Because of the cells being removed during the manufacturing process, no viruses may be transmitted. Additionally, because of the acellular nature of this membrane, no inflammatory reactions or rejection will occur. The inert allograft, when used as a membrane, acts as an architectural framework that allows for fibroblast migration and vascularization. AlloDerm is an acellular dermal matrix originally developed in 1994 to be used as a skin allograft for burn patients.[34] It has been used in the medical and dental literature as an allograft for various procedures because of its ability to rapidly vascularize and to increase soft tissue thickness. In the dental literature, AlloDerm has been successfully used for root coverage, thickening of soft tissues, and GBR.[35,36] AlloDerm GBR is a thinner version (thickness ranges from 0.5 to 0.9 mm) of the original AlloDerm product (thickness ranges from 0.9–1.6 mm), specifically designed for GBR. AlloDerm GBR has been successfully used as a barrier membrane and has also been shown to significantly increase soft tissue thickness by 45% and 73% from baseline at 6 and 9 months, respectively (baseline 0.55 ± 0.16 mm to 0.80 ± 0.26 mm at 6 months and 0.95 ± 0.28 mm at 9 months; $P < 0.0033$), when used as a barrier membrane for GBR of horizontal alveolar ridge deficiencies.[37,43] (Fig. 36.40 A, B, and C).

Sizing and Positioning of Membranes

The selection of the membrane type is one of the most important aspects of bone regeneration protocol. The choice of a specific type of barrier membrane is directly related to the ultimate success of the regenerative process. With numerous resorbable and nonresorbable membranes available, each one has specific properties that either help or hinder the isolation properties of the procedure. These properties relate ultimately to the workability of the material and the longevity of its protection of the underlying graft particles.

The size of the membrane must be large enough to completely cover the entire graft site after the bulk of the graft has been placed in the recipient site. As the membrane is then stretched over the graft, it must be wide enough and long enough to guarantee that all of the graft particles will be isolated from any soft tissue or bacterial ingrowth. Experience indicates that the minimum membrane will be 20 × 20 mm and in almost all large graft sites, use of a 20 × 40 mm membrane will be needed. Attempting to piecemeal two or three small membranes together is not only difficult, but also introduces another variable into the concept of graft isolation over an extended time frame. The most efficient way to trim and shape a large piece of dermal matrix or connective tissue is to wet a tongue depressor in saline and then use this as a "cutting board" for the membrane (Fig. 36.41).

Positioning of membranes around teeth is very critical to reduce complications. The use of d-PTFE requires a minimum of 2 mm between the edge of the membrane and the side of an adjacent root surface. d-PTFE membranes with titanium struts should be trimmed in a manner that prevents a lateral extension of the strut

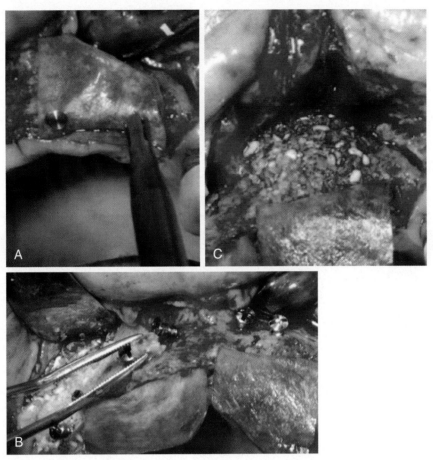

• **Fig. 36.39** Pericardium Membrane. (A) Fixation of membrane. (B) Autogenous bone being placed under tent screws. (C) Final veneer graft of allograft bone.

in the region of the coronal aspect of the graft site. Titanium struts that are positioned close to the interproximal root surfaces will often lead to membrane exposure and a compromised graft volume in the region. Newer d-PTFE membranes are designed to keep these lateral extensions located away from these critical regions. Specific elimination of all sharp edges or rough margins is critical in the elimination of membrane perforation through thin regions of the overlying flap. GBR techniques using titanium mesh require 2 mm of clearance from the root of a tooth because of similar issues.

When using resorbable membranes around teeth, the 2-mm rule is not a critical factor, and resorbable membranes can be placed directly against the roots of the adjacent teeth without causing a membrane failure. Acellular dermal matrix does not need to be separated from root surfaces, keeping in mind that this same membrane is used in routine periodontal procedures for root coverage. The only complication with placing resorbable membranes directly against natural roots is related to primary wound closure in the root proximity. Membranes must be smooth, and they should allow the overlying flap to be adapted evenly around the neck of a tooth root.

Initial Placement of Membrane

After preparation of the recipient site, the barrier membrane may be initially fixated. The initial fixation may be completed either apically or on the lingual aspect of the ridge. Fixation of the membrane before placing the particulate graft assures that

the membrane will not shift after the bulk of the graft has been placed and that it defines the apical extent of the graft itself. In situations where tacks cannot be used the membrane can be fixed both apically and palatally/lingually with sutures. It should be kept in mind that definition of this space is established by the membrane. If the thickness of the graft narrows as the graft extends toward the apex of the regenerative site, the thickness of the bony support of the implant itself will also be reduced. In that instance an apical fenestration often occurs, introducing one of a number of variables that can complicate the predictability of an implant over time (Figs. 36.42 and 36.43).

Step 7: Space Maintenance

Aside from the soft tissue exclusion and clot stability, space maintenance is key to the success of the GBR process. The creation and continued unmoving support of the graft "space" can be accomplished with membranes supported by tenting screws/pins, titanium-reinforced membranes, molded titanium mesh, block grafts, dental implants, or the bulk of particulate graft material.[44–48] Most of the new techniques in GBR protocols require specific support of this area where bone is needed. Simply filling the defect space with bone particles has been shown to greatly limit the final bone volumes, and definition of the actual shape of the ridge is really not predictable. As this protected "free zone" is defined, possibilities of successful development of new bone have been greatly improved.

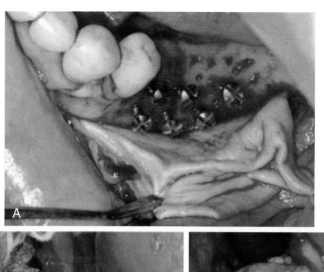

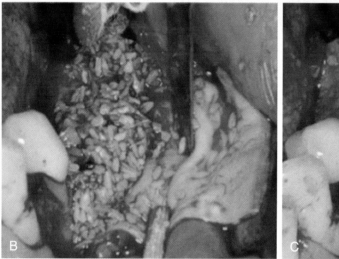

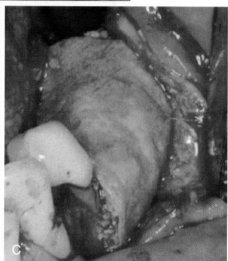

• **Fig. 36.40** Collagen Membranes. (A) Bone screws placed in defect area. (B) Collagen membrane hydrated and fixated with tacks. (C) Site grafted and membrane positioned over graft.

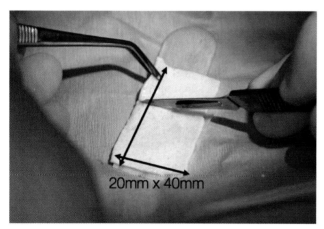

• **Fig. 36.41** Modification of membrane to encompass defect using a #15 blade.

Space Maintenance Options

1. **d-PTFE integrated with titanium struts**
2. **Titanium Mesh**
3. **Tent Screws**

Tent Screw Technique

To support the membrane support and prevent collapse of the graft in most particulate membrane techniques, tenting screws are used. The principle of tenting screws utilizes the "head" of the screw for vertical and horizontal support. This support system literally creates the surface countour of the membrane and bone graft material, which allows for the bone regeneration process to proceed in a predictable manner.

Size of Fixation Screws. Bone fixation screws on the market today are generally non-resorbable screws that either have threads from the head to the tip of the screw or a smooth neck with 3 mm of thread design at the tip of the screw.[47,48,50,51] Use of resorbable screws has been described, and this possibility gives the surgeon the option to avoid a reentry procedure to remove the fixation screws.[41] As the variety of fixation screws is explored, choices of screws with large-head diameters are preferred. The wide head is important with this technique because the primary purpose of the screw is to support the membrane during the complete bone maturation process. If the head of the screw perforates through the membrane, the vertical support will be lost and the particulate graft is subject to pressure and micromovement. When support is lost, the final volume and consistency of the matured ridge will be altered.

Use of narrow-diameter (small) screw heads that are used in block grafting procedures was found to periodically result in compromised and decreased bone growth. Most likely, the membrane will lose its vertical support after the small screw head perforates through the membrane.

Ideally, bone fixation screws with a shaft diameter of 1.5 mm are recommended instead of thicker screws because it decreases the

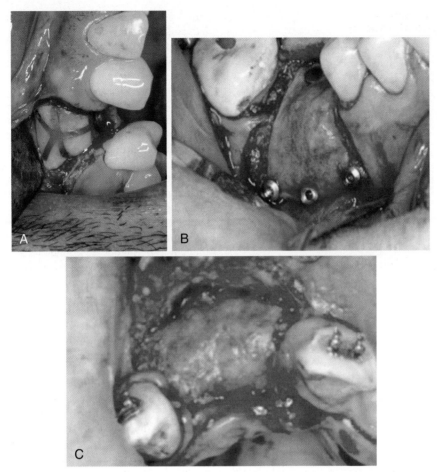

• **Fig. 36.42** Membrane Placement in Proximity to Teeth. (A) Titanium-reinforced membrane. (B) Extended collagen membrane. (C) Acellular matrix.

overall post-grafting bone volume when larger-diameter screw shafts are used. Most screws today are self-threading and are easily inserted into decortication holes. The most common length of tent screws is approximately 6 mm, however the clinician should anticipate screw lengths of 10 -12 mm for larger osseous defects (Fig. 36.44).

Tent Screw Numbers. The amount of support required to maintain the spatial dimensions of the graft site determine the number and positioning of these screws. Screws are anchored in the recipient site as needed to form a dome over the graft site that replicates the height of bone needed for ideal implant placement. Ultimately the tenting screws act as "tent poles" to support the membrane, decrease graft mobility, and relieve external pressure on the graft.[49] Placement of simple membranes over graft materials without defining space maintenance will usually lead to variable postoperative bone volumes and often deficient bony support on the facial and lingual aspect of the coronal aspects of the implant platform (i.e., membrane collapse) (Fig. 36.45).

Tent Screw Positioning. The positioning of the screws should be planned in a manner that will result in a dome shape that is formed by the "heads of the screws" matching the required contour of the final ridge form. The use of multiple screws in this technique creates very specific ridge forms that cannot be attained with unsupported membranes. Screws are placed 3 to 4 mm apart to allow solid bone formation between the screws. Basically, the number and position of tent screws is directly related to the size and the required contour of the bone graft.

Clinical situations where screws have been placed too close together periodically demonstrate weaker zones of bone formation which may result in difficult implant positioning. This can be important because lateral forces are placed on mature bone graft sites during implant osteotomy preparation and implant placement. Postoperative bony ridges using this specific technique have been found to easily tolerate the lateral forces of bone spreaders and wide body implants without any significant problems related to flaking or granular bony ridge forms. The only problem encountered with respect to screw positioning has been related to screw positions that were too close to the crest of the ridge. In these situations, an osteotomy diameter can encroach on the unfilled screw hole and the thin fragment of bone can become detached (Figs. 36.46 A, B, C, and D) (Figs. 36.47 A, B, C, and D).

Care should also be exercised in placing tent screws in approximation to adjacent teeth. The location and trajectory of adjacent tooth roots should be determined to prevent screw placement into a tooth root. Ideally, post-operative radiographs should be taken to verify ideal positioning in relation to tooth roots.

Step 8: Bone Graft Placement

The success of a bone graft is very dependent on the proper application of the basic principles of bone development. This has been emphasized as surgeons attempt to regenerate large bony defects that require development of a viable graft that can be far from the recipient bone, where all of the regenerative components originate.

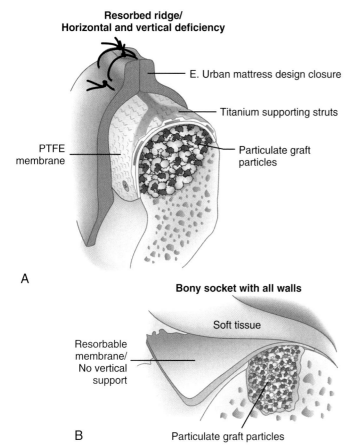

Resorbed ridge/
Horizontal and vertical deficiency

E. Urban mattress design closure

Titanium supporting struts

PTFE membrane

Particulate graft particles

A

Bony socket with all walls

Soft tissue

Resorbable membrane/ No vertical support

B   Particulate graft particles

• **Fig. 36.43** Resorbable vs. Non-resorbable membrane (A)This figure represents a nonresorbable dense polytetrafluoroethylene (d-PTFE) barrier membrane (provided by Osteogenics Biomedical) that has titanium supporting struts to prevent collapse into the regenerative space fill the underlying space with a bony matrix that can be replaced with viable bone as the regenerative process is completed. (B) This figure demonstrates the use of a resorbable barrier membrane with no supporting components. In this situation the membrane functions as a protective layer that prevents ingrowth of soft tissue into the underlying space. Membranes should generally be elevated above the ridge deficiency with screws or titanium to prevent collapse into the space or shifting of the graft particles.

This is even more important in vertical regeneration because the graft particles contact the host bone only at the base of the defect, and the other three sides of the graft are totally separated from this natural source of cells for angiogenesis and cellular ingrowth.

Prior to placement of the graft material, the recipient site should be free of soft tissue remnants, bone decorticated, and initial fixation of the membrane should be completed. When placing graft material into a bony defect, ideally a systematic layered approach should be utilized consisting of three layers which is dependent on the size and location of the graft site.

Layer # 1: Autograft (Optional)

The first layer of the guided bone regeneration graft is comprised of autogenous bone. Autogenous bone is usually indicated in any bony defect which requires horizontal bone growth of greater than 3 mm or in all cases of vertical regeneration. Autogenous bone harvesting today is typically harvested from any exposed region of cortical/cancellous bone present in the oral cavity. In the maxilla, donor sites are often available apical to most implant sites and in the tuberosity area. In the mandible, in the lateral aspect of the

ramus provides a bountiful source of cortical bone which may be harvested via numerous techniques.

Ramus Graft Harvest

Incision and Reflection. The incision for harvesting a graft in the ramus region starts at the level of the occlusal plane and proceeds down the external oblique ridge a short distance until it extends medially to the distal buccal aspect of the second molar or that same region if the area is edentulous. The incision continues anteriorly, following the crest of the ridge or following the sulcus to the distal aspect of the first molar or premolar, where a vertical release is usually prepared. The incision should always be located lateral to the retromolar pad to avoid any possible damage to the lingual nerve. The flap is reflected laterally to expose the cortical bone distal to the terminal molar and a minimal exposure of the lateral aspect of the ramus.

Ramus Harvesting Techniques. To harvest cortical bone from the ramus, numerous techniques are available;

Lateral Ramus Block: A cortical block may be harvested from the ramus and broken into smaller cortical particles. The amount of surface area obtained from smaller particles is much greater than what could be obtained by fixating an entire harvested block. The harvested block is processed by breaking the block into small pieces using double-action rongeurs. Use of large particles is not recommended, and complete destruction of the block with a bone mill has also not produced the results found with reasonable sized particles. The preparation of dense cortical bone has always presented a challenge in block grafting when an irregularly surfaced cortical graft needs to be trimmed and reshaped for adaptation in a graft site. In the case of particulate grafting, the complete piece of cortical bone must be broken into small pieces before it can be used. Control of the graft particles during this process is critical because loose particles can be easily lost or contaminated as the graft is processed. Autogenous bone harvests are challenging, and loss of critical bone particles or blocks can cause unnecessary time delays and patient discomfort if additional bone needs to be harvested to replace a contaminated block.

The particulate grafting technique described in this chapter requires that a piece of a cortical block be completely broken up into small particles that are then packed into irregular bony defects. These small particles tend to "shoot out" of the rongeurs if they are not carefully contained. The best way to eliminate the loss of these cortical particles is to fill a clear, shallow glass beaker or bowl with saline. The block is then submerged in the saline, and double-action rongeurs are used to break it up into the particle size needed for the procedure. The saline slows escaping particles in the same manner that water slows the movement of a bullet that is fired into water. The bone is typically broken up into 1 × 2 mm particles for placement in the graft site. (Figs. 36.48).

Scraping Technique: Another option of obtaining autogenous bone is removing cortical bone chips from the external oblique ridge. A double action rongeur may be used to remove small fragments from the exposed bone. The scrapings may be placed into a sterile surgical bowl with sterile saline. Another option of obtaining cortical chips is with the use of specific manufactured "scrapers", which not only harvest the bone, but also collect it within the scraper device. And lastly, piezosurgery units may be used with dedicated scraper tips. (Fig. 36.49).

Trephine Technique: The use of trephine burs (i.e. cylindrical end-cutting burs) have been advocated to harvest bone from the ramus area. These end-cutting burs that are available in various diameters, with the 6–8 mm trephine being the most popular for

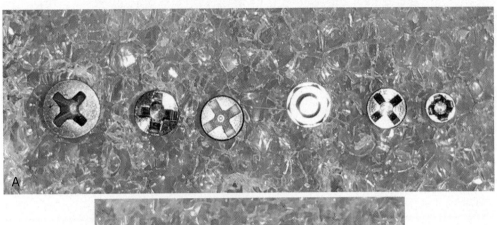

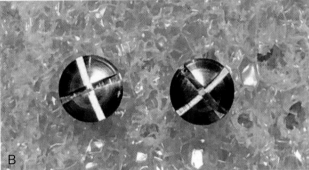

• **Fig. 36.44** Tent Screw Size (A) Older generation tent screws of various diameters and head size, (B) Newer tent screws with larger, convex head which allow for more ideal space maintenance.

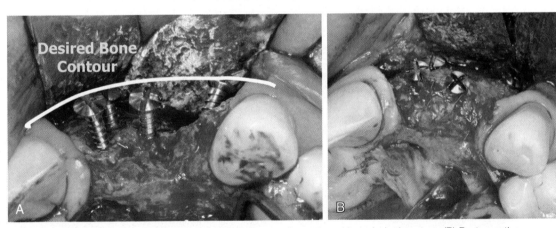

• **Fig. 36.45** (A). Tent screws used to stabilize membrane to achieve desired contour. (B) Postoperative results of bone growth to ideal contours.

harvesting bone from the ramus. One half of the trephine bur is placed over the external oblique bony ridge, while the other half is lateral to the bone and above the reflected masseter muscle, which is elevated off the anterior lateral aspect of the ramus. The trephine bur is used with an angled surgical drill at 2,000 rpm with copious saline irrigation, to a depth of approximately 5–8 mm, making sure the cuts are above and lateral to the position of the inferior alveolar nerve (IAN), artery and vein. The IAN position should be identified via a CBCT exam survey.

Ramus Recipient Site Closure. After removing the harvested donor bone the donor site is filled with a double layer of collagen tape before closing the wound with a combination of interrupted and mattress sutures. This closure is monitored as each suture is tied to confirm that there is no flap tension. The use of Vicryl or Teflon (Cytoplast) sutures is recommended to allow the implant clinician the opportunity to remove the sutures when he or she feels the wound

has adequately healed. Due to the nature of soft tissue in the ramus region, overlapping tissue margins can contribute not only to postoperative opening of wounds, but also to a lengthy recovery process.

Additional Harvest Sites. Maxillary Tuberosity Donor Site: The maxillary tuberosity offers a variable amount of trabecular bone, which is dependent on the extent of maxillary bone atrophy and maxillary sinus pneumatization. The cancellous nature of the bone allows it to be molded into the extraction socket. The tuberosity should be evaluated with a CBCT survey to determine the maxillary sinus location and the amount of host bone present.

Tori: The use of cortical bone harvested from lingual tori has been shown to produce excellent results. This is dense cortical bone, and large amounts of bone can be harvested from the typical lingual donor site. The use of Piezosurgery techniques allows the tori to be separated from the mandible without the threat of injury to underlying anatomic regions. There has been no noted difference

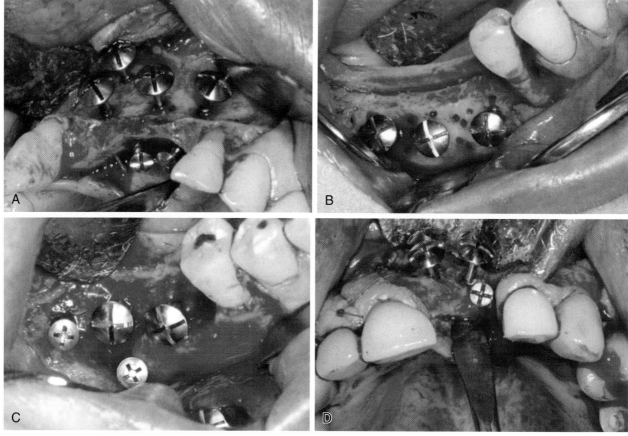

• **Fig. 36.46** (A to D) Screw placement literally determines the final contours of the augmented graft site. The screw head should never be placed higher than the level of the adjacent interproximal bone. When large head screws are used on the buccal aspect, the uppermost edge should be angled slightly to prevent its sharp edge from perforating the membrane. The best location for the largest diameter screw heads is lower down in the graft site where lateral support is needed.

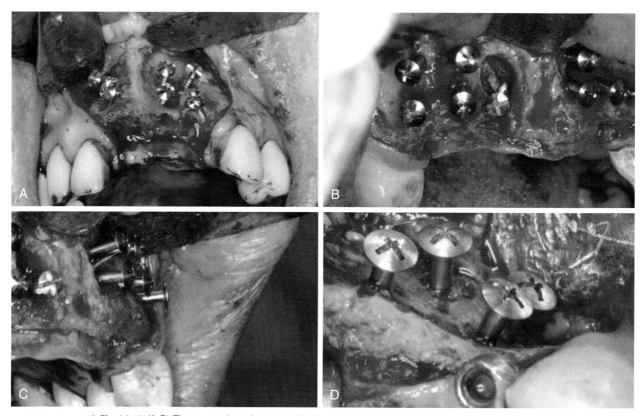

• **Fig. 36.47** (A-D) The screws have been used in these varied surfaced defects to define a smooth final ridge contour that will allow implant placements in proper locations specified by the restorative wax-up.

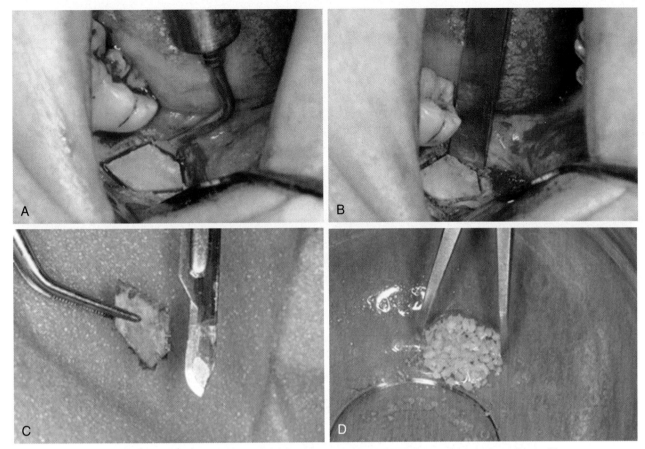

• **Fig. 36.48** Ramus Autograft Harvest With Piezosurgery Unit. (A) Piezo cuts made in ramus bone. (B) Block removed. (C) Harvested block. (D) Block bone made into particulate chips.

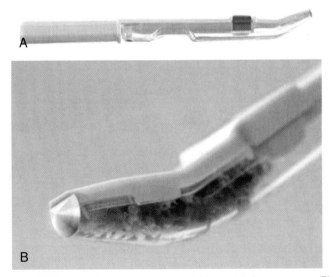

• **Fig. 36.49** Alternative Bone Scraper. (A) Disposable bone scraper. (B) Harvested bone inside scraper.

in the final graft quality when tori were used as the donor source in regeneration cases (Fig. 36.50).

Placement of Layer # 1. The small autograft chips or small particulate pieces are placed directly on the host bone surrounding the bone screws. Because of the extensive nature of grafts requiring autogenous bone, at least 50% of the graft volume should be made up of this autogenous bone, with allograft compromising the second layer. Graft particles are transferred from the bowl to the graft site with cotton forceps or a Molt curette. A bone or amalgam plugger with a small end can be used to manipulate the particles between the various screws. This process fills most of the defect and voids, regardless of the topography of the recipient site. It should be kept in mind that the volume of this graft is clearly defined by the levels of the heads of the bone screws. The screws have been positioned in a manner that defines the outermost borders of the desired bony ridge, corresponding to the requirements of the restorative plan and the needed sites for implant placement (Fig. 36.51).

Particulate Graft Material Options. There are many optional techniques and materials for use in regenerative graft procedures. Successful application of these techniques requires that the clinician have a comprehensive understanding of the various types of bone grafts and bone substitutes available, and the inherent advantages and disadvantages of each material. The ideal characteristics of a bone substitute include biocompatibility, low incidence of infection and immunogenicity, predictable maintenance of space over time, and the ability to be replaced entirely with new, viable bone growth. To comprehend the concept of bone regeneration and to select the ideal bone graft material, the implant clinician should have a strong understanding of bone biology.

Allograft Bone. Allogenic bone is harvested from an individual of the same species and transplanted to a genetically different individual. Allografts are considered to be one of the best sources for supplementation of an autograft or as an alternative to an autograft. Allografts are available in many different preparations, with the most common being FDBA and demineralized FDBA (DFDBA). Although their biological properties vary, they

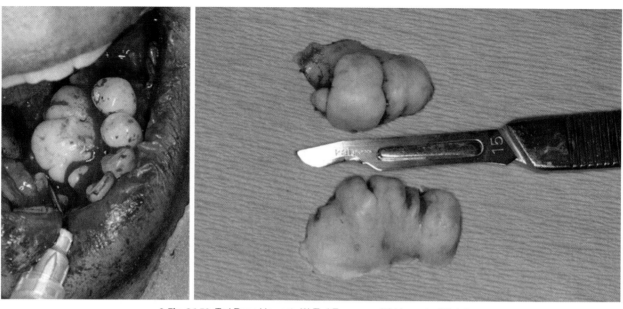

• **Fig. 36.50** Tori Bone Harvest: (A) Tori Exposure (B) Harvested Tori.

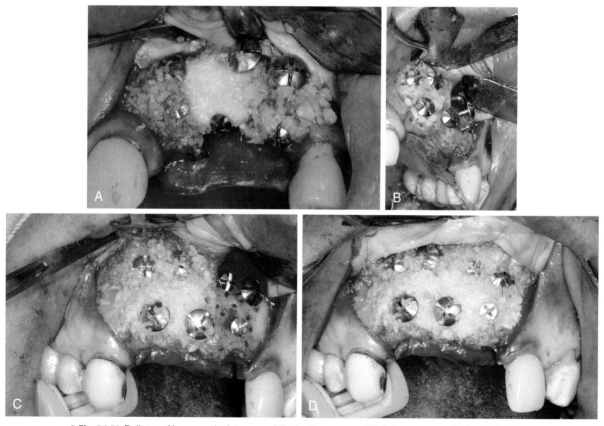

• **Fig. 36.51** Delivery of bone particulate around the tenting screws: (A) Autogenous cortical particles have been placed around the screws on each side of the defect. The allograft application has been started in the center region and it will then be placed over the autogenous particles. (B) Autogenous bone particles have been placed around the fixation screws and the screw lengths are visible in the adjacent region where graft has not been positioned yet. (C) The allograft is placed over the autogenous bone on the right side before the layers are started on the opposite side. (D). The particulate has been placed over the entire recipient site and the membrane is ready to be drawn over the entire region.

generally exhibit osteoconductive qualities with reduced osteoinductive properties found in DFDBA. FDBA and DFDBA offer the advantage of decreased patient morbidity secondary to the elimination of the need for a second surgical site.

Allografts undergo extensive and rigorous processing procedures. First, allografts are processed by freeze-drying the graft at approximately –15°C to –20°C, allowing for easier handling and a decreased antigenicity. The main drawbacks of freeze-dried bone include the potential risk for cross-infection and the possibility of immunologic reactions because of its protein content. The possibility of disease transmission cannot be completely eliminated; however, there are no documented cases of disease transmission related to the use of allografts in dentistry after completion of more than 1 million cases in a 25-year period.[57] In addition, allografts have been related to variations in sample quality related to age and the health variations of the donor. These variations in the regenerative properties of a specific sample indicate the possible importance of using a sample from a single donor rather than a donor pool. Allografts are primarily osteoconductive materials, with some reduced osteoinductive properties in demineralized bone matrix preparations.

Types of Allografts. The most common allografts used in implant dentistry have varying characteristics. For example:

- DFDBA is osteoconductive and osteoinductive. The material consists of highly processed bone with at least 40% of the mineral content of the bone matrix being removed by 0.5 to 0.6 M hydrochloric acid until the calcium content is reduced to less than 2%.[58] This allows for increased availability of matrix-associated BMPs or growth factors that allow the graft to become osteoinductive.

- FDBA is an allogenic bone that does not undergo the demineralization process. Also referred to as "mineralized" because the mineral content has not been reduced, FDBA has the same BMP content in its organic matrix. However, it does not have the same osteoinductive capability as DFDBA. FDBA has been shown to be a better scaffold for osteoconduction than DFDBA, which allows for superior space maintenance.[59] Eventually osteoclasts break down the mineral content of FDBA until demineralization occurs, inducing new bone formation and a prolonged protein release.

Particle Form and Size. The allograft particle form and size contribute to the predictability of bone regeneration.

- **Ideal particle form:** Allografts are available in three particle forms: cortical, cancellous, and cortico-cancellous. Cortical allografts are associated with an increased density and greater space maintenance properties, subsequently allowing a slower resorption rate. Cancellous chips are advantageous because they allow for osteoconductive scaffolding and deposition of osteoblasts while also allowing a faster resorption rate. The cortico-cancellous mixture allows for the benefits of both cancellous and cortical bone.

- **Ideal particle size:** The particle size of the allograft material is very important in the bone regeneration process, because a particle size that is too small (less than 125 μm) leads to fast resorption with inconsistent bone formation. A larger particle size (greater than 1000 μm) restricts resorption and may be sequestered or result in delayed healing. Studies have shown an ideal particle size for predictable bone regeneration to be approximately 250 to 1000 μm.[60]

Xenografts. Xenografts are bone grafts originating from a different species. Most commonly, xenografts are derived from bovine (cattle) origins, with less common sources including equine (horses) and porcine (pigs). The most common xenografts are natural hydroxyapatite (HA) derived from animal bone and anorganic bone matrix produced from bovine sources. Xenogenic bone grafts exhibit excellent osteoconductive properties and act as a scaffold for newly deposited bone. Although xenografts are available in greater supply than allograft materials, they have been shown to exhibit elevated inflammatory responses, along with a slow and inconsistent resorption process. Consideration must also be given to the risk for cross-contamination with bovine spongiform encephalopathy or porcine endogenous retroviruses. Unfortunately it has been shown to be difficult to adequately screen xenografts for the possibility of a viral presence[61] (Fig. 36.52).

Alloplasts. Because of the remote possibility of disease transmission from allografts and xenografts, some in the literature have advocated alternative bone substitute options. Alloplasts, which are synthetic, are a biocompatible option for the implant clinician. Alloplasts have the advantage of relatively no immunogenic responses, and there is no risk for disease transmission. These materials have been shown to be osteoconductive, with an interconnecting pore system that serves as a scaffold for the migration of bone-forming cells.[62] Unfortunately many alloplastic grafts do not allow the graft material to be replaced with vital bone cells, which results in nonvital bone at the implant interface.

Types of Alloplasts. A wide range of synthetic materials for allografts have been developed, such as synthetic HA, β-tricalcium phosphate, calcium-phosphate cements, and glass ceramics.

- HA is the basic component of inorganic bone and exhibits a similar chemical composition to natural bone. HA is most commonly processed from natural reef coral skeletons or homogenized calcium-phosphate powder. It is not only biocompatible and osteoconductive, but also has excellent space-maintaining qualities. However, synthetic HA has shown unpredictable and slow degradation after approximately 1 to 2 years.[63]

- Tricalcium phosphate has a calcium-to-phosphate ratio of 1.5, which is much lower than HA and results in less compressive strength. Calcium phosphates resorb 10 to 20 times faster than HA, and their macroscopic mechanical properties are inadequate for load-bearing surfaces because of their inherent brittleness. Because of the fast biodegradation rate, this bone can be unpredictable and is not consistent with adequate bone deposition.

- Carbonate apatite with collagen has been shown to resemble bone more than any other calcium phosphate available. The inorganic content of bone contains approximately 7% carbonate by weight.[64] Studies have shown that carbonate apatite exhibits a more controlled resorptive pattern, as well as excellent osteoconductivity and biocompatibility.[65] When carbonate apatite is combined with collagen, the biological stability and strength are increased, which allows the scaffolds to act as a delivery vehicle for growth factors and living cells for bone formation.[66] Scanning electron microscopy studies have shown that the highly porous and interconnected structure ensures a biological environment that is conducive to cell attachment, proliferation, angiogenesis, and tissue growth.[67]

- Bioactive glasses are ceramic substitutes that are reinforced by oxides—sodium oxide, calcium oxide, phosphorus pentoxide, and silicon dioxide—and exhibit questionable mechanical strength. They are absorbable and have no risk for disease transmission or immune responses. The bioactive ceramics exhibit improved mechanical properties relative to bioactive glass, but they are still brittle enough to fracture when subjected to cyclic loading. To improve their resistance to fracture, methods of incorporating stainless-steel and zirconia fibers have been performed. Studies have shown questionable efficacy of bioactive glasses with respect to osteoconduction qualities and the ability to bond to tissues (bioactivity).[68]

Layer # 2 Summary. The second layer of the graft is ideally made up of particulate allograft that is placed over the top of the autograft (i.e. or 100% allograft for smaller defects < 3 mm). The allograft should veneer over the screw heads, however care should be exercise to not "overfill" the graft site. The recommended allograft bone type is either 70% mineralized / 30% demineralized or a cortical/cancellous mixture of mineralized bone. It is highly recommended that the ridge be overdeveloped rather than underdeveloped. Excessive overfilling of the graft site may lead to difficult tissue closure and increases the possibility of incision line opening.

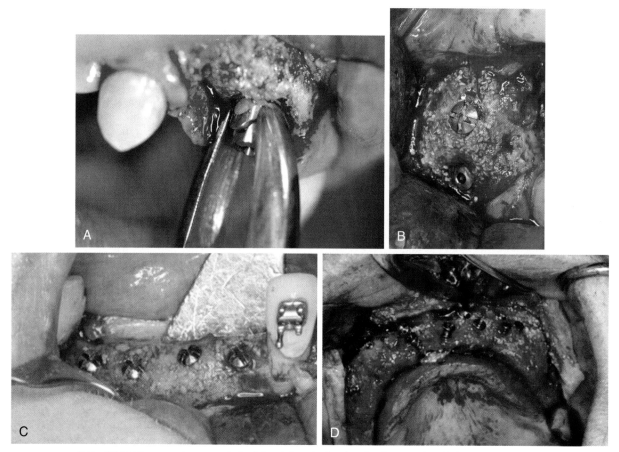

• **Fig. 36.52** There can be very substantial variations in the density of matured graft sites, depending on what type of graft was used initially. The delayed turn-over of bovine particulate can greatly affect the density when an implant is placed before the complete substitution cycle has been completed. (A) PepGen15. (B) OsteoGraf 300/FDBA. (C) 90% autogenous/FDBA. (D) Mix of autogenous/bovine/FDBA.

Layer # 3: Final Implant Placement

After the graft material (Layers # 1 and # 2) is ideally positioned, the membrane (previously fixated apically or lingually) is stretched over the graft site. The membrane should be of sufficient size to totally encompass the entire graft. The goal of the membrane fixation is to not allow any movement, which could negatively affect the wound healing. In most cases, the final fixation is on the palatal aspect of the ridge with two tacks. Additional fixation can be used as needed in large graft sites to limit membrane movement.

Bone Growth Factors

Bone growth factors can be a significant part of the bone-grafting process as they may enhance the formation and mineralization of bone. In addition, bone growth factors may induce undifferentiated mesenchymal cells to differentiate into bone cells that trigger a cascade of intracellular reactions for the release of additional bone growth and cell-enhancing factors. These growth factors actually bind to specific receptors on the surface of target cells directing a more timely healing process. More than 50 known growth factors have been identified and categorized according to their specific contributions to the functions in bone healing. The two most common bone growth factor techniques utilize blood concentrates and recombinant human Bone Morphogenetic Protein-2.

Blood Concentrates. Most blood concentrates used in implant dentistry today are direct derivatives of platelets. The platelet, also called a thrombocyte, are blood cells that are primarily involved in the blood clotting process. A unique secondary function of a platelet is to release a wide range of growth factors that enhance collagen production, cell mitosis, blood vessel growth, cell recruitment, and cell differentiation.[69]

The two most utilized and studied platelet concentrates in implant dentistry today are platelet-rich plasma (PRP) and platelet-rich fibrin (PRF). The first-generation blood concentrate, platelet-rich plasma, was first introduced by Marx in 1998. His studies showed bone maturity to be twice as effective with the use of PRP in grafted sites, and the addition of PRP increased bone density up to 30% in healed sites.[70]

A second-generation blood substitute, platelet-rich fibrin, was first described by Choukroun in 2001. This concentrate has been shown to exhibit a much simpler processing protocol in comparison to PRP. PRF is very effective in the release of important growth factors present in platelets, such as platelet-derived growth factor (PDGF), transforming growth factor beta (TGF-ß), insulin-like growth factor (IGF), fibroblast growth factor (FGF), and epithelial growth factor (EGF). [71] (Box 36.9) Multiple clinical studies have shown increased soft tissue healing, enhanced healing of grafted bone, promotion of angiogenesis, and faster wound healing.[72–74]

The internal organization make-up of platelet rich fibrin is rather unique as it contains three adhesive molecules (fibrin, fibronectin, and vitronectin) that result in a highly elastic, matricial mesh architecture. This complex three-dimensional structure allows for a longer release of growth factors. As the platelets degranulate, a sustained release of growth factors may range from a time period of one to four weeks.[75]

1. **Platelet-derived growth factor (PDGF)**
   - Stimulates fibroblast mitogenesis and collagen synthesis
2. **Transforming growth factor beta (TGF-ß)**
   - Enhances wound healing via endothelial angiogenesis
3. **Insulin-like growth factors (IGF)**
   - Enhances rate and quality of wound healing via bone matrix formation and cell replication
4. **Epithelial growth factor (EGF)**
   - Increases angiogenesis and epithelial mitogenesis
5. **Fibroblast growth factor (FGF)**
   - Increases angiogenesis, epithelialization, and fibroblasts
6. **Vascular Endothelial Growth Factor (VEGF)**
   - Increases endothelial growth factor and angiogenesis

PRF is an autologous fibrin matrix that incorporates platelets, leukocytes, cytokines, and circulating stem cells that are gradually released to accelerate physiologic healing. It is easily obtained and does not require any biochemical blood handling.[52] After drawing blood and placing in a centrifuge for 12 minutes, the coagulation cascade will be triggered. The end result is a fibrin clot in the middle layer, situated between the acellular platelet-poor plasma and the red blood cells. When this fibrin clot (PRF) is used as a membrane, it will help isolate and protect the wound while serving as a matrix to accelerate healing. When the PRF is mixed with the graft material (allograft), the fibrin clot acts as a biological connector between all of the elements of the graft, while also acting as a matrix that initiates angiogenesis, stem cell accumulation, and migration of osteoprogenitor cells to the graft. Thus the synergistic effects of the fibrin matrix and growth factors allow for the enhanced healing of the hard and soft tissues. Studies have shown that PRF with freeze-dried bone allograft (FDBA) heals faster than FDBA alone.[53]

The second-generation blood concentrate platelet rich fibrin (PRF) has been shown to be advantageous in comparison to platelet rich plasma (PRP):

- Is naturally polymerized and requires no chemical use
- Requires a conventional, single spin centrifuge
- Has a slower release of growth factors
- Is more efficient with cell migration and proliferation
- More advantageous fibrin network that stores cytokines and growth factors
- Better healing properties
- Less disposables required resulting in less expense

Platelet Rich Fibrin Uses. With bone augmentation procedures, PRF may be used as either a membrane or added to the particulate bone grafting material. Studies have shown that PRF is advantageous in healing during regenerative procedures either as a membrane or when added to particulate bone.[76] Because the PRF membrane resorbs rather fast (~ 7 days), it is not the most ideal membrane to be used to prevent soft tissue invasion. Therefore, usually the PRF membrane is placed over the primary membrane (e.g. collagen) to aid in hard and soft tissue healing (Figs. 36.53).

Recombinant human bone morphogenetic protein-2. Recombinant human bone morphogenetic proteins (rhBMPs) are a group of sequentially arranged amino acids and polypeptides that are osteoinductive proteins, acting to initiate, stimulate, and amplify bone morphogenesis. BMPs stimulate mesenchymal stem cells to induce bone formation via differentiation to osteoblasts, which form and mineralize new bone. BMP-2 has been purified,

sequenced, and cloned, and is marketed as rhBMP-2 (recombinant human bone morphogenetic protein-2; Infuse; Medtronic, Inc., Minneapolis, Minn.). Infuse bone graft consists of two components: a 1.5 mg/mL concentration of rhBMP-2 and an absorbable collagen sponge. Studies have shown rhBMP-2 with titanium mesh to be an effective treatment for augmentation of the deficient bony ridge before implant placement.[54] The new bone formed by rhBMP-2 has been shown to be similar to native bone and can withstand the stresses of implant placement and prosthetic function.[55]

Step 9: Closure

The final closure of the bone graft site is one of the most important steps of the grafting process. Ideally, a tension-free flap adaptation is the key to predictable results. If a poor suturing technique is used, incision line opening may result, which significantly increases the morbidity of the procedure. Therefore, meticulous principles should be adhered to with respect to a tension-free flap, ideal suture technique, and the close post-operative evaluation of the surgical site.

The type of suture selected should include a high tensile strength material. The most common suture materials used today include vicryl (absorbable) or PTFE (nonmabsorbable). The primary principle of wound closure in GBR cases is attaining a completely "tension-free" closure over the submerged graft. Specific attention must be directed to proper approximation of the margins of the flap to confirm there is no overlapping of the tissue flaps.

Usually the combination of horizontal mattress and interrupted sutures are used to close these graft sites. One of the primary advantages of using the horizontal mattress sutures is the ability to "evert" the tissue margins. By everting the margins of the flap outward, the connective tissue layers will be approximated against each other. A flap closure that "overlaps" two flaps is actually placing the connective tissue layer of the first flap over the epithelial layer of the adjacent flap. This type of poor approximation leads to at best a weak suture line and most often an open margin postoperatively. Additional interrupted sutures may be used to approximate all edges of the wound. The vertical incisions may be closed with 5-0 Chromic, as they may greatly reduce the post-op formation of tissue scars.

(Fig. 36. 54). (Fig. 36.55 A, B, and C) (Fig. 36. 56).

Postoperative Treatment

Provisional Restoration

The successful maturation of a bone graft site requires that the area be completely protected from micromovement of the isolating membrane and the underlying graft material. A successful graft is totally dependent on blood clot adhesion, capillary ingrowth, and the introduction of associated growth factors for predictable healing. It has been estimated that micromovement of 25 μm over a graft site can decrease the final graft volume as much as 40%. Therefore, disruption of any kind will consistently yield compromised results in mature graft development, if not full graft failure.

The most common source of daily pressure on a site occurs when the patient's transitional appliance has contact with the surface of the graft site. If possible, a fixed bonded transitional bridge should be placed over the graft site because it totally prevents contact with the underlying graft site. If this is not possible and the patient insists on a temporary prosthesis, plans for a carefully constructed removable partial denture should be formulated. A transitional prosthesis (flipper or removable partial

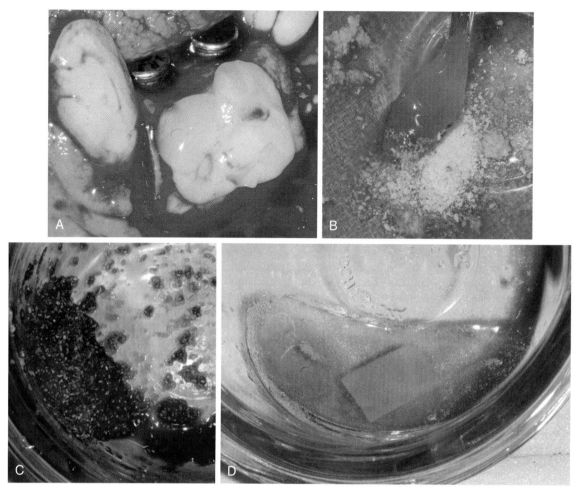

• **Fig. 36.53** (A) PRF used as a secondary membrane over the primary membrane, (B) PRF may be added to the graft material, (C) Sticky Bone, (D) Platelet Poor Plasma may be used to hydrate the primary (collagen) membrane

denture) must be modified to eliminate any significant contact with the graft site. If a removable prosthesis is absolutely necessary, all buccal flanges should be removed, and if possible, the acrylic should be altered to create regions of support on the lingual surfaces of the adjacent teeth. Occlusal rests should be used, or in cases where this is not possible, there must be good adaptation of the prosthesis to direct the forces to alternative stress-bearing areas (i.e., tissue areas away from the graft site that take the pressure off the graft site).

Essix appliances allow temporary replacement of teeth in narrow span regions, allowing long-term prostheses to be fabricated after the initial healing process has been completed. However, the Essix appliance does have disadvantages related to esthetics, fracture, wear issues, and discoloration. The Snap-On Smile appliance (Den-Mat Holdings, LLC) has been used successfully over longer-span edentulous regions with more pleasant esthetics that and increases patient acceptance (Figs. 36.57) (Fig. 36. 58) (Fig. 36.59).

Development of Ideal Bone Density in Regeneration Sites

The sole purpose of ridge augmentation and bone grafting is to develop a dense, stable volume of bony support for implants of appropriate sizes and numbers that are placed in the locations specified by the restorative plan. The quality and density of the

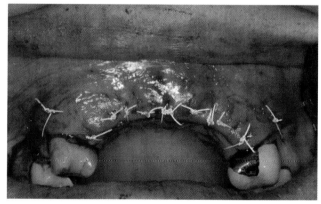

• **Fig. 36.54** Bone Graft Suturing. Polytetrafluoroethylene (PTFE) sutures over ridge with minimal tension from the vertical release incisions.

final graft development are important because a weak and granular implant osteotomy site is more susceptible to crumbling during implant insertion. These granular ridges can also resorb when the implant is loaded and stress is placed on the coronal aspect of the implant-bone interface. As clinicians plan augmentation procedures, they must understand the limitations of the materials that they are using and the techniques that are going to be used.

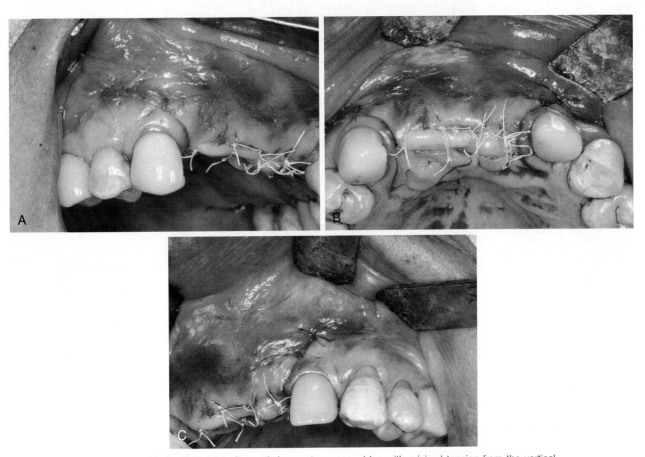

• **Fig. 36.55** (A, B, C) Polytetrafluoroethylene sutures over ridge with minimal tension from the vertical release incisions.

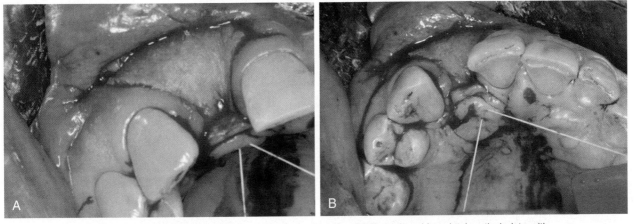

• **Fig. 36.56** Alternative Lingual Suture Membrane Fixation. (A) Tack placed in palatal cortical plate with suture started through the palatal flap, passing below the flap and back through the membrane. (B) The suture is then passed back from beneath the flap and out again.

Misch[56] created a system of bone densities for implants, ranging from D1 (hardest) to D4 (softest/most porous). These divisions encompass the acceptable ranges for the placement and rigid fixation of implants. Successful regeneration procedures develop a final osteotomy site that provides adequate bone volume in a dense, firm, manageable form that has a large number of vital bone cells that will easily integrate with the titanium implant body.

Success in bone grafting requires a thorough knowledge of the variety of grafting materials that are available and their capacity to be readily replaced with vital bone on a timely basis. The ultimate goal is a clear understanding of the concepts of osteoinduction and osteoconduction, which is critical for predictable grafting success. It is easy in the incorporation of regeneration into a practice routine to simply open a bottle of bone for use in a surgical procedure, instead of preparing to open a second site for a cortical bone harvest. Unfortunately, the characteristics of different types of bone graft vary greatly and in the long term this can significantly affect the volume and quality of the regenerated bone. It is vitally important that the clinician have a strong understanding

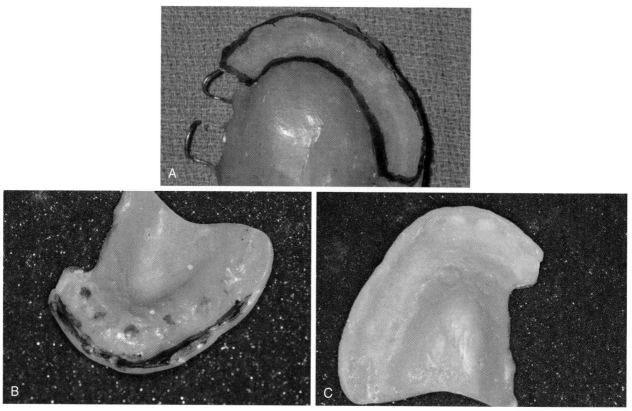

• **Fig. 36.57** Interim Prosthesis Modification. (A and B) The buccal flange and the grafted area should be modified to remove any possible pressure areas. (C) Post adjusted prosthesis showing minimal flange and ridge area relieved.

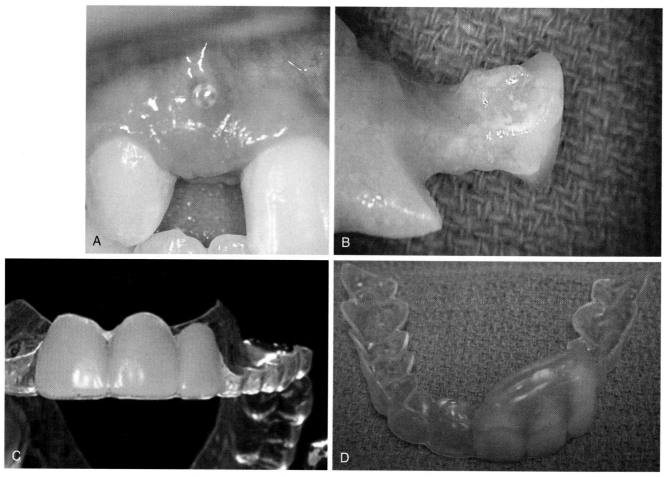

• **Fig. 36.58** Interim Prosthesis-Related Pressure. (A) Fixation screw exposed with associated bone loss (B) caused by interim prostheses with protrusion placing pressure on graft. (C) Essix appliances allow temporary replacement of teeth in narrow span regions. However, the Essix appliances do have disadvantages in respect to limited esthetics, fractures, and discoloration. If adjusted properly, it will not allow any pressure on the graft site. (D) Essix appliance with added acrylic that encompasses the soft tissue defect and potentially may place undue pressure on the grafted area.

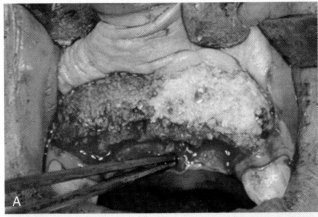

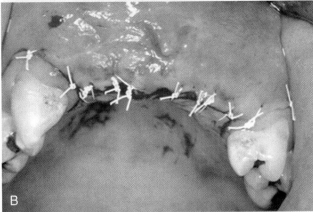

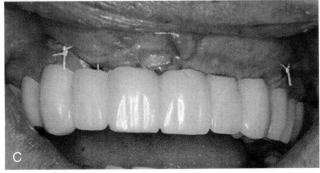

• **Fig. 36.59** Alternative Interim Prosthesis. (A) Large grafting site. (B) Final closure of ridge augmentation. (C) Placement of Snap-On Smile over the closed graft site to protect augmentation site during the healing process.

• BOX **36.10** **GBR Bone-Grafting Options**

1. **Autogenous Grafts:** a graft removed from one anatomic location and placed in another location in the same individual
   Donor sites: tuberosity, ramus, symphysis, iliac crest, etc. (coagulum, particulate, block grafts)
   Indications: used as the 1st layer in GBR procedures which require > 3 mm of bone growth (horizontal) or vertical bone growth
2. **Allograft:** grafts taken from the same species—human cadaver
   a. **Osteoinductive Allografts:** grafting materials that provide a biological stimulus (proteins and growth factors) that induce the progression of mesenchymal stem cells and other osteoprogenitor lineage. (Example: Demineralized Freeze Dried Bone Allograft {DFDBA})
   b. **Osteoconductive Allografts:** relatively inert filling materials that integrate with new forming bone. Osteoconduction is the process that permits osteogenesis when cells already committed to bone formation are also present in a closed environment.
   (Example: Mineralized Freeze-Dried Bone Allograft {FDBA})
   Indications: used as 2nd layer for grafts > 3 mm or as sole grafting material for grafts < 3 mm
      Options: 1. 70% FDBA / 30 DFDBA
            2. 100% FDBA (Cortico-Cancellous)
3. **Xenograft:** osteoconductive graft from another species
   (Examples: Bovine {Bio-Oss, Bio-Oss porcine, and equine)
   Indications: rarely used in GBR protocols
4. **Alloplast:** osteoconductive—a chemically or naturally derived nonanimal material
   (Examples: Hydroxyapatite, Bioglass, calcium sulfate)
   Indications: rarely used in GBR protocols
5. **Biologics:** cell-based therapies, growth factors, and osteoconductive matrices, that clinically enhance bone regeneration
   (Example: Emdogain, recombinant human bone morphogenetic protein-2, platelet-rich plasma, platelet-rich fibrin)
   Indications: elective use, however highly recommended in larger graft cases

and foundation of the use and indications of the available bone grafting materials (Box 36.10).

Graft Maturation Healing Times

As time frames for graft maturation are considered, it must be kept in mind that this whole approach to grafting is a "substitution" process where the grafted bone is eventually going to be replaced with newly developed natural bone. For adequate healing the graft must be given sufficient time to resorb and for new bone to be regenerated in its place. This process varies considerably as different graft types are considered. A common issue with clinicians early in their learning curve is trying to use a "fixed" healing time period for all particulate grafts.

Ideally many factors must be taken into consideration when determining the healing time. One of the most important

factors is the number of remaining walls of bone that surround the recipient site. In general the larger the number of walls surrounding the graft, the shorter the healing time. The second factor is the use of autogenous bone within the graft. The more autogenous bone used, the shorter is the healing time. The quantity of allograft is a significant factor because the greater the amount of allograft, the longer the required healing period. This is directly tied to the time needed for adequate angiogenesis. The type of bone used is also significant with the healing time: autogenous (fast), allograft (moderate), xenograft (slow), and alloplast (slow to unpredictable bone turnover). Lastly, systemic diseases such as diabetes, hyperparathyroidism, thyrotoxicosis, osteomalacia, osteoporosis, and Paget's disease may all affect the healing response. (Box 36.11)

In summary, it is always best to err on the side of safety and allow for more bone healing time. For most cases involving graft sites composed entirely of allograft, 6 to 8 months is recommended when graft volumes are less than 4 mm in dimension. In similar sites with larger graft volumes (>4 mm), 6 to 10 months is highly recommended. Premature reentry into the graft may initiate many complications. In cases of poor or delayed healing, the quality of bone will be very weak and granular, similar to D5 bone. This type of bone is very soft and prone to overpreparation, ultimately resulting in a poor bone-implant contact. If this situation is encountered, the surgical implant placement protocol should be altered with underpreparation of the osteotomy, osseodensification techniques and/or the use of osteotomes. The concepts of ridge remodeling after loading should be seriously considered, and placement of additional layers of xenograft with membrane coverage should be used. Overall, patience in graft maturation is critically important.

Bone-Grafting Complications

Incisive Canal Involvement in Regeneration Sites

Implant restorations in the anterior maxillary region present one of the most difficult challenges in dentistry today. The combination of esthetic demands, biomechanical/functional issues, and phonetic challenges require implant placement in ideal positions. The incisive foramen is the exit point of the nasopalatine canal, where the terminal branch of the descending palatine artery and nasopalatine nerve pass into the oral cavity. The proximity of the incisive foramen and the path of the canal must be evaluated in all maxillary incisor implant treatment plans because there can be significant variations in the size, position, and angulation of the nasopalatine canal and the exiting foramen. As the bone around the maxillary central incisors resorbs, the zone of available bony support moves palatally, frequently encroaching on the incisive foramen.

Defining the dimensions and pathway of the nasopalatine canal with CBCT imaging allows the surgeon to decide whether implants can be placed within the required restorative space or whether augmentation will be needed for ideal placement. This is particularly important in cases involving immediate implants because the lingual angulation of the immediate implant osteotomy could potentially fenestrate into the incisive canal. A fenestration in the side of an osteotomy allows neural/fibrous tissue invasion into the osteotomy, retarding bone growth and rigid fixation of the implant.

Axial CBCT images provide the most accurate view of the size, shape, and location of the canal in respect to the possible implant sites. Use of CBCT cross sections and three-dimensional images can also help determine the positions and dimensions of this important anatomic variant. The clinician must be aware of a possible widening of the canal above the level of the foramen, creating a fenestration between the canal and the osteotomy in the more apical regions of the osteotomy. As the cross sections of the CBCT are reviewed, the possible presence of a nasopalatine cyst should be ruled out, and edentulous arches should be reviewed for an enlarged foraminal dimension, as is often noted. The positions of implants in central incisor regions where the foramen is involved should be adjusted distally where an FP-1 restoration does not require a specific placement. This slight adjustment distally prevents fenestration on the mesiopalatal line angle, where this deficiency most likely will occur.

Severe bone resorption on the facial aspect of the maxilla reduces the ridge thickness to surprising extents, often leaving only a thin ridge that is positioned well to the palatal aspect of the required location for a central incisor implant. It should be kept in mind that a line between the cingula of the two cuspids passes directly over the incisal foramen. Subsequently, if an implant is placed this far palatally, the emergence profile will originate at a significantly proclined angle and the complete restoration will be palatally positioned. Cases such as this require that the seriously deficient ridge be regenerated before implant placement.

Regions that are determined to be deficient will require facial augmentation using techniques that are capable of generating sufficient lateral/vertical bone volume for proper implant placement and restorative success. Cases where the implant can be moved slightly in a distal direction can sometimes prevent the need for major augmentation. Another option in a FP-3, RP-4, or RP-5 case is the obliteration and grafting of the nasopalatine canal, which can aid in providing significant bone volume for implant placement into vital bone and potentially creating a better ridge consistency on maturation. (Fig. 36.60)

Releasing the Tissue Flap From Underlying Tenting Screws

Flap reflection is a basic procedure that is common in all surgical applications. Correct tissue manipulation allows the flap to be released and reflected without tearing or damaging the underlying periosteal layer. The use of bone fixation screws in particulate grafting techniques creates a complicated situation for flap reflection because the fibrous tissue layer of the periosteum surrounds the head of the screw and any exposed portion of the neck of the screw. As the flap is reflected away from a screw insertion site, this fibrous layer must be released before the flap can continue to be drawn away from the region.

This binding attachment cannot be easily drawn over the screw heads, and there is a potential to create perforations or tears in the flap as it is released. Flap reflection in this situation starts with a simple full-thickness crestal incision that is prepared over the graft site. Flap release is initiated with a sharp curette that is used to release the flap and to reflect the periosteum, scraping side to side until the full flap can be elevated. As the flap is released, the bone fixation screws must be freed from the thick layer of fibrous tissue that adheres to the screw head. A #12 scalpel maybe used to sever the fibrous layer over the screw, and a sharp curette is then used to continue the flap release until another screw is encountered. Once the flap has been completely released, the fixation screws are accessible for removal before placing the implants (Fig. 36.61).

Exposure of the Bone Fixation Screw During the Healing Process

Bone fixation screws in regeneration sites sometimes become exposed during the healing process, potentially leading to bacterial invasion around the neck of the screw. Careful attention to the time lines of the screw exposure and the type of regenerative process is important in these situations. It is not uncommon for the tissue covering the heads of the fixation screws to become very thin. This paper-thin tissue allows the color and contour of the screw heads to be visible and palpable. This is of no significant concern, and the only precaution is directed to relief of any removeable appliance that could be placing pressure on the

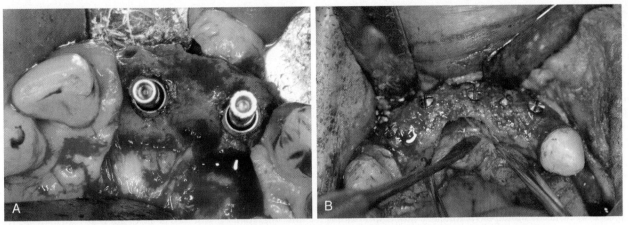

• **Fig 36.60** Incisive Canal Approximation (A) Two implants in # 8 and # 9 positions after significant bone augmentation, note that even with augmentation, implant placement impinging on incisive canal, (B) After extensive maxillary grafting, anatomical limitations of the incisive canal contraindicates implant placement.

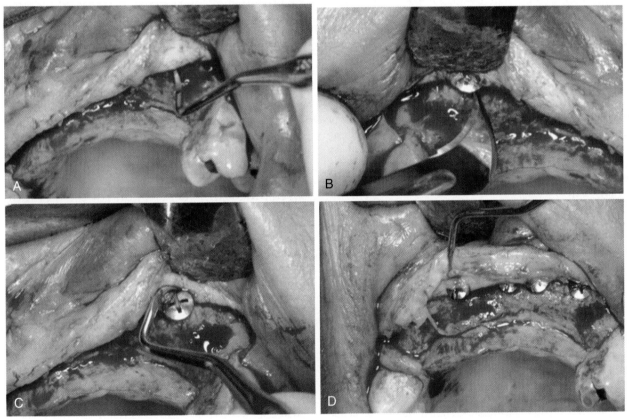

• **Fig. 36.61** Bone Screw Removal. (A and B) The flap has been completely released and the fixation screws are accessible for removal (before placing the implants). (C and D) Bone must be removed from inside the screws before attempting removal with either a 12 blade or periodontal scaler.

already tender and thin tissue. If at any time the actual head perforates through the tissue, it should be considered for removal.

Exposure of fixation screws in particulate grafting occurs when the head of the screw works its way through the overlying membrane and eventually perforates through the thin layer of the mucosa that covers the graft site. This typically happens when the screw head has a thin diameter that perforates through the membrane and eventually through the tissue. Particulate grafting techniques use these fixation screws to support the membrane and to define the shape of the desired bony contours. The use of a

screw with a "wide head" is found to be important for predictable results. The type of membrane used for graft isolation also makes a significant difference when perforation of the screw through the membrane is a concern. Acellular dermal matrix and pericardium tend to be very resistant to membrane perforation during the healing process, whereas collagen membranes are soft when moistened and tend to perforate and tear if strain is placed on the hydrated membrane. Perforation of a membrane allows the ingress of foreign matter and fibrous soft tissue cells into the graft site, causing a disruption in the bone regeneration process. If the head of the screw pushes through the soft tissue and is exposed, bacterial contamination may result, potentially leading to graft infection and possible failure.

The head of the bone fixation screws should have a wide and smooth diameter that provides enough surface area to support the membrane and to limit abrasion against the overlying mucosal layer. A small head will tend to work its way through a membrane when it is placed under tension or where a delicate membrane is being used. The typical bone fixation screw has a diameter of 1.5 mm, and the head of the screw should be as wide as possible. Newer generations of fixation screws have been designed specifically for membrane grafting, and they provide a very wide surface area for even support of a membrane. These larger heads also support such a large surface that the actual number of fixation screws can be reduced significantly.

Exposed screw heads should be maintained with chlorhexidine rinses until the surrounding soft tissue has healed. It is recommended that the screws in particulate techniques be removed at this time to eliminate the possibility of contamination of the graft through the opening around the shaft of the screw. If the screw is preventing pressure on the graft in respect to the use of a removable prosthesis, retention of the screw could be considered. Under no circumstances should efforts be made to cover the screw by repositioning the soft tissue (Fig. 36.62).

Incision Line Opening in Bone-Grafting Sites

Maintenance of complete soft tissue coverage over healing bone-grafting sites is one of the most important principles that must be observed for predictable grafting success. Any time that the healing graft site is exposed to the oral flora during the healing process, there will be some type of compromised change in the final graft site volume and in its overall integrity. Incision line opening with compromised graft results can often be a major limiting factor in successful implant placement.

Incision line opening can compromise even the most carefully planned regeneration site, and most of these graft sites will require additional grafting at a later time if an actual complication develops. An open incision line introduces numerous potential complications into the healing process. First, the introduction of microorganisms into a graft site through an open incision can lead to an infection in the healing graft site. Exposure of the graft particles and the presence of purulence is an indication of impending failure of the graft. The infection reduces the pH in the graft site, causing a breakdown of the graft particles and eventually compromising the resulting ridge volume. Second, an open incision line may allow exposure and breakdown of the barrier membrane, contributing to fibrous tissue ingrowth into the graft site. Lastly, there exists a potential for particulate graft materials to escape the graft site, resulting in an inadequate bone volume in the final proposed implant site.

The most important concept in maintaining incision line integrity is consistent tension-free wound closure. This protective seal can be most effectively managed from the standpoint of overall flap management throughout the surgical procedure. A clinician's experience in manipulation of soft tissue affects this aspect of bone regeneration more than any other part of bone regeneration surgery. As the clinician gains more experience in delicate tissue management and begins to understand the maintenance of a tension-free flap closure, problems with graft and membrane exposure will become an uncommon occurrence.

All regeneration sites require that the overlying tissue flap be stretched over the wide bulk of the graft at the completion of the procedure. Unfortunately there is a finite distance that a tissue flap can be freely stretched, and at this point the wound closure is placed under tension. Even though pressure can be exerted on the stiches to force closure of the wound, the incision line is put under an unreasonable amount of stress. The continual tension and pressure will eventually lead to necrosis of the tissue around the sutures, leading to an open incision postoperatively.

The inner surface of a reflected flap is lined with the periosteum: a thin, dense binding layer of tissue that cannot be stretched. The tissue directly below the periosteum is very loose mobile tissue full of elastic fibers. This disparity in tissue types can predictably be neutralized with a shallow incision through the dense periosteal layer. This "tissue release" is accomplished by preparing a clear and continuous releasing incision through the periosteum, exposing the underlying elastic layers of tissue that can then be released for expansion of the flap over the enlarged graft site. As this incision perforates the periosteal layer, the two edges clearly separate, allowing the elastic tissue below the periosteum to stretch. A sharp pair of Metzenbaum scissors is then placed into the space below the periosteum, and as the scissor tips are opened, the tissue easily releases and the edges separate further. This is repeated until the complete flap is stretched over the graft site and 5 mm beyond the opposite flap margin.

In the event of an incision line opening, the patient should be placed on a frequent monitoring protocol to observe the status of the graft material and any grafting hardware present. The oral microflora must be managed with the use of daily chlorhexidine rinses. The clinician must not attempt to suture the site again because healing margins along incision lines feature tissue that cannot, at that time, support the pressure of another suture under tension (Figs. 36.63 and 36.64).

High Mucogingival Junction Following Ridge Augmentation

Major ridge augmentation requires that the soft tissue flap be stretched over the enlarged graft site. Through the process of extending this tissue laterally over a large and bulky graft, the mucogingival junction is elevated to a level that often surrounds the abutment with mucosa. Various approaches are available to prevent or repair this deficiency of keratinized tissue, but the addition of pre-surgical procedures to an already involved series of surgical appointments often prevents implant teams from coping with this situation.

The simplified approach is to place a very wide autologous tissue graft from the palate over the mucosal region prior to the actual augmentation procedure. The main complaint about this approach is the fact that palatal grafts like this have a whiter color after the graft is placed and it really does not match the thin and pink color of anterior restorative sites. Those grafts are better indicated for use in posterior regions.

The best method available in this situation was described by Dr. Esteban Urban who recommends releasing the loose mucosal tissue with a split thickness flap, leaving the underlying periosteum and fibrous tissue intact. The released mucosal flap is sutured apically with multiple 5-0 Chromic sutures, creating an exposed zone of exposed tissue from the top of the ridge to the newly sutured tissue. A thin strip of palatal tissue is removed, and it is sutured along the apical suture line to fixate the repositioned tissue. This technique will ultimately prevent relapse of the mucosal tissue level. A large piece of mucograft (i.e. resorbable collagen matrix - Geistlich Mucograft®) is placed over the exposed periosteum and

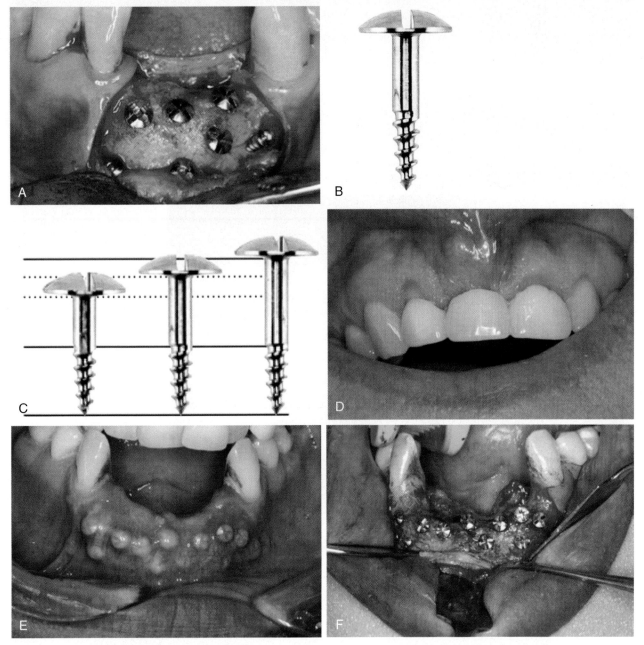

• **Fig. 36.62** Membrane Tent Screws. (A) Larger screw heads are more likely to grow bone than smaller screw heads. Note the lack of bone around the small-headed screw on the far right side of the photo. (B) Wide-head bone screw. (C) Tent screws are available in various width shanks and lengths. (D) As the graft heals and the membrane resorbs, the head of the fixation screws are often visible through the thin mucosa covering the healing graft site. This is not a complication, and no special treatment is necessary. (E) Screw perforation through thin tissue. (F) Screw removal before implant placement.

sutured with chromic sutures. This arrangement of tissue, mucograft, and tissue graft create a predictable zone of keratinized tissue on the facial aspect of the implant restoration and the addition of the mucograft basically eliminates any discomfort related to the repositioning of the mucosal flap. (Fig. 36.65 A, B, C, D, and E)

Graft Infection

Graft materials resorb rapidly at a lower pH condition, with HA crystals dissolving at pH 5.5 or less. Infectious environments may contain a pH of 2 or less, which can cause the rapid dissolution of

a graft. Infection may be caused by lack of aseptic surgical technique, incision line opening, or infection from adjacent dental sources. The presence of a localized infection in a bone graft will cause dissolution of the graft material, contributing to graft failure. The severity of this failure can vary depending on the duration of the infection and the onset of the contamination.

The use of proper surgical technique is vital in the prevention of surgical contamination. Preoperative antibiotic regimens, chlorhexidine scrubs, and aseptic technique will limit bacterial contamination at the time of surgery. Proper suture technique and flap design are grafting fundamentals that

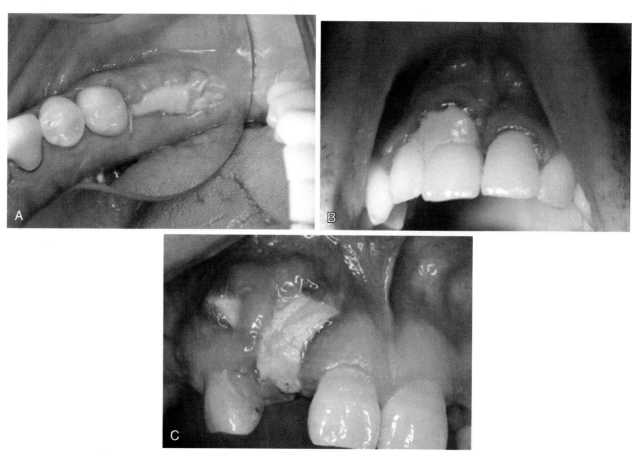

• **Fig. 36.63** Membrane Exposure. (A) Acellular dermis exposure. (B) Collagen membrane exposure. (C) Dense polytetrafluoroethylene exposure through buccal mucosa and residual ridge. All membrane exposures should be maintained as long as possible.

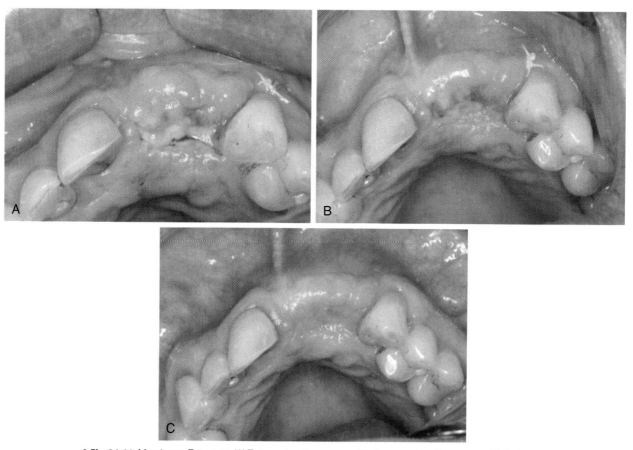

• **Fig. 36.64** Membrane Exposure. (A) Two weeks after surgery. (B) Three weeks after surgery. (C) By keeping the area clean with chlorhexidine, at 5 weeks postoperative closure is obtained.

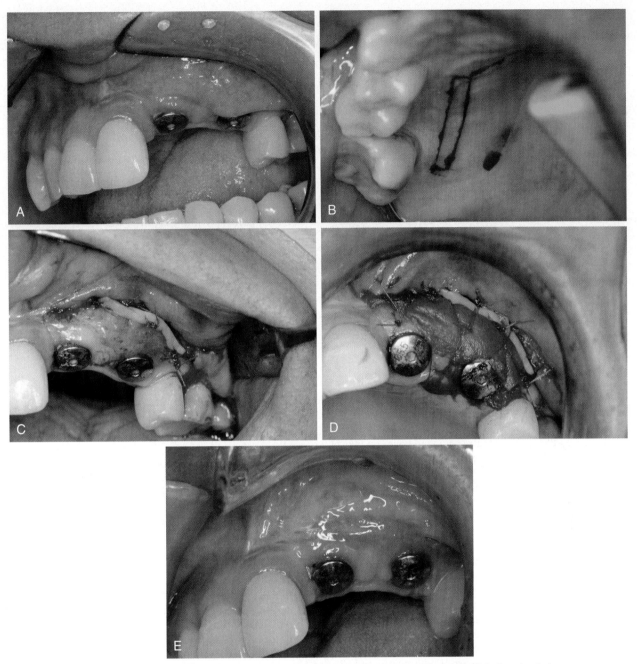

• **Fig. 36.65** High mucosal attachment in the restorative space of the prosthesis: (A). Note the elevated mucogingival junction, particularly on the distal implant. (B). Free Tissue harvest. (C). Split thickness release of the mucosa, with apical fixation using 5 0 Chromic sutures. (D). Fixation of the free tissue graft at the depth of the newly defined vestibule. The exposed tissue between the tissue graft and the top of the ridge is covered with "Mucograft". (E). Three week post operative image is graft site with new zone of keratinized attachment.

prevent incision line opening that can also expose the graft to the oral microflora. Lastly, the clinician should ensure that all space maintenance components (nonresorbable membranes, titanium mesh, tenting screws) are free from sharp edges that may perforate the mucosa postoperatively, allowing the ingress of bacteria into the graft.

Postoperative examinations must be routinely scheduled, especially during the initial stages of wound healing. The patient must be instructed in hygiene techniques that minimize strain on the incision line, and postoperative chlorhexidine rinses can be used to manage the bacterial microflora. If incision line opening occurs, the patient must be placed on a chlorhexidine rinsing protocol to keep the graft site clean until the granulation is complete. If the patient experiences purulence from the site or general malaise, antibiotic protocols must be commenced immediately. Nonresorbable membranes should be maintained for at least 6 weeks unless the site becomes infected. If this occurs, the membrane should be removed before the situation advances.

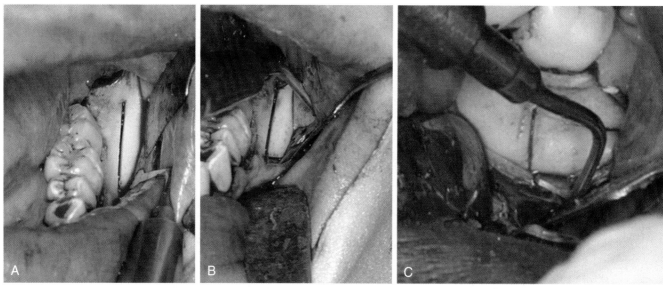

• **Fig. 36.66** Piezoelectric Handpiece Trauma. (A and B) The shaft of the handpiece (A) and the insert (B) should not be allowed to contact the soft tissue because soft tissue burns or trauma may result. (C) Ideal position of handpiece and insert with no contact to adjacent tissues.

Ultrasonic Piezosurgery-Related Tissue Injury

The use of ultrasound technology in dentistry first began in the 1950s, and newer Piezosurgery units have been developed using low-frequency ultrasound (10–60 kHz) for the selective cutting of bone. Traditional bone drilling with motorized drills is easily available to clinicians; however, cutting bone with a drill can generate excessive amounts of heat in dense bone, potentially damaging the surrounding tissue. A surgical drill that comes in contact with blood vessels, nerves, or sinus membranes can also cut or damage adjacent vital structures. The use of Piezosurgery in implant surgery has been a welcome alternative to motorized drills in many applications. At the lower ultrasonic frequencies used for Piezosurgery, surgical inserts cut through hard, mineralized bone but do not damage the surrounding soft tissue or generate high amounts of heat. Piezosurgery has been especially useful in implant surgery, where bone must be cut in close proximity to a nerve or blood vessel.

As Piezosurgery has been performed, it has been reported by practitioners that the inserts should not be allowed to function while in direct contact with the soft tissue flap. Earlier surgical units were reported to "heat up the insert tip" during use, and irritations or burns on the soft tissue flap were sometimes detected. This altered tissue issue has not been evident in updated Piezosurgery units, but careful attention must be directed to protection of surrounding soft tissue during ultrasonic insert use. Instructors describe this as an abrasive phenomenon caused by the rapid ultrasonic movement of the tip against the soft tissue. Care must be taken to keep the tissue flap away from the ultrasonic inserts.

Development of any abrasive or burn-type lesion should be treated symptomatically, just as any other oral burn or abrasive lesion would be treated. If there are any signs of more serious damage, more involved treatment may require appropriate referrals for wound care (Figs. 36.66 A, B, and C and 36.67).

Summary

To satisfy the ideal goals of implant dentistry, the hard and soft tissues need to be present in ideal volume and quality. After tooth loss, the resorption of the alveolar process occurs so often that augmentation procedures are often necessary to restore the hard and soft tissues. This becomes especially significant when the edentulous areas are in the esthetic zone. Augmentation procedures not only enhance the final esthetic result, but also will make a more predictable biomechanical foundation to minimize possible complications. In implant dentistry today, there exist a vast array or procedures and protocols to augment deficient implants sites. This chapter presented an overview of the indications for guided bone regeneration techniques along with a classification of differing ridge morphology that will allow the clinician to understand the predict ability and difficulty based on the bony ridge deficiency. The following images demonstrate the regenerative potential of current approaches to bone augmentation. Jensen and Terheyden[78] in 2009 reviewed 108 articles and concluded that the mean average of particulate grafting with a membrane was 2.6mm and 24.4% required additional grafting post operatively. As the concept of "Space Maintenance" has been explored over recent years, techniques and barrier materials have improved significantly, changing the ability of surgeons to regenerate ridge defects. The following cases are examples of the ability of these techniques to regenerate large amounts of bone in critical regions. These are not a few "rare cases" that have been cherry picked for this publication. Careful application of the principles described in this chapter have demonstrated similar results on a very predictable basis (Box 36.12 and Figs. 36.68-36.72).

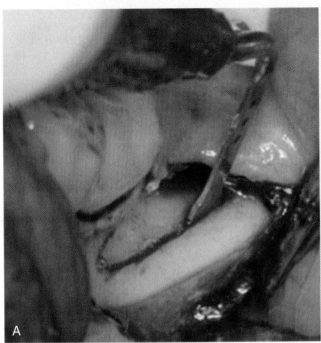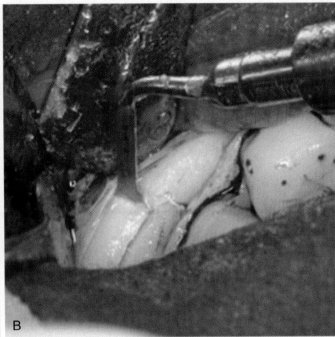

• **Fig. 36.67** Ideal Retraction. (A) The piezoelectric inserts are separated from the surrounding soft tissue with "Pritchard retractors" and wide flap access. (B) Two retractors retract the tissue, whereas the piezo insert prepares the bone.

• **BOX 36.12 Guided Bone Regeneration Protocol**

Step 1: Incision
a. Position—ideally bisect the attached tissue; if compromised keratinized tissue, incision should be made more to the lingual
b. Broad based—release incisions should always be broad based to maintain adequate blood supply to allow for ideal healing
c. Papilla sparing—when possible around adjacent natural teeth, incisions should be made maintaining the papilla; this reduces the chance of altering or losing the papilla and the development of a "black triangle"

Step 2: Reflection
A full-thickness reflection is recommended. The amount of reflection is related to development of adequate exposure to the graft site for placement of bone grafts and barrier membranes. It is also important in preparation of the site for tension-free primary closure.

Step 3: Removal of Recipient Site Soft Tissue
It is imperative that all soft tissue is removed from the recipient site because soft tissue remnants will prevent bone formation. This may be accomplished in various ways including: (1) hand instrument removal, (2) small round burs (#8 carbide), or (3) laboratory straight handpiece burs (carbide, diamond).

Step 4: Decortication
The recipient site should be decorticated to increase bleeding (angiogenesis) and to allow bone growth factors to enter the area, enhancing bone formation. When decorticated, bleeding must be visible through the decortication sites. Cross-cut fissure burs or small, round burs may be used to perforate the cortical plate.

Step 5: Tissue Release
It is imperative the tissue is prepared prior to graft placement to prevent disruption of the graft material. Therefore, the flap is prepared to minimize any tension on the incision line. Ideally, the facial flap should extend a minimum of 5 mm over the lingual flap. There are two techniques which include (1) periosteal release - # 15 blade, and (2) blunt dissection – Metzunbaum scissors.

Step 6: Membrane Placement
a. Membrane selection—the type of membrane will depend on the shape and volume of bone required, the predictability of soft tissue closure (resorbable vs. nonresorbable), and the experience of the surgeon.
b. Hydration—most membranes will need to be hydrated to allow for proper placement and to minimize the possibility of poor closure
c. Fixation—the membrane should be apically fixated with tacks or sutures to minimize movement. Usually the facial/buccal tacks are placed before grafting. This initial stabilization of the membrane allows the site to remain undisturbed after graft placement. It is highly recommended to fix the membrane on the lingual/palatal aspect with tacks or sutures.
d. Adequate periosteal release over the graft site—the tissue should be released enough for the flap to be stretched freely, allowing tension-free closure. Ideally the facial flap should extend a minimum of 5 mm beyond the lingual flap.

Step 7: Space Maintenance
For predicatble bone growth, the space must be maintained to allow the bone grafting material to heal undisturbed. Placement of a support system (tenting screws, polytetrafluoroethylene (PTFE) membrane with titanium, titanium mesh) must be used. Collapse of the graft site will result in compromised bone growth.

Step 8: Graft Material Placement
a. **Autogenous:** Usually, autogenous bone is recommended when bone growth of greater than 3 mm is required. When indicated, autograft should be the first layer (against the host bone). The autograft shavings should cover the complete recipient bed below the screws.

Continued

• BOX 36.12 Guided Bone Regeneration Protocol—cont'd

b. **Allograft:** The allograft should be placed as the second layer in larger bone graft cases (> 3 mm). For smaller graft cases, 100% allograft may be used (i.e. 70% FDBA / 30 DFDBA or 100% FDBA Cortico-Cancellous). The particulate bone should be densely packed to avoid air spaces which tend to harbor bacteria.

• After the bone graft is placed, the membrane is drawn completely over the graft material with 2 to 3 mm of overlap over native bone to limit exposure of the particulate during the healing process. The membrane should be fixated (on the free end) with tacks or sutures. In situations where the membrane cannot be fixated, it can be tucked under the lingual flap and the coronal surface can be included in the closure sutures to limit movement. If platelet-rich fibrin or platelet-rich plasma is being used, it should be placed over the membrane (in between the tissue and membrane).

Step 9: Closure

a. *Suture selection:* The most ideal sutures for tissue closure are Vicryl (resorbable) or PTFE (Cytoplast, nonresorbable). The PTFE suture allows adjustment of the suture tension as the knot is being tied, and results in minimal inflammation around a healing incision line.

b. *Primary sutures:* the crest or ridge area should be closed first with a tension-free suture line. Mattress sutures should be placed at intervals that distribute the pressure on the incision over a large surface area. Mattress suture evert the tissue flaps, thereby decreasing the possibility of incision line opening. Interrupted sutures may be used between the mattress sutures. A common mistake is to close the vertical releasing incisions first, thereby placing tension on the crestal suture line.

c. *Secondary sutures:* After the crestal area has been closed, the releasing incisions may be closed passively. Care should be exercised not to place too much tension on the releasing flaps, thereny limiting tension on the crestal sutures.

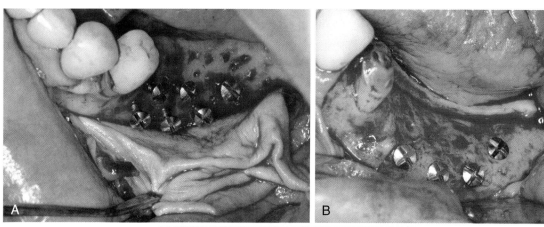

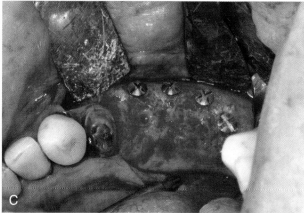

• **Fig. 36.68** (A – C) Posterior mandible augmentation for horizontal regeneration using autogenous , mineralized freeze-dried bone allograft, and GBR acellular dermis membrane.

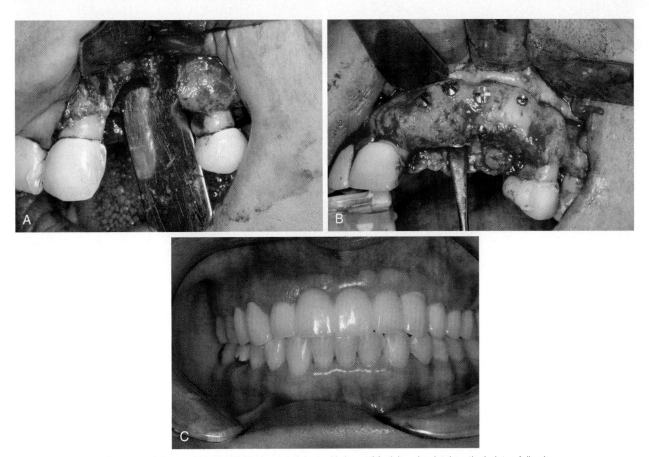

• **Fig. 36.69** Advanced Vertical & Horizontal defect with loss of facial and palatal cortical plates following the loss of two implants. (A) Flap reflection showing the severe destruction caused by two failed implants. (B) The final ridge form following ridge augmentation with autogenous bone and allograft/acellular dermis, (C) Final Prosthesis

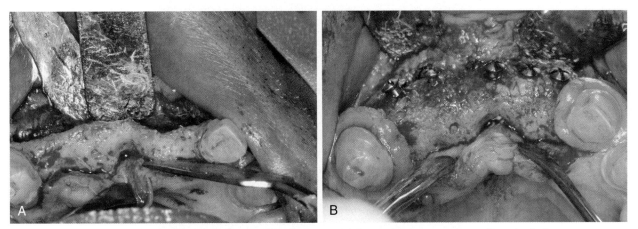

• **Fig. 36.70** Maxillary Anterior Horizontal Augmentation; (A) Exposed defect, note the papilla saving incision design, (B) Post-op bone augmentation healing.

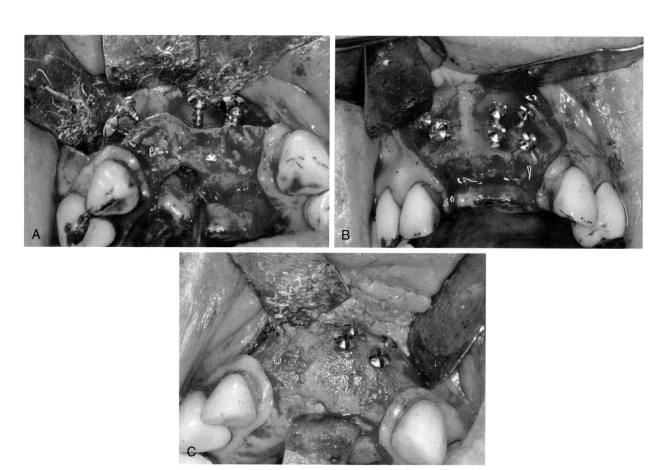

• **Fig. 36.71** Maxillary Anterior Augmentation (A). Anterior regeneration using space maintenance for site development. (Autogenous bone, FDBA and Acellular dermis). (B). Post-augmentation ridge form

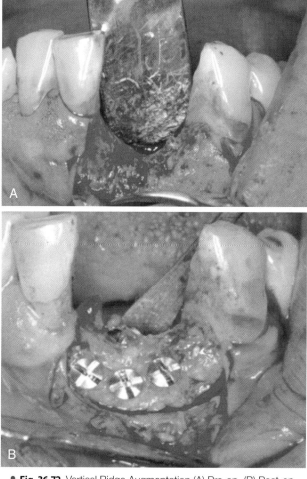

• **Fig. 36.72** Vertical Ridge Augmentation (A) Pre-op, (B) Post-op.

References

1. Schropp L, Wenzel A, Kostopoulos L, Karring T. Bone healing and soft tissue contour changes following single-tooth extraction: a clinical and radiographic 12-month prospective study. *Int J Periodontics Restorative Den.* 2003;23:313–323.
2. Clementini M, Morlupi A, Canullo L, et al. Success rate of dental implants inserted in horizontal and vertical guided bone regenerated areas: a systematic review. *Int J Oral Maxillofac Surg.* 2012;41:847–852.
3. Hammerle CH, Jung RE, Feloutzis A. A systematic review of the survival of implants in bone sites augmented with barrier membranes (guided bone regeneration) in partially edentulous patients. *J Clin Periodontol.* 2002;29(3):226–231, discussion 232–223.
4. McAllister BS, Haghighat K. Bone augmentation techniques. *J Periodontol.* 2007;78:377–396.
5. Jensen SS, Terheyden H. Bone augmentation procedures in localized defects in the alveolar ridge: clinical results with different bone grafts and bone-substitute materials. *Int J Oral Maxillofac Implants.* 2009;24:218–236.
6. Nevins M, Mellonig JT. The advantages of localized ridge augmentation prior to implant placement: a staged event. *Int J Periodontics Restorative Den.* 1994;14:96–111.
7. Liu J, Kerns DG. Mechanisms of guided bone regeneration: a review. *Open Dent J.* 2014;8:56–65.
8. Van der Weijden F, Dell'Acqua F, Slot DE. Alveolar bone dimensional changes of post-extraction sockets in humans: a systematic review. *J Clin Periodontol.* 2009;36(12):1048–1058.
9. Hof M, Tepper G, Semo B, Arnhart C, Watzek G, Pommer B. Patients' perspectives on dental implant and bone graft surgery: questionnaire-based interview survey. *Clin Oral Implants Res.* 2014;25(1):42–45.
10. Cook DR, Mealey BL, Verrett RG, et al. Relationship between clinical periodontal biotype and labial plate thickness: an in vivo study. *Int J Periodontics Restorative Dent.* 2011;31(4).
11. Ryan CD, Mealey BL, Verrett RG, et al. Relationship between clinical periodontal biotype and labial plate thickness: an in vivo study. *Int J Periodontics Restorative Dent.* 2011;31(4):344–354.
12. Linkevicius T, Apse P, Grybauskas S, Puisys A. Influence of thin mucosal tissues on crestal bone stability around implants with platform switching: a 1-year pilot study. *J Oral Maxillofac Surg.* 2010;68(9):2272–2277.
13. Dahlin C, Buser D, Dahlin C, Schenk R, eds. *Guided Bone Regeneration in Implant Dentistry.* Chicago. IL: Quintessence Publ; 1994. Scientific Background of guided bone regeneration.
14. Chou AH, LeGeros RZ, Chen Z, Li Y. Antibacterial effect of zinc phosphate mineralized guided bone regeneration membranes. *Implant Dent.* 2007;16(1):89–100.
15. Nishibori M, Betts NJ, Salama H, Listgarten MA. Short-term healing of autogenous and allogeneic bone grafts after sinus augmentation: a report of 2 cases. *J Periodontol.* 1994;65(10):958–966.
16. Pitaru S, Tal H, Soldinger M, Grosskopf A, Noff M. Partial regeneration of periodontal tissues using collagen barriers. Initial observations in the canine. *J Periodontol.* 1988;59(6):380–386.
17. Fiorellini JP, Buser D, Riley E, et al. Effect on bone healing of bone morphogenetic protein placed in combination with endosseous implants: a pilot study in beagle dogs. *Int J Periodontics Restorative Dent.* 2001;21:41–47.
18. Melcher AH, Accurs GE. Osteogenic capacity of periosteal and osteoperiosteal flaps elevated from the parietal bone of the rat. *Arch Oral Biol.* 1971;16:573–580.
19. Zhang Y, Zhang X, Shi B, Miron RJ. Membranes for guided tissue and bone regeneration. *Annals of Oral & Maxillofacial Surg.* 2013;1(1):10.
20. Pellegrini G, Pagni G, Rasperini G. Surgical approaches based on biological objectives: GTR versus GBR Techniques. *Int J Dent.* 2013;521–547.
21. Dahlin C, Linde A, Gottlow J, Nyman S. Healing of bone defects by guided tissue regeneration. *Plast Reconstr Surg.* 1988;81:672–676.
22. Buser D, Dula K, Hirt HP, Schenk RK. Lateral ridge augmentation using autografts and barrier membranes: a clinical study with 40 partially edentulous patients. *J Oral Maxillofac Surg.* 1996;54:420–432, discussion 432–423.
23. Chiapasco M, Abati S, Romeo E, Vogel G. Clinical outcome of autogenous bone blocks or guided bone regeneration with e-PTFE membranes for the reconstruction of narrow edentulous ridges. *Clin Oral Implants Res.* 1999;10:278–288.
24. Simion M, Dahlin C, Rocchietta I, et al. Vertical ridge augmentation with guided bone regeneration in association with dental implants: an experimental study in dogs. *Clin Oral Implants Res.* 2007;18:86–94.
25. Pocket Dentistry [internet]. Barrier Membranes for Guided Bone Regeneration. [updated 2015 Jan 5; cited 2017 Dec 28]. Available from: https://pocketdentistry.com/3-barrier-membranes-for-guided-bone-regeneration/#end_en139.
26. Rispoli L, Fontana F, Beretta M, Poggio CE, Maiorana C. Surgery guidelines for barrier membranes in guided bone regeneration (GBR). *J Otolaryngol Rhinol.* 2015;1(2):1–8.
27. Buser D, Dula K, Hess D, et al. Localized ridge augmentation with autografts and barrier membranes. *Periodontol.* 1999;2000:151–163. 19.
28. Trombelli L, Farina R, Marzola A, et al. GBR and autogenous cortical bone particulate by bone scraper for alveolar ridge augmentation: a 2-case report. *Int J Oral Maxillofac Implants.* 2008;23:111–116.
29. Simion M, Baldoni M, Rassi P, Zaffe D. A comparative study of the effectiveness of e-PTFE membranes with and without early exposure during the healing period. *Int J Periodontics Restorative Dent.* 1994;14(2).
30. Machtei EE. The effect of membrane exposure on the outcome of regenerative procedures in humans: a meta-analysis. *J Periodontol.* 2001;72(4):512–516.
31. Bartee BK, Carr JA. Evaluation of a high-density polytetrafluoroethylene (n-PTFE) membrane as a barrier material to facilitate guided bone regeneration in the rat mandible. *J Oral Implantol.* 1995;21(2):88–95.
32. Fontana F, Santoro F, Maiorana C, et al. Clinical and histologic evaluation of allogeneic bone matrix versus autogenous bone chips associated with titanium-reinforced e-PTFE membrane for vertical ridge augmentation: a prospective pilot study. *Int J Oral Maxillofac Implants.* 2008;23(6).
33. Buser D, Dula K, Belser U, et al. Localized ridge augmentation using guided bone regeneration. 1. Surgical procedure in the maxilla. *Int J Periodontics Restorative Den.* 1993;13:29–45.
34. Feuille F, Knapp CI, Brunsvold MA, Mellonig JT. Clinical and histologic evaluation of bone-replacement grafts in the treatment of localized alveolar ridge defects. Part 1: mineralized freeze-dried bone allograft. *Int J Periodontics Restorative Dent.* 2003;23:29–35.
35. Sterio TW, Katancik JA, Blanchard SB, et al. A prospective, multicenter study of bovine pericardium membrane with cancellous particulate allograft for localized alveolar ridge augmentation. *Int J Periodontics Restorative Dent.* 2013;33:499–507.
36. Fowler EB, Breault LG, Rebitski G. Ridge preservation utilizing an acellular dermal allograft and demineralized freeze-dried bone allograft: Part II. Immediate endosseous implant placement. *J Periodontol.* 2000;71:1360–1364.
37. Wainwright DJ. Use of an acellular allograft dermal matrix (AlloDerm) in the management of full-thickness burns. *Burns.* 1995;21:243–248.
38. Pocket Dentistry. Barrier membranes for guided bone regeneration. [updated 2015 Jan 5; cited 2017 Dec 28]. https://pocketdentistry.com/3-barrier-membranes-for-guided-bone-regeneration/#end_en139.
39. Luitaud C, Laflamme C, Semlali A, et al. Development of an engineering autologous palatal mucosa-like tissue for potential clinical applications. *J Biomed Mater Res B Appl Biomater.* 2007;83(2):554–561.

40. Yamada M, Kubo K, Ueno T, et al. Alleviation of commercial collagen sponge- and membrane-induced apoptosis and dysfunction in cultured osteoblasts by an amino acid derivative. *Int J Oral Maxillofac Implants.* 2010;25(5):939–946.

41. Rispoli L, Fontana F, Beretta M, Poggio CE, Maiorana C. Surgery guidelines for barrier membranes in guided bone regeneration (GBR). *J Otolaryngol Rhinol.* 2015;1(2):1–8.

42. Rothamel D, Schwarz F, Sager M, Herten M, Sculean A, Becker J. Biodegradation of differently cross-linked collagen membranes: an experimental study in the rat. *Clin Oral Implants Res.* 2005;16(3):369–378.

43. Schwarz F, Rothamel D, Herten M, et al. Immunohistochemical characterization of guided bone regeneration at a dehiscence-type defect using different barrier membranes: an experimental study in dogs. *Clin Oral Implants Res.* 2008;19(4):402–415.

44. McAllister BS, Haghighat K. Bone augmentation techniques. *J Periodontol.* 2007;78:377–396.

45. Griffin TJ, Cheung WS, Hirayama H. Hard and soft tissue augmentation in implant therapy using acellular dermal matrix. *Int J Periodontics Restorative Dent.* 2004;24:352–361.

46. Polimeni G, Koo KT, Qahash M, et al. Prognostic factors for alveolar regeneration: effect of a space-providing biomaterial on guided tissue regeneration. *J Clin Periodontol.* 2004;31:725–729.

47. Le B, Burstein J, Sedghizadeh PP. Cortical tenting grafting technique in the severely atrophic alveolar ridge for implant site preparation. *Implant Dent.* 2008;17:40–50.

48. Le B, Rohrer MD, Prasad HS. Screw "tent-pole" grafting technique for reconstruction of large vertical alveolar ridge defects using human mineralized allograft for implant site preparation. *J Oral Maxillofac Surg.* 2010;68:428–435.

49. Caldwell GR, Mealy BL. A prospective study: alveolar ridge augmentation using tenting screws, acellular dermal matrix and combination particulate grafts. A Thesis for Master of Science in Periodontics—The University of Texas Health Science Center at San Antonio Graduate School of Biomedical Sciences. May 2013

50. Hempton TJ, Fugazzotto PA. Ridge augmentation utilizing guided tissue regeneration, titanium screws, freeze-dried bone, and tricalcium phosphate: clinical report. *Implant Dent.* 1994;3:35–37.

51. Simon BI, Chiang TF, Drew HJ. Alternative to the gold standard for alveolar ridge augmentation: tenting screw technology. *Quintessence Int.* 2010;41:379–386.

52. Choukroun J, et al. Platelet-rich fibrin (PRF): a second-generation platelet concentrate. Part IV: clinical effects on tissue healing. *Oral Surg Oral Med Oral Pathol Oral Radiol Endod.* 2006;101(3):e56–e60.

53. Choukroun J, et al. Platelet-rich fibrin (PRF): a second-generation platelet concentrate. Part V: histologic evaluations of PRF effects on bone allograft maturation in sinus lift. *Oral Surg Oral Med Oral Pathol Oral Radiol Endod.* 2006;101(3):299–303.

54. Misch CM. Bone augmentation of the atrophic posterior mandible for dental implants using rhBMP-2 and titanium mesh: clinical technique and early results. *Int J Periodontics Restorative Dent.* 2010;31(6):581–589.

55. Boyne PJ, Lilly LC, Marx RE, et al. De novo bone induction by recombinant human bone morphogenetic protein-2 (rhBMP-2) in maxillary sinus floor augmen- tation. *J Oral Maxillofac Surg.* 2005;63:1693–1707.

56. Misch CE. Bone density: a key determinant for treatment planning. In: *Contemporary Implant Dentistry.* St. Louis: Mosby; 2008:130–146.

57. Sanz M, Vignoletti F. Key aspects on the use of bone substitutes for bone regeneration of edentulous ridges. *Dent Mater.* 2015;31(6):640–647.

58. Boyce T, Edwards J, Scarborough N. Allograft bone: the influence of processing on safety and performance. *Orthop Clin North Am.* 1999;30(4):571–581.

59. Piattelli A, Scarano A, Corigliano M, Piattelli M. Comparison of bone regeneration with the use of mineralized and demineralized freeze-dried bone allografts: a histological and histochemical study in man. *Biomaterials.* 1996;17(11):1127–1131.

60. Shapoff CA, Bowers GM, Levy B, Mellonig JT, Yukna RA. The effect of particle size on the osteogenic activity of composite grafts of allogeneic freeze-dried bone and autogenous marrow. *J Periodontol.* 1980;51(11):625–630.

61. Jacobsen G, Easter D. *Allograft vs. Xenograft: Practical Considerations for Biologic Scaffolds.* Musculoskeletal Transplant Foundation; 2008.

62. Barrack RL. Bone graft extenders, substitutes, and osteogenic proteins. *J Arthroplasty.* 2005;20(4 2):94–97.

63. Esposito M, Grusovin MG, Rees J, et al. Effectiveness of sinus lift procedures for dental implant rehabilitation: a Cochrane systematic review. *Eur J Oral Implantol.* 2010;3(1):7–26.

64. LeGeros RZ. Calcium phosphates in oral biology and medicine. *Monogr Oral Sci.* 1991;15:1–201.

65. Suh H, Park JC, Han DW, Lee DH, Han CD. A bone replaceable artificial bone substitute: cytotoxicity, cell adhesion, proliferation, and alkaline phosphatase activity. *Artif Organs.* 2001;25(1):14–21.

66. Peter M, Binulal NS, Nair SV, Selvamurugan N, Tamura H, Jayakumar R. Novel biodegradable chitosan-gelatin/nano-bioactive glass ceramic composite scaffolds for alveolar bone tissue engineering. *Chem Eng J.* 2010;158(2):353–361.

67. Salim S, Ariani MD. In vitro and in vivo evaluation of carbonate apatite-collagen scaffolds with some cytokines for bone tissue engineering. *J Indian Prosthodont Soc.* 2015;15(4):349–355.

68. Chan C, Thompson I, Robinson P, Wilson J, Hench L. Evaluation of Bioglass/dextran composite as a bone graft substitute. *Int J Oral Maxillofac Surg.* 2002;31(1):73–77.

69. Wang H, Boyapati L. "PASS" principles for predictable bone regeneration. *Implant Dent.* 2006;15(1):8–17.

70. Kiran NK, Mukunda KS, Tilak Raj TN. Platelet concentrates: a promising innovation in dentistry. *J Dent Sci Res.* 2011;2:50–61.

71. Marx RE, Carlson ER, Eichstaedt RM, Schimmele SR, Strauss JE, Georgeff KR. Platelet-rich plasma: growth factor enhancement for bone grafts. *Oral Surg Oral Med Oral Pathol Oral Radiol Endod.* 1998;85(6):638–646.

72. Choukroun J, Diss A, Simonpieri A, et al. Platelet-rich fibrin (PRF): a second-generation platelet concentrate. Part IV: clinical effects on tissue healing. *Oral Surg Oral Med Oral Pathol Oral Radiol Endod.* 2006;101(3):e56–e60.

73. Choukroun J, Diss A, Simonpieri A, et al. Platelet-rich fibrin (PRF): a second-generation platelet concentrate. Part IV: clinical effects on tissue healing. *Oral Surg Oral Med Oral Pathol Oral Radiol Endod.* 2006;101:56–60.

74. Kang YH, Jeon SH, Park JY, et al. Platelet-rich fibrin is a Bioscaffold and reservoir of growth factors for tissue regeneration. *Tissue Eng Part A.* 2011;17:349–359.

75. Dohan DM, Choukroun J, Diss A, et al. Platelet-rich fibrin (PRF): a second-generation platelet concentrate. Part I: technological concepts and evolution. *Oral Surg Oral Med Oral Pathol Oral Radiol Endod.* 2006;101:e37–e44.

76. Kobayashi E, Flückiger L, Fujioka Kobayashi M. Comparative release of growth factors from PRP, PRF, and advanced-PRF. *Clin Oral Investig.* 2016;20(9):2353–2360.

77. Montanari M, Callea M, Yavuz I, Maglione M. A new biological approach to guided bone and tissue regeneration. *Case Reports.* 2013 (2013): bcr2012008240.

78. Storgard JS, Hendrik T. Bone augmentation procedures in localized defects in the alveolar ridge: clinical results with different bone grafts and bone-substitute materials. In: *Database of Abstracts of Reviews of Effects (DARE): Quality-assessed Reviews [Internet].* UK: Centre for Reviews and Dissemination; 2009.

37

Maxillary Sinus Anatomy, Pathology, and Graft Surgery

RANDOLPH R. RESNIK AND CARL E. MISCH

The posterior maxilla has been described as one of the most challenging and complex intraoral regions that confronts the implant clinician. There exist many treatment planning and patient factors that contribute to these problems in this area, which in many cases require the clinician to have additional training and an increased skill set:

- Poor bone density
- Compromised available bone
- Increased pneumatization of the maxillary sinus
- Increased crown height space
- Ridge position shifts toward lingual (medial)
- Difficult access because of anatomic location
- Increased biting force
- Requirement of wider diameter implants and increased number

Before discussing the various treatment options of the posterior maxilla, it is imperative that the implant clinician have a strong foundation for maxillary sinus anatomy, anatomic variants, pathology, and a comprehensive understanding of the various treatment approaches.

Maxillary Sinus Anatomy

The maxillary sinuses were first illustrated and described by Leonardo Da Vinci in 1489 and later documented by the English anatomist Nathaniel Highmore in 1651.[1] The maxillary sinus, or antrum of Highmore, lies within the body of the maxillary bone and is the largest and first to develop of the paranasal sinuses (Fig. 37.1). Adult maxillary sinuses are pyramid-shaped, air-filled cavities that are bordered by the nasal cavity. There is much debate about the actual function of the maxillary sinus. Possible theorized roles of the sinus include weight reduction of the skull, phonetic resonance, participation of warming humidification of inspired air, and olfaction. A biomechanical adaptation of the maxillary sinus directs forces away from the orbit and cranial cavity when a force is delivered to the midface.

Development and Expansion of the Maxillary Sinus

A primary pneumatization occurs at approximately 3 months of fetal development by an outpouching of the nasal mucosa within the ethmoid infundibulum. At that time, the maxillary sinus is a bud situated at the infralateral surface of the ethmoid infundibulum between the upper and middle meatus. Prenatally, a secondary pneumatization occurs. At birth, the sinus is still an oblong groove on the mesial side of the maxilla just above the germ of the first deciduous molar.[2]

At birth, the sinus cavities are filled with fluid. Postnatally and until the child is 3 months old the growth of the maxillary sinus is closely related to the pressure exerted by the eye on the orbit floor, the tension of the superficial musculature on the maxilla, and the forming dentition. As the skull matures, these three elements influence its three-dimensional (3D) development. At 5 months, the sinus appears as a triangular area medial to the infraorbital foramen.[3]

During the child's first year, the maxillary sinus expands laterally underneath the infraorbital canal, which is protected by a thin bony ridge. The antrum grows apically and progressively replaces the space formerly occupied by the developing dentition. The growth in height is best reflected by the relative position of the sinus floor. At 12 years of age, pneumatization extends to the plane of the lateral orbital wall, and the sinus floor is level with the floor of the nose. During later years, pneumatization spreads inferiorly as the permanent teeth erupt. The adult sinus has a volume of approximately 15 mL (34 mm height x 33 length x 23 mm width). The main development of the antrum occurs as the permanent dentition erupts and pneumatization extends throughout the body of the maxilla and the maxillary process of the zygomatic bone. Extension into the alveolar process lowers the floor of the sinus approximately 5 mm. Anteroposteriorly, the sinus expansion corresponds to the growth of the midface and is completed only with the eruption of the third permanent molars when the young person is about 16 to 18 years of age.[4]

In the adult, the sinus is pyramid shaped with consisting of four bony walls, the base of which faces the lateral nasal wall and the apex of which extends toward the zygomatic bone (Fig. 37.2). The floor of the maxillary sinus cavity is reinforced by bony or membranous septa, joining the medial or lateral walls with oblique or transverse buttress-like webs. They develop as a result of genetics and stress transfer within the bone over the roots of teeth. These have the appearance of reinforcement webs in a wooden boat and

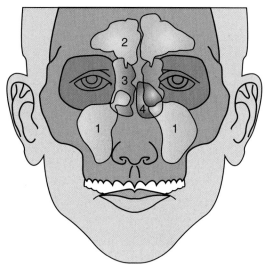

● **Fig. 37.1** Maxillary sinus *(1)* is the largest of the four paranasal sinuses. The initial maxillary sinus formation is completed at age 16 to 18 years. *2, Frontal sinus; 3, ethmoid sinus; 4, sphenoid sinus.*

rarely divide the antrum into separate compartments. These elements are present from the canine to the molar region and tend to disappear in the maxilla of the long-term edentulous patient when stresses to the bone are reduced. Karmody found that the most common oblique septum is located in the superior anterior corner of the sinus or infraorbital recess (which may expand anteriorly to the nasolacrimal duct).[5] The medial wall is juxtaposed with the middle and inferior meatus.

Although the maxillary sinus maintains its overall size while the teeth are present, an expansion phenomenon of the maxillary sinus occurs with the loss of posterior teeth.[6] The antrum expands in both inferior and lateral dimensions. This expansion may even invade the canine eminence region and proceed to the lateral piriform rim of the nose. The dimension of available bone height of the posterior maxilla is greatly reduced as a result of dual resorption from the crest of the ridge and pneumatization of the sinus after the loss of teeth. The sinus expansion is more rapid than the crestal bone height changes. As a result of the inferior sinus expansion, the amount of available bone in the posterior maxilla greatly decreases in height (Fig. 37.3). The maxillary sinus tends to enlarge with age, as well as with edentulism, which further

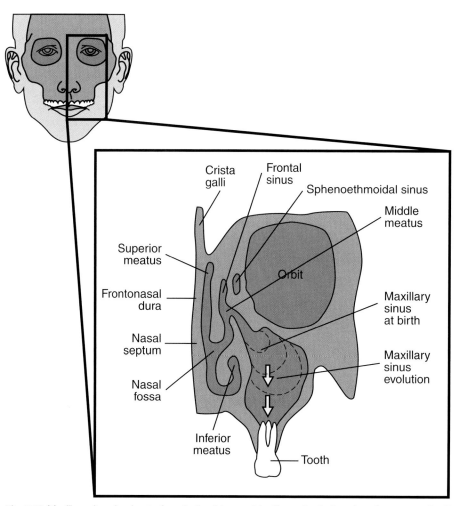

● **Fig. 37.2** Maxillary sinus begins to form in the fetus and by 5 months is the size of a pea, under the eye, and close to the ostium for drainage. By 16 years of age, the maxillary sinus has four thin, bony walls around it. The superior wall separates it from the floor of the orbit. The medial wall contains the ostium to drain the sinus and separates it from the nasal fossa. The lateral wall forms the maxillary bone below the zygomatic arch. The floor of the antrum rests above the roots of the teeth.

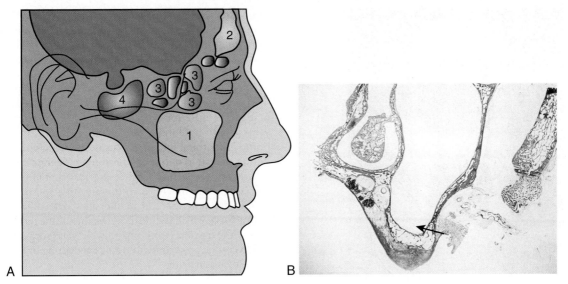

• **Fig. 37.3** (A) The fourth expansion phenomenon of the maxillary sinus occurs with the loss of the posterior teeth. The anterior portion of the sinus may expand to the piriform rim of the nose. The inferior expansion may approach the crest of the ridge. *1,* Maxillary sinus; *2,* frontal sinus; *3,* ethmoid sinus; *4,* sphenoid sinus. (B) Coronal section of the posterior region of the edentulous human maxilla. Note expansion of the sinus floor inferiorly far below the level of the floor of the nose. The alveolar ridge bone is markedly atrophied, whereas the ridge submucosa has become fibrotic. Stained with Rescorcin Fuchsin stain and counterstained with Ban Gieson. (Courtesy Mohamed Sharawy, Augusta, Georgia.)

decreases the amount of available bone. In addition to the diminished quantity, bone in the posterior maxilla often is softer and of poorer quality. Radiographs typically reveal sparse trabeculations, and the tactile experience of drilling in this bone resembles a Styrofoam type of material (D4 Bone).

After normal sinus expansion, with periodontal disease and tooth loss increasing the bone loss, inadequate bone will result between the alveolar ridge crest and the floor of the maxillary sinus. In most cases, bone quantity will be compromised for implant placement. The limited available bone is compounded by a decrease in bone density and the shifting of the residual ridge in a medial direction. Therefore this area of the maxilla is often reported with an increased incidence of implant malpositioning and morbidity.

Bone Resorption Process

The maxilla generally has a thinner cortical plate facially compared with any region of the mandible, and very minimal cortical bone is present on the ridge. In addition, the trabecular bone in the posterior maxilla is finer (less dense) than other dentate regions. When maxillary posterior teeth are lost, an initial decrease in bone width at the expense of the labial bony plate results. The width of the posterior maxilla has been shown to decrease at a more rapid rate than in any other region of the jaws.[7] The resorption phenomenon is accelerated by the loss of vascularization of the alveolar bone and the existing fine trabecular bone type. However, because the initial residual ridge is inherently wide in the posterior maxilla, even with a significant decrease in the width of the ridge, adequate-diameter root-form implants (~5mm) usually can be placed. However, as the resorption process continues, the residual ridge continues to progressively shift toward the palate until the ridge is significantly resorbed into a medially positioned narrower bone volume.[8] This results in the buccal cusp and central fossa of the final restoration being cantilevered facially to satisfy esthetic requirements at the expense of biomechanics in the moderate to severe atrophic ridges. This cantilevered part

of the prosthesis is usually in the form of a ridge lap pontic area, which in most cases results in hygiene difficulties.

Resultant Poor Bone Density

In general, the bone quality is poorest in the posterior maxilla, compared with any other intraoral region.[9] A literature review of clinical studies reveals that the poorest bone density may decrease implant loading survival by an average of 16%, and it has been reported as low as 40%.[10] The cause of these failures is related to several factors. Bone strength is directly related to its density, and the poor-density bone of this region is often 5 to 10 times weaker, compared with bone found in the anterior mandible. Bone densities directly influence the bone-to-implant contact percentage (BIC), which accounts for the force transmission to the bone. The BIC is least in D4 bone, and the stress patterns in this bone migrate farther toward the apex of the implant (Fig. 37.4). As a result, bone loss is more pronounced and also occurs along the implant body, rather than only crestally, as in other denser bone conditions. D4 bone also exhibits the greatest biomechanical elastic modulus difference compared with titanium under load.[11] Earlier studies and surgical protocols did not take into consideration the poor BIC in this area.

In the posterior maxilla, the deficient osseous structures and an absence of cortical plate on the crest of the ridge is often observed, which further compromises the initial implant stability at the time of insertion. The labial cortical plate is thin, and the ridge is often wide. As a result, the lateral cortical BIC to stabilize the implant is often insignificant. The implant placement protocol often uses bone compression (osseodensification) rather than bone extraction (removal) to create the implant osteotomy to compensate for these deficiencies. If the surgical protocol is not modified, the initial healing of an implant in D4 bone will be compromised.

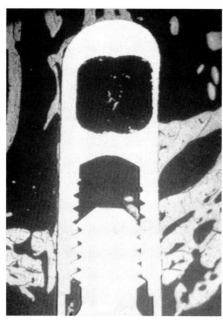

• **Fig. 37.4** Bone–implant contact percent is often reduced in the posterior maxilla because the quality of bone is poorer than other regions of the mouth. This histologic slide depicts the numerous areas of no bone contact at the implant interface.

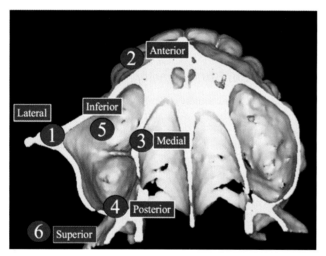

• **Fig. 37.5** Maxillary sinus is comprised of six walls that contain significant anatomic and vital structures, which are important in the placement of implants. *1*, Lateral, *2*, anterior, *3*, medial, *4*, posterior, *5*, inferior, *6*, superior.

Bony Walls

The maxillary sinus features six bony walls, each of which contain important anatomic structures that play a significant role in the treatment of the maxillary posterior region. The implant clinician must have a strong understanding and foundation of the bony walls associated with the posterior maxilla in the preoperative assessment before surgical procedures (Fig. 37.5)

Anterior Wall

The anterior wall of the maxillary sinus consists of thin, compact bone extending from the orbital rim to just above the apex of the cuspid. With the loss of the canine, the anterior wall of the antrum may approximate the crest of the residual ridge. Within the anterior wall and approximately 6 to 7 mm below the orbital rim, with anatomic variants as far as 14 mm from the orbital rim, is the infraorbital foramen (Fig. 37.6A). The infraorbital nerve runs along the roof of the sinus and exits through the foramen. The infraorbital blood vessels and nerves lie directly on the superior wall of the maxillary sinus and within the sinus mucosa.

Tenderness to pressure over the infraorbital foramen or redness of the overlying skin may indicate inflammation of the sinus membrane from infection or trauma, which may contraindicate graft surgery until resolution. In patients exhibiting anatomic variants of the infraorbital foramen, neurosensory impairment may occur during retraction of this area, leading to neurapraxia type injuries. The use of worn, sharp-edged retractors should be avoided when reflecting tissue superiorly in this area to avoid potential injuries. Within the anterior wall of the sinus, the thinnest part is the canine fossa, which is directly above the canine tooth. The anterior wall of the maxillary sinus may also serve as surgical access during Caldwell-Luc procedures to treat a preexisting or post–sinus graft, pathologic condition.

Superior Wall

The superior wall of the maxillary sinus coincides with the thin inferior orbital floor. The orbital floor slants inferiorly in a mediolateral direction and is convex into the sinus cavity.

A bony ridge is usually present in this wall that houses the infraorbital canal, which contains the infraorbital nerve and associated blood vessels. Dehiscence of the bony chamber may be present, resulting in direct contact between the infraorbital structures and the sinus mucosa.

Ocular symptoms may result from infections or tumors in the superior aspects of the sinus region and may include proptosis (bulging of the eye) and diplopia (double vision). When these problems occur, the patient is closely supervised, and a medical consult is advised to decrease the risk of severe complications that may result from the spread of infection in a superior direction. Superior-spreading infections may lead to significant ocular problems or brain abscesses. As a result, when ocular or cerebral symptoms appear, aggressive therapy to decrease the spread of infection is indicated. Overpacking the maxillary sinus with bone graft material during a sinus graft may result in pressure against the superior wall if a sinus infection develops (see Fig. 37.6B).

Posterior Wall

The posterior wall of the maxillary sinus corresponds to the pterygomaxillary region, which separates the antrum from the infratemporal fossa. The posterior wall usually has several vital structures in the region of the pterygomaxillary fossa, including the internal maxillary artery, pterygoid plexus, sphenopalatine ganglion, and greater palatine nerve. The posterior wall should always be identified radiographically because when the wall is not present, a pathologic condition (including neoplasms) is to be suspected (see Fig. 37.6C).

Common donor sites to obtain autogenous bone for sinus augmentation procedures include the tuberosity area. Special consideration should be taken for the posterior extent of the tuberosity removal. Aggressive tuberosity removal may lead to bleeding in the infratemporal fossa (pterygoid plexus), resulting in life-threatening situations.

It should be noted that pterygoid implants placed through the posterior sinus wall and into this region may approach vital structures, including the maxillary artery. A blind surgical technique to place a pterygoid implant through the posterior wall may have increased surgical risk. However, they are of benefit primarily

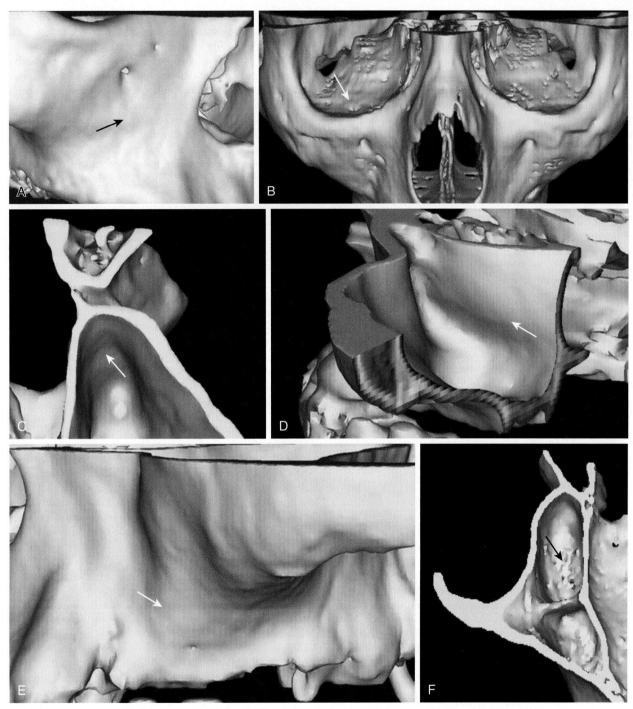

• **Fig. 37.6** Six bony walls of the maxillary sinus. (A) Anterior. (B) Superior. (C) Posterior. (D) Medial. (E) Lateral. (F) Inferior.

when third or fourth molars are needed for prosthetic reconstruction or sinus grafts are contraindicated and available bone posterior to the antrum is present.

Medial Wall

The medial wall of the antrum coincides with the lateral wall of the nasal cavity and is the most complex of the various walls of the sinus. On the nasal aspect, the lower section of the medial wall parallels the lower meatus and floor of the nasal fossa; the upper aspect corresponds to the middle meatus. The medial wall is usually vertical and smooth on the antral side (see Fig. 37.6D).

The main drainage avenue of the maxillary sinus is through the maxillary ostium. The primary ostium is located in the superior aspect of the sinus medial wall and drains its secretions via the ethmoid infundibulum through the hiatus semilunaris into the middle meatus of the nasal cavity. The infundibulum is approximately 5 to 10 mm long and drains via ciliary action in a superior and medial direction. The ostium diameter averages 2.4 mm in health; however, pathologic conditions may alter the size to vary from 1 to 17 mm.[12]

The maxillary ostium and infundibulum are part of the anterior ethmoid middle meatal complex, the region through which the frontal and maxillary sinuses drain, which is primarily responsible for mucociliary clearance of the sinuses to the nasopharynx. As a result, obstruction in one or more areas of the complex will usually result in rhinosinusitis or lead to morbidity of the graft or implant. Patency of the maxillary ostium is most crucial preoperatively and postoperatively during maxillary graft sinus surgery to prevent infection and morbidity of the graft. Evaluating the patency of the ostium via cone beam computerized tomography (CBCT) is easily accomplished with evaluation of serial cross-sectional images. The patency of the ostium must be ascertained before surgery to prevent or minimize postoperative complications. This is easily verified via coronal or cross-sectional images on CBCT surveys. Of utmost importance when performing any procedure involving the maxillary sinus, the patency of the ostium must be maintained throughout the postoperative period. If ostium patency is compromised, increased morbidity of the implant or graft will occur because the mucociliary action of the maxillary sinus will be compromised.

Smaller, accessory or secondary ostia may be present that are usually located in the middle meatus posterior to the main ostium. These additional ostia are most likely the result of chronic sinus inflammation and mucous membrane breakdown. They are present in approximately 30% of patients, ranging from a fraction of a millimeter to 0.5 cm, and are commonly found within the membranous fontanelles of the lateral nasal wall.[13] Fontanelles are usually classified either as anterior fontanelles (AFs) or posterior fontanelles (PFs) and are termed by their relation to the uncinated process. These weak areas in the sinus wall are sometimes used to create additional openings into the sinus for treatment of chronic sinus infections. Primary and secondary ostia may, on occasion, combine and form a large ostium within the infundibulum.

Lateral Wall

The lateral wall of the maxillary sinus forms the posterior maxilla and the zygomatic process. This wall varies greatly in thickness from several millimeters in dentate patients to less than 1 mm in an edentulous patient. A CBCT examination will reveal the osseous thickness of the lateral wall, which is crucial in defining the osteotomy location and preparation technique. Patients exhibiting increased parafunction forces will have thicker lateral walls (see Fig. 37.6E). The lateral wall thickness of the maxilla has been noted to be extremely variable, with some cases being nonexistent. This will lead to an increased possibility of membrane perforation, even occurring on reflection. In contrast, the lateral wall may be very thick, which is usually seen with patients that exhibit parafunction and have just recently lost the posterior teeth. In these situations, lateral wall sinus grafting becomes very difficult because of the cortical thickness. The lateral wall houses the intraosseous anastomosis of the infraorbital and posterior superior alveolar artery, which may lead to a bleeding complication because this area is the site for osteotomy preparation of the lateral wall sinus graft procedure.

Inferior Wall

The inferior wall or floor of the maxillary sinus is in close relationship with the apices of the maxillary molars and premolars. The teeth usually are separated from the sinus mucosa by a thin layer of bone; however, on occasion, teeth may perforate the floor of the sinus and be in direct contact with the sinus lining. Studies have shown that the first molar has the most common dehiscent tooth root, occurring up to approximately 30% to 40% of the time.[14] In dentate patients the sinus floor is approximately at the level of

the nasal floor. In the edentulous posterior maxilla the sinus floor is often 1 cm below the level of the nasal floor (see Fig. 37.6F).

Radiographically, the sinus inferior floor morphology is easily seen via 3D imaging. The floor is rarely flat and smooth; the presence of irregularities and septa should be determined and their exact locations noted. Irregular floors are most often seen after teeth are extracted, leaving residual bony crests that increase risk of perforation because of the difficulty in membrane reflection. In some cases, the bony crests are not even seen on the CBCT evaluation.

Complete or incomplete bony septa may exist on the floor in a vertical or horizontal plane. Approximately 30% of dentate maxillae have septa, with three-fourths appearing in the premolar region. Complete septa separating the sinus into compartments are very rare, occurring in only 1.0% to 2.5% of maxillary sinuses.[15] The presence of septa complicate lateral wall sinus graft procedures, which leads to an increased likelihood of membrane perforation.

Ostiomeatal Complex

The ostiomeatal unit is composed of the maxillary ostium, ethmoid infundibulum, anterior ethmoid cells, hiatus semilunaris, and the frontal recess, which encompasses the area of the middle meatus. This common channel allows for air flow and mucociliary drainage of the frontal, maxillary, and anterior ethmoid sinuses. Blockage in this area leads to impaired drainage of the maxillary, frontal, and ethmoid sinuses, which may result in rhinosinusitis and postoperative complications after implant or grafting procedures.

Radiographic identification of the ostiomeatal complex and related structures must be evaluated to prevent potential postoperative complications. Pathology or variations within the ostiomeatal complex may lead to postoperative sinus graft morbidity or implant complications caused by compromised mucociliary drainage (alteration of normal sinus physiology) of the maxillary sinus.

Blood Supply and Sensory Innervation

The vascular supply in the maxillary sinus is a vital part of the healing and regeneration of bone after a sinus graft and healing of a dental implant. The blood supply to the maxillary sinus is derived from the maxillary artery, which emanates from the external carotid artery. The maxillary artery supplies the bone surrounding the sinus cavity and also the sinus membrane. Branches of the maxillary artery, which most often include the posterior superior alveolar artery and infraorbital artery, form endosseous and extraosseous anastomoses that encompass the maxillary sinus. The formation of the endosseous and extraosseous anastomoses in the maxillary sinus is termed the double arterial arcade. Studies have shown vascularization of postgraft material to depend on the intraosseous and extraosseous anastomoses, along with the blood vessels of the Schneiderian membrane, which is supplied by the posterior superior alveolar artery and the infraorbital artery along the lateral wall.[16]

There exist different factors that alter the vascularization in this area. With increasing age, the number and size of blood vessels in the maxilla decrease. As bone resorption increases, the cortical bone becomes thin, resulting in less vascularization. As the lateral wall becomes thinner, the blood supply to the lateral wall and lateral aspect of the bone graft comes primarily from the periosteum, resulting in a compromised vascularization to the region.

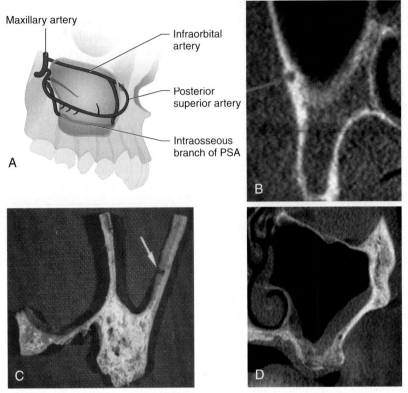

• **Fig. 37.7** Blood supply of the maxillary sinus. (A) Extraosseous and intraosseous anastomosis, which is made up of the infraorbital and posterior superior artery. (B) Cross-sectional cone beam computerized tomography image depicting intraosseous anastomosis *(arrow)*. (C) Intraosseous notch *(arrow)* containing the intraosseous anastomosis, which comprises the posterior superior artery and infraorbital artery. (D) Posterior lateral nasal artery location in the medial wall of the maxillary sinus. *PSA,* Posterior Superior Artery.

Extraosseous Anastomosis

The extraosseous anastomosis is found in approximately 44% of the population and is usually in close approximation to the periosteum of the lateral wall.

The extraosseous anastomosis is superior to the endosseous unit, which is approximately 15 to 20 mm from the dentate alveolar crest. To minimize vascular trauma to the extraosseous anastomosis, surgical and anatomic considerations should be addressed. Ideally, vertical incisions should be made as short as possible to decrease the possibility of blood vessel damage. It is crucial to gain adequate access to the lateral aspect of the maxilla, and the periosteum should be reflected full thickness with great care. Haphazard reflection may lead to severing or damage to the anastomosis, with resultant postoperative edema. Severing of the extraosseous anastomosis may result in significant increased bleeding during the surgical procedure. This intraoperative complication may give rise to impaired visibility for the clinician, along with increased surgery duration. Additionally, postoperative complications such as pain, edema, and ecchymosis may result from the severing of these blood vessels. If trauma to these vessels occurs, direct pressure or the use of electrocautery may be used. However, electrocautery may potentially cause membrane damage or necrosis. If severe bleeding occurs, curved Kelly hemostats are used to clamp the bleeding vessel, followed by ligature placement. A slowly resorbable suture with high tensile strength such as Vicryl is recommended.

Intraosseous Anastomosis

The intraosseous anastomosis is found within the lateral wall of the sinus, which supplies the lateral wall and the sinus membrane. In an edentulous maxilla with posterior vertical bone loss, the endosseous anastomosis may be 5 to 10 mm from the edentulous ridge. The endosseous artery has been shown to be observed on CBCT scans in approximately one-half of the patients requiring a sinus graft.[17] However, anatomic cadaver studies have shown the prevalence to be 100%.[17] In 82% of cases, the most common anatomic location was observed between the canine and second premolar region.[18] However, with a long-term edentulous patient with a thin lateral wall, the artery may be atrophied and almost nonexistent.

Surgical, radiographic, and anatomic considerations should be addressed to minimize trauma to these blood vessels. The CBCT radiographic identification is extremely important in identifying these blood vessels before surgery so preparation may be made. Radiographically, smaller anastomoses will not be seen if the pixel size (~1.0 mm) is less than one-half the size of the anastomosis vessel. Studies have shown that the use of a 0.3 or 0.4 CBCT pixel size for radiographic evaluation will most likely show the smaller anastomoses.[19]

Studies have shown that in 20% of lateral wall osteotomies significant bleeding complications may occur,[20] mainly because the anastomosis is greater than 1.0 mm in diameter. It has been shown that vessels larger than 1.0 mm are more problematic and associated with significant bleeding, whereas smaller vessels (<1.0 mm) are usually insignificant and easily managed (Fig. 37.7; Box 37.1).

In most cases, bleeding is a minor complication and of short duration; however, in some instances it may be significant and difficult to manage. To control bleeding, there are many possible treatments: (1) the patient should be repositioned into an upright position and pressure applied with a surgical gauze; (2) electrocautery may be used, although this may lead to membrane necrosis and perforation, with possible migration of graft material; (3) a second window may be made proximal to the bleeding source to gain access to the bleeding vessel, especially if location cannot be obtained from the original window; and (4) cutting the bone and vessel with a high-speed diamond with no irrigation (which cauterizes the vessel).

Posterior Lateral Nasal Artery

A posterior lateral nasal artery (branch of the sphenopalatine artery that also rises from the maxillary artery) supplies the medial aspect of the sinus cavity. The medial and posterior walls of the maxillary sinus mucosa receive their blood supply from the posterior lateral nasal artery.

During sinus graft surgery the clinician may be in close approximation to this artery when elevating the membrane off the medial wall. Care should be exercised to minimize trauma to this area because aggressive reflection of the membrane may result in trauma to the blood vessel or perforation into the nasal cavity.

Trauma to this artery may cause significant bleeding in the sinus proper and also within the nasal cavity. Because the medial sinus wall is very thin (usually one-half the thickness of the lateral wall), aggressive membrane reflection may result in trauma, leading to bleeding issues.

Sphenopalatine/Infraorbital Arteries

The sphenopalatine artery is also a branch of the maxillary artery and enters the nasal cavity through the sphenopalatine foramen, which is near the posterior portion of the superior meatus of the nose.

As the sphenopalatine artery exits the foramen, it branches into the posterior lateral nasal artery and the posterior septal artery.[21] Additionally, the infraorbital artery enters the maxillary sinus via the infraorbital fissure in the roof of the sinus and ascends cranially into the orbital cavity. Because of the anatomic locations of these blood vessels, it is rarely a concern with respect to sinus graft surgery.

The sphenopalatine and infraorbital blood vessels are usually not problematic for bleeding complications during lateral-approach sinus elevation surgery because of their anatomic locations. However, incorrect incision locations and aggressive reflection may damage the blood vessels. If bleeding does occur, it is usually easily controlled with pressure and local hemostatic agents.

Maxillary Sinus Mucosa

The epithelial lining of the maxillary sinus is a continuation of the nasal mucosa and is classified as a pseudostratified, ciliated columnar epithelium, which is also called the respiratory epithelium.

The epithelial lining of the maxillary sinus is much thinner and contains fewer blood vessels than the nasal epithelium. This accounts for the membrane's pale color and bluish hue. Five primary cell types exist in this tissue: (1) ciliated columnar epithelial cells, (2) nonciliated columnar cells, (3) basal cells, (4) goblet cells, and (5) seromucinous cells. The ciliated cells contain approximately 50 to 200 cilia per cell. In a healthy maxillary sinus the cilia cells assist in clearing mucus from the sinus and into the nasopharynx. The nonciliated cells compose the apical aspect of the membrane, contain microvilli, and serve to increase surface area. These cells have been theorized to facilitate humidification and warming of inspired air. The basal cell's function is similar to that of a stem cell that can differentiate as needed. The goblet cells in the maxillary sinus produce glycoproteins that are responsible for the viscosity and elasticity of the mucus produced. The maxillary sinus contains the highest concentration of goblet cells compared with the other paranasal sinuses. The maxillary sinus membrane also exhibits few elastic fibers attached to the bone (no tenacious attachment is usually present), which simplifies elevation of this tissue from the bone during grafting procedures. The thickness of the sinus mucosa in health varies, but it is generally 0.3 to 0.8 mm.[22] In smokers, it varies from very thin and almost nonexistent to very thick, with a squamous type of epithelium.

Radiographically, normal, healthy paranasal sinuses reveal a completely radiolucent (dark) maxillary sinus. Any radiopaque (whitish) area within the sinus cavity is abnormal, and a pathologic condition should be suspected. The normal sinus membrane is radiographically invisible, whereas any inflammation or thickening of this structure will be radiopaque. The density of the diseased tissue or fluid accumulation will be proportional to varying degrees of gray values.

Maintaining the integrity of the sinus membrane is crucial in decreasing postoperative complications, including loss of graft material and the possibility of infection.

Many factors may alter the physiology of the sinus mucosa, such as viruses, bacteria, and foreign bodies (implants). Care should be taken to minimize membrane perforations during surgery. If perforations occur, appropriate repair treatment protocols should be followed.

Maxillary Sinus Mucociliary Clearance

Normal mucociliary flow is crucial to maintaining the healthy physiology of the maxillary sinus. In a healthy sinus an adequate system of mucus production, clearance, and drainage is maintained. The key to normal sinus physiology is the proper function of the cilia, which is the main component of the mucociliary transport system. The cilia move contaminants toward the natural ostium and then to the nasopharynx. The cilia of the columnar epithelium beat toward the ostium at approximately 15 cycles per minute, with a stiff stroke through the serous layer, reaching into the mucoid layer. They recover with a limp reverse stroke within the serous layer. This mechanism slowly propels the mucoid layer toward the ostium at a rate of 9 mm per minute and into the middle meatus of the nose.[22]

In health, mucoid fluid is transported toward the ostium of the maxillary sinus and drains into the nasal cavity, eliminating inhaled small particles and microorganisms. This mucociliary transport system is an active transport system that relies heavily on oxygen. The amount of oxygen absorbed from the blood is not adequate to maintain this drainage system; additional oxygen has to be absorbed from the air in the sinus. This is why the patency of the ostium is crucial in maintaining the normal transport system.

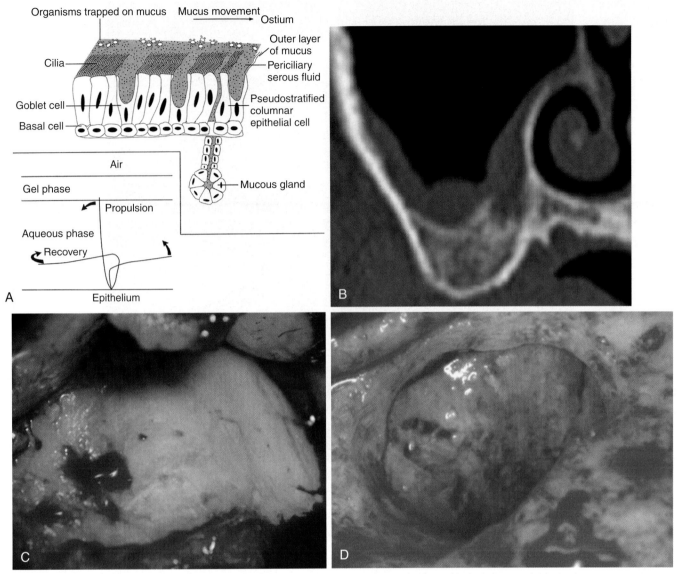

• **Fig. 37.8** Maxillary sinus membrane (Schneiderian Membrane). (A) The pseudostratified columnar epithelium cells have 50 to 200 cilia per cell that beat toward the ostium to help clear 1 L of mucus from goblet and mucous glands each day from the sinus. In health, the mucous has two layers: a bottom serous layer and top mucoid layer. The cilia beat with a stiff stroke in the mucoid layer toward the ostium and a relaxed recovery stroke within the serous layer. (B) Cross-sectional image depicting an inflamed Schneiderian membrane. If the sinus membrane is of normal thickness, it will not be visible on a radiograph. (C) Clinical image depicting the thinness of the lateral wall and show through *(dark blue)* of the Schneiderian membrane. (D) Bluish hue of the membrane after lateral wall window preparation.

Various elements may decrease the number of cilia and slow their beating efficiency. Viral infections, pollution, allergic reactions, and certain medications may affect the cilia in this way. Genetic disorders (e.g., dyskinetic cilia syndrome) and factors such as long-standing dehydration, anticholinergic medications and antihistamines, cigarette smoke, and chemical toxins also can affect ciliary action[23] (Fig. 37.8).

An alteration in the sinus ostium patency or the quality of secretions can lead to disruption in ciliary action, which may result in rhinosinusitis. For clearance to be maintained, adequate ventilation is necessary. Ventilation and drainage are dependent on the ostiomeatal unit, which is the main sinus opening. Ciliary movements of ciliated epithelial cells dictate clearance of the maxillary sinus. It is important to maintain the patency of the maxillary ostium and the ostiomeatal complex in the postoperative period to minimize the possibility of complications.

The physiologic mucociliary transport system may be compromised by abnormalities in the cilia, which include a decrease in overall ciliary number and poor coordination of their movement. This altered physiology may result in an increased morbidity of implant placement or bone graft healing. Therefore it is crucial that the mucociliary drainage mechanism be maintained throughout the postoperative treatment period. This is most likely accomplished with good surgical technique, evaluation and treatment of prior drainage issues, and strict adherence to the use of pharmacologic agents (e.g., antibiotics, corticosteroids).

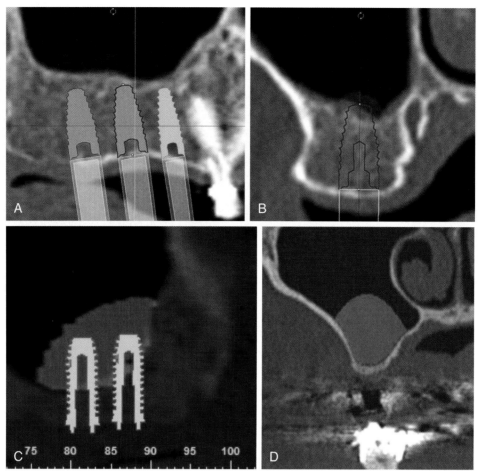

• **Fig. 37.9** Subantral augmentation classification. (A) SA-1: implant placement that does not extend into the maxillary sinus proper. (B) SA-2: implant placement that elevates the sinus membrane approximately 1 to 2 mm without bone grafting. (C) SA-3: implant placement and simultaneous bone grafting by either a crestal or lateral-wall approach. (D) SA-4: lateral wall sinus augmentation with delayed implant placement.

Maxillary Sinus Bacterial Flora

There is much debate on the bacterial flora of the maxillary sinus. Maxillary sinuses have been considered to be generally sterile in health; however, bacteria can colonize within the sinus without producing symptoms. In theory, the mechanism by which a sterile environment is maintained includes the mucociliary clearance system, immune system, and the production of nitric oxide within the sinus cavity. In recent endoscopic studies, normal sinuses were shown to be nonsterile, with 62.3% exhibiting bacterial colonization. The most common bacteria cultured were *Streptococcus viridans, Staphylococcus epidermidis,* and *S. pneumoniae.*[24] The culture findings for secretions in acute maxillary sinusitis yielded high numbers of leukocytes, *S. pneumoniae,* or *S. pyogenes,* with *Haemophilus influenzae* being recovered from the purulent exudates with lower numbers of staphylococci. Other reports have indicated the bacterial flora of the maxillary sinus consists of nonhemolytic and alpha hemolytic streptococci, as well as *Neisseria* spp. Additional microorganisms identifiable in various quantities belong to staphylococci, *Haemophilus* spp., pneumococci, *Mycoplasma* spp., and *Bacteroides* spp. This is important to note because the sinus graft procedure often violates the sinus mucosa, and bacteria may contaminate the graft site, leading to postoperative complications.

The implant clinician must understand the importance of reducing the bacterial count and possible microorganisms that may initiate infections in the maxillary sinus. A strict aseptic technique should be adhered to during any surgical procedures that invade the maxillary sinus proper. This will minimize the possibility of bacterial colonization within the graft, which may lead to increased morbidity. The type of bacteria inhabiting the sinus is very important because it dictates what antibiotic is prescribed preoperatively, postoperatively, and therapeutically in case of infection. The most common bacteria present in the sinus must be susceptible to the specific antibiotic to prevent infection and decrease the morbidity of the graft. The antibiotic selected should not be the clinician's "favorite"; instead it should be the most ideal antibiotic, which is specific for the involved bacteria. Ideally, Augmentin (875/125 mg) has been shown to be most effective antibiotic for bacterial infections in the maxillary sinus.

Maxillary Sinus: Clinical Assessment

To establish adequate osseous morphology for the placement of endosteal implants in the resorbed maxillary posterior region, various grafting techniques have been developed to increase bone volume. In 1987 Misch[25] developed four different categories for the treatment of the posterior maxilla (termed subantral [SA]) as SA-1 through SA-4 and was later modified and updated by Resnik in 2017 (Fig. 37.9). The SA-1 posterior maxilla allows implant placement inferior to the sinus cavity, without penetration into

TABLE 37.1	Preoperative and Postoperative Physical Examination
Site	Signs of Infection
Inferior wall	Bulge in hard palate, ill-fitting denture, loose teeth, hypesthesia or nonvital teeth, bleeding, palatal erosion, oroantral fistula
Medial wall	Nasal obstruction, nasal discharge, epistaxis, cacosmia, visible mass in nostril
Anterior wall	Swelling, pain, skin changes
Posterior wall	Midface pain, hypesthesia of one-half of face, loss of function of lower cranial nerves
Superior wall	Diplopia (double vision), proptosis (eye bulging out), chemosis, pain or hypesthesia, decreased visual acuity

the sinus proper. Because the sinus floor is not altered, a preexisting sinus pathology or anatomic variant will be less likely to affect the healing process. As such, if the patient has a preexisting maxillary sinus condition or develops a sinus infection after implant placement, then implants are not at risk of becoming contaminated. However, the SA-2 to SA-4 surgical procedures do alter the sinus membrane and sinus floor. With these treatment options, a thorough preoperative evaluation is completed to rule out any existing pathologic condition in the maxillary sinus. In this way, the risk of possible mucus or bacteria contaminating the graft and creating a bacterial smear layer on the implant is reduced. Therefore the possibility of impaired bone formation during healing is reduced. In addition, because of the proximity of the maxillary sinus to numerous vital structures, postoperative complications can be very severe and even life-threatening.

Pathologic conditions associated with the paranasal sinuses are common ailments and afflict more than 31 million people each year. Approximately 16 million people will seek medical assistance related to sinusitis; yet sinusitis is one of the most commonly overlooked diseases in clinical practice. Potential infection in the region of the sinuses may result in severe complications. Infections in this area have been reported to result in sinusitis, orbital cellulitis, meningitis, osteomyelitis, and cavernous sinus thrombosis. In fact, paranasal sinus infection accounts for approximately 5% to 10% of all brain abscesses reported each year.[26]

A physical examination of the maxillary sinus evaluates the middle third of the face for the presence of asymmetry, deformity, swelling, erythema, ecchymosis, hematoma, or facial tenderness (Table 37.1). Nasal congestion or obstruction, prevalent nasal discharge, epistaxis (bleeding from the nose), anosmia (the loss of the sense of smell), and/or halitosis (bad breath) are noted.

The clinical examination for maxillary rhinosinusitis concerns the regions surrounding the maxillary antrum. The examination is conducted to assess each wall surrounding the maxillary sinus separately. The infraorbital foramen on the facial wall of the antrum is palpated through the soft tissue of the cheeks or intraorally to determine whether tenderness or discomfort is present. The intraoral examination assesses the floor of the antrum by alveolar ulceration, expansion, tenderness, paresthesia, and oroantral fistulae. The eyes are examined to evaluate

the superior wall of the sinus for proptosis, pupillary level, lack of eye movement, and diplopia. The nasal fluids may be used to evaluate the medial wall of the sinus by asking the patient to blow the nose in a waxed paper. The mucus should be clear and thin in nature. A yellow or greenish tint or thickened discharge indicates infection. Infected maxillary sinuses typically are symptomatic, which can exhibit exudate in the middle meatus and may be inspected with a nasal speculum and headlight (rhinoscopy) through the nares. The methods of examination of the infected maxillary sinus may include transillumination, nasoendoscopy, bacteriology, cytology, fiberoptic antroscopy, and radiography CBCT, or magnetic resonance imaging [MRI]).

Maxillary Sinus Radiographic Evaluation

Various radiographic techniques have been used in implant dentistry to evaluate the maxillary posterior region. In the early days of oral implantology, evaluation of this area was limited to 2-dimensional (2D) radiographs. However, these types of radiographs have inherent disadvantages that are affected by magnification and distortion, which leads to errors in diagnosis and treatment planning. Currently, this anatomic area is evaluated mainly by the use of 3D radiographic techniques (CBCT) or medical CT because they have become more accurate and efficient, with a significant reduced radiation.

Cone Beam Computerized Tomography

CBCT surveys have allowed the implant clinician to evaluate anatomic structures, anatomic variants, and pathologies more accurately. Many software programs are available that allow combining 3D images with computer software and allow an accurate assessment of the maxillary sinus. Because visualization of the maxillary sinus and surrounding structures are crucial for the proper diagnosis and treatment planning, it is highly suggested the implant clinician utilize CBCT anytime procedures involve the maxillary sinus.

Presently, no radiographic modality provides more information about the paranasal sinuses than CBCT. This type of radiography provides much more detailed information about the anatomy and pathologic condition of the sinuses compared with 2D radiography. Studies have concluded that CBCT is the best option for viewing the surrounding osseous structures and pathologic condition in the maxillary sinuses.[27,28]

The maxillary sinus can be evaluated with most CBCT images, including reformatted axial, panoramic, cross-sectional, sagittal, and 3D images. Most physicians use the coronal radiographs to evaluate the paranasal sinuses. The implant clinician must have a clear understanding of the CBCT radiographic anatomy and the pathologic conditions associated with the posterior maxilla and maxillary sinus regions.

Normal Anatomy

Maxillary Sinus Membrane (Schneiderian Membrane)

A CBCT scan of normal, healthy paranasal sinuses reveals a completely radiolucent (dark) maxillary sinus. Any radiopaque (whitish) area within the sinus cavity is abnormal, and a pathologic condition should be suspected. The normal sinus membrane is radiographically invisible, whereas any inflammation or thickening of this structure will be radiopaque. The density of the diseased tissue or fluid accumulation will be proportional to varying degrees of gray values.

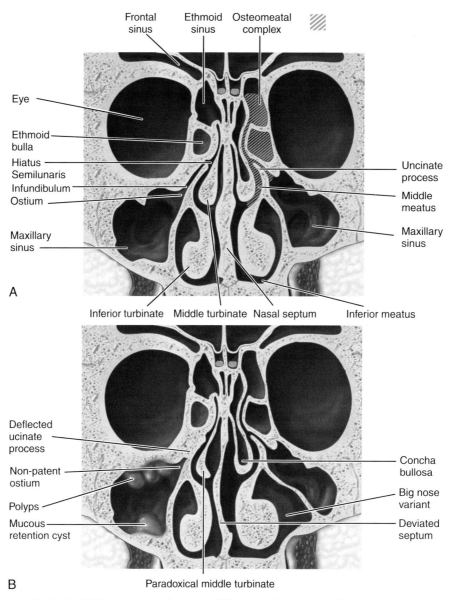

• **Fig. 37.10** (A) Normal paranasal anatomy. (B) Paranasal pathology and anatomic variants.

Ostiomeatal Complex

The ostiomeatal unit is composed of the maxillary ostium, ethmoid infundibulum, anterior ethmoid cells, and the frontal recess. The main drainage avenue of the maxillary sinus is through the ostium. The maxillary ostium is bounded superiorly by the ethmoid sinuses and inferiorly by the uncinate process. The uncinate process is a bony knifelike projection that is attached inferiorly to the inferior turbinate and posteriorly has a free margin. Drainage continues through the ostium into the infundibulum, which is a narrow passageway leading into the middle meatus. The middle meatus is the radiolucent space bounded by the middle and inferior turbinates.

Nasal Cavity

Within the nasal cavity, three nasal turbinates or conchae (superior, middle, and inferior) exist and are small downward projections of bone. Between the turbinates is a space or recess termed a meatus. The respiratory epithelium covers the turbinates and meatus and warms, moistens, and cleans the air that is respirated into the lungs.

The nasal septum is the bony partition that creates a barrier between the right and left sides of the nasal cavity. Obstructions within any aspect of the nasal system predispose the area to pathologic conditions (Fig. 37.10).

Maxillary Sinus: Anatomical Variants

Numerous anatomic variants arise that can predispose a patient to postsurgical complications. When these conditions are noted, a pharmacologic protocol may need to be altered and/or implants may be placed after the sinus graft has matured, rather than predisposing them to an increased risk by inserting them at the same time as the sinus graft. As stated previously, patency of the ostium is paramount to maintain drainage. Preexisting skeletal and bony abnormalities of the ostiomeatal complex may compromise the patency of the maxillary ostium, thereby, predisposing patients to maxillary rhinosinusitis.

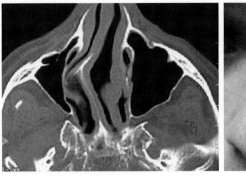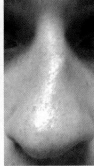

• **Fig. 37.11** Nasal septum deviation is a common variant. Extreme cases may obstruct the ostiomeatal unit and increase the risk of sinusitis after a sinus graft.

Nasal Septum Deviation

A nasal septum deviation is a very common anatomic variant, occurring in as much as 70% of the population older than 14 years. This bony variant in extremes may cause obstruction of the ostiomeatal unit, which results in inflammation from air turbulence, causing increased mucosal drying and particle deposition. If the deviation is long-standing, then atrophy of the middle turbinate may occur, resulting in narrowing of the ostiomeatal complex (Fig. 37.11).[29]

Timmenga and colleagues[30] evaluated 45 patients who received 85 sinus grafts with endoscopy postsurgery. Of the 45 patients, five were found to have sinusitis postsurgery; all five of those patients had a nasal deviation or oversized turbinate. Therefore when these conditions are observed, consideration should be given to not place the implant at the same time as the sinus graft, and the recommended preoperative and postoperative pharmacologic protocol is especially warranted.

Middle Turbinate Variants

The middle turbinate plays a significant role in proper drainage of the maxillary sinus. A concha bullosa is a pneumatization within the middle turbinate and may occlude the ostiomeatal complex, compromising adequate drainage. This variant is seen in approximately 4% to 15% of the population (Fig. 37.12).[31] Another variant in this anatomic structure is a paradoxically curved middle turbinate, which presents a concavity toward the septum, decreasing the size of the meatus. This also predisposes the patient to a higher incidence of sinus disease.

Uncinate Process Variants

The uncinate process is a projection of the ethmoid bone which is located in the wall of the lateral nasal cavity. This bony process is an important anatomic structure in the patency of the ostium. A deflected uncinate process (either laterally or medially) can narrow the ethmoid infundibulum, affecting the ostiomeatal complex. Perforations may also be present within the uncinate process, leading to communication between the nasal cavity and ethmoid infundibulum. In addition, the uncinate process may be pneumatized. Although this is rare, it may compromise adequate clearance and drainage of the maxillary sinus.

Supplemental Ostia

A supplemental ostium or secondary ostia may occur between the maxillary sinus and the middle meatus, which is often found in

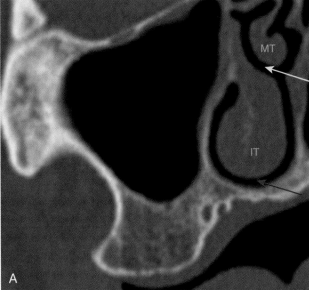

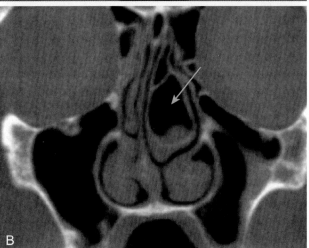

• **Fig. 37.12** (A) Nasal cavity anatomy: inferior turbinate *(IT)*, middle turbinate *(MT)*, inferior meatus *(red arrow)*, middle meatus *(yellow arrow)*. Note the paradoxical middle turbinate. (B) Coronal image depicting concha bullosa (arrow) and deviated septum.

the posterior fontanelles (PF). This may be found in approximately 18% to 30% of individuals. Because these secondary openings are usually located posterior and inferior to the natural ostium, they may predispose the patient to sinusitis by the recirculation of infected secretions from the primary meatus back into the sinus cavity. On occasion, these secondary ostia may be encountered during the elevation of the medial wall of the antrum before placement of the sinus graft. When observed, a piece of collagen is placed over the site to prevent graft material from entering the nasal cavity.

Maxillary Hypoplasia

Hypoplasia of the maxillary sinus may be a direct result from trauma, infection, surgical intervention, or irradiation to the maxilla during the development of the maxillary bone. These conditions interrupt the maxillary growth center, producing a smaller than normal maxilla. A malformed and positioned uncinate process is associated with this disorder, leading to chronic sinus drainage problems. Most often, these patients have adequate bone

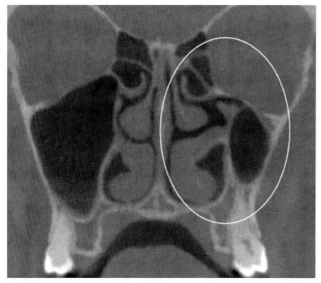

• **Fig. 37.13** Maxillary hypoplasia. Coronal cone beam computerized tomographic view of an abnormally small sized maxillary sinus

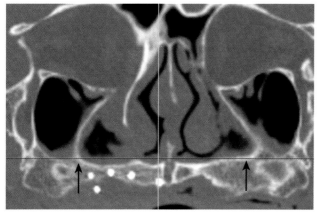

• **Fig. 37.14** Inferior meatus pneumatization (big nose variant). Cone beam computerized tomographic panoramic image depicting the abnormally large nasal cavity extending into the molar area.

height for endosteal implant placement, and a sinus graft is not required to gain vertical height (Fig. 37.13).

Inferior Turbinate and Meatus Pneumatization (Big-Nose Variant)

Misch had observed, on rare occasion, that the inferior third of the nasal cavity pneumatizes within the maxilla and resides over the alveolar residual ridge. An evaluation of 550 computerized tomography (CT) scans of complete or partially edentulous maxillae found this condition in 18 patients (3% incidence). When the patient has this condition, the maxillary sinus is lateral to the edentulous ridge. When inadequate bone height is present below this structure, a sinus graft does not increase available bone height for an implant. This condition is difficult to observe on a two-dimensional panoramic radiograph. If unaware, then the implant can be placed into the nasal cavity above the residual ridge and even penetrate the inferior turbinate. A sinus graft is contraindicated with this patient condition because the sinus is lateral to the position of the implants. Instead, in most cases an onlay graft is required to increase bone height (Fig. 37.14).

Maxillary Sinus Pathology

A pre-existing, pathologic, maxillary sinus condition may be a relative or absolute contraindication for many procedures that will alter the sinus floor before or in conjunction with sinus grafting and/or implant insertion. The risk of postoperative infection is elevated and may compromise the health of the implant and the patient. Therefore pathologic conditions, either preoperative or postoperative, of a maxillary sinus should be evaluated, diagnosed, and treated.

Pathologic conditions of the maxillary sinus may be divided into four categories: (1) inflammatory lesions, (2) cystic lesions, (3) neoplasms, and (4) antroliths and foreign bodies. Studies have shown that 20% to 45% of the asymptomatic population has a subclinical pathologic condition in the maxillary sinus. The author has evaluated approximately 2000 prospective candidates for maxillary sinus augmentation procedures at the Misch International Implant Institute for signs of pathology. The results concluded 38.7% of asymptomatic patients had maxillary sinus pathologic conditions on CBCT scan evaluation. Manji and colleagues evaluated 275 patients and concluded that 45.1% were classified as exhibiting sinus pathology (i.e., 56.5% had mucosal thickening (≥5 mm), 28.2% with polypoidal thickening, 8.9% partial opacification and/or air/fluid level, and 6.5% complete opacification).[32] Because of this increased incidence, it is highly recommended that a thorough radiographic evaluation be completed on all prospective sinus elevation patients.

Inflammatory Disease

Inflammatory conditions can affect the maxillary sinus from odontogenic and nonodontogenic causes.

Odontogenic Rhinosinusitis (Periapical Mucositis)

Odontogenic sinusitis describes a type of sinus disease in which radiographic, microbiologic, and/or clinical evidence indicates it is of a dental origin (i.e., from a tooth). The close proximity of the roots of the maxillary posterior teeth to the floor of the sinus suggest any inflammatory changes in the periodontium or surrounding alveolar bone may result in pathologic conditions in the maxillary sinus.

Etiology. Odontogenic sinusitis is usually the result of an infected tooth (e.g., periapical abscess, cyst, granuloma, periodontal disease) that causes an expansile lesion within the floor of the sinus. Periapical inflammation has been shown to be capable of affecting the sinus mucosa, with and without perforation of the cortical bone of the sinus floor. Infection and inflammatory mediators are capable of spreading directly or via bone marrow, blood vessels, and lymphatics to the maxillary sinus, causing an inflammatory response.[33] Additional etiologic factors include sinus perforations during extractions and foreign bodies (e.g., gutta-percha, root tips, amalgam). Odontogenic rhinosinusitis is often polymicrobial, with anaerobic streptococci, *Bacteroides* spp., *Proteus* spp., and coliform bacilli involved. Studies have shown 10% to 40% of all rhinosinusitis sinusitis cases may have an underlying dental pathology.[34,35]

Radiographic Appearance. The radiographic evaluation of patients with odontogenic sinusitis will most commonly demonstrate a unilateral maxillary sinusitis. A unilateral maxillary odontogenic sinusitis is often overlooked on CBCT scans because they are frequently asymptomatic. Involvement of the ostiomeatal complex may result in extension to adjacent paranasal sinuses (e.g., ethmoid, frontal, sphenoid), ranging from 27% to 60% among patients with odontogenic sinusitis.[36] Odontogenic sinusitis has been shown to exhibit bilateral involvement in 20% of

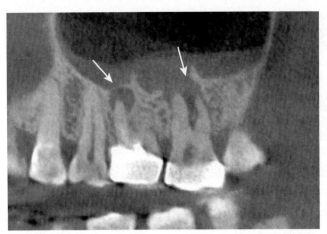

• **Fig. 37.15** Odontogenic rhinosinusitis. Cone beam computerized tomographic panoramic view showing molar roots extending into the maxillary sinus, resulting in inflammation of the sinus membrane. Note the communication between the maxillary molar roots and the maxillary sinuses.

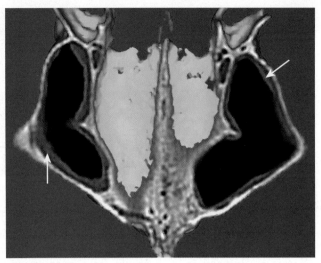

• **Fig. 37.16** Mild mucosal thickening. Three-dimensional axial view showing bilateral mucosal thickening (gray area surrounding the bony walls of the maxillary sinus).

patients. In some cases, a slight thickening of the sinus membrane may be present adjacent to the offending tooth.[37] Usually the radiographic appearance will be a radiopaque band that follows the contours of the sinus floor.

Differential Diagnosis. Odontogenic sinusitis may be confused with acute rhinosinusitis sinusitis; however, acute rhinosinusitis is almost always symptomatic. Mild mucosal thickening from a non-odontogenic origin (e.g., smoking, allergy) may also show similar radiographic signs. However, the nonodontogenic origin may be confirmed from lack of radiographic evidence of a diseased or painful tooth.

Treatment. Before any type of sinus augmentation or implant placement into the sinus, the tooth or teeth involved should be treated periodontally, endodontically, or extracted. After intraoral soft tissue healing and resolution of the pathologic condition (i.e., a minimum of 6 weeks), the bone graft and/or implant may be performed with minimal morbidity. The removal of unhealthy teeth decreases sinus membrane thickening, but most of the time it does not completely resolve it. In addition, epithelial metaplasia with the ciliated mucosa changing to simple cuboidal and stratified squamous keratinized tissue may result. Therefore, depending on the severity, in some cases the mucosal thickness may remain because of the change in epithelia structure and metaplasia changes[6] (Fig. 37.15).

Mild Mucosal Thickening (Nonodontogenic)

Sinus membrane thickening has been shown to be present in approximately 46.7% of patients, with equal distribution between healthy and unhealthy natural teeth.[38] The most common area for the mucosal thickening has been shown to be in the midsagittal sinus region, which is adjacent to the first and second molars. In the literature, it is accepted that mucosal thickening greater than 2 mm is considered a pathologic sinus membrane.[39-42]

Etiology. Local odontogenic issues, such as periapical pathology, periodontal disease, and the health of the adjacent dentition, have been shown to be the etiologic factor in the inflammatory response to the sinus membrane in approximately 50% of cases.[43] However, nonodontogenic factors such as smoking,[44] allergies, sinus congestion, mold, and air pollution may aggravate the sinus mucosa, resulting in mild thickening. Chronic inflammatory conditions may result in altered bacterial flora, along with mucociliary clearance and cilia changes.

Radiographic Appearance. On a CBCT image, usually thickened mucosa will appear as a radiopaque widened membrane. Thickened mucosa can easily be seen when evaluating axial images.

Treatment. Usually no treatment is necessary because mild mucosal thickening is asymptomatic. Studies have shown that slight mucosal thickening allows for sinus grafting procedures to be completed with a decreased incidence of membrane perforation (Fig. 37.16).

Acute Rhinosinusitis

A nonodontogenic pathologic condition may also result in inflammation in the form of sinusitis. The most common type of sinusitis is acute rhinosinusitis (i.e., sinusitis symptoms of less than 3 months). The signs and symptoms of acute rhinosinusitis are rather nonspecific, making it difficult to differentiate from the common cold, influenza type of symptoms, and allergic rhinitis. However, the most common symptoms include purulent nasal discharge, facial pain and tenderness, nasal congestion, and possible fever.

Acute maxillary rhinosinusitis results in 22 to 25 million patient visits to a physician in the United States each year, with a direct or indirect cost of $6 billion. Although four paranasal sinuses exist in the skull, the most common involved in rhinosinusitis are the maxillary and frontal sinuses.[45]

Etiology. An inflammatory process that extends from the nasal cavity after a viral upper respiratory infection often causes acute maxillary sinusitis. Microbiological cultures have shown the most common pathogens causing acute rhinosinusitis are *S. pneumoniae*, *H. influenzae*, and *Moraxella catarrhalis*. These pathogens include approximately 20% to 27% β-lactamase–resistant bacteria. *S. aureus* has also been cited, with the microbiology of acute rhinosinusitis. However, this pathogen is usually only seen in nosocomial (hospital-induced) sinusitis and is unlikely to be seen in an elective sinus graft patient.

The most important factor in the pathogenesis of acute rhinosinusitis is the patency of the maxillary ostium.[46,47] Local predisposing causes of sinusitis include inflammation and edema associated with a viral upper respiratory tract infection or allergic rhinitis. As a consequence, mucous production within the sinus may be abnormal in quality or quantity, along with a compromised

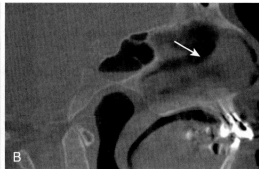

• **Fig. 37.17** Acute rhinosinusitis. (A and B) Flat radiopaque (gray) line within the maxillary sinus, which is termed an air-fluid level and consistent with acute rhinosinusitis.

mucociliary transport. In an occluded ostium, an accumulation of inflammatory cells, bacteria, and mucus exists. Phagocytosis of the bacteria is impaired with immunoglobulin (Ig)-dependent activities decreased by the low concentration of IgA, IgG, and IgM found in infected secretions.

The oxygen tension inside the maxillary sinus has significant effects on pathologic conditions. When the oxygen tension in the sinus is altered, resultant sinusitis occurs. Growth of anaerobic and facultative organisms proliferate in this environment.[48] Many factors may alter the normal oxygen tension within the sinuses. A direct correlation exists between the ostium size and the oxygen tension in the sinus. In patients with recurrent episodes of sinusitis, oxygen tension is often reduced, even when infection is not present. As a consequence, a history of recurrent acute rhinosinusitis is relevant to determine whether a bone graft or dental implant may be at increased risk of morbidity.

Radiographic Appearance. The radiographic hallmark in acute rhinosinusitis is the appearance of an air-fluid level. A line of demarcation will be present between the fluid and the air within the maxillary sinus. If the patient is radiographically positioned supine, then the fluid will accumulate in the posterior area; if the patient is upright during the imaging survey, the fluid will be seen on the floor and horizontal in nature. Additional radiographic signs include smooth, thickened mucosa of the sinus, with possible opacification. In severe cases, the sinus cavity may fill completely with supportive exudates, which gives the appearance of a completely opacified sinus. With these characteristics, the terms pyocele and empyema have been applied.

Treatment. Because acute rhinosinusitis is one of the most common health problems today, patients having sinus grafting procedures should be well screened for a past history and current symptoms. Even though acute rhinosinusitis is a self-limiting disease, a symptomatic patient should be treated and cleared by their physician before any grafting procedures. These patients are also more prone to postoperative rhinosinusitis. As a result, a sinus graft is performed and given a longer healing period before placement of an implant. In addition, the suggested antibiotic coverage may be altered and extended, both before and after the sinus graft procedure (Fig. 37.17).

Chronic Rhinosinusitis

Chronic rhinosinusitis is a term used for a sinusitis that does not resolve in 3 months and also has recurrent episodes. It is the most common chronic disease in the United States, affecting approximately 37 million people. Symptoms of chronic rhinosinusitis are associated with periodic episodes of purulent nasal discharge, nasal congestion, and facial pain.

Etiology. As maxillary rhinosinusitis progresses from the acute phase to the chronic phase, anaerobic bacteria become the predominant pathogens. The microbiology of chronic rhinosinusitis is very difficult to determine because of the inability to acquire accurate cultures. Studies have shown that possible bacteria include *Bacteroides* spp., anaerobic gram-positive cocci, *Fusobacterium* spp., and aerobic organisms (*Streptococcus* spp., *Haemophilus* spp., *Staphylococcus* spp.).[49] A Mayo Clinic study showed that in 96% of patients with chronic rhinosinusitis, active fungal growth was present.[50]

Radiographic Appearance. Chronic rhinosinusitis may appear radiographically as thickened sinus mucosa, complete opacification of the antrum, and/or sclerotic changes in the sinus walls (which give the appearance of denser cortical bone in the lateral walls).

Treatment. Medical evaluation and clearance by an experienced physician in sinus pathology (e.g., otolaryngologist [ENT]) is highly recommended for patients with chronic maxillary rhinosinusitis before any sinus grafting, because significant bacterial resistance and fungal growth is highly probable. Fungal infections are often difficult to treat and control, and serious complications may result in postoperative sinus graft patients. In many chronic rhinosinusitis patients, a sterile and nonpathologic sinus is difficult to obtain, contraindicating (absolute) sinus grafting and/or implants.

Allergic Rhinosinusitis

Etiology. Allergic sinusitis is a local response within the maxillary sinus caused by an irritating allergen in the upper respiratory tract. Therefore allergens may be a cause of acute or chronic rhinosinusitis. This category of sinusitis may be the most common form, with 15% to 56% of patients undergoing endoscopy for sinusitis showing evidence of allergy. Allergic rhinosinusitis often leads to chronic sinusitis in 15% to 60% of patients.[51] The sinus mucosa frequently becomes irregular or lobulated, with resultant polyp formation.

Radiographic Appearance. Polyp formation related to allergic sinusitis is usually characterized by multiple, smooth, rounded, radiopaque shadows on the walls of the maxillary sinus. Most commonly, polyps initially are located near the ostium and are easily observed on a CBCT scan. In advanced cases, ostium occlusion, along with displacement or destruction of the sinus walls, may be present with a radiographic image of a completely opacified sinus.

Treatment. When patients have a history of allergic rhinosinusitis, special attention must be given to a patent ostium, bacterial resistance, and close postoperative supervision. Polyps, if enlarged or too numerous, may be required to be removed before the sinus

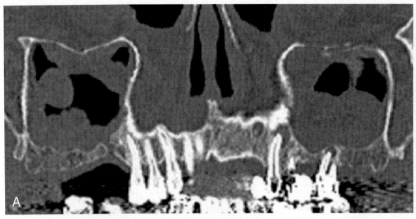
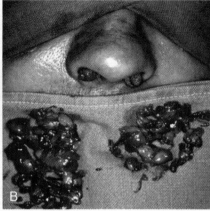

• **Fig. 37.18** Allergic rhinosinusitis. (A) Bilateral polypoid inflammation consistent with allergic rhinosinusitis. (B) Polyp removal on a patient with chronic allergic rhinosinusitis. Unfortunately the polyps have a high incidence of recurrence, and in many cases this contradicts implant treatment.

graft. This may be performed through an anterior Caldwell-Luc approach or by an endoscopic procedure via the maxillary ostium.

Allergic sinusitis patients often have a greater risk of complications related to an increase in allergen production. Because sinus grafting is an elective procedure, the time of year for the surgery may be altered to decrease the postoperative infection risk. For example, if hay fever or a grass allergy is related to the patient's sinusitis, then the sinus graft surgery should be performed in the season or seasons that have least risk to aggravate the sinus mucosa (i.e., winter or fall). In severe cases of polyposis, any procedure violating the sinus proper may be an absolute contraindication (Fig. 37.18).

Fungal Rhinosinusitis (Eosinophilic Fungal Rhinosinusitis)

Granulomatous rhinosinusitis is a very serious (and often overlooked) disorder within the maxillary sinus. Patients who exhibit signs of fungal rhinosinusitis may indicate an extensive history of antibiotic use, chronic exposure to mold or fungus in the environment, or history of immunosuppression. Fungal rhinosinusitis has been categorized into five types: acute necrotizing (fulminant), chronic invasive, chronic granulomatous invasive, fungal hall (sinus mycetoma), and allergic. The first three types are classified as tissue-invasive and the last two are noninvasive fungal rhinosinusitis.[52]

Etiology. Fungal infections are usually caused by aspergillosis, mucormycosis, or histoplasmosis. Chronic rhinosinusitis patients should always be evaluated for granulomatous conditions because a high percentage of fungal growth exists in this patient population. Of concern in these patients is eosinophils are activated that release major basic protein (MBP) into the mucus, which attacks and destroys the fungus. However, this may result in the membrane being irritated and possibly irreversibly damaged, which allows bacteria to proliferate. Three possible clinical signs may differentiate fungal rhinosinusitis from acute or chronic rhinosinusitis; however, a positive diagnosis requires mycological and histologic studies.[53]

1. No response to antibiotic therapy
2. Soft tissue changes in sinus associated with thickened reactive bone, with localized areas of osteomyelitis
3. Association of inflammatory sinus disease that involves the nasal fossa and facial soft tissue

Radiographic Appearance. Granulomatous rhinosinusitis is extremely variable and may appear radiographically as mild

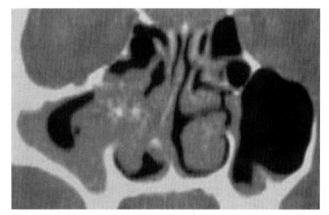

• **Fig. 37.19** Fungal rhinosinusitis. Coronal cone beam computerized tomographic image of fungal rhinosinusitis, which has the radiographic appearance of an opacified sinus with localized highly densified areas.

thickening (less common) to complete opacification (more common) of the sinus. The majority of sinuses show complete opacification with hyperdense areas.[54] Extension beyond the maxillary sinus to other sinuses is common and expansion and erosion of a sinus wall may be present.

Treatment. Patients with a history or current knowledge of fungal rhinosinusitis should be referred to their physician or an ENT for treatment and surgical clearance (i.e., in most cases clearance will not be given because fungal rhinosinusitis is rarely curable). Treatment usually involves debridement and therapy with an antifungal agent, such as amphotericin B (Fig. 37.19).

Cystic Lesions

Cystic type lesions are a common occurrence in the maxillary sinus. They may vary from microscopic lesions to large, destructive, expansile pathologic conditions. Cystic lesions may include pseudocysts, retention cysts, primary mucoceles, and postoperative maxillary cysts.

Pseudocysts (Mucous Retention Cyst)

The most common cysts in the maxillary sinus are mucous retention cysts. After much controversy, in 1984, Gardner[55] distinguished these cysts into two categories: (1) pseudocysts and (2)

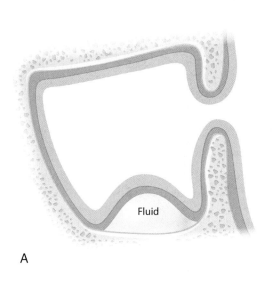

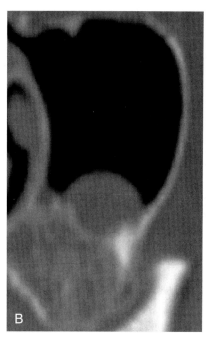

• **Fig. 37.20** Pseudocyst. (A) Diagram showing fluid accumulation underneath the membrane. (B) Radiograph showing the dome-shaped characteristics of a pseudocyst.

retention cysts. Pseudocysts are more common and of much greater concern during sinus graft surgery, compared with retention cysts. Pseudocysts recur in approximately 30% of patients and are often unassociated with sinus symptoms. As a consequence, many physicians do not treat this condition. However, when their size is larger (approximately >10 mm in diameter), pseudocysts may occlude the maxillary ostium during a sinus graft procedure and increase the risk of postoperative infections. Studies have shown successful bone graft and implant placement in maxillary sinuses with pseudocysts.[56]

Etiology

A pseudocyst is caused by an accumulation of fluid beneath the periosteum of the sinus mucosa. This elevates the mucosa away from the floor of the sinus, giving rise to a dome-shaped lesion. Pseudocysts have also been termed mucosal cysts, serous cysts, and nonsecreting cysts. Pseudocysts are not true cysts because they lack an epithelial lining; however, they are surrounded by fibrous connective tissue.[57] The cause of the fluid is thought to result from sinus mucosa bacterial toxins or from odontogenic causes (Fig. 37.20).

Radiographic Appearance

Pseudocysts are depicted radiographically as smooth, homogenous, dome-shaped, round to ovoid, well-defined radiopacities. Pseudocysts do not have a corticated (radiopaque) marginal perimeter and almost always located on the floor of the sinus cavity. In some cases, pseudocysts may encompass the entire maxillary sinus, making diagnosis difficult because it may be radiographically similar to rhinosinusitis.

Treatment

Pseudocysts are not a contraindication for sinus graft surgery, unless their approximate size increases the possibility of occluding the maxillary ostium. If a large pseudocyst (i.e., greater than 8 mm) is present, then the elevation of the membrane during a sinus graft may raise the cyst to occlude the ostium. In addition, on elevation

or placement of the grafting material, the cyst may be perforated, allowing fluid within the cyst to contaminate the graft. Large cysts of this nature should be drained and allowed to heal before or in conjunction with sinus elevation surgery. Most often, an ENT physician should evaluate to determine any intervention. If a pseudocyst is less than 8 mm, then less concern is needed and the fluid may be drained in conjunction with sinus grafting, depending on the surgeon's experience in the treatment of this condition. Caution should be exercised to prevent membrane perforation. A strict recall evaluation of this area during the follow-up period of the sinus graft surgery is in order because reoccurrence of pseudocysts is common.

Retention Cysts

Retention cysts may be located on the sinus floor, near the ostium, or within antral polyps. Because they contain an epithelial lining, researchers consider them to be mucous secretory cysts and "true" cysts. Retention cysts are often microscopic in size.

Etiology

Retention cysts result from partial blockage of seromucinous gland ducts located within the connective tissue underlying the sinus epithelium. As the secretions collect, they expand the duct, producing a cyst that is encompassed by respiratory or cuboidal epithelium. They may be caused by sinus infections, allergies, or odontogenic reasons.

Radiographic Appearance

Retention cysts are usually very small and not seen clinically or radiographically. In rare instances, they may achieve adequate size to be seen in a CT image and may resemble the appearance of a small pseudocyst.

Treatment

No treatment for retention cysts exist before or in conjunction with a sinus graft and/or implant insertion.

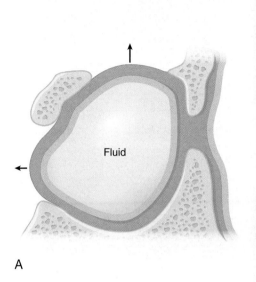

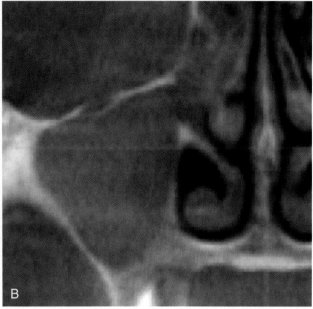

• **Fig. 37.21** Primary maxillary sinus mucocele. (A) Diagram showing expansive nature of a primary maxillary sinus mucocele. (B) Radiograph showing the initial stage of complete opacification and later stages including expansion of the bony plates.

Primary Maxillary Sinus Mucocele

A primary mucocele is a cystic, expansile, destructive lesion that may include painful swelling of the cheek, displacement of teeth, nasal obstruction, and possible ocular symptoms.[58] The primary mucocele is more commonly found in the ethmoid sinus (45.5%) versus the maxillary sinus (18.3%).[59]

Etiology

The primary mucocele arises from blockage of the maxillary ostium by fibrous connective tissue. Because of the compromised drainage, the mucosa expands and herniates through the antral walls. This mucocele is classified as a cyst because it is lined by antral epithelium, which contains mucin.

Radiographic Appearance

In the early stages, the primary mucocele involves the entire sinus and appears as an opacified sinus. As the cyst enlarges, the walls become thin and eventually perforate. In the late stages, destruction of one or more surrounding sinus walls is evident.

Treatment

Surgical removal of this cyst is indicated prior to any bone augmentation procedures (Fig. 37.21).

Secondary Maxillary Sinus Mucocele (Postoperative Maxillary Cyst)

A postoperative maxillary cyst of the maxillary sinus is a cystic lesion that usually develops secondary to a previous trauma or surgical procedure in the sinus cavity. It also has been termed a surgical ciliated cyst, postoperative maxillary sinus mucocele, or a secondary mucocele.[60-62] Secondary mucoceles occur most commonly in the maxillary sinus (86%) versus the ethmoid sinus (7.1%).[59]

Etiology

A postoperative maxillary cyst is a direct result of trauma or past history of surgery within the maxillary sinus. The cyst is derived from the antral epithelium and mucosal remnants that previously were entrapped within the prior surgical site. This separated mucosa results in an epithelium-lined cavity in which mucin is secreted. The antrum becomes divided by a fibrous septum in which one part drains normally, whereas the other part is composed of the mucocele. It is relatively rare in the United States; however, it constitutes approximately 24% of all cysts in Japan. At least three reported cases exist of a postoperative maxillary cyst forming after a sinus graft procedure, including one by the author of this chapter.[63]

Radiographic Appearance

The cyst radiographically presents as a well-defined radiolucency circumscribed by sclerosis. The lesion is usually spherical in the early stages, with no bone destruction. As it progresses, the sinus wall becomes thin and eventually perforates. In later stages, it will appear as two separated anatomic compartments.

Treatment

Surgical ciliated cysts should be enucleated before any bone augmentation procedures. If observed after the sinus graft, then the cysts should be enucleated and regrafted in the site (Fig. 37.22)

Neoplasms

Etiology

Primary malignant tumors within the maxillary sinus are usually caused by squamous cell carcinomas or adenocarcinomas. Signs and symptoms of malignant disease are related to the surrounding sinus wall that the tumor invades and includes swelling in the cheek area, pain, anesthesia or paresthesia of the infraorbital nerve (e.g., anterior wall), and visual disturbances (e.g., superior wall). These tumors in the sinus are usually nonspecific and give a variety

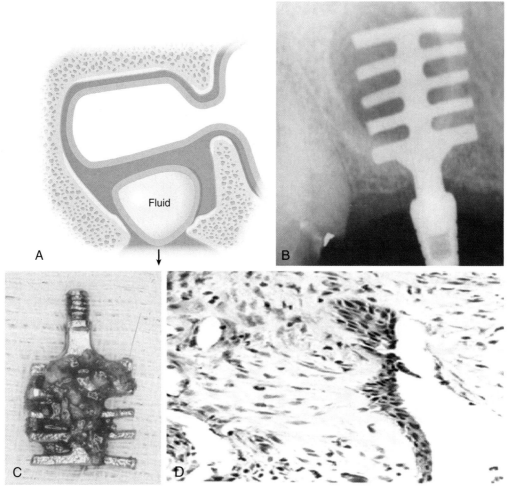

• **Fig. 37.22** Secondary maxillary sinus mucocele. (A) Diagram showing cystic nature of a secondary mucocele, which divides the sinus into two compartments. (B) Radiograph of blade implant with well-defined radiolucency around the implant. (C) Blade implant removed with associated pathology. (D) Histology revealing a secondary maxillary sinus mucocele.

of consequences, including opacified sinuses; soft tissue masses in the sinus; and sclerosis, erosion, or destruction of the walls of the sinus. Sixty percent of squamous cell carcinomas of the paranasal sinuses are located in the maxillary sinus, usually in the lower one-half of the antrum. Clinical signs in the oral cavity reflect the expansion of the tumor and an increased mobility of the involved teeth. Invasion of the infratemporal fossa is also possible.[1]

Radiographic Appearance

Radiographic signs of neoplasms may include various-sized radiopaque masses, complete opacification, or bony wall changes. A lack of a posterior wall on a panoramic radiograph should be a sign of possible neoplasm (Fig. 37.23).

Treatment

Any signs or symptoms of a lesion of this type should be immediately referred for medical consultation. Sinus graft surgery is absolutely contraindicated while this condition exists.

Antroliths and Foreign Bodies

Maxillary sinus antroliths are the result of complete or partial encrustation of a foreign body. These masses found within the maxillary sinus originate from a central nidus, which can be endogenous or exogenous.[64]

Etiology

The majority of endogenous sources are from dental origin, including retained roots, root canal sealer, fractured dental instruments, and dental implants. Additionally, bone spicules, blood, and mucus have been reported to cause antroliths.[65] Reports in the literature of exogenous sources include paper, cigarettes, snuff, and gluc.[66] Although most antroliths are asymptomatic, they often are associated with sinusitis.

Radiographic Appearance

The radiographic appearance of a maxillary antrolith resembles either the central nidus (e.g., retained root) or appears as a radiopaque, calcified mass within the maxillary sinus (Fig. 37.24).

Differential Diagnosis

Because the calcified antrolith is composed of calcium phosphate ($CaPO_4$), calcium carbonate salts, water, and organic material, it will be considerably more radiopaque than an inflammatory or cystic lesion.[67] The central nidus of the antrolith is similar to its usual radiographic appearance.

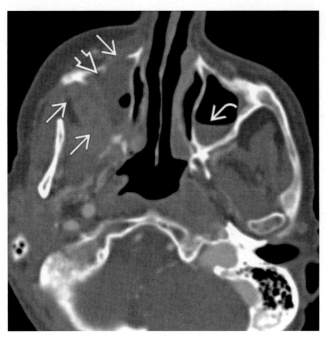

• **Fig. 37.23** Axial contrast-enhanced computerized tomography (bone window) shows almost complete radiopacification of the right maxillary sinus by squamous cell carcinoma. There is destruction of the walls of the sinus and an air-fluid interface in the left sinus. (From Koenig LJ, et al. *Diagnostic Imaging: Oral and Maxillofacial.* 2nd ed. Philadelphia, PA: Elsevier; 2017.)

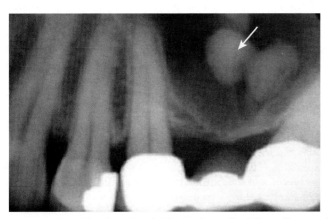

• **Fig. 37.24** Antroliths. Any object left in the sinus will calcify and is termed an antrolith. Antroliths usually will result in mucociliary clearance issues.

Treatment

Before sinus augmentation and implant placement, the antrolith should be surgically removed. If sinusitis exists, then the sinus cavity should be allowed to heal completely before sinus augmentation procedures. A nonsymptomatic condition may have the antrolith removed and sinus graft performed at the same surgery, only if the sinus membrane is not compromised.

Miscellaneous Factors That Affect the Health of the Maxillary Sinus

Smoking

The use of tobacco is one of the main factors that may lead to an increased morbidity after sinus graft procedures. Smoking is known to be associated with an increased susceptibility to allergies and infections because it interferes with ciliary function and secretory immunity of the nasorespiratory tract. In the maxillary sinus, this may have direct effects on both immune exclusion and suppression because IgA and IgM responses are reduced, whereas IgE responses are increased. Smoking is believed to interfere with bone graft healing because it reduces local blood flow by increasing peripheral resistance and causing an increased platelet aggregation. By-product chemicals of smoking, such as hydrogen cyanide and carbon monoxide, have been shown to inhibit wound healing, as does nicotine, which inhibits cellular proliferation. Tobacco may interfere directly with osteoblastic function, and strong evidence exists of decreased bone formation in smokers. In addition, smokers have a significant reduction of bone mineral content. Bone mineral density can be reduced two to six times in a chronic smoker. Overall, smoking may contribute to poor available bone quality and poor healing capacity resulting from vascular and osteoblastic dysfunction.[68]

There exist many clinical studies with smoking and sinus graft procedures. Klokkevold evaluated the success rate of dental implants placed in the posterior maxilla; it showed a 7% greater failure rate compared with nonsmokers.[69] Lindquist showed that smokers can also suffer detrimental effects around successfully integrated maxillary implants, with a significantly greater bleeding index, greater mean peri-implant pocket depth, more frequent peri-implant inflammation, and radiographically greater mesial and distal bone loss.[70] Olson and colleagues found an association between dental implants placed in augmented maxillary sinuses and history of smoking.[71] Widmark reported a higher failure rate in smokers after rehabilitation of severely resorbed maxillae with and without bone graft.[72] Schwartz-Arad and colleagues evaluated 212 implants in the posterior maxilla, resulting in a 95.5% success rate with nine failures. Of the nine failures, five were in patients that smoked.[73]

In summary, smoking is not an absolute contraindication for sinus graft procedures. However, patients should be instructed to cease smoking before and after sinus graft procedures because of the literature-based studies showing a higher risk of wound dehiscence, graft infection and/or resorption, and a reduced probability of osseointegration. It is recommended, however, that if a decision to proceed with surgery has been made, then patients refrain from smoking at least 15 days before surgery (i.e., the time it takes for nicotine to clear systemically) and 4 to 6 weeks after surgery. Moreover, smokers should sign a detailed informed consent in which risks connected to smoking are clearly defined and explained.

Relative and Absolute Contraindication to Maxillary Sinus Graft Procedures

In general contraindications for implant surgery also apply to sinus graft procedures. However, additional specific and local conditions may exist that increase morbidity. Several conditions related to the maxillary sinus are a concern, but they are not necessarily contraindications to the sinus graft procedure. The implant clinician, after evaluation of the CBCT scan and evaluation of the maxillary sinus, will in some cases need further medical evaluation before proceeding with procedures that may invade the sinus proper. There exists a wide variation in the severity of the possible pathologic conditions that may be present in the maxillary sinus. For example, a patient may have a mild deviated septum. Because it does not affect the mucociliary clearance of the maxillary sinus

• BOX 37.2 **Absolute versus Relative Contraindications**

Relative contraindications:
1. Limited anatomic/structural impairments of the sinus or nasal walls that are correctable (i.e., deviated septum)
2. Inflammatory/infectious processes that are treatable
3. Foreign bodies
4. Oroantral fistulas

Absolute contraindications:
1. Anatomic/structural impairments of the sinus or nasal walls that are noncorrectable.
2. Inflammatory/infectious processes that cannot be resolved (i.e., chronic rhinosinusitis)
3. Fungal or granulomatous diseases of the nasosinus.
4. Benign/malignant neoplasms of the nasosinus.

• BOX 37.3 **Medical Consultation: Otolaryngologist (ENT)**

No referral
1. Mild mucosal thickening
2. Small cyst (<8 mm)
3. History of mild Sinusitis with no radiographic evidence of pathology

Referral recommendation
1. Air-fluid Level
2. Cyst (~ >8 mm)
3. Primary/secondary mucocele
4. Polyps
5. Opacified sinus
6. Chronic sinusitis (MRSA, fungal)
7. Bony wall expansion /destruction
8. Previous trauma
8. Foreign body in sinus
10. Early learning curve

ENT, Ear, nose, and throat (otolaryngologist); MRSA, methicillin-resistant Staphylococcus aureus.

and there is no associated pathology, no medical consultation by an ENT is warranted. However, if a deviated septum is present and severe, resulting in a nonpatent ostium, an ENT referral would be highly recommended.

A list of relative and absolute contraindications is listed in Boxes 37.2 and 37.3.

Reduction of Sinus Graft Complications

Even though sinus graft procedures have high success rates, these procedures tend to have a higher risk of infection than implant placement surgery because the patient is predisposed to infections originating from the oral surgical procedure (i.e., intraoral infection originating from the surgical site) or from the sinus graft procedure (i.e., infection within the sinus proper). Therefore a surgical environment that includes a strict aseptic technique including intraoral and extraoral scrubbing with chlorhexidine, scrubbing and draping the patient, and gowning the doctor and assistant should be considered in addition to sterile gloves and sterile instruments. The risk of postoperative sinus infection is generally less than 5% when these procedures and a preoperative and postoperative pharmacologic regimen are used.[73,74]

Prophylactic Medications

Systemic Antimicrobial Medications
The risks of bacterial contamination before and after sinus graft procedures are much different than routine implant surgical procedures. Therefore the pharmacologic protocol for sinus graft procedures should be effective against the organisms in this surgical site. The recommended pharmacologic regimen includes a prophylactic antibiotic, anti-inflammatory medications, and antimicrobial rinses.

Compared with routine dental implant surgery, sinus augmentation has a greater chance of morbidity because of the possible additional routes of infection. Bacterial invasion may originate from different sources such as (1) intraoral surgery, (2) bone graft material, and (3) bacteria from the sinus cavity. Additionally, it has been well documented that the inclusion of foreign bodies (e.g., implants, autografts, allografts) increases infection rates.[75,76] Because a greater chance of infection and morbidity exists with this type of surgical procedure, a strict antibiotic protocol is of benefit. Antibiotic medications have been shown to significantly reduce the number of sinus graft or implant failures caused by infection.[77]

Following the principles of prophylactic antibiotic administration, the antibiotic should be effective against the bacteria most likely to cause infection. The most likely contaminating organisms after intraoral surgery are primarily streptococci, anaerobic gram-positive cocci, and anaerobic gram-negative rods. *S. pneumoniae, H. influenzae,* and *M. catarrhalis* are the three most common pathogens found within the maxillary sinus that may lead to acute sinus infections.[78] *S. aureus* is not common with acute episodes; however, it has been shown to have a significant role in causing chronic rhinosinusitis disease, along with anaerobic bacteria. The organisms associated with infection in general oral surgical procedures include α-hemolytic streptococci and *S. viridans.*[79] Therefore a pharmacologic protocol should be effective against these organisms.

When evaluating various classes of antibiotic medications used for treatment of maxillary sinus infections, the antibiotic class of choice is the β-lactam antibiotic drugs. With the wide range of possible routes of bacterial invasion and types of bacteria, the antibiotic drug must be broad spectrum to account for all these possibilities. However, bacterial resistance has become a significant problem in the treatment of these pathogens. Bacterial resistance is initiated by two common mechanisms: (1) production of antibiotic-inactivating enzymes (*S. aureus, H. influenzae,* and *M. catarrhalis*) and (2) alteration in target site (*S. pneumoniae*). Studies have shown the following resistance (i.e., β-lactamase production) results[80]:

H.influenzae: 36.8%
M.catarrhalis: 98%
S.pneumoniae: 28.6%

Because of the high rate of bacterial resistance, amoxicillin (the drug of choice for many years) is no longer recommended for antibiotic prophylaxis for the sinus graft surgery. Instead, amoxicillin-clavulanate (Augmentin) is used because the addition of clavulanic acid enhances amoxicillin's activity against the β-lactamase–producing strains of bacteria.

The patient with a history of nonanaphylactic allergic reaction to penicillin may take cefuroxime axetil (Ceftin) as an alternative.[81] Ceftin is a second-generation cephalosporin that possesses good potency, efficiency, and strong activity against resistant *S. pneumoniae* and *H. influenzae.* If a patient has a true history of anaphylactic reaction to penicillin, recurrent sinus infections, or a recent history of antibiotic use, then doxycycline may be used. In the past, the quinolone class of antibiotics (e.g., Levaquin, Avelox) have been used with excellent success because they exhibit superior activity against most types of involved bacteria. However, recently the Food and Drug Administration (FDA) has recommended the adverse effect of tendon damage does not warrant its routine use anymore.

Maximum effectiveness of prophylactic antibiotic drugs occurs when the antibiotic is in adequate concentrations in the tissue before bacterial invasion is initiated. Because the sinus mucosa has limited blood supply when infection and inflammation is present, poor antibiotic blood levels are achieved. Therefore to combat possible bacterial invasion from the sinus surgery, antibiotic medications should be administered at least 1 full day (24 hours) before surgery and extended for approximately 5 days after surgery.

Local Antibiotic Medications

The antibiotic concentration within a blood clot of the sinus graft depends on the systemic blood titer. After the clot stabilizes, further antibiotic drugs do not enter the area until revascularization.[82] The bone graft is a dead space with minimum blood supply and absence of protection by the host's cellular defense mechanisms. This leaves the graft prone to infections that would normally be eliminated by either the host defenses or the antibiotic. The osteogenic induction of autografts and allografts is greatly retarded when contaminated with infectious bacteria.[83] To ensure adequate antibiotic levels in an SA graft, it is recommended to add antibiotic to the graft mixture.[84,85] This local antibiotic may protect the graft from early contamination and infection. Numerous studies have shown that an antibiotic added to graft material has no deleterious effects on bone growth. Antibiotic drugs such as penicillin, cephalosporin, and clindamycin, even in high concentrations, have not been found to be destructive to bone-inductive proteins.[86]

The locally delivered antibiotic should have efficacy against the most likely organisms encountered. Because the incidence of allergy is so high with β-lactam antibiotic drugs, the parenteral form of cefazolin (Ancef) is recommended. If there exists a true allergy to penicillin (i.e., anaphylactic), then Cleocin may be used as an alternative. Orally administered capsules and tablets should not be used within the graft because they contain fillers that interfere with bone regeneration.

Clinical experience indicates that less risk of infection exists when preoperative and postoperative antibiotic drugs are used both orally and in the graft. Because infection considerably impairs bone formation for patients undergoing sinus graft procedures, oral antibiotic coverage is continued for approximately 5 days after the surgery. Recommended antibiotic drugs are shown in Box 37.4.

Oral Antimicrobial Rinse

An additional antimicrobial medication used with respect to sinus augmentation surgery is chlorhexidine gluconate. This category of antimicrobial rinse has been shown to successfully decrease infectious episodes and minimizes postoperative complications from the incision line.[87] Gentle oral rinses of chlorhexidine gluconate 0.12% should be used twice daily for 2 weeks after surgery or until the incision line is completely healed.[88]

Glucocorticoid Medications

Sinus augmentation surgery usually results in increased postoperative inflammation. Therefore a pharmacologic regimen

---

> **• BOX 37.4 Recommended Prophylactic Antibiotic Drugs for Sinus Grafting Procedures**
>
> **Systemic Antibiotic Prophylaxis**
> 1. Augmentin (amoxicillin-clavulanic acid) (825 mg/125 mg), one tablet bid starting 1 day before surgery and 5 days after surgery
>
> **Non-anaphylactic allergy to penicillin**
> 2. Ceftin (cefuroxime axetil) (500 mg), , one tablet bid starting 1 day before surgery and 5 days after surgery
>
> **Anaphylactic allergy to penicillin**
> 3. Doxycycline (100 mg), one tablet bid starting 1 day before surgery and 5 days after surgery
>
> **Local Antibiotic in Graft**
> 1. Ancef (Cefazolin 1 gm): Dilute with 2 mL saline (500 mg/mL)
>   a. 0.2 mL or 100 mg: add to collagen membrane
>   b. 0.8 mL or 400 mg: add to graft material
> 2. Clindamycin 150 mg/1 mL
>   a. 0.2 mL or 30 mg: add to collagen membrane
>   b. 0.8 mL or 120 mg: add to graft material
>
> *bid, Twice a day.*

> **• BOX 37.5 Glucocorticoid Protocol**
>
> **Dexamethasone (4 mg) × 6 tablets**
> - Two tablets (8 mg) in the morning, the day before surgery
> - Two tablets (8 mg) in the morning of surgery
> - One tablet (4 mg) in the morning, the day after surgery
> - One tablet (4 mg) in the morning, the second day after surgery

---

is recommended to decrease postoperative edema. Glucocorticoids have been well documented to decrease inflammation of the soft tissue and minimize postoperative pain, swelling, and incision line opening. In addition, the clinical manifestations of surgery on the sinus mucosa also can be decreased by use of a glucocorticoid medication.[89] Therefore the usual surgical protocol for most implant surgeries, including sinus grafts, includes a short-term dose of dexamethasone (Decadron) (Box 37.5). To ensure patency of the ostium and minimize inflammation in the sinus before surgery, steroid medications are initiated 1 full day before surgery. This medication should also be extended 2 days postoperatively because edema peaks at 2 to 3 days postsurgery.

Decongestant Medications

Sympathomimetic drugs that influence α-adrenergic receptors have been used as therapeutic agents for the decongestion of mucous membranes. Both systemic and topical decongestant medications are useful in reopening a blocked sinus ostium and facilitating drainage. Oxymetazoline 0.05% (Afrin or Vicks Nasal Spray) and phenylephrine 1% are useful topical decongestant medications. The vasoconstrictor action of oxymetazoline lasts approximately 5 to 8 hours, which is preferred compared with 1 hour for phenylephrine. However, decongestant drugs have many disadvantages. Topical decongestant drugs can cause a rebound phenomenon and the development of rhinitis medicamentosa if used more than 3 to 4 days. The effectiveness of the topical decongestant is markedly enhanced by proper position of the patient's head during administration of the drug. It should also be noted that the pulse amplitude and blood flow in the sinus mucosa is reduced with decongestant drugs, such as oxymetazoline. This may, in turn, decrease the defense mechanism within the tissues.[90]

As a consequence of the medical and local risks of decongestant medications, the modified sinus graft pharmacologic protocol no longer recommends the prophylactic use of decongestant medications.

Analgesic Medications

In most cases, sinus graft procedures usually require very minimal postoperative analgesic coverage. If a narcotic is required, any analgesic combination containing codeine, such as Tylenol 3, is prescribed postoperatively because codeine is a potent antitussive, and coughing may place additional pressure on the sinus membrane and introduce bacteria into the graft. The patient is instructed to cough (if necessary) with the mouth open so excessive air pressure does not occur through the ostium.

Cryotherapy

With sinus elevation procedures, postoperative inflammation in the posterior maxilla is very common because of the extent of tissue reflection. Because postoperative swelling can adversely affect the incision line, measures should be taken to minimize this condition. Application of cold dressings and cold oral liquids, along with elevation of the head and limited activity for 2 to 3 days, will help minimize the swelling. The applied cold dressing and liquids will cause vasoconstriction of the capillary vessels, reducing the flow of blood and lymph, resulting in a lower degree of swelling. Ice or cold dressings should only be used for the first 24 to 48 hours. After 2 to 3 days, heat may be applied to the region to increase blood and lymph flow, which helps to clear the area of the inflammatory consequences. This also assists in the reduction of ecchymosis that may have occurred from the bleeding and tissue reflection.

Aseptic Technique

Because of the extent of tissue reflection, technique sensitivity of sinus surgery, and need for asepsis, oral or conscious sedation is usually recommended for sinus graft procedures. After sedation and adequate infiltration anesthesia (i.e., posterior and middle alveolar nerve, greater palatine nerve) are obtained, the patient is prepared for surgery. Preparation of the surgical site is important in sinus manipulation surgery to reduce contamination by the patient's own normal flora. The oral cavity cannot become a sterile environment for surgery. However, intraoral preparation before surgery may significantly reduce the bacterial count in the mouth. Studies reveal a significant reduction in bacteremia during extractions and implant surgery complications after preparation with antiseptic mouth rinse.[89,90]

Iodophor compounds (Betadine) are a most effective antiseptic. However, because the iodine is complexed with organic surface-active agents, it has been shown to inhibit the osteoinduction of allograft bone. Therefore the use of 0.12% chlorhexidine gluconate (Peridex) scrub and rinse is most often used as intraoral preparation of the surgical site requiring a bone graft. Extraoral presurgical scrubbing of the skin should also be performed with chlorhexidine antiseptics prior to surgery.

Surgical Treatment of the Maxillary Sinus: History

In the early 1970s, Tatum began to augment the posterior maxilla with autogenous rib bone to produce adequate vertical bone for implant support.[91,92] He found that onlay grafts below the existing alveolar crest would decrease the posterior intradental height significantly, yet very little bone for endosteal implants would be gained. Therefore in 1974 Tatum developed a modified Caldwell-Luc procedure for sinus augmentation (SA) grafting. The crest of the maxilla was infractured to elevate the maxillary sinus membrane. Autogenous bone was then added in the area previously occupied by the inferior third of the sinus. Endosteal implants were inserted in this grafted bone after approximately 6 months. Implants were then loaded with final prostheses after an additional 6 months.

In 1975 Tatum developed a lateral-approach surgical technique to elevate the sinus membrane and place implants simultaneously. The implant system used was a one-piece ceramic implant, and a permucosal post was required during the healing period. Early ceramic implants were not designed adequately for this procedure, and results with the technique were unpredictable. In 1981 Tatum developed a submerged titanium implant for use in the posterior maxilla and achieved predictable results.

From 1974 to 1979, the primary graft material for sinus grafts was autologous bone. In 1980 Tatum[55,93] further expanded the application of the SA augmentation technique with a lateral maxillary approach and the use of synthetic bone. The same year, Boyne and James first reported on the sinus graft technique using autogenous bone for SA grafts.[60] Most of the publications in the 1980s were anecdotal or based on very small sample sizes.

Treatment Classifications for the Posterior Maxilla

In 1984, Misch[61] organized a treatment approach to the posterior maxilla based on the amount of bone below the antrum, and in 1986 he expanded the treatment approach to include the available bone width that was related to implant design. In 1987 Misch included the technique of the sinus floor elevation through the implant osteotomy before implant placement.[62] He reported on 170 sinus graft cases, with two complications and an uneventful resolution.

In the Misch SA classification, the treatment modality is dependent on the available bone height between the floor of the antrum and the crest of the residual ridge in the region of the ideal implant locations. The SA protocol also suggested a surgical approach, bone graft material, and a time table for healing before prosthetic reconstruction. In 1995 Misch[94] modified his 1987 classifications to include the lateral dimension of the sinus cavity; this dimension was used to modify the healing period protocol because smaller width sinuses (0–10 mm) form bone faster than larger width (>15 mm) sinuses. The Division A–width ridge was also increased to 6 mm to permit more bone to encompass the implant on each side. In 2017 Resnik modified the Misch classification to include alternative treatment options with short implants, crestal grafting approaches, and treatment plan modifications based on force-related factors, which are detailed in Box 37.6 (Figs. 37.25–37.28).

Surgical Technique

Subantral Option One: Conventional Implant Placement

The first Misch SA treatment option, SA-1, occurs when sufficient bone height is available to permit the placement of endosteal implants following the usual surgical protocol, with no maxillary sinus involvement. Because the quality of bone in the posterior maxilla often is D3 or D4 bone, bone compaction or osseodensification to prepare the implant site is common. This technique permits a more rigid initial insertion of the implant and also increases the BIC.

Required Bone Dimensions

In the abundant bone volume (Division A),the minimum ideal bone height for the SA-1 is related to the associated force factors. Under favorable conditions, a minimum of 8 mm of bone is required from the crest of the ridge to the inferior floor of the sinus for the placement of an 8-mm implant. The literature has concluded that short implants (8 mm) have been shown to be successful in the posterior maxilla. If multiple implants are placed, then ideally the implants should be splinted for force distribution. For unfavorable conditions, greater than 10 mm of bone is required in height to allow for placement of an implant so it does not invade the maxillary sinus. This will allow an implant of 10 mm in length to be placed that will allow for a greater insertion torque and BIC. Therefore the implant will be less likely to have force-related effects that may

---

• BOX 37.6   Force-Related Factors

Favorable Conditions
- Good quality of bone (D2/D3 bone) with the presence of cortical bone present
- Minimal occlusal force factors
- No parafunction
- Ideal crown/implant ratio

Unfavorable Conditions
- Poor quality of bone (D3/D4 bone) with no cortical bone present
- Increased occlusal force factors
- Parafunctional forces present
- Poor crown/implant ratio

---

cause micromovement during the healing phase and poorer healing (Fig. 37.29).

Because the maxillary sinus proper is not invaded during an SA-1 approach, it is less critical if preexisting pathology in the sinus is present. However, if pathology is present that warrants medical referral, then this should be completed before any implant placement. Therefore in general the sinus pathologic contraindications for sinus graft surgery do not apply for implant insertion when adequate bone is present below the sinus for implants of adequate size to support the load of the prosthesis. Although a common axiom in implant dentistry is to remain 2 mm or more from an opposing landmark, this is not necessary in the SA region.

Narrower bone volume patients (Division B) in SA-1 may be treated with osteoplasty or augmentation to increase the width of bone. The insertion of smaller surface area implants (as small-diameter root-form implants) are not suggested because the forces are greater in the posterior regions of the mouth, and the bone density is less than in most regions. In addition, the narrow ridge is often more medial than the central fossa of the mandibular teeth and will result in an offset load on the restoration, which will increase the strain to the bone. However, multiple narrow diameter implants may be placed to support one tooth (i.e., two narrow diameter implants to support one molar).

Osteoplasty in the SA-1 posterior maxilla may change the SA category if the height of the remaining bone is sufficient to allow for adequate bone postosteoplasty. Augmentation for width may be accomplished with bone spreading, membrane grafting, or autogenous grafts. Larger diameter implants are often required in the molar region, and bone spreading to place wider implants is the most common approach when the bone density is poor. If less than 2.5 mm of width is available in the posterior edentulous region (C–w), then the most predictable treatment option is to increase width using onlay autogenous bone grafts. After graft maturation the area is reevaluated to determine the proper treatment plan classification.

Endosteal implants in the SA-1 category are left to heal in a nonfunctional environment for approximately 4 to 8 months (depending on bone density and force factors) before the abutment post(s) are added for prosthodontic reconstruction. Care is taken to ensure that the implants are not traumatized during the initial healing period. Progressive loading during the prosthetic phases of the treatment is suggested in D3 or D4 bone (Box 37.7).

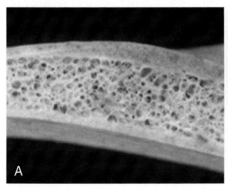
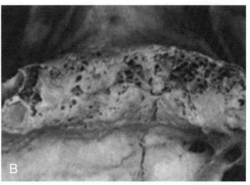

• **Fig. 37.25** Bone quality. (A) Thick cortical bone and a dense cancellous bone, which is consistent with a D2 type of bone, (B) No cortical bone present, with very fine trabecular bone, which is usually consistent with D4 bone and mainly found in the posterior maxilla.

Subantral Option Two: Sinus Lift and Simultaneous Implant Placement

The second SA option in the Misch SA classification, SA-2, is selected when the intended implant length is 1 to 2 mm greater than the vertical bone present (Fig. 37.30). In this technique, 1 to 2 mm may be achieved via elevating the sinus membrane without bone grafting. Tatum[95] originally developed this technique in 1970, and Misch[96] first published it in 1987. Summers[97]

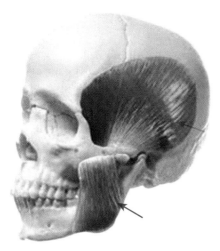

• **Fig. 37.26** Force factors. The posterior maxilla is very susceptible to force-related issues because of strong muscles such as the temporalis (green) and masseter (red).

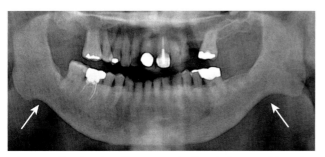

• **Fig. 37.27** Parafunction. Forces are significantly increased in patients who exhibit parafunction. In this radiograph, the prominent antegonial notch is consistent with parafunctional forces and masseter hypertrophy.

published a similar procedure in 1994, 24 years after Tatum's first presentation.

Because the SA-2 surgical approach modifies the floor of the maxillary sinus, a preexisting pathologic condition of the sinus should not be present because it may affect the implant site by retrograde infection.

This technique is reserved for 8 to 10 mm of host bone below the sinus in which an implant is placed via an osteotome technique that elevates the membrane approximately 1 to 2 mm with the use of no grafting. Ideally, an 8-mm implant is used with caution in these cases.

Rationale

In some situations, a longer implant may be required for prosthetic support and initial fixation. Worth and Stoneman[98] have reported a comparable phenomenon of bone growth under an elevated sinus membrane called a "halo formation". They observed the natural elevation of the sinus membrane around teeth with periapical disease. The elevation of the membrane resulted in new bone formation once the tooth infection was eliminated. In an article by Palma and colleagues[99] the elevation of the sinus membrane in implant insertion, with or without a graft material below the mucosa, gave similar results in primates regarding implant stability or BIC after healing. As a result of the autologous bone present above the apical portion of the implant with an SA-2 technique, and the sinus floor fracture (which increases the regional accelerated phenomenon of bone repair and formation), new bone formation over the implant apex is predictable.

Incision and Reflection

In an edentulous posterior maxilla, a full-thickness incision is made on the crest of the edentulous ridge from the tuberosity to the distal of the canine region. A vertical, lateral relief incision is made at its distal and anterior extension of the crestal incision for approximately 5 mm. If minimal attached tissue exists on the crest of the ridge, which is more often observed in the premolar region, then the primary incision is made more palatal to place more keratinized tissue on the facial aspect. When teeth are present in the region, the crestal incision extends at least one tooth beyond the edentulous site. If one tooth is missing, the reflection is similar to a single-tooth replacement option, and even a direct (flapless technique) may be used.

A full-thickness palatal flap is first reflected because the palatal dense cortical plate facilitates soft tissue reflection. Special attention is given to avoid the pathway of the greater palatine artery or to remain completely subperiosteal so that this structure remains

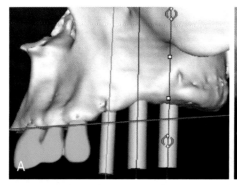
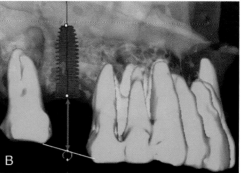

• **Fig. 37.28** Crown/implant ratio. The maxillary posterior region often is confronted with a an increased interocclusal space because of the vertical and horizontal bone resorption. (A) Three-dimensional image showing the apical positioning of implants caused by vertical bone resorption. (B) Cone beam computerized tomography interactive treatment planning evaluating the increased crown height space.

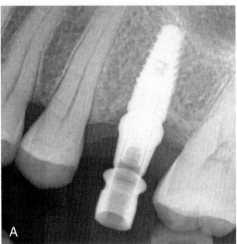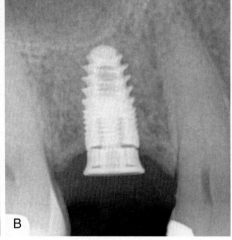

• **Fig. 37.29** SA-1 (A and B) Treatment plan which includes implant placement below the maxillary sinus proper.

• **BOX 37.7 SA-1 Requirements**

- **Favorable conditions:** >8 mm host bone (implant approximately 8 mm in length or greater)
- **Unfavorable conditions:** >10 mm host bone (implant approximately 10 mm in length or greater)

---

within the soft tissue. The labial mucosa is reflected off the edentulous ridge, rather than elevating the tissue from the bone. The crest should not be used to leverage the tissue because the ridge may have minimal cortical bone and a perforation may result. This could result in damage to the residual ridge or possibly even penetrate the sinus or nasal cavity. Once the tissue is reflected, the width of the available bone is evaluated to ensure that it is greater than 6-7 mm wide and allows the placement of Division A root-form implants.

Osteotomy and Sinus Elevation (SA-2)

The endosteal implant osteotomy is prepared as determined by the density of bone protocol, which is usually D3 or D4 bone. The depth of the osteotomy is approximately 1 to 2 mm short of the floor of the antrum. When in doubt of the height dimension, the osteotomy should err on a shorter length. The implant osteotomy is prepared to the appropriate final diameter, short of the antral floor, by approximately 1 mm.

A flat-end or cupped-shape osteotome is selected for the infracture of the sinus floor. Usually in D3 bone, an osteotome of the same diameter as the final osteotomy is selected. In D4 bone, an osteotomy one to two sizes smaller than the final implant size maybe used, performing an osseodensification technique. The osteotome is inserted and tapped firmly in 0.5- to 1.0-mm increments beyond the osteotomy until reaching its final vertical position, up to 2 mm beyond the prepared implant osteotomy. A slow elevation of the sinus floor is less likely to tear the sinus mucosa. This surgical approach compresses the bone below the antrum, causes a greenstick-type fracture in the antral floor, and slowly elevates the unprepared bone and sinus membrane over the broad-based osteotome. If the osteotome cannot proceed to the desired osteotomy depth after tapping, then it is removed and the osteotomy is prepared again with rotary drills an additional 1 mm in depth. The osteotome is then reinserted to attempt the greenstick fracture of the antral floor.

Care should be exercised when removing the osteotomes from the osteotomy site. The osteotome should never be luxated

because this will increase the width of the final osteotomy, leading to less insertion torque. Once the osteotome prepares the implant site, the implant may then be threaded into the osteotomy and extended up to 2 mm above the floor of the sinus. The implant is slowly threaded into position so the membrane is less likely to tear as it is elevated. The apical portion of the implant engages the more dense bone on the cortical floor, ideally with bone over the apex, and an intact sinus membrane. The implant may extend 0 to 2 mm beyond the sinus floor, and the 1 mm of compressed bone covering over the implant apex results in as much as a 3-mm elevation of the sinus mucosa (Fig. 37.31). Ideally, the implant design should include a convex apex with no apical openings as this design will be less likely to cause a membrane perforation.

Modified SA2 Techniques

Rosen and associates[100,101] developed a modification to the SA-2 treatment approach for use at the time of an extraction of a maxillary molar. The technique is indicated when the maxillary molar is extracted, the surrounding walls of bone are intact, and no periapical pathologic condition is present. The crest of the ridge to the antral floor should be 7 mm or more in height. Once the tooth is extracted and the surrounding bony walls confirmed, a modification of the SA-2 technique is in order. A 5- to 6-mm trephine bur is used in the center of the extraction site and prepares the bone 1 to 2 mm below the antral floor. A 5- to 6-mm-diameter, flat-ended or cup-shaped osteotome and mallet intrudes the core of bone 2 mm above the sinus floor, creating 9 mm or more of vertical bone. A socket graft may be used within the extraction socket but is not pushed into the surgical space of the sinus because it may perforate the sinus mucosa. After 4 months, an implant may be inserted.

Some authors have used the SA-2 sinus lift procedure to gain more than 2 mm of implant vertical height. However, these blind surgical techniques increase the risk of sinus membrane perforation.

The success of the intact sinus membrane lift cannot be confirmed before or at the time of implant placement. Attempts to "feel" the elevation of the membrane from within an 8-mm-deep implant osteotomy may cause tearing of the sinus lining.

Attempting to elevate the sinus mucosa more than 2 mm through an implant osteotomy 3 to 4 mm wide and 8 mm deep is not predictable. Reiser and colleagues[102] reported that when the sinus elevation was 4 to 8 mm in cadavers, almost 25% resulted in sinus perforation. The implant osteotomy sinus floor

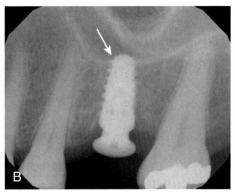

• **Fig. 37.30** SA-2. (A) Radiograph depicting an SA-2 (maxillary second premolar) and SA-1 (maxillary first molar). (B) SA-2 implant that includes implant insertion with penetration into the maxillary sinus proper 1 to 2 mm without bone grafting.

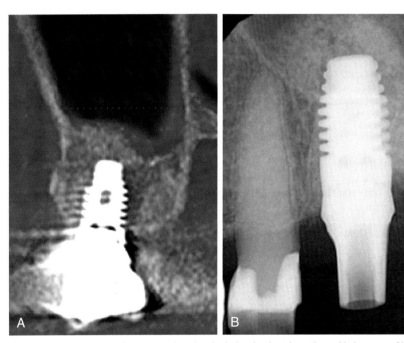

• **Fig. 37.31** (A) SA-3 crestal. Treatment plan that includes implant insertion with bone grafting via the crestal (osteotomy) approach gaining approximately 3 to 4 mm of height. (B) Lateral wall. Treatment plan that includes implant insertion with bone grafting via the lateral-wall approach gaining more than 4 mm of height (i.e., amount of height is determined by size of lateral wall).

technique is often attempted because of the perceived ease of surgery of an SA-2 technique versus a lateral-wall or transcrestal approach.

Complications

If a sinus membrane perforation occurred during the initial implant placement procedure, then bone height growth is less likely to occur. This is the primary reason why only **0 to 2 mm** of additional bone height is attempted with this technique. However, even when membrane perforation occurs and/or no bone grows around the apical end of the implant, the SA-2 technique is of benefit because the apical end of the implant is surrounded by denser bone. This enhances rigid fixation during healing and increases BIC, leading to improved loading conditions. If inadequate bone is formed around the apical portion of an implant, then a progressive-loading protocol for D4 bone is suggested during prosthetic reconstruction (Box 37.8).

> • **BOX 37.8** **SA-2 Requirements**
>
> - **Favorable conditions:** (>8 mm host bone, ideally 10-mm implant)
> - **Unfavorable conditions:** (>10 mm host bone, ideally 12-mm implant)

Subantral Option Three: Sinus Graft with Immediate Endosteal Implant Placement

The third approach to the maxillary posterior edentulous region, SA-3, is indicated when at least 5 mm of vertical bone and sufficient width are present between the antral floor and the crest of the residual ridge in the area of the intended prosthesis abutment (Fig. 37.32).

A residual height of 5 mm for the SA-3 category has been selected for two main reasons: (1) this height (in adequate bone width and quality) can be considered sufficient to allow primary stability of implants placed at the same time as the sinus graft procedure, and (2) because of the amount of residual bone (5mm), greater blood supply is present, which allows for more predictable and faster healing.

Anesthesia

Infiltration anesthesia has been used with success for sinus graft surgeries in the past; however, more profound regional anesthesia is achieved by blocking the secondary division of the maxillary nerve (V2). The sinus graft surgery often requires the reflection of the soft tissue extending to the zygomatic process. In addition, several branches of the maxillary division of the fifth cranial nerve innervate the sinus mucosa. As such, a V2 block is advantageous for patient comfort, and this achieves anesthesia of the hemimaxilla, side of the nose, cheek, lip, and sinus area.

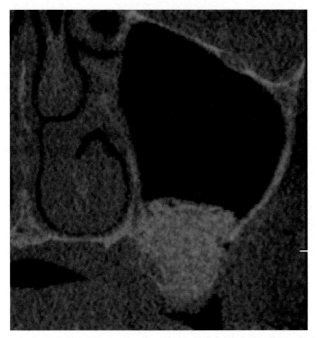

• **Fig. 37.32** SA-4. Treatment plan that includes bone grafting via the lateral-wall approach with no implant placement. Implant placement is delayed according to the healing of the sinus graft sites.

Two options exist for V2 block anesthesia: (1) high and within the pterygomaxillary tissue behind the posterior wall of the maxilla or (2) at the depth of approximately 1 inch with a long-gauge needle within the greater palatine foramen (Fig. 37.33). The first method is easier to perform but may injure the pterygoid plexus or the maxillary artery and result in hematoma, or it may fail to reach the proper landmark. With the second option, it is more difficult to locate the foramen and negotiate up the canal. It may also injure the greater palatine artery or nerve. Too deep an administration with a greater palatine approach may result in the penetration of the orbit floor. Possible sequelae include periorbital swelling and proptosis, diplopia, retrobulbar block with dilated pupil, corneal anesthesia, motionless eye, retrobulbar hemorrhage, and optic nerve block with transient loss of vision. However, the success rate is greater, and the clinical risks appear minimal. Therefore most often, the first attempt for block anesthesia is within the greater palatine foramen; if unsuccessful, then the high posterior approach is used. Prevention of these complications is ensured by reduction of the needle depth measurement for smaller patients and the strict application of the technique. Proper angulation during soft tissue penetration prevents possible entrance into the nasal cavity through the medial wall of the pterygopalatal fossa.

Infiltration anesthesia is first administered to the posterior and middle alveolar nerve and greater palatine nerve. Scrubbing, gowning, and draping of the patient is next. Then after the infiltration is effective, the V2 block is administered. A long-acting anesthetic such as bupivacaine 0.5% (Marcaine) is preferred. Block anesthesia with these agents is longer acting than infiltration in the maxilla.[103]

The greater palatine foramen is found using an open-bore instrument (i.e., the handle of a mouth mirror with the mirror portion removed). Pressure is applied with this instrument along the palatal tissue, at the union of the residual ridge and hard palate, in the region of the second molar. Most often, the open-bore handle will feel and recede into the foramen. Slight pressure for a few seconds then marks the tissue over the opening of the foramen. A long, 1.5 inch needle is introduced into the foramen from the opposite side of the mouth and negotiates the canal for approximately 1 inch.

Surgical Approaches

There exist two options for grafting the sinus along with simultaneous implant placement.

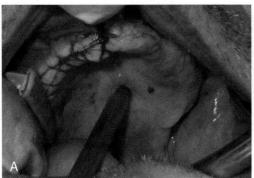 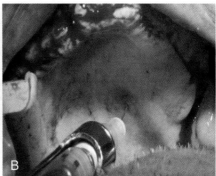

• **Fig. 37.33** Anesthesia, V2 block. (A) Greater palatine foramen approach through the greater palatine foramen located 1 cm medial and adjacent to the second molar teeth. (B) Cotton swab may be pressed at the junction of the hard palate and the maxillary alveolar process until it falls into the foramen depression. The needle is advanced perpendicular until bone is contacted slowly at an angle of 45 degrees to the long axis of the hard palate.

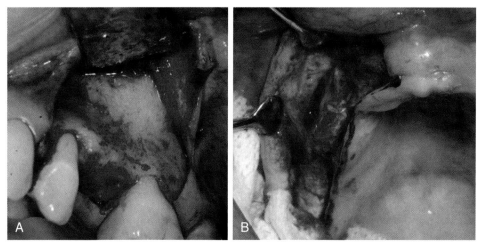

• **Fig. 37.34** Incision/reflection. Full-thickness reflection is necessary to expose the lateral wall. (A) For a single-tooth sinus augmentation, usually the incision extends one tooth on each side of the edentulous site. (B) For a large SA4 edentulous area, the anterior incision must extend 5-10 mm anterior to the anterior wall (approximately distal of cuspid) and posteriorly to the tuberosity.

Lateral Wall. A Tatum lateral maxillary wall approach is performed by performing an osteotomy over the lateral wall of the maxillary sinus, infracturing the window, elevating the sinus membrane and window, grafting to the medial wall, and then placing the implant (SA-3).

Incision and Reflection. A crestal incision is made on the palatal aspect of the maxillary posterior edentulous ridge from the tuberosity to one tooth anterior to the anterior wall of the maxillary sinus, leaving at least 2 mm of attached tissue on the facial aspect of the incision. Because ridge resorption occurs toward the midline at the expense of the buccal dimension, the incision is made with awareness of the greater palatal artery, which proceeds close to the crest of the ridge in the severely atrophic maxilla. If bleeding from the palatal flap occurs, then a hemostat may be used to constrict the blood vessels distal to the bleeding, pressure may be applied over the greater palatine foramen with a blunt instrument, or electrocoagulation at the bleeding site may be used.

A vertical relief incision is made on the distal of the incision to enhance surgical access to the maxillary tuberosity. A broad-base anterior vertical relief incision is also made at least 10 mm anterior to the anterior vertical wall of the sinus. This may result in the incision being made over the distal aspect of the first bicuspid or canine. The facial soft tissue flap is designed, following general principles, with a base wider than the crest to ensure proper blood supply. The palatal portion of the flap is first reflected, followed by the facial crestal tissue, which is reflected off the crest.

The facial full-thickness mucoperiosteal flap is reflected to expose the complete lateral wall of the maxilla and a portion of the zygoma. The facial flap should be reflected to provide complete vision and access to the maxillary lateral wall. The superior aspect of the flap should never approach the infraorbital foramen because aggressive reflection of the facial flap may cause a neuropraxia type of nerve impairment and damage to this nerve structure. The reflected labial tissue can be sutured to the cheek mucosa, carefully avoiding the parotid duct. All fibrous and soft tissue should be removed from the lateral-wall access site to avoid soft tissue contamination of the bone graft. Entrapping soft tissue within the sinus may lead to formation of a secondary mucocele or surgical ciliated cyst. A moist 4 x 4 gauze or a 2-4 molt with a scraping motion easily removes this tissue (Fig. 37.34).

Access Window. The overall design of the lateral-access window is determined after the review of the CBCT scan, which helps determine the thickness of the lateral wall of the antrum, the position of the antral floor from the crest of the ridge, the posterior of the anterior wall in relationship to the teeth (if present), the presence of septa on the floor and/or walls of the sinus, and any associated pathology within the maxillary sinus.

The outline of the Tatum lateral-access window is scored on the bone with a rotary handpiece under copious cooled sterile saline. It is often easier to perform this step at 50,000 rpm (1:1 handpiece), but it is possible even at 2000 rpm, depending on the lateral-wall bone thickness. There exist multiple techniques to score the sinus window: (1) carbide bur (No. 6 or No. 8), (2) diamond bur, (3) bone removal burs (e.g., Dask bur), or (4) Piezosurgery units. With experience, the first bur is usually a No. 8 round carbide, which scratches the bone and designs the overall window dimension. This bur is followed with a No. 8 round diamond, which "polishes" away the bone within the groove made by the carbide bur. A No. 8 round diamond bur for the entire process is of benefit for an early learning curve because carbide burs "chatter" more and may tear the sinus membrane if the bur inadvertently comes in contact with it.

The inferior score line of the rectangular access window on the lateral maxilla is placed approximately 1 to 2 mm above the level of the antral floor (i.e., which in an SA-3 is >5 mm from the crest). If the inferior score line is made at or below the level of the antral floor, then infracture of the lateral wall will be impossible because the score line will be over host bone. If the inferior score line is made too high (>4 mm) above the sinus floor, then a ledge above the sinus floor will result in a blind dissection of the membrane on the floor, which may also lead to perforation.

The most superior aspect of the lateral-access window should be approximately 2-3 mm above the planned implant length (i.e., 12-mm implant would require the window to be 15 mm from the ridge crest). A soft tissue retractor placed above the superior margin of the lateral-access window (i.e., always maintained on bone, not soft tissue) helps retract the facial flap and prevents the retractor's inadvertent slip into the access window, which may damage the underlying membrane of the sinus.

The anterior vertical line of the access window is scored approximately 1 to 2 mm from the anterior sinus border. The

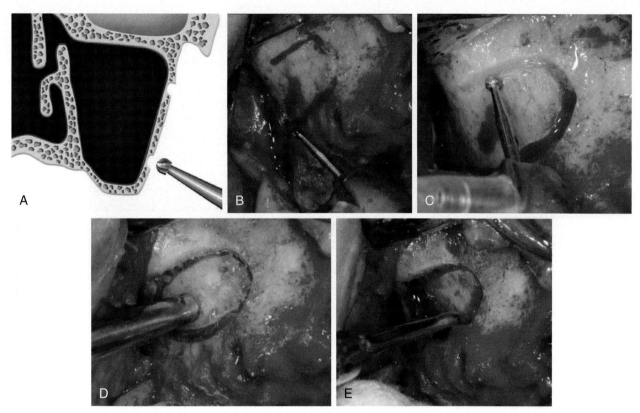

• **Fig. 37.35** Window preparation. (A) Window osteotomy should be made just through the cortical bone. (B) Initially, an outline form should be completed with a round carbide (No. 8), (C) Final preparation should be completed through the cortical bone with a round diamond (No. 8). (D and E) Osteotomy is complete when the window is free 360°.

distal vertical line should be made approximately 5 mm distal to the most posterior planned implant site (i.e., this will allow for adequate space if the implant position is changed more distally). If the patient is fully edentulous, the distal vertical line should be made approximately 5 mm distal to the first molar position. If the sinus access window outline is difficult to determine in relation to the sinus cavity, then it should err over the antrum rather than over the bone around this structure.

In general, a larger access window offers many advantages, including easier access, less stress on the membrane during initial elevation, and ease of additional membrane elevation with instruments because of the direct access that facilitates graft placement. The corners of the access window should always be rounded, not right or acute angles. If the corner angles are too sharp, then membrane perforation may occur from the use of a surgical curette at the corner or during the infracture of the lateral wall. Once the lateral-access window is delineated, the rotary bur continues to scratch the outline with a paintbrush stroke approach under cooled sterile saline irrigation, until a bluish hue is observed below the bur or hemorrhage from the site is observed. The expansion of the maxillary sinus after tooth loss pushes the arteries of the membrane to the outside of the structure and just below the surrounding bone. Therefore either the bluish hue of the membrane or bleeding in the area are signs of approaching the sinus membrane. This observation should be achieved circumferentially around the access window. The access window should not be overprepared in depth because direct contact with the membrane with rotary burs may cause a perforation (Fig. 37.35).

Complications

Endosseous Anastomosis. It should be noted that the largest blood vessel in the lateral wall is from an endosseous anastomosis from the posterior superior alveolar and the infraorbital artery. However, when the lateral wall is very thin in the edentulous patient, the anastomosis will atrophy and become nonexistent. The anastomosis has been shown to be located approximately 15 to 20 mm from the alveolar crest.

The horizontal lines of the access window should ideally not be positioned directly over this structure. The vertical lines of the access window often cut through the artery. Because the blood supply may be from either direction, both vertical access lines may have bleeding. This is rarely a concern for vision or blood loss during the procedure. If intraosseous bleeding is a problem, then the high-speed diamond used to score the window may be used without irrigation and polish the bleeding site, which cauterizes the vessel from the heat on the bony wall. Electrocautery may also be used on this vessel, if necessary. A hemostat maybe used; however, care should be exercised to avoid fracturing the lateral wall and/or perforating the sinus mucosa. Elevating the head and a surgical sponge applied to the site for a few minutes also aides in the control of hemorrhage.

Sinus Membrane Elevation. The first step in elevating the window is to ensure that the lateral window is completely "free" from the host bone. A flat-ended metal punch (or mirror handle) and mallet may be used to gently infracture the lateral-access window from the surrounding bone while still attached to the thin sinus membrane. The flat-ended punch is first positioned in the center of the window. If light tapping does not greenstick fracture the bone, then the flat-ended punch is placed along the periphery of the access window and tapped again. If the window does not separate easily, then the punch is rotated so that only an edge comes in contact with the scored line. This decreases the surface area of the punch against the score line and increases the

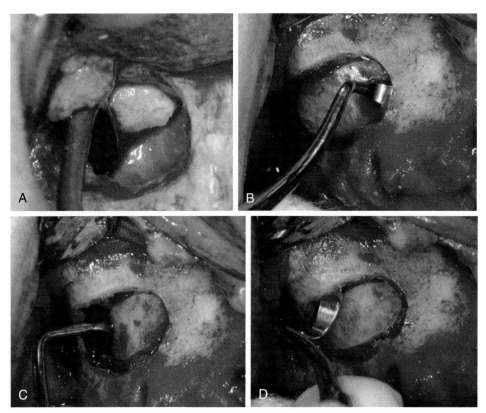

• **Fig. 37.36** Sinus membrane reflection. (A) Membrane reflection starts on the floor, (B) is extended to the anterior wall, (C) extended to the posterior, (D) and then to the superior. Curette should always be maintained on the bone to prevent perforation.

stress against the bone. Another light tap with the mallet will most likely cause greenstick fracture of the bone along the scored line. If this still does not free the window, then further scoring of the bone with the handpiece and diamond bur is indicated, and the tapping procedure is repeated.

A short-bladed soft tissue curette designed with two right-angle bends is introduced along the margin of the window (i.e., Salvin Sinus Curette No. 1). The curved portion is placed against the window, whereas the sharp edge is placed between the sinus membrane and the margin of the inner wall of the antrum for a depth of 2 to 4 mm. The curette should always stay on the bone and be used in a scraping motion. If any sharp edges of bone remain on the bone's margin, then they may be flicked off with the curette. The curette is slid along the bone margin 360 degrees around the access window. This ensures the release of the membrane from the surrounding walls of the sinus without tearing from the sharp bony access margins. The sinus membrane may be elevated from the antral walls easily because it has few elastic fibers and is not attached to the cortical wall. Specially designed and shaped curettes are available to facilitate this surgical maneuver. A larger curved periosteal or sinus membrane elevator is then introduced through the lateral-access window along the inferior border (i.e., Salvin Sinus Curette No. 2). Once again, the curved portion is placed against the window, and the sharp margin of the curette is dragged along the floor of the antrum while elevating the sinus membrane. The curette should always be maintained on the bony floor to avoid a membrane perforation. The curette is never blindly placed into the access window. The implant clinician should see and/or feel the curette against the antral floor or sinus walls at all times. Once the mucosa on the antral floor is elevated, the lateral, distal, and medial wall of the sinus is addressed. The

curette is pushed against the bone that easily reflects the membrane. The sinus membrane is inspected for perforations or openings into the antrum proper.

It is easier to gain direct vision and access to the distal portions of the antrum than the anterior portions when the sinus area expands beyond the access window. Therefore whenever the periosteal elevator or curette cannot stay against the bone with good access in the anterior area, the access window should be increased in size toward the anterior. A Kerrison rongeur or a second window similar to the initial score-and-fracture technique may be used to expand the size of the access window.

The periosteal elevators and curettes further reflect the membrane off the anterior vertical wall, floor, and medial vertical wall. It is better to err on the high side to ensure that ideal implant height may be placed without compromise (i.e., always maintaining a patent ostium). The lateral-access window is positioned as part of the superior wall of the graft site, once in final position. The SA space has the original sinus floor as the base; the posterior antral wall, medial antral wall, and anterior antral wall as its sides; and the lateral-access window and elevated sinus mucosa as its superior wall (Figs. 37.36 and 37.37).

Sinus Graft: Layered Approach.

Top Layer: Collagen and Antibiotic. A resorbable collagen membrane (Oratape) soaked with a parental form of antibiotic (Ancef 0.2 mL) is then prepared (Box 37.9). The collagen and antibiotic are placed onto the elevated antral floor region and attach to the sinus mucosa on the superior part of the graft site. The collagen is a carrier for the antibiotic to decrease the risk of postoperative infection. In addition, in case of membrane tearing or separation of the sinus mucosa (with or without the awareness of the clinician), the collagen membrane seals the opening (Fig. 37.38). It is imperative that a portion of the membrane be left

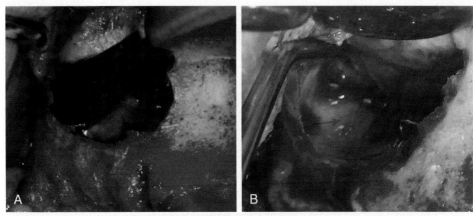

• **Fig. 37.37** Window elevation. (A and B) The window should not be "intruded" but elevated. When complete, the lateral wall will be at 90 degrees and the medial bone exposed (green arrow).

• BOX 37.9   Sinus Graft Layered Technique

1. **Top layer (superior)**
   a. Collagen membrane
   b. Local antibiotic (Ancef)
2. **Middle layer (intermediate)**
   a. 70% mineralized freeze-dried bone allograft
   b. 30% demineralized freeze-dried bone allograft
   c. Platelet-rich fibrin from 10 mL of whole blood
   d. Antibiotic (Ancef 500 mg/mL)
3. **Bottom layer (inferior)**
   a. Autogenous bone, tuberosity*

*Dependent on the amount of host bone present

---

outside of the sinus, preventing "intrusion" of the entire membrane into the sinus during bone placement.

Second Layer: Sinus Graft Materials. The second layer of the sinus graft layered approach is the most abundant and consists of the allograft bone grafting material. Many materials have been proposed in single or combination mixes, including mineralized and demineralized freeze-dried bone,[104,105] β-tricalcium phosphate (β-TCP),[106] xenograft hydroxyapatite (HA) (bovine anorganic bone), and calcium carbonates (bioactive glass).[107] In addition, more recent research has focused on combining "traditional" bone substitutes with bone growth factors.[108] Each graft material used in the sinus graft technique presents a similar, yet distinct, biological approach to the healing process.

What Type of Graft Material? Autogenous bone for years has been considered the gold standard of grafting material. Tatum first developed and reported the use of autogenous bone for sinus grafts in the 1970s, and Boyne[109,110] and James first published the information in 1980. In primates (*Macaca fascicularis*), Misch[111,112] found the use of iliac crest or tail bone in sinus grafts produced bone slightly denser than typical in the region, as evidenced from histology sections harvested at the reentry procedure. Similar findings have been observed during case series studies, with patients undergoing sinus grafts with autologous bone from the iliac crest or intraoral donor sites.[113]

It is interesting to note that sinus grafts in the literature that have used 100% autogenous bone have lower success rates than sinus grafts with synthetic substitutes (e.g., Del Fabbro and colleagues[114] reported 87.70% versus 95.98%).[115] Many additional studies have concluded that 100% autogenous bone results in less

bone formation that a composite type of graft. Hallman and colleagues showed that sinuses grafted with 100% xenograft compared with 100% autogenous exhibited greater healing and higher implant survival rates.[116] Froum and colleagues reported that if 20% autogenous bone was added to other bone substitutes, a greater mean vital bone formation was found.[117]

Demineralized freeze-dried bone (DFDB) has been shown to be osteoinductive, which is capable of inducing undifferentiated mesenchymal cells to form osteoblasts. The mechanism for this process appears to relate to the bone morphogenic protein (BMP) found primarily in cortical bone. In animal and human studies, DFDB allograft (DFDBA) powder used alone in sinus grafts did not provide satisfactory results. Bone was present but not in sufficient volume as the graft material originally placed. Speculation exists that the material resorbs more rapidly than the bone formation process, resulting in less bone formation. In addition, studies have shown that DFDB, when placed into an area of low-oxygen tension (hypoxic or hypocellular tissue), results in fibrous or cartilage tissue rather than bone.[118] Other authors have observed similar conclusions on the poor performance of DFDB used alone in animal and human studies.[119] At the Sinus Graft Consensus Conference,[14] high success rates were reported for all materials and combinations, with the exception of DFDB when used alone.

Mineralized freeze-dried bone allografts (FDBAs) are an allogenic bone that does not undergo the demineralization process. FDBA has the same BMP content in its organic matrix; however, it does not have the same osteoinductive capability as DFDBA. FDBA has been shown to be a better scaffold (osteoconduction) than DFDBA, which allows for superior space maintenance.[120] Eventually, osteoclasts breakdown the mineral content of FDBA until demineralization occurs, inducing new bone formation and a prolonged protein release.

Cammack and colleagues examined mineralized and demineralized freeze dried allograft used in sinus augmentation procedures and found no statistical significance between the two bone substitutes. A histomorphometric study by Froum and colleagues[121] at 26 to 32 weeks after grafting evaluated mineralized cancellous bone allograft (MCBA) and anorganic bovine bone material (ABBM) for sinus augmentation. Bilateral sinus grafts, one filled with MCBA and the other with ABBM, were compared. The average vital bone content of the MCBA was 28.25%, compared with the ABBM of only 12.44%. Therefore mineralized corticocancellous bone of approximately 250 to 1000 μm is advantageous for

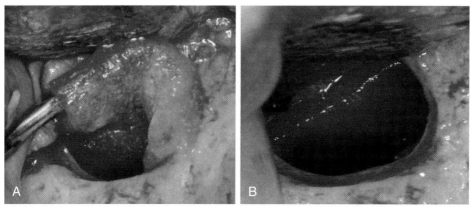

• **Fig. 37.38** Top layer. (A and B) Fast-resorbing collagen (e.g., Collatape) is used with antibiotic as the top layer. The collagen membrane should be positioned to the medial wall and with a small segment exposed outside the superior aspect of the window. A longer acting collagen may be used if a known membrane perforation is present.

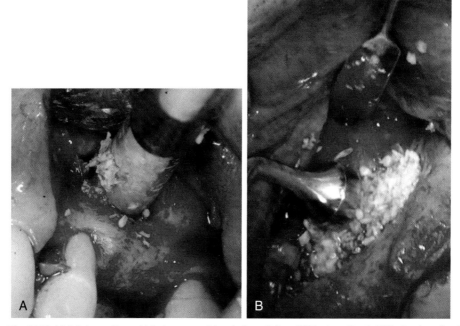

• **Fig. 37.39** Middle layer. The middle layer consists of allograft (i.e., 70% mineralized, 30% demineralized) plus antibiotic. (A) Allograft syringed into the sinus proper. (B) Packing of the sinus with a packer.

bone graft material because it fulfills space maintenance requirements and allows for cell migration.[122]

Allograft bone material is available in three particle forms: cortical, cancellous, and corticocancellous. Cortical allografts are associated with an increased density and greater space maintenance properties, which allow for slower resorption. Cancellous chips are advantageous because they allow for osteoconductive scaffolding and deposition of osteoblasts while being faster resorbing. Ideally, the use of corticocancellous bone is advantageous because it allows for both the benefits of cancellous and cortical bone to be used in the grafting process.

The ideal particle size of the allograft material is very important in the bone regeneration process because too small (<125 μm) particle size leads to fast resorption, with an inconsistent bone formation. A larger particle size (>1000 μm) restricts resorption and may be sequestered or result in delayed healing. Studies have

shown an ideal particle size for predictable bone regeneration to be approximately 250 to 1000 μm.[123]

In addition to the mineralized bone, bone graft factors in the form of platelet-rich fibrin may be used. Whole blood is drawn (approximately 10 ml) from the patient and placed into a centrifuge for 10 to 15 minutes at 3000 rpm. The blood is separated by the centrifuge into three layers: (1) red blood cells, (2) platelet-rich fibrin (PRF), and (3) platelet-poor plasma (PPM). The PRF layer contains many growth factors that are involved in the cascade of bone mineralization.[124] The PRF is added to the bone substitutes, along with a local antibiotic to be added into the sinus proper. A parenteral form of antibiotic is used rather than a tablet form because oral antibiotic drugs often have fillers in the product that are not osteoconductive. The most common antibiotic is Ancef 500 mg/mL, and 0.8 mL of solution is added to the graft (Fig. 37.39).

Summary: 2nd Layer. The second layer of the lateral-wall sinus graft will consist of the following:

1. a. 70% mineralized FDBA, 30% demineralized DFDBA
   OR
   b. Mineralized FDBA: (Corticocancellous)
      - Particle Size = 250–100 μm
      - Approximately 250–1000 μm
2. PRF
3. Local antibiotic (Ancef)

These materials are mixed in a surgical bowl and filled into a bone grafting syringe or 1 cc hypodermic syringe. When placing the graft material, insert the syringe into the sinus proper in approximation to the medial wall and material is extruded as the syringe is removed. The grafting material should be deposited in an anterior and inferior direction. This will ensure material raises the lateral window instead of intrusion toward the medial wall. Intrusion will lead to lack of bone formation near the medial wall and may affect implant placement and post-sinus mucociliary function. By extruding the material in the anterior direction, bone graft material will be placed into the anterior segment of the sinus incorporating graft material in contact with the anterior wall and increasing blood supply for healing. The material should be condensed with a serrated packer, and packing pressure should be firm but not excessive. Inadequate pressure will result in air-spaces, which may predispose the graft to future infection. Excessive condensation may lead to perforation of the membrane and extrusion of material into the sinus proper.

Bottom Layer

Regional Acceleratory Phenomenon. The third or bottom layer will consist of multiple steps to enhance bone growth. First, especially if little bleeding is present from the sinus floor and the anterior wall, a sharp instrument (e.g., scaler, curette) is used to scratch the bone. This trauma will initiate the regional acceleratory phenomenon (RAP), which introduces more growth factors into the site and starts the angiogenesis process. The blood vessels allow migration of osteoclasts and osteoblasts that resorb and replace the graft with live, viable bone. In addition, the blood vessels provide blood supply to the autologous bone portion of the graft, which is required for initial osteogenesis. The medial wall should not be scratched because it is very thin and perforation may occur.

Autogenous Bone. The second part of the third layer is the use of autogenous bone. Osteogenic material is capable of producing bone, even in the absence of local undifferentiated mesenchymal cells. Autogenous bone predictably exhibits this activity in the sinus graft. Misch has performed reentry of more than 1500 sinus grafts (at implant placement) accompanied by more than 50 human histologic sections and 18 primate sinus grafts and histology. A consistent histologic and clinical finding is that bone grows into the augmentation region from the surrounding walls of the maxillary antrum in which the sinus membrane was elevated.[125] In other words, the bone growth came from the surrounding walls of bone, similar to an extraction socket. The last regions to form bone are usually the center of the lateral-access window and the region under the elevated sinus membrane. In fact, no new bone at time intervals up to 12 months was found to grow immediately under the sinus membrane.

The most common harvest site for the lateral-wall approach is the maxillary tuberosity on the same side of the patient that the sinus is being augmented. In this way, an additional surgical site is not required, which decreases morbidity to the patient. Additional sources of bone to be added to the graft site may be any bone fragments from implant osteotomy sites, bone cores over the roots of anterior teeth, sinus exostoses, and cores from the mandibular symphysis or ramus region. The autogenous bone is placed on the original bony floor in the area most indicated for implant insertion. A blood supply from the host bone can be established earlier to this grafted bone and maintains the viability of the transplanted bone cells and the osteogenic potential of the transplanted bone growth factors. Autogenous bone represents an important component of the sinus graft, and is of more importance in an SA-4 approach compared with an SA-3, which has more host bone present (Fig. 37.40).

The harvest of the tuberosity bone is initiated with the exposure of the tuberosity bone; however, care should be exercised to not extend the incision to the hamular notch area because this may result in potential bleeding episodes. Once there is full-thickness reflection of the tuberosity bone, double-action rongeurs may remove small pieces of the mainly cancellous bone. The tuberosity bone is usually soft and therefore is compressed to form more cells per volume. Usually, rotary burs or bone chisels are not recommended because this reduces the amount of bone grafted and increases the possibility of perforation into the sinus proper. Additional autogenous bone may be harvested intraorally or extraorally, as indicated on a case-by-case basis (Fig. 37.41).

The autogenous bone is then placed on the floor by making small spaces with a curette within the allograft material. Ideally, a space should be made to the medial wall because it is advantageous for autograft chips to be placed in approximation to the medial wall. After placement of the autogenous bone, the grafted area is veneered with the allograft material to fill any voids that are present.

Implant Insertion. A review of the literature by Del Fabbro and colleagues[126] notes success rates of implants placed at the same time as the graft have a survival rate of 92.17%, whereas a delayed implant insertion has a survival rate of 92.93%. The 5 to 10 mm of initial bone height in an SA-3 posterior maxilla, the cortical bone on the residual crest, and the cortical-like bone on the original antral floor may stabilize an implant that is inserted at the time of the graft and permit its rigid fixation. Therefore when the conditions are ideal for the SA-3 sinus graft, the implant may be inserted at the same appointment. When inserting implants into an SA-3 sinus graft, the sinus should always be completely filled prior to implant placement. Attempting to graft after implant insertion is very difficult and will lead to voids. When preparing the osteotomy into the grafted sinus, a finger rest should be maintained so that control of the handpiece is maintained upon perforation into the sinus. Care should be exercised to not extend the osteotomy into the grafted material. This will result in dispersion of the graft material. Penetration though the inferior floor should only be approximately 1 mm, as there will be no resistance from the graft material when placing the implant. In most cases, the osteotomy will be underprepared to allow for osseodensification (D4 bone). Implant placement is more accurate when inserted with a handpiece (Figs. 37.42 and 37.44).

The advantage of the SA-3 technique is the decreased treatment time because the implant and sinus graft are completed at the same time. In addition, there exist several disadvantages of immediate implant placement compared with delaying implant placement (i.e., SA-4 approach):

1. The individual rate of healing of the graft may be assessed during the healing period, while the implant osteotomy is being prepared and the implant inserted. The healing time for the implant is no longer arbitrary, but it is more patient specific.
2. Under ideal conditions, postoperative sinus graft infections occur in approximately 3% to 5% of patients, which is greater than the percentage for implant placement surgery or intraoral onlay

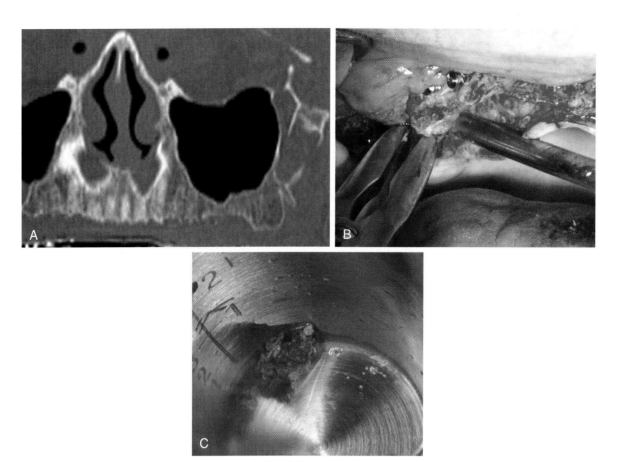

• **Fig. 37.40** Autogenous bone harvest. (A) Usually because of access, the maxillary tuberosity is the most ideal location for autogenous harvest. (B) Harvest can be completed with a double-action rongeur. (C) Usually large autogenous pieces may be obtained without penetration into the maxillary sinus.

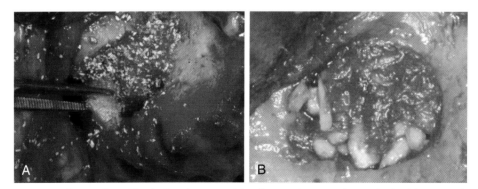

• **Fig. 37.41** Bottom layer. The bottom layer consists of any autogenous bone obtained because the importance of autogenous bone is inversely proportional to the amount of host bone present. (A) harvested bone placed into window. (B) Final bone packing of autogenous bone.

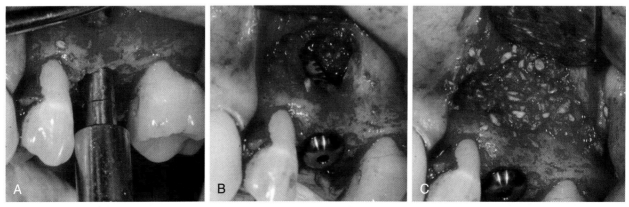

• **Fig. 37.42** SA-3 implant placement. (A) After lateral-wall sinus grafting, the osteotomy is completed, usually after the initial surgical drill, osteotomes are used to widen the osteotomy. (B) Implant placement into graft material. (C) Final veneer grafting over implant site.

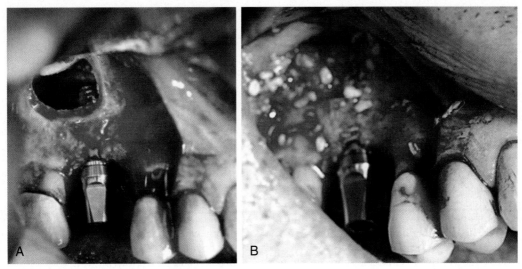

• **Fig. 37.43** Membrane. (A) Collagen membrane positioning over the lateral window (i.e., may use platelet-rich fibrin over collagen). (B) Final suturing of surgical site.

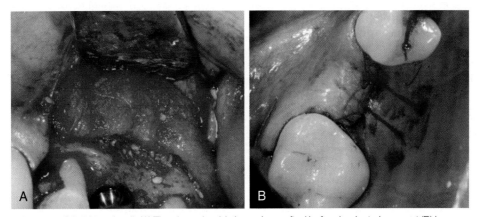

• **Fig. 37.44** SA-3 lateral wall. (A) The sinus should always be grafted before implant placement (B) because grafting is difficult to complete after implant is placed (i.e., cannot graft on medial aspect of implant).

bone grafts. If the sinus graft becomes infected with an implant in place, then a bacterial smear layer may develop on the implant and make future bone contact with the implant less predictable. The infection is also more difficult to treat when the implants are in place and may result in greater resorption of the graft as a consequence. If the infection cannot be adequately treated, then the graft and implant must be removed. Therefore a decreased risk of losing the graft and implant exists if a postoperative infection occurs with a delayed implant insertion. Some reports in the literature indicate a slightly higher failure rate of implants when inserted simultaneously compared with a delayed approach.

3. Blood vessels within the graft are required to form and remodel bone. An implant in the middle of the sinus graft does not provide a source of blood vessels. It may even impair the vascular supply.

4. Bone width augmentation may be indicated in conjunction with sinus grafts to restore proper maxillomandibular ridge relationships and/or increase the implant diameter in the molar region. Augmentation may be performed simultaneously with the sinus graft. As a result, larger diameter implants may be placed with the delayed technique.

5. The bone in the sinus graft is denser with the delayed implant placement. As such, implant angulation and position may be improved because it is not dictated by existing anatomic limitations at the time of the sinus graft.

6. The clinician may access the sinus graft before implant insertion. On occasion, the sinus graft underfills a region, and the lack of awareness of the condition during implant insertion at the same time results in an implant placed in the sinus proper, rather than the graft site.

7. On reentry to a sinus graft, it is not unusual to observe a crater-like formation in the center of the lateral-access window, with soft tissue invagination. If the implant is already in place, then it may be difficult to remove the soft tissue and assess its precise extent. When soft tissue is present at a delayed implant insertion, the region is curetted and replaced with a bone graft before implant placement. The healing time for the implant is related to the developing bone assessed at the delayed surgery, not an arbitrary period that may be, on occasion, too brief.

Membranes. After implant placement, a thin layer of graft material may be veneered over teh lateral access opening. A resorbable membrane (e.g., Collatape) is then placed over the lateral-access window (Fig. 37.43). A membrane will delay the invasion of fibrous tissue into the graft and will enhance the repair of the lateral bony wall. A nonresorbable membrane should not be used because reentry would be required and the possibility of postoperative sinus infection will increase. A bacterial smear layer may accumulate in the nonresorbable material and contribute to the infection process. Rarely will a resorbable membrane become infected.

PRF may be used as a double membrane by placement over the lateral collagen membrane to increase the amount of growth factors for bone formation and to increase the growth factors for tissue healing. If inadequate PRF is available because it was used in the second layer of the graft, then PPP may be used because platelets are present but in lower quantities. Froum and colleagues[127] evaluated sinus grafts with barrier membranes over the lateral-access wall compared with no barrier membrane. All sinus graft combinations in the study demonstrated higher vital bone percentage on the cores when a barrier membrane was used. Misch observed a higher vital bone percentage even when collagen was used over the lateral-access site compared with no collagen. Tarnow and colleagues completed a split-mouth design study with bilateral sinus grafts, with or without covering the lateral window with a membrane. Histologic samples revealed a higher percentage of bone with a membrane (25.5%) compared with no membrane (19.9%).[128]

Soft Tissue Closure. The soft tissues and periosteum should be reapproximated for primary closure without tension, with care to eliminate graft particles in the incision line. Because of the access window grafting, along with the double layer membrane, it is often necessary to stretch the tissue to allow for tension-free closure. Therefore the facial flap must often be expanded, which usually can be completed by periosteal release incisions. A tissue pickup holds the facial flap to the height of the mucogingival tissues junction. The flap is then elevated, and a No. 15 blade is used to incise the tissue 1 mm deep through the periosteum above the mucoperiosteum. Tissue scissors are then introduced into the incision parallel to the facial flap at a depth of 3 to 5 mm. A blunt dissection under the flap releases the periosteum and muscle attachments to the base of the facial flap. The flap may then be advanced over the graft site to the palatal tissues.

It should be noted that horizontal vascular anastomoses are located lateral to the maxilla, within the soft tissue (extraosseous anastomosis), and approximately 20 mm above the crest of the ridge. A blunt dissection does not violate these vessels. No tension should exist on the facial flap with primary closure of the site. Interrupted horizontal mattress or a continuous suture (3-0 polyglycolic acid [PGA]) may be placed. Suturing is more critical with this procedure than with many other implant placements. Incision line opening may contribute to infection, contamination, or loss of graft materials. The borders and flange of an overlaying soft tissue–borne denture or partial denture are aggressively relieved to eliminate pressure against the lateral wall of the maxilla.

Crestal Approach. The second option for an SA-3 sinus augmentation and implant placement is the use of the crestal approach. This approach has become more popular for reducing complications from lateral-wall sinus augmentation procedures. The crestal approach sinus augmentation uses an osteotome to break through the floor and then graft below the sinus membrane. The following are the five steps used in the procedure:

Step 1: A conventional full-thickness flap with crestal incision is completed to gain access to the bony ridge. A pilot drill is used to perform the initial osteotomy 1 to 2 mm short of the sinus floor. The exact measurement of the available bone is completed via CBCT images. Incrementally larger surgical drills or osteotomes should be used to widen the osteotomy, at least one drill short of the final implant width.
Step 2: A small diameter osteotome is inserted into the prepared site to compress the sinus floor using a surgical mallet. A slight

"give" will occur when the bone is breached. A periapical radiograph may be taken to verify positioning. Incremental wider osteotomes are inserted to expand and to obtain vertical expansion of the bone height to accommodate the implant diameter.
Step 3: After the last osteotome is used, bone graft material is slowly introduced into the osteotomy site. First, a PRF coagulant maybe placed into the osteotomy site. This will allow for enhanced soft tissue healing via penetration through the collagen membrane to increase bone growth. Second, collagen is tapped into position to elevate the membrane. A small piece of collagen (i.e., approximately 1½ larger than the osteotomy hole) is placed into the osteotomy site, with the last osteotome. The collagen will act as a buffer between the bone graft material and the sinus membrane. The collagen is less likely to perforate the membrane.
Step 4: The graft material is slowly introduced into the sinus osteotomy with a bone graft spoon or an amalgam carrier. The sinus floor is then elevated by repeated increments of bone graft material and placed into position with an osteotome.
Step 5: Once the osteotomy is widened and sinus membrane is elevated to the desired height, the implant may be inserted.

This SA-3 crestal technique has the advantage of surgical simplicity, which decreases possible surgical morbidity. The main disadvantage of this technique is the unknown perforation of the sinus membrane. Ideally, the sinus membrane integrity should be maintained during the procedure. The limitations of this technique include elevating the membrane approximately 3 to 4 mm. If greater height is required, the lateral-wall approach may be used (Figs. 37.45 and 37.46; Box 37.10).

Subantral Option Four: Sinus Graft Healing and Extended Delay of Implant Insertion

In the fourth option for implant treatment of the posterior maxilla, SA-4, the SA region for future endosteal implant insertion is first augmented, then after sufficient healing, implant placement is completed. This option is indicated when less than 5 mm remains between the residual crest of bone and the floor of the maxillary sinus (Fig. 37.47). In addition, if an SA-3 approach is warranted because only 5 mm of bone is present, but pathology is present, it is often advantageous to complete an SA-4 technique. The SA-4 corresponds to a larger antrum and minimal host bone on the lateral, anterior, and distal regions of the graft because the antrum generally has expanded more aggressively into these regions. The inadequate vertical bone in these conditions decreases the predictable placement of an implant at the same time as the sinus graft, and less recipient bone exists to act as a vascular bed for the graft. In addition, in most cases, less autologous bone exists in the tuberosity for harvesting, and fewer septa or webs will exist in the sinus (and typically exhibit longer mediodistal and wider lateromedial dimensions). Therefore the fewer bony walls, less favorable vascular bed, minimal local autologous bone, and larger graft volume all mandate a longer healing period and slightly altered surgical approach.

The Tatum lateral-wall approach for sinus graft is performed as in the previous SA-3 procedure without the implant insertion (Fig. 37.48). Most SA-4 regions provide better surgical access than their SA-3 counterparts because the antrum floor is closer to the crest, compared with the SA-3 posterior maxilla. However, in Division D maxillae, it is usually necessary to expose the lateral maxilla and the zygomatic arch. The access window in the severely atrophic maxilla may even be designed in the zygomatic arch. In general, the medial wall of the sinus membrane is elevated approximately

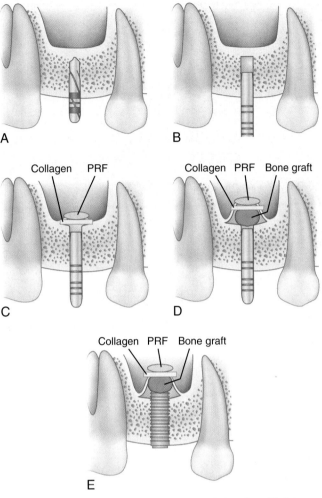

• **Fig. 37.45** Crestal approach. (A) Step 1: Initial osteotomy short of sinus floor. (B) Osteotome used to widen osteotomy. (C) Platelet-rich fibrin and collagen membrane placement. (D) Allograft material placement. (E) implant placement.

12 mm from the crest so that adequate height is available for future endosteal implant placement. The combination of graft materials used and their placement are identical to the SA-3 technique lateral-wall approach. However, because less autogenous bone is often harvested from the tuberosity, an additional harvest site may be required, most often above the roots of the maxillary premolars or from the mandible (i.e., ascending ramus).

The width of the host site for most edentulous posterior maxillae is Division A. However, when Division C–w to D exists, a membrane or onlay graft for width is indicated. When the graft cannot be secured to the host bone, it is often better to perform the sinus graft 6 to 9 months prior to the autogenous graft for width. After the graft maturation, the implants may be inserted (Box 37.11).

Vascular Healing of Graft

Healing of the sinus graft takes place by several vascular routes, including the endosseous vascular anastomosis and the vasculature of the sinus membrane from the sphenopalatine artery. In mildly resorbed ridges, the host bone receives its blood supply from both centromedullary and mucoperiosteal vessels. However, as age and the resorption process increases, the bone gradually becomes totally dependent on the mucoperiosteum for the blood supply. The periphery of the graft is mainly supplied by vessels of the sinus

membrane and by intraosseous vascular bundles. The central portions of the graft receive blood from collateral branches of the endosseous anastomosis. The extraosseous vascular anastomosis may enter the graft from the lateral-access window.

Many local variables are related to sinus graft maturation, including healing time, the volume of the SA graft, the distance from the lateral to medial wall (small, average, or large), and the amount of autologous bone in the multilayered approach, all of which relate to the speed and amount of new bone formation.

The time of evaluation of the sinus graft is perhaps the greatest variable of all. Froum and colleagues[129,130] evaluated a sinus graft from the same patient at 4 months, 6 months, 12 months, and 20 months. The amount of new bone continuously increased, compared with the amount of graft material in the antrum. In addition, the additional time allowed the graft to mature into a load bearing type of bone. In summary, the more time that elapsed from sinus graft to implant loading, the more vital bone was available to support the occlusal load.

The type of bone graft material used in the sinus graft may affect the rate of bone formation. Bone formation is fastest and most complete within the first 4 to 6 months with autogenous bone, followed by the combination of autogenous bone, porous HA, and DFDB (6–10 months); alloplasts only (i.e., TCP) may take 24 months to

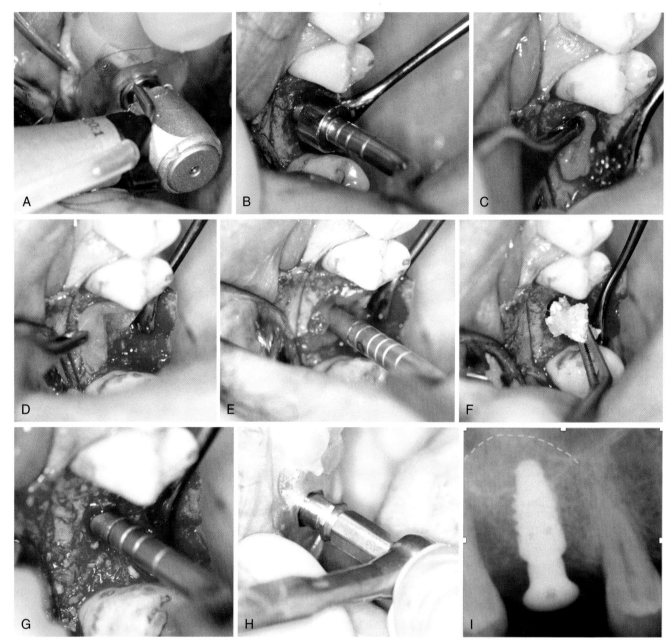

● **Fig. 37.46** Crestal approach. (A) Initial osteotomy completed via fully guided template 1 mm short of the sinus floor, (B) Sequential osteotomes are used to infracture sinus floor, (C) Placement of PRF plug, (D) Collagen membrane placed over osteotomy site, (E) Osteotome used to elevate collagen membrane, (F) Bone allograft placed into osteotomy site in increments, (G) Osteotomes elevate graft material, (H) Implant placement, (I) Final implant with graft material.

● **BOX 37.10** **SA-3 (Crestal Approach) Requirements**

- **Favorable conditions:** (>5 mm host bone, Implant size < 4mm greater than host bone)
- **Unfavorable conditions:** (>8 mm host bone, Implant size < 4mm greater than host bone)

form bone. The time required before implant insertion for SA-4 or implant uncovery is dependent on the volume of the sinus graft. Most healed sinus augmentations (i.e., especially SA-4) will be the D4 type of bone; therefore osseodensification surgical approach and progressive bone loading techniques should be strictly followed.

Postoperative Instructions

The postoperative instructions are similar to those for most oral surgical procedures. Rest, ice, pressure, and elevation of the head are particularly important. Strict adherence to the pharmacologic protocol as mentioned previously is vital to decrease postop morbidity is of major importance. Although smoking is not an absolute contraindication for sinus grafting, smoking during the healing period may negatively affect the healing and increase the possibility of postoperative infections.

Blowing the nose and/or creating negative pressure while sucking through a straw or cigarettes should also be eliminated for the 2 weeks after surgery. Block and Kent[131] reported on a patient who lost the entire sinus graft 2 days after surgery from

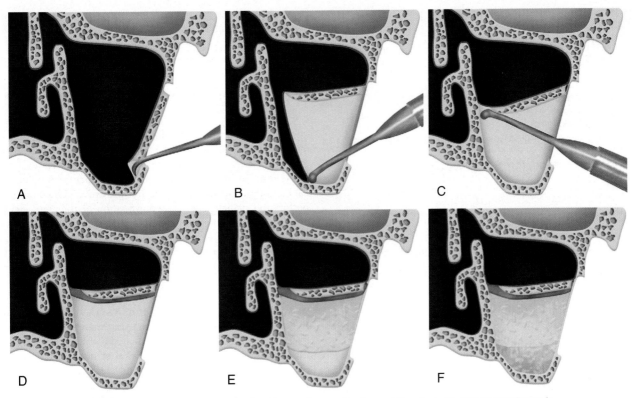

• **Fig. 37.47** SA-4. (A) Membrane elevation starting on the floor of the sinus. (B and C) Membrane is reflected to the medial wall. (D) First layer (superior) is collagen with antibiotic. (E) Second layer (middle) allograft bone. (F) Third layer (floor), which is comprised of autogenous bone.

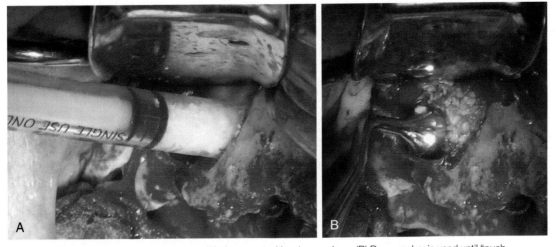

• **Fig. 37.48** SA-4. Bone placement (A) placement with a 1-cc syringe. (B) Bone packer is used until "push-back" is obtained.

• BOX 37.11 SA-4 Requirements

• **Favorable or unfavorable conditions:** <5 mm host bone

blowing the nose. Sneezing, if it occurs, should be done with the mouth open to relieve pressure within the sinus. Swelling of the region is common, but pain is usually less severe than after anterior implants in an edentulous mandible. In addition, the patient should be warned against lifting and pulling on the lip to observe the surgical site or during oral hygiene procedures to reduce the

risk of incision line opening. The patient should be notified that small bone particles or synthetic bone found in the mouth or expelled from the nose with bleeding is not unusual (Box 37.12).

Implant Insertion

The implant surgery at reentry after successful sinus grafts is similar to SA-1, with a few exceptions. The periosteal flap on the lateral side is elevated to directly allow inspection of the previous access window of the sinus graft. The previous access window may appear completely healed with bone, soft and filled with loose graft material, or with cone-shaped fibrous tissue in-growth (with the base of the cone toward the lateral wall).

• BOX 37.12 Sinus Graft Postoperative Instructions

1. Do not blow your nose.
2. Do not smoke or use smokeless tobacco.
3. Do not take in liquids through a straw.
4. Do not lift or pull on lip to look at sutures (stitches).
5. If you must sneeze, then do so with your mouth open to avoid any unnecessary pressure on the sinus area.
6. Take your medication as directed.
7. You may be aware of small granules in your mouth for 2 to 3 days after surgery.
8. Bleeding from the nostril may be present for the first 24 hours after surgery.

• BOX 37.13 Membrane Perforations

- Small (<2 mm) fast-resorbing collagen (e.g., Collatape, Oratape)
- Medium (2–4 mm) regular collagen (e.g., OraMem)
- Large (>4 mm) longer acting collagen (e.g., Renovix, OraMem Extend)

If the graft site on the lateral-access wall appears clinically as bone, then the implant osteotomy and placement follow the approach designated by the bone density. If soft tissue has proliferated into the access window from the lateral-tissue region, then it is curetted and removed. The region is again packed to a firm consistency with autologous bone from the previously augmented tuberosity and mineralized freeze-dried bone. The implant osteotomy may then be prepared and the implant placed a the D4 bone protocol. Additional time (6 months or more) is allowed until the stage II implant uncovery is performed and progressive bone loading is used during prosthetic reconstruction. The time interval for stage II uncovery and prosthetic procedures after implant insertion of a sinus graft is dependent on the density of bone at the reentry of implant placement. The crest of the ridge and the original antral floor may be the only cortical bone in the region for implant fixation. The most common bone density observed for a sinus graft reentry is D3 or D4. Most often, mineralized bone graft (or xenograft) material in the sinus graft has not converted to bone. The tactile sense and the CBCT evaluation interpret the mineralized graft material as a denser bone type; therefore a tactile or radiographic D3 bone may actually be D4-like bone. It is prudent to wait longer (rather than shorter) for implant uncovery. An SA-4 sinus graft has a recommended healing time at least 4 to 6 months for implant insertion and another 4 to 8 months for implant uncovery. Therefore the overall graft maturity time is 4 to 10 months for SA-3, and SA-4 healing time is 8 to 14 months before prosthetic reconstruction. Progressive loading after uncovery is most important when the bone is particularly soft and less dense. Inadequate bone formation after the sinus graft healing period of SA-4 surgery is a possible, but uncommon, complication.

Intraoperative Complications Related to Sinus Graft Surgery

Membrane Perforations

The most common complication during sinus graft surgery is tearing or creation of an opening in the sinus membrane (Box 37.13). This has several causes, which include a preexisting perforation, tearing during scoring of the lateral window, existing or previous pathologic condition, and elevation of the membrane from the bony walls. According to studies, membrane perforations occur about 10% to 34% of the time. It has been reported with a higher frequency in smokers. If membrane perforation occurs more often than this, then the clinician should give consideration to alter or reevaluate the surgical technique used in sinus grafting.

Sinus membrane perforation usually does not affect the sinus graft. However, in a report of the Sinus Consensus Conference, analysis of failed sinus grafts found 48% (79 of 164 failures) were attributed to sinus membrane perforations.[130] In an endoscopic evaluation after sinus grafts, macrolaceration of the sinus membrane resulted in a typical sinusitis appearance, even when clinical conditions of infection were not present.[132] Once the tear or perforation is identified, the continuation of the sinus elevation procedure is modified. The sinus membrane should be elevated off the bony walls of the antrum, despite the mucosal tear. If a portion of the membrane is not elevated away from a sinus wall, then the graft material will be placed on top of the membrane, preventing the bone graft from incorporating with the bony wall.

The perforation of the sinus membrane should be sealed to prevent contamination of the graft from the mucus and contents of the sinus proper and to prevent the graft material from extruding into the sinus proper. When graft materials enter the sinus proper, they may become sources for infection or may migrate and close off the ostium to the nasal cavity and create an environment for an infection.

Numerous studies have shown a very low probability of sinus infections after perforations in the sinus membrane. Jensen and colleagues[133] reported that graft maturation occurred and no sinus infections were observed despite a 35% incidence of sinus perforation during the procedure in 98 patients.

The surgical correction of a small perforation is initiated by elevating the sinus mucosal regions distal from the opening. Once the tissues are elevated away from the opening, the membrane elevation with a sinus curette should approach the tear from all sides so that the torn region may be elevated without increasing the opening size. The antral membrane elevation technique decreases the overall size of the antrum, thus "folding" the membrane over on itself and resulting in closure of the perforation. A piece of resorbable collagen membrane (e.g., Collatape) is placed over the opening to ensure continuity of the sinus mucosa before the sinus bone graft is placed. The collagen will stick to the membrane and seal the SA space from the sinus proper.

If the sinus membrane tear is larger than 6 mm and cannot be closed off with the circumelevation approach, then a resorbable collagen membrane with a longer resorption cycle (e.g., Renovix, BioMend), may be used to seal the opening.

The remaining sinus mucosa is first elevated as described previously. A piece of collagen matrix is cut to cover the sinus tear opening and overlap the margins more than 5 mm. It should be noted that when a sinus tear occurs, it is sealed with a dry collagen membrane so that it may be rotated into the lateral-access opening, gently lifted to the mucosal tissue around the opening, and allowed to stick to the mucosa. Once the opening is sealed, the sinus graft procedure may be completed in routine fashion. However, care should be taken when packing the sinus with graft material. After a perforation, the graft is easily pushed through the collagen-sealed opening and into the sinus proper. The graft material is then gently inserted and pushed toward the sinus floor and sides but not toward the top of the graft. A sinus perforation may cause an increased risk of short-term complications. A greater bacterial penetration risk exists into the graft material through the torn membrane. In addition, mucus may invade the graft and affect the amount of bone formation. Graft material may leak through the tear into the sinus proper, migrate to and through the ostium, and be eliminated through the nose or obstruct the ostium and prevent the normal sinus drainage. Ostium obstruction is also possible from swelling of the membrane related to the surgery. These conditions increase the risk of infection. However, despite these potential complications, the risk of the infection is low (less than 5%); therefore the sinus graft surgery should continue, and the patient should be monitored postoperatively for appropriate treatment (Figs. 37.49 and 37.50).

Antral Septa

Antral septa (i.e., also termed buttresses, webs, and struts) are the most common osseous anatomic variants seen in the maxillary sinus. Underwood,[134] an anatomist, first described maxillary sinus septa in 1910. He postulated that the cause of these bony projections derived from three different periods of tooth development and eruption. Krennmair and colleagues[135] further classified these structures into two groups: primary structures, which are a result of the development of the maxilla, and secondary structures, which arise from the pneumatization of the sinus floor after tooth loss.

Misch[136] postulated that septa might be bone reinforcement pillars from parafunction when the teeth were present. He noticed these structures occur more often in SA-3 sinuses and after a shorter history of tooth loss. Long-term edentulous sites and SA-4 sinuses have fewer septa. The prevalence of septa has been reported to be in the range of 33% of the maxillary sinuses in the dentate patient and as high as 22% in the edentulous patient.[137] The septa may be complete or incomplete on the floor, depending on whether they divide the bottom of the sinus into compartments. The septa may also be incomplete from the lateral wall or, the medial wall, or it should extend from the floor.

The shape of an incomplete maxillary sinus septum often resembles an inverted gothic arch that arises from the inferior or lateral walls of the sinus. In rare instances, they may divide the sinus into two compartments that radiate from the medial wall toward the lateral wall.

The most common location of septa in the maxillary sinus has been reported to be in the middle (second bicuspid–first molar) region of the sinus cavity. CBCT scan studies have shown that 41% of septa are seen in the middle region, followed by the posterior region (35%) and the anterior region (24%). For diagnosis and evaluation of septa, CBCT scans are the most accurate method of radiographic evaluation.[138] Panoramic radiography has been shown to be very inaccurate, with a high incidence of faulty diagnoses.

Sinus septa may create added difficulty at the time of surgery. Maxillary septa can prevent adequate access and visualization to the sinus floor; therefore inadequate or incomplete sinus grafting is possible. These dense projections complicate the surgery in several ways. After scoring the lateral-access window in the usual fashion, the lateral-access window may not greenstick fracture and rotate into its medial position. The strut reinforcement is also more likely to tear the membrane during the releasing of the access window. The sinus membrane is often torn at the apex of the buttress during sinus membrane manipulation because difficulty exists in elevating the membrane over the sharp edge of the web, and the curette easily tears the membrane at this position. However, because septa are mainly composed of cortical bone, immediate implant placement may engage this dense bone, allowing for strong intermediate fixation. Moreover, septa allow for faster bone formation because they act as an additional wall of bone for blood vessels to grow into the graft.

Management of Septa Based on Location

The use of CBCT radiographs before sinus graft surgery permits the surgeon to observe and plan the necessary modifications to the sinus graft procedure as a result of the septa. The modification to the surgery is variable depending on its location. The septa may be in the anterior, middle, or distal compartment of the antrum. When the septum is found in the anterior section, the lateral-access window is divided into sections: one in front of the septa and another distal to

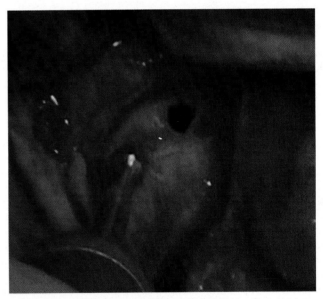

• **Fig. 37.49** Maxillary sinus perforation from window outline osteotomy.

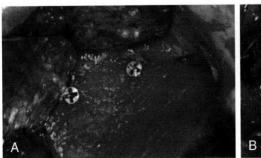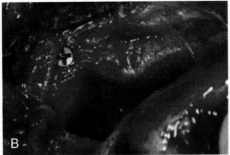

• **Fig. 37.50** Perforation repair. (A and B) Extended collagen membrane fixated on the superior aspect of the sinus cavity.

the structure. This permits the release of each section of the lateral wall after tapping with a blunt instrument. The elevation of each released section permits investigation into the exact location of the septa and to continue the mucosal elevation.

The mucosal tissue may often be elevated from the lateral walls above the septa. The curette may then slide down the side walls and release the mucosa from the bottom half of the septum on each side. The sinus curette should then approach the crest of the buttress from both directions, up to its sharp apex. This permits elevation of the tissue over the web region without tearing the membrane. When the strut is located in the middle region of the sinus, it is more difficult to make two separate access windows within the direct vision of the clinician. As a result, one access window is made in front of the septa. The sinus curette then proceeds up the anterior aspect of the web, toward its apex. The curette then slides toward the lateral wall and above the septal apex. The curette may then slide over the crest of the septum approximately 1 to 2 mm. A firm, pulling action fractures the apex of the septum. Repeated similar curette actions can fracture the web off the floor. Once the septum is separated off the floor, the curette may proceed more distal along the floor and walls. When the septum is in the posterior compartment of the sinus, it is often distal to the last implant site. When this occurs, the posterior septum is treated as the posterior wall of the sinus. The sinus membrane manipulation and sinus graft are placed up against and anterior to the posterior septum (Figs. 37.51–37.53).

Bleeding

Bleeding from the lateral-approach sinus elevation surgery is rare; however, it has the potential to be troublesome. Three main arterial vessels should be of concern with the lateral-approach sinus augmentation. Because of the intraosseous and extraosseous anastomoses that are formed by the infraorbital and posterior superior alveolar arteries, intraoperative bleeding complications of the lateral wall may occur. The soft tissue vertical-release incisions of the facial flap in a resorbed maxilla may sever the extraosseous anastomoses. The extraosseous anastomosis on average is located 23 mm from the crest of the dentate ridge; however, in the resorbed maxilla, it may be within 10 mm of the crest. When this artery is severed, significant bleeding has been observed. These vessels originate from the maxillary artery and have no bony landmark to compress the vessel. Therefore vertical release incisions in the soft tissue should be kept to a minimum height with delicate reflection of the periosteum. Hemostats are usually difficult to place on the facial flap to arrest the bleeding. Significant pressure at the posterior border of the maxilla and elevation of the head to reduce the blood pressure to the vessels usually stops this bleeding. The elevation of the head may reduce nasal mucosal blood flow by 38%.[139,140]

The vertical component of the lateral-access wall for the sinus graft often severs the intraosseous anastomoses of the posterior alveolar artery and infraorbital artery, which is on average approximately 15 to 20 mm from the crest of a dentate ridge. Methods to limit this bleeding, which is far less of a risk, have been addressed and include cauterization by the handpiece and diamond bur without water, electrocautery, or pressure on a surgical sponge while the head is elevated (Fig. 37.54).

The third artery of which the implant surgeon should be cautious is the posterior lateral nasal artery. This artery is a branch of the sphenopalatine artery that is located within the medial wall of the antrum. As it courses anteriorly, it anastomoses with terminal branches of the facial artery and ethmoidal arteries. A significant bleeding complication may arise if this vessel is severed during elevation of the membrane off the thin medial wall.

Epistaxis (active bleeding from the nose) is a common disorder; however, it has been reported that 6% of patients who experience this in the general population require medical treatment to control and stop the hemorrhage because it lasts longer than 1 hour. Treatment options to treat epitasis include nasal packing, electrocautery, and the use of vasoconstrictive drugs. Vessel ligation and/or endoscopic surgery are necessary on rare occasions.

The most common site (90%) of nasal bleeding is from a plexus of vessels at the anteroinferior aspect of the nasal septum and the anterior nasal cavity (which is anterior to the sinus cavity and within the anterior projection of the nose). The posterior nasal cavity accounts for 5% to 10% of epitasis events and is in the region of the sinus graft. If the orbital wall of the sinus is perforated, or if an opening into the nares is already present from a previous event, then the sinus curette may enter the nares and cause bleeding. The arteries involved in this site are composed of branches of the sphenopalatine and descending palliative arteries, which are branches of the internal maxillary artery. The posterior half of the inferior turbinate has a venous network called the Woodruff plexus. Lavage of the nares with warm saline and oxymetazoline decongestant sprays provides excellent vasoconstrictive activity to treat the condition. A cotton roll with silver nitrate or lidocaine with 1:50,000 epinephrine may also be effective.

Bleeding from the nose may also be observed after sinus graft surgery. Placing a cotton roll, coated with petroleum jelly with dental floss tied to one end, within the nares may obtund nose bleeding after the surgery. After 5 minutes the dental floss is gently pulled and removes the cotton roll. The head is also elevated, and ice is applied to the bridge of the nose. If bleeding cannot be controlled, then reentry into the graft site and endoscopic ligation by an ENT surgeon may be required (Figs. 37.55 and 37.56).

Short-Term Postoperative Complications

Short-term complications are defined as those that occur within the first few months after surgery.

Incision Line Opening

Incision line opening is uncommon for this procedure because the crestal incision is in attached gingiva and usually is at least 5 mm away from the lateral-access window. Routinely, the soft tissue requires release before primary approximation and suturing. Because a collagen membrane is placed over the window, the soft tissue will usually not approximate without tension unless the surgeon expands the facial flap by releasing the periosteum above the mucogingival junction (where the tissue becomes thicker). Incision line opening occurs more commonly when lateral-ridge augmentation is performed at the same time as sinus graft surgery, or when implants are placed above the residual crest and covered with the soft tissue. It may also occur when a soft tissue–supported prosthesis compresses the surgical area during function before suture removal.

The consequences of incision line opening are delayed healing, leaking of the graft into the oral cavity, and increased risk of infection. However, if the incision line failure is not related to a lateral onlay graft and is only on the crest of the ridge and away from the

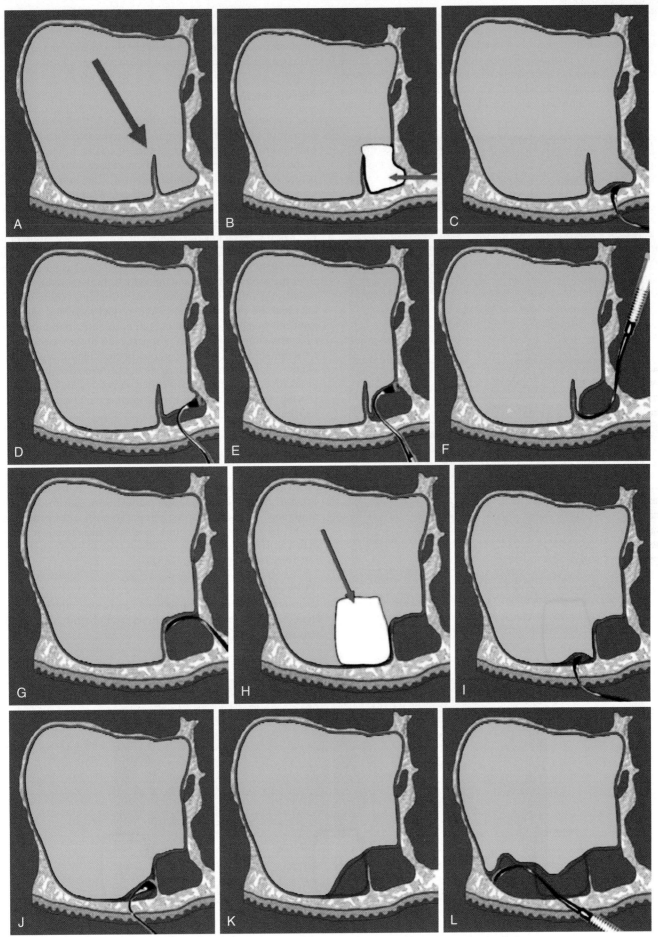

• **Fig. 37.51** Large septum in center of sinus. (a) Septum. (B) Window made anterior to septum. (C) Membrane is elevated off of floor. (D–G) Membrane is exposed anteriorly, posteriorly and to the medial wall. (H) Posterior window is outlined. (I–L) Membrane exposed on second window allowing for grafting around the septum.

sinus access window, then the posterior crestal area is allowed to heal by secondary intention. During this time, a soft tissue–borne prosthesis should be aggressively relieved, with no reline material in contact with the ridge. If incision line opening includes a portion of a nonresorbable membrane (i.e., for lateral-ridge augmentation), then the membrane should be cleaned at least twice daily with an oral rinses of chlorhexidine.

Nerve Impairment

The infraorbital nerve is of concern in sinus elevation surgery because of its anatomic position. This nerve enters the orbit via the inferior orbital fissure and continues anteriorly. It lies in a groove in the orbital floor (which is also the maxillary sinus superior wall) before exiting the infraorbital foramen. The infraorbital nerve exits the foramen approximately 6.1 to 7.2 mm from the orbital rim. Note that anatomic variants have been reported to include dehiscence and malpositioned infraorbital foramina, along with the nerve transversing the lumen of the maxillary sinus rather than coursing through the bone within the sinus ceiling (orbital floor). Malpositioned nerves have been reported as far as 14 mm from the orbital rim in some individuals. In the severely atrophic maxilla, the infraorbital neurovascular structures exiting the foramen may be close to the intraoral residual ridge and should be avoided when performing sinus graft procedures to minimize possible nerve impairment. This is of particular concern on soft tissue reflection and the bone preparation of the superior aspect of the window. Special considerations should be taken during reflection of the superior flap, and sharp-ended retractors should be avoided. Usually, those most at risk have a small cranial base (i.e., elderly females).

Complication

Because the infraorbital nerve is responsible for sensory innervations to the skin of the molar region between the inferior border of the orbit and the upper lip, iatrogenic injury to this vital structure can result in significant neurosensory deficits of this anatomic area. Most often the nerve is not severed, and a neuropraxia results. Even though this injury is sensory and there is no motor deficit, patients usually have a difficult time adapting to this neurosensory impairment (Fig. 37.57).

Management

If an infraorbital nerve impairment occurs, the implant clinician should immediately follow the clinical and pharmacologic neurosensory impairment protocol.

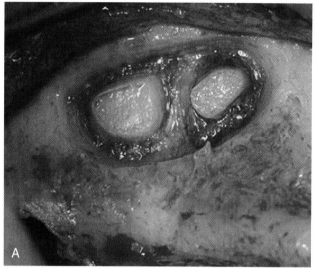
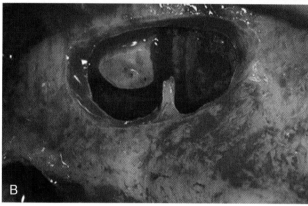

• **Fig. 37.52** Clinical image of septum. (A) Two windows bisecting the septum. (B) Both windows reflected exposing the septum.

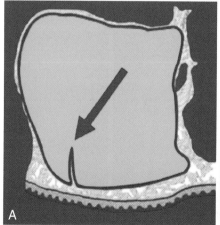
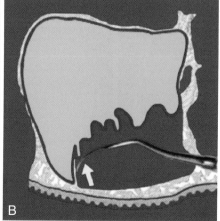

• **Fig. 37.53** Septum in posterior part of sinus. (A) Maxillary septum found on the floor in the posterior of the sinus. (B) An access window and curette elevates the mucosa anterior to the septum. The posterior septa is used as a posterior wall to contain the graft material.

Revision Surgery

When failure or compromise of the sinus graft occurs, reentry procedures are sometimes required to correct deficits. Failed or compromised sinus grafts result in altered soft and hard tissue characteristics, mainly the formation of adhesions of the Schneiderian membrane to the buccal flap. This results in difficulty with reflecting the buccal flap during the reentry procedure. Studies have shown that separation of the adhesions from the sinus mucosa led to a 47% perforation rate. In addition, it has been shown that altered characteristics of the Schneiderian membrane result in a nonflexible thick fibrotic membrane. In some cases, in which voids are present but have difficult access, regrafting procedures may need to be accomplished via a closed approach through the osteotomy site.[101]

Treatment Implications

Because of access issues, along with the higher perforation rate and fibrotic changes in the Schneiderian membrane, patients need to be informed of a higher postoperative complication rate involving questionable reentry bone growth and implant success. If reentry is necessary, usually bony adhesions and bony fenestrations of the lateral walls will be present.

The combination of fibrotic changes of the Schneiderian membrane, increased chance of perforation, and altered sinus physiology lead to a high complication rate. The continuation of the sinus mucosa and oral mucosa make reentry revision surgery problematic and difficult. This will require the separation of the oral and sinus mucosa to gain access to the sinus proper (Fig. 37.58).

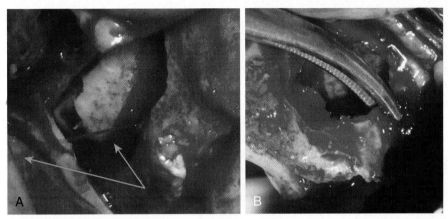

• **Fig. 37.54** Intraosseous anastomosis. (A) Significant bleed from anastomosis (B) controlled by crushing bony area in which bleeding originated.

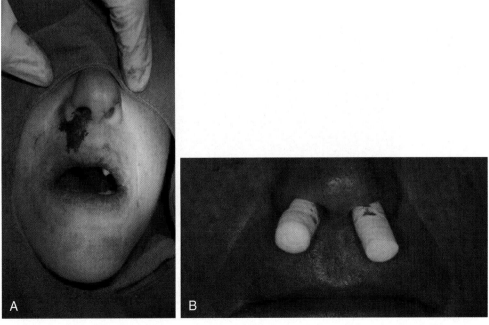

• **Fig. 37.55** Nasal bleeding. (A) Nasal bleeding immediately postop (B) usually may be controlled by gauze pressure packs.

Edema

Because of the extent of tissue reflection and manipulation, sinus graft surgery often results in significant edema. The resultant postoperative swelling can adversely affect the incision line, leading to greater morbidity.

Prevention

The use of good surgical technique that involves careful reflection and retraction will decrease the amount of postoperative edema.

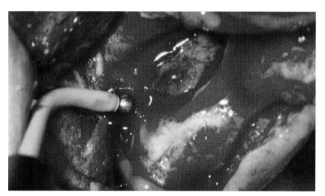

• **Fig. 37.56** Bleeding control. Bleeding may be controlled by electrocautery.

The greater the surgery duration, the greater is the chance of edema. Caution should be used to decrease the amount of surgical duration and should not exceed the patient's tolerance. To minimize edema, corticosteroid use is used 1 day before and 2 days after surgery. This short-term prophylactic steroid use will allow for adequate blood levels to combat edema, which usually will peak at 48 to 72 hours. Dexamethasone is the ideal drug of choice because of its high antiinflammatory potency.

Cryotherapy

Application of an ice pack, along with elevation of the head and limited activity for 2 to 3 days, will help minimize the postoperative swelling. This cryotherapy will cause vasoconstriction of the capillary vessels, reducing the flow of blood and lymph and resulting in a lower degree of swelling. Ice or cold dressings should only be used for the first 24 to 48 hours. After 2 to 3 days, heat (moist) may be applied to the region to increase blood and lymph flow to help clear the area of the inflammatory consequences. This will also help reduce the possibility of ecchymosis that may result.

Ecchymosis

Sinus graft surgery also increases the possibility of bruising or ecchymosis. Because of the extent of reflection, bone preparation,

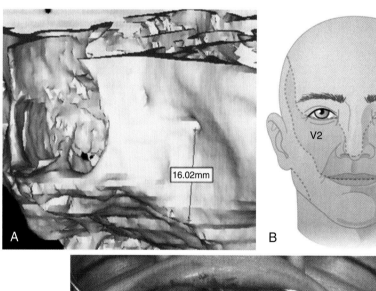

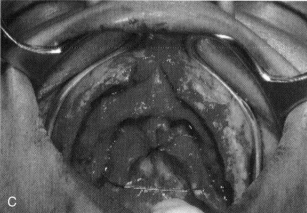

• **Fig. 37.57** Nerve impairment. (A) Infraorbital foramen anatomic variants that are close to the residual ridge. (B) V2 sensory impairment. (C) Special broad-based retractor which minimizes trauma to the infraorbital nerve.

and the highly vascular surgical area, ecchymosis will occur more often with this procedure compared with other implant related surgeries.

Etiology

The etiology of ecchymosis includes the following: blood vessels rupture → red blood cells die and release hemoglobin → macrophages degrade hemoglobin via phagocytosis → production of bilirubin (bluish-red) → bilirubin is broken down to hemosiderin (golden-brown).

Prevention

In most cases, ecchymosis will not be able to be completely prevented; however, the goal should be to minimize the extent of bruising. Additionally, good surgical technique, shorter surgical duration, the avoidance of anticoagulant analgesics, and postoperative cryotherapy all aid in the control of this phenomenon. Patients should always be informed of the possibility of ecchymosis. This is easily accomplished by having it be part of the postoperative instructions (Fig. 37.59).

Pain

Minimal discomfort and pain is usually associated with sinus graft surgery. However, if narcotics are indicated, any analgesic combination containing codeine, such as Tylenol 3, is prescribed postoperatively because codeine is a potent antitussive, and coughing

may place additional pressure on the sinus membrane and introduce bacteria into the graft. The patient is instructed to cough (if necessary) with the mouth open to minimize possible air pressure changes within the sinus cavity.

Oroantral Fistulae

Oroantral fistulae may develop postoperatively, especially if the patient has a history of past sinus pathology or infection. Small oroantral fistulae (<5 mm) usually will close spontaneously after treatment with systemic antibiotic drugs and daily rinses with chlorhexidine. However, larger fistulae (>5 mm) will normally require additional surgical intervention (Fig. 37.60). Larger fistulae are associated with an epithelialized tract, which is the result of the fusion of the sinus membrane mucosa to the oral epithelium. When this occurs, patients will most likely complain of fluids entering the nasal cavity on eating or drinking. Caution should be exercised in using the Valsalva maneuver (i.e., nose blowing test) to confirm the presence of an oroantral fistula at the time of surgery. The patient is asked to pinch their nostrils together to occlude the nose. The patient blows gently to see if air escapes into the oral cavity via the sinus. This is not recommended because this test may create an opening or make a small opening larger. The Valsalva maneuver may be used postoperatively to diagnose a suspected communication.

Management

Closure of oroantral fistulae can be accomplished by using broad-based lingual or facially rotated flaps (Figs. 37.61 and 37.62). Buccal flaps to close the fistula may be more difficult after a sinus graft because of the location of the graft site. In addition, the buccal tissue is very thin, and rotated or expanded buccal flaps usually result in loss of vestibular depth. Before the initiation of the flap design, the soft tissue around the fistula is excised and the sinus floor curetted to ensure direct bone contact. A tension-free rotated

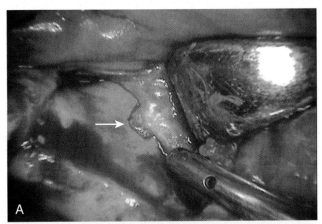
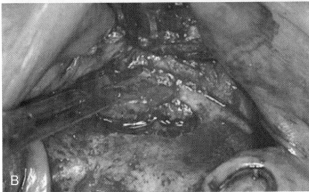

• **Fig. 37.58** Revision surgery. (A) Postoperative infections often result in the sinus and nasal epithelium being continuous, (B) Reentry into sinus requires incising the tissue to separate the oral and nasal epithelium.

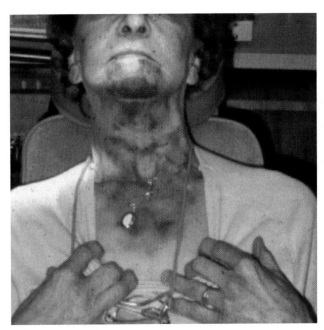

• **Fig. 37.59** Postoperative edema and ecchymosis. One of the most common postoperative complications is edema and ecchymosis, which often may extend into the mandible and neck area.

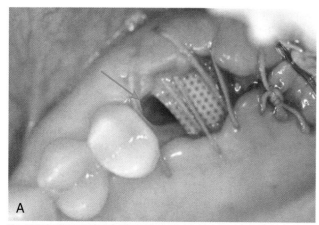

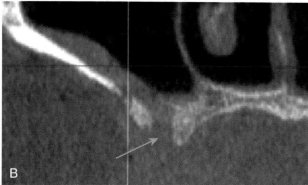

• **Fig. 37.60** Oroantral fistula: (A) Postoperative fistula resulting from poor wound healing. (B) Radiograph showing communication between the sinus and oral cavity.

flap is then made for complete covering of the communication. For oroantral closure after sinus graft procedures, a lingual flap is recommended because of the abundance of keratinized mucosa with an adequate blood supply. Flap designs include island flaps, "tongue-shaped" flaps, or rotational and advanced flaps, depending on the size of the exposure. A key to closing the oroantral opening is the dissection of the buccal flap lateral to the fistula. An incision that extends 15 mm anterior and posterior to the fistula is of benefit. The fistula then has an elliptical incision on each side of the opening. The core of tissue and the fistulous tract are excised. The facial flap is undermined and expanded well into the tissues of the cheek. The palatal aspect of the incision is adjacent to the tongue-shaped flap. Placement of the incision for the pedicle flap should be split thickness and take into account the location and depth of the greater palatine artery. Once the attached palatal pedicle graft is rotated to the lateral and attached to the facial flap, horizontal mattress sutures are placed to invert the flap to achieve a watertight seal. Sutures with high tensile strength (Vicryl) should be used and allowed to remain in place for at least 2 weeks (Fig. 37.63).

Post-Operative Infection

When evaluating postsurgical infectious complications after sinus graft procedures, the implant clinician must differentiate the type, location, and etiology of the infectious episode. The infection may originate within the graft site or may originate in the maxillary sinus proper. It could also be a combination of both (Table 37.2). Very few studies have evaluated these different processes. Postsurgically, there exist many reports with varying results

(approximately 0%–27%) on the incidence of infection leading to acute rhinosinusitis.[141] Postoperative infections after sinus graft surgery may result from the following:

• **Acute rhinosinusitis:** infection within the sinus proper
• **Graft site:** infection within the graft area
• **Combination infection**: from acute rhinosinusitis and graft site

Graft Site Infections

Etiology of Graft Site Infection

The graft site may become infected from many sources: (1) preexisting site bacteria, (2) bacterial contamination of the surgical site, (3) graft material, (4) surgical technique, (5) bacterial contamination from acute rhinosinusitis, (6) lack of systemic and local prophylactic antibiotics, and (7) systemic, mediation, or lifestyle factors (Fig. 37.64).

Additionally, studies have shown a direct correlation between an increased infection rate with simultaneous implant placement and with simultaneous ridge augmentation.

One such study showed that simultaneous ridge grafting increased the infection rate significantly (15.3%) versus sinus grafting alone (3%).[142] Most often, the infection begins more than 1 week after surgery, although it may begin as soon as 3 days later.

Diagnosis

The most common sign of graft site infection is swelling, pain, dehiscence, or exudate near or including the grafting surgical site. Patients may complain of poor taste and loss of graft particles in their mouth. Incision line opening is a common sequalae with exudate discharge. Graft site infections usually occur within days to weeks of the surgery and are less common as a late infection. Initially, the infection may start as a graft site infection (localized to the graft), which then leads to an acute maxillary rhinosinusitis (Fig. 37.65).

Treatment

Although the incidence of infection after the procedure is usually low, the damaging consequences on osteogenesis and the possibility of serious complications require that any infection be aggressively treated. In case of postoperative infection, it is recommended that the clinician perform a thorough examination of the area by palpation, percussion, and visual inspection to identify the area primarily affected. Infection will usually follow the path of least resistance and is observed by changes in specific anatomic sites to which it spreads.[143]

Early, aggressive treatment is crucial for graft site infections to prevent the loss of graft or extension of the infection into the sinus proper, causing an acute rhinosinusitis or spread of infection to other vital areas. Initially, systemic antibiotics along with antimicrobial rinses should be used. If infection persists, debridement and drainage should be completed, along with the use of sterile saline and chlorhexidine. A Penrose drain may also be used in cases that do not respond to systemic antibiotics. In some instances, oroantral fistulae result after infection cessation (see the section "Oroantral Fistulae").

Antibiotic treatment in the maxillary sinus, both prophylactically and therapeutically, is much different than for most oral surgical procedures. When selecting antibiotic medications for sinus infections, a variety of factors must be evaluated. These include the most common type of pathogens involved, antimicrobial resistance, pharmacokinetic and pharmacodynamic properties, and

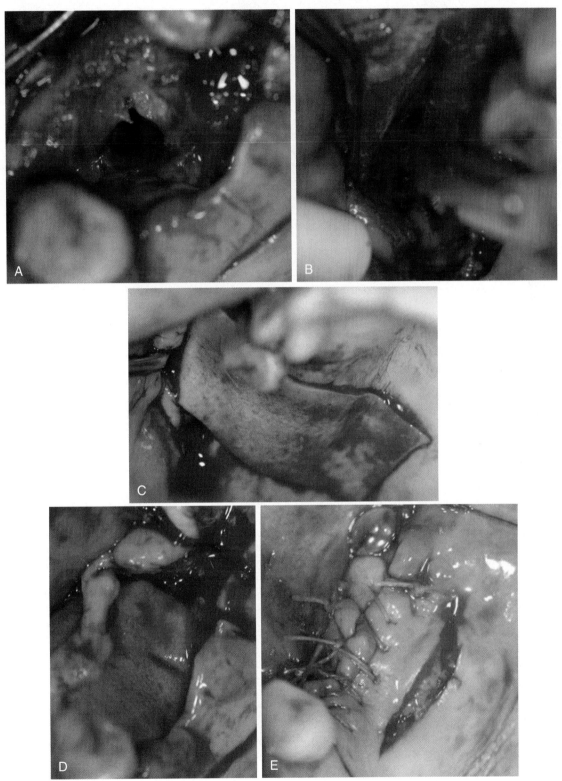

• **Fig. 37.61** Oroantral fistula repair. (A) oroantral fistula, (B) flap extension for tension-free closure, (C) Extended collagen membrane, (D) Membrane positioned, (E) Lateral sliding flap to obtain primary closure.

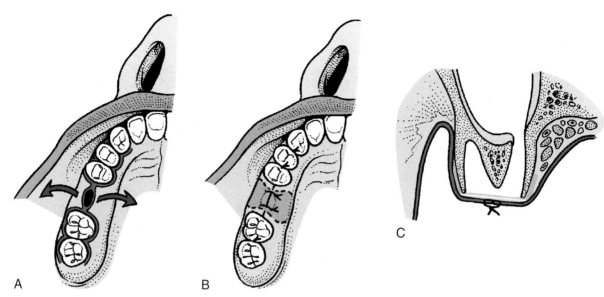

• **Fig. 37.62** Membrane-assisted closure of oroantral communications. (A) Oroantral fistula in the right maxillary alveolar process in the region of the missing first molar, which is to be closed with subperiosteal placement of alloplastic material such as gold or titanium foil or a resorbable collagen membrane. Facial and palatal mucoperiosteal flaps are developed. Extension of the flaps along the gingival sulcus one or two teeth anterior and posterior allows some stretching of the flap to facilitate advancement for closure over the defect. The fistulous tract is excised. Osseous margins must be exposed 360 degrees around the bony defect to allow placement of the membrane beneath the mucoperiosteal flaps. The flap is supported on all sides by underlying bone. (B) Closure. Ideally, the flaps can be approximated over the defect. In some cases, a small gap between the flaps will heal over the membrane by secondary intention. Even if the intraoral mucosa does not heal primarily, the sinus lining usually heals and closes, and the membrane is then exfoliated or resorbed, and mucosal healing progresses. (C) Cross-section of membrane closure technique. Buccal and palatal mucoperiosteal flaps are elevated to expose osseous defect and large area of underlying alveolar bone around the oroantral communication. The membrane overlaps all the margins of the defect, and the facial and palatal flaps are sutured over the membrane. (From Hupp JR, et al. *Contemporary Oral and Maxillofacial Surgery.* 5th ed. St Louis, MO: Elsevier; 2009.)

the tissue (sinus) penetration of the various antibiotic drugs. The antibiotic medication of choice should be effective against respiratory and oral pathogens while exhibiting known activity against resistant strains of the common pathogens. Two such factors are used when evaluating sinus antibiotic medications: (1) the minimum inhibitory concentration (MIC) and (2) the concentration of antibiotic drugs penetrating inflamed diseased sinus tissue. The MIC is the lowest concentration of the antimicrobial agent that results in the inhibition of growth of a microorganism. The MIC is usually expressed by MIC 50 or MIC 90, meaning that 50% or 90% of the microbial isolates are inhibited, respectively. Previous studies and treatment modalities used amoxicillin as the first drug of choice. However, with the increasing prevalence of penicillinase- and β-lactamase–producing strains of *H. influenzae* and *M. catarrhalis*, along with penicillin-resistant strains of *S. pneumoniae*, other alternative antibiotic drugs should be selected.

β-Lactam Medications. The most common β-lactam antibiotic drugs used in the treatment of rhinosinusitis and graft site infections are penicillin (amoxicillin, Augmentin) and cephalosporin (Ceftin, Vantin). Amoxicillin has been the drug of choice for years to combat the bacterial strains associated with rhinosinusitis and infections in the oral cavity. However, its effectiveness has been questioned recently because of the high percentage of β-lactamase–producing bacteria and penicillin-resistant *S. pneumoniae.* Augmentin (amoxicillin-clavulanate) has the added advantage of activity against β-lactamase bacteria. It has been

associated with a high incidence of gastrointestinal side effects. However, with the dosing regimen (twice a day [bid]), these complications have been significantly decreased. Two recommended cephalosporin medications have also been suggested to treat rhinosinusitis: cefuroxime axetil (Ceftin) and cefpodoxime proxetil (Vantin). Other cephalosporin drugs fail to achieve adequate sinus fluid levels against the causative pathogens. Ceftin and Vantin have good potency and efficacy, while exhibiting strong activity against resistant *S. pneumoniae* and *H. influenzae.*

Macrolide Medications. Macrolide drugs are bacteriostatic agents that include erythromycin, clarithromycin (Biaxin), and azithromycin (Zithromax). Macrolide medications have good activity against susceptible pneumococci; however, with the increasing rate of macrolide resistance, their use in combating sinus pathogens is becoming associated with a high likelihood of clinical failure. These antibiotic drugs are very active against *M. catarrhalis,* although their activity on *H. influenzae* is questionable. These antibiotic medications are not suggested to treat postoperative sinus infections.

Lincosamide Medications. Clindamycin (Cleocin) is the primary lincosamide drug used in clinical practice today that is considered to be bacteriostatic. However, in high concentrations, bactericidal activity may be present. Clindamycin is mainly used for the treatment of gram-positive aerobes and anaerobes. With acute sinus disease, clindamycin is usually not indicated because it exhibits no activity against

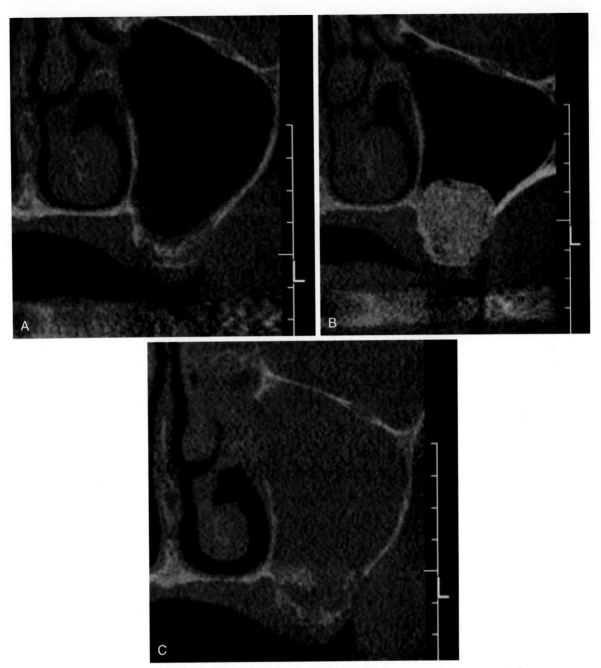

• **Fig. 37.63** Postsinus graft infection. (A) Preoperative radiograph. (B) Postoperative sinus augmentation. (C) 4-week postop with graft site infection and acute rhinosinusitis.

H. influenzae and *M. catarrhalis.* This drug may be used in chronic sinus conditions because anaerobic organisms play a much larger role in the disease process.

Tetracycline-Derived Medications. Doxycycline (Vibramycin) is a bacteriostatic agent with adequate activity against penicillin-susceptible pneumococci and *M. catarrhalis.* This drug does not exhibit any activity against penicillin-resistant bacteria and is not effective against *H. influenzae.* However, doxycycline may be used as an alternative antibiotic for the treatment of acute rhinosinusitis infections.

Sulfonamide Medications. The most common sulfonamide drug, trimethoprim-sulfamethoxazole (Bactrim) is bacteriostatic. Recently a high rate of resistance to these drugs has been seen with *S. pneumoniae, H. influenzae, M. catarrhalis,* and other sinus

pathogens. This drug should not be considered to treat postoperative infections unless a culture and sensitivity test has been performed and susceptibility is shown.

Metronidazole Medication. Metronidazole is the most important member of the nitroimidazole group. It is bactericidal and is effective against gram-positive and gram-negative anaerobic bacteria. Its main use would be in the treatment of chronic sinus (not acute) conditions. The medication should be used with another antibiotic drug to be effective against aerobic bacteria.

Antibiotic Conclusion. In the evaluation of different antibiotic drugs used for the treatment of pathologic conditions of the sinus, meticulous analysis of the activity against the most common pathogens must be evaluated. With all of the antibiotic medications evaluated, amoxicillin-clavulanate, and cefuroxime axetil

TABLE 37.2	**Types of Postoperative Sinus Infections**		
	Acute Rhinosinusitis	**Graft Site Infection**	**Combination**
Etiology	• Preexisting pathology • Nonpatent ostium • Anatomic variants • Graft overfill • Postsurgery physiologic alteration • Spread of infection from graft site • History of chronic rhinosinusitis • Preexisting odontogenic or allergic rhinosinusitis	• Preexisting pathology • Oral pathogen contamination • Untreated periodontitis • Perforation • Lack of asepsis • Long duration surgery • Simultaneous ridge augmentation • Simultaneous implant placement • Lack of prophylactic medication • Lack of local graft antibiotics • Systemic diseases, smoking/alcohol	Primary site could be sinus proper or graft site
Bacteria	Aerobic gram-positive cocci (*Streptococcus pneumoniae*) Aerobic gram-negative rods (*Haemophilus influenzae*) (*Staphylococcus epidermidis, Streptococcus viridans, Branhamella catarrhalis*)	Aerobic gram-positive cocci (*S. viridans*) Aerobic gram-positive cocci (*Staphylococcus aureus*) Aerobic gram-negative rods (*Bacteroides*) Aerobic gram-positive cocci (peptostreptococcus)	Any combination of pathogens
Prevention	CBCT: Confirmation of ostium patency Confirmation of no pathology or anatomic variants Prophylactic medications	Prophylactic medication Good surgical technique Aseptic technique Short surgical duration No membrane perforation	Any combination of preventive measures
Symptoms	Mild: Facial pain/edema Congestion Nasal drip/blockage Cough Severe: Significant facial pain/edema Fever Headache Proptosis/diplopia Malaise	Site pain/edema Incision line opening Exudate Bad taste Bleeding Intraoral swelling	Any combination of symptoms
Ideal antibiotic	β-Lactam	β-Lactam Lincosamide	β-Lactam
Initial treatment	Antibiotic: 1. Augmentin 2. Ceftin Nasal saline	Antibiotic: 1. Augmentin 2. Clindamycin Chlorhexidine	Antibiotic: 1. Augmentin 2. Ceftin Nasal saline/rinse
Secondary treatment	Referral, especially if cerebral/ocular symptoms	Debridement/irrigation Possible culture	Debridement Possible culture Referral, especially if cerebral/ocular symptoms

CBCT, Cone beam computerized tomography.

show excellent MIC 90 blood levels against the most common pathogens associated with sinus infections.

Decongestant Medications. Recent recommendations in the medical literature state that nasal decongestants (sympathomimetic drugs) should not be used except in severe cases of congestion and infection. Nasal decongestants have been shown to impair blood flow, decreasing antibiotic levels to the site. Additionally, it may cause a rebound phenomenon and the development of rhinitis medicamentosa. This rebound phenomenon has been theorized to occur as a negative feedback vasodilation after repeated introductions of the sympathomimetic (vasoconstricting) drug.

Saline Rinses. An important treatment for the patient with the presence of acute rhinosinusitis and graft infections is the use of saline rinses with a bulb syringe or a squeeze bottle in the nostril used to lavage the sinus through the ostium. The nasal saline rinse has a long history for treatment of sinonasal disease. Hypertonic and isotonic saline rinses have proven to be effective against chronic rhinosinusitis. These techniques of nasal irrigation have been evaluated, with the best option of a positive-pressure irrigation using a squeeze bottle that delivers a gentle stream of saline to the nasal cavity (NeilMed's Sinus Rinse; NeilMed Pharmaceuticals Inc.). The syringe or squeeze bottle should not seal the nasal

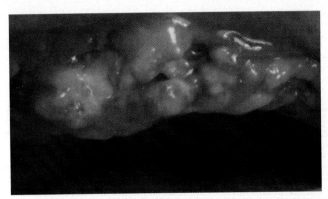

• **Fig. 37.64** Graft site infection showing exudate and incision line opening.

opening because this may force bacteria up toward the ethmoidal sinus. Instead, a gentle lavage with sterile saline rinses the sinus and flushes out the mucus and exudate. Ideally, the head is placed down and forward so that the saline can reach the ostium in the superior and anterior portion of the sinus. The course of therapy should continue for at least 7 days.[144] Another option is the Neti Pot, which is very common among chronic rhinosinusitis patients (Fig. 37.66).

Acute Rhinosinusitis Infections

Etiology of Acute Rhinosinusitis

There are two causes of acute maxillary rhinosinusitis after sinus graft surgery: (1) preexisting maxillary sinus pathology or (2) progression of sinus graft surgery to involve the maxillary sinus proper (Fig. 37.67).

Diagnosis

Maxillary rhinosinusitis is a complication that arises when the patient postoperatively complains of any of the following symptoms: (mild) headache, pain, or tenderness in the area of the maxillary sinus; rhinorrhea; or (severe) fever, headache, or ocular symptoms. Studies have supported the fact that patients who had predisposing factors for rhinosinusitis were more at risk of developing postoperative transient rhinosinusitis.

The wide range of reported percentages (3%–20%) may be the result of different methods used for diagnosis (i.e., clinical, radiographic, endoscopic). Cases of maxillary sinusitis after dental implant surgery have rarely been reported in the dental literature. However, recently in the medical literature, numerous cases of minor to severe complications after sinus surgery have been documented. Although very infrequent, severe infections may lead to more severe complications, such as orbital cellulitis, optic neuritis, cavernous sinus thrombosis, epidural and subdural infection, meningitis, cerebritis, blindness, osteomyelitis, and, although rare, brain abscess and death.[145]

Treatment

If infection occurs postoperatively, treatment must be aggressive because of the possible complications that may arise to close anatomic structures. Systemic antibiotic therapy is the first line of treatment, along with close observation of symptoms. Recent medical literature discourages the use of systemic decongestants and highly recommends the use of saline lavage and rinses. Systemic decongestants have been shown to impair site antibiotic

delivery and also have a high degree of rebound effect (rhinitis medicamentosa).

If symptoms are not alleviated with antibiotic and decongestant medications, possible referral to the patient's physician or ENT is warranted. Emergency consultation should be considered if the patient complains of a severe headache that is not relieved by mild analgesics, as well as persistent or high fever, lethargy, visual impairment, or orbital swelling.

The authors highly recommend that a professional association with an ENT be obtained. Because the possible morbidity of these infections and causative pathogen is not easily determined, referral is sometimes needed. Additionally, if mild sinus symptoms persist or signs of severe infection are present, immediate referral is recommended. Resolution of these conditions has been accomplished with the use of antibiotic drugs, endoscopic treatment, or Caldwell-Luc procedures (Fig. 37.68).

Combination (Graft Site Infections/Acute Rhinosinusitis)

Etiology

The etiology of a combination infection can either be initiated from the graft site or the sinus proper.

Diagnosis

The diagnosis for a combination type infection can parallel a combination of graft site symptoms and/or acute rhinosinusitis.

Treatment

The treatment of a combination type infection should include the use of a β-lactam antibiotic (e.g., Augmentin) followed by the use of debridement and nasal saline rinses. If ocular or cerebral symptoms persist, or the patient does not respond to antibiotic treatment, referral is recommended.

The most current, comprehensive study on the treatment of sinus disease involves guidelines established by the Sinus and Allergy Health Partnership, Centers for Disease Control and Prevention, and the FDA in 2000. With this information as a guide, the following recommendations for antibiotic use in the treatment of infections after sinus graft are suggested (Box 37.14).

Spread of Infection

Because of the anatomic and topographic location of the maxillary sinus, infections from oral or sinus pathogens may spread quickly to adjacent sites.

Sinus-related pathologic conditions are the most common cause of orbital infection, accounting for 60% to 84% of cases. Because of the seriousness of ocular infections, early diagnosis and aggressive treatment is paramount.

Various routes may predispose this area to infection from the maxillary sinus and include the following:
1. The venous plexus of the maxillary sinus drains through the posterior wall into the deep facial vein, through the pterygoid plexus, and finally into the cavernous sinus.
2. Veins also perforate the osseous roof of the maxillary sinus, entering the orbit through the superior and inferior ophthalmic vein. These veins also are connected to the pterygoid plexus and cavernous sinus.

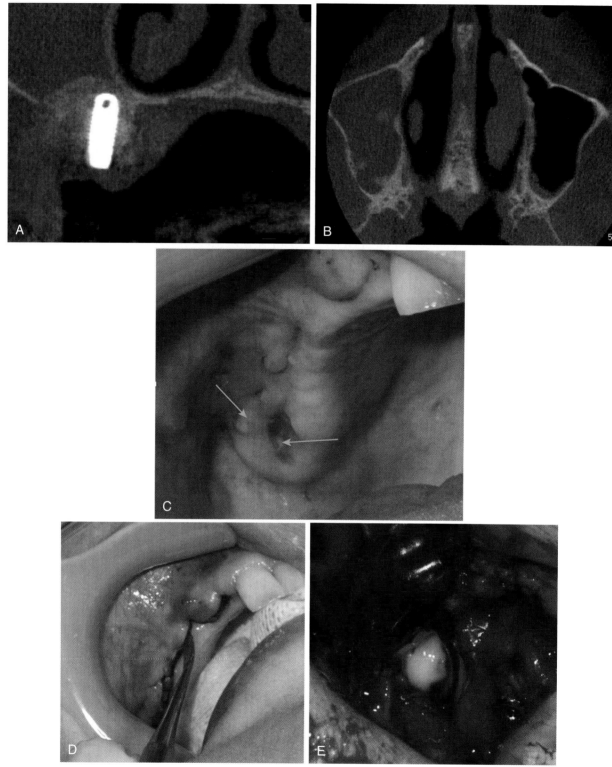

• **Fig. 37.65** Postgraft infection. (A) Cone beam computerized tomographic (CBCT) coronal image showing implant with associated infection. (B) Axial CBCT image showing a completely opacified sinus. (C) Intraoral view of draining fistula tracts *(green arrows)*. (D) Incision and drainage. (E) Exudate and infected tissue removal.

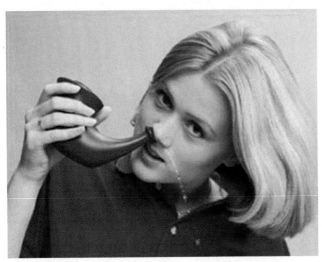

• **Fig. 37.66** Neti Pot. Used for nasal irrigation resulting in flushing out the nasal passages.

3. Additionally, numerous veins perforate the anterior wall that drain into the superior ophthalmic vein and into the cavernous sinus. From the cavernous sinus, drainage through the deep middle cerebral vein communicates with the white substance of the brain's superficial venous system.

Because of the elaborate maxillocerebral venous anastomoses, spread of infection from the maxillary sinus may result in possible sequelae such as brain abscesses, intraorbital abscesses, orbital cellulitis, cavernous sinus thrombosis, and osteomyelitis.

Implant Penetration Into the Sinus

Bränemark and colleagues[146] reported on animal histologic studies and 44 clinical cases of implants penetrating the maxillary sinus. They reported success rates comparable to other maxillary implants, and no postoperative signs or symptoms were found with these implants. An animal study by Boyne[147] led to the same conclusion. The assumption was that direct connection between hard and soft tissues to the integrated implant created a barrier to the migration of microorganisms. However, it should be noted these animals do not have the same incidence of maxillary sinusitis comparable to humans.

It is possible that an implant that penetrates the sinus floor may contribute to a source of periodic sinusitis because a bacterial

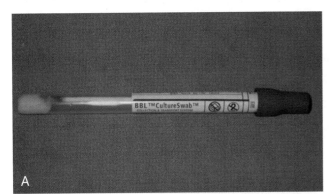

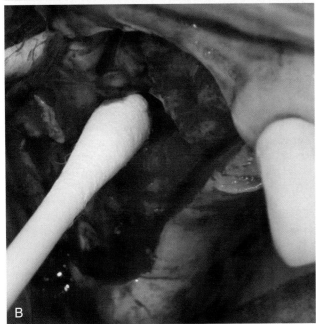

• **Fig. 37.67** Culture and sensitivity. In some cases of rhinosinusitis, a culture and sensitivity test may be administered. (A) Swab sealed and sent to laboratory for culture and sensitivity testing.(B) Culture swab placed into the infected site.

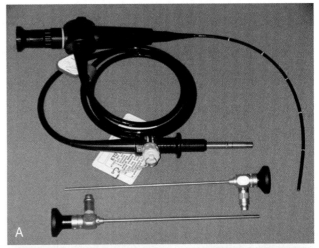

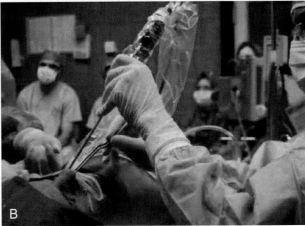

• **Fig. 37.68** Functional endoscopic sinus surgery (FESS). (A) FESS scope. (B) Surgical placement of FESS.

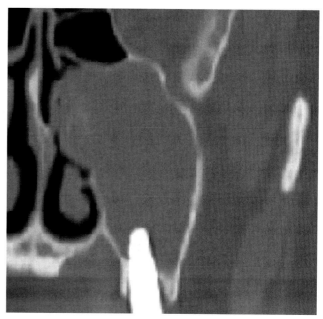

• **Fig. 37.69** Implant penetration into sinus. Coronal image showing implant placement into maxillary sinus leading to a completely opacified maxillary sinus.

smear layer would be difficult to remove through regular phagocytic activity. When this is suspected, removal of the implant or an apicoectomy of the implant apex, from a lateral-access window, may be of benefit (Fig. 37.69).

Overfilling of the Sinus

The goal of the sinus graft is to obtain sufficient vertical height of bone to place endosteal implants with long-term success. The maximum length requirement of an implant with adequate surface of design is rarely more than 15 mm, and as a result, the goal of the initial sinus graft is to obtain at least 16 mm of vertical bone from the crest of the ridge. This usually means the bottom one-half of the sinus is filled with graft material because most sinuses approximate 35 mm in height. A CBCT scan of the sinus before surgery may be used to estimate the amount of graft material required for the ideal volume of sinus graft material. Care should be given to the amount of graft material placed into the sinus. Overfilling the sinus can result in blockage of the ostium, especially if membrane inflammation or the presence of a thickened sinus mucosa exists.

The majority of sinus graft overfills do not have postoperative complications. If, however, a postoperative sinus infection occurs without initial resolution, reentry and removal of a portion of the graft and changing the antibiotic protocol may be appropriate (Fig. 37.70).

Postoperative Cone Beam Computerized Tomographic Mucosal Thickening (False Positive for Infection)

Immediate postoperative radiographs may reveal significant mucosal thickening within the sinus. The clinician should not determine this to be infection unless the previously mentioned signs of infection are noted. Normally, elevation of the sinus mucosa and bone grafting does alter the overall maxillary sinus environment by reducing the size of the sinus and repositioning the mucociliary transport system. In spite of this, only short-term clearance impairment exists, resulting in only subclinical effects on the sinus physiology. However, in cases of preoperative sinusitis histories, elevation surgery may predispose a patient to sinus-related complications. It has been shown that these procedures do alter the microbial environment. Studies reveal at 3 months after surgery, positive sinus cultures were present compared with cultures taken for the same patients preoperatively. However, after 9 months the cultures were similar to the preelevation results. The key is maintenance of the ostiomeatal opening between the maxillary sinus and the nasal cavity.

Migration of Implants

In 1995 the first case of a displaced (migrated) implant into the maxillary sinus was documented. Since then, an increased number of reports are coming to light, documenting an ever-increasing problem. Reports have shown that implants migrating from the maxillary sinus have been found in the sphenoid sinus, ethmoid sinus, orbit, nasal cavity, and anterior cranial base.

Etiology

The etiology of implant displacement or migration from the maxillary sinus includes many possibilities. The timing of

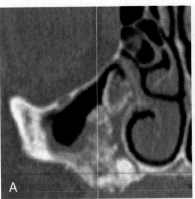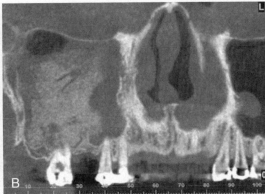

• **Fig. 37.70** Overfilling of the sinus. (A) Cone beam computerized tomographic coronal scan image depicting excess graft material occluding the maxillary ostium. (B) Significant overfill of maxillary sinus leading to an acute rhinosinusitis.

implants ending up in the maxillary sinus proper varies from intraoperative displacement to migration years later. Many etiologic factors have been suggested, according to the timing (early versus late) (Table 37.3).

Prevention

For early migration/displacement complications, most likely the cause is surgical error or incorrect treatment planning. When evaluating late migration/placement complications, the majority of issues are a direct result of postoperative prosthetic errors (too early loading) or factors that are precipitated by lack of integration or minimal bone at the implant interface.

Management

The management of displaced or migrated implants into the maxillary sinus should be treated with urgency. Leaving implants in the maxillary sinus may lead to acute rhinosinusitis complications. Additionally, implants left in the maxillary may become calcified (antrolith) or become displaced into other anatomic areas (e.g., sinuses, orbit, nasal cavity, brain).

The patients should be referred as soon as possible for removal via a Caldwell-Luc approach or endoscopy (functional endoscopic sinus surgery [FESS]) (Figs. 37.71–37.77).

Postoperative Fungal Infection

Fungal infection after sinus bone grafting is rarely reported; however, with the increased number of sinus graft procedures being performed, inevitably more will be reported in the literature. Fungal sinusitis is a destructive, invasive disease that is mostly caused by *Aspergillus*. *Aspergillus* spp. is a fungus of the Ascomycetes class, which is one of the most commonly encountered in the human environment. In the diagnosis of fungal sinusitis, there exist two forms: noninvasive and invasive. The invasive form is rare and is almost always associated with immunocompromised patients. Erosion and osseous destruction occurs that may be fatal. However, this form has not been associated with dental implants or sinus graft surgery.

Case studies have shown postoperative complications after sinus graft surgery[148] and overextension of root canal filling involving the noninvasive form. This type of fungus growth is also

TABLE 37.3	**Migration of Dental Implants**	
Early	**Late**
• Poor initial stability	• Too early loading
• Overpreparation of osteotomy site	• Changes in intranasal or intrasinus pressure
• Poor quality of bone	• Peri-implantitis
• No crestal cortical bone	• Autoimmune reaction
• Implant placement into sinus without bone graft	
• Incorrect treatment planning	
• Surgical inexperience	
• Untreated antral preparation	
• Postoperative sinus infection	
• Immediate placement implants	

termed fungus balls or aspergilloma and is associated with immunocompetent patients.

Diagnosis

Usually, the patient will present with clinical symptoms of frontal headache, orbicular pain, nasal congestion, and bleeding, with signs of chronic rhinosinusitis. Radiographically, a distinctly increased soft tissue density mass (radiopacity) is seen on CBCT scans.

Management

Referral to an ENT for evaluation and confirmation of diagnosis. Usually, treatment involves surgical removal via Caldwell-Luc or FESS techniques because systemic antimycotic drugs are ineffective.

Summary

In the past, implant treatment in the posterior maxilla was reported as the least predictable region for implant survival. Causes cited include inadequate bone height, poor bone density, and high occlusal forces. Past implant modalities attempted to avoid this region, with procedures such as excessive cantilevers from anterior implants or excess numbers of pontics when implants are placed anterior and posterior to the antrum.

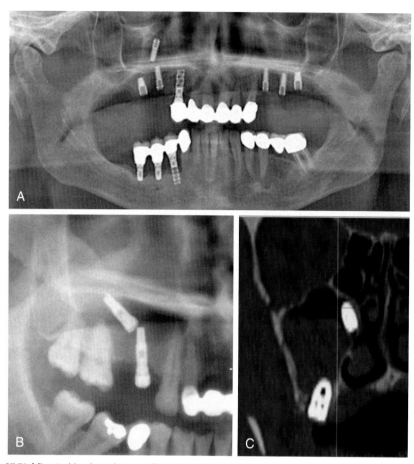

• **Fig. 37.71** Migrated implants into maxillary sinus. (A and B) Implants displaced into maxillary sinus. (C) Implant obstructing the maxillary ostium.

The maxillary sinus may be elevated and SA bone regenerated to improve available bone height. Tatum began to develop these techniques as early as the mid-1970s.[3] Misch[149] developed four options for treatment of the posterior maxilla in 1984 based on the height of bone between the floor of the antrum and the crest of the residual bone. These options were further modified to reflect the width of available bone, once adequate height was obtained. Root-form implants of adequate size are indicated in the posterior maxilla. The higher forces and less dense bone often require larger diameter implants.

It is the observation of the authors, using the sinus graft procedures described in this chapter for more than 30 years, in clinical practice, universities, and private implant institutes, that the sinus graft procedure is more than 97% effective. This region of the mouth predictably grows more bone in height than any other intraoral region. However, an organized approach needs to be completed with respect to patient selection, pathology evaluation, pharmacologic management, and surgical and prosthetic protocol to increase success and decrease potential morbidity of the procedures.

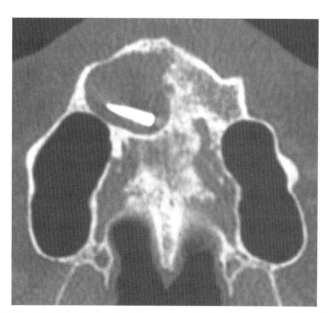

• **Fig. 37.72** Migrated implant into nasal cavity. Implant that was displaced into the maxillary sinus and eventually eroded through the medial wall of sinus into the nasal cavity.

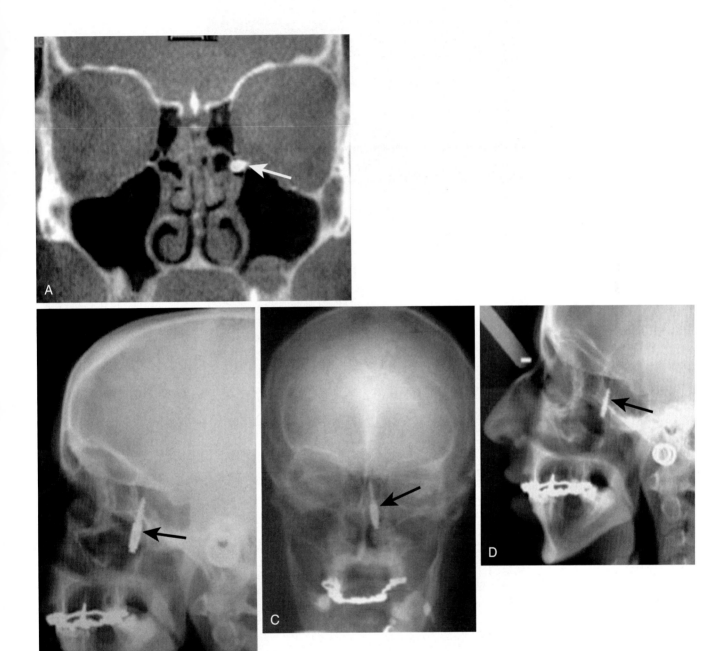

• **Fig. 37.73** Migrated implants. (A) Ethmoid sinus. (B–D) Migrated implant into sphenoid sinus. (A, From Haben M, Balys R, Frenkiel S. Dental implant migration into the ethmoid sinus. *J Otolaryngol.* 2003;32:342–344, 2003; B–D, From Felisati G, Lozza P, Chiapasco M, et al. Endoscopic removal of an unusual foreign body in the sphenoid sinus: an oral implant. *Clin Oral Implants Res.* 2007;18:776–780.)

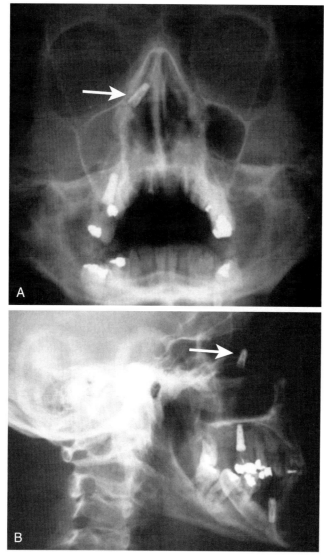

• **Fig. 37.74** (A and B) Migrated implants into the orbital area. (From Griffa A, Viterbo S, Boffano P. Endoscopic-assisted removal of an intraorbital dislocated dental implant. *Clin Oral Implants Res.* 2010;21:778–780.)

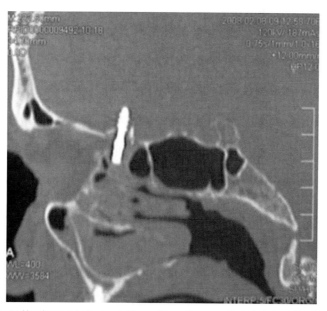

• **Fig. 37.75** Migrated implants anterior cranial base. (From Cascone P, et al. A dental implant in the anterior cranial fossae. *Int J Oral Maxillofac Surg.* 2010;39:92–93.)

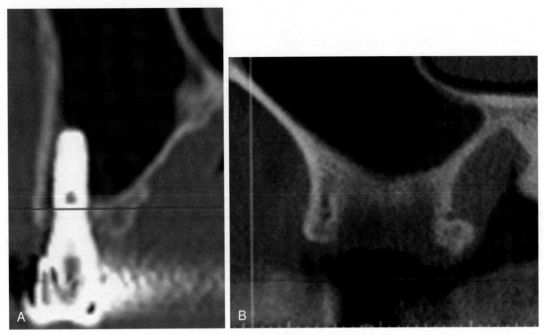

• **Fig. 37.76** Etiology of displaced/migrated implants. (A) Implant placement into maxillary sinus without bone grafting. (B) Implant placement into sites with poor bone density, therefore compromised primary stability.

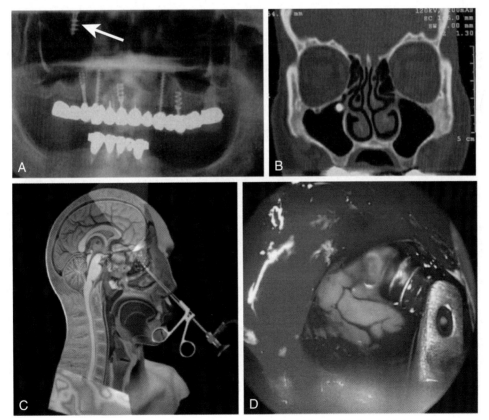

• **Fig. 37.77** (A) Panoramic radiograph depicting migrated dental implant in the right sinus. (B) Coronal image showing implant in the maxillary ostium area. (C) Functional endoscopic sinus surgery (FESS) approach to retrieve implant. (D) Removal of implant from sinus cavity. (From Chiapasco M, Felisati G, Maccari A, et al. The management of complications following displacement of oral implants in the para-nasal sinuses: a multicenter clinical report and proposed treatment protocols. *Int J Oral Maxillofac Surg.* 2009;38(12):1273–1278.)

References

1. Blitzer A, Lawson W, Friedman WH, eds. *Surgery of the Paranasal Sinuses*. Philadelphia: WB Saunders; 1985.
2. Lang J, ed. *Clinical Anatomy of the Nose, Nasal Cavity and Paranasal Sinuses*. New York: Thieme; 1989.
3. Anon JB, Rontal M, Zinreich SJ. *Anatomy of the Paranasal Sinuses*. New York: Thieme; 1996.
4. Stammberger H. History of rhinology: anatomy of the paranasal sinuses. *Rhinology*. 1989;27:197–210.
5. Karmody CS, Carter B, Vincent ME. Developmental anomalies of the maxillary sinus. *Trans Am Acad Ophthalmol Otol*. 1977;84:723–728.
6. Hinni ML, McCaffrey TV, Kasperbauer JL. Early mucosal changes in experimental sinusitis. *Otolaryngol Head Neck Surg*. 1993;107:537.
7. Pietrokovski J. The bony residual ridge in man. *J Prosthet Dent*. 1975;34:456–462.
8. Misch CE. Divisions of available bone in implant dentistry. *Int J Oral Implantol*. 1990;7:9–17.
9. Misch CE. Bone character: second vital implant criterion. *Dent Today*. 1988;7:39–40.
10. Goodacre JC, Bernal G, Rungcharassaeng K, et al. Clinical complications with implants and implant prostheses. *J Prosthet Dent*. 2003;2:121–132.
11. Misch CE, Qu Z, Bidez MW. Mechanical properties of trabecular bone in the human mandible: implications for dental implants treatment planning and surgical placement. *J Oral Maxillofac Surg*. 1999;57:700–706.
12. Misch CE. *C Ontemporary Implant Dentistry*. 3rd ed. St Louis: Mosby; 2008.
13. Rice DH, Schaefer SD. *E Ndoscopic Paranasal Sinus Surgery*. 3rd ed. Philadelphia: Lippincott Williams & Wilkins; 2003.
14. Kilic C, Kamburoglu K, Yuksel SP, Ozen T. An assessment of the relationship between the maxillary sinus floor and the maxillary posterior teeth root tips using dental cone-beam computerized tomography. *Eur J Dent*. 2010;4(4):462.
15. Ulm CW, Solaur P, Krennmar G, et al. Incidence and suggested surgical management of septa in sinus lift procedures. *Int J Oral Maxillofac Implants*. 1995;10:462–465.
16. Traxler H, Windisch A, Geyerhofer U, et al. Arterial blood supply of the maxillary sinus. *Clin Anat*. 1999;12(6):417–421.
17. Elian N, Wallace S, Cho SC, et al. Distribution of the maxillary artery as it relates to sinus floor augmentation. *Int J Oral Maxillofac Implants*. 2005;20:784–787.
18. Nicolielo LFP, Van Dessel J, Jacobs R, et al. Presurgical CBCT assessment of maxillary neurovascularization in relation to maxillary sinus augmentation procedures and posterior implant placement. *Surg Radiol Anat*. 2014;36(9):915–924.
19. Apostolakis D, Bissoon AK. Radiographic evaluation of the superior alveolar canal: Measurements of its diameter and of its position in relation to the maxillary sinus floor: a cone beam computerized tomography study. *Clin Oral Implants Res*. 2014;25:553–559.
20. Zijderveld SA, van den Bergh JP, Schulten EA, ten Bruggenkate CM. Anatomical and surgical findings and complications in 100 consecutive maxillary sinus floor elevation procedures. *J Oral Maxillofac Surg*. 2008;66:1426–1438.
21. Solar P, Geyerhofer U, Traxler H. Blood supply to the maxillary sinus relevant to sinus floor elevation. *Clin Oral Implants Res*. 1999;10:34–44.
22. Morgensen C, Tos M. Quantitative histology of the maxillary sinus. *Rhinology*. 1977;15:129.
23. Scadding GK, Lund VJ, Darby YC. The effect of long-term antibiotic therapy upon ciliary beat frequence in chronic rhinosinusitis. *J Laryngol Otol*. 1995;109:24–26.
24. Jiang RS, Liang KL, Jang JW. Bacteriology of endoscopically normal maxillary sinuses. *J Larynogol Otol*. 1999;113:825–828.
25. Misch CE. Maxillary sinus augmentation for endosteal implants: organized alternative treatment plans. *Int J Oral Implantol*. 1987;4:49–58.
26. American Academy of Otolaryngology—Head and Neck Surgery. Fact sheet: 20 questions about your sinuses. Available at: http://www.entnet.org/healthinfo/sinus/sinus_questions.cfm. Accessed October 7, 2007.
27. Zinreich SJ, Kennedy DW, Rosenbaum AE, et al. Paranasal sinuses: CT imaging requirements for endoscopic surgery. *Radiology*. 1987;163:769–775.
28. McGowan DA, Baxter PW, James J. *The Maxillary Sinus and its Dental Implications*. Oxford: Butterworth-Heinemann; 1993.
29. Bolger WE, Butzin CA, Parsons DS. Paranasal sinus bony anatomic variations and mucosal abnormalities: CT analysis for endoscopic surgery. *The Laryngoscope*. 1991;101:56–64.
30. Timmenga MN, Marius N. *Maxillary Sinus Floor Elevation Surgery: Effects on Maxillary Sinus Performance [doctoral DisserTation]*. Groningen, The Netherlands: University of Groningen; 2003.
31. McKenzie M. *Manual of Diseases of the Nose and Throat*. London: Churchill Livingstone; 1980.
32. Manji A, Faucher J, Resnik RR. Suzuki JB Prevalence of maxillary sinus pathology in patients considered for sinus augmentation procedures for dental implants. *Implant Dent*. 2013;22(4):428–435.
33. Maxillary BW. Sinusitis of dental origin. *Am J Orthod Oral Surg*. 1943;29:133–151.
34. Melen I, Lindahl L, Andreasson L, Rundcrantz H. Chronic maxillary sinusitis: Definition, diagnosis and relation to dental infections and nasal polyposis. *Acta Otolaryngol (Stockh)*. 1986;101:320–327 ([PubMed]).
35. Puglisi S, Privitera S, Maiolino L, et al. Bacteriological findings and antimicrobial resistance in odontogenic and non–odontogenic chronic maxillary sinusitis. *J Medical Microbiology*. 2011;60:1353–1359.
36. Saibene AM, Pipolo GC, Lozza P, et al. Redefining boundaries in odontogenic sinusitis: a retrospective evaluation of extramaxillary involvement in 315 patients. *Int Forum Allergy Rhinol*. 2014;4:1020–1023.
37. Saibene AM, Vassena C, Pipolo C, et al. Odontogenic and rhinogenic chronic sinusitis: a modern microbiological comparison. *Int Forum Allergy Rhinol*. 2015;6:41–45.
38. Block MS, Dastoury K. Prevalence of sinus membrane thickening and association with unhealthy teeth: a retrospective review of 831 consecutive patients with 1,662 cone-beam scans. *J Oral Maxillofacial Surg*. 2014;72(12):2454–2460.
39. Bornstein MM, Wasmer J, Sendi P, et al. Characteristics and dimensions of the schneiderian membrane and apical bone in maxillary molars referred for apical surgery: a comparative radiographic analysis using limited cone beam computed tomography. *J Endod*. 2012;38:51.
40. Janner SF, Caversaccio MD, Dubach P, et al. Characteristics and dimensions of the schneiderian membrane: a radiographic analysis using cone beam computed tomography in patients referred for dental implant surgery in the posterior maxilla. *Clin Oral Implants Res*. 2011;22:1446.
41. Maillet M, Bowles WR, McClanahan SL, et al. Cone-beam computed tomography evaluation of maxillary sinusitis. *J Endod*. 2011;37:753.
42. Pazera P, Bornstein MM, Pazera A, et al. Incidental maxillary sinus findings in orthodontic patients: a radiographic analysis using cone-beam computed tomography (CBCT). *Orthod Craniofac Res*. 2011;14:17.
43. Rege IC, Sousa TO, Leles CR, et al. Occurrence of maxillary sinus abnormalities detected by cone beam CT in asymptomatic patients. *BMC Oral Health*. 2012;12:30.
44. Bascom R, Kesavanathan J, Fitzgerald TK, et al. Sidestream tobacco smoke exposure acutely alters human nasal mucociliary clearance. *Environ Health Perspect*. 1995;103:1026.

45. American Academy of Otolaryngology—Head and Neck Surgery. Fact sheet: 20 questions about your sinuses. Available at: http://www.entnet.org/healthinfo/sinus/sinus_questions.cfm. Accessed October 7, 2007.
46. Daley DL, Sande M. The runny nose infection of the paranasal sinuses. *Infect Dis Clin North Am.* 1988;2:131.
47. Zinreich SJ, Messerklinger W, Drettner B. The obstruction of the maxillary ostium. *Rhinology.* 1967;5:100–104.
48. Aust R, Drettner B. Oxygen tension in the human maxillary sinus under normal and pathological conditions. *Acta Otolaryngol.* 1974;78:264.
49. Bolzer WE, Kennedy DW. Changing concepts in chronic sinusitis. *Hosp Pract.* 1992;27:20.
50. Ponikau JU, Sherris DA, Kern EB. The diagnosis and incidence of allergic fungal sinusitis. *Mayo Clin Proc.* 1999;74:877–884.
51. Beninger MS, Mickleson SA. Functional endoscopic sinus surgery, morbidity and early results. *Henry Ford Hosp Med J.* 1990;38:5.
52. Chakrabarti A, Das A, Panda NK. Overview of fungal rhinosinusitis. *Indian J Otolaryngol Head Neck Surg.* 2004;56(4):251–258.
53. Dufour X, Kauffmann-Lacroix C, Ferrie JC, et al. Paranasal sinus fungus ball: epidemiology, clinical features and diagnosis. A retrospective analysis of 173 cases from a single medical center in France, 1989-2002. *Med Mycol.* 2006;44:61–67.
54. Mukherji SK, Figueroa RE, Ginsberg LE, et al. Allergic fungal sinusitis: CT findings. *Radiology.* 1998;207(2):417–422.
55. Gardner, David G. "Pseudocysts and retention cysts of the maxillary sinus." *Oral surgery, oral medicine, oral pathology.* 1984;58(5):561–567.
56. Oh JH, An X, Jeong SM, Choi BH. Crestal Sinus augmentation in the presence of an antral pseudocyst. *Implant Dent.* 2017;26(6):951–955.
57. Harar RP, Chadha NK, Rogers G. Are maxillary mucosal cysts a manifestation of inflammatory sinus disease? *J Laryngol Otol.* 2007;121(8):751–754.
58. Kudo K, et al. Clinicopathological study of postoperative maxillary cysts. *J Jpn Stomatol Soc.* 1972;21:250–257.
59. Lee KC, Lee NH. Comparison of clinical characteristics between primary and secondary paranasal mucoceles. *Yonsei Med J.* 2010;51(5):735–739.
60. Boyne PJ, James RA. Grafting of the maxillary sinus floor with autogenous marrow and bone. *J Oral Surg.* 1980;38:613–616.
61. Misch CE. Divisions of available bone. *Contemporary implant dentistry.* 1993;1:125–128.
62. Misch CE. Treatment planning for the edentulous posterior maxilla. In: Misch CE, ed. *Contemporary Implant Dentistry.* 2nd ed. St Louis: Mosby; 1999.
63. Misch CM, Misch CE, Resnik RR, Ismail YH, Appel B. Postoperative maxillary cyst associated with a maxillary sinus elevation procedure: a case report. *J Oral Implantol.* 1991;17(4):432–437.
64. Blaschke FF, Brady FA. The maxillary antrolith. *Oral Surg Oral Med Oral Pathol.* 1979;48:187–191.
65. Evans J. Maxillary antrolith: a case report. *Br J Oral Surg.* 1975;13:73–77.
66. Crist RF, Johnson RI. Antrolith: report of case. *J Oral Surg.* 1972;30:694–695.
67. Karges MA, Eversol LR, Poindexter BJ. Report of case and review of literature. *J Oral Surg.* 1971;29:812–814.
68. Levin L, Schwartz-Arad D. The effect of cigarette smoking on dental implants and related surgery. *Implant Dent.* 2005;4:357–361.
69. Klokkevold PR, Ham TJ. How do smoking, diabetes and periodontitis affect outcomes of implant treatment? *Int J Oral Maxillofac Implants.* 2007;22:173–202.
70. Lindquist LW, Carlsson GE, Jemt T. Association between marginal bone loss around osseointegrated mandibular implants and smoking habits: a 10-year follow-up study. *J Dent Res.* 1997;10:1667–1674.
71. Olson JW, Dent CD, Morris HF, Ochi S. Long-term assessment (5 to 71 months) of endosseous dental implants placed in the augmented maxillary sinus. *Ann Periodontol.* 2000;5:152–156.
72. Widmark G, Andersson B, Carlsson GE, Lindvall AM, Ivanoff CJ. Rehabilitation of patients with severely resorbed maxillae by means of implants with or without bone grafts: a 3- to 5-year follow-up clinical report. *Int J Oral Maxillofac Implants.* 2001;16:73–79.
73. Schwartz-Arad D, Herzberg R, Dolev E. The prevalence of surgical complications of the sinus graft procedure and their impact on implant survival. *J Periodontol.* 2004;75(4):511–516.
74. Barone A, Santini S, Sbordone L, et al. A clinical study of the outcomes and complications associated with maxillary sinus augmentation. *Int J Oral Maxillofac Implants.* 2006;21:81–85.
75. Peterson LJ. Antibiotic prophylaxis against wound infections in oral and maxillofacial surgery. *J Oral Maxillofac Surg.* 1990;48:617–620.
76. Olson M, O'Connor M, Schwartz ML. Surgical wounds infection: a 5 year prospective study of 10,193 wounds at the Minneapolis VA Medical Center. *Ann Surg.* 1984;199:253.
77. Dent CD, Olson JW, Farish SE, et al. The influence of preoperative antibiotics on success of endosseous implants up to and including stage II surgery: a study of 2641 implants. *J Oral Maxillofac Surg.* 1997;55(suppl 115):19–24.
78. Lebowitz AS. Antimicrobic therapy in rhinologic infection. In: Goldsmith J, ed. *The Principles and Practice of Rhinology.* New York: John Wiley & Sons; 1987.
79. Mulliken JB, Glowacki J, Kaban LB, et al. Use of demineralized allogenic bone I implants for the correction of maxillocraniofacial deformities. *Ann Surg.* 1981;194:366–372.
80. Jacobs MR, Felmingham D, Appelbaum PC, et al. The Alexander Project 1998-2000: susceptibility of pathogens isolated from community-acquired respiratory tract infection to commonly used antimicrobial agents. *J Antimicrob Chemother.* 2003;52:229–246.
81. Snydor A, Gwaltney J, Cachetto DM, et al. Comparative evaluation of cefuroxime axetil and cefaclor for treatment of acute bacterial maxillary sinusitis. *Arch Otolaryngol Head Neck Surg.* 1989;115:1430.
82. Gallagher DM, Epker BN. Infection following intraoral surgical correction of dentofacial deformities: a review of 140 consecutive cases. *J Oral Surg.* 1980;38:117–120.
83. Urist MR, Silverman BF, Buring K, et al. The bone induction principle. *Clin Orthop Relat Res.* 1967;53:243–283.
84. Mabry TW, Yukna RA, Sepe WW. Freeze-dried bone allografts combined with tetracycline in the treatment of juvenile periodontitis. *J Periodontol.* 1985;56:74–81.
85. Beardmore AA, Brooks DE, Wenke JC, et al. Effectiveness of local antibiotic delivery with an osteoinductive and osteoconductive bone-graft substitute. *J Bone Joint Surg Am.* 2005;87:107–112.
86. Petri WH. Osteogenic activity of antibiotic-supplemented bone allografts in the Guinea pig. *J Oral Maxillofac Surg.* 1984;42:631–636.
87. Lambert PM, Morris H, Ochi S. The influence of 0.12% chlorhexidine digluconate rinses on the incidence of infectious complications and implant success. *J Oral Maxillofac Surg.* 1997;55(suppl 5):25–30.
88. Ragno JR, Szkutnik AJ. Evaluation of 0.12% chlorhexidine rinse on the prevention of alveolar osteitis. *Oral Surg Oral Med Oral Pathol.* 1991;72:524–526.
89. Falck B, Svanholm H, Aust R. The effect of xylometazoline on the mucosa of human maxillary sinus. *Rhinology.* 1990;28:239–477.
90. Ragno JR, Szkutnik AJ. Evaluation of 0.12% chlorhexidine rinse on the prevention of alveolar osteitis. *Oral Surg Oral Med Oral Pathol.* 1991;72:524–526.
91. Tatum OH. *Lecture Presented at Alabama Implant Study Group.* Birmingham: Ala; 1977.
92. Tatum OH. Maxillary and sinus implant reconstruction. *Dent Clin North Am.* 1986;30:107–119.

93. Tatum Jr OH, Lebowitz MS, Tatum CA, et al. Sinus augmentation: rationale, development, long term results. *N Y State Dent J.* 1993;59:43–48.
94. Misch CE. Divisions of available bone in implant dentistry. *Int J Oral Implantol.* 1990;7:9–17.
95. Tatum H Jr. Maxillary and sinus reconstructions. *Dent Clin North Am.* 1986;30:207–229.
96. Misch Carl E. Contemporary implant dentistry. *Implant Dentistry.* 1999;8(1):90.
97. Summers RB. Maxillary implant surgery: the osteotome technique. *Compend Cont Educ Dent.* 1994;15:152–162.
98. Worth HM, Stoneman DQ. Radiographic interpretation of antral mucosal changes due to localized dental infection. *J Can Dent Assoc.* 1972;38:111.
99. Palma VC, Magro-Filho O, de Oliveria JA, et al. Bone reformation and implant integration following maxillary sinus membrane elevation: an experimental study in primates. *Clin Implant Dent Relat Res.* 2006;8:11–24.
100. Rosen Paul S, Robert Summers, Jose R. Mellado, Leslie M. Salkin, Richard H. Shanaman, Manuel H. Marks, Paul A. Fugazzotto. The bone-added osteotome sinus floor elevation technique: multicenter retrospective report of consecutively treated patients. *International Journal of Oral and Maxillofacial Implants.* 1999;14(6):853–858.
101. Mardinger O, Moses O, Chaushu G, et al. Challenges associated with reentry maxillary sinus augmentation. *Oral Surg Oral Med Oral Pathol Oral Radiol Endod.* 2010;110(3):287–291.
102. Reiser GM, Rabinovitz Z, Bruno J, et al. Evaluation of maxillary sinus membrane response following elevation with the crestal osteotome technique in human cadavers. *Int J Oral Maxillofac Implants.* 2001;16:833–840.
103. Malamed SF. Techniques of maxillary anesthesia. In: Malamed S, ed. *Handbook of Local Anesthesia.* 3rd ed. St Louis: Mosby; 1990.
104. Whittaker JM, James RA, Lozada J, et al. *Histological response and clInical Evaluation of Heterograft and Allograft Materials in the Elevation of the Maxillary Sinus of the Preparation of Endosteal Implant Sites.*
105. Hurzeler MB, Quinones CR, Kirsch A, et al. Maxillary sinus augmentation using different grafting materials and dental implants in monkeys, part III. *Clin Oral Implants Res.* 1997;8:401–411.
106. Nishibori M, Betts NJ, Salama H, et al. Short term healing of autogenous and allergenic bone grafts after sinus augmentation—a report of 2 cases. *J Periodontol.* 1994;65:958–966.
107. Furusawa T, Mizunuma K. Osteoconductive properties and efficacy of resorbable bioactive glass as a bone grafting material. *Implant Dent.* 1997;6:93–101.
108. Wiltfang J, Schiegel KA, Schultze-Mosgau S, et al. Sinus floor augmentation with beta-tricalciumphosphate (beta-TCP): does platelet-rich plasma promote its osseous integration and degradation. *Clin Oral Implants Res.* 2003;12:213–218.
109. BOYNE Philip J. Grafting of the maxillary sinus floor with autogenous marrow and bone. *J. Oral Surg.* 1980;38:613–616.
110. Tatum Jr OH. Sinus Augmentation. *Statistical evaluation of.* 1993;15:1979–1994.
111. Misch CE, Dietsh F. Subantral augmentation in Macaca fascicularis—pilot study, Am Acad implant dent 40th Mtg Abs. *J Oral Implantol.* 1991;17:340.
112. Misch CE. Maxillary sinus left with subantral augmentation. In: Misch CE, ed. *Contemporary Implant Dentistry.* St Louis: Mosby; 1993.
113. Moy PK, Lundgren S, Holmes RE. Maxillary sinus augmentation: histomorphometric analysis of graft materials for maxillary sinus floor augmentation. *J Oral Maxillofac Surg.* 1993;51:857–862.
114. Del Fabbro M, Testori T, Francetti L, et al. Systematic review of survival rates for implants placed in the grafted maxillary sinus. *Int J Periodontics Restorative Dent.* 2004;24:565–577.
115. Tidwell JK, Blijdorp PA, Stoelinga PJW, et al. Composite grafting of the maxillary sinus for placement of endosteal implants. *Int J Oral Maxillofac Surg.* 1992;21:204–209.
116. Hallman M, Sennerby L, Lundgren S. A clinical and histologic evaluation of implant integration in the posterior maxilla after sinus floor augmentation with autogenous bone, bovine hydroxyapatite, or a 20:80 mixture. *Int J Oral Maxillofac Implants.* 2002;17(5):635–643.
117. Froum SJ, Tarnow DP, Wallace SS, et al. Sinus floor elevation using anorganic bovine bone matrix (OsteoGraf/N) with and without autogenous bone: a clinical, histologic, radiographic, and histomorphometric analysis-part 2 of an ongoing prospective study. *Int J Periodontics Restorative Dent.* 1998;18(6):528–543.
118. Loukota RA, Isaksson SG, Linner EL, et al. A technique for inserting endosseous implants in the atrophic maxilla in a single stage procedure. *Br J Oral Maxillofac Surg.* 1992;30:46–49.
119. Nishibori M, Betts NJ, Salama H, et al. Short term healing of autogenous and allergenic bone grafts after sinus augmentation—a report of 2 cases. *J Periodontol.* 1994;65:958–966.
120. Piattelli A, Scarano A, Corigliano M, Piattelli M. Comparison of bone regeneration with the use of mineralized and demineralized freeze-dried bone allografts: a histological and histochemical study in man. *Biomaterials.* 1996;17:1127–1131.
121. Froum SJ, Wallace SS, Elian N, et al. Comparison of mineralized cancellous bone allograft (Puros) and anorganic bovine bone matrix (Bio-Oss) for sinus augmentation: histomorphometry at 26 to 32 weeks after grafting. *Int J Periodontics Restorative Dent.* 2006;26:543–551.
122. Cammack GV, Nevins M, Clem D3, Hatch JP, Mellonig JT. Histologic evaluation of mineralized and demineralized freeze-dried bone allograft for ridge and sinus augmentations. *Int J Periodontics Restorative Dent.* 2005;25(3):231–237.
123. Block MS, Finger I, Lytle R. Human mineralized bone in extraction sites before implant placement: Preliminary results. *J Am Dent Ass.* 2002;133(12):1631–1638.
124. Nevins M, Kirker Head C, et al. Bone formation in the goat maxillary sinus induced by absorbable collagen sponge implants impregnated with recombinant human bone morphogenetic protein-2. *Int J Periodontics Restorative Dent.* 1996;16:9–19.
125. Vlassis JM, Hurzeler MB, Quinones CR. Sinus lift augmentation to facilitate placement of non submerged implants—a clinical and histological report. *Pract Periodontics Aesthet Dent.* 1993;5:15–23.
126. Del Fabbro M, Testori T, Francetti L, et al. Systematic review of survival rates for implants placed in the grafted maxillary sinus. *Int J Periodontics Restorative Dent.* 2004;24:565–577.
127. Froum SJ, Wallace SS, Elian N, et al. Comparison of mineralized cancellous bone allograft (Puros) and anorganic bovine bone matrix (Bio-Oss) for sinus augmentation: histomorphometry at 26 to 32 weeks after grafting. *Int J Periodontics Restorative Dent.* 2006;26:543–551.
128. Tarnow DP, Wallace SS, Froum SJ, et al. Histologic and clinical comparison of bilateral sinus floor elevations with and without barrier membrane placement in 12 patients: part 3 of an ongoing prospective study. *Int J Periodontics Restorative Dent.* 2000;20(2):117–125.
129. Froum SJ, Wallace SS, Tarnow DP, Cho SC. Effect of platelet-rich plasma on bone growth and osseointegration in human maxillary sinus grafts: three bilateral case reports. *International Journal of Periodontics and Restorative Dentistry.* 2002;22(1):45–54.
130. Jensen OT, Leonard BS, Block MS, et al. Report of the sinus Consensus Conference of 1996. *Int J Oral Maxillofac Implants.* 1998;13(suppl):11–30.
131. Block MS, Kent JN. Maxillary sinus grafting for totally and partially edentulous patients. *J Am Dent Assoc.* 1993;124:139.
132. Aimetti M, Romagnoli R, Ricci G, et al. The effect of macrolacerations and microlacerations of the sinus membrane as determined by endoscopy. *Int J Periodontics Restorative Dent.* 2001;21:581–589.
133. Jensen J, Sindet-Petersen S, Oliver AJ. Varying treatment strategies for reconstruction of maxillary atrophy with implants: results in 98 patients. *J Oral Maxillofac Surg.* 1994;52:210–216.

134. Underwood Arthur S. An inquiry into the anatomy and pathology of the maxillary sinus. *Journal of anatomy and physiology.* 1910;44(4):354.

135. Krennmair G, Ulm CW, Lugmayr H, et al. The incidence, location and height of maxillary sinus septa in the edentulous and dentate maxilla. *J Oral Maxillofac Surg.* 1999;57:667–671.

136. Misch CE. Dental Implant Prosthetics. St. Louis. *Mosby Inc.* 2005;211:223.

137. Kim MJ, Jung UW, Kim CS, et al. Maxillary sinus septa: prevalence, height, location and morphology: a reformatted computed tomography scan analysis. *J Periodontol.* 2006;77:903–908.

138. Lee WJ, Lee SJ, Kim HS. Analysis of location and prevalence of maxillary sinus septa. *Journal of periodontal & implant science.* 2010;40(2):56–60.

139. Gurr P, Callahan V, Baldwin D. Laser-Doppler blood flowmetry measurement of nasal mucosa blood flow after injection of the greater palatine canal. *J Layngol Otol.* 1996;110:124–128.

140. Flanagan D. Arterial supply of maxillary sinus and potential for bleeding complication during lateral approach sinus elevation. *Implant Dent.* 2005;14:336–339.

141. Guerrero JS. Lateral window sinus augmentation: complications and outcomes of 101 consecutive procedures. *Implant Dent.* 2015;24(3):354–361.

142. Barone A, Santini S, Sbordone L, et al. A clinical study of the outcomes and complications associated with maxillary sinus augmentation. *Int J Oral Maxillofac Implants.* 2006;21(1):81–85.

143. Sandler NA, Johns FR, Braun TW. Advanc structures in the management of acute and chronic sinusitis. *J Oral Maxillofac Surg.* 1996;54:1005–1013.

144. Olson DEL, Rosgon BM, Hilsinger RL. Radiographic comparison of three nasal saline irrigation. *The Laryngoscope.* 2002;112:1394–1398.

145. Smith D, Goycollea M, Meyerhoff WL. Fulminant odontogenic sinusitis. *Ear Nose Throat J.* 1979;58:411.

146. Brånemark PI, Adell R, Albrektsson T, et al. An experimental and clinical study of osseointegrated implants penetrating the nasal cavity and maxillary sinus. *J Oral Maxillofac Surg.* 1984;42:497–505.

147. Boyne PJ. Analysis of performance of root form endosseous implants placed in the maxillary sinus. *J Long Term Eff Med Implants.* 1993;3(2):143–159.

148. Sohn DS, Lee JK, Shin HI, et al. Fungal infection as a complication of sinus bone grafting and implants: a case report. *Oral Surg Oral Med Oral Pathol Oral Radiol Endod.* 1993;107(3):375–380.

149. Misch Carl E. *Contemporary implant dentistry.* 2nd edition. Saint Louis: Mosby; 1999.

38

Intraoral Autogenous Bone Grafting

C. STEPHEN CALDWELL AND CARL E. MISCH

Treatment plans in implant dentistry in the past used existing bone volume to determine the location and type of implant and restorations were adapted to accommodate irregularities related to implant locations. In abundant bone (Division A), endosseous root form implants were inserted; in bone of moderate width (Division B), blade implants were placed; and in inadequate height of bone (Division C–h), subperiosteal implants were the treatment of choice.

Treatment planning has dramatically changed. The final prosthesis type and design is first determined, followed by determining the ideal implant positions, numbers, and sizes. The available bone is often inadequate to provide the foundation required for a predictable treatment plan. As a consequence, bone grafting has become a more frequent solution for achieving long-term success.

In addition to the biomechanical and functional needs significant esthetic considerations need to be included in planning a case. Bone grafting is often indicated to allow placement of an implant in the proper location for an ideal esthetic result. In addition, the soft tissue drape often requires enhancement in the esthetic zone as the bone foundation sets the tone for the soft tissue drape. Therefore when ideal crown contours (FP-1) and soft tissue are desired, bone augmentation is an important aspect of the treatment plan. As a result of biomechanical-based foundations and esthetic desires, a primary diagnostic consideration for implant prostheses is the available bone in the edentulous span. The placement of endosteal dental implants requires adequate bone volume at the desired locations for ideal prosthetic support. With insufficient bone volume, several surgical techniques may be used to reconstruct the deficient ridge in preparation for implant placement, including bone spreading (ridge splitting), bone growth factors, particulate grafting (allograft, xenograft, alloplast), and autogenous grafting (intraoral or extraoral donor sites).

The number of key factors present and the geometry of a bony defect are important considerations in the selection of a modality for ridge augmentation.[1] In general the fewer the number of remaining bony walls, the greater is the need for osteopromotive techniques. Although allografts and guided bone regeneration techniques have been used predictably in slight-to-moderate bone regeneration (primarily for inadequate width in the horizontal dimension), these methods have limitations and have been found to produce less favorable results in the treatment of larger bone deficiencies.[2-13] Ideally the most predictable bone graft material possesses osteoconductive, osteoinductive, and osteogenic properties. The only type of bone-grafting material that maintains all three of these regenerative properties is autogenous (autologous) bone. Therefore autologous cortical/trabecular bone grafts may be considered and have been proved to be highly successful for the repair of moderate-to-severe alveolar atrophy and bone defects (Fig. 38.1).[14-28]

History of Autogenous Bone Grafts

The use of iliac crest autologous bone blocks with osteointegrated implants was initially described by Brånemark et al.[29] and is now an accepted procedure in oral and maxillofacial rehabilitation. Although the iliac crest is often used in oral and maxillofacial reconstruction with dental implants,[30-34] there are many disadvantages related to harvesting bone from the ilium. The surgery is far more aggressive than intraoral techniques and it must be performed in a hospital setting under general anesthesia. This ultimately will increase patient cost, and complications from the surgery, such as neurosensory and gait disturbances are increased.[35] As an alternative to the iliac crest, there are multiple autogenous donor graft sites that originate intraorally; these include the mandibular symphysis, mandibular ramus, and maxillary tuberosity.

In the literature the mandibular symphysis was one of the first intraoral donor sites reported. Early case reports described its use in the repair of intraoral birth defects, such as cleft palates.[36,37] In 1992 Misch et al.[38] expanded the indications for use of the mandibular symphysis and ramus block bone grafts with endosteal dental implants. In the repair of localized alveolar defects of the jaws, bone grafts harvested from the intraoral sites known to offer several advantages.[20,38-41] The main advantage of intraoral versus extraoral donor grafts is their convenient surgical access and lower morbidity. The proximity of donor and recipient sites can reduce operative and anesthesia time, making them ideal for outpatient implant surgery. In addition, patients report minimal donor site discomfort compared with bone harvested from the iliac crest or other extraoral donor sites.[19,20,38-45] Bone harvested from the maxillofacial region appears to have inherent biological advantages in bone graft augmentation. This may be attributed to the embryologic origin of the donor bone.[43,46-51] The majority of bones in the human skeleton are of endochondral origin (from a cartilaginous precursor). With the exception of alveolar bone and the mandibular condyles, the maxilla and body of the mandible develop intramembranously.[52] It has been demonstrated that membranous

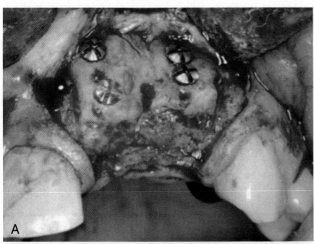

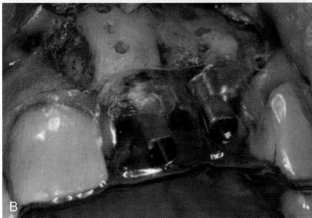

• **Fig. 38.1** Autogenous Bone Grafting: (A) Clinical image depicting block grafting to a large defect in the maxillary left central and incisor area. (B) Post-graft healing allows for ideal placement's of dental implants.

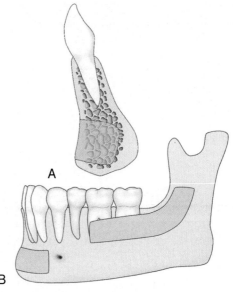

• **Fig. 38.2** (A) The symphysis block graft is usually harvested approximately 5 mm below the roots of the anterior teeth and extends to the lingual plate. (B) The symphysis and ramus region are two of the most popular sites that are harvested for intraoral defects.

bone grafts show less resorption in comparison with endochondral bone grafts.[46,47,49,53-56] Although cancellous grafts revascularize more rapidly than cortical grafts,[14] cortical membranous grafts revascularize more rapidly than endochondral bone grafts, with a thicker cancellous component.[48,57] Early revascularization of membranous bone grafts results in an improved maintenance of graft volume.[48,56-58] It is also theorized that bone of ectomesenchymal origin, such as the mandible, has a better potential for incorporation in the maxillofacial region because of a biochemical similarity in the protocollagen of the donor and recipient bone.[59] More recent research suggests that grafted bone independent from its embryogenic origin will mimic the properties of the recipient bone.[60] The inductive capacity of cortical grafts is explained by their higher concentration of bone morphogenetic proteins.[60-62] Bone from the maxillofacial skeleton contains increased concentrations of growth factors, which may lead to a greater capacity for bone repair and graft retention.[63] Another hypothesis is that the improved survival of craniofacial bone grafts is simply caused by their three-dimensional structure.[64,65] Because these grafts have a thicker cortical volume, they resorb at a slower rate.[53,54,57,66] In bone graft reconstruction, an emphasis has been placed on the transplantation of viable osteoprogenitor cells from cancellous marrow grafts, because the majority of osteoblasts are present in cancellous bone.[18] However, because of significant graft resorption associated with cancellous block grafts from endochondral

donor bone, they are not the primary donor bone in reconstruction of mandibular discontinuity defects and ridge augmentation for soft tissue–supported prostheses.[16,18,55-57,67,68] In contrast, corticocancellous block grafts harvested from the ilium have greater bone volume compared with particulate cancellous grafts.[57] When endosteal implants are surgically placed in corticocancellous bone, it has been observed that bone resorption is slower. This may be because of the microarchitecture of the bone graft (i.e., cortical compared with cancellous).

Cortical bone harvested from the mandible exhibits slower graft resorption and excellent graft incorporation into the host bone compared with cancellous bone grafts.[57] This is due to the vast amounts of osteocytes, growth factors, and bone morphogenetic protein contained in cortical bone. This facilitates angiogenesis and osteoblast migration into the graft site.[69-72] It has also been shown that the dense structure of the cortical grafts offers improved implant stability and interfacial stress transmission on implant loading.[73-75] When used in block bone grafting, the results have been consistent, with excellent graft stability.[19-23,25,26,38-45,76-91] Mandibular block bone grafts may be harvested from the residual ridge, symphysis, body, and ascending ramus (Fig. 38.2).

Preoperative Evaluation of Recipient Site

A preoperative, comprehensive evaluation of the host graft site is extremely important. The implant clinician must identify any esthetic concerns, the graft dimensions needed to reconstruct the osseous deficiency or zone of atrophy, the soft and hard tissue topography, and the periodontal and endodontic health of the adjacent teeth.[38,92,93] The host site should ideally be evaluated in width, height, and length. In general the most predictable bone augmentation sites require only the width dimension and extend for one tooth. This provides mesiodistal and apical walls of host bone. A one-tooth span provides ease

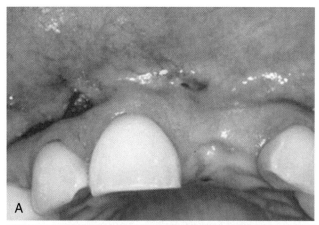

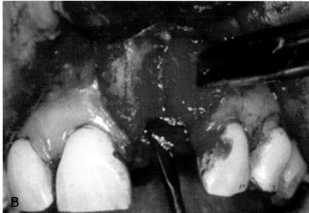

• **Fig. 38.3** Clinical evaluation of the underlying bone is often misleading. (A) Clinical evaluation of edentulous site. (B) After mucoperiosteal flap, tissue is reflected to reveal significant bony defect.

of soft tissue manipulation and minimal risk for incision line opening. The least predictable bone graft sites are more than four teeth in length and require more than 5 mm of height and width of bone (Fig. 38.3).

The implant clinician must always take into consideration the final prosthesis in the treatment planning of osseous defects. When an FP-1 prosthesis is the treatment of choice, the adjacent teeth next to the host graft site should ideally have bone on the roots to a level within 2 mm of the cement-enamel junction. When a bone graft is placed adjacent to a tooth root (rather than bone), the graft most often resorbs to the level of the existing bone on the adjacent tooth root. Therefore in a one-intratooth defect, a line drawn from each bone level on the adjacent roots is the maximum bone height that can be predictably expected.

In selection of the donor bone for a graft site the graft recipient site needs to be evaluated in terms of width and height graft requirements. When greater than 4 mm of donor bone graft width is required (C-w bone volume), the mandibular symphysis is the preferable donor site because of the corticocancellous nature of the graft. When donor graft requirements are less than 4 mm in width, the ascending ramus of the mandible should be considered (Division B to B-w bone volume). When considering atrophy in the vertical dimension, the symphysis of the mandible is a good source of bone because of the greater volume of bone that can be acquired.

An accurate radiographic assessment is imperative for complete assessment of the osseous defect. Ideally preoperative

imaging studies should include a cone beam computed tomographic (CBCT) scan because they have become the standard of care in preoperative implant surgical planning and in the evaluation of the recipient and donor sites.[94-96] Mounted study casts on a semiadjustable articulator of the patient's jaws allow the implant team to fully evaluate the anatomy of the jaws and teeth that cannot be fully appreciated while examining the oral cavity. In addition to mounted study models, a diagnostic wax-up of the reconstructed jaw and dentition will help to determine graft dimensions such as width, height, and implant positioning in relation to the opposing dentition. From this information, surgical templates may be fabricated with respect to the ideal implant position in relation to the position of the final prosthesis (Fig. 38.4).[38,41,94,95]

Preparation of Recipient Site

The recipient graft site should be clinically evaluated before bone harvesting is initiated. This assessment allows the clinician to obtain accurate graft dimensions that are required to reconstruct osseous defects or zones of atrophy in preparation for future implant placement. Soft tissue incisions to expose the recipient site are made within attached keratinized tissue. In an edentulous ridge the soft tissue incision is made slightly lingual to the gingival crest to reduce the risk for incision lines opening from jaw movement and postsurgical edema. When harvesting a monocortical block of bone, vertical releasing incisions are made anterior and posterior to the crestal incision line to provide good visualization of the surgical site and ease of graft harvest, and to avoid tearing of the soft tissue flap. The soft tissue reflection of the flap distal to the graft site may be a full- or split-thickness reflection to facilitate soft tissue healing and reduce incision line opening (Figs. 38.5 and 38.6).

Selection of Intraoral Donor Site

After the recipient site has been reviewed, the selection of the donor site can be determined. The severity of the defect basically determines if this graft can be taken from the ramus or in major defects, from the mandibular symphysis. In minor defects where cancellous bone is applicable, bone form the maxillary tuberosity can be considered. It is always preferable to use autogenous bone as the graft material in this type of case.

Mandibular Symphysis Donor Site

Anatomy

The mandibular symphysis describes the area in the midline of the mandible where the two lateral halves of the mandible fuse at an early period of life. The median ridge divides and encloses the triangular eminence or mental protuberance. The base of the protuberance is depressed in the center and is raised on either side to form the mental tubercle. The most inferior aspect of the mandibular symphysis is termed the "menton," and this area serves as the origin of the geniohyoid and genioglossus muscles (Fig. 38.7). Because the average interforaminal distance is greater than 4 cm, the symphysis is ideal for recipient sites that require large intraoral grafts. In general the symphysis has proven to be a good graft choice for graft reconstruction cases that require graft sizes of four or more teeth, especially when both vertical and horizontal deficiencies are present.

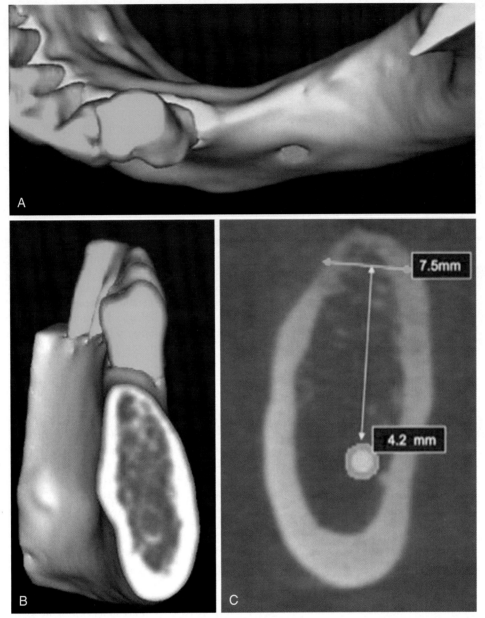

• **Fig. 38.4** Cone Beam Computed Tomographic Evaluation of Edentulous Space. (A) Three-dimensional image of edentulous site showing compromised width. (B) Cross section of compromised bone. (C) Cross section showing accurate height and width measurements.

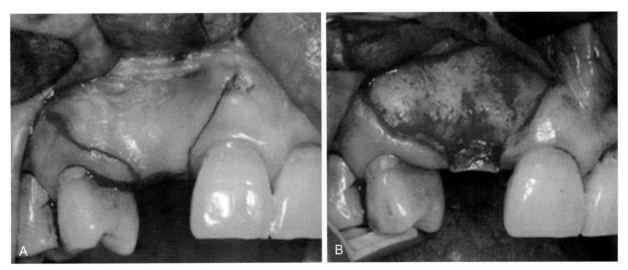

• **Fig. 38.5** Papilla-Sparing Incision. (A) Broad-based incision maintaining the papilla. (B) Full reflection revealing the bony defect that will dictate the donor site graft.

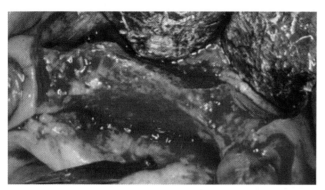

• **Fig. 38.6** Larger trapezoid flap exposing large undercuts on facial and lingual.

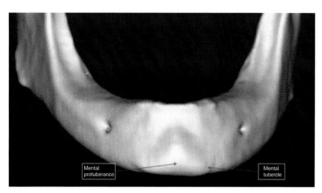

• **Fig. 38.7** Mandibular symphysis anatomy showing the mental protuberance and the mental tubercle.

Radiographic Evaluation

As part of the treatment planning process, CBCT imaging studies are recommended to evaluate the symphysis to determine the anatomic bone morphology, which includes the approximate length of the mandibular teeth, the distance between the mental foramina, and the vertical height of bone between the root apices and the inferior border of the mandible. CBCT imaging allows comprehensive three-dimensional visualization of the graft site, avoidance of unwanted complications, especially violation of the floor of the mouth with its highly vascular structures (e.g., sublingual and submental arteries). CBCT imaging is superior to plain film radiographs (e.g., panoramic) because it can provide the clinician with anatomic information in three dimensions that are not available on two-dimensional films. However, intraoperative periapical radiographs may be used to ascertain the apical location of the incisor teeth to prevent injury to the roots of the anterior teeth.

It is imperative to determine the buccal-lingual dimension of available bone throughout the symphysis area. Great care should be exercised to avoid hourglass mandibles because perforation of the lingual plate may lead to fracture or damage to blood vessels. The width of the mandible in the midline is usually the greatest dimension and decreases toward the mental foramen area. Mandibular symphysis width is several millimeters narrower in the region of the premolar and canines, compared with the midline (Fig. 38.8).

The average dimension of the anterior mandible between the mental foramina is approximately 44 mm, with African American males having the greatest distance, followed by white males, and African American females.[97] It is recommended that all osteotomy cuts remain a minimum of 5 mm from the anterior aspect of the mental foramen to avoid injury to the mental neurovascular bundle and mental nerve. In a study by Montazem et al.,[98] dentate cadaver mandibular blocks were harvested from the mandibular symphysis to evaluate the maximum bone quantity without causing damage to the mental nerve. When two symmetric blocks were measured from each site, the average was 21 × 10 × 7 mm, the largest was 25 × 13 × 9 mm, and the smallest measured 21 × 6.5 × 6 mm.[98] Therefore the mandibular symphysis is an ideal donor site for harvesting cortico-cancellous blocks (Fig. 38.9).

Anesthesia

The anterior symphyseal region of the mandible is innervated by the mandibular branch of the fifth cranial nerve (V3) and cervical nerves from C-3 and C-4. Bilateral dental or Akinosi (closed-mouth) blocks with lidocaine 2% (1:100,000 epinephrine) and Marcaine 0.5% (1:200,000 epinephrine) can be used to obtain V3 innervation anesthesia. Infiltration anesthesia is then performed anterior and inferior to the mental foramen and in the midline at the base of the mental protuberance.

Incision and Reflection

Surgical access to the symphysis is accomplished using crestal or vestibular incisions. When incisor teeth are present, a vestibular approach is recommended as reflection of the soft tissue around the anterior teeth may result in tissue recession and root exposure soft tissue healing.[99] In addition, a vestibular incision is less traumatic and results in reduced postoperative discomfort. However, the vestibular incision will usually result in more intraoperative bleeding and the highest risk for incision line opening, but the least risk for soft tissue changes around the teeth and root exposure after healing. It also creates much simpler access to the symphysis area and allows for easier suturing of the incision line. Limiting the distal extent of the vestibular incision to the canine tooth area (i.e., mesial of the canine) will reduce the incidence of mental nerve neurosensory impairment.[38,39,44] When there is a high mucogingival junction (MGJ) or high muscle attachments, a sulcular incision may be indicated because a vestibular incision would have a higher incidence of incision line opening. In addition, sulcular incisions are advantageous when less than 4 mm of keratinized gingival height is found around the lower anterior teeth because incision line opening is a greater risk. This is often seen when the mentalis muscle is large and parafunctional forces in this region exist. The sulcular incision carries the least risk for incision line opening after healing but has an increased risk for root exposure. The sulcular approach is also the most time consuming approach from the standpoint of suturing (Fig. 38.10).

Using a scalpel or electrocautery, an incision is made through the mucosa and periosteum down to the symphysis bone between the bilateral canine teeth. Using a periosteal elevator, the soft tissue flap is reflected (full-thickness) off of the anterior mandible. Full-thickness reflection is required so that no soft tissue remains on the donor bone that could interfere with healing (Figs. 38.11 and 38.12).

To avoid ptosis of the chin, it is recommended that soft tissue dissection to the inferior border of the mandible be avoided. This limited reflection prevents complete reflection of the mentalis muscle from its lower attachment to the bone.

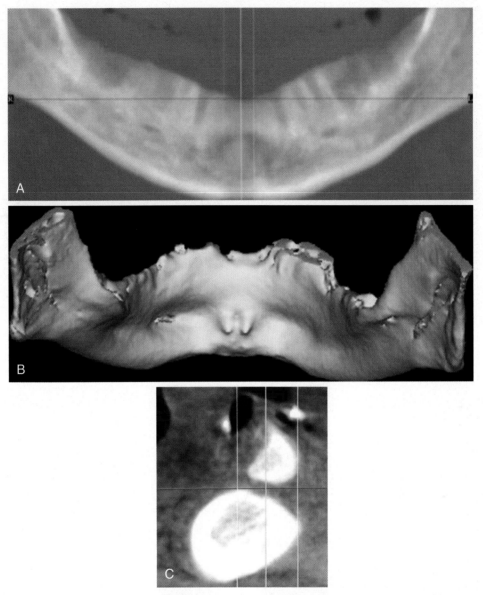

• **Fig. 38.8** Cone Beam Computed Tomography Evaluation. (A) It is very important not to solely treatment plan the anterior mandible via the two-dimensional or three-dimensional panoramic image. (B) Three-dimensional image depicting hourglass anatomy. (C) Cross section showing severe undercuts.

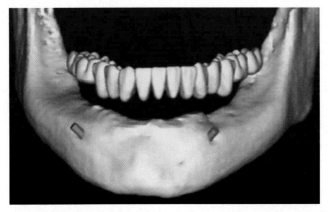

• **Fig. 38.9** The average interforaminal distance between the mental foramen is greater than 44 mm, and accurate measurements should be determined before graft harvesting.

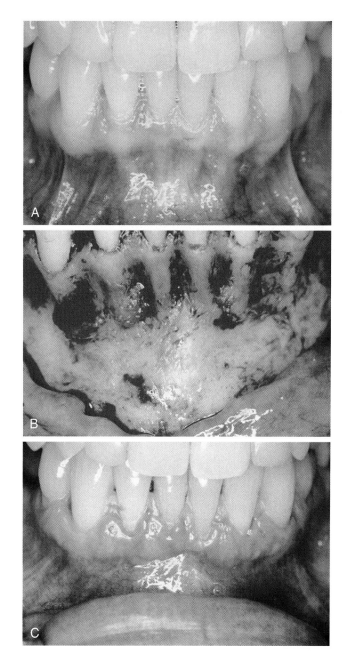

• **Fig. 38.10** (A) Sulcular incisions are usually made in the anterior mandible for a symphysis harvest when the keratinized tissue is less than 4 mm in height or when a heavier musculature is observed. (B) The incision extends distal to the canines, and a vertical release incision is made anterior and above the height of the mental foramen. A full-thickness mucoperiosteal flap reflection exposes the symphysis for the harvest. (C) A sulcular incision has less risk for postoperative incision line opening; however, there is a greater risk for root exposure after healing.

Donor Site Osteotomy Harvest

After the symphysis is exposed, the osteotomy for the graft harvest is planned. The dimensions of the block bone graft are determined by the size of the host bone defect. The osteotomies may be performed with a surgical fissure bur (557, 702—straight 1:1 handpiece), oscillating saw, or Piezotome unit. In general the Piezosurgery unit allows more efficient and bone-saving osteotomy cuts (Fig. 38.13).

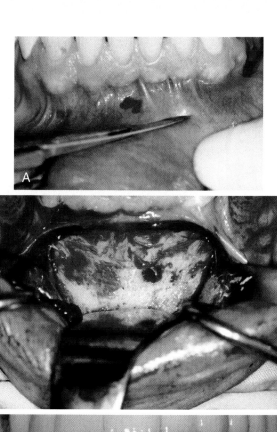

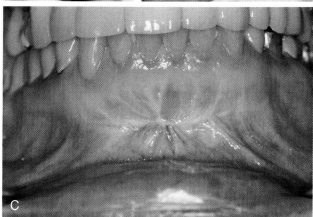

• **Fig. 38.11** (A) A vestibular incision is made 5 to 10 mm below the muco-gingival junction when 4 to 9 mm of keratinized tissue height is observed on the facial of the mandibular anterior teeth. (B) The incision extends to the distal of the canines, and a vertical release incision is made for approximately 10 mm (above the height of the mental foramen). A full-thickness mucoperiosteal reflection exposes the mandibular symphysis. (C) Vestibular incisions often heal with scar formation.

Piezotome surgery (Acteon Corp.) is a technology that uses a modulated ultrasonic frequency to cut or sever mineralized tissue. This ultrasonic surgery technique uses microoscillations (i.e., 60–200 m/sec at 25–29 kHz) to cut hard tissue, without damaging soft tissue. With this type of surgical modality, precision cuts can be prepared and greater bone graft quantities can be harvested on a predictable basis. In addition, visibility is improved because a cavitation effect is created from the irrigation/cooling solution that is used. Numerous studies have shown the ultrasonic bone cutting technique to be more favorable than conventional rotary instruments.[100]

The harvesting of the symphysis block includes four different osteotomy cuts: (1) superior, (2) inferior, (3) right vertical, and (4) left vertical (Figs. 38.14 and 38.15).

Superior Cut. The superior bone cut is usually made first and is dictated by the location of the mandibular incisor and canine teeth. To avoid root injury of the incisor teeth, when harvesting blocks of bone from the symphysis, it is recommended to remain a minimum of 5 mm apical to the apices of the incisor and canine teeth. Usually the canine teeth are much longer than the incisor teeth (i.e., incisors: ~12–14 mm, canines: ~16 mm).[101] The angulation of the superior cut is slightly converging (i.e., with respect to the lingual plate) because this will minimize injury to the tooth roots and allow for easier removal of the bone. The depth of the osteotomy should always be through the labial cortex; however,

it should never be extended lingually to the lingual cortical plate (Fig. 38.16).

Inferior Cut. The inferior bone cut is often the most difficult to perform because access is always difficult and challenging. Care should be exercised not to compromise the inferior border of the mandible because this may cause iatrogenic fracture of the symphysis area and possibly create a discontinuity defect. The horizontal inferior osteotomy should be at least 5 mm or more superior to the inferior border of the mandible, and the lingual cortical plate should be preserved so that the lingual plate does not fracture off during the harvest.

Vertical Cuts. Bilateral vertical cuts are made to connect the horizontal superior and inferior cuts. The location of these cuts must be at a minimum 5 mm anterior to each mental foramen. The presence of an anterior loop should always be evaluated and when present, proper modification to the location of the cuts should be adjusted. As the horizontal and vertical cuts are connected, care should be taken to make sure all four cuts are completely through the cortical plates and that they each connect with the adjacent cut. Small islands of intact bone can prevent the block from freely being removed from the donor site. (Fig. 38.17).

Block Removal

Block removal from the symphysis is usually completed with a straight/curved bone chisel and mallet or a Potts elevator. The chisel/elevator is usually placed in one of the vertical cut areas, and an elevated force is applied to verify movement of the block. If no movement of the block is present, the osteotomies may be deepened slightly and reverification that all cuts are continuous. The chisel can be used with the mallet; however, the mandible should be stabilized to prevent any damage to the temporomandibular joint. Ideally the patient should maintain his or her teeth in maximum intercuspation.

After block removal, cancellous bone may be available (i.e., determined by CBCT cross-sections) to harvest to supplement

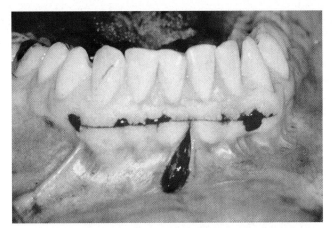

• **Fig. 38.12** When there exists an abundant amount of attached keratinized tissue on the facial aspect of the mandibular anterior teeth, an incision in the keratinized tissue is of benefit. The incision is made to the distal of the canines. In this case a midline vertical incision was made, because the symphysis harvest was limited in size.

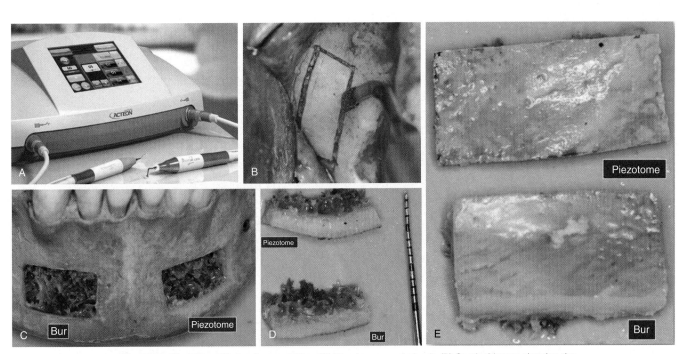

• **Fig. 38.13** Piezotome (Acteon) versus Bur. (A) Piezotome surgical unit. (B) Surgical image showing the superior osteotomy cut with the Piezotome. (C) Cadaver study showing a more ideal osteotomy with a Piezotome surgery unit in comparison with a bur. (D and E) Harvested block comparing the Piezotome and bur.

any voids in the block graft. Bone curettes of varying sizes will allow for the available cancellous bone to be removed from the donor site.[102] Care must be exercised not to perforate the lingual cortical plate. In some cases, because of the size of the block or the acute angle of the symphysis, the block outline may require sectioning into two sections. This will allow for easier block removal because two blocks of bone can be harvested from the symphysis instead of one large block of bone. Another option is to maintain a section of bone in the midline of the symphysis because this will decrease the risk for altering the postoperative appearance of the chin, especially when the patient has a prominent chin point. After the bone block is harvested, the defect can be filled with a particulate graft material (e.g., microporous hydroxyapatite and a collagen membrane) to minimize the possibility of a defect and to help to restore the contour of the mandible (Fig. 38.18; Boxes 38.1 and 38.2).

Closure

If a vestibular incision is used, a two-layered soft tissue closure is recommended for suturing. The periosteum is first closed with resorbable suture (e.g., 4–0 or 5–0 Vicryl), as well as the mentalis muscle and vestibular mucosa. This is followed by the outer tissue closure with a high tensile strength suture material (e.g., Vicryl, PTFE). To allow for ease of closure, the patient should bite into the centric occlusion, which also decreases tension on the flap. Postoperative pressure dressings in the form of pressure

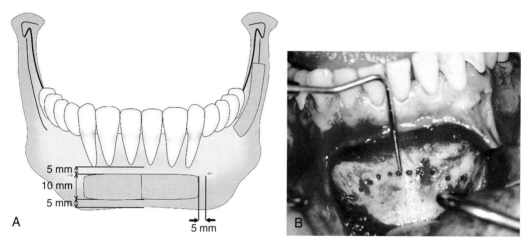

• **Fig. 38.14** (A) The guidelines for the symphysis block harvest are usually 5 mm from each mental foramen, 5 mm below the roots of the anterior teeth, and 5 mm from the inferior border of the mandible. (B) The superior osteotomy for the bone block is made 5 mm from the apex of the mandibular anterior teeth. The block margin slopes down in the canine region because of the longer roots.

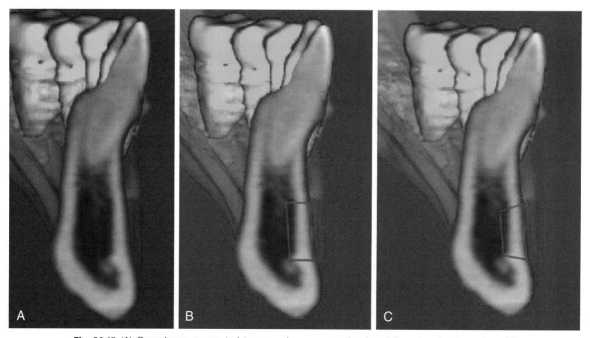

• **Fig. 38.15** (A) Cone beam computed tomography cross section in midline showing buccal and lingual contours. (B) Osteotomy cuts should not be perpendicular to the outer buccal plate because block removal will be difficult. (C) Osteotomy cuts should converge toward the lingual to allow for easier removal.

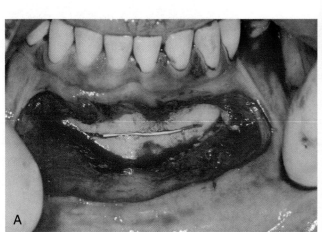
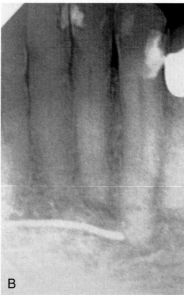

• **Fig. 38.16** (A) When in doubt on the location of the superior cut, a radiopaque material may be placed in the osteotomy and evaluated radiographically. (B) The radiograph reveals the initial osteotomy is too close to the canine root and should be 6 mm more apical in this region.

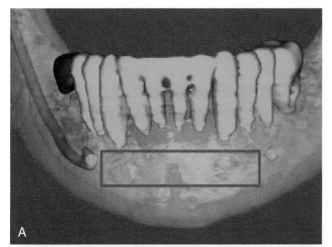

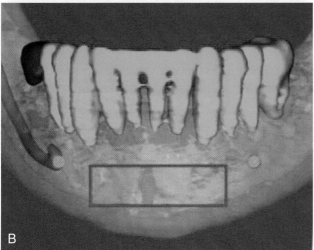

• **Fig. 38.17 Symphysis Graft Outline.** (A) Outline too close to mental foramen and apical regions of the teeth. (B) Ideal outline with ideal space from the mental foramen and teeth roots.

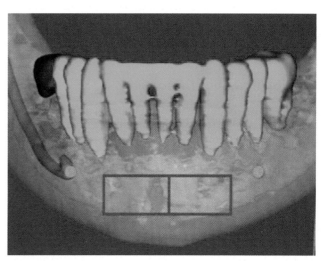

• **Fig. 38.18** In some cases, involving large blocks, the bone should be sectioned in half to allow for easier removal.

• BOX 38.1 Symphysis Bone Graft

Indications
- Horizontal and vertical ridge augmentation
- Thicker graft required (corticocancellous)
- Maximum: 0.7 × 1.5 × 6 cm

Advantages
- Easy access
- Can obtain large amount of cancellous bone
- Usually a corticocancellous graft

Disadvantages
- Altered sensation of mandibular anterior teeth
- Inferior alveolar nerve damage
- Patient cosmetic concerns
- More challenging closure
- Greater possibility of incision dehiscence

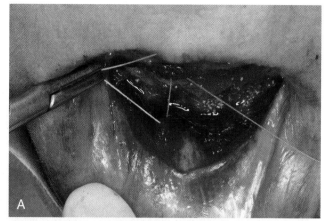

• BOX 38.2   **Symphysis Graft Osteotomy Technique**

Incision: vestibular—depending on access, slightly apical to mucogingival junction from mesial of cuspid to mesial of cuspid; an alternative incision is a sulcular incision
Superior: 5 mm below apices of anterior teeth
Inferior: 5 mm superior to the inferior border of mandible
Vertical: 5 mm anterior to mental foramen
Bone harvest: chisel and mallet, or Potts elevator

---

tapes placed over the skin of the chin can reduce the development of hematoma formation, incision line dehiscence, and infection (Figs. 38.19 and 38.20).

Alternative Symphysis Procedures

If a large monocortical bone block is not indicated, circular-shaped bone cores ranging from 4 to 10 mm in diameter may be harvested with a trephine bur for use in alveolar augmentation.[103] Trephine burs of varying diameters can remove bone cores of different lengths down to the lingual cortex of the mandible. A Molt curette or other instrument is then used to recover the bone core. It is critical that the bone cores be fixated and immobilized during the healing phase to avoid nonunion of the bone core to the native host mandible. After 4 to 6 months of bone healing, dental implants can usually be surgically placed into the grafted bone. After an additional 3-month healing period, the implants may be prosthetically restored.

Mandibular Ramus Donor Site

A second intraoral autogenous donor graft site that may be used is the mandibular ramus. The mandibular ramus has many advantages as a potential donor site. This area allows sufficient amounts of bone to be harvested for graft reconstruction and provides easy access to the ascending ramus, patient discomfort is less compared with the symphysis graft, and there is reduced risk for neurosensory disturbances from injury to the inferior alveolar neurovascular bundle. The primary disadvantage with the use of ramus grafts is that access may be difficult in some cases and the quantity of bone is limited (i.e., mainly in width).

Anatomy

The mandibular ramus is the second largest part of the mandible (i.e., mandibular body is the largest), and it extends cranially from the angle of the mandible and away from the body at approximately 110 degrees. The ramus is quadrilaterally shaped and is made up of two surfaces, four borders, and two processes.

Anatomic Surfaces:
1. Lateral surface: It is relatively flat and is defined by the internal and external oblique ridges, and the Masseter muscle attachment encompasses much of the surface.
2. Medial surface: The medial surface includes the entrance to the mandibular foramen and the inferior alveolar vessels and nerve. The lingula is the surrounding prominent ridge that gives attachment to the sphenomandibular ligament. The mylohyoid groove runs obliquely downward and forward, and is the location for mylohyoid vessels and nerve. The internal pterygoid inserts behind the mylohyoid groove.

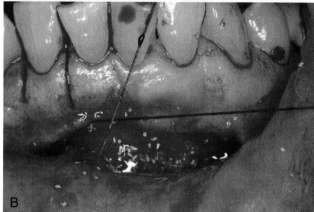

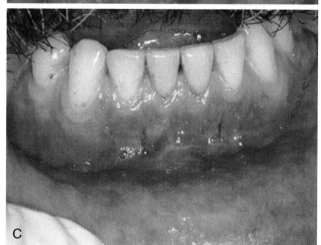

• Fig. 38.19 Vestibular Closure. (A) Use of a "two layer" closure in a chin graft site limits excess tension on the healing wound as the mentalis muscle is flexed. The mentalis can be sutured to its remnants if they are visible or it can be anchored with sutures that pass from the muscle, through the interproximal tissue, around an incisor, and back through the adjacent interproximal papilla to then draw the muscle to its proper level. This is completed on both sides of the symphysis. (B) A second suture line is used to approximate the mucosal layer of the vestibule. Assuring that there is not any tension on the sutured wound. (C) Post operative photo showing a matured vestibular block graft donor site.

Anatomic Borders:
1. Inferior border: The lower border is a thicker part of the mandible, which is continuous with the inferior border of the mandible. The lower border junctions with the posterior

border at the angle of the mandible (gonial angle). The masseter muscle attaches laterally, and the internal pterygoid attaches medially.

2. Anterior border: It is continuous with the oblique line and is thin at the crest.

3. Posterior border: It is thicker and is covered by the parotid gland.

4. Superior border: This is a thin bone that makes up two processes, the coronoid and condylar. The mandibular notch is a deep concavity that separates the two processes.

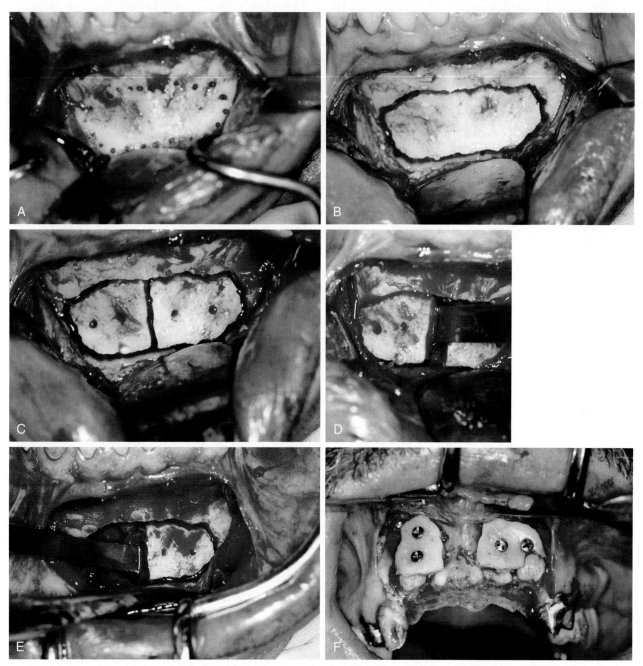

• **Fig. 38.20** (A) The inferior osteotomy is planned and is usually 5 mm above the inferior border of the mandible when a harvest is primarily for an increased width of bone. (B) A fissure bur may be used to connect the dots of the planned bone block. (C) The block is usually designed to be harvested in two pieces. (D) After an osteotome is used to ensure the osteotomy is made up to the lingual plate, the chisel is angled to shear the one block from this landmark. (E) The second bone block is easier to harvest because the bone chisel can slide along the lingual plate with direct access. (F) The bone blocks are positioned in key implant regions, with at least two fixation screws.

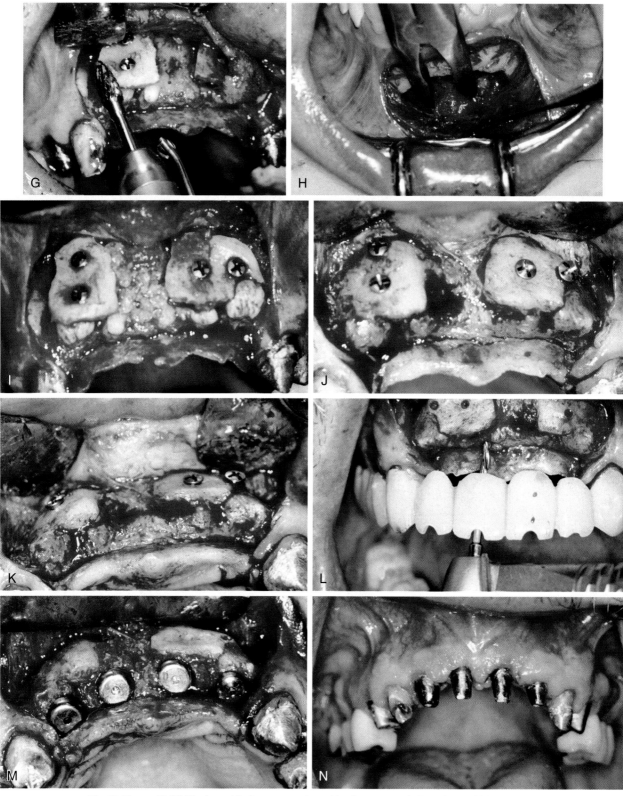

● **Fig. 38.20, cont'd** (G) The bone blocks are recontoured in situ to smooth the edges, which might perforate the soft tissue flaps. (H) Additional particulate bone may be harvested from the symphysis with a rongeur or trephine bur. (I) The particulate bone is placed between the blocks and in any voids between the host bone and blocks. (J) A reentry into the host site after 5 months. (K) The block grafts usually exhibit less resorption compared with the particulate graft (in the center). (L) A drill guide is used to position the implants into the graft site. (M) Four implants are positioned in the grafted site. (N) After 4 months of healing the abutments are inserted and the prosthesis may be fabricated.

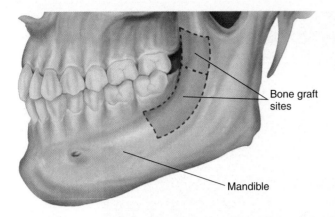

• **Fig. 38.21** The ramus and posterior body may be used as a bone block harvest site.

Anatomic Processes:

1. Coronoid process: This is a thin, triangular eminence that allows attachment to the masseter and temporalis muscle.
2. Condylar process: The condylar process ends with the condyle, which is the articular surface for articulation with the *articular disk* of the *temporomandibular joint* (Fig. 38.21).

Radiographic Evaluation

Clinical evaluation of the ascending ramus is ideally evaluated via CBCT technology. With the various CBCT views available to evaluate the ramus area, the amount of bone available for grafting, along with the location of the inferior alveolar nerve canal, may be determined. The anteroposterior length of the external oblique and prosthetic "buccal shelf" ranges from no presence from the third to first molar, to a dominant projection lateral to the body of the mandible. An index finger may be placed on the external oblique ridge of the ascending ramus and lateral aspect of the mandible. Often a ledge is palpable lateral to the second molar region and begins to disappear at the medial of the first molar. The wider the "ledge" lateral to the molars or body of an edentulous mandible, the wider the ramus block bone that can be harvested. Some mandibles have almost no "buccal shelf," whereas others are very significant (i.e., ~7 mm). Most often the buccal shelf disappears at the mid-first molar region to the anterior and to the third molar region on the posterior aspect. The ramus length is variable, with the most common vertical limit below the coronoid process, because this structure is so very thin that a block section would remove the entire segment. When determining the location of the graft site, there exist three anatomic variables that require clinical and radiographic evaluation.

1. The first variable includes the buccal-lingual mandibular canal position. Although the buccolingual position of the mandibular canal is variable within the body of the mandible, the distance from the canal to the medial aspect of the buccal cortical plate (medullary bone thickness) has been found to be greatest at the distal half of the first molar.[104] Therefore when larger grafts are planned, the anterior vertical bone cut may be made in this area. The vertical bone cuts are progressively deepened until bleeding from the underlying cancellous bone is visible, which will allow for a safe distance from the mandibular canal.[105,106]
2. The second variable is the distance from the external oblique and ramus to the inferior alveolar canal. The mean anteroposterior

width of the ramus is 30.5 mm, with the mandibular foramen located about two-thirds of the distance from the anterior border.[105] A CBCT scan is ideally used to assess and evaluate these bony dimensions. The lingula on the medial ramus is the entry point of the inferior alveolar nerve, and its location is variable. It may be at the occlusal plane (most often), above the occlusal plane, or below the occlusal plane. The lingula may be in the anterior third of the ramus, the middle third, or the distal third of the width of the ramus. As a general rule the higher and farther forward the lingula, the closer the inferior alveolar canal is adjacent to the external oblique ridge. As a result the ramus block harvest must be located lateral to the inferior alveolar canal and is usually less than 3 mm thick. The lower and more distal the lingual is in the ramus on the CBCT, the lower the inferior alveolar canal is to the external oblique. As a result the ramus block may be as much as 6 mm in width.
3. The third variable is the width of the posterior ramus. In general, females have a thinner ramus body and width compared with males. Because of these anatomic variables, a rectangular block of cortical bone 3 to 6 mm in thickness may be harvested from the ramus.[106] The length of the rectangular graft may range from 1 to 3.5 cm, and the height approximately 1 cm.[20,44,107] Such anatomic dimensions may correct width deficiencies involving a span of three to four teeth.

Although use of the coronoid process as an autologous graft has been reported,[108-110] the amount of bone for ridge augmentation is negligible considering the potential postoperative disability of a coronoidectomy.[111,112] However, such anatomic size and shape may be used as a veneer graft to gain additional ridge width. The anatomic proximity makes the ramus well suited for augmentation to the posterior mandible inadequate in width (Fig. 38.22).[42]

Incision and Reflection

The surgical procedure to harvest a block bone graft from the ramus is similar to performing a sagittal split ramus osteotomy.[106,113-119] With a scalpel, an incision is initiated on the midcrest of the ridge in the posterior edentulous patient, beginning at the base of the retromolar pad. Caution should always be exercised to avoid the retromolar pad in the incision design because this may result in neurosensory impairment issues (i.e., paresthesia, anesthesia, or dysphasia caused by injury of the lingual nerve, the chorda tympani nerve, and a sympathetic branch of the parasympathetic nerve to the submandibular gland with the lingual nerve).

Initiating the incision on the ascending ramus no higher than the level of the occlusal plane minimizes the possibility of severing the buccal artery or exposing the buccal fat pad.[106] The incision continues anteriorly into the buccal sulcus of the molar teeth or posterior ridge area. When making the incision in this area, often a minor bleeding issue may result. At the height of the occlusal plane, the buccal artery crosses the ascending ramus of the mandible. The maxillary artery traverses anteriorly and laterally to the retromolar pad. If severed, profuse bleeding is observed, which is usually treated with hemostats to clamp the vessel on the lingual aspect of the incision.

A mucoperiosteal flap is reflected from the mandibular body, exposing the lateral aspect of the ramus. The attachment of the buccinator muscle is observed first. A periosteal elevator is placed medial to this structure and directly on the bone of the external oblique and along the ramus. The flap is elevated

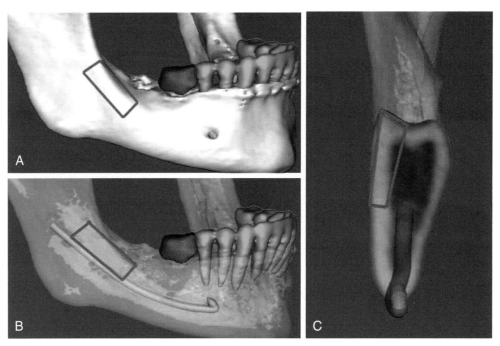

• **Fig. 38.22** Ramus Bone Graft. (A) Outline of four major osteotomy cuts. (B) Translucent outline of donor site and its relationship to the inferior alveolar canal. (C) Cross-sectional view of graft site.

superiorly along the external oblique ridge. After the facial flap is reflected the incision in the midramus may be extended to the attachment of the temporalis muscle. The periosteal elevator slides along the ramus 15 mm deep, down the ramus toward the first premolar region, and identifies the mental foramen. The host site is reflected and prepared for receiving the block graft (Fig. 38.23).

Donor Site Osteotomy Harvest

Superior Cut. The width of the ramus and the external oblique lateral of the mandibular body are identified. A straight handpiece and a small, round drill (No. 2–4) or a thin flat insert on a Piezosurgery unit punctures the bone 3 to 6 mm (i.e., dependent on the bony thickness as per the CBCT survey) from the lateral aspect of the ramus and external oblique for the superior cut. The holes should allow at least 3 mm of bone on the lingual of the ramus and 2 mm of bone adjacent to the molar teeth (when present). The length of the graft is determined, as dictated by the host site (previously reflected and prepared). The penetrating holes, just through the cortical bone, are then connected with a fissure bur (No. 557 surgical length) or Piezosurgery unit. The depth of the osteotomy should ideally be greater than 2 mm above the mandibular canal (Fig. 38.24).

Vertical Cuts. The anterior vertical cut may then be made and begins in relation to the existence and width of the buccal shelf (extend oblique ridge) of the mandible. Usually the mid-first molar is in the position of the anterior vertical cut. After the vertical osteotomy approximates the position of the inferior alveolar nerve, the osteotomy is limited to the thickness of the buccal cortical plate, usually 2 to 3 mm in thickness. The osteotomy is progressively deepened until bleeding bone from the osteotomy is observed. The anterior osteotomy is usually 10 to 12 mm in length. The posterior osteotomy is then completed, which is usually above and lateral to the inferior alveolar nerve (in front of

the lingula on the lingual of the ramus). The posterior osteotomy may be full thickness through the cortical plate to the horizontal osteotomy. Because the mandibular canal in this region is usually inferior or posterior, the osteotomy is made through the entire depth of the cortex (Figs. 38.25 and 38.26).

Inferior Cuts. The inferior osteotomy will connect the posterior, and anterior vertical cuts may be performed with an oscillating saw, large, round bur (No. 8) in a straight handpiece, or a right angled insert with a Piezosurgery unit. This cut is usually the most difficult because access and visibility are limited. With the inferior cut a shallower cut is made into the cortex to create a line of fracture. This inferior cut with a drill should not be made completely through the cortex, because it may be located in close proximity to the mandibular canal. The piezosurgery tip allows preparation of a more defined cut and it does not have the danger of damaging the nerve if it happens to come in contact with any vital structure.

Ideally the superior, anterior, and posterior vertical, and inferior cuts should be made continuous so ease of harvesting is accomplished. A thin chisel is gently tapped along the entire length of the external oblique osteotomy, taking care to parallel the lateral surface of the ramus to avoid inadvertent injury to the inferior alveolar nerve. A wider wedge chisel or Potts elevator may then be inserted and levered to pry the bone block segment free and complete the greenstick fracture of the graft from the ramus. After removal of the block, any sharp edges around the ramus are smoothed with a bur or file. A hemostatic dressing (collagen, gelatin sponge, oxidized cellulose) may be placed into the donor area, and closure of the site may be completed after fixation of the graft to the receptor site (Boxes 38.3 and 38.4).

Alternative Ramus Procedures

An alternative option from obtaining a ramus block is the harvesting of bone cores with trephine burs. The cores can be fixated if large enough or ground down to small particulate pieces that can

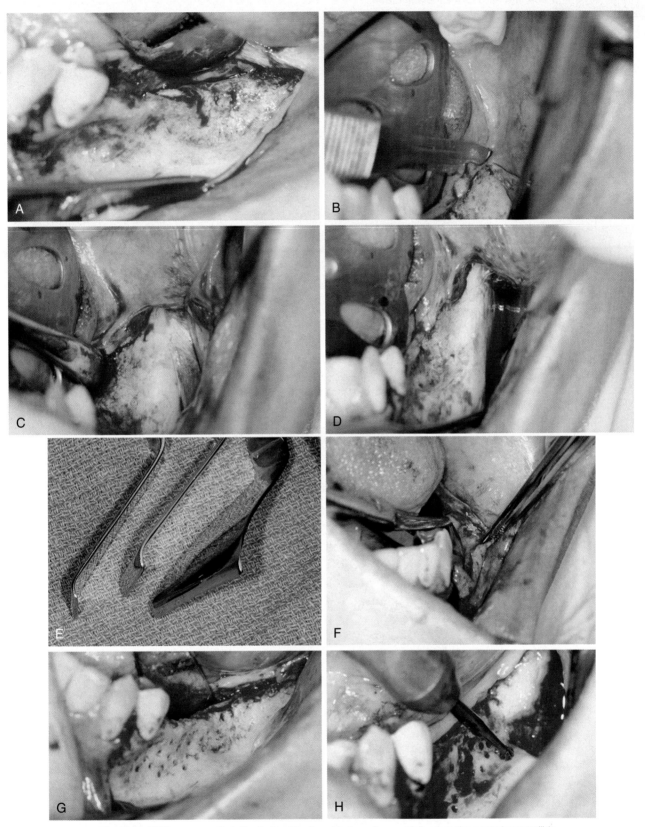

• **Fig. 38.23** (A) The ramus site is the first option for a block graft, especially when the posterior mandible requires augmentation. The incision in an edentulous posterior mandible starts at the retromolar pad and continues to the first premolar. (B) After the full-thickness posterior mucoperiosteal flap is reflected, the incision is extended lateral to the retromolar pad and directly over the bone of the ascending ramus to the height of the occlusal plane. (C) The facial flap is reflected, and the attachment of the buccinator muscle is identified. (D) A periosteal elevator slides along the lateral aspect of the ramus, under the masseter muscle, for a depth of 15 mm. The incision is extended along the ascending ramus when the donor block requires additional length. (E) Ramus retractors are shaped to retract the masseter and curved to allow the preparation of the block at the inferior margin. (F) The facial flap is advanced. Metzenbaum tissue scissors are used in a blunt dissection to create the submucosal space. (G) The host site is prepared for the graft with small holes through the cortical plate, 3 to 5 mm apart. (H) The host site is prepared with a round bur to create a wall of bone at the apical region of the graft.

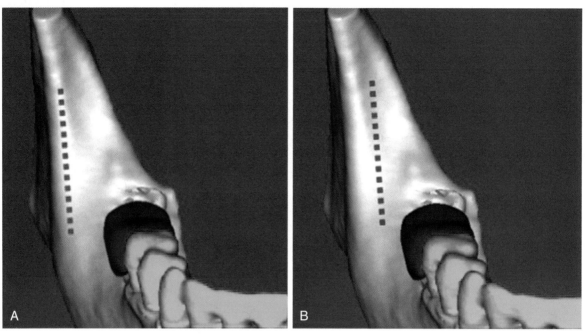

● **Fig. 38.24** Superior Osteotomy Cuts. (A) Too close to the lateral border, which would result in too thin of a graft. (B) Ideal position that allows for a wider graft.

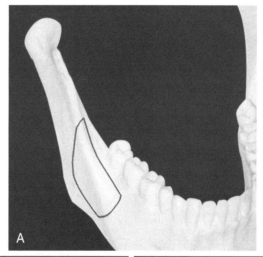

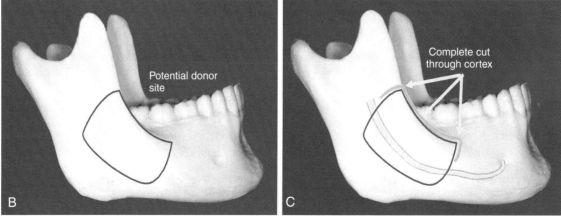

● **Fig. 38.25** (A) The ramus donor site is lateral to the molars (buccal shelf region) and extends up the ascending ramus. (B) The ramus donor site uses the outer cortical bone of the ramus and posterior body of the mandible. (C) The top portion of the ramus donor block (green line) is usually above and lateral to the position of the inferior alveolar nerve complex.

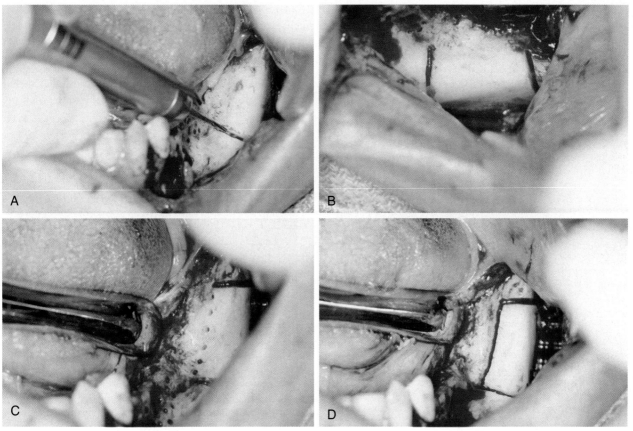

• **Fig. 38.26** (A) The anterior vertical cut is made with a straight handpiece and a fissure bur or oscillating saw. The position is often at the mid-first molar region. The cuts 5 mm above the inferior alveolar nerve (IAN) complex are full thickness. (B) The posterior vertical cut is often above and lateral to the lingual and IAN, and therefore may be made full thickness along the lateral ramus to the superior block margin. The width of the bone block on the superior margin is designed with a small, round bur and ranges from 3 to 6 mm in width from the lateral border. (C) The superior osteotomy is made through the cortical bone and may extend to within 5 mm of the posterior IAN. The horizontal dimension of the ramus block determines the width of the donor site and is related to the amount of bone needed and the anatomy of the donor site. (D) A fissure bur connects the pilot holes of the horizontal cut. This cut is through the cortical plate and may proceed to 2 mm above the IAN.

Indications
- Horizontal and vertical ridge augmentation
- Three to four tooth edentulous sites (maximum size = 3 × 5 cm)

Advantages
- Allows for largest average surface area of intraoral grafts
- No esthetic concerns
- Decreased pain and discomfort
- Decreased chance of incision dehiscence

Disadvantages
- Inferior alveolar and lingual nerve injury
- Access may be difficult
- Trismus

Incision:
Initiates at the level of the occlusal plane in the ascending ramus (medial to the external oblique ridge)
Extends anteriorly, avoiding the retromolar pad
Superior: on external oblique ridge along anterior border of the mandibular ramus (approximately one-third width of the mandible)
Anterior: distal half of the first molar
Posterior: superior aspect of the external oblique ridge (level of occlusal plane)
Inferior: ~10 mm in height

Tuberosity Donor Site

The maxillary tuberosity has been shown to be a viable intraoral donor source for autogenous bone and a source of osteoprogenitor cells.[77,120] The tuberosity bone, although variable in the amount of bone that can be harvested, has been shown to be advantageous in maxillary sinus grafting and ridge augmentation procedures. The cancellous nature of this bone allows it to be shaped and molded.

be used with a membrane graft. Small bone chisels can be used to remove the bone cores. It is hard to collect large volumes of bone using a trephine and harvesting of blocks is probably better suited for most involved graft sites (Figs. 38.27 and 38.28).

Tuberosity grafts may be used as a particulate graft, or in some cases a block graft (Fig. 38.29).

Anatomy

The maxillary tuberosity is defined as the bone at the lower part of the infratemporal surface of the maxilla. It is a rounded eminence that is especially prominent after growth of the third molars. The quality of bone in the maxillary tuberosity is usually considered a very poor type of bone, usually a D4 bone with fine trabeculae and minimal to no cortical bone. The thicker soft tissue in the tuberosity area can be extremely misleading, which frequently results in a misrepresentation of the amount of available bone. The anatomic limitations of this area include the maxillary sinus, pterygoid plates, adjacent teeth when present, and the greater palatine canal.

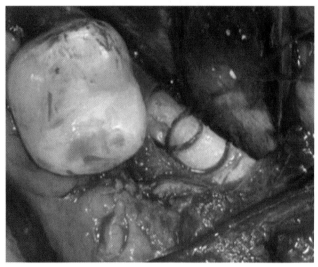

• **Fig. 38.27** The ramus is exposed and bone cores are obtained via trephine burs.

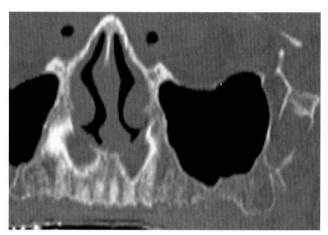

• **Fig. 38.29** Cone beam computed tomographic panoramic view depicting a significant amount of tuberosity bone available for grafting.

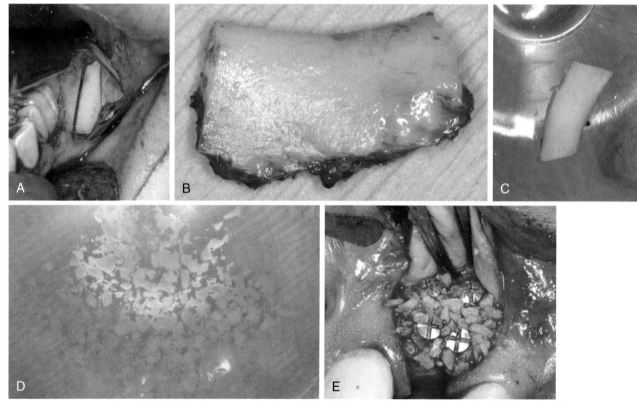

• **Fig. 38.28** (A) Autogenous ramus harvest block. (B) Harvested cortical ramus block. (C) Block stored in sterile saline. (D) Block reduced to particulate fragments. (E) Particulate fragments placed in the donor site. (*From Caldwell CS. Bone grafting complications. In: Resnik RR, Misch CE, eds.* Misch's Avoiding Complications in Oral Implantology. *St. Louis, MO: Elsevier; 2018.*)

Radiographic Analysis

Ideally a CBCT examination will reveal the quantity of bone present below the sinus. It is imperative to make an accurate assessment of the bone quantity because exposing the maxillary sinus after graft removal may lead to increased complications (Fig. 38.30).

Incision and Reflection

The incision to expose the maxillary tuberosity consists of a crestal incision and a posterior vertical release (45 degrees) from the posterior part of the tuberosity. The incision should never extend onto the lingual contour of the posterior tuberosity or into the hamular notch area because this area is associated with an increased possibility of bleeding episodes. It is important to incise to the bone because in some cases the tissue can be very thick.

Donor Site Osteotomy Harvest

After reflection of a mucoperiosteal flap the bone may be harvested from the tuberosity with a double-action rongeur or chisel. Removing the graft with a chisel will allow the harvesting of a larger piece of bone; however, a greater chance of perforation into the maxillary sinus is possible (Fig. 38.31; Boxes 38.5 and 38.6).

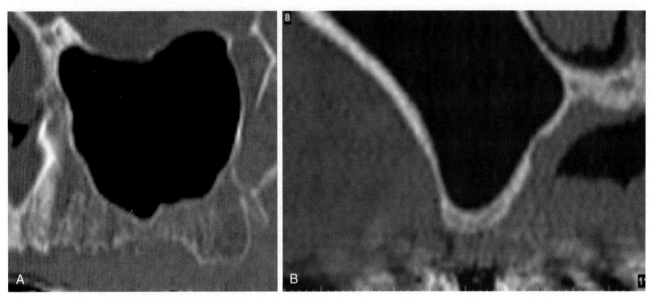

• **Fig. 38.30** Cone Beam Computed Tomographic Cross Section. (A) Significant amount of bone for grafting. (B) Minimal amount of bone present that would likely result in a communication with the maxillary sinus.

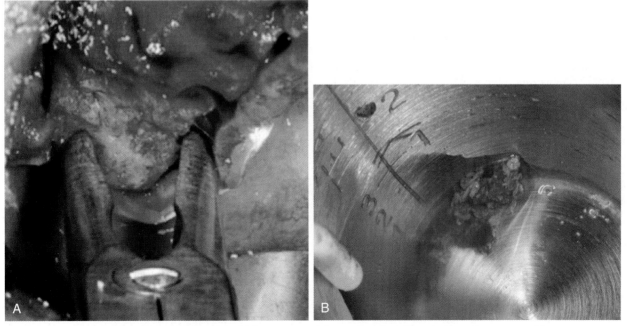

• **Fig. 38.31** Tuberosity Harvest. (A) Bone removed from tuberosity with a double-action rongeur. (B) Tuberosity bone cores after harvest.

• BOX 38.5 **Tuberosity Bone Graft**

Indications
- Socket grafting, sinus augmentation, small bony defects
- Approximately 1–3 mL

Advantages
- Allows for largest average surface area of intraoral grafts
- No esthetic concerns
- Decreased pain and discomfort
- Decreased chance of incision dehiscence

Disadvantages
- Entry into maxillary sinus
- Oral-antral fistula
- Bleeding (posterior-superior alveolar, pterygoid plexus)
- Hematoma

• BOX 38.6 **Tuberosity Graft Osteotomy Technique**

Incision: midcrestal incision from first molar to posterior extent of ridge (short of hamular notch)
Bone harvest: double-action rongeur, chisel and mallet, Piezosurgery

---

Block Graft Preparation

Fixation of the Block Graft

Once the monocortical block of bone has been harvested, the recipient site is ready to receive the graft. It cannot be overstressed that for successful graft survival at the recipient site, complete soft tissue coverage must be present that is passive and tension free. If the soft tissue flap has extensive tension, the incision lines will open, resulting in graft exposure and eventual infection of the graft that will result in loss of the bone graft.

Soft Tissue Preparation

The soft tissue dissection beyond the graft recipient site will help to avoid soft tissue incision line opening and graft exposure. With most bone grafts, soft tissue closure may be challenging. Misch developed a submucosal space technique that helps in overcoming this potential complication. The technique reflects a full-thickness flap over the graft site and at least 5 mm above the height of the MGJ. The periosteum and soft tissues 5mm above the MGJ remain on the bone and are not reflected. The facial flap is then lifted 3 to 5 mm above the depth of the MGJ and using a scalpel, an incision through the periosteum 1 to 2 mm deep and parallel to the crestal incision extends over and beyond the vertical releasing incision. After the incision is made through the periosteum, pointed tissue scissors (i.e., Metzenbaum scissors) may be introduced into the periosteal incision for 10 to 15 mm or more, parallel to the surface mucosa, with the blades of the scissors closed, so the facial flap thickness is 3 to 5 mm. The tissue scissors are then opened with blunt dissection, which allows the muscles to be separated from the flap and creates a submucosal space. With the periosteum, tissues and muscles attached to the bone are on one side, and a 3- to 5-mm-thick facial flap is on the other side.

With this technique the facial flap may now advance the depth of the submucosal space 10 mm or more. This technique greatly increases the ability to advance the soft tissue flap over a large block graft. The advantage of the submucosal space technique is that a split-thickness flap is created and maintains the muscles on the periosteum, which is attached to the bone above the contours of the host site. Because the muscle attachments are the primary source of vascularization to the periosteum and host bone, vascularity remains undisturbed. Muscle healing is a primary cause of flap retraction and incision line opening. Because the muscles are no longer attached to the facial flap and the flap may be advanced more than 10 mm, there is no tension on the incision line, which reduces the risk for incision line opening. One complication of the soft tissue procedures to improve graft coverage is the loss of vestibular depth. The reduced vestibular depth is rarely an esthetic concern, and when the restoration is implant retained, the prosthesis does not rely on a valve seal for primary retention (as in a complete denture). Advancement of the facial flap for graft coverage may also result in a reduction in keratinized mucosa over the facial aspect of the gingival crest. In some cases, soft tissue or acellular dermis grafts may be necessary, or the attached mucosa may be repositioned facially at the stage II implant uncovery surgery (Fig. 38.32).

Preparation of the Recipient Site

The next step in graft reconstruction is preparation of the lateral and crestal surfaces of the host and grafted bone using a small-diameter drill equal to or smaller than the drill size of bone screws used to fixate the donor bone (i.e., ~1.4-mm diameter). The rationale for this procedure is to facilitate angiogenesis at the graft site.

Drill perforations are 3 to 5 mm apart in the entire area of the graft and host site. Perforations are created under copious amounts of saline and penetrate both the facial and lingual plates of bone in the region of the graft, especially when augmentation is desired on both sides of the residual ridge. This procedure increases the availability of osteogenic cells, accelerates revascularization, increases the regional acceleratory phenomenon, and improves graft union[96,121,122] (Figs. 38.33 and 38.34).

Fixation of the Block Graft

After the block of bone has been harvested, it can be stored in sterile saline solution or immediately fixated to the host bone. Minimal time should elapse before placement of the block on the host bone.[123,124] When placing the bone graft onto the host bone, the cancellous portion of the graft should be in contact with the host bone.[81,125,126] Because the graft should passively rest on the host bone, the host bone and harvested block of bone need to be contoured before graft fixation.[127,128] The edges of the block of bone can be smoothed with a small, round bur to create a fine, smooth surface that blends in with the surface of the host bone when fixated with rigid fixation screws. Particulate cancellous bone can then be used to fill in any voids between the host bone and harvested block of bone.

When preparing the harvested block of bone, the drill holes on the surface of the block graft are slightly larger than the diameter of the rigid fixation screws. This permits the rigid fixation screws to compress the block graft directly up against the host bone while the screw is threaded completely through both cortices (Fig. 38.35). The outer thread of the fixation screw is usually 1.4 to 2.0 mm in diameter, with a V-shaped thread design. This allows the screw to thread into the host bone during fixation of the graft to the host bone, and removal of the screw at the time of implant placement 4 to 6 months after the graft has remodeled to

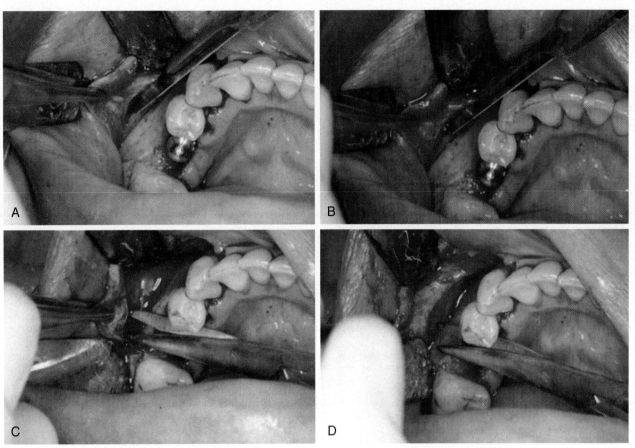

• **Fig. 38.32** Tissue Preparation for Tension-Free Closure.(A and B) Periosteal release technique with a scalpel. (C and D) Blunt dissection that stretches the periosteum with the use of blunted scissors.

the jaw. The head of the fixation screw should be 2.2 mm or more in diameter and flat so that it can compress the donor block graft against the host bone.

A lag fixation screw design should not be used. A lag screw design has smooth metal for 5 to 10 mm below the screw head, and the apical half of the screw has threads. When the screw is placed through the block of bone and host bone, the technique is effective in rigidly fixating the block of bone to the host bone (Fig. 38.36). However, when the screw is removed before implant placement, it has been observed that newly regenerated osseous tissue has formed around the smooth portion of the lag screw. This may present problems in removal of the lag screw. While removing the lag screw, the surgeon may have to tap the graft while the screw is being removed. This could lead to loosening of the bone graft from the host bone.

There are many rigid fixation screw kits that can be used in bone graft procedures available to the clinician. It is recommended that the clinician use self-tapping threaded screws with the tip of the screw pointed and not blunt, to allow penetration into bone. Screw kits come in a variety of screw diameter sizes. The two most commonly used to rigidly fixate the block of bone to the host bone are 2.0- and 1.6-mm-diameter screws. After the bone graft has been harvested the next step is stabilizing the graft passively to the host bone and rigidly fixating the graft with the use of rigid fixation screws, plates, or stainless-steel wires. If using rigid fixation screws, two or more screws are required to fixate the graft to the host bone that avoids movement. When using only a single rigid fixation screw, the block of bone may not be rigidly fixated to the host bone. If the graft is not rigidly

fixated to the host bone, the graft may rotate and move, which will lead to a fibrous union.

The screws are ideally secured to both the facial and the lingual cortical plates. Therefore with bicortical stabilization the osteotomy screw holes must penetrate both facial and lingual cortices. In most cases the host site will need to be altered to allow a passive fit for the graft. This is easily accomplished with a small, round carbide (No. 6, No. 8). In addition, the block may be altered with a pear-shaped carbide because the block should have no sharp edges. After recontouring, the donor block of bone is slightly recessed into the host bone 1 to 2 mm, and there should exist no micromovement. With completion of the bone graft procedure, the soft tissues are reapproximated and closed with sutures. After a graft healing period of 4 to 6 months, dental implants may be placed into the graft site.

Membranes and Block Grafts

The use of membranes over autogenous block grafts is controversial in the literature. Chaushu et al.[129] reported soft tissue complications, including membrane exposure (42 [30.7%] of 137), incision line opening (41 [30%] of 137), and perforation of the mucosa over the grafted bone (19 [14%] of 137). Infection of the grafted site occurred in 18 (13%) of 137 bone grafts. Gielkens et al.[130] conducted a metaanalysis to investigate the effects of barrier membranes on onlay autogenous grafts. They concluded after a vast systemic review that the available studies are too weak to support the use of membranes. Therefore at this time there are insufficient data to support the use or nonuse of barrier membranes with respect to bone resorption.

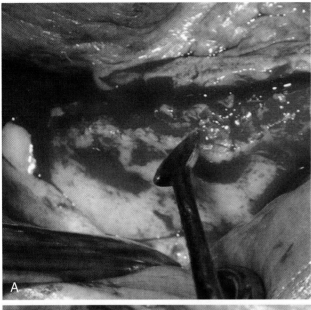

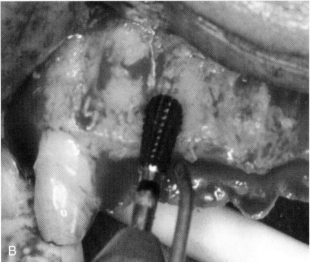

● **Fig. 38.33** Soft Tissue Removal. (A) Soft tissue removed with a sharp periosteal elevator. (B) Course carbide in a 1:1 straight handpiece.

Maturation and Integration of Block Grafts

In most cases, a radiographic survey (e.g. periapical, bite-wings, CBCT) is obtained to evaluate healing approximately 3–4 months after the initial surgery. In conjunction with the radiographic assessment, a clinical examination should be used to evaluate the changes in the grafted ridge contour as well as the tiassue health. Once healing is complete, tissue reflection access is obtained to remove any bone screws and allow for ideal implant placement. The autogenous graft should be evaluated for any mobility, which usually is indicative of bone graft failure. (Fig. 38.37, Fig. 38.38).

Comparison of Intraoral Bone-Grafting Donor Sites

A comparison of intraoral donor sites for onlay grafting before implant placement was reported by Misch.[44] The volume of the symphyseal donor grafts was almost twice as great as ramus sites (1.74

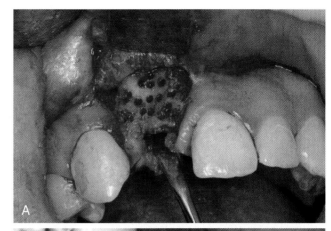

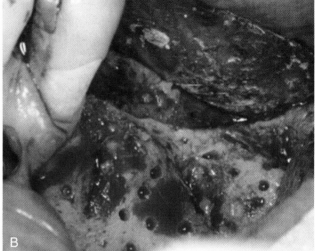

● **Fig. 38.34** Recipient Site Decortication. (A) Decortication holes that initiate angiogenesis to heal the graft. (B) Must have bleeding through the decortication holes for the growth factor release.

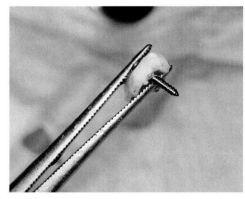

● **Fig. 38.35** A lag screw approach is used to fixate the block. The screw slides through the block, and the screw head is larger than the hole in the block.

versus 0.9 cm³). The ramus was primarily a cortical graft, whereas the symphysis block was cortical/trabecular. However, the ramus and symphysis donor sites have similar success rates. Aloy-Prósper et al.[131] in a systemic review showed the success and survival rates of implants placed into vertical and horizontal defect ridges treated with intraoral block grafts. They concluded that placing implants into block grafts versus native bone had similar success rates.

Clavero et al.[120] compared the morbidity and amount of complications with ramus and symphysis donor sites. They determined although the symphysis has better accessibility, the ramus donor site allows for a greater amount of harvested bone, with higher bone density and more cortical content, together with fewer complications.

Gultekin et al.[132] studied the difference in bone loss between autogenous block grafts and guided bone regeneration (GBR). They concluded that both the block graft group and GBR group provided sufficient volume of bone for implant placement. However, the GBR group did show greater bone resorption in comparison with the autografts.

Yates et al.[133] compared the harvested volume of the ramus versus the symphysis and also the associated morbidity. They determined that the ramus can provide the greatest volume of bone and significantly less morbidity in comparison with symphysis bone grafting (Table 38.1).

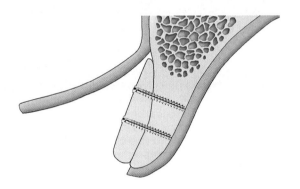

• **Fig. 38.36** The screw should fixate each bone block. The screws should engage the lingual plate of the host site.

Postoperative Care and Instructions

An increase in incision line opening has been associated with postoperative smoking and diabetes in patients with autografts.[26,134] Patients should stop smoking at least 3 days before surgery and at a minimum until the incision line has healed. It is imperative that the graft be immobilized during healing and there exists no external pressure on the graft. Removable soft tissue–borne prostheses should not be worn or should be adjusted to prevent graft loading. The flange area of a removable prosthesis should be completely removed, and the edentulous ridge area is generously relieved, which requires the patient to use denture adhesive for prosthesis retention. However, the denture adhesive should not be placed over the incision line. The patient is instructed to use the provisional removable prosthesis for cosmetic appearance only rather than function.

Careful postoperative follow-up is necessary to inspect the bone graft region and eliminate pressure areas from an overlying prosthesis. More favorable provisional solutions are tooth-borne fixed or removable partial dentures, resin-bonded bridges, or denture teeth bonded to the adjacent dentition.[135] The use of transitional implants to support a fixed-interim prosthesis during the healing phase may be considered for patients less tolerant of removable provisional restorations.[136,137]

Complications

Symphysis Graft Complications

Incision Line Opening

Many factors predispose the symphysis donor site to incision line opening. If a vestibular incision is used, a two-layered suture technique is recommended. A suture with a high tensile strength should be used (e.g., Vicryl, PTFE) to maintain the integrity of the incision line. The patient should be instructed not to pull on the lower lip to evaluate the surgical site because this will increase the chances of incision dehiscence. Misch[138] determined that

TABLE 38.1	Comparison of Intraoral Donor Sites			
Criteria	**Symphysis**	**Ramus**	**Tuberosity**
Surgical access	Good	Fair to good	Fair to good
Patient cosmetic concern	High	Low	Low
Graft shape	Thick	Thin veneer	Thin to thick
Graft morphology	Cortico-cancellous	Cortical	Cancellous
Graft size (cm)	5–15	5–10	~5
Graft resorption	Minimal	Minimal	Moderate
Healed bone quality	D1, D2	D1, D2	D3, D4
Donor Site Complications			
Postoperative pain/edema	Moderate	Minimal	Minimal
Neurosensory: teeth	Common (temporary)	Uncommon	Uncommon
Neurosensory: tissue	Uncommon (temporary)	Uncommon	Uncommon
Incision dehiscence	Occasional (vestibular)	Uncommon	Uncommon

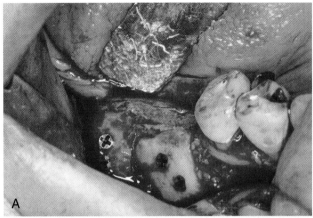

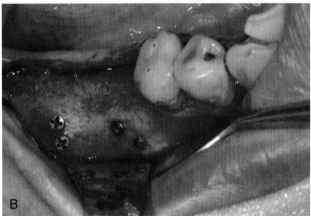

• **Fig. 38.37** (A). Two blocks of cortical bone have been fixated on the lateral aspect of the posterior mandibular ridge with fixation screws. Medullary particulate has been used to fill the voids around the block grafts. (B). The mineralized block grafts after five months of healing. Note the smooth surface of the final graft and the nature of the intertwined recipient site and the grafted blocks.

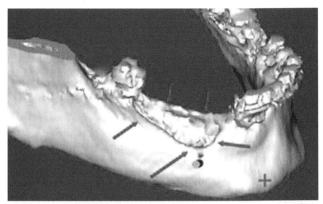

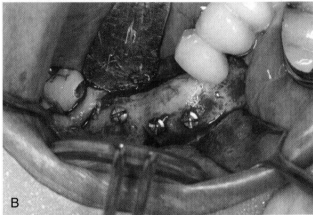

• **Fig. 38.38** (A). This 3 D image shows the severe bony defect resulting from removal of a blade implant. This vertical defect extends to the level of the mandibular canal. (B). Five month postop matured block graft site that was supplemented with particulate around the remaining defects. Note the density of the final bony structure.

dehiscence of the donor site occurred in 10.7% of anterior mandibles because of function of the mentalis muscle, and no incision line opening was found in the posterior mandible or ramus donor sites.

Neurosensory Impairment

Neurosensory deficits of the third branch of the trigeminal nerve are rare in association with symphysis grafts. However, it is a common sequela to have neurosensory changes in the mandibular anterior teeth. Because the second terminal branch of the inferior alveolar nerve (incisive branch) terminates in the anterior mandibular area, it is not uncommon to sever this section of the nerve during osteotomy preparation. However, because the incisive nerve is only a sensory nerve to the incisor teeth, this usually results in only a "dullness" in sensation. Hoppenreijs et al.[139,140] showed a negative pulpal response in 16% of patients after a symphysis graft, with total resolution in 6 to 12 months.

Usually a neurosensory impairment of the mandibular anterior teeth does not result in a painful sensation, but it is disruptive, causing patients to generally describe the incisors as having a "woody feeling." This series of complications can usually be avoided by refraining from aggressive harvesting of medullary bone surrounding the donor site.

Studies have shown the incidence of neuropraxia after the harvesting of block grafts from the ramus versus the symphysis. After 18 months, more than 50% of the patients with harvest sites in the symphysis still had altered sensation. None of the patients in the ramus donor group reported any symptoms at 18 months.[141]

The superior portion of the harvest site should be prepared at least 5 mm below the level of the incisor root tips to prevent a neurosensory impairment. Care must be taken to avoid the longer roots of the cuspids as each end of the harvest pattern is prepared. Aggressive harvesting of the medullary portion of the symphysis should be minimized in the superior aspects if possible to limit damage to neural pathways through the region. Most importantly, complete patient education must be conducted "before" the surgery informing the patient about potential sensory changes that could occur. The patient should be aware that he or she could feel a dullness or "woody" feeling of the mandibular anterior teeth after surgery. This can be temporary or a permanent condition, but it has never been described as a particularly annoying feeling. Rarely is there an indication for endodontic therapy, as the vitality of the teeth returns to normal.

Bleeding Episodes

When a cortical graft and the surrounding medullary bone are harvested in the symphyseal region, the underlying neurovascular components are often compromised. These disruptions to the nerves and blood vessels may be accompanied by possible significant bleeding immediately after the graft harvest.

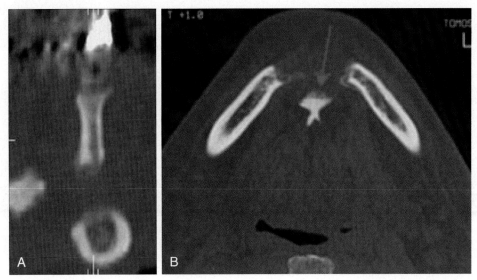

● **Fig. 38.39** (A) Cross-sectional image depicts fractured symphyseal plate from poor patient selection of a symphysis graft. (B) Axial view. (*From Cordaro L, Rossini C, Mijiritsky E. Fracture and displacement of lingual cortical plate of mandibular symphysis following bone harvesting: case report.* Implant Dent. *2004;13:202-206.*)

The incisive nerve is the second terminal branch of the inferior alveolar nerve that provides innervation to the mandibular teeth. The incisive nerve path between the mental foramina has been known to be a safe zone for bone harvesting because of the lack of vital structures that can be affected by grafts taken from this region. A thorough understanding of the neurologic and vascular anatomy in this region is critical for the prevention of complications during and after surgery in the symphyseal region. Aggressive graft harvesting in this area may give rise to a lingual plate perforation, which leads to possible significant bleeding issues and airway management complications.

The sublingual arteries may also cause significant bleeding if the lingual plate is perforated. The incisive neurovascular bundle is found to join other vascular structures in the midsymphyseal region. The genioglossus muscle attaches to the genial tubercle in the midline, and the sublingual artery courses through the lingual foramen at the genial tubercle. The lingual artery is approximately 1 to 2 mm in diameter, and cross-sectional views clearly show its anastomosis with the incisive canal at this point.

The preparation of a grafting osteotomy in the midline can potentially resect these blood vessels if they fall in the path of the vertical preparation. If this occurs, the sectioned extension of the lingual artery can prolapse back into the floor of the mouth. The severed vessel may release arterial blood flow in the sublingual space, potentially raising the tongue to a point that compromises the airway. Immediate emergency intervention to maintain the airway is critical, and in some cases this requires use of a tracheostomy until the blood flow has been controlled (Fig. 38.39).

Ptosis

One of the main patient concerns when confronted with the prospect of symphysis grafting is a change in facial or soft tissue appearance. The idea of having a permanent bony chin defect or ptosis contributes to a patient's apprehension regarding this procedure.

The main concern of patients after a symphysis graft is a postoperative change in the soft tissue contour of the chin. In the literature there exists no evidence of a statistically significant incidence of dehiscence or chin ptosis after a symphysis graft. To minimize the possibility of ptosis, avoid degloving the mentalis muscle by maintaining the facial and inferior aspects of the mandible and the lingual aspect of the inferior border of the mandible during flap refection. In addition, to prevent lower lip height reduction and vermilion zone inversion, the integrity of the periosteum to the inferior reflection should not be deeper than one-third of the total distance from the vermilion border to the MGJ. An extraoral bandage or pressure dressing may be used postoperatively for support and to help with compression of the wound.

Ramus Graft Complications

Neurosensory Deficit

Patients have also shown less concern with bone removal from the ramus area, and augmentation of this donor site is unnecessary. Although vestibular incision dehiscence has occurred with symphysis grafts, it is usually not a common occurrence in the ramus donor site. Patients are less able to discern neurosensory disturbances in the posterior buccal soft tissues compared with the lower lip and chin. Although the incision along the external oblique ridge may injure the long buccal nerve, reports of postoperative neurosensory deficit in the buccal mucosa are less frequent and will most likely go unnoticed by the patient.[142,143] In contrast with the teeth superior to the symphysis donor site, patients have reported minimal altered sensation in their molar teeth.[44,144]

Damage to the inferior alveolar neurovascular bundle could also occur during harvesting of the graft in the ramus area of the mandible. When using bone chisels or elevators, the instruments must parallel the lateral surface of the ramus to avoid a nerve impairment. If the inferior ramus cut is below the level of the inferior alveolar canal, graft separation should not be completed until it can be verified that the neurovascular bundle is not trapped within the graft. Although nerve injury to the inferior alveolar nerve is low, patients should be aware of this risk during the consultation before surgery.

On occasion the inferior alveolar nerve is identified and directly observed when the block graft is removed from the ramus. When this occurs, dexamethasone (Decadron) 4 mg (1 cc) may be placed

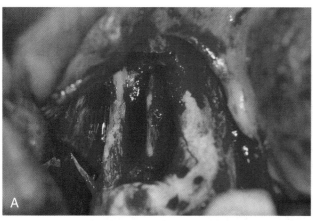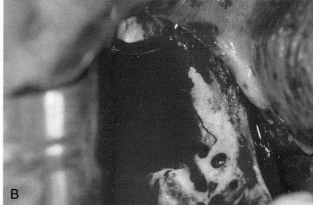

• **Fig. 38.40** (A) On occasion the inferior alveolar nerve complex can be identified after the block is removed. (B) When this occurs, dexamethasone (Decadron) 4 mg (1 cc) may be used directly on the nerve to reduce inflammation.

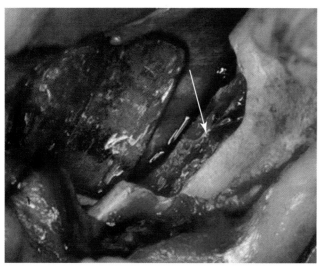

• **Fig. 38.41** Large donor graft site leading to exposure of the inferior alveolar nerve (arrow) with associated neurosensory impairment. *(From Caldwell CS. Bone grafting complications. In: Resnik RR, Misch CE, eds.* Misch's Avoiding Complications in Oral Implantology. *St Louis, MO: Elsevier; 2018.)*

directly on the nerve for 30 seconds to reduce inflammation and edema. A second dose of 4 mg (1 cc) then is applied for an additional 30 seconds. A collagen sponge may be placed over the site, but hydroxyapatite or graft material is not indicated (Figs. 38.40 and 38.41).

Bone Graft Complications

Incision Line Opening in Bone-Grafting Sites

Maintenance of complete soft tissue coverage over healing bone-grafting sites is one of the most important principles that must be observed for predictable grafting success.

Anytime that the healing graft site is exposed to the oral flora during the healing process, there will be some type of compromised change in the final graft site volume and in its overall integrity. Incision line opening with compromised graft results can often be a major limiting factor in successful implant placement.

Incision line opening can compromise even the most carefully planned regeneration site, and most of these graft sites will require additional grafting at a later time if an actual complication develops. An open incision line introduces numerous potential complications into the healing process. First, the introduction of microorganisms into a graft site through an open incision leads to an infection in the healing graft site. Exposure of the block graft and accompanied graft particles accompanied by the presence of purulence is an indication of impending failure of the graft. The infection reduces the pH in the graft site, causing a breakdown of the graft and eventually compromising the resulting ridge volume. Second, an open incision line may allow exposure and breakdown of any barrier membranes, contributing to fibrous tissue ingrowth into the graft site. Lastly, there exists a potential for particulate graft materials that have been packed around the circumference of the block to escape the graft site, resulting in an inadequate bone volume in the final proposed implant site.[145]

Tension-free tissue coverage is the most critical variable in preventing incision line opening. A clinician's experience in manipulation of soft tissue affects this aspect of bone regeneration more than any other part of bone regeneration surgery. As the clinician gains more experience in delicate tissue management and begins to understand the maintenance of a tension-free flap closure, problems with graft and membrane exposure will become an uncommon occurrence.

The inner surface of a reflected flap is lined with the periosteum: a thin, dense layer of tissue that cannot be stretched. It is impossible to stretch the soft tissue flap over a graft site without first severing this layer of tissue. This "tissue release" is accomplished by preparing a clear and continuous releasing incision through the periosteum, exposing the underlying elastic layers of tissue that can then be released for expansion of the flap over the enlarged graft site. As this incision perforates the periosteal layer, the two edges clearly separate, allowing the elastic tissue below the periosteum to stretch. A sharp pair of Metzenbaum scissors is then placed into the space below the periosteum, and as the scissor tips are opened, the tissue easily releases and the edges separate farther. This is repeated until the complete flap is stretched over the graft site and 5 mm beyond the opposite flap margin.

In the event of an incision line opening, the patient should be placed on a frequent monitoring protocol to observe the status

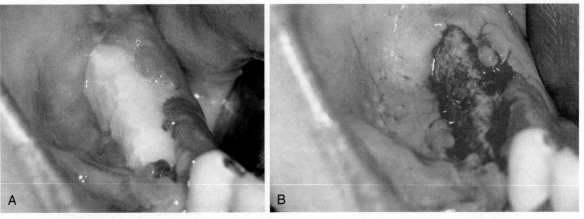

• **Fig. 38.42** (A) Incision line opening or block dehiscence is a complication of block bone grafts. (B) The soft tissue should not be resutured over the graft that dehisces during the first few months. Instead, the block is recontoured so the bone above the tissue margins is removed. The area is left to heal by secondary intention.

of the graft material and any grafting hardware present. The oral microflora must be managed with the use of daily chlorhexidine rinses. The clinician must not attempt to suture the site again because healing margins along incision lines feature tissue that cannot, at that time, support the pressure of another suture under tension.

If graft dehiscence occurs, the wound should be allowed to heal by secondary intention. Resuturing an incision line opening is rarely successful and will usually result in a larger dehiscence. The block graft may be recontoured with a diamond bur to reduce the bulk of exposed bone. The bone above the margins of the surrounding tissue is ground off, which also removes the biofilm. This procedure is repeated every 2 to 4 weeks until the site is closed (Figs. 38.42 and 38.43).

Mobility of the Block

Mobility of an autogenous graft during the healing process will almost always result in a graft failure. Mobility of the block prevents proper integration of the newly forming bone, and eventually it will lead to soft tissue invasion between the block and the recipient site. Rigid fixation of the block graft to the recipient bone site is critical for success in the regenerative process. Although regeneration with block grafting is related to the concept of "barrier by bulk," micromovement will often contribute to a weak bond between the cortical graft and the recipient site. This will potentially cause the block to separate from the ridge as pressure is placed on the interface between the native bone and the integrated block as a result of the implant being inserted into the osteotomy. The most common cause for graft mobility is insufficient fixation or pressure from a prosthesis postoperatively.

Initial fixation of a block graft must be attained when the block is originally placed in the recipient site. Any movement of the block during the healing process will disrupt the formation of a stable clot around the migrating cells, and a loose block will not integrate into the host bone. Ideally two fixation screws should be used in every block graft, eliminating any micromovement of the block during the healing process.

The recipient site should be prepared for close approximation of the surface of the block graft to the recipient site. The block should be inlaid into the recipient site, and particles of medullary bone or allograft should be packed around the circumference,

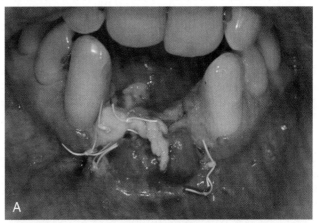

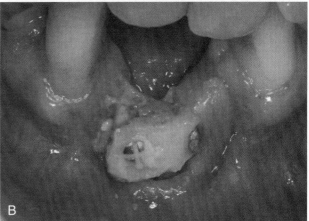

• **Fig. 38.43** Consequences of Resuturing an Incision Line Opening. (A) Incision line opening 2 weeks after surgery and treated with resuturing. (B) Six weeks postresuturing showing significant incision line opening.

filling any discrepancies. The temporary prosthesis should be adjusted to prevent any contact with the graft site, and the buccal flange should be removed on any removable appliance to limit micromovement.

Fixation screws should be engaged into the underlying bone enough to provide rigid support of the graft. A longer shaft on the supporting screw may be necessary to obtain ridge fixation in soft bone. The screws should have a self-threading tip, and the preparation hole should be prepared deep enough to prevent the shaft of the screw from bottoming out in dense cortical bone. Excess insertion pressure on a screw passing into very dense bone without adequate depth preparation can contribute to the head of the screw snapping off during its insertion. Most updated fixation screws have a pointed self-threading screw tip that helps with screw insertion.

If micromovement of the block graft occurs during surgery, the block should be removed and the screws should be replaced with longer or wider fixation screws. If the movement occurs during the healing phase, the block should be monitored carefully; however, most likely it will need to be removed (Fig. 38.44).

Soft Tissue Irritation From an Overextended Fixation Screw

Bone fixation screws are routinely placed in the bony ridge for various reasons during implant-related surgery. It is not uncommon to discover the end of a screw extending beyond the lingual or palatal cortical plate. When this occurs, there is a potential for the overextended screw to cause discomfort. Overextended screws can be a source of irritation to the thin soft tissue on the lingual aspect of the mandible. The movement of the thin mucosa and tongue against the sharp point of the screw can cause quite a bit of discomfort. This is not usually an issue in the maxilla, where the thicker nature of the palatal tissue acts as a protective buffer.

To prevent this complication, screw placement should be followed by both a visual inspection of the opposing surface of cortical bone and a digital review of any potential problems areas that will need correction. The only way to treat an overextended screw involves reflection of a flap to provide access for removal of the overextension or removal of the complete screw. Screw removal is not usually a reasonable solution because that would require reflection of the tissue overlying the maturing graft site and disruption of the graft as the screw is removed (Fig. 38.45).

Implant Placement

Because mandibular donor grafts exhibit minimal resorption, predictable gains in bone volume allow implant placement in most planned sites. A staged treatment plan with implant placement after graft healing is the preferred method of reconstruction. Reports on simultaneous implant insertion during bone graft placement have revealed complications, such as block graft fracture, wound dehiscence with exposure of implants and graft, and a higher implant failure rate compared with a staged approach.[38-40,46,55,146] In addition, diminished bone contact has been found around titanium implants placed simultaneously with autologous grafts.[12,30,85,147] A staged surgery permits implant placement for ideal prosthetic alignment without the concern of graft fixation or remodeling. Staging the implant placement also provides an improved vascularity of the transplanted bone as the exposed surface area is increased and unimpeded by an inert biomaterial.[53,148] It also allows for any unanticipated increase in graft resorption and should provide a more stable foundation. The implant-bone interface should be improved, because the implant surface is in close contact with the already incorporated bone graft. Autologous bone grafts offer an improved quality

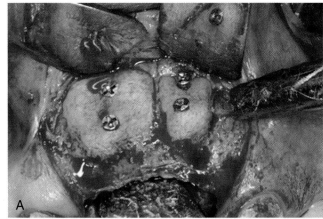
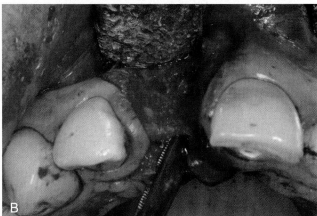
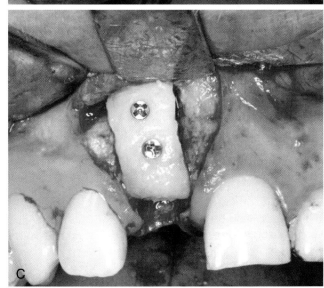

• **Fig. 38.44** Prevention of Graft Mobility. (A) Two screws need to be placed to prevent micromovement during healing. (B) The donor site needs to be prepared to minimize "rocking" of the graft when fixated. (C) Block graft securely fits into host site. (*From Caldwell CS. Bone grafting complications. In: Resnik RR, Misch CE, eds.* Misch's Avoiding Complications in Oral Implantology. *St Louis, MO: Elsevier; 2018.*)

of bone at earlier healing times compared with allogeneic bone grafts or guided bone regeneration techniques.[38,58,87,149-151] The density of healed block mandibular bone grafts has been found to be D1 to D2 regardless of the original quality of the recipient site.[38,44,58] An appropriate drilling sequence for dense bone and

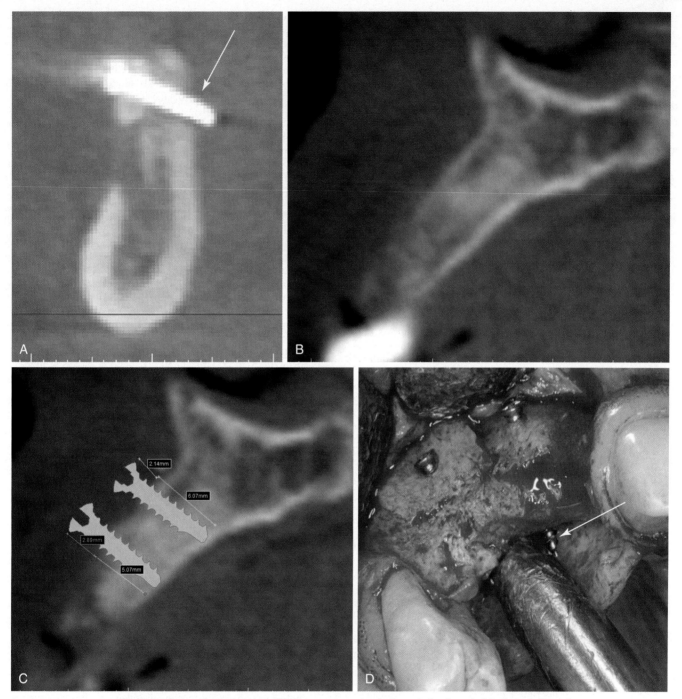

• **Fig. 38.45** Screw Overextension. (A) When screw extends through the lingual plate (arrow), this will often result in pain and discomfort for the patient. (B) Preoperative evaluation for fixation screw. (C) Ideally the fixation screw should exhibit bicortical stabilization, and the length measurements may be determined via cone beam computed tomographic measurements. (D) The protruding tip of this fixation screw has been visualized. (*From Caldwell CS. Bone grafting complications. In: Resnik RR, Misch CE, eds.* Misch's Avoiding Complications in Oral Implantology. *St. Louis, MO: Elsevier; 2018.*)

tapping may be necessary for atraumatic implant placement. The implant surgery activates bone formation and induces interfacial remodeling with bone maintenance, even in unloaded conditions.[152,153] After integration a progressive bone loading of the implants is recommended.[154] Additional graft resorption after implant insertion has not been noted radiographically on loaded cases.[155-158]

Summary

Autologous bone grafts are the only type of graft material that heals via osteogenesis, osteoinduction, and osteoconduction. Bone harvested from the maxillofacial region offers several advantages in the reconstruction of the residual ridge for implant placement. Intraoral donor sites require only one operational field, which decreases the surgical and anesthetic time. Larger block bone grafts may be harvested from the mandibular symphysis, body, or ramus area. Particulate autograft may be harvested from the maxillary tuberosity, extraosseous tori, ridge osteoplasty, extraction sites, implant osteotomy, and bone collection devices. These grafts require a short healing period and exhibit minimal resorption, while maintaining their dense quality. The morbidity of graft harvest is low, and complications usually result in only temporary debilitation. The use of these techniques allows the placement of implants in ideal positions for optimal esthetics and functional support.

References

1. Misch CE, Dietsh F. Bone grafting materials in implant dentistry. *Implant Dent.* 1993;2:158–167.
2. Buser D, Bragger U, Lang NP, et al. Regeneration and enlargement of jaw bone using guided tissue regeneration. *Clin Oral Implant Res.* 1990;1:22–32.
3. Lekholm U, Becker W, Dahlin C, et al. The role of early vs. late removal of GTAM membranes on bone formation around oral implants placed in immediate extraction sockets: an experimental study in dogs. *Clin Oral Implant Res.* 1993;4:121–129.
4. Palmer RM, Floyd PD, Palmer PJ, et al. Healing of implant dehiscence defects with and without expanded polytetrafluoroethylene membranes: a controlled clinical and histological study. *Clin Oral Implant Res.* 1994;5:98–104.
5. Jovanovic SA, Schenk RK, Orsini M, et al. Supracrestal bone formation around dental implants: an experimental dog study. *Int J Oral Maxillofac Implants.* 1995;10:23–31.
6. Pinholt EM, Haanaes HR, Donath K, et al. Titanium implant insertion into dog alveolar ridges augmented by allogenic material. *Clin Oral Implant Res.* 1994;5:213–219.
7. Becker W, Lekholm U, Dahlin C, et al. The effect of clinical loading on bone regenerated by GTAM barriers: a study in dogs. *Int J Oral Maxillofac Implants.* 1994;9:305–313.
8. Lang NP, Hammerle CHF, Bragger U, et al. Guided tissue regeneration in jawbone defects prior to implant placement. *Clin Oral Implant Res.* 1994;5:92–97.
9. Simion M, Baldoni M, Rossi P, et al. A comparative study of the effectiveness of e-PTFE membranes with and without early exposure during the healing period. *Int J Periodont Rest Dent.* 1994;14:167–180.
10. Simion M, Trisi P, Piatelli A. Vertical ridge augmentation using a membrane technique associated with osseointe-grated implants. *Int J Periodont Rest Dent.* 1994;14:497–511.
11. Fritz ME, Malmquist J, Koth D, et al. The use of guided bone regeneration to fill large mandibular defects in monkeys: a pilot study. *Int J Oral Maxillofac Implants.* 1994;9:644–652.
12. Becker W, Schenk R, Higuchi K, et al. Variations in bone regeneration adjacent to implants augmented with barrier membranes alone or with demineralized freeze-dried bone or autologous grafts: a study in dogs. *Int J Oral Maxillofac Implants.* 1995;10:143–154.
13. Caplanis N, Sigurdsson TJ, Rohrer MD, et al. Effect of allogeneic, freeze-dried, demineralized bone matrix on guided bone regeneration in supra-alveolar peri-implant defects in dogs. *Int J Maxillofac Implants.* 1997;12:634–642.
14. Hammack BL, Enneking WF. Comparative vascularization of autogenous and homogenous bone transplants. *J Bone Joint Surg.* 1960;42A:811.
15. Male AJ, Gasser J, Fonseca RJ, et al. Comparison of onlay autologous and allogenic bone grafts to the maxilla in primates. *J Oral Maxillofac Surg.* 1983;42:487–499.
16. Boyne PJ. Performance of bone grafts in reconstructive surgery. In: Williams EF, ed. *Biocompatibility of Tissue Analogs.* Boca Raton, Fla: CRC Press; 1985:(2).
17. Burchardt H. Biology of bone transplantation. *Orthop Clin North Am.* 1987;18:187–195.
18. Marx RE. Biology of bone grafts. *Oral Maxillofac Surg Knowl Update.* 1994;1:3–17.
19. Cordaro L, Amade DS, Cordaro M. Clinical results of alveolar ridge augmentation with mandibular block bone grafts in partially edentulous patients prior to implant placement. *Clin Oral Implants Res.* 2002;13:103–111.
20. Misch CE. Use of mandibular ramus as a donor site for onlay bone grafting. *J Oral Implantol.* 2000;26:42–49.
21. Proussaefs P, Lozada J, Kleinman A, Roaher MD. The use of ramus autogenous block grafts for vertical alveolar ridge augmentation and implant placement: a pilot study. *Int J Oral Maxillofac Implants.* 2002;17:238–248.
22. Proussaefs P, Lozada J. The use of intraorally harvested autogenous block grafts for vertical alveolar ridge augmentation: a human study. *Int J Periodontics Rest Dent.* 2005;25:351–363.
23. Proussaefs P. Clinical and histologic evaluation of the use of mandibular tori as donor site for mandibular block autografts: report of three cases. *Int J Periodont Res Dent.* 2006;26:43–51.
24. Schwartz-Arad D, Levin L. Multitier technique for bone augmentation using intraoral autogenous bone blocks. *Implant Dent.* 2007;16:5–12.
25. Schwartz-Arad D, Levin L. Intraoral autogenous block onlay bone grafting for extensive reconstruction of atrophic maxillary alveolar ridges. *J Periodontol.* 2005;76:636–641.
26. Schwartz-Arad D, Levin L, Sigal L. Surgical success of intra-oral autogenous block onlay bone grafting for alveolar ridge augmentation. *Implant Dent.* 2005;14:131–138.
27. Garg AK, Morales MJ, Navarro I, et al. Autogenous mandibular bone grafts in the treatment of the resorbed maxillary anterior alveolar ridge: rationale and approach. *Implant Dent.* 1998;7:167–176.
28. Cranin AN, Katzap M, Demirdjan E, et al. Autogenous bone ridge augmentation using the mandibular symphysis as a donor. *J Oral Implantol.* 2001;27:43–47.
29. Brånemark PI, Lindstrom J, Hallen O, et al. Reconstruction of the defective mandible. *Scand J Plast Reconstr Surg.* 1975;9:116–128.
30. Breine U, Brånemark PI. Reconstruction of alveolar jaw bone. *Scand J Plast Reconstr Surg.* 1980;14:23–48.
31. Keller EE, van Roekel NB, Desjardins RP, et al. Prosthetic-surgical reconstruction of the severely resorbed maxilla with iliac bone grafting and tissue-integrated prostheses. *Int J Oral Maxillofac Implants.* 1987;2:155–165.
32. Listrom RD, Symington JM. Osseointegrated dental implants in conjunction with bone grafts. *Int J Oral Maxillofac Surg.* 1988;17:116–118.
33. Kahnberg KE, Nystrom L, Bartholdsson L. Combined use of bone grafts and Brånemark fixtures in the treatment of severely resorbed maxillae. *Int J Oral Maxillofac Implants.* 1989;4:297–304.
34. Misch CE, Dietsh F. Endosteal implants and iliac crest grafts to restore severely resorbed totally edentulous maxillae: a retrospective study. *J Oral Implantol.* 1994;20:100–110.
35. Joshi A, Kostakis GC. An investigation of post-operative morbidity following iliac crest graft harvesting. *Br Dent J.* 2004;196:167–171.
36. Sindet-Pedersen S, Enemark H. Reconstruction of alveolar clefts with mandibular or iliac crest bone grafts: a compa-rative study. *J Oral Maxillofac Surg.* 1990;48:554–558.
37. Borstlap WA, Heidbuchel KLWM, Freihofer HPM, et al. Early secondary bone grafting of alveolar cleft defects: a comparison between chin and rib grafts. *J Cranio Max Fac Surg.* 1990;18:201–205.
38. Misch CM, Misch CE, Resnik R, et al. Reconstruction of maxillary alveolar defects with mandibular symphysis grafts for dental implants: a preliminary procedural report. *Int J Oral Maxillofac Implants.* 1992;7:360–366.

39. Jensen J, Sindet-Pedersen S. Autogenous mandibular bone grafts and osseointegrated implants for reconstruction of the severely atrophied maxilla: a preliminary report. *J Oral Maxillofac Surg.* 1991;49:1277–1287.

40. Jensen J, Sindet-Pedersen S, Oliver AJ. Varying treatment strategies for reconstruction of maxillary atrophy with implants: results in 98 patients. *J Oral Maxillofac Surg.* 1994;52:210–216.

41. Misch CM, Misch CE. The repair of localized severe ridge defects for implant placement using mandibular bone grafts. *Implant Dent.* 1995;4:261–267.

42. Misch CM. Ridge augmentation using mandibular ramus bone grafts for the placement of dental implants: presentation of a technique. *Prac Periodont Aesth Dent.* 1996;8:127–135.

43. Aalam AA, Nowzari H. Mandibular cortical bone grafts part 1: anatomy, healing process, and influencing factors. *Compend Contin Educ Dent.* 2007;28:206–212.

44. Misch CM. Comparison of intraoral donor sites for onlay grafting prior to implant placement. *Int J Oral Maxillofac Implants.* 1997;12:767–776.

45. Misch CM. Enhance maxillary implant sites through symphysis bone graft. *Dent Implant Update.* 1991;2:101–104.

46. Smith JD, Abramson M. Membranous vs. endochondral bone autografts. *Arch Otolaryngol.* 1974;99:203.

47. Zins JE, Whitaker LA. Membranous vs endochondral bone autografts: implications for craniofacial reconstruction. *Plast Reconstruct Surg.* 1983;72:778.

48. Kusiak JF, Zins JE, Whitaker LA. The early revascularization of membranous bone. *Plast Reconstr Surg.* 1985;76:510–514.

49. Lin KY, Bartlett SP, Yaremchuk MJ, et al. The effect of rigid fixation on the survival of onlay bone grafts: an experimental study. *Plast Reconstruct Surg.* 1990;86:449–456.

50. Rabie ABM, Dan Z, Samman N. Ultrastructural identification of cells involved in the healing of intramembranous and endochondral bones. *Int J Oral Maxillofac Surg.* 1996;25:383–388.

51. Miller NA, Penaud J, Kohler C, et al. Regeneration of bone graft donor sites. *Clin Oral Implants Res.* 1999;10:326–330.

52. Avery JK. Development of cartilages and bones of the facial skeleton. In: Avery JK, ed. *Oral Development and Histology.* New York: Thieme Medical Publishers; 1994.

53. Marx RE. The science of reconstruction. In: Bell WH, ed. *Modern Practice in Orthognathic and Reconstructive Surgery.* Philadelphia: WB Saunders; 1992.

54. Shirota T, Ohno K, Motohashi M, et al. Histologic and microradiologic comparison of block and particulate cancellous bone and marrow grafts in reconstructed mandibles being considered for dental implant placement. *J Oral Maxillofac Surg.* 1996;54:15–20.

55. Lu M, Rabie AB. Quantitative assessment of early healing of intramembranous and endochondral autogenous bone grafts using micro-computed tomography and Q-win image analyzer. *Int J Oral Maxillofac Surg.* 2004;33:369–376.

56. Lu M, Rabie AB. Macroarchitecture of rabbit mandibular defects grafted with intramembranous or endochondral bone shown by micro-computed tomography. *Br J Oral Maxillofac Surg.* 2003;41:385–391.

57. Ozaki W, Buchman SR. Volume maintenance of onlay bone grafts in the craniofacial skeleton: micro-architecture versus embryologic origin. *Plast Reconstr Surg.* 1998;102:291–299.

58. Glowacki J. In: discussion of Kusiak JF, Zins JE, Whitaker LA: *The early revascularization of membranous bone. Plast Reconstr Surg.* 1985;76:515.

59. Rosenthal AH, Buchman SR. Volume maintenance of inlay bone grafts in the craniofacial skeleton. *Plast Reconstr Surg.* 2003;112:802–811.

60. Sharawy M, El-Shazly D, Um IW, et al. Fate of allogeneic cranial bone grafted to rabbit mandible (abstract 1015). *J Dent Res.* 1996;75.

61. Takikawa S, Bauer TW, Kambic H, et al. Comparative evaluation of the osteoinductivity of two formulations of human demineralized bone matrix. *J Biomed Mater Res A.* 2003;65:37–42.

62. Martin GJ, Boden SD, Titus L, et al. New formulations of demineralized bone matrix as a more effective bone graft alternative in experimental posterior lateral lumbar spine arthrodesis. *Spine.* 1999;24:637.

63. Finkleman RD, Eason AL, Rakijian DR, et al. Elevated IGF-II and TGF-B concentrations in human calvarial bone: potential mechanism for increased graft survival and resistance to osteoporosis. *Plast Reconstr Surg.* 1994;93:732–738.

64. Hardesty RA, Marsh JL. Craniofacial onlay bone grafting: a prospective evaluation of graft morphology, orientation and embryonic origin. *Plast Reconstr Surg.* 1990;85:5–14.

65. Manson PN. Facial bone healing and bone grafts: a review of clinical physiology. *Clin Plast Surg.* 1994;21:331–348.

66. Alberius P, Gordh M, Linberg L, et al. Influence of surrounding soft tissues on onlay bone graft incor-poration. *Oral Surg Oral Med Oral Pathol.* 1996;82:22–33.

67. Lew D, Marino AA, Startzell JM, et al. A comparative study of osseointegration of titanium implants in corticocancellous block and corticocancellous chip grafts in canine ilium. *J Oral Maxillofac Surg.* 1994;52:952–958.

68. Wong RW, Rabie AB. A quantitative assessment of the healing of intramembranous and endochondral autogenous bone grafts. *Eur J Orthod.* 1999;21:119–126.

69. Buser D, Dula K, Belser UC, et al. Localized ridge augmentation using guided bone regeneration. II. Surgical procedure in the mandible. *Int J Periodont Rest Dent.* 1995;15:11–29.

70. Roberts WE, Garetto LP, DeCastro RA. Remodeling of devitalized bone threatens periosteal margin integrity of endosseous titanium implants with threaded or smooth surfaces: indications for provisional loading and axially directed occlusion. *J Ind Dent Assoc.* 1989;68:19–24.

71. Schenk RK. Bone regeneration: biologic basis. In: Buser D, Dahlin C, Schenk RK, eds. *Guided Bone Regeneration in Implant Dentistry.* Chicago: Quintessence; 1994.

72. Buser D, Dula K, Hirt HP, et al. Lateral ridge augmentation using autografts and barrier membranes: a clinical study with 40 partially edentulous patients. *J Oral Maxillofac Surg.* 1996;54:420–432.

73. Misch CE. Density of bone: effect on treatment plans, surgical approach, healing and progressive bone loading. *Int J Oral Implantol.* 1990;6:23–31.

74. Sennerby L, Thomsen P, Ericson LE. A morphometric and biomechanic comparison of titanium implants inserted in rabbit cortical and cancellous bone. *Int J Oral Maxillofac Implants.* 1992;7:62–71.

75. Bidez M, Misch CE. Issues in bone mechanics related to oral implants. *Implant Dent.* 1992;1:289–294.

76. Collins TA. Onlay bone grafting in combination with Brånemark implants. *Oral Maxillofac Surg Clin North Am.* 1991;3:893–902.

77. ten Bruggenkate CM, Kraaijenhagen HA, van der Kwast WA, et al. Autogenous maxillary bone grafts in conjunction with placement of I.T.I. endosseous implants: a preliminary report. *Int J Oral Maxillofac Surg.* 1992;21:81–84.

78. Rosenquist JB, Nystrom E. Occlusion of the incisal canal with bone chips. *Int J Oral Maxillofac Surg.* 1992;21:210–211.

79. Bahat O, Fontanesi RV, Preston J. Reconstruction of the hard and soft tissues for optimal placement of osseointegrated implants. *Int J Periodont Rest Dent.* 1993;13:255–275.

80. Collins TA, Nunn W. Autogenous veneer grafting for improved esthetics with dental implants. *Compend Contin Educ Dent.* 1994;15:370–376.

81. Becker W, Becker BE, Polizzi G, et al. Autogenous bone grafting of bone defects adjacent to implants placed into immediate extraction sockets in patients: a prospective study. *Int J Oral Maxillofac Implants.* 1994;9:389–396.

82. Becker W, Becker BE, Caffesse R. A comparison of demineralized freeze-dried bone and autologous bone to induce bone formation in human extraction sockets. *J Periodontol.* 1994;65:1128–1133.

83. Raghoebar GM, Batenburg RHK, Vissink A, et al. Augmentation of localized defects of the anterior maxillary ridge with autogenous bone before insertion of implants. *J Oral Maxillofac Surg.* 1996;54:1180–1185.

84. Friberg B. Bone augmentation at single-tooth implants using mandibular grafts: a one-stage surgical procedure. *Int J Periodont Rest Dent.* 1995;15:437–445.

85. Lustmann J, Lewinstein I. Interpositional bone grafting technique to widen narrow maxillary ridge. *Int J Oral Maxillofac Implants.* 1995;10:568–577.

86. Lazzara R. Transplantation of a preosseointegrated implant from the mental area to a maxillary sinus graft. *Int J Periodont Rest Dent.* 1995;15:539–547.

87. Williamson RA. Rehabilitation of the resorbed maxilla and mandible using autogenous bone grafts and osseointegrated implants. *Int J Oral Maxillofac Implants.* 1996;11:476–488.

88. Triplett RG, Schow S. Autologous bone grafts and endosseous implants: complementary techniques. *J Oral Maxillofac Surg.* 1996;54:486–494.

89. Boyne PJ. Bone grafts: materials. In: Boyne PJ, ed. *Osseous Reconstruction of the Maxilla and the Mandible: Surgical Techniques Using Titanium Mesh and Bone Mineral.* Chicago: Quintessence; 1996.

90. von Arx T, Hardt N, Wallkamm B. The TIME technique: a new method for localized alveolar ridge augmentation prior to placement of dental implants. *Int J Oral Maxillofac Implants.* 1996;11:387–394.

91. Chiapasco M, Zaniboni M, Rimondini L. Autogenous onlay bone grafts vs. alveolar distraction osteogenesis for the correction of vertically deficient edentulous ridges: a 2-4 year prospective study on humans. *Clin Oral Implant Res.* 2007;18:432–440.

92. Garber DA, Belser UC. Restoration-driven implant placement with restoration-generated site development. *Compend Contin Educ Dent.* 1995;16:796–804.

93. Mecall RA, Rosenfeld AL. The influence of residual ridge resorption patterns on fixture placement and tooth position in the partially edentulous patient. Part III. Presurgical assessment of ridge augmentation requirements. *Int J Periodont Rest Dent.* 1996;16:323–337.

94. Rosenfeld AL, Mecall RA. The use of interactive computed tomography to predict the esthetic and functional demands of implant-supported prostheses. *Compend Contin Educ Dent.* 1996;17:1125–1144.

95. Sarment DP, Misch CE. Scannographic templates for novel preimplant planning methods. *Int Mag Oral Implan.* 2002;4:16–22.

96. Albrektsson T. Repair of bone grafts: a vital microscopic and histologic investigation in the rabbit. *Scand J Plast Reconstr Surg.* 1980;14:1–12.

97. Cutright B, Quillopa N, Schubert W. An anthropometric study of the key foramina for maxillofacial surgery. *J Oral Maxillofac Surg.* 2003;61:354–357.

98. Montazem A, Valauri DV, St-Hilaire H, et al. The mandibular symphysis as a donor site in maxillofacial bone grafting: a qualitative anatomic study. *J Oral Maxillofac Surg.* 2000;58:1368–1371.

99. Gapski R, Wang HL, Misch CE. Management of incision design in symphysis graft procedures: a review of the literature. *J Oral Implant.* 2001;26. 13243-13142.

100. Suer BT, Yaman Z. Harvesting mandibular ramus bone grafts using ultrasonic surgical device: report of 20 cases. *J Dent Oral Disord Ther.* 2014;2(1):5.

101. Nelson Stanley J. *Wheeler's Dental Anatomy, Physiology and Occlusion-E-Book.* Elsevier Health Sciences; 2014.

102. Buhr W, Coulon JP. Limits of the mandibular symphysis as a donor site for bone grafts in early secondary cleft palate osteoplasty. *Int J Oral Maxillofac Surg.* 1996;25:389–393.

103. Kaufman E, Wang PD. Localized vertical maxillary ridge augmentation using symphyseal bone cores: a technique and case report. *Int J Oral Maxillofac Implants.* 2003;18:293–298.

104. Rajchel J, Ellis E, Fonseca RJ. The anatomical location of the mandibular canal: its relationship to the sagittal ramus osteotomy. *Int J Adult Orthod Orthognath Surg.* 1986;1:37.

105. Smith BR, Rajchel JL. II. Anatomic considerations in mandibular ramus osteotomies. In: Bell WH, ed. *Modern Practice in Orthognathic and Reconstructive Surgery.* Philadelphia: WB Saunders; 1992.

106. Hall HD. Intraoral surgery. In: Bell WH, ed. *Modern Practice in Orthognathic and Reconstructive Surgery.* Philadelphia: WB Saunders; 1992.

107. Gungormus M, Yavuz MS. The ascending ramus of the mandible as a donor site in maxillofacial bone grafting. *J Oral Maxillofac Surg.* 2002;60:1316–1318.

108. Wood RM, Moore DL. Grafting of the maxillary sinus with intraorally harvested autogenous bone prior to implant placement. *Int J Oral Maxillofac Implants.* 1988;3:209–214.

109. Wheeler S, Holmes RE, Calhoun CJ. Six-year clinical and histologic study of sinus-lift grafts. *Int J Oral Maxillofac Implants.* 1996;11:26–34.

110. Berry RL, Edwards RC, Paxton MC. Nasal augmentation using the mandibular coronoid as an autogenous graft: report of case. *J Oral Maxillofac Surg.* 1994;52:633–638.

111. McLoughlin PM, Hopper C, Bowley NB. Hyperplasia of the mandibular coronoid process: an analysis of 31 cases and a review of the literature. *J Oral Maxillofac Surg.* 1995;53:250–255.

112. Koury ME. Complications of mandibular fractures. In: Kaban LB, Pogrel MA, Perrott DH, eds. *Complications in Oral and Maxillofacial Surgery.* Philadelphia: WB Saunders; 1997.

113. Trauner R, Obwegeser H. The surgical correction of mandibular prognathism and retrognathia with consideration of genioplasty. Part I. Surgical procedures to correct mandibular prognathism and reshaping of the chin. *Oral Surg.* 1957;10:677.

114. DalPont G. Retromolar osteotomy for correction of prognathism. *J Oral Surg.* 1961;19:42.

115. Hunsuck EE. Modified intraoral splitting technique for correction of mandibular prognathism. *J Oral Surg.* 1968;26:250.

116. Epker BN. Modifications in the sagittal osteotomy of the mandible. *J Oral Surg.* 1977;35:157.

117. Bell WH, Schendel SA. Biologic basis for modification of the sagittal ramus split operation. *J Oral Surg.* 1977;34:362.

118. Heggie AAC. The use of mandibular buccal cortical grafts in bimaxillary surgery. *J Oral Maxillofac Surg.* 1993;51:1282–1283.

119. Jensen J, Reiche-Fischel O, Sindet-Pedersen S. Autogenous mandibular bone grafts for molar augmentation. *J Oral Maxillofac Surg.* 1995;53:88–90.

120. Clavero J, Lundgren S. Ramus or chin grafts for maxillary sinus inlay and local onlay augmentation: Comparison of donor site morbidity and complications. *Clin Implant Dent Relat Res.* 2003;5:154.

121. Whitaker LA. Biological boundaries: a concept in facial skeletal restructuring. *Clin Plast Surg.* 1989;16:1.

122. Nyman S, Lang NP, Buser D, et al. Bone regeneration adjacent to titanium dental implants using guided tissue regeneration. A report of two cases. *Int J Oral Maxillofac Implants.* 1990;5:9–14.

123. Marx RE, Snyder RM, Kline SN. Cellular survival of human marrow during placement of marrow cancellous bone grafts. *J Oral Surg.* 1979;37:712–718.

124. Steiner M, Ramp WK. Short-term storage of freshly harvested bone. *J Oral Maxillofac Surg.* 1988;46:868–871.

125. Thompson N, Casson JA. Experimental onlay bone grafts to the jaws: a preliminary study in dogs. *Plast Reconstr Surg.* 1970;46:341–349.

126. Knize D. The influence of periosteum and calcitonin on onlay bone graft survival. *Plast Reconstr Surg.* 1974;53:190–199.

127. Fonseca RJ, Clark PJ, Burkes EJ, et al. Revascularization and healing of onlay particulate autologous bone grafts in primates. *J Oral Surg.* 1980;38:572–577.

128. Dado DV, Izquierdo R. Absorption of onlay bone grafts in immature rabbits: membranous versus endochondral bone and bone struts versus paste. *Ann Plast Surg.* 1989;23:39–48.

129. Chaushu G, Mardinger O, Peleg M. Analysis of complications following augmentation with cancellous block allografts. *J Periodontol.* 2010;81(12):1759–1764.

130. Gielkens PF, Bos RR, Raghoebar GM. Is there evidence that barrier membranes prevent bone resorption in autologous bone grafts during the healing period? A systematic review. *Int J Oral Maxillofac Implants.* 2007;22(3):390–398.

131. Aloy-Prósper A, Peñarrocha-Oltra D, Peñarrocha-Diago MA, et al. The outcome of intraoral onlay block bone grafts on alveolar ridge augmentations: a systematic review. *Med Oral Patol Oral Cir Bucal.* 2015;20(2):e251.

132. Gultekin BA, Bedeloglu E, Kose TE, et al. Comparison of bone resorption rates after intraoral block bone and guided bone regeneration augmentation for the reconstruction of horizontally deficient maxillary alveolar ridges. *BioMed Res Int.* 2016.

133. Yates DM, Brockhoff II HC, Finn R, Phillips C. Comparison of intraoral harvest sites for corticocancellous bone grafts. *J Oral Maxillofac Surg.* 2013;71(3):497–504.

134. Jones JK, Triplett RG. The relationship of smoking to impaired intraoral wound healing. *J Oral Maxillofac Surg.* 1992;50:237–239.

135. Misch CM. The extracted tooth pontic-provisional replacement during bone graft and implant healing. *Pract Periodont Aesth Dent.* 1998;10:711–718.

136. Schnitman PA, Wohrle PS, Rubenstein JE. Immediate fixed interim prostheses supported by two-stage threaded implants. Methodology and results. *J Oral Implantol.* 1990;16:96–105.

137. Salama H, Rose LF, Salama M, et al. Immediate loading of bilaterally splinted titanium root-form implants in fixed prosthodontics—a technique reexamined: two case reports. *Int J Periodont Rest Dent.* 1995;15:345–361.

138. Misch CM. Comparison of intraoral donor sites for onlay grafting prior to implant placement. *Int J Oral Maxillofac Implants.* 1997;12:767–776.

139. Hoppenreijs TJM, Nijdam ES, Freihofer HPM. The chin as a donor site in early secondary osteoplasty: a retrospective clinical and radiological evaluation. *J Cranio Maxillofac Surg.* 1992;20(3):119–124.

140. Borstlap WA, Stoelinga PJ, Hoppenreijs TJ, van't Hof MA. Stabilisation of sagittal split advancement osteotomies with miniplates: a prospective, multicentre study with two-year follow-up. Part I. Clinical parameters. *Int J Oral Maxillofac Surg.* 2004;33(5):433–441.

141. Miller RJ, Edwards WC, Boudet C, Cohen JH. Revised Maxillofacial Anatomy: the mandibular symphysis in 3D. *Int J Dent Implants Biomaterials.* 2009;2:1–7.

142. Hendy CW, Smith KG, Robinson PP. Surgical anatomy of the buccal nerve. *Br J Oral Maxillofac Surg.* 1996;34:457–460.

143. Nkenke E, Radespiel-Troger M, Wiltfang J, et al. Morbidity of harvesting of retromolar bone grafts: a prospective study. *Clin Oral Implants Res.* 2002;13:513–521.

144. Silva FM, Cortez AL, Moreira RW, et al. Complications of intraoral donor site for bone grafting prior to implant placement. *Implant Dent.* 2006;15:420–426.

145. Fontana F, Maschera E, Rocchietta I, Simion M. Clinical classification of complications in guided bone regeneration procedures by means of a nonresorbable membrane. *Int J Periodontics Restorative Dent.* 2011;31(3):265–274.

146. Koole R, Bosker H, Noorman van der Dussen F. Secondary autogenous bone grafting in cleft patients comparing mandibular (ectomesenchymal) and iliac crest (mesenchymal) grafts. *J Cranio Max Fac Surg.* 1989;17:28–30.

147. Nystrom E, Kahnberg KE, Albrektsson T. Treatment of the severely resorbed maxillae with bone graft and titanium implants: histologic review of autopsy specimens. *Int J Oral Maxillofac Implants.* 1993;8:167–172.

148. Buser D, Dula K, Belser U, et al. Localized ridge augmentation using guided bone regeneration. I. Surgical procedure in the maxilla. *Int J Periodont Rest Dent.* 1993;13:29–45.

149. Simion M, Dahlin C, Trisi P, et al. Qualitative and quantitative comparative study on different filling materials used in bone tissue regeneration: a controlled clinical study. *Int J Periodont Rest Dent.* 1994;14:199–215.

150. Simion M, Fontana F. Autogenous and xenogeneic bone grafts for the bone regeneration: a literature review. *Minerva Stomatol.* 2004;53:191–206.

151. Pansegrau KJ, Friedrich KL, Lew D, et al. A comparative study of osseointegration of titanium implants in autogenous and freeze-dried bone grafts. *J Oral Maxillofac Surg.* 1998;56:1067–1073.

152. Roberts EW. Bone tissue interface. *J Dent Educ.* 1988;52:804–809.

153. Chen J, Chen K, Garetto LP, et al. Mechanical response to functional and therapeutic loading of a retromolar endosseous implant used for orthodontic anchorage to mesially translate mandibular molars. *Implant Dent.* 1995;4:246–258.

154. Misch CE. Early crestal bone loss etiology and its effect on treatment planning for implants. *Postgrad Dent.* 1995;2:3–16.

155. Hall MB. Marginal bone loss around Brånemark fixtures in bone grafts used for augmentation. *J Oral Maxillofac Surg.* 1990;48:117.

156. Ozkan Y, Ozcan M, Varol A, et al. Resonance frequency analysis assessment of implant stability in labial onlay grafted posterior mandibles: a pilot clinical study. *Int J Oral Maxillofac Implants.* 2007;22:235–242.

157. Sjostrom M, Lundgren S, Milson H, et al. Monitoring of implant stability in grafted bone using resonance frequency analysis. A clinical study from implant placement to 6 months of loading. *Int J Oral Maxillofac Surg.* 2005;34:45–51.

158. Sethi A, Kaus T. Ridge augmentation using mandibular block bone grafts: preliminary results of an ongoing prospective study. *Int J Oral Maxillofac Implants.* 2001;16:378–388.

39

Extraoral Bone Grafting for Implant Reconstruction

DAVID J. DATTILO

Introduction

The pool of patients that are eligible for dental implant reconstruction has expanded widely since Brånemark's research first hit the world of dentistry in the early 1980's. Extensive research in bone biology, coupled with newer and proven bone grafting techniques, leaves almost no patient outside the boundaries of eligible recipients. This includes patients with large bony defects resulting from trauma, resection from pathologic lesions, and congenital deformities, which would be classified as division E in the Misch-Judy classification of available bone and prosthetic options.[1,2] Procedures designed to provide large quantities of bone harvested from outside of the facial region that were previously used to only restore continuity and primitive function now are expected to reproduce vertical and horizontal dimensions for ideal placement of implant fixtures for the support of multiple prosthetic designs.

These new demands on the implant surgeon make the evaluation of the recipient defect, both dimensions and biologic environment, as well as the appropriateness of the potential donor site bone quality, of paramount importance. For instance, loss of bone from treatment of neoplastic or other pathologic processes represents far greater reconstructive challenges than loss of bone from trauma or infection. Other factors important to deciding the type and quantity of bone graft required to be harvested for larger defects is the presence of systemic diseases and the possible exposure to therapeutic doses of ionizing radiation. Success rates of bone grafts in irradiated jaws have been found to be lower by significant amounts, as well as complication rates of 81.3%.[3] The rich cellular components that make autogenous grafts the "gold standard" of implant-supported bone grafts, along with techniques such as hyperbaric oxygen treatment, platelet-rich plasma, and the use of engineered growth factors such as bone morphogenetic protein (BMP), all act to combat and hopefully overcome any hostile environment to provide a healthy osseous base for the placement of dental implants.

The four major anatomic areas for harvesting of free autogenous bone that will be discussed in this chapter include the cranium, the anterior and posterior iliac crest, and the tibial plateau. The necessity required for the proverbial Mother of these inventive techniques was primarily provided by the multiple facial injuries sustained by American and German soldiers during World War I and II. Surgeons from both countries, when faced with such large deformities caused by the latest in wartime ballistics, searched the body for the largest reservoirs of bone that could be used to fill these functional and cosmetic defects. Surgical researchers Wolff, Moss, Tessier, Boyne, and Marx then took these procedures and investigated the details of bone graft healing and the interaction between the bone and the recipient soft tissue bed.[7,8] These initial autogenous bone grafts, however, were characterized by rapid and advanced bone resorption, which sometimes reached 30% to 90% in the best of conditions.[9,10] With the advent of endosteal implants used in conjunction with autogenous grafts, research began reporting the maintenance of the grafted bone and the prevention of this rapid bone resorption.[11,12] Surgeons placing extraoral autogenous bone grafts, when used in conjunction with endosteal implants, can now expect to maintain better than 90% of the initial grafted segment.

Autogenous free bone grafts harvested from these four donor sites and their subsequent recipient sites have other unique biologic qualities that contribute to their appropriate use for dental implant support. Calvarium and mandibular bone are of intramembranous origin formed through the progressive differentiation from primordial mesenchymal cells to stem cells to osteocytes, while the maxilla, anterior and posterior iliac crest and the tibia are formed through endochondral ossification through the transformation and replacement of already formed cartilage.

Early studies comparing these two types of grafts on animal models revealed superiority of intramembranous bone grafts taken from the skull to endochondral bone grafts taken from the ilium or the rib.[4,5] At one year, the intramembranous grafts appeared to maintain the original grafted volume, whereas the endochondral grafts were decreased in volume by 75%. These findings appeared to be counterintuitive because the higher cancellous bone content of the endochondral grafts would seem to welcome a much faster revascularization than the more cortical intramembranous bone. Follow up studies actually showed a more rapid revascularization of these membranous grafts with complete ingrowth of vessels from the host bone and periosteum at 14 days whereas the endochondral bone still showed significant areas of necrotic bone and areas of resorption.[6]

Ironically, it appears the mechanism of revascularization of both the intramembranous and endochondral grafts proceeds along the same pathway borrowing similarities from both mechanisms with the grafted bone acting as the matrix (osteoconduction) that

Medical Illustration Drawing	Source	Cortical	Cancellous
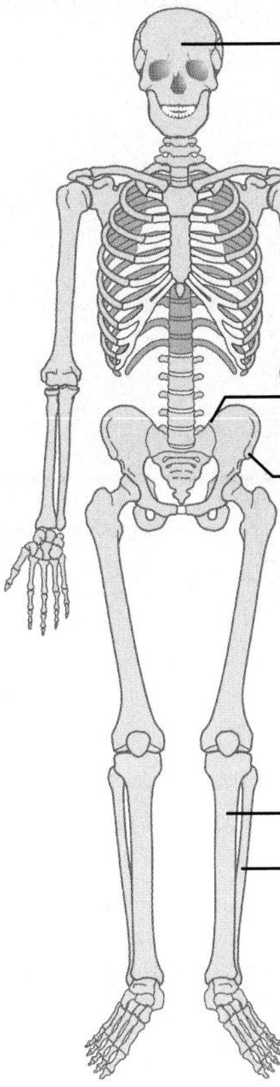	Cranium	Large area on bilateral parietal regions	Minimal
	Posterior iliac crest	5x5 cm Cortico-cancellous blocks	100–125cc's Morcilized bone
	Anterior iliac crest	3x5 cm Cortico-cancellous blocks	50cc's Morcilized bone
	Tibia	None	24–40cc's Cancellous bone
	Fibula	Maximum of 26cm in length and 3cm in width of vascularized bicortical bone	

• **Fig. 39.1** Extraoral autogenous donor sites with the resultant quantity of cortical and cancellous bone.

is subsequently replaced by osteoid generated by viable osteogenic cells (osteogenesis) with regulation from grafted growth factors (osteoinduction).

Each of the four major donor sites for free autogenous grafts are unique in their ability to provide one or both of the essential structural elements of bone, which include the strong and rigid cortical or the softer but more cellular and regenerative cancellous. These two bone types also differ in the process in which they regenerate new bone. The calvarial graft is predominantly cortical bone and used in areas in which maintenance of a particular dimension is essential for a longer term, bone grafts from the iliac crest provide both cortical and cancellous bone in different quantities, and the tibial plateau is useful for obtaining quantities of cancellous bone only (Fig. 39.1).

All of these grafts can be augmented with a number of different supplemental materials, regenerated blood products, and exogenous growth factors, which may assist in turning these grafted sites into the ideal bone quality to support future implant placement.

Finally, in spite of all of the positive science and technology supporting the potential regenerative capacity of free autogenous grafts, there will always be instances in which the size of the defect, or the lack of sufficient soft tissue cover and blood supply, or both, prevent the use of this technique. For the sake of completeness, the end of this chapter will discuss the use of the vascularized composite bone grafts. Originally used to augment the largest of facial defects with less than optimum cosmetic and functional results, this procedure also has progressed and improved along with the rise in dental implant technology to refine the technique

and provide more than an acceptable osseous base for an implant-supported prosthesis.

Extraoral Donor Bone Graft Sites

Calvarial Graft

The prospect of having bone harvested from the skull (calvarial), which is an area so close to one of the most vital structures of the human body, makes most patients cringe at the possibilities of such a dangerous procedure. The reality is quite the opposite. Of all of the extraoral bone grafting procedures discussed in this chapter, the split-thickness calvarial graft offers a very convenient option of unlimited bone with the least amount of postoperative morbidity. Access incisions are hidden inside the hairline and postoperative pain is minimal. For implant-guided reconstruction, the donor site lies close to the recipient site, therefore the procedure is not prolonged significantly more than an intraoral grafting procedure. The cortical nature and volume of the outside table with the intervening diploe of cancellous bone provide wide possibilities of shape, contour, and stability for reconstruction of any potential dental implant site. This bone is particularly useful for onlay grafting to augment the atrophic mandible and maxilla (Fig. 39.2).

Tessier, in his landmark publication in 1982, first championed the use of full- and split-thickness cranial grafts for the reconstruction of congenital deformities in children and young adults.[13] For the purposes of site preparation for the placement of dental implants, the use of the split-thickness graft will more than suffice.

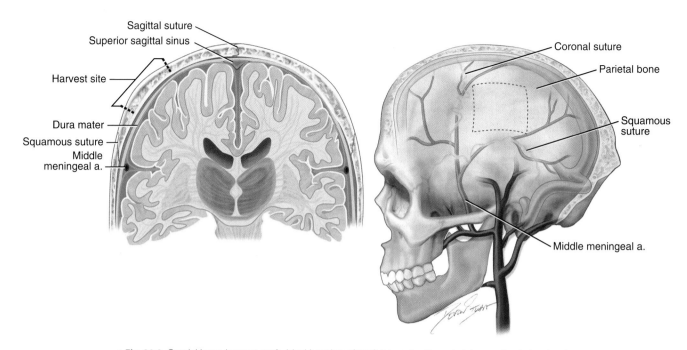

• **Fig. 39.2** Cranial bone harvest graft. Ideal location of graft harvest with underlying anatomic landmarks. (From Kademani D, Tiwana P, eds. *Atlas of Oral & Maxillofacial Surgery.* Philadelphia, PA: Elsevier; 2015.)

The parietal bone, just above the insertion of the temporalis muscle, is the ideal spot for harvesting because of its thickness and its relative isolation from vital structures both above and below the cranial vault. The thickness of the parietal bone can vary from 3 to 12 mm, and any site less than 6 mm is a contraindication because of the possibility of dura exposure and possible tear. This procedure is also contraindicated in children less than 9 years of age because of the underdevelopment of the diploic space.[14] It is also recommended that surgeons choose the nondominant hemisphere side of the cranium, although postharvest magnetic resonance imaging (MRI) studies of the underlying brain did not detect any abnormalities, even in cases when there was a full-thickness breach.[15]

Anatomy and Technique

Incision design and placement is dependent on the amount of graft required for the reconstruction. For a large graft, a bicoronal incision is marked off in the hair bearing the scalp 4.0 cm posterior to the anterior hairline to hide the resultant scar and to expose as much of the parietal surface as possible. For smaller grafts, incisions may be made directly over the donor sight (Fig. 39.3).

The hair is washed and prepped, however, it is not shaved. Local anesthetic with vasoconstrictor is injected along the planned incision site. It is imperative to wait the mandatory time (5–7 minutes) to allow the anesthetic vasoconstriction in this very vascular area to be effective. Electrocautery may be used from the dermis layer down to the bone so as to not disturb the hair follicles. Raney clips are then placed on both sides of the incision to help control further bleeding. Bone incisions are then outlined with a surgical marker or electrocautery, making sure all boundaries are behind the coronal suture and well away from the midline to avoid the superior sagittal sinus. The superior incision should be placed 2.0 cm lateral to the superior sagittal sinus, and the inferior extent of the incision should be 2.0 cm above the squamoparietal suture to avoid the middle meningeal artery. This area, the middle to posterior region of the parietal bone, has been shown to exhibit the thickest bone with the most developed diploic space.[16] For the

purposes of grafting for implant site preparation, ideal graft measurements can be separated into 1 to 1.5 × 3 to 4 cm to prevent fracture of the graft during harvesting.

With presurgical data from computerized tomography (CT) or cone beam CT (CBCT) scans indicating the approximate thickness of the skull, the initial osteotomies are initiated with a small Steiger bur or a Piezo saw down to the underlying diploe. Copious irrigation during the osteotomy is important so that the temperature of the bone is not increased this close to the cranial contents and to maintain the cellular vitality of the bone graft as best as possible. The outer edge of the initial osteotomy is then beveled down with an egg-shaped bur to provide a better access angle to allow a curved osteotome into the appropriate plane of the underlying diploe (Fig. 39.4). Beveling around additional sides of the initial graft may be necessary to avoid breaching the internal table. Once the initial graft of a multiple graft donor site is elevated cleanly, the remaining segments can be lifted much easier having already established the appropriate plane and angle between the outer and inner table.

After the grafts have been removed and placed in saline, hemostasis is obtained and the wound is closed in layers. Various cements, putties, and bone substitutes are available to reestablish the contour of the cranium and obtain hemostasis from the cut edges of the bone. Closure of the periosteum and galea are performed with resorbable sutures, and the skin can be closed with staples as long as attention is paid to eversion of the scalp margins. Drains are rarely necessary.

Complications

1. *Alopecia along the incision line.* This is caused by the use of electrocautery and prolonged use of Raney clips, causing ischemic hair follicle injury. Scars caused by this can be minimized by using a zigzag incision design.
2. *Bleeding from the harvest site.* This can be controlled by the use of surgical hemostatic agents such as topical microfibrillar collagen (Avitine) and the use of bone wax or bone cement packed

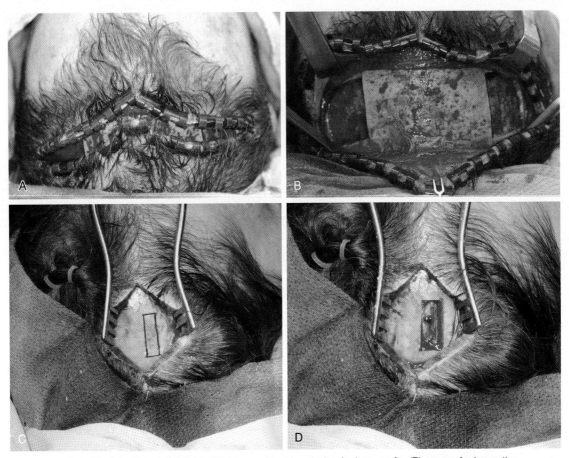

• **Fig. 39.3** Calvarian graft incision. (A) Bicoronal incision design for large grafts. (B) access for harvesting grafts from both sides of the parietal cranium. (C) Smaller incision design. (D) Bone graft harvest for single site.

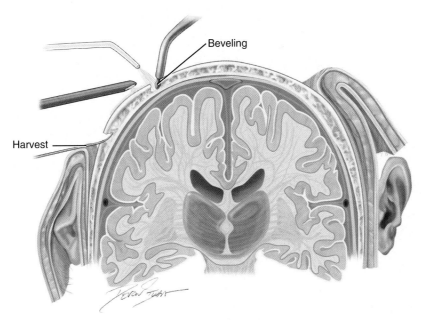

• **Fig. 39.4** Calvarian osteotomy. Beveling the osteotomy to prevent perforation of inner table while raising outer table graft. (From Kademani D, Tiwana P, eds. *Atlas of Oral & Maxillofacial Surgery.* Philadelphia, PA: Elsevier; 2015.)

into the diploic spaces and along the base of the bed. If bone cement is used, make sure that the exogenic heat caused by the chemical setup of the material does not come into contact with the bed until it has dissipated.

3. *Inner table perforations.* Small inner table perforations with no evidence of a dural tear are of no consequence and can be covered with any selection of softer fillers. If a small tear exists, then the tear will need to be sutured closed to prevent a cerebrospinal fluid leak. If the tear is large and no immediate means of closure is at hand, then a neurosurgical consult is necessary.

4. *Bleeding from major vessels.* These are very rare occasions, however, if a misadventure would result in copious bleeding from the central sagittal sinus and continuous pressure with surgical packing is indicated. Because this is venous blood, the hemostatic control should not result in any brain or scalp ischemia. If the middle meningeal artery on the inferior border of the temporal border is cut, then an immediate neurosurgical consult is necessary because this could result in an epidural hematoma.

Case Study

A 32-year-old male with a history of congenital absence of multiple maxillary and mandibular teeth presents for implant reconstruction. The patient had previous orthognathic surgery to correct a class III maxillary atrophic deformity. CT scans revealed severe alveolar bone atrophy of all four quadrants (Fig. 39.5).

Through a bicoronal approach, split-thickness outer table grafts were harvested from the parietal bone from the right and the left cranium. The grafts were placed with two-point fixation in an onlay fashion throughout the maxilla and mandible. Additional particulate bone pulverized from the unused grafts was used to fill in areas between the fixated grafts (Fig. 39.6).

At 6 months the grafted sites were exposed for removal of fixation screws and placement of implant fixtures. Note the minimal change and resorption of the original grafts that is emblematic of the high-density cortical grafts of the cranium. Surgical guide splints were fabricated before the uncovering for implant placement (Figs. 39.7 and 39.8; Boxes 39.1 and 39.2).

Iliac Crest Bone Graft

The ilium is historically the most popular donor site for facial bone grafting because of the high volume of cancellous and cortical bone. The corticocancellous block harvested from the ilium provides the "best of both worlds" in bone grafting by combining the high cellular transfer of the cancellous matrix with the BMP-rich structural support of the cortical bone (Fig. 39.9).

The anterior ilium may yield up to 50 cc of bone for augmentation. This amount can reconstruct a 5.0-cm segmental defect of the mandible using the following equation: 1.0 cm requires 10.0 cc of bone. For the purposes of implant site preparation, this is usually sufficient; however, if larger division E deformities exist, then the posterior ilium may be used. The posterior iliac crest can be harvested for donor bone when more significant volumes are necessary for the grafting of a facial defect. The posterior iliac crest provides the same quality and ratio of cancellous and cortical bone but in quantities approaching 100 ml of cancellous bone and a maximum of a 5 × 5-cm cortical block.[17]

The success of endosseous implants placed in iliac crest grafted sites is well documented. In a retrospective study by Misch published in 1994 and updated in 1999, a total of 1364 implants

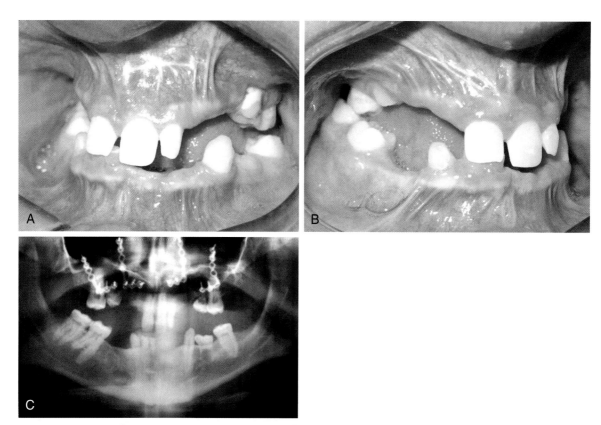

• **Fig. 39.5** Clinical and radiographic images of patient with diffuse atrophic maxillary and mandibular bony areas from multiple congenitally missing teeth. (A) Left lateral image. (B) Right lateral image. (C) Panoramic image.

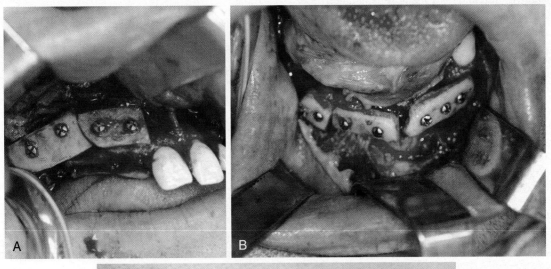

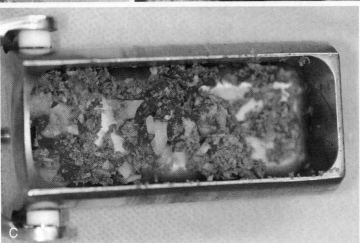

• **Fig. 39.6** (A) Cortical onlay grafts to maxilla. (B) Cortical onlay grafts to mandible. (C) Morselized cortical bone for augmenting areas between grafts.

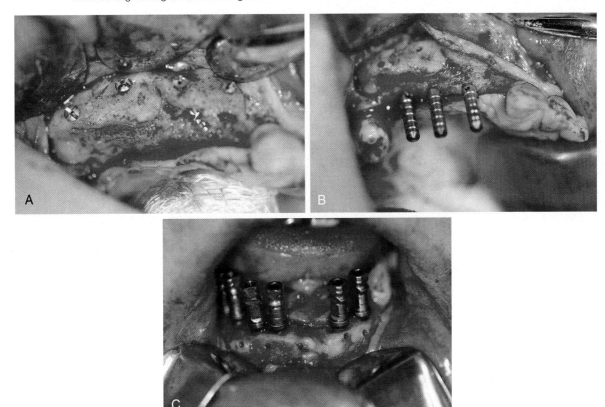

• **Fig. 39.7** (A) Uncovered grafts at 6 months. (B) Placement of maxillary implants. (C) Placement of mandibular implants.

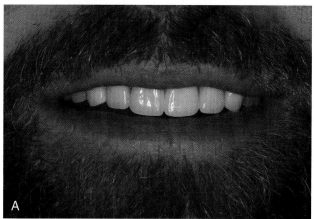

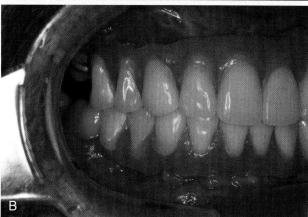

- **Fig. 39.8** (A) Final image, frontal at rest. (b) Final prosthesis.

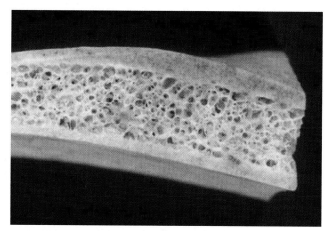

- **Fig. 39.9** Cross section of iliac crest showing inner and outer table of cortical bone with a large area of cellular-rich cancellous bone in between.

TABLE 39.1	Iliac Crest Grafts Study (1984–2005)	
	Patients	**Arches**
Male patients	36	42
Female patients	146	179
Total	182	221

• BOX 39.1 Calvarian Graft: Indications and Advantages

1. Easy access with minimal postoperative pain or morbidity
2. Onlay grafts of primarily cortical bone; can be morselized into particulate graft
3. For vertical and horizontal ridge augmentation of maxilla and mandible
4. Large quantity of bone

• BOX 39.2 Calvarian Graft: Contraindications and Cautions

1. Metabolic bone diseases such as osteopetrosis, osteogenesis imperfecta, Paget disease
2. Radiation to the skull
3. Children under 8 years old
4. Male pattern baldness
5. Previous skull trauma or surgery

---

placed in iliac crest bone grafts (940 maxillary and 424 mandibular) in either an immediate or delayed fashion revealed an overall survival rate of 96.7%[18] (Table 39.1).

The diversity of the iliac crest bone makes it useful not just in large segmental defects but also in routine C–w and C–h defects, which may benefit from the presence of the greater osteogenic potential of the autogenous bone, such as larger unilateral or bilateral sinus lift procedures. As with any bone graft, the success

depends on adherence to basic surgical principles that call for rigid immobilization with screw fixation of the blocks and a rigid basket-type containment membrane (space maintenance) for all cancellous-only grafts, with minimal external pressure throughout the healing period (Box 39.3).

The disadvantages of both the anterior and the posterior iliac crest grafts include the use of a distant site from the oral cavity. This may require the use of two surgical teams or an increased surgical time for a single team with meticulous attention to maintaining separate fields to prevent cross-contamination from the oral cavity. In the case of the posterior iliac crest the surgical time can be doubled because the patient needs to be turned to the prone position for harvest. Contraindications to the use of the anterior or posterior ilium would be the presence of a hip prosthesis to reduce any risk of hardware failure or infection (Box 39.4).

Anatomy and Technique

The surgeon needs to first palpate the anatomic landmarks of the iliac crest, which can be difficult in obese patients, but it is absolutely necessary to prevent damage to local sensory nerves that overlay the anterior ilium. From posterior to anterior the landmarks include the iliohypogastric, the subcostal, and the lateral femoral cutaneous nerves. The iliohypogastric nerve arises from the dorsal rami of L1 and L2 (lumbar vertebrae) and passes directly over the midcrest and is in most cases unavoidable. The subcostal nerve arises from the dorsal ramus of T12 over the edge of the anterior superior spine to innervate the skin of the groin. The lateral femoral cutaneous nerve will also sometimes deviate from its usual course under the inguinal ligament in 2.5% of the population and also pass over the same area of the anterior ilium.[19] Therefore the anterior superior iliac spine (ASIS) is first marked and the crest is then palpated to the widest portion to the iliac tubercle. The incision is then marked 2 cm lateral to the iliac crest and 2 cm posterior to the ASIS to reduce injury to these two important sensory nerves[19,20] (Fig. 39.10).

The subcutaneous tissue and the subperiosteal plane is then infiltrated with local anesthesia and vasoconstrictor. After appropriate prepping and draping, the incision is made through skin down to the superficial abdominal facia or Camper and Scarpa fascia. Once through this fascial layer, the crest is easily palpated and the fibers from the medial external oblique and the lateral tensor fascia lata muscle are separated. A periosteal incision can now be made with electrocautery between these two muscles. Continuing to stay at least 1.5 cm posterior to the ASIS, subperiosteal dissection is performed to obtain access to the crest, as well as the medial wall under the iliacus muscle. Free cancellous bone can then be harvested through cortical windows created through the crest and corticocancellous blocks obtained by further exposure down the medial wall elevating the iliacus muscle. Blocks can be harvested via osteotomies

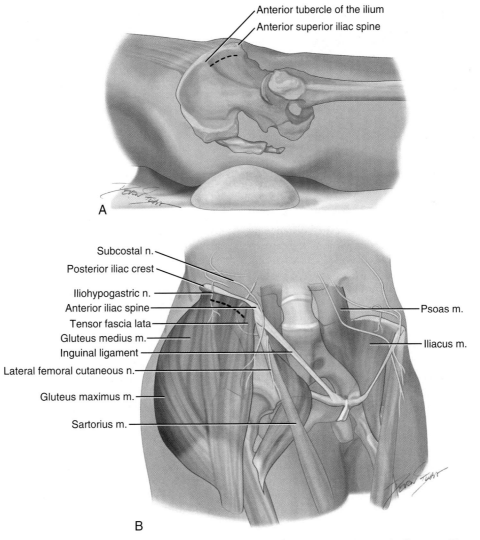

Anterior tubercle of the ilium
Anterior superior iliac spine

A

Subcostal n.
Posterior iliac crest
Iliohypogastric n.
Anterior iliac spine
Tensor fascia lata
Gluteus medius m.
Inguinal ligament
Lateral femoral cutaneous n.
Gluteus maximus m.
Sartorius m.
Psoas m.
Iliacus m.

B

• **Fig. 39.10** (A) Lateral view demonstrating placement of a soft roll to elevate the anterior iliac crest. The incision *(dashed line)* is placed lateral to the crest and posterior to the anterior iliac spine. (B) Anterior view of the anterior iliac crest shows the relationships of the muscular and neural structures as they relate to the proposed incision *(dashed line)*. Although not typically visualized during harvest, the iliohypogastric nerve may be encountered with posterior extension of the incision. (From Kademani D, Tiwana P, eds. *Atlas of Oral & Maxillofacial Surgery.* Philadelphia, PA: Elsevier; 2015.)

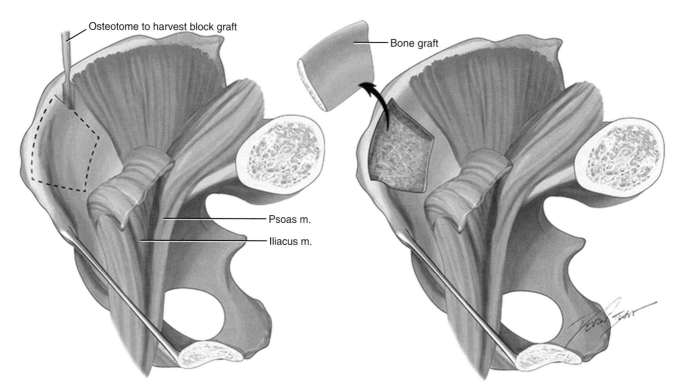

Osteotome to harvest block graft

Bone graft

Psoas m.

Iliacus m.

• **Fig. 39.11** Harvesting of a corticocancellous block from the medial aspect of the anterior ilium after reflection of the iliacus muscle. An osteotome or saw can be used for the corticotomies in the suggested design. After retrieval of the block, the exposed underlying cancellous bone can be harvested using bone curettes and gouges. (From Kademani D, Tiwana P, eds. *Atlas of Oral & Maxillofacial Surgery.* Philadelphia, PA: Elsevier; 2015.)

through the medial wall down to the cancellous layer. A parallel incision is then made to the first cut at a desired distance no more than 4 to 5 cm from the first cuts. Ninety-degree incisions are then made to connect these cuts on the inferior and superior margins. With the use of an osteotome the cortical cancellous blocks are lifted away carefully to not penetrate the posterior wall (Fig. 39.11).

After the block graft has been elevated, additional cancellous bone for augmentation of the graft can be curettaged from the sides and the base of the graft bed. Closure of the periosteum and fascial layers is performed after hemostasis of the bone edges and any soft tissue adjacent to the donor site. Drains are not usually necessary. The use of long-acting local anesthetics can be used to help in postoperative pain control and to encourage early ambulation.

The technique for posterior iliac harvest differs from the anterior iliac in many ways; however, the most obvious way is the prone positioning of the patient. Either before or after exposure of the recipient site, all extraoral or intraoral wounds need to be packed and isolated from contamination while the patient is turned and the graft harvested. Incisions should be first marked beginning at least 1 cm lateral to the posterior superior iliac spine to avoid the sacroiliac ligament and then extended 5 to 6 cm laterally. After local and hemostatic infiltration, an incision is made through skin and taken down to the superior iliac spine. Unlike the anterior technique, grafts are harvested from the lateral cortex

by elevating the gluteal musculature with the superior cut being just below the crest of the ridge to avoid ilium fractures caused by weakening (Fig. 39.12).

In children both the anterior and posterior iliac crests act as ossification sites and not true growth centers. The cartilaginous crest should be kept intact, and any grafts, cortical or cancellous, should be harvested from below this border.

Complications

1. *Seroma.* A common complication surrounding the incision site usually caused by over activity in the early postoperative course. Initial aspiration and placement of drain if it continues to recur.
2. *Bleeding and hematoma.* A stable hematoma can arise from persistent oozing from the harvest bone beds. Hematomas can be prevented with fibrillary collagen packing or bone wax at the bone edges. Normally they will reabsorb. An expanding hematoma caused by an active bleeder is a much more serious situation and, as in pelvic fractures, could result in a large amount of blood loss before its presence is identified. The patient should be treated for any signs of hypovolemic shock, and the wound should be reexplored to identify and control the bleed.
3. *Postoperative paresthesia of the thigh.* Also known as meralgia paresthetica, this is a temporary paresthesia of the distribution of the lateral femoral cutaneous nerve, which could be caused

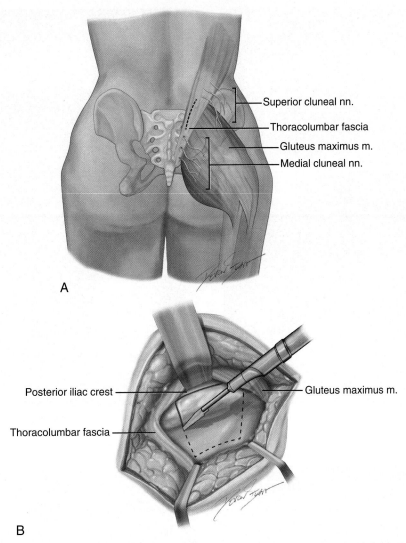

• **Fig. 39.12** (A) Outline demonstrating incision design of posterior iliac crest harvest in relation to superior cluneal and medial cluneal nerves. (B) Outline of osteotomies. (From Kademani D, Tiwana P, eds. *Atlas of Oral & Maxillofacial Surgery.* Philadelphia, PA: Elsevier; 2015.)

by pressure on the nerve from a hematoma of the iliacus muscle at the harvest site of the anterior table or pressure from retraction of the anterior flap. Permanent anesthesia could be the result of a poorly placed incision.

4. *Postoperative pain.* This is helped by long-acting local anesthetics with intravenous (IV) and analgesics by mouth (PO), and aggressive physical therapy to get the patient up and walking.

5. *Abdominal perforation.* This is a very rare occurrence of an anterior table harvest caused by the protection from surrounding musculature. Overweight patients may be at higher risk because anatomy is unclear, and over aggressive use of rotary instruments for bone harvest may exist. An immediate general surgery consult is indicated (see Table 39.1).

Case Study 1: Corticocancellous Morcellized Graft

A 28-year-old female with a history of basal cell nevus syndrome presented with right-sided swelling of her face. CT scan and Panorex revealed a multilocular radiolucent lesion encompassing the body and ascending ramus of the left mandible. Biopsy confirmed the presence of a diffuse spread of an odontogenic keratocyst (Fig. 39.13).

The patient was taken to the operating room for resection of the lesion, which required disarticulation of the condyle and was immediately reconstructed with an anterior iliac crest bone graft through an external facial incision. The corticocancellous blocks were placed in a bone mill and collagen-soaked sponges of BMP were placed into the rigidly fixated bone crib (Fig. 39.14).

At 20 weeks with the CT scan showing good consolidation of bone, the implant fixtures were placed. At 4 months the dental implants (Fig. 39.15) were uncovered and restored. At 5 years the grafted area continued to show good consolidation, continued support for the implant fixtures, and no recurrence of the cystic tumor (Fig. 39.16).

Case Study 2: Corticocancellous Block Grafts

A 53-year-old female with an atrophic maxilla prefers a fixed prosthesis to articulate against a partially dentate mandible, very

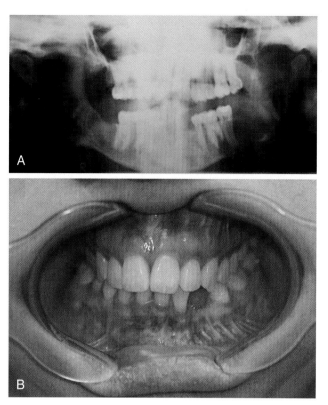

• **Fig. 39.13** (A) Large keratocyst of left mandible. (B) Preresection occlusion.

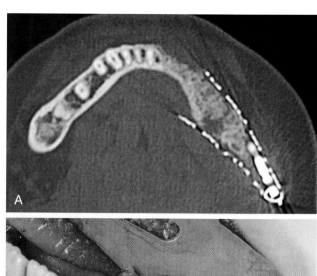

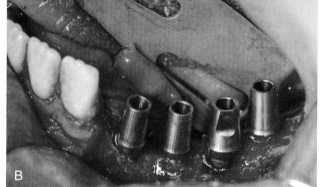

• **Fig. 39.15** (A) Computerized tomography of consolidated graft at 20 weeks. (B) Placement of implant fixtures.

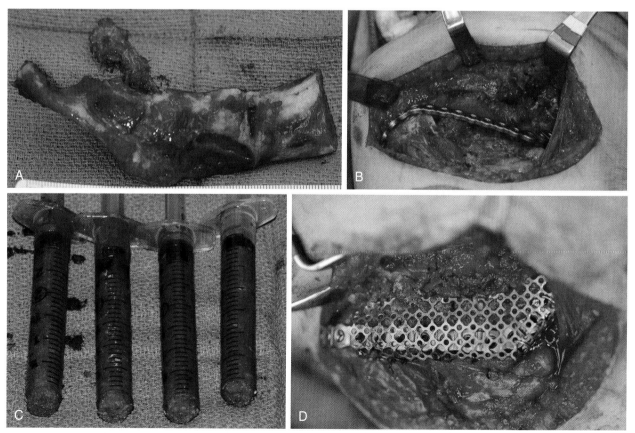

• **Fig. 39.14** (A) Resected specimen. (B) Prefabricated reconstruction plate and condylar prosthesis in place. (C) Morcellized corticocancellous bone in syringes. (D) Bone graft packed into retaining crib.

narrow bone in the anterior, and low-lying sinus floors on the posterior bilaterally (Fig. 39.17).

Corticocancellous strips were then harvested from the inner table of the anterior iliac crest. Bilateral sinus lifts were performed using cancellous bone from the residual harvest bed. The harvested blocks were then cut appropriately and then rigidly fixated as onlay grafts (Fig. 39.18). Additional cancellous bone was used to augment the rigidly fixated grafts, and the surgical site was closed in a tension-free fashion. The bone grafts were allowed to heal and consolidate for 6 months. A full denture prosthesis was fabricated for the patient for the interim period. The site was reopened, the fixating screw removed, and eight implant fixtures were placed (Fig. 39.19). After integration of the implants a fixed hybrid prosthesis was fabricated.

Tibial Bone Graft

The proximal tibial metaphysis provides an excellent source of cancellous bone. The quantity that may be harvested is close to or equal to that of the anterior ilium. The tibial graft has a low complication rate and is technically easy to perform. Comparison of tibial versus iliac crest grafts in secondary alveolar cleft reconstruction showed similar bone densities at 6 months.[21] Tibial bone grafts are most commonly used for maxillary sinus lift procedures and augmentation of existing bone for the placement of implant fixtures.[22] The rather low morbidity and easy surgical access allows skeletally mature adults to have the surgery completed on an outpatient basis. Because of possible damage to developing epiphyseal growth plates, this procedure is not recommended for children or adolescents; however, several authors have reported the safe and successful use of these grafts for alveolar cleft grafting in children.[23]

As with the ilium grafting sites, it is recommended to avoid sites that have had previous surgery with orthopedic hardware or prosthetic joint replacements. It is also prudent to avoid using this procedure on patients that apply large amounts of force to the tibia on a repetitive basis, such as runners and other active athletes.

Anatomy and Technique

After placing support under the leg and rotating it to provide better access, the surgeon marks out a 2- to 3-cm incision site over the skin of the anterolateral aspect of the leg directly over the Gerdy tubercle, which is lateral to the tuberosity. Catone and colleagues[24] described the incision as angled, with its cephalic limit superior and medial to the tibialis anterior muscle origin and extending lateral to the patellar ligament. After incising through the subcutaneous and fascial layers of the iliotibial tract, the periosteum is reflected to expose the cortex of the tibial metaphysis. With the use of an end-cutting bur, a window is cut into the cortex approximately the size of a dime. This cortical layer is very thin and usually is of little use to the graft and is not replaced. Bone curettes are then used to remove the cancellous bone in all directions and down the shaft of the tibia. Careful attention in harvesting in the superior direction is taken so that the joint space is not entered. A thrombin-soaked collagen sponge can then be placed in the donor site for hemostasis, and the wound is closed in layers with the iliotibial tract closed, followed by the skin and subcutaneous tissue (Fig. 39.20).

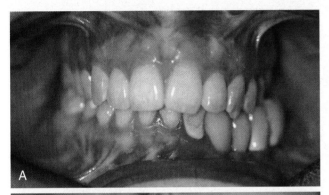

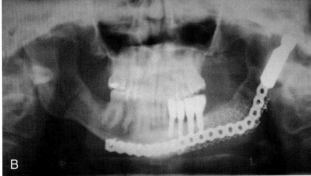

• **Fig. 39.16** (A) Final restored occlusion. (B) Final Panorex of restored segment showing consolidated graft with implants.

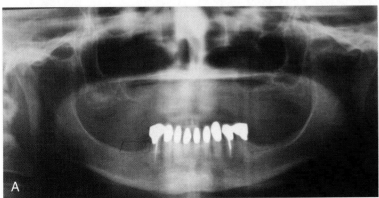

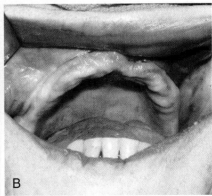

• **Fig. 39.17** (A) Preoperative panoramic image. (B) Clinical photo of atrophic maxillary ridge.

An alternative medial approach has been described[25] with similar soft tissue and bony osteotomies to harvest the donor graft. This approach, however, does not transect the iliotibial tract, resulting in less soft tissue covering the bony donor site and creating the potential for wound breakdown after closure (Box 39.5).

Postoperatively the patient can bear weight as tolerated with no vigorous physical activity for 6 weeks. Local wound care with periodic elevation of the site to prevent swelling is recommended. Routine analgesia of hydrocodone or acetaminophen is usually adequate.

Complications

1. *Ankle swelling.* Swelling and ecchymosis is caused by the natural lymphatic drainage system of the lower leg. In most cases, this will spontaneously resolve.
2. *Knee joint entrance or tibia fracture.* This is caused by over aggressive harvesting of bone in a superior direction. Initial treatment would be splinting of the leg with staphylococcal antibiotic coverage, followed by orthopedic surgical consult (Box 39.6).

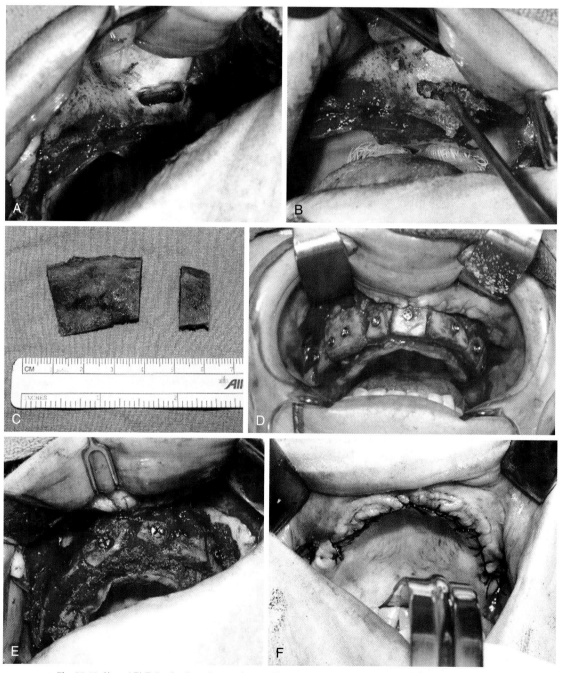

• **Fig. 39.18** (A and B) Full reflection of posterior maxilla, osteotomy, and bone grafting of the sinus floor. (C) Bone block harvested from iliac crest. (D) Segmented bone blocks fixated to maxilla. (E) Cancellous bone packed around cortical grafts. (F) Final closure.

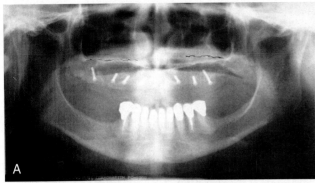

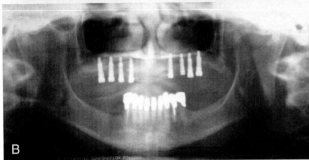

• **Fig. 39.19** (A) Panorex at 6 months before implant placement. (B) Final position of implants.

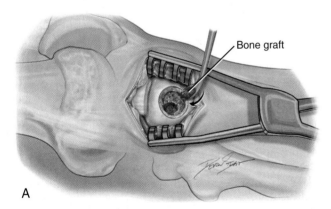

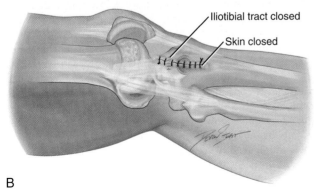

• **Fig. 39.20** (A) Exposed osteotomy over the Gerdy tubercle and curettage of underlying bone. (B) Layered closure of incision (delete 123–1) caption. (From Kademani D, Tiwana P, eds. *Atlas of Oral & Maxillofacial Surgery.* Philadelphia, PA: Elsevier; 2015.)

• BOX 39.5 Tibial Graft: Advantages and Indications

1. Cancellous grafts of 25–40 cc
2. Sinus grafts
3. Socket grafts and ridge preservation
4. Minimal postoperative pain
5. Outpatient procedure.

• BOX 39.6 Tibia Graft: Disadvantages and Cautions

1. Contraindicated in metabolic bone disease, history of knee surgery or osteomyelitis
2. Caution in growing child, rheumatoid arthritis, or bisphosphonate history

---

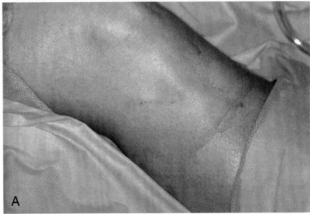

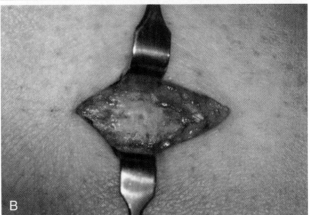

• **Fig. 39.21** (A) Incision design over tubercle. (B) Exposure of underlying cortex.

Case Study

A 56-year-old female presented with large edentulous maxillary posterior space for implant reconstruction. A low-lying sinus floor precluded implant placement without sinus grafting. The patient was given an IV deep sedation, and the intraoral and right knee sites were prepped and draped and kept isolated from each other throughout the procedure. A 4-cm incision was designed and infiltrated with local anesthesia just blow the Gerdy tubercle on the right leg (Fig. 39.21).

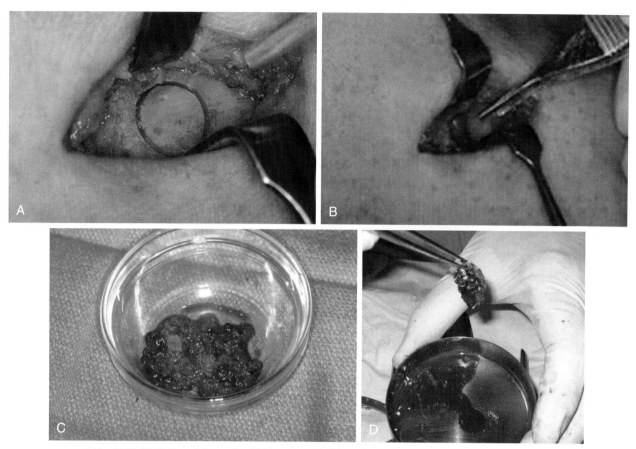

• **Fig. 39.22** (A) Outline of donor site. (B) Bone harvested from donor site. (C) Preparation of with platelet-rich plasma (PRP). (D) Donor bone mixed with PRP.

The anterior wall of the tibial plateau was exposed and hemostasis obtained. With the use of a small round bur a circular bone incision was made and the thin cortical cap removed. Then, 24 cc of cancellous bone was curetted out of the site and mixed with strips of platelet-rich fibrin and packed into the sinus floor bed. Enough supportive bone was available to place immediate implants at the time of surgery (Figs. 39.22 and 39.23).

Vascularized Composite Graft: The Fibula

As mentioned previously, when the bed for a bone graft is compromised by radiation therapy, lack of blood supply, extensive length of the defect, or just the compromised medical condition of the patient, a vascularized composite graft may be indicated. These grafts differ from the free autogenous grafts because they do not depend on the recipient's local environment to aid in the regeneration and consolidation of new bone. These composite grafts bring their own blood supply with them and maintain normal physiologic function within all of the transferred tissues. This will include a certain amount of soft tissue that helps to cover and protect these bone grafts in compromised receptor sites. The downside of these grafts is the increased procedure time and the sometimes unavailable expertise of a microvascular surgeon. Technical complications include larger defects at the donor sites and the inability of the surgeon to construct a bony bed that is any different from the anatomic dimensions of the grafted bone. In the past, this bone stock, while providing excellent reconstruction of the continuity defect, did not always provide the best base for an implant-supported prosthesis. As the reconstructive surgeon and implantologist worked together over the years and realized the limitations of both, most of these problems have been resolved. These advances in cooperation between the surgeon and the implantologist is no better evidenced than in the emergence of the computer-aided design (CAD)/computer-aided manufacturing (CAM) technology, producing three-dimensional models for both the harvest and the implant placement, which has decreased treatment time from months to days.

Since the composite bone grafts were introduced in the late 1970s many donor sites have been recommended. In 1989 Hidalgo introduced the osteocutaneous fibula free flap for use in mandibular reconstruction, with 12 cases measuring defects averaging 13.5 cm.[26] Since then the fibula free flap has become the gold standard for reconstruction of large mandibular defects because of its consistency in size, its vascular pedicle length, and its ability to provide a reliable skin paddle with the bone flap. Its segmental blood supply also allows for in situ osteotomies, which aids in better anatomic reconstruction (Box 39.7).

Regarding quality of bone for osseointegration, Frodel and Moscoso, in two separate studies, compared the bone stock and thickness as it relates to the placement of endosseous implants in the four commonly used vascularized donor sites: the iliac crest, scapula, fibula, and radius. Although the iliac crest was found to have greater amount of bone stock, the results did not achieve statistical significance and the testing relied mostly on clinical observation.[27,28]

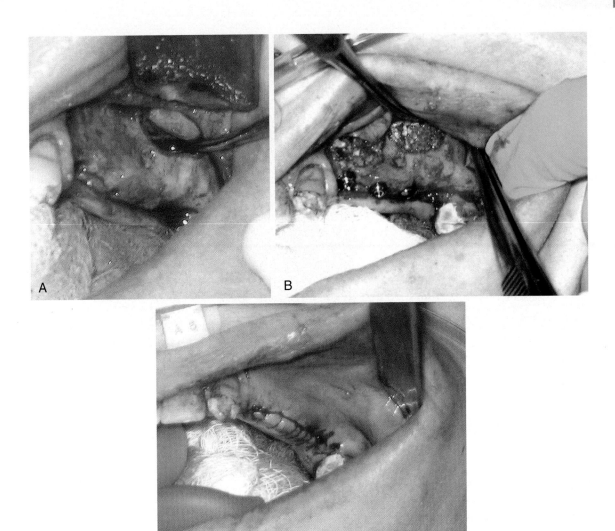

• **Fig. 39.23** (A) Maxillary sinus prepared for graft. (B) Lateral wall sinus augmentation. (C) Final wound closure.

• **BOX 39.7** **Vascularized Composite Graft: Advantages and Indications**

1. Reconstruction defects with poor tissue vascularity and questionable soft tissue coverage
2. Reconstruction of defects larger than 6 cm
3. Postcancer reconstruction with provision of protective skin paddle
4. Can withstand postsurgical radiation
5. Failed large free bone grafted segments
6. Can withstand immediate placement of dental implants

The first histologic study of the bone implant interface in a human vascularized graft was reported by Dattilo and colleagues in 1995.[29] This study showed that although the implant had successfully integrated into the iliac crest grafted bone and was clinically stable, the surrounding bone resembled the fine trabecular pattern of D4 density most commonly found in areas of the posterior maxilla (Fig. 39.24A). Sumi and coworkers in 2001 published a similar study using fibula graft and found the interface and surrounding bone to be more dense and cortical,

resembling the D1 and D2 of the anterior native mandible[30] (see Fig. 39.24B–C). This amount of bone density that has been shown to increase the stability and longevity of implants gives the fibula another distinct advantage over the other composite grafts (Box 39.8).

Anatomy and Technique

A detailed description of the surgical approach and harvest of this graft is beyond the scope of this chapter. However, a basic knowledge of the anatomic contents and its harvest is important for the implant surgeon to know, as well as the limitations and benefits of its use. The graft is harvested via a lateral approach through the intermuscular septum of the peroneus longus and peroneus brevis muscles. Dissection is taken to the anterior compartment for dissection of the vascular pedicle. The composite graft is based off the peroneal artery, which is a branch of the popliteal artery Fig. 39.26. During this dissection of the feeding vasculature, the anterior tibial artery and the deep peroneal nerve need to be identified and retracted medially to prevent injury. The diameter of the peroneal artery is 1 to 2.5 mm and matches well with the facial artery and vein, which are the most common vessels used for anastomosis in the receptive bed

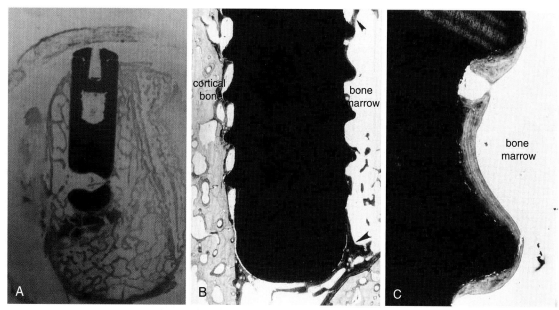

• **Fig. 39.24** (A) Implant interface with iliac crest composite graft with the fine trabecular pattern of predominantly cancellous bone. (B) Implant interface with fibula graft with dense cortical bone on left cortex side and fine cortical interface on marrow side. (C) Closeup of cortical bone formation on marrow side with no intervening fibrous tissue. (A, From Dattilo D, et al. Interface analysis of hydroxyapatite-coated implants in a human vascularized iliac bone graft. *Int J Oral Maxillofac Implants.* 1995;10(4):405–409. B and C, From Sumi Y, Hasewaga T, Osamu M, et al. Interface analysis of titanium implants in a human vascularized fibula bone graft. *J Oral Maxillofacial Surg.* 2001;59(2):213–216.)

• **BOX 39.8** Vascularized Composite Graft: Disadvantages and Cautions

1. Contraindicated if previous femoral artery graft in place
2. Previous fracture
3. Caution in metabolic bone disease

---

region. Of maximum importance is the careful dissection of the eight perforating vessels along the fibula, which are most commonly located along the junction of the middle third and distal third of the fibula. The vascularized bone is accompanied by portions of the peroneus longus, peroneus brevis, and the tibialis posterior muscle. The composition of the graft can change, however, depending on the position of perforating vessels to the skin and musculature (Fig. 39.25). Dissection down to the fibula and subsequent resection is performed while the vascular pedicle is still intact. The available fibula can have a width between 1.0 and 3.0 cm and a length of up to 26 cm; however, at least 5.0 to 8.0 cm is needed to be left on the superior and inferior portion to maintain stability to the ankle and knee joint. It is at this point that CAD/CAM-generated cutting guides can be used to perform the initial resection and subsequent segmental osteotomies using the rich blood supply to this graft.[31] Custom-generated plates also can be placed at this time, as well as placement of endosseous dental implants, before separating the blood supply (Fig. 39.26).

Only after all of this is completed will the microvascular surgeon resect the peroneal artery and venous complex and reapproximate it up to the receptor bed in the upper or lower jaw. A prefabricated plate, also generated from the custom CAD/CAM models, can now rigidly fixate the composite graft in place.

Complications

1. *Thrombosis of the arterial (pale flap) and venous (blue flap).* This will result in necrosis of the flap if local measures or the reanastomosis procedure fails.
2. *Wound Infection.* Treat this with antibiotics and local wound care.
3. *Compartment syndrome.* This is rare but serious. It is caused by internal pressure on donor site tissue. Immediate surgical intervention is indicated.

Case Study 1: Fibula Reconstruction with Immediate Placement and Loading of Implants

A 34-year-old male with a multiloculated lesion of the anterior mandible extending from #18 to #29 with tissue diagnosis of ameloblastoma (Fig. 39.27). Virtual surgical planning (VSP) using CAD/CAM images to fabricate surgical cutting guides, custom rigid fixation plates, and custom models were used to determine implant placement and positioning for immediate placement of interim prosthesis. At surgery, custom cutting guides were used for resection of the tumor at predetermined positions (Fig. 39.28). At surgery the pedicle flap was exposed through the lateral approach and the fibula was osteotomized at the specific length needed using cutting cones provided by virtual planning models. Guides also were provided by the virtual planning models (Fig. 39.29). Because of the unique segmental blood supply of the fibula, separate osteotomies could be made to form the necessary curvature as dictated by the presurgical models. The implants are placed and the custom plate is fastened to the graft before the in situ graft is released from the peroneal vascular blood supply. The peroneal vein and artery is then released and reanastomosed to the facial artery and vein near the reception site of the graft after the anterior segment is rigidly fixated to the right and left proximal segments of the mandible. The interim denture is then fixated to the

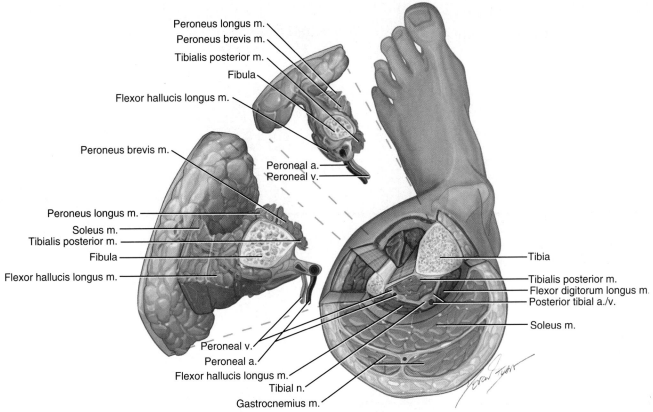

Peroneus longus m.
Peroneus brevis m.
Tibialis posterior m.
Fibula
Flexor hallucis longus m.

Peroneus brevis m.

Peroneal a.
Peroneal v.

Peroneus longus m.
Soleus m.
Tibialis posterior m.
Fibula
Flexor hallucis longus m.

Tibia
Tibialis posterior m.
Flexor digitorum longus m.
Posterior tibial a./v.

Soleus m.

Peroneal v.
Peroneal a.
Flexor hallucis longus m.
Tibial n.
Gastrocnemius m.

• **Fig. 39.25** Cross-sectional anatomy of the leg showing two possible sizes of osteocutaneous grafts. The upper smaller graft has septocutaneous vascular perforators running through the crural septum between the peroneus longus and brevis muscles and gastrocnemius muscles. The larger graft is necessitated when the perforators are identified partially through the flexor hallucis longus muscle requiring harvesting of parts of this muscle. (From Kademani D, Tiwana P, eds. *Atlas of Oral & Maxillofacial Surgery.* Philadelphia, PA: Elsevier; 2015.)

transoral implants. Implants placed in the bicortical vascularized graft routinely measure greater than 35 ncm of torque to allow placement of immediate prostheses (Figs. 39.30–39.33).

Case Study 2: Double-Barrel Fibula Graft with Immediate Placement of Implants

The double-barrel technique is used to increase the height of the reconstructed mandible. This is a 52-year-old male with a pathologic fracture of the mandible caused by osteoradionecrosis (Fig. 39.34). The wide excision of the necrotic bone was planned and the guides were fabricated to complete the graft and the implants in one surgery.

The custom plate and the fibula models were used to first resect the bone at the proper dimension and also to osteotomize the fibula in situ at the proper length. The dental implants were placed with guides into the upper segment before detaching the graft from the peroneal blood supply (Fig. 39.35). The graft is brought up to the jaw and folded on itself, maintaining the blood supply to double the height. The inferior segment is secured to the custom plate to reapproximate the natural contour of the jaw, and the upper segment has more freedom to be rotated and secured in a position that is best suited for a good functional occlusion (Fig. 39.36).

Finally both segments are secured and covered with portions of the soft tissue pedicle to secure its survival. The implants are uncovered in 4 months and restored. Sometimes it is necessary to debulk thick intraoral soft tissue pedicles and perform grafted vestibuloplasties to create a more healthy, soft tissue environment around the implants (Fig. 39.37).

Summary

The revolution in oral reconstruction brought about by the introduction of dental implants has revived the art and science of bone regeneration and grafting in dentistry. From the reconstruction of major jaw deformities to the augmentation of the smallest defect around a single tooth a bone graft is almost always considered to improve the environment of an implant fixture and help ensure its longevity.

The autogenous bone from the donor sites described in this chapter provide the three major qualities of a successful graft: osteoconduction, osteoinduction, and osteogenesis. The transfer of viable primitive mesenchymal and osteoblastic cells, as well as the growth factors (BMP) place the autogenous bone graft well above any of the allografts yet developed. Pain, deformity, and complications at the harvesting site are the

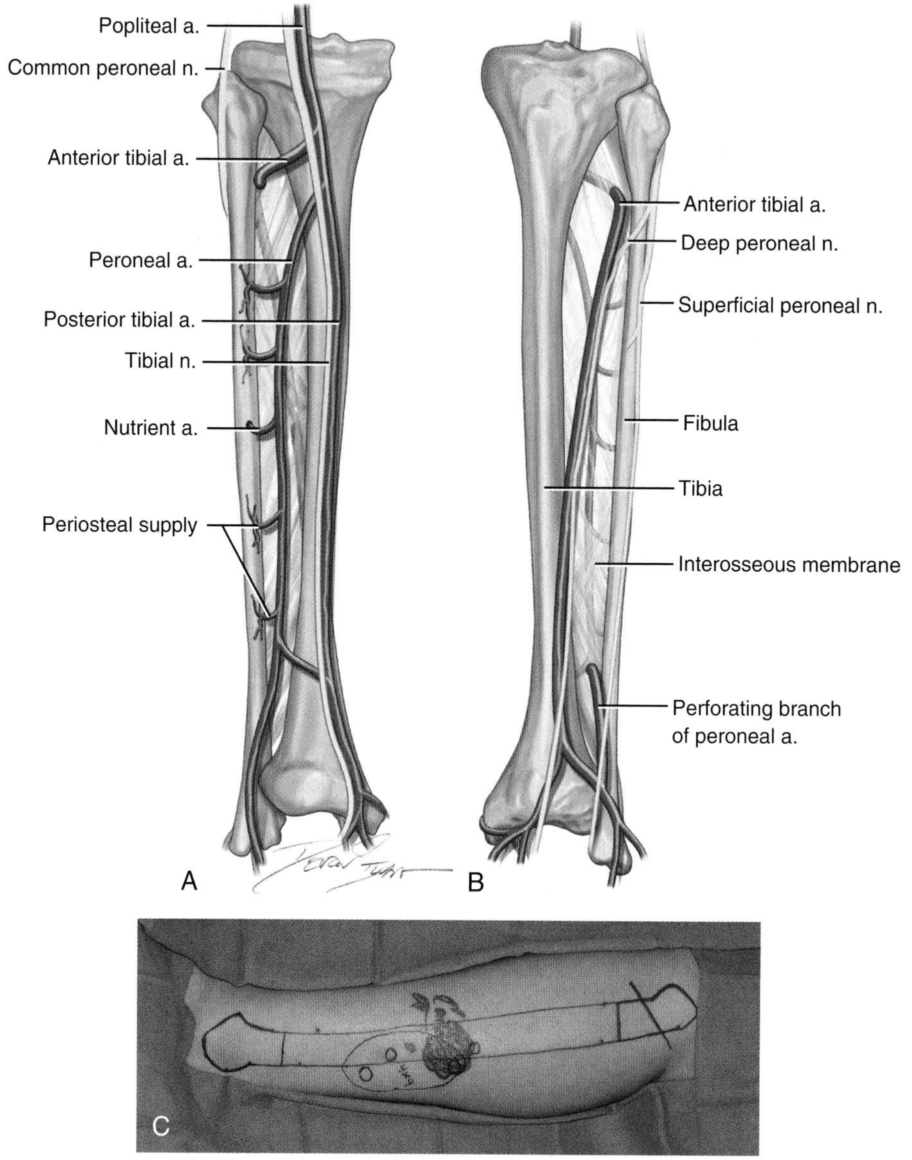

• **Fig. 39.26** (A) Anterior view of left leg. The common peroneal nerve crosses the fibular neck, dividing into the superficial and deep peroneal nerves. The anterior tibial vessel descends with the deep peroneal nerve along the anterior medial aspect of the interosseous membrane. The distal aspect of the peroneal artery passes through the interosseous membrane into the anterior compartment. (B) Posterior view of left leg. The popliteal artery branches into the anterior tibial artery, which branches into the anterior tibial artery and the posterior tibial artery, which branches into the peroneal artery, which provides the blood supply to the fibula through a nutrient artery and numerous periosteal vessels. (C) Fibula illustrated with 6 cm marked from the fibular head and lateral malleolus. Peroneal nerve illustrated inferior to the fibular head. Perforators marked in circles and a 4 × 9-cm skin paddle is drawn out (Courtesy of Fayette Williams DDS, MD.). (From Kademani D, Tiwana P, eds. *Atlas of Oral & Maxillofacial Surgery.* Philadelphia, PA: Elsevier; 2015.)

usual arguments for using alloplastic or nonautogenous substances as replacements. In a report published in 2005 a group of renowned craniofacial surgeons presented a survey of their combined 25-year experience with cranial, tibial, crest, and rib grafts. In 20,000 cases reviewed, less than 1% of complications were noted in any one area of bone harvest. The authors' conclusions were that the often heard statement that an alloplastic material was used to "spare the patient the added time and complications of harvesting and autogenous graft" is, in fact, not a reasonable argument for a well-trained surgeon and may

actually cause a failure or a compromised result at the reconstructed site.[32]

VSP will no doubt be a strong influence in the future of extraoral autogenous grafting for the implant patient. From the fabrication of custom cutting guides for resection, harvesting, and placement of larger grafts to the fabrication of immediate implant-borne prosthesis, these new computerized technologies will continue to promote and maintain the extraoral autogenous bone graft as the gold standard of dental implant reconstruction.

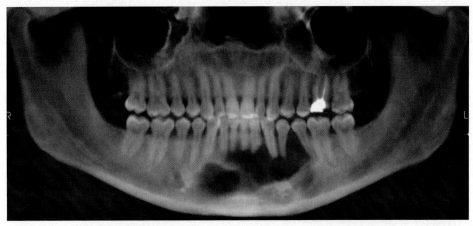

• **Fig. 39.27** Panorex showing radiolucency involving anterior mandible and dentition. (Courtesy of Fayette Williams DDS, MD.)

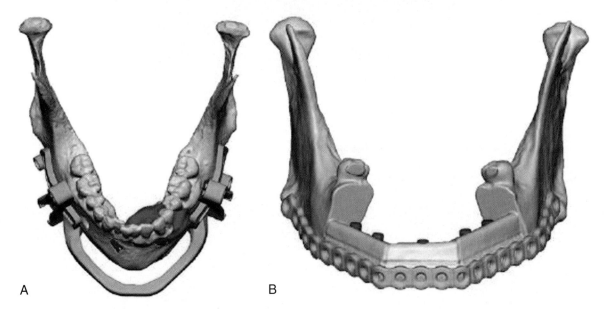

A   B

• **Fig. 39.28** (A) Computer-aided design (CAD)/computer-aided manufacturing (CAM) images of a cutting guide for resection of tumor and (B) custom reconstruction plate and guide for implant placement. (Courtesy of Fayette Williams DDS, MD.)

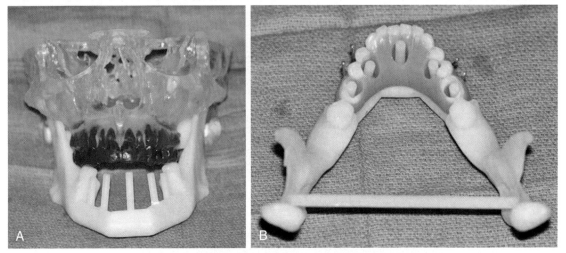

• **Fig. 39.29** (A and B) Computer-aided design (CAD)/computer-aided manufacturing (CAM) generated models for fabrication of immediate prosthesis. (Courtesy of Fayette Williams DDS, MD.)

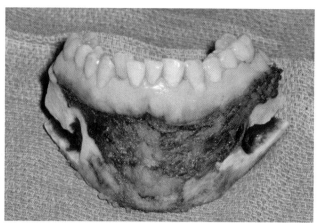

• **Fig. 39.30** Surgical specimen of anterior mandible. (Courtesy of Fayette Williams DDS, MD.)

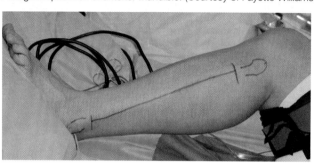

• **Fig. 39.31** Incision designed on the lateral left leg over the intermuscular septum between the soleus and peroneus longus muscle. (Courtesy of Fayette Williams DDS, MD.)

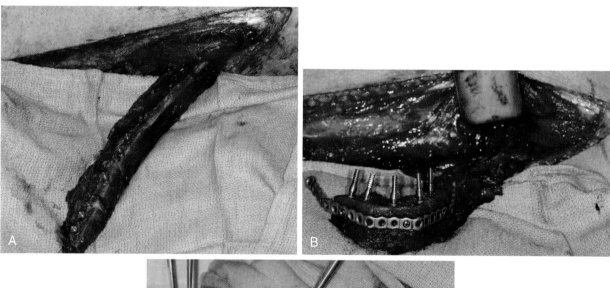

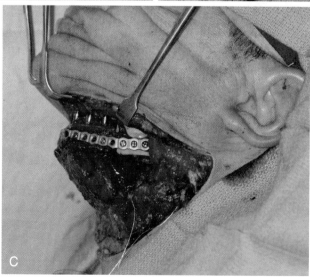

• **Fig. 39.32** (A) segmental osteotomies and dental implant placement of the graft in situ (Courtesy of Fayette Williams DDS, MD). (B) Custom plate used to shape graft for placement (Courtesy of Fayette Williams DDS, MD). (C) Graft placed and fixated to mandible and reanastomosis of vessels begins (Courtesy of Fayette Williams DDS, MD).

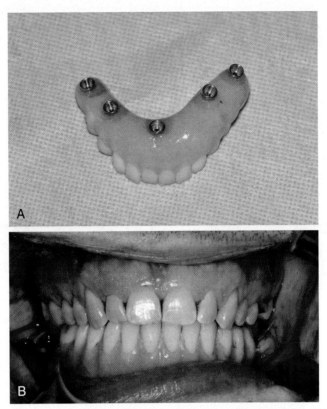

• **Fig. 39.33** (A) Prefabricated custom prosthesis from Computer-aided design (CAD)/computer-aided manufacturing (CAM) models (Courtesy of Fayette Williams DDS, MD). (B) Final occlusion before leaving the operating room (Courtesy of Fayette Williams DDS, MD).

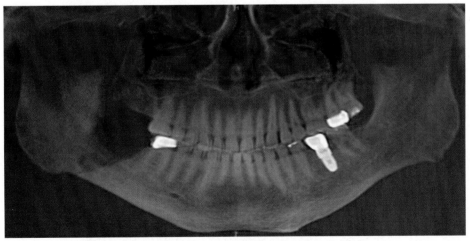

• **Fig. 39.34** Panorex of pathologic fracture (Courtesy of Fayette Williams DDS, MD).

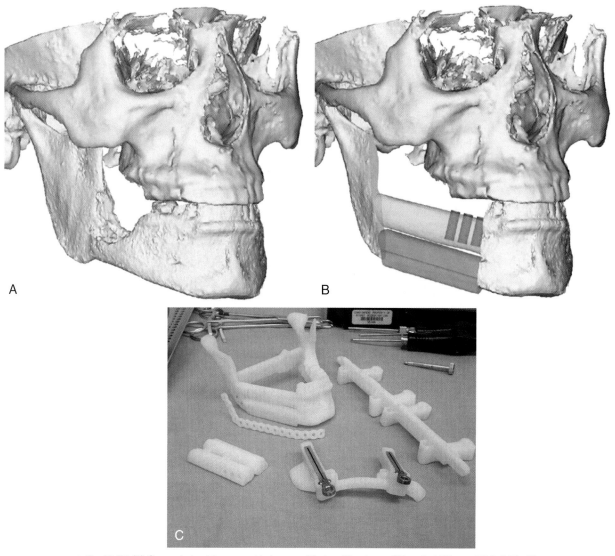

• **Fig. 39.35** (A) Computerized tomographic image of lesion (Courtesy of Fayette Williams DDS, MD). (B) Virtual Surgical image of extent of resection and planned folded fibula graft (Courtesy of Fayette Williams DDS, MD). (C) Computer-aided design (CAD)/computer-aided manufacturing (CAM) (Courtesy of Fayette Williams DDS, MD).

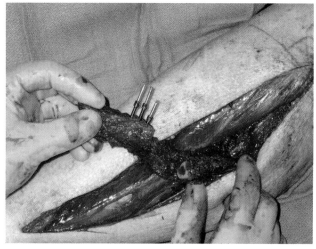

• **Fig. 39.36** Fibula graft osteotomized in half in situ with dental implants place in superior portion.

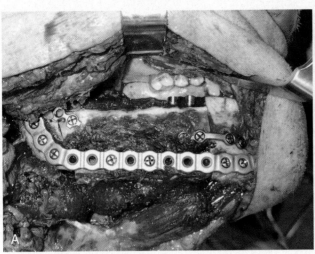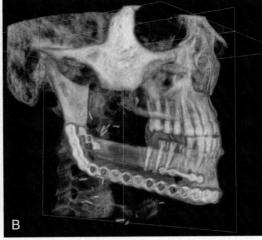

• **Fig. 39.37** (A) Double layered fibula secured with custom reconstruction plate and superior portion with smaller position plates (Courtesy of Fayette Williams DDS, MD). (B) Six-week computerized tomography scan to check position. (Courtesy of Fayette Williams DDS, MD.)

References

1. Misch CE. Divisions of available bone in implant dentistry. *Int J Oral Implantol.* 1990;7:9–17.
2. Misch CE. Prosthetic options in implant dentistry. *Int J Oal Implantol.* 1991;7:17–21.
3. Shugaa-Addin B, Al-Shamiri HM, Al-Maweri S, Tarakji B. The effect of radiotherapy on survival of dental implants in head and neck cancer patients. *J Clin Exp Dent.* 2016;8(2):e194.
4. Smith JD, Abramson M. Membranous vs endochondral bone autografts. *Arch Otolaryngol.* 1974;99:203–205.
5. Zins JE, Whitaker LA. Membranous versus endochondral bone: Implications for craniofacial reconstruction. *Plas Reconstr Surg.* 1983.
6. Kusiak JF, Zins JE, Whitaker A. The early revascularization of membranous bone. *J Plas Reconstr Surg.* 1985.
7. Oppenheimer AJ, Ton L, Buchman SR. Craniofacial bone grafting: wolff's law revisited, craniomaxillofac. *Trauma Reconstr.* 2008;1:49.
8. Tessier P, Kawamoto H, Matthews D, et al. Autogenous bone grafts and bone substitutes: tools and techniques. A 20,000 case experience in maxillofacial and craniofacial surgery. *Plast Reconstr Surg.* 2005;116:6s.
9. Wang J, Waite D, Steinhauser E. Ridge augmentation: and evaluation and follow-up report. *J oral Surg.* 1976;34:66–602.
10. Curtis T, Ware W, Beirne OR, et al. Autogenous bone grafts for atrophic edentulous mandibles, a final report. *J Prosthet Dent.* 1987;57:73–78.
11. Verhoeven JDW, Cune MS, Teriou M, et al. The combined use of endosteal implants and iliac crest onlay grafts in the severely atrophic mandible: a longitudinal study. *Int J Oral Maxillofac Surg.* 1997;26:351–357.
12. MalchiodiL QA, D'Addona A, et al. Jaw reconstruction with grafted autologous bone:early insertion of osseointegrated implants and early prosthetic loading. *J Oral Maxillofac Surg.* 2006;64:1190–1198.
13. Tessier P. Autogenous bone grafts taken from the calvarium for facial and cranial applications. *Clin Plast Surg.* 1882;9:531.
14. Koenig WJ, Donovan JM, Pensler JM. Cranial bone grafting in children. *Plast Reconstr Surg.* 1995;95:1–4.
15. Fearson JA. A magnetic resonance imaging investigation of potential subclinical complications after in situ cranial bone graft harvest. *Plast Reconstr Surg.* 2000;105:1935–1939.
16. Moreira-Gonzalez A, Papay FE, Zins JE. Calvarial thickness and its relation to cranial bone harvest. *Plast Reconstr Surg.* 2006;117:1964.
17. Zouhary KJ. Bone grafting from distant sites: concepts and techniques. *Oral Maxillofac Surg Clin North Am.* 2010;22:301.
18. Misch CE. Extraoral autogenous donor bone grafts for endosteal implants. In: Misch CE, ed. *Contemporary Implant Dentistry.* 2nd ed. St Louis: Mosby; 1999.
19. Mischkowski RA, Selbach I, Neugebauer J, et al. Lateral femoral cutaneous nerve and iliac crest bone grafts: anatomical and clinical considerations. *Int J Oral Maxillofac Surg.* 2006;35:366.
20. Kademani D, Keller E. Iliac crest grafting for mandibular reconstruction. *Atlas Oral Maxillofac Surg Clin North Am.* 2006;14:161.
21. Sivarajasingam V, Fell G, Morse M, Shepaherd JP. Secondary bone grafting of alvelarclefts: a densitometric comparison of iliac crest and tibial bone grafts. *Cleft Palate Craniofac J.* 2001;38:11–14.
22. Peysakhov D, Ferneini EM, Bevilacqua RG. Maxillary sinus augmentation with autogenous tibial bone graft as an in office procedure. *J Oral Implantol.* 2012;38:50.
23. Walker TW, Modayil PC, Cascarini L, et al. Retrospective review of donor site complications after harvest of cancellous bone from the anteriomedial tibia. *Br J Oral Maxillofac Surg.* 2009;47:20.
24. Catone GA, Reimer BL, McNeir D, Ray R. Tibial autogenous cancellous bone as an alternative donor site in maxillofacial surgery: a preliminary report. *J Oral Maxillofac Surg.* 1992;50:1258.
25. Herford AS, King BJ, Becktor J. Medial approach for tibial bone graft: anatomic study and clinical technique. *J Oral Maxillofac Surg.* 2003;61:358.
26. Hidalgo DA. Fibula free flap: a new method of mandibular reconstruction. *Plast Reconstr Surg.* 1989;84(1):71.
27. Frodel JL, Funk GF, Capper DT, et al. Osseointegrated implants: a comparative study of bone thickness in four vascularized bone flaps. *Plast Recontruc Surg.* 1993;92:449–455.
28. Moscoso JF, Keller J, Genden E. Vascularized bone flaps in oromandibular reconstruction. *Arch Otolaryngol Head Neck Surg.* 1994;120:36–43.
29. Dattilo DJ, Misch CM, Arena S. Interface analysis of hydroxyapatite-coated implants in a human vascularized iliac bone graft. *Int J Oral Maxillofac Implants.* 1995;10:405–409.
30. Sumi Y, Hasegawa T, Miyaishi O, Ueda M. Interface analysis of titanium implants in human vascularized fibula bone graft. *J Oral Maxillofac Surg.* 2001;59:213–216.
31. Tepper O, Hirsch D, Levine J, Garfein E. The new age of three-dimensional virtual surgical planning in reconstructive plastic surgery plastic a reconstructive. *Surgery.* 2012.
32. Tessier P, Kawamoto H, Posnick J, Raulo Y, Tulasne F, Wolfe SA. Complications of harvesting autogenous bone grafts: a group experience of 20,000 cases. *Plast Reconsr Surg.* 2005;116:5.

40

The Use of Botox and Dermal Fillers in Oral Implantology

RANDOLPH R. RESNIK AND AMANDA M. SHEEHAN

The field of oral implantology is constantly changing because of the advances in technology and science. With a better understanding of the dynamic relationships of the soft tissues surrounding the orofacial complex, the use of injectable botulinum toxins (BTXs) and dermal fillers has become an integral part of dentistry. With respect to oral implantology, dental implant clinicians are in a unique position to evaluate and treat patients with these products. These pharmacologic agents may be used to control parafunctional habits, help restore function, relieve pain, and supplement facial esthetics in conjunction with implant prosthetic procedures. Currently, the two most popular treatments used in conjunction with oral implantology procedures include the use of injectable neurotoxins (BTX) and injectable dermal fillers (hyaluronic acid).

Injectable Neurotoxin (Botulinum Toxin)

Botulinum toxin, first used in humans in the 1970s, has become very popular in dentistry. In 2002 Botox was approved in the United States for cosmetic treatment and for the treatment of excessive forces from hyperfunctional muscle activity. There exist eight different serotypes of BTX (i.e., designated as A to H), with some being purified for therapeutic injections into hyperactive muscles. Today, botulinum toxin type A (BTX-A; purified isolate from fermentation of the bacterium *Clostridium botulinum*) is the most potent and widely used serotype in clinical practice. BTX-A is a stable compound that is present in a vacuum-dried powder that currently is marketed under three different brand names: Botox, Dysport, and Xeomin. They all contain the same active ingredient of BTX-A; however, they differ in their formulation: onabotulinum toxin A (Botox), abobotulinum toxin A (Dysport), and incobotulinumtoxin A (Xeomin).

Mechanism of Action

In general, BTX-A blocks the neuromuscular transmission by inhibiting the release of acetylcholine from motor nerve terminals, which results in a reduction of muscle contractions. Acetylcholine is a neurotransmitter that is responsible for muscle contractions. The muscle inhibition occurs in multiple steps (binding, internalization, translocation, and cleavage) by BTX-A cleaving to a protein (SNAP-25), which is an integral part of acetylcholine docking and release from vesicles in the nerve endings. When injected intramuscularly, BTX-A produces a chemical denervation of the muscle, which results in a reduction of muscle activity (Fig. 40.1).[1]

The effects of the botulinum neurotoxins are temporary because the nerve terminals will recover back to their normal function. Initially axonal sprouts arise from the affected nerve in response to growth factors from the inactive muscle. The axonal sprouts form new immature synapses to the injected muscle, which allows neuromuscular transmission to return to normal.

How Supplied and Preparation

In the United States BTX-A is manufactured as a purified neurotoxin complex supplied as a white powder in sterile glass vials. Each vial contains either 50, 100, and 200 units (U) of BTX-A, with an expiration date of 2 years when stored properly at –5°C to –20°C. The BTX-A vial should always be refrigerated until use. Because of its powder form, the BTX-A must be reconstituted with 0.9% NaCl sterile saline solution. Most commonly, BTX-A is supplied in a 100-U vial that is usually diluted with 2 or 4 mL of saline, which results in a 5.0/2.5-U BTX-A per 0.1 mL solution. Commonly the dilution is dictated by the muscle or region being treated, or by the clinician's preference. Usually a 1.0-mL tuberculin syringe with a 26- to 30-gauge needle is used to draw up the required solution for administration.[2] Once opened and reconstituted, the solution must be used within 24 hours because the BTX-A and diluent contain no preservatives. The solution should be stored in a refrigerator at 2°C to 8°C (36°F–46°F). If preservatives are used, the shelf-life is significantly increased. Hexsel et al.[3] have shown that refrigerated, reconstituted BXT-A can be used for up to 6 weeks without loss of efficacy (Table 40.1 and Fig. 40.2).

Generalized Botulinum Toxin Type A Injection Technique/Dose

In general, injections should be made perpendicular to the skin surface and intramuscularly into the belly of the muscle. However, in some situations a more customized injection pattern may be required.

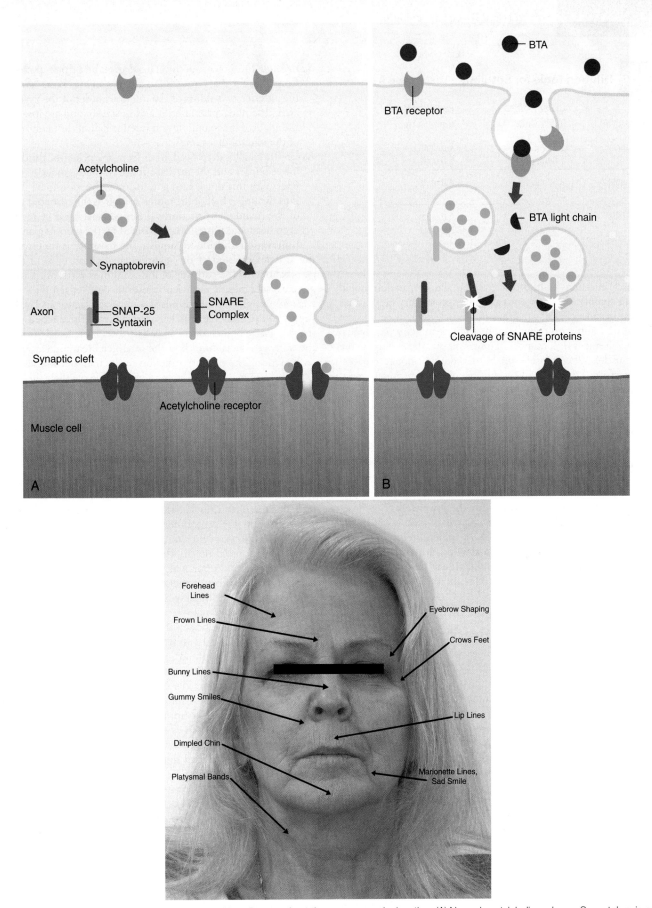

• **Fig. 40.1** (A and B) Diagram depicting the action of botulinum toxin at the neuromuscular junction. (A) Normal acetylcholine release. Synaptobrevin and VAMP-2 (not shown) on the surface of the vesicle containing acetylcholine joins with SNAP-25 and syntaxin on the internal axonal surface. This forms a complex that allows fusion of the vesicle with the membrane to release acetylcholine into the synaptic cleft. Acetylcholine binds to its receptor on the surface of the muscle cell, opening voltage-gated sodium channels that result in membrane depolarization. (B) Action of botulinum toxin. Botulinum toxin type A (BTA) is internalized by the axon when bound by its receptor on the cell surface. The light chain of the toxin is taken up and cleaves the SNARE proteins before the acetylcholine vesicles can bind. The result is a lack of acetylcholine release into the synaptic cleft and subsequent paralysis of the muscle. (C) Common facial anatomic areas for Botox injections. (A and B: From Miller J, Clarkson E. Botulinum toxin type a: review and its role in the dental office. Dent Clin North Am. 2016;60:509-521.)

TABLE 40.1	Dilution Table for Botulinum Toxin Type A	
BTX-A VIAL	**Diluent Added (0.9% NaCl)**	**Resulting Dose (Units/0.1mL)**
50 units	1.25 mL	4.0 units
	1.0 mL	5.0 units
100 units	2.50 mL	4.0 units
	2.0 mL	5.0 units
200 units	5.0 mL	4.0 units
	4.0 mL	5.0 units

For muscle injections in the orofacial region, skin preparation should always be completed using aseptic alcohol wipes and dry sterile gauze sponges. In most clinical situations the muscles should be injected bilaterally to minimize complications from asymmetry or unequal nerve involvement (i.e., number of units will vary depending on the target muscle). When considering the ideal dosing amount, the total number of units will depend on the area of interest, muscle mass, and strength and gender of the patient. In general, men will require more units than women. Care should be taken when choosing the dilution being used because higher dilution may result in further migration of the BTX-A and may result in unwanted effects.

Duration of Action

The U.S. Drug Administration recommends an injection frequency of once every 3 months with the lowest effective dose. In some patients multiple injections may over time result in the development of antibodies to BTX-A, which results in effect reduction and inactivating the toxin activity. However, in general the length of efficacy varies among individuals and is dependent on the patient's metabolism of the toxin and the use or activity of the muscle being treated.

Botulinum Toxin Type A Uses in Implant Dentistry

1. Parafunctional habits
2. Temporomandibular joint syndrome/temporomandibular dysfunction (TMJ/TMD)
3. Excessive tissue display (gummy smile)

Parafunctional Habits

Masseter Muscle Hyperactivity

A common sequela of patients with parafunction is masseter hypertrophy. The masseter muscle is one of the primary muscles of mastication. When the masseter muscle is hyperactive or overused, the facial appearance often enlarges and results in a negative cosmetic impact with altered facial lines. Muscle function is also altered, which results in excessive force being placed on the teeth/implants. Studies have shown a significant reduction in masseter muscle volume with an average reduction in mass of 22% and up to approximately 35% reduction after the continued use of BTX-A[4] (Figs. 40.3 and 40.4).

Anatomy. The masseter muscle is a thick quadrilateral muscle that consists of two heads: (1) superficial and (2) deep.

Superficial: The larger superficial head arises by a thick aponeurosis from the maxillary process to the zygomatic bone and from the anterior two-thirds of the inferior border of the zygomatic arch. The fibers pass inferior and posterior, and are inserted in the angle of the mandible and inferior half of the lateral surface of the mandibular ramus.

Deep: The smaller deep head arises from the posterior third of the lower border and the medial surface of the zygomatic arch. Its fibers pass in a downward and forward direction to be inserted into the upper half of the ramus as high as the coronoid process of the mandible. Anteriorly the superficial head conceals the deep head and posteriorly is covered by the parotid gland.

Innervation and Blood Supply. The masseter is innervated by the anterior division of the mandibular division (V3) of the trigeminal nerve. The pathway of innervation is gyrus precentralis > genu capsula interna > nucleus motorius nervi trigemini > nervus trigeminus > nervus mandibularis > musculus masseter. The blood supply to the masseter muscle is derived from three blood vessels: the masseteric branch of the maxillary artery, the facial artery, and the transverse facial branch of the superficial temporal artery.

Function. The primary function of the masseter muscle is elevation of the mandible. The masseter muscle parallels the medial pterygoid muscle; however, it is significantly stronger and its superficial fibers can be responsible for protrusive movements.[5]

Botox Technique. Injection into the masseter muscle for the treatment of masseter hypertrophy was first discussed by von Lindern et al.[6] They suggested injections into the zygomatic arch and mandibular angle. However, this method revealed a higher risk for injection into the parotid gland, which led to significant complications. Hu et al.[7] determined a safe zone for injection sites into the masseter muscle. They recommended the safest entry point to be in the central compartment of the masseter muscle as to avoid injections into the parotid gland and the mandibular branch of the facial nerve. The parotid gland is located superficial and at the posterior margin of the muscle. Branches of the facial nerve also run superficial to the muscle. The delineation of the "safe zone" is a line drawn from the lower ear to the angle of the mouth (superior margin). The anterior extent is determined by palpation and the posterior extent is the posterior angle of the mandible (Fig. 40.4). The inferior border is delineated by the inferior border of the mandible.

Mapping Injection Sites. An outline of the muscle needs to be completed to determine the maximum areas of contraction and tension points of the masseter muscle. Initially a line is drawn with a removable skin marker from the lateral commissure (corner of the mouth) to the bottom of earlobe (small pointed eminence of the external ear that projects over the meatus). The inferior border of the mandible is outlined, and the anterior and posterior borders of the muscle are marked. The patient is asked to clench his or her teeth, and the maximum contraction points are documented and marked. Skin markings can easily be removed with alcohol swabs.

Injection Technique. Two syringes of reconstituted 25 U of BTX-A are drawn up in into syringes and approximately 5 U is injected deep into the belly of the muscle at each tension point. In most cases the needle is inserted perpendicular to the skin surface (Fig. 40.5).

Studies. Many studies have shown the successful reduction in masseter hypertrophy via BTX-A injections.[7-10] With multiple injections, concomitant reduction in gross masseter size has been shown to be up to 40%.[8] Rafferty et al.[11] showed masseter-induced bite force reduction of up to 85% at week 3 after injections and 65% less at week 7. However, clenching returned to

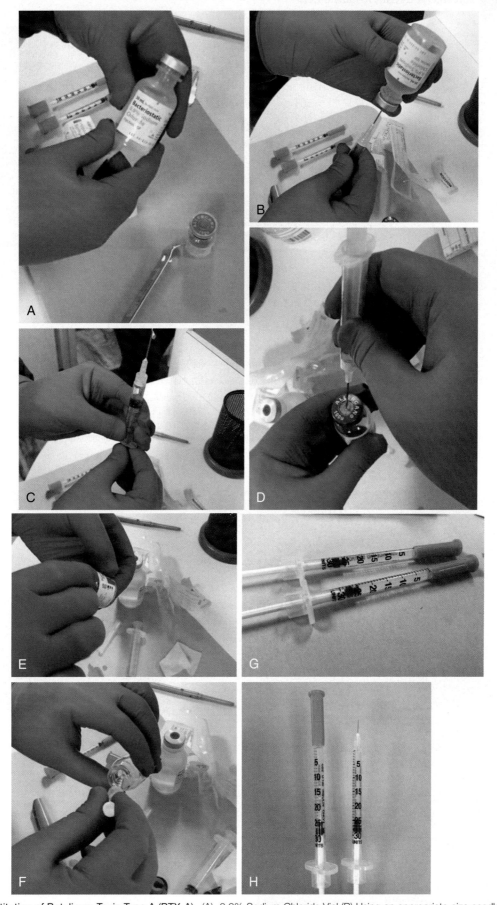

• **Fig. 40.2** Reconstitution of Botulinum Toxin Type A (BTX-A). (A) 0.9% Sodium Chloride Vial (B) Using an appropriate-size needle and syringe, draw up 1, 1.25 or 2.5 mL of 0.9% preservative sterile saline. (C) Invert needle and tap side to expel any air bubbles. (D) Insert the needle and slowly inject the saline into the BTX-A. Vacuum must be present in the vial, which demonstrates that sterility of the vial is intact. (E) Remove the syringe, then gently mix the vial with the saline by rotating the vial. Record the date and time of reconstitution on the label. (F) Using a small tuberculin syringe draw up the required amount of solution; angle the needle into the bottom corner of the vial to allow for full extraction of solution. Do not completely invert the vial and expel any air bubbles in the syringe barrel. (G and H) Final syringes with BTX-A solution are ready for injection.

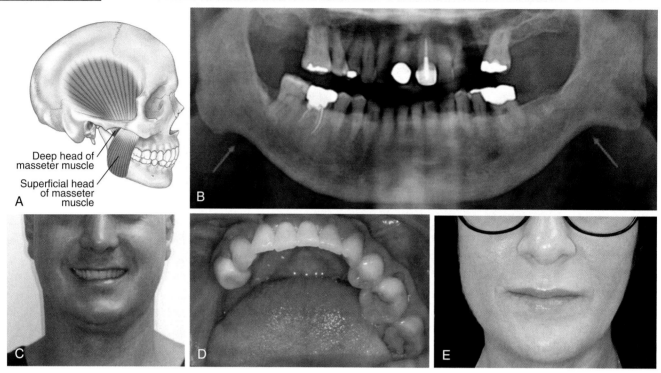

• **Fig. 40.3** Masseter Hypertrophy. (A) Masseter muscle. *(From Nanci A. Ten Cate's Oral Histology: Development, Structure, and Function. 9th ed. St. Louis, MO: Elsevier; 2018.)* (B) Radiograph depicting large antegonial notch resulting from the excessive force on the angle of the mandible. (C) Enlarged facial appearance from hypertrophied muscle. (D) Image of patient with missing dentition in lower left. (E) Resultant hypertrophy of right masseter and atrophy of left masseter.

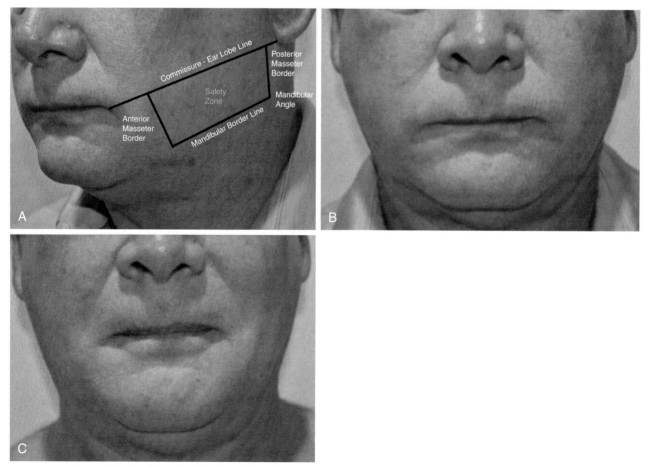

• **Fig. 40.4** Masseter Muscle. (A) Injection boundaries. (B) Masseter hypertrophy. (C) Reduction of masetter mass after Botox injections.

baseline values faster as the result of other muscles compensating. Van Zandijcke and Marchau[12] described in 1990 the use of 100 U of BTX-A injections to the temporalis and masseter muscles in patients with brain injuries. The mean duration of response was approximately 19 weeks and mean peak effect (abolishment

of grinding) was approximately 3.5 weeks. In general the targeted musculature usually adapts to the injections, and frequency of injections usually decreases because of the atrophy of the muscles.

Complications. Injections in the masseter muscle area are relatively safe with minimal side effects. Inaccurate injection location

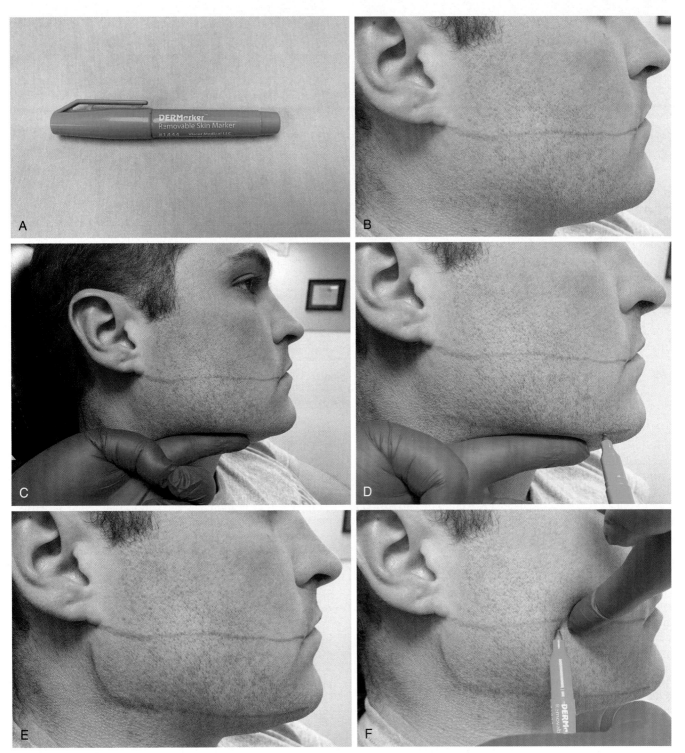

• **Fig. 40.5** Masseter Mapping and Injection Technique. (A) Skin Marker, (B) Commissure—ear lobe line drawn. (C) Inferior border of mandible trajectory evaluated. (D) Inferior border points marked. (E) Inferior border and posterior border points connected. (F) Anterior masseter muscle border marked.

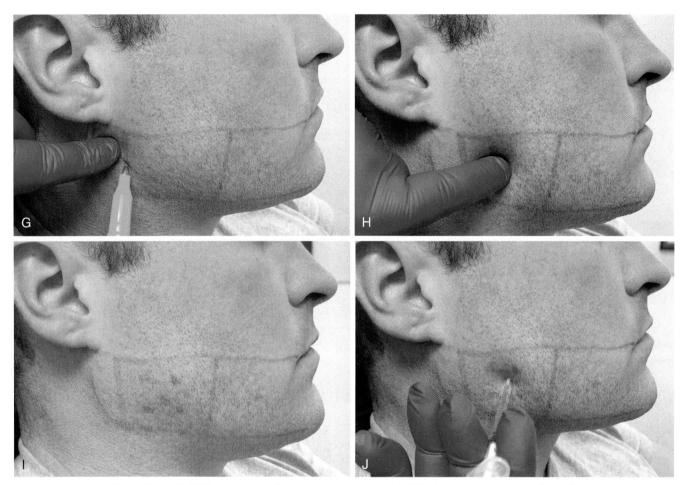

Fig. 40.5, cont'd (G) Posterior masseter muscle border marked. (H) Tension points determined. (I and J) Injection of 5 units deep into the belly of the muscle at each point.

or too high injection volume may lead to excessive swelling, bruising, facial muscle weakness, and xerostomia. Postoperatively, patients may report a "thicker" saliva and usually this is related to higher doses and injections into the parotid gland. Injections made too far anteriorly may lead to BTX-A diffusion into adjacent muscles, leading to smile alteration (Fig. 40.6).

Temporalis Muscle

The temporalis muscle (also called the *temporal muscle*) is considered a muscle of mastication and arises from the temporal fossa.

Anatomy. The temporalis muscle is a broad, fan-shaped muscle of mastication on the lateral aspect of the skull. It arises from the temporal fossa, which is a large depression on the lateral aspect of the skull. A temporal fascia completely covers the surface of the muscle. The muscle fibers converge as they descend through a space between the zygomatic arch and end with the temporalis tendon. The temporalis tendon is considered a very thick tendon that inserts at the coronoid process of the mandible (Fig. 40.7).

Innervation and Blood Supply. The third division of the mandibular branch of the trigeminal nerve innervates the temporalis muscle by the deep temporal nerves. The deep temporal branches of the maxillary artery, along with the middle temporal artery, contribute to the blood supply of the muscle.

Function. The temporalis muscle is considered the strongest muscle of mastication. It can be divided into two functional parts, the anterior and posterior. The anterior temporalis runs vertically and is responsible for elevation of the mandible. The posterior temporalis runs horizontally, and contraction results in retrusive movements of the mandible.[13]

Botox Technique

Mapping Injection Sites. The anterior, posterior, and superior extent of the temporalis muscle is marked with a skin marker. As the patient clenches his or her teeth, the maximum areas of contraction and/or tension points are marked within the boundaries.

Injection Technique. The injection technique for the temporalis muscle usually consists of two injections, superficial and deep, according to the location of the areas of maximum contraction. The superficial injections are positioned into the thinner upper portions of the temporalis muscle in a fan shape. The deeper injection involves the split of the superficial temporalis fascia, which is located approximately 1.5 mm superior to the zygomatic arch[15] (Figs. 40.8 and 40.9).

Duration. When BTX-A is injected for parafunctional habits in temporalis muscles, patients appear to require repeated injections at approximately 5 months. Other studies have shown injections to be repeated every 6 months.[14]

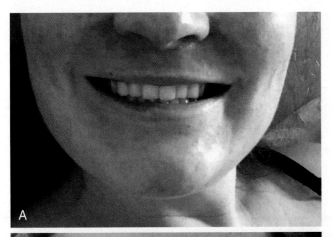

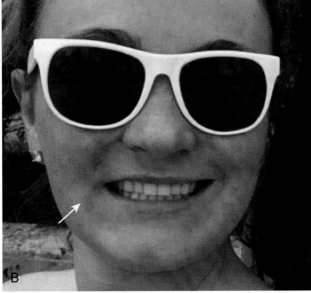

• **Fig. 40.6** Smile Alteration Complication: (A) Normal smile, (B) Smile alteration resulting from injection on the right side which was too medial, which inadvertently diffused and affected the Risorius muscle. Note the constricted smile on the right side.

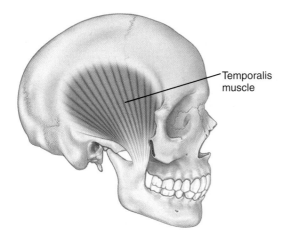

• **Fig. 40.7** Temporalis Muscle. *(From Nanci A.* Ten Cate's Oral Histology: Development, Structure, and Function. *9th ed. St. Louis, MO: Elsevier; 2018.)*

Temporalis muscle

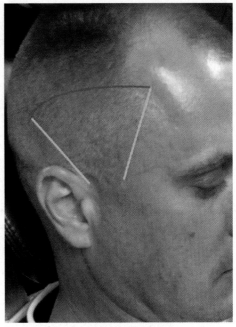

• **Fig. 40.8** Temporalis Muscle Boundaries.

Temporomandibular Joint Syndrome (TMJ)/ Temporomandibular Dysfunction (TMD) Pain

The use of BTX-A has been shown to treat TMJ or TMD complications, with the injection of the masseter and temporalis muscles. Guarda-Nardini et al.[16] demonstrated the use of Botox in the treatment of decreasing myofascial pain symptoms in bruxers, compared with saline injections. Baker et al.[17] evaluated the use of masseter and temporalis injections for patients exhibiting chronic masticatory myofascial pain dysfunction. Results showed a decrease in overall pain and overall maximum voluntary opening.

Success rates are variable in the treatment of patients with TMJ. Studies have reported that BTXs used for the treatment of TMD disorders may cause dysphagia[18] or temporal drooling.[19] However, in both of these reports greater than 100 U was administered.

Temporomandibular Dysfunction/Temporomandibular Joint Technique

The TMD/TMJ BTX-A technique is very similar to the traditional masseter and temporalis muscle techniques, with the only difference being dictated by myofascial trigger points. To determine the location of injections for TMD/TMJ technique, myofascial trigger points must be located. Trigger points are hyperirritable areas within the fascia surrounding the muscle, which may differ from areas of maximum contraction. Usually in TMD/TMJ cases, one or more trigger points are generally present, which on palpation will cause transmission of pain along the muscle or neuronal tracks. Disruption of the trigger points have been reported to bring short- and long-term pain relief.[20]

1. Palpate for two trigger points in the masseter and mark with a skin marker.
2. Palpate for three trigger points in the temporalis and mark with tissue pen.

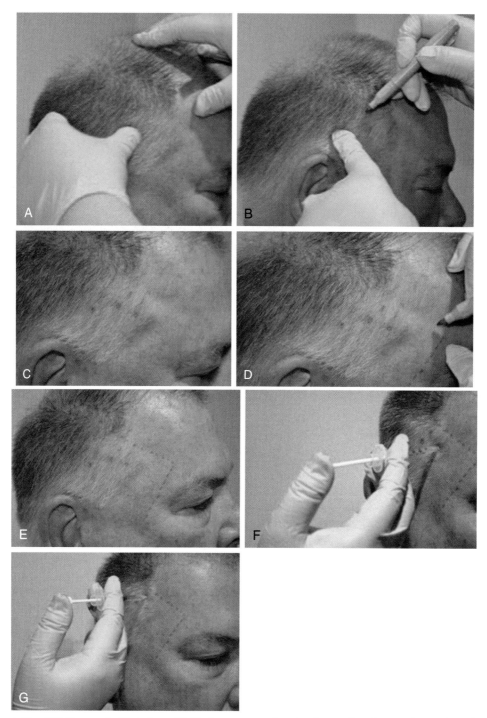

• **Fig. 40.9** Temporalis Technique. (A) Maximum areas of contraction and/or trigger points evaluated while the patient clenches his teeth. (B) Trigger points are marked with skin marker. (C) Final tension points. (D) Anterior and superior borders are marked. (E) Final boundary outline and tension points. (F and G) Five units of botulinum toxin type A per injection point.

3. Clean injection areas with alcohol wipes.
4. Using four tuberculin syringes, draw up (2) 20-U syringes and (2) 25-U syringes.
5. Inject 10 U into each trigger point in the masseter.
6. Inject 12.5 U into temporalis anterior fan, 7.5 U into the middle, and 5 U into the temporalis posterior fan. (Fig. 40.10).

Excessive Tissue Display (Gummy Smile)

In the rehabilitation of the dental implant patient, clinicians are often confronted with excessive display of maxillary gingival tissue on smiling. The "gummy smile" results in difficulty in restoring patients because of nonideal esthetics and displeasure

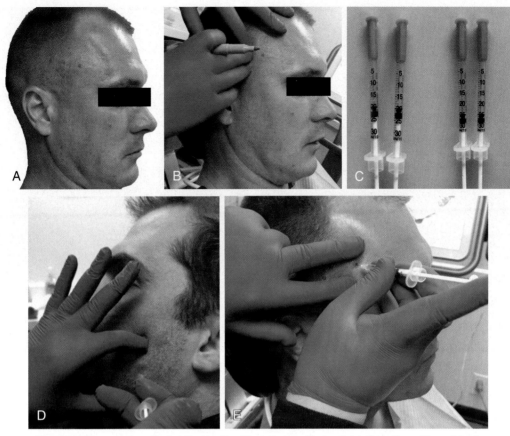

• **Fig. 40.10** Temporomandibular Dysfunction/Temporomandibular Joint Technique: Clean Injection Areas With Alcohol Wipes. (A and B) Palpate for (A) two trigger points in the masseter and (B) three trigger points in the temporalis, and mark with tissue pen. (C) Using four tuberculin syringes, draw up (2) 20-U syringes and (2) 25-U syringes. (D) Inject 10 U into each trigger point in the masseter. (E) Inject 12.5 U into anterior fan, 7.5 U into the middle, and 5 U into the posterior fan of the temporalis muscle.

in the prosthesis-tissue junction. Caution should be exercised with the treatment of gummy smiles because vertical maxillary excess is historically treated surgically by means of maxillary impaction via a Le Fort 1 osteotomy procedure. For patients exhibiting delayed passive eruption, gingivectomies are the ideal treatment. Botox can be used for correction of hyperfunctional upper lip elevator muscles. Therefore, before treatment, it is crucial that the etiology of the gummy smile be ascertained.

Kokich et al.[21] described an excessive gingival-to-lip distance of 4 mm or more, which they classified as "unattractive" by laypeople and dental professionals. Excessive gingival display has been shown to have a prevalence rate of approximately 11% of the population, with more women displaying excessive gingiva than men, with a 2:1 female:male ratio.[22,23,24]

There exist two types of smiles in the literature, the "social" and the "enjoyment" smile. The social smile is a voluntary, unstrained and static facial expression that is usually used as a greeting. The lip component is due to the muscular contraction of the elevator muscles of the lip. In contrast, the enjoyment smile is involuntary and usually results from laughter or pleasure. The upper and lower lip elevator and depressor muscles are responsible for the full expansion of the lips, which show maximum anterior tooth display.[25] A cosmetic smile has been defined as displaying less than 2 mm of the gum tissue. Any smile showing more than 2 mm is classified as a gummy smile or excessive gingival display.[26] When treating these patients, it is imperative to have a

preoperative photo of their enjoyment smile showing their maximum lip movement, to properly assess the needs and outcome of the BTX-A treatment. In summary, a thorough intraoral and extraoral examination is imperative because the excessive gingival display may be treated with BTX-A only when it caused by hypermobility of the lip, not when the excessive gingival display is the result of the position of the maxilla (skeletal position) or a short upper lip (Fig. 40.11).

Etiology

In the production of a smile, many muscles are involved, including orbicularis oris, levator labii superioris alaeque nasi (LLSAN), levator labii superioris (LLS), zygomaticus major (ZM), and depressor septi nasi muscle. In cases of true hyperfunctional upper lips, the primary muscle responsible for the hyperactivity with resultant excess display of gingiva is the LLSAN. The LLSAN is translated from the Latin as the "lifter of the upper lip and wing of the nose." This muscle originates from the upper frontal process of the maxilla and inserts into the skin of the lateral nostril and upper lip. Its main action involves elevation of the upper lip and is also involved in dilation of the nostrils and creation of associated deep nasolabial folds (Fig. 40.12 and Box 40.1).

Injection Technique

Hwang et al.,[27] at Yonsei University College of Dentistry, have proposed an injection point for the treatment of a gummy smile,

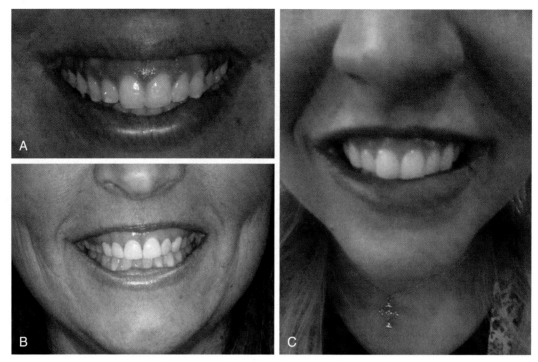

• **Fig. 40.11** (A–C) Excess tissue "gummy smiles" examples.

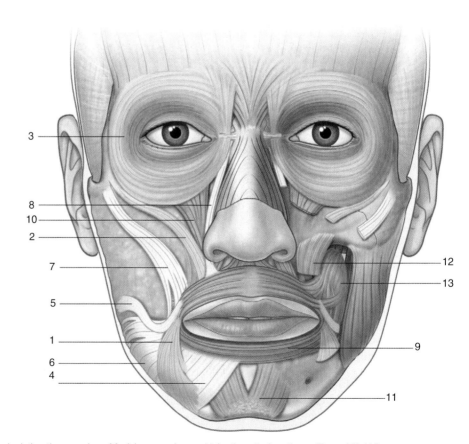

Layer 1
1. Depressor anguli oris
2. Zygomaticus minor
3. Orbicularis oculi

Layer 2
4. Depressor labii inferioris
5. Risorius
6. Platysma
7. Zygomaticus major
8. Levator labii superioris
   alaeque nasi

Layer 3
9. Orbicularis oris
10. Levator labii superioris

Layer 4
11. Mentalis
12. Levator anguli oris
13. Buccinator

• **Fig. 40.12** Image depicting the muscles of facial expression and injection site locations. *(From Afifi AM, Djohan R. Anatomy of the head and neck. In: Neligan PC, ed.* Plastic Surgery. Vol. 3: Craniofacial, Head and Neck Surgery. *3rd ed. London: Elsevier; 2013.)*

• BOX 40.1   Facial Muscles Anatomy and Function

Orbicularis Oris Muscle
Origin: maxilla and mandible
Insertion: skin around the lip
Function: muscle encircling the mouth is a sphincter muscle and is responsible for closing the mouth; it is known as the "kissing muscle," because it is used to pucker the lips

Levator Anguli Oris Muscle
Origin: maxilla inferior to the infraorbital foramen
Insertion: modiolus
Function: lifts the upper lip

Zygomaticus Major Muscles
Origin: zygomatic bone
Insertion: orbicularis at modiolus
Function: works with the risorius muscle to assist in laughing and smiling by lifting the corners of the mouth

Zygomaticus Minor Muscles
Origin: malar surface of the zygomatic bone
Insertion: orbicularis oris
Function: draws the upper lip backward, upward, and outward and is used in smiling

Levator Labii Superior Muscle
Origin: medial infraorbital margin
Insertion: skin and muscle of the upper lip
Function: elevates the lip

Levator Anguli Muscle
Origin: maxilla
Insertion: modiolus
Function: elevates the angle of the mouth medially

Levator Labii Superior Alaeque Nasi Muscle
Origin: nasal bone
Insertion: nostril and upper lip
Function: dilates the nostril and elevates the upper lip and nose

Depressor Anguli Oris Muscle
Origin: tubercle of mandible
Insertion: modiolus of mouth
Function: depresses angle of mouth

Depressor Labii Inferior Muscle
Origin: oblique line of mandible between symphysis and mental foramen
Insertion: integument of the lower lip, orbicularis oris, modiolus
Function: depression of the lower lip

Risorius Muscle
Origin: parotid fascia
Insertion: modiolus
Function: retracts the angle of the mouth to produce a smile

Buccinator Muscle
Origin: alveolar processes of maxilla and mandible
Insertion: fibers of orbicularis oris
Function: compresses the cheeks against the teeth

---

which is named the Yonsei point. The Yonsei point is located at the center of a triangle formed by LLS, LLSAN, and zygomaticus minor muscles. The merger of these muscles can be felt by palpating lateral to the nose while smiling and is roughly 1 cm lateral to the ala of the nose and 3 cm superior from the lateral oral commissure. Hwang et al.[27] have recommended a dose of 3 U at each injection site (bilaterally).

Achieving ideal outcomes for the treatment of excessive tissue display is extremely technique sensitive, with excess treatment often occurring in transverse elongation and dysfunctional animation of the maxillary lip. Therefore clinicians early on their learning curve should treat these areas cautiously and gradually, with multiple low-dose treatments over a longer time period in lieu of a single bolus in one appointment.[28] Ideally the lip at rest and high lip line should be documented with photographs by measuring from the gingival zenith to the inferior border of the upper lip. Patients with natural asymmetry to their smile may need different amounts of BTX-A on each side to achieve an ideal smile level. The asymmetry should be reevaluated at a 2-week interval, and more BTX-A can be added to the hyperactive side (Figs. 40.13 to 40.15).

Facial asymmetry corrected with Botox should be over a 4-week period, with approximately 2 U administered bilaterally at the initial visit and 1 U administered 2 weeks later. This technique usually will result in a more symmetric smile.

Duration. The duration of action of BTX-A is not permanent, lasting on average for 6 months with a range of 4 to 8 months.[29] In most cases, BTX-A needs to be administered approximately two to three times a year, depending on how much muscle activity

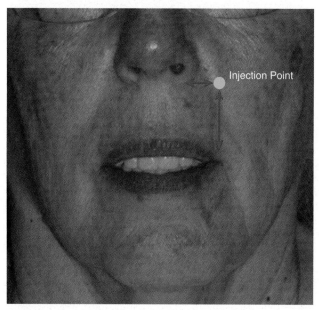

• **Fig. 40.13** Yonsei Point. Is located 1 cm lateral to the ala of the nose and 3 cm superior to the oral commissure.

is present. The therapeutic effects will usually appear in 24 to 72 hours and peak in 1 to 4 weeks, with a decline after 3 to 4 months.[30]

Studies. Polo[22] showed favorable results with a mean gingival exposure reduction of 5.2 mm. Although the amount of

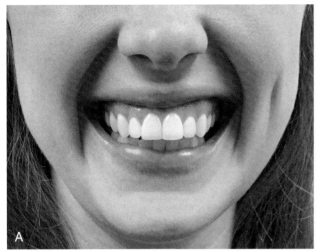

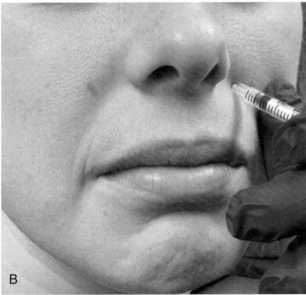

• **Fig. 40.14** Gummy Smile Injection Points (Yonsei). (A) Gummy smile, (B) Yonsei injection points.

gingival display increased from 2 weeks to 24 weeks, the amount of original display had not returned at 24 weeks. Park et al.[31] showed a mean reduction in masseter thickness of up to 2.9 mm, measured at 3 months postoperatively. With multiple injections, eventual atrophy of the masseter muscle resulted in requiring less frequent doses, with a recommended recall of 4 to 6 months.

Complications. In the treatment of the gummy smile, many complications may arise consisting of asymmetries, lip sagging, lip protrusion, exaggerated lip elongation, and interference with speech. As stated, the clinician must be able to distinguish hyperfunctional upper lips from other causes of gummy smiles. For instance, attempts to treat maxillary excess conditions with BTX-A may lead to unnatural results from the excessive loss of function needed to prevent gingival display. When short clinical crowns are present, tissue alteration in the form of a gingivoplasty should be completed to obtain esthetic crown lengthening. In general, vertical maxillary excess cases are usually treated with a maxillary impaction via Le Fort I osteotomy.

Generalized Botulinum Toxin Type A Postoperative Instructions

Postoperative care is very important with BTX-A patients because deviation from the following instructions may lead to increased complications:

1. Patients should be instructed not to touch or massage the injected areas for a minimum of 4 hours. This will prevent the dispersion of BTX-A into adjacent sites and allow the BTX-A to penetrate the targeted area for ideal effect.
2. Patients should restrict physical activity for a minimum of 24 to 48 hours because this will minimize inflammation.
3. Patients should avoid alcohol and smoking. Excessive perspiration (e.g., exercise, sauna) should be avoided because tissue healing may be affected.
4. Patients should be instructed to refrain from lying down for at least 4 hours after injections in the face because this may alter the dispersion of the BTX-A.
5. Patients should be educated on potential bruising, redness, and swelling, which are common after the injections. These side effects usually will resolve within 7 to 10 days.
6. Patient education is important on expectations because results may not be immediate. Usually changes will be seen as early as 3 to 7 days, with maximum results after 14 days.

Generalized Contraindications to Botox

Generalized contraindications to Botox include[32]:
- Psychologically unstable patients or patients who have questionable motives and unrealistic expectations
- Individuals who are dependent on intact facial movements and expressions for their livelihood (e.g., actors, singers, musicians, and other media personalities)
- Patients afflicted with a neuromuscular disorder (e.g., myasthenia gravis, Eaton-Lambert syndrome, tardive dyskinesia, stroke)
- Individuals who are allergic to any of the components of BTX-A or BTX-B (i.e., BTX, human albumin, saline, lactose, and sodium succinate) or eggs
- Patients who are currently taking specific medications that may interfere with neuromuscular impulse transmission and may potentiate the side effects of BTX (e.g., aminoglycosides, penicillamine, quinine, and calcium blockers); drug classes that have been shown to affect BTX-A include anticholinergic drugs, muscle relaxants, other botulinum neurotoxin products, dopamine-blocking drugs, and some over-the-counter vitamins such as vitamin E, fish oils, Omega 3 fatty acids, and coenzyme Q_{10}
- Pregnant or lactating individuals (BTXs are classified as pregnancy category C drugs)
- Patients with presence of infection at the proposed injection site

Generalized Complications to Botox

Generalized complications to Botox include:
- Migration of BTX-A into associated muscles near the injection site
- Headache or flu-like symptoms
- Discomfort or pain at injection site

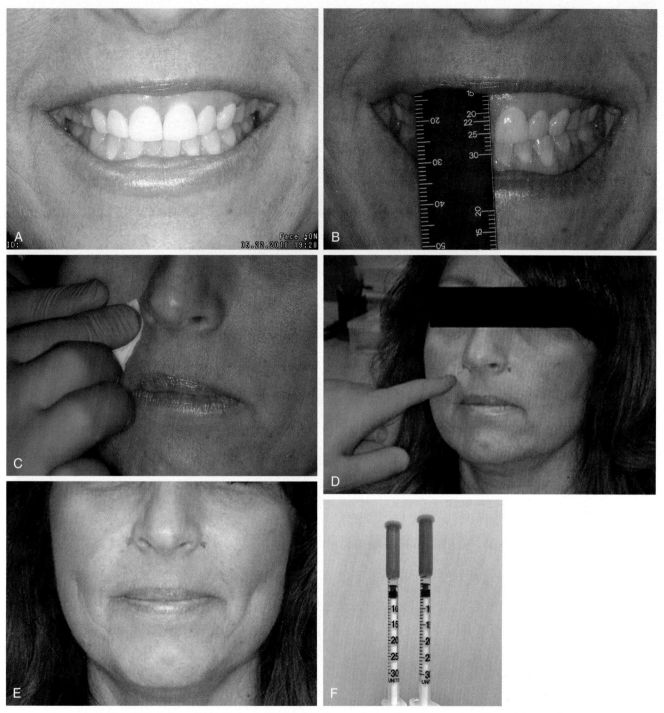

• **Fig. 40.15 Gummy Smile Technique.** (A and B) Have patient smile as large as possible and document with photos. (C) Injection site is cleaned with alcohol wipe. (D) Palpate for the levator labii superioris alaeque nasi muscle and mark with tissue pen bilaterally. (E) Have patient smile and verify vertical movement of marked areas. (F) Draw up two separate tuberculin syringes with 1 to 2 U of BTX-A.

- Spread of BTX-A toxin effects, which spread to unwanted muscle or anatomic areas; this is most likely a result of the incorrect injection site or too great a volume administered
- Breathing or swallowing complications that may occur immediately or weeks after injections
- Swelling, rash, headache, local numbness, pain at injection site, bruising, respiratory problems, or allergic reactions
- Antibiotics have been shown to shorten the length of duration of BTX-A

Injectable Fillers

Another pharmacologic agent that is becoming increasingly popular in implant dentistry is dermal fillers. In the past, injectable fillers such as liquid silicone and bovine collagen were used to replace or enhance the volume of subcutaneous tissue. However, these products exhibited a high incidence of allergic and foreign body reactions. Today, many fillers without the side effects that were associated with the earlier agents are on the market. These

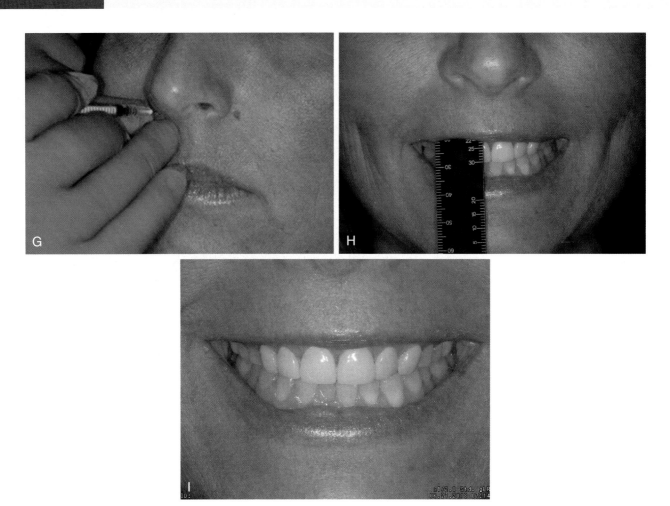

Fig. 40.15, cont'd (G) Inject 1 to 2 units into levator labii superioris alaeque nasi muscle bilaterally by inserting needle halfway the depth of the needle. (H and I) After 2 weeks the patient should be evaluated for symmetry and adjusted if needed.

newer filler products are classified as either "permanent" (e.g., polymethylmethacrylate [PMMA], calcium hydroxyl appetite, and expanded polytetrafluoroethylene) or "nonpermanent" (e.g., collagen or hyaluronic acid). Currently, the most commonly used fillers in dentistry are hyaluronic acid products such as Juvéderm (Allergan) and Restylane (Medicis).[33] These filler products have the advantage of being supplied in various viscosities, are easy to handle, have safe antigenicity, and effects can be reversed or dissolved using hyaluronidase (reversal agent) (Table 40.2).

Significant advances in the injectable dermal filler markets have led to a growing interest and increased usage. These minimally invasive injectable procedures have been geared toward the treatment of facial aging and facial enhancement; however, they are becoming more popular in dental implant-related areas. Approximately 3 million soft tissue procedures were performed in the United States in 2016, of which the majority were of hyaluronic acid–based fillers.[34]

With respect to dental implant patients, many patients are at an advanced age, with associated facial aging symptoms. Therefore the implant clinician must consider the benefits of rejuvenation techniques for maximizing the cosmetic outcomes in association with the implant procedures. In today's implant practice, the standard is for the implant dentist to consider the benefits of facial volume restoration when performing implant surgery on patients who may benefit from these products.

Hyaluronic acid fillers have become popular in the United States and global markets because they are user friendly, are stable at room temperature, are available in single preloaded syringes that require no preparation, are relatively inexpensive, and have the ability to be reversed with hyaluronidase. Additional advantages include they exhibit longer duration of action in comparison with collagen preparations and require no allergy testing.

Hyaluronic acid is an anionic, simple nonsulfated glycosaminoglycan widely found throughout connective, epithelial, and neural tissues. The natural hyaluronic acid contributes to tissue repair via cell hydration and lubrication. With age, the hyaluronic acid in the skin decreases, which results in decreased dermal hydration. If the skin is exposed to excessive ultraviolet B rays, cells within the dermis will induce the loss of hyaluronic acid from dermal tissue, resulting in photoaging.

Hyaluronic acid has a large particle size that leads to its inherent hydrophilic nature, thus allowing it to retain large amounts of water (can absorb up to 1000 times its molecular weight). When injected under the skin the hyaluronic acid fillers attract and bind water, thus providing volume to the skin. Because of its nonimmunogenic nature, it is devoid of many of the allergenic collagen fillers that were prevalent in the past.

The modern hyaluronic acid–based fillers are created by crosslinking the hyaluronic acid chains by conjugation with butanediol

TABLE 40.2	Available Dermal Fillers	
Material	**Brand Name**	**Duration and Biodegradability**
Autologous fat		Temporary and biodegradable
Hyaluronic acid	*Restylane®, Restylane Perlane®, Restylane Lipp®, Restylane Touch®, Restylane Vital®* Macrolane® 20, 30	
	Juvederm Ultra 1, 2, 3®, Juvederm Voluma® Hylaform®, Hylaform Plus®, Hylaform Fineline® Others: Rofilan Forte®, Matridur®, Puragen®, Glytone®, Isogel®, Prevelle®, etc	Temporary and biodegradable
Collagen	Zyplast®/Zyderm® (bovine) Cosmoderm®/Cosmoplast® (human) Evolence®, Permacol®, Fibroquel® (porcine)	Temporary and biodegradable
Calcium hydroxylapatite	*Radiesse®*	Semipermanent and biodegradable
Poly L-lactic acid	Sculptra®/New Fill®	Semipermanent and biodegradable
β-Tricalcium phosphate with hyaluronic acid	Atlean®	Semipermanent and biodegradable
Polyacrylamide gel	Aquamid® Bio-Alcamid®	Permanent and not biodegradable
Polymethyl methacrylate	Arteplast®, Artecoll®, Artefill®	Semipermanent and not biodegradable
	Dermalive®/ Dermadeep®	
Dimethylsiloxane polymers	Silicone	Permanent and not biodegradable

From Carruthers A, Carruthers J. *Botulinum Toxin: Procedures in Cosmetic Dermatology Series.* St. Louis, MO: Elsevier; 2018.

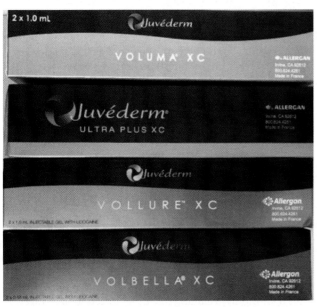

• **Fig. 40.16** Available Dermal Fillers (Allergan, Irvine, Calif.).

diglycidyl ether. The cross-linked hyaluronic acid may be processed in various ways that yield homogeneous gels (the Juvéderm family) or suspensions of particles in gel carriers (NASHA Restylane). Therefore, each type of hyaluronic acid filler contains varying amounts of hyaluronic acid and through the various cross-linking processes, different properties of gels and varying degradation rates result (Fig. 40.16).

Mechanism of Action

The use of hyaluronic acid stimulates cell proliferation, migration, angiogenesis, and reepithelialization, and reduces collagen and scar formation.[35] In comparison with collagen injections, hyaluronic acid products do not require preinjection testing and produce relatively reproducible, longer-lasting results.[36]

How Supplied and Preparation

Currently, there are three major companies, Allergan, Medicis, and Merz, that have multiple hyaluronic acid fillers on the market. There is no universal filler that is appropriate for every application or for every patient. It is important to understand the physical properties of the fillers and how they interact for predictable clinical outcomes. Each of the major brands have multiple hyaluronic acid options in their lines that are specifically designed for different treatment sites. It is important to properly understand and follow the indications for usage for each hyaluronic acid filler being used. Some of the more common dermal fillers include:

Restylane (Sub-Q, Uppsala, Sweden) was the first hyaluronic acid product sold in the United States. Restylane is supplied as a gel with a particle size of 400 µm. This product is most commonly used to treat nasolabial folds, the lips, and the oral commissures. It can also be used for cheek augmentation and to improve deformities of the chin and prejowl sulcus. However, it is not generally used for the treatment of fine lines.

Perlane (Sub-Q, Uppsala, Sweden) is a hyaluronic acid product of nonanimal origin. It has a large particle size (1000 µm) and is used to treat moderate-to-severe wrinkles and folds. This product contains 0.3% lidocaine to decrease injection discomfort.

Juvéderm (Allergan Inc., Santa Barbara, Calif.) has many advantages over Restylane. It is usually softer and produces fewer lumps in the skin when injected close to the surface. Juvéderm is popular in correcting slight or moderate nasolabial folds in patients with fine skin. It is also used for lip enhancement and to treat minor defects in facial contours. Juvéderm has multiple

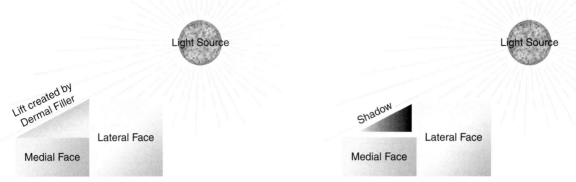

• **Fig. 40.17** Photo of general indications for dermal fillers. (*From Aicken M. Dermal filler doses. Aesthetics. 2017;4:41. © Aesthetics Media Ltd*)

sublines of products with different viscosities. One of their recent products is Juvéderm Volbella, which is a soft, smooth gel used to increase lip fullness and correct perioral lines. Another popular Juvéderm product is Juvéderm Voluma, which is used for the cheek area and for midfacial volume loss. Juvéderm Vollure is commonly used in nasolabial folds and perioral restoration.

Restylane Lipp (Allergan Inc., Santa Barbara, Calif.) is a specific hyaluronic acid gel that is designed for lip augmentation. The benefit of this material is that it lasts approximately 12 months; however, it must be homogenously distributed. Injecting excessive volume may lead to the inability of massage to redistribute the material.

BELOTERO® (Merz) is a high-quality hyaluronic acid dermal fillers with patented CPM® (Cohesive Polydensi ed Matrix) technology that integrates easily to smooth various tissues. It is mainly used for wrinkles or fine lines as well as restoring facial volume.

Versa (Revanesse) hyaluronic acid is for nasolabial folds in mid to deep dermis.

Indications

The main indication for the use of dermal fillers is for facial rejuvenation. Another popular area to use Dermal fillers are used to correct volume deficiencies to enhance facial contours. One of the most common areas is the nasolabial fold, which forms a pronounced furrow as patients age. Specifically, in implant dentistry the use of dermal fillers for black triangles is becoming increasingly popular. In addition, with respect to implant prosthetics, because of hard and soft tissue loss, dermal fillers are being used for lip augmentation, facial augmentation, and commissures for the treatment of angular cheilitis or a downturned smile (Fig. 40.17).

General Technique

A definite learning curve exists when injecting dermal fillers. It is imperative the clinician obtain adequate training and practice in performing these procedures. Depending on the anatomic area, there exists a variation in the amount of injected material, along with the depth and angle of injection. In addition, the clinician must understand the ideal dermal filling agent specific to the area of treatment. The viscosity of the material selected will dictate the gauge of needle used to deliver the dermal filler, with 30 gauge being the most commonly used. Lighter body materials often used in the lips may use a 32 gauge, while heavier bodied materials may require a 27 gauge. Microcannulas have grown increasingly popular because they yield advantages such as fewer injection points, leading to less trauma to the tissue and blood vessels.

Injection Technique

There exist two general techniques for injecting dermal fillers into tissue:

Retrograde technique: Needle is advanced and syringe plunger is depressed as the needle is withdrawn.

Anterograde technique: Plunger is depressed as soon as needle is placed subdermally so the filler elevates the subcutaneous tissues, which reduces the incidence of vascular perforation.

Specifically, there are a number of detailed injecting techniques that have been developed over the years. Each of the following techniques allow for a tailored approach which is specific for the anatomic location and clinical outcome expected. Some of the more common techniques include linear threading, fanning, serial puncturing, or cross-hatching. A combination of multiple techniques is often used.

1. *Linear threading:* The full length of the needle is inserted into the tissue and the filler is injected as the syringe is slowly retracted. This technique results in the filler remaining in the location of the injection, therefore not spreading or dissipating throughout the tissue. The linear threading or "tunneling" technique is ideal for straight, narrow lines and wrinkles.
2. *Serial puncture:* Multiple injections are placed serially along the length of the treatment so the filler will merge in a continuous line. This technique is usually indicated for small, fine lines and wrinkles.
3. *Fan technique:* One line of the filler material is injected by the linear threading technique; then the direction is changed and injected along a new line.
4. *Cross-hatching:* The linear threading technique is used at the periphery of the treatment area; the needle is withdrawn and is inserted adjacent to the first site and the procedure is repeated. This method is carried out continuously at right angles to the original line (Fig. 40.18).

Duration of Action

In general, temporary dermal fillers usually last from 6 to 12 months; however much variation exists depending on the treatment location, patient's anatomy, and muscle use. Newer temporary fillers are coming onto the market that have longer durations, ranging from 18 months to 24 months.

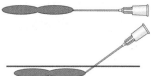
1. Linear threading technique

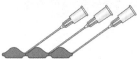
2. Serial puncture technique

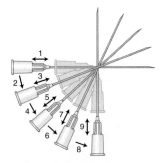
3. Fan technique

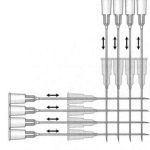
4. Cross-hatching technique

• **Fig. 40.18** Dermal Filler Techniques. (1) Linear threading; (2) serial puncture; (3) fan; and (4) cross-hatching.

Permanent Fillers

With the scope of procedures increasing with soft tissue augmentation, an increasing demand for permanent fillers is becoming more prevalent. The U.S. Food and Drug Administration defines permanent fillers as materials that are composed of nonabsorbable or permanent materials.[9] Permanent fillers are advantageous in providing long-term results; however, they carry the potential for irreversible complications. Therefore these agents require clinicians with experience and a higher level of expertise. Currently, in the United States, the available permanent fillers are PMMA and liquid injectable silicone. The use of liquid injectable silicone and PMMA is advantageous because they require no maintenance procedures that result in increased inconvenience, cost, and pain. The main disadvantage of permanent fillers is that they cannot be reversed or removed easily. The postoperative side effects associated with permanent fillers tend to be far greater than temporary fillers. A second disadvantage of permanent fillers is their lack of adaptability or modification as facial tissues change shape.[37]

Dermal Filler Use in Implant Dentistry

1. Black triangle
2. Lips
3. Face/cheek augmentation because of midfacial volume loss
4. Commissure (downturned smile and angular cheilitis)

Black Triangles

The soft tissues adjacent to a dental implant ideally need to be in harmony with adjacent teeth and/or implants. Unfortunately, especially in the maxillary anterior region, it is not uncommon for there to be a lack of papilla tissue (black triangle), resulting in non-ideal esthetic and functional issues. Papilla tissue may be lost from trauma, tooth loss, lack of adjacent contact area, or associated bone loss. The reconstruction of interdental papilla is a complicated and difficult periodontal treatment. There exist very limited options in the surgical treatment of this problem. To

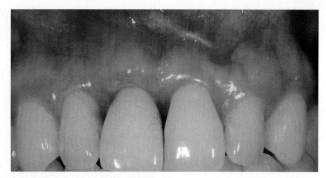
• **Fig. 40.19** Black Triangle. Maxillary anterior between #8 and #9 resulting in an unesthetic result.

further complicate the situation, food particles often accumulate in the space and create esthetic issues (Fig. 40.19).

Etiology

In anterior regions of the dentition, the interdental papilla is usually of a pyramidal form, whereas in the posterior regions the papillae are more flattened in the buccolingual direction. Tarnow et al.[38] have shown that the level of the bony crest to the contact area has a direct correlation between the presence or absence of interproximal papillae. Their results showed when there was 5 mm or less from the contact area to the crestal bone, 100% of the time papillae were present. When the distance was 6 mm or greater than 7 mm, respectively, 56% or 27% of the time papillae were present. Other studies have shown papillae decrease with increasing distance between adjacent roots and have become more prominent with increasing distance from the contact area to the alveolar crest.[39]

Tarnow, in a second study, showed increased crestal bone loss when the interimplant distance was less than 3 mm.[40] Therefore papilla loss would occur when implants adjacent to each other are placed too close. However, many additional factors are significant in determining whether papillae are present, which include tooth size and shape, implant/tooth position, periodontal status, tissue biotype, and possible prosthesis overhang/misfit.

Nordland and Tarnow[41] have proposed a classification using three reference points that include the contact point, facial and apical extent of cement-enamel junction (CEJ), and interproximal extent of CEJ. From these criteria a classification was reported with four descriptions of papilla:

Normal: interdental papilla occupies embrasure space to the apical part of the interdental contact point
Class I: tip of interdental papilla occupies space between the interdental contact point and the most coronal part of the CEJ
Class II: tip of interdental papilla lies at or apical to the CEJ but coronal to the apicalmost part of the CEJ on facial aspect
Class III: tip of interdental papilla lies at level with or apical to the facial CEJ

Injection Technique. A hyaluronic gel is injected 2 to 3 mm apical to the tip of the papilla. The tissue is entered with the needle until bone is contacted. The needle is slightly pulled back and material is deposited to plump up the papilla. A gentle massage and molding of the filler is completed, ideally with a cotton swab. Approximately 0.1 to 0.15 ml of product is used routinely per papilla treated (Fig. 40.20). Usually, papillary injected need to be repeated every 6 months.

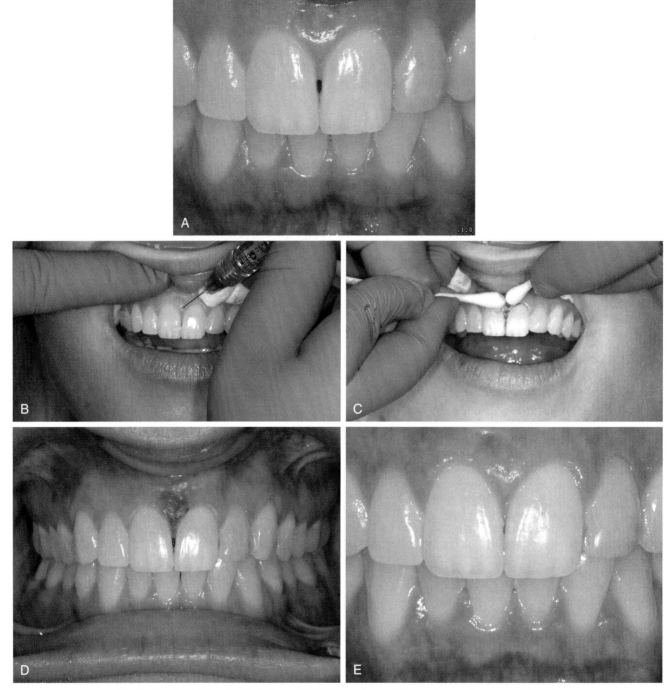

• **Fig. 40.20** Black Triangles Technique. (A) Obtain a photo of the black triangle area as a baseline. Anesthetize area to be treated via local infiltration. (B) Inject hyaluronic acid dermal filler into papilla with the bevel of the needle down and angled in the direction that the papilla needs to be bulked. (C) Shape papilla using cotton-tip applicators. Often multiple appointments are needed to achieve ideal outcome. (D) Immediate post-operative view. (E) 2-week post-operative view after two treatments.

Lips

When evaluating patients for comprehensive dental care involving dental implants, the lips are an often overlooked anatomic area. Lips are an essential part of the facial symmetry of the patient and esthetics. In society today patients are more esthetically conscious and view lips as needing to be fuller and more pronounced. When the vermilion lip is thin, facial harmony may be disrupted. With

the aging process, there becomes a less exposed vermilion, consisting of increased loss of vermilion bulk and length.

Anatomy

The lips are referred to as the "Labium superius oris" (upper) and "Labium inferius oris" (lower). The anatomy of the upper lip extends from the base of the nose superiorly to the nasolabial folds laterally and inferiorly to the free edge of the vermilion border.

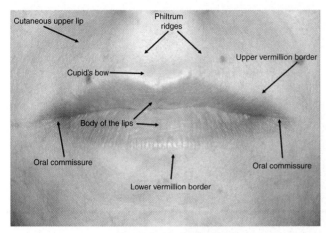

• **Fig. 40.21** Lip Anatomy.

The vermilion border is defined as the junction of the lips and the skin, and the area with the borders is termed the *vermilion zone*.

The vermilion border of the upper lip is known as the "Cupid's bow." Along the upper vermilion/skin border, two elevations of the vermilion form the Cupid's bow, which are raised vertical columns of tissue that form a midline depression called the *philtrum*.[42] The fleshy protuberance in the center of the upper lip is the tubercle, which is also known as the pro-cheilon (Fig. 40.21).

Most Common Lip Issues

The most common patient complaint concerning the lips is a deflating vermilion, mainly from insufficient volume. Usually female lips are fuller and bulge forward in comparison with male lips. The most ideal approach to lip augmentation depends on the deficiency and the patient's esthetic expectations. Most commonly the upper lip is treated more often than the lower. In general, genetically thin lips are treated with a deeper-placed filler, followed by volume correction with a superficial filler arch. When cosmetic enhancement is required, a superficially placed filler for expansion of the vermilion is ideal.[42]

Injection Technique

Jacono[43] has postulated a classification of 15 anatomic lip zones that is used to direct fillers for lip augmentation and to customize lip contour and size. This intended technique allows for better direction of the filler placement to create more fullness and maintain shape. He maintains five major zones within the lip region: vermilion/white roll, subvermilion, peristomal, philtral column, and commissural. The subvermilion corresponds to the dry mucosal lip, and the peristomal at the junction of dry and wet mucosal lip. The vermilion/white roll can be further subdivided in the upper lip to include lateral, Cupid's bow apical, and central philtral zones, whereas the lower lip vermilion is divided into medial and lateral zones. The subvermilion is subdivided into medial and lateral zones, and the peristomal into medial and lateral zones (Fig. 40.22).

1. Anesthesia is completed with an infraorbital block on the maxilla and a mental or inferior alveolar on the mandibular arch.
2. Different techniques are advocated for lip filler placement. The serial puncture and linear threading are usually used when applying the antegrade or retrograde method. The choice of one technique over another is usually personal preference of the clinician.

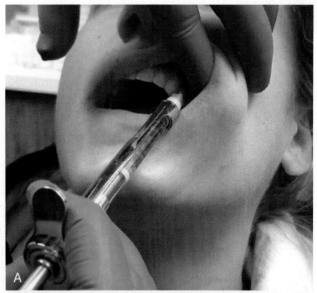

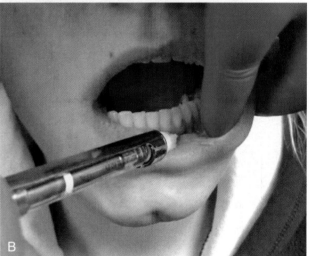

• **Fig. 40.22** Lip Injection Anesthesia. (A) Maxillary infraorbital injection. (B) Mandibular mental nerve block.

3. Medium-depth fillers are usually used for lip augmentation, such as: (1) Restylane, (2) Juvéderm Ultra, and (3) Esthélis Basic with the use of a 30-gauge needle or a 27-gauge cannula (Fig. 40.23).

Lip Injection Complications Complications

The most common complications from lip filler injections include post-injection lumps and nodules. Improper technique or over-aggressive injection may lead to irregularity or lumpiness, which usually occurs when overcorrection is completed. If the filler product is placed too superficial, beading can occur, leaving an unesthetic result. If large nodules or lumps are present, hyaluronidase injections may be used to dissolve the product. Herpetic labialis reactivation may be prevented with oral antivirals (acyclovir, famciclovir, or valaciclovir) (Fig. 40.24).

Face

There are two common areas in the face that directly impact esthetics with dental implant patients. These include the nasolabial folds and marionette lines, which become more prominent

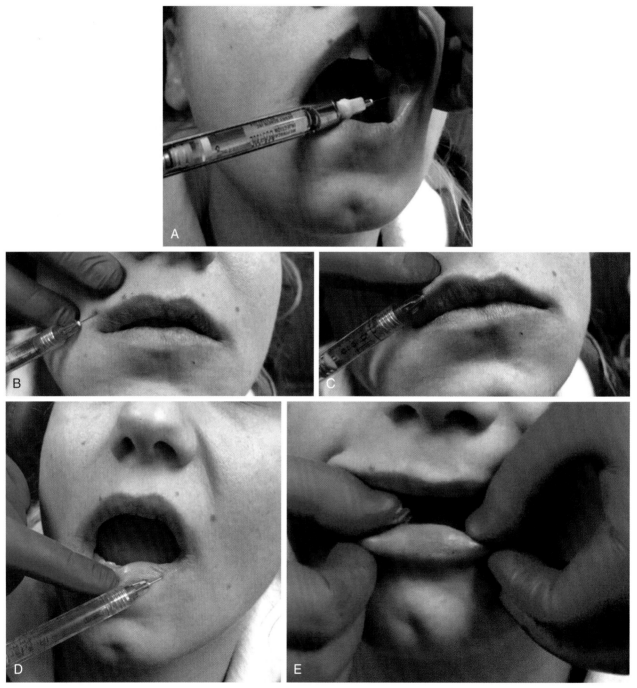

● **Fig. 40.23** **Lip Technique.** The lip augmentation is initiated by anesthetizing the upper and lower lips with bilateral Gordon Modified infraorbital blocks, mental blocks, (A) infiltration lateral to commissure of the mouth. (B, C, and D) Generally, begin by outlining the lips by injecting the subvermilion border starting at the commissure by placing retrograde threads. (E) Massage the outline using Vaseline to smooth.

continued

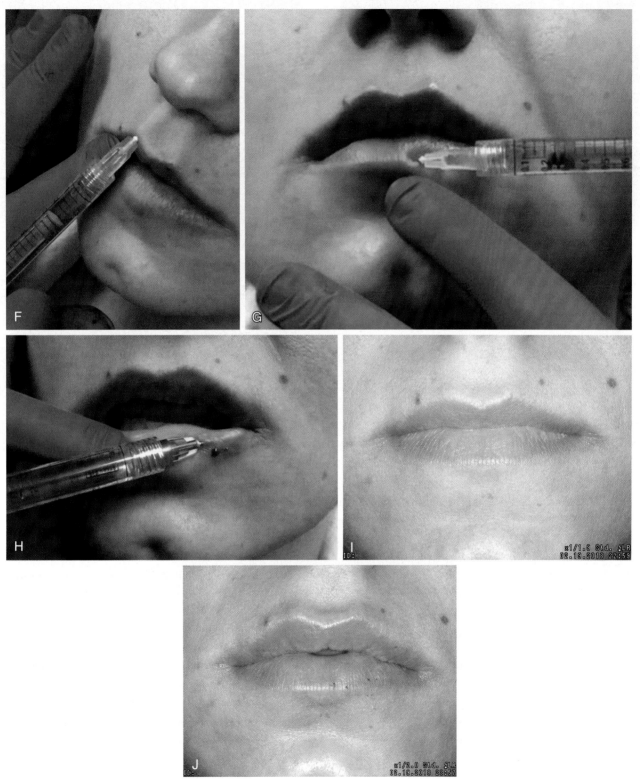

Fig. 40.23, cont'd (F). After the outline is completed, place two linear threads through the philtrum columns. Massage to smooth using cotton-tip applicator. (G- H) Assess for asymmetries and correct with threading or serial punctures. (I and J) Fill the lower and upper body of the lips to your liking. Massage well to smooth any irregularities.

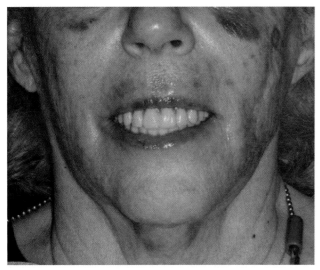

• **Fig. 40.24** Lip Complications: Edema and Ecchymosis.

with the aging process and loss of teeth/bone. The problem with these areas is the loss of volume and that they develop folds that become unesthetic. The darks lines associated with these areas are from a "shadow," which results from an elevated lateral component and less elevated medial area (i.e., a step is present between the two tissue areas)[44] (Fig. 40.25).

Goal of Facial Fillers

Basically, the goal of facial fillers is reduction of the "steps," which will reduce the loss of the shadow and the appearance of the lines.

Nasolabial Folds/Nasolabial Crease

As patients age, the vertical lines at the corner of the mouth become more evident. The zygomatic retaining ligaments become lax and the malar soft tissue migrates downward along the direction of the Zygomaticus Muscles (ZM), which results in bulging against the nasolabial crease. The skin lateral to the crease will stretch and become redundant, which results in the formation of a prominent nasolabial fold.[45]

Anatomic Area. The nasolabial folds include two skin folds that are located from the side of the nose to the corners of the mouth, which is made up of bulging fat pads. Basically this is the area that separates the cheek from the upper lip. The extent of the fold is at the junction of the nasal alar, the cheek, and the upper lip. As the fold progresses inferiorly, it will be in either a straight, convex, or concave shape and ends below and lateral to the corner of the mouth.[46] This anatomic area has been termed "smile" or "laugh" lines.[47] When patients smile, multiple muscles are responsible for the accentuation of the fold. The ZM muscle will pull the cheeks superior and laterally, and the orbicularis oris muscle pulls the upper lip inferiorly and medially. The levator anguli oris will contract, which results in the skin fold crease deepening and becoming more prevalent. The nasolabial crease, or sulcus, is the facial line between the upper lip and cheek, extending from the alae nasi to the lip commissure.

Injection Technique. In the treatment of nasolabial folds, volume of material is paramount to restoring contour. Usually a thicker dermal filler material is utilized deeper into the tissue space. If superficial placement of a thinner dermal filler is used, lack of contour will result with minimal longevity. Most commonly, the retrograde linear threading technique is used along

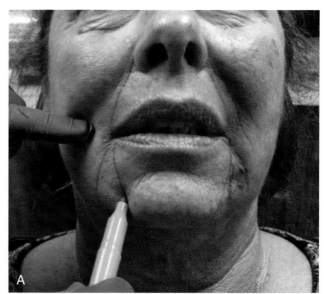

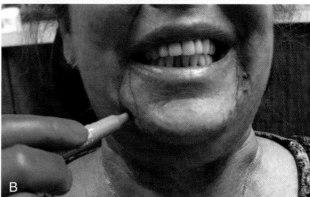

• **Fig. 40.25** (A and B) Dermal filler sites within the facial area.

the nasolabial fold. Caution should always be exercised in staying medial to the fold while depositing the product. If filler is injected laterally, deepening of the fold will occur resulting in esthetic issues.

Complication. Caution should be exercised in injecting in the subcutaneous layer lateral to the ala because the angular artery is most commonly located and the risk for vascular occlusion is higher (Fig. 40.26).

Marionette Lines

Marionette lines are associated with advancing age and are dependent on facial structure and anatomy. They are bilateral extensions of the nasolabial crease, which are directed inferiorly.

Anatomic Area. The marionette lines are formed mainly from the depressor anguli oris muscle and platysma muscle.

Injection Technique. The filler is ideally placed inferiorly in the subcutaneous layer and dermis in the oral commissure. To achieve a tissue eversion, inject in a fanning direction, which forms a tent pole effect. The use of the filler in the depressor anguli oris and mentalis and platysma below the mandibular margin allows the lateral oral commissure to elevate, restoring a more harmonious expression.

Complications. Injecting above or lateral to the lines will increase the shadowing effect by increasing the step (Fig. 40.27).

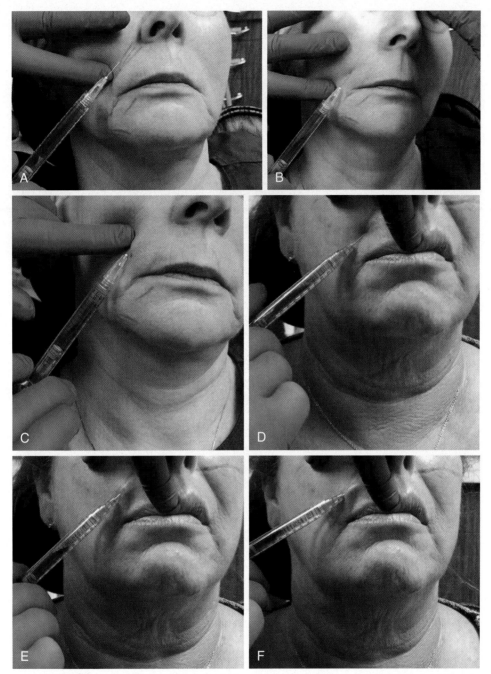

• **Fig. 40.26** Nasolabial Fold. (A) Nasolabial fold marked with skin marker. (B) Using the anterograde linear threading technique, dermal fillers are extruded along the nasolabial fold. (C and D) Be sure to stay medial to the fold while depositing product because extending laterally will result in deepening the fold. (E and F) Final medial injections.

Angular Cheilitis

Angular cheilitis is diagnosed by the presence of redness, inflammation, maceration, and fissuring of the oral commissures. Patients usually describe a painful, burning area at the corners of the mouth. In many cases mastication is impacted and range of opening is compromised.

Etiology. The etiology of angular cheilitis is multifactorial and involves many conditions that promote a moist environment within the oral commissure area. Deficiencies in iron, riboflavin

(B$_2$), folate (B$_9$), cobalamin (B$_{12}$), or zinc have been associated with this disorder. In addition, a decrease in vertical dimension from tooth loss, bone resorption, or inability to wear prostheses leads to the development of angular cheilitis. In almost all cases *Candida albicans* contributes to the pathophysiology of angular cheilitis.

Injection Technique. Therapeutic use of dermal fillers in the lips and perioral structures has become increasingly popular in implant dentistry (Fig. 40.28). Treatment of the lips and perioral structures

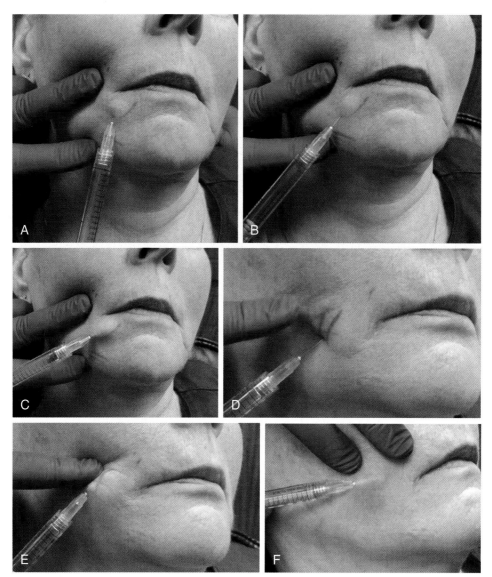

• **Fig. 40.27** Marionette lines follow the line down from the nasal labial fold, ensuring that you stay medial to the fold again. (A) Fan across in an upward vector to lighten the marionette lines (B–D). Follow with fanning or cross-hatching above the marionette lines in an upward direction (E and F). Massage well to eliminate any bumps from the product.

yields various practical dental improvements in orthognathic soft tissue profile, retention of removable prosthetics, proper phonetics, asymmetric smiles, and loss of soft tissue profile due to missing teeth. In treating the oral commissures a significant decrease in angular cheilitis has been noted. Injection of dermal fillers has been shown to restore the commissure anatomy and decrease the sulcus area to minimize recurrence. However, the clinician must investigate all possible etiologies of the angular cheilitis and treat accordingly. Nutritional deficiencies and a collapsed vertical dimension of occlusion have been associated with angular cheilitis. Anticandidal treatment may be used alone or in conjunction with dermal filler treatment. The injection technique for angular cheilitis includes having the patient opening wide, and injection of dermal filler directly into the commissure with a linear thread technique. The threading or fanning technique may be used also under the lower lip in an upward vector to increase elevation of the tissue.

Reversals for Dermal Fillers

Dermal fillers are advantageous because they exhibit reversibility with an enzyme, hyaluronidase. Hyaluronidase is a naturally occurring protein in the body and will catabolize hyaluronic acid usually within 24 hours through hydrolysis. This reversal agent is mainly used when overcorrection or misplacement of the dermal filler occurs.

Complications With Dermal Fillers

Dermal fillers are associated with complications, some that can be quite severe. A through medical history is advised before injecting dermal fillers. A history of hypertrophic scars or keloids may contraindicate the procedure. A history of herpes simplex infections may require premedication with valacyclovir

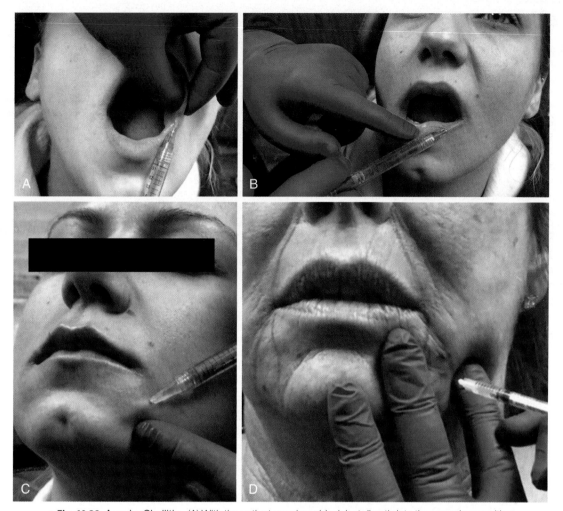

• **Fig. 40.28 Angular Cheilitis.** (A) With the patient opening wide, inject directly into the commissure with a linear thread. (B) Follow with linear thread in the lower lip line. Massage lip to smooth. (C) Optional fanning below to fill any depressions. (D) Often this treatment is done in combination with injecting the depressor anguli oris with botulinum toxin type A.

or other antivirals before lip injections. Patients who take anticoagulant therapy or certain vitamins should be treated with caution because of increased risks associated with bleeding and bruising.

The most common complication of dermal fillers includes an asymmetric appearance caused by too much material being injected into a particular site. Clinicians should always attempt to undertreat specific areas because overtreatment is extremely difficult to remedy.

More common local complications appear as redness, inflammation, and bruising. This often occurs secondarily from trauma caused by the injections. Erythema usually resolves within hours; however, edema may last for multiple days. Edema may be reduced by minimizing the number of injection sites, using epinephrine-containing anesthetics, and applying ice/cold compresses after the procedure. It has been suggested that using a product such as arnica (homeopathic herb) may reduce the effects of the trauma from the injections.

Injection to the proper angle and depth is of utmost importance; being too superficial may result in the "Tyndall effect," where the skin appears bluish at the injection site. Tissue necrosis may also occur if the filler occludes a blood vessel. In the event of suspected tissue necrosis, immediate reversal with hyaluronidase is advised and close postoperative care is imperative.

Complications[48]

Early Onset (Immediate > 15 Days)
Due to the procedure, not filler related
    Erythema
    Pain bruising
    Swelling at injection site
    Infection (viral or bacterial) can be related to filler due to biofilm
Due to filler behavior and placement technique
    Overcorrection
    Misplacement
    Hypersensitivity (type IV reaction)
    Vascular occlusion
    Granuloma

Late Onset (> 15 days)
Due to the procedure, not filler related
    Chronic infection
    Itching
Due to filler behavior and placement technique
    Skin discoloration
    Nodules (product accumulation)
    Hypertropic scarring
    Hypersensitivity (type IV reaction)

Conclusion

The use of Botox and dermal fillers have been shown through the literature to be valuable adjuncts in implant dentistry. These pharmacologic agents are successful in treating many facial and maxillofacial musculature dysfunctions as they provide an overall conservative, minimally invasive treatment approach. Most notably, Botox may be indicated for the treatment of parafunctional habits that may be detrimental to the overall dental implant success. In addition, the use of Botox in the treatment of various temporomandibular joint syndrome/temporomandibular dysfunction (TMJ/TMD) disorders and excessive tissue display (gummy smiles) have been shown to successful. The use of dermal fillers have become popular for facial and cheek soft tissue augmentation as well as for the treatment of angular cheilitis. With respect to dental implants, papilla loss leading to the formation of black triangles may be treated with dermal fillers leading to the reversal of the open spaces. Therefore, with the advances of technology and science, the use of Botox products as well as dermal fillers are becoming more popular and have become a mainstay in implant dentistry.

References

1. Binder WJ, Blitzer A, Brin MF. Treatment of hyperfunctional lines of the face with botulinum toxin A. *Dermatol Surg.* 1998;24:1198–1205.
2. Delcanho R. Botox injections. In: Selvaratnam P, Niere K, Zuluaga Maria, eds. *Headache, Orofacial Pain and Bruxism.* Churchill Livingstone; 2009:347–356.
3. Hexsel DM, De Almeida AT, Rutowitsch M, et al. Multicenter, double blind study of the efficacy of injections with botulinum toxin type A reconstituted up to six consecutive weeks before application. *Dermatol Surg.* 2003;29:523–529.
4. Kim HJ, Yum KW, Lee SS, et al. Effects of botulinum toxin type A on bilateral masseteric hypertrophy evaluated with computed tomographic measurement. *Dermatol Surg.* 2003;29(5):484–489.
5. Fehrenbach M, Herring SW. *Illustrated Anatomy of the Head and Neck.* 4th ed. Philadelphia: Saunders; 2012:97.
6. von Lindern JJ, Niederhagen B, Apple T, et al. Type A botulinum toxin for the treatment of hypertrophy of the masseter and temporal muscles: an alternative treatment. *Plast Reconstr Surg.* 2001;107:327–332.
7. Hu KS, Kim ST, Hur MS, et al. Topography of the masseter muscle in relation to treatment with botulinum toxin type A. *Oral Surg Oral Med Oral Pathol Oral Radiol Endod.* 2010;110:167–171.
8. Al-Ahmad HT, Al-Qudah MA. The treatment of masseter hypertrophy with botulinum toxin type A. *Saudi Med J.* 2006;27(3):397–400.
9. Clark GT. The management of oromandibular motor disorders and facial spasms with injections of botulinum toxin. *Phys Med Rehabil Clin North Am.* 2003;14(4):727–748.
10. Rijsdijk BA, Van ESRJ, Zonneveld FW, et al. Botulinum toxin type A treatment of cosmetically disturbing masseteric hypertrophy. *Ned Tijdschr Geneeskd.* 1998;142(10):529–532.
11. Rafferty KL, Liu ZJ, Navarrete AL, et al. Botulinum toxin in masticatory muscles: short-and long-term effects on muscle, bone, and craniofacial function in adult rabbits. *Bone.* 2012;50(3):651–662.
12. Van Zandijcke M, Marchau MM. Treatment of bruxism with botulinum toxin injections. *J Neurol Neurosurg Psychiatry.* 1990;53(6):530.
13. Scheid RC, Woelfel JB. *Woelfel's dental anatomy: its relevance to dentistry.* Philadelphia: Lippincott Williams & Wilkins; 2007:41.
14. Bas B, Ozan B, Muglali M, Celebi N. Treatment of masseteric hypertrophy with botulinum toxin: a report of two cases. *Med Oral Patol Oral Cir Bucal.* 2010;15(4):649–652.
15. Schwartz Marvin, Freund Brian. Treatment of temporomandibular disorders with botulinum toxin. *Clin J pain.* 2002;18(6):S198–S203.
16. Guarda-Nardini L, Manfredini D, Salamone M, et al. Efficacy of botulinum toxin in treating myofascial pain in bruxers: a controlled placebo pilot study. *Cranio.* 26:126–135.
17. Baker, J. S., & Nolan, P. J. (2017). Effectiveness of botulinum toxin type A for the treatment of chronic masticatory myofascial pain: A case series. *The Journal of the American Dental Association,* 148(1), 33–39.
18. Tan EK, Jankovic J. Treating severe bruxism with botulinum toxin. *J Am Dent Assoc.* 2000;131:211–216.
19. Monroy PG, Da Fonseca MA. The use of botulinum toxin-a in the treatment of severe bruxism in a patient with autism: a case report. *Spec Care Dentist.* 2006;26:37–39.
20. Sinha Aditya, Hurakadli Megha, Yadav Pramod. Botox and derma fillers: the twin face of cosmetic dentistry. *Int J Contemp Dent Med Rev.* 2015.
21. Kokich Vincent O, Asuman Kiyak H, Peter Shapiro A. Comparing the perception of dentists and lay people to altered dental esthetics. *J Esthet Restor Dent.* 1999;11(6):311–324.
22. Polo M. Botulinum toxin type A (Botox) for the neuromuscular correction of excessive gingival display on smiling (gummy smile). *Am J Orthod Dentofacial Orthop.* 2008;133(2):195–203.
23. Peck S, Peck L. Selected aspects of the art and science of facial esthetics. *Sem Orthod.* 1995;1(2):105–126.
24. Al-Jabrah, Osama, Raghda Al-Shammout, Waddah El-Naji, Mahasen Al-Ajarmeh, and Abdel-Hakeem Al-Quran. "Gender differences in the amount of gingival display during smiling using two intraoral dental biometric measurements." *Journal of Prosthodontics: Implant, Esthetic and Reconstructive Dentistry* 19, no. 4 (2010): 286–293.
25. Ackerman MB, Ackerman JL. Smile analysis and design in the digital era. *J Clin Orthod.* 2002;36(4):221–236.
26. Nasr MW, Jabbour SF, Sidaoui JA, et al. Botulinum toxin for the treatment of excessive gingival display: a systematic review. *Aesthet Surg J.* 2015;36(1):82–88.
27. Hwang WS, Hur MS, Hu KS, et al. Surface anatomy of the lip elevator muscles for the treatment of gummy smile using botulinum toxin. *Angle Orthod.* 2009;79(1):70–77.
28. Miller J, Clarkson E. Botulinum toxin type A: review and its role in the dental office. *Dent Clin North Am.* 2016;60(2):509–521.
29. Grover S, Malik V, Kaushik A, et al. A future perspective of botox in dentofacial region. *J Pharm Biomed Sci.* 2014;04(05):525–531.
30. Clark GT, Stiles A, Lockerman LZ, et al. A critical review of the use of botulinum toxin in orofacial pain disorders. *Dent Clin N Am.* 2007;51:245–261.
31. Park NY, Ahn KY, Jung DS. Botulinum toxing type a treatment for contouring of the lower face. *Dermatol Surg.* 2003;29(5):477–483.
32. Patel D, Mehta F, Trivedi R, et al. Botulinum toxin and gummy smile-A review. *IOSR J Dent Med Sci.* 2013;4(1):1–5.
33. Freund B, Finkelstein I, Ko G. Review of the applications of botulinum toxin and tissue fillers in dental practice. *Oral Health.* 2014.
34. https://www.plasticsurgery.org/documents/News/Statistics/2016/top-five-cosmetic-plastic-surgery-procedures-2016.pdf.
35. Chen J, Abatangelo G. Functions of hyaluronan in wound repair. *Wound Repair Regen.* 1999;7(2):79–89.
36. Rohrich RJ, Ghavami A, Crosby MA. The role of hyaluronic acid fillers (Restylane) in facial cosmetic surgery: review and technical considerations. *Plast Reconstr Surg.* 2007;120(suppl 6):41S–54S.
37. Carruthers J, Carruthers A. Soft tissue augmentation, fourth edition. *Procedures in Cosmetic Dermatology Series.* Elsevier; 2018.
38. Tarnow D, Elian N, Fletcher P, et al. Vertical distance from the crest of bone to the height of the interproximal papilla between adjacent implants. *J Periodontol.* 2003;74:1785–1788.

39. Cho HS, Jang HS, Kim DK, et al. The effects of interproximal distance between roots on the existence of interdental papillae according to the distance from the contact point to the alveolar crest. *J Periodontol*. 2006;77:1651–1657.

40. Tarnow, Dennis, Nicolas Elian, Paul Fletcher, Stuart Froum, Ann Magner, Sang-Choon Cho, Maurice Salama, Henry Salama, and David A. Garber. "Vertical distance from the crest of bone to the height of the interproximal papilla between adjacent implants." *Journal of periodontology* 74, no. 12 (2003): 1785–1788.

41. Nordland WP, Tarnow DP. A classification system for loss of papillary height. *J Periodontol*. 1998;69:1124–1126.

42. Luthra A. Shaping lips with fillers. *J Cutan Aesthet Surg*. 2015;8(3):139.

43. Jacono AA. A new classification of lip zones to customize injectable lip augmentation. *Arch Facial Plast Surg*. 2008;10(1):25–29.

44. Guyuron B, Michelow B. The nasolabial fold: a challenge, a solution. *Plastic Reconstr Surg*. 1994;93(3):522–529.

45. Weinzweig J. *Plastic Surgery Secrets Plus*. Elsevier;2010. 498–505.

46. Zufferey J. Anatomic variations of the nasolabial fold. *Plastic Reconstr Surg*. 1992;89(2):225–231.

47. Pogrel MA, Shariati S, Schmidt B, et al. The surgical anatomy of the nasolabial fold. *Oral Surg Oral Med Oral Pathol, Oral Radiol Endod*. 1998;86(4):410–415.

48. Carruthers A, Carruthers J. *Botulinum Toxin: Procedures in Cosmetic Dermatology Series*. Elsevier; 2018.

PART VIII

Dental Implant Maintenance

41

Peri-Mucositis and Peri-Implantitis Diagnosis, Classification, Etiologies, and Therapies

JON B. SUZUKI AND KEVIN R. SUZUKI

Implant dentistry has evolved into an evidence-based, clinical science with well-documented research to validate previously unsupported clinical practice procedures. Significant efforts that focus on the biology and biomechanics of implant dentistry have helped to develop and refine clinical techniques based on peer-reviewed findings. However, despite improved and predictable clinical successes in implantology, peri-implant diseases have been diagnosed with increasing incidence. The evolution of research and understanding of biologic concepts in implant dentistry and implant rescue has caused many areas of debate and controversy. Innovative theories have been developed that have resulted in technique modifications. Science has spurred implant dentistry to new pinnacles of success, which is highly based upon essential principles of periodontal regeneration.

The tremendous expansion of knowledge in implant dentistry has created new ideas and terminology that is redefined based on new applications to implant dentistry. In many instances new research may contradict established paradigms. It may be challenging for clinicians to select correct protocols, procedures, armamentarium, and techniques. As materials and techniques are further investigated, dogma may undergo criticism and controversy. Experienced clinicians consistently introduce and refine techniques and instruments to maintain clinical excellence as technology and research advance.

One area of expansion of knowledge and views relates to the maintenance of dental implants. Early research explored techniques and instruments that were current for the methods and materials of that era. Although many of those implants are still in function in patients today, research and advances in technology have given us newer materials, implant design, and protocols to maintain dental implant health.

An understanding of the mucoepithelial implant attachment is essential before commencing maintenance procedures. Controversies and parameters for probing and crestal bone loss are important for clinicians to recognize. There are anatomic and histologic differences between the attachment apparatus of teeth compared with implants that are osseointegrated. The bacterial plaque biofilm on these implant-tissue attachments may be significant to clinical success.

When the clinician understands the parameters of implants and teeth, specific maintenance plans may be established for the patient to minimize the possibility of developing peri-implant disease. Clinicians should inform patients of expectations and outcomes during treatment, and demonstrate oral hygiene options appropriate during each stage. Patients need to recognize the importance of maintenance protocols, and clinicians should assess compliance to home care routines. Patients also should be competent to perform home maintenance. These strategies would certainly minimize risks for peri-implant disease and implant failures.

As the acceptance of and demand for dental implants increase, the need to understand the importance of maintenance as it relates to long-term implant success also increases. The role of the dental hygienist in implant maintenance and care as well as diagnosing peri-implant disease is increasing and becoming more defined.

Implants and associated prostheses are much different from natural teeth and may require adjunctive procedures and instruments for professional and patient care. Complications may arise when clinicians fail to comprehend these differences, because they may adversely impact the implant's outcome, increasing the morbidity of treatment. The techniques and protocols used must be effective at removing biofilms and accretions, and procedures performed by patients and clinicians should avoid damage to the components of the implant, abutment, restoration, and associated tissue.

Establishment and maintenance of the soft tissue seal around the transmucosal portion of the implant enhances the success of an implant. This barrier is fundamentally a result of appropriate wound healing and connection of epithelial attachments. The maintenance of healthy peri-implant tissues contributes to implant success and minimizes peri-implant disease. In addition, tissues free of inflammation and a biofilm-controlled implant sulcus will support the patient's general and oral health.

Peri-implant Disease

One important, but often neglected, component of comprehensive dental implant treatment is the postprosthetic evaluation and treatment of peri-implant issues. There are many conflicting opinions and controversies on the diagnosis and treatment of these complications. Failure to effectively and promptly diagnose and treat peri-implant disease with dental implants leads to an increase in implant and prosthetic failure.

Dental professionals are initially trained to have a firm understanding of the disease processes associated with the natural dentition. A variety of tests, indices, and radiographic signs are used to determine the health of a natural tooth. Dental implants and their related prostheses have fundamentally different relationships to the oral environment than teeth, and these differences necessitate a change in diagnostic protocol for the determination of health. Failure to understand these processes may lead to undiagnosed disease states and potential morbidity of the implant system.

The implant clinician must have a strong understanding of the anatomic and histologic differences between natural dentition and the dental implant as they pertain to periodontal structures. By having this foundation, the clinician may appreciate these necessary differences and will be better equipped to effectively diagnose peri-implant disease processes. With the increase in the number of dental implants being placed each year, a resultant increase in the incidence of peri-implant disease has been seen. Two conditions of peri-implant disease are ***peri-implant mucositis*** and ***peri-implantitis***.[1] The 6th European Workshop on Periodontology in 2008 concluded that peri-implant diseases are infectious in nature and are defined by "changes in the level of crestal bone, presence of bleeding on probing, and/or suppuration; with or without deepening of the peri-implant pockets."[2]

In differentiation between these two peri-implant conditions, both have been shown to be localized around implants and demonstrate features similar to adult chronic periodontal disease.[3] These conditions may be analogous to gingivitis (peri-mucositis) and periodontitis (peri-implantitis). However, biologic differences exist between the natural teeth and implants. Basically, peri-implant tissues are more susceptible to infections, due to differences in soft tissue attachment and biofilms that may advance to the alveolar-implant complex (see discussion in Chapter 42).[4]

Gingivitis is a bacteria-induced inflammation involving the region of the marginal gingiva above the crest of bone and adjacent to a natural tooth. The most common forms are associated with plaque and may be classified as: (1) acute necrotizing, (2) ulcerative, (3) hormonal, (4) drug induced, or (5) spontaneously occurring.[5] These categories may also relate to the gingival tissues around an implant.[6,7] The classification of gingivitis and periodontitis has currently been updated by the American Academy of Periodontology.[8]

The bacteria responsible for gingivitis around a tooth may affect the epithelial attachment, without loss of connective tissue attachment. Because the connective tissue attachment of a tooth extends an average of 1.07 mm above the crestal bone, at least 1 mm of protective barrier above the bone is present. In contrast, no connective tissue attachment zone exists around an implant because there is an absence of connective fibers that extend into the implant surface. Therefore no connective tissue barrier exists to protect the crestal bone around an implant.[9]

Periodontitis around teeth is characterized by apical movement of junctional epithelium and periodontal attachment, coupled with loss of alveolar bone. Bacteria are thought to be responsible by stimulating the body's immune response, which results in an

• **BOX 41.1   Common Bacteria Associated With Pocket Depths**

Shallow
- Gram-positive facultative cocci, rods
- Gram-negative anaerobic cocci, rods
- Motile rods
- Spirochetes
- Black-pigmented bacteroides
- Fusobacterium

Deep
- Vibrios organisms

overall resorptive effect on the periodontal attachment apparatus. The American Academy of Periodontology (2018) recognizes stages of periodontitis: stage 1, stage 2, stage 3, and stage 4. Former specific subtypes[10] for each category such as adult chronic periodontitis, rapidly progressive periodontitis, localized juvenile, and prepubertal periodontitis are now encompassed within stage 1, stage 2, and stage 3 of periodontitis.

In contrast with teeth, early crestal bone loss around an implant body prosthetically may not always be caused by pathogens. In many cases, the associated bone loss may result from stress factors too great for the immature, incompletely mineralized bone-implant interface or an extension of the biologic width onto a smooth metal crest module.[11] Therefore, an implant may exhibit early crestal bone loss with a different mechanism or cause, compared with natural teeth. However, bacteria in some cases may be the primary factor, because anaerobic bacteria have been observed in the microgap between the implant and the abutment or in the sulcus of implants. This is especially evident when sulcus depths are greater than 5 mm (Box 41.1).[12] A systematic review[13] highlights potential etiologies of early crestal bone loss around recently osseointegrated implants.

In summary, periodontal disease that develops around dental implants has been classified into two separate entities: peri-implant mucositis and peri-implantitis. Peri-implant mucositis is defined as a reversible inflammatory reaction in the peri-implant tissues surrounding an implant. Peri-implantitis is defined as an inflammatory reaction, with loss of supporting bone around an implant (Fig. 41.1).

The Role of Biofilm in Peri-Implant Disease

The oral biofilm originates from bacteria and saliva, which result in sticky masses of bacteria with a polysaccharide matrix that accumulate on hard and soft surfaces in the oral cavity. The bacterial and biofilm formation may adhere to any implant surfaces in the oral cavity and have been reported to result in pocket formation and loss of the supporting bone.[14-16] Di Giulio et al.[17] determined that biofilm is one of the major causes of implant failure. The Consensus of the 7th European Workshop on Periodontology stated that peri-implant infections are always caused by plaque and its by-products (i.e., biofilm).[18]

The role of biofilms has been heavily studied and has been reported to be responsible for approximately 65% of peri-implant diseases.[19] After exposure of the implant surface to the oral cavity, a pellicle is formed in less than 30 minutes.[20] The pellicle is derived from the saliva, various bacteria present in the oral cavity, and also host tissue products. After formation of the pellicle, bacterial attachment occurs by cell-to-cell adhesion on the implant surface.[21] Most bacteria use biofilm as the primary method of growth, because they facilitate nutrient exchange and prevent competing microorganisms.[22] Studies have shown the process of biofilm colonization is the same on teeth as with dental implants.[23]

Therefore the most ideal solution to prevent microbial infections is to decrease the colonization of bacteria on implant surfaces. Unfortunately, many characteristics (e.g., material, surface roughness) of prosthetic and implant surfaces directly affect the bacterial adhesion and biofilm formation.[24]

For reversal of the peri-implant disease process, the biofilm must be removed with mechanical debridement or chemical obliteration. If not removed, mature plaque will form. It has been shown that bacteria will migrate from teeth to implants and from implant to implant. Similar to teeth, clinical findings of failing implants include inflammation, pocket formation, and progressive bone loss.[25]

The microorganisms may initiate an inflammatory release of cytokines that will enhance accumulation of neutrophils to the implant lesion. This process will continue to attract more leukocytes and continue to facilitate more peri-implant tissue damage and inflammation.[26,27] If the inflammation progresses, it will lead to peri-implantitis, with the characteristic feature of bone loss around the implant. If left untreated, stromal tissue cells may also propagate, leading to an increase in infiltrates of proinflammatory cells that promotes further tissue breakdown,[28-30] which may eventually lead to loss of osseointegration, implant mobility, and ultimately implant failure.[31-33] In addition to the results of a systematic review, there is evidence that the pathogens *Prevotella intermedia*, *Campylobacter rectus*, *Aggregatibacter actinomycetemcomitans*, and *Treponema denticola* have been implicated in the pathogenesis of peri-implantitis.[34,35]

Current chemotherapeutics cannot penetrate thick biofilm, because rough surfaces have been found to hold more biofilm than smooth surfaces.[36] Bacterial deposits produce exotoxins and lipopolysaccharides (endotoxins) that inhibit fibroblast and osteoblastic growth, and thus prevent proximal regeneration onto the implant surface. Although it is impossible to guarantee 100% sterility of exposed implant surfaces, the body is capable of removing small amounts of bacterial deposit via host defense mechanisms.[37]

Carefully removing macrodeposits of plaque biofilm and irrigating with antimicrobial solution is generally sufficient to allow a favorable environment for new attachment formation. It is recommended that patients complete a full-mouth debridement to reduce bacterial colonies, including plaque biofilms on exposed implant surfaces (Box 41.2).

Peri-implant Mucositis

Peri-implant mucositis is an inflammatory condition of the soft tissue surrounding an implant, which is similar to gingivitis around natural teeth. In both animal and human studies, peri-implant mucositis has been shown clinically and histologically to be comparable to gingivitis around natural teeth.[184] This has been defined

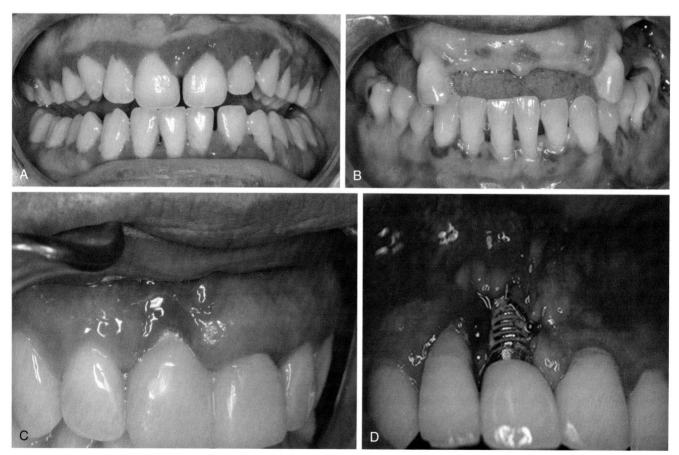

• **Fig. 41.1** (A) Spongiotic gingivitis exhibiting erythematous marginal tissue with cyanotic tissue. (B) Periodontitis: mandibular anterior exhibiting severe horizontal bone loss. (C) Peri-mucositis: erythematous buccal gingiva with associated bleeding around implant crown. (D) Peri-implantitis: significant bone loss with erythematous tissue with significant plaque accumulation. (*From Suzuki JB, Misch CE. Periodontal and maintenance complications. In: Resnik RR, Misch CE, eds.* Misch's Avoiding Complications in Oral Implantology. *St. Louis, MO: Elsevier; 2018.*)

as a reversible condition with no loss of attachment or bone loss. The prevalence rate of peri-implant mucositis (bleeding on probing and no loss of bone) in systemic reviews has been shown to be approximately 30% of implants and 47 % of patients.[38] However, other studies have reported the incidence to be as high as 80% of patients and 50 % of implants observed. Ferreira et al. reported a prevalence of 64.6% at the patient level and 62.6% at

implant level.[39] Clinically, bleeding on peri-implant probing with mucositis may be present without suppuration. If peri-mucositis is allowed to progress, peri-implantitis may result, which includes loss of bone and possible loss of osseointegration, similar to loss of attachment and bone with periodontitis. The relationship between plaque accumulation and peri-implant mucosal inflammation has been proven through numerous studies (Fig. 41.2).[40-42]

BOX 41.2 Bacteria and Etiology of Peri-Implant Mucositis

Bacteria

Prevotella intermedia
Porphyromonas gingivalis
Aggregatibacter actinomycetemcomitans
Tannerella forsythia (formerly Bacteroides forsythus)
Treponema denticola
Prevotella nigrescens
Fusobacterium nucleatum

Etiology

- Poor Oral Hygiene
- Poor Compliance with Supportive Procedures
- Poor Prosthesis Design
- Poor Fit of Prosthesis
- Non-ideal Implant Position
- Lack of Non-Keratinized Peri-Implant Mucosa
- Retained Cement

Etiology

Most cases of peri-implant mucositis are due to poor oral hygiene, inability to clean the implant or prosthesis, nonideal implant position, poor fit of the prosthesis, and retained cement. Poorly placed implants or overcontoured prostheses may lead to difficulty or inability to properly clean the implants (Fig. 41.3). In addition, peri-implant mucositis may also be caused by titanium alloy hypersensitivity. Most dental implants today are covered by a titanium dioxide layer that gives the implant a high surface energy that facilitates the interaction between the host tissues and the dental implant. When the implant becomes exposed to the oral environment, a lower surface energy may provoke a type IV hypersensitivity reaction that may contribute to peri-implant mucositis.[43]

Prevention

Because of the high prevalence of peri-implant mucositis, it is imperative that the clinician be able to assess the risk profile of each patient and integrate these considerations when treatment

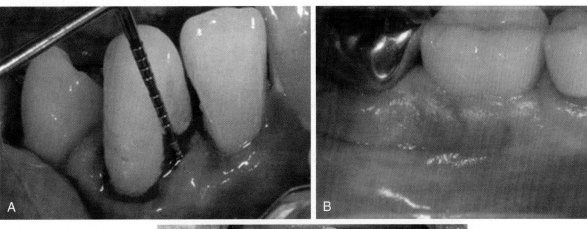
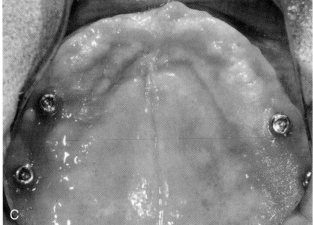

Fig. 41.2 Peri-mucositis. (A) Bleeding on probing without bone loss with a diagnosis of peri-mucositis. (B) Inflammation on the buccal aspect of the mandibular first molar implant. (C) Maxillary overdenture causing peri-mucositis and fungal infections.

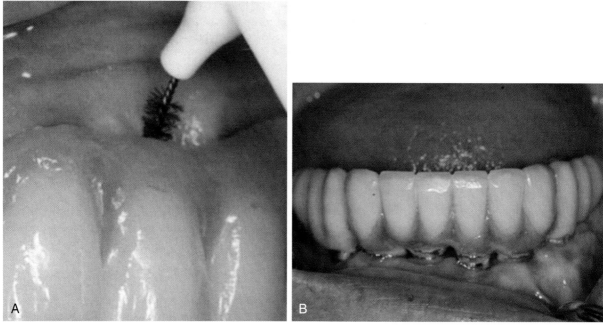

• **Fig. 41.3** Prosthesis-Related Peri-mucositis. (A) Hygiene difficulty because of an (B) When prostheses are fixed, usually hygiene will be more difficult.

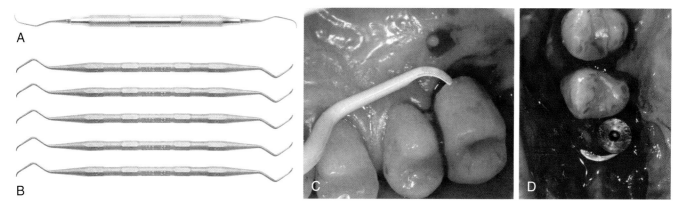

• **Fig. 41.4** (A) Titanium curette. (B) Carbon-reinforced curette. (C) Teflon/plastic. (D) Steel curette. (*A and B, Courtesy Salvin Dental Specialties, Inc., Charlotte, N.C.*)

planning is initiated. A consensus report by the Academy of Periodontology has shown risk factors to include poor oral hygiene, history of periodontal disease, smoking, retained cement, and occlusal disharmonies. Therefore, a comprehensive medical history should be evaluated for any risk factors and the patient should be informed of possible associated complications.

Tobacco smoking leads to the end product of nicotine and nornicotine that increases cytokine levels and reactive oxygen species. Increased smoking has been shown to result in increased levels of alveolar bone loss with dental implants.[44] Diabetes mellitus has also been shown to increase the risk for peri-implant disease compared with healthy individuals.[45] This is due to elevated blood sugar levels that compromise wound healing and the host immune system.

Management

Peri-implant mucositis is a reversible inflammatory process. However, if not treated properly, the persistent inflammatory condition may progress to peri-implantitis that results in irreversible bone loss. In most cases peri-implant mucositis is a precursor for the development of peri-implantitis.[46]

Nonsurgical (closed debridement) mechanical debridement to remove plaque and calculus from the implant surface using mechanical instruments such as scalers and curettes coupled with antimicrobial rinse therapies is the primary therapeutic approach for peri-implant mucositis.[47]

In a systematic review, nonsurgical mechanical debridement is effective in the management of peri-implant mucositis. Use of antiseptics increased the observed outcomes.[48] It is crucial to implement a comprehensive patient and professional oral hygiene program to manage peri-implant mucositis. Power brushes, interproximal and irrigation power devices, dentifrices, and antimicrobials have been shown to be highly effective in the management of peri-implant mucositis.

Professional Mechanical Debridement

For the removal of supragingival and subgingival biofilm and bacteria, debridement of the exposed implant surface and implant abutment must be completed. There exist many different debridement systems.

Curettes. The selection of scalers for titanium implant debridement is important to minimize surface changes after treatment. Various types of curettes are available for debridement procedures (Fig. 41.4):

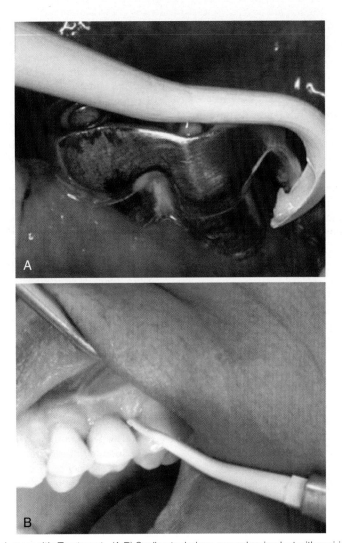

• **Fig. 41.5** Peri-mucositis Treatment. (A,B) Scaling technique around an implant with peri-implant inflammation.

- Titanium-coated curettes are specifically made for dental implant debridement because they have a similar hardness to the titanium surface and will not scratch or mar the surface.
- Carbon-fiber curettes are softer than the implant surfaces and will not damage the implant surface. These types of curettes are prone to fracture.
- Teflon curettes are similar to carbon-reinforced curettes and will not scratch the surface of the implant.
- Plastic curettes have been advocated as the instrument of choice to prevent damage from the implant surface.
- Stainless-steel curettes are much harder than titanium alloy and are not recommended for use around dental implants because they may alter the implant surface.[49]
- Amorphous resin scalers come with unfilled or filled resin. Unfilled resin scalers have no reinforcements for shape or stiffness, whereas filled resin fillers may use materials such as silica, graphite, or glass. These scalers have replacement tips on stainless-steel handles.
- Titanium brush burs insert into implant motors. They have a variety of shapes, allowing them to adapt around the implant or prosthesis surface circumferentially, around a single surface, and for groove cleaning. Brushes are used at 600 rpm and adapted against the implant surface to remove debris.

Hasturk et al. evaluated six different types of scaler materials to scratch surfaces of different brands of implants abutments, and they were compared with scanning electron microscopy. The results showed glass-filled resin curettes caused the most scratches, whereas the unfilled resin scalers had the least surface alteration. However, these studies are on smooth titanium abutments and not on the rough implant surface.[50]

There may not be clinical relevance regarding whether curettes scratch implant surfaces. Anastassiadis et al. reported that metal scalers do not readily scratch cementum; it is questionable that a titanium implant surface, which has a higher Mohs hardness, should be of any concern.[51]

Furthermore, scalers as a whole may be effective in removing large calculus particles or granulation tissues but are rather ineffective trying to navigate the perimeter and grooves of an exposed implant surface. For that reason, curette material may not be a significant concern, but rather the activity of curetting may be (Fig. 41.5).

Ultrasonic Devices

Ultrasonic devices with special polyetheretherketone-coated tips have been used to debride the implant surface. This tip is made of a plastic material with a stainless-steel core. This ultrasonic device allows the debridement of plaque and calculus, while leaving a smooth and clean surface.

Although metal tips are not recommended, plastic tips may be at an increased risk of shredding when cleaning around implant grooves and threads. Tips made of PEEK material (Hu-Friedy, Chicago, Ill.) have been shown to be resistant to shredding and may be considered (Fig. 41.6).

Antimicrobials

Antiseptics are defined as antimicrobial substances that are non-damaging to living tissue/skin while reducing the possibility of infection, sepsis, or putrefaction. Several types of antiseptics are ready for dental use: chlorhexidine 0.12% or 0.2%, cetylpyridinium chloride, sodium hypochlorite 1.0%, hydrogen peroxide 3.0%, citric acid 40.0%, Ethylenediamine tetraacetic acid (EDTA) 24%, povidone-iodine 10%, and phenols/essential oils.[52,53]

For management of peri-mucositis, several qualities are needed for antiseptics to be effective: biofilm penetration, long substantivity, tissue biocompatibility, and low resistance. Removal of macrodeposits should be performed with scalers first.

Chlorhexidine applied on a cotton pellet and burnished against a machined surface has shown a 92.9% *Porphyromonas gingivalis* endotoxin reduction.[54] Povidone-iodine has high antiseptic capability but has a highly irritating effect if any residue comes in contact with an osseous structure. Several of the antiseptics and their effectiveness on *Staphylococcus epidermidis*, *Candida albicans*, and *S. sanguinis* have been investigated. Although sodium hypochlorite was most effective in the reduction of all three bacterial biofilms, it has the highest tissue toxicity. Hydrogen peroxide was active against only *C. albicans*, whereas chlorhexidine gluconate and phenols/essential oils had activity against only *Streptococcus sanguinis* and *C. albicans*[55] (Fig. 41.7).

Patient At-Home Mechanical Debridement

Implant patients must understand their role in maintaining their dental implants and implant prosthesis. An individualized home care assessment and protocol must be developed for each patient, and it must be customized according to the tissue condition, implant position, and type of prosthesis. Home care devices that have been shown to be safe around implant surfaces include toothbrushes (manual or powered), floss (e.g., plastic, braided nylon, coated, stiffened ends to clean under pontic areas, and dental tape). In addition, oral irrigators, interdental brushes, and end-tuft brushes may be used. (See Chapter 42 for a complete list of home care aids.) A strong home care regimen may significantly reduce the amount and composition of subgingival microbiota around teeth. This reduction most likely will translate to a decreased risk for periodontal disease initiation or recurrence. Furthermore, the decreased prevalence of periodontal pathogens in supragingival plaque decreases potential reservoirs of these species.[63]

Peri-implantitis

The American Academy of Periodontology has defined peri-implantitis as an "inflammatory reaction associated with the loss of supporting bone beyond initial biologic bone remodeling

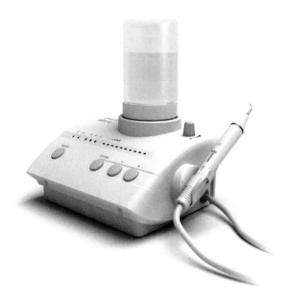

• **Fig. 41.6** Ultrasonic scalers may be used to treat peri-mucositis.

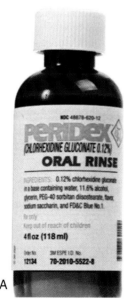
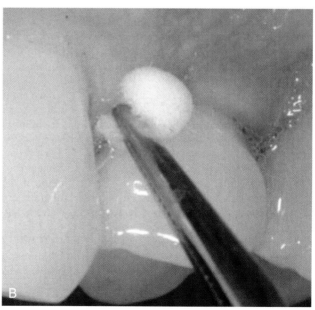

• **Fig. 41.7** (A) Chlorhexidine: used as a rinse or locally applied (Peridex; 3M ESPE Dental Products, St. Paul, Minn.). (B) Local application of chlorhexidine to implant surface.

• BOX 41.4   Clinical Symptoms Associated With Peri-Implantitis

- Vertical bone loss (radiographic, probing, or both)
- Peri-Implant pockets
- Bleeding on probing
- Exudate
- Mucosal swelling
- Erythema
- Usually no associated pain

around an implant in function."[64] Peri-implantitis has been shown to exhibit similar microbial flora as chronic periodontitis. Although there is no consensus regarding microorganisms, Perez-Chaparro et al.[65] identified three commonly occurring pathogens associated with peri-implantitis: *Porphyromonas gingivalis*, *Treponema denticola*, and *Tannerella forsythia*. The dental implant may exhibit all the signs of peri-implant diseases, including exudate, increased pocket depths, and crater-like osseous defects, which are strictly localized around the implant. If left untreated, significant bone loss, infection, and mobility could result, leading to loss of implant osseointegration. Additional clinical signs include radiographic vertical bone loss greater than 2 mm, bleeding on probing (with or without exudate), mucosal swelling and erythema, and an absence of pain (Box 41.4). The crestal bone loss may be induced by stress, bacteria, or a combination of both. A systematic review on peri-implantitis[66] identifies acknowledged etiologies and related causes of peri-implantitis.

After bone loss from stress or bacteria occurs, the sulcular crevice deepens and a decrease in oxygen tension is present. Anaerobic pathogenic bacteria may become the primary promoters of the continued bone loss. An exudate or abscess indicates exacerbation of the peri-implant disease and possible accelerated bone loss. Studies have shown the prevalence rate of peri-implantitis has been found in 28% to 56% of subjects and 12% to 43% of implant sites (Fig. 41.9).[67]

Etiology

Peri-implantitis has been associated with a gram-negative anaerobic microbiota, similar to that found in severe periodontitis around natural teeth.[68] Peri-implantitis encompasses similar clinical signs of peri-implant mucositis, but loss of bone and attachment is observed. A stabilized implant that continues to exhibit loss of bone levels is indicative of peri-implantitis.

Biofilm

Although bacterial biofilm insult is identified as the main cause of peri-implant mucositis, peri-implantitis is considered to be initiated by stress factors caused by poor biomechanical forces. In addition, several other etiologic factors exist, such as poor implant placement, poor oral hygiene, residual cement, host response, poor implant surface, unfavorable osseous density, untreated periodontitis, alcohol excess, smoking, untreated endodontic lesions, diabetes, among others. Monje et al.,[69] in a systemic review, confirmed that peri-implantitis may be prevented with a strong peri-implant maintenance program, along with a comprehensive patient, clinical, and implant-related evaluation. They concluded a minimum recall and hygiene program be tailored to the patient's risk profiling and at a minimum of a 5- to 6-month interval.

Occlusal Stress

Unfavorable stress factors can initiate crestal bone loss, and bacterial biofilm challenges may further enhance the rate of osseous destruction. In recent studies, bacterial biofilms attached onto the surface of implants were shown to create a highly acidic environment that causes corrosion, pitting, cracking, etc.[70] Furthermore, recent studies have shed light on the release of titanium ions from the implant surface, which results in a significant increase in a local inflammatory response[71] (Table 41.1).

History of Periodontitis

Most long-term studies and systemic reviews have concluded that patients with a history of periodontitis had a higher incidence of peri-implantitis in comparison with periodontally healthy patients.[72,73] Papantonopoulos et al.[74] have reported on two implant phenotypes that are directly related to peri-implantitis. A peri-implantitis-susceptible phenotype was associated with fewer teeth and younger age, and was predominantly in the mandible. A peri-implantitis-resistant phenotype was mainly found in the maxilla.[74]

Smoking/Tobacco Use

Although many conflicting studies exist on the relationship between smoking and peri-implantitis, most reports have shown statistically significant differences between smokers and nonsmokers. Rinke et al.[75] reported that smokers had an approximate odds ratio of 31.58 in development of peri-implantitis. The overall peri-implantitis rate in their study population was 11.2% and as high as 53% for patients who smoked and had a history of periodontitis.

Diabetes

The relationship between diabetes and periodontal disease is well established. Poorly controlled diabetes has also been associated with peri-implantitis.[76,77] Venza et al.[78] reported that the long-term prognosis for dental implants is more favorable when the patient's glycosylated hemoglobin (HbA_{1c}) is less than 7%.

Canullo et al.[79] proposed an evidence-based classification for different clinical subtypes of peri-implantitis, including: (1) surgically triggered peri-implantitis, (2) prosthetically driven peri-implantitis, and (3) plaque-induced peri-implantitis. They state that these three subtypes of peri-implantitis are separate, different entities that may be distinguished with predictive profiles. In addition, various risk factors can act synergistically with a clinical scenario, which make the causative factors more difficult (Table 41.2).[79]

Prevention

Home Care

An effective oral hygiene program is paramount to minimize peri-implant disease. This has been shown through various studies. Direct correlations between poor oral hygiene and peri-implant bone loss in a 10-year follow-up study were reported.[80] Other studies have shown a correlation with poor oral hygiene and a higher plaque score.[81] In addition, patients who have lost their teeth to periodontal disease are more susceptible to peri-implantitis.[82]

Professional Care

Thorough periodontal charting and review is essential. Patients with periodontitis must have this pathologic condition controlled before implant placement. Patients who do not demonstrate the

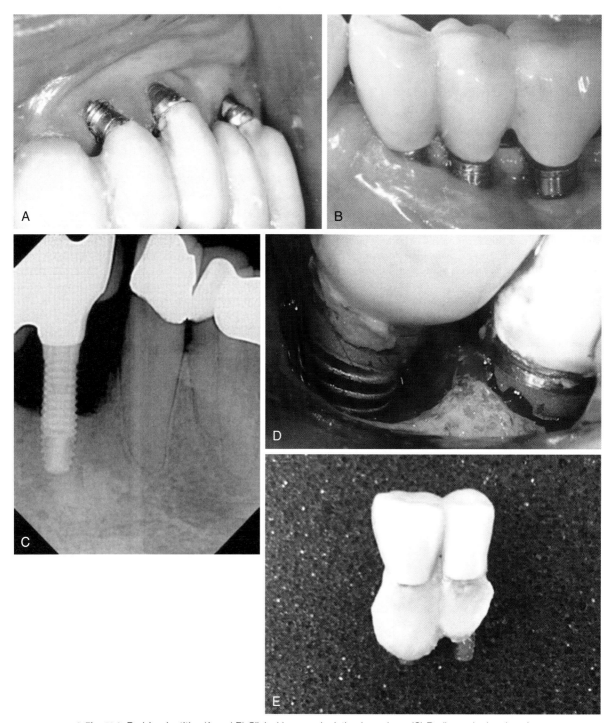

• **Fig. 41.9** Peri-Implantitis. (A and B) Clinical images depicting bone loss. (C) Radiograph showing significant bone loss around implant. (D) Cratering bone loss. (E) Implant failure caused by calculus formation.

ability to maintain oral hygiene need to be educated and put on stringent professional care regimens.

Prosthetic Design

A thoroughly evaluated cone beam computed tomography scan study with favorable biomechanical design for prosthetics is mandatory. Ideal implant position is paramount to allow for a properly designed prosthesis that is cleansable.

Cementation Technique

The meticulous use of cements when delivering a prosthesis is imperative, or the clinician can choose to use a screw-retained prostheses. If a cementable prosthesis is utilized, the clinician must take precautions to prevent retainment of cement. Conventional cementable techniques that are normally used for natural teeth are not recommended (See Fig. 41.5).

TABLE 41.1	Human Studies on Peri-Implantitis Treatment			

Author	Procedure	Number of Patients and Implants and Time of Follow Up	Treatment	Outcome
Leonhardt et al 2003	Access surgery	9 patients 26 implants 60 months	Systemic antibiotics (according to micro-biologic analysis) + access surgery + decontamination of the implant surface using 10% hydrogen peroxide 0.2% CHX 2× a day rinse	Healing: 58% of the implants 7 implants lost 4/19 ongoing bone loss 6/19 bone gain Mean gingival bleeding was reduced from 100%–5% Disease progression at 2 other implants
Romeo et al 2007	Apically repositioned flap surgery + implant surface modification Resective surgery	19 patients 38 implants (11 hollow screw and 7 solid screw) 12–24–36 months	Systemic antibiotics (amoxicillin for 8 days) + full mouth disinfection 9 patients with resective surgery and 10 with resective surgery and modification of surface topography Implant surface decontamination with metronidazole gel, tetracycline hydrochloride, and saline	Radiographic assessment: Implantoplasty is an effective treatment procedure Significantly better results w/apical reposition flap surgery + implant surface modification
Behneke et al 1997	Bone grafts and bone graft substitutes surgery • Nonsubmerged	10 patients 14 implants 6 months–2 years	Irrigation with iodine + systemic antibiotics (Ornidazole 500 mg × 2 for 7 days) Implant surface treated with air powder and irrigation with saline 7 implants with 2–3 wall defects got bone chips and 7 implants with 1 wall defect got bone blocks	Clinical: (6 months/14 implants) BI: 2.4–0.3 PD: 5.9–2.3 mm Clinical: (2 years/5 implants) BI: 2.4–0.4 PD: 5.9–2.5 mm Radiographic: (3–12 months/14 implants) Average bone fill: 3 mm
Behneke et al 2000	Bone grafts and bone graft substitutes surgery • Nonsubmerged	25 implants 6 months to 3 years	Irrigation with iodine for 1 month + debridement with mucoperiosteal flap surgery Implant surface decontamination with air abrasive instruments for 30 seconds + saline irrigation + 7 bone chips and 18 bone blocks (Metronidazole 400 × 2 for 7 days)	Clinical: (1 year/18 implants) PD: 5.3–2.2 mm Clinical: (3 year/10 implants) PD: 5.3–1.6 mm Radiographic: (1 year/18 implants) Mean bone fill: 3.9 mm Radiographic: (3 year/10 implants) Mean bone fill: 4.2 mm
Aughtun et al 1992	Barrier membranes • Nonsubmerged	12 patients 15 implants 6–12 months	ePTFE membrane + systemic antibiotics (tetracycline 200 mg × 1 for 12 days) + implant detoxification (air powder) + irrigation with saline	Clinical: PI: 1.9–1.0 BI: 1.1–1.1 PD: 5.2–4.1 mm Radiographic Mean bone loss: 0.8 mm Minor improvements on soft tissue conditions Membrane exposure
Jovanovic et al 1992	Barrier membranes • Nonsubmerged	7 patients 10 implants 6 months to 3 years	ePTFE membrane + systemic antibiotics (Tetracycline 250 mg × 4 for 7 days) + implant detoxification (air-powder + chloramine T + saline irrigation)	Clinical: PI: 1.7–0.6 GI: 2.1–0.3 PD: 6.8–4.1 mm All clinical signs improved Radiographically: 7 defects showed bone fill 3 defects: no bone fill

Continued

TABLE 41.1	Human Studies on Peri-implantitis Treatment—cont'd			
Author	Procedure	Number of Patients and Implants and Time of Follow Up	Treatment	Outcome
Khoury and Buchmann 2001	Grafting materials + barrier membranes	25 patients 41 implants 36 months	Systemic antibiotics Group 1 (12 implants): detoxification with chlorhexidine irrigation + citric acid + hydrogen peroxide + saline + bone blocks and particulate bone Group 2 (20 implants): treatments as group 1 + ePTFE Group 3 (9 implants): treatments as group 1 + collagen membrane (submerged)	Clinical: 1: PD reductions: 5.1 mm 2. PD reductions: 5.4 mm 3. PD reductions: 2.61 mm Radiographic: 2.4 mm bone fill 2.8 mm bone fill 1.9 mm bone fill 58.6% of the barrier treated implant sites were compromised by early post therapy complications The additional application of barriers does not improve the overall treatment outcomes 3 years following therapy
Mattout et al 1995	With and without grafting material	19 patients	23 defects: ePTFE alone 11 defects: ePTFE + DFDBA + hydrated tetracycline Postoperative: 0.1% CHX + amoxicillin 500 mg (2× for 8 days)	Mean success rate 68% for the membrane group and 90% for the membrane + bone allograft
Schwarz et al 2006	Grafting materials + barrier membranes • Nonsubmerged	22 patients 22 implants 6 months	Granulation tissue removed + implant surface debridement with plastic curettes + irrigation with saline Group 1: Nanocrystalline HA Group 2: Bovine xenograft + resorbable collagen membrane	Clinical: 1: PD: reductions: 2.1 mm 2. PD: reductions: 2.6 mm "In both groups, radiologic observation revealed a decreased translucency within the intrabony component of the respective peri-implant bone defect." Additionally, both treatments resulted in clinically reductions in PD and gains of CAL at 6 months after surgery
Schwarz et al 2008	Grafting materials + barrier membranes • Nonsubmerged	22 patients 2 years	Group 1: Access flap surgery + nanocrystalline hydroxyapatite Group 2: Access flap surgery + natural bone mineral + collagen membrane	2 patients in NHA: severe pus formation at 12 months Clinically: PD: Group 1: 1.5 ± 0.6 mm Group 2: 2.4 ± 0.8 mm CAL gains: Group 1: 1.0 ± 0.4 mm Group 2: 2.0 ± 0.8 mm Both treatments showed efficacy over 2 years. Natural bone mineral + collagen membrane showed better clinical improvements
Roos- Jansaker et al 2007a	Grafting materials + barrier membranes • Nonsubmerged	36 patients 65 implants 12 months	Systemic antibiotic (amoxicillin 375 × 3 + metronidazole 400 mg × 2) for 10 days starting 1 day before surgery Debridement of the granulation tissue, implant surface decontamination with hydrogen peroxide and irrigated with saline Group I: Bone substitute + resorbable membrane Group 2: Bone substitute but no membrane	Group 1: PD reduction: 2.9 mm Mean bone fill: 1.5 mm Group 2: PD reduction: 3.4 mm Mean bone fill: 1.4 mm

TABLE 41.1   Human Studies on Peri-implantitis Treatment—cont'd

Author	Procedure	Number of Patients and Implants and Time of Follow Up	Treatment	Outcome
Roos-Jansaker et al 2007b	Grafting materials + barrier membranes Submerged	12 patients 16 implants 12 months	Systemic antibiotics (amoxicillin 375 × 3 + metronidazole 400 mg × 2) for 10 days starting 1 day before surgery. Debridement of granulation tissue. Implant surface decontamination with hydrogen peroxide and irrigation with saline Bone substitute + resorbable membrane	Clinical and radiographic improvements were observed. PD reduction: 4.2 mm Mean bone fill: 2.3 mm
Haas et al 2000	Diode Laser treatment during surgery	17 patients 24 implants 3–9.5 months	Implant surface decontamination with curettage + laser + defect filled with autogenous bone + ePTFE membrane + systemic antibiotics for 5 days	Radiographically: 3 months from time of membrane removal: 21.8% 9.5 months: mean bone gain: 36.4%
Bach et al 2000	Diode Laser treatment during surgery	30 patients 5 years	Group 1: Scaling + 1.5% CHX + open flap debridement, apical repositioning the flap + osseous augmentation and/or mucogingival corrections Group 2: Treatments as group 1 + laser decontamination with diode laser (810 nm w/6 W)	Group 1: 18 months: no increased PD, BOP or sign of inflammatory process 2 years: 2 patients with increase PD, BOP and clinical sign of inflammation 4 years: 5 patients with increase PD, BOP and clinical sign of inflammation Between 3 and 5 years: 4 implants removed Group 2: 3 years: no relapse 5 years: 5 patients with increase PD and clinical signs of inflammation No implant removed Significant reduction of gram-negative, anaerobic bacteria in laser group than conventional group
Dortbudak et al 2001	Diode laser treatment during surgery	15 patients 15 implants	Implant surface: Curettage + rinsing with saline for 1 minute, then stained with toluidine Half of the implants further treated with diode laser for 1 minute	TBO alone results in a significant bacterial reduction of *P. intermedia* and AA on plasma flame-sprayed contaminated implant surfaces, while a combined treatment leads to a reduction to AA, *P. gingivalis*, and *P. intermedia*. Complete elimination of bacteria was not achieved
Romanos and Nentwig 2008	CO_2 laser + bone augmentation + membrane	15 patients 27.10 ± 17.83 months	Open flap debridement w/ titanium curettes + CO_2 laser (2.84 ± 0.83 watts) for 1 minute Bone augmentation (bovine or autogenous bone) and collagen membrane No systemic antibiotics	PI: Preoperative: 1.01 ± 1.37 Postoperative: 0.98 ± 1.20 BI: Preoperative: 2.76 ± 0.35 Postoperative: 1.03 ± 0.85 PD: Preoperative: 6.00 ± 2.03 mm Postoperative: 2.48 ± 0.63 mm Keratinized tissue BI: Preop: 2.30 ± 1.45 mm Postop: 2.41 ± 1.39 mm

Continued

TABLE 41.1	Human Studies on Peri-implantitis Treatment—cont'd			
Author	Procedure	Number of Patients and Implants and Time of Follow Up	Treatment	Outcome

Deppe et al 2007	CO_2 laser + bone augmentation	32 patients 73 implants 4 months and 5 years	Group 1 (19 implants): Soft tissue resection + conventional decontamination
			Group 2 (15 implants): Treatment as group 1 + βTCP + autogenous bone grafts
			Group 3 (22 implants): Soft tissue resection + CO_2 laser decontamination
			Group 4 (17 implants): Treatment as group 3 + βTCP + autogenous bone
				3 implants lost in group 1
				4 implants lost in group 2
				2 implants lost in group 3
				4 implants lost in group 4
				Beginning of hygiene phase
				PI:
				  Group 1: 1.8 ± 1.2
				  Group 2: 1.4 ± 1.2
				  Group 3: 1.4 ± 0.9
				  Group 4: 2.6 ± 0.5
				BI:
				  Group 1: 2.7 ± 0.9
				  Group 2: 2.3 ± 1.4
				  Group 3: 2.8 ± 1.2
				  Group 4: 3.3 ± 0.6
				PD:
				  Group 1: 6.2 ± 1.8
				  Group 2: 5.1 ± 1.7
				  Group 3: 5.7 ± 1.4
				  Group 4: 5.7 ± 1.4
				Immediately before surgery
				PI:
				  Group 1: 0.7 ± 0.8
				  Group 2: 0.9 ± 0.4
				  Group 3: 0.7 ± 0.8
				  Group 4: 0.5 ± 0.6
				BI:
				  Group 1: 0.7 ± 0.8
				  Group 2: 0.5 ± 0.8
				  Group 3: 0.6 ± 0.3
				  Group 4: 1.2 ± 0.6
				PD:
				  Group 1: 5.1 ± 1.3
				  Group 2: 4.8 ± 1.4
				  Group 3: 6.1 ± 1.6
				  Group 4: 5.0 ± 1.3
				4 months
				PI:
				  Group 1: 0.6 ± 0.7
				  Group 2: 0.6 ± 0.6
				  Group 3: 0.8 ± 0.6
				  Group 4: 0.5 ± 0.4
				BI:
				  Group 1: 0.9 ± 0.5
				  Group 2: 0.6 ± 0.6
				  Group 3: 0.7 ± 0.6
				  Group 4: 0.9 ± 0.8
				PD:
				  Group 1: 3.2 ± 0.9
				  Group 2: 2.4 ± 0.7
				  Group 3: 2.1 ± 1.3
				  Group 4: 1.0 ± 0.7
				5 years

TABLE 41.1	Human Studies on Peri-implantitis Treatment—cont'd			
Author	Procedure	Number of Patients and Implants and Time of Follow Up	Treatment	Outcome
				PI: Group 1: 0.8 ± 0.8 Group 2: 1.1 ± 0.8 Group 3: 1.0 ± 1.3 Group 4: 1.2 ± 1.3 BI: Group 1: 1.1 ± 1.2 Group 2: 2.1 ± 1.4 Group 3: 1.8 ± 1.1 Group 4: 1.9 ± 1.0 PD: Group 1: 4.3 ± 1.2 Group 2: 2.5 ± 1.1 Group 3: 3.4 ± 1.5 Group 4: 2.5 ± 1.4 Treatment of peri-implantitis may be accelerated by using a CO_2 laser + soft tissue resection Long-term results in augmented defects, no difference between laser and conventional decontamination
Froum et al 2012	Regenerative approach Biologics + bone + membrane	51 implants 38 patients 3–7.5 years	Systemic antibiotics (2000 mg amoxicillin or 600 mg clindamycin) 1 hr before surgery and continue 500 mg amoxicillin tid or clindamycin 150 mg qid for additional 10 days Surface decontamination w/ bicarbonate powder for 60 seconds (air abrasive device), 60-second irrigation with sterile saline, tetracycline (50 mg/mL with cotton pellets or brush for 30 seconds, then second bicarbonate air abrasion 60 seconds, application of 0.12% CHX for 30 seconds, then 60 seconds reirrigation with sterile saline + enamel matrix derivatives + anorganic bovine bone soaked in platelet derived growth factor for at least 5 minutes or mineralized freeze-dried bone + collagen membrane or subepithelial CT graft at area (<2 mm KG) Group 1: Greatest defect depth radiographically Group 2: Greatest bone loss on the facial of implant	•No implant lost •PD reduction: Group 1: 5.4 mm Group 2: 5.1 mm •Bone level gain: Group 1: 3.75 mm Group 2: 3 mm

AA, Aggregatibacter actinomycetemcomitans; *BI*, Bleeding index; *BOP*, Bleeding on probing; *BTCP*, Beta Tricalcium Phosphate; *CAL*, Clinical attachment level; *CHX*, Chlorhexidine; *DFDBA*, Demineralized freeze-dried bone allograft; *ePTFE*, expanded polytetrafluoroethylene; *GI*, Gingival Index; *HA*, Hydroxyapatite; *KG*, Keratinized gingiva; *NHA*, Nanocrystalline Hydroxyapatite; *PD*, Probing depth; *PI*, Plaque index; *TBO*, toluidine-blue-O.

From Suzuki JB, Misch CE. Periodontal and maintenance complications. In: Resnik RR, Misch CE, eds. *Misch's Avoiding Complications in Oral Implantology*. St. Louis, MO: Elsevier; 2018.

Control of Parafunctional Forces

An occlusal guard is crucial in preventing unfavorable occlusal stress. The night guard is adjusted to be on a flat plane occlusion to disperse stress. Careful discussion should be conducted with the dental laboratory to convey the desired design for successful clinical outcomes.

Management

The objective of treatment for peri-implantitis is for osseous regeneration of the implant-bone defect. However, such treatment has been challenging because the implant surface needs to be detoxified, along with modifying the soft and hard tissues. This may involve nonsurgical and surgical treatment.

TABLE 41.2	Predictive Profiles Associated With Peri-Implantitis[223,224]	
Risk Factor	**Predictive Profiles**	
Type 1: surgical factors	• Presence of plaque associated with orovestibular and mesiodistal implant malpositioning • Failed bone reconstruction	
Type 2: prosthetic factors	• Plaque associated with retained cement remnants • Nonideal finish line margin (≥2 mm below soft tissue margin) • Occlusal overloading • Prosthesis material fracture • Abutment screw loosening • Implant fracture	
Type 3: plaque-induced	Generalized bone-level recession associated with plaque accumulation, without any surgical/prosthetic complication	

Nonsurgical Management of Peri-Implantitis

Nonsurgical treatment of peri-implant mucositis is often successful. In contrast, the nonsurgical treatment for peri-implantitis is not as predictable. This is most likely due to the inability to remove the bacterial biofilm from the exposed implant surface. Such difficulty has been especially observed with rough surface dental implants.[83] A systematic review illustrated that implant surfaces and diameter are potential risk factors for bone loss and peri-implantitis.[84]

The nonsurgical treatment of peri-implantitis usually involves the debridement and detoxification of implant surfaces, similar to the treatment of peri-implant mucositis. However, the issue that arises is that these exposed surfaces usually have concurrent subgingival pockets.

Low-Abrasive Amino Acid Glycine Powder. Low-abrasive amino acid glycine powder has been shown to be an effective treatment for removing biofilm without damaging the implant surface, and hard and soft tissues of the periodontium. This technique uses a special handpiece with a plastic tube nozzle with three orthogonally oriented holes. An air-powder mixture with reduced pressure is expelled through the nozzle, which prevents the formation of air emphysema complications. The nozzle is moved in a circumferential movement around the implant surface.[85]

Although more extensive studies need to be conducted as to technique efficacy, glycine powder can be incorporated into a treatment regimen. The clinician should be careful to use the powder only in areas where access is available, including a posttreatment rinse to remove any residue. This modality is best used in cases with a buccal dehiscence and/or horizontal bone loss without crater or infrabony pocketing. An air-powder unit (Hu-Friedy, Chicago, Ill.) that adapts to a slow-speed handpiece is available and may be used effectively (Fig. 41.10).

Ultrasonic Devices. For treatment of peri-implantitis, tip modifications (i.e., carbon fiber, silicone, or plastic) must be used. Care must be exercised not to use metal tips as they may alter the implant surface. Ultrasonic devices should be used only when plastic tips are available. Irrigation and meticulous cleaning are recommended in treatment for either open flap debridement or closed flap irrigation.

Lasers. One of the newer and least invasive methodologies to treat peri-implant mucositis and peri-implantitis involves the use of laser photonic energy, a coherent form of infrared or visible light, usually of a single wavelength. Lasers have been used effectively for decades in oral implantology in second-stage recovery of implants through the ablation and vaporization of overlying soft tissue.[86]

Laser Protocols. Similar to their use in treating periodontal disease, lasers provide different treatment approaches for peri-implantitis: nonsurgical, surgical, antimicrobial photodynamic therapy, and photobiomodulation.

• *Nonsurgical:* In the nonsurgical modality, lasers are used adjunctively to help remove calculus, reduce inflammation and remove diseased soft tissue, and reduce subgingival pathogens. Using different types of lasers, such as the diode, Nd:YAG (neodymium-doped yttrium aluminum garnet), erbium, or carbon dioxide laser, the laser beam is directed at the inflamed soft tissue within the sulcus, using noncontact overlapping strokes to disrupt the biofilm, reduce the microbial population, and decontaminate the pocket epithelium. Erbium lasers have also been shown to remove calculus from the implant surface.[87-95]

• *Surgical:* Minimally invasive laser-assisted surgical techniques involve removal of diseased epithelial lining. More invasive surgical procedures involve conventional elevation of a full-thickness flap for surgical access, followed by laser-assisted degranulation, surface debridement and decontamination, and osseous tissue removal or recontouring. As indicated, bone augmentation may be performed through placement of bone-grafting material.[96-103]

• *Antimicrobial Photodynamic Therapy:* Antimicrobial photodynamic therapy in periodontology is a light-based approach to terminating bacteria. A photoactivatable substance (photosensitizer) is applied to the targeted area (i.e., within the sulcus) and then activated by laser light. Singlet oxygen and other cytotoxic reactive agents are produced to reduce periodontopathogens.[104-109]

• *Photobiomodulation:* is a form of light therapy that uses nonionizing forms of light, including lasers in the visible and infrared spectrum. The nonthermal technique is used to elicit photophysical and photochemical events. In implantology, it is used to promote wound healing and tissue regeneration. It has also been shown to increase osteoblastic proliferation, collagen deposition, and bone neoformation.[110-115]

Although laser-based peri-implantitis treatment techniques are generally positive, some studies indicate adjunctive use of lasers have limited or no extra beneficial effect compared with conventional treatment methodologies. Additional well-designed, long-term, randomized controlled trials are needed to verify the clinical and microbiologic outcomes of laser use.[116-118]

Assurance of positive therapeutic outcomes is facilitated by an informed clinical technique, prudent use of proper laser operating parameters, and awareness of all laser wavelengths. However, when used inappropriately, laser energy can adversely alter implant surfaces and/or induce undesirable temperature increases, which may be detrimental to implant health[119-122] (Fig. 41.11).

In 2014 a human clinical study consisting of 16 patients was published, using a pulsed 1064-nm Nd:YAG laser (PerioLase MVP-7; Millennium Dental Technologies, Cerritos, Calif.). The technique introduced is known as the Laser-Assisted Peri-Implantitis Protocol (LAPIP) to manage patients with peri-implantitis[123] without the use of bone augmentation (Fig. 41.12). (LAPIP is

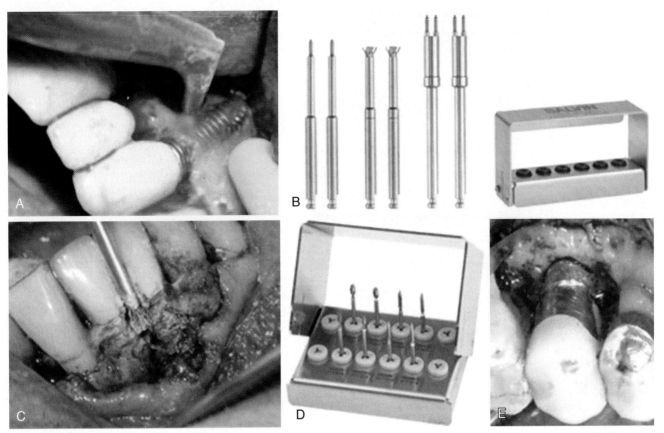

• **Fig. 41.10** (A) Low-Abrasive Powder. Hu-Friedy glycine powder jet used to debride titanium implant surfaces, (B) Titanium Brushes, (C) Clinical image of titanium brushes applying detoxification agent, (D) Implantplasty Kit for removal of implant threads, (E) Implant with threads removed.

a registered trademark of Millennium Dental Technologies, Inc., Cerritos, Calif.)

The clinicians used a modification of a well-defined surgical procedure, the Laser-Assisted New Attachment Protocol (LANAP), used for treating periodontitis. This technique was defined as a minimally invasive surgical therapy that may be appropriate for multiple periodontal defects and possibly as a first line of management of periodontal disease.[124] In two recent histologic studies, the LANAP has shown evidence of new attachment and tissue regeneration.[125,126] Based on this evidence, in 2016 the U.S. Food and Drug Administration granted marketing clearance for the PerioLase MVP-7 Laser for a first-of-its-kind clinical indication for use: periodontal regeneration, that is, true regeneration of the attachment apparatus (new cementum, new periodontal ligament, and new alveolar bone) on a previously diseased root surface when used specifically in the LANAP.

For the treatment of peri-implantitis, the LAPIP follows the step-by-step sequence defined in the LANAP procedure, but with a reduced light dose (energy) around implants.

1. Surgical probings are performed under local anesthesia to record the depths of all bony defects around the implant. Pocket depth and phenotype help to determine the amount of laser energy to be delivered during the ablation and hemostasis applications.
2. The laser fiber is then inserted into the periodontal pocket, oriented in a prescribed fashion, and the laser is activated at particular settings to ablate (remove) the diseased epithelial lining and granulomatous tissue, to denature pathologic proteins, and to create bacteria antisepsis.

3. Ultrasonic scalers are used to remove foreign substances (including calculus and cement) from the implant surfaces.
4. Bone is modified, removed, reshaped, and decorticated in a prescribed manner to stimulate the release of blood, stem cells, and growth factors from the bone.
5. The laser is then used again at specifically adjusted settings in hemostasis mode to form a thick, stable fibrin clot, activate growth factors, and upregulate gene expression.
6. Coronal soft tissue is approximated against the implant using finger pressure to achieve adhesion. No sutures are used because this is a flapless procedure.
7. Removal of occlusal interference is performed to reduce traumatic forces and mobility.

The technique has been shown to produce healing in an environment conducive to true regeneration of new alveolar bone. Reosseointegration of the implant is anticipated.

The study analyzed 16 cases, 9 females and 7 males, with an average age of 54 years and a range of 32 to 79 years. Median time that had elapsed between the date of implant placement and the date of LAPIP treatment was 4 years (3 months to 16 years). Follow-up data ranged from 8 to 36 months after LAPIP treatment. All clinicians reported control of the peri-implantitis infection, reversal of bone loss, and rescue of the incumbent implant.

Radiographic evidence combined with three-dimensional geometric modeling was used to estimate the rate of addition of new bone to the alveolar crest. The rate of bone deposition was determined to be 14.9 mm^2 in cross-sectional area per year. In two cases, new bone deposition was observed at rates of 0.62 and 1.6 mm^3 per month, respectively. Complete recovery (resolution of

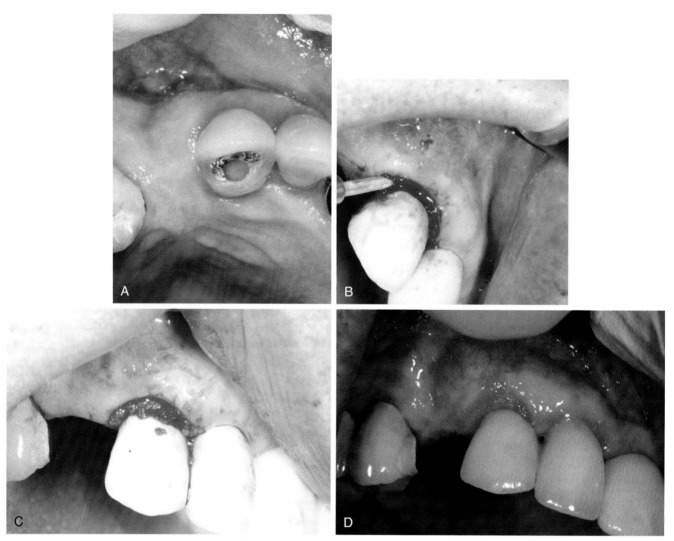

• Fig. 41.11 Laser Treatment. (A) Initial evaluation of peri-implantitis. (B) Laser tip activated around sulcular margins of implant. (C) Immediate postsurgical appearance. (D) Two weeks postoperatively with granulation tissue re-forming around implant collar. (*From Suzuki JB, Misch CE. Periodontal and maintenance complications. In: Resnik RR, Misch CE, eds. Misch's Avoiding Complications in Oral Implantology. St. Louis, MO: Elsevier; 2018.*)

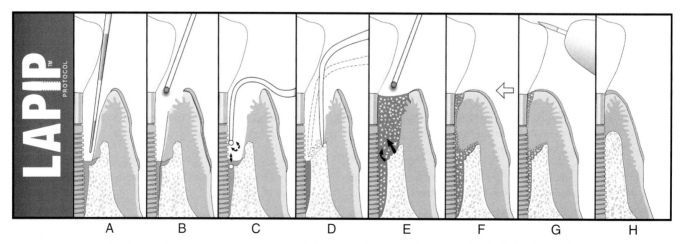

• Fig. 41.12 Artists sketch of sequence of clinical steps for Laser-Assisted Peri-Implantitis Protocol (LAPIP) procedure using the PerioLase MVP-7 pulsed neodymium-Yttrium Aluminum garnet (Nd:YAG) laser. (permission from Millenium, Cerritos, CA USA and From Suzuki JB. Salvaging implants with an Nd:YAG laser: a novel approach to a growing problem. Compend Contin Educ Dent. 2015;36:756-761.)

peri-implantitis) averaged 1 to 3 years, depending on the size of the initial lesion. Analysis of collected data revealed that bone deposition is not linear. Large defects healed more rapidly at first, but the rate slowed as the defect diminished. A modest trend was shown for larger lesions to heal more rapidly.

Although the results of this clinical study appear promising, further study of the predictability and effectiveness of the LAPIP technique is warranted. The effectiveness of the 1064-nm Nd:YAG laser wavelength in achieving its successful clinical outcomes with the LAPIP protocol may be attributed to a variety of factors.[127] These include the Nd:YAG laser's ability to:

- selectively remove inflamed pocket epithelium, with no significant damage to underlying connective tissue,[128-131]
- reduce pathogenic microorganisms in the periodontal pocket,[132-136]
- produce an antiinflammatory effect,[137-140] and
- stimulate alveolar bone growth at the cellular level.[141-144]

Whether used adjunctively or as the primary instrument, lasers offer the field of oral implantology a number of safe and effective clinical applications for the treatment of peri-implant mucositis and peri-implantitis. Techniques range from nonsurgical and surgical uses, to antimicrobial photodynamic therapy and photo biostimulation. Additional investigations will further determine the underlying mechanisms of their action. Proper training and scrupulous adherence to specific laser-based protocols will help assure favorable therapeutic patient outcomes.

Laser settings are specific to each individual laser according to manufacturers' protocols. Care should be exercised to cover all exposed surfaces (i.e., each exposed thread) for the detoxification process. Use of regenerative material (allografts and extended resorbable membranes) is highly recommended. Tissues are modified and sutured to reapproximate tissue for tension-free primary closure.

It is critical to limit time exposure of the implant surface with the laser application to avoid overheating or charring. This may increase implant morbidity and possibly lead to premature loss of the implant because of bone disintegration.

Locally Applied Antibiotics. The recommended locally applied antibiotic (LDA) during surgical implant rescue is tetracycline at 50 mg/mL solution. Tetracycline capsules can be opened and mixed with small amounts of saline solution to create a paste. This paste is burnished onto implant surfaces for 60 seconds, then thoroughly rinsed with saline. Tetracycline is bacteriostatic, as it targets the 30s ribosomal subunit in the messenger RNA translation complex of bacterial protein synthesis. Because tetracycline has an inhibitory effect on matrix metalloproteinases, the tetracycline paste needs to be completely removed. A study with pure tetracycline application showed reosseointegration after 4 months.[56] It is highly recommended to incorporate tetracycline in surgical rescue therapy for peri-implantitis.

Tetracycline capsules (two 500-mg capsules) may be mixed with a few drops of saline to form a viscous consistency. It should stay gelled when applied to exposed implant surfaces during surgery. The mixture is allowed to sit on the implant surface for 1 minute, then is thoroughly rinsed off. It allows proximal contact of antibiotics to implant surface colonies and may assist in success in treatment of peri-implantitis.

Another option of local antibiotic administration is with minocycline, which is a tetracycline derivative. Minocycline is manufactured in an encapsulated microsphere of poly(lactic-coglycolic acid), a biodegradable polymer called Arestin (OraPharma, Warminster, Pa.).[57] The subgingival application of minocycline microspheres has been shown to maintain therapeutic levels for 14 days. Williams et al.[58] reported on a 9-month study that showed the

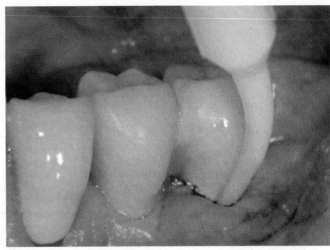

● **Fig. 41.8** Locally Applied Antibiotic. Arestin placed into the sulcus area for the treatment of peri-mucositis.

● **BOX 41.3** Antibiotic Prescription Formulation

Amoxicillin 500 mg tid (three times per day), total of 21 capsules
Metronidazole 250 mg, 21 tablets tid, until all consumed by the patient
Minocycline (Arestin) applied subgingivally around implants with pockets

therapeutic efficacy of minocycline microspheres in significantly reducing probing depth in conjunction with scaling. Oringer et al.[59] concluded that minocycline microspheres induce a potent short-term reduction in the gingival crevicular fluid molecular markers of bone resorption (Fig. 41.8).

Systemic Antibiotics. The use of systemic antibiotics has been established for management of periodontitis.[60] However, peri-mucositis treatment studies with use of systemic antibiotics are lacking. It is known that patients with periodontitis are three times more likely to experience peri-implantitis, but the bacterial colonies found in peri-implantitis and periodontitis share few characteristics. Still, many studies have demonstrated the most effective antibiotic combination is amoxicillin and metronidazole.

Metronidazole is bactericidal to anaerobic organisms and disrupts DNA synthesis. It has been shown to be especially effective against *A. actinomycetemcomitans, P. gingivalis,* and *P. intermedia.*[61] The combination of amoxicillin and metronidazole has also been shown to have long-term effects against *A. actinomycetemcomitans*[62] (Box 41.3).

For patients who are allergic to amoxicillin, alternative systemic antibiotics are clindamycin, ciprofloxacin, metronidazole, or azithromycin. Local drug delivery systems such as minocycline (Arestin, off U.S. Food and Drug Administration label) may be considered.

Surgical Management of Peri-Implantitis

Although nonsurgical treatment of peri-implantitis may be effective in some cases, the majority of cases require a more invasive approach to ensure an effective treatment outcome. There are various surgical techniques (see later) to treat peri-implantitis, depending on the final objective.[145] Surgical management is completed with curettes, specialized titanium brushes with an implant handpiece, and/or a glycine polishing handpiece. Along with mechanical decontamination, a chemical decontamination process should be followed, using compounds such as doxycycline/tetracycline or citric acid. The flaps are then

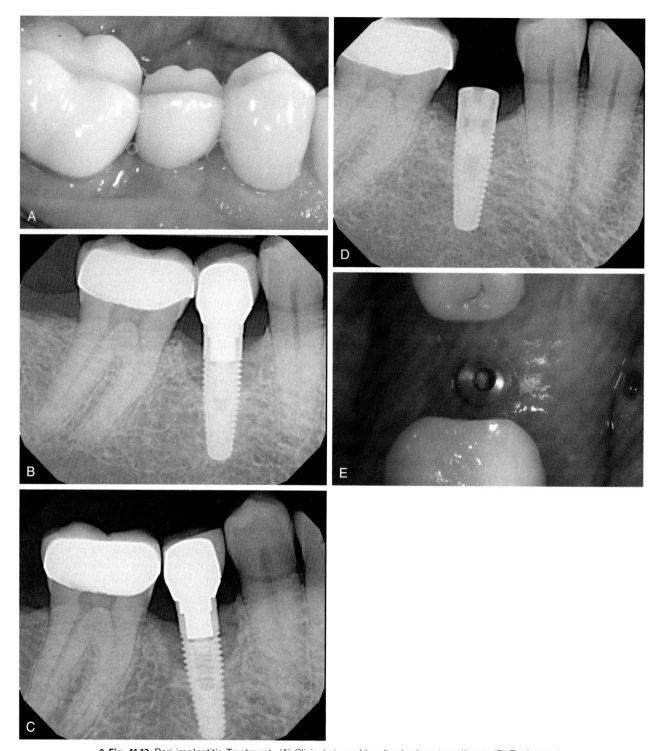

• **Fig. 41.13** Peri-implantitis Treatment. (A) Clinical view of localized edematous tissue. (B) Radiograph depicting circumferential bone loss. (C) Three months post-LANAP treatment. (D and E) Nine months post-LANAP treatment. (*Courtesy Allen Honigman, DDS*)

reapproximated in their original position, using horizontal mattress sutures, which adapt tissue around the implant while creating a ferrule effect. Interrupted sutures will also serve this purpose (Fig. 41.13).

It is possible to also complete a subepithelial tissue augmentation while performing the access flap debridement. Simultaneous tissue grafting with debridement had a significant reduction of bleeding on probing, pocket depth, and clinical attachment loss at a 6-month postoperative evaluation.[146]

1. Sulcular incision around desired dentition being careful to extend at least one tooth mesial and one tooth distal in anticipation to the area of treatment
2. Full-thickness flap reflection is complete past the mucogingival junction on both buccal and palatal/lingual if necessary
3. Implants are detoxified with tetracycline paste, EDTA, or citric acid, cleaned with curettes and titanium brushes
4. Air powder glycine to further clean implant threads previously exposed

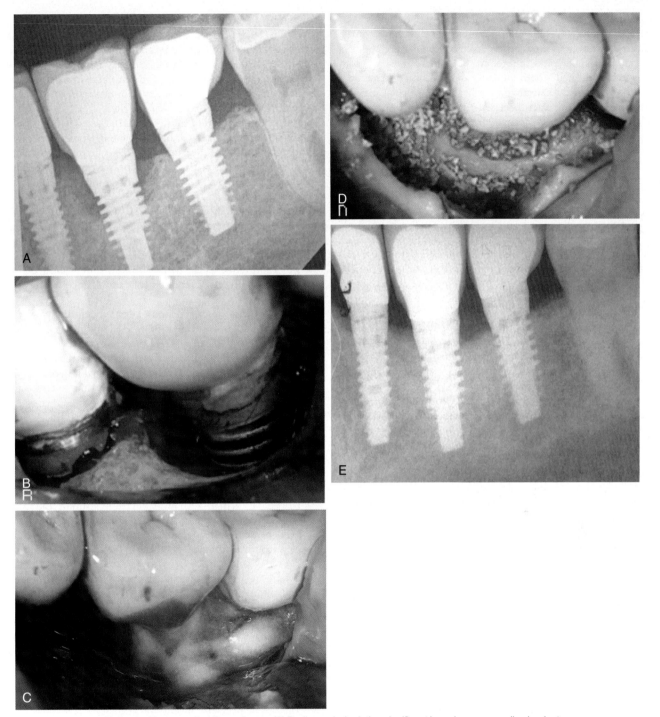

• **Fig. 41.14** Regenerative Procedures. (A) Radiograph depicting significant bone loss surrounding implant in the first molar position. (B) Full-thickness reflection showing extent of defect with retained cement. (C) Detoxification with tetracycline hydrochloride, after removal of cement. (D) Augmentation with allograft. (E) Postoperative radiograph 2 years postoperatively. (*Courtesy Dr. Nolen Levine.*)

5. Flaps are readapted over osseous structure and should be in relatively similar position
6. Horizontal mattress sutures or interrupted sutures may be used, being cautious not to exert excess tension, which causes bunching of tissues; tissue does not have to be completely approximated; new tissue will form and granulate in the wound site

Heitz-Mayeld et al.[147] reported on a 12-month prospective study with antiinfective surgical therapy outcomes for peri-implant disease. Thirty-six patients with moderate to advanced

peri-implantitis had access flap disinfection, followed with a combination of systemic antibiotics (amoxicillin and metronidazole). At 1 year, 92% of patients had stable crestal bone height, and all had a marked reduction of probing depth. On probing, 47% had complete resolution of bleeding.[147]

Regenerative Procedures. For peri-implantitis cases where a crater-like defect is present, regeneration is recommended (Fig. 41.14). Even though regeneration is an ideal treatment modality for all peri-implantitis cases, there are criteria that must be fulfilled to allow successful treatment. In a similar principle to bone regeneration for natural teeth, the greater number of osseous walls remaining in a defect, the better the anticipated clinical outcomes.

Also, the prosthesis must be free from any premature contacts that may introduce excessive force to the implant interface. Ideally, especially in single-tooth implant cases, removal of the crown would be performed to ensure proper healing. A sulcular incision is performed from one tooth mesial to one tooth distal of the implant. A full-thickness mucoperiosteal flap is reflected to gain adequate access to defect. Thorough removal of granulation tissue is vital. Mechanical debridement is then initiated. A titanium brush with a small tip may be needed to access the implant surface if the osseous crater around the implant has little access.

After thorough mechanical debridement, freeze-dried bone allograft may be packed in with a resorbable membrane. Soft tissue augmentation may also be included, which will enhance healing. Flap advancement is usually indicated to achieve soft tissue primary closure around implants. A high tensile suture material suture is recommended to ensure the flap does not open prematurely. Implants should be free from any pressure or premature contacts that may introduce excessive force to the implant interface. Ideally, especially in single-tooth implant cases, any occlusal prematurities should be removed.

In addition to the steps listed earlier, enamel matrix protein, platelet-derived growth factor, and human allograft or bovine xenograft in conjunction with a collagen membrane or subepithelial tissue graft was suggested to enhance regeneration. Systematic reviews on the merits of clinical regeneration, of platelet concentrates[148] and bone marrow aspirates have been published recently.[149]

Regenerative Technique

1. Sulcular incision is made around the clinical site with one tooth mesial and one tooth distal.
2. Full-thickness mucoperiosteal flap is reflected past the mucogingival junction to ensure enough tension release from flap tissue. It is essential to produce adequate release so there is minimal tension when closing the flap. Inadequate reflection will result in incision line opening, which will increase morbidity of the graft.
3. The bone surface is curetted to clean and remove all soft tissue remnants. Bone surface is curetted, being careful to remove all remnants of soft tissue. Detoxification:
   a. Tetracycline paste, EDTA, or citric acid is applied to the exposed surface for 30 to 60 seconds.
   b. Rinse with sterile saline for 30 seconds.
4. A full-thickness flap is reflected to gain adequate access to the defect and implant threads. Thorough removal of granulation tissue is critical. Bone graft of choice (i.e., ideally an autograft or allograft) is placed on defect.
5. A resorbable membrane (extended resorbable collagen membrane: 4–6 months) is then draped over bone graft, being careful to cover 3 mm past all edges of bone graft.
6. Tissue tension is reduced via tissue-stretching techniques. Flaps are sutured (i.e., high-tensile strength suture material [polyglycolic acid (PGA) sutures, 4–0]), being careful to provide tension-free closure to produce maximal contact between tissue edges (primary closure) (Fig. 41.15).

Apically Repositioned Surgical Technique. This surgical technique is used for implants that have generalized horizontal bone loss greater than one to two threads. An internal bevel incision or sulcular incisions circumscribing buccal and lingual contours of the implant are made. Two vertical incisions are added on the mesial and distal of the dental implant, creating a pyramidal flap. The clinician should recognize the importance of the blood supply of the flap, and a wide base is necessary to ensure the sulcular

margin of the flap does not slough. On the lingual/palatal a gingivectomy may be performed at the level of the anticipated final gingival height. Submarginal incisions may be performed in cases where keratinized gingival tissue is adequate (e.g., palate). Ideally a partial-thickness flap is recommended because it will improve apical flap adaptation. Full-thickness flaps elevation technique may be easier in difficult-to-access clinical sites.

Once reflected, similar treatment as the access flap may be vital. Granulation tissue needs to be completely removed, followed by thorough cleaning of implant surfaces. A chemical detoxification can similarly be performed. A decision may be made to remove implant threads with a handpiece if significant loss of osseous support is present and regeneration is unlikely. The final flap is sutured to the underlying periosteal tissue if a split-thickness flap was used. If a full-thickness flap was performed, it can be adapted apically via individual interrupted sutures. The goal is to readapt tissue back onto remaining osseous support to minimize thickness of a soft tissue collar, thereby minimizing probing depth. Steps of Flap Access, Debridement, and Resective Surgery are described below:

1. Sulcular incision is made around desired dentition, being careful to extend at least one tooth mesial and one tooth distal in anticipation to the area of treatment.
2. Full-thickness flap reflection is complete past the mucogingival junction on both buccal and palatal/lingual if necessary.
3. Osseous recontouring is complete at this time to create a positive architecture.
4. Implants are detoxified with tetracycline paste, EDTA, or citric acid, cleaned with curettes and titanium brushes.
5. Air-powder glycine treatment of exposed implant threads is performed.
6. Flaps are readapted over remaining osseous structure and should be apical in comparison with the original flap position.
7. Horizontal mattress sutures or interrupted sutures can be used, being careful not to exert too much tension that causes bunching of tissues. Tissues do not have to be completely approximated. New tissue will form and granulate in the wound site (Table 41.3).

Platelet Concentrate Growth Factors. In implant dentistry the two most common platelet concentrates are termed under the general acronyms of PRP (platelet-rich plasma) or PRF (platelet-rich fibrin). These products are often considered growth factors and used in regenerative medicine. Although protocols vary, most platelet concentrates are blood extracts from a whole blood sample that is processed via centrifugation. The processing technique separates the blood components into usable (e.g., fibrinogen/fibrin, platelets, growth factors, and leukocytes in liquid plasma) or unusable (e.g., red blood cells).[150]

The use of platelet concentrates (e.g., PRP and PRF) for the treatment of peri-implant defects has been widely researched, with varying results. Unfortunately, the literature on this topic is controversial and conclusions are extremely variable.

Platelet-Rich Plasma. PRP with and without bone substitutes has been studied with the treatment of peri-implant defects. In various dog research models, most researchers have not found beneficial results with PRP alone,[151] in combination with xenograft bone,[152-154] and with guided bone regeneration procedures.[155] In general the literature as a whole has not shown a significant benefit in the treatment of peri-implant defects. Simonpieri et al.,[156] in a comprehensive review, stated that PRP does not show conclusive results. A possible reason for this is that natural bleeding from the surgery site is sufficient to saturate the area with blood growth factors and allow for increased healing ability.

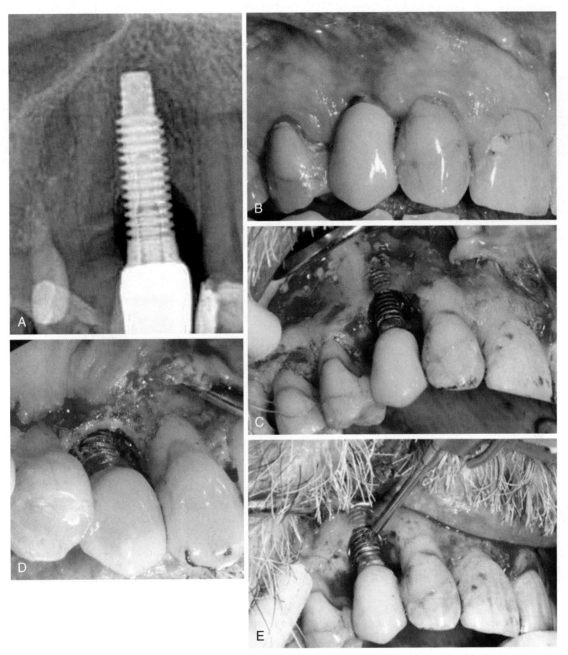

• **Fig. 41.15** Treatment of Peri-implantitis. (A) Maxillary right canine exhibiting bone loss and peri-implantitis. (B) Clinical view. (C) Full-thickness reflection depicting the circumferential and buccal bone loss. (D) Lingual view of defect and thread removal. (E) Removal of soft tissue remnants with titanium brush.

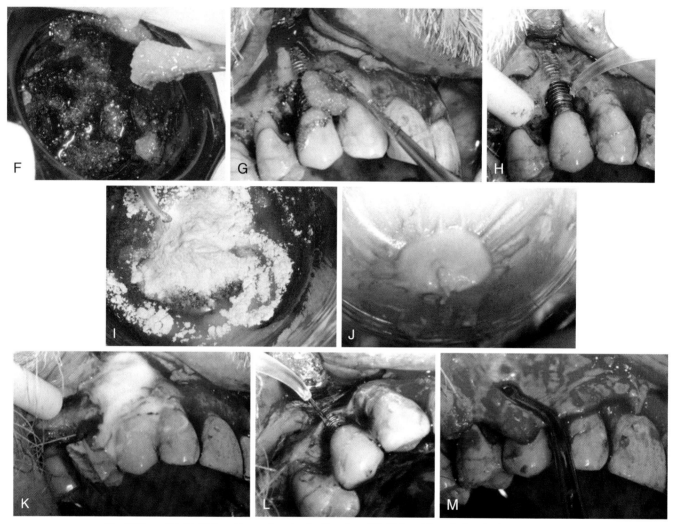

Fig. 41.15, cont'd (F) Citric acid powder mixed with saline. (G) Citric acid applied to implant surface for detoxification. (H) Irrigation with saline. (I) Tetracycline paste. (J) Tetracycline mixed with saline. (K) Tetracycline paste applied to implant surface. (L) Irrigation with saline. (M) Tissue tension evaluated.

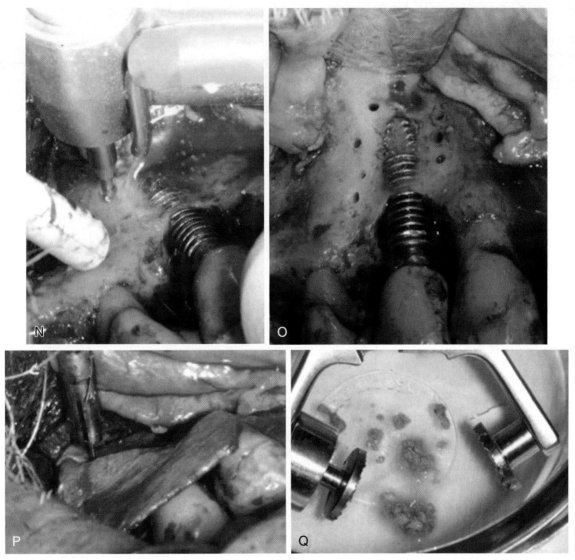

Fig. 41.15, cont'd (N) Decortication. (O) Confirmation of bleeding from cortical holes. (P) Acellular dermis modified and placed with tacks. (Q) Autograft harvested from tuberosity.

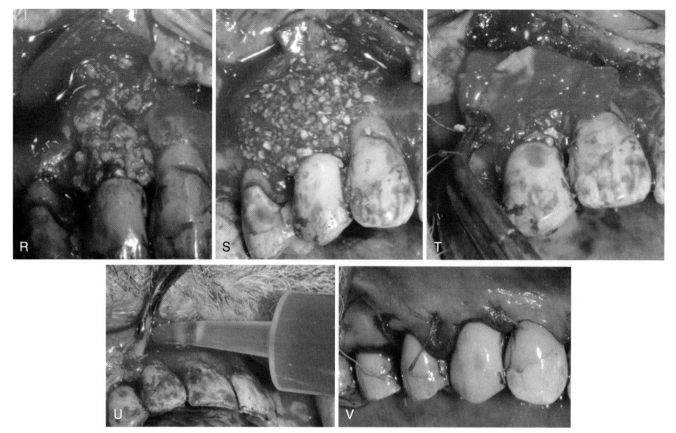

Fig. 41.15, cont'd (R) Autograft placed as first layer. (S) Allograft placed as second layer. (T) PRF membrane placed over acellular dermis. (U) Platelet-rich fibrin syringed under flap. (V) Final closure.

Platelet-Rich Fibrin. In contrast, PRF is used as a "generic" name for the second-generation platelet concentrates, which are derivatives of PRP. The original protocol by Dohan, Choukroun, et al.[157] used no anticoagulants and was termed L-PRF (leukocyte- and platelet-rich fibrin). Later, they have been modified to include advanced-PRF (A-PRF) and injectable-PRF (i-PRF), as well as several other groups of products.

The L-PRF fibrin matrix contains mostly platelets and leukocytes (e.g., lymphocytes). The L-PRF clot is created without blood modification (i.e., no anticoagulants) and is the result of the natural coagulation process during centrifugation.[158] Because of its strong fibrin network and bone growth cell factors (leukocytes, platelet aggregates, circulating stem cells), the L-PRF clot has been shown to have beneficial results, with bone substitutes in the filling of peri-implant defects.

With respect to bone regeneration and treatment of defects, L-PRF has been shown to be beneficial when added to bone substitute material.[159] Also, when L-PRF is used as a regenerated membrane, increase soft tissue healing is seen. Numerous studies have confirmed increased benefits of soft tissue stimulation and promotion of gingival remodeling.[160,161] The L-PRF has also been shown to regulate the interactions between the bone and soft tissue, thereby promoting healing and remodeling of the tissue.[162]

Because peri-implantitis involves an inflammatory and bacteria-laden defect, the exposed implant surface is contaminated with a bacterial biofilm and altered surface characteristics. The titanium oxide surface is destroyed with peri-implant disease,

new bone growth can be initiated only after complete decontamination of the implant surface. Therefore, if the contaminated surface is not restored, bone grafting will most likely not be successful. Multiple protocols have been suggested to clean (i.e., detoxify) the implant surface. Although dependent on the type of implant surface, the use of PRF in the bone regeneration technique has been shown to heal compromised peri-implant defects.[163]

Protocol.
1. A full-thickness reflection is completed to expose the osseous and mucogingival defect. Debridement is completed to remove nonvital hard tissue, together with granulation tissue.
2. The implant surface is then detoxified with citric acid, EDTA, and/or tetracycline paste. A titanium brush may be used with a latch-type handpiece to aid in the decontamination process.
3. A whole blood sample is collected in a 10-mL tube without an anticoagulant.
4. The blood sample is immediately centrifuged for 12 minutes at approximately 2700 rpm. Because there is no anticoagulant, the platelets are activated and trigger the coagulation cascade when they contact the tube walls. There will exist three distinct layers: (1) top layer—platelet-poor plasma (PPP); (2) middle layer—PRF; and (3) bottom layer—red blood cells.
5. The fibrinogen is transformed into a fibrin network via the circulating thrombin. The resultant fibrin clot is located in the center of the tube, which is concentrated with acellular plasma and platelets.

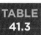

TABLE 41.3 Treatment of Peri-mucositis and Peri-implantitis

Peri-Mucositis

Patient Self-Administered

Plaque Control

- Toothbrushes (manual or powered)
- Toothpastes
- Antimicrobial rinses
- Flossing/oral irrigators
- Topical application of gel
- Systemic antibiotics
- Probiotic *Lactobacillus reuteri*–containing tablets

Professional

Mechanical plaque control
- Hand instruments
- Powered instruments

Chemical plaque control
- Local delivery of antibiotics
- Chlorhexidine (antimicrobials)
- Phosphoric acid
- Ozone, oxygen, and saline solution

Mucogingival debridement

Prosthesis alteration

Peri-Implantitis

Non-Surgical

Mechanical instruments
- Nonmetal instruments
- Rubber cups
- Air abrasive

- Metal instruments
- Burs

Adjunctive treatments
- Microbiologic test
- Local antimicrobials
- Systemic antimicrobials

Disinfect titanium surfaces
- Antiseptics
- Chemical
- Air polishing
- Laser

Mucogingival debridement

Prosthesis alteration

Surgical

- Open flap debridement
- Surface decontamination
- Regenerative approaches
- Biologics
- Guided tissue regeneration
- Guided bone regeneration
- Systemic antibiotics

Retrograde Peri-implantitis (Maintenance and Prevention)

Patient self-administered preventive regimens

Supportive periodontal therapy/maintenance (professionally)
- Mechanical nonsurgical therapy
- Mucogingival Debridement
- Prosthesis Alteration

Adapted from Suzuki JB, Misch CE. Periodontal and maintenance complications. In: Resnik RR, Misch CE, eds. *Misch's Avoiding Complications in Oral Implantology.* St. Louis, MO: Elsevier; 2018.

6. The acellular plasma (PPP), which is the top layer, may be removed with a pipette into a syringe. The PRF fibrin clot is then placed into a PRF box and processed into a membrane. The liquid part (PRF) of the PRF box is then collected and placed in with the graft material. If additional liquid is indicated for the graft material, the acellular plasma (PPP) may be added, as a small number of platelets are present in this concentrate.

7. After grafting the defect, the PRF membrane is placed over the defect. If a second membrane is used (e.g., collagen), then the membrane may be moistened with acellular plasma.

8. The soft tissue flaps are approximated and closed with a high-tensile-strength suture material (e.g., Vicryl, polytetrafluoro-ethylene [PTFE]).

In conclusion, the L-PRF technique is a simple, effective, and nonexpensive technique to enhance the soft and hard tissues around peri-implant defects. When added to the bone substitute material, there exist immune and antibacterial properties that benefit the healing process.[164,165] The use of L-PRF as a membrane allows the peri-implant defect to create a healthy, thick, and stable soft tissue interface for increased soft tissue health.

Suzuki-Resnik Peri-Implant Disease Protocol

To simplify the treatment of peri-implant disease and maintenance protocols, Suzuki and Resnik have formulated a comprehensive treatment regimen. This consists of four protocols with associated detailed step-by-step regimen.

PROTOCOL 1:

< 3mm probing depths
No Plaque or No Bleeding on Probing (BOP)

Treatment

- Maintain Regular Home Care
- 3 - 6 month hygiene recall

PROTOCOL 2: (Peri-Implant Mucositis)

< 3mm probing depths
Plaque presence / Bleeding on Probing (BOP)
   Or

3 – 5 mm probing depths
Plaque presence / Bleeding on Probing (BOP)

Treatment

- Follow **Treatment Regimen A**
- Increase Hygiene Recall Frequency (~ 3 months)
- Increase Home Care Education
- If no resolution, proceed to Protocol 3

PROTOCOL 3: (Peri-Implantitis)

> 5 mm probing depths
Plaque presence / Bleeding on Probing
Crestal Bone Loss > 2 mm

Treatment

- Follow **Treatment Regimen A, B, C, & D**
- Increase Hygiene Recall Frequency (~ 3 months)
- Increase Home Care Education
- Rx

PROTOCOL 4: Implant Mobility

Pain upon function
Bone loss > 50% of implant length
Uncontrolled exudate

Treatment

- Follow **Treatment Regimen E**

Peri-Implant Disease Treatment Regimen

Treatment Regimen A: Mechanical Closed Debridement (Acceptable Instrumentation)

- Resin, Titanium, Graphite, Carbon-Fiber, and Gold-tipped instruments can be used to remove deposits
- Prophy Cup/Brush
- Air-Polisher with Glycine Powder (Hu-Friedy), Prophy Jet (Dentsply)
- Cavitron (use blue implant tip)
- Rx: Chlorhexidine (0.12%, 0.2%) or cetylpyridinium chloride
- Check Occlusion

Treatment Regimen B: Antiseptic Therapy

- Subgingival antiseptic irrigation (0.12%, 0.2% Chlorhexidine) is added to the mechanical therapy
  - Irrigate intracrevicularly to disrupt and dislodge the biofilm, then thoroughly debride the implant surface with a curette. Irrigate a 2nd time to rinse out the debris and further detoxify the subgingival area. Pressure is then applied for one minute to obtain intimate soft tissue/restoration contact.
- Alternative Antiseptic; diluted sodium hypochlorite (NAOCl).
  - Diluted (.25%) NAOCl solution = one teaspoon (5ml) of standard 6% household bleach (Clorox) and diluting it with 4 oz (125ml) of water.
- Check Occlusion, possible occlusal guard

Treatment Regimen C: ANTIBIOTICS

- Add systemic and/or local antibiotic treatment

Systemic : **Amoxicillin, Metronidazole (500 mg, 3 times/daily for 8 days)**

   Alternative: Clindamycin, Augmentin, Tetracycline, Bactrim, Ciprofloxacin

Local : **Tetracycline**

   Alternative: , Doxycycline, Minocycline spheres (Arestin®)

Treatment Regimen D: SURGERY (Access, Open Debridement, Bone Graft, Closure)

Step 1: Access Flap, Open Debridement with Hand Instruments, Implantoplasty (Salvin Bur Kit)

Step 2: Detoxify With:
- 1. Apply **0.12% or 0.2% Chlorhexidine** with cotton pellet for 60 sec. (rinse with saline)
  +
- 2a. Apply **20-40% Citric Acid** with cotton pellet or spatula or titanium brushes (Salvin) for 60 sec.(rinse with saline)
  OR
- 2b. Apply **Tetracycline Paste** with titanium brushes (Salvin) for 60 sec. (rinse with saline)
  - Other Detoxification Agents: EDTA, Hydrogen Peroxide, 0.25% NAOCl
  - Er:YAG laser
  (diode laser alone results in an unacceptable increase in implant body temperature)

Step 3: Bone Graft with Mineralized/Demineralized (70/30) + Autograft (if indicated)

Step 4: Cross-Linked Collagen (Extended Collagen)

Step 5: Tension-Free Closure with Vicryl (PGA) or PTFE sutures

Treatment Regimen E: IMPLANT REMOVAL

Lack of Keratinized Tissues

Lack of a zone of keratinized gingiva around teeth and oral implants is now recognized as serving an important clinical function for implant health. Direct clinical evidence confirms the need for nonmobile keratinized tissue next to natural teeth. However, the tooth with the least amount of keratinized tissue is often the mandibular first premolar.[166] Yet this tooth is rarely the first tooth lost from periodontal disease. If all other periodontal indices are normal, the amount or absence of keratinized gingiva has little to do with the expected longevity of the tooth. In longitudinal studies, the lack of adequate keratinized and attached tissue does not compromise the long-term health of soft and hard tissue, as long as patients maintain good oral hygiene.[167,168]

Many clinicians consider keratinized attached gingiva important to maintaining gingival health.[169] Mucogingival considerations in restorative dentistry have been considered.[170] They concluded that if subgingival restorations were to be placed in areas of minimal keratinized gingiva with less than optimal plaque control, augmentation to widen the zone of keratinized tissue may be warranted.

Although keratinized tissue around a tooth may not be mandatory for long-term health, a number of benefits are present with keratinized mucosa. The color, contour, and texture of the soft tissue drape should be similar around implants and teeth when in the esthetic zone. The interdental papillae should ideally fill the interproximal spaces. A high smile line often exposes the free gingival margin and interdental papillae zones. The keratinized tissue is more resistant to abrasion. As a result, hygiene aids are more comfortable to use, and mastication is less likely to cause discomfort.

The degree of gingival recession appears related to the absence of keratinized gingiva. Root sensitivity and esthetic concerns may be associated with gingival recession. From a restorative dental aspect, keratinized mucosa is more manageable during the retraction and impression-making process. Subgingival margin placement is improved, as is long-term stability in the presence of keratinized tissue. Many of these benefits directly apply to the soft tissue around an implant.

Natural teeth have two primary types of tissue: attached, keratinized gingiva and unattached, nonkeratinized mucosa. The type of tissue around a dental implant is more varied than natural teeth. After bone loss in the maxilla, excess tissue is often found, and the tissue is usually keratinized, unattached gingiva. An implant

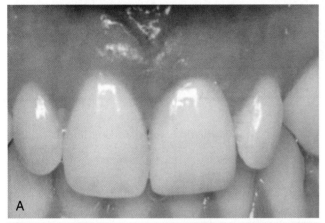

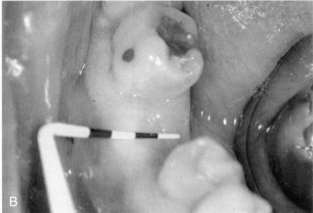

• **Fig. 41.16** Ideal Keratinized Tissue. (A) Healthy tissue surrounding implant. (B) Preoperative evaluation measuring the amount of attached tissue.

placed in the region may also have keratinized, unattached tissue. The tissues around the implant may also be similar to most natural teeth, surrounded by keratinized, attached gingiva (Fig. 41.16). The tissues may be nonkeratinized, unattached mucosa, more often in the mandible after bone height loss or after a bone graft and flap advancement to approximate the gingiva (Fig. 41.17). The nonkeratinized tissue may also be attached when acellular dermal matrix tissue (Oracell; Salvin Dental Specialities) is positioned under the periosteum and bounds the overlying tissues to the bone. In theory, structural differences in implants compared with teeth make them more susceptible to the development of inflammation and bone loss when exposed to plaque accumulation or microbial invasion (e.g., less vascular supply, fewer fibroblasts, lack of connective tissue attachment, cementation).[171]

Some reports indicate that the lack of keratinized tissue may contribute to implant failure. Kircsch et al. reported the most important criterion for implant health in the posterior mandible was related to the absence or presence of keratinized gingiva.[172] In this report mobile, nonkeratinized mucosa exhibited greater probing depths, which was histologically confirmed. A study in monkeys found that an absence of keratinized mucosa increases the susceptibility of peri-implant regions to plaque-induced destruction.[173]

The presence of keratinized tissue next to an implant presents some unique benefits, compared with natural teeth. Keratinized gingiva has more hemidesmosomes; the junctional epithelial attachment zone may be of benefit when in keratinized tissue. Whereas the orientation of collagen fibers in the connective tissue zone of an implant may appear perpendicular to the implant surface, these fibers in mobile nonkeratinized tissue run parallel to the surface of the implant.

Mobile mucosa may disrupt the implant-epithelial attachment zone and contribute to an increased risk for inflammation from plaque (Fig. 41.18).[174] In addition to the general advantages of keratinized tissue stated for teeth, keratinized tissue around implants may also be beneficial in several other ways. In a two-stage protocol the implant is less likely to become exposed during the healing process. The formation of an interdental/implant papillae is completely unpredictable with mobile nonkeratinized tissues. When the nonkeratinized tissue is mobile, several reports state that this is unsatisfactory.

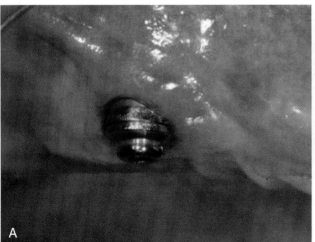

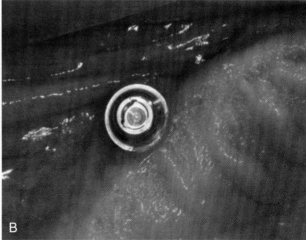

• **Fig. 41.17** (A and B) Implants placed to retain a lower overdenture that are malpositioned with minimal attached tissue present. In these type of cases, the tissue will usually remain irritated, inflamed, and painful.

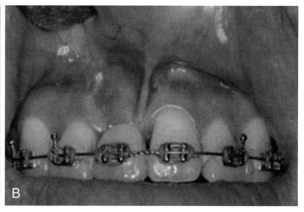

• **Fig. 41.18** (A and B) Maxillary implants with inadequate attached tissue.

A classification of attached gingiva and surgical alternatives to improve soft tissue types in edentulous sites for implant placement is critical for long-term implant survival.[175] Ideal adequate keratinized tissue should be established clinically before implant placement, especially in the posterior regions.

Interestingly, the studies that have advocated for the need for keratinized mucosa around dental implants have primarily investigated implants with rough surfaces. Failure of rough-surface implants (e.g., hydroxyapatite-coated and plasma-sprayed cylinder-shaped implants) has been related to a lack of keratinized mucosa.[176]

A meta-analysis reported 20% fewer instances of peri-implantitis in smooth-surface implants compared with rough-surface implants.[177] Another benefit of keratinized tissue is the clinical ease of treatment to reduce pocket depths if crestal bone loss occurs. Probing depths of 6 mm or more are more often associated with anaerobic bacteria. If the implant is out of the esthetic zone, a gingivectomy to reduce pocket depth is predictable. An apically positioned flap with nonkeratinized mucosa is less predictable and is more difficult to perform.

The significance of keratinized mucosa in the maintenance of dental implants with different surface conditions cannot be underestimated. All 69 patients and 339 implants in the study had implant restorations for at least 3 years, and as long as 24 years, with an average of 8.1 years. Bleeding index, modified plaque index, gingival index, probing depth, width of attached keratinized mucosa, and amount of attached mucosa were recorded. In addition, average annual bone loss was calculated, using past and present radiographs. Gingival inflammation and plaque accumulation were significantly higher in patients with less than 2 mm of keratinized mucosa or 1 mm of attached mucosa. The surface condition of the implant was not statistically significant in this study, although the smooth implants with less than 2 mm of keratinized mucosa were less stable than other groups relative to the soft tissue profile.

In this study the average annual bone loss was not influenced by the amount of keratinized or attached mucosa or the type of implant surface configuration (smooth versus rough). The greatest amount of bone loss was observed with rough implants in keratinized mucosa of less than 1 mm, but the difference was not statistically significant. The presence of keratinized mucosa was most significantly advantageous in the soft tissue health of posterior implants, as indicated by the gingival index. Posterior implants, even in the presence of keratinized tissue, had a 3.5-fold higher annual bone loss than anterior implants in this study (0.14 versus 0.04 mm). Implant location appears to be more important than the presence or absence of keratinized mucosa.

In most clinical situations attached keratinized gingiva is more desirable. A fixed prosthesis (FP-1) in the esthetic zone requires keratinized mucosa to develop the soft tissue drape around the implant restorations. Mandibular overdentures also benefit from a vestibule and zone of nonmobile keratinized tissue around the implant abutments to minimize the possibility of painful tissue.

Management of Lack of Keratinized Tissue

Several surgical techniques to increase the amount of keratinized tissue around dental implants have been described in the literature:
1. Autogenous free gingival graft
2. Autogenous subepithelial connective tissue graft
3. Allogenic soft tissue grafts from human cadavers (e.g., Oracell; Salvin Dental)
4. Xenogenic soft tissue grafts from animals

Augmentation can be completed before surgery, concurrent with surgery, or after implant surgery. The most ideal time to graft is before surgery.

Presurgical Augmentations
1. A trapezoidal flap is reflected from the desired areas of grafting.
2. Full-thickness mucoperiosteal flap is the design of choice.
3. Autogenous or acellular dermal matrix (Oracell; Salvin Dental) is modified to the desired dimensions.
4. PGA or chromic suture is used (5–0 recommended) to secure allogenic dermal matrix (AlloDerm) to the recipient site.
5. Flap is modified to be tension free and pulled over to cover acellular dermal matrix and sutured with 4–0 or 5–0 with PGA or PTFE sutures (Fig. 41.19).

Concurrent Augmentation
The steps for concurrent augmentation are as follows:
1. The full-thickness flap is reflected at the site of desired implant position (one tooth mesial and one tooth distal).
2. After implant placement and/or bone augmentation, autogenous or acellular dermal matrix is layered over the augmentation site.
3. It is critical to have abundant tissue release (i.e., tension-free closure) to allow coverage of soft tissue over bone graft.
4. The flap is sutured with no tension and secured for primary intention healing with 4–0 or 5–0 with PGA or PTFE sutures (Figs. 41.20 and 41.21).

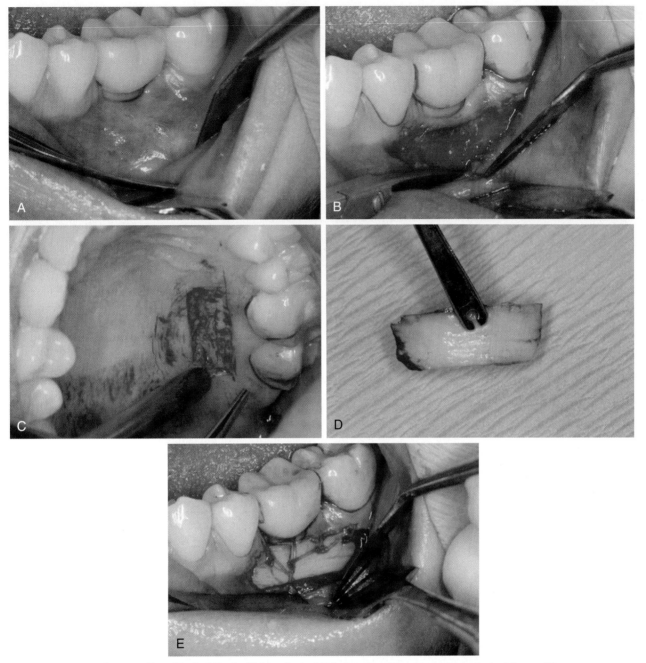

• **Fig. 41.19** Free Gingival Graft. (A) Mandibular left first molar with compromised attached tissue. (B) Recipient site modified. (C) Palatal graft removed. (D) Palatal tissue graft. (E) Tissue graft sutured in place.

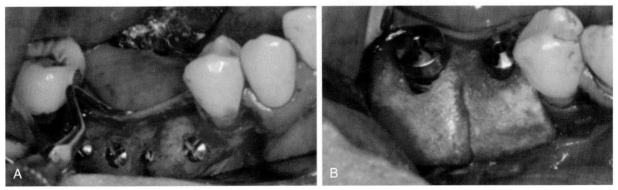

• **Fig. 41.20** Acellular Dermis. (A) Bone graft with inadequate attached tissue. (B) Acellular dermis placed around implant healing abutments.

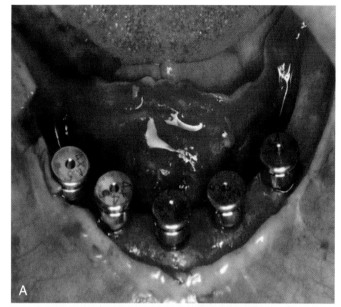

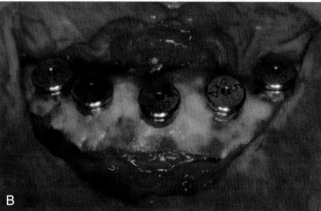

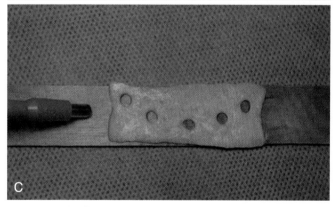

• **Fig. 41.21** Acellular Dermis. (A) Five implants placed in the anterior mandible. (B) Dermis modified to fit over healing abutments. (C) Dermis placed over implants and healing abutments.

Post-implant Tissue Augmentation

After the soft tissue flap has healed, the soft tissue augmentation can be performed during the abutment change appointment or uncovery appointment (3 months of healing). The steps are as follows:

1. A full-thickness flap is reflected, being wide enough to cover the size of the autogenous or acellular dermal matrix membrane.

2. Dermal matrix is ideally positioned and sutured to neighboring attached tissue (chromic 5–0).
3. The flap is advanced over the matrix, being careful to cover the entire allograft tissue (5–0 sutures are preferred).

Retained Cement Peri-implant Disease

Cemented implant prostheses are used in implant dentistry because of the lower cost, relative simplicity, more passive fit, improved esthetics, and similarity to traditional prosthetics. However, with all of these advantages comes a significant disadvantage, the retention of postoperative cement. The retained cement has been shown to harbor bacteria (similar to calculus with a natural tooth), which leads to peri-implant disease (Fig. 41.22).

During implant restoration cementation, it is possible that excess cement can become extruded into the gingival sulcus around the implant. The presence of cement in the sulcus has been shown to cause complications such as discomfort, inflammation, soft tissue swelling, and bleeding or exudate on probing.[178] It has been reported that cement can extrude at the implant abutment-interface when subgingival margins are present. Subgingival cement associated with an implant is more difficult to remove compared with a natural tooth, and various instruments used for this purpose have been shown to result in damage to implant abutments.[179] It has been proposed that any mass of foreign material present adjacent to a dental implant has the potential to negatively impact health and survival of the implant. The specific material itself may determine how a disease process can manifest. Further, the use of cements intended for natural teeth may not be appropriate for use with implant restorations.[180]

Studies suggest that excess cement has been shown to be a possible cause of implant failure.[181] Incidence of excess cement extrusion into peri-implant soft tissues and its adverse effects are well documented in the literature.[182,183] Cement retains microbial flora similar to organisms responsible for inflammatory periodontal diseases. The surface of retained cement has a rough topography, making removal of these microbes difficult, and can also result in accumulation significant enough to form a peri-implant biofilm similar to natural teeth.[185,186] Clinical studies that have analyzed retained methacrylate-based cement samples from patients for bacterial colonization have shown a strong tendency for bacterial invasion by pathogens and opportunistic species.[187] Remnant cement from implant restorations has been associated with consequences of increased bleeding on probing, suppuration, and peri-implant attachment loss.[188] It is the formation of a peri-implant biofilm that can cause the initiation and progression of peri-implant mucositis and peri-implantitis diseases.[189-191] Peri-Implantitis has been documented in several studies with a prevalence rate that ranges from 6% to as high as 47% of patients who have implants and have been followed over periods of 9 to 14 years.[192-194]

The problem of excess cement has been associated with greater than 80% of cases of peri-implant disease. No particular difference or correlation could be associated with the type of cement used to lute the restoration in regard to either the presence of disease or treatment response (when comparing resin cement, resin-modified glass ionomer, zinc polycarboxylate, and glass ionomer). Further, the presence of cement retention and inflammation was not dependent on the type of implant surface; titanium plasma–sprayed or sand-blasted large-grit acid-etched surfaces and titanium dioxide–blasted surfaces were

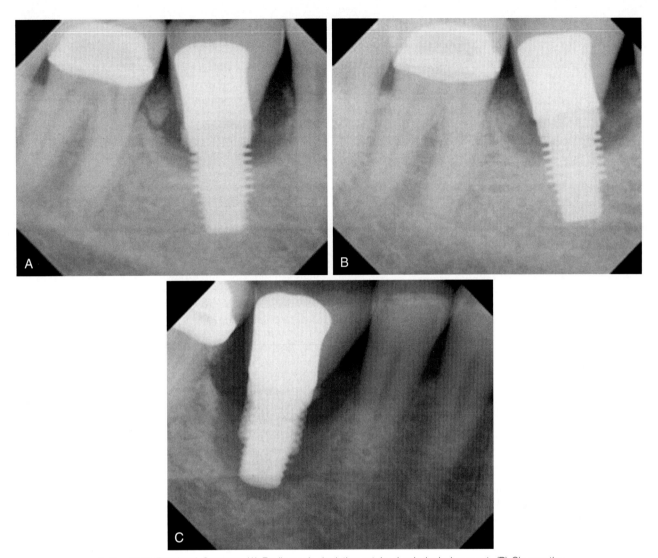

• **Fig. 41.22** Retained Cement. (A) Radiograph depicting retained subgingival cement. (B) Six months postoperatively. (C) Cement retention leading to failure of implant.

compared.[195] In cases where cement is inadvertently left as an overhang or expressed into the peri-implant tissues, it should be detected and removed.

Etiology

The etiology of cement-retained peri-implantitis is as follows:

Cement: The retained cement acts as a nidus for bacterial accumulation and proliferation. The roughened surface of the cement inhibits the hygienic removal of the bacteria, which leads to peri-implant disease. Cement acts the same way as the etiologic factor in periodontal disease.

Sulcus-Teeth Versus Implant: Around natural teeth the junctional epithelium and connective tissue attachment insert perpendicularly into the cementum, which tends to prevent the flow of excess cement into the sulcus. In contrast, the connective tissue around dental implants runs parallel, with no attachment into the implant surface. The flow of cement is not restricted, and it easily migrates apically (Fig. 41.23).

Submucosal Margins: Margins of implant restorations are often placed more than 2 mm subgingivally for a better emergence profile and esthetics. However, studies have shown the deeper the margins, the more difficult the removal of cement. In margins that are greater than 1.5 mm subgingivally, it is almost impossible to remove the cement totally.[197]

Location: Retained cement may attach to the following: (1) crown, (2) abutment, and (3) bone. If the cement is pushed into the sulcular area and reaches the bone, significant chronic issues will arise (Fig. 41.24).

Timing: Perhaps one of the most interesting, yet troubling aspects of cement-associated peri-implant disease is the range of time that can and has historically passed before obvious signs of an inflammatory disease response is evident during clinical detection. Wilson and Thomas[196] have shown that the time it takes for retained cement to become problematic and to eventually be diagnosed is in a range of 4 months to 9.3 years, with an average of 3 years. Another group showed detection ranging from several weeks to 4 years postcementation. This documented that delayed detection in inflammatory signs of peri-implant disease indicates a premise that cemented implant restorations should be examined periodically for disease.[199]

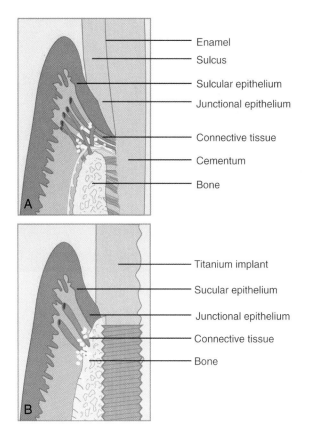

Radiographic Evaluation: Several techniques are described in the literature to locate excess cement around implant restorations. These include use of a dental endoscope and an invasive method of open flap debridement for direct observation.[200,201] Radiographic examination has been shown to be effective at detecting excess cement overhangs in tooth-supported restorations and can serve as a less invasive method of detection for cement-retained implant-supported restorations.[202,203] Radiographic examination is valuable in cement detection only if the luting agent has a high-enough radiodensity level.[204]

It is significant to note that with respect to restoration luting cements and radiopacity, there is no currently established minimum radiopacity standard (however, there is currently a national standard radiopaque value mandated for all endodontic sealer cements; American National Standards Institute/ADA specification No. 57). Therefore there is a broad range of radiographic visibility for restorative luting cements from having a highly radiopaque appearance to being completely undetectable.[205] Ideally, the luting agent should be more radiographically dense than the titanium alloys. Cements that are zinc based (i.e., Fleck's, Temp-Bond, Tempbond NE) have been shown to be most readily detectable radiographically with the higher gray level values. Studies have shown that many non-zinc-based cements are not detected radiographically, such as self-adhesive resin cement (RelyX Unicem), resin cement (Improv and Premier Implant Cement), glass ionomer (RelyX), and calcium hydroxide (Dycal). Being able to evaluate the presence of excess cement and then determining whether removal is indicated is crucial to facilitate appropriate restorative protocols.[206] After restoration cementation, residual excess cement has the highest likelihood of detection at the interproximal aspects. It is at these sites where the accumulation of the bulk of excess cement produces the effect of an enhanced radiopacity described by one group as the "peripheral egg shell effect."[207]

• **Fig. 41.23** Different Attachment Systems for Implant Versus Tooth. (A) Circular fibers attach into the cementum, minimizing the possibility of cement retention. (B) Because an endosseous implant does not contain an attachment system with the tissue, retained cement can be easily extruded into the sulcular area. (*From Resnik RR. Fixed prosthodontics complications. In: Resnik RR, Misch CE, eds.* Misch's Avoiding Complications in Oral Implantology. *St. Louis, MO: Elsevier; 2018; adapted from LeBeau J. Maintaining the long-term health of the dental implant and the implant-borne restoration.* Compend Contin Educ Oral Hyg. *1997;3:3–10.*)

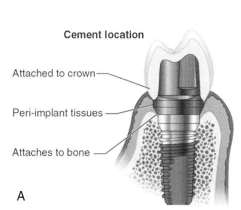

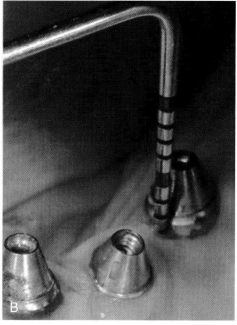

• **Fig. 41.24** Cement Attachment Location. (A) Retained cement may adhere to the crown/abutment, peri-implant tissues, or the bone. (B) Implant with deep pathologic pocket associated with retained cement.

Type of cement: Many types of cement are used today in implant dentistry to retain implant-supported crowns. Agar et al.[208] have shown that cement with resin components is the most difficult to remove from the abutment surface after cementation. Cements containing zinc have been shown to be ideal for cementing implant crowns because they are the easiest to see radiographically. Zinc phosphate is a well-known popular cement choice, which makes retrievability difficult. In addition, because of its solubility in the oral environment, a dry field is definitely needed. Provisional cements are also popular in cementing implant crowns because they allow for retrieval. However, because provisional cements exhibit weaker retentive strengths, uncementation of the implant prosthesis may be problematic.

Cememt Thickness: There is a large variation in the radiographic detection ability of cements. Some cements have a very high radiographic density, which allows for detection on radiographs. However, many cannot be detected, even at greater thickness ($\approx$2 mm).

Cementation technique: A common reason for retained cement is the cervical cementation technique, which usually parallels the technique for cementation on natural teeth.

Most clinicians place an excessive amount of cement within the internal surface of the crown, which leads to extrusion in the sulcular area.

Prevention

Supragingival Margins. Excess retained cement may be minimized by designing the abutment margins supragingivally. However, dentists are reluctant to place the margins at this level, especially if the crowns are in the esthetic zone. Studies have shown margins placed 1 mm supragingival or at the gingival margins allow for ease of cement removal without a decreased chance of retention.[209]

Ideal Application of Cement. Controlling the amount of cement that is placed in the implant crown will allow for a decreased possibility of cement retention. Clinicians are reluctant to use a small amount of cement because this translates into the possibility of leakage and loss of retention.

Excess cement may lead to improper seating, alteration of occlusion, and difficulty in cement removal. Ideally a uniform thickness of 40 μm over the intaglio surface is ideal; however, in a clinical setting, this is very difficult. The internal surface of the crown may sometimes be irregular, and unequal flow patterns may exist between parallel and nonparallel surfaces.

Additional factors that complicate ideal cementation are the cement's flow properties, viscosity, dimensional stability, and wettability of the surfaces.

Screw-Retained Prostheses. Although screw-retained implant prostheses have the disadvantages of higher cost and compromised esthetics in some cases, the lack of cement is a significant advantage.

Implant Abutment Modification. To reduce the amount of excess cement, studies have shown that modification of the abutment leads to less pressure and extruded cement. Ideally the abutment should be vented with two 0.75-mm radius vent holes, placed 3 mm apical to the occlusal area of the abutment and 180 degrees apart. This technique by Wadhwani et al.[210] has been shown to limit the amount of cement extruded into the gingival sulcus of implant-retained crowns.

Techniques

Various techniques to reduce retained cement have been discussed in the literature. A popular technique is the abutment copy technique, which uses Teflon tape inside the intaglio surface before copying the abutment with a polyvinyl siloxane material. The cement-filled final implant crown is seated on the copied abutment for excess cement removal before it is quickly transferred intraorally to be fully seated. This technique minimizes the possibility of retained cement; however, it has limitations when cementing a multiple splinted implant prosthesis[211] (Fig. 41.25).

The Resnik technique (lubrication technique) uses water-soluble petroleum jelly placed on the outer surfaces of the crown or prosthesis and below the implant margin (i.e., sulcular area). A controlled cementation technique is utilized which controls the amount of cement used and also allows for the removal of excess cement prior to final cementation. The advantage of this technique allows for the prevention of cement from adhering to the crown, sulcus, or underlying bone (Box 41.5 and Fig. 41.26).

Removal of Retained Implant Cement

Even the most diligent and skilled implant clinician may leave residual cement in the sulcular area of implant crowns. The importance of postoperative appointments for implant patients after cementation of the restoration cannot be overemphasized. Regular maintenance is extremely crucial for cement-retained crowns. Possible symptoms that may warrant an evaluation for retained cement are localized inflammation, bleeding on probing, exudate, progressively increased probing depths, and radiographic bone loss.

Nonsurgical

Nonsurgical treatment includes regular curettage with hand instruments. It should be noted it is very difficult to remove all cement non-surgically.

Surgical

In many cases, surgical access is necessary for complete cement removal, which includes flap, curettage, and detoxification with possible grafting. In cases of peri-implant disease the detection and removal of excess cement have frequently (76% of afflicted patients) resulted in resolution of clinical inflammatory signs in as little as a month posttreatment. This was possibly due to removal of cement irritants causing both bacterial and mechanical insult. Some authors advocate hand scalers, piezoelectric, and magnetostrictive mechanical devices (along with the benefit of a dental endoscope instrument for direct visualization of cement deposits)[212] (Fig. 41.27).

Peri-implant Mucosal Hyperplasia

The gingival overgrowth results in extreme difficulty for the patient to maintain adequate hygiene and for the clinician in performing debridement. When gingival overgrowth is associated with radiographic bone loss, the resultant periodontal pockets are expressed as "true" periodontal pockets. If there is no associated bone loss, the pockets are termed "pseudo" pockets or gingival pockets.[213]

Gingival hyperplasia may also result in an esthetic issue for the patient. This will require surgical intervention to reduce the tissue. In addition, gingival hyperplasia may make it impossible for a prosthesis to be completely seated (i.e., bar overdenture) or give rise to chronic tissue soreness.

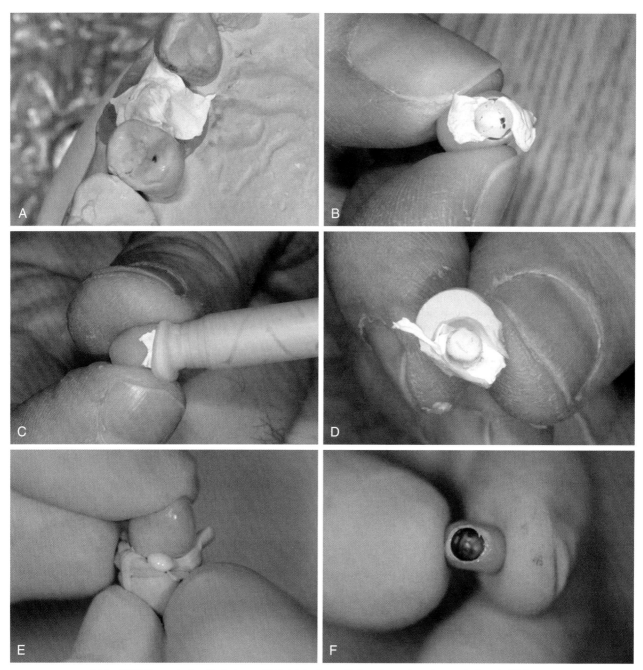

• **Fig. 41.25** Cementation Technique. (A) Polytetrafluoroethylene tape placed over abutment. (B) Crown inserted onto abutment. (C) Polyvinyl impression material added to the internal surface of the crown to make an abutment duplicate. (D) Internal surface of crown: abutment inserted onto implant in the mouth. (E) Cement added to crown and placed on polyvinyl abutment duplicate. (F) Excess cement removed, then inserted onto abutment in mouth.

• **BOX 41.5** Cementation Technique (Resnik Technique)

Step 1: Apply water-soluble petroleum jelly to the outer margin of the crown with a 1-mL tuberculin syringe.

Step 2: Seal the abutment screw (cotton ball, Teflon tape) without sealing the entire access.

Step 3: Place a thin layer of petroleum jelly 360 degrees with a 1 mL tuberculin syringe within the sulcus and around the implant.

Step 4: Apply a thin layer (≈40 μm) of cement to the intaglio surface of the crown abutment.

Step 5: Seat crown, remove crown, remove excess cement adhered to the outer margin surface, and remove any sulcular excess cement and petroelum jelly with a brush.

Step 6: Reseat crown, evaluate for any excess cement.

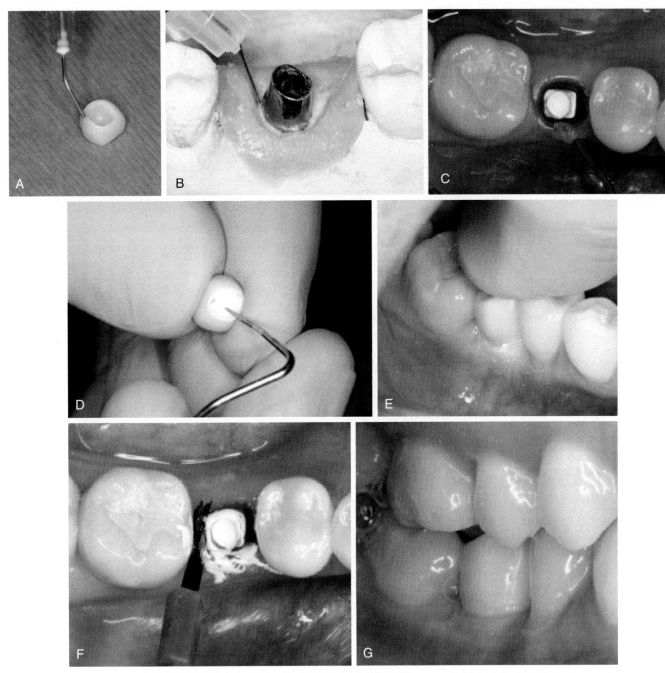

• **Fig. 41.26** Alternative Cementation Technique. (A) Outside of the crown is lubricated with water-soluble petroleum jelly. (B) Illustration-Water-soluble jelly placed within the sulcus with a 1-mL tuberculin syringe. (C) Clinical image after sulcular lubricant placed, (D) Cement is placed into the internal surface of the crown. (E) Crown is inserted into mouth. (F) Crown is removed and excess cement is removed with a brush. (G) Crown is reinserted onto abutment.

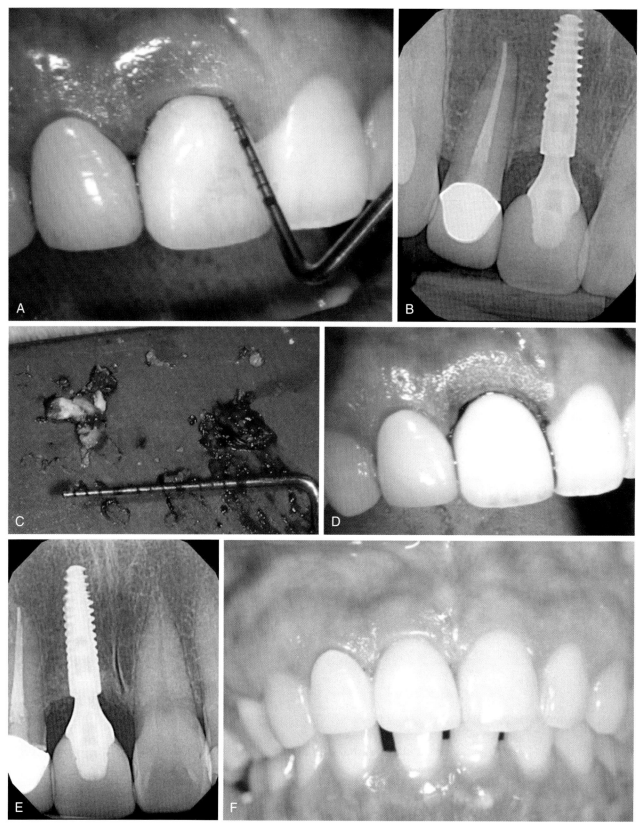

• **Fig. 41.27** Retained Cement. (A) Implant restoration in function for 6 months with persistent signs of peri-implant mucositis. (B) Radiographically evident manifestation of remnant cement at the restorative margin. (C) Excess cement after instrumentation with titanium and plastic curettes. (D) Peri-implant tissues immediately after instrumentation. (E) Radiograph demonstrating excess cement has been removed. (F) Condition of peri-implant tissues at 6-week reevaluation appointment.

Etiology

After clinical diagnosis of implant-related gingival overgrowth, potential etiologies must be identified, such as hormonal, medication induced, allergy induced, or patient-related habits. Various hormonal factors (e.g., related to pregnancy or puberty) and medications have been associated with the gingival overgrowth. Medications such as phenytoin (i.e., Dilantin), immunosuppressants (e.g., cyclosporine), calcium channel blockers, and amphetamines have been associated with gingival hyperplasia.

Gingival overgrowth has also been associated with patient habits such as mouth breathing. Allergy-induced hyperplasia is also becoming more prevalent in implant dentistry. With the use of titanium alloys for the fabrication of the dental implants and abutments, exacerbated allergic reactions are becoming a more common problem. Nickel (Ni), combined with titanium or in the final prosthesis, may exacerbate and cause an acute allergic reaction. Aluminum (Al) and beryllium (Be) have been associated with eczema and soft tissue reactions that result in gingival overgrowth.

Prevention

If a patient is considered to be at high risk for implant-related gingival hyperplasia (e.g., because of medications), he or she should be instructed to maintain meticulous oral hygiene. In addition, a more frequent recall protocol (four times per year) should be implemented that includes debridement. The prosthesis should be evaluated and maintained with a minimum of 1 mm of space between the tissue and the prosthesis, for ease of cleaning and prevention of prosthesis-induced irritation.

Management

The treatment of peri-implant hyperplasia should begin with conventional periodontal therapies to reduce plaque biofilm and inflammation. The surgical management of implant gingival overgrowth may require gingivectomy (if adequate keratinized gingiva is present) or apically positioned flaps (without adequate keratinized gingiva).

The use of 0.12% or 0.2% chlorhexidine twice per day has been shown to be successful in reducing tissue overgrowth and bacteria counts. When gingival hyperplasia is present around implants associated with overdentures, care should be exercised to minimize further enlargement (Fig. 41.28).

Commonly, practitioners will relieve the denture so the path of insertion does not cause irritation or mucosal injury. This may lead to inadequate thickness of acrylic, predisposing the prosthesis to fracture. Ideally the tissue enlargement should be reduced and the causative agent identified and treated accordingly. It is important to note that even with meticulous care and removal of etiology, gingival overgrowth may recur. Communication with the patient is key to avoid misunderstanding (Box 41.6).

Implant Quality Scale

The criteria for success in implant dentistry remain complex. Most clinical studies reporting success and failure do not qualify the type of success achieved. Instead, the term *success* primarily has been used interchangeably with survival of the implant. The term *failure* has been used to indicate the implant is no longer present in the mouth. Nearly all reports in the prosthetic literature also report survival as success.

What is success for a natural tooth? In the periodontal literature a quality of health is presented, and well-established guidelines

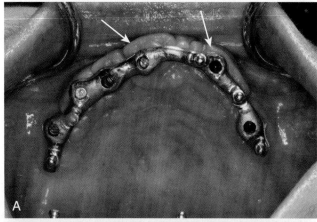

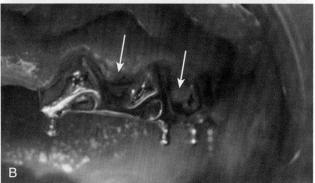

• **Fig. 41.28** Hyperplasia. (A and B) Hyperplastic tissue growth surrounding existing implant prosthesis resulting in home care difficulty. (*From Suzuki JB, Misch CE. Periodontal and maintenance complications. In: Resnik RR, Misch CE, eds.* Misch's Avoiding Complications in Oral Implantology. *St. Louis, MO: Elsevier; 2018.*)

• BOX 41.6 Pharmacologic Agents That Cause Gingival Hyperplasia

Anticonvulsants
Phenytoin
Phenobarbital
Lamotrigine
Vigabatrin
Ethosuximide
Topiramate
Primidone

Calcium channel blockers
Nifedipine
Amlodipine
Verapamil

Immunosuppressant drugs
Cyclosporine

Systemic factors
Pregnancy
Puberty
Vitamin C deficiency
Leukemia
Neoplasms (fibromas, papillomas, carcinomas)

based on clinical criteria describe the ideal health of natural teeth. The general term *success* in implant dentistry should be replaced with the concept of quality of health, with a health-disease continuum describing the status of implants.

TABLE
41.4 **Implant Quality Scale**

Implant Quality Scales	Clinical Conditions	Suzuki-Resnik Protocol
Success (optimal health) Osseointegration/Stage 0 osseoseparation	No pain or tenderness upon function 0 mobility <2 mm radiographic bone loss from initial surgery PD < 4 mm No suppuration No BOP	Protocol 1
Survival (satisfactory health) Stage I osseoseparation Peri-mucositis	No pain 0 mobility <2 mm radiographic bone loss from initial surgery Peri-mucosal inflammation PD ± 4 mm (bleeding and/or suppuration on probing)	Protocol 2
Survival (potentially compromised) Stage II osseoseparation Early peri-implantitis	No pain 0 mobility 2–4 mm radiographic bone loss PD ± 4 mm (bleeding and/or suppuration on probing) Peri-mucosal inflammation Bone loss <25% of the implant length	Protocol 2 or Protocol 3
Survival (compromised health) Stage III osseoseparation Moderate peri-implantitis	Variable pain 0 mobility Peri-mucosal inflammation PD ≥6 mm (bleeding and/or suppuration on probing) Bone loss 25%–50% of the implant length	Protocol 3
Failure (clinical failure) Stage IV osseoseparation Advanced peri-implantitis	Peri-mucosal inflammation Pain upon function PD >8 mm (bleeding and/or suppuration on probing) Bone loss >50% of the implant length Mobility Uncontrolled exudate Maybe no longer in mouth	Protocol 4
Others (such as retrograde peri-implantitis)	Variable peri-mucosal inflammation Radiographically: periapical lesion around implant Clinical: pain, tenderness, fistula formation or swelling	Surgical reentry and revision or removal of implant

BOP, bleeding on probing; *PD*, probing depth; *SPT*, supportive periodontal therapy.

From Suzuki JB, Misch CE. Periodontal and maintenance complications. In: Resnik RR, Misch CE, eds. *Misch's Avoiding Complications in Oral Implantology*. St. Louis, MO: Elsevier; 2018. Data from Suzuki JB, Hsiao YJ, Misch CE. Personal communication, 2017.

Success criteria for endosteal implants have been proposed previously.[214-218] The Misch scale proposes management modalities corresponding to different treatment levels.[219]

The most recent Suzuki-Misch-Hsiao implant health scale was published in Resnik and Misch's *Avoiding Implant Complications* (2017).[220] The Suzuki-Misch-Hsaio scale presented implant quality of health based on clinical evaluation (Table 41.4). This quality of health scale allows the implant dentist to evaluate an implant using the listed criteria, place it in the appropriate category, and then treat the implant accordingly. The prognosis also is related to the quality scale.

Ideal clinical conditions for natural teeth include absence of pain, less than 0.1 mm of initial horizontal mobility under lateral forces of less than 100 g, less than 0.15 mm of secondary mobility with lateral forces of 500 g, absence of observed vertical mobility, periodontal probing depths of less than 2.5 mm, radiographic crestal bone height 1.5 to 2.0 mm below the cementoenamel junction, intact lamina dura, no bleeding on probing, no exudate, and absence of recession or furcation involvement on multirooted teeth.

The American Dental Association CDT (2018) has defined five periodontal types for diagnosis and treatment of natural teeth.[221,222] The American Dental Association's categories of disease do not simply indicate success or failure but rather a range from health to disease. This classification allows a clinical approach to treatment in each category. A similar scale for implants has been established as an aid to diagnosis and treatment that also proposes management approaches according to the signs and symptoms.

Group I: Optimum Health

Group I represents implant success with optimum health conditions. No pain is observed with palpation, percussion, or function. No mobility is noted in any direction with loads less than 500 g of implant movement (IM). Less than 2.0 mm of crestal

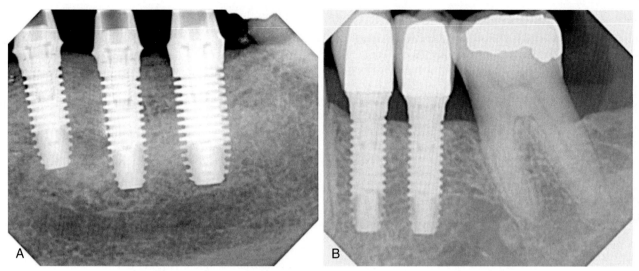

• **Fig. 41.29** Group I: Optimum Health. (A and B) Ideal implants with no associated bone loss.

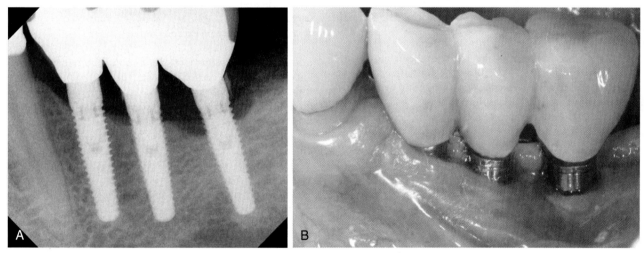

• **Fig. 41.30** Group II: Satisfactory Health. (A and B) Implants exhibit satisfactory health and are stable, but tenderness is observed on palpation, percussion, or function.

bone has been lost since the placement of the implant. This bone loss is typically a result of the implant biologic width below the abutment connection and surface of the implant. The implant has no history of exudate, and no radiolucency is present around the implant body. The probing depth is equal to or less than 5 mm and is stable after the first year. Ideally the bleeding index is 0 to 1. Group I implants follow a normal maintenance program every 6 months. The prognosis is very good to excellent (Fig. 41.29).

Group II: Satisfactory Health

Group II implants exhibit satisfactory health and are stable. No tenderness is observed on palpation, percussion, or function. No observable implant mobility was present in the horizontal or vertical direction with loads less than 500 g. Crestal radiographic bone loss is observed between 2 and 4 mm from implant placement. The most common cause is the early loading bone loss related to the amount of occlusal force and the density of the bone. No pain is observed. Probing depths may be as much as 5 to 6 mm because of the original tissue thickness and marginal bone loss, but are stable. Bleeding on probing index is often 1 or even 2. These implants may be considered to have peri-implant mucositis. The treatment indicated for group II implants consists of a stress reduction protocol for the implant system, shorter intervals between hygiene appointments (e.g., 3 months), reinforcement of oral hygiene instructions, annual radiographs until the crestal bone has stabilized, and gingivoplasty or sulcus reduction procedures where indicated. The prognosis is good to very good depending on the depth of the implant sulcus.

For pockets less than 6 mm in depth, the following can be concluded:

1. Mechanical therapy alone or combined with chlorhexidine results in the clinical resolution of peri-implant mucositis lesions.
2. Histologically both treatments result in minimal inflammation compatible with health.
3. The mechanical effect alone is sufficient to attain clinical and histologic resolution of mucositis lesions (Fig. 41.30).

Group III: Compromised Survival

Group III implants are classified as compromised survival and exhibit a slight-to-moderate peri-implantitis and compromised health status. Peri-implantitis is defined as an inflammatory process affecting the tissue around an implant that results in loss of supporting bone.

Group III implants are characterized by radiographically evident vertical bone loss, peri-implant pocket, bleeding on probing (plus occasional suppuration), and mucosal swelling and redness but no pain on function.

These implants warrant more aggressive clinical therapy. No pain is apparent in function, but tenderness may be slight on percussion or function. No vertical or initial horizontal mobility (IM-0) is evident. Greater than 4 mm of crestal bone loss has occurred since implant insertion but less than half the length of the implant. Greater than 7 mm and increasing probing depths are also present, usually accompanied by bleeding when probing. Exudate episodes may have lasted more than 1 to 2 weeks and may be accompanied by a slight radiolucency evident around a crestal region of the implant.

Group III implants warrant aggressive surgical and prosthetic intervention. Stress factors are also addressed. The prosthesis may be removed in nonesthetic regions. If a bar (used to support and retain an overdenture) is present, it may be removed during the surgical therapy. Modification of the occlusal scheme and methods to decrease the forces in the afflicted regions after hard and soft tissue surgical treatment include decreasing cantilever length, occlusal adjustment, and occlusal splint therapy.

In cases of rapid bone changes, the prosthesis design may be modified completely from a fixed to a removable restoration to stress relief and soft tissue support. Additional implants to support the restoration may be indicated, especially if the patient is unwilling to wear a removable prosthesis.

Systemic and topical antibiotics and local chemical agents such as chlorhexidine are indicated in the presence of exudate.

However, this method is usually of short-term benefit if the causative agents of implant failure are not eliminated.

Surgical management most often consists of soft tissue removal or exposure of a portion of the implant. Bone grafts may be used together with these approaches around the implant. A three-step approach is implemented for this category in the following order: (1) antimicrobial therapy (local or systemic), (2) stress reduction, and (3) surgical intervention.

The prognosis is good to guarded, depending on the ability to reduce and control stress after the surgical corrections have improved the soft and hard tissue health (Fig. 41.31).

Group IV: Clinical Failure

Group IV of implant health is clinical or absolute failure. The implant should be removed under any of these conditions: (1) pain on palpation, percussion, or function; (2) greater than 0.5 mm of horizontal mobility; (3) any vertical mobility; (4) uncontrolled progressive bone loss; (5) uncontrolled exudate; (6) more than 50% bone loss around the implant; (7) generalized radiolucency; or (8) implants surgically placed but unable to be restored (sleepers). Implants that are surgically removed or exfoliated are also in the category of failure.

This category also includes implants surgically removed or exfoliated and no longer in the mouth. The remaining edentulous area often is treated with autogenous, synthetic, or other substitute bone graft materials to replace the missing bone. After the favorable bony conditions are augmented, implants may be inserted again with a good prognosis.

The terminology for implant failure often is confusing, with different terms describing similar situations. Terminology for implant failure using the time period of failure has been suggested as a primary criterion. Many implant failures are not described ideally by the time of the complication and are not addressed in this nomenclature.

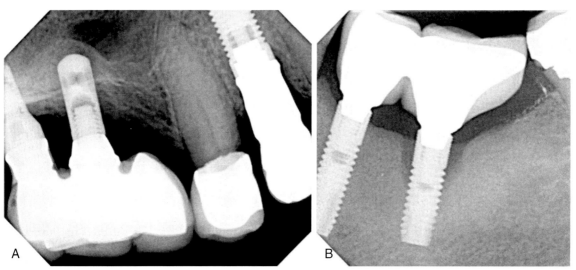

• **Fig. 41.31** Group III: Compromised Survival. (A and B) Implants are classified as compromised survival and exhibit a slight-to-moderate peri-implantitis and compromised health status.

Occasionally the patient will not permit removal of the implant. Regardless of whether the patient returns for implant removal, the implant is recorded as a failure in all statistical data. The patient should be warned against the irreversible damage to the surrounding bone with implants retained in this condition. Consideration should be given to their removal because future treatment may be compromised (Fig. 41.32).

Conclusion

Once the surgical and prosthetic phases of implant therapy have been completed, the work of the clinician is not over. Patients must be educated regarding proper maintenance of their implant-supported restorations, and routine examinations should be performed to monitor overall health. Many differences exist in the biology of natural teeth compared with implant-supported restorations as they pertain to periodontal status. It is critically important that the implant clinician recognize these differences, properly diagnose disease states, and effectively manage these problems should they arise. By understanding the etiologies of the various peri-implant disease states, a clinician can work with the patient to build an effective protocol of prevention (Figs. 41.33 and 41.34).

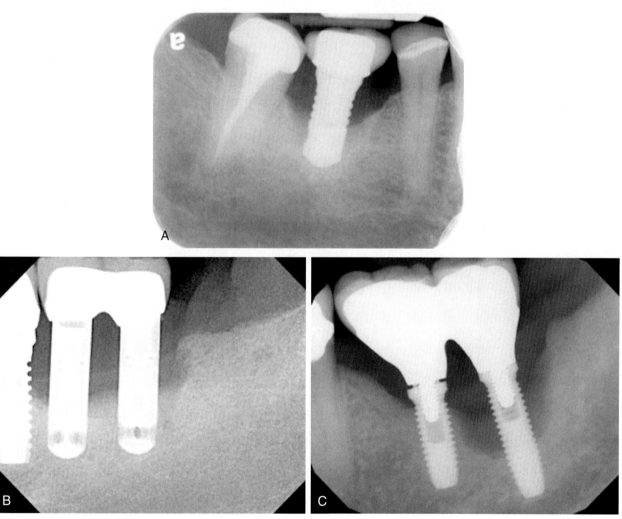

• **Fig. 41.32** Group IV: Implant Failure. (A–C) Implants are deemed absolute failures.

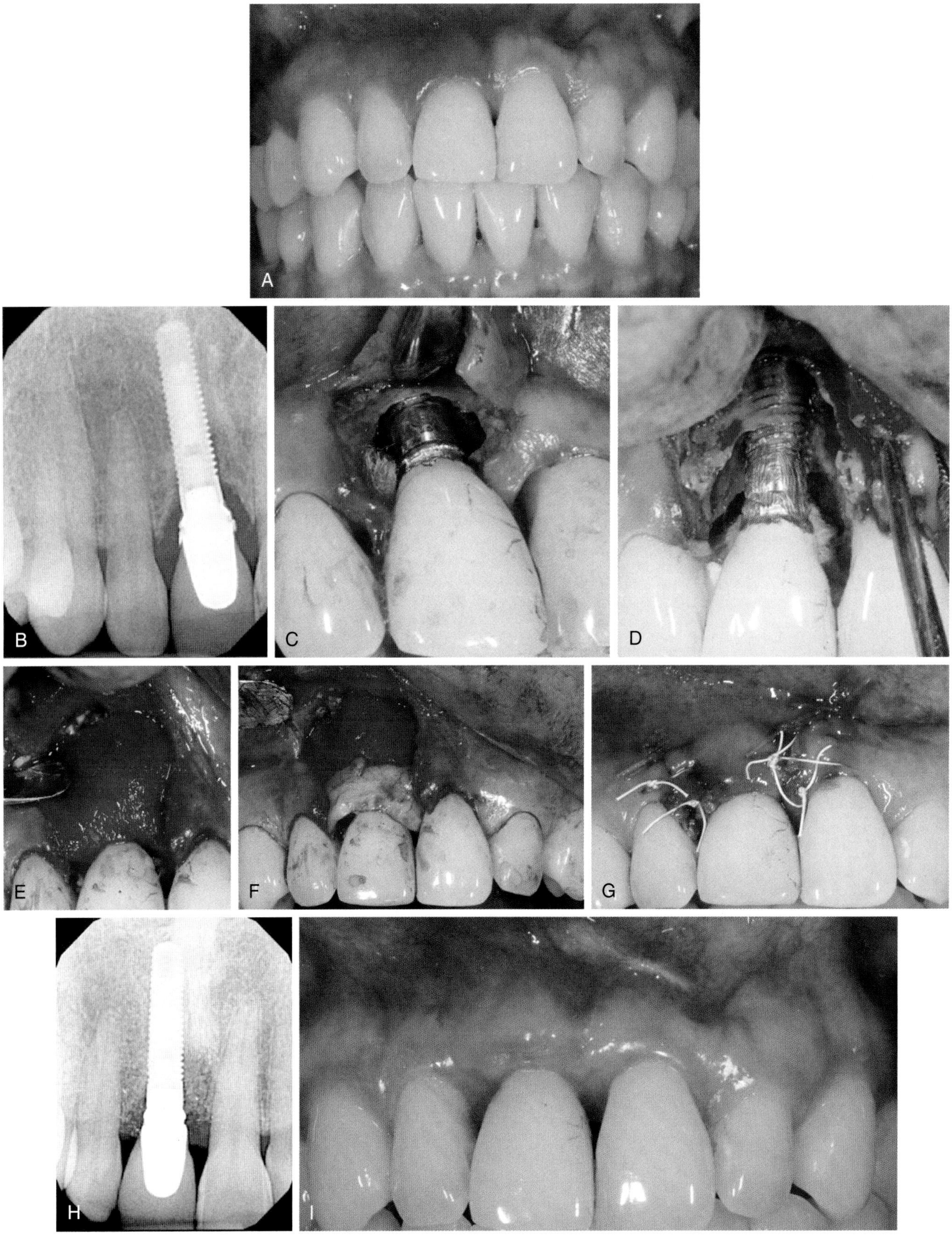

• **Fig. 41.33** Peri-implant Disease Protocol. (A) Maxillary right central incisor implant with associated bone loss and poor tissue health. (B) Radiographic evidence of peri-implant disease. (C) Tissue reflection revealing osseous defect. (D) Implantoplasty (removal of surface threads) and detoxification. (E) Bone grafting and collagen membrane placed. (F) Subepithelial connective tissue graft. (G) Final closure. (H) Immediate postoperative radiograph. (I) One-year follow-up.

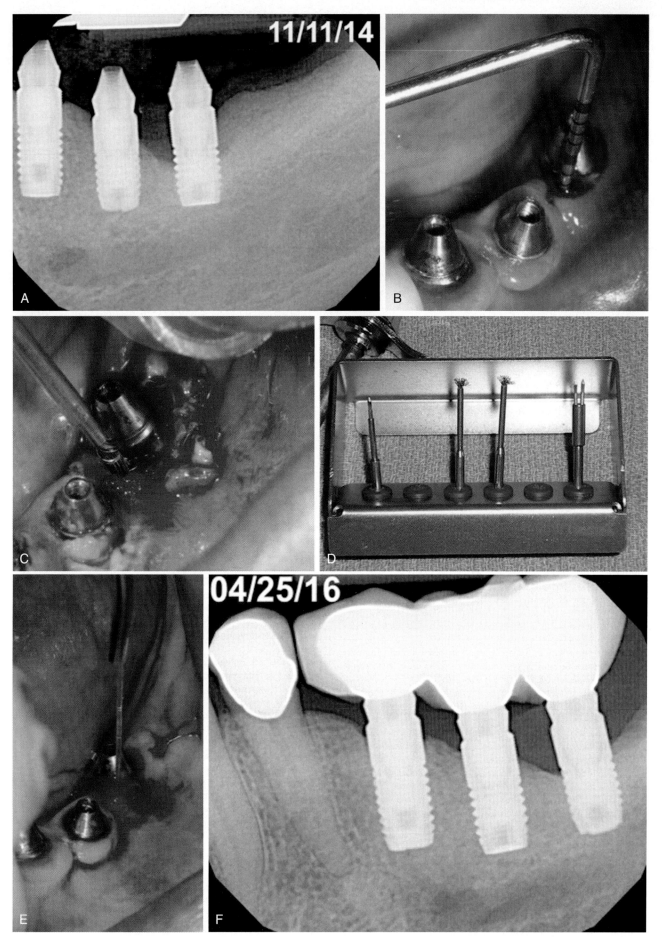

• **Fig. 41.34** Peri-implant Disease Protocol. (A) Mandibular left first molar bone loss. (B) Bleeding on probing. (C) Implant threads detoxified and titanium brushes used to remove soft tissue remnants. (D) Titanium brushes (Salvin Dental Specialties). (E) Laser treatment. (F) Two years postoperatively.

References

1. American Academy of Periodontology. Academy report: peri-implant mucositis and peri-implantitis: a current understanding of their diagnoses and clinical implications. *J Periodontol.* 2013;84:436–443.
2. Mombelli A, Lang NP. The diagnosis and treatment of peri-implantitis. *Periodontology.* 2000;17:63–76. 1998.
3. Lindhe J, Meyle J. Peri-implant diseases: consensus report of the sixth European workshop on periodontology. *J Clin Periodontol.* 2008;35:S282–S285.
4. Mombelli A, Muller N, Cionca N. The epidemiology of peri-implantitis. *Clin Oral Implants Res.* 2012;23(suppl 6):67–76.
5. Suzuki JB. *Diagnosis and classification of the periodontal diseases; in Dent Clin N Amer.* Philadelphia: Saunders; 1988
6. Albrektsson T, Canullo L, Cochran D, et al. "Peri-Implantitis": a complication of a foreign body or a man-made "disease." Facts and fiction. *Clin Implant Dent Relat Res.* 2016;18(4):840–849.
7. Salvi GE, Lang NP. Diagnostic parameters for monitoring peri-implant conditions. *Int J Oral Maxillofac Implants.* 2004;19(suppl):116–127.
8. American Academy of Periodontology. New periodontitis and peri-implantitis classification. *J Periodontol.* 2018;89(suppl 1):S1–S8.
9. Poli PP, Cicciu M, Beretta M, et al. Peri-implant mucositis and peri-implantitis: a current understanding of their diagnosis, clinical implications and a report of treatment using a combined therapy approach. *J Oral Implantol.* 2017;43:45–50.
10. Suzuki JB. Oral microbiology and immunology; in *Medical Microbiology.* Patrick Murray, ed., CV Mosby Co., St. Louis, MO. 1990.
11. Oh TJ, Yoon J, Misch CE, et al. The causes of early implant bone loss: myth or science. *J Periodontol.* 2002;73:322–333.
12. Rams TE, Roberts TW, Tatum Jr H, et al. The subgingival microflora associated with human dental implants. *J Prosthet Dent.* 1984;5:529–534.
13. Ting M, Craig J, Balkin BE, Suzuki JB. Peri-implantitis: a comprehensive overview of systematic reviews. *J Oral Implantology.* 2018;44(3):225–247.
14. Mombelli A, van Oosten MA, Schurch Jr E, Land NP. The microbiota associated with successful or failing osseointegrated titanium implants. *Oral Microbiol Immunol.* 1987;2(4):145–151.
15. Costerton JW, Stewart PS, Greenberg EP. Bacterial biofilms: a common cause of persistent infections. *Science.* 1999;284(5418):1318–1322.
16. Patel R. Biofilms and antimicrobial resistance. *Clin Orthop Relat Res.* 2005;437:41–47.
17. Di Giulio M, Traini T, Sinjari B, et al. Porphyromonas gingivalis biofilm formation in different titanium surfaces, an in vitro study. *Clin Oral Implants Res.* 2016;27(7):918–925.
18. Lang NP, Berglundh T. Working group 4 of seventh european workshop on periodontology. *Periimplant diseases: where are we now.* 2011:178–181.
19. Renvert S, Roos-Jansaker AM, Claffey N. Non-surgical treatment of periimplant mucositis and peri-implantitis: a literature review. *J Clin Periodontol.* 2008;35:305–315.
20. Furst MM, Salvi GE, Lang NP, et al. Bacterial colonization immediately after installation on oral titanium implants. *Clin Oral Implants Res.* 2007;18:501–508.
21. Costerton JW, Montanaro L, Arciola CR. Biofilm in implant infections: its production and regulation. *Int J Artif Organs.* 2005;28:1062–1068.
22. Socransky SS, Haffajee AD. Dental biofilms: difficult therapeutic targets. *Periodontol.* 2000;2002(28):12–55.
23. Violant D, Galofré M, Nart J, Teles RP. In vitro evaluation of a multispecies oral biofilm on different implant surfaces. *Biomed Mater.* 2014;9(3):035007.
24. de Avila ED, Avila-Campos MJ, Vergani CE, et al. Structural and quantitative analysis of a mature anaerobic biofilm on different implant abutment surfaces. *J Prosthet Dent.* 2016;115(4):428–436.
25. Ata-Ali J, Flichy-Fernandez AJ, Alegre-Domingo T, et al. Clinical, microbiological, and immunological aspects of healty versus peri-implantitis tissue in full arch reconstruction patients: a prospective cross-sectional study. *BMC Oral Health.* 2015;15:43.
26. Kinane DF. Aetiology and pathogenesis of periodontal disease. *Ann R Australas Coll Dent Surg.* 2000;15:43–50.
27. Javed F, A-Hezaimi K, Salameh Z, et al. Proinflammatory cytokines in the crevicular fluid of patients with peri-implantitis. *Cytokine.* 2011;53:8–12.
28. Perez-Chaparro PJ, Goncalves C, Figueiredo LC, et al. Newly identified pathogens associated with periodontitis: a systematic review. *J Dent Res.* 2014;93:846–858.
29. Klinge B, Meyle J. Peri-implant tissue destruction. The Third EAO Consensus Conference 2012. *Clin Oral Implants Res.* 2012;23(suppl 11):203–213.
30. Agarwal S, Suzuki JB, Riccelli AE. Role of cytokines in the modulation of neutrophil chemotaxis in localized juvenile periodontitis. *J Periodontal Res.* 1994;29(2):127–137.
31. Klinge B, Meyle J. Peri-implant tissue destruction. The Third EAO Consensus Conference 2012. *Clin Oral Implants Res.* 2012;3(suppl 11):203–213.
32. Rosen P, Clem D, Cochran D, et al. Peri-implant mucositis and peri-implantitis: a current understanding of their diagnoses and clinical implications. *J Periodontal.* 2013;84:436–443.
33. Faggion Jr CM, Listl S, Tu YK. Assessment of end-points in studies on peri-implant treatment. *J Dent.* 2010;38:443–450.
34. Persson GR, Renvert S. Cluster of bacteria associated with peri-implantitis. *Clin Implant Dent Relat Res.* 2014;16:783–793.
35. Hutlin M, Gustafsson A, Hallstrom H, et al. Microbiological findings and host response in patients with peri-implantitis. *Clin Oral Implants Res.* 2002;13:349358.
36. Mombelli A, Muller N, Cionca N. The epidemiology of peri-implantitis. *Clin Oral Implants Res.* 2012;23(suppl 6):67–76.
37. Suzuki JB. Immunology of the periodontal diseases: in Periodontics. Grant DA, Stern IB, and Listgarten M, eds. CV Mosby Co., St. Louis, MO. 1987.
38. Lee C-T, Huang Y-W, Zhu L, Weltman R. Prevalences of peri-implantitis and peri-implant mucositis: systematic review and meta-analysis. *J Dent.* 2017;62:1–12.
39. Ferreira SD, Silva GLM, Cortelli JR, Costa JE, Costa FO. Prevalence and risk variables for peri-implant disease in Brazilian subjects. *J Clin Periodontol.* 2006;33:929–935.
40. Zitzmann NU, Berglundh T, Marinello CP, Lindhe J. Experimental peri-implant mucositis in man. *J Clin Periodontol.* 2001;28:517–523.
41. Salvi GE, Aglietta M, Eick S, Sculean A, Lang NP, Ramseier CA. Reversibility of experimental peri-implant mucositis compared with experimental gingivitis in humans. *Clin Oral Implants Res.* 2012;23:182–190.
42. Meyer S, Giannopoulou C, Courvoisier D, Schimmel M, Müller F, Mombelli A. Experimental mucositis and experimental gingivitis in persons aged 70 or over. Clinical and biological responses. *Clin Oral Implants Res.* 2017;28(8):1005–1012.
43. Sennerby L, Lekholm U. The soft tissue response to titanium abutments retrieved from humans and reimplanted in rats. A light microscopic pilot study. *Clin Oral Impl Res.* 1993;4:23–27.
44. Atieh MA, Alsabeeha NH, Faggion CM, Duncan WJ. The frequency of peri-implant diseases: a systematic review and meta-analysis. *J Periodontol.* 2013;84(11):1586–1598.
45. Javed F, Romanos GE. Impact of diabetes mellitus and glycemic control on the osseointegration of dental implants: a systematic literature review. *J Periodontol.* 2009;80:1719–1730.
46. Costa FO, Takenaka-Martinez S, Cota LO, et al. Peri-implant disease in subjects with and without preventive maintenance: a 5-year follow-up. *J Clin Periodontol.* 2012;39(2):173–181.
47. Trejo PM, Bonaventura G, Weng D, et al. Effect of mechanical and antiseptic therapy on peri-implant mucositis: an experimental study in monkeys. *Clin Oral Implants Res.* 2006;17:294–304.

48. Renvert S, Roos-Jansaker AM, Claffey N. Non-surgical treatment of peri-implant mucositis and peri-implantitis: a literature review. *J Clin Periodontol.* 2008;35:305–315.

49. Fakhraver B, Khocht A, Jefferies SR, Suzuki JB. Probing and scaling instrumentation on implant abutment surfaces: an in vitro study. *Impl Dent.* 2012;21(4):311–316.

50. Bassetti M, Schär D, Wicki B, et al. Anti-infective therapy of peri-implantitis with adjunctive local drug delivery or photodynamic therapy: 12-month outcomes of a randomized controlled clinical trial. *Clin Oral Implants Res.* 2014;25(3):279–287.

51. Hasturk H, Nguyen DH, Sherzai H, et al. Comparison of the impact of scaler material composition on polished titanium implant abutment surfaces. *J Dent Hyg.* 2013;87(4):200–211.

52. Anastassiadis PM, Hall C, Marino V, et al. Surface scratch assessment of titanium implant abutments and cementum following instrumentation with metal curettes. *Clin Oral Investig.* 2015;19(2):545–551.

53. Sánchez-Garcás M, Gay-Escoda C. Peri-implantitis. *Med Oral Pathol Oral Cir Bucal.* 2004;9:63–74.

54. Dennison DK, Huerzeler MB, Quinones C, Caffese RG. Contaminated implant surfaces: an in vitro comparison of implant surface coating and treatment modalities for decontamination. *J Periodontol.* 1994;65(10):942–948.

55. Faria G, Cardoso CR, Larson RE, et al. Chlorhexidine-induced apoptosis or necrosis in L929 fibroblasts: a role for ndoplasmic reticulum stress. *Toxicol Appl Pharmacol.* 2009;234(2):256–265.

56. Hall EE, Meffert RM, Hermann JS, et al. Comparison of bioactive glass to demineralized freeze-dried bone allograft in the treatment of intrabony defects around implants in the canine mandible. *J Periodontol.* 1999;70(5):526–535.

57. Norowski Jr PA, Bumgardner JD. Biomaterial and antibiotic strategies for peri-implantitis: a review. *J Biomed Mater Res B Appl Biomater.* 2009;88(2):530–543.

58. Williams RC, Paquette DW, Offenbacher S, et al. Treatment of periodontitis by local administration of min ocycline microspheres: a controlled trial. *J Periodontol.* 2001;72:1535–1544.

59. Oringer RJ, Al-Shammari KF, Aldredge WA, et al. Effect of locally delivered minocycline microspheres on markers of bone resorption. *J Periodontol.* 2002;73(8):835–842.

60. Loesch WJ. Nonsurgical treatment of patients with periodontal disease. *Oral Surg Oral Med Oral Pathol Oral Radiol Endod.* 1996;81:533–543.

61. Guerrero A, Griffiths GS, Nibali L, et al. Adjunctive benefits of systemic amoxicillin and metronidazole in non-surgical treatment of generalized aggressive periodontitis: a randomized placebo-controlled clinical trial. *J Clin Periodontol.* 2005;32(10):1096–1107.

62. Pavicic M, Van Winkelhoff AJ, Dougué NH, et al. Microbiological and clinical effects of metronidazole and amoxicillin in Actinobacillus actinomycetemcomitans associated periodontitis: a 2-year evaluation. *J Clin Periodontol.* 1994;21(2):107–112.

63. Haffajee AD, Smith C, Torresyap G, et al. Efficacy of manual and powered toothbrushes (II). Effect on microbiological parameters. *J Clin Periodontol.* 2001;28(10):947–954.

64. Poli Pier P, Cicciu M, Beretta M, Maiorana C. "Peri-implant mucositis and peri-implantitis: a current understanding of their diagnosis, clinical implications, and a report of treatment using a combined therapy approach. *J Oral Implantol.* 2017;43(1):45–50.

65. Perez-Chaparro PJ, Duarte PM, Shibli JA, et al. The current weight of evidence of the microbiologic profile associated with peri-implantitis: a systematic review. *J Periodontol.* 2016;87:1295–1304.

66. Ting M, Craig J, Balkin BE, Suzuki JB. Peri-implantitis: a comprehensive overview of systematic reviews. *J Oral Implantol.* 2018;44(3):225–247.

67. Mir-Mari J, Mir-Orfila P, Figueiredo R, Valmaseda-Castellón E, Gay-Escoda C. Prevalence of peri-implant diseases. A cross-sectional study based on a private practice environment. *J Clin Periodontol.* 2012;39(5):490–494.

68. Renvert S, Roos-Jansaker AM, Lindahl C, et al. Infection at titanium implants with or without a clinical diagnosis of inflammation. *Clin Oral Implants Res.* 2007;18:509–516.

69. Monje A, Aranda L, Diaz KT, et al. "Impact of maintenance therapy for the prevention of peri-implant diseases: a systematic review and meta-analysis". *J Dent Res.* 2016;95(4):372–379.

70. Rodrigues DC, Valderrama P, Wilson TG, et al. Titanium corrosion mechanisms in the oral environment: a retrieval study. *Materials.* 2013;6:5258–5274.

71. Wachi T, Shuto T, Shinohara Y, et al. Release of titanium ions from an implant surface and their effect on cytokine production related to alveolar bone resorption. *Toxicology.* 2015;327:1–9.

72. Karoussis IK, Salvi GE, Heitz–Mayfield LJ, Brägger U, Hämmerle CH, Lang NP. Long–term implant prognosis in patients with and without a history of chronic periodontitis: a 10–year prospective cohort study of the ITI® Dental Implant System. *Clin Oral Implants Res.* 2003;14(3):329–339.

73. Roos–Jansåker A, Renvert H, Lindahl C, Renvert S. "Nine–to fourteen–year follow–up of implant treatment. Part III: factors associated with peri–implant lesions". *J Clin Periodontol.* 2006;33(4):296–301.

74. Papantonopoulos G, Gogos C, Housos E, Bountis T, Loos BG. Prediction of individual implant bone levels and the existence of implant "phenotypes". *Clin Oral Implants Res.* 2017;28(7):823–832.

75. Rinke S, Ohl S, Ziebolz D, Lange K, Eickholz P. Prevalence of peri-implant disease in partially edentulous patients: a practice–based cross–sectional study. *Clin Oral Implants Res.* 2011;22(8):826–833.

76. Nguyen–Hieu T, Borghetti A, Aboudharam G. Peri–implantitis: from diagnosis to therapeutics. *J Investig Clin Dent.* 2012;3(2):79–94.

77. Venza I, Visalli M, Cucinotta M, et al. Proinflammatory gene expression at chronic periodontitis and peri–implantitis sites in patients with or without type 2 diabetes. *J Periodontology.* 2010;81(1):99–108.

78. Venza I, Visalli M, Cucinotta M, et al. Proinflammatory gene expression at chronic periodontitis and peri–implantitis sites in patients with or without type 2 diabetes. *J Periodontology.* 2010;81(1):99–108.

79. Canullo L, Tallarico M, Radovanovic S, Delibasic B, Covani U, Rakic M. Distinguishing predictive profiles for patient–based risk assessment and diagnostics of plaque induced, surgically and prosthetically triggered peri–implantitis. *Clin Oral Implants Res.* 2016;27(10):1243–1250.

80. Lindquist LW, Carlsson GE, Jemt T. Association between marginal bone loss around osseointegrated mandibular implants and smoking habits: a 10-year follow-up study. *J Dent Res.* 1997;76:1667–1674.

81. Wen X, Liu R, Li G, et al. History of periodontitis as a risk factor for long-term survival of dental implants: a meta-analysis. *Int J Oral Maxillofac Implants.* 2014;29:1271–1280.

82. Sgolastra F, Petrucci A, Severino M, et al. Periodontitis, implant loss and peri-implantitis. A meta-analysis. *Clin Oral Implants Res.* 2015;26:e8–e16.

83. Renvert S, Polyzois I, Claffey N. How do implant surface characteristics influence peri-implant disease? *J Clin Periodontol.* 2011;38(suppl 11):214–222.

84. Ting M, Jefferies SR, Xia W, Engqvist H, Suzuki JB. Classification and effects of implant surface modification on the bone: human cell-based in-vitro studies. *J Oral Implantol.* 2017;43:58–83.

85. Petersilka GJ, Steinmann D, Haberlein I, et al. Subgingival plaque removal in buccal and lingual sites using a novel low abrasive air-polishing powder. *J Clin Periodontol.* 2003;30:328–333.

86. Martin E. Lasers in dental implantology. *Dent Clin North Am.* 2004;48(4):999–1015.

87. Coluzzi DJ, Aoki A, Chininforush N. Laser treatment of periodontal and peri-implant disease. Chapter 14. In: Coluzzi DJ, Parker

SPA, eds. *Lasers in Dentistry – Current Concepts.* Switzerland: Springer: Cham; 2017:293–316.

88. Bach G, Neckel C, Mall C, Krekeler G. Conventional versus laser-assisted therapy of peri-implantitis: a five-year comparative study. *Implant Dent.* 2000;9(3):247–251.

89. Schwarz F, Sculean A, Rothamel D, Schwenzer K, Georg T, Becker J. Clinical evaluation of an Er:YAG laser for nonsurgical treatment of peri-implantitis: a pilot study. *Clin Oral Implants Res.* 2005;16(1):44–52.

90. Schwarz F, Bieling K, Bonsmann M, Latz T, Becker J. Nonsurgical treatment of moderate and advanced peri-implantitis lesions: a controlled clinical study. *Clin Oral Investig.* 2006;10(4):279–288.

91. Persson GR, Roos-Jansåker AM, Lindahl C, Renvert S. Microbiologic results after non-surgical erbium-doped:yttrium, aluminum, and garnet laser or air-abrasive treatment of peri-implantitis: A randomized clinical trial. *J Periodontol.* 2011;82(9):1267–1278.

92. Roncati M, Lucchese A, Carinci F. Non-surgical treatment of peri-implantitis with the adjunctive use of an 810-nm diode laser. *J Indian Soc Periodontol.* 2013;17(6):812–815.

93. Al-Falaki R, Cronshaw M, Hughes FJ. Treatment outcome following use of the erbium, chromium:yttrium, scandium, gallium, garnet laser in the non-surgical management of peri-implantitis: a case series. *Br Dent J.* 2014 24;217(8):453–457.

94. Renvert S, Lindahl C, Roos Jansåker AM, Persson GR. Treatment of peri-implantitis using an Er:YAG laser or an air-abrasive device: a randomized clinical trial. *J Clin Periodontol.* 2011;38(1):65–73.

95. Abduljabbar T, Javed F, Kellesarian SV, Vohra F, Romanos GE. Effect of Nd:YAG laser-assisted non- surgical mechanical debridement on clinical and radiographic peri-implant inflammatory parameters in patients with peri-implant disease. *J Photochem Photobiol B.* 2017;168:16–19.

96. Do JH, Klokkevold PR. Supportive implant treatment. Chapter 83 in: In: Newman MG, Takei HH, Klokkevold PR, Carranza FA, eds. *Carranza's Clinical Periodontology.* 12th ed. St. Louis: Elsevier; 2015:805–812.

97. Deppe H, Horch HH, Neff A. Conventional versus CO_2 laser-assisted treatment of peri-implant defects with the concomitant use of pure-phase beta-tricalcium phosphate: a 5-year clinical report. *Int J Oral Maxillofac Implants.* 2007;22(1):79–86.

98. Romanos GE, Nentwig GH. Regenerative therapy of deep peri-implant infrabony defects after CO_2 laser implant surface decontamination. *Int J Periodontics Restorative Dent.* 2008;28(3):245–255.

99. Azzeh MM. Er,Cr:YSGG laser-assisted surgical treatment of peri-implantitis with 1-year reentry and 18-month follow-up. *J Periodontol.* 2008;79(10):2000–2005.

100. Badran Z, Bories C, Struillou X, Saffarzadeh A, Verner C, Soueidan A. Er: YAG laser in the clinical management of severe peri-implantitis: a case report. *J Oral Implantol.* 2011;37:212–217.

101. Schwarz F, John G, Mainusch S, Sahm N, Becker J. Combined surgical therapy of peri-implantitis evaluating two methods of surface debridement and decontamination. A two-year clinical follow up report. *J Clin Periodontol.* 2012;39(8):789–797.

102. Papadopoulos CA, Vouros I, Menexes G, Konstantinidis A. The utilization of a diode laser in the surgical treatment of peri-implantitis. A randomized clinical trial. *Clin Oral Investig.* 2015;19(8):1851–1860.

103. Valente NA, Andreana S. Treatment of peri-implantitis using a combined decontaminative and regenerative protocol: case report. *Compend Contin Educ Dent.* 2018;39(2):96–101.

104. Takasaki AA, Aoki A, Mizutani K, et al. Application of antimicrobial photodynamic therapy in periodontal and peri-implant diseases. *Periodontol 2000.* 2009;51(1):109–140.

105. Haas R, Baron M, Dörtbudak O, Watzek G. Lethal photosensitization, autogenous bone, and e-PTFE membrane for the treatment of peri-implantitis: preliminary results. *Int J Oral Maxillofac Implants.* 2000;15(3):374–382.

106. Dörtbudak O, Haas R, Bernhart T, Mailath-Pokorny G. Lethal photosensitization for decontamination of implant surfaces in the treatment of peri-implantitis. *Clin Oral Implants Res.* 2001;12(2):104–108.

107. Thierbach R, Eger T. Clinical outcome of a nonsurgical and surgical treatment protocol in different types of peri-implantitis: a case series. *Quintessence Int.* 2013;44(2):137–148.

108. Bombeccari GP, Guzzi G, Gualini F, Gualini S, Santoro F, Spadari F. Photodynamic therapy to treat periimplantitis. *Implant Dent.* 2013;22(6):631–638.

109. Bassetti M, Schär D, Wicki B, et al. Anti-infective therapy of peri-implantitis with adjunctive local drug delivery or photodynamic therapy: 12-month outcomes of a randomized controlled clinical trial. *Clin Oral Implants Res.* 2014;25(3):279–287.

110. Anders JJ, Lanzafame RJ, Arany PR. Low-level light/laser therapy versus photobiomodulation therapy. *Photomed Laser Surg.* 2015;33(4):183–184.

111. Pinheiro ALB, Marques AMC, Soares LGP, Barbosa AFS. Bone biomodulation. Chapter 25. In: de Freitas PM, Simões A, eds. *Lasers in Dentistry. Guide for Clinical Practice.* Ames, Iowa: John Wiley & Sons; 2015:196–206.

112. Khadra M. The effect of low level laser irradiation on implant-tissue interaction. In: vivo and in vitro studies. *Swed Dent J.* 2005;(suppl 172):1–63.

113. García-Morales JM, Tortamano-Neto P, Todescan FF, de Andrade Jr JC, Marotti J, Zezell DM. Stability of dental implants after irradiation with an 830-nm low-level laser: a double-blind randomized clinical study. *Lasers Med Sci.* 2012;27(4):703–711.

114. Tang E, Khan I, Andreana S, Arany PR. Laser-activated transforming growth factor-β1 induces human β-defensin 2: implications for laser therapies for periodontitis and peri-implantitis. *J Periodontal Res.* 2017;52(3):360–367.

115. Torkzaban P, Kasraei S, Torabi S, Farhadian M. Low-level laser therapy with 940 nm diode laser on stability of dental implants: a randomized controlled clinical trial. *Lasers Med Sci.* 2018;33(2):287–293.

116. Romanos GE, Weitz D. Therapy of peri-implant diseases. Where is the evidence? *J Evid Based Dent Pract.* 2012;12(suppl 3):204–208.

117. Aoki A, Mizutani K, Schwarz F, et al. Periodontal and peri-implant wound healing following laser therapy. *Periodontol 2000.* 2015;68(1):217–269.

118. Mizutani K, Aoki A, Coluzzi D, et al. Lasers in minimally invasive periodontal and peri-implant therapy. *Periodontol. 2000.* 2016;71(1):185–212.

119. Kilinc E, Rothrock J, Migliorati E, Drukteinis S, Roshkind DM, Bradley P. Potential surface alteration effects of laser-assisted periodontal surgery on existing dental restorations. *Quintessence Int.* 2012;43(5):387–395.

120. Stübinger S, Homann F, Etter C, Miskiewicz M, Wieland M, Sader R. Effect of Er:YAG, CO_2 and diode laser irradiation on surface properties of zirconia endosseous dental implants. *Lasers Surg Med.* 2008;40(3):223–228.

121. Geminiani A, Caton JG, Romanos GE. Temperature increase during CO_2 and Er:YAG irradiation on implant surfaces. *Implant Dent.* 2011;20(5):379–382.

122. Geminiani A, Caton JG, Romanos GE. Temperature change during non-contact diode laser irradiation of implant surfaces. *Lasers Med Sci.* 2012;27(2):339–342.

123. Nicholson D, Blodgett K, Braga C, et al. Pulsed Nd:YAG laser treatment for failing dental implants due to peri-implantitis. In: Rechmann P, Fried D, eds. *Lasers in dentistry XX, Proc.* Bellingham, WA: SPIE; 8929.

124. Kao RT, Nares S, Reynolds MA. Periodontal regeneration – Intrabony defects: a systematic review from the AAP regeneration workshop. *J Periodontol.* 2015;86(suppl):S77–S104.

125. Yukna RA, Carr RL, Evans GH. Histologic evaluation of an Nd:YAG laser-assisted new attachment procedure in humans. *Int J Periodontics Restorative Dent.* 2007;27(6):577–587.

126. Nevins ML, Camela M, Schupbach P, Kim S-W, Kim DM, Nevins M. Human clinical and histologic evaluation of laser-assisted

new attachment procedure. *Int J Periodontics Restorative Dent.* 2012;32(5):497–507.

127. Suzuki, Jon B. Salvaging Implants with an Nd:YAG Laser: a novel approach to a growing problem. compendium. Nov/Dec 2015.

128. Gold SI, Vilardi MA. Pulsed laser beam effects on gingiva. *J Clin Periodontol.* 1994;21(6):391–396.

129. Ting CC, Fukuda M, Watanabe T, Sanaoka A, Mitani A, Noguchi T. Morphological alterations of periodontal pocket epithelium following Nd:YAG laser irradiation. *Photomed Laser Surg.* 2014;34(12):649–657.

130. Harris DM, Yessik M. Therapeutic ratio quantifies antisepsis: ablation of porphyromonas gingival/s with dental lasers. *Lasers Surg Med.* 2004;35(3):206–213.

131. Giannelli M, Bani D, Viti C, et al. Comparative evaluation of the effects of different photoablative laser irradiation protocols on the gingiva of periodontopathic patients. *Photomed Laser Surg.* 2012;30(4):222–230.

132. Cobb CM, McCawley TK, Killoy WJ. A preliminary study on the effects of the Nd:YAG laser on root surfaces and subgingival microflora in vivo. *J Periodontol.* 1992;63(8):701–707.

133. McCawley TK, McCawley MN, Rams TE. LANAP immediate effects in vivo on human chronic periodontitis microbiota. *J Dent Res.* 2014;93 (spec issue A):Abstract 428.

134. de Andrade AKP, Feist IS, Pannuti CM, Cai S, Zezell DM, De Micheli G. Nd:YAG laser clinical assisted in class II furcation treatment. *Lasers Med Sci.* 2008;23(4):341–347.

135. Giannini R, Vassalli M, Chellini F, Polidori L, Dei R, Giannelli M. Neodymium:yttrium aluminum garnet laser irradiation with low pulse energy: a potential tool for the treatment of peri-implant disease. *Clin Oral Implants Res.* 2006;17(6):638–643.

136. Gonçalves F, Zanetti AL, Zanetti RV, et al. Effectiveness of 980-nm diode and 1064-nm extra-long-pulse neodymium-doped yttrium aluminum garnet lasers in implant disinfection. *Photomed Laser Surg.* 2010;28(2):273–280.

137. Gómez C, Domínguez A, García-Kass AI, García-Nuñez JA. Adjunctive Nd:YAG laser application in chronic periodontitis: clinical, immunological, and microbiological aspects. *Lasers Med Sci.* 2011;26(4):453–463.

138. Qadri T, Poddani P, Javed F, Tunér J, Gustafsson A. A short-term evaluation of Nd:YAG laser as an adjunct to scaling and root planing in the treatment of periodontal inflammation. *J Periodontol.* 2010;81(8):1161–1166.

139. Giannelli M, Bani D, Tani A, et al. In: vitro evaluation of the effects of low-intensity Nd:YAG laser irradiation on the inflammatory reaction elicited by bacterial lipopolysaccharide adherent to titanium dental implants. *J Periodontol.* 2009;80(6):977–984.

140. Javed F, Kellesarian SV, Al-Kheraif AA, et al. Effect of Nd:YAG laser-assisted non-surgical periodontal therapy on clinical periodontal and serum biomarkers in patients with and without coronary artery disease: a short-term pilot study. *Lasers Surg Med.* 2016;48(10):929–935.

141. Arisu HD, Türköz E, Bala O. Effects of Nd:YAG laser irradiation on osteoblast cell cultures. *Lasers Med Sci.* 2006;21(3):175–180.

142. Chellini F, Sassoli C, Nosi D, et al. Low pulse energy Nd:YAG laser irradiation exerts a biostimulative effect on different cells of the oral microenvironment: "An in vitro study". *Lasers Surg Med.* 2010;42(6):527–539.

143. Kim IS, Cho TH, Kim K, Weber FE, Hwang SJ. High power-pulsed Nd:YAG laser as a new stimulus to induce BMP-2 expression in MC3T3-E1 osteoblasts. *Lasers Surg Med.* 2010;42(6):510–518.

144. Kim K, Kim IS, Cho TH, Seo YK, Hwang SJ. High-intensity Nd:YAG laser accelerates bone regeneration in calvarial defect models. *J Tissue Eng Regen Med.* 2015;9(8):943–951.

145. Romanos E, Javed F, Delgado-Ruiz RA, et al. Peri-implant Diseases. A review of treatment interventions. *Dent Clin N Am.* 2015;59:157–178.

146. Schwarz F, Sahm N, Becker J. Combined surgical therapy of advanced peri-implantitis lesions with concomitant soft tissue volume augmentation. A case series. *Clin Oral Implants Res.* 2014;25(1):132–136.

147. Heitz-Mayfeld LJA, Salvi GE, Mombelli A, et al. Anti-infective surgical therapy of peri-implantitis. A 12-month prospective clinical study. *Clin Oral Impl Res.* 2012;23:205–210.

148. Ting M, Tadepalli NS, Kondaveeti R, Braid SM, Lee CYS, Suzuki JB. Intra-Oral applications of platelet concentrates: a comprehensive overview of systematic reviews. *J Interdiscipl Med Dent Sci.* 2018;6:233. https://doi.org/10.4172/2376-032X.1000233.

149. Ting M, Afshar P, Adhami A, Braid SM, Suzuki JB. Maxillary sinus augmentation using chairside bone marrow aspirate concentrates for implant site development: a systematic review of histomorphometric studies. *Int J Implant Dent.* 2018.

150. Dohan Ehrenfest DM, Rasmusson L, Albrektsson T. Classification of platelet concentrates: from pure platelet-rich plasma (P-PRP) to leucocyte- and platelet-rich fibrin (L-PRF). *Trends Biotechnol.* 2009;27:158–167.

151. Casati MZ, de Vasconcelos Gurgel BC, Goncalves PF, et al. Platelet-rich plasma does not improve bone regeneration around peri-implant bone defects—a pilot study in dogs. *Int J Oral Maxillofac. Surg.* 2007;36(2):132–136.

152. Sanchez AR, Eckert SE, Sheridan PJ, Weaver AL. Influence of platelet-rich plasma added to xenogeneic bone grafts on bone mineral density associated with dental implants. *Int J Oral Maxillofac Implants.* 2005;20(4):526–532.

153. Sanchez AR, Sheridan PJ, Eckert SE, Weaver AL. Regenerative potential of platelet-rich plasma added to xenogenic bone grafts in peri-implant defects: a histomorphometric analysis in dogs. *J Periodontol.* 2005;76(10):1637–1644.

154. Sanchez AR, Sheridan PJ, Eckert SE, Weaver AL. Influence of platelet-rich plasma added to xenogeneic bone grafts in periimplant defects: a vital fluorescence study in dogs. *Clin Implant Dent Relat Res.* 2005;7(2):61–69.

155. de Vasconcelos Gurgel BC, Goncalves PF, Pimentel SP, et al. Platelet-rich plasma may not provide any additional effect when associated with guided bone regeneration around dental implants in dogs. *Clin Oral Implants Res.* 2007;18(5):649–654.

156. Simonpieri A, Del Corso M, Vervelle A, et al. Current knowledge and perspectives for the use of platelet-rich plasma (PRP) and platelet-rich fibrin (PRF) in oral and maxillofacial surgery part 2: Bone graft, implant and reconstructive surgery. *Curr Pharm Biotechnol.* 2012;13(7):1231–1256.

157. Dohan DM, Choukroun J, Diss A, Dohan SL, Dohan AJ, Mouhyi J, et al. Plateletrich fibrin (PRF): a second-generation platelet concentrate. Part I: technological concepts and evolution. *Oral Surg Oral Med Oral Pathol Oral Radiol Endod.* 2006;101:e37e44.

158. Pradeep AR, Shetty SK, Garg G, Pai S. Clinical effectiveness of autologous platelet-rich plasma and Peptide-enhanced bone graft in the treatment of intrabony defects. *J. Periodontol.* 2009;80(1):62–71.

159. Simonpieri A, Del Corso M, Sammartino G, Ehrenfest DMD. The relevance of Choukroun's platelet-rich fibrin and metronidazole during complex maxillary rehabilitations using bone allograft. Part I: a new grafting protocol. *Implant Dent.* 2009;18(2):102–111.

160. Del Corso M, Sammartino G, Dohan Ehrenfest DM. Re: "Clinical evaluation of a modified coronally advanced flap alone or in combination with a platelet-rich fibrin membrane for the treatment of adjacent multiple gingival recessions: a 6-month study". *J Periodontol.* 2009;80(11):1694–1697.

161. Choukroun J, Diss A, Simonpieri A, et al. Plateletrich fibrin (PRF): a second-generation platelet concentrate. Part IV: clinical effects on tissue healing. *Oral Surg Oral Med Oral Pathol Oral Radiol Endod.* 2006;101(3):e56–60.

162. Dohan Ehrenfest DM, Diss A, Odin G, Doglioli P, Hippolyte MP, Charrier JB. In vitro effects of Choukroun's PRF (platelet-rich fibrin) on human gingival fibroblasts, dermal prekeratinocytes, preadipocytes, and maxillofacial osteoblasts in primary cultures.

Oral Surg Oral Med Oral Pathol Oral Radiol Endod. 2009;108(3): 341–352.

163. Choukroun J, Simonpieri A, Del Corso M, Mazor Z, Sammartino G, Dohan Ehrenfest DM. Controlling systematic perioperative anaerobic contamination during sinus-lift procedures by using metronidazole: an innovative approach. *Implant Dent.* 2008;17(3):257–270.

164. Bielecki TM, Gazdzik TS, Arendt J, Szczepanski T, Krol W, Wielkoszynski T. Antibacterial effect of autologous platelet gel enriched with growth factors and other active substances: an in vitro study. *J Bone Joint Surg Br.* 2007;89(3):417–420.

165. Cieslik-Bielecka A, Bielecki T, Gazdzik TS, Arendt J, Szczepanski T. Autologous platelets and leukocytes can improve healing of infected high-energy soft tissue injury. *Transfus Apher Sci.* 2009;41(1):9–12.

166. Ainamo J, Löe H. Anatomical characteristics of gingiva. A clinical and microscopic study of the free and attached gingiva. *The J Periodontol.* 1966;37(1):5–13.

167. Wang HL, Greenwell J. Surgical periodontal therapy. *J Periodontal.* 2001;25:89–99.

168. Porter JA, Von Fraunhofer JA. Success or failure of dental implants: a literature review with treatment considerations. *Gen Den.* 2004;53:423–432.

169. Padial-Molina M, Suarez F, Rios HF, et al. Guidelines for the diagnosis and treatment of peri-implant diseases. *Int J Periodontics Restorative Dent.* 2014;34:e102–111.

170. Vargas-Reus MA, Memarzadeh K, Huang J, et al. Antimicrobial activity of nanoparticulate metal oxides against peri-implantitis pathogens. *Int J Antimicrob Agents.* 2012;40:135–139.

171. Waal Y, Raghoebar GM, Huddleston-Slater JJ, et al. Implant decontamination during surgical peri-implantitis treatment: a randomized, double-blind, placebo-controlled trial. *J Clin Periodontal.* 2013;40:186–195.

172. Kirsch A, Ackermann KL. The IMZ osteointegrated implant system. *Dent Clin North Am.* 1989;33:733–791.

173. Warrer K, Buser D, Lang NP, et al. Plaque-induced peri- implantitis in the presence or absence of keratinized mucosa: an experimental study in monkeys. *Clin Oral Implants Res.* 1995;6:131–138.

174. Choukroun J, Diss A, Simonpieri A, et al. Platelet-rich fibrin (PRF): a second generation platelet concentrate. Part V: histologic evaluation of PRF effects on bone allograft maturation in sinus lift. *Oral Surg Oral Med Oral Pathol Oral Radiol Endod.* 2006 e;101:229.

175. He L, Lin Y, Hu X, et al. A comparative study of platelet-rich fibrin (PRF) and platelet-rich plasma (PRP) on the effect of proliferation and differentiation of rat osteoblasts in vitro. *Oral Surg Oral Med Oral Pathol Oral Radiol Endod.* 2009;108:707–713.

176. Meffert RM, Langer B, Fritz ME. Dental implants: a review. *J Periodontol.* 1992;63:859–870.

177. Esposito M, Coulthard P, Thomsen P, Worthington HV. The role of implant surface modifications, shape and material on the success of osseointegrated dental implants. *A Cochrane systematic review.* 2005.

178. Pauletto N, Lahiffe BJ, Walton JN. Complications associated with excess cement around crowns on osseointegrated implants: a clinical report. *Int J Oral Maxillofac Implants.* 1999;14:865–868.

179. Agar JR, Cameron SM, Hughbanks JC, Parker MH. Cement removal from restorations luted to titanium abutments with simulated subgingival margins. *J Prosthet Dent.* 1997;78:43–47.

180. Wadhwani CPK, Schwedhelm ER. The role of cements in dental implant success, part 1. *Dentistry Today.* 2013:1–11.

181. Gapski R, Neugeboren N, Pemeraz AZ, Reissner MW. Endosseous implant failure influenced by crown cementation: a clinical case report. *Int J Oral Maxillofac Implants.* 2008;23:943–946.

182. Pauletto N, Lahiffe BJ, Walton JN. Complications associated with excess cement around crowns on osseointegrated implants: a clinical report. *Int J Oral Maxillofac Implants.* 1999;14:865–868.

183. Gapski R, Neugeboren N, Pomeranz AZ, Reissner MW. Endosseous implant failure influenced by crown cementation: a clinical case report. *Int J Oral Maxillofac Implants.* 2008;23:943–946.

184. Pontoriero R, Tonelli MP, Carnevale G, Mombelli A, Nyman SR, Lang NP. Experimentally induced peri-implant mucositis. A clinical study in humans. *Clin Oral Implants Res.* 1994;5:254–259.

185. Berglundh T, Lindhe J, Marinello C, Ericsson I, Liljenberg B. Soft tissue reaction to de novo plaque formation on implants and teeth. An experimental study in the dog. *Clin Oral Implants Res.* 1992;3:1–84.

186. Lang NP, Berglundh T, Heitz-Mayfield LJ, Pjetursson BE, Salvi GE, Sanz M. Consensus statements and recommended clinical procedures regarding implant survival and complications. *Int J Oral Maxillofac Implants.* 2004;19(suppl):150–154.

187. Korsch M, Walther W, Marten SM, Obst U. Microbial analysis of biofilms on cement surfaces: an investigation in cement-associated peri-implantitis. *J Appl Biomater Funct Mater.* 2014;12(2):70–80.

188. M1 Korsch, Robra BP, Walther W. Predictors of excess cement and tissue response to fixed implant-supported dentures after cementation. *Clin Implant Dent Relat Res.* 2013.

189. Augthun M, Conrads G. Microbial findings of deep periimplant bone defects. *Int J Oral Maxillofac Implants.* 1997;12:106–112.

190. Salcetti JM, Moriarty JD, Cooper LF, et al. The clinical, microbial, and host response characteristics of the failing implant. *Int J Oral Maxillofac Implants.* 1997;12:32–42.

191. Leonhardt A°, Berglundh T, Ericsson I, Dahle´n G. Putative periodontal pathogens on titanium implants and teeth in experimental gingivitis and periodontitis in beagle dogs. *Clin Oral Implants Res.* 1992;3:112–119.

192. Roos-Jansa°ker AM, Lindahl C, Renvert H, Renvert S. Nine- to fourteen-year follow-up of implant treatment. Part II: Presence of peri-implant lesions. *J Clin Peri- odontol.* 2006;33:290–295.

193. Marrone A, Lasserre J, Bercy P, Brecx MC. Prevalence and risk factors for peri-implant disease in Belgian adults. *Clin Oral Implants Res.* 2012.

194. Koldsland OC, Scheie A, Aass AM. Prevalence of peri-implantitis related to severity of the disease with different degrees of bone loss. *J Periodontol.* 2010;81:231–238.

195. Thomas GW. The positive relationship between excess cement and peri-implant disease: a prospective clinical endoscopic study. *J Periodontol.* 2009;80:1388–1392.

196. Wilson TG, Jr. "The positive relationship between excess cement and peri-implant disease: a prospective clinical endoscopic study". *J Periodontol.* 2009;80(9):1388–1392.

197. Present S, Levine RA. Techniques to control or avoid cement around implant-retained restorations. *Compendium.* 2013;34(6): 432–437.

198. Pauletto N, Lahiffe BJ, Walton JN. Complications associated with excess cement around crowns on osseointegrated implants: a clinical report. *Int J Oral Maxillofac Implants.* 1999;14:865–868.

199. Daubert DM, Weinstein BF, Bordin S, Leroux BG, Flemming TF. Prevalence and predictive factors for peri-implant disease and implant failure: a cross-sectional analysis. *J Periodontol.* 2015;86(3):337–347.

200. Pauletto N, Lahiffe BJ, Walton JN. Complications associated with excess cement around crowns on osseointegrated implants: a clinical report. *Int J Oral Maxillofac Implants.* 1999;14:865–868.

201. Gapski R, Neugeboren N, Pomeranz AZ, Reissner MW. Endosseous implant failure influenced by crown cementation: a clinical case report. *Int J Oral Maxillofac Implants.* 2008;23:943–946.

202. O'Rourke B, Walls AW, Wassell RW. Radiographic detection of overhangs formed by resin composite luting agents. *J Dent.* 1995;23:353–357.

203. Soares CJ, Santana FR, Fonseca RB, Martins LR, Neto FH. In vitro analysis of the radiodensity of indirect composites and ceramic inlay systems and its influence on the detection of cement overhangs. *Clin Oral Investig.* 2007;11:331–336.

204. Rosenstiel SF, Land MF, Crispin BJ. Dental luting agents: a review of the current literature. *J Prosthet Dent.* 1998;80:280–301.

205. Wadhwani CPK, Schwedhelm ER. The role of cements in dental implant success, part 1. *Dentistry Today.* 2013;1–11.

206. Wadhwani C, Hess T, Faber T, Piñeyro A, Chen CSK. A descriptive study of the radiographic density of implant restorative cements. *J Prosthet Dent.* 2010;103:295–302

207. Wadhwani C, Rapoport D, La Rosa S, et al. Radiographic detection and characteristic patterns of residual excess cement associated with cement retained implant restorations: a clinical report. *J Prosthet Dent.* 2012;107:151–157.

208. Agar JR, Cameron SM, Hughbanks JC, Parker MH. Cement removal from restorations luted to titanium abutments with simulated subgingival margins. *J Prosthet Dent.* 1997;78:43–47.

209. Linkevicius T, Vindasiute E, Puisys A, Peciuliene V. The influence of margin location on the amount of undetected cement excess after delivery of cement-retained implant restorations. *Clin Oral Implants Res.* 2011;22(12):1379–1384.

210. Wadhwani C, Piñeyro A, Hess T, et al. Effect of implant abutment modification on the extrusion of excess cement at the crown-abutment margin for cement-retained implant restorations. *Int J Oral Maxillofac Implants.* 2011;26(6):1241–1246.

211. Wadhwani C, Piñeyro A. Technique for controlling the cement for an implant crown. *J Prosthet Dent.* 2009;102:57–58.

212. Wilson TG. The Positive relationship between excess cement and peri-implant disease: a prospective clinical endoscopic study. *J Periodontol.* 2009;80:1388–1392.

213. Suzuki JB. Diagnosis and classification of the periodontal diseases. *Dent Clin North Am.* 1988;32(2):195–216.

214. Schnitman PA, Shulman LB. Recommendations of the consensus development conference on dental implants. *J Am Dent Assoc.* 1979;98:373–377.

215. Cranin AN, Silverbrand H, Sher J, et al. The requirements and clinical performance of dental implants. In: Smith DC, Williams DF, eds. *Biocompatibility of Dental Materials.* Boca Raton, FL: CRC Press; 1982:42–45 (4).

216. McKinney RV, Koth DC, Steflik DE. Clinical standards for dental implants. In: Clark JW, ed. *Clinical Dentistry.* Harperstown, PA: Harper and Row; 1984:78–81.

217. Albrektsson T, Zarb GA, Worthington P, et al. The long-term efficacy of currently used dental implants: a review and proposed criteria of success. *Int J Oral Maxillofac Implants.* 1986;1:1–25.

218. Albrektsson T, Zarb GA. Determinants of correct clinical reporting. *Int J Prosthodont.* 1998;11:517–521.

219. Misch CE. Implant quality scale: a clinical assessment of the health-disease continuum. *Oral Health.* 1998;88:15–25.

220. Suzuki JB, Misch CE. Peri Implantitis. Chapter 18. In: Resnik R, Misch CE, eds. *Avoiding Implant Comoplications.* USA: Elsevier – Mosby St. Louis; 2017.

221. Council on Dental Care Programs. Reporting periodontal treatment under dental benefit plans. *J Am Dent Assoc.* 1988;17:371–373.

222. Council on Dental Care Programs. Reporting periodontal treatment under dental benefit plans. *J Am Dent Assoc.* 1988;17:371–373.

223. Canullo L, Tallarico M, Radovanovic S, Delibasic B, Covani U, Rakic M. Distinguishing predictive profiles for patient–based risk assessment and diagnostics of plaque induced, surgically and prosthetically triggered peri–implantitis. *Clinical oral implants research.* 2016;27(10):1243–1250.

224. Marco T, Canullo L, Wang HL, Cochran DL, Meloni SM. "Classification systems for peri-implantitis: a narrative review with a proposal of a new evidence-based etiology codification". *Int J Mol Sci.* 2018;33(4).

42

Implant Maintenance: Long-Term Implant Success

JON B. SUZUKI AND DIANA BRONSTEIN

The maintenance of endosseous implants has evolved over many decades, from trial and error of various anecdotal supportive therapy methods to evidence-based protocols. These newer maintenance protocols allow for the implant clinician to implement individualized patient care of the peri-implant tissues.[1,2] With patients understanding the benefits of dental implants, the dental profession is moving away from traditional prosthetics and integrating the latest dental implant technologic advances into treatment plans. Therefore in the future, a greater need will be required by the implant clinician to integrate a comprehensive systemic and supportive protocol to maintain the success and longevity of the implant prosthesis.[3]

Prevention of peri-implant disease is now an accepted fundamental cornerstone of effective and predictable treatment strategies. The preventive approach commences with ideal and realistic case selection, preoperative patient education, and control of risk factors associated with increased implant complication incidence.[4] The lifelong professional implant maintenance protocol must be communicated to and acknowledged by the patient as part of his or her presurgical educational process. Patients at a higher risk for the development of peri-implantitis need to be identified and monitored with a stricter maintenance protocol. In addition, because of the inherent differences between implants and teeth, patient education is crucial on the specifics of hygiene with respect to the dental implants and the type of prosthesis.[5]

Anatomy of Peri-implant Hard and Soft Tissues

The implant clinician must have a strong foundation for the relationship between the peri-implant tissues and the signs of disease so that early detection and definitive treatment may be rendered. If a disease process goes undiagnosed, hard and soft tissues complications may lead to an increased morbidity of the implants or associated prosthesis. When evaluating the hard and soft tissues surrounding a dental implant, many differences exist between the natural teeth and dental implants. The support system of natural teeth is much better designed to reduce biomechanical forces to the crestal bone region, thereby reducing the possibility of peri-implant disease. Because of the periodontal membrane, nerve and blood vessel complex, and occlusal material (enamel), occlusal overload is far less in comparison with dental implants.[6]

Soft Tissue Differences

For a natural tooth the surrounding soft tissue has an average biological width of 2.04 mm between the depth of the sulcus and the crest of the alveolar bone.[7] It should be noted that the biological "width" is actually a height dimension with a greater range in the posterior region compared with the anterior and may be greater than 4 mm in height.[8] With natural teeth the biologic width is composed of a connective tissue attachment (1.07 mm average) above the bone and a junctional epithelial attachment (0.97 mm average) at the sulcus base, with the most consistent value among individuals being the connective tissue attachment.

The connective tissue attachment zone of the "biological width" around a tooth will prevent penetration into the sulcus and allows gingival fibers of the connective tissue attachment zone to establish direct connection with the cementum of the natural tooth. It acts as a physical barrier to the bacteria in the sulcus to the underlining periodontal tissues. Eleven different gingival fiber groups comprise the connective tissue attachment zone observed around a natural tooth and tissue: dentogingival (coronal, horizontal, and apical), alveologingival, intercapillary, transgingival, circular, semicircular, dentoperiosteal, transseptal, periosteogingival, intercircular, and intergingival.[9] At least six of these gingival fiber groups insert into the cementum of the natural tooth: the dentogingival (coronal, horizontal, and apical), dentoperiosteal, transseptal, circular, semicircular, and transgingival fibers. In addition, some crestal fibers from the periodontal fiber bundles also insert into the cementum above the alveolar bone, forming a true attachment to the tooth. Clinically this attachment will prevent a periodontal probe from invading the periodontal ligament (PDL) space and minimize the ingress of bacteria (Fig. 42.1).

In comparison, the sulcular regions around an implant are very similar in many respects. The rete peg formation within the attached gingiva and the histologic lining of the gingiva within the sulcus are similar in implants and teeth.[10] A free gingival margin forms around a tooth or implant, with nonkeratinized sulcular epithelium and the epithelial cells. At the base, junctional epithelial cells are present for both. However, a fundamental difference characterizes the base of the gingival complex around teeth. Whereas a tooth has two primary regions that make up the biological width, an implant has only one (Fig. 42.2).

The biological seal for an implant, which is analogous to the epithelial attachment of the tooth, is needed to protect

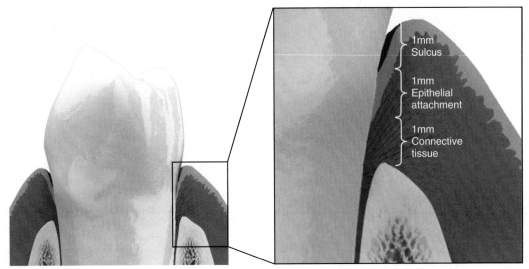

● **Fig. 42.1** The biologic width for a natural tooth is approximately 1 mm of connective tissue above the bone and 1 mm of epithelial attachment between the sulcus and the connective tissue. *(From Misch CE. An implant is not a tooth: a comparison of periodontal indices.* Dental Implant Prosthetics. *2nd ed. St. Louis, MO: Mosby; 2015.)*

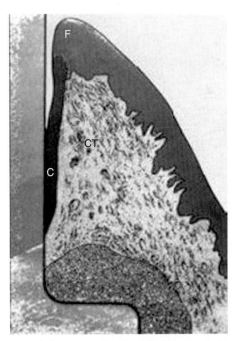

● **Fig. 42.2** The soft tissue around an implant (I) has a sulcular region very similar to a tooth. A free gingival margin (F) with nonkeratinized sulcular epithelium and cells at the base (C) has junctional epithelial attachment above the bone (B). *CT,* Connective tissue.

the implant-bone interface against bacterial irritants, as well as mechanical trauma such as restorative materials, prosthesis design, and occlusal forces. Cochran et al.[11] has reported the biologic width to be 3.3 mm for dental implants, but unlike the biological width dimension for teeth, they also included the sulcus depth. In a typical implant gingival region, only two of the gingival fiber groups are found around a tooth (circular and periosteogingival fibers), and no periodontal fibers are present.[12] These fibers do not insert into the implant body below the abutment margin as they do into the cementum of natural teeth.[13] Instead, the collagen fibers around an implant

run parallel to the implant surface, not perpendicular, as with natural teeth.[14] Hence the implant has only a junctional epithelial "attachment" system. The gingival and periosteal fiber groups are responsible for the connective tissue attachment component of the biological width around teeth, and these are not present around the transosteal region of an implant. The "biological width" around the abutment-implant connection should not be similarly compared with the connective tissue attachment of a tooth. The biological seal around dental implants may to some degree prevent the migration of bacteria and endotoxins into the underlying bone. However, an attachment component of the biological width similar to the one found with natural teeth is not present with dental implants (Fig. 42.3).

Tooth Versus Implant Movement

A natural tooth exhibits normal physiologic movements in vertical, horizontal, and rotational directions. The amount of movement of a natural tooth is related to its surface area and root design. Therefore the number and length of the roots; their diameter, shape, and position; and the health of the PDL primarily influence a tooth's mobility. A healthy tooth normally exhibits zero clinical mobility in a vertical direction. Studies have shown the actual initial vertical tooth movement to be approximately 28 μm and is the same for anterior and posterior teeth.[15] The vertical movement of a rigid implant (i.e., integrated) has been measured as 2 to 3 μm under a 10-lb force and is due mostly to the viscoelastic properties of the underlying bone (i.e., bone density at the bone-implant interface).[16]

Muhlemann[17] found that horizontal tooth movement may be divided into initial mobility and secondary movement. The initial mobility is observed with a light force, occurs immediately, and is a consequence of the PDL. Initial horizontal tooth mobility is greater than initial vertical movement. A very light force (500 g) horizontally moves the tooth. The initial horizontal mobility of a healthy, "nonmobile" posterior tooth is less than that of an anterior tooth and ranges from 56 to 75μm, which is two to nine times the vertical movement of the tooth.

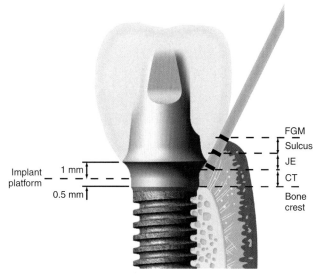

FGM
Sulcus
JE
CT

Implant platform

1 mm

0.5 mm

Bone crest

• **Fig. 42.3** An implant has no connective tissue fibers in the connective tissue zone that insert into the implant. The peri-implant probe penetrates the sulcus, junctional epithelial attachment (JE), and most of the connective tissue zone. *CT,* Connective tissue; *FGM,* free gingival margin. *(From Misch CE. An implant is not a tooth: a comparison of periodontal indices. Dental Implant Prosthetics. 2nd ed. St. Louis, MO: Mosby; 2015.)*

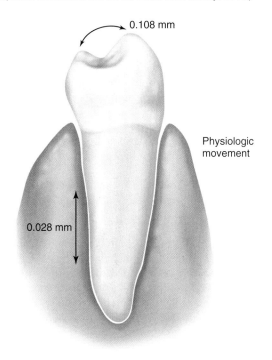

0.108 mm

Physiologic movement

0.028 mm

• **Fig. 42.4** The physiologic movement of a tooth has been measured as 28 μm in the apical direction and up to 108 μm in the horizontal direction. *(From Misch CE. An implant is not a tooth: a comparison of periodontal indices. Dental Implant Prosthetics. 2nd ed. St. Louis, MO: Mosby; 2015.)*

Initial horizontal mobility is even greater in anterior teeth and ranges from 70 to 108 μm in health[18] (Fig. 42.4).

The secondary tooth movement described by Muhlemann[17] occurs after the initial movement, when greater forces are applied. When an additional force is applied to the tooth, a secondary movement is also observed, which is related directly to the amount of force. The secondary tooth movement is related to the viscoelasticity of the bone and measures as much as 40 μm under considerably greater force (Fig. 42.5).

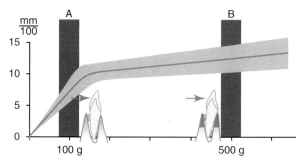

A   B

$\frac{mm}{100}$

15

10

5

0

100 g   500 g

• **Fig. 42.5** A secondary horizontal movement of a tooth occurs after the initial tooth movement when a greater force is applied and is related to the deformation of the alveolar bone. *(From Misch CE. An implant is not a tooth: a comparison of periodontal indices. Dental Implant Prosthetics. 2nd ed. St. Louis, MO: Mosby; 2015.)*

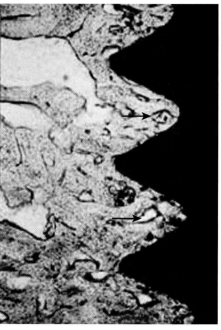

• **Fig. 42.6** Osseointegration is a histologic term that describes a direct bone-implant contact at the level of magnification of a light microscope.

When evaluating implant movement, "rigid fixation" indicates the absence of clinical mobility of an implant tested with vertical or horizontal forces less than 500 g. Rigid fixation is a clinical term, and osseointegration is a histologic term. Osseointegration is defined as bone in direct contact with an implant surface at the magnification of a light microscope (Fig. 42.6). Over the years these two terms have been used interchangeably, and implant abutment support is most predictable with rigid fixation. Lack of implant mobility (IM) does not always coincide with a direct bone-implant interface. However, when observed clinically, rigid fixation usually means that at least a portion of the implant is in direct contact with bone, although the percentage of bone contact cannot be specified. A mobile implant indicates the presence of connective tissue between the implant and bone.

Increased tooth mobility may be caused by occlusal trauma or bone loss. Increased tooth mobility alone is not a criterion of periodontal health or pathology. Unlike a tooth, for which mobility is not a primary factor for longevity, mobility is a primary determining factor for implant health. Rigid fixation is also an excellent indicator of the implant health status because it is an easy, objective test. As such, rigid fixation is usually the first clinical criterion and the most important when evaluating a dental implant.

Past techniques to evaluate primary stability and mobility of dental implants have included percussion and mobility tests with mirror handles. However, these techniques were very subjective and were associated with inaccurate results. In implant dentistry today, the most common technique to assess the stability of dental implants is the use of resonance frequency analysis (RFA). Resonance frequency analysis (RFA) is a non-invasive, reliable, and clinically acceptable technique developed by Meredith in 1996.[19] This technique includes magnetic pulses being sent to a small metal post that is temporarily attached to the implant. As the post vibrates, the probe reads the resonance frequency which is translated into a value termed implant stability quotient (ISQ). The ISQ value is evaluated via a scale that ranges from 1 to 100, with high values indicating increased stability. Usually, acceptable ranges of stability lie between 55 – 85 ISQ, with values below 55 indicating possible mobility of the implant.[20] This technology is advantageous as measurements may be taken at the time of implant placement and used as a baseline for future measurements in the evaluation of the health of the dental implant. The Penguin RFA® (Glidewell Direct; Irvine, Calif.) is commercially available which uses re-usable multi-pegs that are implant specific. In addition, this device is cordless which is very user friendly for the clinician. When evaluating mobility of the implant, ideally the prosthesis should be removed, which allows for the multi-pegs to be directly inserted into the implant body.

Evaluating the mobility of the prosthesis does not allow for an accurate assessment of dental implant health as the associated mobility is most commonly from a loose abutment screw (Box 42.1 and Fig. 42.7).

A natural tooth with primary occlusal trauma exhibits an increase in clinical mobility and radiographic PDL space. After the cause of trauma is eliminated, the tooth may return to zero clinical mobility and a normal radiographic appearance. This scenario is not predictable around an implant. The implant clinician should not restore an implant with any clinical mobility, because the risk for failure is great. However, after the prosthesis is completed and IM-1 develops, the risk is small to evaluate the implant for a few months and decrease almost all stress during this time frame. Implants with slight detectable mobility of approximately 0.1 mm of horizontal movement (IM-1), similar to the mobility of a healthy central incisor, on occasion may return to rigid fixation and zero mobility. However, to reachieve rigid fixation, the implant should be taken completely out of occlusion for several months and strictly monitored. The return of rigid fixation of an implant is far greater if no mobility is noted before the implant is placed into function.

An implant with horizontal movement greater than 0.5 mm (IM-3) is at much greater risk than a tooth. A root form implant with greater than 0.5 mm horizontal mobility (IM-3) or any vertical mobility (IM-4) should be removed to avoid continued bone loss and future compromise of the implant site or adjacent teeth (Table 42.1).

Maintenance Protocol

Medical and Dental Histories

The first step in the maintenance protocol is to update the patient's medical and dental histories. This is a mandatory component of the maintenance protocol and is crucial in determining whether there presently exist any concomitant conditions that would predispose the patient to peri-implant disease.

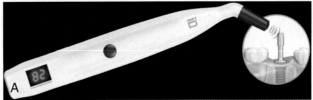

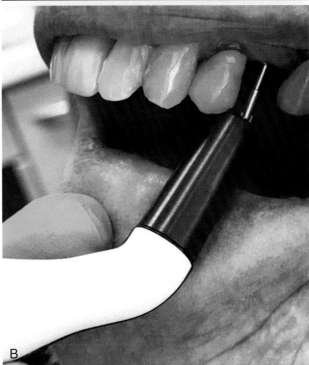

• **Fig. 42.7** (A, B) Penguin Resonance Frequency Analysis Unit (Aseptico) which measures the ISQ (Implant Stability Quotient) implant stability using reusable, calibrated MulTipegs.

• **BOX 42.1** Mobility Measurements[97]

Scale	Description
0	Absence of clinical mobility with 500 g in any direction
1	Slight detectable horizontal movement
2	Moderate visible horizontal mobility up to 0.5 mm
3	Severe horizontal movement greater than 0.5 mm
4	Moderate-to-severe horizontal and any visible vertical movement

Medical History

Medical conditions may change during the maintenance phase (i.e., after implant prosthesis completion) of treatment that have a direct impact on the morbidity and success of the implants or prosthesis. It is imperative the patient relates any updates to his or her medical history because many systemic conditions may affect the long-term prognosis of dental implants and the prosthesis.

1. Xerostomia: The lack of saliva (i.e., dry mouth) is caused by hypofunction of the salivary glands and may be caused by numerous medications and systemic conditions. Most commonly, autoimmune conditions may result in xerostomia, as well as many medications, especially if given concurrently.

TABLE 42.1	Comprehensive Differences Between Natural Teeth and Dental Implants	
	Natural Teeth	**Dental Implants**
Interface	Periodontal membrane	Direct bone
Junctional epithelium	Hemidesmosomes and basal lamina (lamina lucida and lamina densa zones)	Hemidesmosomes and basal lamina (lamina lucida and lamina densa, and sublamina lucida zones)
Connective tissue	12 groups: six insert perpendicular to tooth surfaces ↓ Collagen, ↑ fibroblasts	Only two groups: parallel and circular fibers; no attachment to the implant surface ↑ Collagen, ↓ fibroblasts
Vascularity	Greater; supraperiosteal and PDL	Less; mainly periosteal
Biologic width	2.04–2.91 mm	3.08 mm
Mobility	+	–
Pain	+/– (tooth may be hyperemic)	–
Attrition	+ Wear facets, abfraction, fremitus	– (~ porcelain fracture, possible screw loosening)
Radiographic changes	+ Increased radiopacity and thickness of cribriform plate	Crestal bone loss
Interference awareness	+ (Proprioception)	– (Osseoperception)
Nonvertical forces	Relatively tolerated	Results in bone loss
Force-related movement	Primary: movement of PDL Secondary: osseous movement	Primary: osseous movement
Lateral force	Apical third of root surface	Crestal bone
Lateral movement	56–108 µm	10–50 µm
Apical movement	25–100 µm	3–5 µm
Tactile sensitivity	High	Low
Signs of overloading	PDL thickening, fremitus, mobility, wear facets, pain	Screw loosening, screw fracture, abutment fracture, implant body fracture, bone loss

PDL, Periodontal ligament.

Xerostomia has been shown to affect the dental biofilm composition and intraoral healing of the soft tissues. Immune cells (e.g., neutrophils) and immune factors (e.g., lysozyme, secretory IgA) are normally delivered and distributed in the oral cavity through the saliva; therefore a lack of saliva may lead to lowered antimicrobial components in the oral cavity.[21-24] Prosthetically, patients who acquire xerostomia after completion of treatment may become compromised. For example, a patient with a soft tissue–borne implant prosthesis (i.e., RP-5 overdenture) may experience soft tissue irritation because of the lack of saliva.

2. Autoimmune diseases: Selected autoimmune diseases have been associated with peri-implantitis. For example, lichen planus causes the hemidesmosomal epithelial attachment to the implant surface to become disabled, leading to peri-implant mucositis and possibly progressing to peri-implantitis.[25] However, long-term implant survival, according to current research, does not seem to be affected.[26] With many autoimmune diseases, patients may lose their manual dexterity, thereby decreasing hygiene ability and also difficulty in removing an attachment-dependent overdenture prosthesis. Some of the more common autoimmune disorders and the associated symptoms that may affect the oral cavity are as follows:
   • Sjogren's syndrome: xerostomia
   • Systemic lupus erythematosus: corticosteroid treatment and immunosuppressive medications

   • Scleroderma: manual dexterity and immunosuppressive medications
   • Rheumatoid arthritis: manual dexterity and immunosuppressive medications
   • HIV: compromised lymphocytes and immunosuppressive medications

3. Bone diseases: Altered bone physiology in conditions such as osteoporosis/osteomalacia/osteopenia, Paget's disease, and fibrous dysplasia may significantly increase the risk for complications for implant patients.[27]

4. Diabetes: Poor diabetic control (i.e., > 7% A_{1c}) correlates the inflammatory markers closer to patients with chronic periodontitis when peri-implantitis is present. Patients with diabetes, especially if uncontrolled, are prone to acquire infections and vascular complications. The healing process is affected by the impairment of vascular function, chemotaxis, and neutrophil function, as well as an anaerobic milieu. Protein metabolism is decreased, and healing of soft and hard tissue is delayed, which may lead to the susceptibility of infection. Neuropathy and impaired nerve regeneration may be altered, as well as angiogenesis.[28]

5. Pregnancy: During the maintenance period, radiographs should be delayed until after birth with pregnant patients. Medical clearance should be obtained if radiographs or procedures need to be performed on an emergency basis.

6. Radiation treatment to the oral cavity: Patients who receive radiation to the oral cavity after implant treatment may suffer from many deficits including oral mucositis, xerostomia, compromised healing, and reduced angiogenesis. This is a direct result of changes in the vascularity and cellularity of hard and soft tissue, damage to the salivary glands, and increased collagen synthesis that results in fibrosis. Therefore patients exhibiting these complications should be treated symptomatically. Patients who presently wear a tissue-borne prosthesis (RP-5) may benefit from changing the final prosthesis to a fixed (non-tissue-bearing) prosthesis.

7. Sleep apnea: Patients who are diagnosed with sleep apnea are often treated with continuous positive airway pressure (CPAP). The CPAP machine uses a hose and mask that delivers constant steady air pressure. CPAP machines may place an increased force on the oral cavity. Therefore if patients are using a CPAP machine, the implant area should be monitored closely.

8. Elderly patients: Elderly patients have been shown to have many issues with adapting to the final implant prostheses. Postinsertion complications such as muscle control, hygiene difficulty, tissue inflammation, and overdenture seating are significant in the older population study. During maintenance visits, patient education should be continuously reenforced.

9. Smoking: The use of tobacco should be closely monitored with implant patients. Studies have shown the detrimental effects of the gases and chemicals (e.g., nitrogen, carbon monoxide, carbon dioxide, ammonia, hydrogen cyanide, benzene, nicotine) released in cigarette smoke. Multiple retrospective studies have shown that smokers experience almost twice as many implant failures compared with nonsmokers, and there exists a strong correlation with peri-implantitis.[29] The negative effects of smoking on the implants/prosthesis should be reenforced at each maintenance visit.

10. Phenytoin (Dilantin): The most common medication to cause peri-implant conditions is phenytoin (Dilantin). Dilantin is associated with a high incidence of gingival overgrowth (hyperplasia) of peri-implant soft tissue, *implant gingival hyperplasia*, *mucosal proliferation*, *proliferative gingivitis*, and *implant-related tissue hyperplasia*, and has been recognized as a significant clinical issue in implant dentistry today. If there is no associated bone loss, the pockets are termed *pseudopockets* or *gingival pockets*. These hyperplasia-induced pockets may harbor pathogenic anaerobic bacteria. The plaque biofilm colonization and maturation in implant pockets initiates inflammation. The resultant hyperplastic tissue is most commonly composed of compact collagenous fibers, fibroblasts, and inflammatory cells. Management of peri-implant gingival overgrowth should include the identification of the etiology (e.g., medication or humoral). If the etiology is determined to be medication induced, consultation with the patient's physician is recommended for possible alternative treatment.

11. Miscellaneous: Epidemiologic and longitudinal studies have found an association of peri-implantitis prevalence with hepatitis and cardiovascular disease.[30] Cardiovascular disease is associated with periodontitis and peri-implantitis through the systemic-inflammatory-mediator link and appears to be an indirect cofactor in patients whose profile identifies them as being predisposed to inflammatory diseases.[31]

Interestingly, genetics has been implicated with aggressive periodontal diseases, which appear to be correlated with peri-implantitis. Studies associate peri-implant disease with the *IL-1* gene polymorphism in smokers.[32]

• BOX 42.2 Loe and Silness Bleeding Index

Normal
0 = mild inflammation, slight color change and edema, no bleeding
1 = moderate inflammation, redness, edema, bleeds on probing
2 = severe inflammation, marked redness and edema ulceration, spontaneous bleeding

Dental History

The dental history update is crucial in determining any changes to the patient's oral condition. Changes in home care practices, along with recent dental treatment, should be documented and evaluated for any impact on the implant prostheses. Of special concern are parafunctional habits (e.g., clenching, bruxism), which if present or worsening may lead to peri-implant diseases or implant failure.

Clinical Evaluation of the Implant(s)/Prosthesis

Soft Tissue Assessment

An overview of the visual signs of gingival inflammation (e.g., redness, edema, alterations of tissue contour, fistula tracts) should be evaluated and documented. Poor tissue tone (i.e., thin, friable, flaccid) surrounding an implant may harbor food, plaque, and calculus, which increases the possibility of inflammation and infection. A gingival health index may be used to evaluate the soft tissue health. The most common bleeding gingival index used for implants is the Loe and Silness gingival index. When used on teeth, this index scores gingival inflammation from 0 to 3 on the facial, lingual, and mesial surfaces of all teeth. The symptom of bleeding comprises a score of at least 2 (Box 42.2). The facial and lingual are already being probed to evaluate bone loss that cannot be seen on a radiograph. Because the bleeding index evaluates inflammation, the Loe and Silness index is adequate for implants, and because fewer implants typically are used to restore a region compared with the presence of natural teeth, one also may evaluate the distal surface when bleeding is present[33] (Fig. 42.8).

Assessment of Home Care

Because the presence of microbial biofilm has been shown to be a leading factor in the pathogenesis of peri-implant disease, the routine assessment of plaque accumulation should be a priority of each maintenance visit. This objective form of plaque monitoring should ideally be performed and documented at each maintenance visit. Consistent use of the same plaque index is paramount because this will allow an easier determination of the presence of a disease process. High plaque scores have been shown to have a direct correlation with peri-implant mucositis and increased probing depths.[34] Mombelli et al.[35] and Lindquist et al.[36] have reported implant-specific plaque indices to be used at dental implant maintenance appointments. Mombelli et al.[35] suggested a numerical scale from 0 to 3, which is dependent on the amount of visible plaque present or by running a probe over the implant surface. Lindquist et al.[36] recommended a similar scale (i.e., 0–2) dependent on the amount of visible plaque (Fig. 42.9 and Box 42.3).

Probing

Probing around dental implants is a controversial topic even though it has been shown in the literature to be a reliable and important factor in determining peri-implant health. The safety of probing, once thought to be detrimental, has been well established

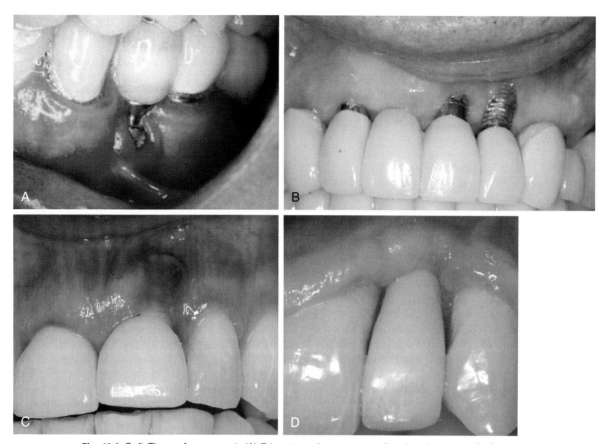

• **Fig. 42.8** Soft Tissue Assessment. (A) Edematous tissue surrounding dental implant. (B) Significant gingival recession leading to exposure of the implant bodies allowing for plaque accumulation. (C) Poor tissue quality resulting from facial bone loss. (D) Soft tissue recession resulting from apical positioned implant which leads to soft tissue loss and resultant black triangles.

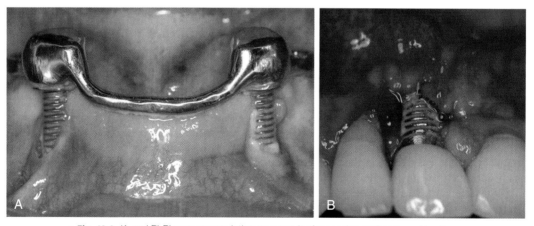

• **Fig. 42.9** (A and B) Plaque accumulation as a result of recession and poor oral hygiene.

and does not jeopardize the integrity of the implant system.[37,38] Etter et al.[39] reported after probing of the implant system, healing of the epithelial attachment will occur approximately 5 days after clinical probing.

The connective tissue zone for an implant has only two fiber groups, and neither of them inserts into the implant. As a result, with an implant, the probe goes beyond the sulcus, through the junctional epithelium attachment, and through the type III collagen connective tissues and reaches closer to the bone.[40] Because the probe penetrates deeper next to an implant compared with a tooth, one should take

care not to contaminate the implant sulcus with bacteria from a diseased periodontal site. To prevent contamination, the dental probe tip may be placed in chlorhexidine after each reading, thereby reducing the possibility of inoculating the sulcular area of the next probed area. In most cases probing depths of 2 to 4 mm have been established as a healthy condition[41] (Figs. 42.10 and 42.11).

In addition, there exists controversy concerning the type of periodontal probe to use with dental implants. Many authors have advocated the use of plastic periodontal probes[42,43]; however, more recent articles have recommended conventional metal

Lindquist Plaque Index

0 = no visible plaque
1 = local plaque accumulation
2 = general plaque accumulation (>25%)

Mombelli Plaque Index

0 = no visible plaque
1 = plaque recognized by probing over smooth margin of implant
2 = visible plaque
3 = abundance of soft matter

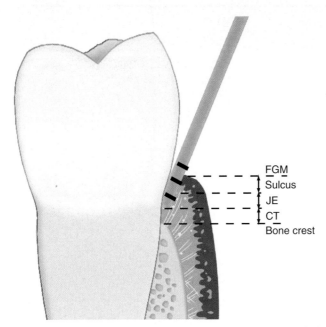

FGM
Sulcus
JE
CT
Bone crest

• **Fig. 42.10** A probe placed into the sulcus of a tooth goes through the sulcus and the epithelial attachment. It is stopped by the connective tissue attachment. The biological width of a natural tooth has a connective tissue zone that inserts into the cementum of the tooth. A periodontal probe will penetrate the sulcus and the junctional epithelial (JE) attachment. *CT,* Connective tissue; *FGM,* free gingival margin. *(From Misch CE. An implant is not a tooth: a comparison of periodontal indices.* Dental Implant Prosthetics. *2nd ed. St. Louis, MO: Mosby; 2015.)*

probes because they do not appear to damage the mucosal attachment or mar the implant surface.[44,45]

Ideally there should be baseline clinical probing depths acquired after the initial insertion of the prosthesis. However, in some cases, because of malpositioned implants or an overcontoured prosthesis, obtaining true probing depths may be difficult. In these cases a more routine radiographic evaluation is indicated to help ascertain peri-implant health.

When bleeding on probing is present, usually this is indicative of positive peri-implant disease. Studies have shown that similar to natural teeth, the absence of bleeding on probing may be interpreted as highly predictive of stability of the peri-implant tissues.[46,47] However, a positive correlation exists with bleeding on probing and histologic signs of inflammation at peri-implant tissue levels.[48]

Care should be exercised to avoid false-positive readings for bleeding on probing depths. Gerber et al.[49] reported that a pressure of approximately 0.15 N should be used to minimize incorrect readings. Probing around dental implants has been shown to be more sensitive to force variation in comparison with natural teeth.[50]

The thickness and the type of tissue may influence the mucosa/epithelium surrounding a dental implant. Van Steenberghe et al.[51] determined that shallow (minimal) probing depths are associated with keratinized tissue, and deeper probing depths are consistent with alveolar mucosa (i.e., movable tissue) surrounding the implant.

On probing the peri-implant tissues, if suppuration is present, the implant clinician should be conscious of the strong evidence of the presence of infection or peri-implant disease. Radiographic evaluation should be immediately completed to determine the etiology of the exudate and the infectious origin.

When evaluating probing depths, greater than 3 mm is not a definite sign of peri-implantitis; peri-implant tissue dimensions are influenced by the implant type and shape, the connections of the multiple components (material and retention mode), and the prosthetic restoration design and configuration. Coveted soft tissue conditioning in the esthetic zone to simulate an interdental papilla can lead to an increase in the distance from the implant shoulder to the mucosal margin of up to 5 mm.[52] Clinical presentations may be misdiagnosed as peri-implantitis when factors such as mucositis and marginal bone remodeling ensue from deep positioning of the implant for more acceptable esthetic outcomes. The diagnosis of peri-implantitis may also be caused by the local anatomic variations.[53]

Controversy surrounds the issue of using bleeding and gingival health as an implant health indicator. Unlike a natural tooth, implant success in the first few years is related more often to biomechanical equilibrium than to gingival health. Compared with a natural tooth, the soft tissue inflammation caused specifically by bacteria may be more restricted to above the crestal bone, because of the lack of a periodontal membrane or fibrous tissue between the implant and the bone interface. As a result the bleeding index may not be as significant when evaluating early implant health status.[54]

Presence of Keratinized Tissue

In recent literature, compelling clinical published reports have correlated peri-implantitis with keratinized gingiva and biotype thickness. A few studies have shown a minimal correlation between keratinized tissue and implant success. However, other reports have shown a lack of keratinized tissue is associated with bone loss,[55] increased plaque accumulation,[56] increased gingival recession,[57] increased gingival inflammation,[58] and a higher frequency of bleeding on probing.[59]

The soft tissue at the implant site has been recognized as a crucial factor in long-term maintenance of healthy implant restorations. The soft tissue quality at the implant site, together with the gingival biotype, is a predisposing factor in a patient's resistance to plaque accumulation and inflammatory-mediated peri-implant disease.[60,61] Unattached, nonkeratinized mucosal tissue is more problematic because implants do not have inserting supracrestal gingival fibers, which serve as a barrier to bacterial insult; Sharpey's fibers run parallel to the implant, leaving only the hemidesmosomal seal of the junctional epithelium at the neck of the implant to protect underlying soft and hard peri-implant structures. During the mastication process, this seal may be broken when the vestibule is shallow and frenum attachment is high, causing excess pressure on the

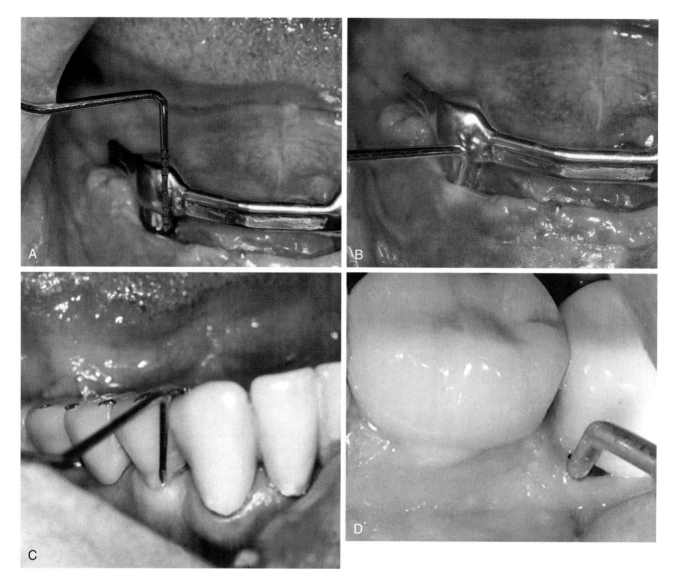

• **Fig. 42.11** Controversies related to probing include the material of the probe and the difficulty in obtaining accurate measurements (A) probing around an implant retaining a bar overdenture; (B) if excessive probing pressure is used, probing depths will be inaccurate and traumatize the tissue; (C) if the prosthesis is overcontoured, difficulty in probing will result; (D) difficulty probing with a plastic probe around the contours of a fixed prosthesis.

tissue. Microbial colonization may then progress to the crestal and peri-implant tissue, which may result in the early stages of peri-implant disease. If plaque control is not adequate around the implants lacking keratinized gingiva, tissue may cause irritation and sensitivity, which may be uncomfortable for the patient.

For the existing soft tissue the quality may be classified as either a thin or a thick biotype. Thin gingival biotype is indicative of thin underlying supporting bone. Thin structures are less vascularized and more prone to recession and resorption in the presence of inflammation. Therefore patients with a thin biotype are more susceptible to peri-implant complications, especially if keratinized tissue is compromised (Box 42.4).

In conclusion, there is increasing literature to support the advantage of keratinized tissue over nonkeratinized tissue. Many authors recommend keratinized mucosa more intensely than others.

In specific clinical instances, attached, keratinized gingiva is more often desirable. For example, a fixed prosthesis (FP-1) in the esthetic zone (anterior maxilla) will require keratinized mucosa to

1. Similar to natural teeth tissue in color, contour, and texture of the soft tissue drape
2. More esthetic, especially when a high smile line exists
3. Keratinized tissue is more resistant to abrasion
4. Maintaining papillae is more predictable if keratinized tissue is present
4. Hygiene aids are more comfortable to use
5. Degree of gingival recession is proportional to the amount of keratinized gingiva
6. Keratinized mucosa is more manageable during the retraction and impression process
7. Long-term tissue stability is greater with keratinized tissue
8. With two-stage implant placement, wound dehiscence is less likely

develop a soft tissue drape around the implant prosthesis. Another prime example is with a mandibular overdenture, which benefits from a stable vestibule and a zone of nonmobile tissue around the

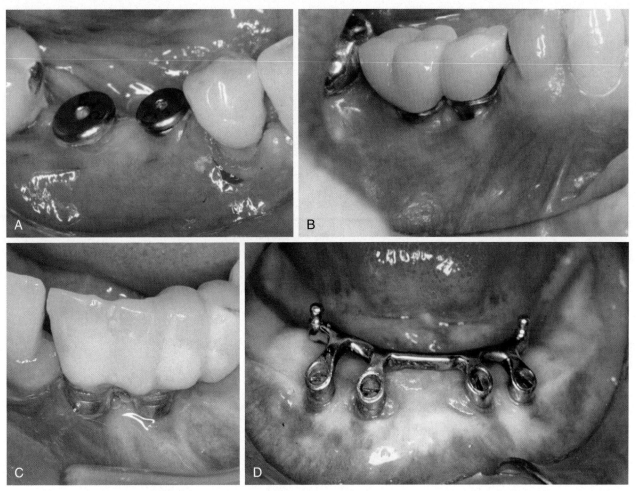

• **Fig. 42.12** Inadequate Keratinized Tissue. (A) Lack of quality attached tissue on facial aspect of the healing abutments. (B and C) Lack of keratinized tissue on facial of final prosthesis. (D) Bar overdenture exhibiting compromised attached tissue because of the facial placement of the implants.

implant abutments. When these conditions exist, it is less likely for patients to exhibit tissue sensitivity. Current recommendations based on clinical experience and current systematic reviews are to evaluate and, if possible, increase deficient sites of inadequate keratinized gingiva around implants prophylactically if peri-implant disease exists[62,63] (Fig. 42.12).

Mobility of Implant/Prosthesis

At each maintenance appointment the mobility of the prosthesis and implants should be evaluated. If mobility exists, the etiology should be ascertained, specifically if it is due to a loose screw or implant failure. Usually if pain is present when the prosthesis is moved in a buccal-lingual and apical direction, then it is most likely due to an implant failure (i.e., unless the tissue is impinging on the tissue, resulting in pain). When implant failure exists, pain will result because of the soft tissue interface. If no pain exists, then usually this is indicative of screw loosening (Fig. 42.13).

Pain/Sensitivity

A component of the maintenance protocol is the determination of any possible subjective findings of pain, tenderness, and sensitivity concerning the patient's peri-implant tissues, implant body, or implant prosthesis. Pain and tenderness are subjective criteria and depend on the patient's interpretation of the degree of discomfort.

Pain is defined as an unpleasant sensation ranging from mild discomfort to excruciating agony. Tenderness is more an unpleasant awareness of the region. An implant rarely is troubled by the subjective criteria of pain or sensitivity after initial healing. In contrast to a natural tooth an implant does not become hyperemic and is not temperature sensitive. If a traumatic occlusion situation is present, rarely will symptoms be present with an implant.

Implant-Related Pain. After the implant has achieved primary healing, absence of pain under vertical or horizontal forces is a primary subjective criterion. Usually, but not always, pain does not occur unless the implant is mobile and surrounded by inflamed tissue or has rigid fixation but impinges on a nerve. The most common condition that causes discomfort from an implant is when a loose implant abutment is entrapping some of the soft tissue in the abutment-implant connection. Usually, after the soft tissue in the region is removed and the abutment is repositioned, the discomfort or pain will subside.

When an implant is mobile, pain may occur early or late in treatment. In either case the condition rarely improves. Pain on loading of rigid implants has been observed more often on immediately loaded implants compared with those healing unloaded for an extended period. Implant sensitivity or mild tenderness rather than pain in a rigid implant is also most unusual and signals a more significant complication for an implant than for a tooth. Tenderness during function or percussion usually implies

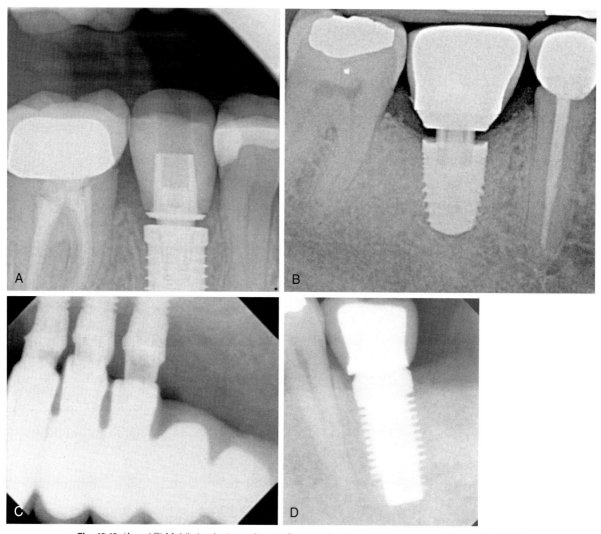

• **Fig. 42.13** (A and B) Mobile implant prostheses diagnosed at the maintenance appointment. (C) Ill-fitting and loose full-arch fixed prosthesis. (D) Ill-fitting prosthesis which may result from loose abutment screw.

healing in the proximity of a nerve or, on rare occasions, bone stress beyond physiologic limits.

On occasion an implant body may fracture from fatigue. Fatigue is related to the amount of force, the number of cycles, the strength of the material, the diameter of the component, and the number of implants splinted together. This condition is similar to a fractured root. In any case, radiographic evidence of the fracture may be difficult to ascertain. Percussion and forces up to 500 g (1.2 psi) with a bite stick are used clinically to evaluate a tooth or implant for pain or discomfort. Percussion and heavy biting on a wood stick associated with pain are clinical indices. In these cases the implant is most often removed, which especially in the mandible (i.e., dense bone) may be difficult (Fig. 42.14).

Abutment-Related Pain. When the abutment-implant connection is not secure, pain may result because of tissue integration into the void. This pain is usually persistent and occurs most often during percussion or function. If this occurs, the prosthesis and abutment should be removed, soft tissue excised, and components repositioned (Fig. 42.15).

Infection-Related Pain. Especially in the early stages of peri-implantitis, pain usually does not present as a primary clinical symptom. Unless active infection with suppuration accompanies sufficient osseous destruction, patients do not experience pain.

Because dental implants do not have a PDL support and its sensory apparatus, low-grade infections and bone resorption are not detected by marginal gingiva. As the disease process begins around an implant, the patient may feel slight irritation, but normally not alarming pain.[64,65] It is recommended that the implant clinician be proactive in evaluating the status of dental implants with the incorporation of a routine maintenance protocol for implant patients.

Occlusion

Ideally, in most fixed implant cases an implant-protected occlusion should be present. Implant-protected occlusion (i.e., canine guidance) should be adhered to so the anterior teeth protect the posterior teeth (i.e., protrusive movements) and the posterior teeth protect the anterior (i.e., centric occlusion).

Traumatic occlusion has been shown to be an etiologic factor in the loss of bone around the peri-implant region. A timed occlusion should always be present, which includes the natural teeth contacting first before the contact of the implant (i.e., to compensate for the PDL compression during occlusal contacts). During light contact, extrathin articulating paper (e.g., shimstock) should be easily pulled through the occlusal contact with an implant. Then during heavy contact, minimal resistance should be present. Miyata et al.[66] reported with monkey studies that bone loss

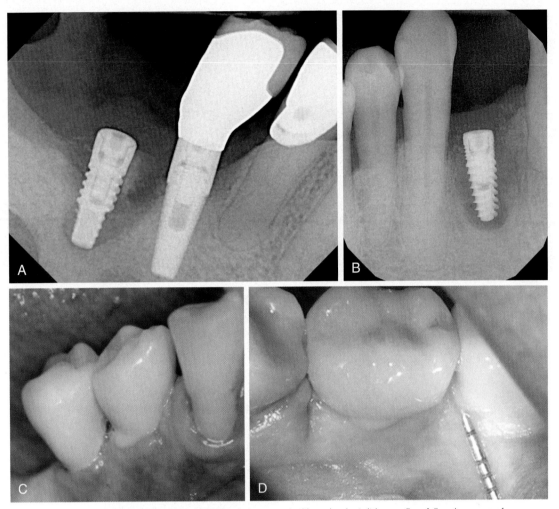

● **Fig. 42.14** Implant Pain. (A and B) If pain is present with an implant, it is usually a failure because of a soft tissue encapsulation; radiographs reveal significant radiolucency surrounding the implant bodies. (C and D) If suppuration is present, usually the patient will be symptomatic.

may occur with an excess occlusal contact of 180 μm, even in the absence of peri-implant inflammation. Therefore it is imperative that the implant clinician evaluate and modify the existing occlusion if necessary, at each appointment (Fig. 42.16).

In addition, the presence of parafunctional habits (e.g., clenching, bruxism) should be documented and treated, most commonly with an occlusal guard. A hard acrylic centric is most commonly used.

Prosthesis

At each maintenance appointment the prosthesis should be evaluated for not only mobility but also any fractures of the prosthesis material (e.g., porcelain, acrylic, zirconia). If material fracture is present, the occlusion should be immediately evaluated and the possibility of replacement is determined. For a removable prosthesis, all implant attachments should be evaluated for mobility and retention.

Radiographic Evaluation of the Implant and Prosthesis

An accurate and thorough radiographic examination should be performed as a routine adjunct to the clinical maintenance examination (Box 41.2). Ideally the radiographic modality used should

be able to standardize the evaluation of the implant interface and bone level. The selection of the radiographic modality is dictated by the number and position of implants, along with the type of prosthesis.

Upon radiographic evaluation the crestal bone region is often the most diagnostic for the ranges of optimum, satisfactory, and compromised health conditions. Radiographic interpretation is one of the easiest clinical tools to use to assess implant crestal bone loss, but has many limitations. However, a two-dimensional radiograph will illustrate only the mesial and distal crestal levels of bone (Fig. 42.17).

When early bone loss occurs, it is most often present on the facial aspect of the implant. The absence of radiolucency around an implant does not indicate bone is present at the interface. Therefore two-dimensional radiographs (i.e., periapical, bitewings, panographic films) may often be misleading on revealing the amount of bone loss. In the mandibular anterior region, as much as a 40% decrease in density is necessary to produce a traditional radiographic difference in this region because of the dense cortical bone.[67] When abundant bone width is present, a V-shaped crestal defect around an implant may be surrounded by cortical bone and, as a result, the radiograph is less diagnostic for bone loss.

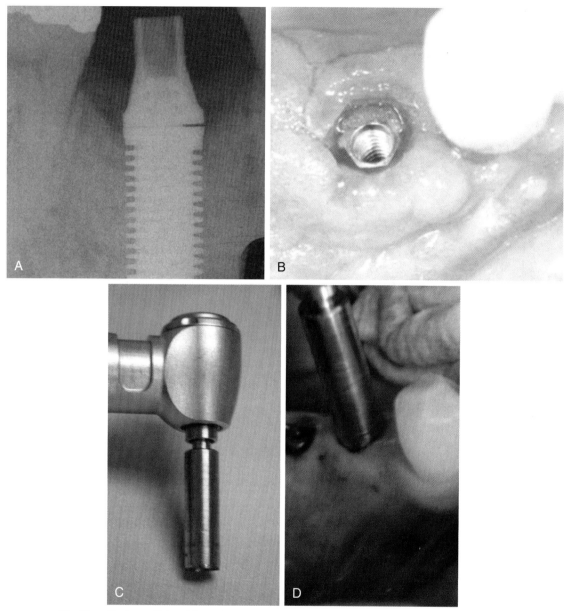

• **Fig. 42.15** Abutment-Related Pain. (A) An incomplete abutment seating will result in tissue growth with resultant pain. (B) After implant is removed, tissue impingement is evident. (C and D) The excess tissue is removed with a latch-type tissue punch.

Radiograph Type

The type of radiograph used in the evaluation of the implant and prosthesis is difficult to generalize. Standardized periapical radiographs are usually recommended as the most common type of radiographic modality in evaluation of dental implants. The long cone paralleling technique should be used to minimize image distortion.[68] Panoramic radiographs exhibit inherent disadvantages, including magnification, distortion, overlapping images, and poor resolution. Therefore panoramic radiographs are not the most ideal radiograph in evaluating bone loss (Fig. 42.18). However, in cases where periapical or bitewing radiographs cannot be obtained, panoramic films may be used.

Cone beam computed tomography (CBCT) scans, although superior to plain film radiographs in the diagnosis and treatment planning phases of implant dentistry, are usually not indicated for routine maintenance unless complications are present.

Studies evaluating the visibility of the buccal plate showed that if the amount of bone present is less than 0.6 mm in thickness, the bone will be invisible on a CBCT image.[69] In addition, CBCT images suffer from beam hardening, which leads to the formation of a radiolucency surrounding the implant. This occurs from a greater number of photons being absorbed (Fig. 42.19). In summary, the type of image modality should be specifically tailored to each individual patient, according to clinical and anatomic circumstances.

Radiograph Accuracy

It is often more difficult to obtain an accurate radiograph of the implant body in comparison with a natural tooth. Most commonly, implants are placed more apical to the apex of the pre-existing natural teeth. As a result the apex of the implant often is located beyond muscle attachments or in regions almost impossible to capture with a parallel radiographic method. A foreshortened image to encompass the apical portion of the implant results in poor display of the crestal bone. An accurate radiograph will show a clear depiction of the threads on the radiograph and a proper angulation. If the implant threads are clear on one side but blurry on the other, the angulation was incorrect by approximately 10%[70] (Fig. 42.20). If both sides of a threaded implant

are unclear, the radiograph is not diagnostic for crestal bone loss assessment because of angulation issues. Ideally the abutment-implant connection should appear as a clear line between the two components. When the top of the implant is placed at the crest of the regional bone, the amount of crestal bone loss is most easy to evaluate (Fig. 42.21).

In addition, the prosthesis should be evaluated for any radiographic changes from the baseline radiographs. Of utmost importance is the fit of the prosthesis because an ill-fitting or loose prosthesis may lead to peri-implant disease. If a space is present between the prosthesis and the abutment, the prosthesis should be immediately evaluated for passivity and mobility.

Radiograph Timing

The most important radiograph for use in the maintenance phase is the postprosthetic baseline radiograph. This radiograph is most often taken at the prosthesis insertion appointment. By this time the "biological width" most likely will have influenced the implant crest module bone level.

In general, implants with machined surfaces or external hex connections are usually subject to an initial remodeling of the bone level. Adell et al.[71] reported an average bone loss of 1.5 mm during the first year and 0.1 mm per year thereafter. However, recent implant design changes have reduced this bone loss with internal connections and platform switching.[72,73]

In most cases an individualized radiographic protocol should be developed based on the number and location of implants, type of prosthesis, and any associated complications. A comprehensive and generalized radiologic protocol was established by Resnik[74] in 2016 (Box 42.5).

Radiographic Crestal Bone Loss

The marginal bone around the implant crestal region is usually a significant indicator of implant health. The cause of crestal bone loss around an implant is multifactorial and may occur at different

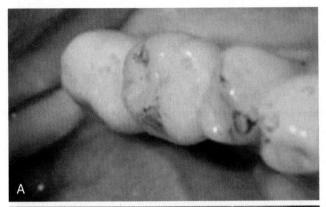
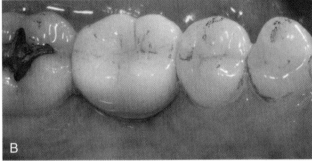

• **Fig. 42.16** Occlusal Contacts. (A) The occlusion should be checked at each maintenance appointment to ensure lack of premature contacts. (B) Ideal occlusion consists of primary contact (i.e., light occlusion) on the natural teeth and light contact on implants during heavy occlusion.

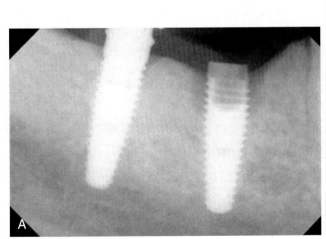
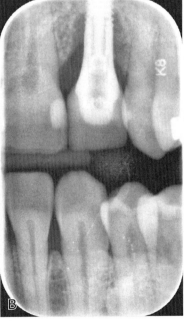

• **Fig. 42.17** (A) Radiograph depicting significant bone loss surrounding the anterior implant; however, this may be misleading because it depicts only the mesial and distal bone levels. (B) Vertical bitewing exhibiting ideal angulation.

time periods: surgical bone loss, initial "biologic width" bone loss, early loading bone loss, intermediate-term bone loss, and long-term bone loss. Each period may be associated with a different cause for the bone loss. Most often the surgical trauma results in minimal bone loss, but on occasion, bone loss may reach several millimeters (Fig. 42.22).

When the abutment is attached to the implant body, approximately 0.5 to 1 mm of connective tissue forms apical to this connection.[75] This associated bone loss may be caused by an "implant biologic width." Initial bone loss during the surgical healing phase may vary for submerged and unsubmerged healing protocols.[76]

After the implant is connected with a permucosal element, the marginal bone may be lost during the first month from: (1) the position of the abutment-implant connection or (2) the crest

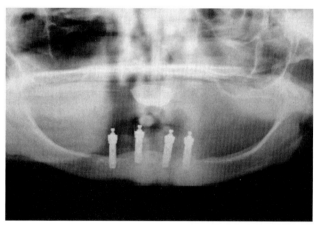

● **Fig. 42.18** Panoramic Image. The determination of the amount of bone loss on a panoramic image is misleading because of the magnification, distortion, overlapping images, and poor resolution.

module design of the implant. The abutment-implant connection may cause 0.5 to 1.0 mm of bone loss when it is at or below the bone. In addition, when smooth metal is present below the abutment-implant connection, additional bone loss will occur in direct relation to the smooth metal region. The bone levels will most often reside at the first thread or at a roughened surface after the first month after permucosal element placement (Fig. 42.23 and Box 42.6).

Diagnosis of Peri-implant Disease

After the clinical and radiographic maintenance examination is complete, a diagnosis of the current peri-implant condition is warranted. In the evaluation of the peri-implant tissues, three possible conditions may exist: (1) healthy condition, (2) peri-implant mucositis, and (3) peri-implantitis.

Healthy Condition

If there exist no signs of inflammation, bleeding, recession, bone loss, or implant/prosthesis mobility, then the patient's implants/prosthesis is determined to be in a "healthy" state (Fig. 42.24 and Box 42.7).

Treatment includes adherence to routine implant maintenance (i.e., usually 3–6 months).

Peri-implant Mucositis

Peri-implant mucositis is defined as a localized inflammation within the soft tissue surrounding the implant bodies. In addition, redness and bleeding on probing may be present. However, the bone level has not changed; therefore no hard tissue recession (i.e., bone loss) has occurred. Peri-implant mucositis is similar to gingivitis with respect to natural teeth (Fig. 42.25).

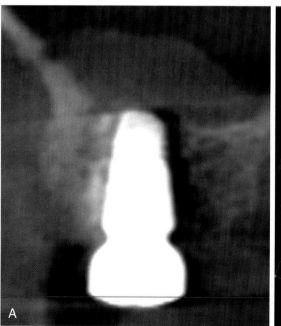
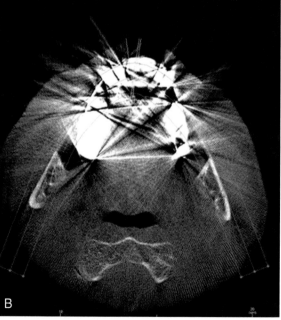

● **Fig. 42.19** Inherent Cone Beam Computed Tomography Disadvantages. (A) Beam hardening resulting in a radiolucency surrounding the implant. (B) Scatter that is caused by the presence metallic objects (e.g., crowns, implants).

Treatment includes remediation of the causative factors of peri-implant mucositis and associated follow-up care.

Peri-implantitis

Peri-implantitis is defined as localized inflammation with concomitant bone loss. In most peri-implantitis cases suppuration and clinical probing depths are present, together with bleeding on probing. On radiographic evaluation, marginal bone loss is present in comparison with the original baseline radiographs (Fig. 42.26).

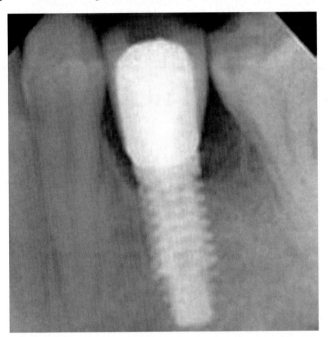

• **Fig. 42.20** On this periapical radiograph the threads are clear. On the right side only, the central ray was not directed completely perpendicular to the implant body but was within 10 degrees. This film is not ideal to ascertain the amount of bone loss.

Treatment includes remediation of the causative factors and usually hard and soft tissue surgical intervention, followed by continued maintenance care.

Frequency of Maintenance Visits

Peri-implant disease may result from opportunistic infections that lead to soft and hard tissue complications; therefore it is mandatory to monitor the peri-implant tissues at regular intervals. If early signs of disease are diagnosed, aggressive intervention may prevent the loss of hard tissue. Zitzman et al.[77] reported that peri-implant mucositis may exhibit apical progression after only 3 months of plaque buildup around implants. Therefore a 3-month maintenance regimen is recommended within the first year of implant placement to evaluate the tissue health and the patient's home care. If after the first year the peri-implant tissues are healthy, then the maintenance interval may be extended to 6 months. However, a stricter recall protocol should be adhered to if the patient does exhibit risk factors or comorbidities.[78]

Patient Home Care

Ideally a home care assessment should be determined before the initiation of dental implant treatment. In partially or completely edentulous patients, usually compromised home care is already present. In addition, during the postsurgical phase of treatment, patients are often lax in their hygiene practices because of fear of causing damage to the surgery site. Therefore it is imperative that the patient be educated on the necessity and need for a comprehensive home care regimen.

When educating patients on home care, various techniques may be used, as long as they are safe and effective. Depending on the type of implant, implant position, location in the oral cavity, and type and size of the prosthesis, various devices along with the frequency may be recommended. No single hygiene device has been shown to be ideal in all situations. There exists a full array of

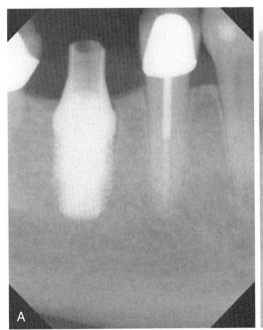
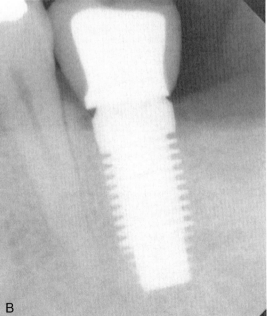

• **Fig. 42.21** (A) Poor angulation resulting in no threads of the implants being seen. (B) Ideal positioning as implant threads on mesial and distal are easily seen.

brushes, floss threading systems, and other devices available to aid patients in their hygiene protocols.

One common mistake often employed by clinicians is to add too many oral hygiene devices for patient home care. Studies have shown that when multiple devices are recommended, patients are more apt to become discouraged and less motivated. However, when a combination of toothbrushing devices, auxiliary aids, and antimicrobial mouthrinses are used, an increased plaque inhibition is seen.[79]

Specific Dentifrices

Manual and Electromechanical Devices

In general most exposed facial and lingual surfaces may be cleaned with a soft, multitufted nylon toothbrush. The implant clinician should recommend to each individual patient which brush angle would be ideal to access all areas within the mouth. The modified Bass technique should be used or a short, horizontal, back-and-forth movement may be incorporated into the hygiene regimen. The brush may be held at a 45-degree angle to the gingival tissue.[80]

Most commonly, patients often prefer electromechanical devices, which have been shown to be superior to manual brushing around dental implants.[81] When using electromechanical devices (i.e., sonic toothbrushes, oscillating-rotating power toothbrushes), especially in difficult-to-access areas, end-tufted brushes and tapered rotary brushes tend to be beneficial. Studies have confirmed the benefits of these devices.[82,83] Rasperini et al.[82] reported

---

• BOX 42.5 Radiograph Timing Protocol

Preoperative

Cone Beam Computed Tomography
- All vital structures identified
- Sinus-related procedures: must confirm patency of ostium and lack of pathology

Intraoperative
- Peri-apical radiograph (PA) after pilot drill during placement to confirm positioning and proximity to vital structures and adjacent teeth
- PA of final placement with cover screw or healing abutment
- PA before uncover surgery (stage 2 procedure)

Prosthetic
- PA to confirm implant is ready to restore
- PA to confirm abutment is seated properly
- PA to confirm proper seating of prosthesis/cement removal (will be baseline for future evaluation radiographs)

Postoperative
- PA once annually for the first 3 years after implant prosthetics to monitor bone level
- Normal (acceptable): <0.2 mm vertical bone loss per year for first 3 years
- After 3 years, PA should be taken every 2 years
  In addition to radiographic evaluation, the following should be evaluated:
- Presence of pain, suppuration
- Implant and/or prosthesis mobility
- Hyperocclusion
- Soft tissue changes (bleeding, recession, hyperplasia)
  In some cases a periapical radiograph cannot be accurately obtained because of positioning issues; therefore a panoramic radiograph may be used as an alternative radiographic modality.

---

a reduction in bleeding (~50% in the first year) and decrease in probing depths (~0.3 mm) with power toothbrushes.

Most manufactured power brushes have soft, interchangeable bristle heads (flattened, rubber cuplike, short and long pointed

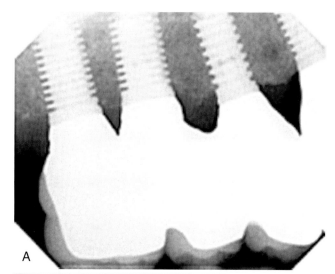

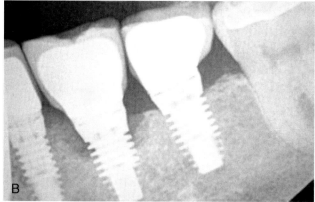

• **Fig. 42.22** Postprosthetic Images. (A) Ideal radiograph showing no signs of bone loss. (B) Image depicting significant early bone loss at first maintenance appointment.

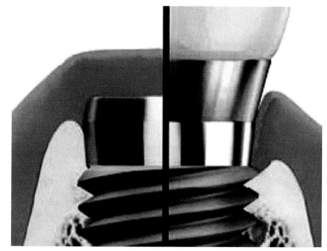

• **Fig. 42.23** When an implant is placed with the abutment connection at the crest of the ridge (left side), after the permucosal abutment is connected the bone is usually lost to the first thread, especially when the crest module is machined or smooth (right side).

BOX 42.6 Etiology of Implant Crestal Bone Loss

Time	Etiology
Surgery	Trauma to bone
Uncovery	"Implant biologic width" related to abutment location and implant crest module design
Early	Occlusal trauma
Intermediate	Bacteria or occlusal trauma
Long term	Bacteria

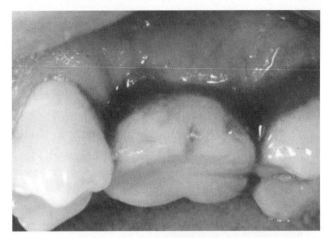

• **Fig. 42.25** Periimplant Mucositis. Molar implant prosthesis exhibiting signs of bleeding; however, no bone loss is present.

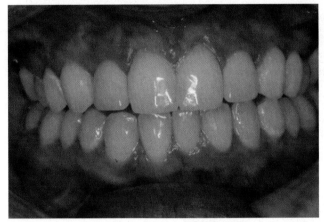

• **Fig. 42.24** Healthy Implant Condition. No signs of inflammation, bleeding, tissue recession, or bone loss (lateral incisors).

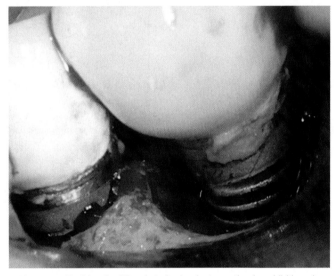

• **Fig. 42.26** Peri-implantitis. Anterior implant prosthesis exhibiting signs of significant recession, inflamed gingival tissue, and plaque accumulation.

BOX 42.7 Healthy Clinical Findings

1. No signs of inflammation (pink, firm peri-implant mucosa)
2. No probing depths (<4 mm)
3. Absence of bleeding on gentle probing (<15 N)
4. No suppuration
5. No pain or sensitivity
6. No radiographic bone changes

in shape) that may be used. The short and long pointed tips are ideal for reaching proximal areas, wide embrasures, and pontic areas under a splinted prosthesis. The hollowed rubber cup may be used on the facial and lingual aspects of the implant and prosthesis (Fig. 42.27).

Toothpaste/Gel

The selection of a toothpaste should be low abrasive as to not scratch the surface of the exposed implant. Dentifrices should be avoided that contain harsh abrasive ingredients, including stain removers and smoker's toothpaste.[84] Selective fluorides may result in etching and roughness on implant surfaces.[85,86]

Interproximal Brushes

With some types of prostheses (e.g., full-arch fixed prosthesis), interproximal brushes with small brush heads may be indicated to gain easier access. Ideally these types of device should be plastic-coated because metal may damage the implant surface.[79] The interdental brush is used to massage the gingival tissue, which results in increased blood flow and healthier tissue. Patients should be

instructed to insert the tip interproximally in an occlusal direction and use a gentle rotary motion against the gingiva[80] (Fig. 42.28).

Floss Aids

Flossing around dental implants is also a controversial topic. Most patients are resistant to flossing their natural teeth, especially if floss threaders are required. Therefore flossing has an inherent disadvantage in patient compliance and also dexterity issues. When flossing around implants, it is often difficult to manipulate and maneuver the floss around a malpositioned implant or an overcontoured/atypical prosthesis. Floss is ideally used interproximally, especially when a splinted prosthesis is present. Thicker floss is available (e.g., "yarnlike") that allows for cleaning around abutments and prostheses, and ease of penetrating hard to reach interproximal areas. Floss may be used in conjunction with chlorhexidine or other antimicrobials to decrease plaque accumulation.

It is imperative that the patient is instructed on the proper technique on flossing around dental implants. Improper or over-aggressive flossing may lead to tissue trauma and resultant peri-implant soft tissue lesions (Fig. 42.29).

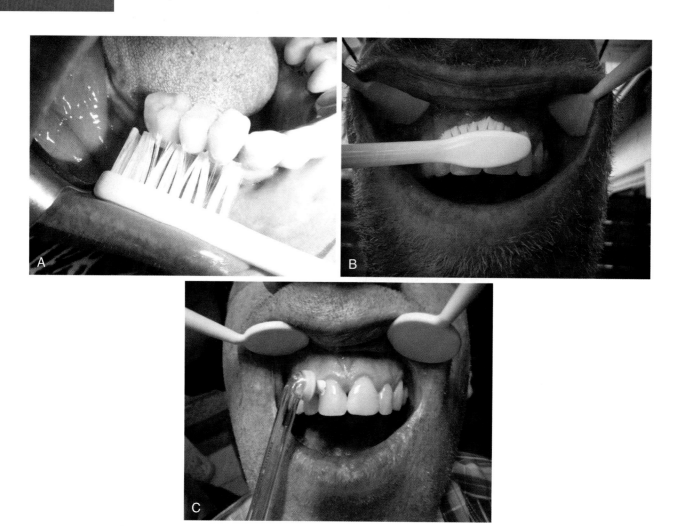

• **Fig. 42.27** (A) Manual brushing around a dental implant (Procter & Gamble, Cincinnati, Ohio). (B) Electro-mechanical toothbrush around a dental implant Philips Sonicare. (C) AirFloss Pro (Philips).

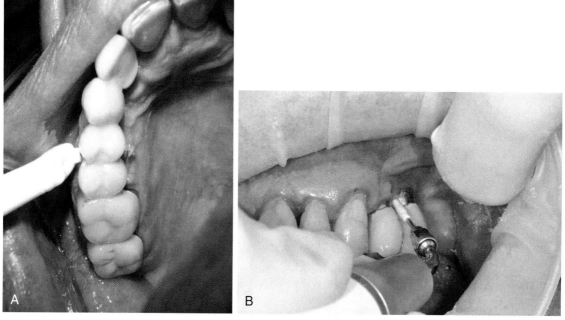

• **Fig. 42.28** (A) Interproximal brush (Sunstar Butler, Chicago, Ill.). (B) Hu-Friedy EMS Piezo implant tip, PIEZON® TECHNOLOGY.

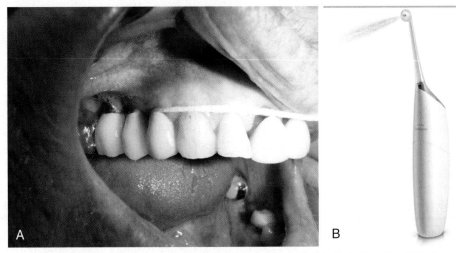

• **Fig. 42.29** (A and B) Floss aids. (B) Microdroplets of air and liquid with AirFloss Pro (Philips).

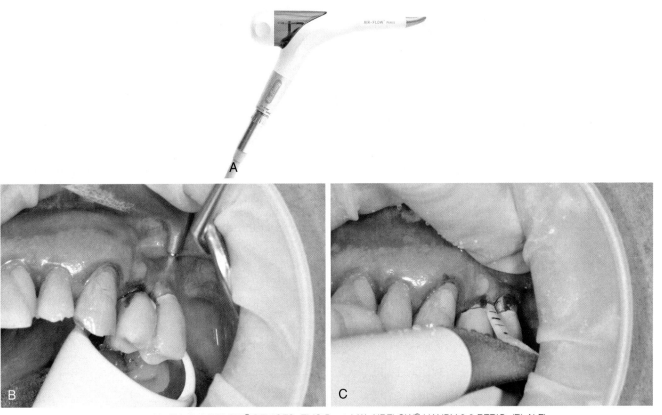

• **Fig. 42.30** Hu-Friedy AIRFLOW® DEVICES, EMS Dental (A) AIRFLOW® HANDY 3.0 PERIO. (B) AirFlow interdental and supragingival. (C) Ideal placement of Hu-Friedy PerioFlow tip into subgingival areas.

Oral Irrigator

The oral irrigator (e.g., Air Floss Pro, Philips) may be beneficial in removing supragingival debris, especially when difficult access exists because of the prosthesis type. Numerous studies have shown an oral irrigator to be superior in reducing gingival bleeding, inflammation, and plaque in comparison with string floss.[87-89] Magnuson et al.[90] found oral irrigators to reduce bleeding around implants by 81% in contrast with 33% for flossing. However, caution must be exercised in using an oral irrigator because excessive force (i.e., high pressure) may damage the junctional epithelium, which may lead to a bacteremia.[91] To minimize complications,

patients should be instructed on the proper use of these devices, mainly using a low to medium speed and angulating the tip to be perpendicular to the long axis of the implant body.

Patients should be instructed to use a nonmetal tip once to twice daily.

An antimicrobial (e.g., chlorhexidine, cetylpyridinium chloride) may be used as an irrigant that decreases the bacterial count in the oral cavity.[92] Studies comparing rinsing with 0.12% chlorhexidine with irrigating with 0.06% chlorhexidine showed the irrigation group to be 87% more effective in reducing gingivitis in comparison with the rinsing group[93] (Fig. 42.30 and Box 42.8).

Antimicrobial Rinses

The regular use of chemotherapeutic agents such as antimicrobial rinses may be used as an adjunct in plaque control. Chlorhexidine gluconate is the most commonly used antimicrobial rinse in implant dentistry because it is safe, inexpensive, and nontoxic. It is very effective because of its substantivity, which is the binding of the medication to the soft tissues and implant surfaces. Studies have shown that a 30-second rinse of chlorhexidine inhibits 90% of oral bacteria for more than 5 hours.[92] Chlorhexidine or cetylpyridinium chloride may be locally applied with a cotton swab or may be used as a rinse twice daily (Fig. 42.31 (B)).

In-Office Debridement

In certain situations a maintenance visit will lead to the need for in-office debridement. When excessive dental plaque and calculus are present, the dental professional must use instruments for proper removal. However, care should be exercised in not damaging the implant or prosthesis. Older implant systems made of commercially pure titanium, which is a softer metal, are easily damaged with conventional instruments. If surface damage results, the titanium oxide surface layer will be altered, which may cause surface corrosion.[94] However, more recent implant designs use titanium alloy, which is far more resistant to surface alteration.

> • **BOX 42.8** **Benefits of Oral Irrigator**[3]
>
> - May clean supragingival, subgingival, and interdental areas
> - May remove supragingival and subgingival plaque (biofilm)
> - Has been shown to be more effective than string floss for dental implants
> - More effective than chlorhexidine with implant care
> - Has been shown to be safe if used properly
> - Easy to use

The use of ultrasonic instrumentation is not recommended with dental implants, unless the stainless steel tips are covered with a protective sleeve. Fig. 42.28 (B) these scalers may disrupt the titanium dioxide surface, which leads to plaque accumulation. These scratches and gouges may be detrimental to long-term health and hygiene practices.[95] Air polishers with bicarbonate particles (e.g., Prophy-Jet) may also be detrimental to the implant surface. Studies have shown alteration of the implant surface may result because random pitting and irregularities within the surface may occur. Therefore air polishers with bicarbonate particles should not be used around implants or the prosthesis.[96]

Low-abrasive amino acid glycine powder has been shown to be an effective treatment for removing biofilm without damaging the implant surface or hard and soft tissues. This piezo instrument (Hu-Friedy, Chicago, Ill.) uses a special handpiece with a plastic tube nozzle with three orthogonally oriented holes. An air-powder mixture with reduced pressure is expelled through the nozzle, which prevents the formation of air emphysema complications. The nozzle is moved in a circumferential movement around the implant surface Fig. 42.30 (A), (B), (C) and Fig. 42.31 (A).

Although more extensive studies need to be conducted as to technique efficacy, glycine powder can be incorporated into a treatment regimen. The clinician should be careful to use the powder only in areas where access is available and a posttreatment rinse can remove any residue. This modality is best used in cases with buccal dehiscence and/or horizontal bone loss without crater or infrabony pocketing.

After debridement procedures a follow-up visit should be scheduled approximately 1 month later. At this appointment the health of the peri-implant tissues should be evaluated together with home care reinforcement. Usually after the 1-month follow-up the patient should be seen on a 3-month recall. If peri-implant health is normal, patients can usually be placed on a 3- to 6-month recall system.

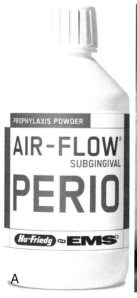
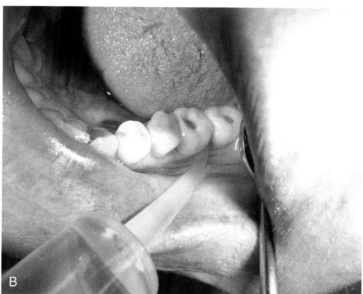

• **Fig. 42.31** Subgingival irrigation therapeuticals. (A) AIRFLOW PERIO POWDER for Hu-Friedy EMS AIRFLOW® THERAPY SYSTEM, prophylaxis powder. (B) Irrigation with Chlorhexidine gluconate in monojet syringe interproximally and subgingivally.

Conclusion

The ongoing maintenance of dental implants is one of the most important factors for long-term health. With increasing numbers of implants being placed each year, it is evident that the prevention of peri-implant disease is paramount to success. An individualized implant maintenance program needs to be implemented that is tailored to the specific patient, the implants, and the prosthesis. Successful implant maintenance depends on many factors, most importantly communication and collaboration between the dental professional and the patient. Peri-implant disease is a prevalent disease; therefore a comprehensive maintenance program is essential to decrease complications. The implant clinician must understand the factors and the need for a systematic maintenance protocol, along with informing his or her patients of the most updated information to ensure longevity of their implants and prosthesis.

References

1. Corbella S, Del Fabbro M, Taschieri S, et al. Clinical evaluation of an implant maintenance protocol for the prevention of peri-implant diseases in patients treated with immediately loaded full-arch rehabilitations. *Int J Dent Hyg.* 2011;9:216–222.
2. Silverstein L, Garg A, Callan D, Shatz P. The key to success: maintaining the long-term health of implants. *Dent Today.* 1998;17: 104, 106, 108–111.
3. Lyle DM. Implant maintenance: is there an ideal approach? *Compend Contin Educ Dent.* 2013;34(5):386–390.
4. Sanz M, Chapple IL. Clinical research on periimplant diseases: Consensus report of Working Group 4. *J Clin Periodontol.* 2012;39:202–206.
5. Glavind L, Attström R. Periodontal self-examination. A motivational tool in periodontics. *J Clin Periodontol.* 1979;6:238–251.
6. Bidez MW, Misch CE. Force transfer in implant dentistry: basic concepts and principles. *J Oral Implantol.* 1992;18:264–274.
7. Gargiulo A, Wentz F, Orban B. Dimensions and relations of the dentogingival junction in humans. *J Periodontol.* 1961;32:261–268.
8. Vacek JS, Gher ME, Assad DA, et al. The dimensions of the human dentogingival junction. *Int J Periodontics Restorative Dent.* 1994;14:154–165.
9. Rateitschak KH. Periodontology. In: Rateitschak KH, Rateitschak EM, Wolf HF, et al., eds. *Color Atlas of Dental Medicine.* 2nd ed. New York: Thieme; 1989.
10. James RA, Schultz RL. Hemidesmosomes and the adhesion of junctional epithelial cells to metal implants: a preliminary report. *J Oral Implantol.* 1974;4:294.
11. Cochran DL, Herman JS, Schenk RK, et al. Biologic width around titanium implants: a histometric analysis of the implanto-gingival junction around unloaded and loaded submerged implants in the canine mandible. *J Periodontol.* 1997;68:186–198.
12. Schroeder A, Pohler O, Sutter F. Tissue reaction to a titanium hollow cylinder implant with titanium plasma sprayed surface. *Schweiz Monatsschr Zahnmed.* 1976;86:713–727.
13. Ericsson I, Lindhe J. Probing at implants and teeth: an experimental study in the dog. *J Clin Periodontol.* 1993;20:623–627.
14. Abrahamsson I, Berglundh T, Lindhe J. The mucosal barrier following abutment disreconnection: an experimental study in dogs. *J Clin Periodontol.* 1997;24:568–572.
15. Parfitt GS. Measurement of the physiologic mobility of individual teeth in an axial direction. *J Dent Res.* 1960;39:608–612.
16. Sekine H, Komiyama Y, Hotta H, et al. Mobility characteristics and tactile sensitivity of osseointegrated fixture-supporting systems. In: Van Steenberghe D, ed. *Tissue Integration in Oral Maxillofacial Reconstruction.* Amsterdam: Excerpta Medica; 1986.
17. Muhlemann HR. Tooth mobility: a review of clinical aspects and research findings. *J Periodontol.* 1967;38:686–708.
18. Rudd KD, O'Leary TJ, Stumpf AJ. Horizontal tooth mobility in carefully screened subjects. *Periodontics.* 1964;2:65–68.
19. Meredith N, Alleyne D, Cawley P. Quantitative determination of the stability of the implant-tissue interface using resonance frequency analysis. *Clin Oral Implant Res* 1996;7:261-7.
20. Sennerby L, Meredith N. Implant stability measurements using resonance frequency analysis: biological and biomechanical aspects and clinical implications. *Periodontology.* 2000, 2008.
21. Antoniazzi RP, Miranda LA, Zanatta FB, et al. Periodontal conditions of individuals with Sjögren's syndrome. *J Periodontol.* 2009;80:419–435.
22. Habbab KM, Moles DR, Porter SR. Potential oral manifestations of cardiovascular drugs. *Oral Dis.* 2010;16:769–773.
23. Smidt D, Torpet LA, Nauntofte B, Heegaard KM, Paedersen AM. Associations between oral and ocular dryness, labial and whole salivary flow rates, systemic diseases and medications in a sample of older people. *Community Dent Oral Epidemiol.* 2011;39: 276–288. 40.
24. Fejerskov O, Escobar G, Jøssing M, Baelum V. A functional natural dentition for all- and for life? The oral healthcare system needs revision. *J Oral Rehabil.* 2013;40:707–722.
25. Hernández G, Lopez-Pintor RM, Arriba L, Torres J, de Vicente JC. Implant treatment in patients with oral lichen planus: a prospective-controlled study. *Clin Oral Implants Res.* 2012;23:726–732.
26. López-Jornet P, Camacho-Alonso F, Sánchez-Siles M. Dental implants in patients with oral lichen planus:a cross-sectional study. *Clin Implant Dent Relat Res.* 2014;16:107–115.
27. Dvorak G, Reich KM, Tangl S, Goldhahn J, Haas R, Gruber R. Cortical porosity of the mandible in an osteoporotic sheep model. *Clin Oral Implants Res.* 2011;22:500–505.
28. March and F, Raskin A, Dionnes-Hornes A, et al. Dental implants and diabetes: conditions for success. *Diabetes Metab.* 2012;38:14–19.
29. Cavalcanti R, Oreglia F, Manfredonia MF, et al. The influence of smoking on the survival of dental implants: a 5-year pragmatic multicenter retrospective cohort study of 1727 patients. *Eur J Oral Implantol.* 2010;4(1):39–45.
30. Marrone A, Lasserre J, Bercy P, Brecx MC. Prevalence and risk factors for peri-implant disease in Belgian adults. *Clin Oral Implants Res.* 2013;24:934–940.
31. Renvert S, Aghazadeh A, Hallstrom H, Persson GR. Factors related to peri-implantitis - a retrospective study. *Clin Oral Implants Res.* 2014;25(4):522–529.
32. Bormann KH, Stühmer C, Z'Graggen M, et al. IL-1 polymorphism and periimplantitis. A literature review. *Schweiz Monatsschr Zahnmed.* 2010;120:510–520.
33. Löe H. The gingival index, the plaque index and the retention index systems. *J Periodontol.* 1967;38(6):610–616, ISSN 0022- 3492.
34. Lekholm R, Adell R, Lindhe J, et al. Marginal tissue reactions at osseointegrated titanium fixtures (II). A cross-sectional study. *Int J Oral Maxillofac Surg.* 1986;15:53–61.
35. Mombelli A, Marxer M, Gaberthuel T, et al. The microbiota of osseointegrated implants in patients with a history of periodontal disease. *J Clin Periodontol.* 1995;22:124–130.
36. Lindquist LW, Rocker B, CarlsonGE. Bone resorption around fixtures in edentulous patients treated with mandibular fixed tissue-integrated prostheses. *J Prosthet Dent.* 1988;59:59–63.
37. Newman MG, Flemmig TF. Periodontal considerations of implants and implant associated microbiota. *Int J Oral Implantol.* 1988;5(1):65–70.
38. Orton GS, Steele DL, Wolinsky LE. The dental professional's role in monitoring and maintenance of tissue-integrated prostheses. *Int J Oral Maxillofac Implants.* 1989;4(4):305–310.
39. Etter TH, Håkanson I, Lang NP, Trejo PM, Caffesse RG. Healing after standardized clinical probing of the perlimplant soft tissue seal: a histomorphometric study in dogs. *Clin Oral Implants Res.* 2002;13(6):571–580.
40. Ericsson I, Lindhe J. Probing at implants and teeth: an experimental study in the dog. *J Clin Periodontol.* 1993;20:623–627.

41. Lang NP, Berglundh T, Heitz-Mayfield LJ, Pjetursson BE, Salvi GE, Sanz M. Consensus statements and recommended clinical procedures regarding implant survival and complications. *Int J Oral Maxillofac Implants.* 2004;19(l):150–154.

42. Heitz-Mayfield LJ. Peri-implant diseases: diagnosis and risk indicators. *J Clin Periodontol.* 2008;35(8 l):292–304.

43. Humphrey S. Implant maintenance. *Dent Clin North Am.* 2006;50(3):463–478.

44. Lindhe J, Meyle J, Group D of European Workshop on Periodontology. Peri-implant diseases: Consensus report of the Sixth European Workshop on Periodontology. *J Clin Periodontol.* 2008;35(8):282–285.

45. Lang NP, Berglundh T. Working group 4 of the Seventh European Workshop on Periodontology. Periimplant diseases: where are we now? – Consensus of the Seventh European Workshop on Periodontology. *J Clin Periodontol.* 2011;38(11):178–181.

46. Jepsen S, Rühling A, Jepsen K, et al. Progressive peri-implantitis. Incidence and prediction of peri-implant attachment loss. *Clin Oral Implants Res.* 1996;7(2):133–141.

47. Luterbacher, Mayfield L, Bragger U, Land NF. Diagnostic characteristics of clinical and microbiological tests for monitoring periodontal and peri-implant mucosal tissue conditions during supportive periodontal therapy (SPT). *Clin Oral Implants Res.* 2000;11(6):521–529.

48. Luterbacher S, Mayfield L, Bragger U, et al. Diagnostic characteristics of clinical and microbiological tests for monitoring periodontal and periimplant mucosal tissue conditions during supportive periodontal therapy (SPT). *Clin Oral Implants Res.* 2000;11:52–59.

49. Gerber JA, Tan WC, Balmer TE, et al. Bleeding on probing and pocket probing depth in relation to probing pressure and mucosal health around oral implants. *Clin Oral Impl Res.* 2009;20(1):75–78.

50. Mombelli A, Buser D, Lang NP, et al. Comparison of periodontal and peri-implant probing by depth force pattern analysis. *Clin Oral Implants Res.* 1997;8:448–454.

51. van Steenberghe D. Periodontal aspects of osseointegrated oral implants modum Branemark. *Dent Clin North Am.* 1988;32:355–370.

52. Gallucci GO, Grütter L, Chuang SK, Belser UC. Dimensional changes of peri–implant soft tissue over 2 years with single–implant crowns in the anterior maxilla. *J Clin Periodontol.* 2011;38:293–299.

53. Mombelli A, Müller N, Cionca N. The epidemiology of peri-implantitis. *Clin Oral Implants Res.* 2012;23(6):67–76.

54. Misch CE, Resnik R. *Misch's Avoiding Complications in Oral Implantology-E-Book.* Elsevier Health Sciences; 2017.

55. Ross-Jansaker AM, Renvert H, Lindahl C, Renvert S. Nine-to fourteen-year follow-up of implant treatment. Part III: factors associated with peri-implant lesions. *J Clin Periodontol.* 2006;33(4):296–301.

56. Bouri Jr A, Bissada N, Al-Zahrani MS, Fadoul F, Nounen I. Width of keratinized gingiva and the health status of the supporting tissues around dental implants. *Int J Oral Maxillofac Implants.* 2008;23(2):323–326.

57. Schrott AR, Jimenez M, Hwang JW, Fiorellini J, Weber HP. Five-year evaluation of the influence of keratinized mucosa on peri-implant soft-tissue health and stability around implants supporting full-arch mandibular fixed prostheses. *Clin Oral Implants Res.* 2009;20(10):1170–1177.

58. Adibrad M, Shahabuei M, Sahabi M. Significance of the width of keratinized mucosa on the health status of the supporting tissue around implants supporting overdentures. *J Oral Implantol.* 2009;35(5):232–237.

59. Chung DM, Oh TJ, Shotwell JL, Misch CE, Wang HL. Significance of keratinized mucosa in maintenance of dental implants with different surfaces. *J Periodontol.* 2006;77(8):1410–1420.

60. Lin GH, Chan HL, Wang HL. The significance of keratinized mucosa on implant health: a systematic review. *J Periodontol.* 2013;84:1755–1767.

61. Gobbato L, Avila-Ortiz G, Sohrabi K, Wang CW, Karimbux N. The effect of keratinized mucosa width on peri-implant health: a systematic review. *Int J Oral Maxillofac Implants.* 2013;28:1536–1545.

62. Bronstein D, Suzuki K, Garashi M, Suzuki JB. Contemporary esthetic periodontics. *StomaEduJ.* 2016;3(2):26–36.

63. Esposito M, Maghaireh H, Grusovin MG, Ziounas I, Worthington HV. Soft tissue management for dental implants: what are the most effective techniques? A Cochrane systematic review. *Eur J Oral Implantol.* 2012;5:221–238.

64. Lang PL, Berglundh T. Working group 4 of the VII E.W.o.P. Peri-implant diseases: where are we now? Consensus of the Seventh European Workshop on Periodontology. *J Clin Periodontol.* 2011;38(11):178–181.

65. Froum S, Rosen P. A Proposed Classification for peri-implantitis. *Int J Periodontics Restorative Dent.* 2012;32(5):533–540.

66. Miyata T, Kobayashi Y, Araki H, Ohto T, Shin K. The influence of controlled occlusal overload on peri-implant tissue. Part 3: a histological study in monkeys. *Int J Oral Maxillofac Implants.* 2000;15(3):415–431.

67. White SC, Pharoah M. *Oral Radiology: Principles and Interpretation.* 5th ed. St Louis: Mosby; 2004.

68. Friedland B. The clinical evaluation of dental implants: a review of the literature, with emphasis on the radiographic aspects. *Oral Implantol.* 1987;13:101–111.

69. Naitoh M. Labial bone assessment surrounding dental implant using cone-beam computed tomography:. *Clin. Oral Impl. Res.* 2012;23:970–974.

70. Gröndahl K, Ekestubbe A, Gröndahl HG. *Radiography in Oral Endosseous Prosthetics.* Goteborg, Sweden: Nobel Biocare AB; 1996.

71. Adell R, Lekholm U, Rockler B, Brånemark PI. A 15-year study of osseointegrated implants in the treatment of the edentulous jaw. *Int J Oral Surg.* 1981;10(6):387–416.

72. Shin YK, Han CH, Heo SJ, Kim S, Chun HJ. Radiographic evaluation of marginal bone level around implants with different neck designs after 1 year. *Int J Oral Maxillofac Implants.* 2006;21(5):789–794.

73. Lazzara RJ, Porter SS. Platform switching: a new concept in implant dentistry for controlling postrestorative crestal bone levels. *Int J Periodontics Restorative Dent.* 2006;26(1):9–17.

74. Resnik RR. *Personal Communication*; 2017.

75. Quirynen M, Naert I, Teerlinck J, et al. Periodontal indices around osseointegrated oral implants supporting overdentures. In: Schepers E, Naert J, Theunier G, eds. *Overdentures on Oral Implants.* Leuwen, Belgium: Leuwen University Press; 1991.

76. Herrmann JS, Cochran DL, Nummikoski PV, et al. Crestal bone changes around titanium implants: a radiographic evaluation of unloaded non-submerged and submerged implants in the canine mandible. *J Periodontol.* 1997;68:1117–1130.

77. Zitzmann N, Berglundh T, Marinello CP, et al. Experimental peri-implant mucositis in man. *J Clin Periodontol.* 2001;28:517–523.

78. Humphrey S. Implant maintenance. *Dental Clin North Am.* 2006;50(3):463–478.

79. Biesbrock AR, Bartizek RD, Gerlach RW, Terézhalmy GT. Oral hygiene regimens, plaque control, and gingival health: a two-month clinical trial with antimicrobial agents. *J Clin Dent.* 2007;18(4):101–105.

80. Kracher CM, Smith WS. Oral health maintenance of dental implants. *Dent Assist.* 2010;79(2):27–35.

81. Esposito M, Worthington H, Coulthard P, et al. Maintaining and reestablishing health around osseointegrated oral implants: a Cochrane systematic review comparing the efficacy of various treatments. *Periodontology.* 2003;33:204–212.

82. Rasperini G, Pellegrini G, Cortella A, et al. The safety and acceptability mucosa in patients with oral implants in aesthetic areas: a prospective. *Implantol.* 1(3):221–228.

83. Vandekerckhove B, Quirynen M, Warren PR, et al. The safety and efficacy of a powered toothbrush on soft tissues in patients with

implant-supported fixed prostheses. *Clin Oral Investig.* 2004;8(4). 26–10.

84. Wingrove S. Focus on implant home care: before, during, and after restoration. *RDH.* 2013;33(9):52–58.

85. Nakagawa M, Matsuya S, Shiraishi T, Ohta M. Effect of fluoride concentration and pH on corrosion behavior of titanium for dental use. *J Dent Res.* 1999;78(9):1568–1572. https://doi.org/10.1177/00220345990780091201.

86. Matono Y, Nakagawa M, Matsuya S, Ishikawa K, Terada Y. Corrosion behavior of pure titanium and titanium alloys in various concentrations of acidulated phosphate fluoride (APF) solutions. *Dent Mat J.* 2006;25(1):104–112.

87. Barnes CM, Russell CM, Reinhardt RA, et al. Comparison of irrigation to floss as an adjunct to tooth brushing: effect on bleeding, gingivitis, and supragingival plaque. *J Clin Dent.* 2005;16(3):71–77.

88. Rosema NA, Hennequin-Hoenderdos NL, Berchier CE, et al. The effect devices on gingival bleeding. *J Int Acad Periodontol.* 2011;13(1):2–10.

89. Sharma NC, Lyle DM, Qaqish JG, et al. Effect of a dental water jet with bleeding in adolescent patients with fixed orthodontic appliances. *Am J.* 2008;133(4):565–571.

90. Magnuson B, Harsono M, Silberstein J, et al. *Water Flosser Vs. Floss: Comparing Reduction in Bleeding Around Implants [Abstract].* Seattle WA: Presented at the International Association for Dental Research Meeting; March 23, 2013.

91. Brough Muzzin KM, Johnson R, Carr P, Daffron P. The dental hygienist's role in the maintenance of osseointegrated dental implants. *J Dent Hyg.* 1988;62(9):448–453.

92. Friedman LA. Oral hygiene for dental implant patients. *Tex Dent J.* 1991;108(5):21–23.

93. Felo A, Shibly O, Ciancio SC, et al. Effects of subgingival chlorhexidine irrigation on peri-implant maintenance. *Am J Dent.* 1997;10(2):107–110.

94. Meffert RM. The soft tissue interface in dental implantology. *J Dent Educ.* 1988;52(12):810–811.

95. Koumjian JH, Kerner J, Smith RA. Implants: hygiene maintenance of dental implants. *Ill Dent J.* 1991;60(1):54–59.

96. Thomson-Neal D, Evans GH, Meffert RM. Effects of various prophylactic treatments on titanium, sapphire, and hydroxyapatite-coated implants: an SEM study. *Int J Periodontics Restorative Dent.* 1989;9(4):300–311.

97. Misch CE. Implant quality scale: a clinical assessment of the health-disease continuum. *Oral Health.* 1998;88:15–25.

Treatment Plan Options

Edentulous Maxilla

1. No treatment
   Disadvantage: Difficulty in eating/speaking, continued bone loss, maintain current prosthesis (ill-fitting)
2. Complete upper denture
   Advantage: Minimal treatment, fast
   Disadvantage: Removable prosthesis disadvantages, difficulty in eating/speaking, palate coverage, continued bone loss
3. Implant-supported overdenture (removable, RP5)
   Advantage: Removable prosthesis that "clips" in, added retention, soft tissue support
   Disadvantage: Full denture with palate, have to remove at night, removable, clips need changed on a regular basis (additional cost), may have associated mobility of prosthesis
4. Implant-supported overdenture (removable, RP4)
   Advantage: Removable prosthesis that clips in, horseshoe shaped (no full palate), no soft tissue coverage, totally implant supported
   Disadvantage: Have to remove at night, removable prosthesis, clips need changed on a regular basis (additional cost)
5. Implant-supported fixed prosthesis (fixed)
   Advantage: Fixed prosthesis (does not come out), increased biting force
   Disadvantage: Usually will need extensive bone grafting and more implants, need for pink porcelain or acrylic because of the amount of bone loss, teeth will be larger (FP-2/FP-3), may not be able to increase soft tissue support, increased expense

Edentulous Mandible

1. No treatment
   Disadvantage: Difficulty in eating/speaking, continued bone loss, maintain current prosthesis (ill-fitting)
2. Complete lower denture
   Advantage: Minimal treatment, fast
   Disadvantage: Removable prosthesis, difficulty in eating/speaking, continued bone loss
3. Implant-supported overdenture (removable, RP5)
   Advantage: Removable prosthesis that clips in, less implants required, soft tissue support
   Disadvantage: Full denture, have to remove at night, removable, clips need changed on a regular basis (additional cost)
4. Implant-supported overdenture (removable, RP4)
   Advantage: Removable prosthesis that clips in, no soft tissue coverage
   Disadvantage: Have to remove at night, removable, clips need changed on a regular basis (additional cost)
5. Implant-supported fixed prosthesis (fixed)
   Advantage: Fixed prosthesis (does not come out), increased biting force

Disadvantage: Usually will require more implants, increased expense, need for pink porcelain or acrylic because of the amount of bone loss, teeth will be larger (FP-2/FP-3), may not be able to increase soft tissue support

Single Tooth Missing

1. No treatment
   Disadvantage: Esthetics, adjacent teeth will move (tilting), supraeruption, decreased mastication, food impaction, continued bone loss, occlusal force
2. Partial denture
   Advantage: Minimal treatment, fast
   Disadvantage: Removable prosthesis, difficulty in eating/speaking, extensive pressure on adjacent teeth/soft tissue which leads to additional tooth loss, poor long-term success rate, increased bone loss, tissue soreness
3. Fixed partial denture
   Advantage: Fast, esthetic, usually no need for hard/soft tissue grafting
   Disadvantage: Alteration of adjacent teeth, higher incidence of decay, increased endodontic treatment, hygiene difficult
4. Implant-supported crown
   Advantage: No alteration of adjacent teeth, higher success rate than fixed partial denture (most studies >90% success rate)
   Disadvantage: Longer treatment time, requires bone quality and quantity, esthetic issues possible

Multiple Missing Teeth

1. No treatment
   Disadvantage: Esthetics, adjacent teeth will move (tilting), supraeruption, decreased mastication, continued bone loss, food impaction, occlusal force
2. Partial denture
   Advantage: Minimal treatment, fast
   Disadvantage: Removable prosthesis, difficulty in eating/speaking, tissue soreness, places extensive pressure on adjacent teeth/soft tissue which leads to additional tooth loss, poor long-term success rate
3. Fixed partial denture (if indicated)
   Advantage: Fast, esthetic
   Disadvantage: Alteration of adjacent teeth, higher incidence of decay, increased endodontic treatment, hygiene difficult
4. Implant-supported crown
   Advantage: No alteration of adjacent teeth, higher success rate than fixed partial denture (most studies >90% success rate)
   Disadvantage: Longer treatment time, requires bone quality and quantity, esthetic issues possible

Index

Note: Page numbers followed by f indicate figures; t, tables; b, boxes